Exercise Physiology
Nutrition, Energy, and Human Performance

NINTH EDITION

Exercise Physiology
Nutrition, Energy, and Human Performance

NINTH EDITION

William D. McArdle

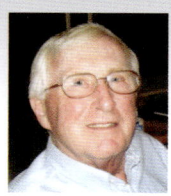

Professor Emeritus
Department of Family, Nutrition,
 and Exercise Science
Queens College of the City University of New York
Flushing, New York

Frank I. Katch

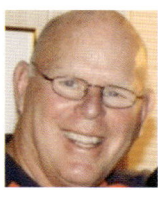

Instructor and Board Member
Certificate Program in Fitness Instruction
UCLA Extension
Los Angeles, California
Former Professor and Chair of Exercise Science
University of Massachusetts
Amherst, Massachusetts

Victor L. Katch

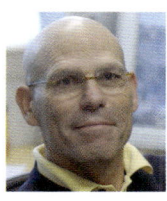

Professor Emeritus
School of Kinesiology
Associate Professor, Pediatric Cardiology
School of Medicine
University of Michigan
Ann Arbor, Michigan

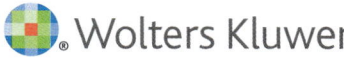

Philadelphia • Baltimore • New York • London
Buenos Aires • Hong Kong • Sydney • Tokyo

Acquisitions Editor: Lindsey Porambo
Development Editors: David Payne, Amy Millholen
Editorial Assistant: Jada Davis
Marketing Manager: Phyllis Hitner
Production Project Manager: David Saltzberg
Design Coordinator: Stephen Druding
Art Director, Illustration: Jennifer Clements
Manufacturing Coordinator: Margie Orzech-Zeranko
Prepress Vendor: Straive

Ninth Edition

Copyright © 2023 Wolters Kluwer.

Copyright © 2015, 2010, 2007, 2001, 1996, 1986, 1981 Wolters Kluwer Health | Lippincott Williams & Wilkins. All rights reserved. This book is protected by copyright. No part of this book may be reproduced or transmitted in any form or by any means, including as photocopies or scanned-in or other electronic copies, or utilized by any information storage and retrieval system without written permission from the copyright owner, except for brief quotations embodied in critical articles and reviews. Materials appearing in this book prepared by individuals as part of their official duties as U.S. government employees are not covered by the above-mentioned copyright. To request permission, please contact Wolters Kluwer at Two Commerce Square, 2001 Market Street, Philadelphia, PA 19103, via email at permissions@lww.com, or via our website at shop.lww.com (products and services).

Selected photographs © 2023 by Fitness Technologies, Inc., and Frank I. Katch and Victor L. Katch. This material is protected by copyright. No photographs may be reproduced in any form or by any means without permission from the copyright holders. For permission to use photographs, contact Fitness Technologies, 5043 Via Lara Lane, Santa Barbara, CA 93111.

Appendices E, F, and L Copyright © 2023 by Frank I. Katch, Victor L. Katch, William D. McArdle, and Fitness Technologies, Inc., 5043 Via Lara Lane, Santa Barbara, CA 93111. No part of these appendices may be reproduced in any manner or by any means without written permission from the copyright holders. To request permission, contact the copyright holders via email at fkatch@mac.com. 5/2022

9 8 7 6 5 4 3 2 1

Printed in Mexico

Cataloging-in-Publication Data available on request from the Publisher

ISBN: 978-1-9751-5999-3

This work is provided "as is," and the publisher disclaims any and all warranties, express or implied, including any warranties as to accuracy, comprehensiveness, or currency of the content of this work.

This work is no substitute for individual patient assessment based upon healthcare professionals' examination of each patient and consideration of, among other things, age, weight, gender, current or prior medical conditions, medication history, laboratory data and other factors unique to the patient. The publisher does not provide medical advice or guidance and this work is merely a reference tool. Healthcare professionals, and not the publisher, are solely responsible for the use of this work including all medical judgments and for any resulting diagnosis and treatments.

Given continuous, rapid advances in medical science and health information, independent professional verification of medical diagnoses, indications, appropriate pharmaceutical selections and dosages, and treatment options should be made and healthcare professionals should consult a variety of sources. When prescribing medication, healthcare professionals are advised to consult the product information sheet (the manufacturer's package insert) accompanying each drug to verify, among other things, conditions of use, warnings and side effects and identify any changes in dosage schedule or contraindications, particularly if the medication to be administered is new, infrequently used or has a narrow therapeutic range. To the maximum extent permitted under applicable law, no responsibility is assumed by the publisher for any injury and/or damage to persons or property, as a matter of products liability, negligence law or otherwise, or from any reference to or use by any person of this work.

shop.lww.com

To my wife, my four children and 14 grandchildren whose lives give meaning to my own.

BILL McARDLE

To Kerry, my best friend and wife of 53 years, and to our 3 children and their families: David and his wife Malia and grandson Cole; Ellen and her husband Sean, and our grandchildren James and Laura; and Kevin and his wife Kate and granddaughter Emily. You all have achieved the honorable with distinction in your personal, academic, and business pursuits. You truly are what makes life worth living!

FRANK KATCH

To my wife Heather; daughters Erika and Leslie; son Jesse; and wonderful grandkids, Ryan, Cameron, Ella, Emery and Jude. I also want to thank all of my graduate students for their continued friendship. "It's been a great adventure."

VICTOR KATCH

Preface

Exercise Physiology: Nutrition, Energy, and Human Performance, ninth edition, represents our attempt to keep pace with the ever-expanding and integrated exercise physiology field. Studies on nutrition, biochemistry, kinesiology, genetics, molecular biology, epidemiology, public health, and the multifaceted fields related to medicine are published in peer-reviewed national and international journals focusing on physical activity, exercise, and human movement. Integrating exercise-related research among different academic disciplines was uncommon in the years prior to the early 1960s. Exercise physiology research began to prosper with increasing frequency as graduate-level programs broadened the interest in the physical activity/exercise sciences and produced young scholars who published their research in high-impact research journals in many different fields.

In this extensive text revision, we continue to highlight "classic" studies for supportive context for the newer findings discussed within the textbook's 33 chapters. As in our prior eight editions, we have visually enhanced text material by upgrading and adding over 1000 new images. An expanded introductory chapter provides the historical perspective for the text material in all chapters.

Ever since our first edition more than four decades ago, new knowledge has exploded about physical activity's physiologic effects in general and the body's specific responses to movement in particular. We initially naively believed that citation frequency for many topic areas had reached a zenith, leveling off during the 10-y decade from 1986 to 1996, but were we ever wrong! Instead, the rate of increase continues to expand exponentially, beyond our wildest expectations. While the increase in research papers has slowed in a few areas to "just" several thousand new publications every few years, other areas have increased tremendously, making it difficult to keep pace. In the molecular biology domain related to physical activity/exercise, for example, what began as only several hundred research papers in 2004 now in September 2022 numbers in the hundreds of thousands every few years. As an example, when searching PubMed for the terms "molecular biology" in February 2022, already 1306 research articles had been published. Refining the search by adding the term "physical activity" yielded 21 new publications. There is no doubt that with expanding interest in physical activity's role tied to the molecular biology domain, the most recent broad and restricted topic areas continue to accelerate unabated.

We admire the early pioneers in the relatively young exercise physiology and sports medicine–related fields. As graduate students in the late 1960s, we never imagined that interest in exercise physiology would increase so dramatically. The exercise physiology textbook we used in our own undergraduate physical education classes included less than about 40% of the topic areas we now review in considerable detail. For example, there was little or no information about different muscle fiber types, no discussion about the intricate biochemical events in aerobic and anaerobic metabolism, and almost no information about genetics' role in physical activity, health, disease and its risks, metabolism, and ergonomics and sports performance/biomechanics. With each passing year, a new generation of scholars committed to studying physical activity and exercise with a scientific approach continued to explore new interrelationships among key drivers related to human adaptation to exercise stress. Some researchers began to study physiologic mechanisms and their effects on physical activity and vice versa, whereas others evaluated individual differences in exercise and sports performance among different populations, from the physically challenged to Olympic-caliber athletes.

At our first scientific conference (American College of Sports Medicine [ACSM] in Las Vegas, 1967), only 13 years after ACSM's inception in 1954, still as graduate students, we rubbed elbows with the "giants" in the field, many of whom were themselves mentored by the leaders of their era. Several hundred ACSM members listened attentively as the superstars of exercise physiology and physical fitness (e.g., Erling Asmussen, Per-Olof Åstrand, Bruno Balke, Elsworth Buskirk, Thomas Cureton, Lars Hermansen, Steven Horvath, Henry Montoye, Bengt Saltin, and Charles Tipton) presented their research and fielded penetrating questions from young graduate students eager to consume the latest scientific information presented by these shining stars.

Sitting under an open tent in the Nevada desert with one of the world's leading physiologists, Dr. David Bruce Dill (then age 74; profiled later in this book's introduction), we listened to his research assistant—a high school student—lecture about temperature regulation in the desert burro. A few hours later, one of us (FK) sitting next to a white-haired older gentleman chatted about his master's thesis project, which involved a practical densitometric method to determine body density in university female tennis and swim team athletes. Only later did an embarrassed coauthor learn that this was Captain Albert R. Behnke, MD (1898–1993; ACSM Honor Award, 1976), modern-day "father" of human body composition assessment whose crucial experiment in diving physiology established standards for decompression and use of mixed gases for deep dives. Dr. Behnke's pioneering hydrostatic weighing studies in 1942 led to the reference man and reference woman model to describe the body's compositional components, and the Somatogram and Body Profile Analysis System based on surface anthropometry. Years later, Dr. Behnke and F. Katch coauthored papers with Victor Katch in body composition measurement techniques.

In our early years, the three of us were indeed fortunate to work with the very best mentors and scholars in our field. William McArdle studied for his PhD at the University of Michigan with the productive physical education scholar Dr. Henry Montoye (ACSM charter member; ACSM President, 1962 to 1963; Citation Award, 1973) and Dr. John Faulkner (ACSM President, 1971 to 1972; Citation Award, 1973; ACSM Honor Award, 1992).

Frank Katch completed his master of science degree at the University of California (UC), Santa Barbara, under the supervision of thesis advisors Dr. Ernest Michael Jr. (former PhD student of pioneer exercise physiologist-physical fitness scientist Dr. Thomas Kirk Cureton from the University of Illinois and "father of the physical fitness movement" in the United States; ACSM Honor Award, 1969) and Dr. Barbara Drinkwater (ACSM President, 1988 to 1989; ACSM Honor Award, 1996). He then completed doctoral studies at the University of California, Berkeley, with Professor Franklin Henry, known for the novel memory-drum movement concept related to exercise specificity, and author of the seminal paper, "Physical Education—an Academic Discipline" (*JOHPER* 1964;35:32), which provided much of the basis of today's current kinesiology programs throughout the world.

Victor Katch completed his master of science thesis at UC Berkeley supervised by Dr. Jack Wilmore (ACSM President, 1978 to 1979; Citation Award, 1984; first *Exercise and Sport Science Reviews* editor, 1973 to 1974) and also was a doctoral student mentored by Dr. Franklin Henry at UC Berkeley.

As the three of us reexamine those earlier times, we realize like many of our former and current colleagues that our academic fortunes prospered because our mentors shared an unwavering commitment to study sport, exercise, and human movement from a strong scientific and physiologic perspective. These scholars (and later colleagues) demonstrated the need for physical educators to become adequately prepared in the exercise sciences, which included not only courses in exercise physiology and training adaptations but also in statistics, public health/epidemiology, fitness management, psychology, sport biomechanics, motor control, tests and measurement, and computer science.

Similar to our text's first edition, published in 1981, this ninth edition reflects our continued commitment to integrate the science gleaned from different fields that form the fabric of our discipline. As an example, proper nutrition links to good health, effective weight control, and optimal physical activity and sports performance, while physical activity participation and exercise training connect to body weight control and optimizing overall good health. We are thankful that the medical establishment and governmental agencies continue to promote physical activity as an important tool to prevent and rehabilitate sedentary-related disease states, including childhood and adult type 2 diabetes, obesity, cancer, and lung, heart, neuromuscular, and endocrine diseases.

We are grateful for the small part we have played in educating more than 450,000 undergraduate and graduate students who have used our textbook over the years. A source of great pride for us is that a dozen or more students who were enrolled in our initial classes and used our first edition text pursued advanced degrees and are now university professors and administrators. The tradition of textbook adoption has been passed on to their students, many of whom serve as aspiring educators at colleges and universities, exercise specialists, personal trainers, physicians and physical therapists, and researchers in allied fields. We are forever indebted to our former teachers and mentors for fostering intellectual curiosity that has not diminished.

To all of you accompanying us on this exciting educational journey, which delivered to us new areas to study such as space exploration, molecular biology, and genetics relating to physical activity and obesity, we end with this fitting quote in Latin attributed to prolific French book and independent journal author, mystic, and astronomer Nicolas Camille Flammarion (1842 to 1925; http://scihi.org/camille-flammarion-popular-astronomy/): "**Ad Veritatem Per Scientiam**" (**To Truth Through Science**). This timely saying is inscribed in gold above the observatory and museum entrance to his Chateau at Juvisy-sur-Orge outside of Paris and honored with a French stamp showing his likeness and observatory.

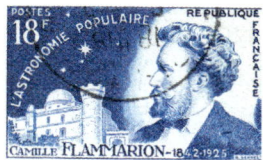

As we approach the culmination of our own satisfying careers, we are counting on you, the next generation of exercise scientists, allied health specialists, and educators, to continue spreading the word about the important role that exercise physiology plays in our society and contributing to the yet-to-be-uncovered truths to thrust the field onward into the decades ahead.

ORGANIZATION

This ninth edition maintains an eight-section structure and an introductory section about the historical origins of exercise physiology. The concluding "On the Horizon" section and its chapter have changed from an addendum to a numbered section and chapter, reflective of molecular biology's rightful place as an established core field within the discipline.

The ninth edition also has undergone a complete art makeover. Most of the existing figures have been redrawn to provide consistency with newly created illustrations. Throughout the text, we have included hundreds of Internet resources (URLs) to provide an expanded Web access to supplement insights about timely text material.

FEATURES

This text's features have been specifically designed to help students facilitate learning. They include the following:

Introduction: A View from the Past. The text's introduction, subtitled "A View from the Past," reflects our continued interest in and respect for the earliest underpinnings interwoven in the field and the direct and indirect contributions from male and female physician-scientists who contributed to the field.

Chapter Objectives. Each chapter opens with a comprehensive summary of learning goals, helping students to become familiar with the materials to be covered in a chapter.

Ancillaries at-a-Glance. A complete list of electronic resources associated with a chapter makes accessing online materials easy; callouts in the text reinforce for students opportunities to broaden their knowledge beyond the text pages.

FYI. The text continues the tradition of FYI (For Your Information) boxes, which provide relatively short inserts of related information, current research, or interesting sidebars germane to the text's topic, ranging from "Music Positively Effects Heart Rate Variability" to "Consuming Excess Calories Produces Fat Gain Regardless of Nutrient Source."

In a Practical Sense. Every chapter highlights practical applications about specific topic areas, ranging from "Waist-to-Hip Girth Ratio to Determine Disease Risk," to "How to Assess and Evaluate One-Repetition Maximum for Bench Press and Leg Press."

Integrative Questions. Open-ended questions encourage students to thoughtfully consider complex concepts.

Expanded Art Program. The full-color art program remains a salient feature of the textbook. Nearly every figure has been revised to make its textual and visual elements "pop" or altered to highlight important teaching points that reinforce text material. New figures have been added to chapters to enhance current and updated content, including the use of new medical illustrations. A new table format clearly organizes essential data.

References, Appendices, and Animations (Available Online). All references, appendices, and animations are available online on Lippincott Connect. Appendices feature valuable information about nutritive values, energy expenditures, metabolic computations in open-circuit spirometry, and more and are cross-referenced in the chapters with special features, such as the one below.

Lippincott® Connect   Appendix C, available on Lippincott Connect, lists Royal Society medals and awards for distinguished and meritorious scientist-researchers.

High-quality animations bring key exercise physiology concepts to life and, likewise, are cross-referenced in the chapters with an icon, as the example feature illustrates:

 See the animation "Sliding Filament Theory" on Lippincott Connect to view this process.

Focus on Research (Available Online). Almost all chapters have a companion online Focus on Research, featuring a key research article from a renowned scientist. These well-designed studies illustrate how "theory comes to life" via the dynamics of well-designed and insightful research.

NEW TO THE NINTH EDITION

The flow of information in this edition remains similar to prior editions. Components of the entire text have been upgraded to reflect current research findings related to the diverse areas of exercise physiology. We have revised almost every figure and supplemented them with high-quality medical illustrations. Within each chapter, while we discuss the contents and meaning relevant to each table, we have placed the tables at the end of each chapter to allow for better text and image/figure flow on the pages. Additionally, we have included hundreds of new Web sites to provide readers access to the abundance of updated information available about the intricacies relevant to topic areas in exercise physiology.

Our current reference lists, available on Lippincott Connect (https://connect.lww.com), include up-to-date research results gleaned from national and international journals related to specific topic areas. An "Additional References" section has been added to the end of each chapter that provides a bibliography of articles that augment the materials already presented in the chapter. We hope you profit from and enjoy this continuation of our journey through the ever-expanding and maturing exercise physiology discipline.

ANCILLARIES: THE TOTAL TEACHING PACKAGE

Exercise Physiology: Nutrition, Energy, and Human Performance, ninth edition, includes additional resources for both instructors and students.

Approved adopting instructors will be given access to the following resources on thePoint:

- Test bank
- PowerPoint presentations
- Image bank of downloadable figures and tables in multiple formats
- LMS cartridges

Students

Students who purchase *Exercise Physiology: Nutrition, Energy, and Human Performance*, ninth edition, have access to the following additional resources, accessible on Lippincott Connect with the scratch-off code provided on this book's inside cover:

- Animations
- References
- Appendices
- Focus on research article abstracts and analysis
- Featured information on microscope technologies, notable events in genetics, Nobel prizes, outstanding female scientists, and much more

Acknowledgments

We feel very fortunate since the first *Exercise Physiology* edition published in 1981 to have cherished colleagues provide topical information about many exercise physiology subject areas. Our introductory chapter (Introduction: A View from the Past) pays homage to influential pioneers in our field, with whom we shared close personal and professional relationships as we began our academic careers. We are honored to have benefitted from collaborations with the very best scholars in the physical education and exercise science academic disciplines in the United States and internationally—and will never forget their encouragement and inspiring influence on us in so many ways.

We acknowledge our master's and senior honors students who worked in our laboratories for their projects and contributed so much to our research and personal experiences: Pedro Alexander, Christos Balabinis, Margaret Ballantyne, Brandee Black, Michael Carpenter, Steven Christos, Roman Czula, Gwyn Danielson, Toni Denahan, Marty Dicker, Sadie Drumm, Peter Frykman, Scott Glickman, Marion Gurry, Carrie Hauser, Margorie King, Peter LaChance, Jean Lett, Maria Likomitrou, Robert Martin, Cathi Moorehead, Susan Novitsky, Joan Perry, Sharon Purdy, Michelle Segar, Debra Spiak, Lorraine Turcotte, Lori Waiter, Stephen Westing, and Howard Zelaznik.

We also dedicate this 9th edition to our former students who earned PhD or master's degrees (and were also co-authors on scientific publications) in physical education, exercise science, physical therapy, or medicine. They have gone on to distinguish themselves as teachers, practitioners, and researchers in areas directly or indirectly related to exercise physiology and the physical fitness fields. They include Denise Agin, Stamitis Agiovlasitis, Doug Ballor, Dan Becque, Geroge Brooks, Barbara Campaigne, Michael Carpenter, Ed Chaloupka, Kenneth Cohen, Edward Coyle, Dan Delio, Julia Chase Delio, Sadie Drumm, Chris Dunbar, Patti Freedson, Roger Glaser, Ellen Glickman, Kati Haltiwinger, Everett Harmon, Jay Hoffman, Tibor Hortobagyi, Gary Kamen, Margorie King, Crandall Jensen, Carol Jones, Jie Kang, Mitch Kanter, Betsy Keller, Marliese Kimmerly, Margorie King, Peter LaChance, George Lesmses, Steve Lichtman, Charles Marks, Robert Mofatt, Karen Nau-White, Steven Ostrove, James Rimmer, Deborah Rinaldi, Stan Sady, Lapros Sidossis, Debra Spiak, Bob Spina, John Spring, Bill Thorland, Michael Toner, Laurel Trager-Mackinnon, Lorraine Turcotte, John Villanacci, Jonnis Vrabis, Nancy Weiss, Arthur Weltman, Nancy Wessingeer, Stephen Westing, Anthony Wilcox, and Linda Zwiren.

With a debt of gratitude, we also thank many colleagues in different disciplines who have been generous with their time by providing valuable insights about chapter content areas (ACSM administrative staff, NASA researchers in exercise physiology, history, and nutritional sciences), Adrian Adams, Pedro Alexander, Fredrick Amuchie, Jose Antonio, Luis Aragon, Francisco Arencibia-Albite, Jerry Ball, Stephen Blair, Walter Block, Susan Bloomfield, Marvin Boluyt, Frank Booth, Katarina Borer, Claude Bouchard, George A. Bray, Edward Burke, David Clarke, H. Harrison Clarke, Tom Colaiezzi, David Costill, Pete Darcy, Jean-Pierre Després, Jonathon Dimes, Rod Dishman, Dee W. Edington, Petter Elvestad, Tom Fahey, Deborah Falla, Harold Falls, Dario Farina, Don Fleming, Carl Foster, Barry Franklin, Larry R. Gettman, Gordon Giesbrecht, Bob Girandola, Carl Gisolfi, R. Donald Hagan, Jay Hertel, Steven Heymsfield, Will Hopkins (http://sportsci.org/), Susan Katz, Gitle Kirkesola, Eve Malakoff-Klein, Wendy Kohrt, William Kraemer, Richard Kreider, Pierre LaGasse, David Lamb, Helen W. Lane, Stuart Lee, Richard Lieber, John Magel, Anssi Manninen, Ernest D. Michael Jr., Pedro Gualberto Morales, Tim Noakes, Roger Palay, Øyvind Pedersen, Michael Pollock, Peter B. Raven, George Q. Rich III, Amnon Rosenthal, Loring Rowell, Corey Rynders, Rudy Schmerl, Richard Schmidt, Gary Schneider, Stephen Seiler, Brian Sharkey, Wayne Sinning, James Skinner, Leon Smith, John F. Spahr, John F. Spahr Jr., Julie Stegman, Walt Thompson, Paul Vanderburgh, Judy Weltman, and Edward Wickland.

We appreciate the creative individuals at Wolters Kluwer Health, Lippincott Williams & Wilkins, who helped to guide this 9th edition through the various production stages from initial manuscript editing, figure creation and art acquisitions through final page-proof editing and cover design. We are grateful to Lindsey Porambo, acquisitions editor and Amy Milholen, in-house Senior Development Editor, for their support in handling critical editing issues in bringing this edition to fruition in a timely manner. We also are thankful for the exceptional technical and creative expertise Jennifer Clements, Art Director/Illustration, provided for creative art contributions for the Introduction and 33 chapters in the pursuit to produce the best art program possible. Thank you to the editorial team Lindsey, Jennifer, Amy, David Payne (freelance Developmental Editor), David Saltzberg, Production Product Manager, Steve Druding, Design Production Manager, and Gayathri Govindarajan, Composition Project Manager, for your hard work, enthusiasm, and commitment to this project.

William D. McArdle
Sound Beach, New York
Frank I. Katch
Santa Barbara, California
Victor L. Katch
Ann Arbor, Michigan

Contents

INTRODUCTION
A View from the Past   **xiv**

PART ONE
EXERCISE PHYSIOLOGY   1

SECTION 1   **Nutrition: The Base for Human Performance**   **3**

CHAPTER 1
Carbohydrates, Lipids, and Proteins   4

PART 1 • CARBOHYDRATES   6
   Carbohydrate Kinds and Sources   6
   Recommended Carbohydrate Intake   11
   Carbohydrates' Role in the Body   11
   Carbohydrate Dynamics During Physical Activity   12
PART 2 • LIPIDS   15
   Lipid Characteristics   15
   Lipid Kinds and Sources   15
   Recommended Lipid Intake   22
   Lipid Dynamics in Physical Activity   25
PART 3 • PROTEINS   28
   About Protein   28
   Protein Categories   29
   Recommended Protein Intake   30
   Protein's Role in the Body   32
   Protein Metabolism Dynamics   32
   Nitrogen Balance   33
   Protein Dynamics During Physical Activity   35

CHAPTER 2
Vitamins, Minerals, and Water   42

PART 1 • VITAMINS   44
   About Vitamins   44
   Vitamin Types   44
   Vitamins' Role in the Body   45
   Defining Nutrient Needs: Dietary Reference Intakes   46
   Vitamin Antioxidant Role   47
   Vitamin-Rich Food Sources   48
   Physical Activity, Free Radicals, and Antioxidants   49
   Does Vitamin Supplementation Provide a Competitive Edge?   50
PART 2 • MINERALS   52
   Mineral Essentials   52
   Mineral Functions   52
   Calcium   53
   Female Athlete Triad   59
   Male Athlete Triad   61
   Phosphorus   62
   Magnesium   62
   Iron   62
   Sodium, Potassium, and Chlorine   66
   Minerals and Exercise Performance   67
PART 3 • WATER   69
   The Body's Water Content   69
   Water's Functions   69
   Water Balance: Intake Versus Output   70
   Physical Activity and Water Requirements   72

CHAPTER 3
Optimal Nutrition for Physical Activity   86

   Nutrient Intake Among the Physically Active   88
   Good Nutrition Essentials   93
   Dietary Guidelines for Americans   93
   Physical Activity and Food Intake   98
   Precompetition Meal   103
   Liquid Meals and Prepackaged Nutrition Bars, Powders, and Drinks   104
   Carbohydrate Feedings Prior to, During, and in Recovery from Physical Activity   106
   High-Glycemic Foods' Possible Role in Obesity   110
   Foods' Insulin Index   111
   Glucose Feedings, Electrolytes, and Water Uptake   112

SECTION 2   **Energy for Physical Activity**   **119**

CHAPTER 4
Food's Energy Value   120

   Measuring Food's Energy Content   122
   Food's Gross Energy Value   124
   Food's Net Energy Value   126
   Calculating a Meal's Energy Value   127

CHAPTER 5
Introduction to Energy Transfer   134

   Energy: The Capacity for Work   136
   Energy Interconversions   137
   Biologic Work in Humans   139
   Enzymes and Coenzymes: Energy Release Rate Alteration   139
   Hydrolysis and Condensation: The Basis for Digestion and Synthesis   143

CHAPTER 6
Energy Transfer in the Body   150

PART 1 • PHOSPHATE BOND ENERGY   152
   Adenosine Triphosphate: The Energy Currency   152
   Phosphocreatine: The Energy Reservoir   154
   Cellular Oxidation   155
   Oxygen's Role in Energy Metabolism   157
PART 2 • ENERGY RELEASE FROM MACRONUTRIENTS   158
   Energy Release from Carbohydrate   160
   Energy Release from Lipid   168
   Energy Release from Protein   172
   The Metabolic Mill: Interrelationships Among Carbohydrate, Lipid, and Protein Metabolism   173

CHAPTER 7
Energy Transfer During Physical Activity   178

   Immediate Energy: The Adenosine Triphosphate-Phosphocreatine System   180
   Short-Term Energy: The Glycolytic (Lactate-Forming) System   180
   Long-Term Energy: The Aerobic System   182

Physical Activity Energy Spectrum 185
Recovery Oxygen Uptake 187

CHAPTER 8
Measuring Energy Expenditure — 194

Measuring the Body's Heat Production 196
Doubly Labeled Water Technique 202
Respiratory Quotient 202
Respiratory Exchange Ratio 205

CHAPTER 9
Energy Expenditure During Rest and Physical Activity — 210

PART 1 • ENERGY EXPENDITURE AT REST 212
Basal and Resting Metabolic Rate 212
Metabolic Size Concept 212
Metabolic Rate: Age and Sex Comparisons 214
Five Factors That Affect TDEE 216
PART 2 • ENERGY EXPENDITURE DURING PHYSICAL ACTIVITY 220
Energy Expenditure Classification for Physical Activities 220
The MET 221
Average Daily Energy Expenditure Rates 221
Energy Cost of Household, Industrial, and Recreational Activities 222
Body Mass Influence 222
Heart Rate to Estimate Energy Expenditure 222

CHAPTER 10
Energy Expenditure During Walking, Jogging, Running, and Swimming — 226

Human Movement Efficiency and Economy 228
Human Movement Efficiency 228
Human Movement Economy 230
Running Energy Expenditure 233
Swimming 239

CHAPTER 11
Individual Differences and Measuring Energy Capacities — 248

Metabolic Capacity and Exercise Performance: Specificity Versus Generality 250
Overview: Exercise Energy Transfer Capacity 250
Anaerobic Function Physiologic and Performance Tests 250
Anaerobic Energy Transfer: The Immediate and Short-Term Energy Systems 251
Anaerobic Energy Transfer: The Short-Term Glycolytic (Lactate-Forming) Energy System 253
Aerobic Energy Transfer: The Long-Term Energy System 258

SECTION 3 Aerobic Energy Delivery and Use — 273

CHAPTER 12
Pulmonary Structure and Function — 274

Ventilation Anatomy 276
Ventilation Mechanics 278
Inspiratory and Expiratory Dynamics 279
Lung Volumes and Capacities 281
Lung Function, Aerobic Fitness, and Physical Performance 283
Pulmonary Ventilation 284
Variations from Normal Breathing Patterns 287
The Respiratory Tract During Cold-Weather Physical Activity 289

CHAPTER 13
Gas Exchange and Transport — 292

PART 1 • GAS PARTIAL PRESSURE, MOVEMENT, AND EXCHANGE 294
Respired Gas Concentrations and Partial Pressures 294
Gas Movement in Air and Fluids 295
Gas Exchange in the Lungs and Tissues 297
PART 2 • OXYGEN TRANSPORT IN BLOOD 299
Oxygen Transport in Physical Solution 299
Oxygen Transport in Hemoglobin 299
P_{O_2} in the Lungs 300
P_{O_2} in the Tissues 303
PART 3 • CARBON DIOXIDE TRANSPORT IN BLOOD 305
Carbon Dioxide Transport in Physical Solution 305
Carbon Dioxide Transport as Bicarbonate 305
Carbon Dioxide Transport in Hb 306

CHAPTER 14
Pulmonary Ventilation Dynamics — 310

PART 1 • PULMONARY VENTILATION 310
Ventilatory Control 310
Ventilatory Regulation During Physical Activity 312
PART 2 • PULMONARY VENTILATION DURING PHYSICAL ACTIVITY 314
Ventilation and Energy Demands During Physical Activity 314
Oxygen Cost of Breathing 317
Does Ventilation Limit Aerobic Power and Endurance Performance? 320
PART 3 • ACID-BASE REGULATION 321
Buffering 321
Intense Physical Activity Effects 323

CHAPTER 15
The Cardiovascular System — 326

Cardiovascular System Components 328
Hypertension 338
Blood Pressure Response to Physical Activity 341
Heart's Blood Supply 345
Myocardial Metabolism 347

CHAPTER 16
Cardiovascular Regulation and Integration — 352

Intrinsic Heart Rate Regulation 354
Extrinsic Regulation of Heart Rate and Circulation 360
Blood Redistribution 365
Integrative Responses During Physical Activity 367
Physical Activity After Cardiac Transplantation 369

CHAPTER 17
Cardiovascular Dynamics During Physical Activity — 372

Measuring Cardiac Output 374
Cardiac Output at Rest 375
Cardiac Output During Physical Activity 376
Cardiac Output Distribution 378
Cardiac Output and Oxygen Transport 380
Cardiovascular Adjustments to Upper-Body Exercise 382

CHAPTER 18
Skeletal Muscle Structure and Function — 388

Skeletal Muscle Gross Structure 390
Skeletal Muscle Ultrastructure 396
Chemical and Mechanical Events During Muscle Action and Relaxation 403
Muscle Fiber Type 409

CHAPTER 19
Neural Control and Human Movement — 420

Neuromotor System Organization 422
Nerve Supply to Muscle 430
Proprioceptors: Specialized Receptors in Muscles, Tendons, and Joints 439

CHAPTER 20
The Endocrine System: Organization and Acute and Chronic Responses to Physical Activity — 448

Endocrine System Overview 450
Endocrine System Organization 450
Resting and Exercise-Induced Endocrine Secretions 455
Exercise Training and Endocrine Function 479
Resistance Training and Endocrine Function 485
Opioid Peptides and Physical Activity 486
Physical Activity and Immune Function 487

PART TWO
APPLIED EXERCISE PHYSIOLOGY — 499

SECTION 4 — Enhancing Energy Transfer Capacity — 501

CHAPTER 21
Training for Anaerobic and Aerobic Power — 502

Exercise Training Principles 504
How Training Impacts the Anaerobic Energy Systems 506
Anaerobic System Changes with Training 506
How Training Impacts the Aerobic System 507
Seven Factors Affecting Aerobic Training Responses 518
Tracking Aerobic Fitness Improvements 525
Maintaining Aerobic Fitness Gains 526
Training Methods 527
Overtraining Considerations 531
Physical Activity and Exercise Training During Pregnancy 533

CHAPTER 22
Muscular Strength: Training Muscles to Become Stronger — 542

PART 1 • STRENGTH MEASUREMENT AND RESISTANCE TRAINING 544
Muscular Strength Development Roots in Antiquity 544
Resistance Training Objectives 548
Muscle Strength Measurement 548
Gender Differences in Muscle Strength 552
Training Muscles to Become Stronger 556
PART 2 • RESISTANCE TRAINING: STRUCTURAL AND FUNCTIONAL ADAPTATIONS 569
Neural and Muscular Adaptations Impact Strength Improvements 569
Comparative Male and Female Training Responses 576
Detraining Effects on Muscle 577
Resistance Training and Metabolic Stress 578
Circuit Resistance Training 578
Muscle Soreness and Stiffness 579

CHAPTER 23
Special Aids to Exercise Training and Performance — 592

An Increasing Challenge to Fair Competition 594
On the Horizon 595

PART 1 • PHARMACOLOGIC AGENTS FOR ERGOGENIC EFFECTS 596
Anabolic Steroids 596
Structure and Action 596
Clenbuterol and Other β_2-Adrenergic Agonists 603
Other Adrenergic Agonists 605
Growth Hormone: Genetic Engineering Now Common in Sports 605
Dehydroepiandrosterone 606
Androstenedione: Benign Prohormone Nutritional Supplement or Potentially Harmful Drug? 608
Amino Acid Supplementation 609
Amphetamines 613
Caffeine 613
Ginseng and Ephedrine 616
Buffering Solutions 618
Anticortisol Compounds: Glutamine and Phosphatidylserine 619
β-Hydroxy-β-Methylbutyrate 620
PART 2 • NONPHARMACOLOGIC APPROACHES FOR ERGOGENIC EFFECTS 621
Red Blood Cell Reinfusion—Blood Doping 621
Hormonal Blood Boosting (EPO) 622
Warm-Up (Preliminary Exercise) 623
Oxygen Inhalation (Hyperoxia) 625
Modifying Carbohydrate Intake 627
Chromium 630
Creatine 632
Medium-Chain Triacylglycerols 636
Pyruvate 637

SECTION 5 — Exercise Performance and Environmental Stress — 645

CHAPTER 24
Physical Activity at Medium and High Altitude — 646

Altitude Stressors 648
Oxygen Loading at Altitude 649
Acclimatization 650
Metabolic, Physiologic, and Exercise Capacity at Altitude 658
Altitude Training and Sea-Level Performance 661
Combined Altitude Stay with Low-Altitude Training 662

CHAPTER 25
Exercise and Thermal Stress — 668

Weather Versus Climate: Time as a Factor 670
PART 1 • THERMOREGULATION MECHANISMS 670
Thermal Balance 670
Hypothalamic Temperature Regulation 671
Thermoregulation in Cold Stress 672
Thermoregulation During Heat Loss 672
How Clothing Impacts Thermoregulation 675
PART 2 • THERMOREGULATION AND ENVIRONMENTAL HEAT STRESS DURING PHYSICAL ACTIVITY 678
Physical Activity in the Heat 678
Rehydration and Hyperhydration to Maintain Fluid Balance 683
Factors That Modify Heat Tolerance 686
Complications from Excessive Heat Stress 689
PART 3 • THERMOREGULATION AND ENVIRONMENTAL COLD STRESS DURING PHYSICAL ACTIVITY 691
Physical Activity in the Cold 691
Cold Acclimatization 693
How Cold Is Too Cold? 694

CHAPTER 26
Sport Diving — 702

- Diving History: Antiquity to the Present 704
- Pressure-Volume Relationships and Diving Depth 712
- Snorkeling and Breath-Hold Diving 712
- Scuba Diving 717
- Special Problems Breathing Gases at High Pressures 720
- Dives to Exceptional Depths: Mixed-Gas Diving 725
- Underwater Swimming Energy Cost 728

CHAPTER 27
Microgravity: The Last Frontier — 734

- The Weightless Environment 736
- The International Space Station's 20th Anniversary 738
- Aerospace Physiology and Medicine Historical Overview 740
- Spaceflight Physiology 748
- Countermeasure Strategies 759
- Overview of Physiologic Responses to Spaceflight 767
- NASA's Ambitious Vision for Future Space Exploration 767
- Practical Benefits from Space Biology Research 774
- Final Words 774

SECTION 6
Body Composition, Energy Balance, and Weight Control — 793

CHAPTER 28
Body Composition Assessment — 794

- Four Limitations in Using the Weight-for-Height Tables 796
- Overweight, Overfat, and Obesity Prevalence 796
- The Body Mass Index: A Popular but Imprecise Clinical Standard 797
- Modeling Human Body Composition 801
- Common Techniques to Assess Body Composition 808
- Average Percentage Body Fat 829
- How to Determine Goal Body Mass 830
- Looking to a Brighter Future 830

CHAPTER 29
Physique, Performance, and Physical Activity — 836

- Physique Status in Champion Athletes 838
- Body Composition in 100-Year-Old Males and Females 855

CHAPTER 30
Overweight, Overfatness (Obesity), and Weight Control — 862

PART 1 • OBESITY 864
- Historical Perspective 864
- Obesity Remains a Global Epidemic 864
- Increased Body Fat: A Progressive Long-Term Process 867
- Physical Inactivity: A Crucial Component for Excessive Fat Accumulation 871
- Excessive Body Fat's Health Risks 872
- Criteria for Excessive Body Fat: How Fat Is Too Fat? 874

PART 2 • WEIGHT CONTROL PRIMARY PRINCIPLES INVOLVE DIET AND PHYSICAL ACTIVITY 882
- Energy Balance: Input Versus Output 882
- Dieting for Weight Control 883
- Factors That Impact Weight Loss 889
- Increase Physical Activity for Weight Control 890
- Regular Physical Activity's Effectiveness 893
- Weight Loss Recommendations for Wrestlers and Power Athletes 897
- Gaining Weight: The Competitive Athlete's Dilemma 898

SECTION 7
Exercise, Successful Aging, and Disease Prevention — 907

CHAPTER 31
Physical Activity, Health, and Aging — 908

- The Graying of America 910
- The New Gerontology 910

PART 1 • PHYSICAL ACTIVITY IN THE POPULATION 913
- Physical Activity Epidemiology 913

PART 2 • AGING AND PHYSIOLOGIC FUNCTION 921
- Age Trends 921
- Trainability and Age 930

PART 3 • PHYSICAL ACTIVITY, HEALTH, AND LONGEVITY 931
- Physical Activity, Health, and Longevity 931
- Regular Moderate Physical Activity Benefits 932

PART 4 • CARDIOVASCULAR DISEASES 934
- CHD Links to Cellular Level Alterations 935
- CHD Risk Factors 937

CHAPTER 32
Clinical Exercise Physiology for Cancer, Cardiovascular, and Pulmonary Rehabilitation — 952

- The Exercise Physiologist in the Clinical Setting 954
- Training and Certification Programs for Professional Exercise Physiologists 954
- Clinical Applications of Exercise Physiology to Diverse Diseases and Disorders 956
- Oncology 956
- Cardiovascular Diseases 960
- Cardiac Disease Assessment 964
- Stress Test Protocols 974
- Cardiovascular Disease and Exercise Capacity 976
- Prescribing PA and Exercise 977
- Cardiac Rehabilitation 979
- Pulmonary Diseases 980
- PA and Asthma 986
- Neuromuscular Diseases, Disabilities, and Disorders 987
- Renal Disease 988
- Cognitive/Emotional Diseases and Disorders 989

SECTION 8
On the Horizon — 1007

CHAPTER 33
Molecular Biology: New Vista for Exercise Physiology in Health, Disease, and Performance — 1008

PART 1 • MOLECULAR BIOLOGY HISTORICAL TOUR 1012
- Revolution in the Biologic Sciences 1014
- The Human Genome 1015
- Nucleic Acids 1017
- How DNA Replicates 1025
- Protein Synthesis: Transcription and Translation 1028
- Mutations 1041

PART 2 • NEW HORIZONS IN MOLECULAR BIOLOGY 1047
- Medically Related Research 1047
- Electrophoresis and Gel Transfer Methods 1054
- Gene Editing 1065

PART 3 • HUMAN PERFORMANCE RESEARCH 1070
- The Future Is Now 1075

Index 1087

Introduction: A View from the Past

Exercise Physiology: Roots and Historical Perspectives

It would be a herculean task to chronicle the rich exercise physiology history from its origins in ancient Asia to the present in an introductory text. We have chosen to present a chronological tour about key exercise science-related topics often not adequately developed in exercise physiology courses or their traditional textbooks. Our overall mission is to keep the history flame alive as students embark on their pursuits in the physical activity sciences. Along the way, we offer snapshots of events and people that profoundly influenced the exercise physiology field. We focus on the development of science-based curriculum in colleges and universities in the early 19th century and how influential, forward-thinking scientists helped incubate these early programs. Their dogged insistence on innovation and experimental rigor propelled disparate fields in medicine and the biological sciences to make rapid strides in creating new knowledge about how nutrition, heat, cold, underwater depth/pressure, altitude, and microgravity environmental stressors impacted physical activity.

Our discussion begins with acknowledging the ancient but tremendously influential Indian, Arabic, and prominent Greek physicians; we highlight some milestones (and ingenious experiments), including the many contributions from Sweden, Denmark, Norway, and Finland that fostered sport and exercise as a respectable scientific field. We discuss an information treasure trove about exercise physiology beginnings in America that we discovered in the archives of Amherst College in Massachusetts and in an anatomy and physiology textbook incorporating a built-in student study guide written by the first American father-son writing team. The father, Edward Hitchcock (1793–1864), was Amherst College President; the son, Edward Hitchcock, Jr. (1828–1911), was an Amherst graduate and Harvard-trained physician who assessed anthropometric and strength measurements for almost every student enrolled at Amherst College for nearly three decades from 1861 to 1889. In 1891, much of what forms the current curricula in exercise physiology (including body composition evaluation by anthropometry and muscular strength by dynamic measurements) began in the first physical education scientific laboratory at Harvard University's prestigious Lawrence Scientific School, which was founded in 1847 and placed into Harvard College and Graduate School of Arts and Letters in 1906 (www.thecrimson.com/article/1948/2/21/lawrence-scientific-school-marked-era-in/). The fortuitous science-oriented curricula began with a $50,000 gift to Harvard College from successful and prominent Massachusetts businessman and politician Abbot Lowell (1792–1855).

Another less formal but still tremendously influential factor affected exercise physiology's development: the publishing of American textbooks during the 19th century on anatomy and physiology, physiology, physiology and hygiene, and anthropometry. Teachers and research scientists interested in physiology-related topics could offer formal coursework to highlight exercise and human movement applications. More than 45 textbooks published between 1801 and 1899 yielded new information about exercise and training's influences on the muscular, circulatory, respiratory, nervous, and digestive systems. These early textbooks offered the beginning framework that would shape the future of exercise physiology's content during the following century.

Professor Roberta Park (1931–2018), distinguished UC Berkeley historian of physical education, exercise science, and sport, chronicled the early contributions of physician and science-oriented physical educators to the emerging field of exercise physiology. She steadfastly believed that physical education (and medicine) should be grounded on a sound scientific foundation and fueled by cutting-edge research. Professor Park is remembered for her many contributions to the field,[54,57,61] particularly a 1994 review about health history, physical fitness, and exercise and sport from 1983 to 1993 published in the *Journal of Sport History*.[56] Two of this textbook's authors (FK and VK) were privileged to receive the guidance of this insightful instructor and mentor, along with Franklin Henry (discussed below). Both individuals helped us to cement our unyielding conviction that physical education and exercise physiology will continue to thrive as an academic discipline in the coming decades.

Well-documented historical chronologies provide context and foster appreciation for the early scholars and educators who paved the way for the current cadre of sports science researchers. These early innovators developed new techniques and methodologies in the health, fitness, sports performance, and physical activity fields that became essential components of the exercise physiology core curriculum.

In the Beginning: Exercise Physiology Origins from Ancient Greece to America in the 1800s

Exercise physiology can be traced to the early civilizations of Greece and Asia Minor, although exercise, sports, games, and health topics concerned even earlier civilizations. These included the Minoan and Mycenaean cultures; the great biblical David and Solomon era; and the civilizations of Assyria, Babylonia, Media, and Persia, including Alexander the Great's empires. The ancient civilizations in Syria, Egypt, Macedonia, Arabia, Mesopotamia and Persia, India, and China referenced personal hygiene, exercise, and training. The ancient Indian physician Sushruta practiced in the 5th century BC and taught medical students about plastic surgery methods, a field he founded, particularly reshaping the nose (rhinoplasty). In India at that time adultery was punished by cutting off the nose—hence he devised methods to restore normal facial features to those who suffered this penalty. Historians remember Sushruta for his scholarship in producing the treatise, *Sushruta Samhita*, 150 years before Hippocrates (www.ancient.eu/sushruta/).[66,74] The Oxford University library houses Sushruta's edited compendium from 600 BC and a 1911 three-volume English translation (http://archive.org/stream/englishtranslati00susruoft#page/n3/mode/2up). He detailed 800 medical procedures and 121 blunt and sharp surgical tools (e.g., knives, scalpels, saws, scissors, forceps for extracting teeth and foreign bodies from the nose and ear, different needles for suturing, and bamboo splints to treat limb fractures; https://storage.googleapis.com/global-help-publications/books/help_hamlynhistoryofmedicine.pdf). He also described various disease states and organ deficiencies including how different exercise modes influenced human health and well-being (www.faqs.org/health/topics/50/Sushruta.html). This forward-thinking ancient healer considered obesity a disease and posited that a sedentary lifestyle contributed significantly to the condition.[74] The Indian **Ayurvedic medicine** ("life knowledge" or holistic healing) system existed centuries before the four most famous Greek physicians—Herodicus (5th century BC), Hippocrates (460–377 BC), Aristotle (384–322 BC), and Claudius Galenus (Κλαύδιος Γαληνός), Anglicized as Galen (AD 131–201)—developed their medical systems.

Herodicus (Ἡρόδικος), a physician and athlete, strongly advocated proper diet in physical training. Galen's birth date is estimated based on a notation he made at age 38 while serving as personal physician to the Roman emperors Marcus Aurelius and Lucius Verus.[27,62]

Image: Alessandro Tomasi

Hippocrates produced 87 treatises on medicine, including several on health and hygiene, during the Golden Age of ancient Greece from about 500 to 300 BC (www.ahistoryofgreece.com/goldenage.htm).[7,47,79] He espoused a profound understanding about human suffering,

Image courtesy Alessandro Tomasi, @ATomasi

emphasizing a doctor's place at the patient's bedside. Today, physicians take either the classical or contemporary Hippocratic Oath (www.nlm.nih.gov/hmd/greek/greek_oath.html) based on his "Corpus Hippocratum" and a wish for his disciples to advocate walking as man's best medicine.

Five centuries after Hippocrates, during the early decline of the Roman Empire, Galen emerged as one of the most renowned and influential physicians who ever lived. His early writings influenced the famous physician Hippocrates, who is considered the "father" of present-day sports medicine and was first to write about preventative medicine.[77,78] A wealthy architect's son Galen was born in Pergamos, an ancient Greek kingdom on Asia Minor's coast and later a Roman province that was renowned for its 50,000-book library (approximately one fourth as many as in Alexandria, the greatest city for learning and education in antiquity) and its medical center at the Temple of Asclepios (http://whc.unesco.org/en/list/491), where Galen studied from AD 152 to 156. Galen implemented and enhanced current thinking about health and scientific hygiene, an area that some might consider "applied" exercise physiology. He taught and practiced the "laws of health," similar to today's sensible health advice—*breathe fresh air, eat proper foods, drink the right beverages, exercise, get adequate sleep, have a daily bowel movement, and control one's emotions*.[7] A prolific writer Galen produced at least 80 sophisticated treatises (and perhaps 500 essays) on topics related to human anatomy and physiology, nutrition, growth and development, exercise's beneficial effects,[9] deleterious sedentary living consequences, and treatments for various diseases, including obesity. His study of obesity, including the *polisarkia* concept (now known as **morbid obesity**), undoubtedly influenced Sushruta.[71] Galen proposed treatments that are commonplace today—diet, exercise, and pharmaceuticals. One of the first "bench physiologists," he conducted original experiments in physiology, comparative anatomy, and medicine and performed dissections on humans, goats, pigs, cows, horses, and elephants. As physician to the Pergamos gladiators, he invented surgical procedures to treat tendons and muscles torn in combat, such as a shoulder procedure depicted in a 1544 woodcut (**FIG. I.1**) by famed Renaissance fresco artist Francesco Salviati (1510–1563). This rendering provides a direct link to Hippocratic surgical practice, which continued through the Byzantine period. Galen followed the tenants of the Hippocratic school of medicine

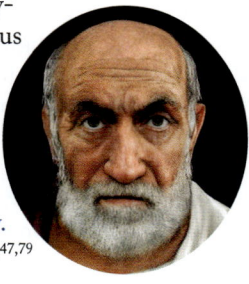

FIGURE I.1. Woodcut by Renaissance artist Francesco Salviati (1510–1563) based on Galen's De Fascius from the first century BC.

Appendix A, available online on Lippincott Connect, provides several influential bibliographies about anatomy and physiology, anthropometry, exercise and training, and exercise physiology.

(https://link.springer.com/article/10.1007/s00381-010-1271-2), believing logical science grounded in experimentation and observation should focus on resolving many disease origins.

Galen wrote detailed descriptions of the forms, kinds, and varieties of "swift" and vigorous exercises, including their proper quantity and duration (**FIG. I.2**). The following quote about exercise from the first complete English translation concerning hygiene summarizes Galen's beliefs about healthful living (*De Sanitate Tuenda*, pp. 53–54):[27]

> To me it does not seem that all movement is exercise, but only when it is vigorous.... The criterion of vigorousness is change of respiration; those movements that do not alter the respiration are not called exercise. .... The uses of exercise, I think are twofold, one for the evacuation of the excrements, the other for the production of good condition of the firm parts of the body.

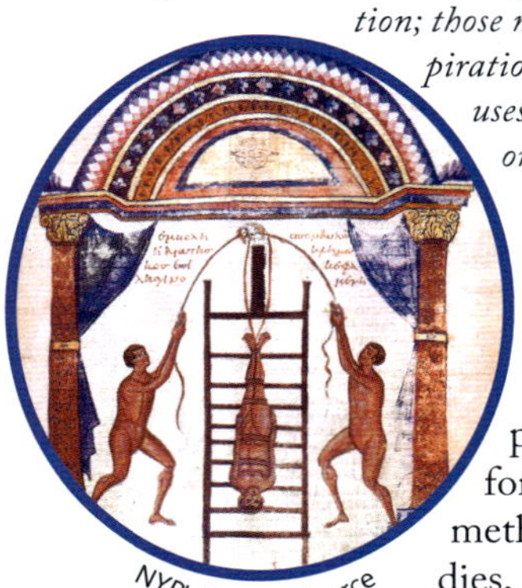

During the early Greek period, the Hippocratic school for physicians devised ingenious methods to treat common maladies, including procedures to reduce pain from dislocated lower lumbar vertebrae, as illustrated in the 11th-century *Commentaries of Apollonius of Chitiron* on the *Periarthron of Hippocrates*. This early Greek surgical "sports medicine" intervention (hanging upside down) treated both injured athletes and the common citizen. Another image shows a procedure to restore a dislocated jaw during a gladiator fight. Note the assistant pushing down on the athlete's head to stabilize it while the practitioner (doctor) uses crude dental tools to restore jaw function, often under numbing opioid influence.

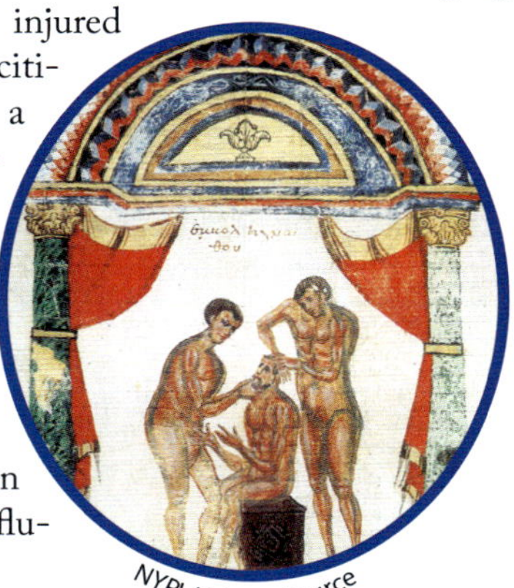

Historians often credit early Greek physicians with the advancements that have led to modern-day medicine, but other influential physicians also contributed, such as in the area of physiology related to the pulmonary circulation. West[75] provides an insightful review of the contributions of Arab physician Ibn al-Nafis (1213–1288), who challenged Galen's long-standing beliefs regarding how blood moved from the heart's right to left sides. He also predicted capillary functions 400 years before Malpighi discovered the pulmonary capillaries. The timeline in **FIGURE I.3** highlights key contributors to medicine, from the time of the ancient Greeks to the Islamic Golden Age, which led to the European Renaissance in the late 1400s and early 1500s. During this period, many physicians, particularly Persian physician Ibn Sina (Avicenna [ca. 980–1037]; www.muslimphilosophy.com/sina/), contributed knowledge about bodily functions to 200 books, including the influential *Shifa* (*The Book of Healing*) and *Al Qanun fi Tibb* (*The Canon of Medicine*).[75]

Book 1 The Art of Preserving Health	
Chapter	Title
I	Introduction
II	The Nature and Sources of Growth and of Disease
III	Production and Elimination of Excrements
IV	Objectives and Hypothesis of Hygiene
V	Conditions and Constitutions
VI	Good Constitution: A Mean Between Extremes
VII	Hygiene of the Newborn
VIII	The Use and Value of Exercise
IX	Hygiene of Breast-Feeding
X	Hygiene of Bathing and Massage
XI	Hygiene of Beverages and Fresh Air
XII	Hygiene of the Second Seven Years
XIII	Causes and Prevention of Excrementary Retardation
XIV	Evacuation of Retained Excrements
XV	Summary of Book 1
Book 2 Exercise and Massage	
I	Standards of Hygiene Under Individual Conditions
II	Purposes, Time, and Methods of Exercise and Massage
III	Techniques and Varieties of Massage
IV	Theories of Theon and Hippocrates
V	Definitions of Various Terms
VI	Further Definitions About Massage
VII	Amount of Massage and Exercise
VIII	Forms, Kinds, and Varieties of Exercise
IX	Varieties of Vigorous Exercise
X	Varieties of Swift Exercises
XI	Effects, Exercises, Functions, and Movements
XII	Determination of Diet, Exercise, and Regime

FIGURE I.2. Table of contents for books 1 and 2 from Galen's *De Sanitate Tuenda (Hygiene)*.

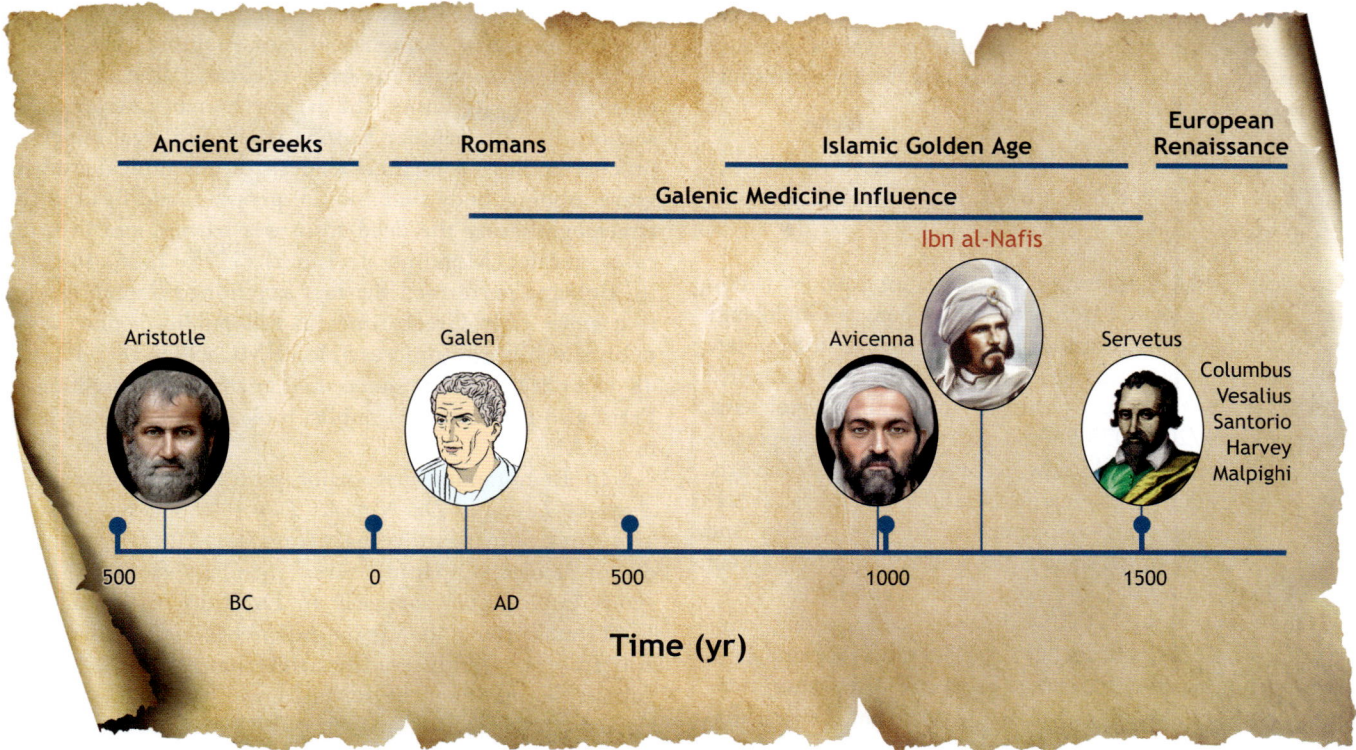

FIGURE I.3. Ancient medicine's Greek and Islamic Golden Age influences.
(Aristotle image courtesy Alessandro Tomasi @ATomasi__; background image: Andrey_Kuzmin/Shutterstock)

The more "modern-day" exercise physiology era includes the Renaissance, Enlightenment, and contributions from European scientific discoveries. In this period, Galen's ideas impacted the writings from pioneer physiologists, anatomists, doctors, and hygiene and health teachers.[52,62,63] Significant contributors include Leonardo da Vinci (1452–1519), Michael Servetus (1511–1564; discovered that blood passes through the pulmonary circulation without moving directly from the right to the left ventricle), Andreas Vesalius (1514–1564), Realdus Columbus (1516–1559; Vesalius' student, who developed concepts about pulmonary circulation and discovered that the heart has two ventricles, not the three postulated by the Galenic School), Santorio Santorio (1561–1636), and William Harvey (1578–1657). We highlight the contributions of da Vinci, Vesalius, Santorio, and Harvey later in this introduction.

In Venice in 1539, Italian physician Hieronymus Mercurialis (1530–1606) published *De Arte Gymnastica Apud Ancientes* (*The Art of Gymnastics Among the Ancients*). This text, heavily influenced by Galen and other early Greek and Latin authors, profoundly shaped subsequent writings about physical training and exercise (then called gymnastics) and health (hygiene). This influence emerged not only in Europe (affecting the Swedish and Danish gymnastic systems), but also the 19th-century gymnastic-hygiene movement in early America. **FIGURE I.4**, redrawn from *De Arte Use Gymnastica*, acknowledges the early Galenic essay, "Exercise with the Small Ball," highlighting his technical rigor about specific strengthening exercises emphasizing rope climbing and discus throwing. Specific sport training helped to prepare athletes for competitions, served as exercises for the "elite" in the population, and was practiced by scribes assigned to well-known mentors in the arts.

Mercurialis favored discus throwing to aid patients suffering from arthritis by improving trunk and arm muscle strength. He advocated rope climbing because it did not pose health problems and was a firm believer in walking, stating that "… a mild pace was good for stimulating conversation, and a faster pace would stimulate appetite and help with digestion." He advocated climbing mountains to help with leg

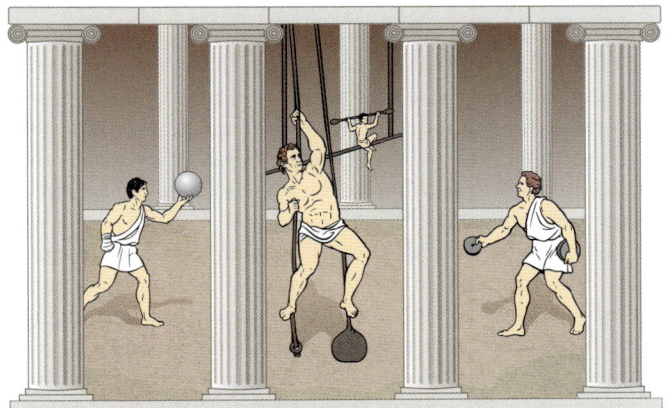

FIGURE I.4. Greek influence of Galen's famous essay, "Exercise with the Small Ball" from Mercurialis's *De Arte Gymnastica Apud Ancientes*, illustrating discus throwing and rope climbing to increase muscle strength.

problems and long jumping (but not during pregnancy) but did not recommend tumbling and handsprings because such movements would produce adverse effects from the intestines pushing against the diaphragm!

Renaissance Period to Nineteenth Century

New ideas formulated during the Renaissance exploded almost every concept inherited from antiquity. Johannes Gutenberg's (ca. AD 1400–1468) printing press, the first to incorporate replaceable, movable type, spread both classic and newly acquired knowledge to the masses (https://makinghistoryrelevant.wordpress.com/2011/07/09/1450-gutenberg-printing-press/). New text materials would now become available for the arts, history, geography, and emerging natural and physical sciences. New educational opportunities for the wealthy and privileged sprang up in universities and colleges throughout Europe (e.g., Bologna, Cambridge, Oxford, and Paris).

The supernatural still influenced discussions concerning physical phenomena, yet prior ideas grounded in religious dogma found a new basis in scientific experimentation. For example, medicine had to confront the new diseases spread by commerce with distant lands. The Black Death plague and other epidemics killed at least 25 million people throughout Europe in just 3 years (1347–1351; www.history.com/topics/middle-ages/black-death). Death from the plague, terrifying and swift, often occurred within 24 hr following symptom onset, which included blood and pus seeping from swelling masses in the armpits and groin followed by fever, chills, vomiting, diarrhea, and excruciating aches and pains.

Medical care became increasingly important at all societal levels as populations expanded throughout Europe and elsewhere. Unfortunately, medical knowledge failed to keep pace. For roughly 12 centuries, physicians, with the exception of the Islamic physicians, made few advances in medicine. Early physician writings had either been lost or preserved only in the Arab world. The devotion given to classical authors allowed the teachings of Hippocrates and Galen to still dominate medical education through the 15th century. Renaissance discoveries greatly modified these approaches. New anatomists went beyond simplistic notions about the four humors—fire, earth, water, air, and their hot, dry, cold, and wet qualities—as they discovered the complexities regarding respiratory, excretory, and circulatory mechanisms.[7,11,80,81]

Once rediscovered, these forgotten ideas caused turmoil. The Vatican banned human dissections, yet a number of "progressive" medical schools continued to engage in such practices, sanctioning one or two cadavers a year or granting official permission to perform an "anatomy" (the old name for a dissection) every 3 years. Performing autopsies helped physicians solve legal questions about a person's death or determine disease origin. In the mid-1200s at the University of Bologna in Italy, every medical student had to attend one yearly dissection, with 20 students assigned to a male cadaver and 30 students to a female cadaver. In 1442, the University of Bologna's Rector required that cadavers for an "anatomy" come from an area located at least 30 miles outside city limits. The earliest human cadaveric dissections in 14th-century Europe relied on illegal means to procure bodies for medical analysis or anatomical study—grave robbing, body snatching of people found dead in the streets, gathering the dead from war battles, and in some cases murder. Mondino de Liuzzi (1275–1326) in 1315 in Bologna performed the first sanctioned human dissection since early Greek times in full public display www.ncbi.nlm.nih.gov/pmc/articles/PMC4582158/pdf/acb-48-153.pdf). The first sanctioned anatomical dissection in Paris, also performed in public, took place 168 years later, in 1483.[45]

In Rembrandt's first major portrait commission, *The Anatomy Lesson of Dr. Nicholas Tulp* (**FIG. I.5**; www.visual-arts-cork.com/famous-paintings/anatomy-lesson-of-doctor-nicolaes-tulp.htm), seven members from the Surgeon's Guild listen intensely to Dr. Tulp on January 31, 1632 (but without "hands-on" experience) as he dissects an arm from a recently executed thief hanged earlier in the day. In the painting, the forceps grasp different arm muscles and tendons to demonstrate the mechanical connection to the fingers of the left hand. The bottom right reveals an open copy from the famous anatomy text *De humani corporis fabrica* by Andreas Vesalius (www.youtube.com/watch?v=DhefUahS55o). This text, by the Belgian pioneer anatomist and physician Vesalius in the 1540s, and later William Harvey's pioneering 1616 lecture on blood flow made anatomic study a central focus in medical education, yet conflicted with the Catholic church's strictures against individual rights violations concerning the dead because the doctrine cherished each person's eventual resurrection. In fact, the church considered anatomic dissections a disfiguring violation of bodily integrity, despite dismembering being a common punishment for criminals. Nevertheless, the close

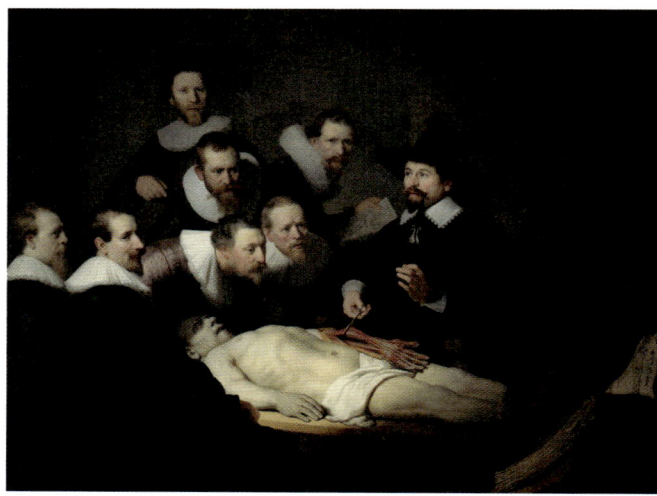

FIGURE I.5. Rembrandt's 1632 *The Anatomy Lesson of Dr. Nicholas Tulp.*
(The Yorck Project: 10,000 Meisterwerke der Malerei.)

cooperation among artists and medical school physicians to portray anatomical dissections became essential in medical education. It also satisfied a public thirst for new information in the emerging field concerning functional anatomy soon to be named "physiology and medicine."

First Appearance of the Term Physiology: A 1552 Medical Textbook

Sixteenth century anatomists played a key role diluting Galenic doctrine about body functioning based on the four humors. Anatomists piercing the veil of how anatomy could explain function fostered a yearning to more fully understand how various systems worked harmoniously based on scientific rationale and direct observation. Salient examples include how muscle contracted and relaxed, how a drop of blood traveled from the heart to the periphery and back again, and how internal chemical reactions could explain fluid exchange, digestion, and heat production from metabolism. Jean Fernel

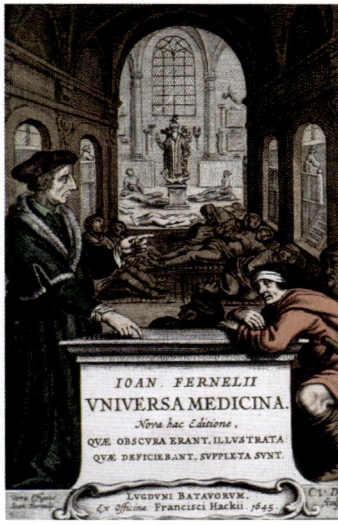

Courtesy National Library of Medicine

(1497–1558), a French physician and professor of medicine at the College de Cornouailles in northern France, coined the term *physiology* in one of his three seminal volumes, *Universa Medicina* (first published 1554; Fernel is depicted in color standing at the left). One of the volumes described diseases (*Pathologia*) and another their treatments (*Therapeutice*). In *Physiologia*, first published in 1552 with 30 subsequent reissues, Fernel posited that "physiology" should describe real-world natural phenomena about biological functions, not the nonnatural ancient Greek humors and natural philosophy that pervaded Galenic medicine for at least 1500 years (www.nature.com/articles/456446b#rightslink). Fernel's new paradigm proposed that the term *physiology* should have essential "truths" as did chemistry and physics, with basic understandings grounded in facts, direct observation, and experimentation. His ideas did not allow for supposition or "nonverifiable animal spirits," which saturated medieval medicine about the body's innermost structures and functions. It was one thing to have anatomists eloquently illustrate body parts, as Vesalius and others did, but it was quite another to explain how body parts like the heart, lungs, kidneys, and blood interacted in a functioning unified body. Fernel's unique propositional framework opened a future avenue for experimentalists to connect form with function and to present a systems approach, not an isolated compartmentalized view, to better understand the new and developing human science—*physiologia*.

First Anatomy Textbook and Human Dissections

In 1316, Mondino de Luzzio (Mondinus; ca. 1270–1326; https://biography.yourdictionary.com/mondino-de-luzzi), a physician and anatomy professor at Bologna, published *Anathomia*, the first book about human anatomy emphasizing dissection. He was first to require teaching systems-oriented anatomy in the medical curriculum (*Anathomia Corporis Humani*; 1316). Human cadavers were foremost in how Mondimus taught anatomy, not Greek and Latin dogma or experiments involving animals to explain human functions. First published in 1478 for mass distribution, *Anathomia* became the most widely used anatomy textbook for the

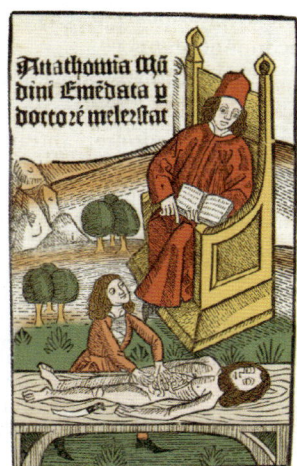

Courtesy National Library of Medicine

next 200 years through 40 editions until the mid-1600s. The 1513 edition preserved the identical inaccurate heart drawing, which included three ventricles, as in the original 1478 edition. By the turn of the 15th century, postmortem anatomic dissections in France and Italy's medical schools were common; they paved the way for Renaissance anatomists whose careful observations and practical experience facilitated connections between human form and function.

First Female Anatomists

Two female faculty from the University of Bologna achieved distinction in anatomy. Laura Caterina Bassi (1711–1778; https://mathshistory.st-andrews.ac.uk/Biographies/Bassi/), the first woman to earn a doctor of philosophy degree and the university's first female professor, specialized in experimental physics and basic sciences. Soon after Bassi, female scholars were allowed to teach in university classrooms. Bassi presented yearly public lectures on physics-related topics (including electricity and hydraulics, correcting telescope distortion, hydrometry, and the relation between a flame and "stable air"). Anna Morandi Manzolini (1717–1774; www.theatlantic.com/health/archive/2012/03/the-lady-anatomist-18th-century-wax-sculptures-by-anna-manzolini/254515/), also professor and chair at the University of Bologna's Anatomy Department, created internal organ wax models and became the

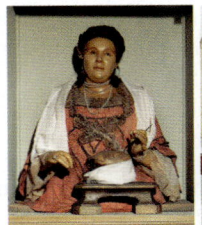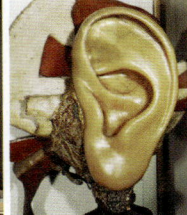

Erich Lessing/Art Resource, NY

anatomy department's chief model maker. The wax self-portrait in the Museum of Human Anatomy at Bologna University (www.youtube.com/watch?v=pTxUXEqqx98) illustrates Manzolini performing an anatomical dissection, clad in the traditional white lab coat, but also dressed in silks with diamonds and pearl jewelry—respectful of her upper social and economic status.

Manzolini produced an ear model that students took apart and reassembled to better understand internal structures. Her abdomen and uterus wax and wood models were used didactically for several hundred years in the medical school.

Other distinguished contributors to the original medical school education included Marcello Malpighi (1628–1694), the father of microscopic anatomy, histology, physiology, and embryology, who studied microscopic tissues and was first to identify capillaries and various kidney structures; physician and skilled anatomist Antonio Maria Valsalva (1666–1723), who coined the term *Valsalva maneuver* and named the Eustachian tube[82] (see Chapter 13); and anatomist Luigi Galvani (1737–1798), a Malpighi student who conducted research in bioelectromagnetics (animal electricity) and discovered that excised frog leg muscle twitched when stimulated by an electric current. Galvani's early experiments paved the way for modern **electrophysiology**.

Progress in understanding human anatomic form eventually led specialists in **physical culture** and hygiene to design exercises to improve overall body strength and training regimens—ever increasing in popularity—that prepared individuals for rowing, boxing, wrestling, competitive walking, and track and field activities and competitions. These exercise specialists and instructors predated today's personal trainers and sports coaches.

Notable European Scientists

The new knowledge explosion in the physical and biologic sciences helped set the stage for future discoveries in human physiology related to states of rest and physical activity.

Leonardo da Vinci (1452–1519)

Da Vinci dissected about 30 human cadavers ranging in age from 2 to 100 years at the hospital of Santa Maria Nuova in Florence (https://www.bbc.com/culture/article/20130828-leonardo-da-vinci-the-anatomist). His realistic drawings presented bodies in different decomposition stages, without use of embalming fluids.

Da Vinci's achievements in anatomy include the following:

- Deduced the nervous system's hierarchical structure, with the brain as a directing command center
- Deduced that the eye's retina was light sensitive, not the lens as previously surmised
- Dissected the fragile eye structures by inventing new thin sectioning methods that included fixing the eye after heating its proteins
- Observed atherosclerotic lesions and deduced their possible role in coronary artery obstruction
- Identified the heart as a muscle "pump," with the arterial pulse corresponding to ventricular contraction
- Developed a system to explain muscular movements by using wires to recreate movements. For example, he determined the mechanics of the biceps brachii muscle and arm action. He explained elbow flexion and hand supination through ulnar twisting action. His detailed drawings with written explanations showed the full arm and its motions, including scapular function.
- Deduced the equal contribution from the mother and father to inherited fetal characteristics

Accurate as Da Vinci's numerous and detailed sketches were, they still preserved Galenic beliefs. Although he never observed pores in the heart's septum, he included them believing they existed because Galen had supposedly "seen" them. Da Vinci first drew accurately the heart's inner structures and constructed valvular function models that showed how the blood flowed only in one direction. This observation contradicted Galen's notion about the ebb and flow of blood among the heart's chambers. Da Vinci could not explain venous and arterial roles in blood flow to and from the heart. It would take another half-century for William Harvey (discussed below) to discover unequivocally that veins return blood to the heart and only arteries conduct blood from the heart to the periphery. Many of Da Vinci's drawings were lost for nearly two centuries and so were unavailable to impact later anatomic experimentation.

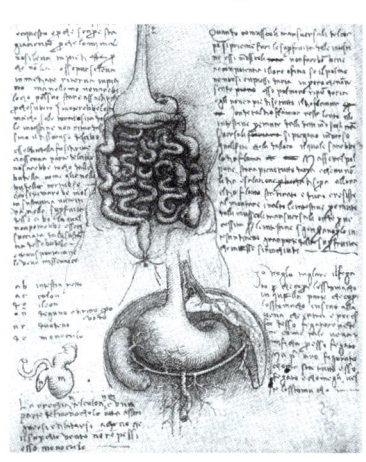

Royal Collection Trust/© Her Majesty Queen Elizabeth II 2021

Da Vinci's artistic technique was influenced by Leon Battista Alberti (1404–1472; https://www.theartstory.org/artist/alberti-leon-battista/life-and-legacy/), a prolific architect who perfected three-dimensional perspectives. This new approach influenced Da Vinci's internal anatomic relationships, as portrayed in his famous idealized nude, *Vitruvian Man*. In his famous drawings of the Vitruvian

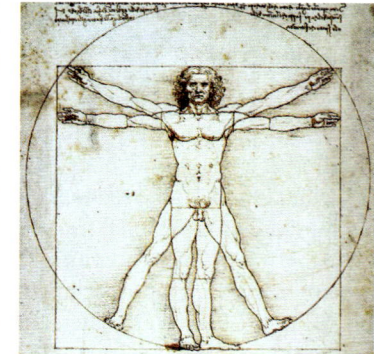

proportions of a man's body, first standing inscribed within a square and then overlaid with spread feet and arms inscribed in a circle, Da Vinci illustrated human proportionality by fusing art with science.

Da Vinci's drawings, although not published during his lifetime, evidently inspired the Flemish physician and anatomist Andreas Vesalius (1514–1564; https://evolution.berkeley.edu/the-history-of-evolutionary-thought/pre-1800/comparative-anatomy-andreas-vesalius/). Vesalius pointed out, based on direct cadaver analyses, that Galen's earlier presumptions about some anatomic relationships had been wrong. Careful reading by scholars verified that Galen based his anatomic observations not on human dissections, but on those of oxen and old-world Barbary macaque monkeys from Algeria and Morocco. Searching for such truths led to Vesalius' publication of his incomparable anatomy text, *De humani corporis fabrica libri septem* (*The Seven Books on the Structure of the Human Body*), commonly known as *Fabrica*.

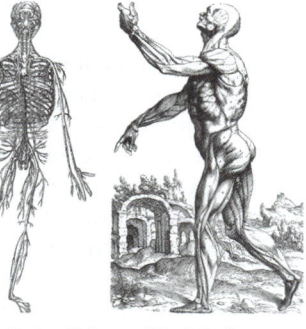

Courtesy National Library of Medicine"

Vesalius's masterful, detailed depiction of human muscular and skeletal architecture, which pared away one muscle layer at a time, revealed the never-before-seen structures beneath. His anatomic drawings show major nerves on the left and the muscular system in action to the right. These three exemplary Renaissance anatomists—Da Vinci, Alberti, and Vesalius—empowered future physiologists and physicians to better understand different body systems with technical accuracy, not just in a way that was purely theoretical or distorted by religious bias.

Albrecht Dürer (1471–1528)

Dürer, a German contemporary of Da Vinci (www.albrecht-durer.org), extended the Italian's concern for ideal dimensions as depicted in Da Vinci's Vitruvian Man by illustrating age-related differences in body segment ratios formulated by 1st century BC Roman architect Marcus Vitruvius Pollio (*De architectura libri decem* [*Ten books on architecture*]). Dürer created a **canon of proportion**, considering total height as unity. For example, in his schema shown for a female, the length of the foot was one sixth of this total, the head one seventh, and the hand one tenth. Relying on his artistic and printmaking skills rather than objective comparison, Dürer made the height ratio between men and women as 17 to 18 (later proved incorrect). Putting Dürer's ideal proportionality ratio into perspective, consider that the ancient Greek physicians

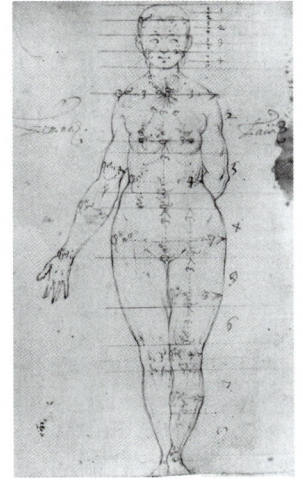

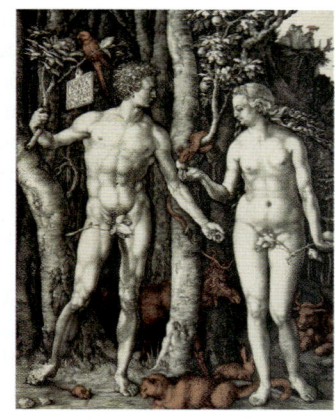

believed the four humors that dominated Galenic medicine actually dictated ideal geometric proportions, not just for humans but for animals. The answer built on the commonly accepted ancient Greek **four humors theory** (www.greekmedicine.net/b_p/Four_Humors.html) and its intrinsic tie to climate. For example, a horse's external proportions and behavior related to the internal proportions of the body's blood humor. As such, each animal's body proportions represented a proportional mix among the four fluid humors related to the climate where the animal lived. In hot and dry lands (such as Asia minor), creatures tended to have an overabundance of yellow bile. In wet and cold lands, such as England and Scotland, the animals had excessive phlegm and thus a **phlegmatic** character. Clearly, the land with the most moderate climate produced the "best" animals. This proportionality theory, originating in ancient Greece, informed Dürer's proportioned illustrations of Adam and Eve in 1542 (www.metmuseum.org/art/collection/search/336222). Nonetheless, Dürer's work inspired American physician Albert Behnke three centuries later in the 1950s to quantify body proportions relative to height into male and female reference body composition standards (see Chapter 28).

Michelangelo Buonarroti (1475–1564)

Michelangelo, like Da Vinci, was a superb anatomist (www.ncbi.nlm.nih.gov/pmc/articles/PMC1279184/). In his drawings, "David" being the most famous, body segments appear in proper proportion (www.michelangelo.org/david.jsp). His famous sculpture clearly shows the veins, tendons, and muscles enclosing a realistic skeleton. His Sistine Chapel frescos often exaggerate musculature (https://theculturetrip.com/europe/italy/articles/michelangelos-must-see-frescoes-in-the-sistine-chapel/); nevertheless, they still convey a scientist's vision of the human body's ideal proportionality.

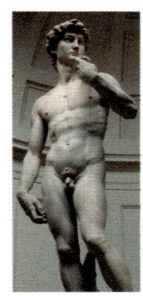

From F. Katch

Andreas Vesalius (1514–1564)

Belgian anatomist and physician Vesalius learned Galenic medicine in Paris but eventually rejected early Greek ideas about human body functions based on his direct cadaver examinations. As his career began, Vesalius authored books on anatomy relying on ancient Greek and Arabic texts but incorporating observations from his detailed dissections.

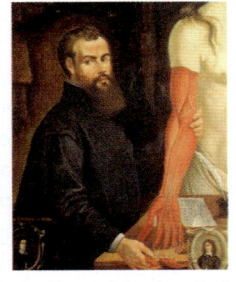

His research culminated in the exquisitely illustrated text first published in Basel, Switzerland, in 1543, *De Humani Corporis Fabrica* (*On the Fabric of the Human Body*), which included a self-portrait showing the exquisite anatomic upper and lower right arm details. Many consider Vesalius's drawings and accompanying 200 woodcuts the best anatomical renderings ever made, ultimately ushering in the modern medicine age (https://hyperallergic.com/712087/500-years-of-drawing-the-human-body/). The same year, he published *Epitome*, a popular abridged version of *De Fabrica* with less text (www.ncbi.nlm.nih.gov/pmc/articles/PMC1520217/), which was translated into English in 1949 (www.ncbi.nlm.nih.gov/pmc/articles/PMC1520217/pdf/califmed00258-0069a.pdf).

Some physicians and clergymen became outraged, fearful that the new science was overturning Galen's time-honored work. Vesalius's treatise accurately rendered bones, muscles, nerves, internal organs, blood vessels (including veins for blood-letting, a popular technique through the ages including Greek antiquity to rid the body of diseases and toxins; medicalantiques.com/medical/Scarifications_and_Bleeder_Medical_Antiques.htm), and the brain. His art differed from Galenic tradition by ignoring what he could not observe directly; hence, several Vesalius drawings contain curious inaccuracies. For example, he drew the inferior vena cava as a continuous vessel; inserted an extra muscle to move the eyeball; and added an extra neck muscle present only in apes. Despite these minor discrepancies, Vesalius clearly attempted to accurately connect form with function. He showed that a muscle could still function after a longitudinal slice was made along the muscle's belly, but a transverse cut prevented its function. Vesalius verified that nerves controlled muscles and stimulated movement, the forerunner to modern muscle contraction theory. His two beautifully illustrated texts overwhelmingly influenced medical education. Their elaborate details about human structures questioned traditional human anatomy theories and emboldened later researchers to explore circulation and metabolism unburdened by misconceptions promoted for over 15 centuries. Vesalius's illuminating and detailed artwork from cadaver dissections hastened future important discoveries in physiology, ushering in modern science and influencing future medical practice.[85]

Santorio Santorio (1561–1636)

A friend of Galileo and professor of medicine at Padua, Italy, Venetian physician Santorio invented innovative exacting devices still in use in clinical medical practice (http://exhibits.hsl.virginia.edu/treasures/santorio-santorio-1561-1636/). Some historians believe that Santorio's body-weighing contraption may have been the first precision medical device. Santorio studied digestion and changes in metabolism by constructing a wooden frame that supported a chair, bed, and worktable.

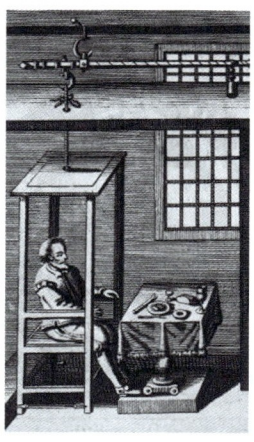

Suspended from the ceiling with scales, the frame recorded daily changes in body weight. For 30 continuous years, Santorio slept, ate, worked, and made love in the weighing contraption to record how much his weight changed as he ate, fasted, or excreted, among other activities. He coined the term "insensible perspiration" to account for body weight differences because he believed weight gain or loss occurred through the pores during respiration. Often depriving himself of food and drink, Santorio determined that daily change in body mass approached 1.25 kg. Santorio's 1614 book about medical aphorisms, *De Medicina Statica Aphorismi*, drew worldwide attention. Although this scientifically trained Italian did not explain the role nutrition played in energy balance (weight gain or loss), Santorio nevertheless inspired later 18th century metabolism researchers by quantifying metabolic effects. Santorio recorded changes in daily body temperature with the first air thermometer, crafted in 1612 as a measuring device. Accuracy was poor because scientists had not yet discovered air pressure's differential effects on temperature. Santorio also measured pulse rate with Galileo's pulsilogium (pulsiometer; http://galileo.rice.edu/sci/instruments/pendulum.html), a device that essentially acted as a stopwatch to monitor a pendulum's oscillation frequencies, which related inversely to the square root of its length. The pulsilogium, composed of a heavy leaden bob and silk cord held by the fingers (top left of inset image), worked by changing the pendulum's length to adjust

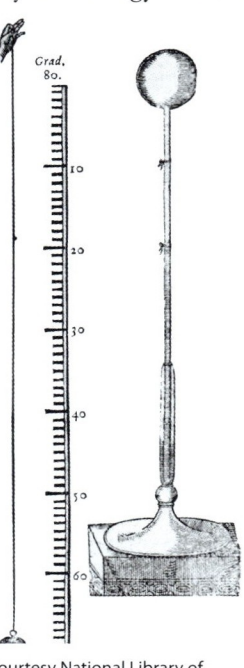

Courtesy National Library of Medicine

oscillation frequency until the periodic oscillation synchronized with the patient's pulse beat.[94] The pulse rate corresponded to the knot's position in the cord alongside a horizontal ruler, with pulse rate measured in length units. Santorio and Galileo, both mathematically minded, jointly invented a wind gauge, a hygrometer to measure ambient humidity, a water current meter to extract bladder stones and remove foreign bodies from the ear, a trocar (sharp surgical device fitted inside a cannula) to surgically drain fluids from cavities, a thermometer, and a device allowing patients to bathe while bedridden consisting of an enclosed vessel containing air that contracted or expanded with temperature fluctuations, forcing water to move up or down a tube.[95]

Ever inventive, Santorio, considered a pioneer physician dedicated to quantifying the science of physical measurement, introduced experimentation into biological science measurement in a Latin treatise published in 1602 or 1603 (*Methodus vitandorum errorum omnium qui in arte medica contingent* [*Methods to avoid errors in medical practice*]). His work led to a better understanding about evidence-based medicine. Santorio made detailed margin notes (*marginalia*) in his books and manuscripts, which later helped to explain his thinking regarding the many topics he wrote about, such as compounds, mixtures, tiny particles (later identified as molecules), and structure of matter.

Santorio surely would be pleased to know that his scientific insights contributed to the soon-burgeoning literature in basic human physiology and, in the 19th and 20th centuries, to modern exercise physiology. He penned this observation almost 400 years ago:

> *In order to commemorate quickly and exactly my knowledge of the pulse of a patient, I have invented the pulsilogium, which makes it possible to measure exactly the beats of the arteries and to compare them with the beats of earlier days. With the help of the pulsilogium, we can monitor at what day and at which hour the pulse deviated in intensity and frequency from its natural state.*

William Harvey (1578–1657)

William Harvey discovered that blood circulates continuously in one direction and, as Vesalius had done before, overthrew at least 1500 years of medical dogma. Animal **vivisection** disproved the ancient supposition that blood moved from the heart's right side to left side through septal pores—structures that even Da Vinci and Vesalius had erroneously acknowledged. Harvey announced his discovery during a 3-day dissection/lecture on April 16, 1616, at the oldest medical institution in England, begun by a Royal Charter from King Henry VIII in 1518—the Royal College of Physicians in London (www.rcplondon.ac.uk/about-rcp/our-history). Twelve years later, he published the details about his insightful experiments in a 72-page monograph, *Exercitatio Anatomica de Motu Cordis et Sanguinis in Animalibus* (*An Anatomical Treatise on the Movement of the Heart and Blood in Animals*; www.bartleby.com/38/3/1000.html), which would become a milestone advance in physiological knowledge about the heart and its role in circulation.

© National Portrait Gallery, London

By combining the new technique of experimentation on living creatures with mathematical logic, Harvey deduced that, contrary to conventional wisdom, blood flowed in only one direction—from heart to arteries and from veins back to the heart. It then traversed to the lungs before completing a circuit and reentering the heart. Harvey publicly demonstrated one-way blood flow by placing a tourniquet around a man's upper arm (see top

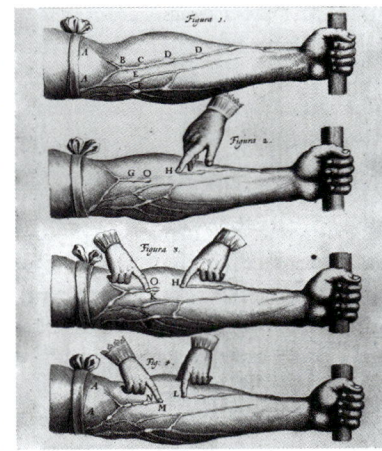
Courtesy National Library of Medicine

of inset image) that constricted arterial blood flow to the forearm and stopped the pulse. By loosening the tourniquet, some blood flowed into the veins. Applying pressure to specific veins forced blood from a peripheral segment where there was little pressure into the previously empty veins. Thus, Harvey proved unambiguously for the first time ever that the heart pumped blood through a closed, unidirectional (circular) system, from arteries to veins and back to the heart. The following was Harvey's conclusion in his magnum opus contribution to medical science (and to all science):

> *It is proved by the structure of the heart that the blood is continuously transferred through the lungs into the aorta as by two clacks of a water bellows to raise water. It is proved by a ligature that there is a passage of blood from the arteries to the veins. It is therefore demonstrated that the continuous movement of the blood in a circle is brought about by the beat of the heart.*[24]

Harvey's experiments with sheep proved mathematically that the blood mass passing through the sheep's heart in a fixed time exceeded what the body could produce—a conclusion identical to that concerning the human heart. Harvey reasoned that if a self-contained constant mass of blood exists, then the large circulation volumes would require a one-way, closed circulatory system. Harvey did not explain *why* the blood circulated, only that it did. He correctly postulated that circulation might distribute heat and nourishment throughout the body. Despite the validity of Harvey's observations, distinguished scientists soundly criticized them in public. Jean Riolan (1577–1657; www.mhs.ox.ac.uk/collections/%20imu-search-page/narratives/?irn=7357&index=0), an ardent Galenist and Parisian-trained physician who chaired the anatomy and botany departments at the University of Paris in the 1640s, maintained that if anatomic findings differed from Galen's, then the body in question must be abnormal and the results faulty.[83] Riolan argued, in concert with early Greek and Galenic medicine, that blood ebbed and flowed like water sloshing in a tube through the veins several times a day to keep the heart in motion as it circulated within it similar to fluid's action on a waterwheel. The heart worked, he posited, with a separate circulation *independently* of the four main body humors—blood, yellow and black bile, and phlegm—and their effect on bodily functions, including control of the psychological realm. Nevertheless, Harvey's epic discovery governed subsequent research on circulation and reversed 1500 years of rigid, religiously inspired dogma.

Giovanni Alfonso Borelli (1608–1679)

Borelli, a protégé of Galileo and Benedetto Castelli (1578–1643) and a mathematician and physicist at the University of Pisa in Italy, used mathematical models to explain how muscles enabled animals to walk, fish to swim, and birds to fly. Well before influential English mathematician and physicist Isaac Newton (1643–1727) published the Laws of Motion, Borelli calculated

Courtesy Wellcome Collection

the forces required to maintain human body equilibrium in various joints, establishing that the body's bony levers magnify motion rather than force. He reasoned that muscles in both humans and animals must produce much larger forces than those resisting the motion for movement to occur, as in running, jumping, swimming, and, for birds, flying. The American Society of Biomechanics presents its most prestigious honor, the coveted Giovanni Borelli Award (https://asbweb.org/society-awards/#:~:text=The%20Borelli%20Award%2C%20the%20most,Borelli%20(1608%2D1679).), for outstanding contributions to the biomechanics field. Borelli's ideas explaining how air entered and exited the lungs, though equally important, were less well known than his work *De Motu Animalium* (*On the Movement of Animals*), first published in 1681, with an English translation in 1989 (www.springer.com/us/book/9783642738142). Borelli observed that lungs filled with air because chest volume increased as the diaphragm moved downward. He deduced that air passed through the alveoli and into the blood, a sharp contrast to Galen's notion that air in the lungs cooled the heart and an advance on Harvey's general observation concerning unidirectional blood flow.

Borelli's accomplished student, Marcello Malpighi (1628–1694; https://www.famousscientists.org/marcello-malpighi/), described blood flowing through microscopic structures (capillaries in the kidneys) and around the lung's terminal air sacs (alveoli). As an example, Malpighi hypothesized based on microscopic studies using the microscope invented by Antonie van Leeuwenhoek (1632–1723) and later improved by Robert Hooke (1635–1703) that urine formation occurred by a filtering mechanism between blood and the kidney's renal tubules. Before Malpighi's pioneering studies, local physicians could not explain how kidney function and urine output related. The image shows the kidney structure of a 2-day-old chick embryo, which Malpighi saw. For his unique contributions, medical historians acknowledge Malpighi as the founder of microscopic anatomy. The Royal Society of London elected him an honorary member for his unique microscopic and other discoveries involving respiration in insects (silkworm) and plant anatomy.

Courtesy National Library of Medicine

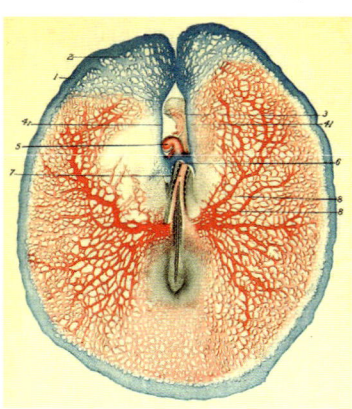

From Lillie FR. The development of the chick; An introduction to embryology. New York: H. Holt & Co., 1908.

Robert Boyle (1627–1691)

Working at Gresham College in London with his soon-to-be-famous student Robert Hooke (1635–1703; www.ucmp.berkeley.edu/history/hooke.html), Boyle devised experiments with a vacuum pump and bell jar to show that combustion and respiration required air. Boyle partially evacuated air from the jar containing a lit candle. The flame soon died. When he removed air from a jar containing a rodent or bird, it became unconscious; recirculating air back into the jar often revived the animal. Compressing the air produced the same results: animals and flames survived longer (www.famousscientists.org/robert-boyle/).

In subsequent experiments, Boyle removed the diaphragm and ribs from a living dog and forced air into its lungs with a bellows. The experiment did not prove that air was essential for life, yet demonstrated that air pressure and volumes alternately contracted and expanded the lungs. He repeated the experiment, this time pricking the lungs so air could escape. Boyle kept the animal alive by forcing air into its lungs, proving that chest movement *per se* maintained airflow, disproving the earlier assertion that lungs affected circulation.

Scientific societies and journals broadcasted these pioneering, insightful discoveries. Boyle belonged to the Royal Society of London (https://royalsociety.org/about-us/history/), chartered in 1663 by King Charles II. The journal *Philosophical Transactions*, first published in 1665, established concepts about scientific priority and peer review process; it remains the world's first and oldest continuously published science journal (https://royalsocietypublishing.org/journal/rstl). One year later in France (1666), Louis XIV approved the first Académie Royale des Sciences (French Academy of Sciences; www.interacademies.org/12179/France), sponsored by Finance Minister Jean-Baptiste Colbert (1619–1683), to preserve French scientific research. It was housed in the Louvre so its staff could undertake studies in physics, chemistry, medicine, agronomy, nutrition and metabolism, and pursue exploratory expeditions to distant lands. In 1603, Italy created its own scientific academy in Rome, which Galileo Galilei joined in 1611. Named the Accademia dei Lincei, it was the first European academy devoted to the natural sciences, which, besides astronomy, chemistry, and mathematics, included entomology and botany (www.lincei.it/en/history). Both French and British societies established journals (*Journal des Scavans* and *Philosophical Transactions of the Royal Society*) and formal meetings to communicate scientific information to an increasingly educated lay public and science-oriented audience fascinated by innovative, fast-paced discoveries.

Stephen Hales (1677–1761)

A renowned English plant physiologist and Royal Society Fellow (http://galileo.rice.edu/Catalog/NewFiles/hales.html), Hales amassed facts from animal experiments regarding blood pressure, the heart's capacity, and blood flow velocity in his text, *Vegetable Statics*, or as translated from Latin, *An Account of Some Statical Experiments on the Sap in Vegetables* (1727).

Courtesy National Library of Medicine

In his well-regarded text, Hales tells how water absorbed air when phosphorus and melted brimstone (sulfur) burned in a closed glass vessel (shown in the image), showing the transfer of "air" released from substances burned in the vessel. Hales measured the air volume either released or absorbed and demonstrated that many common substances contained air. His experiments proved that chemical changes occurred in solids and liquids in calcination (oxidation during combustion). Hales developed an idea suggested by Newton in 1713 that provided the first experimental evidence that the nervous system played a role in muscle contraction.

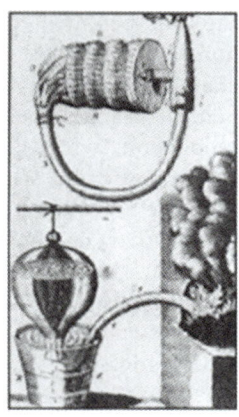

Hales discovered a previously unknown connection between the spinal cord and subsequent reflex actions that allowed him to prove his assertions regarding the nervous system. Hales attached a goose's trachea to a living horse's carotid artery to observe the force required to pump the horse's blood. Hales determined that the muscle blood pressure was too low to impact movement. Instead, he suggested that electrical impulses had coordinated the movement. In decapitated frogs, nerve action continued without brain involvement, thus indicating that nervous system remnants interacted in some way with the spinal cord. Later experiments by Scottish physician Robert Whytt (1716–1766; unconscious reflexes), Swiss anatomist and experimental physiologist Albrecht von Haller (1708–1777; muscle irritability), and Italian physiologist Luigi Galvani (1737–1798; animal electricity) laid the foundations for **neurology**, a new discipline in the medical field.

James Lind (1716–1794)

Trained in Edinburgh, Lind entered the British Navy as a Surgeon's Mate in 1739. During an extended trip in the English Channel in 1747 on the 50-gun, 960-ton H.M.S. *Salisbury* (www.ncbi.nlm.nih.gov/pmc/articles/PMC539665/), Lind conducted a decisive experiment that would change the course of naval medicine and be recognized as the first controlled clinical trial. Lind knew that scurvy often killed two thirds of a ship's crew. Their diet included 1 lb 4 oz of cheese biscuits daily, 2 lb of salt beef twice weekly, 2 oz of dried fish and butter thrice weekly, 8 oz of peas 4 days per week, and 1 gallon of beer daily. Deprived of vitamin C, sailors fell prey to scurvy ("the great sea plague"; www.medicalnewstoday.com/articles/155758.php). By adding vitamin C–rich fresh fruit to their diet, Lind fortified their immune systems so that British sailors no longer perished

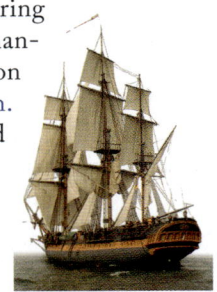

James Steidl/Shutterstock

on extended voyages. From Lind's *Treatise on the Scurvy* (1753) comes the following poignant excerpt[38,72]:

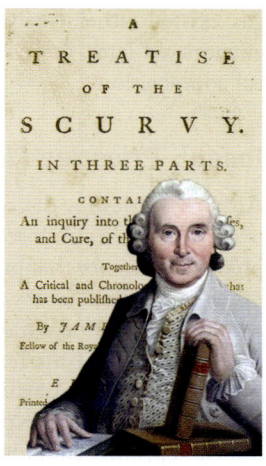

Courtesy James Lind Library

> On the 20th of May, 1747, I selected 12 patients in the scurvy, on board the Salisbury at sea. Their cases were as similar as I could have them. They all in general had putrid gums, the spots and lassitude, with weakness of their knees.... The consequence was, that the most sudden and visible good effects were perceived from the use of oranges and lemons; one of those who had taken them, being at the end of 6 days fit for duty. The spots were not indeed at that time quite off his body, nor his gums sound; but without any other medicine than a gargle for his mouth he became quite healthy before we came into Plymouth which was on the 16th of June. The other was the best recovered in his condition; and being now pretty well, was appointed nurse to the rest of the sick.... Next to oranges, I thought the cyder had the best effects. It was indeed not very sound. However, those who had taken it, were in a fairer way of recovery than the others at the end of the fortnight, which was the length of time all these different courses were continued, except the oranges. The putrification of their gums, but especially their lassitude and weakness, were somewhat abated, and their appetite increased by it.

Lind published two other texts: *An Essay on Preserving the Health of Seamen in the Royal Navy* (1757) and *Essay on Diseases Incidental to Europeans in Hot Climates* (1768). Easily available, his books were translated into German, French, and Dutch. Lind's landmark emphasis on the crucial importance of dietary supplements antedates modern practices. His treatment regimen defeated scurvy, but 50 years had to pass with many more lives lost before the British Admiralty required all ships to provide fresh citrus fruit for regular consumption during both short (several months) and extended (1 year or more) voyages (www.jameslindlibrary.org/illustrating/articles/james-lind-and-scurvy-1747-to-1795).

Joseph Black (1728–1799)

After graduating from medical school in Edinburgh, Black became a chemistry professor at Glasgow University (www.chem.gla.ac.uk/~alanc/dept/black.htm). His *Experiments Upon Magnesia Alba, Quicklime, and Some Other Alcaline Substances* (1756) determined that air contained carbon dioxide gas. He observed that carbonate (lime) lost half its weight after burning. Black reasoned that removing air from lime treated with acids produced a new substance he named "fixed air," or carbon dioxide ($CaCO_3 = CaO + CO_2$). Black's discovery that gas existed either freely or combined with other substances encouraged later, more refined experiments on gases' chemical composition.

Joseph Priestley (1733–1804)

Although Priestley discovered oxygen by heating red mercury oxide (HgO) in a closed vessel, he stubbornly clung to the phlogiston theory that previously had misled other scientists (www.acs.org/content/acs/en/education/whatischemistry/landmarks/josephpriestleyoxygen.html). Dismissing Lavoisier's (1743–1794) proof that respiration produced carbon dioxide and water, Priestley continued to believe in an immaterial constituent (**phlogiston**) that supposedly escaped from substances upon burning. He lectured at the Royal Society about oxygen in 1772 and published *Observations on Different Kinds of Air* in 1773. Elated by his discovery in 1774, Priestley failed to grasp two facts that later research confirmed: (1) the body requires oxygen and (2) cellular respiration produces the end product carbon dioxide.

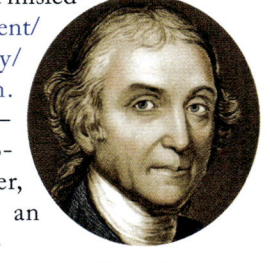

Courtesy National Library of Medicine

Karl Wilhelm Scheele (1742–1786)

In one of history's great coincidences, Scheele, a Swedish pharmacist, discovered oxygen independently of Priestley and Lavoisier (discussed below) (www.britannica.com/biography/Carl-Wilhelm-Scheele). Unfortunately for Scheele, the other two were first to publish their findings and so received the discovery's scientific acclaim, which shattered the long-held notion concerning phlogiston. Scheele published his work on oxygen in 1777, titled *Chemische Abhandlung von der Luft und dem Feuer* (*Chemical Treatise on Air and Fire*). An accomplished chemist, he discovered that heating mercuric oxide released "fire-air" (oxygen) and that burning other substances in fire air produced violent chemical reactions. When different mixtures contacted air inside a sealed container, air volume decreased by 25% and could not support combustion. Scheele named the gas that extinguished fire "foul air." In a memorable experiment, he added two bees to a glass jar immersed in limewater containing fire air to absorb carbon dioxide. After a few days, the bees remained alive, but the level of limewater had risen in the bottle and become cloudy. Scheele observed that a single bee would live twice as long as two bees under the same experimental conditions. With oxygen present, limewater replaced all the volume inside the container (actually a glass milk bottle). Scheele concluded that fixed air replaced the fire air to sustain the bees, but at the end of 8 days the bees perished despite ample honey within the bees' mini-chamber at the top of the bottle. Scheele blamed their demise on phlogiston, which he believed was incompatible with life.

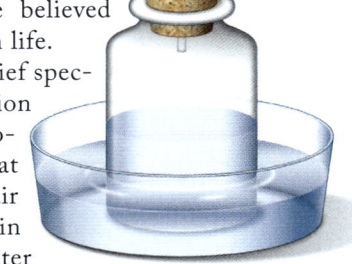

The prevalent belief speculated that combustion stopped without phlogiston present. What Scheele called foul air (phlogisticated air in Priestley's day) later became known as nitrogen gas. In a twist of irony, Scheele refused to accept Lavoisier's explanations concerning respiration. Although Scheele adhered to the phlogiston theory, his experimental work in chemistry continued. In addition to oxygen, he discovered chlorine, manganese, silicon, glycerol, silicon tetrafluoride, hydrofluoric acid, and copper arsenite (later named *Scheele's green* in his honor). The prestigious Royal Swedish Academy of Sciences (founded by naturalist Carl Linnaeus [1707–1778] in 1739; www.kva.se/en/) elected Scheele in 1775 as the first and only pharmacy student elected into that society.

Henry Cavendish (1731–1810)

Henry Cavendish and his contemporaries Black and Priestley began to identify carbohydrate, lipid, and protein constituents (www.nndb.com/people/030/000083778/). *On Factitious Air* (1766) describes a highly flammable substance, later identified as hydrogen, that was liberated when acids combined with metals. *Experiments in Air* (1784) showed that "inflammable air" (hydrogen) when combined with "dephlogisticated air" (oxygen) produced water. Cavendish performed meticulous calculations using a sensitive **torsion balance** invented in 1750 by English scientist and Anglican Church clergyman John Michell (1724–1793; www.cambridge.org/core/journals/british-journal-for-the-history-of-science/article/john-michell-and-henry-cavendish-weighing-the-stars/C8B1F6C4913649A6B992FFD5AB3D3269) to precisely measure the gravitational constant G by computing the Earth's mass as 5.976×10^{24} kg to an accuracy within 1% of modern computations. The landmark 1798 Cavendish experiment (https://sciencedemonstrations.fas.harvard.edu/presentations/cavendish-experiment) played a pivotal role in contemporary rocketry design and future space exploration (see Chapter 27). In 1757, Cavendish received the Copley Medal from London's Royal Society for his many "first" discoveries in chemistry.

Antoine Laurent Lavoisier (1743–1794)

Lavoisier ushered in present concepts in physiology concerning metabolism, nutrition, and exercise (www.sciencehistory.org/historical-profile/antoine-laurent-lavoisier). His discoveries in respiration chemistry and human nutrition were as essential to these fields as Harvey's discoveries were to circulatory physiology and medicine (www.youtube.com/watch?v=AE0kuHKoitE&t=87s). Lavoisier paved the way for energy balance studies by recognizing for the first time that the elements involved in metabolism—carbon, hydrogen, nitrogen, and oxygen—neither appeared suddenly nor disappeared mysteriously. He discovered that only oxygen participates in animal respiration and the "caloric" liberated during respiration was itself the combustion source. In the early 1770s, Lavoisier was first to conduct experiments on human respiration with his colleague and collaborator, chemist and physiologist Armand Séguin (1767–1835). They studied the influence of muscular work on metabolism. A contemporary painting shows the seated Séguin as he depresses a pedal while a copper mask, the forerunner of modern respiration headgear to measure oxygen uptake, captures the expired air (**FIG. I.6**). In image A, a physician takes Séguin's pulse to determine the separate effects of exercise and food consumption. For several hours before the experiment, Séguin abstained from food to avoid digestion's confounding influence on metabolism. Resting metabolism without food in a cold environment increased by 10%; it increased 50% due solely to food, 200% with exercise, and 300% by combining food intake with exercise. Lavoisier's wife Marie, a proponent of science and fierce advocate for her husband's work, sits at a table taking notes (she also drew the sketch). Image B shows Lavoisier's essential laboratory equipment, which is preserved at the Musee des Arts et Metiers in Paris. In a letter written to a friend dated November 19, 1790, Lavoisier told about his four important findings:[44]

> *(1) The quantity of oxygen absorbed by a resting man at a temperature of 26°C is 1200 pouces de France (1 cubic pouce = 0.0198 L) hourly. (2) The quantity of oxygen required at a temperature of 12°C rises to 1400 pouces. (3) During the digestion of food, the quantity of oxygen amounts to from 1800 to 1900 pouces. (4) During exercise, 4000 pouces and over may be the quantity of oxygen absorbed.*

These discoveries, fundamental to prevailing energy balance concepts, could not protect Lavoisier from the intolerance of his orthodox countrymen. The Jacobean tribunal beheaded him in 1794 at age 50 along with 27 codefendants. Yet once more, thoughtless resistance to innovative science temporarily delayed the triumph of truth over rigid dogma. Lavoisier, exonerated several years posthumously, now has his many accomplishments enshrined on architectural masterpieces—the Louvre's façade of the *Cour Napoléo* and his engraved name on the Eiffel Tower as one of France's greatest mathematicians, scientists, and engineers. After his death, Italian born mathematician Joseph-Louis Lagrange (1736–1813; https://mathshistory.st-andrews.ac.uk/Biographies/Lagrange/) stated, "It took them only an instant to cut off that head, and a hundred years may not produce another like it."

Lazzaro Spallanzani (1729–1799)

An accomplished Italian physiologist (and Catholic priest), Spallanzani debunked spontaneous generation as he studied animal fertilization and contraception (www.whonamedit.com/doctor.cfm/2234.html). His famous digestion study describes refined regurgitation experiments similar to those of French entomologist and scientist René-Antoine Ferchault de Réaumur

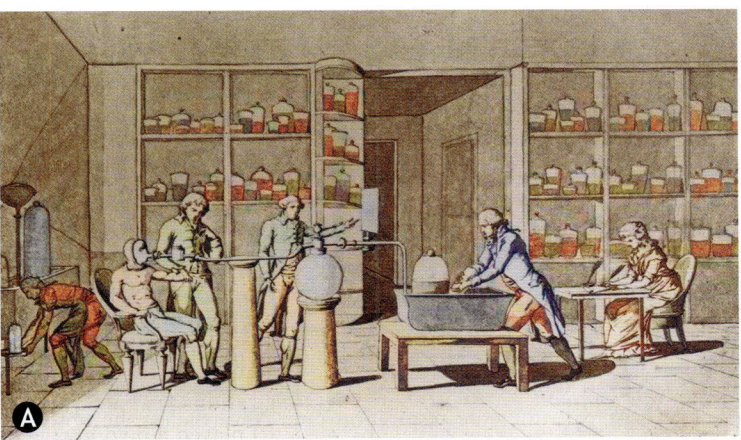
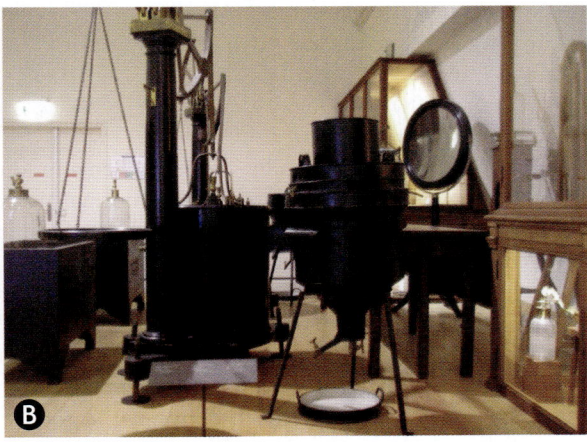

FIGURE I.6. (**A**) Lavoisier supervises the first "true" exercise physiology experiment (heart rate and oxygen uptake measured as the seated subject at the far left breathes through a copper pipe while pressing a foot pedal to increase external work). Sketched by Madame Lavoisier (sitting at the right taking notes). (**B**) Lavoisier's laboratory from the mid-1700s can be visited at Musee des Arts et Metiers in Paris, France, at 160 rue Reaumur.
(Image B © Frank Katch.)

(1683–1757; https://embryo.asu.edu/pages/lazzaro-spallanzani-1729-1799; *Digestion in Birds* (1752). Spallanzani recovered partially digested food from the gizzard of a common scavenger kite, a medium-sized raptor. Birds in perforated containers were fed food with a piece of string attached. After a few hours, he recovered the container's string to determine the food's composition. After perfecting this method, he conducted a self-experiment by swallowing a sponge tied to the end of a string and then regurgitating it. He determined that the sponge absorbed a substance that dissolved bread and various animal tissues, thus indirectly observing how gastric juices function. Spallanzani also was first to perform *in vitro* fertilization in frogs and artificial insemination in dogs. His animal experiments proved that heart, stomach, and liver tissues consume oxygen and liberate carbon dioxide, even in creatures without lungs. This novel idea that respiration and combustion took place within the tissues appeared posthumously in 1804. A century later, this phenomenon would be called *internal respiration*.[2]

Science Source

Nineteenth Century Discoveries in Metabolism and Physiology

Lavoisier's untimely death did not terminate fruitful nutrition and medical research. During the next half-century, scientists discovered carbohydrate, lipid, and protein's chemical composition, further clarifying the current concept known as the **energy balance equation**.[14]

A French chemist and Lavoisier's contemporary, Claude Louis Berthollet identified the "volatile substances" associated with animal tissues (https://biography.yourdictionary.com/claude-louis-berthollet). The image shows Berthollet holding a glass tube during a visit to Lavoisier's laboratory (circa 1770s). Among his many discoveries, Bertholett identified nitrogen as a by-product when ammonia gas burned in oxygen. He demonstrated that normal tissues did not contain ammonia. He believed that hydrogen united with nitrogen during fermentation to produce ammonia. In 1865, Berthollet took exception to Lavoisier's ideas about how much heat was liberated when the body oxidizes an equal weight of carbohydrate or lipid. According to Berthollet, "the quantity of heat liberated in the incomplete oxidation of a substance equaled the difference between the total caloric value of the substance and that of the products formed." We pay tribute to Berthollet and Lavoisier for devising the system for naming chemical compounds still in use today. In 1789, Berthollet was elected a prestigious Royal Society of London Fellow.

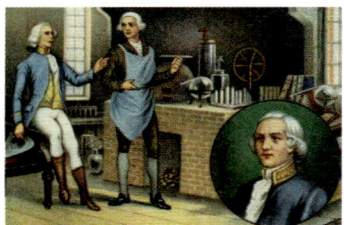

Joseph Louis Proust (1755–1826)

Proust proved that a pure substance isolated in the laboratory or found in nature would always contain the same elements in the same proportions (www.lindahall.org/joseph-proust/). Known as the "Law of Definite Proportions," Proust's ideas about the chemical constancy of a substance provided an important milestone for future nutritional explorers to follow, helping them to analyze the major nutrient components, and thereby calculate energy metabolism from measured oxygen uptake.

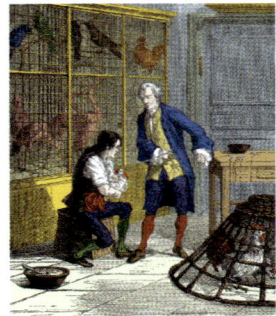

Courtesy National Library of Medicine

Louis-Joseph Gay-Lussac (1778–1850)

In 1810, Gay-Lussac, a pupil of Berthollet, analyzed the chemical composition for 20 animal and vegetable substances (www.nndb.com/people/885/000100585/). He placed the vegetable substances into one of three categories depending on their hydrogen-to-oxygen atom proportions. William Prout (1785–1850) in his classification of the three basic macronutrients accepted Gay-Lussac's identification of saccharine, which was later identified as carbohydrate. Gay-Lussac published 148 articles, mostly in organic chemistry, with colleagues in diverse fields, which included Justis Liebig. Gay-Lussac's adventuresome exploits included solo ascents to 23,000 ft in some of the first hot air balloons, in which he took flight from the Louvre in Paris to determine the air's composition at cold, high altitudes and to study the Earth's magnetic field.

William Prout (1785–1850)

Following up on studies by Lavoisier and Séguin on muscular activity and respiration, Prout, an Englishman and multifaceted physician who conducted research in chemistry, meteorology, and physiology, measured the carbon dioxide exhaled by men exercising to self-imposed fatigue. Moderate physical activity (walking naturally) raised carbon dioxide production to an eventual plateau. This observation predated steady-rate exercise gas exchange kinetics. Prout could not determine the exact carbon dioxide amount respired because no instrumentation existed to measure respiration rate. Nevertheless, he observed that carbon dioxide concentration in expired air decreased dramatically during fatiguing effort (www.sciencedirect.com/science/article/pii/S0187893X15000130).

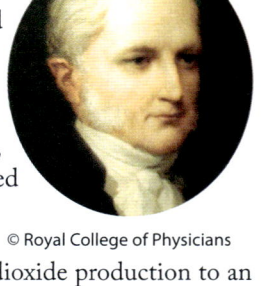

© Royal College of Physicians

A prolific scientist Prout published five books and forty research papers in physiology. His respiration studies were thought provoking for the time. Prout believed the effects on respiration included inhaled air temperature, muscular exertion and digestive system status in moderate-to-intense activity, and body temperature. Based on hundreds of self-experiments with special apparatuses he constructed, Prout concluded that levels of oxygen uptake and carbon dioxide produced differed over a 24-hr period; they peaked at 10 AM and 2 PM, were lowest at 8.30 PM, and remained stable thereafter for another 12 hr.

François Magendie (1783–1855)

In 1821, François Magendie founded the first journal devoted to experimental physiology (*Journal de Physiologie Expérimentale*), a field he literally created and is considered a founding father of. The next year, in his most noteworthy contribution, he discovered that anterior spinal nerve roots control motor activities and posterior roots control sensory functions (called Magendie Law).[84,93]

Courtesy Wellcome Collection

In 1825, he published an influential text, *Anatomy and Physiology of the Nervous System*, highlighting experimental details concerning nerve function. For example, he explained the origin, composition, and cerebrospinal fluid circulation in normal and pathological animal vivisection experiments, often in public, and how cranial nerves functioned. He also was first to prove that the cerebellum governed an animal's equilibrium. His other contributions include articles ranging from human and comparative anatomy to hydrophobia (older term describing fear of rabies). Magendie's accomplishments were not limited to neural physiology. Unlike other physiologists, who claimed tissues obtained their nitrogen from the air, Magendie argued that food consumed provided the nitrogen. To prove his point, he studied animals subsisting on nitrogen-free diets (https://academic.oup.com/jn/article/133/3/638/4688006). In an 1816 experiment related to nutrition and weight control, Magendie was first to illuminate the *empty calorie concept* described in *Précis élementaire de Physiologie*.[96] Despite his momentous scientific contributions, contemporary rivals in England vigorously disputed in print Magendie's claim to be the first to describe these important experimental phenomena. Rather, they accused him of stealing the seminal ideas from an established Scottish anatomist, Sir Charles Bell (1774–1842), who was working in a similar field. In France, Magendie's live animal dissections were severely criticized as needless torture and animal cruelty (calling him the "prince of vivisection"). In a twist of irony, Claude Bernard's wife, Marie Françoise Martin (1819–1901), herself an anti-vivisectionist and staunch animal rights supporter, detested her husband's approach to vivisection and criticized his lack of administering anesthesia to the animals as inhumane. She later established an anti-vivisection society. The publicity given to 19th century vivisection procedures resulted in the British 1876 Cruelty to Animals Act.[97] Recall that many famous scientific experimentalists, from Galen and Aristotle to Vesalius and Harvey, and Hales to Magendie, practiced vivisection in the name of science for societal good. Current practice relies on mice, rats, dogs, and other animals with adherence to regulations to ensure humane and responsible animal research methods (www.nyu.edu/research/resources-and-support-offices/).

William Beaumont (1785–1853)

One of the most fortuitous experiments in medicine began on June 6, 1822, at Fort Mackinac in upstate Michigan (www.ncbi.nlm.nih.gov/books/NBK459/). As fort surgeon, William Beaumont tended the accidental shotgun wound that perforated the abdominal wall and stomach of young French Canadian Samata St. Martin, a voyager who transported goods and passengers by canoe to and from trading posts for the American Fur Company begun by America's first millionaire, John Jacob Astor (1763–1848; www.legendsofamerica.com/we-johnjacobastor/). The wound healed after 10 months but continued to provide new insights concerning digestion. St. Martin's wound formed a small natural "valve" that led directly into the stomach. Beaumont turned St. Martin on his left side, depressed the valve, and then inserted a tube the size of a quill pen or a wing feather from a large bird 5 or 6 inches into the stomach.

Courtesy New York Public Library

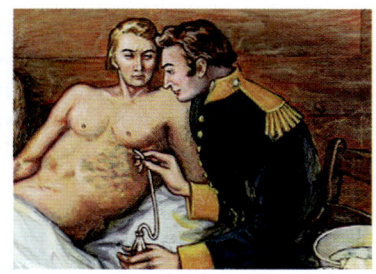

From V. Katch

From 1825 to 1833, he began two kinds of digestive process experiments. First, he observed the fluids discharged by the stomach when different foods were eaten (*in vivo*); second, he extracted samples of the stomach's content and put them into glass tubes to determine the time required for "external" digestion (*in vitro*).

Beaumont revolutionized concepts concerning digestion. For centuries, the stomach was thought to produce heat that somehow "cooked" foods. Alternatively, the stomach was portrayed as a mill, a fermenting vat, or a stew pan. Beaumont published the first experimental results on St. Martin in the *Philadelphia Medical Recorder* in January 1825, and full details in *Experiments and Observations on the Gastric Juice and the Physiology of Digestion* (1833).[24] Beaumont ends his treatise with a list of 51 inferences based on his 238 separate experiments. Although working away from the main centers of medicine on the East Coast, Beaumont used findings culled from the writings of influential European scientists.[98] For example, Jean Baptiste van Helmont (1577–1644), a Flemish physician, was credited as first to prescribe an alkaline indigestive cure.[27] Observing the innards of birds, he reasoned that digestive tract acid could not alone decompose meats and that other substances ("ferments," now known as digestive enzymes) must break down food. Even with their information, Beaumont still followed the scientific method, basing all his inferences on direct experimentation. Beaumont's accomplishment is even more remarkable because the United States, unlike England, France, and Germany, provided no research facilities or "labs" to explore experimental medicine. Little was known about the physiology of digestion. Yet Beaumont, a "backwoods physiologist,"[14] inspired future studies about gastric emptying, intestinal absorption, electrolyte balance, rehydration, and nutritional supplementation with "sports drinks."

Michel Eugene Chevreul (1786–1889)

During his long life, Chevreul carried on a 200-year family tradition by studying chemistry and biology. His classic 1823 chemistry text, *Recherches Chimiques sur les Corps Gras d'origine Animale* (*Chemical Research on Animal Fats*), described how he discovered the biologically important fatty acid category (http://www.ahistoryofgreece.com/goldenage.htm). In 1813, he discovered a new fatty acid, "acide margarique," which was subsequently patented in 1869 by French chemist Hippolyte Mège-Mouriès (1817–1880) by churning beef tallow with milk to create the now ubiquitous butter substitute, margarine (originally known as *oleomargarine*; https://lipidlibrary.aocs.org/resource-material/the-history-of-lipid-science-and-technology/hippolyte-m%C3%A8ge-(1817-1880)). In other organic experiments, Chevreul was the first to show that lard consisted of two main lipids (a solid he called *stearine* and the other a liquid he called *elaine*). Chevreul demonstrated that sugar from a diabetic's urine resembled cane sugar (and also smelled "sweet," an age-old diagnostic clue heralding diabetes).

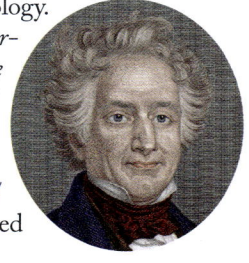
Courtesy National Library of Medicine

Jean Baptiste Boussingault (1802–1884)

A French chemist and agricultural scientist, Jean Baptiste Boussingault's studies concerning animal nutrition (jn.nutrition.org/content/84/1/1.full.pd) paralleled future human nutrition studies. Among his scientific-related accomplishments, he calculated the effects for calcium, iron, and other nutrient substances' nitrogen contribution to energy balance. He also conducted the first crop rotation scientific analysis and determined selected foods' wheat gluten content. In 1836, he established the first agricultural research station in Alsace, France. Here, scientists worked with farmers, ranchers, suppliers, processors, and others involved in food production and agriculture. His pioneering agricultural chemistry work in South America (Colombia) led him to recommend adding iodine to counteract neck swelling from thyroid gland enlargement (goiter). Boussingault also proved that the carbon within a plant came from atmospheric carbon dioxide and that a plant derived most of its nitrogen from soil nitrates, not directly from the atmosphere, as previously believed.

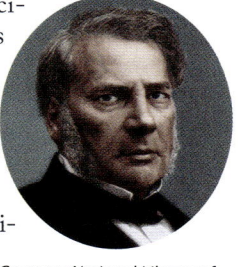
Courtesy National Library of Medicine

Gerardus Johannes Mulder (1802–1880)

A professor specializing in analytical chemistry at Utrecht University, Netherlands, Gerardus Johannes Mulder analyzed albuminous substances he named "proteine" in an 1838 French publication, knowing full well Berzelius had previously coined the term. He postulated a general protein radical identical in chemical composition to plant albumen, casein, and animal fibrin. He maintained that carbon, hydrogen, nitrogen, oxygen, and varying sulfur and phosphorus amounts were basic building blocks for these substances. He also proved that "proteine" would contain substances other than nitrogen available only from plants. Because animals consume plants, substances from the plant kingdom, later called amino acids, served to build animal tissues. Unfortunately, an influential German chemist, Justus von Liebig (1803–1873) attacked Mulder's theories about protein so vigorously they became marginalized within the scientific community. Despite the academic controversy, Mulder strongly advocated society's role in promoting quality nutrition. He asked, "Is there a more important question for discussion than the nutrition of the human race?" Mulder urged people to observe the "golden mean" by eating neither too little nor too much food. This dictum follows the Goldilocks principle from the children's book, *Goldilocks and the Three Bears*, with Goldilocks preferring porridge neither too hot nor too cold, but just right. He established minimum standards for his nation's food supply, which he believed should become compatible with optimum health. In 1847, he proposed these specific recommendations—each day, laborers should consume 100 g protein, and those doing routine work about 60 g. He prescribed 500 g carbohydrate as starch and included "some" lipid without specifying an amount (www.encyclopedia.com/topic/Gerardus_Johannes_Mulder.aspx).

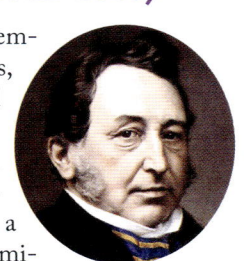

Justus von Liebig (1803–1873)

Embroiled in professional controversies throughout his life, German organic chemist Justus von Liebig still managed to established a large chemistry laboratory in Giesen, Germany, that attracted numerous graduate students, including Carl von Voit, many achieving international reputations for pioneering discoveries in the emerging chemical industry. Liebig developed unique equipment to analyze inorganic and organic substances. He restudied alkaloid (protein) compounds previously discovered by Mulder and concluded that muscular exertion by farm horses or humans required mainly proteins, not just carbohydrates and lipids. Liebig's influential *Animal Chemistry* (1842) text communicated his ideas about energy metabolism.

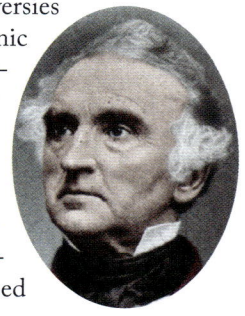
Courtesy National Library of Medicine

Liebig dominated chemistry. Until the 1850s, his theoretical pronouncements about dietary protein's relation to muscular activity were 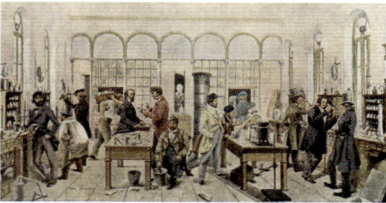 usually accepted without critique by other scientists. Despite his assertions, Liebig never carried out a physiologic experiment or performed nitrogen balance studies on animals or humans. Liebig, ever-so arrogant, demeaned physiologists, believing them incapable of commenting on his theoretic calculations unless they themselves achieved his expertise level.

Liebig made substantial technical improvements to chemical assessment, as for example, an 1830 apparatus to determine the carbon (C), hydrogen (H), and oxygen (O_2) organic substance contents. He also developed innovative glass instruments and weighing techniques using combustion analysis to penetrate a compound's organic molecule structure. In his work with mineral nutrients to determine how plants grow, Liebig identified nitrogen, phosphorus, and potassium as essential nutrients. His experiments revealed that the atmosphere supplies plants with carbon, hydrogen, and water. In other chemistry products related to nutrition, Liebig advocated baking powder to make lighter bread, delved into coffee making chemistry, and developed a breast milk alternative.

By midcentury, a relatively unknown chemist Johannes Wislicenus (1835–1903) and well-established physiologist Adolf Fick (1829–1901) challenged Liebig's unyielding dogma regarding protein's role during exercise. Their simple experiment measured changes in urinary nitrogen while climbing Mr. Falhourn, a well-known alpine mountain resort in Switzerland. They determined by direct measurement that the body's protein supply could not have provided all the hike's energy needs. This insightful experiment discredited Liebig's principle assertion that protein played a pivotal role in supplying energy for vigorous physical activity.

Although erroneous, Liebig's notions about protein as a primary exercise fuel worked their way into popular writings. By the turn of the 20th century, an idea that survives today seemed unassailable: athletic prowess requires a large protein intake. He lent his name to two commercial products: *Liebig's Infant Food*, advertised as a replacement for breast milk, and *Liebig's Fleisch Extract* (meat extract), 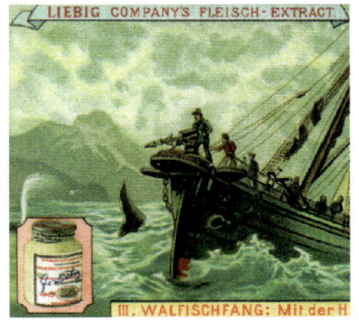 which supposedly conferred special bodily benefits. Liebig argued that consuming his extract and meat would help the body perform additional "work" to convert plant material into useful substances. Liebig was an influential chemist of his time and afterward, his many honors including images of himself and his products appearing on stamps and currency. Even today, fitness magazines and literally thousands of Web sites across social media regularly promote protein supplements to achieve peak exercise performance with little "hard" evidence besides anecdotal confirmation. Whatever the merit of Liebig's claims, debate continues, building on the metabolic studies of W. O. Atwater (1844–1907), F. G. Benedict (1870–1957), and R. H. Chittenden (1856–1943) in the United States and M. Rubner (1854–1932) in Germany.[14]

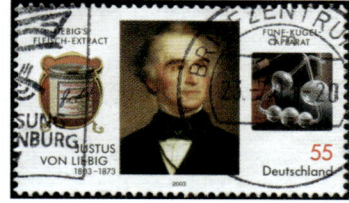
YANGCHAO/Shutterstock

Henri Victor Regnault (1810–1878)

With his colleague Jules Reiset, Henri Regnault, chemistry and physics professor at the University of Paris (and Justis von Liebig's former mentor), used closed-circuit spirometry (Chapter 8) to determine the respiratory quotient (RQ; carbon dioxide production ÷ oxygen uptake) in dogs, insects, silkworms, earthworms, and frogs. In experiments conducted in 1849, they placed animals in a sealed, 45-L bell jar surrounded by a water jacket. A potash solution filtered the carbon dioxide gas produced during respiration. Water rising in the glass receptacle forced oxygen into the bell jar to replace the quantity consumed during energy metabolism. A thermometer recorded temperature, and a manometer measured chamber pressure variations. For dogs, fowl, and rabbits deprived of food, the RQ was lower than when the same animals consumed meat. Regnault and Reiset reasoned that starving animals subsist on their own tissues. Foods never were completely destroyed during metabolism because urea and uric acid were recovered in the urine. London's Royal Society awarded Regnault the Rumford medal in 1848 for "outstandingly important recent discovery in the thermal or optical properties field made by a scientist working in Europe" (www.nndb.com/honors/428/000072212/), joining prior English inductees chemist and inventor Humphrey Davy (1778–1829) in 1816 and physicist Michael Faraday (1791–1867) in 1846. Regnault established relationships between body size and metabolic rate. These ratios preceded the **surface area law** and **allometric scaling** procedures now applied in medicine, human nutrition, pharmacology, kinesiology, and the other exercise and health-related disciplines.

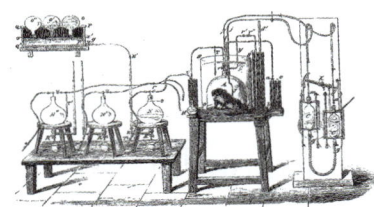
Courtesy Max Planck Institute for the History of Science, Berlin/Virtual Lab

Claude Bernard (1813–1878)

Claude Bernard, often acclaimed as the most distinguished physiologist and experimental 19th century scientist, succeeded Magendie as professor of medicine at the Collège de France (www.famousscientists.org/claude-bernard/). Bernard interned in medicine and surgery before serving as laboratory assistant (*préparateur*) to 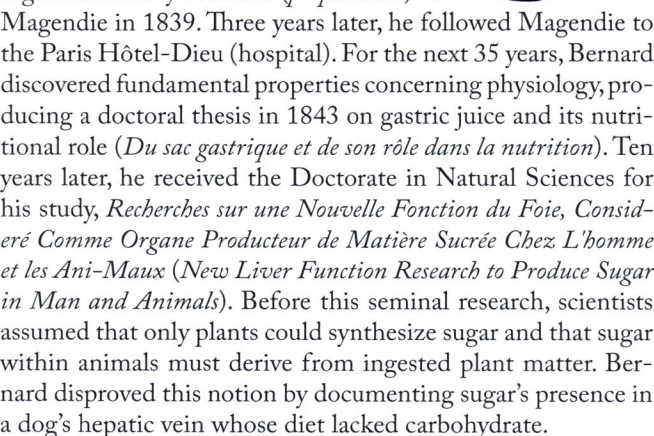 Magendie in 1839. Three years later, he followed Magendie to the Paris Hôtel-Dieu (hospital). For the next 35 years, Bernard discovered fundamental properties concerning physiology, producing a doctoral thesis in 1843 on gastric juice and its nutritional role (*Du sac gastrique et de son rôle dans la nutrition*). Ten years later, he received the Doctorate in Natural Sciences for his study, *Recherches sur une Nouvelle Fonction du Foie, Consideré Comme Organe Producteur de Matière Sucrée Chez L'homme et les Ani-Maux* (*New Liver Function Research to Produce Sugar in Man and Animals*). Before this seminal research, scientists assumed that only plants could synthesize sugar and that sugar within animals must derive from ingested plant matter. Bernard disproved this notion by documenting sugar's presence in a dog's hepatic vein whose diet lacked carbohydrate.

Bernard's experiments profoundly impacted medicine:

- Discovered pancreatic secretions' role in lipid digestion (1848)
- Discovered a new liver function—"internal glucose secretion" into the blood (1848)
- Induced diabetes by puncturing the brain's fourth ventricle floor (1849)
- Discovered local skin temperature elevation during cervical sympathetic nerve surgery (1851)
- Produced sugar by washing excised liver (1855) and glycogen isolation (1857)
- Demonstrated that curare blocked motor nerve endings (1856)
- Demonstrated that carbon monoxide blocked erythrocyte respiration (1857)

Bernard's work also influenced other sciences.[24] His discoveries in chemical physiology spawned physical chemistry and biochemistry, which a century later spawned molecular biology. 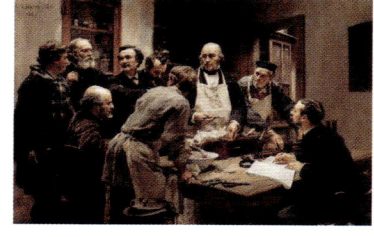 His contributions to regulatory physiology inspired the next generation to understand how metabolism and nutrition impacted exercise. Bernard's influential *Introduction à L'étude de la Médecine Expérimentale* (*The Introduction to the Study of Experimental Medicine*, 1865) illustrates the self-control that enabled his success despite external disturbances related to politics. Bernard urged researchers to vigorously observe, hypothesize, and then test their hypothesis. In the last third of his text, Bernard shares his strategies for verifying results. His disciplined approach remains valid, and exercise physiologists and their students will appreciate reading this meaningful treatise (www.ncbi.nlm.nih.gov/pmc/articles/PMC195131/). Bernard is remembered in the historically important painting by French naturalist artist Leon Augustin Lhermitte (1844–1925) "The Lesson of Claude Bernard" (1889) or "Session at the Vivisection Laboratory." Here, for his medical students, Bernard performs a rare vivisection while wearing his traditional white lab coat. Musée Claude Bernard displays Bernard's many laboratory tools and papers (www.agglo-villefranche.fr/musee-claude-bernard.html). In retrospect, it would be hard to disagree that Bernard became France's greatest representative in early 19th century scientific efforts.

Edward Smith (1819–1874)

Edward Smith, physician, medical writer, public health advocate, and social reformer, fought to promote better living conditions for Britain's lower class, including prisoners. He believed that, during their incarceration at Brixton Prison in inner South London, inmates suffered maltreatment because they received no additional food while toiling on the exhausting "penal treadmill," a unique exercise device invented by renowned British civil engineer Sir William Cubitt (1785–1861), whose steps resembled a Victorian steamship's side paddle wheels. Narrow steps approxi-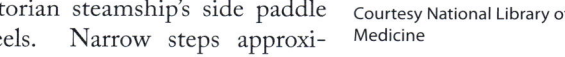

Courtesy National Library of Medicine

mately 7.5 inches apart were attached to a cylinder approximately 6 feet in diameter connected by two large cast iron wheels. The device, first invented as a way to assist farmers in crop production and harvesting, was not contemplated as a punishment device. As a person put one's weight on the step, it depressed the wheel, forcing the person to step onto the step above. In essence, the treadwheel represented an "everlasting staircase." For the larger devices in the prisons, there would be 18 to 25 positions on the wheel, each separated by a wooden partition so each prisoner had no contact with or view of adjacent prisoners and could only view a wall as they walked in silence for 6 hr daily, taking 15 min on the wheel followed by a 5-min rest, for a total of 4 work hours three times weekly. Smith calculated that each man traveled the equivalent 2.3 km/1.43 mi up a steep hill. He also determined that if the inmates were fed the planned 93% carbohydrate diet, they would fail to perform the required hard physical labor and more likely resort to bad prison behaviors. There were 39 treadmills in England's prisons in 1895, but these were 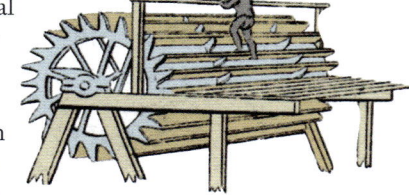 abolished 7 years later when Britain outlawed their use during incarcerations. Not unexpectedly, a treadwheel installed in

Bellevue County penitentiary in New York City in 1822 also was discontinued as punishment and used instead to grind 40 to 60 corn bushels daily for prison meals. At the time, the prison warden commented, "… when the treadmill is combined with solitary confinement, the two punishments furnish the most salutary punishment and the most powerful detriment from crime that the lenient spirit of our laws admits" (www.earlyamericancrime.com/prisons-and-punishments/failure-of-the-treadmill). Slave owners in Charleston, South Carolina, also could rent treadwheels to punish runaway slaves (www.uh.edu/engines/epi374.htm), and the treadwheels used in the West Indies and Jamaican prisons made conditions intolerable and often fatal for inmates, both males and females, who if refusing to climb had their hands lashed to an overhead bar to induce compliance (Paton, 2004).

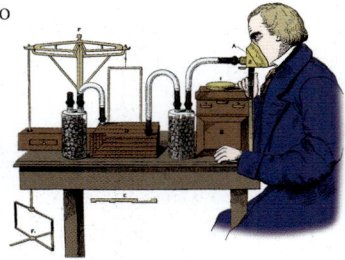

Courtesy Max Planck Institute for the History of Science, Berlin/Virtual Lab

Curious about the strenuousness of treadwheel exercise, Smith conducted studies on himself. He constructed a closed-circuit apparatus (facemask with inspiratory and expiratory valves) to measure carbon dioxide production while climbing at Brixton prison.[24] He expired 19.6 more carbon grams while climbing for 15 min and resting for 15 min than he expired while resting. Smith estimated that if he climbed and rested for 7.5 hr, his daily total carbon output would increase 66%. Smith analyzed four prisoners urine over a 3-wk period to show that urea output related to the ingested foods' nitrogen content, whereas carbon dioxide output more closely related to exercise intensity.

Smith inspired two German researchers to validate the prevailing idea that protein alone powered muscular contraction. Adolf Eugen Fick (1829–1901), discoverer of the **Fick principle** named in his honor during research as a physiologist at the University of Zurich, and relatively unknown German chemistry professor Johannes Wislicenus (1835–1903) questioned whether protein, carbohydrate, or lipid oxidation supplied the energy for muscular effort. In 1864, they climbed Mt. Faulhorn in the Swiss Alps, a 8796-ft/2681-m elevation to the hotel summit. Prior to the climb, they eliminated protein from their diet, reasoning that nonprotein nutrients would have to supply them with energy. They collected their urine before and immediately after the ascent and the following morning. They calculated the external energy equivalent to climb 1956 m/6420 ft (about 75% to the summit) by multiplying body mass by the vertical distance. This external energy requirement *exceeded* protein catabolism reflected by nitrogen in the urine. Therefore, they concluded that the energy from protein breakdown hardly contributed to the exercise energy requirement. These findings posed a serious challenge and decisive blow to Liebig's claim that muscular effort depended on protein as the primary energy source to power the walk (www.ncbi.nlm.nih.gov/pmc/articles/PMC5906749/). When applied to today's exercise physiology studies at even low-to-moderate altitude, the Fick and Wislicenus experiment should be remembered for its originality and pursuit of new knowledge as a forerunner to the current sports physiology and exercise nutrition fields.

Health and Hygiene Influences in the United States

In the United States by the early 1800s, European science-oriented physicians and experimental anatomists and physiologists strongly promoted ideas about health and hygiene.[25,26] Prior to 1800, only 39 first edition, American-authored medical books had been published, a few medical schools had been started in the 13 colonies (College of Philadelphia, 1765; Harvard Medical School, 1782), seven medical societies existed (the New Jersey State Medical Society being the first in 1766[7,10]), and only one medical journal existed (*Medical Repository*, published in 1797; https://www.nejm.org/doi/full/10.1056/NEJM199712253372617). Outside the United States, 176 medical journals were being published in the British Isles and European continent, but by 1850, the number of published books in the United States increased to 117.[70]

Medical journal publications in the United States had increased tremendously during the first half of the 19th century, concurrent with a steady growth in scientific contributions, yet European influences still inspired United States medical thinking and practice.[49] This influence directly impacted the "information explosion" through books, magazines, newspapers, and "health salesmen," who, during public barnstorming travels, hawked endless tonics, elixirs, and other potions to optimize health and cure debilitating disease. The "hot topics" in early 19th century America included nutrition and dieting (called slimming in England), general information about exercise and its bodily effects, how to best develop overall fitness, training (or gymnastic) exercises for recreation, and sport preparation relating to personal health and hygiene.[27]

By the middle of the 19th century, fledgling United States medical schools began to graduate their own students, many of whom assumed leadership positions in the academic world and allied medical sciences. Interestingly, physicians had the opportunity to either teach in medical school and conduct research (and write textbooks) or become associated with physical education and hygiene departments. There, they would supervise physical training programs for the student and athlete.[46] Elizabeth Blackwell (1821–1910) was the first woman to earn a medical degree in the United States, graduating from Geneva Medical College in upstate New York (now Hobart and Williams College) in 1849, and the first female doctor of medicine in the modern era. She was a staunch advocate for women's rights in medical education and, in her early medical career, physical education for girls.

Within this framework, we begin the discussion about early physiology and exercise physiology pioneers with Austin Flint, Jr., MD, a respected physician and physiologist and successful textbook author. His writings provided reliable information for those wishing to place their beliefs about exercise in general and its health benefits on a scientific footing.

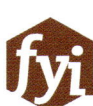

Seventy Years of Influential American Textbooks Published From 1801 to 1871 on Anatomy and Physiology, Exercise and Training, Health, Physical Education, and Medicine

The image below presents the first 70 years of influential American textbooks on anatomy and physiology, anthropometry, exercise, training, and health and medicine published from 1801 through the Civil War period to 1871 that shaped exercise physiology content during the next century and beyond. On Lippincott Connect (Appendix A) is a more complete book listing on these areas up to 1947.

Year	Author and Text
1801	Willich AFM. *Lectures on Diet and Regimen: Being a Systematic Inquiry into the Most Rational Means of Preserving Health and Prolonging Life: Together with Physiological and Chemical Explanations, Calculated Chiefly for the Use of Families, in Order to Banish the Prevailing Abuses and Prejudices in Medicine*. New York: T and J Sworos, 1801.
1831	Hitchcock E. *Dyspepsy Forestalled and Resisted, or, Lectures on Diet, Regimen, and Employment*. 2nd ed. Northampton: J.S. & C. Adams, 1831.
1833	Beaumont W. *Experiments and Observations on the Gastric Juice and the Physiology of Digestion*. Pittsburgh: F.P. Allen, 1833.
1839	Carpenter WB. *Principles of Physiology, General and Comparative*. London: John Churchill, 1839. 4th ed. 1854.
1842	Carpenter WB. *Principles of Human Physiology*. London: Churchill, 1842.
1843	Carpenter WB. *Principles of Human Physiology, with Their Chief Applications to Pathology, Hygiene, and Forensic Medicine. Especially Designed for the Use of Students*. Philadelphia: Lea & Blanchard, 1843, Numerous reprints and editions; 9th ed, 1881 (London): 4th American ed., 1890.
1843	Combe A. *The Principles of Physiology Applied to the Preservation of Health, and to the Improvement of Physical and Mental Education*. New York: Harper & Brothers, 1843.
1844	Dunglison R. *Human Health: The Influence of Atmosphere and Locality; Change of Air and Climate; Seasons; Food; Clothing; Bathing and Mineral Springs; Exercise; Sleep; Corporeal and Intellectual Pursuits, on Healthy Man; Constituting Elements of Hygiene*. Philadelphia: Lea & Blanchard, 1844.
1846	Warren JC. *Physical Education and the Preservation of Health*. Boston: Wiliam D. Ticknor, 1846.
1848	Cruder C. *Anatomy and Physiology Designed for Academies and Families*. Boston: Benjamin B. Mussey and Co., 1848.
1852	Ehickwell E. *The Laws of Life, with Special Reference to the Physical Education of Girls*. New York: George P. Putnam, 1852.
1854	Stokes W. *Diseases of the Heart and Aorta*. Philadelphia: Lindsay, 1854.
1855	Combe A. *The Physiology of Digestion, Considered with the Relation to the Principles of Dietetics*. Philadelphia: Harper and Brothers, 1855.
1856	Beecher C. *Physiology and Calisthenics for Schools and Families*. New York: Harper and Brothers, 1856.
1859	Flint A. *The Clinical Study of the Heart Sounds in Health and Disease*. Philadelphia: Collins, 1859.
1860	Hitchcock E, Hitchcock E Jr. *Elementary Anatomy and Physiology for Colleges, Academies, and Other Schools*. New York: Ivison, Phinney & Co., 1860.
1863	Ordronaux J. *Manual of Instruction for Military Surgeons, on the Examination of Recruits and Discharge of Soldiers*. New York: D. Van Nostrand, 1863.
1866	Flint A. *A Treatise on the Principles and Practice of Medicine; Designed for the Use of Practitioners and Students of Medicine*. Philadelphia: H.C. Les, 1866; 56th edition, 1884.
1866	Flint A. *The Physiology of Man; Designed to Represent the Existing State of Physiological Science as Applied to the Functions of the Human Body. Vol. I. Introduction; The Blood; Circulation; Respiration*, 1866. Vol. II. Digestion; Absorption; Lymph and Chyle (1867). Vol. III. Secretion; Excretion; Ductless Glands; Nutrition; Animal Heat; Movement; Voice and Speech (1870). Vol. IV. Nervous System (1873). Vol. V. Special Senses; Generation (1874). New York: D. Appleton and Company.
1866	Huxley TH. *Lessons in Elementary Physiology*. London: Macmillan and Co., 1866.
1866	Lewis D. *Weak Lungs and How to Make Them Strong*. Boston: Ticknor and Fields, 1866.
1869	Dalton JC. *A Treatise on Physiology and Hygiene; for Schools, Families, and Colleges*. New York: Harper & Brothers, 1869.
1869	Gould BA. *Investigations in the Military and Anthropological Statistics of American Soldiers*. Published for the U.S. Sanitary Commission. New York: Hurd and Houghton, 1869.
1871	Flint A. *On the Physiological Effects of Severe and Protracted Muscular Exercise; with Special Reference to Its Influence Upon the Excretion of Nitrogen*. New York: D. Appleton & Co., 1873.

Background image: fotografermen/Shutterstock

Lippincott® Connect Appendix A, available online on Lippincott Connect, provides several influential bibliographies about anatomy and physiology, anthropometry, exercise and training, and exercise physiology, including Dr. Austin Flint's contributions.

Austin Flint, Jr., MD: American Physician-Physiologist

Austin Flint, Jr., MD (1836–1915), an American pioneer physician-scientist, contributed significantly to the burgeoning physiology literature. Dr. Flint came from a family with a long lineage of physicians, beginning with his great-great-grandfather Edward Flint (1733–1818) and continuing with his son Austin Flint III (1868–1955)—six generations, all well-schooled in the scientific method (Mehta et al., 2000).

Flint served as physiology and physiological anatomy professor in New York's Bellevue Hospital Medical College and chaired the Department of Physiology and Microbiology from 1861 to 1897. In 1858, he received the American Medical Association's prize for basic research on the heart, and his medical school thesis titled "The Phenomena of Capillary Circulation" was published in 1878 in the *American Journal of the Medical Sciences*.

Flint's textbooks were characterized by his admiration for other scholars' work. This included the work of noted French physician Claude Bernard (1813–1878); the celebrated observations of Dr. William Beaumont; and William Harvey's momentous discoveries about the heart's one-way blood circulation.

In 1866, he published what would become the first volume of a classic textbook in a five-volume set, *The Physiology of Man; Designed to Represent the Existing State of Physiological Science as Applied to the Functions of the Human Body. Vol. 1; Introduction;*

The Blood; Circulation; Respiration. Eleven years later, Flint published *The Principles and Practice of Medicine*, which synthesized his first five volumes with meticulously organized sections and supporting documentation in the book's 987 pages.

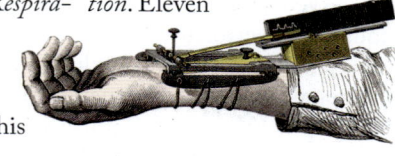
Courtesy Wellcome Collection

The text included four lithograph plates and 313 detailed woodcut anatomic illustrations documenting the body's major systems, along with important physiological principles. In addition, he illustrated equipment to record physiologic phenomena, including French physician and physiologist Étienne-Jules Marey's (1830–1904) early cardiograph for registering the pulse wave form and frequency, Marey's sphygmograph to record pulse measurements—the forerunner of current cardiovascular instrumentation[86,87] (www.woodlibrarymuseum.org/museum/marey-sphygmograph/)—and colleague Jean Baptiste Chauveau's (1827–1917) mechanical devices to measure intracardiac pressures, with which he pioneered cardiac catheterization techniques.

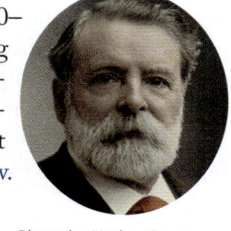
Photo by Nadar; Courtesy Wellcome Collection

Dr. Flint was a careful writer. This was a refreshing approach, particularly because so many "authorities" in physical training, exercise, and hygiene in the United States and abroad were uninformed and unscientific about exercise and its possible role in health care. In his 1877 textbook, Flint wrote about many exercise-related topics. The following examples from Flint's 1877 book present the flavor of exercise physiology as an emerging science in the late 19th century:

- Determining pulse differences with posture changes in men and women
- How age and sex affected heart action
- Exercise intensity influence on heart function and pulse rate
- Respiratory function during and immediately following muscular exercise
- Lavoisier's comments on oxygen uptake and carbon dioxide production during light-to-moderate physical activity

As noted above, Flint acknowledged and supported the work of many colleagues in his own work; likewise, his work influenced many others, including Étienne-Jules Marey, Thomas Cureton, and Earnest Phillip Boas. Marey's advanced sphygmograph revolutionized hospital care because the device popularized the "Graphic Method" in physiology applied to medicine. This enabled researchers and physicians to obtain preservable and quantifiable physiological records. Marey also invented pneumatic devices (tambor) for transmitting pressure changes to a stylus and a specialized pressure device to measure atrial and ventricular changes during the cardiac cycle.

Thomas Cureton (1901–1993; see below), a physical fitness researcher at the University of Illinois (Urbana) exercise physiology laboratory, repurposed Marey's sphygmograph to conduct numerous experiments with the "Cameron heartometer," now a cardiac measuring device to accurately measure and permanently record systolic and diastolic blood pressure, pulse rate, heart action force and character, and extremity circulation. The new adaptation used lights actuated by the pulse rather than by sound. Cureton's studies focused on exercise training programs and how they impacted cardiovascular responses to exercise in children, adults, and athletes.

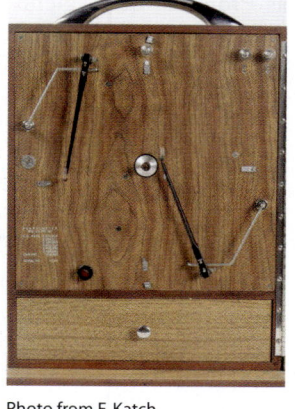
Photo from F. Katch

Nonetheless, it would not be until the next century that the first electronic cardiotachometer would be developed and used to conduct human experiments. Ernst Phillip Boas (1891–1955), an American physician who specialized in heart pathology and physiology and was a founding member of the New York Heart Association, and colleagues invented and patented this device in 1928 (https://sova.si.edu//record/NMAH.AC.0881; https://pubmed.ncbi.nlm.nih.gov/14392453/). Boas's distinguished medical career in New York City included directing Montefiore and Mount Sinai Hospitals and serving as professor of cardiology at Columbia University's College of Physicians and Surgeons and its Teachers College. As an administrator, Boas fought against race prejudice and championed appointing African American physicians and nurses to hospital staffs in the New York City boroughs. Boas advocated for universal health care and equal medical services distribution.

Through his textbooks, Austin Flint, Jr., also influenced Edward Hitchcock, Jr., MD, the first medically trained and scientifically oriented physical education professor in the United States (discussed in more detail in the following section). Hitchcock quoted Flint about the muscular system in his "Health Lectures Syllabus," required reading for all students enrolled at Amherst College for 44 consecutive years, from 1861 to 1905.

The Amherst College Connection

Two physicians, father and son, pioneered the American sports science movement. Edward Hitchcock, DD, LLD (1793–1864), served as professor of chemistry and natural history and, from 1845 to 1854, president at Amherst College. Edward Hitchcock, Jr. (1828–1911), his son, who graduated from Amherst in 1849 and Harvard Medical School in 1853, assumed his father's duties teaching anatomy at Amherst in 1861, after his father convinced the college president at the time to allow it. Dr. Hitchcock, Jr., was officially appointed on August 15, 1861,

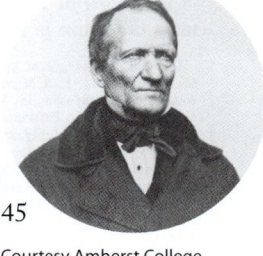
Courtesy Amherst College

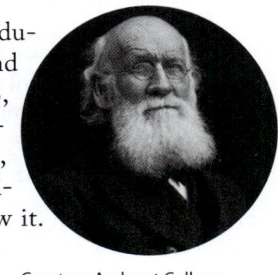
Courtesy Amherst College

as Professor of Hygiene and Physical Education with full academic rank in the Department of Physical Culture at an annual salary of $1000, a position he held almost continuously until 1911. This was the second such academic appointment in physical education to a college or university in the United States.

Early Physical Education Professor

Although Edward Hitchcock, Jr., is often accorded the distinction of being the first physical education professor in the United States, John D. Hooker was actually first appointed to this position at Amherst College in 1860 but resigned in 1861 from poor health, with Hitchcock replacing him. The original idea to create a physical education department with a professorship had been proposed in 1854 by William Augustus Stearns, DD (1805–1876), the fourth president of Amherst College, who considered physical education instruction essential for maintaining students' health and preparing them physically, spiritually, and intellectually. Other institutions were slow to adopt this concept; the next physical education department in America would not be created for another 25 years, in 1879. In 1860, the Barrett Gymnasium at Amherst College was completed and served as the training facility where all students were required to perform systematic exercises for 30 min 4 days weekly. The gymnasium included a laboratory with scientific apparatus (e.g., spirometer, strength and anthropometric equipment) and a piano to provide rhythm during the exercises. Hitchcock reported to the trustees that in his first year he recorded the students' "vital statistics," including age, weight, height, chest and forearm size, lung capacity, and muscular strength. The Hitchcocks geared their textbook to college physical education. They listed the topics covered in numerical order by subject and paid considerable attention to the physiology of species other than humans. The text included questions at the bottom of each page concerning the topics under consideration, making the textbook a primitive study guide or workbook, not an uncommon pedagogic feature in other physiology texts of the time (e.g., Cuder, 1848; Appendix A online).

FIGURE I.7 shows sample pages on muscle structure and function from the Hitchcock and Hitchcock text.

From 1865 to approximately 1905, the Hitchcocks' Health Lectures syllabus (38-page pamphlet, *The Subjects and Statement of Facts Upon Personal Health Used for the Lectures Given to the Freshman Classes of Amherst College*) was essential in the required curriculum.

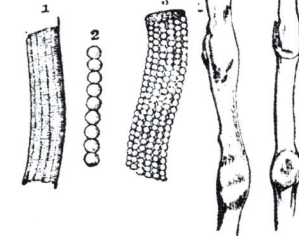
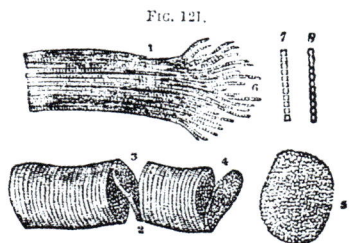

FIGURE I.7. Sample pages from Hitchcock and Hitchcock textbook.
(Reproduced from Hitchcock E, Hitchcock E Jr. *Elementary Anatomy andv Physiology for Colleges, Academies, and Other Schools*. New York: Ivison, Phinney & Co.; 1860:132, 137. Materials courtesy of Amherst College Archives and permission of the Trustees of Amherst College, 1995.)

Body Build Assessment by Anthropometry

From 1861 (just before the outbreak of the Civil War) to 1888, Dr. Hitchcock, Jr., obtained from almost every Amherst College student the following measures: 6 segmental height measures, 23 girths (measured with a cloth anthropometric measuring tape similar to those in use today), 6 breadths, 8 lengths, 8 muscular strength measures (assessed with force-measuring devices similar to the image shown—a crude, spring-loaded hand dynamometer to define "grip strength"), lung capacity (with a spirometer), and pilosity (body hair).

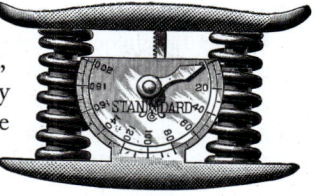

Courtesy Amherst College

In 1889, Dr. Hitchcock and Hiram H. Seelye, MD (a colleague in the physical education and hygiene department and Amherst college physician from 1884 to 1896), published a 37-page anthropometric manual that included five tables of students' anthropometric statistics recorded since 1861. This resource also provided detailed descriptions for taking anthropometric measurements, eye testing, and basic lung and heart examinations before muscular strength testing. In the manual's last section, Dr. Seelye wrote detailed instructions for using the various gymnasium apparatus to remedy round or stooping shoulders, increase chest size and lung capacity, and strengthen and enlarge the muscles of the arms, abdomen, back, thighs, calves, legs, and ankles. The Hitchcock and Seelye manual, the first in the United States to analyze body size and strength from detailed measurements, influenced other physical education departments at Yale, Harvard, Wellesley, and Mt. Holyoke colleges to include anthropometry in their regular physical education and hygiene curriculum.[6]

Early Anthropometry Assessment

Probably unknown to Hitchcock was the 1628 manuscript from the famous early text, *L'Académie de l'Espée*,[65] which appeared at a time when European anatomists and physiologists made important discoveries in science. Recall that proportionality theory from the Italian anatomists and artists impacted ideas about ideal body size and shape. Had Hitchcock's contemporaries known about early attempts to link anthropometric assessment with sport success, they might have more readily included anthropometry in their college curriculum. However, it was not until 67 years after Hitchcock began taking anthropometric measurements at Amherst and 37 years following Harvard's establishment of a physical education scientific laboratory (in 1891) that anthropometric measurements were first made of Olympic athletes, at the 1928 Amsterdam Olympic Games. One elite athlete measured in Amsterdam, Ernst Jokl (1907–1997) from South Africa, represented the German team in the 400-m run and 400-m hurdles. He later became team physician for the United States Olympic Committee (specializing in internal medicine and neurology) and physical education professor at the University of Kentucky in 1952, where he directed the rehabilitation center. Through writing 261 research publications and authoring or editing 27 books (including *Sudden Death of Athletes* [Thomas, 1985]), Jokl spearheaded efforts to raise sports medicine to national and international distinction in its formative years. Jokl, a charter and founding American College of Sports Medicine member (and UNESCO's International Council of Sport and Physical Education; www.icsspe.org/) advanced basic and applied sports science research, including anthropometry. Thus, Hitchcock's visionary ideas about anthropometry's application finally achieved international recognition—physique assessment integrated with physiology and exercise performance are now commonplace in exercise physiology laboratories. Kinanthropometry describes prevailing applied anthropometry. First established at the Physical Activity Sciences International Congress in conjunction with the 1976 Montreal Olympic Games,[64] this definition of this term was refined in 1980[65] to be the study of human size, shape, proportion, composition, maturation, and gross function to promote understanding about human movement dynamics.

From F. Katch

Early Advances in Data Collection and Measurement Techniques

The early interest in anthropometric measurement demonstrated that engaging in daily, vigorous physical activity produced desirable results, particularly for muscular development and its quantification. Almost no early physical education scientists applied statistics to assess training outcomes. Applying prevailing anthropometric analysis methods to the original

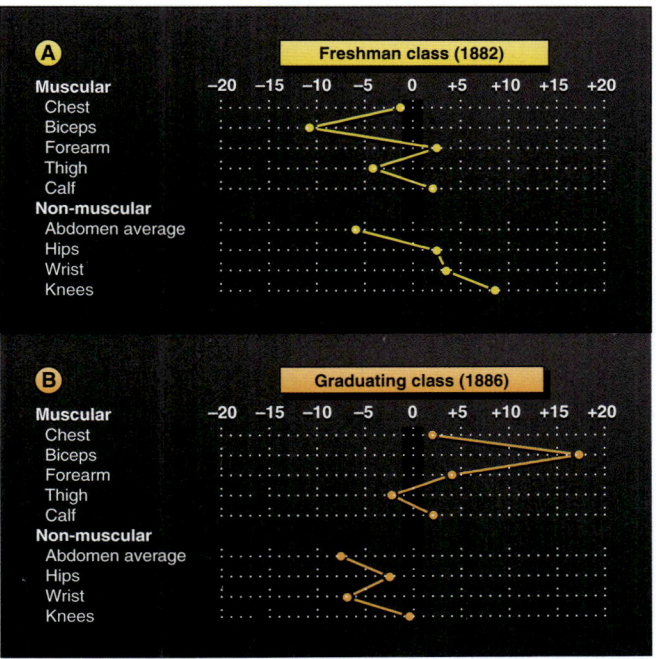

From F. Katch

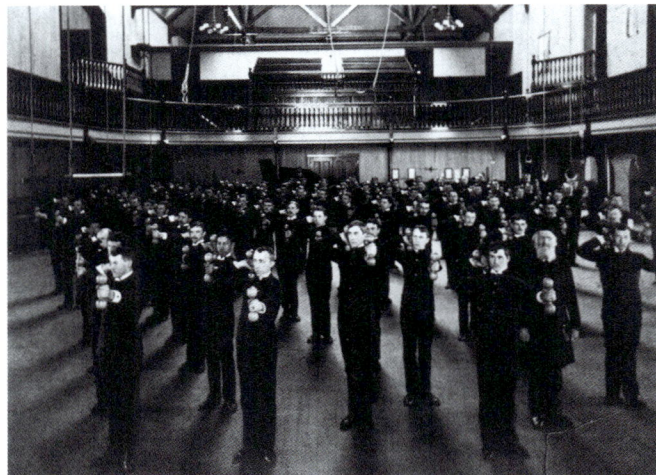

Courtesy Amherst College

Hitchcock data allows us to expand our conclusions about the students who entered Amherst College in 1882 and graduated 4 years later. The accompanying image that displays Behnke's body profile analysis reveals how the average student changed in physical dimensions over 4 years as screened by Behnke's reference standards (presented in Chapter 28). Note the dramatic increase in biceps girth and decreases in the nonmuscular abdomen and hip regions. Average body mass as freshmen in 1882 averaged 59.1 kg/130 lb (stature, 171.0 cm/67.3 in), whereas body mass for the graduating class 4 years later increased 5.5 kg/11.3 lb and stature by 7.4 cm/2.9 in. This image shows Dr. Edward Hitchcock, Jr. (second from right with beard) observing students performing barbell exercises in the Amherst College Pratt Gymnasium. Training to improve strength and better define muscular development included exercises with Indian clubs or barbell swinging and other strengthening modalities with the horizontal bar, rope and rings, dipping machine, inclined presses with weights, pulley weights, and rowing machine. The Hitchcock anthropometric and strength studies were acknowledged in the first formal American textbook on anthropometry, published in 1896 by Jay W. Seaver, MD (1855–1915), physician and lecturer on personal hygiene at Yale University for two decades and later at the Chautauqua Physical Education School, New York, where he taught muscular and nervous systems physiology and anthropometry to prospective physical education teachers. His classic 1906

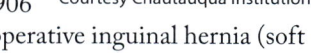

Courtesy Chautauqua Institution

publication on treatment of nonoperative inguinal hernia (soft tissue abdominal or bladder protrusion through a weak point in the abdominal wall; *Arch Physiol Therapy* Vol III, No. II) was based on data from over 20,000 male students at Yale who had this medical condition before entering college. Poorly conditioned individuals developed inguinal hernia in the inner groin region from violent-effort exercise, trauma, vigorous coughing, or lifting heavy objects. Seaver speculated that because men reported such conditions in their family, inheritance must play a role in developing the condition, with surgical repair the most frequently performed general surgery to treat persistent pain and discomfort for this protruding bulge.

While Hitchcock conducted anthropometric studies at the college level, the military managed the first detailed anthropometric, spirometric, and muscular strength measurements on Civil War soldiers in the early 1860s, published by Gould in 1869 (see the bibliographies in Appendix A online). The specially trained military anthropometrists used the *andrometer* to secure the soldier's physical dimensions to the nearest 1/10th inch to fit their uniforms. The idea for fitting uniforms on soldiers had begun in Britain in the early 1850s, when the government commissioned a Scottish tailor who invented the andrometer to accurately determine soldiers' clothing size. This special measuring device was first

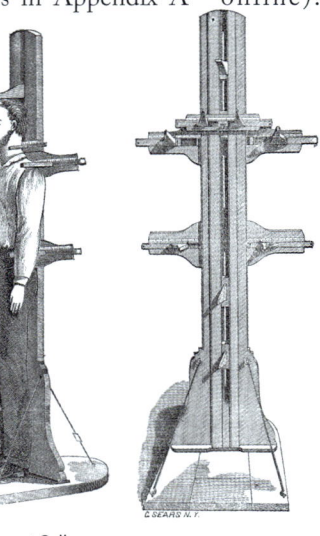

Courtesy Amherst College

used in the early 1860s by the United States Sanitary Commission at numerous military installations along the Atlantic seaboard (e.g., Fort McHenry, Baltimore; Naval Rendezvous, New York City; marine barracks, Brooklyn Navy Yard; bases in South Carolina, Washington, D.C., Detroit, New Orleans). Special "sliders" allowed for reliable measurement of stature; neck, shoulders, and pelvis breadth; and leg length and height to the knees and crotch. Each examiner practiced for 2 days to perfect measurement technique before assignment to a military installation. Data were compiled on 15,781 Whites, Blacks, and Indians between ages 16 and 45 years. These early studies served as prototypes for later military studies about muscular strength and the perceived relevance to battlefield performance. Exercise physiology laboratories worldwide train students in both simple (e.g., skinfolds, girths, body profile) and more complex techniques (e.g., underwater weighing, dual-energy x-ray absorptiometry, ultrasound), which are described in Chapter 28.[63,76]

The inset figure illustrates a mechanical device to evaluate lower body muscular strength more advanced than the one used at Amherst College in mandated military studies conducted 4 years following the Civil War. The testing procedure required the person to stand on the movable lid of a wooden packing box and grasp the rounded adjustable handle. He then lifted straight up with a maximum effort, and the highest score from three trials represented maximum leg strength. Other dynamometers also assessed muscular strength. According to Pearn (www.ncbi.nlm.nih.gov/pubmed/357684), Courtesy Amherst College

the Graham-Desaguliers dynamometer, developed in London in 1763, accurately measured muscular force without synergistic muscles imparting a false testing advantage. In Paris 35 years later, in 1798, a French civil engineer Edme Régnier (1751–1823) improved the dynamometer to measure targeted muscle group isometric force.

The primary use of dynamometer, although used for many purposes in farming (i.e., testing a bridled work horse pulling strength and force generated by motors and machines), was to record human strength, primarily in contests among strongmen (www.gilai.com/article_31/The-History-of-the-Regnier-Dynamometer). François Péron (1775–1810), a French naturalist and explorer, was reportedly the first person to document use of Régnier's dynamometer to measure indigenous people's strength during Australian explorations from 1800 to 1804 (www.portrait.gov.au/people/francois-auguste-peron-1775).

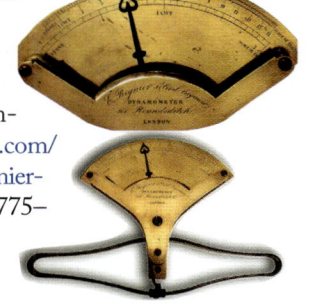

From Pearn J. (1978). Two early dynamometers. An historical account of the earliest measurements to study human muscular strength. J Neurol Sci. Jun; 37(1-2): 127-34.

Edmond Desbonnet (1867–1953), who championed interest in physical culture in Europe and abroad (https://physicalculturestudy.com/2016/12/13/edmond-desbonnet-la-gymnastique-des-organes-c-1900/), recorded students' training progress and made strength measurements to promote interest in what is now called *physical education* by measuring professional and amateur strongmen and wrestlers.

Desbonnet promoted strength development at his Parisian physical culture exercise clubs (e.g., l'Halterophile Club de France; translated from French to English; https://en.wikipedia.org/wiki/Edmond_Desbonnet) and in popular but expensive physical culture salons (gyms) in Europe frequented by society's elite. Ahead of his time by well over 100 years, Desbonnet created advertising posters and published articles in physical culture magazines that incorporated photographs of muscular men and women to appeal to strength development aficionados. European researchers also used testing devices to compare the overall muscular strength among different races. The device illustrated predates various American-made strength-measuring equipment used by physical education faculty at Amherst (Edward Hitchcock), Harvard (Dudley Allen Sargent; 1849–1924), and Yale (Jay Webber Seaver; 1855–1915).

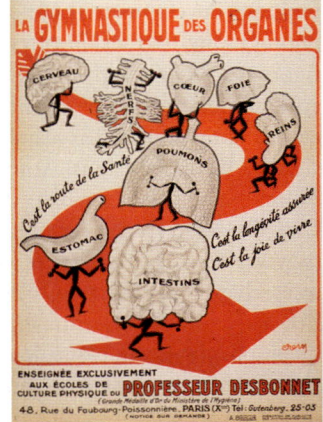

Courtesy National Library of Medicine

Spirometer Evolution in Fitness Assessment

In addition to strength assessment procedures, **spirometers** manufactured by many American and European manufacturers beginning in the early 1800s assessed patient's lung function, particularly vital capacity in hospitals, the military, and athletic events. When World War I began, the first American-made spirometers were designed to undergo the rough usage inseparable from transportation by army trains or on military railroads. Subjects breathed into the spirometers through a mouthpiece connected to flexible rubber tubing. The inset image shows a military-grade "dry" spirometer with mouthpiece and flexible tubing. The front dial recorded lung volumes, with readings expressed in cubic centimeters.

The "water spirometer" or "breath meter," invented by English physician John Hutchinson (1811–1861; www.pftforum.com/history/gallery/hutchinson-spirometer/), who had an aptitude in mechanical engineering, had no graphic breathing record. The patient or observer had to turn a stopcock at expiration's end to confine the air inside the chamber until the value could be read on a graduated scale calibrated in cubic inches. Hutchinson's 1846 precision spirometer, based on an original concept by Scottish tool designer and steam engine inventor James Watt in 1790 (1736–1819; www.bbc.co.uk/history/historic_figures/watt_james.shtml), included twin pulleys and counterweights, a U-tube manometer on the inside to adjust the counterweights so the inside pressure remained the same as that on the outside, and an attached thermometer to correct the gas volume to standard conditions. Volumes, measured manometrically, adjusted atmospheric pressure and corrected room temperature deviation above or below 15.6°C/60°F. For example, if a person expelled 206 cu in, the conversion (cu in × 16.41) would transpose to 3380 mL. Hutchinson, well trained at University College, London Medical School for integrating scientific procedures into medical practice, had been Sir Charles Bell's (1774–1842) celebrated student, anatomist, physiologist, and neurologist and one of the first to describe a neurological disturbance later named to honor him (**Bell's palsy**). Hutchinson and several others posited that height, not body weight, positively related to vital capacity (taller people have larger vital capacities). During that period in medical diagnosis, the prevailing ideas had not yet unraveled the true interrelationships among poor lung function and adverse health outcomes. For his many hospital patients, Hutchinson routinely recorded over 140,000 vital capacity measurements.

In 1842, he made measurements on the American boxing "giant" Charles Freeman (1821–1845), who was in London

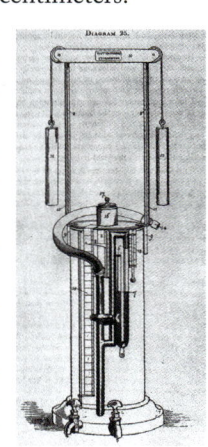

Courtesy Wellcome Collection

National Galleries Scotland

to fight the British bare-knuckle champion "Big Ben" Caunt (1815–1861). Almost 7 ft/83.8 in and weighing 271 lb (converted from stones; 1 stone = 14 lb), his vital capacity was 7.12 L/434 cu in. When Freeman became ill 2 years later, his vital capacity had decreased to 5.65 L, and he died a year later without apparent clinical disease despite reducing body weight by 14 kg/30 lb. Upon autopsy, the diagnosis for death was **phthisis** (tuberculosis).

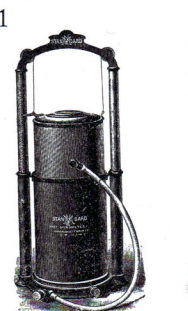
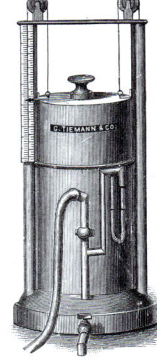

Courtesy Amherst College

Hitchcock used a similar Hutchinson water spirometer, in which expired gas volume moved through the spirometer following inspiration and expiration into a curved, upside-down bell atop a known water volume with numerous variations and improvements over at least the next 60 years. It served as the prototype for most current electronic spirometers (see Chapter 8). Of note is a complete timeline of the spirometer's development and its variations, which mentions Dutch biologist and microscopist Jan Swammerdam's (1637–1680) experiment with dogs the first "gasometer" description in a scholarly French journal by Antoine-Laurent Lavoisier (www.pftforum.com/history/timeline/). The discussion also focuses on a "field gas meter" from a large study of Civil War soldiers based on Hutchinson's original spirometer (designed in the 1840s) and future refinements by other physicians and researchers through the 1900s and beyond.

Hitchcock's Strength-Measuring Methods

The images show Kellogg's universal dynamometer strength-testing device (circa 1897–1901), acquired by Dr. Hitchcock in 1897 to assess the strength of the bilateral forearm, latissimus dorsi, deltoid, pectoral, and shoulder "retractor" muscles. Trunk measurements included the anterior trunk and anterior and posterior neck regions. The measurements also included leg extensors and flexors and thigh adductors.[94] The device included a lever controlled by a piston and cylinder above a mercury column in a closed glass tube. Water kept the oil in the cylinder protected from contact with mercury in the cylinder, and various attachments allowed different muscle groups to push on the lever. Hitchcock determined total body strength as a composite

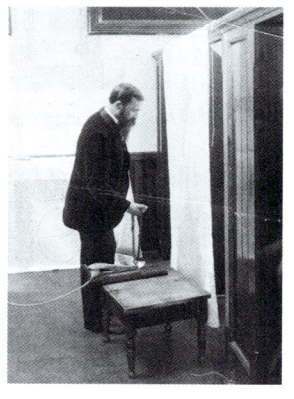

Courtesy Amherst College

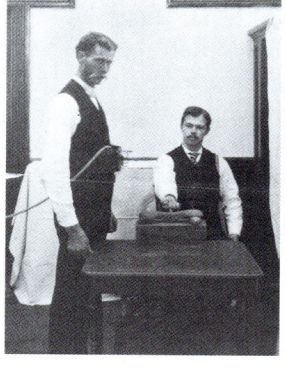

Courtesy Amherst College

body weight score multiplied by dip and pull test scores and back, legs, and average forearm and lung scores. Hitchcock believed that the total strength score remained an arbitrary and relative measure, believing a better comparison method would be desirable. He did not favor lifting a dead weight against gravity unless the lift related in some way to overall body size and dimensions. In Chapter 28, we discuss a practical "normalization" allometric statistical method to compare different body sizes and shapes.

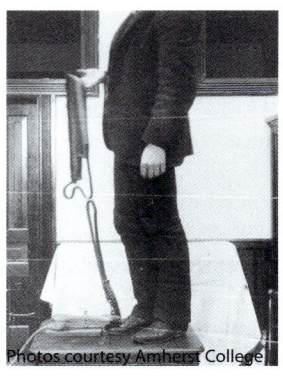

Photos courtesy Amherst College

The First United States Exercise Physiology Laboratory and Degree Program

The first formal exercise physiology laboratory in the United States, established in 1891 at Harvard University, housed a newly created Department of Anatomy, Physiology, and Physical Training at the Lawrence Scientific School.[25,44]

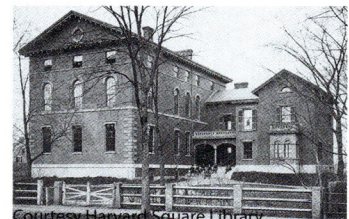

Courtesy Harvard Square Library

Several instructors in the initial undergraduate bachelor of science degree program in Anatomy, Physiology, and Physical Training who started at the same time were Harvard-trained physicians, including physiologist Henry Pickering Bowditch (1840–1911), renowned professor of physiology and Harvard Medical School's Dean. His many achievements included the all-or-none cardiac contraction principle, the treppe, muscular contraction staircase phenomenon, neural reflex (knee jerk) control, child growth and physique developmental standards in boys and girls assessed by photography, and vision physiology. Bowditch, known for his rigorous scientific and laboratory training, brought his expertise and training to the new scientific school program. His Parisian connections included researchers we previously chronicled—Claude Bernard, Louis-Antoine Ranvier, and Étienne-Jules Marey—and his German connections, Carl Ludwig and Carl von Voit. Each year, the American Physiological Society (www.physiology.org/professional-development/awards/researchers/bowditch?SSO=Y) awards the Henry Pickering Bowditch Award Lectureship for original and outstanding accomplishments in physiology.

Bowditch recruited another distinguished Harvard Medical School physiologist, William Townsend Porter (1862–1949), who had a chemistry background from his

German education, to teach at the Lawrence School. Porter founded the *American Journal of Physiology* (www.physiology.org/; first issue published in 1898 with Porter's contribution on isolated mammalian heart tissue; 1898;1:511). In 1901, Porter established the Harvard Apparatus Company in arrangement with Harvard University to produce high-quality laboratory equipment at affordable prices for teaching and physiological research. Porter introduced physiological experiments in his classes, focusing on student experiments with animal coronary circulation with emphasis on acute vessel occlusion.

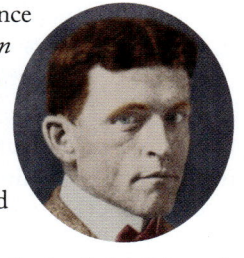

Courtesy National Library of Medicine

George Wells Fitz: Important Contributions

The major influencer in creating the new departmental major, George Wells Fitz, MD (1860–1934), recruited top scientists to join the faculty in Harvard's new program. Fitz vociferously supported a strong, science-based curriculum in preparing the "new breed" of physical educator. The archival records show that the new major required these science-oriented courses: exercise physiology, zoology, animal and human morphology, anthropometry, applied anatomy and animal mechanics, medical chemistry, comparative anatomy, remedial exercises, physics, gymnastics and athletics, physical education history, and English. Physical education students took general anatomy and physiology courses in the medical school; after 4 years, graduates could enroll as second-year medical students and graduate in 3 years with an MD degree. Dr. Fitz taught the physiology of exercise course based on his text, *Principles of Physiology and Hygiene*; thus, we believe he was one of the first medically trained persons to formally teach such a course. It included experimental investigation and original work and thesis, including laboratory study 6 hr weekly. The course prerequisites included general physiology at the medical school or its equivalent. The course provided training in experimental methods related to exercise physiology. Fitz also taught a more general course, Elementary Physiology of the Hygiene of Common Life, Personal Hygiene, and Emergencies (one lecture and one laboratory section weekly for a year or three times a week for 6 months). The lecture notes for the course subsequently were published as *Principles of Physiology* textbook.

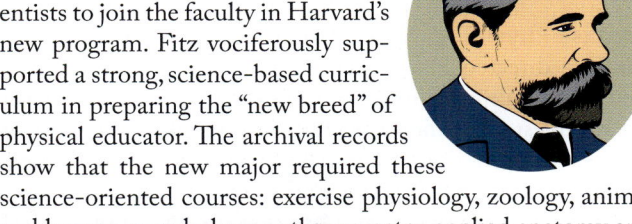

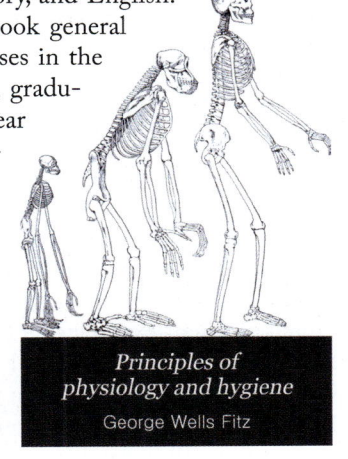

Fitz also taught a course titled Remedial Exercises. The Correction of Abnormal Conditions and Positions. Course content included spinal curvature deformities (and specialized exercise-corrective effects) and "selection and application of proper exercises, and in diagnosing cases when exercise is unsuitable." Several Fitz's scientific publications dealt with spinal deformities; one study, published in the *Journal of Experimental Medicine* in 1896 ("A Study of Types of Respiratory Movements"; volume 1, issue 4) concerned breathing mechanics. In addition to the remedial exercise course, students took a required course, Applied Anatomy and Animal Mechanics. Action of Muscles in Different Exercises. This thrice-weekly course, the forerunner of current biomechanics courses, was taught from 1879 to 1889 by assistant physical training professor Dr. Dudley Allen Sargent (1849–1924; Yale Medical School, 1878).

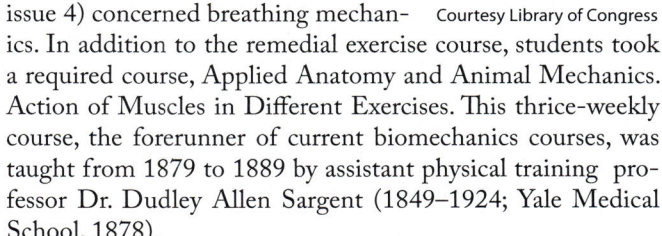

Courtesy Library of Congress

Its prerequisite was medical school general anatomy or its equivalent. Sargent believed that true body strength and physique, assessed by anthropometry and strength measuring equipment, could only be developed by exercising on his newly designed and commercially promoted weight and pulley machines, not the traditional equipment in typical gymnasia with boxing rings, standard rings, and high bars (www.starkcenter.org/igh/igh-v8/igh-v8-n2/igh0802c.pdf). In the course, students were required to read his book, *Handbook of Developing Exercises* (Boston: Franklin Press, Rand, Avery, & Co., 1886), a primer that guided students through all strengthening exercises practiced in Harvard's Hemenway gymnasium. The new state-of-the art facility, donated by Boston philanthropist and public official Augustus Hemenway (1852–1931), opened in 1878 and was enlarged in 1895, with the final design influenced by the most popular gymnasium in Paris in the early 1880s. Before a student could use the gymnasium, Sargent analyzed physique status by anthropometry (girths, breadths, lengths) to determine muscle development along with the individual's body weight, height, and limb measures. Sargent believed a physique examination dictated the person's immediate needs to perform efficiently on his mechanical machines in the gymnasium. To this end, each student received instruction about how to use the machines, which included general and seven "special" recommendations labeled A to G about exercise as described in the inset image from his *Handbook of Developing Exercises*.

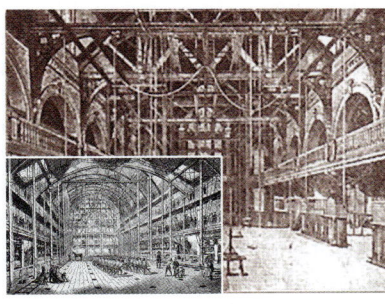

Exercise Physiology Research Laboratory. By the year 1900, nine men had graduated from the program with bachelor of science degrees, with the stated aim of becoming gymnasium directors or physical training instructors. A secondary aim was to prepare students with the necessary knowledge

EXERCISE, General.

When the muscles have been for a long time inactive, begin with light movements, and continue exercise for fifteen or twenty minutes only the first day. Increase the time and amount gradually, never reaching a maximum until nearly through training. Leave off exercise as gently as you begin. Never try to do your best in running, jumping, etc., or at feats of strength, until thoroughly warmed and limbered up. Do not exercise within two hours after eating, nor within a half-hour before.

If much heated and fatigued, a gentle rubbing-down will tend to keep up the surface circulation, and prevent taking cold.

EXERCISE, Special.

A. Exercise between four and six P.M. daily.

B. Take no exercise before breakfast. Exercise between nine and ten P.M., if convenient.

C. Exercise between eleven A.M. and one P.M.

D. Exercise slowly and deliberately, and take frequent intervals of rest. Do not run, row, ride horseback, or play lawn-tennis.

E. Exercise vigorously, fill the lungs frequently, and do not rest until the allotted task is finished.

F. Reduce exercise one-half during examinations, or while doing an unusual amount of brain-work.

G. When subjected to unusual mental or emotional excitement, increase the time and amount of exercise, using chiefly the muscles of the lower extremities.

Courtesy National Library of Medicine

about the science of exercise and future entry into medical school.

With departmental activities in full operation, its outspoken and critical director spoke frankly about academic topics. For example, Dr. Fitz reviewed a new physiology text (*American Text-Book of Physiology*, edited by American physiologist William H. Howell (1860–1945, PhD, MD, LLD, ScD) published in the March 1897 issue of *American Physical Education Review* (Vol. II, No. 1, p. 56). The review praised Dr. Howell's inclusion of content contributed by outstanding physiologists and critiqued an 1888 French book by Fernand Lagrange, which some writers consider the first exercise physiology text. The following is Fitz's review:

> No one who is interested in the deeper problems of the physiology of exercise can afford to be without this book [referring to Howell's Physiology text], and it is to be hoped it may be used as a text-book in the normal schools of physical training. These schools have been forced to depend largely on Lagrange's "physiology of exercise" for the discussion of specific problems, or at least for the basis of such discussions.
>
> The only value Lagrange has, to my mind, is that he seldom gives any hint of the truth, and the student is forced to work out his own problems. This does very well in well-taught classes, but, Alas! for those schools and readers who take his statements as final in matters physiological. We have a conspicuous example of the disastrous consequences in Treve's contribution of the "Cyclopaedia of Hygiene on Physical Education," in which he quotes freely from Lagrange and rivals him in the absurdity of his conclusions.

Fitz-Directed Harvard Influence Ends. For unknown reasons, but coinciding with Fitz's untimely Harvard departure in 1899, the department changed its curricular emphasis (the term *physical training* was dropped from the department title), thus terminating at least temporarily this unique higher education experiment. Park's scholarly presentation discusses the reasons Fitz departed Harvard.[50] His untimely withdrawal certainly was unfortunate for future exercise physiology students. In his 1909 textbook, *Principles of Physiology and Hygiene* (New York: Henry Holt and Co.), the title page listed the following about Fitz's affiliation: "Sometime Assistant Professor Physiology and Hygiene and Medical Visitor, Harvard University." This acknowledgment with the word "sometime" hints at Fitz's obvious displeasure with his former employer!

Exercise Physiology Expansion into Scientific Training. The Fitz-directed Harvard legacy between 1891 and 1899 focused on training young scholars to begin their careers with the strongest scientific basis regarding the health benefits of exercise and physical training. Unfortunately, it would take another quarter century before the next generation of science-oriented physical educators (led not by physical educators but by world-class physiologists, several of which we profile in later sections—Nobel laureate A. V. Hill and 1963 ACSM Honor Award recipient and renowned physiologist David Bruce Dill) would once again integrate robust science physiology and training into the physical education curriculum.

Many individuals contributed to the explosion of new scientific knowledge related to exercise physiology. For 40 years, Russian-born research scientist Peter V. Karpovich (1886–1985) directed the Physiological Research Laboratory at Springfield College in western Massachusetts. In his distinguished career, he wrote and published 150 articles, book chapters, and monographs dealing with fitness and exercise (salient examples include swimming biomechanics, artificial respiration, physical activity caloric expenditure, weightlifting, flexibility, warm up, and footwear studies. His influential and best-selling textbook, *Physiology of Muscular Activity* (Philadelphia: W.B. Saunders, 3rd ed., 1948), first coauthored with Edward C. Schneider (1874–1954) in 1948 and then published under sole authorship in 1953, was translated into five languages and went through eight editions.

Karpovich directed the Physical Fitness Laboratory in the Army's Aviation Medicine School, Randolph Field, Texas, from 1942 to 1945. He worked with the United States Army Quartermaster Research and Development Command in Natick, Massachusetts, on soldiers' clothing and footwear projects. In 1966, he and son George received a patent for a rotary **electrogoniometer** to measure forearm rotation during arm movements—with subsequent

First Course Taught in Exercise Physiology

Dr. Charles Tipton, former ACSM President and recipient of ACSM's Honor and Citation Awards, researched and determined who taught the first college-level/university-level course in exercise physiology and when and where it was offered. Here are his written thoughts on the matter after spending time researching the question in the archives of both Harvard University and Springfield College. Tipton has previously written an historical perspective of our field (Tipton, CM. "Historical Perspective: Origin to Recognition." *ACSM's Advanced Exercise Physiology*. Baltimore: Lippincott Williams & Wilkins, 2006: 11–38).

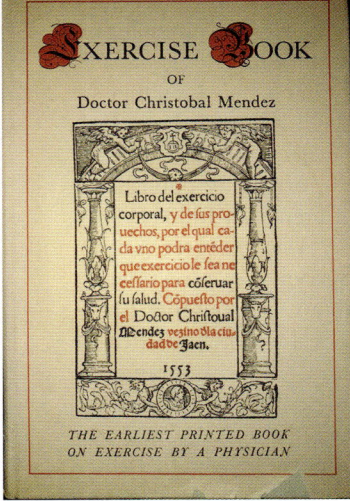

The first textbook concerning exercise and physiology was penned in Latin in 1553 by Spanish trained physician Cristóbal Méndez (1500–1561; "El Libro del Ejercicio Corporal y Sus Provechos" [*Book of Bodily Exercise*]).[1] In North America, an 1855 article by physician William H. Byford (1817–1890) for the first time used the words "physiology of exercise." Byford lamented that physicians were indifferent to the health benefits of exercise while encouraging them to become better informed and to initiate research on the subject.[2] Physicians Edward Hitchcock, Jr. (1828–1911) of Amherst College and Dudley A. Sargent (1849–1924) of Harvard University, likely included physiology of exercise topics in their physical education courses. Nevertheless, it was not until 1892–1893 or 1893–1894 that courses listed as the Physiology of Exercise were officially listed in an institutional Catalogue. In Harvard's 1892–1893 Catalogue, the Department of Anatomy, Physiology and Physical Training offered a formal course in Experimental Physiology, in which the Physiology of Exercise was listed as an integral component with physician George Wells Fitz (1896–1934) as instructor.[3] During the 1893–1894 school year, senior students majoring in physical education at the International Young Men's Christian Association (YMCA) Training School in Springfield, Massachusetts, were enrolled in a Physiology of Exercise course with physician Luther Halsey Gulick, Jr. (1865–1928) responsible for teaching the course.[4] Unfortunately, no catalogue information stated which semester the course was taught. There is no official record of the assigned text for the Harvard students, but it is known that at Springfield College, the required text for the Luther Halsey Gulick, Jr., MD (1865–1918) course was the 1889 Fernand LaGrange text translated from the French edition, *The Physiology of Bodily Exercise*.[5]

Sources:
Byford WH. On the physiology of exercise. *AM J Med Sci*. 1855;30:32.
LaGrange F. *Physiology of Bodily Exercise*. New York: D. Appleton; 1889.
Méndez C. *The Book of Bodily Exercise (1553)*. Baltimore: Waverly Press; 1960. Dr. Francisco Guerra of Yale University's History of Medicine Department translated the text from the original Méndez work, the earliest physician published book on exercise, and reproduced it to look like when it was published in Spain about 500 years ago.

---

publications using the apparatus on different limbs in humans and animals.

In May 1954, Peter Karpovich and his wife, Dr. Josephine L. Rathbone (1899–1989), together with graduate student Charles M. Tipton (1927–2021), became American Federation of Sports Medicine founding members before it transformed into the American College of Sports Medicine (ACSM; www.acsm.org). Karpovich served as ACSM's fifth president (1961–1962). He trained outstanding graduate students in exercise physiology who established their own productive laboratory research programs and professional service (e.g., Charles M. Tipton, ACSM President, 1974–1975; Howard Knuttgen, ACSM President, 1973–1974; Loring B. Rowell, ACSM Honor Award). Tipton, himself, would go on to serve as advisor to 23 PhD students and to receive ACSM's Citation and Honor Awards and the National Academy of Kinesiology Clark W. Hetherington Award.

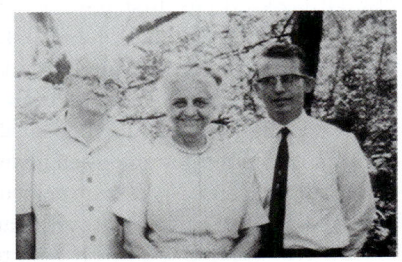

From F. Katch

Exercise Studies in Research Journals

Another notable event occurred in 1898 contributing to exercise physiology growth—publication of three articles about physical activity in the *American Journal of Physiology's* first volume. William T. Porter, noted physiologist from the St. Louis College of Medicine and Harvard Medical School, contributed research articles to the new journal, which was founded by Russel Chittenden and 28 comembers (with 21 medical school graduates) in 1887, and served as editor until 1914.[12] The next four volumes, from 1898 to 1901, contained six additional articles about exercise physiology from research laboratories at Harvard Medical School, Massachusetts Institute of Technology, University of Michigan, and the Johns Hopkins University. The American Physiological Society, publisher of the *American Journal of Physiology*, went on to found the *Physiological Reviews* journal (physrev.physiology.org) in 1921 and today publishes 15 different journals covering research in physiology and related fields,

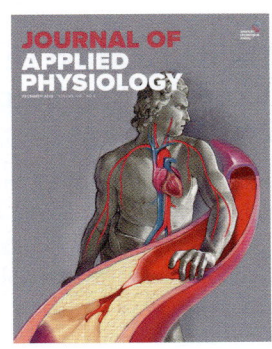

© The American Physiological Society

including the *Journal of Applied Physiology* (www.the-aps.org/), which routinely focuses on exercise-related topics. Appendix A, available online at Lippincott Connect, provides bibliographies from influential publications about anatomy and physiology, anthropometry, exercise and training, and exercise physiology. The list includes two articles from the *Annual Review of Physiology*, Nobel Laureate A. V. Hill's first 1922 muscle contraction mechanism review article, and female physiologist and ACSM Citation Award recipient Francis Hellebrandt's (1901–1992; MD) classic 1940 review concerning exercise physiology studies and rehabilitation medicine.

The German applied physiology publication *Internationale Zeitschrift fur angewandte Physiologie einschliesslich Arbeitsphysiologie* (1929–1973; now the *European Journal of Applied Physiology* [www.springer.com/journal/421/]), a significant exercise physiology research journal, published hundreds of articles in numerous disciplines related to exercise physiology. The *Journal of Applied Physiology* (www.jap.physiology.org) was first published in 1948. Its initial volume contained the now-classic paper on ratio expressions using physiologic data with reference to body size and function by British child-growth and development researcher-pediatrician James M. Tanner, MD (1920–2010; *A History of the Study of Human Growth*, 1981), a must-read for exercise physiologists. Volume 1 of the journal *Medicine and Science in Sports* (now *Medicine and Science in Sports and Exercise* [MSSE; www.journals.lww.com/acsm-msse/toc/1969/03000]), which was published in 1969, featured research in the emerging exercise sciences and sports medicine domains.

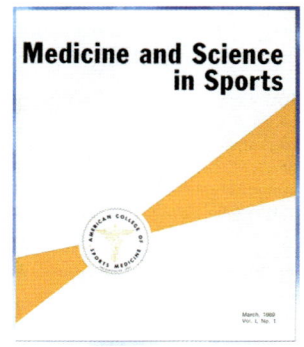

Distinguished Female Pioneer in Exercise Physiology and Rehabilitation Medicine

Francis Anna Hellebrandt (1901–1992) achieved notoriety for directing the University of Wisconsin Medical School's Exercise Physiology Laboratory in 1930 and later the Motor Learning Laboratory in 1957. Her main goal was to encourage women physical education majors to pursue graduate studies in exercise physiology. Her devotion to such a singular task at that time had a broad and overarching impact on the field, quite aside from her outstanding interdisciplinary research, which focused mainly on basic and applied muscle physiology, muscle pathology, and sports skill acquisition sequencing (https://onlinelibrary.wiley.com/doi/full/10.1016/j.pmrj.2013.06.004; www.ncbi.nlm.nih.gov/pubmed/10797891).

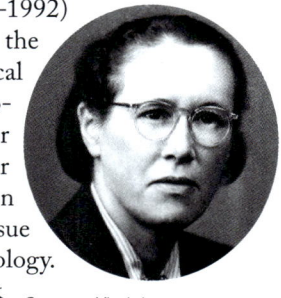

Courtesy Virginia Commonwealth University

First Published Exercise Physiology Textbook?

Who published the first bona fide exercise physiology textbook? Authors of several early exercise physiology texts nominate as "first" Fernand Lagrange's English translation, *The Physiology of Bodily Exercise*, originally published in French in 1888.[6,73,76]

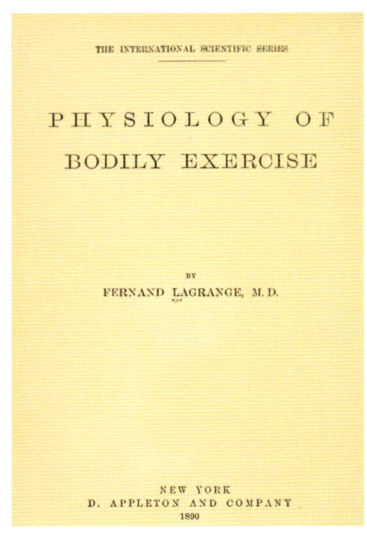

We disagree with Berryman's assessment about the relative historical importance attributed to Lagrange's original text.[6] To deserve such historical recognition, we believe that the work should meet these three criteria:

1. Provide sound scientific rationale for major concepts
2. Provide summary information (based on experimentation) about important prior research in a particular topic area (e.g., contain scientific references to research in the area)
3. Provide sufficient "factual" information about a topic area to achieve academic legitimacy

After reading the Lagrange book in its entirety, we came to the same conclusion as did George Wells Fitz in his early 1900s review. Fitz summarized that it was a popular book about health and exercise with a "scientific" title. In our opinion, the book is *not* a legitimate "scientific" exercise physiology textbook based on any reasonable criteria of the time. Despite Lagrange's assertion that his book focused on physiology applied to exercise and not hygiene and exercise, it is informed by a 19th-century hygienic perspective, not rigorous science. We believe Fitz would accept our evaluation.

Much information was available to Lagrange from existing European and American physiology textbooks about the biology of the digestive, muscular, circulatory, and respiratory systems, including some limited information on physical training, hormones, basic nutrition, chemistry, and muscular contraction. Admittedly, this information was relatively scarce, but well-trained physiologists Austin Flint, William H. Howell (1848–1896; first physiology professor in the Johns Hopkins Medical School), John C. Dalton (1825–1889; first physiology professor in America), and William B. Carpenter (1813–1885; textbook writer and experimentalist) had already produced high-quality textbooks that contained detailed information about physiology in general, with some reference to muscular exercise.[49] We can appreciate why Fitz was so troubled by the kudos given to the Lagrange book. By comparison, the two-volume text by Howell, *An American Text-Book of Physiology*, was impressive; this edited volume contained articles from acknowledged American physiologists. The Howell textbook represented a high-level physiology text even by today's standards. For context, Howell joined the physiology department at the University of Michigan, Ann Arbor, and in 1889 taught the first required physiology course in any medical school in the United States.[99] He then devoted his career at Hopkins Medical School, publishing 55 papers, most dealing with problems in blood physiology (coagulation, hemophilia, thromboplastin) and pathology. Howell, an American Physiological Society charter member, read the first paper at the Society's initial meeting. Fitz was well aware how the high scholarly standards of physiologists such as Howell, Dalton, and Carpenter contributed to excellence in the newly emerging physiology literature, not only from their publications, but in textbook publishing and student mentoring.

We assert that in his quest to provide the best possible science to teach his physical education and medical students, Fitz could not tolerate a book that did not live up to his high expectations, which is presumably why the Lagrange book was not adopted for any Harvard course. It certainly would not have been adopted for any course taught at the developing University of Michigan or John Hopkins Medical Schools. The Lagrange book in total contained fewer than 20 reference citations, and most were ascribed to French research reports or were based on personal accounts and observations from friends performing exercise. Such anecdotal reports must have given Fitz "fits."

Lagrange, an accomplished writer shown in the inset image, wrote extensively on exercise. The *Physiology of Bodily Exercise* text was first published in 1888 in French, with different language translations through 1898, and then into English. Lagrange was not a scientist but rather an accomplished writer for popular journals about sports, exercise, and fitness devoted to the **physical culture movement**. Bibliographic information about Lagrange is limited in the French and American archival records, a further indication validating his relative obscurity as a scholar in an academic field. As far as we know, there have been no citations of his work in any physiology text or published scientific article. For these reasons, we contend the Lagrange book does not qualify as the first exercise physiology textbook. Instead, we posit that this title go to Scottish physician Andrew Combe's text, *The Principles of Physiology Applied to the Preservation of Health, and to the Improvement of Physical and Mental Education* (read online at https://archive.org/stream/principlesofphys1835comb#page/n5/mode/2up), first published in quantity in the third 1834 edition (but years earlier in limited distribution), about 65 years before Lagrange. Combe, a forward thinker, provided intimate details about the physiologic systems gleaned from the available English and European literature. The text contained insightful discussions about exercise effects on bone, principles of "aerobic" and "endurance" training, and how different strengthening exercises related to physical performance. Had Combe lived during the Lagrange era, he certainly could have produced a bona fide "first" textbook legitimately titled, *The Physiology of Bodily Exercise*.

Portrait: Royal College of Physicians of Edinburgh

Other Early Exercise Physiology Research Laboratories

In 1902, Scottish-American industrialist, steel and business magnate, and philanthropist Andrew Carnegie (1835–1919; www.history.com/topics/19th-century/andrew-carnegie) funded the Nutrition Laboratory at the Carnegie Institute in Washington, D.C. (www.carnegiescience.edu/legacy/findingaids/CIW-Administration-Records.html). This laboratory functioned as an independent research organization to generate new knowledge in emerging fields (e.g., genetics, Earth's magnetic properties [terrestrial magnetism], embryology). A new laboratory, focused on nutrition and energy metabolism, opened in 1908 and hired researcher Francis G. Benedict as its first director. Also in the United States, George Williams College (1923) has the distinction as the first physical education research laboratory to study exercise physiology, followed by the University of Illinois (1925) and Springfield College (1927). Nevertheless, the real impact in exercise physiology research with many other research specialties occurred in 1927 within the 800-square foot Harvard Fatigue Laboratory, created in the basement of Harvard University Business School's Morgan Hall.[36] During the next two decades, this laboratory's outstanding work established exercise physiology legitimacy on its own merits as an important area to study three main physical stressors—heat, altitude, and exercise training (https://pubmed.ncbi.nlm.nih.gov/9696994/).

Another exercise physiology laboratory, created in 1934, was the Laboratory of Physiological Hygiene at the University of California, Berkeley.[60] The syllabus for the Physiological Hygiene course (taught by professor Frank Lewis Kleeberger [1904–1993]), which served as a precursor contemporary exercise physiology course, contained 12 laboratory experiments.[51] Several years later, Dr. Franklin M. Henry (1904–1993; ACSM Honor Award) assumed laboratory responsibilities (https://senate.universityofcalifornia.edu/_files/inmemoriam/html/franklinmhenry.html). In 1950, Henry created a 74-page, single-sided mimeographed and stapled, copyrighted book sold at the University's Associated Students Store, titled *Physiology of Work. The Physiological Basis of Muscular Exercise*.

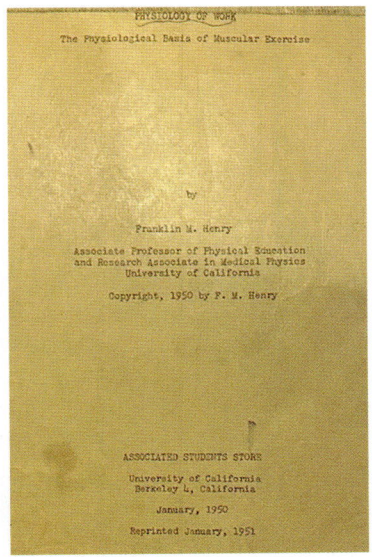

From F. Katch

A revised edition was published in 1963 and updated in 1968 to include a chapter on muscle contraction theory. Undergraduate and graduate students used Henry's original and later revised 1950 laboratory manual, *The Physiological Basis of Muscular Exercise*, in the exercise physiology course for at least the next 20 years.[95] The brief preface stated:

> In order to explain the physiology of work and exercise, it has seemed to the author that it is first necessary to come to some reasonable understanding of the nature of work itself and the mechanisms whereby the raw energy sources supplied to the body are converted into the force of muscle tension. Since oxygen uptake, carbon dioxide production, the transport of these gases and the temporary and final disposal of the products of metabolism assume such a crucial role in the process of muscular work it has also seemed important to treat these topics from a fundamental point of view. With these basic factors understood, the mechanism of oxygen debt comes more clearly into focus. ... While this approach has made necessary the inclusion of a certain amount of preliminary explanation that the more sophisticated reader will be able to pass over, it does have the merit of forcing concentration on the physiological significance of the work mechanism rather than complex details that sometimes lend themselves all to readily to chemical symbolism. F. M. H.

From F. Katch

Henry published experiments in various physiology-oriented journals, as for example, *Journal of Applied Physiology, Annals of Internal Medicine, Aviation Medicine, War Medicine,* and *Science*. Henry's first research project, which was published in 1938, when he was a faculty member in the University's Physical Education Department, concerned the validity and reliability of the pulse-ratio test of cardiac efficiency[29,30,31]; a later paper dealt with predicting aviators' bends, a serious concern during wartime.

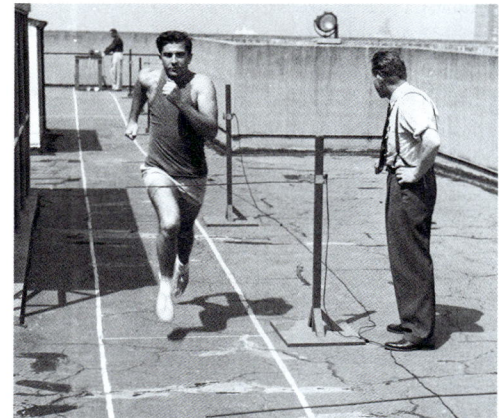

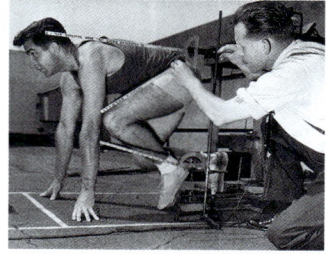 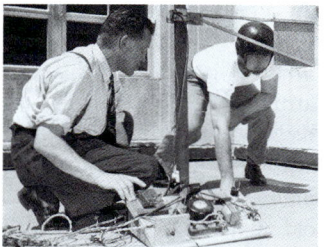

Henry applied his training in experimental psychology to exercise physiology topics, including individual differences in the fast and slow oxygen uptake and recovery curve components during light- and moderate-cycle ergometer exercise; muscular strength; cardiorespiratory responses during steady-rate exercise; intense exercise fatigue assessment; endurance performance determinants; and neural control factors related to human motor performance. The images here show Professor Henry supervising 50-yard sprints (at 5-yd intervals) on the Harmon Gymnasium roof. This study[31] was prompted by A. V. Hill's 1927 observations concerning the muscular contraction "viscosity" factor. At the bottom left, Henry makes limb and trunk anthropometric measurements on a sprinter to assess the sprint start force-time characteristics to better understand the theoretical equation underlying sprint running velocity,[32] while the bottom right image shows evaluation of an initial "explosive" blocking movement from a crouch position in a football lineman.[48]

Henry is remembered for his perceptive experiments regarding motor task specificity-generality and "Memory-Drum Theory" of neuromotor reaction and physical performance (*J Mot Behav.* 1986;18:77). Henry's pivotal paper, "Physical Education as an Academic Discipline" (*Quest.* 1978;29:13), ignited the way for physical education departments to change their emphasis to become more science oriented, with in-depth study of exercise physiology, biomechanics, exercise biochemistry, motor control, and ergonomics.[53] Henry's paper created a transformation across the United States and Canada as traditional physical education departments struggled to either maintain their pedagogical ideals to train students for teaching careers or break from this original model and create an alternative academic field with a strong, basic sciences emphasis.

Harvard Fatigue Laboratory Contributions (1927–1946)

Many outstanding 20th century scientists with an interest in exercise associated with the Harvard Fatigue Laboratory. Lawrence J. Henderson, MD (1878–1942), renowned chemist and Harvard Medical School biochemistry professor, established this soon-to-be acknowledged renowned research facility. David Bruce Dill (1891–1986), a Stanford PhD in physical chemistry, served as the first and only scientific director. This image of Dill shows him analyzing expired air samples using the Haldane apparatus (see Chapter 8) during a 1935 high altitude expedition to the summit camp of **stratovolcano** Aucanquilcha in the Chilean Andes (6100 m/20,000 ft). The experiments investigated exercise effects on respiratory and circulatory functions, blood chemistry, and higher and lower altitude effects on mental functions.

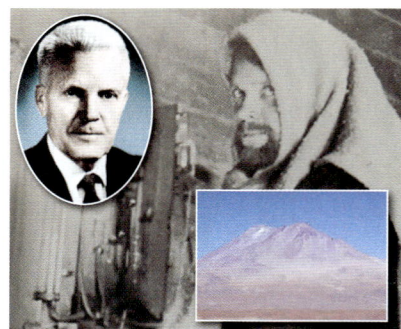

Background photo National Library of Medicine

While at the Fatigue Laboratory, Dill changed his academic interest as a biochemist to an experimental physiologist. He remained an influential driving force in the laboratory's numerous scientific accomplishments.[20] His early academic association with Boston physician Arlen Vernon Bock (who studied at the famous Cambridge [England] Physiological Laboratory with high-altitude physiologist Sir Joseph Barcroft [1872–1947][5] [www.encyclopedia.com/science/dictionaries-thesauruses-pictures-and-press-releases/barcroft-joseph] and Dill's closest friend for 59 years) and contact with 1922 Nobel laureate Archibald Vivian (A.V.) Hill (for discoveries related to muscle's heat production) allowed Dill to successfully coordinate research efforts with scientists from 15 different countries. Hill convinced Bock to write Bainbridge's *Physiology of Muscular Activity*, 3rd edition. Bock, in turn, invited Dill to coauthor the book republished in 1931.[19] Over a 20-year period, at least 352 research papers, numerous monographs,[37] and a book[20] were published in areas of basic and applied exercise physiology, including methodological refinements for blood chemistry analysis and simplified methods to analyze expired air's fractional concentrations.[18] Research at the Fatigue Laboratory before its closure[21] included short-term responses and chronic physiologic adaptations to exercise with exposure to altitude, heat, and cold. In the experiment shown here to determine changes in metabolic and cardiovascular function during different cold stress durations ranging from 30 min to hours wearing different clothing, subjects sat quietly in an environmental chamber, one person in normal clothing and shoes, the other in a military-style parka, undergarments, and special cold weather boots.

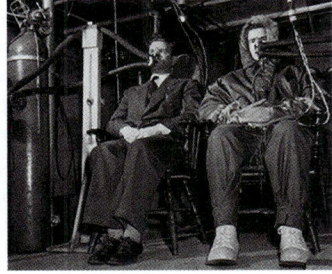

From F. Katch

As in the first exercise physiology laboratory established at Harvard's Lawrence Scientific School in 1892,[50] Harvard's Fatigue Laboratory demanded scholarship excellence. Many Fatigue Laboratory scientists profoundly impacted other exercise physiologists in the United States and abroad. Noteworthy were Ancel Keys (1904–2004), who established the Laboratory of Physiology and Physical Education (later renamed the Laboratory of Physiological Hygiene; https://lphes.umn.edu/) at the University of Minnesota, and Henry L. Taylor (1912–1983). Keys and Taylor were mentors to exercise physiologist Elsworth R. Buskirk (1925–2010), formerly at the National Institutes of Health and later the Noll Physiological Research Center at Pennsylvania State University (originally the Pennsylvania State Human Performance Laboratory and Noll Laboratory;[13] http://noll.psu.edu/#hplh); Robert E. Johnson at the Human Environmental Unit at the University of Illinois; Sid Robinson (1902–1982; the first to receive a PhD from the Harvard Fatigue Laboratory) at Indiana University; Robert C. Darling (1908–1998) at the Department of Rehabilitation Medicine at Columbia University; Harwood S. Belding (1909–1973), who started the Environmental Physiology Laboratory at the University of Pittsburgh; C. Frank Consolazio (1924–1985) U.S. Army Medical Research and Nutrition Laboratory at Denver; Lucien Brouha (1899–1968), who headed the Fitness Research Unit at the University of Montreal and then worked at the Dupont Chemical Company in Delaware; and Steven M. Horvath (1911–2007), established the Institute of Environmental Stress at the University of California, Santa Barbara (https://journals.physiology.org/doi/full/10.1152/advan.00118.2013), working with visiting scientists and mentored graduate students in the Departments of Biology and Ergonomics and Physical Education. After the Fatigue Laboratory was forced to close in 1946, Dill continued as deputy director of the U.S. Army Chemical Corps Medical Laboratory in Maryland from 1948 to 1961. Thereafter, he worked with and is shown in this image testing middle-distance runner and 1928 Olympian and Harvard Fatigue Laboratory-trained physiologist Sid Robinson (1902–1982) at Indiana University's physiology department laboratory (https://biology.indiana.edu/alumni-giving/robinson-scholarship.html). Dill then started the now considerably expanded Desert Research Institute at the University of Nevada (www.dri.edu), conducting basic and applied research on the physiologic responses of humans and animals to hot environments that culminated in a book on the topic.[22]

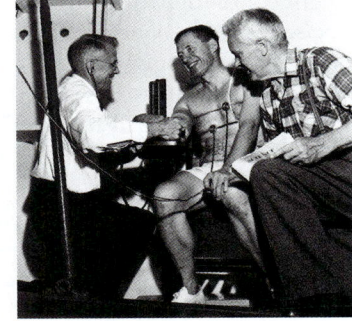

Courtesy Indiana University

The scholarly group associated with the Harvard Fatigue Laboratory mentored the next generation's students who continue to make significant contributions to the exercise physiology field. The monograph by Horvath and Horvath[36] and Dill's[21] chronology represent the most historically direct information sources about the Harvard Fatigue Laboratory; recent studies[23,67] and an edited textbook with 36 research contributors, *History of Exercise Physiology*, by Charles Tipton (see above) have chronicled its research contributions in a separate chapter with 76 references.

Exercise physiology continued to expand after the Fatigue Laboratory closed. Subsequent research efforts probed the full range involving physiologic functions. **TABLE I.1** summarizes these early investigations' depth and breadth.

TABLE I.1 Investigations at the Harvard Fatigue Laboratory

Physiologic Research Methodology Textbook

In 1949, the Research Section of the Research Council of the Research Section of the American Association for Health, Physical Education, and Recreation (AAHPER; an American Association for the Advancement of Physical Education outgrowth created in 1885; now called Society of Health and Physical Educators-SHAPE) published the first textbook devoted to physical education research methodology.[1] Thomas Cureton, PhD (1901–1992; 1969 ACSM Honor Award; see below), a pioneer physical fitness researcher, established and directed the exercise physiology research laboratory at the University of Illinois in 1944 (https://distributedmuseum.illinois.edu/exhibit/physical-fitness-research-laboratory/). Cureton appointed University of California (UC) professor Franklin Henry to chair the committee to write the research methods chapter. The other committee members were respected scientists in their own right and included Anna Espenshade (1905–1973; PhD in psychology from UC Berkeley, specialist in motor development and motor performance during growth[58,59]); Pauline Hodgson (UC Berkeley PhD in physiology who completed postdoctoral work at the Harvard Fatigue Laboratory); Peter V. Karpovich (1896–1975; originated the Physiological Research Laboratory at Springfield College; www.digitalcommonwealth.org/search/commonwealth-oai:6395w908k); Arthur H. Steinhaus, PhD (1897–1970; directed the research laboratory at George Williams College, and 1 of the 11 American College of Sports Medicine founders and research physiologist who authored an important review article [*Physiological Reviews*, 1933] about chronic exercise effects); and eminent Berkeley physiologist Hardin Jones, PhD (1914–1978; Donner Medical Physics Research Laboratory; https://oac.cdlib.org/findaid/ark:/13030/tf9n39p0k0/entire_text/).

The distinguished committee's book chapter represents a research methodology hallmark in exercise physiology. The 99 references, many key articles in this then-embryonic field, covered such exercise-related topics as "heart and circulation, blood, urine and kidney function, work, lung ventilation, respiratory metabolism and energy exchange, and alveolar air."

Another masterful research methods compendium published 14 years later, *Physiological Measurements of Metabolic Functions in Man*, by C. F. Consolazio (1913–1976) and colleagues, provided complete details about specific exercise physiology measurement techniques.[18] Sections contained material previously published from the Harvard Fatigue Laboratory one year before its closing in 1946[35] and from another 1951 text concerning metabolic methods.[17]

The Nordic Connection (Denmark, Sweden, Norway, and Finland)

Denmark and Sweden significantly impacted the robust physical education history as an academic subject field. In 1800, Denmark became the first European country to require military-style gymnastics training in the public school curriculum. Since then, Danish and Swedish scientists have made outstanding contributions to research in both traditional physiology in general and exercise physiology specifically.

Danish Influence

In 1909, the University of Copenhagen endowed the equivalent of a Chair in Anatomy, Physiology, and Theory of Gymnastics.[47] The first docent Johannes Lindhard, MD (1870–1947), teamed

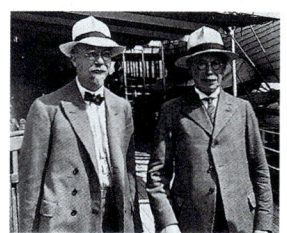

with August Krogh 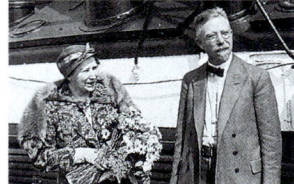 (1874–1949, Nobel Prize recipient specializing in physiological chemistry and precision glass design and construction) to conduct many of the now classic exercise physiology experiments (www.nobelprize.org/search/?s=krogh). For example, Krogh and Lindhard investigated lung's gas exchange, pioneered studies about lipid and carbohydrate's relative oxidation contribution to exercise, measured blood flow redistribution during different exercise intensities, and assessed cardiorespiratory dynamics in exercise (including cardiac output using nitrous oxide gas and acetylene gas, methods studied extensively in the modern era by professors August Krogh and Johannes Lindhard in the early 1900s, and Arthur Grollman [1901–1980] and colleagues in the late 1920s; www.physiology.org/doi/abs/10.1152/ajplegacy.1929.88.3.432?journalCode=ajplegacy).

By 1910, August Krogh and his wife Marie Krogh, MD (1874–1943), had devised ingenious, decisive experiments[40–43] proving how pulmonary gas exchange of oxygen occurred by diffusion and not by oxygen secretion from lung tissue into the blood during exercise or altitude exposure, as postulated by Scottish physiologist Sir John Scott Haldane (1860–1936) and Englishman James Priestley (see above).[28] By 1919, August Krogh had published multiple experiments concerning the mechanism explaining oxygen diffusion and transport, with three in the 1919 *Journal of Physiology*. The early experimental details appear in Krogh's 1936 textbook,[40] but he also was prolific in many other science areas.[39–42] In 1920, he received the Nobel Prize in Physiology or Medicine for discovering the mechanism dictating capillary blood flow control in frog resting and exercising muscle. To honor his prolific achievements, which included 300 scientific articles, the Institute for Physiologic Research in Copenhagen was named after him. We highly recommend the book by comparative physiologist Knut Schmidt-Nielsen (1915–2007), himself a prolific researcher with doctoral degrees in dentistry, odontology, physiology, and 275 research publications, and his wife Bodil Schmidt-Nielsen (1918–2015). Krogh's youngest of four children, also a prolific researcher and the American Physiological Association's first female president (1975). These two superstars in their own right chronicle the numerous incomparable contributions of August and Marie Krogh to science and exercise physiology.[68]

Three other Danish researcher-physiologists—Erling Asmussen (1907–1991 shown at left; ACSM Citation Award, 1976 and ACSM Honor Award, 1979), Erik Hohwü-Christensen (1904–1996; ACSM Honor Award, 1981; in center), and Marius Nielsen (1903–2000; at right)—conducted original exercise physiology studies.[16] These "three musketeers," as

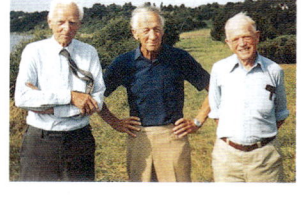

Krogh referred to them, published regularly in top journals from the 1930s to the 1970s. Asmussen, initially an assistant in Johannes Lindhard's laboratory, became a productive researcher specializing in muscle fiber architecture and mechanics. He also published papers with Nielsen and Christensen on applied muscular strength and performance interactions, ventilatory and cardiovascular response to posture and exercise intensity changes, maximum working capacity in arm and leg exercise, changes in muscle's oxidative response during exercise, positive and negative work comparisons, hormonal and core temperature response during different exercise intensities, and respiratory function with decreased oxygen partial pressure. His high level of scholarship is evident in his classic muscular exercise review article that cites his own studies with Danish physiologist and coworker Marius Nielsen (1903–2000) (plus 75 references from other Scandinavian researchers).[2] Nielsen's classic 1938 study concerned temperature regulation during constant load exercise at temperatures ranging from 5°C (41°F) to 36°C (96.8°F). His research revealed that variation in rectal temperature remained essentially unchanged despite wide ambient temperature changes. Asmussen's grasp about biologic functions in exercise remains as relevant today as it was 65 years ago when he placed exercise physiology firmly within the realm of biologic science:

> *The physiology of muscular exercise represents a classic, almost purely descriptive science. Research in many related domains in exercise physiology chronicles how the human organism adapts itself to the stresses and strains of the environment, thereby providing meaningful knowledge for athletes, trainers, industrial human engineers, clinicians, and workers in rehabilitation on the working capacity of humans and its limitations. But the physiology of muscular exercise also is part of its big brother in general biological science—physiology, which attempts to explain how living organisms function by chemical and physical laws that govern the inanimate world. It's important role in physiology considers muscular exercise more than most other conditions, taxes the functions to their maximum. Respiration, circulation, and heat regulation only idle in the resting state. Tracking physiology through successive stages of increasing work intensities allows for a better understanding of the resting condition. How the organism responds to exercise stress illuminates how organisms adapt to disease or how to eliminate its effects by mobilizing its regulatory mechanisms.[2]*

Christensen became Lindhard's student in Copenhagen in 1925. Together with Krogh and Lindhard, Christensen published an important 1936 review describing physiologic dynamics during maximal exercise.[15] In his 1931 thesis, Christensen reported on cardiac output by use of a modified Grollman acetylene method; body temperature and blood sugar concentration during intense cycling exercise; arm and leg exercise comparisons; and training effects. Christensen used oxygen uptake and the respiratory quotient to describe how diet, training state, and exercise intensity and duration affected carbohydrate and lipid use. For an historical perspective, the "carbohydrate loading" concept (see Chapter 2) was first proposed in 1939! Other notable studies included core temperature and blood glucose regulation during light-to-intense exercise at various ambient temperatures. A study by Christensen and Nielsen in 1942 used **finger plethysmography** to study regional blood flow (including skin temperature) during brief constant-load cycle ergometer exercise.[15] Experiments published in 1936 by physician Olé Bang (1901–1988), inspired by his mentor Ejar Lundsgaard, described blood lactate's fate during different exercise intensities and durations.[4] The Christensen, Asmussen, Nielsen, and Hansen experiments were conducted at the Laboratory for the Theory of Gymnastics at the University of Copenhagen. Today, the August Krogh Institute (www1.bio.ku.dk/english/) carries out basic and applied research in exercise physiology.

Since 1973, Swedish-trained scientist Bengt Saltin (1935–2014) shown here taking a gastrocnemius muscle biopsy, and in the other image (hand on hip), supervising an experiment at the August Krogh Institute, Copenhagen, Denmark. Besides Asmussen, Saltin was one of the few Nordic researchers to receive the ACSM Citation Award (1980) and ACSM Honor Award (1990). Saltin's mentor was Per-Olof Åstrand (1922–2015; see below). He also served as professor and director of the Copenhagen Muscle Research Centre at the University of Copenhagen in Denmark.

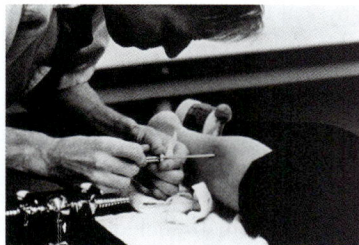
Courtesy David Costill

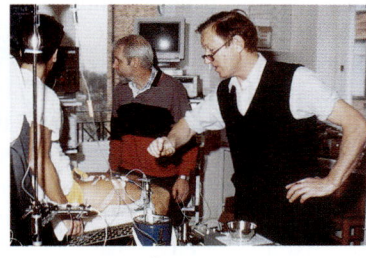
Courtesy Per-Olof Åstrand

Swedish Influence

Swedish exercise physiology can be traced to Per Henrik Ling (1776–1839) who in 1813 became Stockholm's Royal Central Gymnastics Institute's first director.[3] Ling, a specialist in fencing, developed "medical gymnastics," a system which in 1820, became important in Sweden's school curriculum based on Ling's anatomy and physiology studies.

Ling's son Hjalmar Ling (1820–1886) also had a strong interest in medical gymnastics and physiology and anatomy, in part owing to his attendance at lectures by French physiologist Claude Bernard in Paris in 1854. In 1866, Hjalmar Ling published a text about body movement— "kinesiology." Based on his philosophy and influence, the physical education graduates from the Stockholm Central Institute were well schooled in the basic biologic sciences, in addition to achieving high proficiency in sports and games. Currently, the College of Physical Education (Gymnastik-Och Idrottshögskolan; www.gih.se/In-English/) and Department of Physiology in

1 Introduction: A View from the Past

the Karolinska Institute Medical School in Stockholm continue to sponsor studies in exercise physiology and related disciplines (https://ki.se/en/startpage).

Per-Olof Åstrand, MD, PhD (1922–2015), the most famous College of Physical Education (1946) graduate presented his doctoral thesis in 1952 to the Karolinska Institute Medical School. Åstrand taught in the Department of Physiology in the College of Physical Education from 1946 to 1977. When the College of Physical Education became a department of the Karolinska Institute, Åstrand served as professor and department head from 1977 to 1987. Christensen served as Åstrand's mentor and supervised his doctoral dissertation, which included data on physical working capacity of both sexes ages 4 to 33 years. This important study—along with collaborative studies with his wife Irma Ryhming—established research that propelled Åstrand to the forefront of experimental exercise physiology for which he achieved worldwide fame. Four papers published in 1960 with Christensen stimulated further studies on physiologic responses to intermittent exercise.

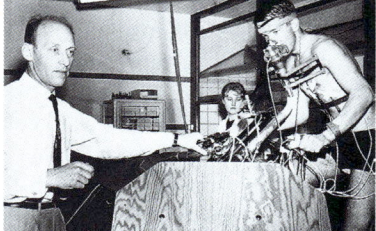
From F. Katch

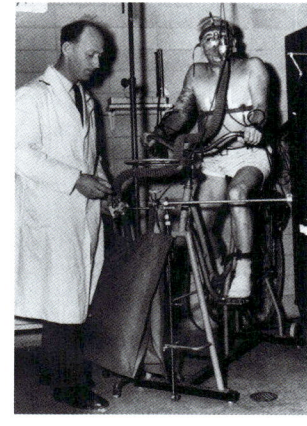
From F. Katch

Åstrand received five honorary doctorate degrees (Université de Grenoble [1968], University of Jyväskylä [1971], Institut Superieur d'Education Physique, Université Libre de Bruxelles [1987], Loughborough University of Technology [1991], and Aristotle University of Thessaloniki [1992]). He was an honorary Fellow of nine international societies, a Fellow of the American Association for the Advancement of Science (for "outstanding career contributions to understanding the physiology of muscular work and applications of this understanding") and received many awards and prizes for outstanding scientific achievements, including the ACSM Honor Award in 1973. Åstrand served on a committee for awarding the Nobel Prize in Physiology or Medicine from 1977 to 1988 and was coauthor with Kaare Rodahl of the *Textbook of Work Physiology* (3rd edition, 1986; translated into seven languages). His English publications number about 200 (including book chapters, proceedings, Scandinavian exercise physiology history,[3] and monographs) and presented invited lectures in approximately 50 countries and 150 different cities outside Sweden. His classic 1974 pamphlet, *Health and Fitness*, distributed 15 to 20 million copies (about 3 million in Sweden)—unfortunately, all without personal royalty! Åstrand mentored many noteworthy exercise physiologists, including "superstars" Bengt Saltin and Björn T. Ekblom.

Further evidence of Saltin's and Åstrand's phenomenal international influence was their annual citation number in the scientific literature during the most productive phase of their academic careers—averaging 15,000 to 20,000 citations *annually* from 1996 to the present! Appendix A, available online at Lippincott Connect, provides influential bibliographies pertaining to anatomy and physiology, anthropometry, exercise and training, and exercise physiology, including contributions to the exercise physiology literature by Saltin and Åstrand in books, book chapters, monographs, and research publications.

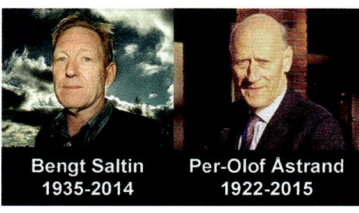
From V. Katch

Two Swedish scientists at the Karolinska Institute, Jonas Bergström (1929–2001; https://academic.oup.com/ndt/article/17/5/936/1818685; left image) and Erik Hultman (1925–2011; www.ncbi.nlm.nih.gov/pmc/articles/PMC3784188/; right image), performed important experiments with the percutaneous needle biopsy procedure that opened new vistas to study muscle fiber type and energetics in exercise. With this procedure, first perfected by Bergström as a doctoral student, it became relatively easy to conduct invasive muscle studies under various exercise conditions, training, and nutritional status. Hultman (muscle biochemist and physiologist) and Bergström (clinical biochemist and kidney specialist), pioneered the first ever human muscle glycogen utilization studies during exercise, and the effects of diet composition and food intake on glycogen restoration following exercise. This research emphasized the central role dietary carbohydrate played in glycogen replenishment—relatively simple dietary strategies we explain in Chapter 1 and universally adopted worldwide by serious endurance athletes. In 1967, Hultman documented ATP degradation and resynthesis during exercise, including muscle phosphocreatine's important role in stabilizing ATP turnover (see Chapter 6). Hultman demonstrated how dietary creatine supplementation positively impacted muscle creatine content to increase physical capacity during intense exercise (see Chapter 23). He published 310 peer-reviewed papers, 45 post-retirement in 1991.

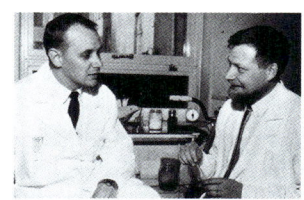

Collaborative work with other Scandinavian researchers (Saltin and Hultman from Sweden and Lars Hermanson [1933–1984] from Norway; see next section) and leading researchers in the United States (e.g., Phillip Gollnick [1935–1991; Washington State University] and David Costill [1936–; image at right, Ball State University]) significantly contributed to the expanding research efforts in physical activity-related topics.

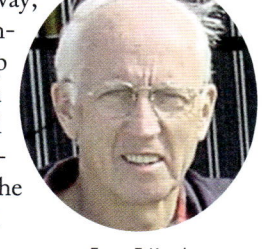
From F. Katch

Norwegian and Finnish Influence

The exercise physiologists trained in the late 1940s analyzed respiratory gases by highly accurate sampling apparatus that measured relatively small carbon dioxide and oxygen quantities in expired air. The analysis method (and analyzer) were developed in 1947 by Norwegian scientist Per Scholander (1905–1980). His micrometer gas analyzer and a larger 1935 version by Haldane-Priestley[69] were memorialized with their names to honor their innovations (see Fig. 8.7).

From F. Katch

Another prominent Norwegian researcher, Lars A. Hermansen (1933–1984; ACSM Citation Award, 1985), an accomplished exercise physiologist at the Institute of Work Physiology (and devoted basketball player at noon lunch breaks), made important contributions before his unexpected passing, including a classic 1969 article, "Anaerobic Energy Release," in the inaugural *Medicine and Science in Sports* volume.[33] Hermansen and colleagues posited that exercising muscle oxidation determines lactate's decline following its rise with workload increases. Other papers included collaborative studies with exercise physiologist colleague Kristian Lange Andersen (1920–), whose seminal work for the WHO included his 1971 opus, "*Fundamentals of Exercise Testing*[34] released in multiple languages worldwide, and 155 scientific publications. In Finland, Martti Karvonen, MD, PhD (ACSM Honor Award, 1991; 1918–2009), from the Physiology Department of the Institute of Occupational Health in Helsinki, is best known for a method to predict optimal exercise training heart rate, the so-called Karvonen Formula. He also conducted studies dealing with exercise performance and its role to prolong longevity. In 1952, Lauri Pikhala, a physiologist, suggested that obesity represented complex physiological and psychological components, not simply physical "unfitness." Ilkka Vuori, starting in the early 1970s, reported on hormone responses to exercise. Paavo Komi (1939–2018), Professor Emeritus from the Department of Biology of Physical Activity at the University of Jyväskylä, was Finland's most prolific researcher, with numerous experiments published in the combined exercise physiology and biomechanics areas (www.jyu.fi/sport/en/biomechanics/biomechanics). In 2001, Komi was honored with the International Olympic Committee's Olympic Order Award, the highest accolade the Olympic Movement bestows for distinguished contributions to support the Olympic ideal related to sport. His leadership contributions included serving the International Council of Sport Science and Physical Education as president from 1990 to 1996 (www.icsspe.org/content/paavo-komi-life-devoted-sport-science). Nordic researchers who received the prestigious ACSM Honor Award (HA) or ACSM Citation Award (CA) include Per-Olof Åstrand (HA, 1973), Erling Asmussen (CA, 1976; HA, 1979), Erik Hohwü-Christensen (HA, 1981), C. Gunnar Blomqvist (CA, 1987), Lars Hermansen (CA, 1985), Matti J. Karvonen (HA, 1991), and Bengt Saltin (CA, 1980; HA, 1990).

From V. Katch

From F. Katch

Other Contributors to Exercise Physiology Knowledge Base

In addition to distinguished American and Nordic applied scientists, many other "giants" in physiology and experimental science made monumental indirect contributions to the exercise physiology knowledge base. The list includes:

Sir Joseph Barcroft (1872–1947). High-altitude research physiologist who pioneered fundamental work concerning hemoglobin functions, later verified by Nobel laureate August Krogh 🌐. Barcroft also performed experiments to determine how cold affected central nervous system function. For up to one hour, Barcroft would lie on a couch without clothing in subfreezing temperatures and record his subjective reactions, and later the physiologic response mechanisms. This image shows Danish physician and physiologist Marie Krogh (1874–1943; August Krogh's wife) collecting data at Barcroft's high altitude experimental station to assess oxygen gas tension.

Christian Bohr (1855–1911). Professor of physiology in the medical school at the University of Copenhagen who mentored August Krogh, and father of nuclear physicist and Nobel laureate Niels Bohr. 🌐 Bohr studied with German physician and physiologist Carl Ludwig (1816–1895) in Leipzig in 1881 and 1883, publishing papers on gas solubility in various fluids, including oxygen absorption in distilled water and in solutions containing hemoglobin. Krogh's careful experiments using advanced instruments (**microtonometer**) disproved Bohr's theory that both oxygen and carbon dioxide were secreted across the lung epithelium in opposite directions based on the time required to equalize gas tension in blood and air.

Sir John Scott Haldane (1860–1936; www.faqs.org/health/bios/55/John-Scott-Haldane.html) conducted research in mine safety, investigating principally the dangerous gases (carbon monoxide), equipment methodology, and pulmonary disease incidence. He participated as a subject in many of his own experiments, as shown in this early 1900 image of him lying supine breathing different gas 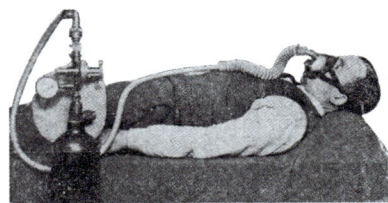 mixture concentrations as a prelude carbon dioxide regulation experiments. He devised a decompression apparatus that deep-sea divers could use for safe ascent. The British Royal Navy and the United States Navy adopted tables based on this work. In 1905, he discovered that carbon dioxide acted on the brain's respiratory center to regulate breathing. In 1911, he and several other physiologists organized an expedition to Pikes Peak, CO, to study high altitude-low oxygen pressure effects. Haldane also showed that combining oxyhemoglobin with ferricyanide rapidly released oxygen to form methemoglobin. The liberated oxygen amount could be accurately calculated from the increased gas pressure in the closed reaction system at constant temperature and volume. Haldane devised a microtechnique to fractionate a mixed gas sample into its component gases (see Chapter 8). Haldane founded the *Journal of Hygiene*. His research, summarized in the prestigious Yale Silliman lectures in 1916 (https://science.sciencemag.org/content/44/1134/419), became the respiratory physiology standard later published into a 1922 text and subsequent 1935 text revision. A tribute to Haldane and his extraordinary accomplishments while living in his Oxford, England home with a well-equipped laboratory on the Oxford University campus is remembered with a blue commemorative plaque near the current Wolfson College site (www.oxfordshireblueplaques.org.uk/plaques/haldane.html).

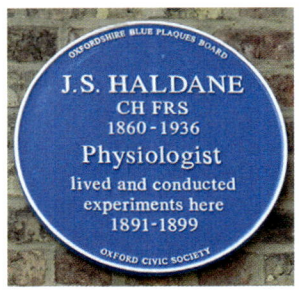

From F. Katch

Otto Meyerhof (1884–1951). Meyerhof's experiments on the energy changes during cellular respiration led to discoveries on lactic acid related to muscular activity, research that led to the Nobel Prize (with A.V. Hill in 1923; www.nobelprize.org/nobel_prizes/medicine/laureates/1922/meyerhof-bio.html). In 1925, Meyerhof painstakingly extracted the enzymes from muscle that convert glycogen to lactic acid. Subsequent research confirmed work done by German physiological chemist Gustav Embden (1874–1933) on carbohydrate metabolism; together they discovered the precise pathways that convert glucose to lactic acid known as the Embden-Meyerhof cycle. While never winning a Nobel Prize, Meyerhof was nominated for one in Chemistry and Physiology or Medicine 12 times in an 8-year period (www.

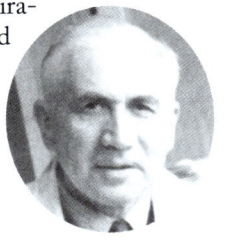

Courtesy University of Pennsylvania

nobelprize.org/nomination/redirector/?redir=archive/show_people.php&id=2780). One of his seminal discoveries involved the chemical fructose diphosphate fermentation (https://link.springer.com/article/10.1007%2FBF01732075).

Nathan Zuntz (1847–1920). In 1886, Zuntz devised the first portable apparatus with Julius Geppert (1856–1937), which made it possible to measure oxygen uptake and carbon dioxide produced during ambulation. This breakthrough in respiratory physiology measurement opened the door to assess respiratory exchange in animals and humans at different altitudes. The device, known by its original name—the "Zuntz-Geppert'schen Respirationsapparat" (Zuntz-Geppert respiratory apparatus) became a standard reference measuring apparatus in emerging exercise physiology and medical/hospital laboratories, which predated computerized instrumentation.

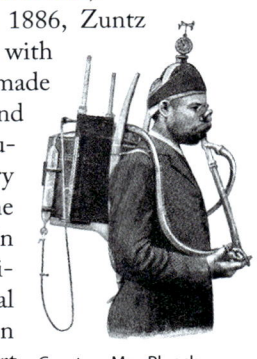

Courtesy Max Planck Institute for the History of Science, Berlin/Virtual Lab

Among other experiments in metabolism, Zuntz proved that carbohydrates served as lipid synthesis precursors, and to achieve proper nutrition, dietary lipids and carbohydrates should not be consumed equally. Zuntz produced 430 research publications in scholarly journals, as for example, experiments with blood and blood gases, circulation, mechanics and respiration chemistry, general metabolism and metabolism of specific foods, energy metabolism and heat production, digestion, and high altitude oxygen supply system prototypes in atmospheric balloons and small climate chambers, which paved the way for future aviation and astronautic systems.[89] Foremost among his many contributions to scientific instrumentation, but less well known, was the first treadmill (Laufband in German) he built in 1889.[88]

Carl von Voit (1831–1908) German physiologist and chemist with a keen interest in dietetics and his talented student *Max Rubner (1854–1932; see next section)* became internationally famous for the proposed isodynamic law related to protein, lipid, and carbohydrate calorific values. This law states that resting heat production remains proportional to the **body surface area**, and consuming food increases heat production. Voit showed that protein breakdown does not increase in proportion to exercise duration or intensity, thus disproving Liebig's assertion that protein served as a primary energy fuel.

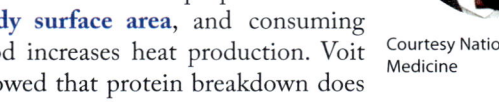

Courtesy National Library of Medicine

Max Rubner (1854–1932), a German physiologist and one of Carl von Voit students. In 1913, he cofounded the Kaiser-Wilhelm Institut für Arbeitsphysiologie (Institute for work physiology), now the *Max Planck Institute of Molecular Physiology* in Dortmund Germany (www.mpi-dortmund.mpg.de/en). His seminal contribution in 1873 published a decade

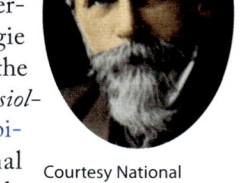

Courtesy National Library of Medicine

later, determined that heat production in warm-blooded animals depended on the animal's body surface area, which in turn was determined by the animal's nutrient intake. This observation extended to studying birds and mammals—overall energy (heat) production in animals maintains a steady body temperature approximately proportional to the animal's surface area. Rubner also argued that larger animals lived longer than smaller animals from their slower metabolism or overall heat production. As a case in point, Rubner calculated a dog's metabolic rate about 2.5 times higher in smaller compared to larger dogs, hence their increased longevity. The early Rubner and von Voit work stimulated future research with a rich literature trying to determine how best to express a physiological measurement to body size–dependent variables—body mass, surface area, lean body mass, or muscle cross-sectional area (see Chapter 22 for further discussion about allometric scaling[90,91]).

Max Joseph von Pettenkofer (1818–1901). Perfected the respiration calorimeter to study human and animal metabolism. The cut-away top calorimeter chamber image shows the entire calorimeter, with a subject sitting in the sealed chamber breathing oxygen in air after entering the chamber (inhalation) and vented air sampled for carbon dioxide concentration (exhalation) to determine respiratory metabolic responses during movement. The schematic image at right shows the full chamber with the gas sampling apparatus, tubing and cylinders with different mixture components.

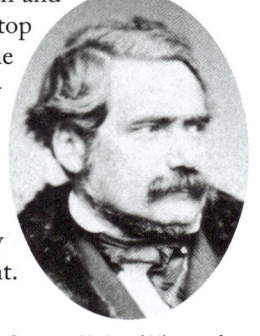
Courtesy National Library of Medicine

Pettenkofer's graduate education working in Justus von Liebig's prestigious Giessen Laboratory in Germany prepared him for a prolific career in practical and theoretical chemistry and public health, the latter benefiting from his tireless efforts to establish a permanent facility—the much-needed Munich *Institute of Hygiene* (www.mvp.uni-muenchen.de/en/home/). This endeavor served as a suitable model for the future Johns Hopkins School Hygiene and Public Health in Baltimore and other United States academic public health programs. Pettenkofer received many awards for his lifetime scientific achievements, notably a stamp to honor his efforts from the former East German republic and other accolades (www.youtube.com/watch?v=7YTNTDjeunQ).

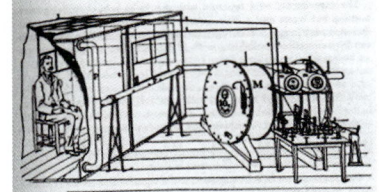
Courtesy National Library of Medicine

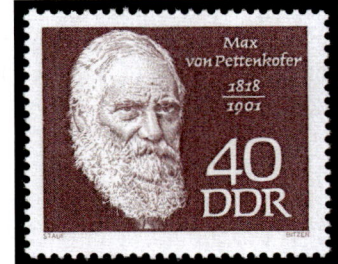

Eduard Friedrich Wilhelm Pflüger (1829–1910). German physiologist who first demonstrated that minute changes in blood gas partial pressures affected the rate of oxygen release across capillary membranes, proving that blood flow alone does not govern how tissues receive oxygen (https://thebiography.us/en/pfluger-eduard-friedrich-wilhelm). Pflüger developed the "respiratory quotient" concept, showing that lung and tissue pulmonary gas exchange results exclusively from gas partial pressure decline stimulated by surplus carbon dioxide buildup and increased oxygen utilization. In 1878, Pflüger created the Institute of Physiology at Bonn, and in 1868, founded *Archiv für die gesamte Physiologie (Pflüger's Archive)*, the most prestigious German physiology journal, editing 130 consecutive volumes. In the emerging nutrition field, Pflüger did not shy away from controversy. For example, he argued that his experiments proved that protein consumption determines protein decomposition (later proved correct) and that protein could not produce glycogen as others had suggested.

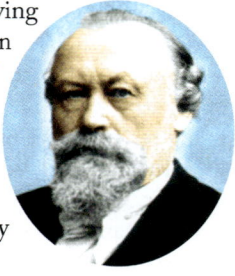
Courtesy National Library of Medicine

Wilbur Olin Atwater (1844–1907; https://specialcollections.nal.usda.gov/guide-collections/wilbur-olin-atwater-papers). Atwater published data about 2600 American food's chemical composition currently in food composition databases (https://ndb.nal.usda.gov/ndb/). His connection to the present appears on today's food labels. His research team in the early 1900s at his Middletown Connecticut laboratory at Wesleyan University determined a food serving's calorie number, including the carbohydrate and lipid percentages. He performed crucial human calorimetric experiments to confirm that the energy conservation law governs matter's transformation in the human body. Many current USDA programs and policies were pioneered by Atwater's meticulous human nutrition experiments, including low-income family dietary and economic needs.

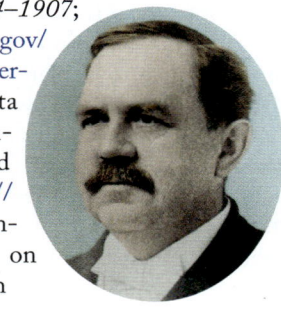
Courtesy National Library of Medicine

Russel Henry Chittenden (1856–1943; www.nasonline.org/publications/biographical-memoirs/memoir-pdfs/chittenden-russell-h-1.pdf). Chittenden received the first PhD in physiological chemistry awarded by an American university. He refocused attention on human's minimal protein requirement at rest or while exercising. He concluded that no debilitation occurred in either normal or athletic young men if protein intake equaled $1.0 \text{ g} \cdot \text{kg}^{-1}$ of body mass. Some scholars regard Chittenden as nutritional biochemistry's founding father in the United States.[12] Chittenden believed that physiological chemistry would give researchers the basic tools to study mechanisms about exercise and its physiology with newly discovered biochemical methods.

Courtesy National Library of Medicine

Frederick Gowland Hopkins 🏅 *(1861–1947*; www.famousscientists.org/frederick-gowland-hopkins/). Awarded the Nobel Prize in 1929 for isolating and identifying the amino acid tryptophan's structure, collaborating with British physiologist Walter Morley Fletcher (1873–1933; mentor to A. V. Hill and Royal Society member) to study muscle chemistry. Their classic 1907 experimental physiology paper incorporated new methods to isolate muscle lactate. Fletcher and Hopkin's chemical methods reduced the muscle's enzyme activity prior to isolating the reactions. They reported that a muscle contracting under low oxygen conditions produced lactate at glycogen's expense. Conversely, oxygen in muscle suppressed lactate formation. The researchers deduced that during muscle contraction, lactate forms from a nonoxidative (anaerobic) process. In contrast, an oxidative (aerobic) process removes lactate with oxygen present during recovery in a noncontracted state.

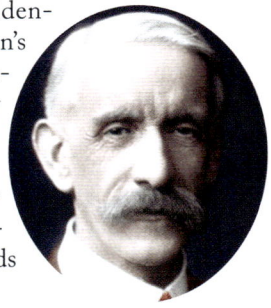
Courtesy National Library of Medicine

Francis Gano Benedict (1870–1957; www.whonamedit.com/doctor.cfm/3319.html). American chemist, physiologist, and nutritionist who conducted exhaustive energy metabolism studies in newborn infants, growing children and adolescents, starving persons, athletes, and vegetarians. Benedict devised "metabolic standard tables" based on sex, age, height, and weight to compare energy metabolism in normal and hospitalized patients. He assisted Atwater in the chemistry department at Wesleyan University over a 12-year period. In all, they conducted over 500 experiments at rest, during exercise, and while dieting using the Atwater-Rosa respiration calorimeter. Their results appeared in six bulletins published by the FDA's Office of Experiment Stations under the general title, *Experiments on the Metabolism of Matter and Energy in the Human Body*. Benedict published studies on alcohol's physiological action (which proved controversial and opposed by temperance organizations), and the effects of exercise and mental effort on energy metabolism. When Atwater died in 1907, Benedict became director at the Nutrition Laboratory in Boston, a post he held for 30 years until retirement. His last monograph, *Vital Energetics, A Study in Comparative Basal Metabolism* (Carnegie Institution Monograph no. 503, 1938), refers to his approximately 400 publications. In 1907, Benedict traveled to Christian Bohr's Copenhagen laboratory, where he collaborated with the then young August Krogh (1920 Nobel Prize in Physiology or Medicine). The following summer in 1908, Benedict accompanied Krogh and his wife Marie to Greenland to study urine output and production in Eskimos at rest and during exercise.

Courtesy National Library of Medicine

Cheng Hanzhang (1897 to ~1950s). A thorough search of Chinese literature by scholars from the Dr. Stephen Hui Research Centre for Physical Recreation and Wellness (in the Sport and Physical Education Department) at Hong Kong Baptist University, Hong Kong, China (https://cprw.hkbu.edu.hk) attempted to answer the question, "What was the earliest book published in China on exercise physiology?" A search of 169 libraries in Taiwan, Hong Kong, and Mainland China determined that Cheng Hanzhang's *Exercise Physiology* text published in 1924 was first, but according to Fu (*J Exerc Sci Fit* 2005;3:61), it may have been first in title but not in content. Cheng, serving as an editor for the influential *Commercial Press* publisher (founded in Shanghai in 1897 and began publishing Chinese books in 1914), also published *Physiology of Gymnastics* five years later in 1929. In 1903, the *Commercial Press* became China's first primary education textbook publisher for books about pedagogy and general exercise. From 1910 to 1950, Cheng translated, proofread, and edited about 30 hygiene, physiology, and medical books, many republished over the next two decades. Cheng clearly was not a scientist nor researcher, but rather the publisher's creative and productive editor. From its founding in 1897, the Commercial Press has published over 50,000 titles in various disciplines, with the mission to promote Chinese education through book publishing.

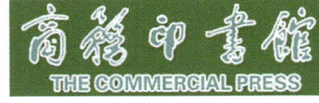

From 1920 to 1940, about 20 general public books were published on exercise, training for different sports, and physical education. Unlike in the United States, there was no formal degree program in kinesiology or the exercise sciences, and no structured research effort by Chinese scientists in exercise in general or exercise physiology specifically. Not surprisingly during this period, no such programs existed because no researchers were trained in the discipline.

Chinese knowledge about the science of exercise came from scientific studies published by Fitz and others from Harvard's 1891 Department of Anatomy, Physiology and Physical Training at the Lawrence Scientific School, and the Harvard Fatigue Laboratory (1927–1946). Scientific efforts in physical education were chronicled in different American histories of physical education in China.[100] The early Chinese fitness movement changed from militaristic bodily exercise to contemporary health considerations. The following quote from the Morris text poses an intriguing question penned in the mid-1920s about China's physical education future:

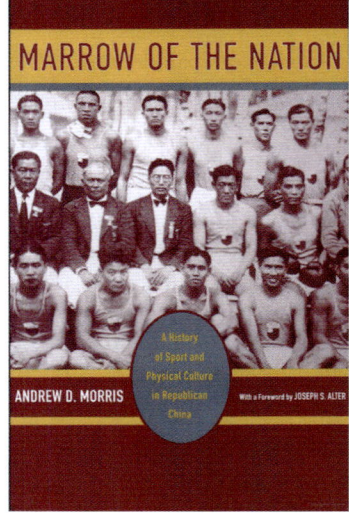
© The Regents of the University of California

Physical education, as has been proved by the majority of civilized nations, is a definite means to afford the human race the knowledge of how to live a happy and active life. Can China follow the same path in which America has built her national physical life?...Or can China afford to live in this twentieth century without adopting any modern physical education system? Gunson Hoh (Hao Gengsheng), *Physical Education in China*, 1926.

Currently, the Society of Chinese Scholars on Exercise Physiology and Fitness (SCSEPF; www.scsepf.org) provides an information forum to stimulate discussion and collaboration among exercise physiologists and fitness professionals. The SCSEPF mission supports the study, practice, and teaching of exercise, and fosters exercise physiology and fitness research in China and abroad. SCSEPF sponsors an Annual Conference, and Elsevier publishes the society's peer-reviewed *Journal of Exercise Science and Fitness* (www.journals.elsevier.com/journal-of-exercise-science-and-fitness). The inset image shows an Asian exercise physiology laboratory featuring the latest in microprocessor technology. The large, overhead curved bars with harness system provides a protective support during data collection for individuals who exercise to maximum at different elevations and speeds.

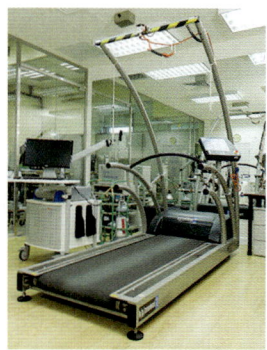

From F. Katch

fyi Christian Muscularity Movement: Lessons from the Victorian Age

Victorian era events during Queen Victoria's 62 year rule from her crowning in 1837 to her death at age 81 in 1901 strongly influence the Christian Muscularity Movement. The granddaughter of King George III, her ascent to the crown occurred at a time of great scientific advances in England. Breakthroughs in scientific endeavors leading to the Movement centered on fierce dedication to achieve excellence in new mechanical instrumentation, and shatter long overdue changes in societal mores. Such events shredded old ideas and led to renewed interest in promoting healthy lifestyles and outward physical appearance: Salient examples include the first electric telegraph perfected (1837); British empire abolishes slavery and frees 800,000 Caribbean slaves (1834); the Peoples Charter in 1838 gave men the right to vote at age 21; establishing the London to Birmingham railroad revolutionized overland travel (1838); Charles Dickens promotes self-awareness and personal development through poems, lectures, and novels (e.g., *Pickwick Papers Great Expectations, A Christmas Carol, David Copperfield, and Tale of Two Cities* [1830s–1860s]; Irish Potato Famine caused one million deaths and devastating sickness in the British Isles, forcing the Queen to repeal the oppressive Corn Laws to reduce tariffs, allowing citizens more expendable income to rehabilitate their worsening health (1845); the Great Exhibition (first World's Fair in 1851) featured technological breakthroughs in farm machinery to enhance crop efficiency, false teeth to curb dental diseases and disfiguration, and kitchen appliances to promote better nutritional practices; mandatory Vaccination Act reduced death and sickness from smallpox (1853); Charles Darwin publishes *On the Origin of Species*, featuring natural selection theory for species survival questioned God's direct involvement in creation (1859), and Alexander Graham Bell's 1876 telephone invention revolutionizes social communication. These Victorian era events coincided with key scientific advances in chemistry and medicine in France, Germany, England, and Scotland, along with the emerging popularity of physique improvement through gymnastic exercise and "strength" training (eventually embraced in the United States). Centuries-old Protestant upbringing and dogma had strained Church teaching about how individuals could live a holy and devout life, yet still foster self-care to promote more masculine, vigorous physical activity through individual and team sports and competitions. Thus, dissatisfaction with a Victorian culture that focused more emphasis on domesticity and sedentary living than new opportunities to refocus healthful living priorities. Protestant leaders at all socio-economic levels promoted competitive sports and physical education activities, including physique development through strength training, to create a Christian muscularity ideal. The muscularity aspect included targeted workout routines with barbells, pulleys, and exercises featuring lifting heavy weights.

Everett Collection/Shutterstock

At the turn of the 20th century, muscle building promotions in magazines and newspapers for home gyms and exercise equipment, along with circus and vaudeville demonstrations and open-air gymnasia in parks and beaches flourished. Eugen Sandow (born Friedrich Wilhelm Müller, 1867–1925; Chapter 22), a pioneer strongman, became a celebrity icon of that era. King George V appointed him Professor of Physical Culture, and he developed training routines for the British army. Sandow became a fierce advocate for physique development and nutritional supplements, spawning a new industry that would later evolve into body building and personal training careers and fitness promotion opportunities. The 1894 poster featured one of Sandow's feats of strength performed at vaudeville shows called the "human dumbbell." A sound mind in a sound body became a rallying cry for a focused obsession to develop physical fitness and lead a more healthful lifestyle.

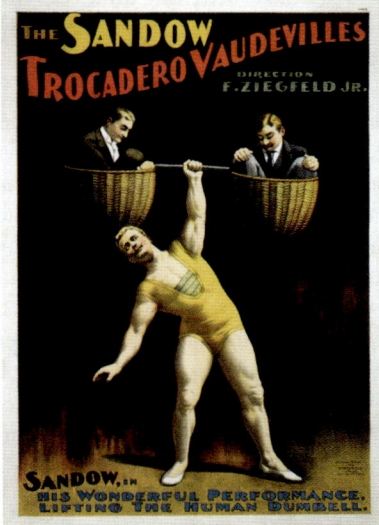

London's Royal Society and New Discoveries

Arguably the oldest scientific English society founded in 1660, London's Royal Society began as a group of 12 physicians and philosophers who studied nature and the physical universe, creating physics and astronomy as natural sciences to advance a discourse about new knowledge discoveries. The Royal Society's motto "*Nullius in verba*" translates as "Take nobody's word for it," which expressed the members' desire to overcome aristocratic authority domination, and foster the importance of facts determined by experiment, not dogma, ritual, and personal opinion. The founders included Christopher Wren (1632–1723; astronomer, English architect who rebuilt 51 churches in London after London's devastating fire in 1666) and Robert Boyle (1627–1691). Weekly meetings viewed experiments

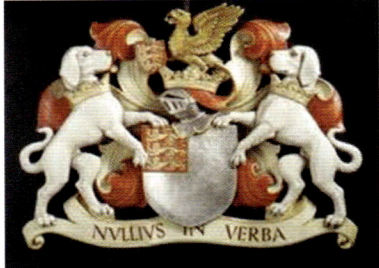

© The Royal Society

and discussed scientific topics developed in England including continental Europe, most notably French scientific advances. In 1662, King Charles II granted the organization its official charter, known formally in 1663 as The Royal Society of London for Improving Natural Knowledge or simply the Royal Society (http://royalsociety.org/about-us/history/; review the societies Philosophical Transactions timeline from its 1665 inception to the present). Under the editorial guidance from Henry Oldenburg (1615–1677) shown in the image, the society soon began publishing *The Philosophical Transactions*, the worlds first devoted to science initially published in March, 1665. A unique feature included peer review, with articles featuring thematic issues. *Philosophical Transactions* celebrated its 360th anniversary in 2020. The *Proceedings of the Royal Society* includes *Series A* publishes research related to mathematical, physical, and engineering sciences, and *Series B* publishes biology-related research. Society Fellowship includes the most eminent engineers, scientists, and technologists from the United Kingdom and British Commonwealth. Each year the Society elects 44 new Fellows, including 8 Foreign Members and up to one Honorary Member from about 700 proposed candidates. In 2020, there were approximately 1700 Fellows and Foreign Members. Within the domain relevant to exercise science, the Members included seven scientists we chronicle in this text, all winning Nobel Prizes in Physiology or Medicine (August Krogh, 1920; Otto Meyerhof, 1922; A.V. Hill, 1922; Frederick Hopkins, 1929; Hans Krebs, 1953; and James Watson and Maurice Wilkins, 1962). Interestingly, this Society's founding in England nearly 400 years ago has a parallel with the relatively new American College of Sports Medicine (ACSM) created by its scientifically productive physical educators and physician ACSM founders who in 1954 realized a common need to elevate scientific inquiry where consolidation among competing groups seemed so logical in the 17th century and again in the 20th century.[8]

Lippincott® Connect — Appendix B, available online on Lippincott Connect, provides details about the Royal Society Medals (Bakerian Medal and Lecture and the Croonian Medal and Lecture).

Accomplished Female Scientists in the Early 20th Century

The triumphs and accomplishments leading to exercise physiology's evolution reveal a glaring omission about female's contributions from the 1850s and continuing for the next 100 years.[55] Many reasons explain this occurrence—but it was not from women's

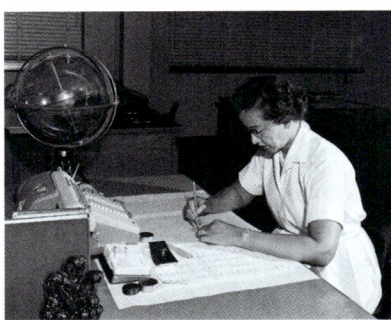

Courtesy NASA via flickr

disinterest in pursuing a scientific career. Rather, females who wished to stand with male colleagues found the going difficult. Opposition included hostility, ridicule, and professional discrimination, typically in chemistry, physics, and medicine, but also in botany, biology, mathematics, molecular biology, and computer science.[92] A few females did break through the almost exclusively male-dominated fields to make significant contributions despite considerable hurdles. The 2016 Academy Award-nominated film, *Hidden Figures*, depicts the struggles of three African-American mathematicians—2015 Medal of Freedom winner and STEM superstar Katherine G. Johnson (1918–; https://obamawhitehouse.archives.gov/blog/2015/11/25/honoring-nasas-katherine-johnson-stem-pioneer), mathematician Dorothy Vaughn (1910–2008), and aerospace engineer Mary Winston Jackson (1921–2005). In 2016 in Vaughn's honor, NASA dedicated Langley's Research Center the *Computational Research Facility*. These trailblazers who overcame racism and gender inequality at NASA devised the mathematical trajectories, launch windows, and return paths for John Glenn's Project Mercury mission, the first to orbit Earth in 1962 (and future Apollo missions reviewed in Chapter 27).

Top scientific community leadership (college presidents, academic deans, curriculum and personnel committees, governing bodies, department heads, and grants and journal review boards) subtly and directly repressed the attempts of women to even enter some fields, let alone achieve parity with male scientists. Subtle discrimination included assignment to underequipped, understaffed, and substandard laboratory facilities; having to teach courses without proper university recognition; disallowing membership on graduate thesis or dissertation committees; and having a male colleague's name appear first (or solo) on research publications, regardless of his contributions. Male "supervisors" typically presented findings from joint conferences and seminars when the woman clearly worked as the lead scientist. Direct suppression included outright refusal to hire women to teach at the university or college level. For those who were hired, many could not directly supervise graduate student research projects. Females also routinely experienced shameful salary inequity (gender pay gap in median salary earnings was 80% in 2017; www.aauw.org/research/the-simple-truth-about-the-gender-pay-gap/).

Nobel Prize in the Sciences

From the creation of the Nobel Prize in 1901, the most esteemed award for monumental discoveries in physics, chemistry, and physiology or medicine has honored 587 men but only 54 females through 2018. The first woman to win a Nobel Prize was Marie Curie (Physics 1903) and again in 1911 (chemistry). Irène Joliot-Curie (Curie's daughter) won the Chemistry Nobel Prize in 1935 with her husband (for discovering artificial radioactivity). The Karolinska Institute in Stockholm selects the Nobel laureates in physiology or medicine (https://ki.se/en/about/the-nobel-prize-in-physiology-or-medicine), and the Swedish Academy of Sciences awards the prizes in chemistry and physics. Considerable controversy has emerged over the years about infighting and politics' role in the selection process. The difference in the gender-specific outstanding scientists pool cannot adequately explain the disparity between male and female Nobel winners. Reading about the 20 female winners lives and times (1901–2019), including others who by all accounts probably deserved the honor, gives a sharper appreciation about the inequity. The 10 female laureates and other three world-class scientists listed through 1997 overcame huge "nonscientific" issues before achieving their eventual scientific triumphs.

In Chapter 33, we pay homage to Rosalind Franklin who surely deserved a Nobel for discovering DNA's unique helical structure, only to be "scooped" when the university laboratory supervisor and colleague surreptitiously showed Watson and Crick, who were visiting for a seminar, Franklin's now famous x-ray crystallography image without her permission while she was on a planned, brief vacation! With this crucial piece of the puzzle they now had "discovered," Watson and Crick quickly realized Franklin's image perfectly unraveled the missing link to be first of many research competitors to identify DNA's structure (another being Caltech professor Linus Carl Pauling [1901–1994], himself a double Nobel Laurette—1954 Chemistry and 1964 Peace Prize). They correctly deduced that DNA must have originated from a helix-shaped molecule, and so the search for DNA's mystery was now resolved. With Franklin away on vacation, they had all the proof they needed to publish the findings. What did they do next? After a few hours celebrating at the now famous Cambridge, England Eagle pub, they literally worked for two days and nights to complete and submit a research paper to *Nature* for "rush" publication. The rest is history—nine years later they received the 1962 Nobel Prize in Physiology or Medicine for "their" ground-breaking contribution to science. Yes, they were indeed first, but their quest

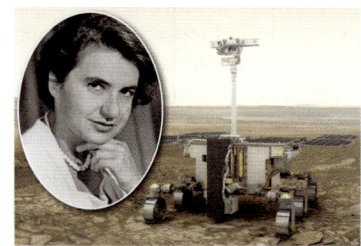

Franklin photo: courtesy National Library of Medicine; Mars rover photo: © ESA/ATG Medialab

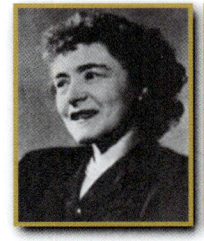
Gerty Radnitz Cori (1896-1954)

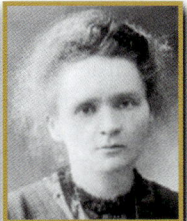
Marie Sklodowska Curie (1867-1934)

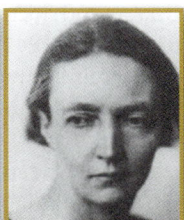
Irene Joliot-Curie (1897-1956)

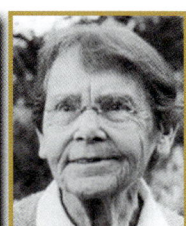
Barbara McClintock (1902-1992)

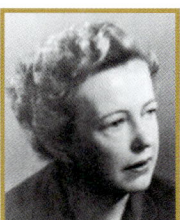
Maria Goeppert Mayer (1906-1972)

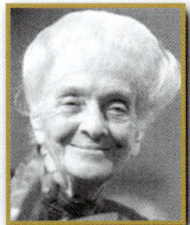
Rita Levi-Montalcini (1909-2012)

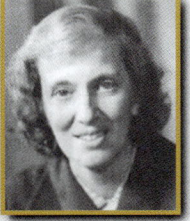
Dorothy Crowfoot Hodgkin (1910-1994)

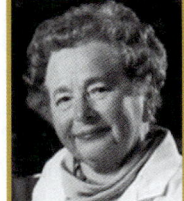
Gertrude B. Elion (1818-1999)

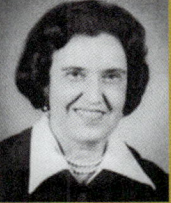
Rosalyn Sussman Yalow (1921-2011)

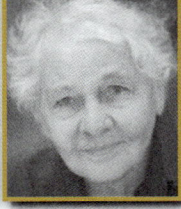
Christiane Nusslein-Volhard (1942)

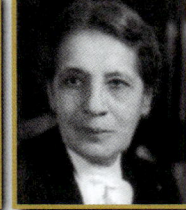
Lise Meltner (1878-1968)

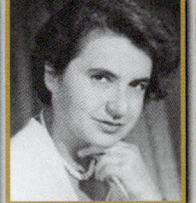
Rosalind Franklin (1920-1958)

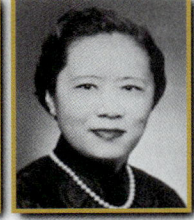
Wu-Chien-Shiung Wu (1912-1997)

Photo credits: Courtesy National Library of Medicine (Cori, Yalow, Franklin); Everett Collection/Shutterstock (Curie); Alamy Stock Photo--Chronicle (Joliot-Curie), MARKA (Levi-Montalcini), Keystone Press (Hodgkin), dpa picture alliance (Nusslein-Volhard); Science Source (McClintock, Mayer, Wu); Wellcome Images/Science Source (Elion); Courtesy Library of Congress (Meltner)

to deduce DNA's secret is not without controversy. Franklin unfortunately died before the Nobel Committee awarded the 1962 Prize, and because only living persons can qualify for a Nobel, her contribution remained ineligible for consideration. To honor her major contribution to scientific discovery on Earth, the European Space Agency in 2019 named the 2022 ExoMars automated rover "Rosalind Franklin," so her namesake will now do the same on the Red Planet Mars (www.youtube.com/watch?v=BNItE7zjhq8).

Lippincott® Connect Appendix C, "Scientific Contributions of Thirteen Outstanding Female Scientists," available online on Lippincott Connect, highlights 13 women pioneers for their perseverance, patience, and unyielding pursuit of excellence in science. Each of the 10 female laureates and the other 3 world-class scientists overcame monumental "nonscientific" issues before achieving their eventual scientific triumphs.

Paying Tribute to the Exercise Physiology Pioneers

We hope the heritage about the exercise physiology pioneers inspires others to strive for excellence in their particular specialties. Successful scientists often must surmount obstacles to achieve success and recognition. The pioneers share common traits—an unyielding passion and uncompromising quest to explore new ground where others had yet to venture. As you progress in your own careers, we hope that you too will experience the pure joy about discovering new exercise physiology truths. Perhaps the female scientists' achievements from outside our field will serve as a gentle reminder to support the next generation scientists and teachers for their accomplishments and passion for their field, regardless of race or gender.

Roots from the Ancients to Modern Times

This introductory section concerning exercise physiology's historical development illustrates that interest in exercise and health had its roots with the ancients. During the 2000 years that followed, the field we now call *exercise physiology* evolved from a symbiotic (albeit, sometimes rocky) relationship among classically trained physicians, academically based anatomists and physiologists, and a small but vocal cadre of physical education innovators. They all struggled to achieve their identity and academic credibility through basic and applied science research and experimentation. The physiologists relied on exercise to study human physiology dynamics; the pioneer physical educators adapted physiology's methodological precision to study human exercise responses.

Dateline 1850s

Beginning in the mid-1850s in the United States, a small but slowly growing effort elevated scientific standards to train physical education and hygiene specialists at the college and university level. The first exercise physiology laboratory created at Harvard University in 1891 contributed to an already burgeoning knowledge explosion in basic physiology, primarily in Britain, Germany, and Nordic countries. Originally, medically trained physiologists made the significant scientific advances in most subspecialties now included in the exercise physiology core curriculum. They studied oxygen metabolism, muscle structure and function, gas transport and exchange, mechanisms concerning circulatory dynamics, digestion, voluntary and involuntary neuromuscular control during physical activity, and adaptations to hostile environments.

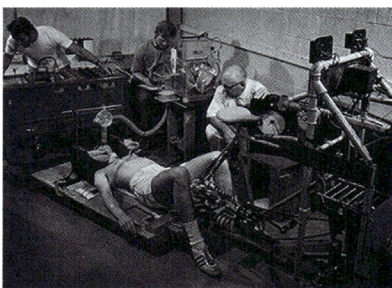
From V. Katch

The exercise physiology domain owes gratitude to the physical fitness pioneers in the United States, spearheaded by Thomas K. Cureton (1901–1993). Cureton often supervised laboratory testing to determine supine cardiac output and oxygen uptake, including minute-by-minute physiological output data following a maximal treadmill test. (www.tandfonline.com/doi/abs/10.1080/02701367.1996.10607920). Cureton, an American College of Sports Medicine charter member (ACSM; 1969 prestigious ACSM Honor Award recipient), served as physical education professor at the University of Illinois at Champaign. Following an initial Springfield College teaching position in Massachusetts in 1929, Cureton trained masters and doctoral degree students over four generations beginning in 1941. Many Cureton graduates attained prestigious exercise physiology teaching and laboratory positions at colleges and universities worldwide.

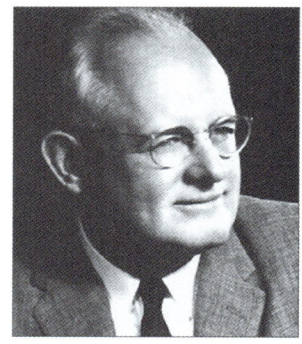

Distinguished Scholars from Other Countries

We have focused on selected early American scientists and physical educators, and other contributors mainly from the Nordic countries and distinguished scholars from other countries. *Claude Bouchard*, Pennington Biomedical Research Center, Baton Rouge, LA (ACSM Citation Award, 1992; ACSM Honor Award, 2002; *John W. Barton*, Sr. Endowed Chair in Genetics and Nutrition); *Oded Bar-Or* (1937–2005), McMaster University, Hamilton, Ontario, Canada (ACSM Citation Award, 1997; ACSM President's Lecture); *Rodolfo Margaria* (1901–1983) and *P. Cerretelli* (1932–2008), Institute of Human Physiology, Medical School of the University of Milan; *M. Ikai*, School of Education, University of Japan; *H. W. Knipping* (1895–1984), Institute of Medicine, University of Cologne, Germany (in 1929, described the "vita maxima," now called the maximal oxygen uptake); *Sir Cedric Stanton Hicks* (1892–1976), Human Physiology Department, University of Adelaide, Australia; *Otto Gustaf Edholm* (1862–1950), National Institute for Medical Research, London; *John Valentine George Andrew Durnin*, Department of Physiology, Glasgow University, Scotland; *Lucien Brohua* (1899–1968), Higher Institute of Physical Education, Faculty of Medicine at the State University of Liège, Belgium, and Harvard Fatigue Laboratory; *Reginald Passmore* (1910–1999), Department of Physiology, University of Edinburgh, Scotland; *Ernst F. Jokl* (1907–1997) (ACSM founder and charter member), Witwatersrand Technical College, Johannesburg, South Africa, and later the University of Kentucky; *L.G.C.E. Pugh* (1909–1994), Medical Research Council Laboratories, London; *Roy Shephard*, School of Physical and Health Education, University of Toronto (ACSM Citation Award, 1991; ACSM Honor Award, 2001); and *C. H. Wyndham* and *N. B. Strydom*, University of the Witwatersrand, South Africa. Many notable German scientific experiments contributed to "early" exercise physiology and sports science during the later 1800s and early 1900s.[35]

A difficult task in acknowledging a long list of noteworthy individuals who contributed to the burgeoning exercise physiology revolution—and by default—failure to mention those who rightly justify thanks that we were lucky enough to begin our graduate studies in the 1960s. We know you too will experience the joy of working with the next generation of committed mentors who will help to chart your future career path.

A Tribute to Our Mentors

In our own undergraduate and graduate studies, we were indeed fortunate to rub shoulders with many national and international "giants" and innovators in physical education and the exercise sciences, and outstanding teachers who tried their best to make us become better scientists and communicators. At the beginning of our graduate studies at the University of California (Frank and Victor Katch) and University of Michigan (William McArdle), we were introduced at the National ACSM annual conferences from 1967 to 2017 to many superstars we respectfully recognize. Their sage advice, encouraging words, and genuine kindness positively impacted our careers, gently pushing us to pursue our passions and greatly exceed our expectations. Thank you Adrian Adams, Per-Olaf Åstrand, Oded Bar-Or, Albert Behnke, Dave Benson, Claude Bouchard, Thomas Cureton, Elwood Craig Davis, Herbert DeVries, Barbara Drinkwater, John JV Durnin, John Faulkner, Harold Falls, Guido Foglia, Franklin M. Henry, Lars Hermansen, Steven Horvath, Paul Hunsicker, Ernst Jokl, Peter Karpovich, Paavo Komi, Jim Lovell and Martin Fettman (astronauts), Ernest Michael, Henry Montoye, Larry Oscai, Roberta Park, Michael Pollock, Paul Ribisl, George Q. Rich, Loring Rowell, Bengt Saltin, Richard Schmidt, Roy Shephard, Wayne Sinning, Charles Tipton, Earl Wallis, Karlman Wasserman, Brian Whipp, and Jack Wilmore.

Concluding Comment

One theme unites the exercise physiology historical adventure—mentoring by visionaries who spent extraordinary time "infecting" students with love for uncovering basic, hard science essentials. These demanding but inspiring relationships developed researchers who, in turn, nurtured the next productive scholars. This applies not only to contemporary exercise physiologists but also to scholars from previous generation. Siegel[71] cites Payne[62] who in 1896 penned the following about William Harvey's 1616 momentous discovery to explain circulatory dynamics, acknowledging past discoveries:

> *No kind of knowledge has ever sprung into being without an antecedent but is inseparably connected with what was known before.... We are led back to Aristotle and Galen as the real predecessors of Harvey in his work concerning the heart. It was the labors of the great school of Greek anatomists ... that the problem though unsolved, was put in such a shape that the genius of Harvey was enabled to solve it.... The moral is, I think, that the influence of the past on the present is even more potent than we commonly suppose. In common and trivial things, we may ignore this connection; in what is of enduring worth we cannot.*

Exercise Physiology Shares a Common Bond

Our historical journey reinforces how current exercise physiology themes share a common bond with what was known and advocated at that time (e.g., the benefits about moderate physical activity, walking as an excellent exercise, the appropriate exercise intensity, training specificity, mental well-being). We end our historical overview with an additional passage that offers astute advice. This is from *A Treatise on Physiology and Hygiene* (New York: Harper & Brothers, 1868), a textbook written 152 years ago by John Call Dalton (1825–1889), MD, the first American-born physiology professor at the renowned Columbia College of Physicians and Surgeons (P&S) in New York City (www.medicalantiques.com/civilwar/Medical_Authors_Faculty/Dalton_John_C.htm). He used live animal operations under ether anesthesia in his physiology classes for medical students, previously taught by recitation only without laboratory experiences.[93] Two hundred and fifty-two years ago in 1767, Columbia P&S became the first institution in the North American Colonies to confer the Doctor of Medicine degree (www.ps.columbia.edu/about-us/history-vagelos-college-physicians-and-surgeons).

Sage Advice in 1869 About Optimal Health for All

Even the "new" thoughts and ideas Dalton penned in 1869 had their roots in antiquity—reinforcing to us the importance to maintain a healthy respect for increasing overall physical activity in our daily lives. Dalton's words are so true today—a common-sense prescription to enjoy optimal health for all.

Courtesy National Library of Medicine

… Running and leaping, being more violent should be used more sparingly … The exact quantity of exercise to be taken is not precisely the same for different persons but should be measured by its effect. It is always beneficial when the natural force of the muscular system requires to be maintained by constant and regular exercise. If all of the muscles, or those of any particular part, be allowed to remain for a long time unused they diminish in size, grow softer, and finally become sluggish and debilitated. By use and exercise, on the contrary, they maintain their vigor, continue plump and firm to the touch, and retain all the characters of their healthy organization. It is very important, therefore, that the muscles should be trained and exercised by sufficient daily use. Too much confinement by sedentary occupation, in study, or by simple indulgence in indolent habits, will certainly impair the strength of the body and injuriously affect the health. Everyone who is in a healthy condition should provide for the free use of the muscles by at least two hours' exercise each day; and this exercise cannot be neglected with impunity, any more than the due provision of clothing and food … The muscular exercise of the body, in order to produce its proper effect, should be regular and moderate in degree. It will not do for any person to remain inactive during the greater part of the week, and then take an excessive amount of exercise on a single day … It is only a uniform and healthy action of the parts that stimulates the muscles and provides for their nourishment and growth … Walking is therefore one of the most useful kinds of exercise has fully employed the muscular powers without producing any sense of excessive fatigue or exhaustion … In all cases, the exercise that is taken should be regular and uniform in degree and should be repeated as nearly as possible for the same time every day.

Yours truly,
JC Dalton

Key Terms

Allometric scaling: Change in human physiologic function(s) related to proportional body size changes

Ayurvedic medicine: World's oldest medical system in India's Vedic Period (c. 5000 BC), translates as "life knowledge" or "life science," incorporates holistic healing with known medical knowledge, herbal remedies, and spiritual concepts to treat and prevent diseases

Bell's palsy: Facial paralysis with inability to control the affected side's facial muscles

Body surface area: The nude, adult human body's total surface area calculated using stature and body mass usually pegged to resting heat production (e.g., total body energy expenditure)

Canon of proportion: Egyptian developed artistic system to draw the human figure based on precise mathematical ratios created ideal proportions using a grid system and length unit known as the anatomical measurement small cubit

Electrogoniometer: Electromechanical device to measure mainly knee, ankle, neck, hand, and hip flexion and extension ranges of motion

Electrophysiology: Voltage changes in the electrical activity in the body's biological macromolecules, cells, tissues, and organs, and how such voltage change impacts physiologic functions

Energy balance equation: Relationship between food calories consumed through food and drink ("energy in") and calories expended for daily energy requirements ("energy out")

Fick principle: An organ's blood flow per unit time from the amount of a marker substance taken up by the organ (e.g., heart's cardiac output), and the marker's arterial and venous concentrations

Finger plethysmography: Infrared photoelectric sensor records changes in finger regional pulsatile blood flow

Four humors theory: Mainstay in medical practice central to the ancient medical teachings of *Hippocrates* and *Galen* who believed four humors represented body liquids—blood, phlegm, black bile, and yellow bile, each respectively associated with air, water, earth, and fire

In vitro: Latin for "within the glass" refers to performing a procedure *outside* a living organism

In vivo: Latin for "within the living" refers to experimentation with a whole, living organism (rather than a partial or dead organism)

Microtonometer: Instrument to determine oxygen and carbon dioxide tensions in arterial blood during arterial puncture by allowing a small air bubble into gaseous equilibrium with a blood sample

Morbid obesity: Body fat percentage exceeds 40%

Neurology: Medicine specialty includes nervous system structure, function, and diseases

Phlegmatic: Relatively unemotional disposition (e.g., tranquil, calm, imperturbable)

Phlogiston: Hypothetical "fire-like" combustible substance (Greek φλόξ flame) proposed by alchemist and physician Johann Joachim Becher (1635–1662) that deposited an ignitable material (oxide) as it burned during breathing to remove the body's phlogiston

Phthisis: Greek term (φθίσις) relating to decay or declining progressive wasting disease, which English and American physicians in the 18th and 19th centuries meant tuberculosis

Physical culture: Originating in mid-19th century Sweden, Germany, France, Czechoslovakia, and England, to promote healthful living combined heavy and light gymnastics/calisthenics, marching, and strength training activities

Physical culture movement: Developed mainly using gymnastics with an emphasis on strength-related skills in the 19th century in Europe, the movement became popular in the United States using specialized strength training apparatus applied to sports, games, dances, and recreational activities

Spirometer: Apparatus measures lung's inspired and expired air volume

Stratovolcano: Highly explosive, dangerous volcano type created from alternate lava and ash layers (e.g., Mt. St. Helens and Mt. Rainier in the United States)

Surface area law: At rest, the heat value of an individual's metabolism remains proportional to the body's surface area

Torsion balance: Force measuring instrument invented in 1750 by English geologist and clergyman John Michell (1724–1793) by precisely measuring the torque on fine twisted wire and equating the torque to the gravitational force between two metal spheres

Vivisection: Performing operations on live animals

References are available online at Lippincott Connect.

Additional References

Aerospace Medicine History. *Aerosp Med Hum Perform*. 2022;93:133.

Askitopoulou H, Vgontzas AN. The relevance of the Hippocratic Oath to the ethical and moral values of contemporary medicine. Part I: The Hippocratic Oath from antiquity to modern times. *Eur Spine J*. 2018;27:1481.

Batlle D. Tribute to Lewis Landsberg: a giant of academic medicine. *Hypertension*. 2022;79:291.

Bem Junior LS, et al. The anatomy of the brain learned over the centuries. *Surg Neurol Int*. 2021;12:319.

Bowes HM, et al. The scaling of human basal and resting metabolic rates. *Eur J Appl Physiol*. 2021;121:193.

Cannon WB. Biographical memoir Henry Pickering Bowditch. 1840–1911. *Natl Acad Sci*. 1922;XV11:180.

Carpenter KJ. Protein cannot be the sole source of muscular energy (Fick, Wislicenus and Frankland, 1866). *J Nutr*. 1997;127:1020S.

Carpenter KJ. Protein requirements of adults from an evolutionary perspective. *Am J Clin Nutr*. 1992;55:913.

Carpenter KJ. The discovery of vitamin C. *Ann Nutr Metab*. 2012;61:259.

Conti AA, Paternostro F. Anatomical study in the Western world before the Middle Ages: historical evidence. *Acta Biomed*. 2019;90:523.

Conti AA. Historical evolution of the concept of health in Western medicine. *Acta Biomed*. 2018;89:352.

Conti AA. Nobel Prizes in Medicine as an overview on XX and XXI centuries biomedicine and health sciences: historical and epistemological considerations. *Acta Biomed*. 2020;91:e2020091.

Cramer P. Rosalind Franklin and the advent of molecular biology. *Cell*. 2020;182:787.

Daneshfard B, et al. Mansur ibn Ilyas Shirazi (1380–1422 AD), a pioneer of neuroanatomy. *Neurol Sci*. 2022;43:2883.

Drobietz M, et al. Who is who in cardiovascular research? What a review of Nobel Prize nominations reveals about scientific trends. *Clin Res Cardiol*. 2021;110:1861.

Elbardisy H, Abedalthagafi M. The history and challenges of women in genetics: a focus on non-western women. *Front Genet*. 2021;12:759662.

Erren TC, et al. Towards a good work-life balance: 10 recommendations from 10 Nobel Laureates (1996–2013). *Neuro Endocrinol Lett*. 2021;42:135.

Estorch M. Eightieth anniversary of Iodine-131: a history of nuclear medicine. *Rev Esp Med Nucl Imagen Mol (Engl Ed)*. 2022;41:66.

Falcetta P, et al. Insulin discovery: a pivotal point in medical history. *Metabolism*. 2022;127:154941.

Falk B, et al. A brief history of pediatric exercise physiology. *Pediatr Exerc Sci*. 2018;30:1.

Fellag Ariouet C. Marie Curie, the international radium standard and the BIPM. *Appl Radiat Isot*. 2021;168:109528.

Frize M. *Laura Bassi and Science in 18th Century Europe: The Extraordinary Life and Role of Italy's Pioneering Female Professor*. Heidelberg: Springer; 2013.

Fye WB. Acute coronary occlusion always results in death—or does it? The observations of William T. Porter. *Circulation*. 1985;71:4.

Giné E, et al. The women neuroscientists in the Cajal School. *Front Neuroanat*. 2019;13:72.

Glancy B, et al. Mitochondrial lactate metabolism: history and implications for exercise and disease. *J Physiol*. 2021;599:863.

Gunga H-C. *Nathan Zuntz. His Life and Work in the Fields of High Altitude Physiology and Aviation Medicine*. New York: Academic Press; 2009.

Hansson N, et al. Why so few Nobel Prizes for cancer researchers? An analysis of Nobel Prize nominations for German physicians with a focus on Ernst von Leyden and Karl Heinrich Bauer. *J Cancer Res Clin Oncol*. 2021;147:2547.

Hartley H. *More Light on Lavoisier. Supplement to a Bibliography of the Works of Antoine Laurent Lavoisier, 1743–1794*. London: Dawsons of Pall Mall; 1965.

Hutchinson J. On the capacity of the lungs and on the respiratory functions, with a view of establishing a precise and easy method of detecting disease by the spirometer. *Med Chir Trans*. 1846;29:137.

Izquierdo M, et al. International exercise recommendations in older adults (ICFSR): expert consensus guidelines. *J Nutr Health Aging*. 2021;25:824.

Jain A. Demise of the stethoscope. *Med J Armed Forces India*. 2022;78:1.

Jouanna J. Hippocrates as Galen's teacher. *Stud Anc Med*. 2010;35:1.

Khuda I, Al-Shamrani F. Stroke medicine in antiquity: the Greek and Muslim contribution. *J Family Community Med*. 2018;25:143.

Kobayashi S, et al. Evolution of microneurosurgical anatomy with special reference to the history of anatomy, surgical anatomy, and microsurgery: historical overview. *Neurosurg Rev*. 2022;45:253.

Konstantinidou S, Konstantinidou E. The thyroid gland in ancient Greece: a historical perspective. *Hormones (Athens)*. 2018;17:287.

Laios K. The thymus gland in ancient Greek medicine. *Hormones (Athens)*. 2018;17:285.

Limneos P, et al. The Asclepian art of medicine and surgery. *Int Orthop*. 2020;44:2177.

Lindinger MI, Ward SA. A century of exercise physiology: key concepts in …. *Eur J Appl Physiol*. 2022;122:1.

Löffler MC, et al. Challenges in tackling energy expenditure as obesity therapy: from preclinical models to clinical application. *Mol Metab*. 2021;51:101237.

Loscalzo J. Hippocrates' First Aphorism: reflections on ageless principles for the practice of medicine. *Perspect Biol Med*. 2016;59:382.

Mackowiak PA. Honoring medicine's fathers. *Am J Med*. 2022;135:264.

Maraldi NM, et al. Anatomical waxwork modeling: the history of the Bologna Anatomy Museum. *Anat Rec*. 2000;261:5.

Martinho DV, et al. Allometric scaling of force-velocity test output among pre-pubertal basketball players. *Int J Sports Med*. 2021;42:994.

Mehta NJ, et al. Austin Flint: clinician, teacher, and visionary. *Tex Heart Inst J*. 2000;27:386.

Morus IR. Out on the fringe: Wales and the history of science. *Br J Hist Sci*. 2021;54:87.

Mukherjee PK, et al. Development of Ayurveda Tradition to trend. *J Ethnopharmacol*. 2017;197:10.

Newfield TP. Syndemics and the history of disease: towards a new engagement. *Soc Sci Med*. 2022;295:114454.

Olmsted JMD. *François Magendie—Pioneer in Experimental Physiology and Scientific Medicine in XIX Century*. New York: Henry Schuman; 1944.

Orfanos CE. From Hippocrates to modern medicine. *J Eur Acad Dermatol Venereol*. 2007;21:852.

Paton D. No Bond but the Law. *Punishment, Race, and Gender in Jamaican State Formation, 1780–1870*. Durham and London: Duke University Press; 2004.

Pope MH. Giovanni Alfonso Borelli—the father of biomechanics. *Spine*. 2005;30:2350.

Portin P. The birth and development of the DNA theory of inheritance: Sixty years since the discovery of the structure of DNA. *J Genet*. 2014;93:293.

Powell JL. Premature rejection in science: the case of the Younger Dry as impact hypothesis. *Sci Prog*. 2022;105:368504211064272.

Prout W. On the quantity of carbonic acid gas emitted from the lungs during respiration, at different times and under different circumstances. *Thomson's Ann Philos*. 1813;2:328.

Qamar S, et al. Stethoscope: an essential diagnostic tool or a relic of the past? *Hosp Pract (1995)*. 2021;49:240.

Rajabnejad MR, et al. Galen: the first cardiac surgeon? *Thorac Cardiovasc Surg*. 2021;69:8.

Sadeghi S, et al. Galen's place in Avicenna's the Canon of Medicine: respect, confirmation and criticism. *J Integr Med*. 2020;18:21.

Salier Eriksson J, et al. Scaling VO$_2$max to body size differences to evaluate associations to CVD incidence and all-cause mortality risk. *BMJ Open Sport Exerc Med*. 2021;7:e000854.

Sánchez-Oro R, et al. Marie Curie: how to break the glass ceiling in science and in radiology. *Radiologia (Engl Ed)*. 2021;63:456.

Santacroce L, et al. Medicine and healing in the Pre-Socratic Thought: a brief analysis of magic and rationalism in ancient herbal therapy. *Endocr Metab Immune Disord Drug Targets*. 2021;21:282.

Sawin CT. Historical note: Jean Baptiste Boussingault (1802–1887) and the discovery (almost) of iodine prophylaxis of goiter. *The Endocrinologist*. 2003;13:305.

Schlick T. Isabella L. Karle: a crystallography pioneer. *DNA Cell Biol*. 2021;40:843.

Shetterly ML. *Hidden Figures: The American Dream and the Untold Story of the Black Women Who Helped Win the Space Race*. New York: HarperCollins Publishers; 2016.

Spriggs EA. John Hutchinson, the inventor of the spirometer—his north country background, life in London, and scientific achievement. *Med Hist*. 1977;21:357.

Sudoł-Szopińska I, Panas-Goworska M. History page: Leaders in MSK radiology, Maria Curie-Skłodowska (1867–1934). *Semin Musculoskelet Radiol*. 2021;25:272.

Teigen LM, et al. Diagnosing clinical malnutrition: perspectives from the past and implications for the future. *Clin Nutr ESPEN*. 2018;26:13.

Thumiger C. Therapy of the word and other psychotherapeutic approaches in Ancient Greek medicine. *Transcult Psychiatry*. 2020;57:741.

Tipton CM, ed. *History of Exercise Physiology*. Champaign: Human Kinetics; 2014.

Tipton CM. Career perspective: Charles M Tipton. *Extrem Physiol Med*. 2015;4:6.

Tipton CM. Living history: Elsworth R, Buskirk. *Adv Physiol Educ*. 2009;33:243.

Tipton CM. Living history: G. Edgar Folk, Jr. *Adv Physiol Educ*. 2008;32:111.

Tipton CM. Sports medicine: a century of progress. *J Nutr*. 1997;127:878S.

Tipton CM. Susruta of India, an unrecognized contributor to the history of exercise physiology. *J Appl Physiol* (1985). 2008;104:1553.

Tipton CM. The emergence of applied physiology within the discipline of physiology. *J Appl Physiol* (1985). 2016;121:401.

Tipton CM. The history of "Exercise is Medicine" in ancient civilizations. *Adv Physiol Educ*. 2014;38:109.

Triarhou LC. Women neuropsychiatrists on Wagner-Jauregg's staff in Vienna at the time of the Nobel award: Ordeal and fortitude. *Hist Psychiatry*. 2019;30:393.

Tyler LG. *John Christopher Draper, Encyclopedia of Virginia Biography, Volume III*. New York: Lewis Historical Publishing Company; 1915.

Voskarides K. Directed evolution. The legacy of a Nobel Prize. *J Mol Evol*. 2021;89:189.

Voswinckel P, Hansson N. Ernst von Leyden (1832–1910): a pioneer in making oncology a respected medical discipline. *J Cancer Res Clin Oncol*. 2021;147:3325.

Weenin JJ. Historical milestones in renal pathology. *Virchows Arch*. 2012;461:3.

West R. A tribute to the dynamic and indelible godfather of sports medicine, Dr. Freddie Fu. *Knee Surg Sports Traumatol Arthrosc*. 2022;30:11.

Wright WF. Early evolution of the thermometer and application to clinical medicine. *J Therm Biol*. 2016;56:18.

Yang J, et al. Physical exercise is a potential "medicine" for atherosclerosis. *Adv Exp Med Biol*. 2017;999:269.

Yapijakis C. Hippocrates of Kos, the father of clinical medicine, and Asclepiades of Bithynia, the father of molecular medicine. Review. *In Vivo*. 2009;23:507.

Table I.1 — Areas of Investigation at the Harvard Fatigue Laboratory that Helped to Establish Exercise Physiology as an Academic Discipline

1. Specificity of the exercise prescription
2. Genetic components of an exercise response
3. Selectivity of the adaptive responses by diseased populations
4. Differentiation between central and peripheral adaptations
5. The existence of cellular thresholds
6. Actions of transmitters and the regulation of receptors
7. Feed-forward and feedback mechanisms that influence cardiorespiratory and metabolic control
8. Matching mechanisms between oxygen delivery and oxygen demand
9. The substrate utilization profile with and without dietary manipulations
10. Adaptive responses of cellular and molecular units
11. Mechanisms responsible for signal transduction
12. The behavior of lactate in cells
13. The plasticity of muscle fiber types
14. Motor functions of the spinal cord
15. The ability of hormonally deficient animals to respond to conditions of acute exercise and chronic disease
16. The hypoxemia of severe exercise

From Tipton CM. Personal communication to F. Katch, June 12, 1995. From a presentation made to the American Physiological Society Meetings, 1995.

PART **One**

Exercise Physiology

Section 1
Nutrition: The Base for Human Performance

Section 2
Energy for Physical Activity

Section 3
Aerobic Energy Delivery and Use

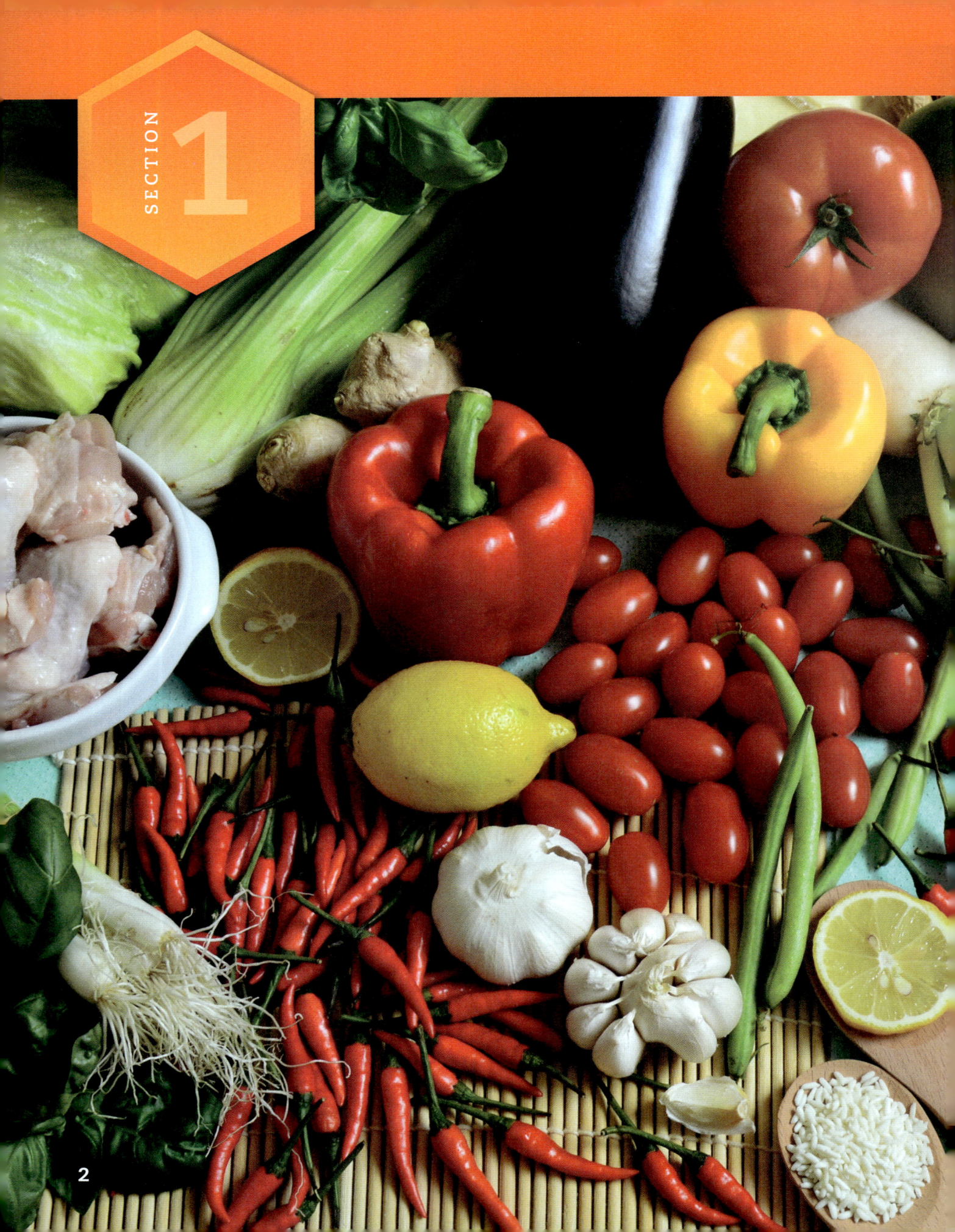

SECTION 1

Nutrition: The Base for Human Performance

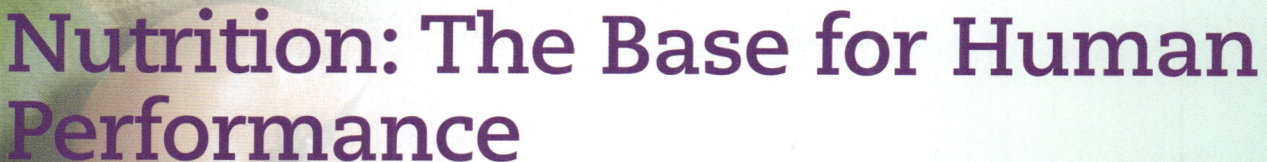

Overview

Nutrition and exercise physiology share natural linkages. Proper nutrition forms the foundation for physical performance—it provides the necessary fuel for biologic work and the chemicals for extracting and using the potential energy found within the fuel source. Nutrients from food also furnish essential elements to repair existing cells and synthesize new tissues.

Some have argued that a "well-balanced" diet readily provides adequate nutrients for physical activity and exercise training, even for the elite athlete, so in-depth nutrition knowledge would offer little value in exercise physiology. Nevertheless, we maintain that studying human movement, energy capacities, and sports performance should highlight the energy sources and the role different nutrients play in energy release and transfer during physical activity. With this knowledge and perspective, the exercise specialist can objectively evaluate claims about how nutritional supplements influence dietary modifications to enhance physical performance. Nutrients provide energy and regulate physiologic processes before, during, and following physical activity to improve human performance linked with dietary modification. Individuals devote considerable time and effort striving to optimize exercise performance, only to fall short from inadequate, counterproductive, and detrimental nutritional practices. The next three chapters present the six nutrient categories—carbohydrates, lipids, proteins, vitamins, minerals, and water—and explore their applicability to exercise physiology and the following five nutrition-related questions:

- What are nutrients?
- Where are nutrients found?
- What are the different nutrient functions?
- What role do nutrients play prior to, during, and following physical activity?
- How does optimal nutrition impact exercise performance and training responsiveness?

CHAPTER 1: Carbohydrates, Lipids, and Proteins

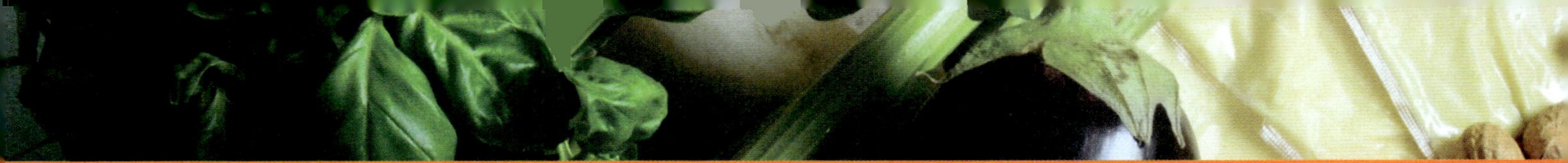

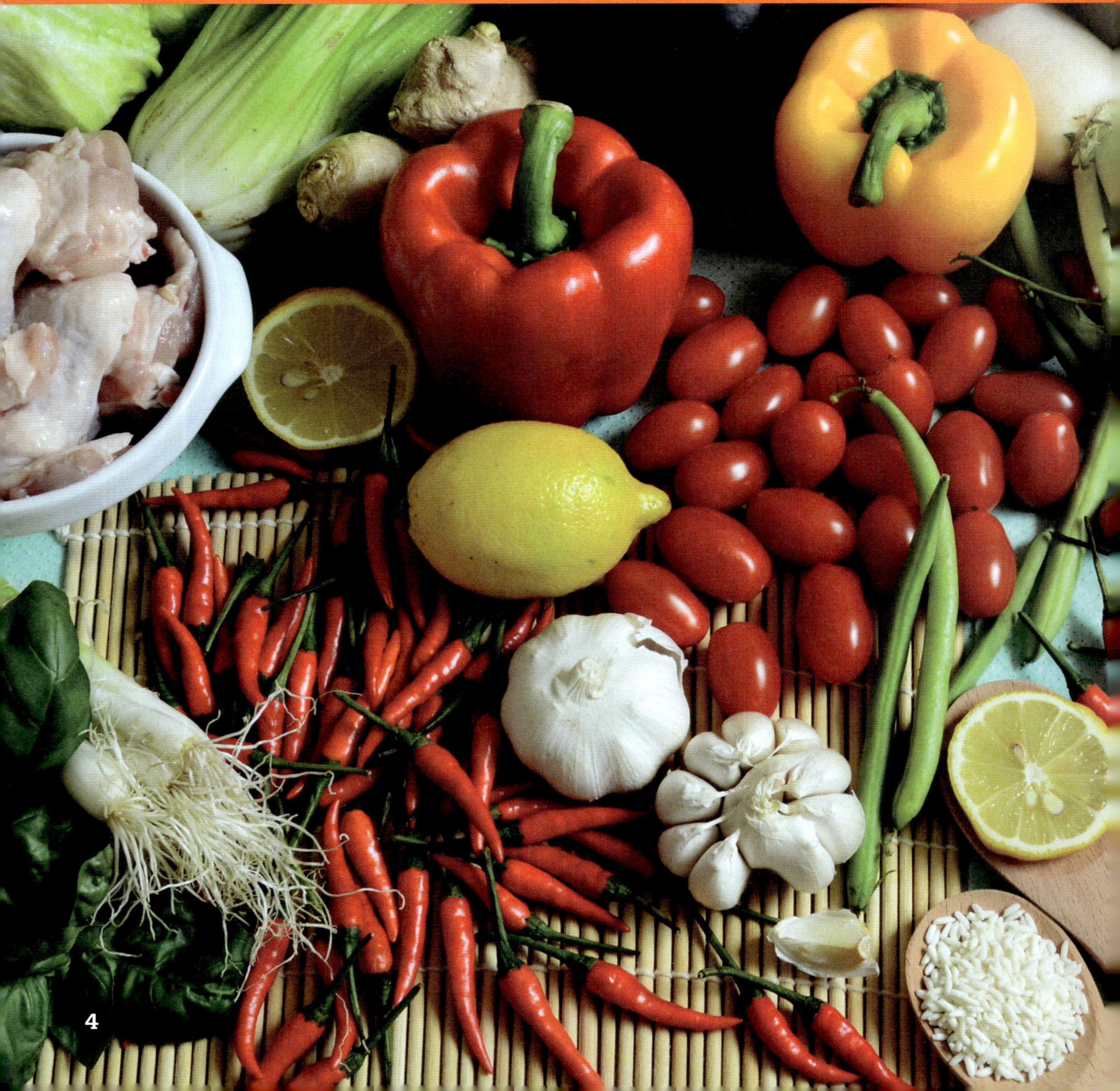

Chapter Objectives

- Distinguish among monosaccharides, disaccharides, and polysaccharides
- Quantify the amount, energy content, and carbohydrate distribution within an average-sized male
- Summarize carbohydrate's four major roles in the body
- Outline carbohydrate metabolism dynamics during various physical activity intensities and durations
- For the different fatty acids (including *trans*- and omega-3 fatty acids), give a food source example, its physiologic functions, and possible role in coronary heart disease
- List major characteristics of high- and low-density lipoprotein cholesterol and discuss how each impacts coronary heart disease
- Make prudent recommendations for dietary lipid intake, including cholesterol, and the different fatty acid types
- Quantify the lipid amount, energy content, and distribution within an average-sized female
- Outline lipid metabolism dynamics during different intensities and durations of physical activity
- Define *essential amino acid* and *nonessential amino acid* and give two food sources for each
- Describe the Recommended Dietary Allowance (RDA) for protein and situations in which an individual might need to increase protein intake above the RDA
- Outline protein's metabolic dynamics in various intensities and durations of physical activity

Ancillaries at-a-Glance

Visit Lippincott Connect to access the following resources.

- References: Chapter 1
- Appendix D: The Metric System and Conversion Constants in Exercise Physiology
- Animations: Alanine-Glucose Cycle, Condensation, Carbohydrate Digestion, Fat Mobilization and Use, General Digestion, Glycogen Synthesis, Hydrolysis, Transamination
- Focus on Research: Protein and Exercise: How Much Is Enough?

The carbohydrate, lipid, and protein nutrients provide energy for bodily functions during rest and physical activity. In addition to their role as biologic fuel, **macronutrient** substances preserve the organism's structural and functional integrity. This chapter discusses each macronutrient's general structure, function, and dietary source. We emphasize why they are important to sustain physiologic function during differing intensities and durations of physical activity.

Part 1 — Carbohydrates

Carbohydrate Kinds and Sources

Carbon, hydrogen, and oxygen atoms combine to form a basic carbohydrate (sugar) molecule in the general formula $(CH_2O)_n$, where n ranges from 3 to 7 carbon atoms with hydrogen and oxygen atoms attached by single bonds. Except for lactose and glycogen from animal origin, plants provide the human diet with carbohydrate, which classify as monosaccharides, oligosaccharides, or polysaccharides. The number of simple sugars linked within these molecules distinguishes each carbohydrate form.

Monosaccharides

Monosaccharides are the basic carbohydrate unit. Glucose, fructose, and galactose represent the three major monosaccharides. **Glucose**, also called dextrose or blood sugar, consists of a 6-carbon (hexose) compound formed naturally in food or in the body through digestion of more complex carbohydrates. **Gluconeogenesis**, the process for making new sugar, occurs primarily in the liver from carbon residues of other compounds (generally amino acids, but also glycerol, pyruvate, and lactate). After the small intestine absorbs glucose, it follows one of three pathways:

1. Becomes available as an energy source for cellular metabolism
2. Forms glycogen for storage in liver and muscles
3. Converts to lipid (triacylglycerol) for later energy use

 See the animation "General Digestion" on Lippincott Connect to view this process.

FIGURE 1.1 illustrates the ring structure for the simple glucose molecule along with other carbohydrates formed in plants from photosynthesis when energy from sunlight interacts with water, carbon dioxide, and the green pigment chlorophyll. Glucose consists of 6 carbon, 12 hydrogen, and 6 oxygen atoms ($C_6H_{12}O_6$). Fructose and galactose, two other simple sugars with the same chemical formula as glucose, have a slightly different C-H-O linkage and are thus different substances with distinct biochemical characteristics.

Fructose (fruit sugar or levulose), the sweetest sugar, occurs in large amounts in fruits and honey. Fructose, like glucose, also serves as an energy source but usually rapidly moves directly from the digestive tract into the blood to primarily convert to lipid but also glucose in the liver. Unlike glucose, which directly metabolizes throughout the body, fructose almost entirely metabolizes in the liver, where it is directed to the liver for glycogen and triacylglycerol synthesis.

Galactose does not exist freely in nature; rather, it combines with glucose to form milk sugar in mammary glands of lactating animals. The body converts galactose to glucose for use in energy metabolism.

Oligosaccharides

Oligosaccharides form when 2 to 10 monosaccharides bond chemically. The major oligosaccharides, the **disaccharides**, or double sugars, form when two monosaccharide molecules combine. Monosaccharides and disaccharides collectively are called **simple sugars**.

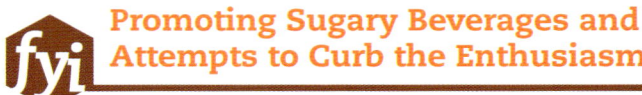

Most soda companies promote their sugary beverages in all media forms, despite strong evidence that such targeted advertising increases risk for obesity, type 2 diabetes, heart disease, fatty liver disease, and other consequential health concerns. In one study, 18- to 40-year-old adults consumed beverages sweetened with high-fructose corn syrup calories for 2 wk (about 25% total daily calorie intake). A dose-response relationship occurred in three important health markers—increased low-density lipoprotein cholesterol, after-meal triacylglycerols, and serum uric acid levels. In June 2016, Philadelphia, PA, become the second American city (Berkeley, CA was first in 2014, followed by San Francisco and Oakland) to impose a 1.5 cents per ounce "soda tax" on both sugar-added and artificially sweetened beverages. The tax added 18 cents to the soda can cost, $1.08 for a six-pack, and $1.02 to a 2-L bottle. The impetus for the tax was to discourage soda drinking to improve overall health, mainly because a shocking 70% of adults and 40% of children were either overweight or obese. The industry lobby vigorously objected to the legislation on grounds of interfering with personal decisions about what and what not to consume. Unfortunately, 1 year after implementing the soda tax, there was no major overall tax impact on Philadelphia's sugar-sweetened sugary drink obsession.

monticello/Shutterstock

Source:
Ma J, et al. Sugar-sweetened beverage, diet soda, and fatty liver disease in the Framingham Heart Study cohorts. *J Hepatol*. 2015;63:462.

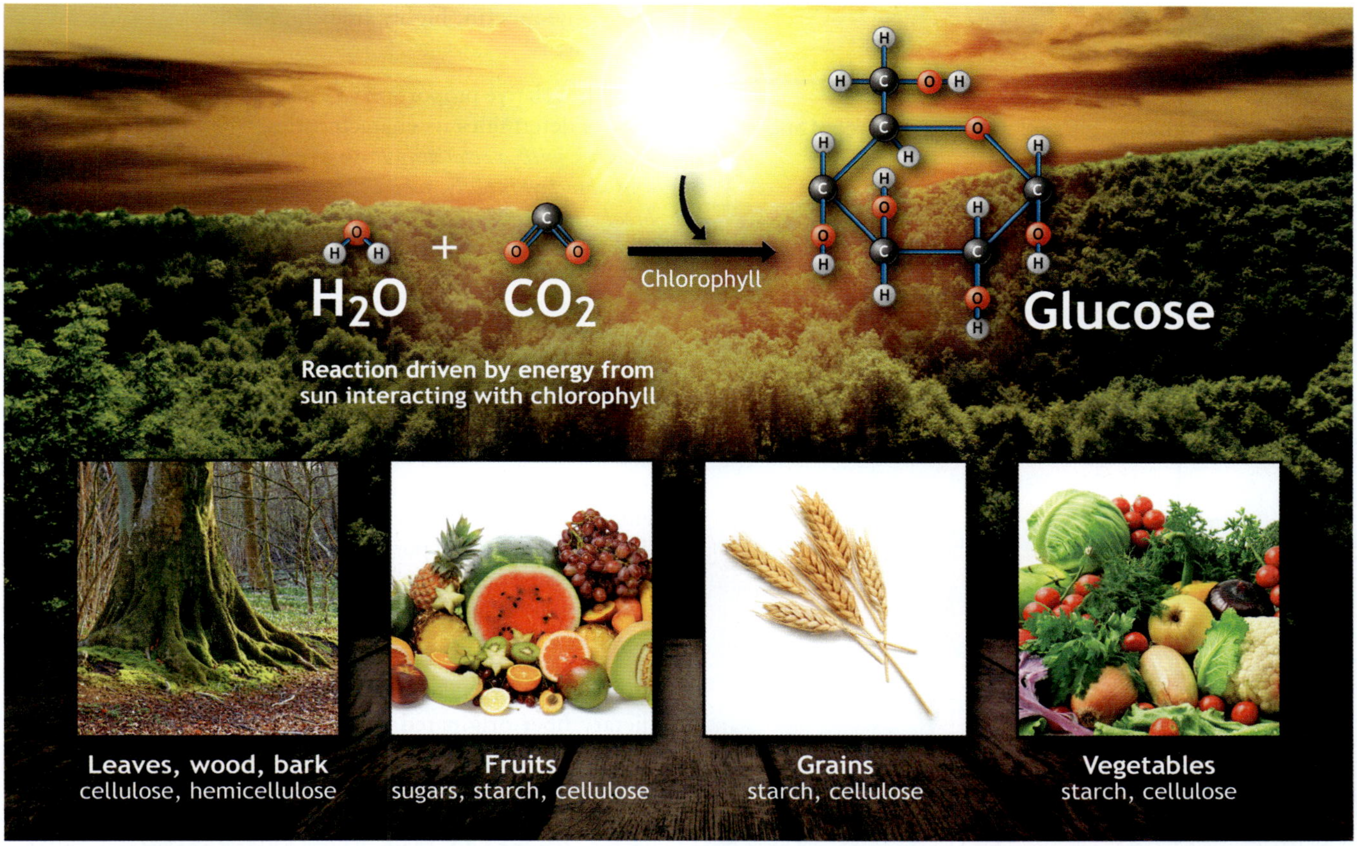

FIGURE 1.1. Simple glucose molecule's three-dimensional ring structure formed during photosynthesis along with other carbohydrate forms created in plants.
(Shutterstock: Derya Draws; aaltair; Serg64.)

Disaccharides all contain glucose. The three principal disaccharides include the following:

1. **Sucrose** (glucose + fructose; also referred to as table sugar), the most common and abundant dietary disaccharide, contributes up to 25% of total calories consumed in the United States. It occurs naturally in most foods that contain carbohydrates, especially beet and cane sugar, brown sugar, sorghum, maple syrup, and honey. Americans consume 17 teaspoons of added sugar (more than one-third cup) each day. It is added to processed sweet drinks, baked goods, candy, ice cream, yogurt, condiments and sauces such as ketchup, and tomato sauce and juice.
2. **Lactose** (glucose + galactose), a sugar *not* found in plants, exists in natural form only in milk as milk sugar. The least sweet disaccharide, lactose, when artificially processed often becomes an ingredient in carbohydrate-rich, high-calorie liquid meals.
3. **Maltose** (glucose + glucose) occurs in beer, breakfast cereals, and germinating seeds. Also called malt sugar, this sugar cleaves into two glucose molecules yet makes only a small contribution to the diet's carbohydrate content.

 See the animation "Digestion of Carbohydrate" on **Lippincott Connect** for a demonstration of this process.

fyi Bad News for Diet Soda and Sugary Soft Drink Lovers

Researchers followed the soft drink consumption for more than 450,000 people from 10 European countries for up to 19 years. No subjects had cancer, diabetes, heart disease, or stroke at the study's start. Individuals who drank two or more 250-mL/8-oz cans (or glasses) of any soda type daily had a higher death risk compared to those drinking less than one can monthly. Those who drank two or more soft drinks had a higher death risk from digestive disorders, and consuming the equivalent diet calorie drinks caused a higher cardiovascular disease death risk. The researchers suggest that high blood sugar and high sugar intake weaken the gut barrier, leading to "leaky gut" and failure for the gut immune system to protect against intestinal inflammation. This functional disturbance alters gut microbiota and increases gut susceptibility to digestive disease risk.

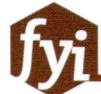
Golubovy/Shutterstock

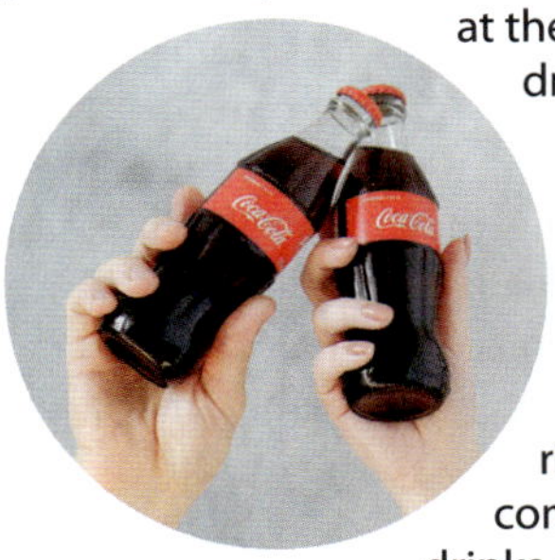

Source:
Malik VS, et al. Long-term consumption of sugar-sweetened and artificially sweetened beverages and risk of mortality in US adults. *Circulation.* 2019;139:2113.

What's in a Name?

Simple sugars with their percentage glucose (green) and fructose (red) content.

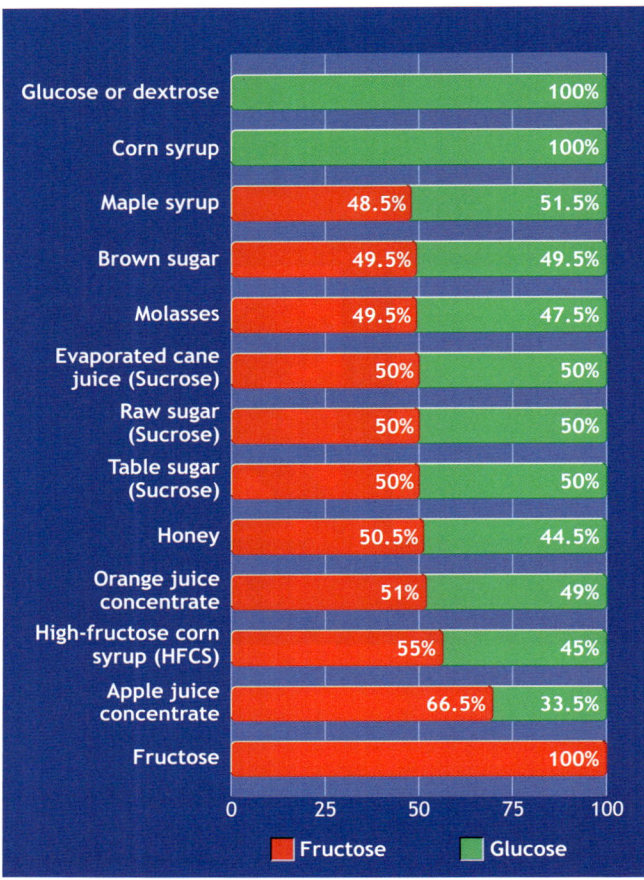

Polysaccharides

Polysaccharide, also termed complex carbohydrate, describes the linkage of three or more (up to thousands) sugar molecules. Polysaccharides form during the chemical process of **dehydration synthesis**, a water-losing reaction that forms a more complex carbohydrate molecule. Plant and animal sources both contribute to these large linked monosaccharide chains.

Plant Polysaccharides

Starch and fiber are the common plant polysaccharide forms.

Starch, the storage carbohydrate form in plants, occurs in seeds, corn, and various bread grains, cereal, pasta, and pastries. Starch exists in two forms displayed in **FIGURE 1.2**.

1. **Amylose**, a long straight chain of glucose units twisted into a helical coil with unbranched bonding of glucose residues (glycosidic linkages) depicted in part A of the figure

2. **Amylopectin**, highly branched monosaccharide linkage (part B)

The relative proportion of each starch form within a plant species determines its characteristics, including "digestibility." *Starches with a relatively large amylopectin amount are digested and absorbed rapidly, whereas starches with high amylose content break down (hydrolyze) at a slower rate.*

 See the animation "Hydrolysis" on Lippincott Connect to view this process.

The term **complex carbohydrate** describes dietary starch, which represents the most important dietary carbohydrate source in the typical U.S. diet, accounting for approximately 50% of total intake. **Fiber**, classified as a nonstarch structural polysaccharide, includes cellulose, the earth's most abundant organic molecule. Fibrous materials resist chemical breakdown by human digestive enzymes. A small portion ferments by bacterial action in the large intestine and ultimately participates in metabolic reactions following intestinal absorption. *Fiber occurs exclusively in plants; it comprises leaves, stems, roots, seeds, and fruit covering structures.*

Fiber Deficiency and Health Implications. Interest in dietary fiber originated from studies that linked high fiber intake, particularly whole-grain cereal fibers, with lower occurrence rates for obesity, systemic inflammation, insulin resistance and type 2 diabetes, hypertension, the metabolic syndrome, digestive disorders, elevated blood cholesterol, colorectal cancer, and heart disease.[1,16,46,48,52,58,82] Americans typically consume about 12 to 15 g of fiber daily, far short of the Food and Nutrition Board of the National Academy of Sciences (www.nationalacademies.org/news/2002/09/report-offers-new-eating-and-physical-activity-targets-to-reduce-chronic-disease-risk) recommendations (38 g for males and 25 g for females up to age 50, and 30 g for males and 21 g for females above age 50).[19]

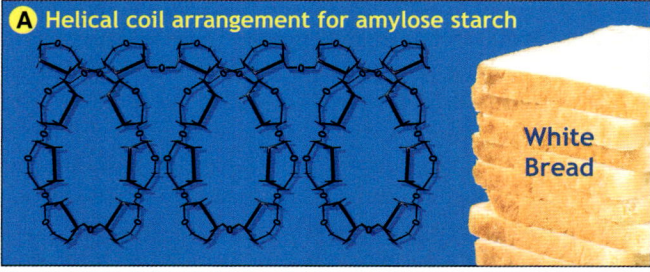

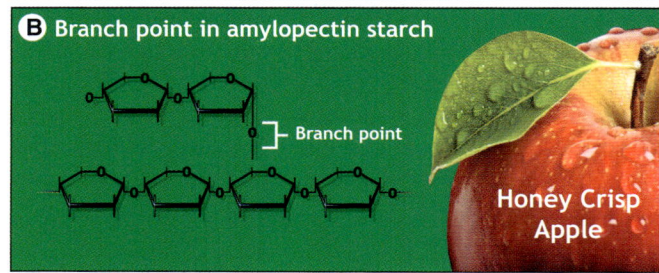

FIGURE 1.2. Two plant starch forms. Straight-chain amylose linkage in white bread (**A**), and highly branched amylopectin molecule in apples (**B**).

Age-Related Recommended Daily Fiber Intake

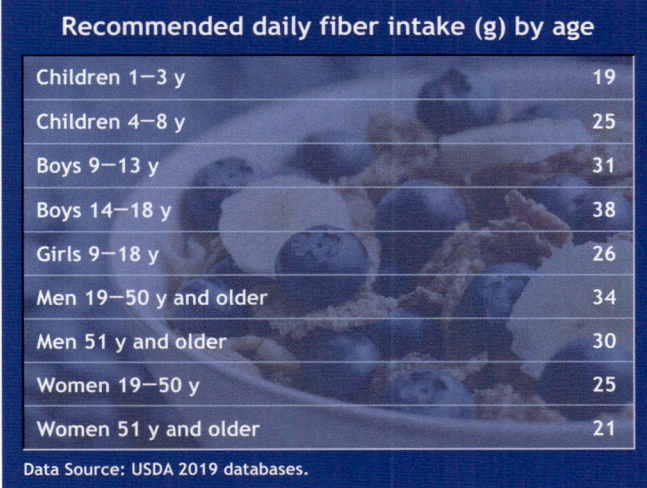

Recommended daily fiber intake (g) by age	
Children 1–3 y	19
Children 4–8 y	25
Boys 9–13 y	31
Boys 14–18 y	38
Girls 9–18 y	26
Men 19–50 y and older	34
Men 51 y and older	30
Women 19–50 y	25
Women 51 y and older	21

Data Source: USDA 2019 databases.

Brian A Jackson/Shutterstock

Lippincott® Connect Appendix D, available online at Lippincott Connect, shows the relationship between metric units and U.S. units, including common work, energy, and power expressions.

Fiber retains considerable water and gives "bulk" to food residues in the intestinal tract. Fiber intake *modestly* reduces serum cholesterol by lowering the low-density lipoprotein profile. Particularly effective are the **water-soluble fibers** (e.g., mucilaginous fibers psyllium seed husk, β-glucan, pectin, and guar gum) present in oats, beans, brown rice, peas, carrots, cornhusks, and many fruits.[31,78] Dietary fiber exerts no effect on high-density lipoproteins (see the section on *High-Density, Low-Density, and Very Low-Density Lipoproteins*). The **water-insoluble fibers** cellulose, many hemicelluloses, and lignin and cellulose-rich wheat bran do not lower cholesterol.

Heart disease and obesity protection may relate to dietary fiber's regulatory role in reducing insulin secretion by slowing the small intestine's nutrient absorption following food intake. Fiber consumption also may confer heart disease protection through beneficial effects on blood pressure, insulin sensitivity, and blood clotting characteristics.[43,79] On the negative side, excessive fiber intake inhibits intestinal absorption for calcium, phosphorus, and iron minerals. *Present nutritional wisdom advocates a daily diet that contains 20 to 40 g fiber (depending on age), with a 3:1 ratio for water-insoluble to soluble fiber.* **TABLE 1.1** lists the fiber content of some common foods.

TABLE 1.1 Total fiber (g) sources in common grains and grain products, nuts and seeds, vegetables and legumes, fruits, and baked goods

Carbohydrates' Physiological Inequality. Different carbohydrate sources have different digestion rates, which possibly explains the link among carbohydrate intake and diabetes and excess body fat. Foods containing dietary fiber slow carbohydrate digestion, minimizing blood glucose surges. In contrast, low-fiber processed starches (and simple sugars in soft drinks) digest quickly and enter the blood at a relatively rapid rate (high glycemic index foods; see Chapter 3). The average American currently consumes 22 to 28 teaspoons of added sugars daily (equivalent to 350 to 440 empty calories)—mostly as high-fructose corn syrup and ordinary table sugar. The blood glucose surge after consuming refined, processed starch and simple sugar has three effects:

1. Stimulates insulin overproduction by the pancreas to accentuate **hyperinsulinemia**
2. Elevates plasma triacylglycerol concentration
3. Accelerates lipid synthesis

Consistently overconsuming simple sugars reduces the body's sensitivity to insulin (i.e., peripheral tissues become more resistant to insulin's effects), requiring progressively more insulin to optimize (lower) blood sugar levels.[65] *Type 2 diabetes occurs when the pancreas fails to produce sufficient insulin. This insensitivity to insulin causes blood glucose to rise.* Individuals should minimize sugary beverage intake, including fruit juices, to lower obesity, diabetes, heart disease, gout, and dental cavity risk. Light-to-moderate physical activity performed regularly improves insulin sensitivity, thereby reducing insulin's requirement for a given glucose challenge, as discussed in Chapter 20.[37]

Added Sugar and the Blood Lipid Profile

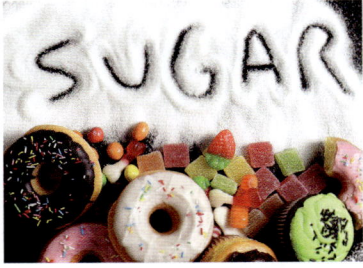

Marcos Mesa Sam Wordley/Shutterstock

Researchers placed 6113 participants from the long-running National Health and Nutrition Examination Survey into five groups based on percentage of total calories consumed as added sugars. Groups ranged in added daily calories from sugar intake from less than 5 (three teaspoons) to 25% or more (46 teaspoons). Sugar intake varied inversely with healthy HDL cholesterol levels (58.7 mg · dL^{-1} [deciliter or 100 mL] in the group consuming the least added sugar to 47.7 mg · dL^{-1} in the group consuming the most). Results varied directly with unhealthy triacylglycerol levels (105 mg · dL^{-1} in the group consuming the least added sugar to 114 mg · dL^{-1} in the group consuming the most). The research was not designed to show cause and effect, but does argue for substituting empty sugar calories with more nutritious foods.

Source:
Welsh JA, et al. Caloric sweetener consumption and dyslipidemia among US adults. *JAMA.* 2010;303:1490.

Glycogen, the Animal Polysaccharide

Glycogen represents the storage carbohydrate within mammalian muscle and liver. It forms as a large polysaccharide polymer synthesized from glucose during **glycogenesis** catalyzed by the enzyme **glycogen synthase**. Irregularly shaped, glycogen ranges from a few hundred to 30,000 glucose molecules linked together, much like a sausage link in a sausage chain, with branch linkages for joining additional glucose units.

See the animation "Glycogen Synthesis" on Lippincott Connect to view this process.

FIGURE 1.3 shows that glycogen biosynthesis involves a four-stage process. *Stage 1.* Adenosine triphosphate (ATP) donates a phosphate to glucose to form glucose 6-phosphate. This reaction involves the enzyme hexokinase. *Stage 2.* Glucose 6-phosphate isomerizes to glucose 1-phosphate by glucose 6-phosphate isomerase. *Stage 3.* The enzyme uridyl transferase reacts uridyl triphosphate (UTP) with glucose-1-phosphate to form uridine diphosphate (UDP)–glucose (a phosphate is released as UTP → UDP). *Stage 4.* UDP-glucose attaches to one end of an existing glycogen polymer. This forms a new bond (known as a glycoside bond) between the adjacent glucose units, with the concomitant UDP release. For each glucose unit added, 2 moles ATP convert to adenosine diphosphate and phosphate.

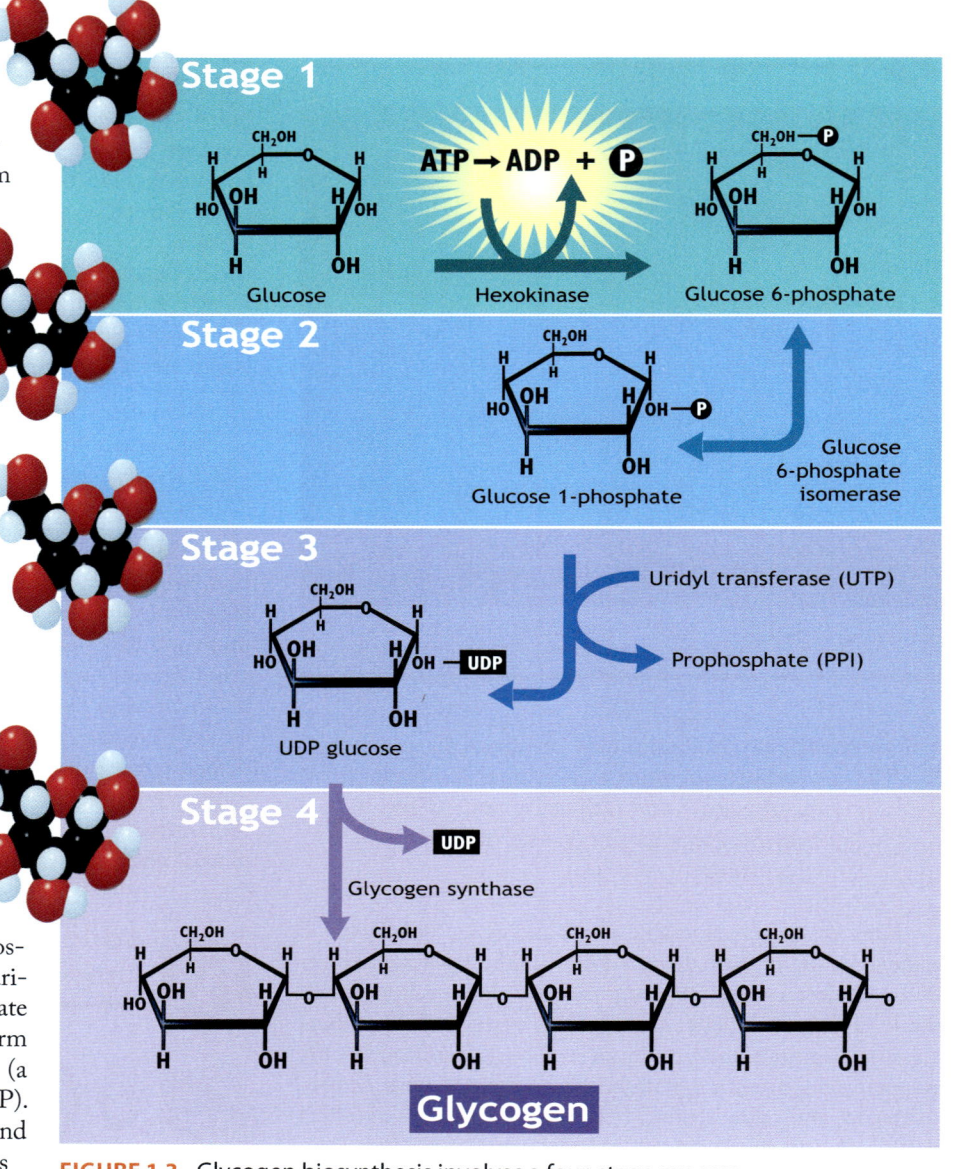

FIGURE 1.3. Glycogen biosynthesis involves a four-stage process.

Glycogen's Storage Capacity. **FIGURE 1.4** illustrates that a well-nourished 80-kg man stores approximately 500 g of carbohydrate. Muscle glycogen accounts for the largest reserve (approximately 400 g, equivalent to 1600 kcal), followed by 90 to 110 g of liver glycogen (highest concentration, representing 3 to 7% of the liver's weight and equivalent to about 400 kcal), with only about 2 to 3 g of plasma glucose (12 kcal). Each glycogen or glucose gram contains approximately 4 calories (kcal) of energy. This means that the average person stores about 2000 kcal as carbohydrate—enough total energy to power a 20-mile continuous run at relatively high intensity.

The body stores comparatively little glycogen, so its quantity fluctuates considerably through dietary modifications. For example, a 24-hr fast or a low-carbohydrate, normal-calorie diet nearly depletes glycogen reserves. In contrast, maintaining a carbohydrate-rich diet for several days almost doubles the body's glycogen stores compared with levels attained with a typical, well-balanced diet. *The body's upper limit glycogen storage averages about 15 g · kg body mass^{-1}, equivalent to 1050 g for a 70-kg/154-lb male and 840 g for a 56-kg/124-lb female.*

Several factors determine glycogen breakdown and resynthesis rate and quantity. During physical activity, intramuscular glycogen provides the muscles' *major* carbohydrate energy source. Concurrently, liver glycogen rapidly reconverts to glucose, regulated by phosphatase enzyme, as an extramuscular glucose supply during physical activity. The term **glycogenolysis** describes this glycogen to glucose reconversion. Liver and muscle glycogen depletion by carbohydrate dietary restriction or intense physical activity stimulates glucose synthesis. This occurs through gluconeogenic metabolic pathways from structural components of other nutrients, particularly proteins.

CHAPTER 1 • Carbohydrates, Lipids, and Proteins

Important Carbohydrate Conversions

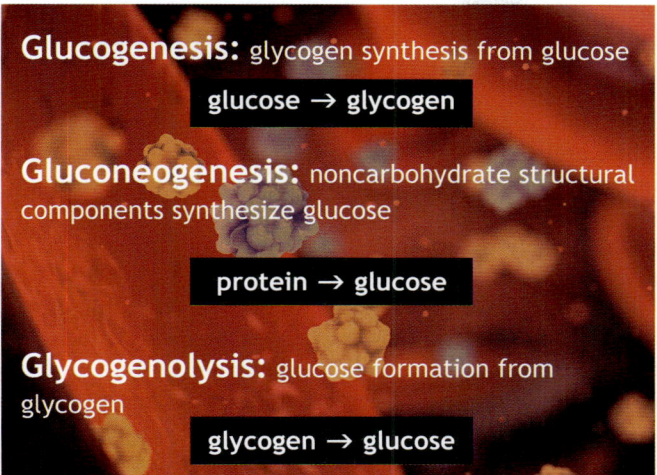

nobeastsofierce/Shutterstock

Hormones play a key role in regulating liver and muscle glycogen stores by controlling circulating blood sugar levels. Elevated blood sugar causes pancreatic beta (β) cells to secrete additional insulin to facilitate cellular glucose uptake and inhibit further insulin secretion. This *feedback regulation* maintains blood glucose at an appropriate physiologic concentration. In contrast, when blood sugar falls below normal, the pancreas's alpha (α) cells secrete **glucagon** to normalize blood sugar concentration. Known as the "insulin antagonist" hormone (http://www.glucagon.com/), glucagon elevates blood glucose by stimulating the liver's glycogenolytic and gluconeogenic pathways. Chapter 20 discusses hormonal regulation in physical activity.

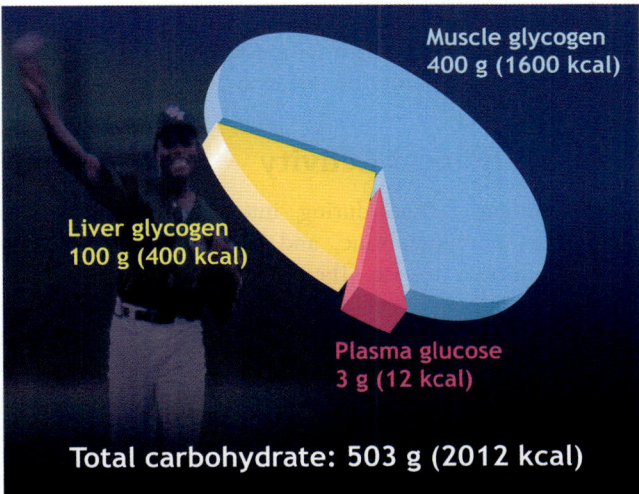

FIGURE 1.4. Total carbohydrate distribution by weight and energy content for liver and muscle glycogen and plasma glucose for an 80-kg man.

Recommended Carbohydrate Intake

No minimum or maximum recommendations exist for total carbohydrate intake. For sedentary 70-kg adults, daily carbohydrate intake typically amounts to about 300 g or between 40 and 50% total caloric intake. *For more physically active people and those involved in exercise training, carbohydrates should equal about 60% of daily calories (400 to 600 g), predominantly as unrefined, fiber-rich fruits, grains, and vegetables. During intense training, carbohydrate intake should increase to 70% total calories consumed or approximately 8 to 10 g · kg body mass^{-1}.*

Nutritious dietary carbohydrate sources include fruits, grains, and vegetables, yet this does not represent the usual carbohydrate intake source for all people. *The typical American consumes about 50% carbohydrate as simple sugars.* This intake arises primarily from sugars as sucrose and high-fructose corn syrup added in food processing. These sugars do not come in a nutrient-dense package characteristically present naturally in fruits and vegetables. High ultra-processed food consumption links to increased overall mortality risk.[81,83]

Carbohydrates' Role in the Body

Carbohydrates serve four important functions related to energy metabolism and exercise performance: energy source, protein-sparer, metabolic primer/ketosis preventer, and central nervous system fuel.

Energy Source

Carbohydrates primarily serve as an energy fuel during intense physical activity. Energy from bloodborne glucose and muscle glycogen catabolism powers a muscle's contractile elements and most other biologic work forms. Sufficient daily carbohydrate intake for physically active individuals maintains the body's relatively limited glycogen stores. *Once cells reach their maximum capacity to store glycogen, excess sugars convert to and store as fat.* Macronutrient interconversion for energy storage explains how body fat can increase when dietary carbohydrate exceeds energy requirements, even with sparse lipid in the diet.

Protein-Sparer

Adequate carbohydrate intake helps to preserve tissue protein. Normally, protein serves a vital role in tissue maintenance, repair, and growth, and to a much lesser degree as a nutrient energy source. Depleting glycogen reserves—as occurs readily in starvation, reduced energy and/or carbohydrate intake, and prolonged, strenuous exercise—dramatically affects the metabolic mixture of fuel for energy. In addition to stimulating lipid catabolism, glycogen depletion triggers glucose synthesis from the labile pool of amino acids (protein). This gluconeogenic conversion offers a metabolic option to augment carbohydrate availability (and maintain plasma glucose levels) even with insufficient glycogen stores. The price paid strains the body's protein levels, particularly muscle protein. In the extreme, this reduces lean tissue mass and adds a solute load on kidneys, forcing them to excrete the nitrogenous by-products from protein breakdown.

INTEGRATIVE QUESTION

What is the rationale for recommending adequate carbohydrate intake rather than excess protein to increase muscle mass through resistance training?

Metabolic Primer/Ketosis Preventer

Components of carbohydrate catabolism serve as "primer" substrate for lipid oxidation. Insufficient carbohydrate breakdown—through either limitations in glucose transport into the cell (e.g., diabetes where insulin production wanes or insulin resistance increases) or glycogen depletion through inadequate diet or prolonged physical activity—causes lipid mobilization to exceed lipid oxidation. Inadequate glycogen catabolism by-products produces incomplete lipid breakdown with accumulation of **ketone bodies**. In excess, ketones increase body fluid acidity to produce the potentially harmful acid condition of **acidosis** or, specifically with regard to lipid breakdown, **ketosis**. Chapter 6 continues the discussion about carbohydrate as a primer for lipid catabolism.

Central Nervous System Fuel

The central nervous system requires an uninterrupted carbohydrate stream to function properly. Under normal conditions, the brain metabolizes blood glucose almost exclusively as its fuel source. In poorly regulated diabetes, during starvation, or with a prolonged low-carbohydrate intake, the brain adapts after about 8 days and metabolizes larger lipid amounts (as ketones) for fuel. Chronic low-carbohydrate, high-fat diets also induce skeletal muscle adaptations to increase lipid use during low-to-moderate physical activity levels while sparing muscle glycogen.

Blood sugar usually remains regulated within narrow limits for two main reasons:

1. Glucose serves as a primary fuel for nerve tissue metabolism.
2. Glucose represents a red blood cell's sole energy source.

At rest and during physical activity, liver glycogenolysis (glycogen-to-glucose conversion) maintains normal blood glucose levels, usually at 100 mg · dL^{-1}. In prolonged marathon running (or similar duration intense activities), blood glucose concentration eventually falls below normal levels from liver glycogen depletion. Simultaneously, active muscle continues to catabolize the available blood glucose. Symptoms of clinically reduced blood glucose (**hypoglycemia**: <45 mg glucose · dL^{-1} blood) include weakness, hunger, mental confusion, and dizziness. This ultimately impairs exercise performance and can contribute to central nervous system fatigue associated with prolonged physical activity. Sustained and profound hypoglycemia can trigger unconsciousness and irreversible brain damage.

Carbohydrate Dynamics During Physical Activity

Biochemical and biopsy techniques (see Chapter 18) and labeled nutrient tracers assess the energy contribution from nutrients during physical activity. Two factors, effort intensity and duration and the exerciser's fitness and nutritional status, largely determine the fuel mixture during physical activity.[10,21]

The liver increases glucose release to active muscle as activity progresses from lower to higher intensity. At the same time, muscle glycogen supplies the predominant carbohydrate energy source during the early exercise stages and thereafter as intensity increases.[26] Compared to lipid and protein use, carbohydrate remains the preferential fuel in intense aerobic activity because it rapidly supplies energy as ATP via oxidative processes. During anaerobic exercise that requires glycolysis, carbohydrate becomes the sole fuel for ATP resynthesis (see Chapter 6). A 3-day diet with only 5% carbohydrate considerably depresses all-out exercise capacity.[41]

Carbohydrate availability in the metabolic mixture controls its energy use. In turn, carbohydrate intake dramatically affects its availability. Blood glucose concentration provides feedback regulation for the liver's glucose output; an increase in blood glucose inhibits hepatic glucose release during physical activity.[29] Carbohydrate availability during exertion helps regulate lipid mobilization and its use for energy.[11,13] As an example, increasing carbohydrate oxidation by ingesting high-glycemic carbohydrates prior to physical activity (with accompanying hyperglycemia and hyperinsulinemia) inhibits two processes:

1. Long-chain fatty acid oxidation by skeletal muscle
2. Free fatty acid (FFA) liberation from adipose tissue

Adequate carbohydrate availability and its increased catabolism inhibit long-chain fatty acid transport into mitochondria, thus controlling the metabolic mixture.

Intense Physical Activity

Neural-humoral factors during intense exercise increase epinephrine, norepinephrine, and glucagon output, while decreasing insulin release. These hormonal responses activate **glycogen phosphorylase** (indirectly by activating cyclic adenosine monophosphate; see Chapter 20) the enzyme that facilitates liver and active muscle glycogenolysis. Think of glycogen phosphorylase as the controller of the glycogen-glucose interconversion to regulate circulating glucose concentration in the bloodstream. Muscle glycogen provides energy without oxygen, so it contributes considerable energy in the first minutes of physical activity when oxygen use fails to meet oxygen demands. As physical activity continues, bloodborne glucose increases its contribution as a metabolic fuel. For

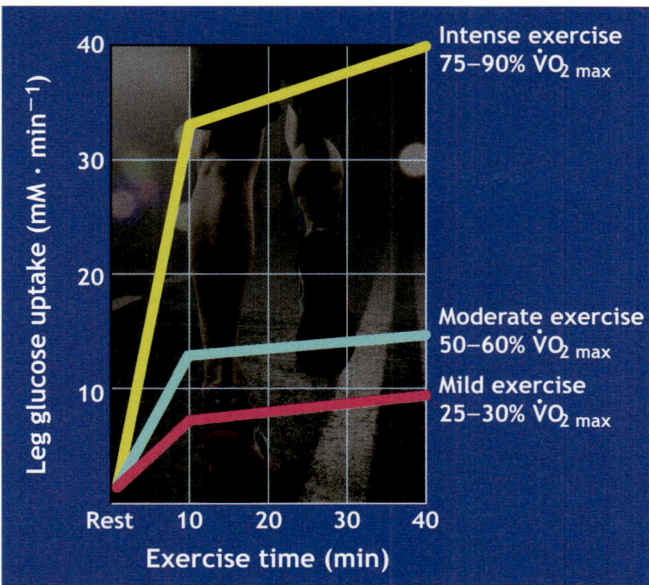

FIGURE 1.5. How exercise duration and intensity affect blood glucose uptake by the leg muscles, with exercise intensity expressed as percentage $\dot{V}O_{2max}$.
(Data from Felig P, Wahren J. Fuel homeostasis in exercise. *N Engl J Med.* 1975;293(21):1078. FOTOKITA/Shutterstock.)

example, blood glucose can supply up to 30% of vigorously active muscles' total energy, with muscle glycogen contributing the remaining carbohydrate energy.

One hour of intense physical activity decreases liver glycogen by about 55%; a 2-hr strenuous workout almost depletes the liver and active muscles' glycogen. **FIGURE 1.5** illustrates that muscles' uptake of circulating blood glucose rises sharply during the initial stage of cycling exercise and continues to increase as cycling continues. After 40 min, glucose uptake rises 7 to 20 times the uptake at rest, depending on exercise intensity. *The selective dependence on carbohydrate metabolism during intense aerobic activity occurs from its energy transfer rate, which is twice that of lipid or protein.*[70] Carbohydrate also generates almost 6% more energy than lipid per liter of oxygen uptake. Chapter 6 discusses carbohydrate's energy release under anaerobic and aerobic conditions.

Moderate and Prolonged Physical Activity

In the transition from rest to moderate intensity activity, active muscle's glycogen stores supply almost all the energy for activity. During the next 20 min, liver and muscle glycogen deliver between 40 and 50% of the energy requirement, with the remainder provided by lipid catabolism with only a limited protein contribution. In essence, the nutrient mixture for energy depends on the *relative exercise intensity* (i.e., percentage $\dot{V}O_{2max}$). During low-intensity activity, lipid is the main energy substrate throughout exercise (see Fig. 1.17). In more intense exercise, liver and muscle glycogen become the prime energy sources. As exercise continues and muscle glycogen decreases, blood glucose becomes the major carbohydrate energy source, while lipid catabolism furnishes an increasingly greater total energy percentage. Eventually, the liver's glucose output fails to keep pace with muscle's glucose use, and plasma glucose concentration decreases. Circulating blood glucose may reach hypoglycemic levels (symptoms usually do not occur until blood glucose concentration lowers to 2.8 to 3.0 mmol·L^{-1} [50 to 54 mg·dL^{-1}]).

FIGURE 1.6 depicts the nutrient metabolic profile during prolonged physical activity in the glycogen-depleted and glycogen-loaded states. As submaximal activity progresses in the glycogen-depleted state, blood glucose levels fall as shown in (A), and circulating FFAs increase dramatically compared with exercise under glycogen-loaded conditions (B). Concurrently, protein's contribution to energy expenditure increases (C). Exercise intensity, expressed as percentage of maximum, also progressively decreases under glycogen-depleted conditions (D). After 2 hr, an exerciser can only maintain about 50% of the initial effort intensity. Reduced power output results directly from the relatively slow rate of aerobic energy release from lipid oxidation, which now becomes the primary energy source. Any of the following potential rate-limiting metabolic processes that precede the citric acid cycle could explain the relatively slower lipid oxidation rate compared with carbohydrate:

1. Adipose tissue FFA mobilization
2. FFA circulatory transport to skeletal muscle
3. Muscle cell FFA uptake

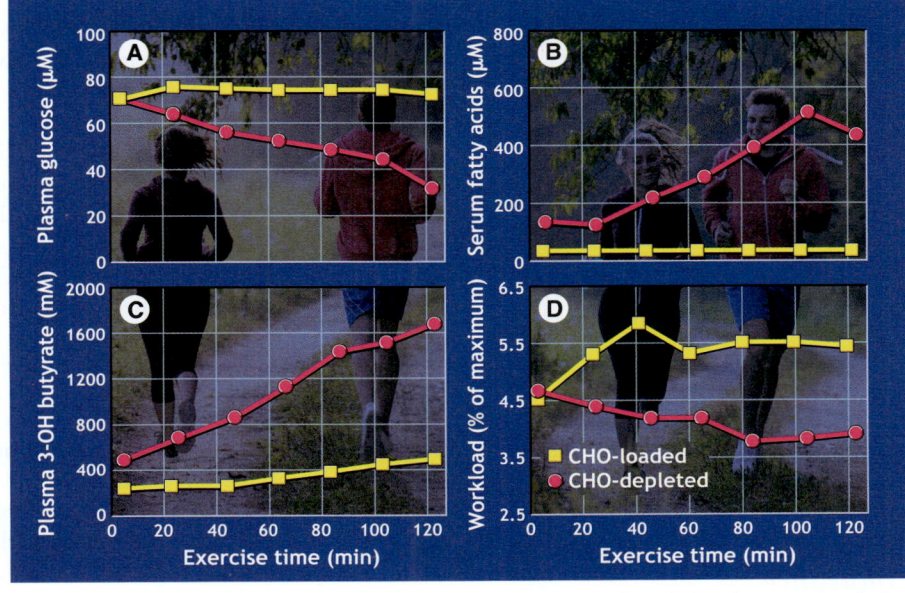

FIGURE 1.6. Nutrient metabolism dynamics during exercise for 2 hr in glycogen-loaded (*yellow*) and glycogen-depleted (*pink*) states.
(Adapted from Wagenmakers AJM, et al. Carbohydrate supplementation, glycogen depletion, and amino acid metabolism. Am J Physiol-Endocrinology and Metabolism 1991;260(6):E883-E890. ©The American Physiological Society (APS). All rights reserved. dotshock/Shutterstock.)

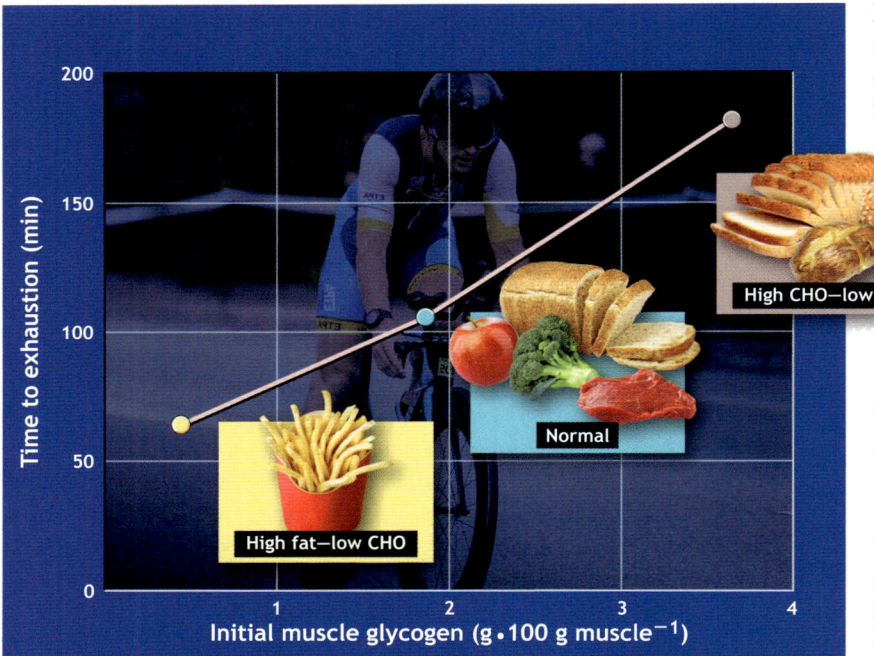

FIGURE 1.7. Classic experiment illustrates how diet composition profoundly affects glycogen reserves and exercise performance.
(Adapted with permission from Bergstrom J, et al. Diet, muscle glycogen and physical performance. *Acta Physiol Scand.* 1967;71:140. Shutterstock: Preto Perola; Joe Gough; Valery121283; Billion Photos; Tim UR; Kyselova Inna; Pineapple studio; Keyur18; Alex Bogatyrev.)

4. Muscle FFA uptake from triacylglycerols in chylomicrons and lipoproteins
5. Fatty acid mobilization from intramuscular triacylglycerols and cytoplasmic transport
6. Fatty acid entry into mitochondria
7. Fatty acid oxidation within mitochondria

Fatigue and Glycogen Availability

Fatigue occurs when physical activity continues to the point that compromises liver and muscle glycogen content, despite sufficient oxygen availability to muscle and an almost unlimited energy supply from stored lipids. Endurance athletes commonly refer to this fatigue sensation as "bonking" or "**hitting the wall**." Inactive muscles maintain their full glycogen content because skeletal muscle lacks the phosphatase enzyme to allow glucose exchange between cells. What remains unclear is why muscle glycogen depletion coincides with fatigue. The answer may relate to three factors:

1. Depressed blood glucose availability for optimal central nervous system function
2. Muscle glycogen's role to "prime" lipid breakdown
3. Slower energy release rate from breakdown of lipid compared to carbohydrate

Diet's Effect on Muscle Glycogen and Endurance

Diet composition profoundly affects glycogen reserves and subsequent exercise performance. **FIGURE 1.7** displays results for a classic experiment illustrating the effects of a high-fat, low-carbohydrate diet, a normal diet, and a high-carbohydrate, low-fat diet on the quadriceps femoris muscle's glycogen content at rest and during endurance exercise on a bicycle ergometer.[3] Six subjects maintained normal caloric intake for 3 days but consumed most of their calories as lipid and 5% or less as carbohydrate (high-fat diet). In the second condition (normal diet), the 3-day diet contained the recommended carbohydrate, lipid, and protein daily percentages. The third diet provided 82% as carbohydrate calories (high-carbohydrate diet). The quadriceps femoris muscle's glycogen content, determined from needle biopsy specimens, averaged 0.63 g glycogen per 100 g wet muscle with the high-fat diet, 1.75 g for the normal diet, and 3.75 g for the high-carbohydrate diet.

Endurance capacity during cycling varied considerably, depending on the diet consumed 3 days before the exercise test. With the normal diet, exercise lasted an average 114 min, whereas endurance averaged only 57 min on the high-fat diet. The high-carbohydrate diet improved endurance performance three times more than did the high-fat diet. Interestingly, fatigue coincided with the same low muscle glycogen level under the three diet conditions. These findings, complemented by other research,[20,24] conclusively demonstrated muscle glycogen's importance to sustain intense physical activity exceeding 1 hr.

A carbohydrate-deficient diet rapidly depletes muscle and liver glycogen and negatively affects performance in short-term anaerobic activity and prolonged intense aerobic activities. These observations apply to individuals who modify their diets by reducing carbohydrate intake below recommended levels. Reliance on starvation diets or other extreme diet forms (e.g., high-fat, low-carbohydrate diets or "liquid-protein" diets) proves counterproductive to optimize exercise performance. Reliance on low-carbohydrate diets makes it difficult from an energy supply standpoint to engage regularly in longer-duration, vigorous activities. Chapter 3 discusses optimal provision for carbohydrate needs prior to, during, and in recovery from strenuous physical activity.

Summary

1. Carbon, hydrogen, oxygen, and nitrogen represent the basic structural units for the body's bioactive substances.
2. Carbon combined with oxygen and hydrogen forms carbohydrates and lipids. Proteins form when carbon, oxygen, and hydrogen combinations bind with nitrogen and minerals.
3. Simple sugars have 3 to 7 carbon atom chains, with hydrogen and oxygen in a 2:1 ratio. Glucose, the most common simple sugar, contains a 6-carbon chain $C_6H_{12}O_6$.

4. Three major carbohydrate classifications include monosaccharides (glucose and fructose), oligosaccharides (disaccharides sucrose, lactose, and maltose), and polysaccharides with three or more simple sugars to create plant starch, fiber, and glycogen.
5. Glycogenolysis describes glycogen reconversion to glucose; gluconeogenesis refers to glucose synthesis, particularly from protein sources.
6. Americans consume 40 to 50% of total caloric intake as carbohydrate, typically as simple sugars and refined starches; these forms of rapidly absorbed carbohydrates may have negative health consequences.
7. Carbohydrate, stored in limited quantity in liver and muscle, serves four important functions: energy source, spares protein breakdown, metabolic primer for lipid catabolism, and uninterrupted central nervous system fuel supply.
8. Muscle glycogen provides the primary energy substrate for anaerobic exercise.
9. The body's glycogen stores (muscle glycogen and glucose from the liver) contribute substantially to energy metabolism in longer-duration endurance-type activities.
10. Lipids contribute 50 to 70% to the total energy requirement during light- and moderate-intensity exercise.
11. Stored intramuscular lipid and lipids from adipocytes supply about 80% of the energy requirements in long-duration physical activities.
12. A carbohydrate-deficient diet quickly depletes muscle and liver glycogen to negatively impact all-out exercise capacity and the sustainability of intense aerobic exercise.
13. Individuals who train intensely should consume between 60 and 70% of daily calories as carbohydrate, predominantly in unrefined, complex form (400 to 800 g; 8 to 10 g · kg body mass^{-1}).
14. With muscle glycogen depletion, physical activity intensity decreases to a level determined by the body's ability to mobilize and oxidize lipid.

Part 2 — Lipids

Lipid Characteristics

A lipid (from the Greek *lipos*, meaning "fat") molecule has identical structural elements as carbohydrate but differs in its linkage and number of atoms. Specifically, the lipid's hydrogen to oxygen ratio considerably exceeds that for carbohydrate. Lipid, the general term for heterogeneous compounds, includes *oils*, *fats*, *waxes*, and *related compounds*. Oils become liquid at room temperature, whereas fats remain solid. Dietary lipid includes 98% triacylglycerol, with about 90% residing in subcutaneous adipose tissue depots. The structural $C_{57}H_{110}O_6$ formula describes the common lipid stearin with an 18.3:1 H:O ratio. Recall that carbohydrate's 2:1 ratio never changes.

Lipid Kinds and Sources

Plants and animals contain lipids in long hydrocarbon chains. Lipids, generally greasy to the touch, remain insoluble in water but soluble in the nonpolar organic solvents acetone, ether, chloroform, and benzene. Lipids belong to one of three main categories:

1. Simple lipids
2. Compound lipids
3. Derived lipids

Simple Lipids

Simple lipids or "neutral fats" consist primarily of *triacylglycerols*—a term preferable to *triglycerides* among biochemists because it describes glycerol acylated by three fatty acids. The fats are "neutral" because at a cell's pH, they have no electrically charged groups. These completely nonpolar molecules have no water affinity. Triacylglycerols constitute the major storage lipid form in fat cells called **adipocytes**. The triacylglycerol molecule contains two different atom clusters. The **glycerol** cluster includes a three-carbon molecule that itself does not qualify as a lipid due to its high water solubility. Three clusters of unbranched carbon-chained atoms, termed **fatty acids**, bond to the glycerol molecule. A carboxyl (–COOH) cluster at one end of the fatty acid chain gives the molecule its acidic characteristics. Fatty acids have straight hydrocarbon chains with as few as 4 carbon atoms or more than 20, with 16 and 18 carbons the most common chain lengths.

Triacylglycerol molecule synthesis or **condensation** produces three water molecules. Conversely, three water molecules attach at the points where the lipid molecule splits during hydrolysis when lipase enzymes cleave the molecule into its constituents. **FIGURE 1.8** illustrates basic molecular structure of a **saturated fatty acid** and **unsaturated fatty acid**. The saturated fatty acid palmitic acid has no double bonds in its carbon chain and contains its maximum available hydrogen atoms (A). Without double bonds, the three saturated fatty acid chains fit together relatively closely to form a "hard" fat (B). The three double bonds in linoleic acid, an unsaturated fatty acid, reduce the number of hydrogen atoms along the carbon chain. Inserting double bonds into the carbon chain prevents close association of the fatty acids, producing a "softer" fat, or an oil. All lipid-containing foods have different proportional mixtures containing saturated and unsaturated fatty acids.

Fatty Acid Carbon Chains

Most naturally occurring fatty acids have an even number chain of carbon atoms that range from 4 to 28, often categorized as short to very long. Fatty acids undergo different

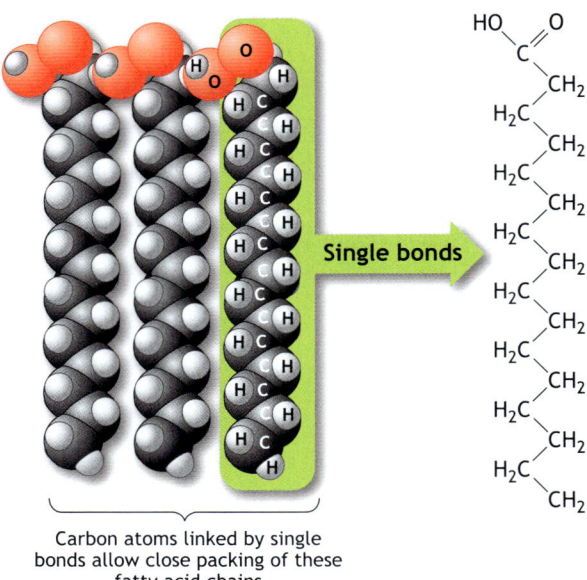

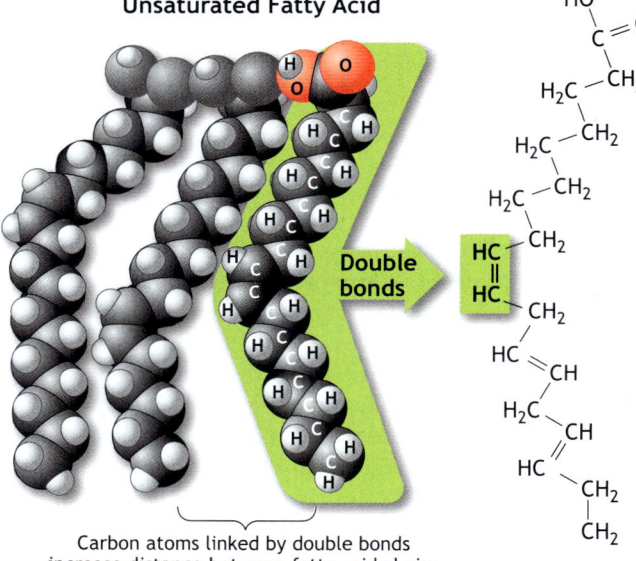

FIGURE 1.8. The major structural difference between saturated **(A)** and unsaturated fatty acids **(B)** are double bonds present or absent among carbon atoms.

- Very long chain fatty acids = greater than 22 carbons (cerotic acid), too long for mitochondrial metabolism, which require breakdown by **peroxisomes** (the small vesicles around cells containing digestive enzymes that break down toxic materials)

SCFA and MCFAs diffuse intact directly from the gastrointestinal tract into the **hepatic portal vein**, readily available for energy use as substrate. LCFAs, in contrast, require **bile salts** for digestion and are incorporated into chylomicrons and transported through lymph for deposit as fat.

 See the animation "Condensation" on Lippincott Connect to view this process.

A saturated fatty acid contains only single covalent bonds among carbon atoms, with all remaining bonds attaching to hydrogen. If the carbon within a fatty acid chain binds the maximum possible number of hydrogens, the fatty acid molecule is said to be "*saturated with respect to hydrogen and termed a saturated fatty acid.*" Saturated fatty acids occur primarily in animal products—beef, lamb, pork, chicken, egg yolk, and dairy fats from cream, milk, butter, and cheese. Saturated fatty acids from the plant kingdom include coconut oil, palm oil, palm kernel oil—often called tropical oils—vegetable shortening, and hydrogenated margarine; commercially prepared cakes, pies, and cookies also contain plentiful amounts of saturated fatty acids.

Unsaturated Fatty Acids

Unsaturated fatty acids contain one or more double bonds along their main carbon chain. Each double bond along the chain reduces the number of potential hydrogen-binding sites; thus, the molecule is said to be "*unsaturated with respect to hydrogen.*" A **monounsaturated fatty acid** contains *one* double bond along the main carbon chain; examples include canola oil, olive oil, peanut oil, and the oil in almonds, pecans, and avocados. A **polyunsaturated fatty acid** contains *two or more* double bonds along the main carbon chain—safflower, sunflower, soybean, and corn oil are examples. All oils provide about 125 calories in 14 lipid grams per tablespoon, with any difference being the oil's fatty acid type. Any nontropical oil represents a good health choice. In contrast, the tropical palm and coconut oils are high in saturated fatty acids and should be avoided. The top in **FIGURE 1.9** lists saturated, monounsaturated, and polyunsaturated fatty acid content in common fats and oils expressed in g per 100 g of lipid. The lower inset table reveals hidden fat percentage by weight of popular foods. Several polyunsaturated fatty acids, most notably linoleic acid (an 18-carbon fatty acid with two double bonds present in cooking and salad oils shown in Fig. 1.8), must originate from dietary sources because they serve as precursors to other fatty acids the body cannot synthesize and are termed **essential fatty acids**. Linoleic acid maintains plasma membrane integrity and sustains growth, reproduction, skin maintenance, and overall body functioning. The heart-healthy omega-3 fatty acids found in fish also are polyunsaturated fats.

metabolic fates depending on their chain length and degree of saturation:

- Short-chain fatty acids (SCFA) = less than 6 carbons (e.g., butyric, acetic, and caprylic acid) in butter and some tropical fats
- Medium-chain fatty acids (MCFA) = 6 to 12 carbons (e.g., lauric and capric acid) in coconut oil, palm kernel oil, and breast milk
- Long-chain fatty acids (LCFA) = 13 to 21 carbons (e.g., palmitic, oleic, and stearic acid) in animals, fish, cocoa, seeds, nuts, and vegetable oils

CHAPTER 1 • Carbohydrates, Lipids, and Proteins

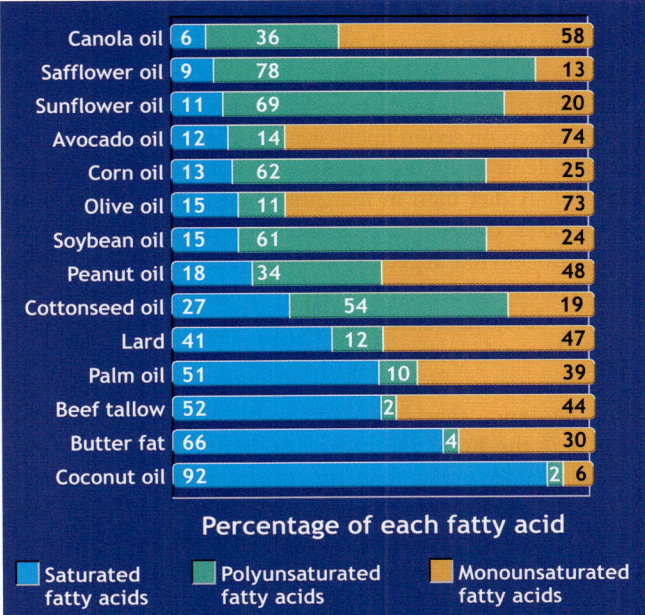

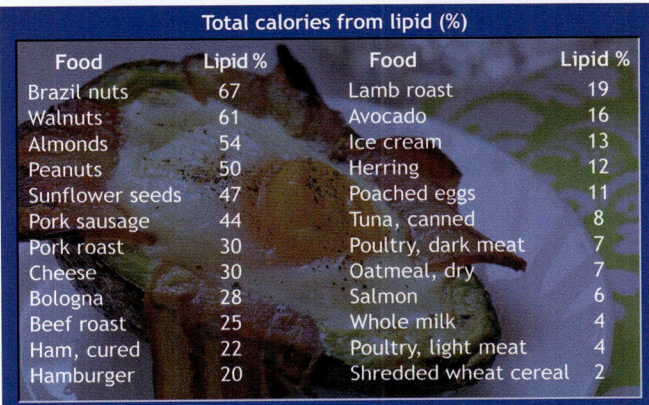

FIGURE 1.9. Diverse fatty acids in common dietary lipid sources (g per 100 g; upper), and hidden total fat percentage in popular foods (lower).
(Data from Food Composition Tables, US Department of Agriculture; https://fdc.nal.usda.gov/. Elena Shashkina/Shutterstock.)

Fatty acids from plant sources generally remain unsaturated and liquefy at room temperature. In contrast, lipids containing longer carbon chains and more saturated fatty acids exist as solids at room temperature; those with shorter carbon chains and more unsaturated fatty acids remain soft. Oils exist as liquids and contain unsaturated fatty acids. The chemical process of **hydrogenation** changes oils to semisolid fats by bubbling liquid hydrogen under pressure into vegetable oil. This reduces the unsaturated fatty acids' double bonds to single bonds so more hydrogens can attach to carbons along the chain. Firmer fat forms because adding hydrogen increases the lipid's melting temperature. Hydrogenated oil behaves as a saturated fat—lard substitutes and margarine are the most common hydrogenated fats.

Triacylglycerol Formation

FIGURE 1.10 outlines the reaction sequence in triacylglycerol synthesis, a process termed **esterification**. Initially, a fatty acid substrate attached to coenzyme A forms fatty acyl-CoA, which then transfers to glycerol to become glycerol 3-phosphate. In subsequent reactions, two additional fatty acyl-CoA join to a single glycerol backbone to form the composite triacylglycerol molecule. Triacylglycerol synthesis increases following a meal for two reasons:

1. Food absorption increases blood's fatty acid and glucose levels
2. Relatively high circulating insulin levels facilitate triacylglycerol synthesis

Triacylglycerol Breakdown

The term *hydrolysis* (more specifically **lipolysis** when applied to lipids) describes triacylglycerol catabolism to yield glycerol and the energy-rich fatty acid molecules. **FIGURE 1.11** shows the lipolysis and triacylglycerol esterification sequences in an adipocyte. This process adds water

fyi Trans Fats: The End for Undesirable Health Benefits

On June 16, 2015, the Food and Drug Administration (FDA) banned partially hydrogenated oils, the primary dietary industrially produced *trans* fat source in processed foods, deeming them not generally recognized as safe. This is consistent with actions by Latvia, Austria, Hungary, and Denmark, countries that have banned or limited total lipid in their food supply to less than 2%. Artificial *trans* fat substances were once touted beginning in the early 1940s as a healthy alternative to 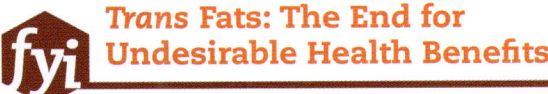 butter and shortenings. *Trans* fats commonly occur in baked goods including packaged cookies, pie crusts, crackers, typical snack foods (e.g., potato, tortilla, and corn chips), deep-fried foods (donuts, frosting, and fried chicken), refrigerated dough, microwave popcorn, nondairy creamers, and stick margarines. The good news is that many fatty acids such as linoleic acid, the main polyunsaturated fatty acid in vegetable oils, nuts, and seeds, associates with a 9% lower coronary heart disease risk and 13% lower mortality risk in a dose-response manner. On January 1, 2010, Tiburon, CA became the first city to ban *trans* fats in food preparation. The FDA estimates that 80% of all *trans* fats have disappeared from U.S. foods. This type of public health action will save over $160 billion over the next two decades in related healthcare costs.

Sources:
Honicky M, et al. Added sugar and trans fatty acid intake and sedentary behavior were associated with excess total-body and central adiposity in children and adolescents with congenital heart disease. *Pediatr Obes.* 2020;15:e12623.
Islam MA, et al. Trans fatty acids and lipid profile: a serious risk factor to cardiovascular disease, cancer and diabetes. *Diabetes Metab Syndr.* 2019;13:1643.
Sloop GD, et al. Perspective: inter-esterified triglycerides, the recent increase in deaths from heart disease, and elevated blood viscosity. *Ther Adv Cardiovasc Dis.* 2018;12:23.

in three distinct hydrolysis reactions shown at the figure's lower portion, with Steps 1 and 2 catalyzed by hormone-sensitive lipase (HSL), and Step 3 by monoglyceride lipase + HSL, which yields a glycerol and fatty acid molecule.[14] Lipolysis predominates under four conditions to yield glycerol and fatty acids:

1. Low-to-moderate–intensity physical activity
2. Low-calorie dieting or fasting
3. Cold stress
4. Depleting glycogen reserves in prolonged endurance activities

Triacylglycerol esterification and lipolysis occur in the cytosol of adipocytes. The fatty acids released during lipolysis can re-esterify to triacylglycerol following their conversion to a fatty acyl-CoA. In addition, they can exit adipocytes to combine with **albumin** for transport to tissues throughout the body. The term **free fatty acid (FFA)** describes this albumin–fatty acid combination.

Lipolysis also occurs in tissues other than adipocytes. Dietary triacylglycerol hydrolysis occurs in the small intestine, catalyzed by pancreatic lipase. The enzyme **lipoprotein lipase** located on capillary walls catalyzes hydrolysis of the triacylglycerols carried by the blood's lipoproteins. Adjacent adipose tissue and muscle cells "take up" the fatty acids released by lipoprotein lipase action, which are resynthesized to triacylglycerol for energy storage.

Trans-Fatty Acids: Unwanted at Any Levels

Trans-**fatty acids** come from the partial hydrogenation of unsaturated corn, soybean, or sunflower oil. A *trans*-fatty acid forms when one hydrogen atom along the restructured carbon chain moves from its naturally occurring same-side position (*cis* position) to the opposite side of the double bond that separates 2 carbon atoms (*trans* position). The richest *trans*-fat sources comprise vegetable shortenings, some margarines, and crackers, candies, cookies, snack foods, fried foods, baked goods, salad dressings, and other processed foods made with partially hydrogenated vegetable oils.

Health concerns about *trans*-fatty acids center on their detrimental effects on serum lipoproteins, overall heart health, and possible role in facilitating cognitive decline with aging in older adults.[5,45,47] A diet high in margarine and commercially baked cookies, cakes, doughnuts, pies, and deep-fried foods prepared with hydrogenated vegetable oils increases low-density lipoprotein cholesterol concentration. Hydrogenated oils, unlike saturated fats, decrease beneficial high-density lipoprotein cholesterol concentration and adversely affect markers of inflammation and endothelial dysfunction.[38,49] In light of strong evidence that *trans*-fatty acids increased heart disease risk,[76] the Food and Drug Administration (FDA; www.fda.gov) mandates that food processors include *trans*-fatty acid amounts on nutrition labels. Keep in mind that current food labeling rules allow products to contain up to 0.5 g *trans* fat and still claim "zero amount."

Lipids: The Good, the Bad, and the Ugly

Subjective terms describe the impact of the various forms of fatty acids in the diet. Unsaturated fatty acids contain one (monounsaturated) or more (polyunsaturated) double bonds along their main carbon chain. They classify as *desirable* because they can lower "unhealthful" LDL cholesterol. In contrast, *undesirable* saturated fatty acids contain only single bonds among carbon atoms; they stimulate the liver's LDL cholesterol production, which ultimately becomes arterial wall plaque. Even more disturbing, partially hydrogenated unsaturated vegetable oil consumption produces *trans*-fatty acids—which not only increase LDL concentration but also lower beneficial HDL cholesterol.

Dietary Lipids

FIGURE 1.12 displays the approximate percentage contribution from

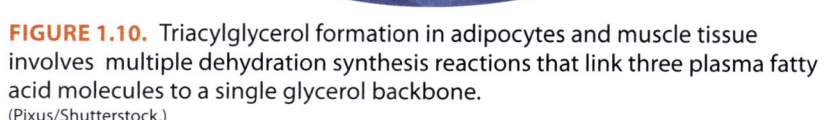

FIGURE 1.10. Triacylglycerol formation in adipocytes and muscle tissue involves multiple dehydration synthesis reactions that link three plasma fatty acid molecules to a single glycerol backbone.
(Pixus/Shutterstock.)

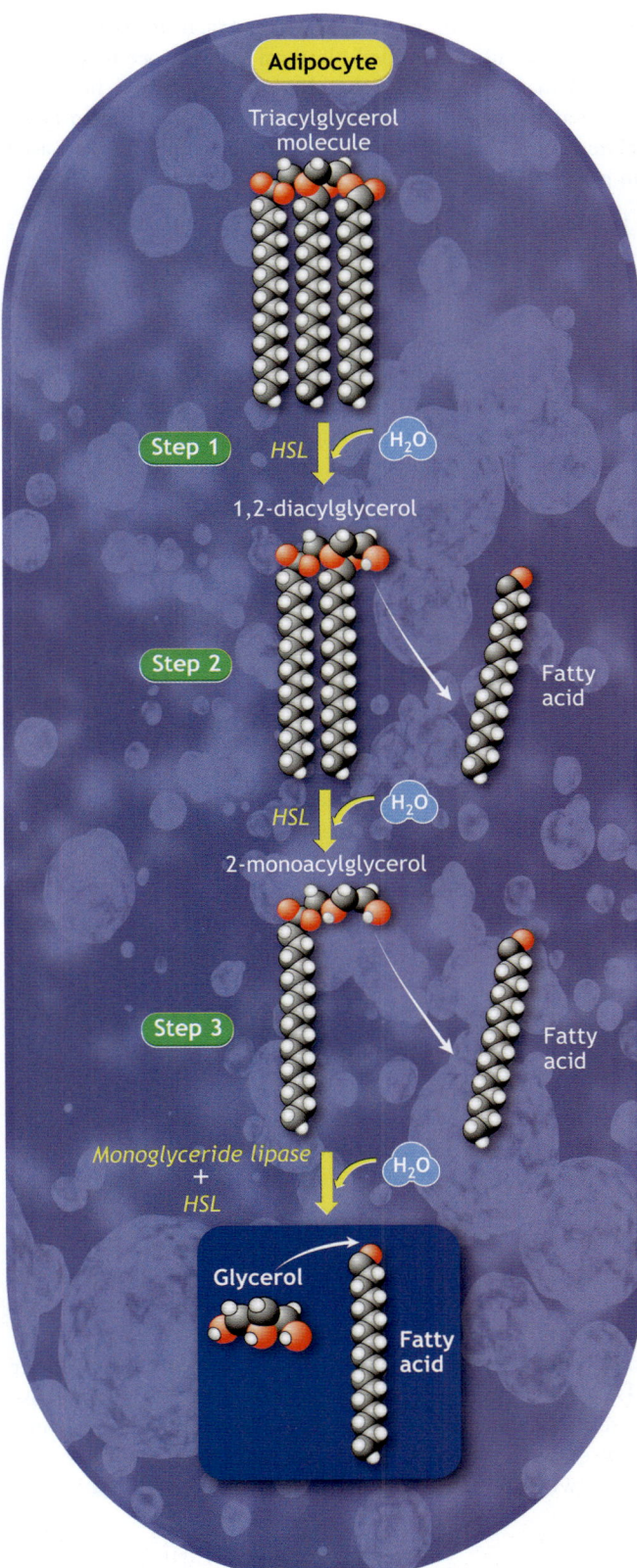

FIGURE 1.11. Triacylglycerol catabolism (lipolysis) to its glycerol and fatty acid components involves a three-step process regulated by hormone-sensitive lipase (*HSL*).
(Pixus/Shutterstock.)

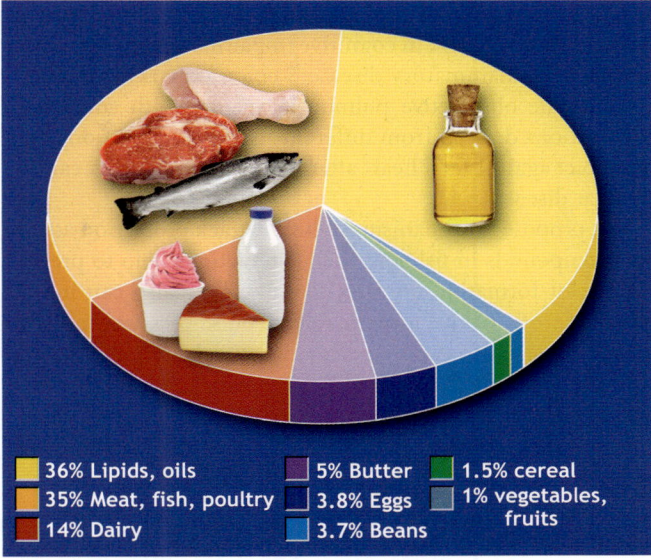

FIGURE 1.12. Contribution from the major food groups to the lipid content in a typical American diet.
(Shutterstock: nexus 7; Cameramannz; saiko3p; M. Unal Ozmen; Elena Schweitzer; Madlen.)

common food groups to the total lipid content of a typical American diet. In the United States, the average person consumes about 15% of total calories as saturated fatty acids daily, a 23 kg/51 lb equivalent when computed on a yearly basis! The relationship between saturated fatty acid intake and coronary heart disease risk has prompted health professionals to recommend two public health strategies:

1. Replacing at least some saturated fatty acids and all *trans*-fatty acids with nonhydrogenated monounsaturated (olive and safflower) and polyunsaturated (soybean, corn, and sunflower) oils, and substitute poultry, nuts, and fish for red meat and cheese
2. Balancing energy intake with regular physical activity to minimize weight gain (and associated LDL increases, HDL cholesterol decreases, and increased insulin resistance and blood pressure) and obtain the health benefits of regular physical activity

From a health standpoint, individuals should consume no more than 10% as saturated fatty acids in the total daily energy intake. This translates to about 300 kcal, or 30 to 35 g for the average young adult male who consumes 3000 kcal daily.

Greenland Eskimos have a low heart disease prevalence. While it is not necessarily a causal factor, they also consume considerable lipids from fish, seal, and whale, foods high in eicosapentaenoic acid and docosahexaenoic acid, two essential long-chain polyunsaturated fatty acids. These oils belong to the **omega-3 fatty acid** family (also termed *n*-3; the last double bond begins 3 carbons from the end carbon), found primarily in oils from shellfish and cold-water herring, anchovies, sardines, salmon, mackerel, and sea mammals. Regular fish intake (minimum two servings weekly, about 8 oz total) benefits the blood lipid profile, particularly plasma triacylglycerols,[39] and overall heart disease risk and mortality rate from ventricular fibrillation and sudden death.[15,34] Additional healthful benefits include improved risk in cognitive impairment and Alzheimer disease,[55,59] inflammatory disease,[80] colon polyps in women,[51] and chronic obstructive pulmonary disease with smoking.[62] Medications derived from different fish oil formulations help to protect against fatal heart attacks, strokes, and other cardiovascular diseases.

A proposed mechanism for heart attack protection asserts that compounds in fish and their interactions help to prevent blood clot formation on arterial walls. They also can inhibit atherosclerotic plaque growth, reduce pulse pressure and total vascular resistance from increased arterial compliance, and stimulate endothelial-derived nitric oxide to facilitate myocardial perfusion[53] (see Chapter 16).

Compound Lipids

Compound lipids (triacylglycerol components combined with other chemicals) represent about 10% of the body's total lipid content. **Phospholipids** contain one or more fatty acid molecules joined with a phosphorus-containing group and several nitrogen-containing molecules. Phospholipids serve four main functions:

1. Interact with water and lipid to modulate fluid movement across cell membranes
2. Maintain cell-structural integrity
3. Play an important blood clotting role
4. Provide structural integrity to nerve fiber's insulating sheath

Other compound lipids include glycolipids (fatty acids bound with carbohydrate and nitrogen) and water-soluble lipoproteins (protein spheres formed primarily in the liver when a protein molecule joins with either triacylglycerols or phospholipids). *Lipoproteins provide the major transportation means for blood lipids.* If blood lipids did not bind to protein, they literally would float to the top like cream in nonhomogenized fresh milk rather than dispersing throughout the vascular system.

High-Density, Low-Density, and Very Low-Density Lipoproteins

Lipoproteins categorize into types according to their size and density and whether they carry **cholesterol** or triacylglycerol. **FIGURE 1.13** illustrates general cholesterol and lipoprotein dynamics in the body, including their transport among the small intestine, liver, and peripheral tissues. The image designated (A) shows that lipoproteins are combined lipid and protein particles that transport cholesterol throughout the body. In (B), lipoproteins transport cholesterol via the bloodstream, and (C) shows that the large VLDL particle attaches to the capillary lining where its cholesterol core is extracted. The smaller LDL particle (D) remains in the blood for transport to the liver for removal, while (E) in the bottom box shows that LDL remains in the blood and travels to the liver for removal. In this case cholesterol excess reduces the lipoprotein receptor number on the liver's cell surface illustrated in (F). With normal blood cholesterol levels shown in (H), arterial walls remain smooth and slippery. High blood cholesterol levels concentrate cholesterol in arterial walls, thereby reducing blood flow. The image at the top right illustrates the four lipoprotein types related to their diameters, with classifications 1 to 4 based on **gravitational density**:

1. **High-density lipoproteins (HDL$_1$ and HDL$_2$).** Produced in the liver and small intestine, these substances contain the highest protein percentage (about 50%) and least total lipid (about 20%), and cholesterol (about 20%) of the lipoproteins.
2. **Low-density lipoproteins (LDLs).** Commonly known as "bad" cholesterol, these normally constitute from 60 to 80% of total serum cholesterol with the greatest affinity for arterial cell walls. LDL delivers cholesterol to arterial tissue where the LDL particles:
   a. Oxidize to alter their physiochemical properties
   b. Deposit inside arterial walls to initiate atherosclerotic plaque development
   c. Contribute to smooth muscle cell proliferation and unfavorable damage that ultimately narrows arteries
3. **Very low-density lipoproteins (VLDLs).** Degraded in the liver to produce LDLs. VLDLs contain the highest lipid percentage (95%), of which about 60% consists of triacylglycerols. VLDLs transport triacylglycerols to muscle and adipose tissue. Under the action of lipoprotein lipase, the VLDL molecule becomes a denser LDL molecule because it then contains fewer lipids. LDLs and VLDLs have the most lipid and fewest protein components.
4. **Chylomicrons.** Emulsified lipid droplets (including long-chain triacylglycerols, phospholipids, and FFAs) exit the intestine and enter lymphatic vessels. The liver metabolizes chylomicrons for storage in adipose tissue. Chylomicrons also transport the fat-soluble vitamins A, D, E, and K.

Unlike LDL, HDL protects against heart disease. HDL acts as a scavenger in **reverse cholesterol transport** by removing it from the arterial wall and delivering it to the liver for incorporation into bile and subsequent excretion via the intestinal tract. LDL and HDL and their specific ratios (e.g., HDL ÷ total cholesterol; LDL ÷ HDL) and subfractions provide more meaningful coronary artery disease risk indicators than total cholesterol *per se*. Regular moderate and intense aerobic exercise and abstinence from cigarette smoking increase HDL, lower LDL, and favorably alter the LDL:HDL ratio.[36,42,64] We discuss these effects more fully in Chapter 31. An online computer program calculates the risk and appropriate cholesterol levels for adults (www.nhlbi.nih.gov/guidelines/cholesterol/index.htm).

Derived Lipids

Simple and compound lipids form **derived lipids**. Cholesterol, considered a lipid, represents the most widely known derived lipid existing *only* in animal tissues. Cholesterol does not contain fatty acids, but rather shares several of a lipid's physical and chemical characteristics.

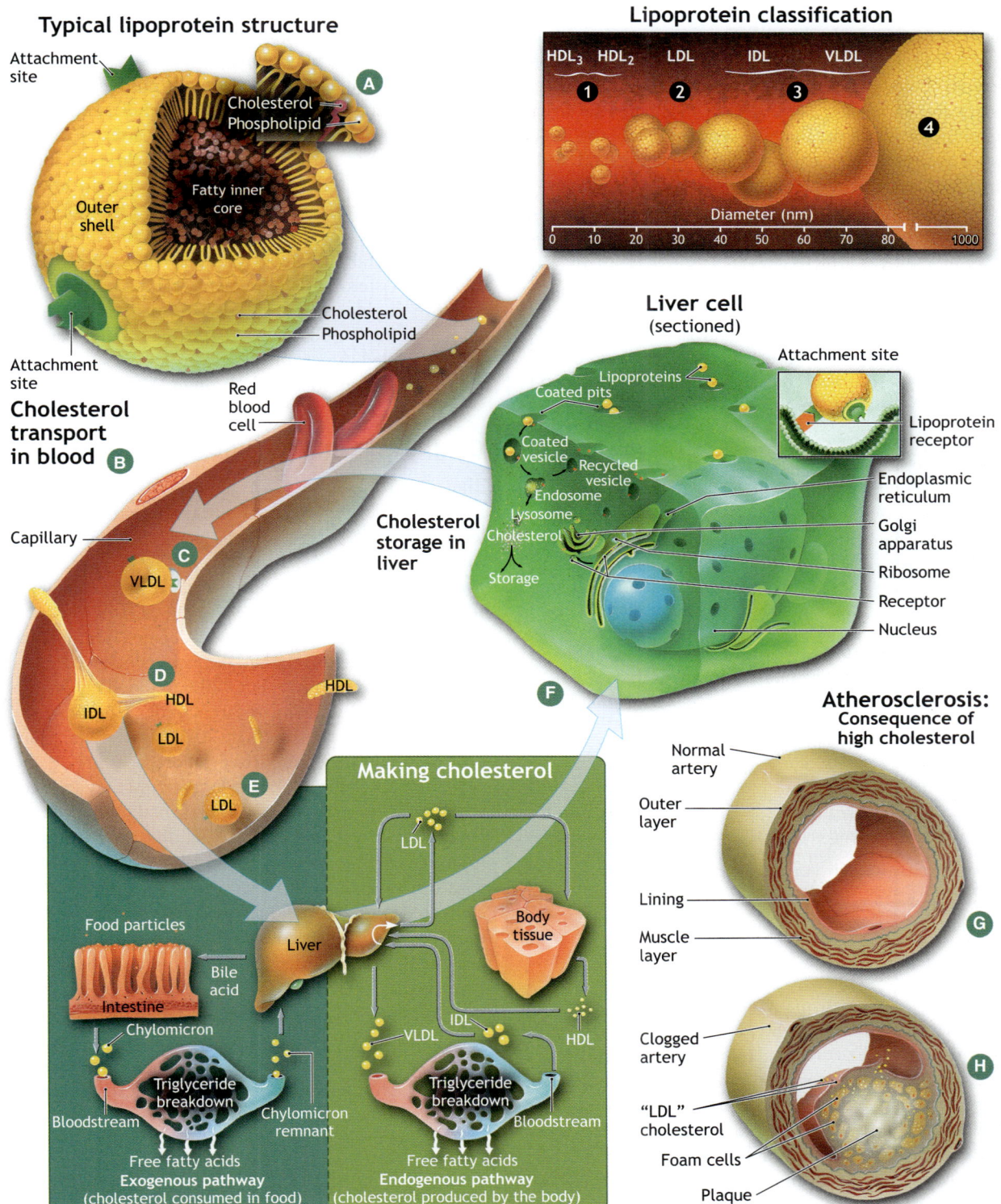

FIGURE 1.13. Cholesterol dynamics in the body. **(A)** Lipoproteins are combined fat and protein particles that transport cholesterol throughout the body. **(B)** Lipoproteins transport cholesterol via the bloodstream. **(C)** The large VLDL particle attaches to the capillary lining where its cholesterol core is extracted. **(D)** The smaller IDL particle remains in the blood for transport back to the liver for removal. **(E)** LDL remains in the blood and travels back to the liver for removal. **(F)** An excess of cholesterol reduces the lipoprotein receptor number on the liver cell surface. **(G)** With normal blood cholesterol levels, arterial walls remain smooth and slippery. **(H)** High blood cholesterol levels concentrate cholesterol in arterial walls, thereby reducing blood flow. Lipoprotein Classification: 1, high density lipoprotein (HDL); 2, low density lipoprotein (LDL); 3, intermediate density lipoprotein (IDL) and very low density lipoprotein (VLDL); 4, chylomicron, dietary cholesterol and triacylglycerol particles absorbed by small intestine.
(Adapted with permission from Anatomical Chart Company. © 2000 Anatomical Chart Company.)

Cholesterol, widespread in animals' plasma membranes, originates either through the diet (*exogenous cholesterol*) or through cellular synthesis (*endogenous cholesterol*). More endogenous cholesterol forms with a diet high in saturated fatty acids and *trans*-fatty acids, which facilitates the liver's LDL cholesterol synthesis. The liver synthesizes about 70% of the body's cholesterol, but other tissues—including the walls of arteries and intestines—also synthesize this compound.

High-Density Lipoproteins and Cancer Risk

A meta-analysis from 24 randomized controlled trials reported that for every 10 mg · dL^{-1} increase in high-density lipoprotein (HDL) cholesterol, cancer risk declined by 36%, with the relationship becoming even stronger after adjusting for demographics and cancer risk factors. The researchers speculated that the HDL molecule (protein ApoA, green; phospholipids, orange with blue cap; cholesterol, orange with violet cap) might exhibit anti-inflammatory and antioxidant effects to reduce cancer risk, or even create beneficial effects from tumor-destroying cells that seek out and destroy abnormal cells. Healthy lifestyle changes that raise HDL levels (nutritious diet, increased physical activity, maintaining healthy body weight, and no smoking) also can reduce chronic risk conditions associated with higher cancer incidence.

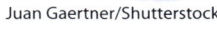
Juan Gaertner/Shutterstock

Sources:
Sultani R, et al. Elevated triglycerides to high-density lipoprotein cholesterol (TG/HDL-C) ratio predicts long-term mortality in high-risk patients. *Heart Lung Circ.* 2020;29:414.
Zhong GC, et al. HDL-C is associated with mortality from all causes, cardiovascular disease and cancer in a J-shaped dose-response fashion: a pooled analysis of 37 prospective cohort studies. *Eur J Prev Cardiol.* 2020;27:1187.

Cholesterol Functions

Cholesterol participates in many bodily functions including building plasma membranes and serving as a precursor in synthesizing vitamin D, adrenal gland hormones, and the sex hormones estrogen, androgen, and progesterone. Cholesterol furnishes a key component for bile synthesis (emulsifies lipids during digestion) and plays a crucial role in forming tissues, organs, and body structures during fetal development.

Egg yolk provides a rich cholesterol source (average about 186 mg per egg), as do red meats and organ meats (liver, kidney, and brain). Shellfish (particularly shrimp), dairy products (ice cream, cream cheese, butter, and whole milk), fast-food breakfasts, and processed meats contain relatively large cholesterol amounts. *Foods from plants contain no cholesterol.*

Cholesterol and Coronary Heart Disease Risk

High total serum cholesterol levels and cholesterol-rich LDL are powerful coronary artery disease predictors. These become particularly potent when combined with other high risk factors like cigarette smoking, physical inactivity, excess body fat, and untreated hypertension. A dietary cholesterol excess in "susceptible" individuals eventually produces **atherosclerosis**, a degenerative process that forms cholesterol-rich deposits (**plaque**) on the medium and larger arteries' inner linings, causing them to narrow and eventually close. Reducing saturated fatty acid and cholesterol intake generally lowers serum cholesterol, yet the effect remains modest for most people.[63,75] Increasing dietary monounsaturated and polyunsaturated fatty acid intake also lowers blood cholesterol, particularly LDL cholesterol.[23,30,38] Frequent walnut consumption may improve the blood lipid profile without causing weight gain or increasing blood pressure. Chapter 31 presents specific recommended values for "desirable," "borderline," and "undesirable" plasma lipid and lipoprotein levels.

Confusion Concerning U.S. Dietary Guidelines

The 2015 Dietary Guidelines Advisory Committee (DGAC) did a complete about-face regarding dietary cholesterol intake by recommending that limits be removed for cholesterol intake from the *2015 Dietary Guidelines for Americans*. This represented a reversal about dietary cholesterol widely circulated since the 1960s. This was not to say that blood cholesterol level was deemed unimportant as a health risk indicator. Rather, the experts believed that dietary intake contributed only about 20% to blood cholesterol level, with the liver supplying the remainder. The newest dietary guidelines were published in 2020, www.dietaryguidelines.gov/2020-advisory-committee-report.

A comprehensive, recent long-term study (about 30,000 adults who self-reported daily food intake for 17 years) challenged these recommendations, finding that eating three to four eggs weekly was associated with a 6% increase in heart disease risk and an 8% increase in all-cause mortality risk compared with eating no eggs (in fact, eating more than four eggs weekly further increased risk). The study focused on eggs because they represented the most common cholesterol-laden food in the American diet. Also, a daily 300-mg cholesterol intake linked to a 17% increased heart disease risk and an 18% increased risk of dying compared without egg consumption. The study's observational nature did not show that eggs and cholesterol *caused* heart disease and death. The researchers concluded that current dietary egg and cholesterol guidelines need re-evaluation.

 See the animation "Fat Mobilization and Use" at Lippincott Connect to view this process.

Recommended Lipid Intake

Recommendations for dietary lipid intake for physically active individuals living in the United States generally follow prudent health-related recommendations for the general population. Dietary lipid currently represents between 34 and 38% total caloric intake equal to about 50 kg/110 lb of lipid consumed yearly. Current recommendations place intake between

20 and 35% depending on lipid type consumed. The American Heart Association (AHA; www.americanheart.org) now encourages Americans to focus more on replacing high-fat foods with fruits, vegetables, unrefined whole grains, fat-free and low-fat dairy products, fish, poultry, and lean meat.[35] Other AHA guideline components include a focus on weight control and addition to the diet of two weekly servings of fish rich in omega-3 fatty acids. A new research line sounds a cautionary note about overconsuming omega-3 fatty acids in supplement form due to increased prostate cancer risk.[7] The American Cancer Society (www.cancer.org) advocates a diet with only 20% total calories from lipid to reduce colon and rectum, prostate, endometrium, and perhaps breast cancer risk. The main dietary cholesterol sources include the same animal food sources rich in saturated fatty acids. Curtailing intake of these foods reduces preformed cholesterol intake and, more importantly, reduces fatty acid intake known to stimulate endogenous cholesterol synthesis.

Diet Versus Drugs to Lower Cholesterol

Food *quality* may surpass total lipid *quantity* in the ongoing battle to lower undesirable blood lipids, as knowledge about what foods exert the greatest beneficial blood lipid effect continues to evolve. Research systematically examined whether foods considered by the FDA (www.fda.gov) to lower blood cholesterol could be incorporated into the diet and produce positive effects in lowering harmful LDL cholesterol. A Canadian study placed 351 citizens with elevated cholesterol into three groups, each assigned different diets for 6 months. Persons on the low–saturated fat (control) diet reduced LDL cholesterol 8 mg $\cdot$ dL^{-1} compared with decreases from 24 and 26 mg $\cdot$ dL^{-2} on diets composed from plant-based lipid and protein—some 13% more than the group eating the low–saturated fat diet.

The cholesterol-lowering effect revealed that dietary changes alone could serve as an alternative to statin medications (e.g., lovastatin, pravastatin, atorvastatin, Zocor, Lipitor, Crestor) that often have undesirable liver and muscular function side effects. This research challenged the idea that simply reducing the diet's saturated fat content from red meat and dairy product sources could deliver the most effective cholesterol-lowering strategy. Mounting evidence supports consuming a cholesterol-lowering diet from healthful plant-based lipid and protein food sources from these four categories:

1. Plant sterol–enriched margarine
2. Peanuts and tree nuts
3. Soy milk, tofu, and soy "meat" products
4. Oats, barley, and other "sticky" or viscous fibers

Energy Source and Reserve

Lipid constitutes the ideal cellular fuel for three reasons:

1. It includes considerable energy per unit weight.
2. It transports and stores easily.
3. It provides a ready energy source.

For a well-nourished individual at rest, lipid provides 80 to 90% of the total energy requirement. Pure lipid's combustion releases about 9 kcal $\cdot$ g^{-1} (38 kJ), more than twice the energy available to the body from an equal quantity of carbohydrate or protein. Recall that triacylglycerol molecule synthesis from glycerol and three fatty acid molecules produces three water molecules. In contrast, when glucose forms glycogen, each glycogen gram stores 2.7 g water. *Lipid exists as a relatively water-free, concentrated fuel, whereas glycogen remains hydrated and heavy relative to its energy content.*

INTEGRATIVE QUESTION

What physiological benefit comes from storing excess calories as lipid compared to an equivalent caloric excess as glycogen?

Lipids account for approximately 15% of the body mass in males and 25% in females. **FIGURE 1.14** illustrates lipids' total mass and energy content in an 80-kg young man. The potential energy stored in the adipose tissue's fat molecules translates to about 108,000 kcal (12,000 g body fat × 9.0 kcal $\cdot$ g^{-1}). A run from downtown San Diego, CA to the convention center in downtown Seattle, WA (assuming about 100 kcal per mile energy expenditure) would deplete the available energy from adipose tissue triacylglycerols (108,000 kcal), intramuscular triacylglycerols (2700 kcal), plasma triacylglycerols (36 kcal), and a minor amount from plasma FFAs (3.6 kcal). Contrast this with the limited 2000-kcal stored carbohydrate reserve that would provide energy for only a 20-mile run! Viewed somewhat differently, the energy reserves from carbohydrate alone could power intense running for about 1.6 hr, whereas exercise would continue for about 75 times longer

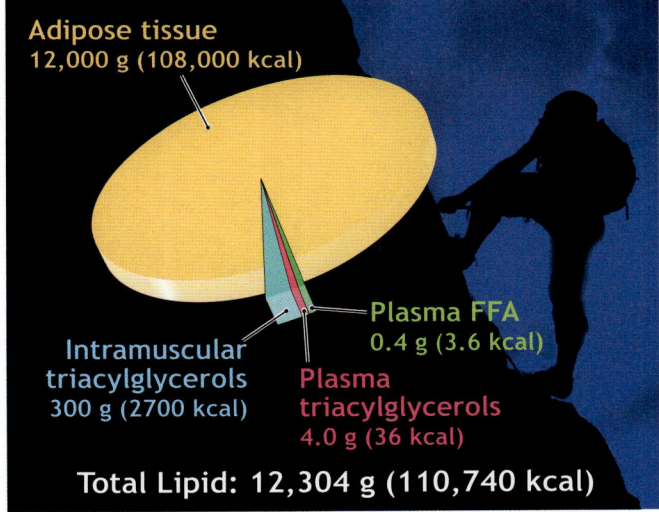

FIGURE 1.14. Total quantity and energy stored in adipose tissue, intramuscular and plasma triacylglycerols, and free fatty acids (*FFA*) within an average young 80-kg male. (David Ionut/Shutterstock.)

or 120 hr from the body's lipid reserves. Lipid as a fuel source also "spares" protein to carry out its tissue synthesis and repair functions.

Protection of Vital Organs and Thermal Insulation

Up to 4% of the body's fat serves to protect against trauma to vital organs such as the heart, liver, kidneys, spleen, brain, and spinal cord. Subcutaneous fat stored just below the skin provides insulation, permitting individuals to tolerate extreme cold.[68] A thicker layer of this insulatory fat benefits deep-sea divers, ocean and channel swimmers, or Arctic inhabitants. In contrast, excess body fat hinders temperature regulation during heat stress, most notably during sustained exercise in air, when the body's heat production can increase 20 times above resting levels. In this case, the insulatory shield from subcutaneous fat retards heat flow from the body. For large-sized American football linemen, excess fat storage provides additional cushioning to protect the participant from the sport's normal traumas. Nonetheless, any possible protective benefit must be weighed against the liability imposed by excess fat's "dead weight" and its impact on energy expenditure, thermal regulation, and subsequent exercise performance.

Vitamin Carrier and Hunger Depressor

Consuming approximately 20 g dietary lipid daily provides a sufficient source and transport medium for the four fat-soluble vitamins A, D, E, and K. Severely reducing lipid intake depresses the body's vitamin level ultimately leading to vitamin deficiency. Dietary lipid also facilitates vitamin A precursor absorption from nonlipid plant sources such as carrots and apricots. After ingesting lipids, it takes about 3.5 hr to empty them from the stomach.

In a Practical Sense

Meet Plant-Based Meats

New nonmeat "meats" are a multibillion-dollar industry prevalent in drive-throughs, fast food eateries, restaurants, and mainstream grocery stores. The alternative meat products can be placed into one of two categories—cell-based protein and plant-based protein.

CELL-BASED PROTEIN MEAT

In cell-based protein, an animal *starter cell,* usually an animal's muscle cell, is extracted and grown in a laboratory culture. In the 6 wk it takes to grow a chicken for slaughter, the cell culture-based process produces the same amount of meatlike protein minus bones and feathers. These protein-cultured "meats" have many names—*slaughter-free, in vitro, vat-grown, lab-grown, cell-based, clean, cultivated,* and *synthetic meat.*

The world's first laboratory-grown burger was cooked and consumed in August 2013. Scientists from Maastricht University in the Netherlands used about 20,000 thin starter-muscle tissue strands from a cow and grew them into muscle strips to replicate the typical real-meat burger.

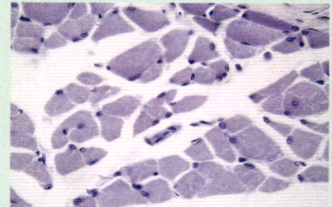
Kallayanee Naloka/Shutterstock

The initial cultured meat growing stage harvests starter cells with rapid cell reproduction rates. The myoblast embryonic progenitor cells differentiate to produce muscle cells (shown in purple stain), and adding nutrients and chemical-growth factors promotes rapid tissue growth so the meat cells can theoretically continue to grow indefinitely. In 2 months, cultured meat production can deliver about 50,000 tons from 10 pork starter-muscle cells!

PLANT-BASED PROTEIN MEAT

For plant-based protein products, protein extracts and isolates from plants combine to create nonmeat protein. In 2020, the two top meatless meat products included **Beyond Meat's** (www.beyondmeat.com) *Beyond Burger* (sold in Carl's Jr, Subway, McDonald's; this company also sells *Beyond Beef,* plant-based ground, and *Beyond Sausage*) and Impossible Foods' *Impossible Burger* (https://impossiblefoods.com/), which is sold in grocery stores and fast-food restaurants (Burger King, Red Robin, White Castle, Umami Burgers, A&W, and Qdoba's).

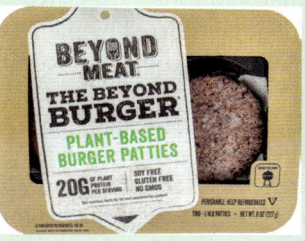
Keith Homan/Shutterstock

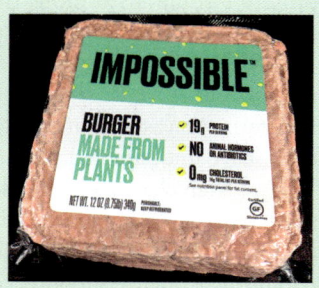
Amy Lutz/Shutterstock

IMPOSSIBLE BURGER, BEYOND BURGER, BEEF BURGER COMPARISONS

The top five Impossible Burger ingredients include water, soy protein concentrate, coconut oil, sunflower oil, and natural flavors. Plant-based heme, called leghemoglobin, inserts into genetically engineered yeast and stimulates more heme production when the yeast ferments.

THE BREAKDOWN

The table presents the nutrition facts and ingredient list for the uncooked Impossible Burger, Beyond Beef, and typical beef burger.

NUTRITION FACTS AND FULL INGREDIENT LIST

Ingredient	Impossible Burger 113 g/4 oz	Beyond Burger 113 g/4 oz	Beef Burger 113 g/4 oz grass-fed; 80% lean)
Calories	240	250	287
Total fat	14 g	18 g	23 g
Saturated fat	8 g	6 g	8.6 g
Cholesterol	0	0	80 mg
Sodium	370 mg	390 mg	75 mg
Total carbohydrates	9 g	3 g	0 g
Dietary fiber	3 g	2 g	0 g
Total sugars	<1 g	0 g	0 g
Protein	19 g	20 g	19 g
Calcium	170 mg (15% DV)	80 mg 6% DV)	20.3 mg (2% DV)
Potassium	610 mg (15% DV)	300 mg (6% DV)	305 mg (6% DV)
Iron	4.2 mg (25%)	(25% DV)	2.1 mg (12% DV)
Ingredients	Water, soy protein concentrate, coconut oil, sunflower oil, natural flavors, 2% or less potato protein, methylcellulose, yeast extract, cultured dextrose, food starch modified, soy leghemoglobin, salt, soy protein isolate, mixed tocopherols (vitamin E), zinc gluconate, thiamine hydrochloride (vitamin B_1), sodium ascorbate (vitamin C), niacin, pyridoxine, and vitamins B_6, B_2), and B_{12}	Water, pea protein isolate, expeller-pressed canola oil, refined coconut oil, contains 2% or less of cellulose from bamboo, methylcellulose, potato starch, natural flavor, maltodextrin, yeast extract, salt, sunflower oil, vegetable glycerin, dried yeast, gum arabic, citrus extract (to protect quality), ascorbic acid (to maintain color), beet juice extract (for color), acetic acid, succinic acid, modified food starch, annatto (for color)	Water, lipids (triacylglycerols), *trans*-fatty acids), proteins (15 different amino acids; essential and nonessential), carbohydrates (glycogen), naturally occurring flavorings, naturally occurring water-soluble and water-insoluble vitamins, naturally occurring minerals

Sources:
https://impossiblefoods.com/burger/, www.beyondmeat.com/products/beyond-beef/, www.nutritionvalue.org/Beef%2C_raw%2C_97%25_lean_meat_%252F_3%25_fat%2C_ground_nutritional_value.html

Sources:
Eshel G, et al. Environmentally optimal, nutritionally aware beef replacement plant-based diets. *Environ Sci Technol.* 2016;50:8164.
Goldstein B. Potential to curb the environmental burdens of American beef consumption using a novel plant-based beef substitute. *PLoS One.* 2017;12:e0189029.

Katz DL. Plant-based diets for reversing disease and saving the planet: past, present, and future. *Adv Nutr.* 2019;10:S304.
Pimentel M. Sustainability of meat-based and plant-based diets and the environment. *Am J Clin Nutr.* 2003;78:660.
Simsa R, et al. Extracellular heme proteins influence bovine myosatellite cell proliferation and the color of cell-based meat. *Foods.* 2019;21:8.

Lipid Dynamics in Physical Activity

Intracellular and extracellular lipid (FFAs, intramuscular triacylglycerols, and circulating plasma triacylglycerols bound to lipoproteins as VLDLs and chylomicrons) supply between 30 and 80% of the energy for physical activity depending on nutritional and fitness status and exercise intensity and duration.[2,44] Increased blood flow through adipose tissue with exercise increases FFA release for delivery and use by muscle. The lipid quantity used for energy in light and moderate activity is three times that compared to resting conditions. As activity becomes more intense, adipose tissue's FFA release fails to increase much above resting levels, leading to a decrease in plasma FFAs. This in turn stimulates increased muscle glycogen use (see Fig. 1.17 later in the chapter).[61] The energy contribution of intramuscular triacylglycerols ranges between 15 and 35%; endurance-trained athletes catabolize the largest quantity, with substantial impairment in use among the obese and/or type 2 diabetics.[32,33,71] Long-term consumption of a high-fat diet induces enzymatic adaptations that enhance lipid oxidation during submaximal physical activity.[40,50] Unfortunately, this adaptation does not translate to improved exercise performance.

The major energy for light-to-moderate physical activity comes from intramuscular triacylglycerols and fatty acids released from triacylglycerol storage sites and delivered to muscle as FFAs. When exercise begins, a transient initial drop in plasma FFA concentration occurs from increased FFA uptake by active muscles. Increased adipose tissue FFA release follows (with concomitant suppression of triacylglycerol formation) from two factors:

1. Sympathetic nervous system hormonal stimulation
2. Decreased plasma insulin levels

In moderate-intensity activity, carbohydrates and lipids supply approximately equal amounts of energy. When this level of activity continues for more than 1 hr, lipid catabolism gradually supplies a greater energy percentage, which coincides with depletion of glycogen reserves. Carbohydrate availability also influences energy use from lipids. With adequate glycogen reserves, carbohydrate becomes the preferred fuel during intense aerobic exercise owing to its more rapid catabolic rate. Toward the end of exercise when glycogen reserves become nearly depleted, lipid, mainly as circulating FFAs, supplies up to 80% of the total energy requirement. **FIGURE 1.15** illustrates the general substrate utilization response during long-duration submaximal cycling exercise. Carbohydrate combustion (reflected by

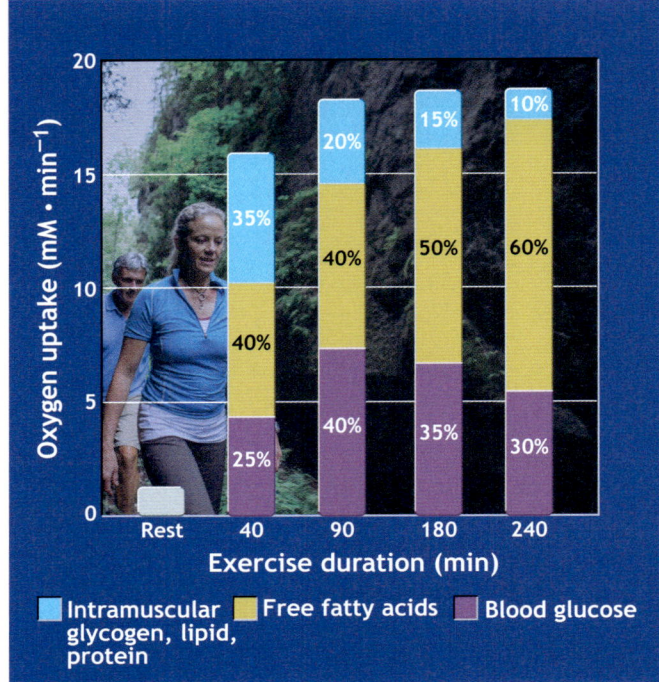

FIGURE 1.16. Generalized percentage contribution from intramuscular glycogen, lipid, protein, free fatty acids, and blood glucose related to oxygen uptake from 40 to 240 min in moderate-intensity physical activity.
(GROGL/Shutterstock.)

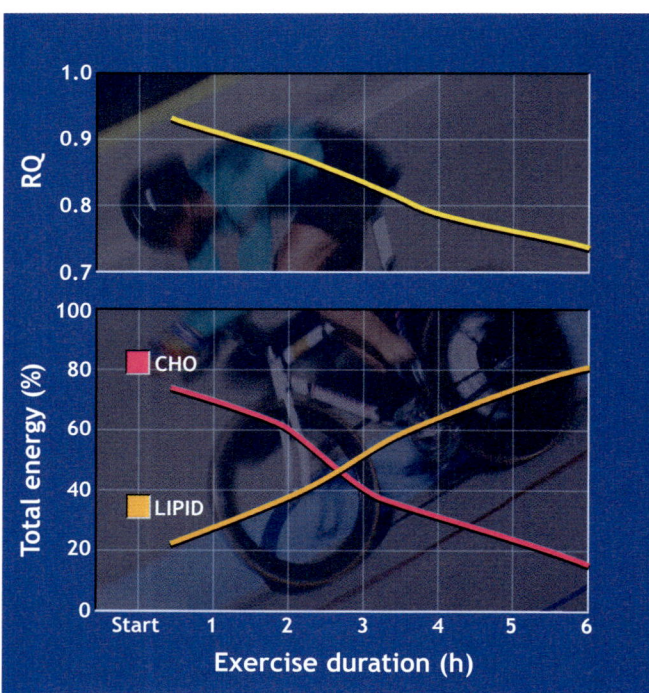

FIGURE 1.15. Respiratory quotient (*RQ*) dynamics during 6-hr-duration submaximal exercise (*top yellow line*). **Bottom figure** illustrates total energy percentage from carbohydrate (*pink line*) and lipid (*orange line*) during the activity.
(Adapted with permission from Edwards HT, et al. Metabolic rate, blood sugar and utilization of carbohydrate. Am J Physiol. 1934;108:203. ©The American Physiological Society (APS). All rights reserved.)

RQ [respiratory quotient]; see Chapter 8) steadily declines during physical activity (top yellow line), with lipid oxidation (orange line) supplying nearly 85% of the total energy. This classic research demonstrated lipid's crucial role in providing an uninterrupted energy supply even with glycogen depletion.

Increased lipid catabolism during prolonged physical activity likely results from a small drop in blood sugar and decreased insulin (a potent inhibitor of lipolysis) and corresponding increased pancreatic glucagon output. Such responses ultimately reduce glucose catabolism and its potential inhibitory effect on long-chain fatty acid breakdown to further stimulate FFA energy liberation. **FIGURE 1.16** plots active muscle's FFA uptake in hours 1 through 4 during moderate physical activity. In the first hour, lipids (including intramuscular lipid) supplied about 50% of the energy requirement, and up to 70% by the third hour.

Exercise intensity governs lipid's contribution to the metabolic mixture.[69,73] **FIGURE 1.17** illustrates lipid dynamics in trained males who exercised between 25 and 85% of maximum aerobic metabolism. During light-to-moderate exercise (≤40% of maximum), lipid provided the main energy source predominantly as plasma FFAs from adipose tissue depots. Increased exercise intensity produced an eventual *crossover* in fuel use balance, as total energy from all lipid breakdown sources remained essentially unchanged. More intense exercise required added energy from blood glucose and muscle glycogen. Total energy from lipids during exercise at 85% maximum did not differ from exercise at 25%.

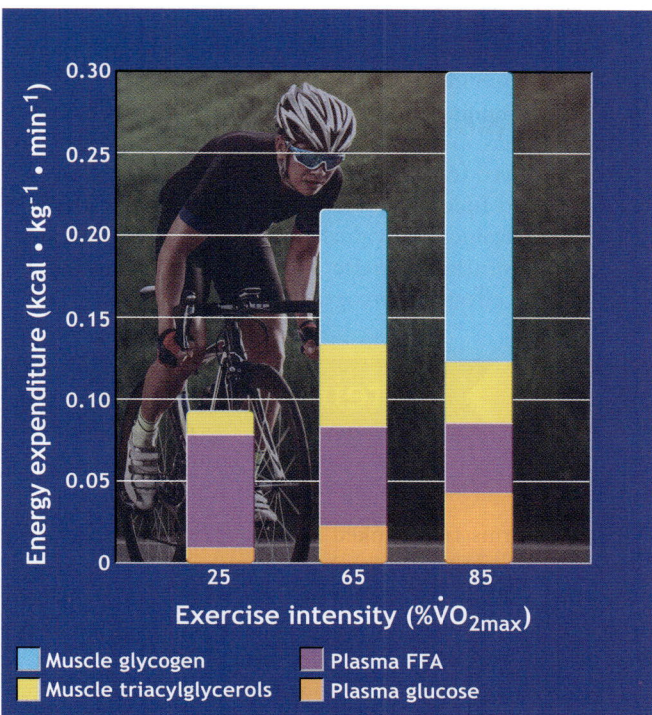

FIGURE 1.17. Energy expenditure related to exercise intensity for steady-state substrates in trained men during cycle ergometer exercise at 25 to 85% maximum capacity.
(Adapted with permission from Romijn JA, et al. Regulation of endogenous fat and carbohydrate metabolism in relation to exercise intensity and duration. *Am J Physiol-Endocrinology and Metabolism*. 1993;265:E380. ©The American Physiological Society (APS). All rights reserved. Patrick Foto/Shutterstock.)

These results confirm the major role that carbohydrate, primarily muscle glycogen, plays as a preferential fuel in intense aerobic exercise.

Regular aerobic exercise training profoundly improves long-chain fatty acid oxidation, particularly from triacylglycerols within active muscle during mild-to-moderate-intensity exercise.[4,26,72] **FIGURE 1.18** illustrates substrate utilization during 2 hr of moderate-intensity exercise before and after endurance training. For a total of 1000 kcal energy expenditure, intramuscular triacylglycerol combustion supplied about 25% of the total energy expenditure before training; this increased to beyond 40% after training. Energy from plasma FFA oxidation decreased from 18% pretraining to about 15% posttraining. Biopsy samples revealed a 41% reduced muscle glycogen combustion in the trained state, which accounted for an overall total energy decrease from all carbohydrate fuel sources (58% pretraining to 38% posttraining). The important point concerns greater FFA uptake and concurrent glycogen conservation by trained compared to untrained limbs at the same moderate absolute exercise level. Seven factors impact training-induced increases in lipid catabolism during physical activity:

1. Facilitated fatty acid mobilization from adipose tissue through increased lipolysis rate within adipocytes
2. Capillary proliferation in trained muscle, increasing the total microvessel number and density for energy substrate delivery
3. Improved FFA transport through the muscle fiber's plasma membrane
4. Increased fatty acid transport within the muscle cell, mediated by carnitine and carnitine acyltransferase
5. Increased mitochondrial size and number
6. Increased enzyme quantity involved in β-oxidation, citric acid cycle metabolism, and electron-transport chain within trained muscle fibers
7. Maintenance of cellular integrity and function (enhances endurance performance independent of conservation of glycogen reserves)

Endurance athletes exercise at a higher absolute submaximal exercise level from improved lipid oxidation capacity before experiencing glycogen depletion's fatiguing effects. This adaptation does not sustain the aerobic metabolism levels generated when oxidizing glycogen for energy. Sustained near-maximal aerobic effort still requires almost total reliance on stored glycogen oxidation for optimal performance.

INTEGRATIVE QUESTION

Why does a high daily physical activity level require regular carbohydrate intake? What "nonexercise" benefits occur from consuming a diet rich in unrefined, complex carbohydrates?

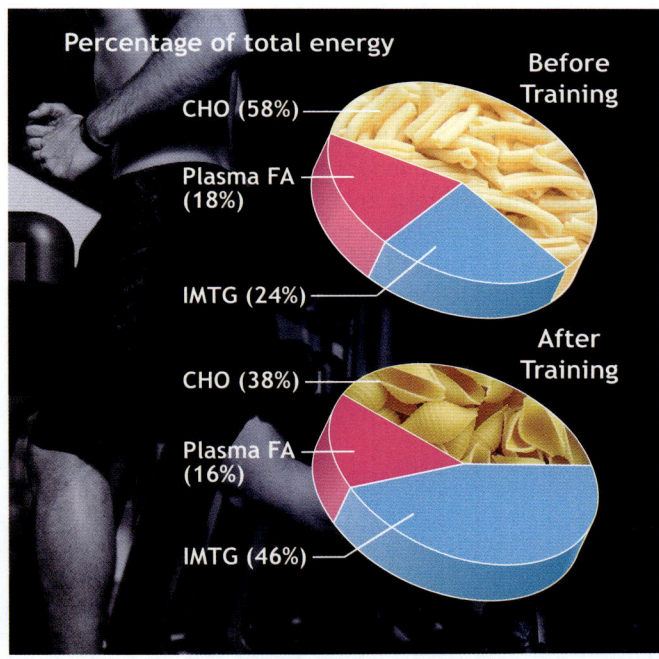

FIGURE 1.18. Percentage of total energy derived from carbohydrate (*CHO*), intramuscular triacylglycerol (*IMTG*), and plasma fatty acid (*FA*) fuel sources during prolonged exercise (8.3 kcal · min⁻¹) before and after endurance training.
(Adapted with permission from Martin WH III, et al. Effect of endurance training on plasma free fatty acid turnover and oxidation during exercise. *Am J Physiol-Endocrinology and Metabolism*. 1993;265:E708. ©The American Physiological Society (APS). All rights reserved. Shutterstock: Jasminko Ibrakovic; AN NGUYEN; bigacis.)

Summary

1. Lipids contain carbon, hydrogen, and oxygen atoms, but with a higher hydrogen-to-oxygen ratio.
2. The formula $C_{57}H_{110}O_6$ describes the lipid stearin. Lipid molecules include 1 glycerol molecule and 3 fatty acid molecules.
3. Lipids, synthesized by plants and animals, classify into three groups: simple lipids (glycerol plus three fatty acids), compound lipids (phospholipids, glycolipids, and lipoproteins) composed of simple lipids combined with other chemicals, and derived lipids (cholesterol), synthesized from simple and compound lipids.
4. Saturated fatty acids contain as many hydrogen atoms as chemically possible; they exist primarily in animal meat, egg yolk, dairy fats, and cheese.
5. A large saturated fatty acid intake elevates blood cholesterol concentration and promotes coronary heart disease.
6. Unsaturated fatty acids contain fewer hydrogen atoms attached to the carbon chain. Unlike saturated fatty acids, double bonds connect carbon atoms.
7. Fatty acids are either monounsaturated or polyunsaturated with respect to hydrogen. Increasing the diet's unsaturated fatty acid proportions protects against coronary heart disease.
8. Lowering LDL blood cholesterol provides significant heart disease protection.
9. Dietary lipid typically provides about 36% of the total energy intake.
10. Prudent recommendations suggest a 30% level or less for dietary lipid, with 70 to 80% as unsaturated fatty acids.
11. Lipids provide the largest nutrient store of potential energy for biologic work.
12. Lipids protect vital organs, provide insulation from the cold, and transport the four fat-soluble vitamins A, D, E, and K.
13. Lipids contribute 50 to 70% to the energy requirement in light-intensity and moderate-intensity physical activity.
14. Stored intramuscular lipid and derived lipid from adipocytes play an important role in prolonged physical activity when circulating FFAs provide more than 80% of the energy requirements.
15. Carbohydrate depletion reduces exercise intensity to a level determined by how well the body mobilizes and oxidizes fatty acids.
16. Aerobic training increases long-chain fatty acid oxidation during mild-to-moderate–intensity exercise, primarily fatty acids derived from triacylglycerols within active muscle.
17. Enhanced lipid oxidation with training spares glycogen to allow trained individuals to exercise at a higher absolute submaximal exercise level before experiencing the fatiguing effects of glycogen depletion.

Part 3 › Proteins

About Protein

A **protein** forms from linked amino acid combinations. An average-sized adult contains between 10 and 12 kg of protein, with skeletal muscle containing the largest quantity (6 to 8 kg), which represents between 60 to 75% of the body's total protein. Humans typically consume about 10 to 15% total calories as dietary protein. During digestion, the small intestine hydrolyzes protein to its amino acid constituents. Most adult's protein content remains remarkably stable, with little amino acid "reserves." Amino acids not used to synthesize protein or other compounds (e.g., hormones) or not available for energy metabolism provide substrate for gluconeogenesis or convert to triacylglycerol for storage in adipocytes.

Structurally, proteins resemble carbohydrates and lipids because they contain atoms of carbon, oxygen, and hydrogen. Protein molecules also contain about 16% nitrogen, along with sulfur and occasionally phosphorus, cobalt, and iron. Just as glycogen forms from many simple glucose subunits linked together, the protein molecule polymerizes from its amino acid "building-block" constituents in numerous complex arrays. **Peptide bonds** link amino acids in chains that take on diverse forms and chemical combinations. Two joined amino acids produce a **dipeptide**, and linking three amino acids produces a **tripeptide**. A **polypeptide** chain contains 50 to more than 1000 amino acids. Humans can synthesize many different protein types. Single cells contain thousands of different protein molecules; some have a linear configuration and some fold into complex shapes having three-dimensional properties. In total, the body contains approximately 50,000 different protein-containing compounds. Each of protein's biochemical functions and properties depends on the specific amino acids sequence as discussed more fully in Chapter 33.

The body's 20 different amino acids each has a positively charged amine group at one end of the molecule and a negatively charged organic acid group at the other end. The amine group has two hydrogen atoms attached to nitrogen (NH_2), whereas the organic acid group (technically termed *carboxylic acid group*) contains 1 carbon atom, 2 oxygen atoms, and 1 hydrogen atom (COOH). The remainder, referred to as the **R group or side chain**, presents in different forms. *The R group's specific structure dictates the amino acid's particular characteristics.* **FIGURE 1.19** illustrates

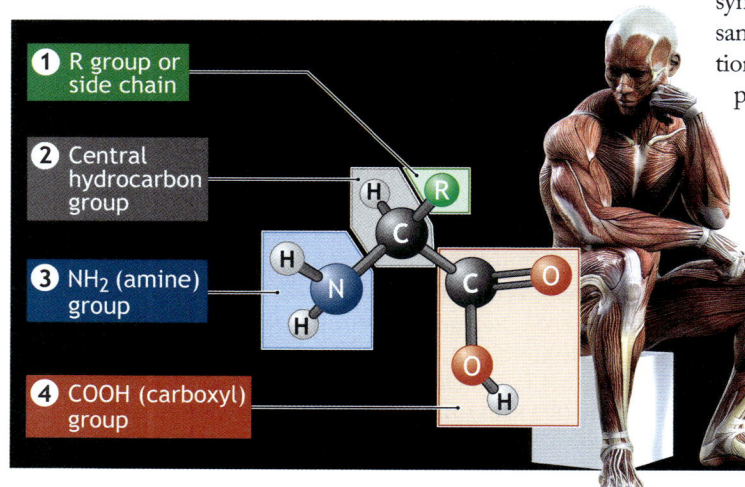

FIGURE 1.19. Four common amino acid features.
(mrjo/Shutterstock.)

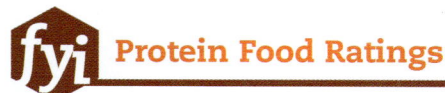 **Protein Food Ratings**

Protein Ratings for Common Foods

Food	Rating
Eggs	100
Fish	70
Lean beef	69
Cow's milk	60
Brown rice	57
White rice	56
Soybean	47
Brewer's hash	45
Whole-grain wheat	44
Peanuts	43
Dry beans	34
White potato	34

Nataly Studio/Shutterstock

four common features about the structure of all amino acids. The potential to combine 20 amino acids produces an almost infinite number of proteins, depending on their amino acid combinations. For example, linking just three different amino acids could generate 20^3 or 8000 different proteins.

Protein Categories

The body cannot synthesize eight amino acids (nine in children and some older adults), so individuals must consume foods that contain them. These make up the **essential amino acids** (also known as indispensable amino acids) *isoleucine, leucine, lysine, methionine, phenylalanine, threonine, tryptophan,* and *valine*. In addition, the body synthesizes cystine from methionine and tyrosine from phenylalanine. Infants cannot synthesize histidine, and children have reduced capability to synthesize arginine. The body manufactures the remaining nine **nonessential amino acids**. The term *nonessential* means these proteins are synthesized from other compounds already in the body at a rate that meets the body's needs for normal growth and tissue repair. It does not mean they are unimportant.

Animals and plants manufacture proteins that contain essential amino acids. An animal-derived amino acid has no health or physiologic advantage over the same amino acid from vegetable origin. Plants synthesize amino acids by incorporating nitrogen from the soil along with carbon, oxygen, and hydrogen from air and water. In contrast, animals have no broad capability for amino acid synthesis; so instead, they consume most of their protein. Synthesizing a specific protein requires appropriate amino acid availability. **Complete proteins**, sometimes referred to as higher-quality proteins, exist in foods containing all essential amino acids in the quantity and correct ratio to maintain nitrogen balance and to provide for tissue growth and repair. An **incomplete protein** lacks one or more essential amino acids. A diet of incomplete protein eventually leads to **protein malnutrition**, whether or not the food sources contain an adequate energy or protein amount.

Protein Sources

Complete protein sources include eggs, milk, meat, fish, and poultry. Eggs provide the optimal mixture of essential amino acids among all food sources; hence, eggs receive the highest quality rating of 100 compared with other foods.

TABLE 1.2 provides some common protein food sources from animal, dairy, and plant categories. Reliance on animal sources for dietary protein accounts for the relatively high cholesterol and saturated fatty acid intake among major industrialized nations.

TABLE 1.2 Protein content for common foods

High-quality protein foods come from animal sources except for the soy isolate proteins such as **tofu**. Vegetables (e.g., lentils, dried beans and peas, nuts, and cereals) remain incomplete in one or more essential amino acids, making their proteins have lower biologic value. It is unnecessary to consume all essential amino acids in a single meal, as once

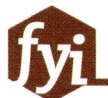 **Plant-Based Diets Reduce Heart Disease Risk**

Researchers with the Physicians Committee for Responsible Medicine (www.pcrm.org/) reviewed multiple observational studies and clinical trials and concluded that plant-based dietary patterns protect against atherosclerosis and decrease the potent heart disease risk markers of blood pressure, blood lipids, and body weight. Specifically, the review concluded that a plant-based diet:

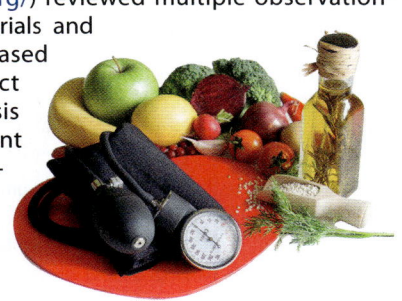
udra11/Shutterstock

- Reduces death risk from cardiovascular disease by 40%
- Reduces coronary heart disease risk by 40%
- Successfully opens fully or partially blocked arteries in up to 91% of patients
- Reduces hypertension risk by 34%
- Associates with a 29 mg · dL^{-1} lower total cholesterol and 23 mg · dL^{-1} lower LDL-C level compared with nonvegetarian diets
- Associates with significant weight loss

believed, as long as balance is maintained over a whole day. *Eating ample grains, fruits, and vegetables supplies all essential amino acids.* Older individuals may benefit from eating good protein sources at each meal throughout the day to support muscle mass and muscle strength maintenance and curtail the inevitable losses brought on by aging.

The Vegan Approach

True vegetarians (**vegans**) consume nutrients from only two sources—the plant kingdom and dietary supplements. In the U.S. population, only 4% consider themselves vegans, yet between 5 and 7% consider themselves "almost-vegans," with nutritional diversity remaining the key for these individuals. For example, a vegan diet contains all essential amino acids if the recommended protein intake contains 60% protein from grain products, 35% from legumes, and 5% from green leafy vegetables.

Many competitive and champion athletes consume diets predominantly from varied plant sources but include some dairy and meat products.[12,54,84-87]

Vegetarian athletes often encounter difficulty planning, selecting, and preparing nutritious meals with a proper amino acid mixture from only plant sources without relying on supplementation. In contrast to diets that rely heavily on animal protein sources, well-balanced vegan and vegetarian-type diets provide abundant carbohydrate crucial for intense, prolonged training. These diets contain little or no cholesterol but abundant

fyi Consume Less Red Meat for a More Healthful Diet

- Red meat consumption relates directly to total mortality and heart disease incidence and strokes, type2 diabetes, and some cancers, particularly colorectal and breast cancer in adolescence and early adult life
- Death rate reduced up to nearly 10% by eating less than half a serving of red meat daily. Meats with the strongest links to cancer include processed meats with added nitrites and nitrates (e.g., cured, smoked, or salted bacon, ham, sausage, hot dogs, and luncheon meats) SofiaV/Shutterstock
- Colorectal cancer risk may link to a high level of nitrite preservatives in processed meats and nitrosamines formed in some vegetables
- On postmortem examination, almost all livestock including poultry contain some antibiotics in their tissues, which may contribute to these drugs' ineffectiveness to fight human infections

Sources:
Bianchi F, et al. Replacing meat with alternative plant-based products (RE-MAPs): protocol for a randomised controlled trial of a behavioural intervention to reduce meat consumption. *BMJ Open*. 2019;9:e027016.
Cases A, et al. Vegetable-based diets for chronic kidney disease? It is time to reconsider. *Nutrients*. 2019;11:1263.
White MC, et al. Prevalence of modifiable cancer risk factors among U.S. adults aged 18-44 years. *Am J Prev Med*. 2017;53:S14.

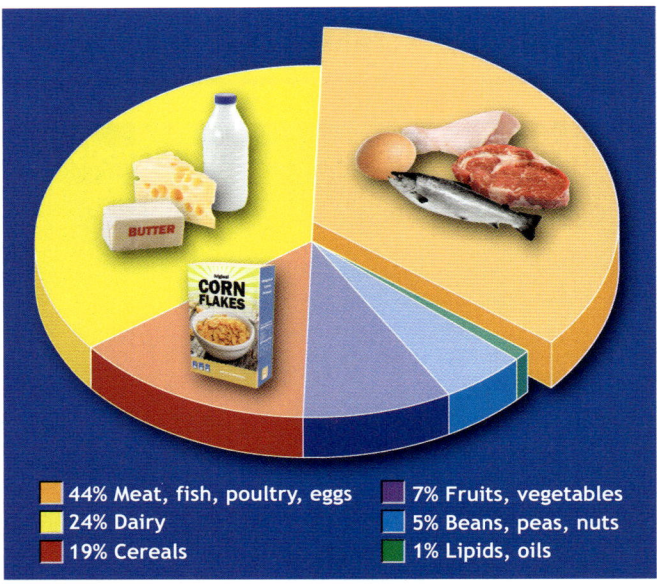

FIGURE 1.20. Contribution from major food sources to the protein content in the typical American diet.
(Shutterstock: Diana Jo Marmont; Elena Schweitzer; Gts; FabrikaSimf; nexus 7; saiko3p; Cameramannz.)

fiber, and rich fruit and vegetable sources of diverse phytochemicals and antioxidant vitamins. A **lactovegetarian diet** provides dairy products such as milk, ice cream, cheese, and yogurt. The lactovegetarian approach minimizes difficulty consuming sufficient protein and increases calcium, phosphorus, and vitamin B_{12} intake. Adding an egg to the diet (**ovolactovegetarian diet**) ensures high-quality protein intake. The pie chart in **FIGURE 1.20** displays protein's major food category contributions to the typical American diet. Note that meat, fish, poultry, and eggs account for the largest percentage contribution (44%), while dairy contributes 24%, with lipids lowest at 1%.

Recommended Protein Intake

Despite many coaches, trainers, and athletes' beliefs, little benefit accrues from consuming excessive protein. *Muscle mass does not increase simply by consuming high-protein foods* from powders, pills, shakes, and specialty meal plans. Elite endurance-trained and resistance-trained athletes' diets often exceed two to five times the recommended intake, usually as meat. This occurs primarily for two reasons:

1. Athletes' diets normally emphasize high-protein foods, an idea from the late 19th century first promoted by German chemist Justus von Liebig (see this text's Introduction).
2. Athletes' caloric intake and energy output surpass those of sedentary counterparts.

If lean tissue synthesis resulted from extra protein consumed by the typical athlete, then muscle mass would increase tremendously, beyond the skeleton's capacity to support the increased mass. For example, consuming an extra 100 g protein (400 kcal) daily would translate to a daily 500-g/1.1-lb increase in muscle mass. This obviously does not happen. Excessive dietary protein either catabolizes directly for energy (following deamination) or recycles as other molecular components, including lipid stored in subcutaneous depots. Excessive dietary protein intake can trigger harmful side effects, particularly strained liver and kidney function from urea elimination.

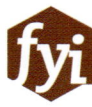 Fact Sheet: FDA's Restaurant Menu Labeling Implementation

The Food and Drug Administration (FDA) wrote the following position statement about Food Labeling practices for restaurants, including chain restaurants: (www.fda.gov/food/food-labeling-nutrition/fdas-implementation-menu-labeling-moving-forward#footnote3):

Nutrition information has been provided to consumers via the labels of most packaged foods for many years. However, before the enactment of the menu labeling laws, nutrition labeling was not generally made available to consumers for foods in restaurants and similar retail food establishments. The Federal Food, Drug, and Cosmetic (FD&C) Act and the Food and Drug Administration's food labeling regulations now require that calorie and other nutrition information be provided in "covered establishments" (chain restaurants or similar retail food establishments) that serve restaurant-type food. At present, the FDA is committed to working flexibly with establishments to help them achieve compliance. We will continue to build on these efforts and our commitment to help inform and educate industry as we move forward in the implementation of menu labeling.

OrelPhoto/Shutterstock

The FD&C Act requires chain restaurants or similar retail food establishments to do the following:

- Post calorie information on menus and menu boards for all standard menu items
- Disclose calorie information on signs adjacent to foods on display and self-service foods that are standard menu items
- Include a succinct statement concerning suggested daily caloric intake and a statement of availability for written nutrition information on menus and menu boards
- Upon a customer's request, have required written nutrition information available on the premises of a chain restaurant or similar retail food establishment

The RDA Represents a Liberal Standard

The **Recommended Dietary Allowance (RDA)** for protein, vitamins, and minerals represents a standard for nutrient intake expressed as a daily average. These guidelines, initially developed in 1943 by the Food and Nutrition Board of the National Research Council/National Academy of Science (https://ods.od.nih.gov/HealthInformation/Dietary_Reference_Intakes.aspx), have been revised periodically.[18] RDA levels represent a liberal yet safe excess to prevent nutritional deficiencies in practically all healthy persons. The online recommendations include 10 macronutrients, 15 vitamins, 21 minerals, body mass index (BMI) calculations, daily caloric needs, and recommended total water intake. The **Estimated Safe and Adequate Daily Dietary Intakes** (ESADDIs) recommendation for certain essential micronutrients (e.g., vitamins biotin and pantothenic acid and trace elements copper, manganese, fluoride, selenium, chromium, and molybdenum) required sufficient scientific data to formulate intake ranges considered adequate and safe, yet insufficient to precisely determine an RDA value. No RDA or ESADDI exists for sodium, potassium, and chlorine; instead, recommendations refer to a minimum requirement for health. The average female consumes 35% more protein than the RDA, while the average male consumes about 65% more than recommended.

We emphasize that the RDA reflects a *population's* nutritional needs over a long time period, and only laboratory measurements can assess a specific individual's requirement. Malnutrition occurs from cumulative weeks, months, and even years of inadequate nutrient intake. Someone who regularly consumes a diet that contains nutrients below the RDA standards may not become malnourished. *The RDA represents a probability statement for adequate nutrition; as nutrient intake falls below the RDA, the statistical probability for malnourishment increases for that person and the probability progressively increases with lower nutrient intake.* In Chapter 2, we discuss the **Dietary Reference Intakes** that represent the current standards for recommended nutrients and other food component intakes.[17]

The data in the unnumbered table list the protein RDAs for adolescent and adult males and females. *On average, 0.83 g protein · kg body mass^{-1} represents the recommended daily intake.* To determine the protein requirement for males and females ages 18 to 65, multiply body mass in kg by 0.83. For a 90-kg man, total protein requirement equals 75 g (90 × 0.83). The protein RDA holds even for overweight persons; it includes an approximate 25% reserve to account for individual differences in the protein requirement for about 97% of the population. Generally, the protein RDA (and the required essential amino acid quantity) decreases with age. In contrast, the protein RDA for infants and growing children equals 2.0 to 4.0 g · kg body mass^{-1}. Pregnant women should increase total daily protein intake by 20 g, and nursing mothers should increase daily intake by an additional 10 g. *A 10% increase in the calculated protein requirement, particularly for a vegetarian-type diet, accounts for dietary fiber's effect to reduce the digestibility of many plant-based protein sources.* Stress, disease, and injury usually increase protein requirements.

Do Athletes Require Greater Protein Intake?

Debate focuses about the possible need for a larger protein requirement for still-maturing adolescent athletes, athletes involved in resistance-training programs that stimulate muscle growth and endurance training regimens that increase protein breakdown, and wrestlers and American football players subjected to recurring tissue microtrauma.[8,67,89] We present additional information about protein balance during physical activity and training in subsequent sections of this chapter.

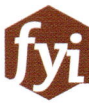

Increased Protein Intake and Strength Training in Older Adults

Recommended protein intake amounts may be too low for older individuals. Two strategies to combat **sarcopenia** with aging would be to consume protein in excess of recommended amounts, and to undertake regular muscle strengthening workouts. Sarcopenia afflicts 15% of people age 65 and older, and 50% above age 80. Synthesizing muscle from protein decreases with age, so increasing high quality protein intake daily would help to minimize sarcopenia and maintain or even increase strength in older adults and the elderly.

karelnoppe/Shutterstock

Sources:
Larsson L, et al. Sarcopenia: aging-related loss of muscle mass and function. *Physiol Rev.* 2019;99:427.
Migliavacca E, et al. Mitochondrial oxidative capacity and NAD$^+$ biosynthesis are reduced in human sarcopenia across ethnicities. *Nat Commun.* 2019;10:5808.

Protein's Role in the Body

Blood plasma, visceral tissue, and muscle represent the three major protein sources in the body. No macronutrient "storage tanks" exist for this macronutrient; all protein sources contribute to building tissue structures or as constituents of metabolic, transport, and hormonal systems. Protein makes up between 12 and 15% of body mass. As would be expected, protein content varies considerably for different cells in different individuals. A brain cell, for example, contains about 10% protein, while red blood cells and muscle cells include up to 20% protein by weight. Also, skeletal muscle's protein content increases somewhat systematically with intense resistance training, but to varying degrees based largely on individual differences in the hormonal response and muscle fiber type. Rapid growth in infancy and childhood triggers tissue anabolism, which accounts for about one third of the protein consumption. Amino acids provide the major building blocks for synthesizing tissue components. Amino acid molecules incorporate into these 12 structural entities:

1. Actin and myosin (muscle microstructures)
2. Cell nucleus (with DNA)
3. Cell plasma membranes
4. Cytoplasmic ribonucleic acid (RNA)
5. Enzymes
6. Epinephrine and norepinephrine (catecholamine hormones)
7. Hair, skin, nails, bones, tendons, ligaments
8. Components of hemoglobin and myoglobin
9. Nicotinamide adenine dinucleotide (NAD) and flavin adenine dinucleotide (FAD)
10. Serotonin (neurotransmitter).
11. Thrombin, fibrin, fibrinogen (blood clotting)
12. Vitamins

Protein Metabolism Dynamics

Dietary protein's main contribution is amino acids, which participate in tissue-building anabolic processes and catabolism of some protein for energy. In well-nourished individuals at rest, protein catabolism contributes between 2 and 5% of the body's total energy requirement. During this process, protein first degrades into its component amino acids. The amino acid molecule then loses its nitrogen (amine group) in the liver (**deamination**) to form urea (H_2NCONH_2). The remaining deaminated amino acid then converts to a new amino acid, converts to carbohydrate or lipid, or catabolizes directly for energy. Urea formed in deamination, including some ammonia, is excreted as urine. Excessive protein catabolism promotes fluid loss because urea must dissolve in water.

Enzymes in muscle facilitate nitrogen removal from certain amino acids (usually alpha-ketoglutarate acid or glutamate; **FIG. 1.21**), with nitrogen passed to other compounds in reversible **transamination** reactions. Transamination occurs when an amine group from a donor amino acid transfers to an acceptor acid to form a new amino acid. The transferase enzyme accelerates the transamination reaction. In muscle, transamination incorporates branched-chain amino acids (BCAAs; leucine, isoleucine, and valine) that generate branched-chain ketoacids (mediated by BCAA transferase). This allows amino acid formation from the non-nitrogen-carrying organic compound pyruvate formed in metabolism. In deamination and transamination, the carbon skeleton of the nonnitrogenous amino acid residue undergoes further degradation during energy metabolism.

FIGURE 1.22 shows the carbon sources from amino acids and the major metabolic paths taken by the deaminated carbon skeletons. Upon removal of their amine group, all amino

Recommended Protein	Male		Female	
	Teen	Adult	Teen	Adult
Daily protein, g · BM^{-1}	0.9	0.8	0.9	0.8
Daily protein, g · average BM^{-1}	59.0	56.0	50.0	44.0

Iulian Valentin/Shutterstock
Syda Productions/Shutterstock

BM, body mass.
Average BM is based on a "reference" male and female. For adolescents (14–18 y), body mass averages 65.8 kg/145 lb for males and 55.7 kg/123 lb for females. For adults, body mass averages 70 kg/154 lb for males and 56.8 kg/125 lb for females.

acids form reactive citric acid cycle intermediates or related compounds. Some larger amino acid molecules (e.g., leucine, tryptophan, and isoleucine—colored green, white, and red, respectively) generate carbon-containing compounds that enter the yellow-coded citric acid cycle's reactions governed by enzymes at different stages to ultimately produce ATP while releasing carbon dioxide and water by-products. Chapter 6 presents a more detailed discussion about energy transfer reactions and citric acid cycle metabolic functions.

Nitrogen Balance

Nitrogen balance occurs when nitrogen intake (protein) equals nitrogen excretion as follows:

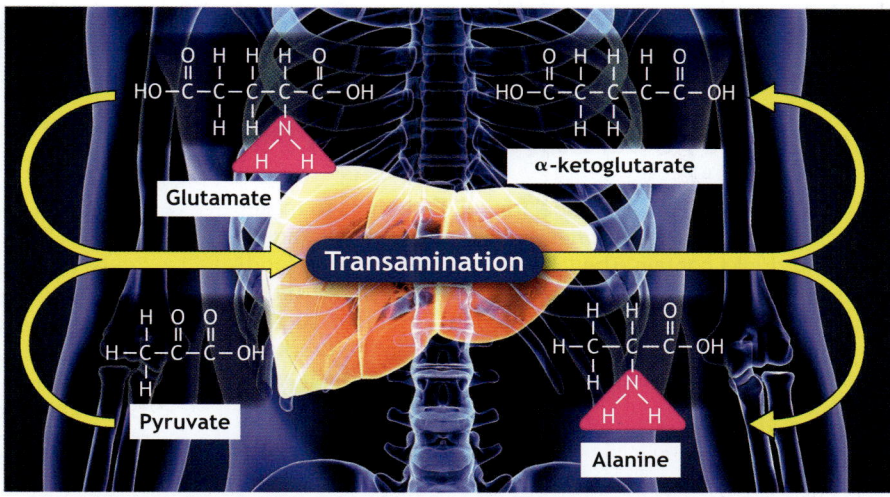

FIGURE 1.21. Transamination provides for intramuscular amino acid synthesis from nonprotein sources. A new amino acid forms when an amine group from a donor group transfers to an acceptor, non-nitrogen-containing acid.
(Life science/Shutterstock.)

$$\text{Nitrogen balance} = N_t - N_a - N_f - N_s = 0$$

where N_t = total nitrogen intake from food; N_u = nitrogen in urine; N_f = nitrogen in feces; and N_s = nitrogen in sweat.

In **positive nitrogen balance**, nitrogen intake exceeds nitrogen excretion to synthesize new tissues from any additional protein. With adequate nutrition, positive nitrogen balance occurs in these conditions:

1. Child growth
2. Pregnancy
3. Recovery from illness
4. Protein synthesis with resistance-exercise training

The body does not develop a protein reserve as it does with lipid storage in adipose tissue or carbohydrate storage as muscle and liver glycogen. Nevertheless, individuals who consume the recommended protein intake have a higher muscle and liver protein content than do individuals who are fed too little protein. Also, muscle protein can be "tapped" to supply additional energy for metabolic functions. In contrast, proteins in neural and connective tissues remain relatively "fixed" because cellular constituents cannot be mobilized for energy without disrupting tissue functions.

Greater nitrogen output than intake, or **negative nitrogen balance**, indicates protein use for energy and possible encroachment from the skeletal muscle's amino acid "storehouse." Interestingly, a negative nitrogen balance occurs even when protein intake exceeds the recommended standard when the body catabolizes protein because of a lack of other energy nutrients. For example, an individual who participates regularly in intense training may consume adequate or even excess protein yet inadequate energy from carbohydrate or lipid. In this scenario, protein increasingly becomes an energy fuel, which creates a negative protein or nitrogen balance and eventual lean tissue loss. The protein-sparing role of dietary carbohydrate and lipid discussed previously becomes important under these conditions:

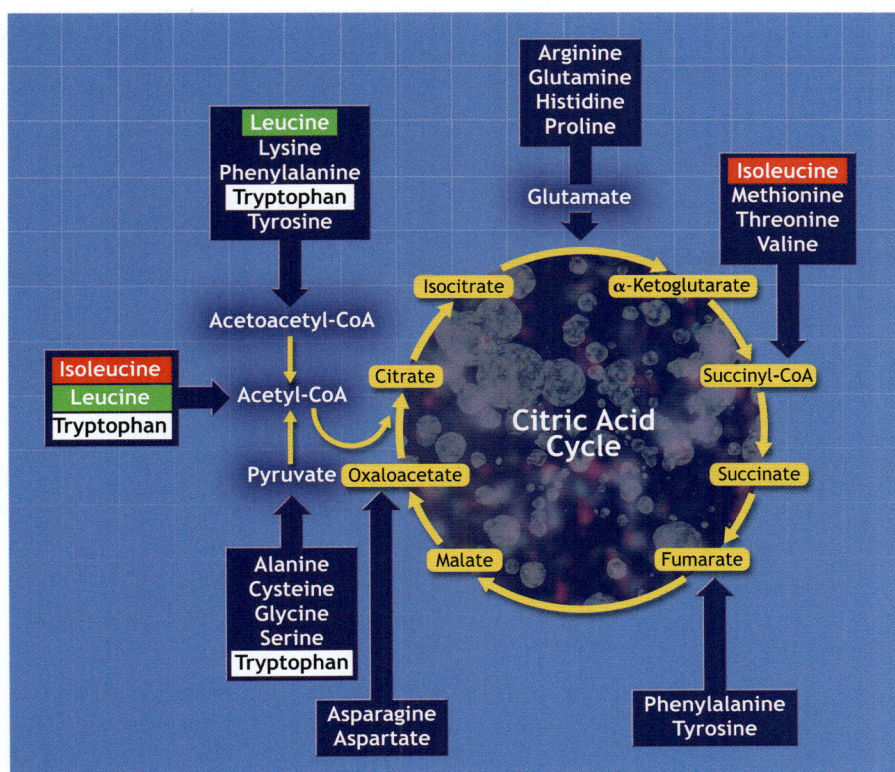

FIGURE 1.22. Major metabolic pathways amino acids follow after deamination or transamination removes the nitrogen group.
(Pixus/Shutterstock.)

In a Practical Sense

The Latest Food Label Nutrition Panel

The revamped nutrition facts label for 2020 attempts to make it easier to see how many calories and added sugars packaged foods and drinks contain. The label is intended to make food choices healthier and safer by adjusting serving size to more realistic levels and specifying the amount of added sugars. The new label lists the quantity of total sugars in the product, including those sugars that are naturally occurring such as in fruits and milk.

The new food label incorporates the following changes:

- Servings per container and serving size are now in larger and/or bolder type.
- Serving sizes have been updated to reflect what people eat and drink today.
- Serving sizes are now based on the amount of food that is customarily eaten at one time and are not a recommendation of how much to eat.
- "Servings per container" now shows the total number of servings in the entire food package or container.
  - The number of calories is now in larger and bolder type.
  - "Calories" refers to the total number of calories, or "energy," supplied from all sources (fat, carbohydrate, protein, and alcohol) in one serving of the food.
  - The "Daily Values" for nutrients have been updated based on new scientific evidence.
  - "% Daily Value (%DV)" shows how much a nutrient in a serving of the food contributes to a total daily diet.
  - The nutrients that are required on the label have been updated.
  - "Added Sugars" is now required on the label and includes sugars that either are added during the processing of foods or packaged as such (e.g., a bag of table sugar) or occur naturally, such as in syrups, honey, and concentrated fruit or vegetable juices.
  - Vitamin D and potassium are also required on the label.
  - Vitamins A and C are no longer required on the label.

Although the ingredient list is not part of the Nutrition Facts label, it is also a helpful tool; it now shows each ingredient in a food by its common or usual name; ingredients are also listed in descending order by weight, so the ingredient that weighs the most is listed first, and the ingredient that weighs the least is listed last.

Side-by-Side Comparison

Original Label

Nutrition Facts	
Serving Size 2/3 cup (55g)	
Servings Per Container 8	
Amount Per Serving	
Calories 230	Calories from Fat 70
	% Daily Value*
Total Fat 8g	12%
Saturated Fat 1g	5%
Trans Fat 0g	
Cholesterol 0mg	0%
Sodium 160mg	7%
Total Carbohydrate 37g	12%
Dietary Fiber 4g	16%
Sugars 12g	
Protein 3g	
Vitamin A	10%
Vitamin C	8%
Calcium	20%
Iron	45%

*Percent Daily Values are based on a 2,000 calorie diet. Your Daily Value may be higher or lower depending on your calorie needs.

	Calories:	2,000	2,500
Total Fat	Less than	65g	80g
Sat Fat	Less than	20g	25g
Cholesterol	Less than	300mg	300mg
Sodium	Less than	2,400mg	2,400mg
Total Carbohydrate		300g	375g
Dietary Fiber		25g	30g

New Label

Nutrition Facts	
8 servings per container	
Serving size	**2/3 cup (55g)**
Amount per serving	
Calories	**230**
	% Daily Value*
Total Fat 8g	10%
Saturated Fat 1g	5%
Trans Fat 0g	
Cholesterol 0mg	0%
Sodium 160mg	7%
Total Carbohydrate 37g	13%
Dietary Fiber 4g	14%
Total Sugars 12g	
Includes 10g Added Sugars	20%
Protein 3g	
Vitamin D 2mcg	10%
Calcium 260mg	20%
Iron 8mg	45%
Potassium 240mg	6%

* The % Daily Value (DV) tells you how much a nutrient in a serving of food contributes to a daily diet. 2,000 calories a day is used for general nutrition advice.

---

1. During periods of tissue growth
2. From the high-energy output and/or tissue synthesis requirements of intense training
3. From the negative nitrogen balance consequences of diabetes, fever, burns, dieting, growth, and steroid administration
4. Semistarvation (several hundred calories below requirements over a protracted period that produces substantial weight loss), and starvation (severe energy intake deficiency, which in the extreme, produces organ damage and eventual death)

Protein breakdown increases only modestly with most modes and intensities of physical activity, yet muscle protein synthesis rises substantially following endurance-type and resistance-type physical activities.[8,57,88] Two factors justify re-examining protein intake recommendations for participants in intense training:

1. Increased protein breakdown during long-term exercise and protracted training
2. Increased protein synthesis in recovery from physical activity

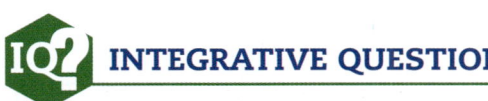

INTEGRATIVE QUESTION

If muscle growth with resistance training occurs primarily from additional protein deposition within the cell, would extra protein consumption above the RDA facilitate muscle growth?

Protein Dynamics During Physical Activity

Current understanding of protein dynamics during physical activity comes from studies that expand the classic method of determining protein breakdown through urea excretion. For example, the release of labeled CO_2 from amino acids injected or ingested increases during exercise in proportion to the metabolic rate.[74] As exercise progresses, plasma urea concentration also increases, coupled with a dramatic rise in sweat's nitrogen excretion, often without any change in urinary nitrogen excretion.[27,60] These observations account for prior conclusions concerning minimal protein breakdown during endurance exercise because prior studies only measured nitrogen in urine. The sweat mechanism serves an important role in excreting nitrogen from breakdown during physical activity (FIG. 1.23). Nonetheless, urea production may not reflect all protein breakdown because oxidation of plasma and intracellular leucine—an essential BCAA—increases during moderate physical activity independent of urea production changes.[6,74]

Figure 1.23 also illustrates that protein's energy use reaches its highest level during exercise in the glycogen-depleted state. This emphasizes carbohydrate's important role as a protein-sparer and indicates how carbohydrate availability affects the demand on protein "reserves" in physical activity. Protein breakdown and gluconeogenesis undoubtedly play a role during endurance physical activity or frequent intense training when glycogen reserves diminish.

Increases in protein catabolism during endurance activities and intense training often mirror the metabolic mixture in acute starvation. With depleted glycogen reserves, gluconeogenesis from amino acid's carbon skeletons largely sustains the liver's glucose output. Augmented protein breakdown reflects the body's attempt to maintain blood glucose for central nervous system functioning. *Athletes in training should consume a high-carbohydrate diet with adequate energy to conserve muscle protein.* The increased protein use for energy and depressed protein synthesis during intense physical activity may partly explain why individuals who resistance-train to build muscle size generally refrain from glycogen-depleting endurance workouts to avoid muscle catabolism and resulting muscle "teardown."

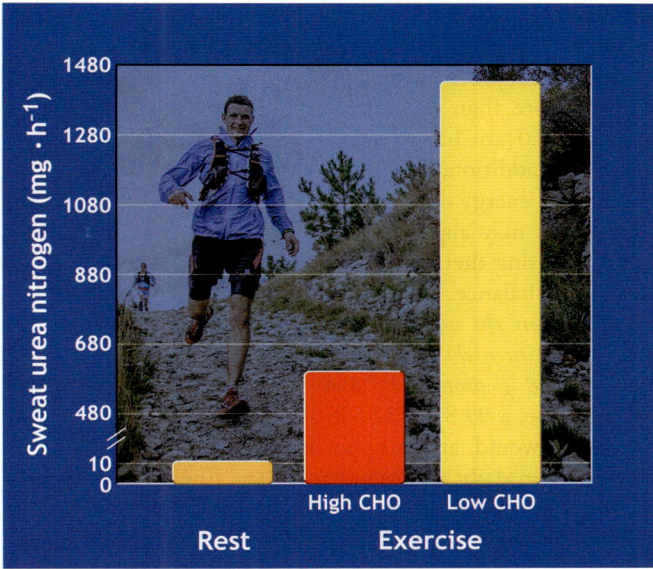

FIGURE 1.23. Urea in sweat excretion at rest and during exercise after carbohydrate loading (high CHO; *red bar*) and carbohydrate depletion (low CHO; *yellow bar*). Low glycogen reserves trigger a larger protein energy contribution assessed by sweat urea.
(Adapted with permission from Lemon PWR, Nagel F. Effects of exercise on protein and amino acid metabolism. *Med Sci Sports Exerc.* 1981;13:141. sportpoint/Shutterstock.)

Modifying Recommended Protein Intake

Research continues to determine whether the initial increased protein demand with arduous training creates a true long-term increase in protein requirement above the RDA. *A definitive answer remains elusive, but protein breakdown above the resting level does indeed occur during endurance and resistance training to a greater degree than previously believed.*[8] Increased protein catabolism occurs to a greater extent when exercising with low carbohydrate reserves and/or low energy or protein intakes.[56,88]

 Removing Nitrogen and Amino Acids

Following deamination (nitrogen removal), the remaining carbon skeletons from either α-keto acid (e.g., pyruvate, oxaloacetate, α-ketoglutarate) follow one of three biochemical routes:

1. **Gluconeogenesis**—18 of 20 amino acids serve as a source for glucose synthesis.
2. **Energy source**—Carbon skeletons oxidize for energy because they form intermediates in citric acid cycle metabolism.
3. **Lipid synthesis**—All amino acids provide potential acetyl-CoA to furnish substrate for fatty acid synthesis.

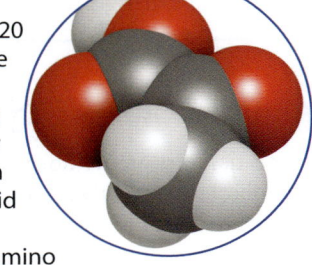

StudioMolekuul/Shutterstock

Unfortunately, research has not pinpointed protein requirements for individuals who resistance-train 4 to 6 hr daily. Their protein needs may average only slightly more than sedentary requirements (perhaps 1.0 to 1.2 g protein · kg body mass^{-1}). In addition, despite increased protein use for energy during intense training, adaptations may augment the body's efficiency in using dietary protein to enhance amino acid balance.

Based on the available evidence, athletes who train intensely should consume between 1.2 and 1.8 g protein · kg body mass^{-1} daily. For example, a 99.8-kg/220-lb American football linebacker would, at the upper end, require 180 g (1.8 × 99.8) protein daily, equivalent to 6.3 oz. The daily value at the lower end would equal 120 g protein (1.2 × 99.8) or 4.2 oz. Protein intake exceeding 1.8 g offers no further advantage to athletes with regard to whole-body protein use.[22] This upper daily value falls within the range typically consumed by physically active males and females, obviating the need to consume supplementary protein.[12] Presleep protein ingestion also may enhance muscle protein synthesis during overnight sleep and boost skeletal muscle's adaptive exercise training responses. When applied during resistance training, presleep protein supplementation facilitates muscle mass and strength increases.[90] In physically active older adults with low habitual dietary protein consumption, larger increases occurred in relative lean body mass and greater fat mass losses in subjects receiving 12-wk daily protein supplementation compared with controls receiving no extra protein.[91] With adequate protein intake, consuming animal protein sources does not facilitate muscle strength or size gains with resistance training compared with protein intake from plant sources.[28] Based on recommendations from the American College of Sports Medicine (www.acsm.org) and American Dietetic Association (www.eatright.org), a reasonable daily protein intake for vegetarian athletes should range between 1.3 and 1.8 g · kg^{-1} body weight.

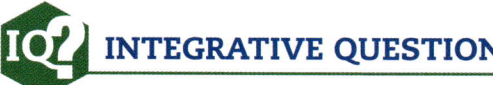

INTEGRATIVE QUESTION

What two questions would an exercise physiologist raise concerning the current protein RDA for those who participate during intense training?

Alanine-Glucose Cycle

Some tissue proteins do not readily metabolize for energy, yet muscle proteins can provide energy for physical activity.[9,25] For example, alanine *indirectly* participates in energy metabolism when exercise energy demand increases. Its release from active leg muscle increases proportionately to exercise severity.[77]

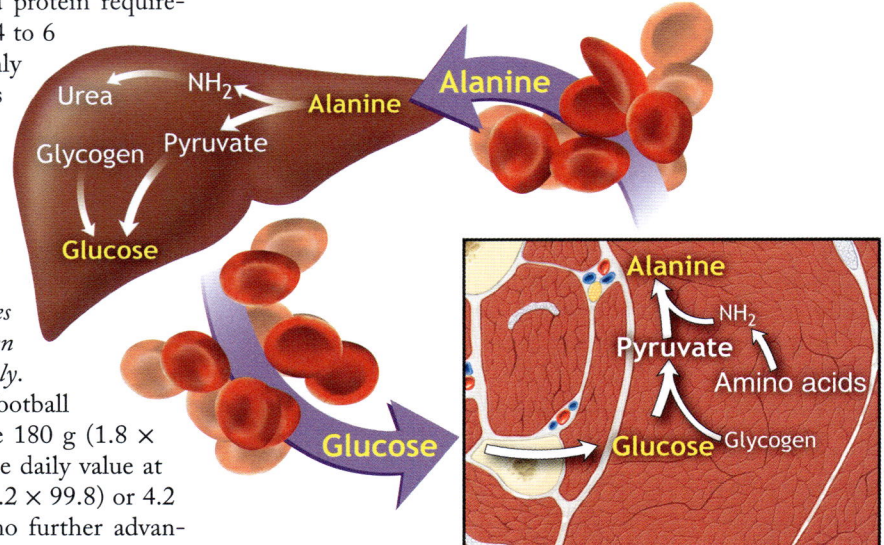

FIGURE 1.24. The alanine-glucose cycle describes alanine synthesis in muscle by glucose-derived pyruvate transamination and release into the bloodstream. Alanine's carbon skeleton reconverts to glucose in the liver, and is released into the bloodstream for uptake by muscle and alanine resynthesis.
(Republished with permission of American Society for Clinical Investigation; permission conveyed through Copyright Clearance Center. From Felig P, Wahren J. Amino acid metabolism in exercising man. *J Clin Invest.* 1971;50:2703.)

Active skeletal muscle synthesizes alanine during transamination from the glucose intermediate pyruvate with nitrogen derived in part from the amino acid leucine. The residual carbon fragment from the amino acid that formed alanine oxidizes for energy within skeletal muscle. Alanine then exits the muscle and deaminates in the liver. During gluconeogenesis, alanine's remaining carbon skeleton converts to glucose, and enters the blood for delivery to active muscle. **FIGURE 1.24** summarizes classic research showing the sequence for the **alanine-glucose cycle**. Alanine, synthesized in muscle from glucose-derived pyruvate via transamination, enters the blood where the liver converts it to glucose and urea. Glucose release into the blood coincides with its subsequent delivery to muscle for energy. During physical activity, increased alanine production and output from muscle helps to maintain blood glucose for nervous system and active muscle needs. After 4 hr of continuous light physical activity, the liver's alanine-derived glucose output accounts for about 45% of the liver's total glucose release. *The alanine-glucose cycle supplies from 10 to 15% of the total exercise energy requirement.* Regular training enhances the liver's glucose synthesis from the carbon skeletons of noncarbohydrate compounds.[66] This facilitates blood glucose homeostasis during prolonged physical activity.

 See the animation "Alanine-Glucose Cycle" at **Lippincott Connect** to view this process.

Summary

1. Proteins differ chemically from lipids and carbohydrates because they contain nitrogen in addition to sulfur, phosphorus, and iron.
2. Subunit amino acid structures form protein. Amino acids contain a side chain (R group) that determines the amino acid's particular chemical characteristics.
3. The body requires 20 different amino acids, each containing an amine group (NH_2) and an organic acid group (carboxylic acid group; COOH).
4. The enormous possible number of protein structures comes from almost unending combinations from 20 different amino acids, each with its own particular structural characteristics.
5. Regular exercise training enhances the liver's glucose synthesis from the carbon skeletons of noncarbohydrate compounds, particularly amino acids.
6. The body cannot synthesize 8 of the required 20 amino acids; the diet must provide these essential amino acids.
7. All animal and plant cells contain protein, complete higher-quality proteins contain all the essential amino acids, and incomplete lower-quality proteins represent the others.
8. Physically active people and competitive athletes can usually obtain the required nutrients predominantly from plant sources.
9. Amino acids serve as protein's building blocks during anabolism (synthesis) of cellular substances, and donate "carbon skeletons" when needed for energy metabolism.
10. The Recommended Dietary Allowance (RDA) represents an excess yet liberal safe level to meet the nutritional needs of practically all healthy persons. For adults, the protein RDA equals 0.83 g·kg^{-1} body weight.
11. Depleting carbohydrate reserves increases protein catabolism during physical activity. Serious athletes must maintain optimal levels of muscle and liver glycogen to maximize athletic performance and maintain muscle mass.
12. Protein serves as an energy fuel to a much greater extent than previously believed. This applies particularly to branched-chain amino acids oxidized in skeletal muscle rather than in the liver.
13. Reexamining the current protein RDA seems justified for athletes who train intensely to account for increased protein breakdown during physical activity, and an augmented protein synthesis in recovery.
14. Increasing daily protein intake to 1.2 to 1.8 g·kg^{-1} body mass daily from food seems a more reasonable alternative than relying on huge intakes from protein powders, high-protein shakes, and high-protein energy bars.
15. Proteins in neural and connective tissues generally do not participate in energy metabolism.
16. The muscle-derived amino acid alanine plays a key role via gluconeogenesis in supporting carbohydrate availability during prolonged physical activity. The alanine-glucose cycle accounts for up to 45% of the liver's glucose release during longer-duration physical activities.

Key Terms

Acidosis: Potentially harmful acidic body fluids

Adipocytes: Technical term for fat cells

Alanine-glucose cycle: Alanine, synthesized in muscle from glucose-derived pyruvate, travels in blood to the liver where it converts to glucose and urea

Albumin: Main globular, water-soluble serum protein made in the liver and transported in human blood to regulate its colloid osmotic pressure

Amylopectin: Highly branched monosaccharide linkage

Amylose: Long, straight glucose chain units twisted into a helical coil

Atherosclerosis: Degenerative process forms cholesterol-rich deposits (plaque) on arteries' inner wall lining causing them to narrow

Bile salts: Primary bile component, a greenish-yellow fluid made by the liver and stored in the gallbladder; helps to digest fats and absorb fat-soluble A, D, E, and K vitamins

Cholesterol: Derived lipid exists only in animal tissue without fatty acids while sharing some lipids' physical and chemical properties

Chylomicrons: Lipoproteins formed when emulsified lipid droplets leave the intestine and enter lymphatic vessels

Complete proteins: Foods that contain all essential amino acids in the correct quantity and ratio to maintain nitrogen balance for tissue growth and repair

Complex carbohydrate: Three up to a thousand sugar molecules linked together

Compound lipids: Fatty acid esters and alcohols (e.g., glycolipids and phospholipids); represent about 10% of body's total lipid content

Condensation: Triacylglycerol molecule synthesis produces three water molecules

Deamination: Forms urea in the liver when an amino acid molecule loses its amine group (nitrogen source)

Dehydration synthesis: Water-losing reaction forms complex polysaccharide molecules

Derived lipids: Simple and compound lipid backbone to synthesize cholesterol steroid compounds

Dietary Reference Intakes (DRI): Quantitative estimates for nutrient intake to plan and assess diets for healthy people; pegged to the reference Recommended Dietary Allowance (RDA), Adequate Intake (AI), Tolerable Upper Intake Level (UL), and Estimated Average Requirement (EAR)

Dipeptide: Protein with two amino acids

Disaccharides: Two combined monosaccharide molecules

Essential amino acids: Eight amino acids (nine in children and some older adults) the body cannot synthesize

Essential fatty acids: Required fatty acids the body cannot synthesize

Esterification: Chemical reactions in triacylglycerol synthesis

Estimated Safe and Adequate Daily Dietary Intakes (ESADDIs): Nutrient intake recommendations considered an adequate yet safe intake range

Fatty acids: Three unbranched carbon-chained atom clusters that bind to a glycerol molecule

Fiber: Nonstarch structural polysaccharide (e.g., plant cellulose)

Free fatty acid (FFA): Albumin + fatty acid

Fructose: Sweetest monosaccharide six-carbon (hexose) compound naturally formed in food

Galactose: Six-carbon (hexose) compound combined with glucose to form milk sugar in lactating animals' mammary glands

Glucagon: "Insulin antagonist" hormone secreted by pancreatic alpha cells to normalize blood sugar concentration by stimulating the liver's glycogenolytic and gluconeogenic pathways

Gluconeogenesis: Process for making new sugar mainly in the liver from primarily amino acids' carbon residues

Glucose: Six-carbon (hexose) compound formed naturally in food often called dextrose or blood sugar

Glycerol: Three-carbon molecule that combines with fatty acids to form the triacylglycerol molecule

Glycogen: Storage carbohydrate form within mammalian muscle and liver

Glycogen phosphorylase: Enzyme that facilitates liver and active muscle glycogenolysis

Glycogen synthase: Enzyme that catalyzes glycogenesis reactions

Glycogenesis: Large polysaccharide glycogen polymer formation synthesized from glucose molecule linkages

Glycogenolysis: Glycogen reconversion to glucose

Gravitational density: High gravitational forces act on lipoprotein particles to determine their density as they float in a liquid medium

Hepatic portal vein: Vein that carries venous blood to the liver from the spleen, stomach, pancreas, and intestines

High-density lipoproteins (HDLs): "Good cholesterol" lipoprotein; contains highest protein percentage (about 50%) and the least total lipid (about 20%) and cholesterol (about 20%)

Hitting the wall: Describes difficulty maintaining endurance exercise despite sufficient oxygen availability and unlimited stored lipid energy supply

Hydrogenation: Changes oils to semisolid lipids by bubbling liquid hydrogen under pressure into vegetable oil by reducing unsaturated fatty acids' double bonds to single bonds to allow more hydrogens to attach to carbons

Hyperinsulinemia: Pancreatic insulin overproduction

Hypoglycemia: Low blood glucose (<45 mg glucose · dL^{-1}); can produce weakness, hunger, mental confusion, and dizziness

Incomplete proteins: Foods that lack one or more essential amino acids required by the body

Ketone bodies: Acetonelike by-products (acetoacetate and β-hydroxybutyrate) from incomplete lipid breakdown

Ketosis: Acidosis from excessive lipid breakdown

Lactose: Glucose + galactose combined

Lactovegetarian diet: Diet that contains dairy but no other animal products

Lipolysis: Lipid chemical breakdown (hydrolysis)

Lipoprotein lipase: Enzyme located on capillary walls that hydrolyzes triacylglycerol

Low-density lipoproteins (LDLs): "Bad cholesterol"; normally carries 60 to 80% total cholesterol, contributing to smooth muscle cell proliferation and artery damage

Macronutrients: Carbohydrate, lipid, and protein nutrients that provide energy for bodily functions during rest and physical activity to preserve an organism's structural and functional integrity

Maltose: Glucose + glucose combined

Monosaccharides: Carbohydrates' basic unit exists as 6-carbon molecule with different carbon, oxygen, and hydrogen configurations to form glucose, fructose, and galactose

Monounsaturated fatty acid: One double bond along the main carbon chain

Negative nitrogen balance: Nitrogen excretion *exceeds* nitrogen intake

Nitrogen balance: Nitrogen intake *equals* nitrogen excretion

Nonessential amino acids: Synthesized from compounds at a rate that meets normal growth and tissue repair needs

Oligosaccharides: Formed when 2 to 10 monosaccharides bond together chemically

Omega-3 fatty acids: Polyunsaturated fatty acids characterized by a double bond three atoms away from the terminal methyl group in the chemical structure

Ovolactovegetarian diet: Diet that contains diary and eggs but no other animal products

Peptide bonds: Linked amino acids chains crucial in protein synthesis

Peroxisomes: Small vesicles without DNA or ribosomes surrounding a single membrane around a cell, which contains digestive enzymes (e.g., catalase) to decompose a cell's toxic substances (hydrogen peroxide) and fatty acids

Phospholipids: Modified triacylglycerols containing one or more fatty acid molecules joined with a phosphorus-containing group and nitrogen-containing molecules

Plaque: Also called an atheroma or atheromatous plaque formed from abnormal macrophage cells or debris accumulation containing lipids, calcium, and fibrous connective tissue in the arterial wall's inner layer

Polypeptide: Long, continuous, and unbranched peptide chain that forms large, bonded amino acid residues

Polysaccharide: Three up to several thousand sugar molecules linked together

Polyunsaturated fatty acid: Contains two or more double bonds along the main carbon chain

Positive nitrogen balance: Nitrogen intake *exceeds* nitrogen excretion

Protein: One or more long nitrogenous organic compound amino acid residue chains

Protein malnutrition: Pathological conditions mostly in children (marasmus and kwashiorkor) arising from insufficient dietary protein

R group or side chain: Amino acid structural component that dictates an amino acid's specific characteristics

Recommended Dietary Allowance (RDA): Recommended nutrient amount for daily consumption to maintain good health

Reverse cholesterol transport: Cholesterol removal by HDL for delivery to the liver for incorporation into bile and subsequent excretion via the intestinal tract

Sarcopenia: Muscle mass loss with aging

Saturated fatty acid: Single covalent bonds along the main carbon chain holds the maximum H atoms as chemically possible

Simple lipids: Glycerol plus three fatty acids (triacylglycerols) called neutral fats

Simple sugars: Monosaccharides and disaccharides

Starch: Storage carbohydrate in plants, seeds, corn, and various bread, cereal, pasta, and pastry grains

Sucrose: Glucose + fructose combined

Tofu: Condensed soy milk that is pressed into solid white blocks

Trans-fatty acids: Partial unsaturated fat hydrogenation when hydrogen atoms along the carbon chain move from naturally occurring *cis* position to the opposite side *trans* position

Transamination: Amine group from a donor amino acid transfers to an acceptor acid to form a new amino acid

Tripeptide: Protein with three amino acids

Unsaturated fatty acid: One or more double bonds along the main carbon chain reduces hydrogen's potential binding site number

Vegan: Person who does not eat any animal products

Very low-density lipoproteins (VLDLs): Transport triacylglycerols to muscle and adipose tissue; contain about 95% lipid, of which about 60% is triacylglycerol

Water-insoluble fibers: Fibers that do not absorb or dissolve in water

Water-soluble fibers: Fibers that absorb or dissolve in water

> References are available online at Lippincott Connect.

Additional References

Abbie E, et al. A low-carbohydrate protein-rich bedtime snack to control fasting and nocturnal glucose in type 2 diabetes: a randomized trial. *Clin Nutr.* 2020;39:3601.

Alcorta A, et al. Foods for plant-based diets: challenges and innovations. *Foods.* 2021;10:293.

Aoyama S, et al. Distribution of dietary protein intake in daily meals influences skeletal muscle hypertrophy via the muscle clock. *Cell Rep.* 2021;36:109336.

Burke LM, et al. Adaptation to a low carbohydrate high fat diet is rapid but impairs endurance exercise metabolism and performance despite enhanced glycogen availability. *J Physiol.* 2021;599:771.

Burke LM. Ketogenic low-CHO, high-fat diet: the future of elite endurance sport? *J Physiol.* 2021;599:819.

Cao J, et al. The effect of a ketogenic low-carbohydrate, high-fat diet on aerobic capacity and exercise performance in endurance athletes: a systematic review and meta-analysis. *Nutrients.* 2021;13:2896.

Costa Leite J, et al. Healthy low nitrogen footprint diets. *Glob Food Sec.* 2020;24:100342.

Gillen JB, et al. Low-carbohydrate training increases protein requirements of endurance athletes. *Med Sci Sports Exerc.* 2019;51:2294.

Ho FK, et al. Associations of fat and carbohydrate intake with cardiovascular disease and mortality: prospective cohort study of UK Biobank participants. *BMJ.* 2020;368:m688.

Kong Z, et al. Affective and enjoyment responses to short-term high intensity interval training with low-carbohydrate diet in overweight young women. *Nutrients.* 2020;12:E442.

Larsen MS, et al. Effects of protein intake prior to carbohydrate restricted endurance exercise: a randomized crossover trial. *J Int Soc Sports Nutr.* 2020;17:7.

Miki AJ, et al. Using evidence mapping to examine motivations for following plant-based diets. *Curr Dev Nutr.* 2020;4:nzaa013.

Paoli A, et al. Effects of two months of very low carbohydrate ketogenic diet on body composition, muscle strength, muscle area, and blood parameters in competitive natural body builders. *Nutrients.* 2021;13:374.

Ravindra PV, et al. Nutritional interventions for improving the endurance performance in athletes. *Arch Physiol Biochem.* 2020;1.

Reynolds AN, et al. Dietary fibre and whole grains in diabetes management: systematic review and meta-analyses. *PLoS Med.* 2020;17:e1003053.

Table 1.1 — Total Fiber Sources in Common Grains and Grain Products, Nuts and Seeds, Vegetables and Legumes, Fruits, and Baked Goods

Food	Serving	Fiber/Serving	Food	Serving	Fiber/Serving
Grains			Corn on cob	1	3.2
Oat bran	1 cup	16.4	Broccoli, raw	1 cup	2.9
Refined white flour, bleached	1 cup	3.4	Black beans	1 oz	2.5
Spaghetti, whole wheat	1 cup	5.0	Green beans, raw, cooked	1 cup	2.5
Penne, whole wheat	1 cup	10.0	Artichoke, raw	1 oz	2.3
Bran muffin	1	4.0	Carrot	1	2.3
Whole-wheat flour	1 cup	15.1	Baked potato	1	2.3
Wheat germ, toasted	1 cup	15.6	Tomato, raw	1	1.8
Couscous	1 cup	8.7	Onions, sliced, raw	1 cup	1.8
Popcorn, air-popped	1 cup	1.3	Lentils, stir fry	1 oz	1.1
Rice bran	1 oz	21.7	Chili w/beans	1 oz	0.9
Millet	1 cup	17.0	**Fruits**		
Corn grits	1 cup	4.5	Avocado	1	22.9
Barley, cooked, whole	1 cup	4.6	Loganberries, fresh	1 cup	9.3
Bulgur wheat	1 cup	25.6	Pear, Bartlett	1	4.6
Rye flour-dark	1 cup	17.7	Figs	2	4.1
Wild rice	1 cup	4.0	Blueberries	1 cup	3.9
All-Bran cereal	1/2 cup	8.5	Strawberries, fresh	1 cup	3.9
Barley	1 cup	31.8	Apple, raw	1	3.5
Oatmeal, cooked	1 cup	4.1	Orange, navel	1	3.4
Grape Nuts	1 cup	10.0	Grapefruit, sections, fresh	1	3.0
Macaroni, cooked enriched	1 cup	2.2	Banana	1	2.3
Rice, white	1 oz	1.5	Pineapple, chunks	1 cup	2.3
Almonds, dried	1 oz	3.5	Grapes, Thompson, seedless	1 cup	1.9
Peanut butter	1 tbsp	1.0	Peach, fresh	1	1.5
Macadamia nuts, dried	1 oz	1.5	Plum, small	1	0.6
Low-fat granola	1 cup	4.5	**Baked Goods**		
Cheerios	1 cup	5.0	Whole-wheat toast	Slice	2.3
Nuts and Seeds			Waffle, homemade	1	1.1
Pumpkin seeds, roasted, unsalted	1 oz	10.2	Pumpkin pie	Slice	5.4
Chestnuts, roasted	1 oz	3.7	Oatmeal bread	Slice	1.0
Peanuts, dried, unsalted	1 oz	3.5	French bread	Slice	0.7
Sunflower seeds, dry	1 oz	2.0	Danish pastry, plain	1	0.7
Walnuts, chopped, black	1 oz	1.6	Fig bar cookie	1	0.6
Vegetables and Legumes			Chocolate chip cookie, homemade	1	0.2
Pinto beans, dry, cooked	1 cup	19.5	White bread	Slice	0.6
Lima beans, fresh, cooked	1 cup	16.0	Pumpernickel bread	Slice	1.7
Black eyed peas, cooked from raw	1 cup	12.2	Rye bread	Slice	1.9
Mixed vegetables (corn, carrots, beans)	1 cup	7.2	Seven-grain bread	Slice	1.7

Data from the United States Department of Agriculture (https://fdc.nal.usda.gov/).

Table 1.2 Protein Content for Common Foods

Food	Serving Size	Protein (g)	Food	Serving Size	Protein (g)
Animal			**Plant**		
Hamburger, cooked	4 oz	30	Chickpeas	0.5 cup	20
Tuna	3 oz	22	Baked beans	1 cup	14
Turkey, light meat	4 oz	9	Tofu	3.5 oz	11
Egg, whole	1 large	6	Lentils	0.5 cup	9
Egg, white	1 large	4	Pasta, dry	2 oz	7
			Peanuts	1 oz	7
Dairy			100% Whole wheat bread	2 slices	6
Cottage cheese, regular	0.5 cup	15			
Yogurt, low fat	8 oz	11	Peanut butter	1 Tbsp	4
Cheese, regular (average for all types)	1 oz	8	Almonds, dry roasted	12	3
Milk, skim	8 oz	8			

CHAPTER 2

Vitamins, Minerals, and Water

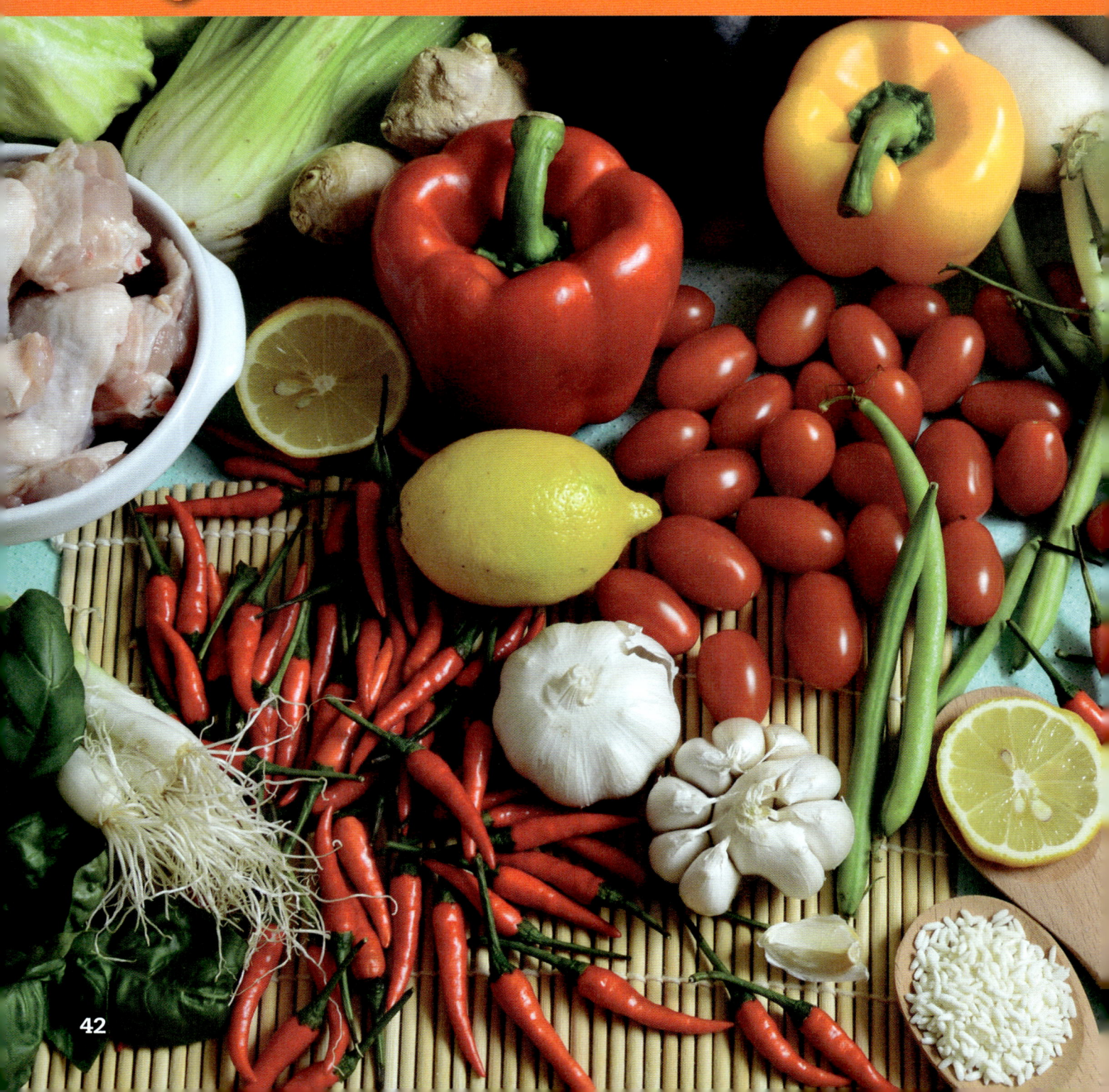

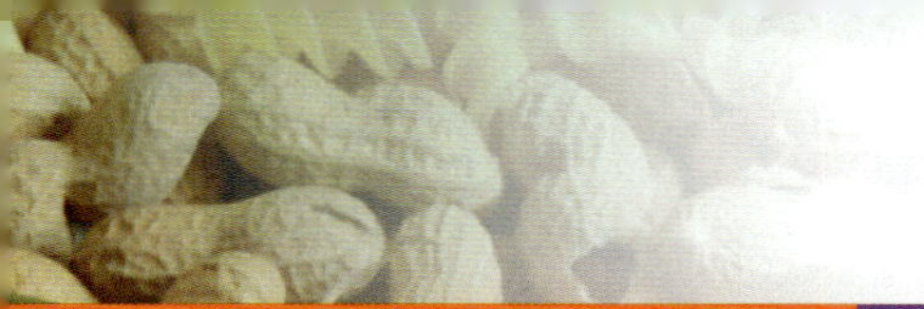

Chapter Objectives

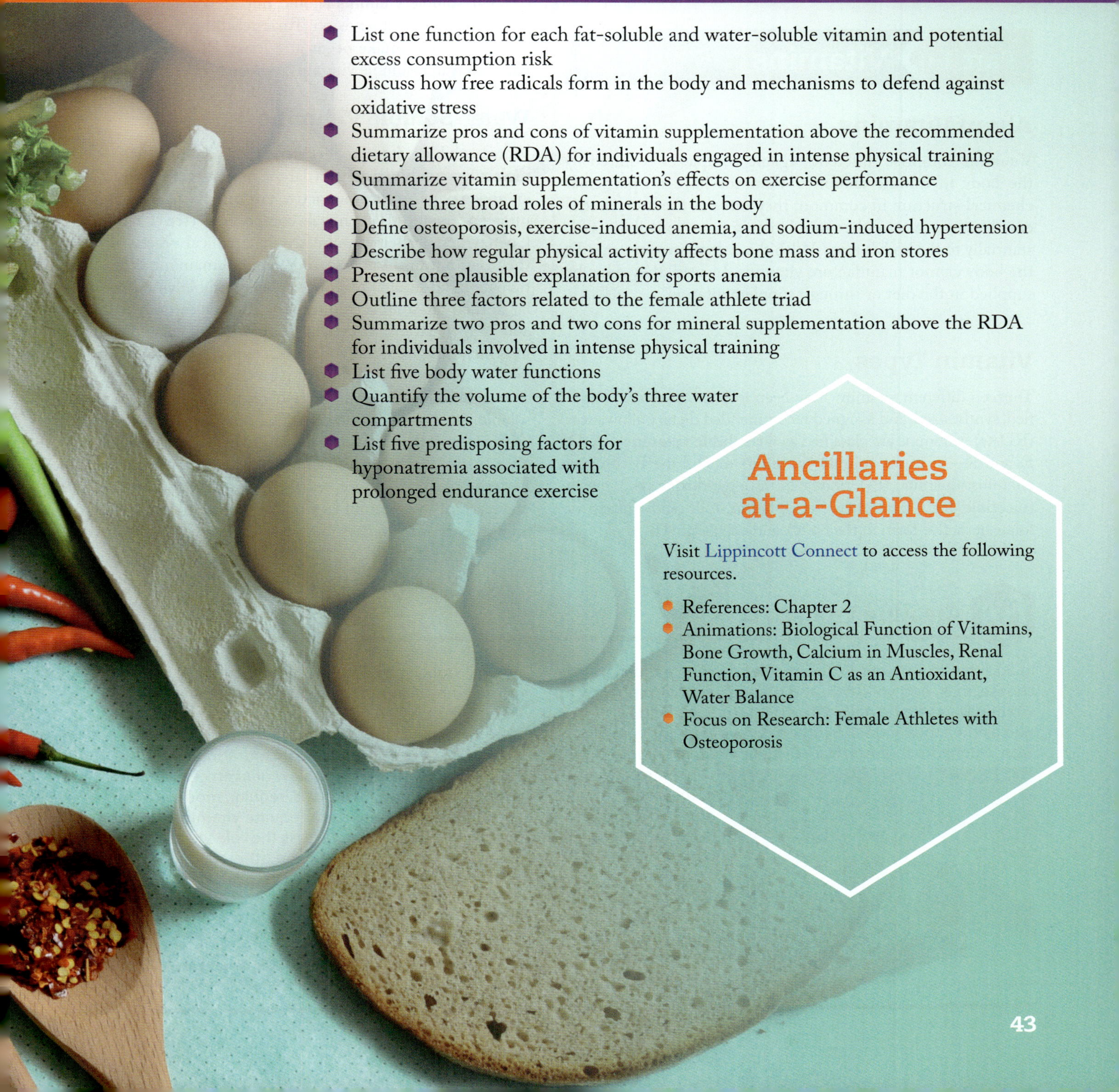

- List one function for each fat-soluble and water-soluble vitamin and potential excess consumption risk
- Discuss how free radicals form in the body and mechanisms to defend against oxidative stress
- Summarize pros and cons of vitamin supplementation above the recommended dietary allowance (RDA) for individuals engaged in intense physical training
- Summarize vitamin supplementation's effects on exercise performance
- Outline three broad roles of minerals in the body
- Define osteoporosis, exercise-induced anemia, and sodium-induced hypertension
- Describe how regular physical activity affects bone mass and iron stores
- Present one plausible explanation for sports anemia
- Outline three factors related to the female athlete triad
- Summarize two pros and two cons for mineral supplementation above the RDA for individuals involved in intense physical training
- List five body water functions
- Quantify the volume of the body's three water compartments
- List five predisposing factors for hyponatremia associated with prolonged endurance exercise

Ancillaries at-a-Glance

Visit Lippincott Connect to access the following resources.

- References: Chapter 2
- Animations: Biological Function of Vitamins, Bone Growth, Calcium in Muscles, Renal Function, Vitamin C as an Antioxidant, Water Balance
- Focus on Research: Female Athletes with Osteoporosis

Effectively regulating all metabolic processes requires delicate blending of food nutrients in the cell's watery medium. **Micronutrients**—small vitamin and mineral quantities—play highly specific roles to facilitate energy transfer and tissue synthesis. The physically active person or competitive athlete need not consume vitamin and mineral supplements if they obtain proper nutrition from a variety of food sources. Such supplementation practices touted by advertising on radio, TV, and print media usually prove physiologically and economically wasteful. Moreover, consuming some micronutrients in excess poses potential health and safety risk.

Part 1 — Vitamins

About Vitamins

Vitamins comprise different organic complexes required by the body in minute amounts. Vitamins have no particular chemical structure in common; they serve as accessory nutrients because they neither supply energy nor contribute substantially to the body's mass. With the exception of vitamin D, the body cannot manufacture vitamins. Instead, they must be supplied in the diet or through supplementation.

Vitamin Types

Thirteen different vitamins have been isolated, analyzed, classified, synthesized, and assigned recommended dietary allowances (RDAs). Vitamins are classified as **fat-soluble vitamins**—A, D, E, and K—or **water-soluble vitamins**—C and the B-complex vitamins: thiamine (B_1), riboflavin (B_2), pyridoxine (B_6), niacin (nicotinic acid), pantothenic acid, biotin, folic acid (folacin or folate, its active form in the body), and cobalamin (B_{12}).

Fat-Soluble Vitamins

Fat-soluble vitamins dissolve and remain in fatty tissues, obviating the need to ingest them daily. It may take years before "unhealthy" symptoms emerge that denote a fat-soluble vitamin deficiency. The liver stores vitamins A, D, and K, whereas vitamin E distributes throughout the body's fatty tissues. Dietary lipids provide the fat-soluble vitamin source; these vitamins travel as part of lipoproteins in the lymph to the liver for dispersion to various tissues. Consuming a true "fat-free" diet would accelerate a fat-soluble vitamin insufficiency.

Fat-soluble vitamins should not be consumed in excess without medical supervision. Toxic reactions to excessive fat-soluble vitamin intake occur at a lower RDA multiple compared to water-soluble vitamins.

Water-Soluble Vitamins

Water-soluble vitamins act largely as **coenzymes**—small molecules combined with a larger protein compound called an apoenzyme to form an active enzyme that accelerates the interconversion of chemical compounds (see Chapter 5). Coenzymes participate directly in chemical reactions; after the reaction runs its course, coenzymes remain intact and participate in additional reactions. Water-soluble vitamins, similar to their fat-soluble counterparts, include carbon, hydrogen, and oxygen atoms. They also contain nitrogen and metallic ions including iron, molybdenum, copper, sulfur, and cobalt.

Water-soluble vitamins disperse in bodily fluids without storage in tissues to any appreciable extent. Generally, a water-soluble vitamin excess intake voids in the urine. Water-soluble vitamins exert their influence for 8 to 14 hr after ingestion; thereafter, their potency decreases in somewhat exponential fashion. For example, the half-life or time required to convert one half of a reactant to a vitamin C product averages approximately 30 min, whereas 9 to 18 days represents thiamine's half-life.

fyi — Creating Vitamin D

In addition to sunlight exposure, dietary sources such as cheese, milk, egg yolk, fish, and orange juice, can supply vitamin D_3, as first detailed in a 1980 study with rat skin as the study model. Synthesizing vitamin D begins with 7-dehydrocholesterol (7-DHC), a molecule highly concentrated in the skin's outer epidermal layer. Ultraviolet radiation (282 to 310 nm UV light) penetrates the skin layer, converting 7-DHC into the vitamin D_3 isomer preD_3.

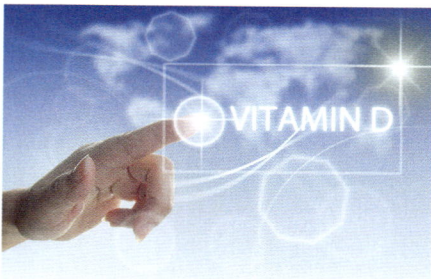
Pixelbliss/Shutterstock

The final stage converts preD_3 into vitamin D_3 at a rate controlled by skin temperature. The reactions continue when a vitamin D–binding protein joins to the newly formed vitamin D for transport in the blood from the reaction site. Vitamin D_3 overconcentration forces the reaction into equilibrium to slow or even cease vitamin synthesis. For most individuals, regular, moderate sun exposure usually produces adequate vitamin D_3 levels. Many studies continue to assess the role vitamin D_3 plays in disease intervention and other medically related applications.

Sources:

Rizzoli R. Vitamin D supplementation: upper limit for safety revisited? *Aging Clin Exp Res*. 2021;33:19.

Janjusevic M, et al. The peculiar role of vitamin D in the pathophysiology of cardiovascular and neurodegenerative diseases. *Life Sci*. 2022;289:120193.

Vitamin D Supplements and Resistance Training Effects

Supplemental vitamin D can improve skeletal muscle function and muscular strength in frail vitamin D–deficient individuals. One experiment studied supplementation's effects on muscle response to resistance training in healthy young and elderly individuals. Healthy untrained young ($n = 20$, age 20 to 30 years) and elderly ($n = 20$, age 60 to 75 years) individuals were assigned randomly to either a 16-wk daily supplement intake of 48 mcg vitamin D + 800 mg calcium (vitamin D group), or 800 mg calcium (placebo group) at a low sunlight latitude. Subjects resistance trained the quadriceps muscle group following an initial 4-wk supplementation period. Changes in muscle cross-sectional area and isometric strength were evaluated, and muscle biopsies determined fiber-type morphology changes and mRNA vitamin D receptor expression, cytochrome p45027B1, and myostatin. No additive effect occurred for vitamin D supplements on either whole muscle hypertrophy or muscle strength compared with placebo. Supplementation accompanied improved muscle quality in the elderly, and fiber-type morphology in the young indicated that vitamin D positively impacted skeletal muscle remodeling.

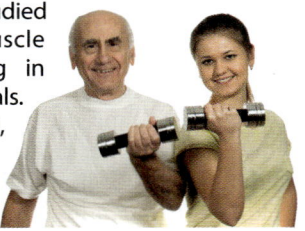
Victorpr/Shutterstock

Sources:
Dadrass A, et al. Anti-inflammatory effects of vitamin D and resistance training in men with type 2 diabetes mellitus and vitamin D deficiency: a randomized, double-blinded, placebo-controlled clinical trial. *J Diabetes Metab Disord*. 2019;18:323.
Mølmen KS, Hamet al. Vitamin D3 supplementation does not enhance the effects of resistance training in older adults. *J Cachexia Sarcopenia Muscle*. 2021;12:5993.

Vitamins' Role in the Body

FIGURE 2.1 summarizes the major biologic functions of vitamins. Vitamins contain no useful energy for the body; instead, they serve as essential links and regulators in metabolic reactions that release energy from food. Vitamins also control tissue synthesis and protect cell's plasma membrane integrity. The water-soluble vitamins play important roles in energy metabolism. For example:

- Vitamin B_1 facilitates the conversion of pyruvate to acetyl-coenzyme A (CoA) in carbohydrate breakdown.
- Niacin and vitamin B_2 regulate mitochondrial energy metabolism.
- Vitamins B_6 and B_{12} catalyze protein synthesis.
- Pantothenic acid, part of coenzyme A (CoA), participates in the aerobic breakdown of carbohydrate, lipid, and protein macronutrients.

- Vitamin C acts as a cofactor in enzymatic reactions, as free radical scavenger in antioxidative processes, and as a component in hydroxylation reactions that provide connective tissue stability and wound healing.
- Vitamins participate repeatedly in metabolic reactions without degradation; the vitamin needs of physically active individuals do not exceed those of sedentary counterparts.

 See the animation "Biologic Function of Vitamins" on **Lippincott Connect** to view this process.

 INTEGRATIVE QUESTION

Should athletes "supercharge" with vitamin supplements to enhance training responses and performance?

Well-balanced meals provide all vitamins in adequate quantity regardless of age and physical activity level. Individuals who expend considerable energy in physical activity generally need not consume special foods or supplements that increase vitamin intake above recommended levels. At high daily physical activity levels, food intake generally increases to sustain the added energy requirements. Additional food from nutritious meals proportionately increases vitamin and mineral intakes. **TABLE 2.1** lists major bodily functions, dietary sources, and symptoms of deficiency or excess for the water-soluble vitamins, while **TABLE 2.2** lists corresponding characteristics for fat-soluble vitamins.

TABLE 2.1 Food sources, bodily functions, and symptoms of deficiency or excess for fat-soluble vitamins

Several vitamin supplementation exceptions exist from difficulty obtaining recommended amounts. For example, foods high in vitamin C and folic acid usually make up only a small part of most Americans' total caloric intake; such food availability also varies by season. Also, different athletic groups have relatively low B_1 and B_6 vitamin intakes, two vitamins prevalent in fresh fruit, grains, and uncooked or steamed vegetables.[44,137] Vegans generally require vitamin B_{12} supplementation because it exists only in foods of animal origin.

TABLE 2.2 Food sources, bodily functions, and symptoms of deficiency or excess for water-soluble vitamins

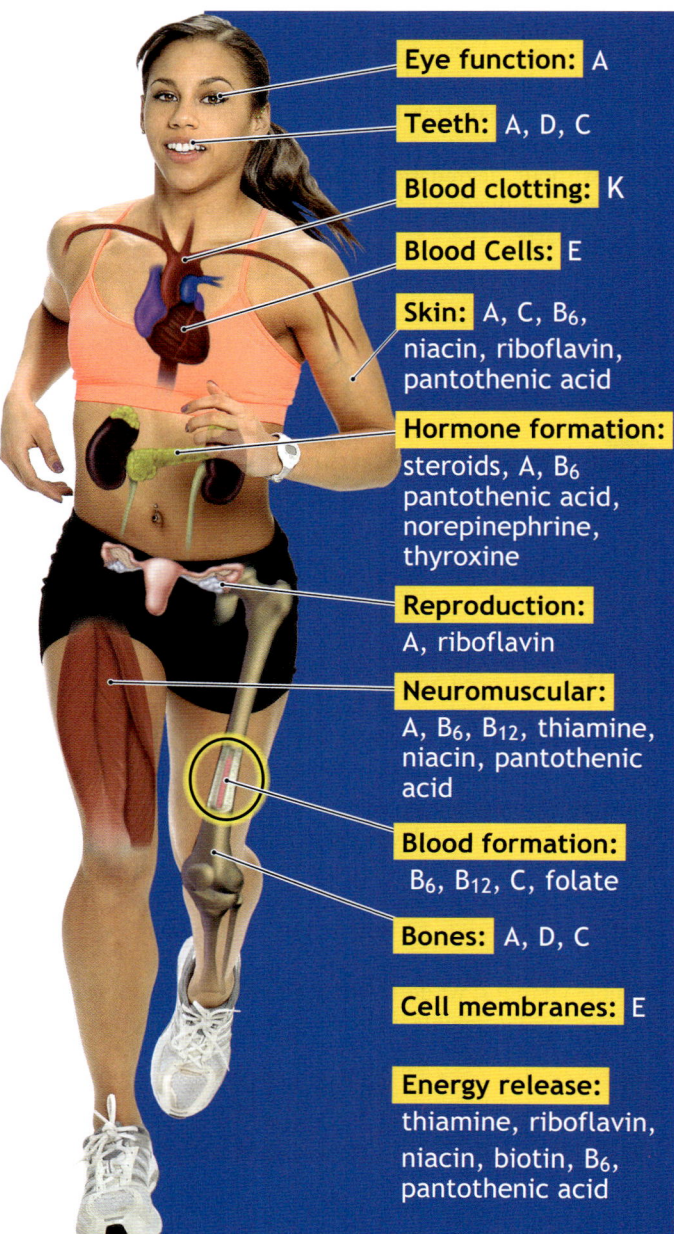

FIGURE 2.1. Vitamins' many biologic functions.
(Gino Santa Maria/Shutterstock)

Defining Nutrient Needs: Dietary Reference Intakes

Controversy surrounding the RDAs caused the National Academy of Medicine (https://nam.edu), formerly the Institute of Medicine (IOM) of the National Academies, to re-examine single standards for specific nutrients. This process led the IOM in cooperation with Canadian scientists to develop the current dietary reference intakes (www.nal.usda.gov/sites/default/files/fnic_uploads/energy_full_report.pdf).

The dietary reference intakes (DRIs) represent an umbrella term encompassing the array of government standards—*RDAs, estimated average requirements, adequate intakes, and the tolerable upper intake levels*—for nutrient recommendations in planning and assessing diets for healthy persons. Recommendations encompass not only daily intakes intended for health maintenance but also upper intake levels to reduce likelihood of harm from excessive intake. The DRIs differ from their predecessor RDAs by focusing more on promoting health maintenance and risk reduction for nutrient-dependent diseases (e.g., heart dysfunctions, diabetes, hypertension, osteoporosis, cancers, and age-related macular degeneration). This contrasts with the traditional criterion of preventing the relatively rare scurvy and beriberi deficiency diseases. In addition to including values for energy, protein, and the micronutrients, the DRIs supply recommendations for the nutritionally important but nonessential plant phytochemical compounds.

The DRIs also include recommendations for gender and life growth and development stages based on age, pregnancy, and lactation. The following define four different sets of DRI values for nutrient and food component intakes:

1. **Estimated average requirement (EAR)**: Average daily nutrient intake level to meet needs of one half the individuals in a particular life-stage and gender group. The EAR provides a useful value to determine inadequate nutrient intake prevalence by the proportion of the population with intakes below this level.
2. Recommended dietary allowance (RDA): The average daily nutrient intake level sufficient to meet the requirement of about 97% of healthy individuals in a particular life-stage and gender group (**FIG. 2.2**). For most nutrients, this value represents the EAR plus 2 standard deviations above the mean level requirement.
3. **Adequate intake (AI)**: Provides an assumed adequate nutritional goal when no RDA exists. It represents a recommended average daily nutrient intake level based on observed or experimentally determined approximations about nutrient intake for apparently healthy persons. The AI proves useful when an RDA cannot be determined and intakes at or above the AI level indicate low risk.
4. **Tolerable upper intake level (UL)**: The highest average daily nutrient intake level likely to pose no adverse health risks to almost all individuals in the specified gender and life-stage group. Risk for adverse effects increase as intake increases above the UL.

TABLE 2.3 Vitamin dietary reference intakes

Most individuals achieve the daily requirement without need for additional supplementation. The mineral iron represents an exception in that most pregnant women require supplements to obtain their increased daily requirement. **TABLES 2.3 AND 2.4** present the DRIs, AIs, and UL values for vitamins.

TABLE 2.4 Tolerable Upper Intake Levels for Vitamins

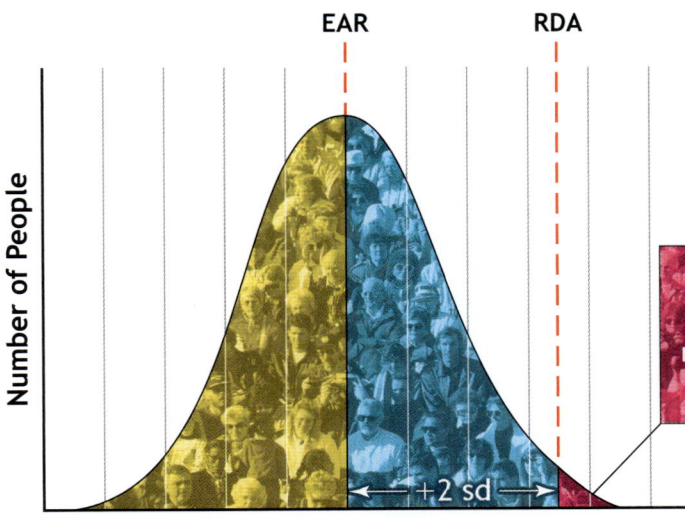

FIGURE 2.2. Theoretical number of persons adequately nourished by a given nutrient intake. Note that in the population, about 3% do not meet the recommended dietary allowance.
(Joseph Sohm/Shutterstock)

Vitamin Antioxidant Role

Most oxygen uptake within mitochondria combines with hydrogen to produce water. Nonetheless, 2 to 5% of oxygen normally forms the reactive oxygen–containing and nitrogen-containing free radical superoxide (O_2^-), hydrogen peroxide (H_2O_2), hydroxyl (OH^-), and nitric oxide (NO), from electron "leakage" along the electron transport chain. A free radical, a highly unstable, chemically reactive molecule or molecular fragment, contains at least one unpaired electron in its outer valence shell. These same radicals are produced by external heat and ionizing radiation and are carried in cigarette smoke, environmental pollutants, and even some medications. Once formed, free radicals interact with other compounds to create new free radical molecules. The new molecules frequently damage two structures:

1. Electron-dense cellular deoxyribonucleic acid (DNA)
2. Lipid-rich cell membranes

In contrast, paired electrons within a molecule represent a more stable electronic state.

Fortunately, cells possess enzymatic and nonenzymatic mechanisms that work in concert to immediately counter potential oxidative damage from a chemical and enzymatic mutagenic challenge. Antioxidants scavenge oxygen radicals or chemically eradicate them by reducing oxidized compounds. For example, when O_2^- forms, the enzyme superoxide dismutase catalyzes its dismutation to form hydrogen peroxide. This enzyme catalyzes the reaction of two identical oxygen molecules to produce two molecules in different oxidation states as follows:

$$O_2^- + O_2^- \xrightarrow[\text{superoxide dismutase}]{2H^+} H_2O_2 + O_2$$

Hydrogen peroxide produced in this reaction breaks down further to water and oxygen in a reaction catalyzed by the catalase enzyme as follows:

$$2H_2O_2 \xrightarrow{\text{catalase}} 2H_2O + O_2$$

 See the animation, "Vitamin C as an Antioxidant" on **Lippincott Connect** to view this process.

Free radical accumulation increases the potential for cellular damage called **oxidative stress** whenever biologically important substances add oxygen to cellular components. These substances include DNA, proteins, and lipid-containing structures—particularly the polyunsaturated fatty acid–rich bilayer membrane that isolates a cell from noxious toxins and carcinogens. Oxidative stress likely acts as a key cell signaling pathway regulator to increase protein breakdown and muscle atrophy during prolonged physical inactivity periods.[126,147] In unchecked oxidative stress, the plasma membrane's fatty acids deteriorate through a chain reaction series termed **lipid peroxidation**. These reactions

 Are Daily Multivitamins Needed?

Physicians who consumed a daily multivitamin supplement over a 12-year period did no better on memory tests than a control group receiving a placebo. In a second study, heart attack patients who received a supplement for 1 to 5 years were no less likely to experience a second attack than patients taking a placebo. A more recent, larger study with 37,193 women aged 45 years and older revealed that multivitamin use over a 16-year period did not associate with reduced short-term or long-term heart attack, stroke, or death risk. As summarized by the paper's lead author: "Taken together, today there is limited evidence to recommend for or against multivitamin use to prevent cardiovascular disease. A healthy diet characterized by ample fruits and vegetables, whole grains and fish, should be consumed to avoid nutritional deficiencies and to prevent chronic diseases."

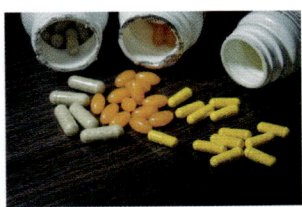
Sirirojo/Shutterstock

Sources:
Edenfield KM. Sports supplements: pearls and pitfalls. *Prim Care*. 2020;47:37.
Goudarzi S, et al. Effect of vitamins and dietary supplements on cardiovascular health. *Crit Pathw Cardiol*. 2020;19:153.
Jacques PF, Rogers G. A beneficial cardiometabolic health profile associated with dietary supplement use: A cross-sectional study. *Int J Vitam Nutr Res*. 2021:1.

incorporate higher than normal oxygen into lipids, thereby increasing the vulnerability of the cell and its constituents. Free radicals facilitate low-density lipoprotein (LDL) cholesterol peroxidation, which leads to cytotoxicity and enhanced coronary artery plaque formation.[96,161] Oxidative stress ultimately increases cellular deterioration associated with advanced aging, disease, and general decline in central nervous system and immune functions.

fyi Typical Nutrient Deficiencies

Over two thirds of Americans fail to meet the estimated average requirement (EAR) for vitamins D, E, and K, and the minerals magnesium and potassium, and about 40% do not meet the EAR for vitamins A and C. In large part, such nutrient inadequacies reflect ingrained dietary patterns that fail to achieve recommended fruit, vegetable, and whole grain consumption guidelines.

Source: Bai Y, et al. Global variation in the cost of a nutrient-adequate diet by population group: an observational study. Lancet Planet Health. 2022;6:e19.

The body cannot deter oxygen reduction and free radical production, but it does provide an elaborate natural defense against its damaging effects. This includes the antioxidant scavenger enzymes catalase, glutathione peroxidase, and superoxide dismutase, and metal-binding protein metalloenzymes.[74] The nutritive, nonenzymatic reducing agents selenium and vitamins A, C, and E and β-carotene also serve important protective functions.[19,50,68,182] The antioxidant chemicals protect the plasma membrane by reacting with and removing free radicals, thus quenching the chain reaction. They also blunt high cellular serum homocysteine's damaging effects (see Chapter 31).[112] A diet with appropriate antioxidant vitamins and other chemoprotective agents in foods consumed, not from supplements, may reduce risk of cardiovascular disease, stroke, diabetes, osteoporosis, cataracts, premature aging, and diverse cancers, including breast, distal colon, prostate, pancreas, ovary, and endometrium.[43,69,111,183]

The **atherosclerosis oxidative modification hypothesis** maintains that mild LDL cholesterol oxidation—similar to butter turning rancid—contributes to plaque-forming, artery-clogging atherosclerotic processes.[37,92,160] One heart disease protection model proposes that antioxidant vitamins inhibit LDL cholesterol oxidation and its subsequent uptake into foam cells embedded in the arterial wall.

A multivitamin may prove beneficial if the diet lacks vitamin B_{12}, vitamin D, or folic acid. Current nutritional guidelines now focus more on consumption of a broad array of food types rather than on supplements of isolated chemicals contained within these foods. Disease protection from a healthful diet links to consuming nutrient-rich fruits, vegetables, whole grains, and lean meat or meat substitutes and low-fat dairy foods.[67]

The National Cancer Institute (www.cancer.gov) encourages the daily intake of five or more fruit and vegetable servings (nine recommended for males), whereas the USDA's Dietary Guidelines recommend two to four fruit and three to five vegetable servings daily.

Vitamin-Rich Food Sources

The following food sources provide rich quantities of vitamins and supply them with nutrient-rich accessory nutrients with potential health-promoting benefits.

- **Vitamin A (carotenoids):** organ meats, carrots, cantaloupe, sweet potatoes, pumpkin, apricots, spinach, milk, collards, eggs
- **Vitamin C:** guava; citrus fruits and juices; red, yellow, and green peppers; papaya; kiwi; broccoli; strawberries; tomatoes; sweet and white potatoes; kale; mango; cantaloupe
- **Vitamin D:** salmon, tuna, sardines, mackerel, oysters, cod liver oil, egg yolks, fortified milk, fortified orange juice, fortified breakfast cereal
- **Vitamin E:** vegetable oils, nuts, seeds, spinach, kiwi, wheat germ
- **Vitamin K:** spinach, kale, collards, Swiss chard, broccoli, romaine lettuce
- **Vitamin B_1 (thiamin):** sunflower seeds, enriched bread, cereal, pasta, whole grains, lean meats, fish, beans, green peas, corn, soybeans
- **Vitamin B_2 (riboflavin):** lean meats, eggs, legumes, nuts, green leafy vegetables, dairy products, enriched bread
- **Vitamin B_3 (niacin):** dairy products, calf's liver, poultry, fish, lean meat, nuts, eggs, fortified bread and cereal
- **Pantothenic acid:** calf's liver, mushrooms, sunflower seeds, corn, eggs, fish, milk, milk products, whole-grain cereal, beans
- **Biotin:** eggs, fish, milk, liver and kidney, milk products, soybeans, nuts, Swiss chard, whole-grain cereal, beans
- **Vitamin B_6:** beans, bananas, nuts, eggs, meat, poultry, fish, potato, fortified bread, and ready-to-eat cereals
- **Vitamin B_{12}:** liver, meat, eggs, poultry, fish (trout and salmon), shellfish, milk, milk products, fortified breakfast cereal
- **Folate (folic acid):** beef liver, green leafy vegetables, avocado, green peas, enriched bread, fortified breakfast cereals

Obtain Vitamins from Food, Not Supplements
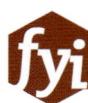

A placebo-controlled 5-year nutritional supplementation trial documented a 7% incident cancer risk (145 events in men and 29 in women) and 2.3% cancer deaths. No association emerged between cancer outcomes and supplementation with B vitamins and/or omega-3 fatty acids. A statistically significant treatment by sex interaction occurred, with no treatment effect on cancer risk among men and increased cancer risk among women for omega-3 fatty acid supplementation. The results suggest that obtaining nutrients from whole foods (not from isolated active substances in supplement form) may explain any positive benefits from these nutrients.

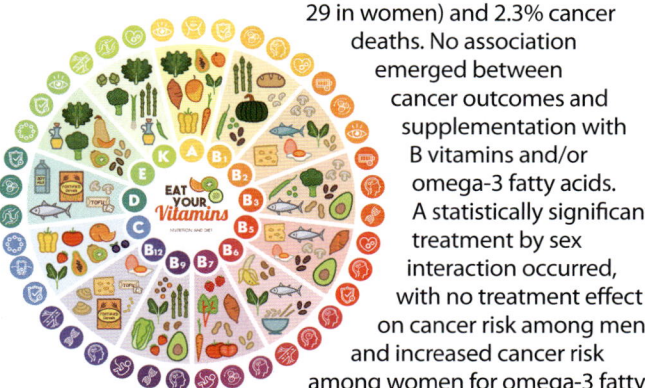

elenabsl/Shutterstock

Sources:
Andreeva VA, et al. B vitamin and/or omega-3 fatty acid supplementation and cancer: ancillary findings from the supplementation with folate, vitamins B_6 and B_{12}, and/or omega-3 fatty acids (SU.FOL.OM3) randomized trial. *Arch Intern Med.* 2012;172:540.
Bakaloudi DR, et al. Intake and adequacy of the vegan diet. A systematic review of the evidence. *Clin Nutr.* 2021;40:3503.

Physical Activity, Free Radicals, and Antioxidants

Physical activity benefits are well documented, yet the possibility for negative effects remains controversial because elevated aerobic exercise metabolism increases reactive oxygen and nitrogen free radical production.[115,120,171] At relatively low cellular levels, free radicals can negatively influence metabolism through signaling mechanisms that maintain cellular balance.[89] Increased free radicals can overwhelm the body's natural defenses to pose a health risk from increased oxidative stress. Free radicals also contribute to muscle injury and soreness from eccentric muscle actions and unaccustomed physical activity (see Chapter 22). Muscle damage releases muscle enzymes and initiates inflammatory cell infiltration into damaged tissues.

An opposing position maintains that free radical production increases during physical activity, yet the body's normal antioxidant defenses remain adequate or concomitantly improve as the natural superoxide dismutase and glutathione peroxidase enzymatic defenses "*up-regulate*" through exercise training adaptations.[125,145,173] Research supports this latter position because the beneficial effects of regular physical activity decrease incidence of heart disease and various cancers related to oxidative stress. Regular physical training also protects against myocardial injury from lipid peroxidation induced by short-term tissue ischemia followed by reperfusion.[35,60,158]

Increased Metabolism During Exercise and Free Radical Production

Exercise produces reactive oxygen species in two ways:

1. By an electron leak in the mitochondria at the cytochrome level to produce excessive superoxide radicals
2. Alterations in blood flow and oxygen supply—underperfusion during intense physical activity followed by substantial reperfusion in recovery—that trigger excessive free radical generation. Reintroducing molecular oxygen in recovery also produces reactive oxygen species that magnify oxidative stress. Some argue that the potential for free radical damage also increases during trauma and stress, from muscle damage, and from environmental pollutants (e.g., smog).

Oxidative stress risk increases with intense physical activity.[2,103,127,184] Exhaustive endurance exercise by untrained persons produces oxidative damage in the active muscles. Intense resistance exercise also increases free radical production, indirectly measured by the lipid peroxidation by-product malondialdehyde.[102] **FIGURE 2.3** illustrates how regular aerobic activity impacts oxidative response, subsequent tissue damage, and protective adaptations.

Oxidative Stress Risk and Antioxidant Supplementation

Two questions arise about the potential for increased oxidative stress with physical activity:

1. Are physically active individuals more prone to free radical damage?
2. Are protective agents with antioxidant properties required in increased amounts in the diets of physically active individuals?

In answer to the first question, the natural antioxidant defenses in well-nourished humans respond adequately to increased physical activity.[174] A single submaximal exercise bout increases oxidant production, yet antioxidant defenses cope effectively in healthy individuals and trained heart transplant recipients.[75,172] Even with multiple exercise bouts performed on consecutive days, the various oxidative stress indices show no antioxidant system impairment.

The answer to the second question remains equivocal.[172] Some evidence indicates that consuming

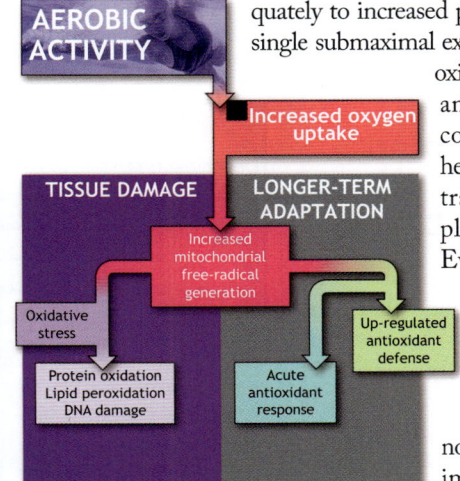

FIGURE 2.3. Adaptations from regular aerobic exercise lessen the likelihood of tissue damage from intense physical activity.

(Jacob Lund/Shutterstock)

exogenous antioxidant compounds either slows activity-induced free radical formation or augments the body's natural defense systems.[35,74] If antioxidant supplementation proves beneficial, vitamin E could be the most important antioxidant related to physical activity and physical training.[27,71]

In one study, vitamin E–deficient animals began training with plasma membrane function compromised from oxidative damage; they reached exhaustion earlier than animals with recommended vitamin E levels. In animals fed a normal diet, vitamin E supplements diminished oxidative damage to skeletal muscle fibers and myocardial tissue caused by training.[55] Humans fed a daily β-carotene, vitamin C, and vitamin E antioxidant mixture had lower serum and breath markers of lipid peroxidation at rest and following physical activity than subjects not receiving supplements. Vitamin E supplementation for 5 months in racing cyclists reduced oxidative stress markers induced by extreme endurance exercise. In another experiment using whole-body resistance training, 2-wk daily vitamin E supplementation with 120 IU decreased free radical interaction with cellular membranes and blunted muscle tissue disruption caused by an intense single exercise bout.[102] In contrast, antioxidant supplementation with vitamins C and E in individuals with no previous vitamin deficiencies did not affect endurance training adaptations.[23,56,180] Thirty-day vitamin E supplementation (1200 IU · d^{-1}) produced a 2.8-fold increase in serum vitamin E concentration without damaging muscle (including postexercise force decrement) or inflammation caused by eccentric muscle actions.[14] Similarly, a 4-wk daily 1000 IU vitamin E supplement produced no effect on biochemical or ultrastructural muscle damage indices in experienced runners after a half marathon.[33]

Recommended vitamin E supplementation ranges between 100 and 400 IU daily but is not without risk. Vitamin E supplementation has produced internal bleeding by inhibiting vitamin K metabolism, particularly in persons taking anticoagulant medication. It also has increased prostate cancer risk among healthy men.[82]

(40%), followed by herbals and botanicals (39%), sports nutrition supplements (28%), and weight management supplements (17%). More than 50% of competitive athletes consume supplements on a regular basis, either to ensure adequate micronutrient intake or to achieve an excess to enhance exercise/sports performance, training responsiveness, and exercise recovery.[26,42,80] Among elite Canadian athletes in predominantly "power-based" sports, 87% declared having taken three or more dietary supplements within the prior 6 months. For athletes, most supplementation was consumed as sports drinks, multivitamin and mineral preparations, carbohydrate bars, protein powder, and meal replacement products.[97] When vitamin-mineral deficiencies appear in physically active people, they most often occur among these three groups:

1. Vegetarians or groups with low-energy intake (e.g., dancers, gymnasts, and weight-class sport athletes) who strive to maintain or reduce body weight
2. Individuals who eliminate one or more food groups from their diet
3. Endurance athletes who overconsume processed foods and simple sugars with low micronutrient density

Vitamins synthesized in the laboratory are no less effective for bodily functions than vitamins from food sources. When deficiencies exist, vitamin supplements reverse deficiency symptoms. When vitamin intake achieves recommended levels, supplements do not improve exercise performance. More than 70 years of research on healthy persons with nutritionally adequate diets does not provide evidence that consuming vitamin (and mineral) supplements improves exercise performance, the hormonal and metabolic responses to exercise, or ability to train arduously and recover from such training.[52,164,170,177]

Protecting Against Upper Respiratory Tract Infections

Moderate physical activity and exercise training heighten immune function, whereas prolonged intense endurance exercise or a strenuous training session transiently suppress

Does Vitamin Supplementation Provide a Competitive Edge?

FIGURE 2.4 displays results from a 2019 survey that found that vitamins and minerals continue as the most commonly consumed supplement category, with 76% of Americans taking these products over a 12-month period (www.crnusa.org/newsroom/dietary-supplement-use-reaches-all-time-high-available-purchase-consumer-survey-reaffirms). Specialty supplements were the second most popular category

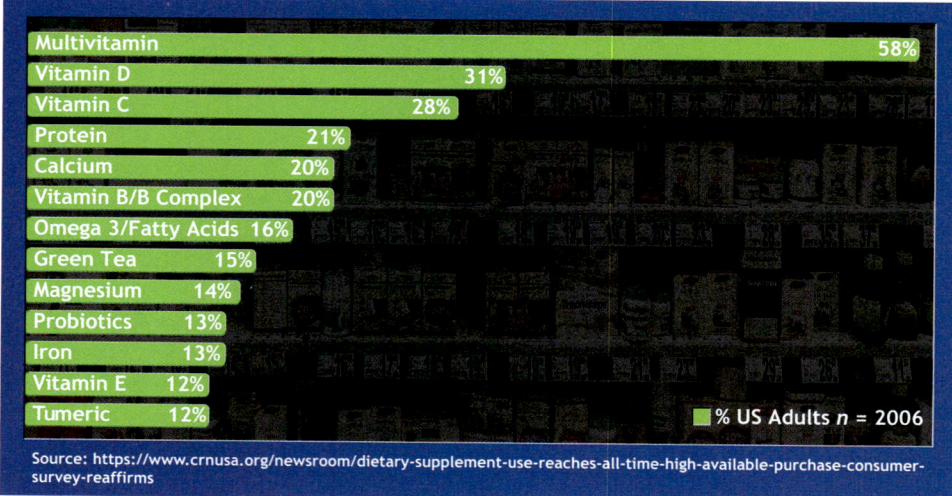

FIGURE 2.4. Ten most popular supplements among U.S. adults. (Radu Bercan/Shutterstock)

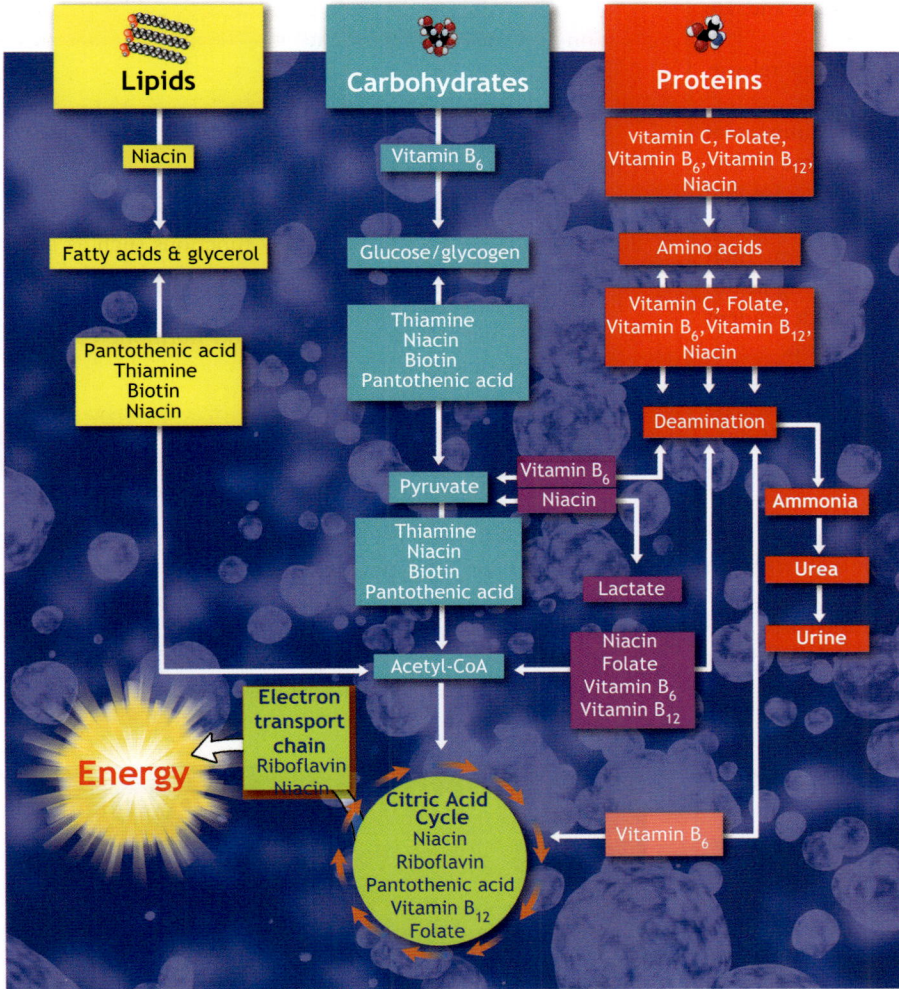

FIGURE 2.5. General schema for water-soluble vitamins' role in carbohydrate, lipid, and protein metabolism.
(Shutterstock: Mitar Vidakovic; Pixus)

Supplementing with vitamin B_6, an essential cofactor in glycogen and amino acid metabolism, did not benefit the metabolic mixture metabolized by women during intense aerobic activity. In general, athletes' status for this vitamin equals reference standards for the population[100] and does not decrease with strenuous physical activity to a level warranting supplementation.[135] For endurance-trained men, taking vitamin B_6 supplementation (20 mg daily) for 9 days provided no ergogenic effect on cycling to exhaustion performed at 70% aerobic capacity.[175] Consuming vitamin D supplements above recommended levels to enhance physical performance remains controversial.[185–187]

Chronic high-potency, multivitamin-mineral supplementation for well-nourished, healthy individuals does not augment aerobic fitness, muscular strength, neuromuscular performance after prolonged running, and general athletic performance.[52,147] In addition to poor effectiveness for B-complex group supplements, no exercise benefits exist for excess vitamins C and E on stamina, circulatory function, or energy metabolism. Short-term daily supplementation with vitamin E (400 IU) produced no effect on normal neuroendocrine and metabolic responses to strenuous exercise or performance time to exhaustion.[148] Vitamin C status, assessed by serum concentrations and urinary ascorbate levels, in trained athletes did not differ from untrained individuals despite large differences in daily physical activity levels.[138] Other investigators report similar findings for other vitamins.[48,136] Active persons typically increase daily energy intake to match their increased energy requirement. As such, a proportionate increase occurs in micronutrient intake in amounts that usually exceed recommended levels.

the body's defense against infectious agents.[118,178] An increased upper respiratory tract infection (URTI) risk occurs within 1 or 2 wk following the exercise stress. Additional vitamins C and E and perhaps carbohydrate ingestion before, during, and following an intense training session can boost the normal immune mechanisms to combat infections.[73,113,117,121] Chapter 20 discusses immune function relationships among physical activity at various intensity levels and durations.

Enhancing Exercise Performance

FIGURE 2.5 illustrates that B-complex and C vitamins play key coenzyme roles to regulate energy-yielding reactions during carbohydrate, lipid, and protein catabolism. They also contribute to hemoglobin synthesis and red blood cell production. The belief that "if a little is good, more must be better" has led many coaches, athletes, fitness enthusiasts, and even a prominent two-time Nobel Prize winner to advocate vitamin supplements above recommended levels (https://cdn.centerforinquiry.org/wp-content/uploads/sites/33/2020/12/22170734/pauling_vitamins.pdf). Nonetheless, the facts do not support such advice for individuals who consume an adequate diet.

Summary

1. Vitamins serve crucial functions in almost all bodily processes, but neither supply energy nor contribute to body mass.
2. With the exception of vitamin D, vitamins are obtained from food or dietary supplementation.
3. Plants synthesize vitamins; animals produce them from precursor provitamins.
4. The 13 known vitamins classify as water soluble or fat soluble.
5. The fat-soluble vitamins include A, D, E, and K, whereas vitamin C and the B-complex vitamins are water soluble.
6. Excess fat-soluble vitamins accumulate in body tissues; when taken in excess, levels can become toxic.

7. Excess water-soluble vitamins remain nontoxic and are excreted in the urine.
8. Vitamins regulate metabolism, facilitate energy release, and play key roles in bone and tissue synthesis.
9. Vitamins A, C, and E and β-carotene serve important protective functions as antioxidants to reduce free radical damage (oxidative stress) and provide heart disease and cancer protection.
10. The dietary reference intakes (DRIs) differ from their predecessor RDAs by focusing more on promoting health maintenance and risk reduction for nutrient-dependent diseases rather than deficiency disease prevention.
11. The DRIs serve as an umbrella term that encompasses the RDAs, estimated average requirements (EARs), adequate intakes (AIs), and tolerable upper intake levels (UIs) for nutrient recommendations to plan and assess diets for healthy individuals.
12. DRI values include recommendations that apply to gender and life stages of growth and development based on age (and during pregnancy and lactation).
13. Physical activity elevates metabolism and increases production of potentially harmful free radicals. A daily diet that encourages antioxidant vitamin and mineral consumption lessens oxidative stress.
14. In well-nourished individuals, the body's natural antioxidant defenses up-regulate in response to increased physical activity.
15. Vitamin supplementation above recommended values does not improve exercise performance or the potential for intense physical training.

Part 2 — Minerals

Mineral Essentials

Approximately 4% of the body's mass consists of 22 mostly metallic elements collectively termed **minerals**. They serve as enzymes, hormones, and vitamin constituents and combine with other chemicals (calcium phosphate in bone, iron in hemoglobin's heme), or exist singularly as, for example, free calcium and sodium in body fluids. The minerals essential to life include 7 **major minerals** (required in amounts >100 mg daily) and 14 minor or **trace minerals** (required in amounts <100 mg daily). Trace minerals account for less than 15 g or 0.02% of total body mass. Excess mineral intake serves no useful physiologic purpose yet can induce toxic effects. Many minerals have established DRIs; a diet that provides this requirement ensures adequate intake for the remaining minerals. Most minerals, major or trace, occur freely in nature—mainly in rivers, lakes, and oceans; in topsoil; and beneath the Earth's surface. Minerals exist in the root system of plants and in the body structures of animals that consume the plants. **TABLE 2.5** presents the DRIs, **TABLE 2.6** lists the UL values, and **TABLE 2.7** lists the major bodily functions, dietary sources, and symptoms of deficiency or excesses.

TABLE 2.5 Mineral dietary reference intakes

Mineral Functions

Minerals serve three broad functions:

1. Provide structure in forming bones and teeth
2. Help to maintain normal bodily functions such as heart rhythm, muscle contractility, neural conductivity, and acid-base balance
3. Regulate metabolism as enzyme and hormone constituents to modulate cellular activity

TABLE 2.6 Tolerable upper intake levels for minerals

FIGURE 2.6 lists participating minerals in catabolic and anabolic cellular processes. Minerals activate reactions that release energy during carbohydrate, lipid, and protein catabolism. They play important roles in nutrient biosynthesis—glycogen from glucose, triacylglycerols from fatty acids and glycerol, and proteins from amino acids. A

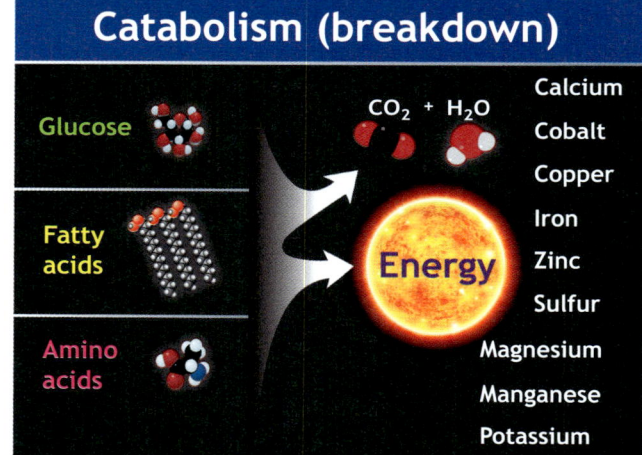
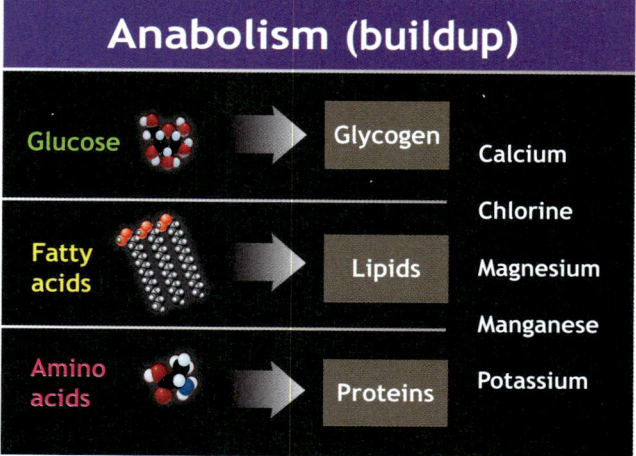

FIGURE 2.6. Minerals that function in macronutrient catabolism and anabolism.

deficiency in one or more essential minerals can disrupt the fine balance between catabolism and anabolism. Minerals also form important hormone constituents. Inadequate thyroxine production from iodine insufficiency, for example, slows the body's resting metabolism. In extreme cases, this could predispose a person to obesity development. Insulin synthesis requires zinc (as do approximately 100 enzymes), whereas chlorine forms the key digestive acid hydrochloric acid.

TABLE 2.7 Food sources, functions, and effects of deficiencies and excesses for important major and trace minerals for healthy adults

The following sections describe specific mineral functions related to physical activity.

Calcium

Calcium, the body's most abundant mineral, combines with phosphorus to form bones and teeth. These two minerals represent approximately 75% of the body's total mineral content equivalent to about 2.5% body mass. In its ionized form (about 1% or 1200 g endogenous calcium), calcium exhibits these nine functions[41,101]:

1. Stimulate muscle
2. Blood clotting
3. Nerve impulse transmission
4. Enzyme activation
5. Calcitriol synthesis (active vitamin D form)
6. Fluid transport across cell membranes
7. Reduce premenstrual syndrome symptoms
8. Reduce colon cancer risk
9. Optimize blood pressure regulation

 See the animation "Calcium in Muscles" on Lippincott Connect to view this process.

Calcium, Estrogen, and Physical Activity

Bone, a dynamic tissue collagen and mineral matrix, exists in a continual state of flux called **remodeling**. Most of the adult skeleton is replaced about every 10 years. Bone-destroying cells called osteoclasts (under parathyroid hormone influence) cause the breakdown or resorption of bone by enzyme action. In contrast, bone-forming osteoblast cells induce bone synthesis. Calcium availability affects bone remodeling dynamics. The two broad bone categories include the following:

1. **Cortical bone**: dense, hard outer layer in the long bone shafts of the arms and legs
2. **Trabecular bone**: spongy, less dense, and relatively weaker bone, most prevalent in the vertebrae and ball of the femur

 See the animation "Bone Growth" on Lippincott Connect to view this process.

Calcium from food or derived from bone resorption maintains plasma calcium levels. Age and gender determine a person's calcium needs. As a general guideline from the National Academy of Medicine (NAM: https://nam.edu/), adolescents and young adults require 1300 mg calcium or the calcium in five 8-oz glasses of milk daily (1000 mg for adults ages 19 to 50 and 1200 mg for those older than age 50). Unfortunately, calcium remains one of the most frequent nutrients lacking in the diets of both sedentary and physically active individuals, particularly adolescent girls. For a typical adult, daily calcium intake only ranges between 500 and 700 mg. Female dancers, gymnasts, and endurance competitors are most prone to calcium dietary insufficiency.[16,108]

Inadequate calcium intake or low calcium-regulating hormone levels cause withdrawal of calcium "reserves" in bone to restore any deficit. Prolonging this restorative imbalance can promote one of two conditions:

1. **Osteopenia**—from the Greek words osteo, meaning "*bone*," and penia, meaning "*poverty*"—a midway condition where bones weaken with increased fracture risk.
2. **Osteoporosis**, literally meaning "porous bones," with bone density more than 2.5 standard deviations below normal for gender. Osteoporosis develops progressively as bone loses its calcium mass or bone mineral content and its calcium concentration or bone mineral density. This deterioration causes bone to progressively become more porous and brittle (**FIG. 2.7**). Eventually, the stresses of normal living cause bone to break, with spine compression fractures occurring most frequently (http://www.nof.org).

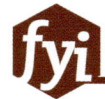 **Osteoporosis Risk Factors**

Normal bone	Osteoporosis
• Advancing age	• Sedentary lifestyle
• Adult fracture history	• Early menopause
• Parent/sibling facture history	• Eating disorder history
• Cigarette smoking	• High animal protein intake
• Slight build or underweight	• Excess sodium intake
• White or Asian female	• Alcohol abuse
• Low dietary calcium before/after menopause	• Vitamin D deficiency

adike/Shutterstock

 **INTEGRATIVE QUESTION**

How do physical activity and calcium intake impact bone health?

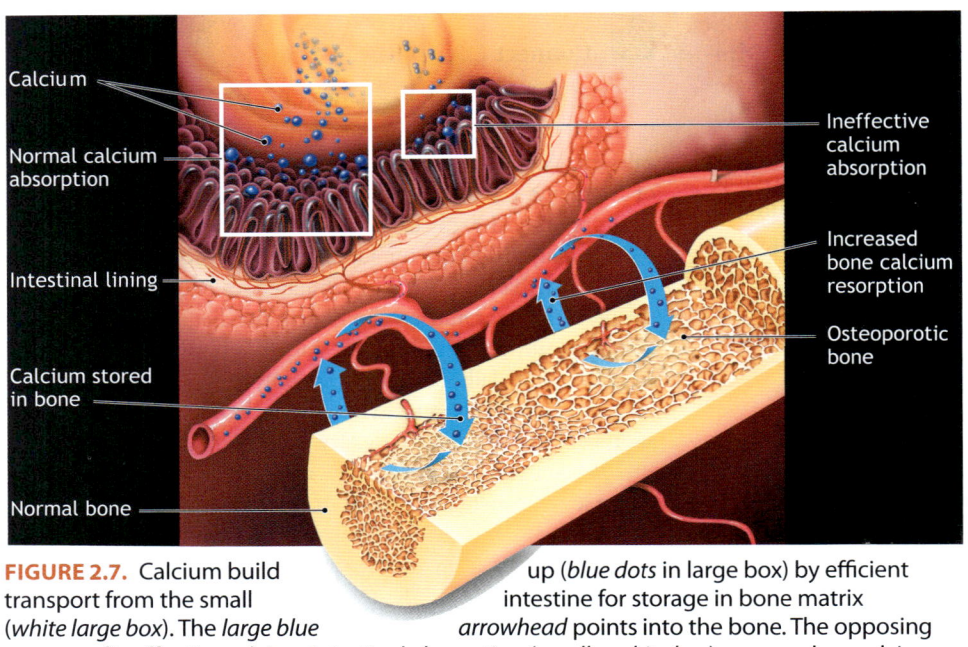

FIGURE 2.7. Calcium build up (*blue dots* in large box) by efficient transport from the small intestine for storage in bone matrix (*white large box*). The *large blue arrowhead* points into the bone. The opposing process of ineffective calcium intestinal absorption (*smaller white box*) occurs when calcium leaches from bones shown by the *large blue arrowhead* pointing into the capillary blood stream, leaving bones brittle with likely fracture occurrence.

Osteoporosis: A Progressive Disease

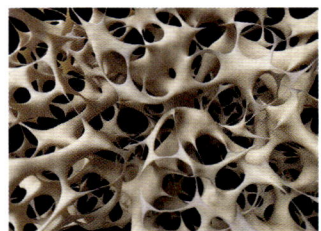

SciePro/Shutterstock

Current estimates indicate that 1 in 4 women and 1 in 18 men aged 65 years and older have osteoporosis, and another 1 in 2 have abnormal bone mass or osteopenia. Between 60 and 80% of susceptibility to osteoporosis links to genetic factors, while 20 to 40% remains lifestyle related. The early teens serve as the prime years to maximize bone mass.[15,107,188] Regular physical activity encourages bone mass gains throughout life's third decade. Osteoporosis for many women begins early in life because the typical teenager consumes suboptimal calcium to support growing bones. This creates an irreversible deficit that cannot be fully eliminated after achieving skeletal maturity. A genetic predisposition can worsen calcium imbalance into adulthood.[53,94,169] Adequate calcium intake, preferably from food and vitamin D supplements (600 international units [IU] daily for most adults and at least 800 IU daily after age 70), helps to maintain normal blood calcium levels and bone mineralization.[18,88,93,94,163,176]

One in two females and one in eight males above age 50 can expect an osteoporosis-related fracture in their lifetime. Increased susceptibility to osteoporosis among older women coincides with menopause and marked decrease in estradiol secretion, the most potent naturally occurring human estrogen (see Chapter 20). Most men normally produce some estrogen with aging—a major reason why older men exhibit relatively lower osteoporosis prevalence. Some circulating testosterone converts to estradiol to help promote positive calcium balance.

Bone Loss Prevention Through Diet

FIGURE 2.8A illustrates that a complex interaction among factors that contribute to bone mass variations.[98,153] Bone mass variation attributable to diet may reflect how it interacts with genetic factors, physical activity patterns, body weight, and drug or medication use (e.g., estrogen therapy). Adequate calcium intake throughout life remains the prime defense against bone loss with age.[15,76] As an example, postmenarchal girls with

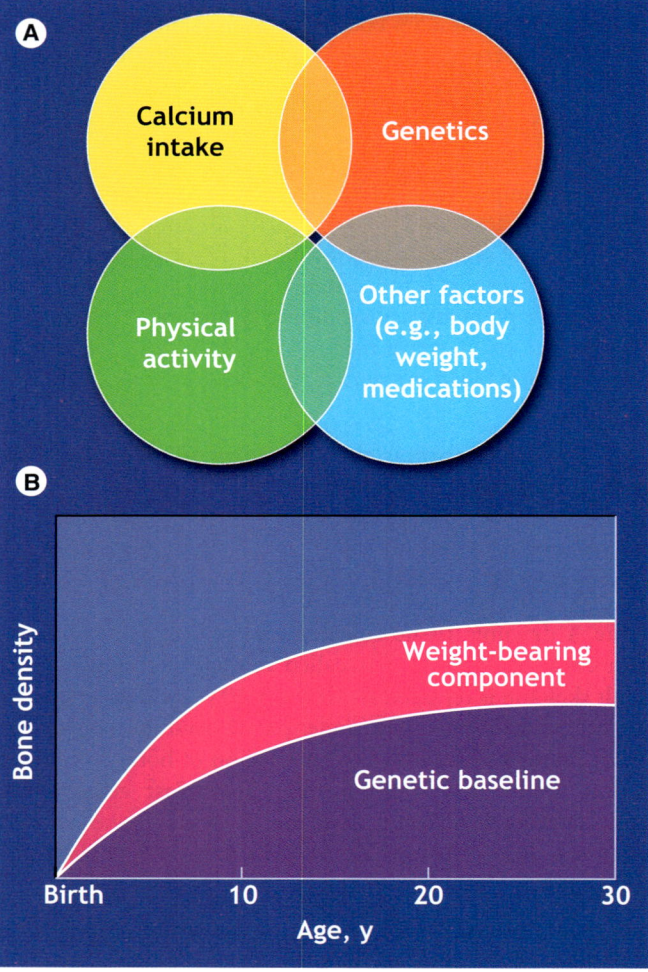

FIGURE 2.8. **(A)** Four intertwined factors impacting variation in bone mass within the population. **(B)** Weight-bearing physical activity augments skeletal mass during growth above the genetic baseline depending on bone mechanical loading.

In a Practical Sense

Milk Products and Health

In the United States, the recommended milk intake (or equivalent cheese, yogurt, or other dairy product) averages three 8-oz (237 mL) servings daily for adults and children 9 years of age or older—an amount substantially higher than the current average adult intake that averages only 1.6 daily servings. The relatively high recommended intake has been justified to meet nutritional requirements for calcium and reduce bone fractures and all-cause mortality risk. Nevertheless, scientists recently have challenged this assertion about milk's health benefits and possible adverse health outcomes.

DAIRY PRODUCT COMPOSITION

TABLE 1 presents human and cow's milk and cheese nutrient composition. To increase milk production, cows have been bred to produce higher insulinlike growth factor 1 (IGF-1) levels, which increases progestins, estrogens, and other hormones levels in milk as they remain pregnant for most of their milking service.

Milk processing has many potential health implications. Pasteurization reduces brucellosis, an infectious disease characterized by higher and lower (undulant) fever swings, sweating, muscle and joint pains, and weakness, tuberculosis, and other pathogen transmissions. Fermentation to produce aged cheese, yogurt, kefir, and other products denatures peptide hormones, alters protein antigens, reduces lactose content, and affects bacterial composition. The fractionation process yields butter, reduced-fat products, and whey protein. Fortification with vitamins A and D can supplement diets with these nutrients.

MILK AND BONE HEALTH

A central rationale for recommending high lifelong milk consumption is that this nutritional behavior will provide calcium's bone health benefits. Such an assumption derives from studies assessing calcium intake and excretion balance in just 155 adults in whom the estimated daily calcium intake needed to maintain balance averaged only 741 mg. Beside the small sample size, these balance studies had other serious limitations, which included 2- to 3-wk short duration with high habitual calcium intake. In other studies, the threshold estimated balance occurred at approximately 200 $mg \cdot d^{-1}$ dietary calcium intake among males with low habitual calcium intakes consistent with the body's adaptation to up-regulate absorption with low dietary intake.

In randomized trials that used bone mineral density as a fracture risk surrogate, daily calcium supplements of 1000 to 2000 mg produced a 1 to 3% greater bone mineral density (BMD) than a placebo. If sustained, this small divergence would be important. However, after 1 year, the rate of BMD change among late perimenopausal and postmenopausal women equaled the placebo value, and upon discontinuing the supplementation, the small difference in BMD disappeared. Because of this transient "beneficial effect" of supplementation, trials lasting 1 year or less can be misleading, and the 2- to 3-wk balance studies to establish calcium requirements have limited relevance to fracture risk. In fact, higher calcium intakes may relate to higher hip fracture rates. **FIGURE 1** shows that countries with the highest milk and calcium intakes have the highest hip fracture rates. This positive association may not be causal, however, because confounding factors (e.g., vitamin D status and ethnicity) could have impacted the findings. Clearly, low dairy consumption tracks with low hip fracture rates across diverse cultures, climates, and economic status. Note that Indonesia and China rank poorly for milk intake yet have the lowest bone fracture rates yearly. To confound the issue, some countries with relatively high dairy consumption also have relatively low hip fracture rates. The United States, Australia, and France, for example, experience relatively low fracture rates with only moderate milk consumption.

MILK AND MORTALITY

When comparing major protein sources from animals or plants, dairy consumption associates with lower mortality than with processed red meat and egg consumption. Similar mortality occurs for unprocessed red meat, poultry, and fish consumption, yet significantly higher than consumption of plant-based protein sources (**FIG. 2**).

HUMAN AND COW'S MILK AND CHEESE NUTRIENT COMPOSITION[a]

Component	Human Milk—8 oz	Whole-Fat Cow's Milk—8 oz	Fat-Free Cow's Milk—8 oz	Cheddar Cheese—37 g
Kilocalories	172	149	83	149
Protein, g	2.5	7.7	8.2	8.0
Total lipid, g	10.0	7.9	0.2	12.3
Saturated fat, g	4.9	4.6	0.1	7.0
Carbohydrate, g	16.9	11.7	12.1	1.1
Calcium, mg	78.0	276.0	289.0	262.0
Potassium, mg	125.0	322.0	381.0	28.0
Phosphorus, mg	34.4	205.0	246.0	167.9

[a]Nutrient composition from U.S. Department of Agriculture (www.usda.org). Cheddar cheese (37 g) remains isocaloric with 237 mL whole milk.
(Africa Studio/Shutterstock)

In a Practical Sense (Continued)

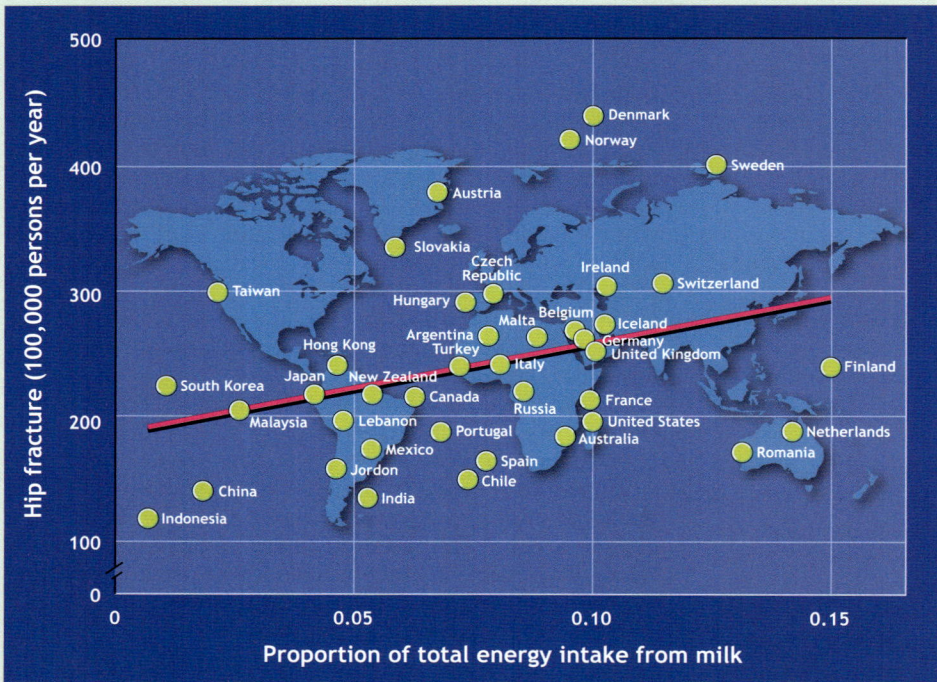

FIGURE 1. Milk consumption as a proportion of total energy intake versus age-standardized hip fractures rates per 100,000 persons per year. Data on national milk intake (including all forms of milk, cheese, and other derived products) are from the United Nations Food and Agriculture Organization and nationally representative hip fracture rates combining males and females standardized to the 2010 world population. (From Willett WC, Ludwig DS. Milk and health. *N Engl J Med.* 2020;382:644. DOI: 10.1056/NEJMra1903547; Copyright © 2020 Massachusetts Medical Society. Reprinted with permission from Massachusetts Medical Society. Map image by T. Lesia/Shutterstock.)

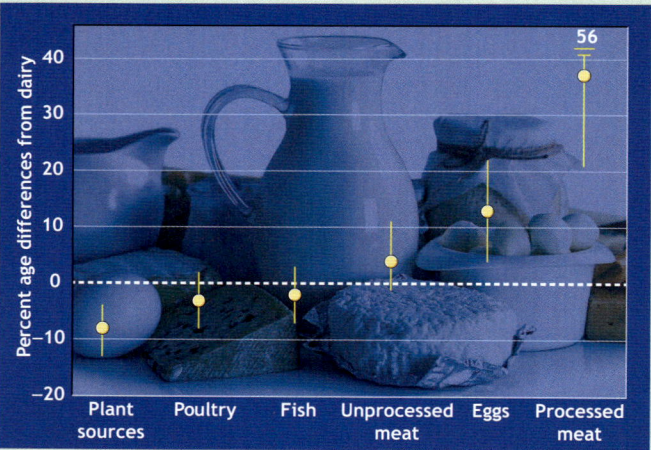

FIGURE 2. Percent age difference in all-cause mortality associated with protein sources. The *colored dashed line* at 0 is the reference mortality value associated with major protein dairy sources. Comparisons reflect 3% of protein energy from each source, with milk corresponding to about 500 g (two 8-oz glasses). Data were recalculated with dairy foods as the comparison based from a 32-year follow-up in 131,342 males and females. Lifestyle, dietary, and other risk factors were statistically adjusted for cardiovascular disease and cancer. (From Willett WC, Ludwig DS. Milk and health. *N Engl J Med.* 2020;382:644. doi: 10.1056/NEJMra1903547. Copyright © 2020 Massachusetts Medical Society. Reprinted with permission from Massachusetts Medical Society. Africa Studio/Shutterstock.)

CONCLUSIONS

The overall evidence in adults does not support high dairy consumption for fracture reduction, the belief that has justified current U.S. nutritional recommendations. Reported health effects from dairy food consumption depend on comparing specific foods or beverages. Dairy foods compare favorably versus processed red meat or sugar-sweetened beverages but compare less favorably with plant-protein sources.

Results for cow's milk consumption in children are less clear because children have greater nutritional requirements for growth. Cow's milk will provide a valuable substitute without availability of mother's milk. In general, overall diet quality dictates optimal milk intake. With low diet quality, especially for children in poor-income environments, dairy foods will improve overall nutrition. In contrast, high milk intake with high-quality diets is unlikely to offer substantial health benefits.

Sources:
Bzikowska-Jura A, et al. The concentration of omega-3 fatty acids in human milk is related to their habitual but not current intake. *Nutrients.* 2019;11:1585.

Wesolowska A, et al. Lipid profile, lipase bioactivity, and lipophilic antioxidant content in high pressure processed donor human milk. *Nutrients.* 2019;11:1972.

Willett WC, Ludwig DS. Milk and health. *N Engl J Med.* 2020;382:644. doi: 10.1056/NEJMra1903547

suboptimal calcium intake who took calcium supplements enhanced bone mineral acquisition.[140] Adolescent girls should consume 1500 mg calcium daily. For middle-aged, estrogen-deprived women following menopause, increasing daily calcium intake from 1200 to 1500 mg improved the body's calcium balance.[11,63,128] Adequate calcium intake and adding animal protein to the diet may reduce hip fracture risk.

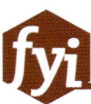

Estrogen's Role in Bone Health

- Increases intestinal calcium absorption
- Reduces urinary calcium excretion
- Inhibits bone resorption
- Decreases bone turnover

Sources:
Ling W, et al. Mitochondrial Sirt3 contributes to the bone loss caused by aging or estrogen deficiency. *JCI Insight.* 2021;6:e146728.
Weivoda MM, et al. miRNAs in osteoclast biology. *Bone.* 2021;143:115757.

Recommended dietary calcium sources include milk and milk products, sardines and canned salmon, kidney beans, and dark green leafy vegetables. Eight ounces of milk or 6 oz yogurt contains 300 mg calcium, and one cup spinach contains 270 mg. Americans spend more than $1 billion a year on calcium supplements hoping to avoid osteoporosis. Nearly 45% of American women, mostly older women, use dietary supplements containing calcium. Calcium supplements can correct dietary deficiencies regardless of whether the extra calcium comes from fortified foods or commercial supplements. For optimal absorption, calcium carbonate should be consumed with meals; calcium citrate may be taken anytime. Calcium citrate causes less stomach upset than other supplement forms and also enhances iron absorption better than calcium gluconate, calcium carbonate, or other highly advertised commercial products. Adequate vitamin D availability facilitates calcium uptake.[187] This vitamin deficiency contributes to osteoporosis with increased fractures risk with falls. Low vitamin D levels may even increase vulnerability to falls. Current recommendations advise against taking a supplement containing more than 1000 mg calcium and 400 IU vitamin D daily to maintain bone health and prevent fractures.

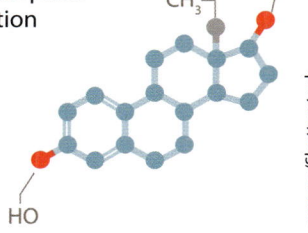

National Academy of Sciences Recommended Daily Calcium Intake

Age (y)	Amount (mg)
1–3	500
4–8	800
9–18	1300
19–50	1000
51 and older	1200

jennyt/Shutterstock

Women at high osteoporosis-related bone fracture risk may benefit from drug therapy. The FDA approved a new Amgen dual-acting drug *Evenity* (romosozumab-aqqg; www.fiercepharma.com/pharma/amgen-s-once-dismissed-osteoporosis-drug-evenity-back-game-after-rosy-fda-panel-vote) in April, 2019, based on a study that assessed about 12,000 women with postmenopausal osteoporosis. This drug gives postmenopausal patients with high fracture risk greater "comfort" against future fractures. The drug contains an antiresorptive compound that slows bone loss and an anabolic agent to facilitate bone accretion.

Calcium supplements should be consumed in moderation as some research has linked excessive intake in supplement form (not food) to increased heart attack and kidney stone risk. Excessive meat, salt, coffee, and alcohol consumption inhibits absorption. Individuals who live and train primarily indoors in northern latitudes should supplement with 200 IU of vitamin D daily.[7,190] Bone matrix formation also depends on vitamin K, prevalent in leafy green and cruciferous vegetables—RDA is 90 mg for women and 120 mg for men.

Physical Activity Benefits

Mechanical loading through regular physical activity slows the skeletal aging rate. Regardless of age or sex, children and adults who maintain an active lifestyle have greater bone mass, bone size, and bone structure than sedentary counterparts.[4,5,62,83,90,159] Former male interscholastic sport participants and female interscholastic power sport competitors have stronger bones than peers even when adjusting for current physical activity levels.[191] Activity's benefits on bone mass accretion, and perhaps bone shape and size, occur primarily during childhood and adolescence when peak bone mass increases to the greatest extent (Fig. 2.8B); benefits may persist beyond activity cessation,[6,59,105,114] often into the seventh and eighth decades of life.[17,84,151] The decline in vigorous physical activity accompanying a sedentary lifestyle with aging closely parallels age-related bone mass loss. In this regard, regular moderate physical activity coincides with more substantial cortical bone measures[144] and a definite lower hip fracture risk in postmenopausal women.[45,141]

Physical activity's osteogenic effect proves most effective during growth in childhood and adolescence and may reduce fracture risk later in life.[15,72,78] Short but vigorous mechanical bone loading with dynamic exercise three to five times a week provides a potent stimulus to maintain or increase bone mass. **FIGURE 2.9** illustrates beneficial effects from resistance training and circuit resistance training, or weight-bearing walking, running, dancing, rope skipping, or gymnastics participation. These activity modes generate a considerable impact load and/or intermittent force against the body's long bones.[39,91,192]

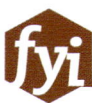 **Vitamin D—More Important Than Previously Believed**

Vitamin D deficiency (defined as blood levels below 20 ng · mL⁻¹) associates with greater knee osteoarthritis risk.

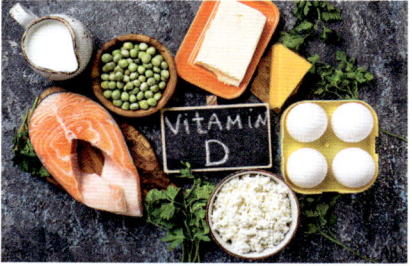

Yulia Furman/Shutterstock

Also, consuming "healthful" vitamin D foods plays a positive role in helping to mitigate risk in breast, colorectal, prostate, gastric, and ovarian cancers, but future, longer-term studies are required to determine whether increased vitamin D present in foods may boost survival for individuals already diagnosed with a malignancy. Vitamin D, intimately involved with immune function, activates disease-fighting T cells. Most studies support the claim that vitamin D–rich foods reduce cancer incidence risk and death.

Source:
Voutsadakis IA. Vitamin D baseline levels at diagnosis of breast cancer: A systematic review and meta-analysis. *Hematol Oncol Stem Cell Ther.* 2021;14:16.

Male and female participants in strength and power activities have as much or more bone mass than endurance athlete counterparts.[132] Volleyball, basketball, and gymnastic activities with relatively high impact and strain on skeletal mass induce the greatest bone mass increases, particularly at weight-bearing sites.[9,30,99,149]

Bone Mass Related to Muscular Strength

Bone mineral density and bone mass relate directly to muscular strength and regional and total lean tissue mass.[32,49,124] Elite teenage weightlifters' lumbar spine and proximal femur bone masses exceed representative values of fully mature reference adults.[29] Eccentric muscle training provides a more potent site-specific osteogenic stimulus than concentric muscle training because greater forces usually occur with eccentric loading.[61] Prior physical activity and sport experiences confer residual effects on an adult's bone mineral density. Exercise-induced bone mass increases achieved during teenage and early-adulthood persist despite their withdrawal from active competition.[81,83]

Site-Specific Muscular Force Effects

Muscle forces acting on specific bones during physical activity, particularly intermittent compression and tension mechanical loading, modify bone metabolism at the stress point.[13,70,79] For example, older cross-country runners' lower limb bones exceed the bone mineral content of less-active counterparts. A baseball player's throwing arm shows greater bone thickness than their less-used, nondominant arm. Likewise, the mineral content of the bone humeral shaft and proximal humerus of the playing arm of a tennis player averages 20 to 25% more than their nondominant arm. Side-to-side difference in nonplayers' arms generally averages only 5%.[83] For females, this positive specific sports training response occurs mostly in players who begin training before menarche.[77] Males who jump trained for 12 months decreased sclerostin blood levels (protein that blocks bone formation), while similarly increasing hormone IGF-1 levels, which supports bone formation.

 **INTEGRATIVE QUESTION**

Why does resistance training the body's major muscle groups offer unique bone mass benefits compared with a typical brisk walking weight-bearing program?

Mechanism for Bone Matrix Increase

Dynamic loading creates hydrostatic pressure gradients within a bone's fluid-filled matrix. Fluid movement within the matrix in response to pressure changes from dynamic activity generates fluid shear stress on bone cells, which initiates a cascade of cellular events to stimulate production of bone matrix

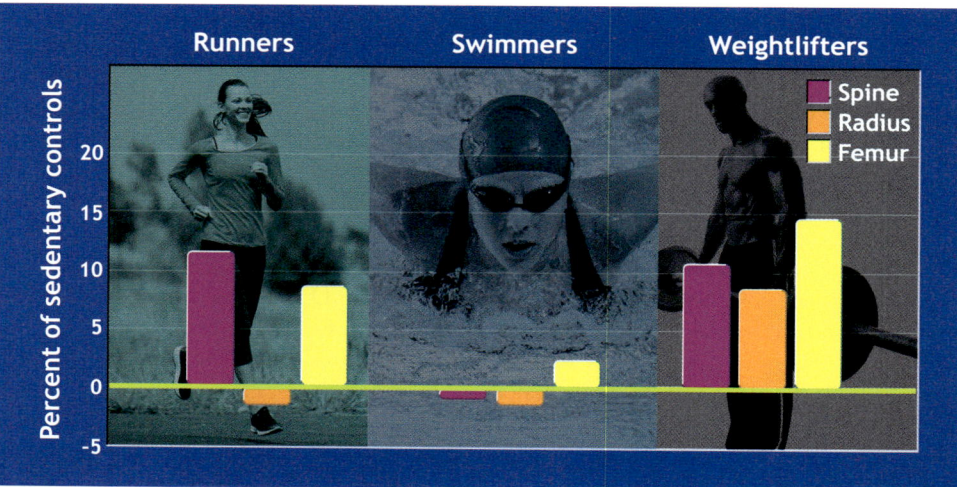

FIGURE 2.9. Beneficial weight-bearing activities on bone mineral density expressed as a percentage of sedentary control values at three skeletal sites for runners, *swimmers*, and *weightlifters*.
(Shutterstock: KieferPix; wavebreakmedia; ARENA Creative)

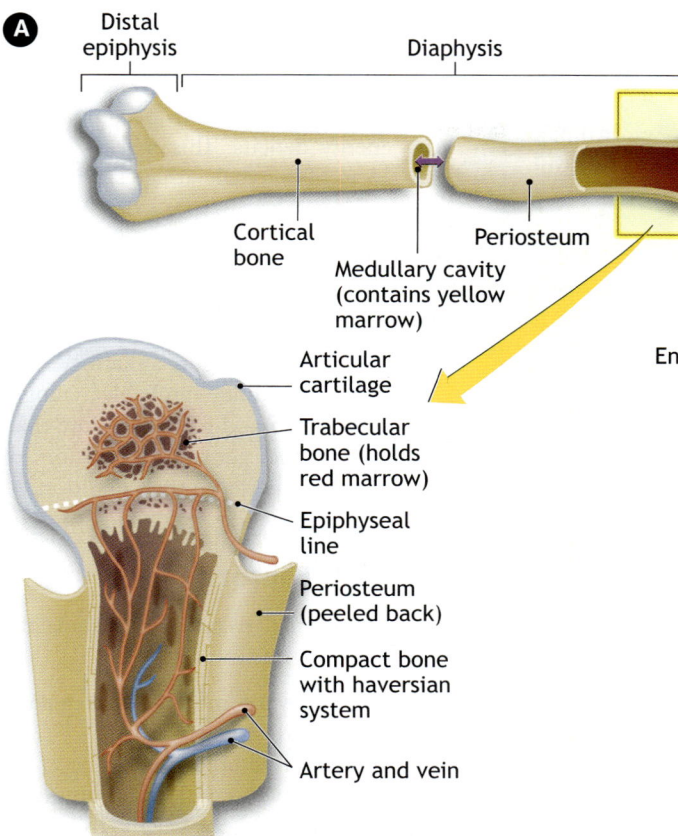

bone mass accretion.[58,87,133] As applied force and strain increase, the number of cycles required to initiate bone formation decrease.[31] Chemicals produced in bone itself also contribute to bone formation. Alterations in bone's geometric configuration to long-term exercise training enhance its mechanical properties.[11] **FIGURE 2.10** shows the typical long bone's anatomic structure and cross-sectional view and depicts bone growth and remodeling dynamics.

Six Principles Promote Bone Health Through Physical Activity

1. Specificity: Physical activity provides a local osteogenic effect.
2. Overload: Progressively increasing exercise intensity promotes continued bone deposition.
3. Initial values: Individuals with the smallest total bone mass have the greatest bone deposition potential.
4. Diminishing returns: As one approaches bone density's biologic ceiling, further density gains require greater physical effort.
5. More not necessarily better: Bone cells desensitize during prolonged mechanical-loading sessions.
6. Reversibility: Discontinuing exercise overload reverses positive osteogenic effects gained through increased physical activity.

Female Athlete Triad

Definition

The **female athlete triad** or triad represents a medical condition observed in physically active girls and women (and some men—see next section) involving one or more of the following components:

1. Low energy availability (EA) with or without disordered eating
2. Menstrual dysfunction
3. Low bone mineral density (BMD)

Female athletes often present with one or more of the three triad components, and early intervention can prevent its progression to serious end points that include clinical eating disorders (EDs), amenorrhea, and osteoporosis.[199–201] The triad model represents each component as the pathological end point for one of the three interrelated spectrums, ranging from a healthy end point to subclinical and, ultimately, clinical conditions. At the continuums "healthy" end (green in **FIGURE 2.11**), each triad component optimizes energy availability to achieve three outcomes:

1. Meeting total energy expenditure requirements
2. Meeting reproductive and bone health needs
3. Maintaining ovulatory menstrual cycles with normal bone mass

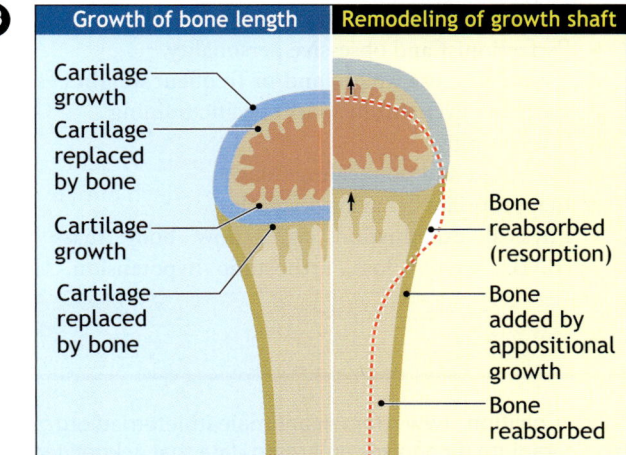

FIGURE 2.10. (A) Anatomic structure and longitudinal long bone view. (B) Bone dynamics during bone growth and continual bone shaft remodeling.

protein.[168] Two factors that regulate mechanosensitivity and subsequent calcium buildup in bone are as follows:

1. Applied force and strain magnitude
2. Repetitive frequency or number of cycles of force application

Owing to bone cells' transient sensitivity to mechanical stimuli, shorter but more frequent high-frequency force periods (mechanical strain) with interspersed rest periods facilitate

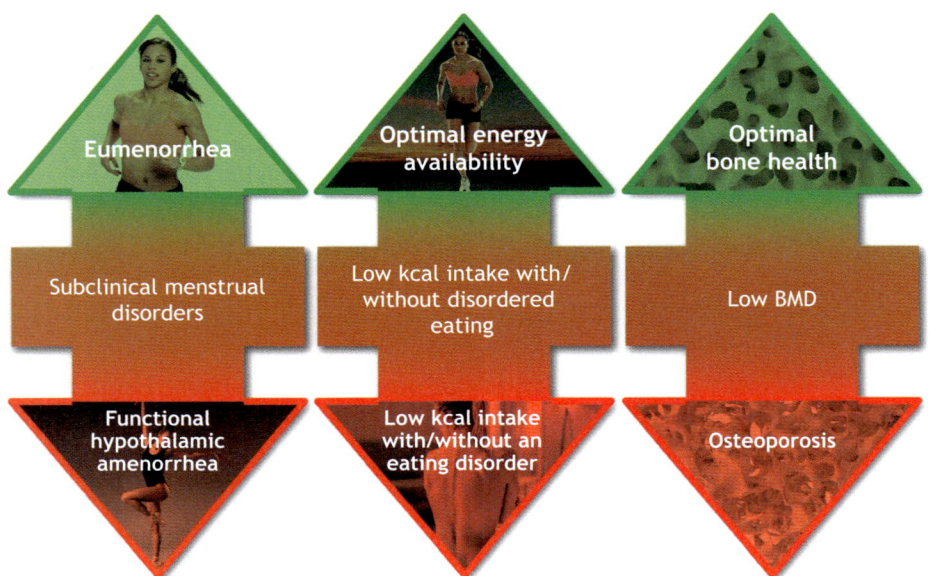

Many female sport participants likely suffer from at least one triad disorder, particularly disordered eating behaviors and accompanying energy deficits. This malady afflicts 15 to 60% female athletes, especially those involved in sports that "silently" promote leanness.[116,166,194,195,202] Amenorrhea's prevalence in body weight–emphasized sports like distance running, gymnastics, ballet, cheerleading, figure skating, and body building—probably ranges between 25 and 65%. No more than 5% of the general population of females experience this condition.

FIGURE 2.11. The female athlete triad spectrum illustrates three inter-related optimal components, shown in *green*, and three corresponding, potentially devastating conditions, depicted in *red*. An athlete's condition can move along each spectrum *arrow* at different rates depending on nutrient intake (dietary factors) and physical activity behaviors.
(Shutterstock: Gino Santa Maria; Olena Yakobchuk; Dmytro Zinkevych; adike)

Risk Factors

Major triad risk factors include the following:

- History of menstrual irregularities and amenorrhea
- Stress fracture history
- Excessive critical comments about eating or weight from parent, coach, or teammates
- Depression history
- Dieting history
- Perfectionist and obsessive personality
- Pressure to lose weight and/or frequent weight cycling
- Early involvement in sport-specific training
- Overtraining
- Recurrent and nonhealing injuries
- Inappropriate behavior of coaches
- Physical examination signs (low body mass index [BMI], weight loss, orthostatic hypotension, lanugo,

At the "unhealthy" continuum's end point (shown in red), each triad component presents the clinical syndrome's end points, including low energy availability with or without disordered eating (energy drain), functional hypothalamic amenorrhea, and osteoporosis.[28,86,95,123,150,193]

 INTEGRATIVE QUESTION

What are some factors that contribute to the female athlete triad, and how might a coach guard against them?

 Female and Male Athlete Triad Coalition

In 1977, the concept female athlete triad was adopted as the official position stand by the American College of Sports Medicine (www.acsm.org). It was updated in 2007 and represented the scientific foundations and clinical conditions affecting physically active women's health. The triad was established using scientifically rigorous research evidence. In its current form, the model argues that low energy availability (energy deficiency), presenting with or without disordered eating behaviors, triggers menstrual disorders, which contributes to poor bone health. The Female Athlete Triad Coalition underwent an official organizational name change in 2019 to become the Female and Male Athlete

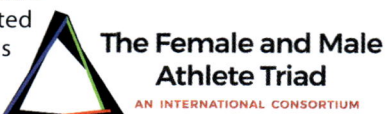

Reprinted with permission from The Female and Male Athlete Triad Coalition (www.femaleandmaleathletetriad.org)

Triad Coalition (www.femaleandmaleathletetriad.org/). This new paradigm recognizes emerging data that acknowledges a similar triadlike model in physically active men. De Souza and colleagues have spearheaded research related to this clinical model, which includes males (Sports Med. 2019;49:125), and other De Souza research modeling about the female athlete triad cited at the end of the chapter (*Br J Sports Med.* 2014;48:289).

Sources:
Logue DM, et al. Low energy availability in athletes 2020: an updated narrative review of prevalence, risk, within-day energy balance, knowledge, and impact on sports performance. *Nutrients*. 2020;12:835.
Moore EM, et al. Examination of athlete triad symptoms among endurance-trained male athletes: a field study. *Front Nutr.* 2021;8:737777.
Nattiv A, et al. American College of Sports Medicine Position Stand. The female athlete triad. *Med Sci Sports Exerc.* 2007;39:1867.

hypercarotenemia), eating disorder signs (e.g., parotid gland swelling and callus on proximal interphalangeal joints [Russell sign])
- Medication history of use of oral contraceptive pills or agents
- Family history of osteoporosis and/or stress fractures

Diagnosis

Following initial risk factor screening, an accurate triad disorder diagnosis depends on a thorough physician's evaluation in concert with other multidisciplinary healthcare team members that include a sports dietitian (registered dietitian, preferably a board-certified dietetics specialist) and a mental health professional. Triad components can be interrelated in that an energy deficiency relates to disordered eating, which plays a causal role in menstrual disturbances. An energy deficiency also associates with **hypoestrogenesis** to produce amenorrhea and low bone density.[199,200]

Bone density relates closely to menstrual regularity and total menstrual cycle number. Premature menstrual cessation removes estrogen's protective effect on bone, making these young women more vulnerable to calcium loss with concomitant bone mass decreases. The most severe menstrual disorders produce the greatest negative effect on bone mass.[24,165] Lowered bone density from extended amenorrhea often occurs at multiple sites, including bone areas regularly subjected to increased force and impact loading during physical activity.[129] The problem worsens in individuals who experience an energy deficit accompanied by low protein, lipid, and energy intakes.[181] In such cases, a poor diet also provides inadequate calcium intake.

Amenorrhea at an early age diminishes regular physical activity's benefits on bone mass. It also increases risk of musculoskeletal injuries and repeated stress fractures during exercise participation.[110] A 5% bone mass loss increases stress fracture risk by nearly 40%. Re-establishing normal menses regains some bone mass but not to levels achieved with normal menstruation. Bone mass often remains permanent at suboptimal levels throughout adult life leaving these women at increased osteoporosis and stress fracture risk, often for years following competitive athletic participation.[38,104]

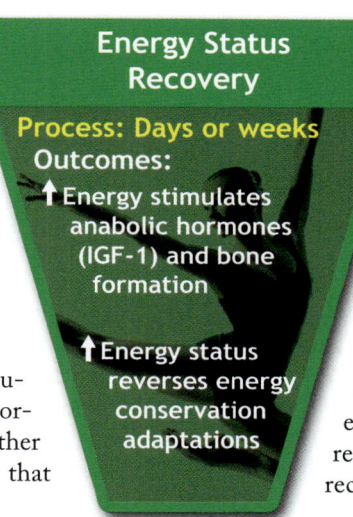

FIGURE 2.12. Conceptual framework for treating the female athlete triad. Energy status stimulates insulinlike growth factor-1 (IGF-1) and improves bone health.
(Sources: World literature[199–203] [cited on Lippincott Connect], and see recent De Souza MJ, et al. citation the end of this chapter. Shutterstock: XiXinXing; Zoriana Zaitseva; YAAV)

Treatment

FIGURE 2.12 displays a framework for treating the female athlete triad. The three triad components recover at different rates with appropriate treatment.[199,202] Energy status recovers after days or weeks of increased energy intake and/or decreased energy expenditure. Menstrual status recovery typically takes months after energy status returns to normal. Full bone mineral density recovery may not occur for many years (if at all) following return to normal for energy intake and menstrual status.[203]

Successful nonpharmacologic athletic amenorrhea treatment typically includes a four-phase behavioral approach plus diet and training interventions:

1. Reduce training intensity 10 to 20%
2. Gradually increase total energy intake
3. Increase body weight 2 to 3%
4. Maintain 1500 mg daily calcium intake

See the animation "Calcium in Muscle" on **Lippincott Connect** to demonstrate this process.

Male Athlete Triad

Similar to females, recent data suggest that a chronic low energy intake of males negatively influences energy metabolism, reproduction, and bone mass, collectively termed the **male athlete triad**.[201,204–207] These three physiologic systems are more robust and resilient to low energy availability in males than in females and thus require more severe energetic perturbations before undesirable responses match those that afflict females.[5,6,8,12,13]

A triadlike syndrome in men appears real but only from limited evidence from well-controlled studies. The concept, **relative energy deficiency in sport (RED-S)**, affects three interrelated components described as low energy availability (energy deficiency) with or without disordered eating, suppressed reproductive functions (low testosterone concentrations and poor semen quality), and impaired bone health.[189,203]

FIGURE 2.13 illustrates the male athlete triad model. The inter-related components of this triad will require additional research documentation to more fully understand the prevalence, dynamics, and consequences of the condition.[189,208]

Phosphorus

Phosphorus combines with calcium to form hydroxyapatite and calcium phosphate—compounds that confer bone and teeth rigidity. Phosphorus serves as an essential intracellular mediator for cyclic adenosine monophosphate (cAMP) and the intramuscular high-energy compounds adenosine triphosphate (ATP) and phosphocreatine (PCr). Phosphorus combines with lipids to form phospholipid compounds, integral to cells' bilayer plasma membrane. The phosphorous-containing phosphatase enzymes regulate cellular metabolism; phosphorous also buffers the acid end products of energy metabolism. Chapter 23 discusses the usefulness of buffering agents to augment intense exercise performance. Athletes usually consume adequate phosphorus, with the possible exception of the low-energy diets of female dancers and gymnasts.[16,108] Rich phosphorus dietary sources include meat, fish, poultry, milk products, and cereals.

Magnesium

Blood contains only about 1% of the body's 20 to 30 g of magnesium, with about half the stores present inside the cells of tissues and organs and with the remainder combined with calcium and phosphorus in bone. About 400 enzymes that regulate metabolic processes contain magnesium, which facilitates muscle and liver glycogen formation from bloodborne glucose. During energy metabolism, magnesium serves as a cofactor in glucose, fatty acid, and amino acid breakdown. Magnesium affects lipid and protein synthesis and contributes to optimal neuromuscular functioning. It acts as an electrolyte and, along with potassium and sodium, helps to regulate blood pressure.

By regulating DNA and ribonucleic acid (RNA) synthesis and structure, magnesium impacts cell growth, reproduction, and plasma membrane integrity. Because of its role as a Ca^{+2} channel blocker, inadequate magnesium could precipitate hypertension and cardiac arrhythmias. Sweating produces only small magnesium losses. Conflicting data concern magnesium supplement's effects on exercise performance and training response.[20,46,167]

The magnesium intake of athletes generally achieves recommended levels, but female dancers and gymnasts have relatively low dietary intakes.[16,108] Rich magnesium sources include green leafy vegetables, legumes, nuts, bananas, mushrooms, and whole grains.

Iron

The body normally contains between 2.5 and 4.0 g (about 1/6 oz) of this trace mineral. Seventy to eighty percent exist in functionally active compounds, predominantly combined with hemoglobin in red blood cells (85% of functional iron). This iron-protein compound increases the blood's oxygen-carrying capacity 65-fold. Iron serves other important exercise-related functions as a **myoglobin** structural component (12% of functional iron), a compound similar to hemoglobin that aids muscle cells' oxygen storage and transport. Small iron amounts also exist in **cytochromes** that facilitate cellular energy transfer. About 20% of the body's iron does not combine in functionally active compounds but rather exists as **hemosiderin** and **ferritin**, which the liver, spleen, and bone marrow store. These stores replenish iron lost from the functional compounds and provide an iron reserve for use during periods of insufficient dietary iron intake. Transferrin, an iron-binding plasma glycoprotein, transports iron from ingested food and damaged red blood cells to tissues in need, particularly the liver, spleen, bone marrow, and skeletal muscles. Plasma transferrin levels reflect current iron intake adequacy.

Physically active individuals should include iron-rich food in their daily diet. Persons with inadequate iron intake, limited iron absorption rates, or unusually high iron loss often develop reduced hemoglobin concentration in red blood cells, commonly known as **iron deficiency anemia**. This medical condition produces general sluggishness, appetite loss, pale skin, sore tongue, brittle nails, infection susceptibility, difficulty keep-

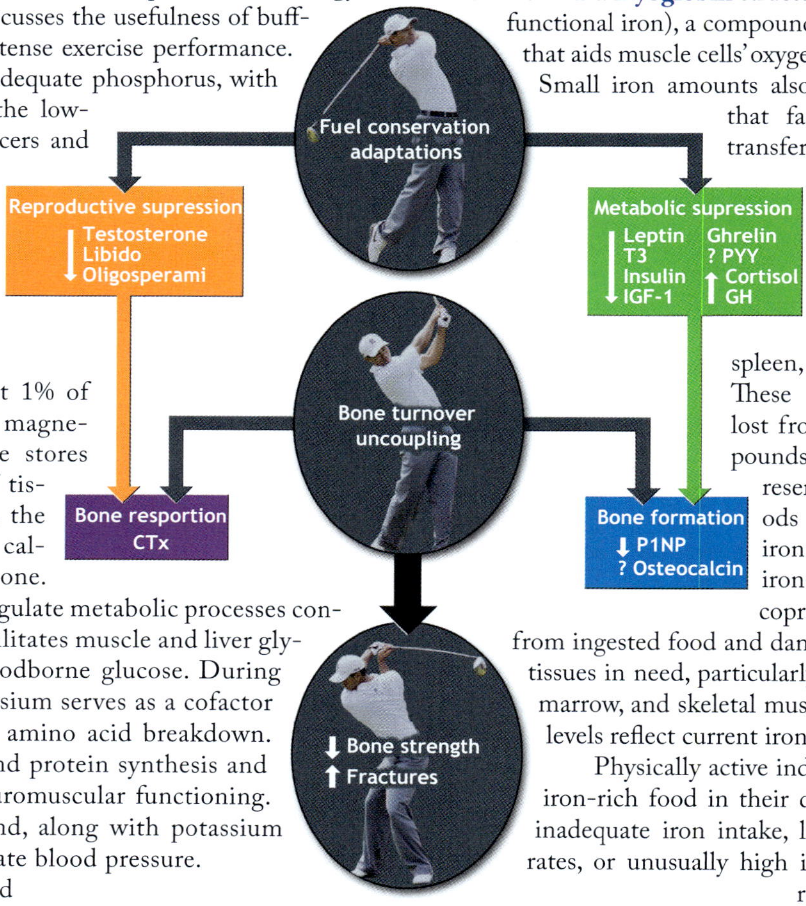

FIGURE 2.13. Conceptual framework for metabolic, reproductive, and bone health in male athletes associated with triadlike female conditions. Changing male athlete's eating patterns and physical activity conditions, robustly reverses metabolic and reproductive suppression from low energy availability than is typical in females. Legend: T3 (total triiodothyronine); PYY (peptide YY); IGF-1 (insulinlike growth factor 1); GH (growth hormone); CTx (C-terminal telopeptide type 1 collagen); P1NP (N-terminal propeptide of type 1 procollagen).
(Sources: World literature[5,6,8,12,13] (refer to chapter references on Lippincott Connect). Brad Thompson/Shutterstock)

ing warm, frontal headaches, dizziness, and reduced capacity to sustain even mild physical activity. "Iron therapy" via controlled blood transfusion usually normalizes the blood's hemoglobin content and subsequent exercise capacity.

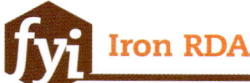

Iron RDA

Recommended Iron RDA	Age, yr	Iron, mg
Children	1–10	10
Males	11–18	12
	19+	10
Females	11–50	15
	51+	10
	Pregnancy	30
	Lactating	30–60

Yulia Furman/Shutterstock

Source:
Food and Nutrition Board, National Academy of Sciences–National Research Council, Washington, DC; www.iom.edu/CMS/3788.aspx

Increased Iron Deficiency Risk in Females

According to the Centers for Disease Control and Prevention (CDC; www.cdc.gov), iron deficiency represents the most common nutritional deficiency and leading cause of anemia in the United States. Insufficient iron intake frequently occurs among young children, teenagers, females of childbearing age, including many physically active females. Between 10 and 13% premenopausal U.S. women suffer from low iron intake, and 3 to 5% are anemic by conventional diagnostic criteria. Six to nine percent of females above age 50 suffer from iron deficiency. Pregnancy can trigger a moderate iron deficiency anemia from the increased iron demands placed on the mother during fetal development.

Iron loss ranges between 15 and 30 mg from the 30 to 60 mL of blood lost during a typical menstrual cycle. This loss requires an additional 5 mg of dietary iron intake daily for premenopausal females and increases the average monthly dietary iron requirement by 150 mg for synthesizing red blood cells lost during menstruation. Approximately 30 to 50% of U.S. females experience dietary iron insufficiency from menstrual blood loss and concomitant low dietary iron intake. The typical iron intake averages 6 mg of iron per 1000 calories consumed, with heme iron providing about 15% of that total.

Fact or Fiction Concerning Exercise-Induced Anemia

Interest in endurance sports, with increased participation by women, has focused research on the influence of intense training on the body's iron status. The term **sports anemia** describes reduced hemoglobin levels approaching clinical anemia (12 g·dL^{-1} blood for females and 14 g·dL^{-1} for males), attributable to physical training. Strenuous training may create an added demand for iron that often exceeds its intake.[196] Depleted iron reserves eventually leads to depressed hemoglobin synthesis and/or reduction in iron-containing compounds within the cell's energy transfer system. Individuals susceptible to an "iron drain" could experience reduced exercise capacity because iron plays a crucial role in oxygen transport and use.

Intense physical training theoretically creates an augmented iron demand from three sources:

1. Sweat
2. Hemoglobin in urine from red blood cell destruction with increased temperature, spleen activity, and circulation rates, from kidney jarring, and mechanical trauma from feet pounding on running surfaces known as foot-strike hemolysis
3. Gastrointestinal bleeding with distance running that is unrelated to age, gender, or performance time

Real Anemia or Pseudoanemia?

Apparent suboptimal hemoglobin concentrations and hematocrits occur more frequently among endurance athletes, supporting the possibility for exercise-induced anemia. However, reduced hemoglobin concentration remains transient, occurring in the early training phase and then returning toward pretraining values. **FIGURE 2.14** illustrates the general response for hematologic variables for high school female cross-country runners during a competitive season. The decrease in hemoglobin concentration generally parallels the disproportionately large expansion in plasma volume with endurance and resistance training[36,54,143] (see Fig. 13.5 in Chapter 13). Several training days increase plasma volume by 20%, while total red blood cell volume remains unchanged. Consequently, total hemoglobin, an important factor in endurance performance, remains the same or increases slightly with training, while hemoglobin concentration decreases in the expanding plasma volume. Despite this hemoglobin dilution, aerobic capacity and exercise performance improve with training.

Mechanical destruction of red blood cells occurs with vigorous physical activity, along with some sweat iron loss. No evidence indicates that these factors strain an athlete's iron reserves and precipitate clinical anemia if iron intake remains at recommended levels. Applying stringent criteria for both anemia and insufficient iron reserves make sports anemia much less prevalent than generally believed. For male collegiate runners and swimmers, no early anemia indications occurred despite large changes in training volume and intensity during the competitive season.[122] For female athletes, iron

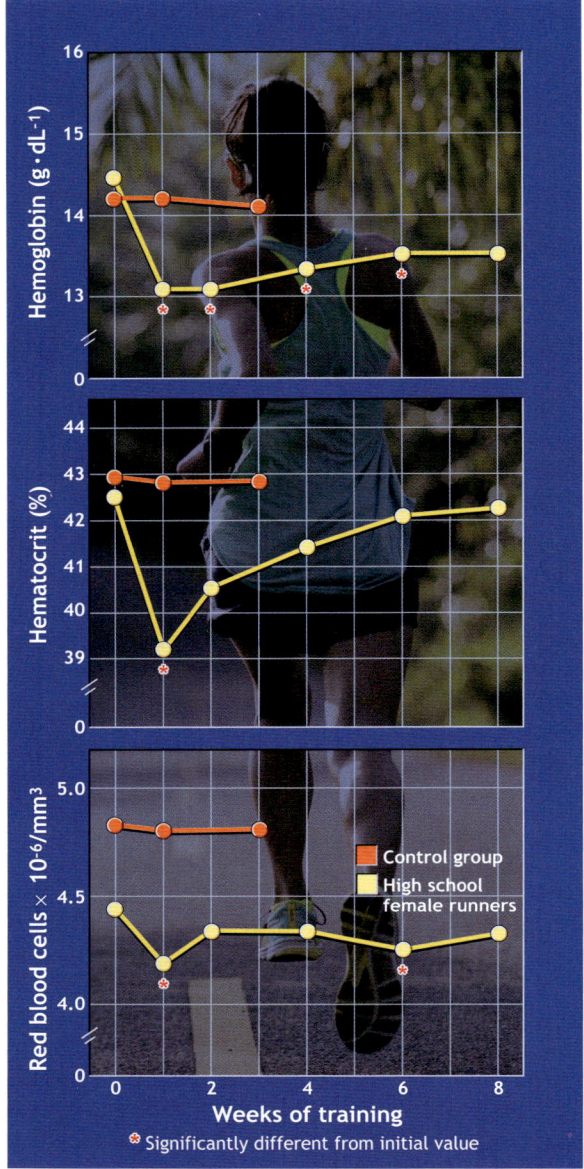

FIGURE 2.14. Hemoglobin, red blood cell count, and hematocrit in female high school cross-country runners and a comparison group during the competitive season.
(Background photo: lzf/Shutterstock)

deficiency anemia prevalence did not differ in comparisons among specific athletic groups or with nonathletic controls.[130]

Should Athletes Take an Iron Supplement?

Any increase in iron loss with training, when coupled with poor dietary habits in adolescent and premenopausal women, strains an already limited iron reserve. This does not mean that all individuals in training should supplement with iron or that dietary iron insufficiency or iron loss caused by physical activity produces sports anemia. It does, however, suggest monitoring an athlete's iron status by periodically evaluating hematologic characteristics and iron reserves, particularly in those who consume iron supplements. Measuring serum ferritin concentration provides useful information about iron reserves. Values below 20 mg · L^{-1} for females and 30 mg · L^{-1} for males indicate depleted reserves.

For healthy individuals whose diets contain the recommended iron intake, excess iron either through diet or supplementation does not increase hemoglobin, hematocrit, or other iron status measures or exercise performance. Potential harm exists from overconsumption or iron overabsorption, particularly with the widespread vitamin C supplement use, which facilitates iron absorption.[47] Iron supplements should not be used indiscriminately. Excessive iron, particularly heme iron, can accumulate to toxic levels and contribute to diabetes, liver disease, and heart and joint damage; it may even promote growth of latent cancers (e.g., colon and prostate) and infectious organisms and create free radicals, which can damage cell membranes, vital proteins, and DNA.

Importance of Iron Source

The small intestine absorbs about 10 to 15% of the total ingested iron, depending on three factors:

1. Iron status
2. Iron's ingested form
3. Meal's nutrient composition

For example, the small intestine usually absorbs 2 to 5% iron from plants (trivalent ferric or nonheme elemental iron),

 Factors Affecting Iron Absorption

Increase Iron Absorption
- Stomach Acid
- Iron in heme form
- High red blood cell demand
- Low body iron stores
- Mean protein factor (MPF) presence
- Vitamin C presence in small intestine

Decrease Iron Absorption
- Phytic acid in dietary fiber
- Oxalic acid
- Polyphenols in tea and coffee
- High body iron stores
- Excess Zn, Mg, Ca taken as supplements
- Decreased stomach acid
- Antacids

jaras72/Shutterstock

whereas iron absorption from animal sources (divalent ferrous or heme) increases to 10 to 35%. Heme iron's presence, which represents between 35 and 55% of iron from animal sources, increases iron absorption from nonheme sources.

Low nonheme iron bioavailability places females on vegetarian-type diets at risk for developing iron insufficiency. They require almost twice the iron as meat eaters (14 mg daily for males and postmenopausal females, and 32 mg · d^{-1} for premenopausal females). Female vegetarian runners have a poorer iron status than counterparts who consume the same iron quantity from predominantly animal sources.[152] Including foods rich in ascorbic acid (vitamin C) in the diet upgrades dietary iron bioavailability. Ascorbic acid prevents ferrous iron oxidation to the ferric form to increase nonheme iron's solubility for absorption at the alkaline pH of the small intestine. The ascorbic acid in one glass of orange juice stimulates a threefold increase in nonheme iron absorption from a typical breakfast meal.[142] Heme iron sources include beef, beef liver, pork, tuna, and clams; oatmeal, dried figs, spinach, beans, and lentils are good nonheme sources. Fiber-rich foods, coffee, and tea contain compounds that interfere with iron and zinc's intestinal absorption.

Functional Anemia

A relatively high nonanemic iron depletion prevalence exists among athletes in diverse sports as well as recreationally active females and males.[34,40,57,146] Low hemoglobin values within the "normal" range often reflect **functional anemia**, or marginal iron deficiency. Depleted iron stores and reduced iron-dependent protein production (e.g., oxidative enzymes) with a relatively normal hemoglobin concentration characterize this condition. Ergogenic effects of iron supplementation on aerobic exercise performance and training responsiveness occur for these iron-deficient athletes.[21,22,197] Physically active but untrained females classified as iron depleted (serum ferritin <16 mg · L^{-1}) but not anemic (Hb >12 g · dL^{-1}) received either iron therapy (50 mg ferrous sulfate) or placebo twice daily for 2 wk.[65] They then completed aerobic training for 4 wk. The iron-supplemented group increased serum ferritin levels with only a small (and nonsignificant) increase in hemoglobin concentration. The improvement in 15-km endurance cycling time in the supplemented group was twice that of females who consumed the placebo (3.4 vs. 1.6 min faster). Women with low serum ferritin levels but with hemoglobin concentrations above 12 g · dL^{-1}, although not clinically anemic, might still be functionally anemic and thus benefit from iron supplementation to improve exercise performance. Similarly, iron-depleted but nonanemic females received either a placebo or 20 mg elemental iron as ferrous sulfate twice daily for 6 wk. **FIGURE 2.15** reveals that iron supplementation attenuated the decreased rate in maximal force measured sequentially during 8 min of dynamic knee extension movements.

Current recommendations support iron supplementation for nonanemic physically active women with low serum ferritin levels. Supplementation in this case exerts little effect on hemoglobin concentration and red blood cell volume. Any

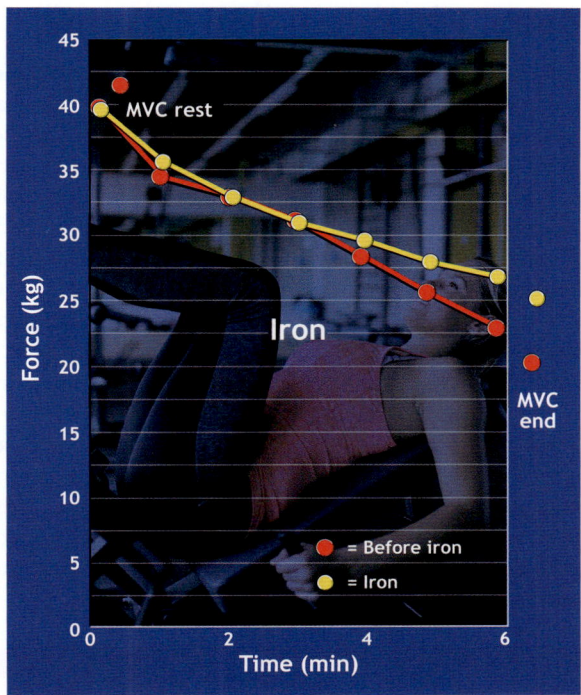

FIGURE 2.15. Maximal voluntary static contractions (MVCs) over the first 6 min of a progressive dynamic knee extension fatigue test before (*red dot*) and after (*yellow dot*) supplementation with either a placebo or iron. MVC end represents the protocol's last MVC, which occurred at different times (average <8 min) for each subject. (NDAB Creativity/Shutterstock)

improved exercise capacity likely occurs from increased muscle oxidative capacity, not the blood's increased oxygen transport capacity.

Genetic Abnormality

Approximately 2 million Americans have a genetic abnormality called **hereditary hemochromatosis** (www.cdc.gov/genomics/disease/hemochromatosis.htm). In the United States, this condition represents the most common single gene disorder afflicting approximately 1 in every 200 to 300 individuals. A person develops hemochromatosis from inheriting the defective gene from both parents. If only one parent passes on the defective gene, the offspring will likely remain a disease carrier without necessarily developing it. Disease symptoms include chronic fatigue, abdominal pain, and menstrual dysfunction. Extreme hemochromatosis can lead to liver cirrhosis or cancer, heart and thyroid disease, diabetes, arthritis, and infertility. Early diagnosis and treatment by reducing the iron load by phlebotomy when medically prudent (e.g., pint of blood withdrawn once or twice weekly until iron levels normalize) can prevent serious complications, which mainly target male Caucasians from Northern European descent. Unlike type 1 diabetes, hemochromatosis remains almost 100% curable, with patients turning asymptomatic if iron levels achieve normal range.

Sodium, Potassium, and Chlorine

Sodium, potassium, and chlorine, collectively termed **electrolytes**, remain dissolved in body fluids as electrically charged particles or ions. Sodium and chlorine represent the chief minerals contained in blood plasma and extracellular fluid, while potassium is the chief intracellular mineral. Electrolytes modulate fluid exchange within the body's fluid compartments, promoting a constant, well-regulated nutrient and waste product exchange between the cell and its external fluid environment. Even moderately low potassium levels (adequate adult intake equals 2600 mg daily for females and 3400 mg for males; a decrease from the prior 4700 $mg \cdot d^{-1}$ requirement) can negatively contribute to salt sensitivity, arterial stiffness, myocardial thickening, and hypertension. Good potassium food sources include bananas, apricots, sweet potatoes, fish, citrus fruits, and nuts. **TABLE 2.8** lists normal values for serum and sweat electrolyte concentrations and the electrolyte and carbohydrate concentrations in popular beverages.

TABLE 2.8 Electrolyte concentrations in blood, serum, and sweat and carbohydrate concentrations in popular beverages

Optimal Sodium Intake

The hormone **aldosterone** conserves sodium in the kidneys under low-to-moderate dietary sodium intake conditions. In contrast, high dietary sodium blunts aldosterone release, with excess sodium voided in the urine to maintain sodium balance throughout a wide intake range. Some individuals cannot adequately regulate excessive sodium intake. For these **salt-sensitive individuals**, abnormal sodium accumulation in bodily fluids increases fluid volume and elevates blood pressure to levels that pose a health risk.

Drugs that interfere with aldosterone action are categorized as **antihypertensives**; they reduce blood pressure by blocking the angiotensin-converting enzyme (ACE), leading to lower aldosterone secretion and action. ACE inhibitor drugs include the generic benazepril (brand name *Lotensin*), captopril (*Capoten*), enalapril (*Vasotec, Epaned*), and lisinopril (*Prinivil, Zestril*; www.medicinenet.com/ace_inhibitors/article.htm). The net ACE inhibitor effect reduces sodium and water retention and simultaneously helps to retain K^+.

Sodium intake in the United States regularly exceeds the recommended 2300 mg Chronic Disease Risk Reduction maximum daily adult level, equivalent to one teaspoon of table salt (NaCl). The sodium in salt constitutes about 40% of the compound. The new adolescent and adult adequate intake value is now reset to 1500 mg. The typical Western diet contains nearly 4000 mg sodium (8 to 12 g tablespoons salt daily), with three quarters from processed food and restaurant meals. This represents 8 times the 500-mg minimum daily sodium requirement. Common sodium-rich dietary sources include monosodium glutamate (MSG), soy sauce, condiments, canned foods, baking soda, and baking powder. Cutting salt intake by 3 g a day could reduce the national yearly heart disease cases by between 60,000 and 120,000 and strokes by 32,000 and 66,000, values on a par with disease reductions observed for declining tobacco use, obesity, and blood cholesterol levels.

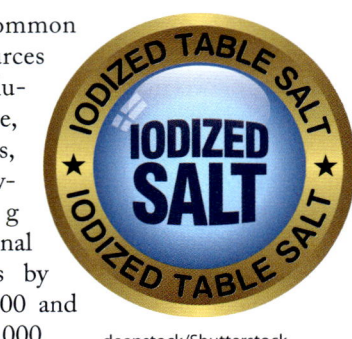

deepstock/Shutterstock

High-Sodium Culprits

The following 10 examples include popular fast-food offerings ranked by sodium content. These foods contain several days' sodium requirement.

1. Outback Steakhouse's Bloomin Onion appetizer (3841 mg)
2. Quiznos' sliced prime rib with mozzarella, roasted peppers, and onions, and mild peppercorn sauce on artisan bread with an au jus side (3610 mg)
3. Burger King's Country Pork Sandwich (3310 mg)
4. Wendy's Hot & Spicy Boneless Wings (2490 mg)
5. Jack in the Box's Deli Trio Grilled Sandwich (2460 mg)
6. Subway's Footlong Black Forest Ham Sub (2400 mg)
7. McDonald's Big Breakfast with Hotcakes and Large Size Biscuit (2260 mg)
8. Chipotle's carnitas burrito, flour tortilla, black beans, guacamole (2240 mg)
9. Taco Bell's Chicken Grilled Stuffed Burrito (2180 mg)
10. Chick-fil-A's Spicy Chicken Deluxe Sandwich (1750 mg)

A Prudent Salt Reduction Strategy

For decades, one low-risk, first-line treatment strategy for high blood pressure attempted to eliminate daily excess dietary sodium, particularly for "salt-sensitive" individuals. If dietary modifications prove ineffective in lowering blood pressure, drug-inducing water-loss diuretics take over as the next defensive stance. Unfortunately, diuretics also produce losses in other minerals, particularly potassium. A potassium-rich diet (e.g., potatoes, bananas, oranges, tomatoes, meat) becomes a patient necessity when using diuretics.

Can Sodium Intake Be Too Low?

A low-sodium diet in conjunction with excessive sweating, persistent vomiting, or diarrhea creates the potential to deplete the body's sodium content to critical levels in a condition termed **hyponatremia**. This potential medical emergency produces muscle cramps, nausea, vomiting, and dizziness, and in the extreme, shock, coma, and death. Chapter 10 provides more detail about fluid intake's crucial role in hyponatremia risk.

Sodium-Induced Hypertension

One first line of defense in treating high blood pressure eliminates excess dietary sodium. Reducing sodium lowers blood pressure via reduced plasma volume depending on the person's responsiveness to NaCl intake.[85] For salt-sensitive individuals, reducing dietary sodium to the low end of the recommended range and upgrading the diet's quality (e.g., minimizing canned and packaged foods and consuming more fresh fruit and vegetables) reduces blood pressure in both normal-weight and obese hypertensives.[1,157,179] Lowering salt intake reduces cardiovascular disease and stroke risk. A 5-g reduction in daily salt intake (about half the 10-g daily intake in some American diets) related to a 23% lower stroke risk and 17% lower cardiovascular disease risk.[162] If dietary constraints do not lower blood pressure, diuretic drugs to induce water loss then become next defense as a strategic option. Unfortunately, diuretics also produce other mineral losses, particularly potassium. A potassium-rich diet should complement diuretic use.

Lower Blood Pressure to Lower Death Risk

The National Institutes of Health (www.nih.gov), with 20,000+ employees and 6000 research scientists, reports that more than 9000 hypertensive men and women aged 50 years and older who received blood pressure–lowering medications significantly reduced systolic blood pressure to either 140 or 120 mm Hg (www.ncbi.nlm.nih.gov/books/NBK279230/). Success achieved at the 120 mm Hg target reduced heart attack, stroke, heart failure risk, and other cardiovascular events by 33% and death risk by 25% compared with the 140 mm Hg target.

Seasontime/Shutterstock

Sources:
Dai H, et al. Global, regional, and national burden of ischaemic heart disease and its attributable risk factors, 1990-2017: results from the Global Burden of Disease Study 2017. *Eur Heart J Qual Care Clin Outcomes.* 2022;8:50.
Hedman K, et al. Peak exercise SBP and future risk of cardiovascular disease and mortality. *J Hypertens.* 2022;40:300.

Minerals and Exercise Performance

Consuming mineral supplements above recommended levels on a long- or short-term basis does not benefit exercise performance or enhance training responsiveness.

Mineral Loss in Sweat

Excessive water and electrolyte loss impairs heat tolerance and physical performance. It also leads to severe dysfunction that culminates in heat cramps, heat exhaustion, or heat stroke. The yearly heat-related deaths during spring and summer football practice provide a tragic illustration about the importance of fluid and electrolyte replacement. An athlete may lose up to 5 kg water from sweating during practice or an athletic event. This corresponds to about 8.0 g salt depletion because each sweat kg (1 L) contains about 1.5 g salt. Despite this potential for mineral loss, replacing water lost through sweating becomes the crucial and immediate need.

Defense Against Mineral Loss

Sweat loss during vigorous physical activity triggers a rapid, coordinated release of the hormones vasopressin and aldosterone and the enzyme renin, which reduce sodium and water loss from the kidneys. Sodium conservation increases even under extreme conditions (e.g., marathon running in warm, humid weather when sweat output can reach $2 \, L \cdot h^{-1}$). Adding salt to the fluid or food ingested usually replenishes electrolytes lost in sweat, while facilitating rehydration. Salt supplements may be beneficial in prolonged activity in the heat when fluid loss exceeds 4 or 5 kg. This can be achieved by drinking a 0.1 to 0.2% salt solution (adding 0.3 tsp table salt per liter water).[3] A mild potassium deficiency can occur with intense exercise training during heat stress; adequate daily food intake usually maintains optimum potassium levels. One cup (8 oz) orange or tomato juice essentially replaces almost all calcium, potassium, and magnesium lost in 3 L (3 kg) of sweat.

Trace Minerals and Physical Activity

Strenuous physical activity increases excretion of the following four trace elements:

1. Chromium: required for carbohydrate and lipid catabolism and proper insulin function and protein synthesis
2. Copper: required for red blood cell formation; influences gene expression and serves as a cofactor or enzyme prosthetic groups
3. Manganese: superoxide dismutase component in the body's antioxidant defense system
4. Zinc: component of lactate dehydrogenase, carbonic anhydrase, superoxide dismutase, and enzymes of energy metabolism, cell growth and differentiation, and tissue repair

Urinary zinc and chromium losses were 1.5- to 2.0-fold higher following a 6-mile run compared to a rest day.[8] Copper and zinc sweat losses also can attain relatively high levels.

Such trace mineral losses with physical activity do not necessarily mean athletes should supplement with these micronutrients. For example, short-term zinc supplementation ($25 \, mg \cdot d^{-1}$) did not benefit metabolic and endocrine responses or endurance performance in eumenorrheic women during intense physical activity.[148] Collegiate football players who supplemented with 200 mg of chromium (as chromium picolinate) daily for 9 wk experienced no beneficial changes in body composition and muscular strength during intense weightlifting compared with a control group that received a placebo.[25] Power and endurance athletes had higher plasma copper and zinc levels than nontraining controls.[134]

In a Practical Sense

The DASH Diet to Lower Blood Pressure with Dietary Intervention

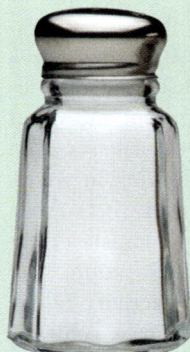

Nearly 50 million Americans have hypertension, a condition that if left untreated, increases stroke and heart attack risk, including kidney failure. Fifty percent of people with hypertension seek treatment, but only about half achieve long-term success. One reason for poor compliance concerns possible side effects of readily available antihypertensive medication. For example, fatigue and impotence often discourage patients from maintaining a chronic medication schedule required by pharmacologic hypertension treatment.

THE DASH APPROACH

Research using **DASH (dietary approaches to stop hypertension**; www.nhlbi.nih.gov/education/dash-eating-plan) demonstrates that this diet lowers blood pressure to almost the same extent as pharmacologic therapy and often more than other lifestyle changes. Two months on the diet reduced systolic pressure by an average of 11.4 mm Hg and diastolic pressure decreased by 5.5 mm Hg. Every 2 mm Hg reduction in systolic pressure lowers heart disease risk by 5% and stroke risk by 8%. The standard DASH diet combined with reduced daily dietary salt intake of 1500 mg produces even greater blood pressure reductions than achieved with the DASH diet only.

NUTRIENT GOALS FOR THE DASH DIET

The table shows daily nutrient goals for the DASH approach for a 2100-kcal intake for a typical 70-kg person. More physically active and heavier individuals should boost their portion size or number of individual items to maintain their weight. Individuals desiring to lose weight or who are lighter or sedentary should eat less but not less than the minimum number of servings for each food group.

DASH DAILY NUTRIENT GOALS: CALORIE CONTRIBUTIONS

Nutrient	Calorie Contribution to 2100-kcal Plan (%)
Total lipid	27%
Saturated fat	6%
Protein	18%
Carbohydrate	55%

DASH DAILY NUTRIENT GOALS: RECOMMENDED AMOUNTS

Nutrient	Recommended Amount
Cholesterol	150 mg
Sodium	2300 mg
Potassium	4700 mg
Calcium	1250 mg
Magnesium	500 mg
Fiber	30 g

Sources:
Djoussé L, et al. DASH score and subsequent risk of coronary artery disease: the findings from million veteran program. *J Am Heart Assoc*. 2018;7:9.
Maddock J, et al. Adherence to a dietary approaches to stop hypertension (DASH)-type diet over the life course and associated vascular function: a study based on the MRC 1946 British birth cohort. *Br J Nutr*. 2018;119:581.
Saglimbene VM, et al. The association of Mediterranean and DASH diets with mortality in adults on hemodialysis: the DIET-HD Multinational Cohort Study. *J Am Soc Nephrol*. 2018;29:1741.
Schwingshackl L, et al. Comparative effects of different dietary approaches on blood pressure in hypertensive and prehypertensive patients: a systematic review and network meta-analysis. *Crit Rev Food Sci Nutr*. 2018;2:1.

---

fyi Consuming Supplements May Not Impact Disease

Think again if you are counting on daily multivitamin multimineral (MVM) pills to ward off chronic cancer or heart disease. Two systematic worldwide literature reviews reported that MVM supplementation in healthy populations had only a modest protective effect on all-cause mortality, including cancer or cardiovascular disease incidence or mortality. Supplementation duration made no difference in disease status. In 2020, Americans purchased over $31 billion on MVM (sales rate increase projected 2 to 3% yearly) with next to a zero chance to impact health status.

Sources:
Fortmann SP. *Vitamin, Mineral, and Multivitamin Supplements for the Primary Prevention of Cardiovascular Disease and Cancer: A systematic Evidence Review for the U.S. Preventive Services Task Force*. Rockville: Agency for Healthcare Research and Quality (US); 2013. Report No.:14-05199-EF-1.
Kim J, et al. Association of multivitamin and mineral supplementation and risk of cardiovascular disease: a systematic review and meta-analysis. *Circ Cardiovasc Qual Outcomes*. 2018;11:e004224.

conejota/Shutterstock

Males and females who train intensely with large sweat production accompanied by marginal nutrition (e.g., wrestlers, endurance runners, ballet dancers, and female gymnasts) should monitor trace mineral intake to prevent an overt deficiency. An excessive intake of one mineral may create a deficiency in another mineral because iron, zinc, and copper interact with each other as they compete for the same carrier during intestinal absorption. For well-nourished athletes and nonathletes, mineral and trace mineral supplementation does not enhance exercise performance or overall health.[197]

Summary

1. Approximately 4% body mass consists of 22 minerals distributed in all body tissues and fluids.
2. Minerals occur freely in nature in rivers, lakes, oceans, and soil. A plant's root system absorbs minerals, which eventually incorporate into the tissues of animals that consume the plants.
3. Minerals function primarily in metabolism as important enzyme constituents.
4. Minerals provide structure to bones and teeth and serve in synthesizing the three biologic macronutrients—glycogen, lipid, and protein.
5. A balanced diet generally provides adequate mineral intake, except in some geographic locations that lack specific minerals in the soil (e.g., iodine in the upper Midwest and Great Lakes regions).
6. Osteoporosis has reached epidemic proportions among older females, which makes adequate calcium intake and regular weight-bearing physical activities and/or resistance training an effective strategy to stress the skeleton and defend against bone loss.
7. Females who train intensely often do not match energy intake to energy output. This reduces body weight and body fat to a point that adversely affects menstruation, which contributes to bone loss at an early age. Restoration of normal menstruation does not fully restore bone mass over the long term.
8. Three inter-related female athlete triad components include energy availability, menstrual status, and bone health. Energy availability and menstrual status directly influence bone health.
9. Similar to females, low energy availability and intense training in males influence metabolism, reproduction, and bone mass, described as the male athlete triad.
10. About 40% of American females of childbearing age suffer from dietary iron insufficiency, which could trigger iron deficiency anemia and negatively disrupt aerobic exercise performance and training.
11. For vegetarian or near-vegetarian females, nonheme iron's relatively low bioavailability increases risk for developing iron insufficiency. Vitamin C in foods or supplements increases intestinal nonheme iron absorption.
12. Regular physical activity probably does not drain the body's iron reserves. If it does, females with the greatest iron requirement and lowest iron intake increase their anemia risk.
13. Periodic iron status assessment should evaluate hematologic characteristics and iron reserves.
14. Excessive sweating produces considerable body water and mineral losses, which require replacement during and following physical activity.
15. Exercise sweat loss usually does not increase mineral requirements above recommended levels.

Part 3 > Water

The Body's Water Content

Water makes up from 40 to 70% body mass, depending on age, gender, and body composition (i.e., differences in lean vs. fat tissue). Water constitutes 65 to 75% of muscle and about 10% of fat weight. Body fat's relatively low water content means individuals with more total fat have a smaller overall percentage of their body weight as water.

FIGURE 2.16 depicts the body's fluid compartments, normal daily body water variation, and specific terminology to describe the various human hydration states. Body mass includes about 55% water in striated muscle, the skeleton, and adipose tissue. For a male and female of equal or similar body mass, the female contains less total body water because her larger adipose tissue content to lower lean body mass ratio differs from her male counterpart. The body contains two fluid "compartments." The **intracellular fluid** compartment refers to fluid inside cells, whereas **extracellular fluid** includes fluids that flow within the microscopic spaces between cells (**interstitial fluid**), as well as lymph, saliva, fluid in eyes, fluid secreted by glands and digestive tract, fluid bathing spinal cord nerves, and fluids excreted by the skin and kidneys. Blood plasma accounts for nearly 20% extracellular fluid (3 to 4 L). Extracellular fluid provides most of the fluid lost through sweating, predominantly from blood plasma. Of the total body water, an average 62% represents intracellular water (26 L of the body's 42 L for an average 80-kg man), with 38% from extracellular sources. Both intracellular and extracellular fluid volumes reflect averages from a dynamic fluid exchange between compartments, particularly in physically active males and females. Moderate-to-intense physical training often increases the percentage water distributed within the intracellular compartment because muscle mass typically increases, with its accompanying large water content. In contrast, an acute exercise bout temporarily shifts fluid from plasma to interstitial and intracellular spaces from increased hydrostatic (fluid) pressure within the circulatory system.

Water's Functions

Water, a remarkably ubiquitous nutrient, serves as the body's transport and reactive medium with many life-sustaining functions. Without water, death occurs within days. Gas diffusion always takes place across water-moistened surfaces. Nutrients

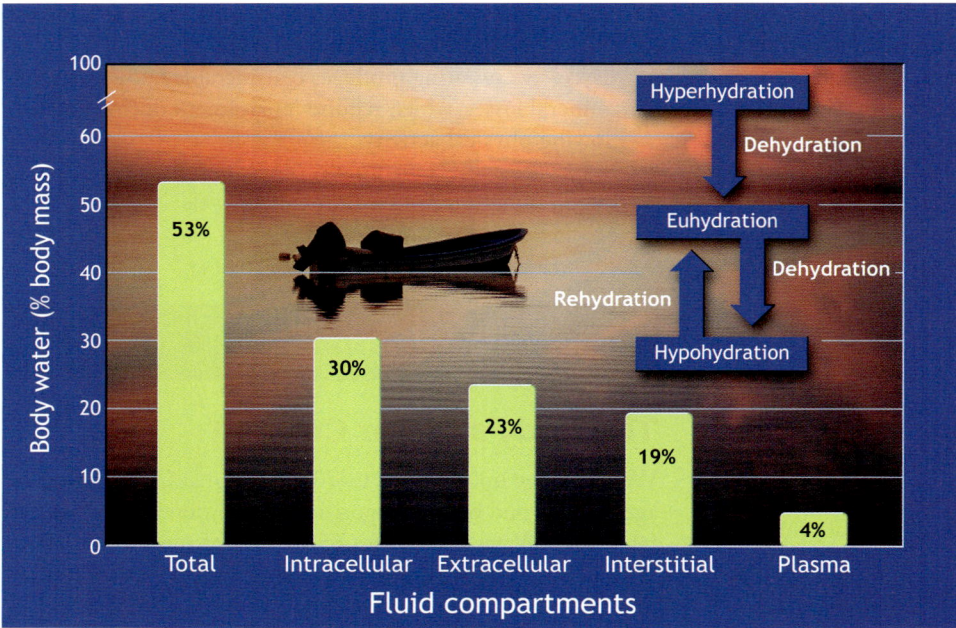

FIGURE 2.16. Fluid compartments, average volumes and total body water and plasma volume variability, and hydration terminology, including the pathway from hyperhydration to euhydration to hypohydration (upper right). Volumes represent an 80-kg man.
(Adapted with permission from Greenleaf JE. Problem: thirst, drinking behavior, and involuntary dehydration. *Med Sci Sports Exerc*. 1992;24:645. HasanZaidi/Shutterstock)

and gases travel in aqueous solution, and waste product residues exit the body through water in urine and feces. Water, in conjunction with proteins, lubricates joints and cushions a variety of "moving" organs such as the heart, lungs, intestines, and eyes. Water is noncompressible, so it provides structure and form to tissues and organs. Water has tremendous heat-stabilizing qualities because it absorbs considerable heat with only small temperature changes. This quality, combined with water's high vaporization point, maintains a relatively stable body temperature during environmental heat stress and the increased internal heat load generated by physical activity. Without water, blood volume decreases causing blood pressure to fall to levels that can precipitate unconsciousness. Without water, digestive and excretory processes deteriorate allowing toxins to accumulate with widespread organ damage and massive organ failure.

Water Balance: Intake Versus Output

The body's water content remains relatively stable over days, weeks, months, and even years. **FIGURE 2.17** displays water intake and output sources.

 See the animation "Water Balance" on Lippincott Connect to view this process.

Water Intake

A sedentary adult in a thermoneutral environment requires about 2.5 L of water daily. For an active person in a warm, humid environment, the water requirement often increases to between 5 and 10 L daily. Three sources provide this water:

1. Foods
2. Liquids
3. Metabolism

As a general rule, the National Academy of Medicine recommends the average female consume about 9.5 cups water daily and for a male about 12 cups daily. This includes fluids (e.g., coffee, tea, juice, soda, milk, alcoholic drinks) but not hidden fluids in food. Environmental heat, humidity, and fitness status influence this requirement. The diet's salt or protein level also affects one's water requirements, with higher intake levels requiring greater water intake.

Water in Foods

Water from foods typically accounts for 20% of recommended total fluid intake. Fruits and vegetables contain considerable water as displayed in the FYI on the next page.

Water from Liquids

The average individual normally consumes 1200 mL (41 oz) water daily. Physical activity and thermal stress increase fluid needs by five or six times this amount. At the extreme, an individual lost 13.6 kg water weight during a 2-day, 17-hr, 55-mile run across Death Valley, California.[131] With proper fluid ingestion, including salt supplements, body weight loss amounted to only 1.4 kg (3.1 lb). In this example, fluid loss and replenishment represented nearly 4 gallons (15.1 L)!

Metabolic Water

The breakdown of macronutrient molecules during energy metabolism forms carbon dioxide and water. This metabolic water provides about 14% of a sedentary person's daily water requirement. Glucose catabolism liberates 55 g of metabolic water, while larger water amounts come from protein (100 g) and lipid (107 g) catabolism. Additionally, each gram of glycogen joins with 2.7 g water when its glucose units link together; glycogen liberates this bound water during its breakdown for energy.

Water Output

The body loses water in four forms:

1. Urine
2. Sweat
3. Water vapor in expired air
4. Feces

Water Loss in Urine

Under normal conditions, the kidneys reabsorb about 99% of the 140 to 160 L of renal filtrate formed each day. Consequently, the daily urine volume the kidneys excrete ranges from 1000 to 1500 mL, or about 1.5 quarts. Elimina-

Foods High in Water Content

Foods high in water content constitute about 22% of the typical American's daily water intake. Contrary to popular lore, little scientific evidence exists for the 64-oz (8 glasses) daily recommendation based on older water consumption survey data. Current recommendations encourage consuming 16 glasses (3.7 L or 16 cups) fluid daily for males and approximately 12 glasses (2.7 L or 12 cups) daily for females.

Payung Jut/Shutterstock

This new evidence applies to individuals living in temperate climates and not engaged in routine, vigorous daily physical activities. High water-containing foods include the following:

- 90 to 99%: fat-free milk, cantaloupe, strawberries, watermelon, lettuce, cabbage, celery, spinach, pickles, squash (cooked)
- 80 to 89%: fruit juice, yogurt, apples, grapes, oranges, carrots, broccoli (cooked), pears, pineapple
- 70 to 79%: bananas, avocados, cottage cheese, ricotta cheese, potatoes (baked), corn (cooked), shrimp
- 60 to 69%: pasta, legumes, salmon, ice cream, chicken breast
- 50 to 59%: ground beef, hot dogs, feta cheese, tenderloin steak (cooked)

Sources:
Tucker MA, et al. Adequacy of daily fluid intake volume can be identified from urinary frequency and perceived thirst in healthy adults. *J Am Coll Nutr.* 2020;39:235.
USDA Food Composition Databases: https://ndb.nal.usda.gov/ndb/

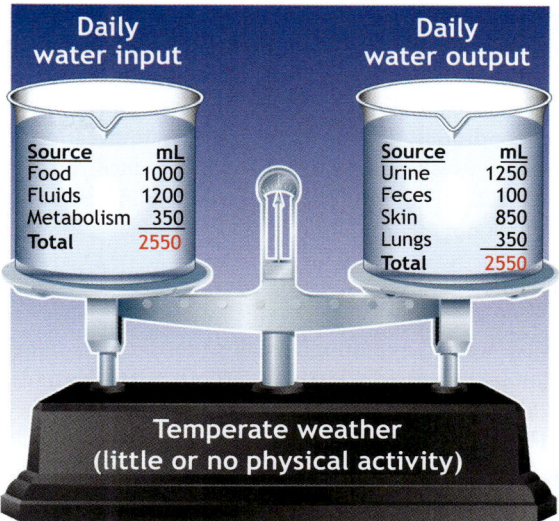

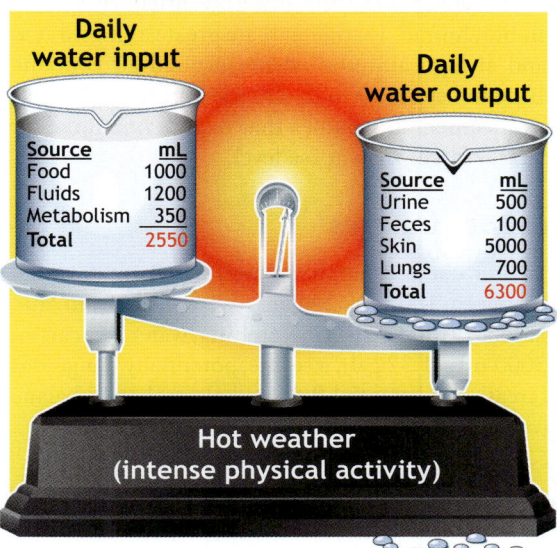

FIGURE 2.17. Water balance in the body. **Top.** Little or no physical activity with thermoneutral (temperate) ambient temperature and humidity. **Bottom.** Moderate-to-intense physical activity in a hot, humid environment.

tion of 1 g of solute by the kidneys requires about 15 mL of water. A portion of water in urine thus becomes "obligated" to rid the body of metabolic by-products such as urea, an end product of protein breakdown. Large protein quantities used for energy (as occurs with a high-protein diet where daily intake exceeds 2.0 g·kg^{-1} body mass) accelerate dehydration during physical activity.

 See the animation "Renal Function" on Lippincott Connect to view this process.

Water Loss in Sweat

On a daily basis, roughly 350 mL of water continually seeps from deeper tissues through the skin to the body's surface as **insensible perspiration**. Water loss also occurs through skin as sweat produced by specialized sweat glands beneath the skin's surface. Evaporation of sweat provides the refrigeration mechanism to cool the body. The body produces 500 to 700 mL of sweat each day under normal thermal and physical activity conditions. This by no means reflects sweating capacity because a well-acclimatized person produces up to 12 L sweat (at a $1 \text{ L} \cdot \text{hr}^{-1}$ rate) during prolonged, intense physical activity in a hot environment.

Water Loss in Vapor

Insensible water loss through small water droplets in exhaled air amounts to between 250 and 350 mL a day from inspired air's complete moistening as it traverses the pulmonary airways. Physical activity also affects this water loss source.[106] For physically active persons, the respiratory passages release 2 to 5 mL of water each minute during strenuous activity, depending on climatic conditions. The lowest ventilatory water losses occur in hot, humid weather and are greatest in cold temperatures and at high altitudes where inspired air contains relatively little moisture. At high altitude mountain climbing and trekking, inspired air volumes that require humidification are considerably larger than at sea level.

Water Loss in Feces

Fecal matter contains approximately 70% water, which produces between 100 and 200 mL water loss from intestinal elimination. With diarrhea or vomiting, water loss can increase up to 5000 mL (1.32 gal), a severe, potentially dangerous condition creating substantial fluid and electrolyte imbalances.

Physical Activity and Water Requirements

Water loss represents the most serious consequence of profuse sweating, which also occurs in a water environment (e.g., vigorous swimming and water polo).

Three factors determine the amount of water lost through sweating:

1. Physical activity intensity
2. Environmental temperature
3. Relative humidity

Relative humidity, the water content in ambient air, affects sweating efficiency in temperature regulation. Ambient air completely saturates with water vapor at 100% relative humidity. This blocks any fluid evaporation from the skin's surface to the air, which minimizes this important avenue for body cooling. Under high humidity, sweat beads on the skin and eventually rolls off without delivering a cooling effect. On a dry day, air can hold considerable moisture and fluid evaporates rapidly from the skin. The sweat mechanism in this environment functions at optimal efficiency to regulate body temperature within a narrow range. Importantly, fluid loss from the vascular compartment strains circulatory function, which ultimately impairs exercise capacity and thermoregulation.

Monitoring body weight changes assessed following urination conveniently quantifies fluid loss during physical activity and/or heat stress. Each 0.45 kg/1 lb body weight loss corresponds to 450 mL/15 oz dehydration.

Hyponatremia

The exercise physiology literature consistently confirms the need to consume fluid before, during, and following physical activity. In many instances, the recommended beverage choice remains plain, cool to cold **hypotonic** water. Still, excessive water intake under certain exercise conditions can be counterproductive and produce the potentially serious medical complication called hyponatremia or "water intoxication," first described in the medical literature among mid-1980s athletes (**FIG. 2.18**).

A sustained low plasma sodium concentration creates an osmotic imbalance across the **blood-brain barrier** allowing for rapid water influx into the brain. The resulting swelling of brain tissue produces cascading symptoms that range from mild (headache, confusion, malaise, nausea, and cramping (classified as exercise-associated hyponatremia [EAH]) to severe (classified as exercise-associated hyponatremic encephalopathy [EAHE]) causing seizures, coma, pulmonary edema, cardiac arrest, and death).[10,51,139,198]

In general, mild hyponatremia exists when serum sodium concentration declines below 135 $\text{mEq} \cdot \text{L}^{-1}$ and serum sodium below 125 $\text{mEq} \cdot \text{L}^{-1}$ triggers severe symptoms. The most conducive conditions for hyponatremia include water overload during ultramarathon-type, continuous activity lasting 6 to 8 h, yet it can occur within only 4 hr as in marathon running.[12,64,66,109]

Mild-to-severe hyponatremia increases in frequency among ultraendurance athletes who compete in hot weather.[156,198] Nearly 30% of athletes competing in the 1984 Ironman Triathlon experienced hyponatremia symptoms, most frequently observed late in the race or during recovery. In more than 18,000 ultraendurance athletes including triathletes, approximately 9% who collapsed during or following competition exhibited hyponatremic symptoms.[119] On average, athletes had consumed fluids with low sodium chloride content (<6.8 $\text{mmol} \cdot \text{L}^{-1}$). The runner with the most severe hyponatremia (serum Na level 112 $\text{mEq} \cdot \text{L}^{-1}$), excreted more than 7.5 L dilute urine during the first 17 h of hospitalization.

INTEGRATIVE QUESTION

How should knowledge about hyponatremia modify conventional recommendations concerning fluid intake prior to, during, and in recovery from long-duration physical activity?

Medical personnel monitored changes in body mass and blood sodium concentration in the 1996 New Zealand Ironman Triathlon participants.[154] For athletes with clinical evidence documenting fluid or electrolyte disturbance, body mass declined 2.5 versus 2.9 kg in athletes not requiring medical care. Hyponatremia accounted for 9% medical abnormalities.

One athlete with hyponatremia (serum Na = 130 mEq·L^{-1}) consumed excessive fluid during the race (16 L; 4.23 gal) and gained 2.5 kg body mass—consistent that fluid overload causes hyponatremia. In an ultradistance multisport triathlon (kayak 67 km/41.6 mi, cycle 148 km/92 mi, and 23.8 km/14.8 mi run), the average competitors' body mass declined 2.5 kg, an amount equal to 3% of initial body mass.[155] No athletes gained weight, and six weighed the same prerace versus postrace; the one athlete who became hyponatremic (serum Na = 134 mEq·L^{-1}) maintained body weight and did not seek medical attention. Serum sodium concentration for the 47 athletes at the finish averaged 139.3 mEq·L^{-1}.

Acclimatization Level Affects Sodium Loss

Sodium concentration in sweat ranges from 5 to 30 mmol·L^{-1} (115 to 690 mg·L^{-1}) in individuals fully acclimatized to the heat to 40 to 100 mmol·L^{-1} (920 to 2300 mg·L^{-1}) in unacclimatized persons. In addition, some individuals produce highly concentrated sweat regardless of their degree of acclimatization. Hyponatremia involves extreme sodium loss through prolonged sweating, coupled with existing extracellular sodium (reduced osmolality) dilution from consuming fluids with low or no sodium (**FIG. 2.18A**). Reduced extracellular solute concentration moves water into cells (Fig. 2.18B), congesting lungs, swelling brain tissue, and adversely affecting central nervous system function.

Several hours of physical activity in hot, humid weather can produce a sweating rate exceeding 1 L·hr^{-1}, with sweat sodium concentrations ranging from 20 to 100 mEq·L^{-1}. Frequently ingesting large plain water volumes draws sodium from the extracellular fluid compartment into the unabsorbed intestinal water. This action further dilutes serum sodium concentration. Vigorous physical activity magnifies the problem because declining renal blood flow with the activity retards urine production, which impedes excess water excretion. Competitive athletes, recreational participants, and occupational workers should be aware of excessive hydration dangers because fluid intake must not exceed fluid loss. Six steps reduce overhydration and hyponatremia risk in prolonged physical activity:

1. Drink 400 to 600 mL (14 to 22 oz) fluid 2 to 3 hr before exercise.
2. Drink 150 to 300 mL (5 to 10 oz) fluid about 30 min prior to physical activity.

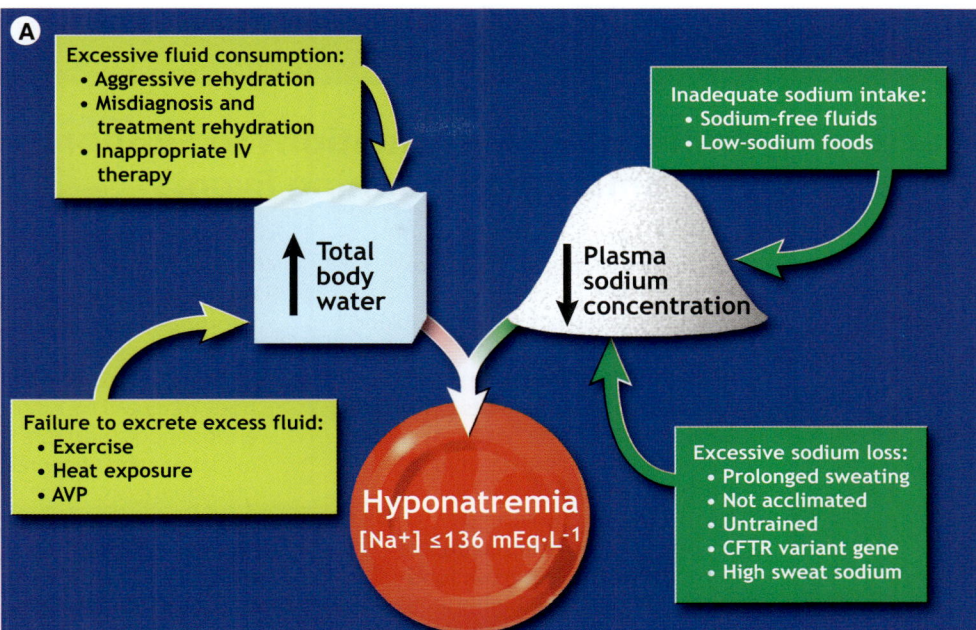

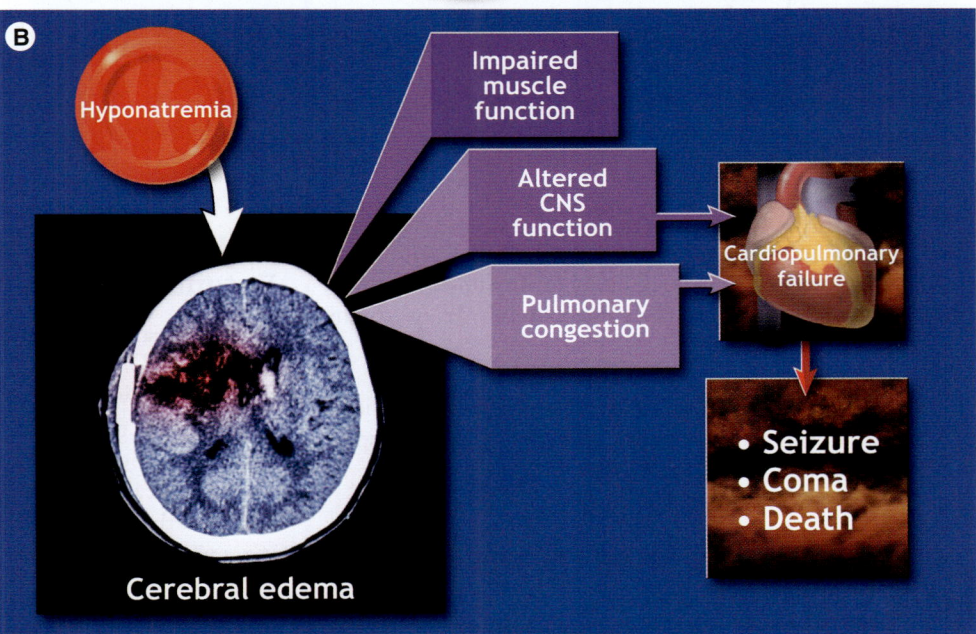

FIGURE 2.18. **(A)** Key factors contributing to hyponatremia (AVP, arginine vasopressin; CFTR, cystic fibrosis transmembrane regulatory gene). **(B)** Hyponatremia's undesirable physiologic consequences can lead to seizure, coma, and ultimately death. CNS, central nervous system. (Adapted with permission from Montain SJ, et al. Hyponatremia associated with exercise: risk factors and pathogenesis. *Exerc Sport Sci Rev.* 2001;29:113. Shutterstock: ArtMediaWorx; Puwadol Jaturawutthichai)

In a Practical Sense

Practical Hydration Recommendations to Support Individualized Strategies in Ultramarathon Running Events

- Initiate exercise in a euhydrated state and avoid pre-exercise hyperhydration.
- "Drink to thirst" during running using "ad libitum" drinking strategies and provided fluids as available.
- Avoid excessive fluid intake volumes; know fluid tolerance limits. Small and frequent drinks limit gastric overload during compromised gastrointestinal function.
- Avoid excessive sodium supplementation during running. Consume sodium based on food cravings. Do *not* use highly visible salt losses as a signal to increase sodium intake.
- With limited access, fluid must be carried by the runner between sources. Consequently, rely on experience or through prior training or laboratory evaluation to assess potential fluid requirements while recognizing that appropriate fluid intake will vary with course topography, ambient conditions, and pacing.
- Determine hydration status from prior fluid intake history and monitoring of body mass, recognizing that some body mass will be lost during prolonged exercise via endogenous fuel store oxidation, water generation with fuel oxidation, and water released bound to glycogen during glycogenolysis.
- When training and/or competing in both dry and humid hot ambient conditions, prior heat acclimatization/acclimation desirably expands plasma volume.
- Oliguria (limited urine output) does not signal dehydration. Avoid urine assessments (e.g., urine color, specific gravity, osmolality) to monitor hydration status.

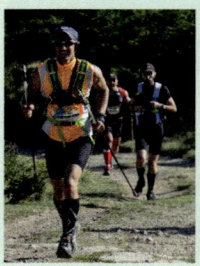
Sanasha chan/Shutterstock

Source:
Costa RJS, et al. Nutrition for ultramarathon running: trail, track, and road. *Int J Sport Nutr Exerc Metab*. 2019;29:130.

---

3. Drink no more than 1000 mL·hr^{-1} (33 oz) plain water spread over 15-min intervals during or after physical activity.
4. Add approximately ¼ to ½ tsp salt per 32 oz to the ingested fluid.
5. Do not restrict dietary salt.
6. Add 5 to 8% glucose to a rehydration drink to facilitate intestinal water uptake by the glucose-sodium transport mechanism

Five Predisposing Factors for Hyponatremia

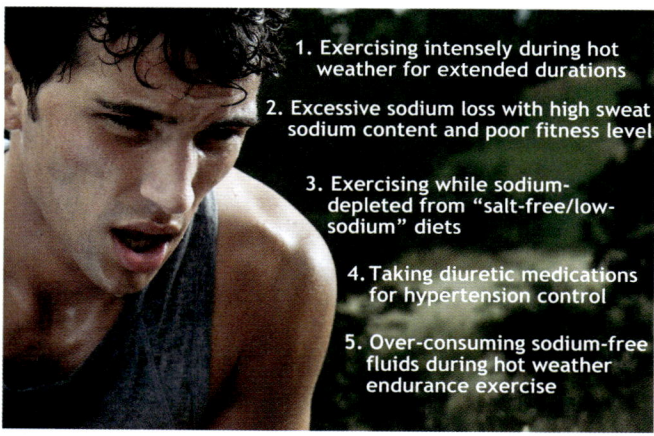

1. Exercising intensely during hot weather for extended durations
2. Excessive sodium loss with high sweat sodium content and poor fitness level
3. Exercising while sodium-depleted from "salt-free/low-sodium" diets
4. Taking diuretic medications for hypertension control
5. Over-consuming sodium-free fluids during hot weather endurance exercise

Rido/Shutterstock

Reducing Overhydration Risk During Extended-Duration Activities

The International Marathon Medical Director's Association (IMMDA; http://immda.org/), USA Track and Field (USATF; www.usatf.org/Home.aspx), and other governing bodies (e.g., Boston Marathon, South African Ironman Triathlons, South African Comrades ultramarathon, and 50 New Zealand walking, minimarathons, marathons, and ultramarathons [www.runningcalendar.co.nz]) provide training guidance and related support to all competitors. The IMMDA guidelines match those adopted at an International Consensus Development Conference in 2015 concerning exercise-associated hyponatremia (EAH; https://bjsm.bmj.com/content/49/22/1432). The ACSM is currently revising its 2007 physical activity guidelines about water consumption during diverse environmental conditions (https://journals.lww.com/acsm-msse/Fulltext/2007/02000/Exercise_and_Fluid_Replacement.22.aspx).[209–211]

Water Intake Guidelines During Endurance Activities

Do not consume an excess of water or sports drinks 2 to 3 hr before an event.

1. Drink 5 to 10 oz plain water 10 to 15 min prior to an event as a fluid excess in the gut does not absorb immediately.
2. During the event, drink only when thirsty, not necessarily at every water station.

3. Drink water from cups along the way (300 to 400 mL an hour equivalent to a normal soda can but no more than 600 mL an hour).
4. Following the event, do not consume large fluid quantities in an attempt to "quickly" replace needed fluid's losses during the event.
5. To reduce dehydration and exercise-associated hyponatremia (EAH) and exercise-associated hyponatremic encephalopathy (EAHE) risk, drink only when truly thirsty, letting "true" thirst dictate fluid intake.
6. Do not consume "salt tablets" during the event or several days before the event, even under hot weather conditions.
7. Do not add "extra" salt to meals or fluids in the days prior to the event. Meals consumed following the event will replace any electrolyte deficits.
8. Do not load up on sports drinks in the days before the event believing that they "build up" electrolyte reserves.

As with any endurance endeavor, do not participate without having devoted weeks or months to structured endurance training. For hot weather events, train under similar hot weather temperature and relative humidity conditions, employing a successful replacement water strategy as during training.

Summary

1. Water makes up 40 to 70% of total body mass.
2. Muscle contains 70% water by weight, while body fat contains 10% water by weight.
3. Total body water occurs intracellularly (62% inside cells) and 38% extracellularly in plasma, lymph, and other fluids.
4. The typical average daily water intake (2.5 L) comes from liquid (1.2 L), food (1.0 L), and metabolic water produced during energy-yielding reactions (0.35 L).
5. Daily water loss in an inactive person comes from urine (1 to 1.5 L), skin as insensible perspiration and sweat (0.85 L), water vapor in expired air (0.35 L), and feces (0.10 L).
6. Food and oxygen are always supplied in aqueous solution, while waste products exit via a watery medium.
7. Water provides structure and form to body tissues and organs and serves a vital role in temperature regulation.
8. Physical activity and exercise training in hot weather increase the body's water requirement, while extreme heat conditions increase fluid needs five or six times above normal requirements.
9. Excessive sweating combined with consuming large water volumes during prolonged activity sets a "perfect storm" for hyponatremia or water intoxication; severe symptoms emerge when serum sodium decreases below 125 $mEq \cdot L^{-1}$.

Key Terms

Adequate intake (AI): Assumed adequate nutritional goal based on nutrient intake estimates in apparently healthy persons when no RDA exists

Aldosterone: Hormone conserves the kidney's sodium in low-to-moderate dietary sodium intake

Antihypertensives: Blood pressure reducing drugs

Atherosclerosis oxidative modification hypothesis: Mild LDL cholesterol oxidation accelerates arterial plaque formation

Blood-brain barrier: Microvasculature endothelial cells that protect the brain from plasma composition fluctuations, circulating neurotransmitters, and other disruptive substances to neural function

Coenzymes: Small molecules combined with a larger protein compound (apoenzyme) to form an active enzyme that accelerates chemical compound interconversions

Cortical bone: Dense, hard outer layer along the arm and leg long bone shafts

Cytochromes: Iron-containing intracellular compounds facilitate energy transfer in metabolic pathways

Dietary approaches to stop hypertension (DASH): Diet rich in fruits, vegetables, whole grains, fish, nuts, beans, and low-fat dairy foods and limited in sugar-sweetened foods and beverages, red meat, and added lipids; lowers blood pressure similarly to pharmacologic therapy and often more than other common lifestyle changes

Electrolytes: Sodium, potassium, and chlorine electrically charged ions dissolved in body fluids

Estimated average requirement (EAR): Average daily nutrient intake level sufficient to meet the requirements for one half of apparently healthy individuals in a particular life-stage and gender group

Extracellular fluid: Interstitial fluid plus lymph, saliva, eye fluids, and gland secretions that bathes the spinal cord and nerves, and skin and kidney fluid excretions

Fat-soluble vitamins: Vitamins A, D, E, and K dissolve and remain in fatty tissues; should not be consumed in excess without medical supervision

Female athlete triad: Syndrome includes eating irregularities, amenorrhea, and osteoporosis; disorders most prevalent in teenage girls involved in sport competition

Ferritin: Stored in the liver, spleen, and bone marrow to replenish iron lost from functional compounds; provides an iron reserve during insufficient dietary iron intake

Functional anemia: Low values for hemoglobin within the "normal" range; also known as marginal iron deficiency

Hemosiderin: Stored in the liver, spleen, and bone marrow to replenish iron lost from functional compounds, which provides an iron reserve during insufficient dietary iron intake

Hereditary hemochromatosis: Genetic disorder when the body builds up excessive iron in the skin, heart, liver, pancreas, pituitary gland, and joints

Hypoestrogenesis: Estrogen deficiency

Hyponatremia: The body's sodium concentration reduces to critically low levels; often called "water intoxication"

Hypotonic: Solution with less solute and more water (lower concentration of solutes) than another solution

Insensible perspiration: Perspiration seeps from deeper tissues; happens before it is perceived or "sensed"

Interstitial fluid: Fluids flowing within microscopic cell spaces among cells

Intracellular fluid: Fluid inside a cell

Iron deficiency anemia: Reduced hemoglobin concentration in red blood cells

Lipid peroxidation: Oxidative degradation of lipids when free radicals remove electrons from cell membrane to cause lipid damage

Major minerals: Minerals required in amounts ≥ 100 mg daily

Male athlete triad: Low energy availability influences metabolism, reproduction suppresses reproductive function, low testosterone concentrations, poor semen quality, and impaired bone health

Micronutrients: Small vitamin and mineral quantities that facilitate energy transfer and tissue synthesis

Minerals: Twenty-two mostly metallic singular or combined elements that serve as enzyme, hormone, and vitamin constituents

Myoglobin: Compound similar to hemoglobin that aids in oxygen storage and transport within muscle cells

Osteopenia: Condition where bones gradually weaken with increased fracture risk

Osteoporosis: "Porous bones" with density greater than 2.5 standard deviations below gender normal

Oxidative stress: Imbalance between reactive oxygen species and how the body detoxifies reactive intermediates and/or repairs resulting tissue and organ damage

Relative energy deficiency in sport (RED-S): Chronic energy deficiency from low energy intake and/or excessive energy output leads to metabolic, reproductive, and bone disorders

Relative humidity: Ratio of water in ambient air at a particular temperature compared to the total quantity of moisture the air could contain expressed as a percentage

Remodeling: Describes bone as a dynamic collagen and mineral tissue matrix existing in a continual flux state

Salt-sensitive individuals: Inadequately regulated excessive sodium intake leads to increased hypertension and cardiovascular disease risk

Sports anemia: Describes reduced blood hemoglobin levels attributable to physical training approaching clinical anemia (12 g·dL^{-1} women; 14 g·dL^{-1} men)

Tolerable upper intake level (UL): Highest average daily nutrient intake level should not pose adverse health effects to individuals in a specified gender and life-stage group

Trabecular bone: Spongy, less dense, and relatively weak bone in the vertebrae and femur ball

Trace minerals: Minerals required in amounts ≤ 100 mg daily

Water-soluble vitamins: Vitamin C and B-complex vitamin coenzymes form an active enzyme to accelerate chemical compound interconversions

> References are available at Lippincott Connect.

Additional References

Aguilo A, et al. Nutritional status and implementation of a nutritional education program in young female artistic gymnasts. *Nutrients*. 2021;13:1399.

Armstrong LE. Rehydration during endurance exercise: challenges, research, options, methods. *Nutrients*. 2021;13:887.

Chao HC, et al. Serum trace element levels and their correlation with picky eating behavior, development, and physical activity in early childhood. *Nutrients*. 2021;13:2295.

Cheng J, et al. Menstrual irregularity, hormonal contraceptive use, and bone stress injuries in collegiate female athletes in the United States. *PMR*. 2021;13:1207.

Edama M, et al. The relationship between the female athlete triad and injury rates in collegiate female athletes. *PeerJ*. 2021;9:e11092.

Gauckler P, et al. Edema-like symptoms are common in ultra-distance cyclists and driven by overdrinking, use of analgesics and female sex—a study of 919 athletes. *J Int Soc Sports Nutr*. 2021;18:73.

Herbert AJ, et al. Bone mineral density in high-level endurance runners: Part A—site-specific characteristics. *Eur J Appl Physiol*. 2021;121:3437.

Hoenig T, et al. Does magnetic resonance imaging grading correlate with return to sports after bone stress injuries? A systematic review and meta-analysis. *Am J Sports Med*. 2021:363546521993807.

Jurov I, et al. Inducing low energy availability in trained endurance male athletes results in poorer explosive power. *Eur J Appl Physiol*. 2022;122:503.

Knechtle B, et al. Vitamin D and stress fractures in sport: preventive and therapeutic measures—a narrative review. *Medicina* (*Kaunas*). 2021;57:223.

Lipman GS, et al. Prospective observational study of weight-based assessment of sodium supplements on ultramarathon performance (WASSUP). *Sports Med Open*. 2021;7:13.

McCubbin AJ, et al. Sports dietitians Australia position statement: nutrition for exercise in hot environments. *Int J Sport Nutr Exerc Metab*. 2020;31:1.

Nguyen VH. School-based nutrition interventions can improve bone health in children and adolescents. *Osteoporos Sarcopenia*. 2021;7:1.

Noel SE, et al. Racial and ethnic disparities in bone health and outcomes in the United States. *J Bone Miner Res*. 2021;36:1881.

Schenk K, et al. Changes in factors regulating serum sodium homeostasis during two ultra-endurance mountain races of different distances: 69 km vs. 121 km. *Front Physiol*. 2021;12:764694.

Statuta SM. The female athlete triad, relative energy deficiency in sport, and the male athlete triad: the exploration of low-energy syndromes in athletes. [Review]. *Current Sports Medicine Reports*. 2020;19:43.

Toro-Román V, et al. Copper concentration in erythrocytes, platelets, plasma, serum and urine: influence of physical training. *J Int Soc Sports Nutr*. 2021;18:28.

Table 2.1 — Food Sources, Bodily Functions, and Symptoms of Deficiency or Excess for Fat-Soluble Vitamins

Vitamin	Dietary Sources	Major Bodily Functions	Deficiency	Excess
Vitamin A (retinol)	Provitamin A (β-carotene) distributed widely in green vegetables; retinol present in milk, butter, cheese, fortified margarine	Rhodopsin constituent (visual pigment) Maintain epithelial tissues; mucopolysaccharide synthesis role	Xerophthalmia (keratinization ocular tissue), night blindness, permanent blindness	Headache, vomiting, peeling skin, anorexia, long bone swelling
Vitamin D (cholecalciferol)	Cod-liver oil, eggs, dairy products, fortified milk, margarine	Promotes growth and bones mineralization Increased calcium absorption	Rickets in children Osteomalacia in adults	Vomiting, diarrhea, weight loss, kidney damage
Vitamin E (tocopherol)	Seeds, green leafy vegetables, margarine, shortening	Antioxidant functions to prevent cell damage	Possible anemia	Relatively nontoxic
Vitamin K (phylloquinone)	Green leafy vegetables; small amounts in cereals, fruits, meats	Important in blood clotting (forming active prothrombin)	Conditioned deficiencies with severe bleeding; internal hemorrhaging	Relatively nontoxic High-dose synthetic forms can cause jaundice

Table 2.2 — Food Sources, Bodily Functions, and Symptoms of Deficiency or Excess for Water-Soluble Vitamins

Vitamin	Dietary Sources	Major Bodily Functions	Deficiency	Excess
Vitamin B_1 (thiamine)	Pork, organ meats, whole grains, nuts, legumes, milk, fruits, and vegetables	Coenzyme (thiamine pyrophosphate) in reactions involving the removal of carbon dioxide	Beriberi (peripheral nerve changes, edema, heart failure)	None reported
Vitamin B_2 (riboflavin)	Widely distributed in foods: meats, eggs, milk products, whole grain and enriched cereal products, wheat germ, green leafy vegetables	Constituent of two flavin nucleotide coenzymes involved in energy metabolism (FAD and FMN)	Reddened lips, cracks at mouth corners (cheilosis), eye lesions	None reported
Niacin (nicotinic acid)	Liver, lean meats, poultry, grains, legumes, peanuts (can be formed from tryptophan)	Constituent of two coenzymes in oxidation reduction reactions (NAD and NADP)	Pellagra (skin and gastrointestinal lesions, nervous mental disorders)	Flushing, burning, and tingling around the neck, face, and hands
Vitamin B_6 (pyridoxine)	Meats, fish, poultry, vegetables, whole grains, cereals, seeds	Coenzyme (pyridoxal phosphate) involved in amino acid and glycogen metabolism	Irritability, convulsions, muscular twitching, dermatitis, kidney stones	None reported
Pantothenic acid	Widely distributed in foods, meat, fish, poultry, milk products, legumes, whole grains	Constituent of coenzyme A, which plays a central role in energy metabolism	Fatigue, sleep disturbances, impaired coordination, nausea	None reported
Folate	Legumes, green vegetables, whole-wheat products, meats, eggs, milk products, liver	Coenzyme (reduced form) involved in transfer of single-carbon units in nucleic acid and amino acid metabolism	Anemia, gastrointestinal disturbances, diarrhea, red tongue	None reported
Vitamin B_{12} (cobalamin)	Muscle meats, fish, eggs, dairy products (absent in plant foods)	Coenzyme involved in single-carbon unit transfer in nucleic acid metabolism	Pernicious anemia, neurologic disorders	None reported
Biotin	Legumes, vegetables, meats, liver, egg yolk, nuts	Coenzymes in fat synthesis, amino acid metabolism, and glycogen (animal starch) formation	Fatigue, depression, nausea, dermatitis, muscle pain	None reported
Vitamin C (ascorbic acid)	Citrus fruits, tomatoes, green peppers, salad greens	Maintains intercellular matrix of cartilage, bone, and dentine; collagen synthesis	Scurvy (degeneration of skin, teeth, blood vessels, epithelial hemorrhages)	Relatively nontoxic Possible kidney stones

Table 2.3 Vitamin Dietary Reference Intakes

Life-Stage Group	Vitamin A (mcg·d⁻¹)[a]	Vitamin C (mg·d⁻¹)	Vitamin D (mcg·d⁻¹)[b,c]	Vitamin E (mg·d⁻¹)[d]	Vitamin K (mcg·d⁻¹)	Thiamin (mg·d⁻¹)	Riboflavin (mg·d⁻¹)	Niacin (mg·d⁻¹)[e]	Vitamin B_6 (mg·d⁻¹)	Folate (mcg·d⁻¹)[f]	Vitamin B_{12} (mcg·d⁻¹)	Pantothenic Acid (mg·d⁻¹)	Biotin (mcg·d⁻¹)	Choline (mg·d⁻¹)[g]
Infants														
0–6 mo	400*	40*	5*	4*	2.0*	0.2*	0.3*	2*	0.1*	65*	0.4*	1.7*	5*	125*
7–12 mo	500*	50*	5*	5*	2.5*	0.3*	0.4*	4*	0.3*	80*	0.5*	1.8*	6*	150*
Children														
1–3 y	300	15	5*	6	30*	0.5	0.5	6	0.5	150	0.9	2*	8*	200*
4–8 y	400	25	5*	7	55*	0.6	0.6	8	0.6	200	1.2	3*	12*	250*
Males														
9–13 y	600	45	5*	11	60*	0.9	0.9	12	1.0	300	1.8	4*	20*	375*
14–18 y	900	75	5*	15	75*	1.2	1.3	16	1.3	400	2.4	5*	25*	550*
19–30 y	900	90	5*	15	120*	1.2	1.3	16	1.3	400	2.4	5*	30*	550*
31–50 y	900	90	5*	15	120*	1.2	1.3	16	1.3	400	2.4	5*	30*	550*
51–70 y	900	90	10*	15	120*	1.2	1.3	16	1.7	400	2.4[h]	5*	30*	550*
>70 y	900	90	15*	15	120*	1.2	1.3	16	1.7	400	2.4[h]	5*	30*	550*
Females														
9–13 y	600	45	5*	11	60*	0.9	0.9	12	1.0	300	1.8	4*	20*	375*
14–18 y	700	65	5*	15	75*	1.0	1.0	14	1.2	400[f]	2.4	5*	25*	400*
19–30 y	700	75	5*	15	90*	1.1	1.1	14	1.3	400[f]	2.4	5*	30*	425*
31–50 y	700	75	5*	15	90*	1.1	1.1	14	1.3	400[f]	2.4	5*	30*	425*
51–70 y	700	75	10*	15	90*	1.1	1.1	14	1.5	400	2.4[h]	5*	30*	425*
>70 y	700	75	15*	15	90*	1.1	1.1	14	1.5	400	2.4[h]	5*	30*	425*
Pregnancy[i,j]														
≤18 y	750	80	5*	15	75*	1.4	1.4	18	1.9	600[f]	2.6	6*	30*	450*
19–30 y	770	85	5*	15	90*	1.4	1.4	18	1.9	600[f]	2.6	6*	30*	450*
31–50 y	770	85	5*	15	90*	1.4	1.4	18	1.9	600[f]	2.6	6*	30*	450*
Lactation														
≤18 y	1200	115	5*	19	75*	1.4	1.6	17	2.0	500	2.8	7*	35*	550*
19–30 y	1300	120	5*	19	90*	1.4	1.6	17	2.0	500	2.8	7*	35*	550*
31–50 y	1300	120	5*	19	90*	1.4	1.6	17	2.0	500	2.8	7*	35*	550*

Note: This table from the DRI reports (see www.nap.edu) presents recommended dietary allowances (RDAs) in **bold type** and adequate intakes (AIs) in regular type followed by an asterisk (*). RDAs and AIs may both be used as goals for individual intake. RDAs are set to meet the needs of almost all (97 to 98%) individuals in a group. For healthy breast-fed infants, the AI is the mean intake. The AI for other life-stage and gender groups covers the needs of all individuals in the group, but lack uncertainty prevents confidence in the percentage of individuals covered by this intake.

[a] As retinol activity equivalents (RAEs). 1 RAE = 1 mcg retinol, 12 mcg β-carotene, 24 mcg α-carotene, or 24 mcg β-cryptoxanthin. To calculate RAEs from REs of provitamin A carotenoids in foods, divide the REs by 2. For preformed vitamin A in foods or supplements and for provitamin A carotenoids in supplements, 1 RE = 1 RAE.
[b] Calciferol. 1 mcg calciferol = 40 IU vitamin D.
[c] In the absence of adequate exposure to sunlight.
[d] As α-tocopherol. α-Tocopherol includes *RRR*-α-tocopherol, the only form of α-tocopherol that occurs naturally in foods, and the 2R-stereoisometric forms of α-tocopherol (*RRR*-α-tocopherol, *RSR*-α-tocopherol, *RRS*-α-tocopherol, and *RSS*-α-tocopherol) that occur in fortified foods and supplements. It does not include the 2S-stereoisometric forms of α-tocopherol (*SRR*-α-tocopherol, *SSR*-α-tocopherol, *SR*-α-tocopherol, and *SSS*-α-tocopherol), also found in fortified foods and supplements.
[e] As niacin equivalents (NE). 1 mg of niacin = 60 mg of tryptophan; 0 to 6 mo = preformed niacin (not NE).
[f] As dietary folate equivalents (DFE). 1 DFE = 1 mcg food folate = 0.6 mcg of folic acid from fortified food or as a supplement consumed with food = 0.5 mcg of a supplement taken on an empty stomach.
[g] AIs have been set for choline, yet there are few data to assess whether a dietary supply of choline is needed at all stages of the life cycle, and it may be that the choline requirement can be met by endogenous synthesis at some of these stages.
[h] Because 10 to 30% of older people may malabsorb food-bound B_{12}, it is advisable for those older than 50 years to meet their RDA mainly by consuming foods fortified with B_{12} or a supplement containing B_{12}.
[i] In view of evidence linking folate intake with fetal neural tube defects, women capable of pregnancy consume 400 mcg from supplements or fortified foods in addition to intake of food folate from a varied diet.
[j] It is assumed that women will continue consuming 400 mcg from supplements or fortified food until their pregnancy is confirmed and they enter prenatal care, normally after the end of the periconceptional period—the critical time for neural tube formation.

Data from Dietary Reference Intakes for Calcium, Phosphorus, Magnesium, Vitamin D, and Fluoride (1997); Dietary Reference Intakes for Thiamin, Riboflavin, Niacin, Vitamin B_6, Folate, Vitamin B_{12}, Pantothenic Acid, Biotin, and Choline (1998); Dietary Reference Intakes for Vitamin C, Vitamin E, Selenium, and Carotenoids (2000); and Dietary Reference Intakes for Vitamin A, Vitamin K, Arsenic, Boron, Chromium, Copper, Iodine, Iron, Manganese, Molybdenum, Nickel, Silicon, Vanadium, and Zinc (2001). These reports may be accessed via www.nap.edu/catalog/dri.

Table 2.4 Tolerable Upper Intake Levels for Vitamins

Life-Stage Group	Vitamin A (mcg·d⁻¹)[b]	Vitamin C (mg·d⁻¹)	Vitamin D (mg·d⁻¹)	Vitamin E (mg·d⁻¹)[c,d]	Vitamin K	Thiamin	Riboflavin	Niacin (mg·d⁻¹)[d]	Vitamin B₆ (mg·d⁻¹)[d]	Folate (mcg·d⁻¹)[d]	Vitamin B₁₂	Pantothenic Acid	Biotin	Choline (g·d⁻¹)	Carotenoids[e]
Infants															
0–6 mo	600	ND[f]	25	ND	ND	ND	ND	ND	ND	ND	ND	ND	ND	ND	ND
7–12 mo	600	ND	25	ND	ND	ND	ND	ND	ND	ND	ND	ND	ND	ND	ND
Children															
1–3 y	600	400	50	200	ND	ND	ND	10	30	300	ND	ND	ND	1.0	ND
4–8 y	900	650	50	300	ND	ND	ND	15	40	400	ND	ND	ND	1.0	ND
Males, Females															
9–13 y	1700	1200	50	600	ND	ND	ND	20	60	600	ND	ND	ND	2.0	ND
14–18 y	2800	1800	50	800	ND	ND	ND	30	80	800	ND	ND	ND	3.0	ND
19–70 y	3000	2000	50	1000	ND	ND	ND	35	100	1000	ND	ND	ND	3.5	ND
>70 y	3000	2000	50	1000	ND	ND	ND	35	100	1000	ND	ND	ND	3.5	ND
Pregnancy															
≤18 y	2800	1800	50	800	ND	ND	ND	30	80	800	ND	ND	ND	3.0	ND
19–50 y	3000	2000	50	1000	ND	ND	ND	35	100	1000	ND	ND	ND	3.5	ND
Lactation															
≤18 y	2800	1800	50	800	ND	ND	ND	30	80	800	ND	ND	ND	3.0	ND
19–50 y	3000	2000	50	1000	ND	ND	ND	35	100	1000	ND	ND	ND	3.5	ND

[a]UL = The maximum level of daily nutrient intake that is likely to pose no risk of adverse effects. Unless otherwise specified, the UL represents total intake from food, water, and supplements. Due to lack of suitable data, ULs could not be established for vitamin K, thiamin, riboflavin, vitamin B₁₂, pantothenic acid, biotin, or carotenoids. In the absence of ULs, extra caution may be warranted in consuming levels above recommended intakes.
[b]As preformed vitamin A only.
[c]As α-tocopherol; applies to any form of supplemental α-tocopherol.
[d]The ULs for vitamin E, niacin, and folate apply to synthetic forms obtained from supplements, fortified foods, or a combination of the two.
[e]β-Carotene supplements are advised only to serve as a provitamin A source for individuals at risk of vitamin A deficiency.
[f]ND, not determinable due to lack of data of adverse effects in this age group and concern with regard to lack of ability to handle excess amounts. Source of intake should be from food only to prevent high levels of intake.

Data from Dietary Reference Intakes for Calcium, Phosphorus, Magnesium, Vitamin D, and Fluoride (1997); Dietary Reference Intakes for Thiamin, Riboflavin, Niacin, Vitamin B₆, Folate, Vitamin B₁₂, Pantothenic Acid, Biotin, and Choline (1998); Dietary Reference Intakes for Vitamin C, Vitamin E, Selenium, and Carotenoids (2000); and Dietary Reference Intakes for Vitamin A, Vitamin K, Arsenic, Boron, Chromium, Copper, Iodine, Iron, Manganese, Molybdenum, Nickel, Silicon, Vanadium, and Zinc (2001). These reports may be accessed via www.nap.edu/catalog/dri.

Table 2.5 Mineral Dietary Reference Intakes

Life-Stage Group	Calcium (mg·d⁻¹)	Chromium (mcg·d⁻¹)	Copper (mcg·d⁻¹)	Fluoride (mg·d⁻¹)	Iodine (mcg·d⁻¹)	Iron (mg·d⁻¹)	Magnesium (mg·d⁻¹)	Manganese (mg·d⁻¹)	Molybdenum (mcg·d⁻¹)	Phosphorus (mg·d⁻¹)	Selenium (mcg·d⁻¹)	Zinc (mg·d⁻¹)
Infants												
0–6 mo	210*	0.2*	200*	0.01*	110*	0.27*	30*	0.003*	2*	100*	15*	2*
7–12 mo	270*	5.5*	220*	0.5*	130*	11*	75*	0.6*	3*	275*	20*	3
Children												
1–3 y	500*	11*	340	0.7*	90	7	80	1.2*	17	460	20	3
4–8 y	800*	15*	440	1*	90	10	130	1.5*	22	500	30	5
Males												
9–13 y	1300	25*	700	2*	120	8	240	1.9*	34	1250	40	8
14–18 y	1300*	35*	890	3*	150	11	410	2.2*	43	1250	55	11
19–30 y	1000*	35*	900	4*	150	8	400	2.3*	45	700	55	11
31–50 y	1000*	35*	900	4*	150	8	420	2.3*	45	700	55	11
51–70 y	1200*	30*	900	4*	150	8	420	2.3*	45	700	55	11
>70 y	1200*	30*	900	4*	150	8	420	2.3*	45	700	55	11
Females												
9–13 y	1300*	21*	700	2*	150	8	240	1.6*	34	1250	40	8
14–18 y	1300*	24*	890	3*	150	15	360	1.6*	43	1250	55	9
19–30 y	1000*	25*	900	3*	150	18	310	1.8*	45	700	55	8
31–50 y	1000*	25*	900	3*	150	18	320	1.8*	45	700	55	8
51–70 y	1200*	20*	900	3*	150	8	320	1.8*	45	700	55	8
>70 y	1200*	20*	900	3*	150	8	320	1.8*	45	700	55	8
Pregnancy												
≤18 y	1300*	29*	1000	3*	220	27	400	2.0*	50	1250	60	13
19–30 y	1000*	30*	1000	3*	220	27	350	2.0*	50	700	60	11
31–50 y	1000*	30*	1000	3*	220	27	360	2.0*	50	700	60	11
Lactation												
≤18 y	1300*	44*	1300	3*	290	10	360	2.6*	50	1250	70	14
19–30 y	1000*	45*	1300	3*	290	9	310	2.6*	50	700	70	12
31–50 y	1000*	45*	1300	3*	290	9	320	2.6*	50	700	70	12

Table presents recommended dietary allowances (RDAs) in **bold type** and adequate intakes (AIs) in ordinary type followed by an asterisk (*). RDAs and AIs may both be used as goals for individual intake. RDAs are set to meet the needs of almost all (97–98%) individuals in a group. For healthy breast-fed infants, the AI is the mean intake. The AI for other life-stage and gender groups is believed to cover the needs of all individuals in the group, but lack of data or uncertainty in the data prevent being able to specify with confidence the percentage of individuals covered by this intake.

Data from Dietary Reference Intakes for Calcium, Phosphorous, Magnesium. Vitamin D, and Fluoride (1997); Dietary Reference Intakes for Thiamin, Riboflavin, Niacin, Vitamin B₅ Folate, Vitamin B₅, Pantothenic Acid, Biotin, and Choline (1998); Dietary Reference Intakes for Vitamin C, Vitamin E, Selenium, and Carotenoids (2000); and Dietary Reference Intakes for Vitamin A, Vitamin K, Arsenic, Boron, Chromium, Copper, Iodine, Iron, Manganese, Molybdenum, Nickel, Silicon, Vanadium, and Zinc (2001).
These reports may be accessed via www.nap.edu/catalog/dri.

Table 2.6 Tolerable Upper Intake Levels[a] for Minerals

Life-Stage Group	Arsenic[b]	Boron (mg·d⁻¹)	Calcium (mg·d⁻¹)	Chromium	Copper (mcg·d⁻¹)	Fluoride (mg·d⁻¹)	Iodine (mcg·d⁻¹)	Iron (mg·d⁻¹)	Magnesium (mg·d⁻¹)[c]	Manganese (mg·d⁻¹)	Molybdenum (mcg·d⁻¹)	Nickel (mg·d⁻¹)	Phosphorus (g·d⁻¹)	Selenium (mcg·d⁻¹)	Silicon[d]	Vanadium (mg·d⁻¹)[e]	Zinc (mg·d⁻¹)
Infants																	
0–6 mo	ND[f]	ND	ND	ND	ND	0.7	ND	40	ND	ND	ND	ND	ND	45	ND	ND	4
7–12 mo	ND	ND	ND	ND	ND	0.9	ND	40	ND	ND	ND	ND	ND	60	ND	ND	5
Children																	
1–3 y	ND	3	2.5	ND	1000	1.0	200	40	65	2	300	0.2	3	90	ND	ND	7
4–8 y	ND	6	2.5	ND	3000	2.2	300	40	110	3	600	0.3	3	150	ND	ND	12
Males, females																	
9–13 y	ND	11	2.5	ND	5000	10	600	40	350	6	1100	0.6	4	280	ND	ND	23
14–18 y	ND	17	2.5	ND	800	10	900	45	350	9	1700	1.0	4	400	ND	ND	34
19–70 y	ND	20	2.5	ND	10,000	10	1100	45	350	11	2000	1.0	4	400	ND	1.8	40
>70 y	ND	20	2.5	ND	10,000	10	1100	45	350	11	2000	1.0	3	400	ND	1.8	40
Pregnancy																	
≤18 y	ND	17	2.5	ND	8000	10	900	45	350	9	1700	1.0	3.5	400	ND	ND	34
19–50 y	ND	20	2.5	ND	10,000	10	1100	45	350	11	2000	1.0	3.5	400	ND	ND	40
Lactation																	
≤18 y	ND	17	2.5	ND	8,000	10	900	45	350	9	1700	1.0	4	400	ND	ND	34
19–50 y	ND	20	2.5	ND	10,000	10	1100	45	350	11	2000	1.0	4	400	ND	ND	40

[a]UL = The maximum level of daily nutrient intake that is likely to pose no risk of adverse effects. Unless otherwise specified, the UL represents total intake from food, water, and supplements. Due to lack of suitable data, ULs could not be established for arsenic, chromium, and silicon. In the absence of ULs, extra caution may be warranted in consuming levels above recommended intakes.
[b]Although the UL was not determined for arsenic, there is no justification for adding arsenic to food or supplements.
[c]The ULs for magnesium represent intake from a pharmacologic agent only and do not include intake from food and water.
[d]Although silicon has not been shown to cause adverse effects in humans, there is no justification for adding silicon to supplements.
[e]Although vanadium in food has not been shown to cause adverse effects in humans, there is no justification for adding vanadium to food and vanadium supplements should be used with caution. The UL is based on adverse effects in laboratory animals, and these data could be used to set a UL for adults but not for children and adolescents.
[f]ND = not determinable due to lack of data of adverse effects in this age group and concern with regard to lack of ability to handle excess amounts. Source of intake should be from food only to prevent high levels of intake.

Data from Dietary Reference Intakes for Calcium, Phosphorous, Magnesium, Vitamin D, and Fluoride (1997); Dietary Reference Intakes for Thiamin, Riboflavin, Niacin, Vitamin B$_6$, Folate, Vitamin B$_{12}$, Pantothenic Acid, Biotin, and Choline (1998); Dietary Reference Intakes for Vitamin C, Vitamin E, Selenium, and Carotenoids (2000); and Dietary Reference Intakes for Vitamin A, Vitamin K, Arsenic, Boron, Chromium, Copper, Iodine, Iron, Manganese, Molybdenum, Nickel, Silicon, Vanadium, and Zinc (2001). These reports may be accessed via www.nap.edu/catalog/dri.

Table 2.7 Food Sources, Functions, and Effects of Deficiencies and Excesses for Important Major and Trace Minerals for Healthy Adults

Mineral	Dietary Sources	Major Bodily Functions	Deficiency	Excess
Major				
Calcium	Milk, cheese, dark green vegetables, dried legumes	Bone and tooth formation, blood clotting, nerve transmission	Stunted growth, rickets, osteoporosis, convulsions	Not reported in humans
Phosphorus	Milk, cheese, yogurt, meat, poultry, grains, fish	Bone and tooth formation, acid-base balance, helps prevent loss of calcium from bone	Weakness, demineralization	Jaw erosion (phossy jaw)
Potassium	Leafy vegetables, cantaloupe, lima beans, potatoes, bananas, milk, meats, coffee, tea	Fluid balance, nerve transmission, acid-base balance	Muscle cramps, irregular cardiac rhythm, mental confusion, loss of appetite; can be life threatening	None if kidneys function normally; poor kidney function causes potassium build up and cardiac arrhythmias
Sulfur	Obtained as part of dietary protein; present in food preservatives	Acid-base balance, liver function	Unlikely to occur with adequate dietary intake	Unknown
Sodium	Common salt	Acid-base balance, body water balance, nerve function	Muscle cramps, mental apathy, reduced appetite	Contributes to high blood pressure
Chlorine (chloride)	Chloride part of salt-containing food; some vegetables and fruits	Important part of extracellular fluids	Unlikely to occur with adequate dietary intake	Contributes to high blood pressure
Magnesium	Whole grains, green leafy vegetables	Activates enzymes involved in protein synthesis	Growth failure, behavioral disturbances	Diarrhea
Trace				
Iron	Eggs, lean meats, legumes, whole grains, green leafy vegetables	Constituent of hemoglobin and enzymes involved in energy metabolism	Iron deficiency anemia (weakness, reduced resistance to infection)	Siderosis; cirrhosis of the liver
Fluoride	Drinking water, tea, seafood	Role in maintaining of bone structure	Higher frequency of tooth decay	Mottling of teeth, increased bone density
Zinc	Widely distributed in foods	Constituent of enzymes involved in digestion	Growth failure, small sex glands	Fever, nausea, vomiting, diarrhea
Copper	Meats, drinking water	Constituent of enzymes associated with iron metabolism	Anemia, bone changes (rare)	Rare metabolic condition (Wilson disease)
Selenium	Seafood, meats, grains	Functions in close association with vitamin E	Anemia (rare)	Gastrointestinal disorders, lung irritations
Iodine (iodide)	Marine fish and shellfish, dairy products, vegetables, iodized salt	Constituent of thyroid hormones	Goiter (enlarged thyroid)	High intake depresses thyroid activity
Chromium	Legumes, cereals, organ meats, fats, vegetable oils, meats, whole grains	Constituent of some enzymes; involved in glucose and energy metabolism	Poorly understood in humans; impaired ability to metabolize glucose	Inhibition of enzymes. Occupational exposures: skin and kidney damage

Table 2.8 — Electrolyte Concentrations in Blood Serum, and Sweat and Carbohydrate Concentrations in Popular Beverages

Substance	Na$^+$ (mEq·L^{-1})[a]	K$^+$ (mEq·L^{-1})	Ca^{++} (mEq·L^{-1})	Mg^{++} (mEq·L^{-1})	Cl$^-$ (mEq·L^{-1})	Osmolality (mOsm·L^{-1})[b]	CHO (g·L^{-1})[c]
Blood serum	140	4.5	2.5	1.5–2.1	110	300	—
Sweat	60–80	4.5	1.5	3.3	40–90	170–220	—
Coca Cola	3.0	—	—	—	1.0	650	107
Gatorade	23.0	3.0	—	—	14.0	280	62
Fruit juice, typical	0.5	58.0	—	—	—	690	118
Pepsi Cola	1.7	Trace	—	—	Trace	568	81
Water	Trace	Trace	—	—	Trace	10–20	—

[a] Milliequivalents per liter.
[b] Milliosmoles per liter.
[c] Grams per liter.

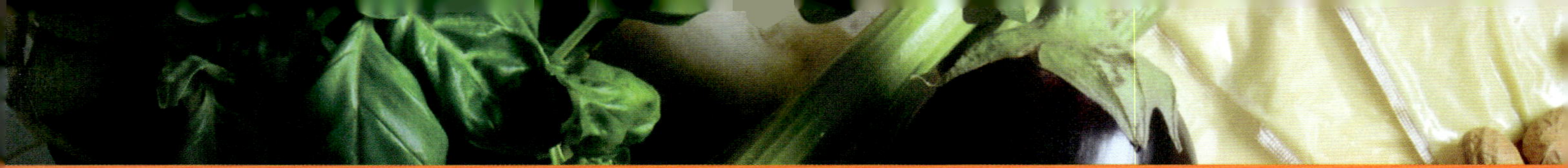

CHAPTER 3

Optimal Nutrition for Physical Activity

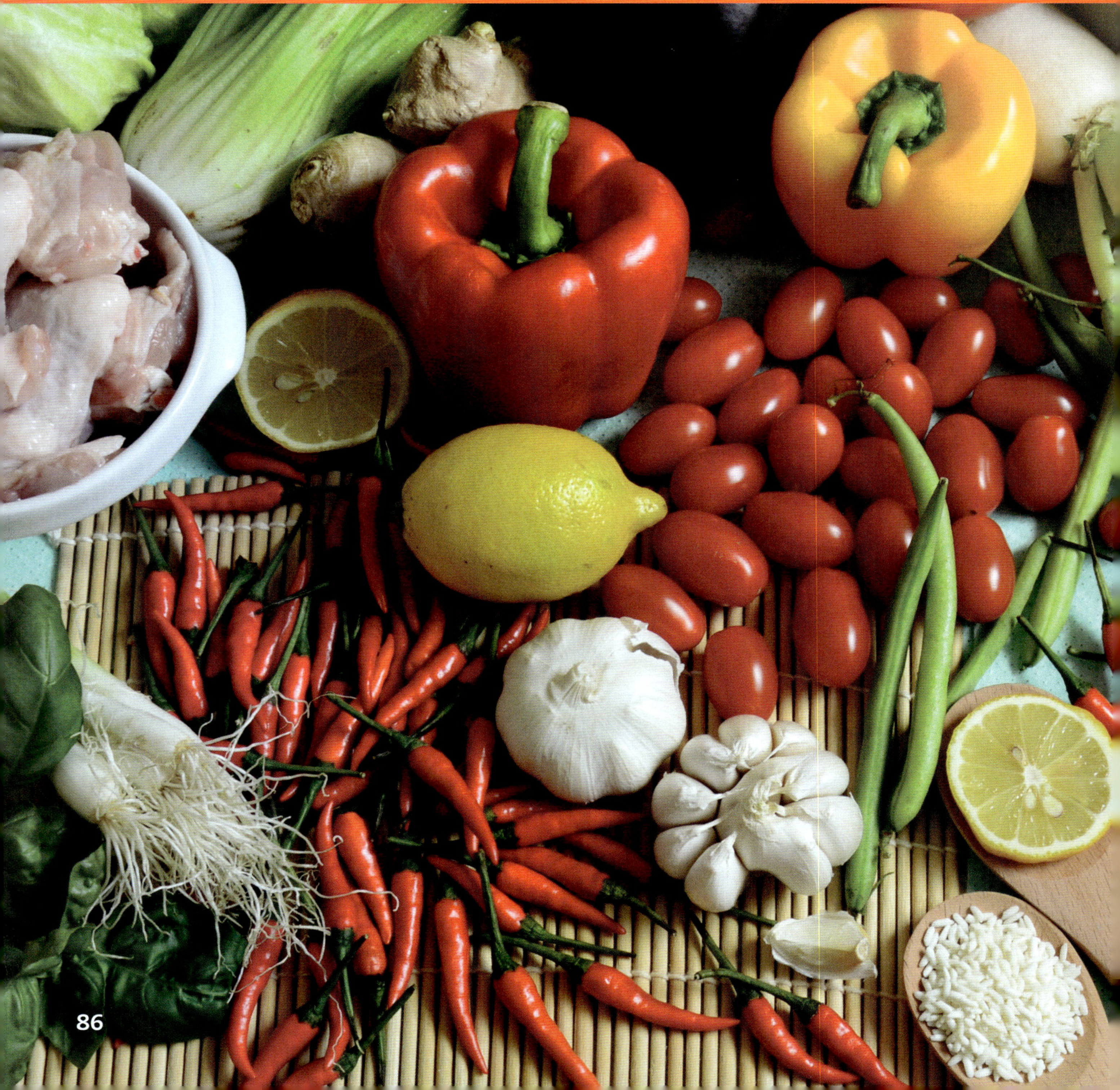

Chapter Objectives

- Compare nutrient and energy intakes in physically active persons with sedentary counterparts
- Provide recommendations for carbohydrate, lipid, and protein intake for individuals who maintain a physically active lifestyle and regularly engage in intense physical training
- Outline the latest MyPlate recommendations
- Give two examples of the energy intakes of athletes who train for competitive sports
- Advise an athlete concerning precompetition meal timing and composition
- Compare and contrast the nutritional purpose and nutrient content among liquid meals, nutrition bars, and nutrition powders and drinks
- Advise endurance athletes about potential negative effects of consuming a concentrated sugar drink within 30 min before competing and how to avoid those effects
- Discuss potential benefits and strategies for carbohydrate intake during intense endurance exercise
- Provide five examples of high-, moderate-, and low-glycemic index foods
- Describe the glycemic index's role in pre-exercise and postexercise glycogen replenishment
- Outline an optimal glycogen replenishment schedule following intense endurance exercise
- Describe foods' insulin index and its importance to athletes
- Describe the ideal sports drink and rationale for its composition
- Give two recommendations for fluid and carbohydrate replenishment during physical activity
- Discuss the controversy concerning high-fat diets for exercise training and endurance performance

Ancillaries at-a-Glance

Visit Lippincott Connect to access the following resources.

- References: Chapter 3
- Animations: Digestion of Carbohydrate, Fat Mobilization and Use, Glycogen Synthesis
- Focus on Research: Potential Effect of Diet on Health Status

An optimal diet supplies required nutrients in adequate amounts for tissue maintenance, repair, and growth without excess energy intake. Less-than-optimal fluid, nutrient, and energy intakes profoundly impact five factors:

1. Thermoregulatory function
2. Substrate availability
3. Physical activity capacity
4. Recovery from physical activity
5. Training responsiveness

Dietary recommendations for physically active individuals must target a particular activity's or sport's energy requirements and its training demands, including individual dietary preferences.[102–106] Various nutrition strategies that include the diet's macronutrient and micronutrient composition as well as total energy intake have been evaluated and/or proposed to reduce the risk of injury and improve recovery time, focusing upon injuries to skeletal muscle, bone, tendons, and ligaments.[107] Nutritional recommendations have focused on the unique requirements of adolescent, female, and masters athletes and those who travel for competition.[108,109] No single food or diet exists for optimal health and exercise performance; careful food intake planning and evaluation must follow sound nutritional guidelines. The physically active person must obtain sufficient macronutrients and energy to replenish liver and muscle glycogen, provide amino acid building blocks for tissue growth and repair, and maintain adequate lipid intake to provide essential fatty acids and fat-soluble vitamins. *In general, individuals who regularly engage in physical activity to keep fit do not require additional nutrients beyond those from a nutritionally well-balanced diet.*[83]

Nutrient Intake Among the Physically Active

Inconsistencies exist among studies that relate diet quality to physical activity level or physical fitness. The discrepancy partly relates to relatively crude and imprecise self-reported physical activity measures, unreliable dietary assessments, and/or small sample size.[34,41,55,59,110,111]

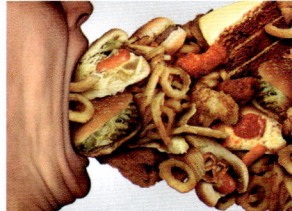

Fisher Photostudio/Shutterstock

Research contrasting nutrient and energy intakes with dietary recommendations for populations classified as low, moderate, and high for cardiorespiratory fitness reveals the following:

1. Increasing physical fitness levels are associated with a progressively lower body mass index (BMI).
2. Remarkably small differences in energy intake relate to physical fitness classification in women and men.
3. Men and women at moderate fitness status consume fewer calories than do those classified as highly fit.
4. A progressively higher dietary fiber intake and lower cholesterol intake occurs across fitness categories.
5. Men and women with higher fitness levels consume diets more closely linked to dietary recommendations for dietary fiber, percentage energy from total lipid, percentage energy from saturated fat, and dietary cholesterol.

Poor Diets and Disease

Lightspring/Shutterstock

About 75% of the U.S. adult population is either overweight or obese with more than 100 million adults classified as prediabetic or diabetic, nearly half the adult population, and the numbers continue to increase. More than 120 million people have cardiovascular disease resulting in nearly 850,000 deaths yearly, or about 2300 deaths on a daily basis. Alarmingly, more Americans now are sick than healthy. The foods regularly consumed—chronically low in essential food categories—contribute to a poor health status. The annual financial costs to healthcare and lost productivity from poor dietary practices remain staggering—cardiovascular disease $351 billion and diabetes $327 billion, with the total yearly obesity cost estimated at $1.72 trillion or 9.3% of the U.S. gross domestic product.

Source:
www.heart.org/en/news/2019/01/31/cardiovascular-diseases-affect-nearly-half-of-american-adults-statistics-show

INTEGRATIVE QUESTION

In what ways do nutritional and energy intake goals for sports training differ from actual competition requirements?

Recommended Nutrient Intake

FIGURE 3.1 illustrates the recommended intakes for protein, lipid, and carbohydrate and the food sources for these macronutrients for a resting daily energy requirement of about 1200 kcal. A total daily energy requirement of about 2000 kcal for females and 3000 kcal for males represents average values for typical young adults. *After meeting basic nutrient requirements as recommended in* **FIGURE 3.1**, *a variety of food sources with emphasis on unrefined complex carbohydrates should supply the extra energy demands for a variety of physical activities during a typical day.*

Protein

As emphasized in Chapter 1, $0.83 \text{ g} \cdot \text{kg}_{BM}^{-1}$ represents the recommended dietary allowance (RDA) for protein intake.

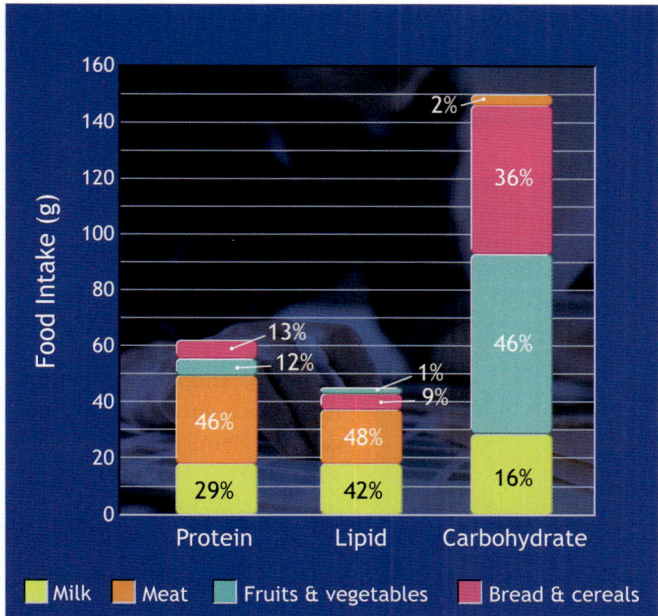

FIGURE 3.1. General recommendations for carbohydrate, lipid, and protein for the three main food categories in a balanced diet to meet average resting daily 1200 kcal energy requirements. Values within bars represent the percentage for group's contribution to the specific macronutrient intake. (TippaPatt/Shutterstock)

A person weighing 77 kg/170 lb would require about 64 g/2.2 oz of protein daily. This recommendation is adequate for most physically active individuals. For example, for older men who consume adequate dietary protein, additional supplementation with 21 g protein after exercise and every night before bed had no additional effect on strength or muscle mass accretion than resistance exercise training without supplementation.[102] Also, in a large randomized trial with functionally limited older men, 1.3 g · kg^{-1} · d^{-1} of protein, which exceeds the RDA, did not increase lean body mass, muscle performance, physical function, or well-being measures or augment anabolic response to exogenous testosterone. For these men, whose usual protein intakes were within recommended levels, their normal protein intake was sufficient to maintain lean body mass.[111]

In general, protein intakes for individuals consuming a typical U.S. diet considerably exceed the protein RDA. For athletes who train intensely, a protein intake between 1.2 and 1.4 g · kg body mass^{-1} adequately meets any added protein-related nutrient demands. Athletes do not necessarily require a protein supplement because their diet typically exceeds by two to four times the protein RDA.

INTEGRATIVE QUESTION

In what situations might a protein intake of twice the recommended dietary allowance still prove inadequate for an individual involved in intense physical training?

Lipid

Precise standards for optimal lipid intake have not been established. Dietary lipid intakes differ depending on personal taste, economic status, geographic influences, and lipid-rich food availability. To promote good health, lipid intake should not exceed 30 to 35% of the diet's energy content and at least 70% should be unsaturated fatty acids. For a Mediterranean-type diet (refer to "Good Nutrition Essentials," later in this chapter rich in monounsaturated and polyunsaturated fatty acids, a 35 to 40% total lipid percentage remains reasonable.

The American Heart Association (www.heart.org) makes three recommendations concerning dietary lipid intake:

1. Consume a diet containing 25 to 35% calories from lipid, primarily polyunsaturated fatty acids.
2. Limit saturated fat intake to less than 7% of total calories consumed.
3. Limit *trans fat* intake to less than 1% of total calories consumed.

Replacing "bad fats" with "good fats" in the diet requires keeping caloric intake in check and not substituting refined carbohydrate foods for foods high in lipid.

High-Fat Diets. Debate centers about the wisdom of maintaining a higher-than-average-fat diet during training or prior to endurance competition.[80,94,101,112] Adaptations to this diet type have consistently shown a shift in substrate use toward higher lipid oxidation during rest and exercise.[7,45,96] High-fat diet proponents argue that increasing daily dietary lipid intake stimulates lipid breakdown and augments lipid catabolism during intense aerobic activities. Any fat-burning enhancement could theoretically conserve glycogen reserves and/or contribute to improved endurance capacity under low glycogen reserve conditions.

 See the animation "Fat Mobilization and Use" on **Lippincott Connect** to view this process.

To investigate possible benefits, endurance capacity was compared between two groups of 10 young men matched for aerobic capacity and fed either a high-carbohydrate diet (65% kcal from carbohydrate) or a high-fat diet (62% kcal from lipid) for 7 wk. The endurance test consisted of pedaling a bicycle ergometer at a predetermined rate. Each group trained for 60 to 70 min at 50 to 85% aerobic capacity, 3 days a week during weeks 1 through 3 and 4 days a week during weeks 4 through 7. Following 7 training wk, the group consuming the high-fat diet switched to the high-carbohydrate diet. **FIGURE 3.2** displays performance for both groups. The endurance performance results were clear—the group consuming the high-carbohydrate diet performed considerably longer after training for 7 wk than the group consuming the high-fat diet (102.4 vs. 65.2 min). When the high-fat diet group switched to the high-carbohydrate diet during week 8, a small 11.5 min improvement in endurance

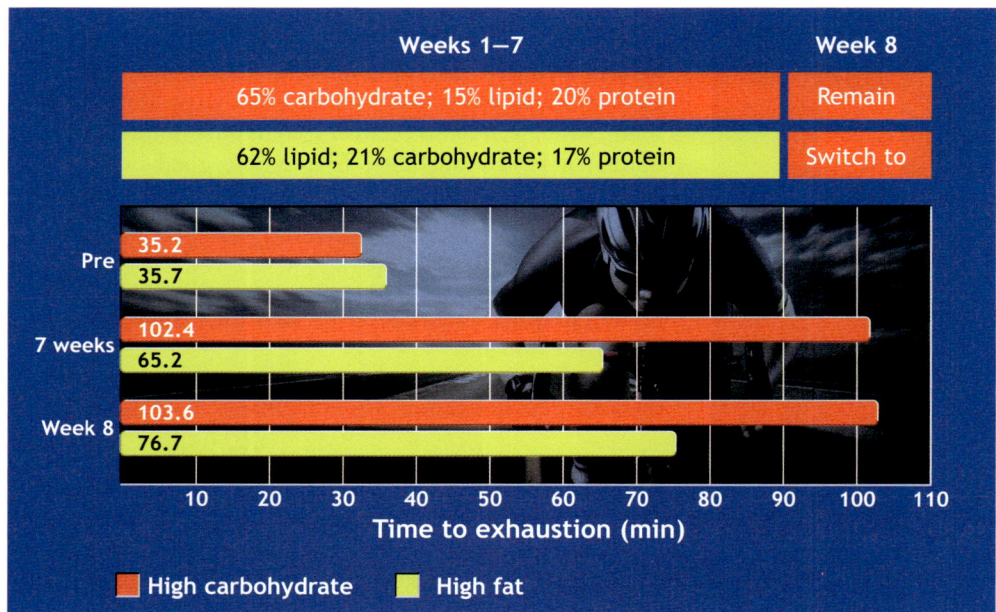

FIGURE 3.2. Effects of high-carbohydrate (CHO) versus high-fat diet on endurance performance in young males.
(Data from Helge JW, et al. Interaction of training and diet on metabolism and endurance during exercise in man. *J Physiol*. 1996;492:293. GoWithLight/Shutterstock.)

occurred. Consequently, total overall improvement in endurance over the 8-wk period achieved 115% for the high-fat diet group, while the group receiving the high-carbohydrate diet improved by 194%. The upper graph shows the percentage macronutrient contribution with the high-carbohydrate and high-fat diets. In essence, the high-fat diet produced *suboptimal* adaptations in endurance performance not fully remedied by switching to a high-carbohydrate diet. For sedentary humans, a low- or high-dietary lipid intake for 4 wk produced no differences in maximal or submaximal aerobic performance.[67]

A high-fat diet may stimulate adaptive responses to augment lipid use, but reliable research has yet to demonstrate consistent training benefits from consuming a high-fat diet. Such a diet can compromise training capacity and increase lethargy, produce fatigue, and elevate perceived exertion ratings.[81,96] The good news indicates that increasing the total lipid calorie percentage to 50% for physically active individuals who maintain a stable body weight and body composition does not compromise selected heart disease risk factors, including plasma lipoprotein profiles.[7,52] Considered in total, credible research does *not* support the popularized idea that reducing carbohydrate while increasing lipid intake above a 30% level produces a more optimal metabolic "zone" to augment endurance performance.[73,85]

Low-Fat Diets. Restricting dietary lipid below recommended levels impairs exercise performance.[38,93] A 20% lipid diet produced poorer endurance than a diet containing about 40% lipid.[64] A low-fat diet blunts the normal plasma testosterone rise following resistance exercise, which may limit such training effects.[97] Consuming low-fat diets during strenuous training creates difficulty in increasing carbohydrate and protein intake enough to provide "substitute" energy to maintain body weight and muscle mass.

Carbohydrate

No health hazard exists when subsisting chiefly on a fiber-rich whole-food plant-based diet, with adequate essential amino acid intake, fatty acids, minerals, and vitamins. The negative end of the nutrition continuum includes low-calorie "semistarvation" diets and other potentially harmful high-fat, low-carbohydrate diets, "liquid-protein" diets, single-food-centered diets, or time-centered diets that restrict food intake to specific feeding times (e.g., only consume foods within a continuous 8-hr period on any given day). Such extremes threaten good health, exercise performance, and training responsiveness.

Prior Creatine Supplementation Enhances Muscle Glycogen Loading

Classic research studies suggest a synergy between glycogen storage and creatine supplementation. Preceding glycogen loading with a creatine loading protocol (20 g creatine daily for 5 d) produced a 10% greater glycogen packing in the vastus lateralis muscle compared with glycogen levels achieved with only glycogen loading. Increases in muscle creatine quantity and cellular volume with creatine supplementation most likely facilitate subsequent muscle glycogen storage.

Sources:
Jensen R, et al. Glycogen supercompensation is due to increased number, not size, of glycogen particles in human skeletal muscle. *Exp Physiol*. 2021;106:1272.
Takahashi Y, et al. Enhanced skeletal muscle glycogen repletion after endurance exercise is associated with higher plasma insulin and skeletal muscle hexokinase 2 protein levels in mice: comparison of level running and downhill running model. *J Physiol Biochem*. 2021;77:469.

A low-carbohydrate diet rapidly compromises glycogen reserves for vigorous physical activity and regular exercise training. Excluding sufficient carbohydrate energy from the diet causes an individual to train in a relative glycogen-depleted state, which can eventually catabolize muscle protein and produce "staleness" to hinder exercise performance.[10,42,57]

 See the animation "Digestion of Carbohydrate" on **Lippincott Connect** to view this process.

Physically active individuals should consume at least 55 to 60% calories as carbohydrates, predominantly fiber-rich, unprocessed grains, beans, fruits, and vegetables. Maintaining a relatively high daily carbohydrate intake often relates more to the considerable energy demands for training than to short-term energy demands of competition.

See the animation "Glycogen Synthesis" on Lippincott Connect to view this process.

Carbohydrate Needs During Intense Training. Training for endurance running, ocean swimming, cross-country skiing, or cycling can produce a chronic fatigue state from successive days of hard training, often related to a gradual depletion in glycogen reserves even with adequate carbohydrate intake. **FIGURE 3.3** illustrates that running 16.1 km or 10 miles three successive days nearly depletes thigh muscle glycogen, even when the runners' diet contained 40 to 60% carbohydrate. By the third day, muscle glycogen was considerably below first day values. Presumably, the body's lipid reserves supplied the predominant energy for running on day 3. The diet must adjust daily carbohydrate intake upward to permit optimal glycogen resynthesis during arduous training but can be gradually reduced concurrent with the decrease in exercise intensity several days before competition.[87,118]

The recommended carbohydrate intake for physically active individuals assumes daily energy intake balances daily energy expenditure. If not, even consuming a relatively large *percentage* of carbohydrate calories will not adequately replenish this important energy reserve. General recommendations for carbohydrate intake range between 6 and 10 g · kg^{-1} · d^{-1}. This amount varies with each individual's daily energy expenditure and physical activity mode. *Individuals who undergo intense endurance training should consume 10 g carbohydrate per kilogram body mass per day to induce protein-sparing and preserve glycogen reserves.* The daily carbohydrate intake for a 46-kg/101-lb athlete who expends about 2800 kcal daily should average 450 g or 1800 kcal. A 68-kg/150-lb athlete should consume 675 g carbohydrate (2700 kcal) daily to sustain a 4200-kcal energy requirement. In both examples, carbohydrates exceed the minimum 55 to 60% total energy intake recommendations with training to optimize physical performance and mood state.[1]

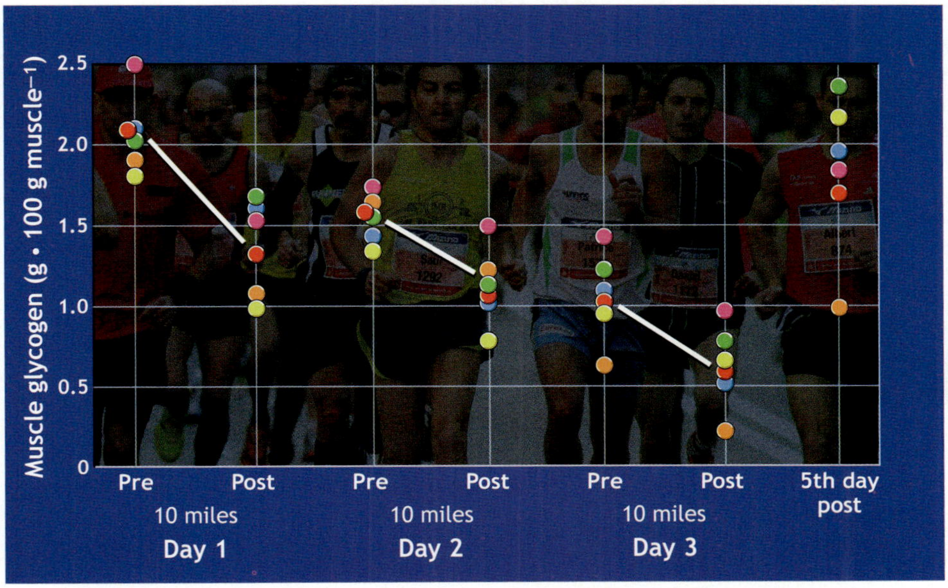

Role of Depleted Carbohydrate. Gradually depleting carbohydrate reserves with repeated strenuous training contributes to the overtraining syndrome. At least 1 to 2 days rest or lighter physical activity combined with a high–complex carbohydrate intake is recommended to reestablish pre-exercise muscle glycogen after exhaustive training or competition. Intense physical activity performed regularly requires a daily upward carbohydrate intake adjustment to optimize glycogen resynthesis and preserve high-quality training. Four guidelines provide nutritional recommendations to reduce athletic fatigue or staleness.

1. Consume easily digested, high-carbohydrate drinks or solid foods 1 to 4 hr before training or competition. Consume about 1 g carbohydrate · kg body mass^{-1} 1 hr prior to activity and up to 5 g carbohydrate · kg body mass^{-1} if the feeding occurs 4 hr prior to activity. A 70-kg/154-lb swimmer, for example, would drink 350 mL/12 oz of a 20% carbohydrate beverage 1 hr before activity, or eat 14 "energy bars," each containing 25 g carbohydrate, spread over the 4-hr period before physical activity.
2. Consume a high-carbohydrate liquid or solid food containing 0.35 to 1.5 g carbohydrate · kg body mass^{-1} · hr^{-1} immediately following physical activity and over the first 4 hr thereafter. A 70-kg/154-lb swimmer could drink a 100 to 450 mL/3.6 to 16 oz of a 25% carbohydrate beverage or one to four energy bars, each containing 25 g carbohydrate, immediately following physical activity and every hour thereafter for 4 hr.
3. Consume a 15 to 25% carbohydrate drink or a solid, high-carbohydrate supplement with each meal. This is achieved by reducing normal food intake by 250 kcal and consuming a high-carbohydrate beverage or solid food containing 250-kcal carbohydrate with each meal.
4. Maintain body glycogen reserves by stabilizing body weight during all training phases by matching energy intake to training's energy demands.

FIGURE 3.3. Changes in muscle glycogen concentration (mean response) for six male subjects before and after each 10-mi/16.1-km run performed on 3 successive days and 5 days after the last run (5th day post).
(Adapted with permission from Costill DL, et al. Muscle glycogen utilization during prolonged exercise on successive days. *J Appl Physiol.* 1971;31:834. ©The American Physiological Society (APS). All rights reserved. Maxisport/Shutterstock.)

In a Practical Sense

Nutritional Assessment Fundamentals: Clinical Signs and Symptoms

Nutritional deficiency usually develops over time, starting at a young age and progressing in stages. An overt deficiency often remains unrecognized until the condition passes the person's "clinical horizon" and moves into a disease state or becomes manifested by acute trauma (e.g., heart attack or type 2 diabetes complications). Nutritional assessment during any developmental deficiency stage provides a basis to identify a problem area and plan a sensible intervention.

In essence, a complete nutritional assessment evaluates a person's nutritional status and nutrient requirements based on interpreting clinical information. The nutritional assessment includes four major areas: dietary intake history, medical history, current review about prior symptoms, and a physical examination that incorporates anthropometric and laboratory data.

ASSESSING DIETARY INTAKE

Four methods provide dietary information.

Method 1: 24-Hour Dietary Recall

This approach involves a person recalling all foods and beverages consumed during the previous 24 hr and includes the approximate portion size and food preparation specifics. Repeat 24-hr recalls that span several days provide a more accurate and reliable estimate for a typical day.

Method 2: Food Diary

With the food diary method, the person records all foods and beverages at the time or as close to the time consumed by brand, weight, and portion size. Typically, the person maintains a food diary for 2 to 7 days.

Method 3: Food Frequency Assessment

A food frequency questionnaire lists various foods and estimates how often they consumed each item. This method does not itemize a specific day's intake. Rather, it provides a typical food consumption pattern.

Method 4: Diet History

A diet history yields general information about a person's dietary patterns including eating habits (meals per day, who prepares meals, and food preparation patterns), food preferences, eating locations, and typical food choices in different situations.

MEDICAL HISTORY

Personal Medical History

A medical history includes immunizations, hospitalizations, surgeries, and acute and chronic injuries and illness—each with nutritional implications. Prescription history and vitamin and mineral supplement use, laxatives, topical medications, and herbal remedies (herbs and other supplements not typically identified as medications) also add valuable information to the total assessment.

Family Medical and Social History

Medical histories that include information about the health/nutrition/exercise status for parents, siblings, children, and spouse can reveal chronic disease risk related to a genetic or social connection. Sociocultural relationships regarding food choices help to understand individual eating patterns and practices. Information about alcohol, tobacco, illicit drugs, and caffeine duration and frequency helps to formulate an effective treatment plan and chronic disease risk.

PHYSICAL EXAMINATION

A nutrition-oriented physical examination focuses on the mouth, skin, head, hair, eyes, fingernails, extremities, abdomen, skeletal musculature, and limb and trunk fat stores. Dry skin, cracked lips, or lethargy may indicate nutritional deficiencies.

NUTRITIONAL INADEQUACY CLINICAL SIGNS AND SYMPTOMS

Organ	Sign/Symptom	Possible Cause
Skin	Pallor	Iron folate, vitamin B_{12} deficiency
	Ecchymosis (purplish patch)	Vitamin K deficiency
	Pressure ulcers/delayed healing	Protein malnutrition
	Hair hyperkeratosis (excess eruption)	Vitamin A deficiency
	Petechiae (minute hemorrhagic spots)	Vitamin A, C, or K deficiency
	Purpura (hemorrhage into skin)	Vitamin C or K deficiency
	Rash/eczema/scaling	Zinc deficiency

Organ	Sign/Symptom	Possible Cause
Hair	Dyspigmentation, easy pluckability	Protein malnutrition
Head	Temporal muscle wasting	Protein-energy malnutrition
Eyes	Night blindness, xerosis	Vitamin A deficiency (pathologic dryness)
Mouth	Bleeding gum	Vitamin C, riboflavin deficiency
	Tongue fissuring (splitting), raw tongue, tongue atrophy (wasting)	Niacin, riboflavin deficiency
Heart	Tachycardia	Thiamin deficiency
Genital/Urinary	Delayed puberty	Protein-energy malnutrition
Extremities	Bone softening	Vitamin D, calcium, phosphorous deficiency
	Bone/joint aches	Vitamin C deficiency
	Edema	Protein deficiency
	Muscle wasting	Protein-energy malnutrition
	Ataxia	Vitamin B_{12} deficiency
Neurologic deficiency	Tetany (muscle twitches, cramps)	Calcium, magnesium
	Paresthesia (abnormal sensation)	Thiamin deficiency
	Lost reflexes (wrist/foot drop)	Thiamin, vitamin B_{12} deficiency
	Dementia	Niacin deficiency

Sources:
Cordellat A, et al. Multicomponent exercise training combined with nutritional counselling improves physical function, biochemical and anthropometric profiles in obese children: a pilot study. *Nutrients.* 2020;12:2723.
Reber E, et al. Nutritional risk screening and assessment. *J Clin Med.* 2019;8:1065.

Good Nutrition Essentials

In the typical "standard American diet," energy-dense but nutrient-poor foods frequently substitute for more nutrient-rich healthful foods. Such a food intake pattern typically includes high-fat, high-sugar foods and large quantities of animal-based proteins. When this dietary pattern persists, it often links to marginal micronutrient intakes, low levels of high-density lipoprotein and high levels of low-density lipoprotein cholesterol, and elevated homocysteine—leading to increased risk for obesity, type 2 diabetes, chronic kidney disease, and coronary heart disease.[117–119]

Dietary Guidelines for Americans

Formulation of the *Dietary Guidelines for Americans* begins initially with the Dietary Guidelines Advisory Committee. These highly acclaimed scientists review current nutrition research and draft a scientific report that the US Department of Agriculture (USDA) and Health and Human Services (HHS) use to develop the final guidelines. The official 2020–2025 *Dietary Guidelines* revisions are expected in early 2021.

In the 1990 National Nutrition Monitoring and Related Research Act, the *Dietary Guidelines for Americans* reflects scientific evidence related to healthful nutrition published jointly by the USDA (www.usda.gov) and HHS (www.hhs.gov) every 5 years. Historically, the *Guidelines* have focused on Americans age 2 years and older, but the USDA 2014 Farm Bill mandated adding information and guidelines for infants and toddlers and pregnant women (www.ers.usda.gov/agricultural-act-of-2014-highlights-and-implications/). The 2020–2025 Guidelines

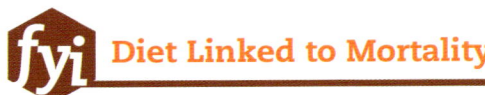

Diet Linked to Mortality

Ten dietary factors link to increased death risk from heart disease, stroke, or type 2 diabetes, conditions described by the term cardiometabolic disease. The table reveals that unhealthful dietary practices like consuming high-sodium foods, fewer nuts and seeds, and processed meats and other poor food choices account for about 45% of annual deaths in the United States. The takeaway message—eat an array of more colorful fruits and vegetables and nuts, seeds, whole grains, polyunsaturated vegetable oils, and omega-3-rich fish, and concurrently minimize consuming foods damaging to health.

Dietary Factors and Increased Mortality	% Annual CMD Deaths
All factors combined	45.4
High sodium intake	9.5
Low nut/seed intake	8.5
High processed meat intake	8.2
Low seafood omega-3 intake	7.8
Low vegetable intake	7.6
Low fruit intake	7.5
High sugar drink intake	7.4
Low whole grain intake	5.9
Low polyunsaturated fat intake	2.3
High unprocessed red meat intake	0.4

Sources:
Huang YQ, et al. Prehypertension and risk for all-cause and cardiovascular mortality by diabetes status: results from the national health and nutrition examination surveys. *Ann Transl Med*. 2020;8:323.
Li Z-H, et al. Associations of habitual fish oil supplementation with cardiovascular outcomes and all-cause mortality: evidence from a large population based cohort study. *BMJ*. 2020;368:m456.
Micha R, et al. Association between dietary factors and mortality from heart disease, stroke, and type 2 diabetes in the United States. *JAMA*. 2017;317:912.

Advisory Committee systematically reviewed more than 270,000 citations, nearly 1500 original research studies, and 33 original systematic reviews. The major themes for the new *Guidelines* include the following:

1. Healthy eating at each life stage (infant, childhood, adolescence, young adults, during pregnancy, mature adulthood, and older adults)
2. The cumulative effects on health over the life span and establishing core elements for a healthy dietary pattern for each life stage
3. Providing a sound framework for meal planning for physically active individuals

Dietary Guidelines Update: 2020–2025

The prior 2015–2020 *Guidelines* identified five principles as overarching guidelines. The new 2020–2025 *Guidelines* suggest modifications and expansion to reflect new evidence. They recognize special nutrient concerns that exist at each life stage to help Americans improve their dietary practices and potentially influence healthful food choices at the next life stage. The guidelines are structured around core foods that meet nutrient needs, associate with health, and reduce chronic disease risk. The five major recommendations are structured to build upon the previous *Guidelines*:

1. **Follow a healthy eating pattern across the life span.**
   a. Introduce the importance of maintaining healthful dietary patterns across each life stage.
      i. Initiate a healthful dietary pattern early in life for infants and young children.
      ii. Follow a healthful dietary pattern appropriate to meet the nutritional needs at each life stage.
      iii. Modify the dietary pattern over the life span to meet the nutritional needs at each life stage.
2. **Focus on variety, nutrient density, and amount.**
   a. Focus on nutritional quality in food choices, portion size, and eating frequency.
   b. For the earliest life stage, focus on breast-feeding and human milk for optimal nutrition, and gradually introduce nutrient-rich complementary foods during infancy's second half.
3. **Limit added sugars and saturated fat calories and reduce sodium intake.**
   a. Limit or replace certain food components. For those who consume alcoholic beverages, lower intakes are healthier than higher intakes and some groups should not drink alcoholic beverages.
      i. Limit foods and beverages that add sugars, saturated fats, alcohol, and salt, and excess energy foods, solid fats, and sodium.
      ii. Replace foods and beverages with added sugars, saturated fats, alcohol, and sodium with more healthful choices.
      iii. During the first 2 years of life, avoid sugar-sweetened beverages.
4. **Shift to healthier food and beverage choices.**
   a. Individuals need to recognize what food and beverage choices are most important to change.
      i. Shift eating patterns to food and beverage choices that have a higher nutrient-to-energy ratio.
      ii. Shift to higher quality food and beverage choices at every age to achieve a more healthful dietary pattern.
5. **Support healthy eating patterns for all individuals.**
   a. To support access to healthful foods and dietary patterns for all Americans, consider cultural, ethnic, and socioeconomic factors that influence food preferences and access to healthful foods and beverages, and important tools and resources for individuals to plan and monitor their diets.

i. Support access to healthful foods and beverages in all food environments for all Americans at all ages.
ii. Promote and support breast-feeding.
iii. Support healthful eating patterns at all ages where people live, learn, work, play, and gather.

The new *Guidelines'* principle message asks individuals to consume a varied but balanced diet. To maintain a healthy body weight, attention must focus on portion size, total calories consumed, and increased daily physical activity. A major goal is to reduce a high-sodium diet with one rich in fruits and vegetables, cereals and whole grains, nonfat and low-fat dairy products, legumes, nuts, fish, poultry, and lean meats, with concomitant caloric reduction in calories from solid fats, added sugars, and refined grains.[4,14,18]

TABLE 3.1 shows the latest relationships among different constituent foods, beverages, and nutrients related to major health outcomes; cardiovascular disease and associated risk factors; overweight and obesity; type 2 diabetes; bone health; colon, lung, breast, and prostate cancers; neurocognitive health; sarcopenia; and all-cause mortality.

TABLE 3.1 Research findings: dietary components associated with health outcomes

The association between dietary patterns and health outcomes reveals remarkable consistency in the findings and their implications. For adults, evidence was considered *moderate* or *strong* among dietary patterns and all health outcomes, except for neurocognitive health, while the evidence was *limited* for prostate and lung cancer. There was insufficient evidence to draw conclusions about dietary patterns and sarcopenia outcomes.

Common dietary pattern characteristics associated with positive health outcomes include higher intake for vegetables, fruits, legumes, whole grains, low- or nonfat dairy, seafood, nuts, and unsaturated vegetable oils, and a lower intake of red and processed meats, sugar-sweetened foods and drinks, and refined grains. Vegetables and fruits were consistently and positively associated with favorable health outcomes, while whole grains were identified in all categories except neurocognitive health. Low- or nonfat dairy, seafood, legumes, and nuts were identified as beneficial components for many but not all favorable outcomes. Detrimental dietary-related health outcomes were associated with higher intakes of red and processed meat, sugar-sweetened foods and beverages, and refined grains. A noteworthy difference from the 2015 Committee report now identifies whole grains with almost the same beneficial outcomes as vegetables and fruits, suggesting that these three plant-based food groups constitute a healthful dietary pattern.

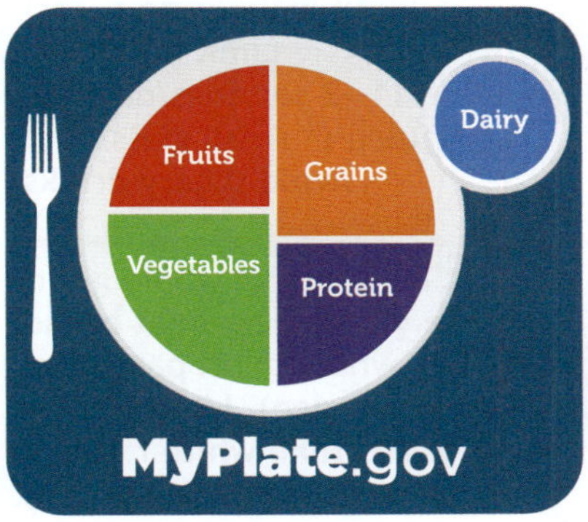

MyPlate: The Healthy Eating Guide

In the first quarter of 2020, the USDA unveiled the revised **MyPlate** icon highlighting nutritional guidelines for healthy eating. The MyPlate strategy, emphasizing more vegetables from all five subgroups, encourages Americans to become healthier in their battle against the **cardiometabolic disorders**, which include abdominal obesity, high fasting triacylglycerols, low HDL cholesterol, and elevated blood pressure.

The MyPlate guide illustrated in **FIGURE 3.4** has different-sized plate portions to symbolize the recommended food groups and builds on the messages from the *Dietary Guidelines for Americans*.[47,49,113] Fruits and vegetables occupy one-half the plate, with vegetables predominating. Grains, particularly whole grains, and proteins make up the other half, with grains taking up a majority from that half. MyPlate eliminates MyPyramid's references to sugars, lipids, or oils. The protein category includes meat, poultry, seafood, eggs, and vegetarian options such as beans and peas, nuts and seeds, and tofu. A smaller blue circle adjoining the plate icon indicates dairy products (a glass of skim or reduced-fat milk, cheese, or yogurt). Daily caloric intake, portion size, lipid intake, and energy expenditure are not represented. Similar to the new *Guidelines*, MyPlate stresses balanced portions among the different food categories (www.ChooseMyPlate.gov).

Seven Suggestions to Improve MyPlate

Shortly following the MyPlate release in 2011, nutrition experts at the Harvard School of Public Health (HSPH) in conjunction with colleagues at Harvard Health Publications unveiled the **Healthy Eating Plate**, a visual guide as a blueprint to eat more healthfully. The Healthy Eating Plate, based on available scientific evidence, showed that a plant-based diet rich in vegetables, whole grains, and healthful lipids and proteins lowered weight

Fruits
- 1–2 cups daily
- One cup raw or cooked fruit or 100% fruit juice; half-cup dried fruit

Vegetables
- 1–3 cups daily
- One cup raw or cooked vegetables or vegetable juice; two cups leafy salad greens

Dairy
- 1.5–3 cups daily
- One cup milk, yogurt, or fortified soy milk; 1.5 ounces natural cheese

Grains
- 3–8 ounces daily
- One slice of bread; half-cup cooked rice, cereal, or pasta; one ounce ready-to-eat cereal

Protein foods
- 2–6.5 ounces daily
- One ounce lean meat, poultry or fish; one egg; tablespoon peanut butter; half-ounce nuts or seeds; quarter-cup beans or peas

FIGURE 3.4. MyPlate, the USDA's current healthy eating guide.

gain and chronic disease risks. Similar to its MyPlate counterpart, the Healthy Eating Plate is easy to understand based on its simplicity—and addresses important deficiencies in MyPlate's details.

Critics argue that MyPlate mixes science with powerful agricultural influences, usually a poor recipe for promoting consumer health. The following MyPlate shortcomings emerge in comparison to the Healthy Eating Plate strategy:

1. Gives no indication about the healthful benefits of whole grains compared to refined grains
2. Gives no indication that some high-protein foods—fish, poultry, beans, nuts—are preferred over red meat and processed meats in lowering chronic disease risk
3. Fails to mention the beneficial role of certain lipids in healthful meal planning
4. Does not differentiate between potatoes and other high-glycemic vegetables that mimic sugar and higher glycemic counterparts
5. Recommends dairy at every meal with little evidence that high dairy intake protects against osteoporosis, and high intakes can be harmful
6. Does not mention sugary drinks' potential negative effects
7. Does not mention regular physical activity as important for overall good health

Healthy Eating Plate

FIGURE 3.5 presents the Healthy Eating Plate, an alternative guide for healthful eating, which addresses deficiencies in the USDA MyPlate recommendations.

The Healthy Eating Plate's main message focuses on diet quality as follows:

- Diet's *carbohydrate type* plays a more important role than carbohydrate *amount* because most vegetable, fruit, whole grain, and bean sources are more desirable than other processed carbohydrate types.
- Avoid sugary beverage drinks, a major extra calorie source with little nutritional value.
- Use healthy oils with meals but does not set a maximum on the calorie percentage people should consume daily from these lipid sources. In this way, the Healthy Eating Plate recommends the opposite of the low-fat message the USDA has endorsed for decades.

The specifics in this alternative plan include six categories:

- **Vegetables**: Eat an abundant variety, but limit potatoes and other high-glycemic starches that similarly raise blood sugar.
- **Fruits**: Choose a "rainbow" of fruit daily.
- **Whole grains**: Choose whole grains (e.g., oatmeal, whole-wheat bread, and brown rice) over refined grains (white bread and white rice).

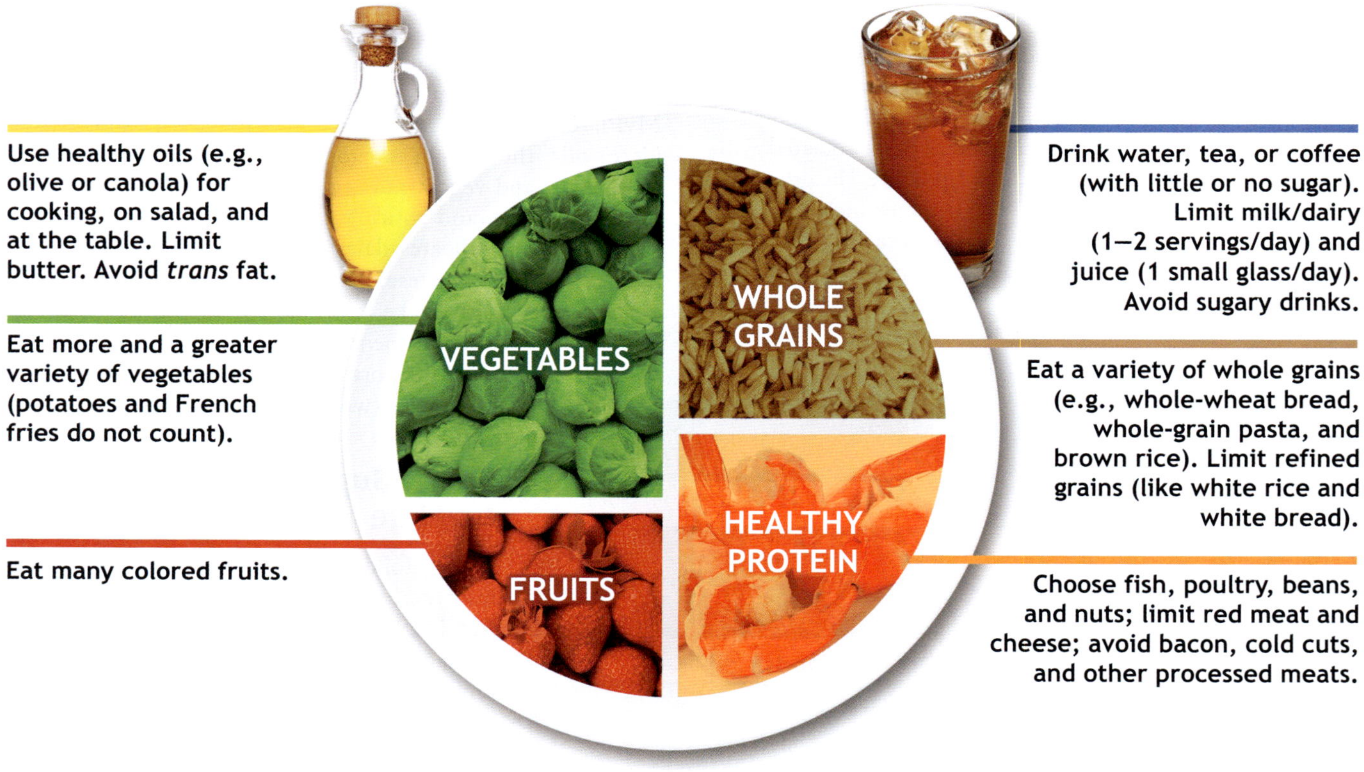

Use healthy oils (e.g., olive or canola) for cooking, on salad, and at the table. Limit butter. Avoid *trans* fat.

Eat more and a greater variety of vegetables (potatoes and French fries do not count).

Eat many colored fruits.

Drink water, tea, or coffee (with little or no sugar). Limit milk/dairy (1–2 servings/day) and juice (1 small glass/day). Avoid sugary drinks.

Eat a variety of whole grains (e.g., whole-wheat bread, whole-grain pasta, and brown rice). Limit refined grains (like white rice and white bread).

Choose fish, poultry, beans, and nuts; limit red meat and cheese; avoid bacon, cold cuts, and other processed meats.

FIGURE 3.5. Example of a healthy eating plate—an alternative to confront deficiencies in the USDA's MyPlate.
(Shutterstock: Alexandr Makarov; InfinityZero; Gcapture; NIPAPORN PANYACHAROEN; uladzimir zgurski; Danny Smythe)

- **Healthful proteins**: Choose fish, poultry, beans, or nuts and consume less red meat and processed meats.
- **Water**: Drink water, tea, or coffee (with little or no sugar). Limit milk and dairy (1 to 2 servings daily) and juice (1 small glass daily) and avoid sugary drinks.
- **Stay active**: Increased physical activity should be integral to everyone's healthy eating program.

Mediterranean Diet Pyramid

The modern Mediterranean diet, first introduced in 1975 by American physiologist and nutrition advocate and research scientist Ancel Keys, PhD, DSc (with his wife Margaret, a trained biochemist who advanced techniques to measure blood cholesterol, coauthored three influential books with Keys) at the University of Minnesota Laboratory of Physiological Hygiene, led to the creation of the **Mediterranean Diet Pyramid** to visually represent a healthful, traditional diet of Mediterranean countries (**FIG. 3.6**). The "real" Mediterranean diet has its origins in the Mediterranean basin (e.g., Nile, Tigris, and Euphrates River areas, home to the ancient Sumerian, Assyrian, Babylonian, and Persian civilizations). This central region became a melting pot for different religions, customs, languages, and foods. This "cradle of society" represented an ancient world time capsule. The historical path from ancient Mediterranean areas to a modern nutritional model now embraced worldwide incorporates all that is good for health based on sound nutrition and a respect for eating habits.

The Mediterranean diet plan emphasizes eight strategies:

1. Substitute olive oil for other lipids and oils including butter and margarine.
2. Make the goal for total lipid less than 25 to over 35% energy (calories), with saturated fat not to exceed 7 to 8%.
3. Include daily low to moderate cheese and yogurt consumption.
4. Consume low to moderate amounts of fish and poultry twice weekly.
5. Emphasize fresh fruit as the typical daily dessert and minimize high-sugar sweets and saturated fats.
6. Reduce red meat consumption to twice monthly (limit to 340 to 450 g/12 to 16 oz).
7. Increase regular physical activity to a level that promotes a healthy weight, fitness, and well-being.
8. Limit moderate wine consumption (1 to 2 glasses daily for men and 1 glass daily for women).

The Mediterranean diet represents no one specific diet but rather a traditional food range that differs in flavor and variety according to geographic region and culture, and protects individuals at high death risk from heart disease, stroke, and metabolic syndrome, presumably from its association with increased antioxidant capacity and low LDL-cholesterol levels.[23,28,65,114] This diet, high in fiber and carbohydrates and foods such as whole grains, nuts, fruits, vegetables, and beans, and limited in red and processed meats, sugary bev-

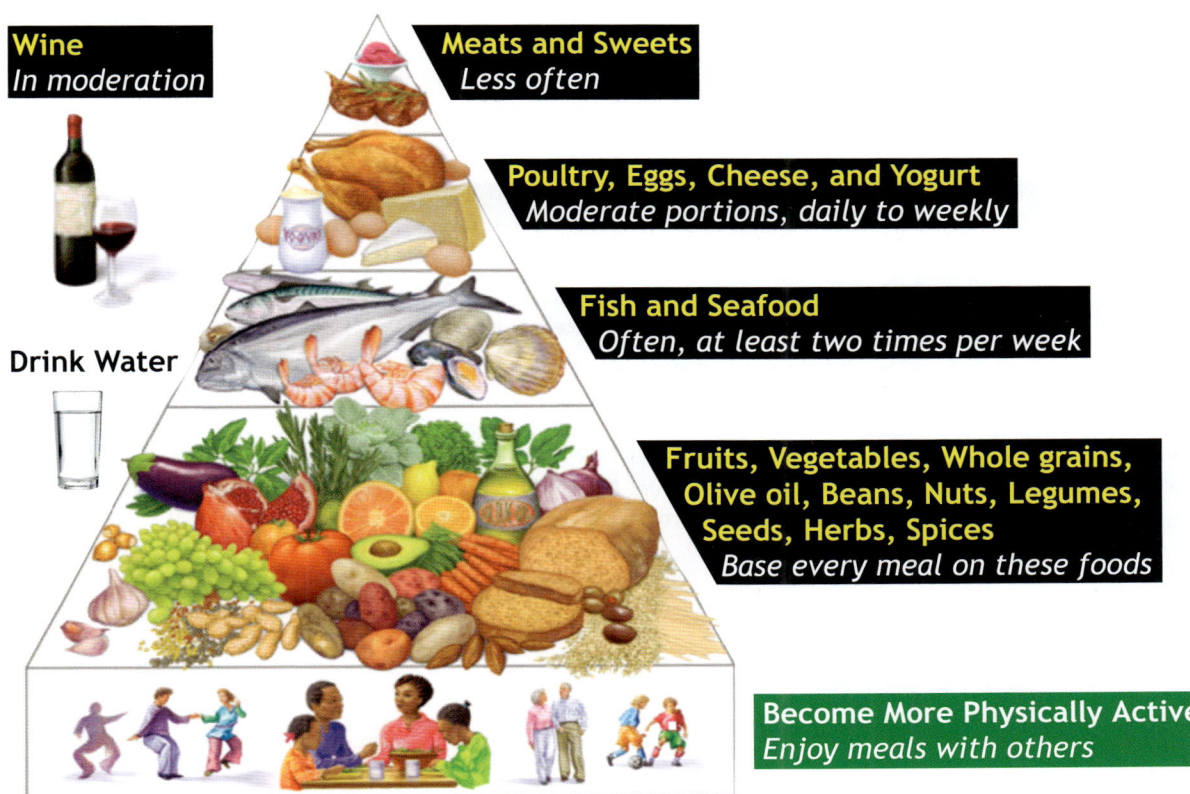

FIGURE 3.6. The Mediterranean diet pyramid.
(Adapted with permission from Oldways Preservation & Exchange Trust, https://oldwayspt.org/. Andrey_Kuzmin/Shutterstock)

erages and sweets, and refined grains and starches, may also promote weight loss and reduce insulin resistance in overweight individuals. Its high monounsaturated fatty acid content (generally olive oil with its associated phytochemicals[79]) helps delay age-related memory loss, decrease cancer risk, and reduce overall morality and frailty in the healthy elderly, a cluster of health problems that rob the elderly of independence and quality of life.[26,51,76,89] The dietary approach may also be effective for improving aerobic exercise performance in less than a week's time.[115] Both Mediterranean Diet Pyramid and Healthy Eating Plate focus on reducing ischemic stroke risk[47] and enhancing cholesterol-lowering drug benefits; they also associate with a reduced damage to small blood vessels in the brain[27,48] and a lower cognitive decline related to Alzheimer disease (the most common dementia form in older adults) and stroke. They may also lower blood pressure and keep the arteries from stiffening in aging. The biggest dietary impact on cancer probably lies in the effect on minimizing overweight and obesity, and risk factors for several cancer forms.

 INTEGRATIVE QUESTION

How would you advise a high school soccer team with diverse ethnic backgrounds and unique food intake patterns about sound nutrition?

Serving Size Versus Portion Size

Confusion exists about serving size and portion size. For example, the USDA defines a standard pasta *serving* as 1/2 cup, whereas the Food and Drug Administration (FDA; www.fda.gov), which regulates food labels, claims 1 cup represents a standard serving. Contrast these sizes with a typical restaurant pasta *portion* that averages about 3 cups—equal to six servings from MyPlate! To add further confusion, most people consider a serving to be the food amount they typically consume (actually a portion), but for the government's presentation, it represents a smaller measurement unit. Picture portions shown in **FIGURE 3.7** are rough size equivalents for popular food items (e.g., for the deck of cards, the 3-oz cooked meat or poultry portion size would equal the size for an actual card deck, not to the illustration size). Within the "real-world" perspective versus government standards, the USDA recommendation to consume 6 to 11 grain or bread daily servings seems *unattainable*. Consider that one serving by government standards represents a relatively small portion size: a 6-oz glass of fruit or vegetable juice; 1 medium-sized orange, banana, or apple; 1 cup salad greens—about fist size; 1 egg; 1 cup milk or yogurt; 1 bread slice; 2 tablespoons peanut butter—about the size of a ping-pong ball; 1/2 cup chopped fruits and vegetables—3 medium asparagus spears, 8 carrot sticks, 1 ear of corn, or 1/4 cup dried fruit like raisins; 3 oz meat, fish, or poultry—about the same size as a playing card deck; 1 teaspoon butter or mayonnaise—the size of a fingertip; or 2 oz cheese—the size equivalent to two thumb widths.

Physical Activity and Food Intake

Balancing energy intake with energy expenditure represents a primary goal for a physically active individual of normal body weight. Energy balance optimizes physical performance and helps to maintain lean body mass, training responsiveness, and immune and reproductive function. The physical activity level represents the most important factor to impact daily energy expenditure.

FIGURE 3.8 illustrates that average energy intakes for U.S. males and females peak between ages 16 and 29 and decline thereafter, with males reporting higher daily energy intakes than females at all ages. Between ages 20 and 29, females consume on average 35% fewer kcal than males on a daily basis (1957 vs. 3025 kcal). Subsequently, the sex difference in energy intake becomes smaller; at age 70, females consume about 25% fewer kcal than males. Comparison data for daily energy intake with aging have remained relatively consistent over the past 30

 2020–2025 Goals and Guidelines for Healthful Eating

Population Goals	Major Guidelines
Overall health eating pattern	• Consume a varied diet with foods from each major food group, emphasizing fruits, vegetables, whole grains, low-fat or nonfat dairy products, fish, legumes, poultry and lean meats • Monitor portion size and number to avoid excess intake
Appropriate body weight (BMI ≤ 25)	• Match energy intact to energy needs • For desirable weight loss, make needed changes to energy intake and expenditure (physical activity) • Limit foots with high sugar content and caloric density
Desirable cholesterol profile	• Limit foods high in saturated fat, *trans* fat, and cholesterol • Substitute with unsaturated fats from vegetables, fish, legumes, and nuts
Desirable blood pressure Systolic <120 mm Hg Diastolic <80 mm Hg	• Maintain a healthy body weight for age and sex • Consume a varied diet emphasizing vegetables, fruits, and low-fat or nonfat dairy products • Limit sodium intake • Limit alcohol intake

Source:
Dietary Guidelines Advisory Committee. 2020. Scientific Report of the 2020 Dietary Guidelines Advisory Committee: Advisory Report to the Secretary of, Agriculture and the Secretary of Health and Human Services. U.S. Department of Agriculture, Agricultural Research Service, Washington, DC.

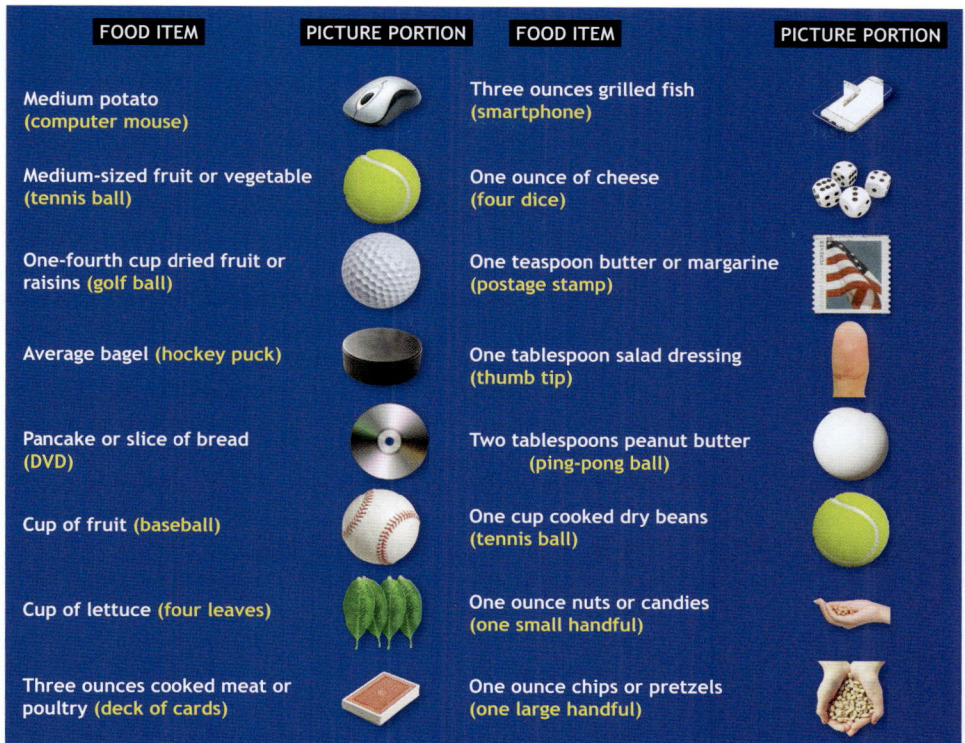

FIGURE 3.7. Popular food items in picture portion size equivalents.
(Shutterstock: AG-PHOTOS; Sashkin; Keattikorn; ALEXEY FILATOV; Dan Thornberg; Tim UR; Bragin Alexey; Zvonimir Atletic; Butterfly Hunter; Yellow Cat; Syda Productions)

years, despite an increase in body fat chiefly in the abdominal-trunk regions for both males and females (see Chapter 30).

Physical Activity Makes a Difference

Individuals who engage regularly in moderate-to-intense physical activity eventually increase daily energy intake to match higher energy expenditure levels. Lumber workers, who expend approximately 4500 kcal daily, unconsciously adjust energy intake to closely balance energy output. Consequently, body mass remains stable despite a relatively large food intake. Athletes' daily food intake in the 1936 Olympics reportedly averaged more than 7000 kcal, or roughly three times the average daily intake. These energy values have justified what many believe an enormous food requirement for athletes in training. These figures likely depict inflated estimates because objective dietary data to support these claims do not exist. Distance runners who train about 100 miles weekly (6-min mile pace at 15 kcal · min^{-1}) probably do not expend more than 800 to 1300 "extra" kcal each day above normal energy requirements to balance their increased energy expenditure. **FIGURE 3.9** presents energy intake data from a large sample representing elite male and female endurance, strength, and team sport athletes in the Netherlands. Daily energy intake for males ranged between 2900 and 5900 kcal; female competitors consumed between 1600 and 3200 kcal. Daily energy intake generally did not exceed 4000 kcal for males and 3000 kcal for females (except for the large energy intakes at the extremes for performance and training). For US Marine Corp male and female recruits, daily energy expenditures averaged 6142 kcal for males and 4732 kcal for females during a 54-hr training exercise.[15]

To complement these observations, elite female swimmers' daily energy expenditure increased to 5593 kcal during high-volume training.[88] This value represents the highest sustained daily energy expenditure reported for female athletes, yet energy intake did not match the increased training demands. It averaged only 3136 kcal, implying a 43% negative energy balance. A negative energy balance in transitioning from moderate to intense training can compromise an athlete's full potential to train and compete.

Tour de France and Other Endurance Activities

FIGURE 3.10 outlines the daily energy expenditure variation for a male competitor during the **Tour de France** professional cycling race. For 3 wk in July, nearly 200 cyclists push themselves over and around the perimeter of France covering 2405 miles, more than 100 miles daily (only 1 day of rest), at an average speed of 24.4 mph. Note the extremely high energy expenditure values and ability to achieve energy balance with liquid nutrition plus normal meals. In this

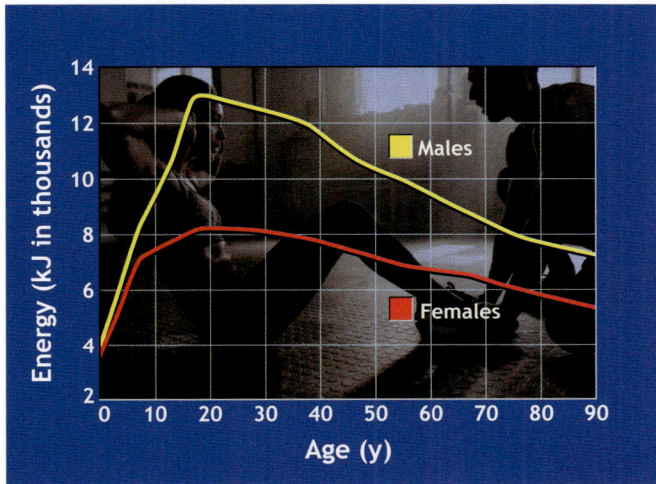

FIGURE 3.8. Average daily energy intake for males and females by age in the U.S. population.
(Jacob Lund/Shutterstock)

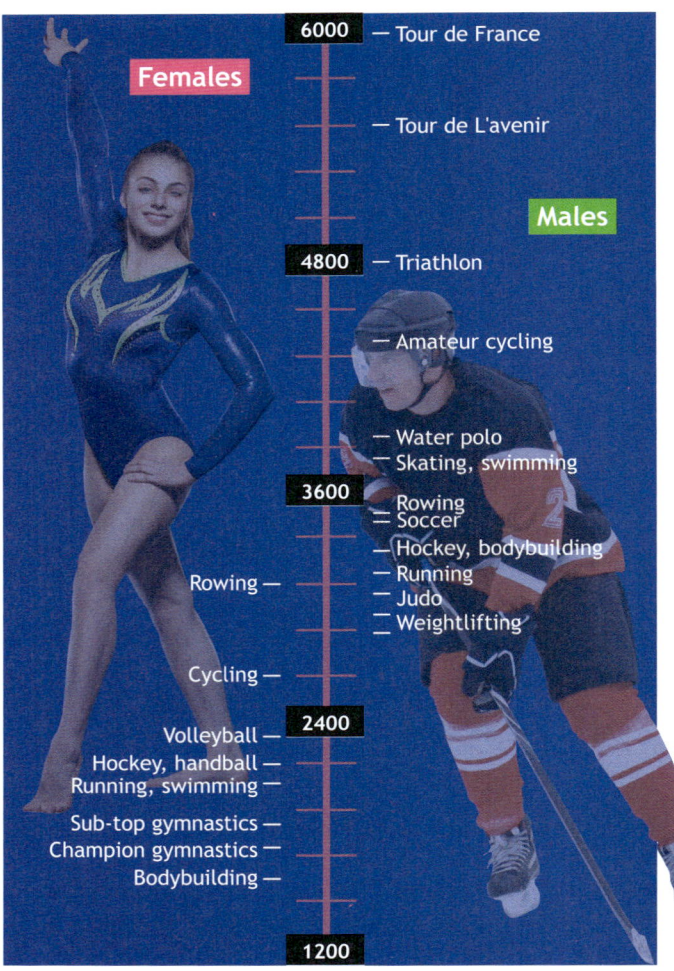

FIGURE 3.9. Daily energy intake (kcal) of elite male and female endurance, strength, and team sport athletes.
(Shutterstock: I T A L O; Skumer)

beware-nutritional-supplements-may-be-contaminated-with-anabolic-steroids], which he publicly admitted to years later. This suggests that such high caloric expenditure levels could have been "contaminated" by the influences of illegal drugs.

Other sport and training activities also require extreme energy output and correspondingly high energy intake, sometimes exceeding 1000 kcal an hour in elite marathoners. Daily energy requirements for world-class cross-country skiers during 1 wk of intense training averaged 3740 to 4860 kcal for women and 6120 to 8570 kcal for men.[75] The values for women agree closely with the 3957 average kcal daily energy expenditure over a 14-day training period for seven elite lightweight female rowers.[40] The doubly labeled water technique (see Chapter 8) evaluated the energy balance for two men who pulled sledges with starting weights of 222 kg/489 lb for 10 hr daily for 95 days during a 2300-km/1400-mi trek across Antarctica.[83] During a 10-day period, one man averaged a 10,654 kcal daily energy expenditure, while his counterpart averaged an extraordinary 11,634 kcal daily output. These values approach the 13,975-kcal theoretical daily energy expenditure ceiling attained by ultra-long-distance runners.[16]

Ultraendurance Competitions

Ultraendurance events are increasingly popular, with significant physiologic challenges that potentially produce relatively large energy deficits during competitions. Caloric deficits have been reported among ultraendurance cyclists in a 16-hr, 384-km/237-mi race.[5] For these athletes, mean energy intake averaged 18.7 MJ/4469 kcal compared with an estimated 25.5-MJ/6095-kcal energy requirement for the race. The functional significance was the negative relationship between energy intake and time to complete the race, which suggests that reducing the energy deficit may be advantageous

grueling sporting event, energy expenditure averaged 6500 kcal daily for nearly 3 wk. Large variations occurred depending on the day's activity level; the daily energy expenditure decreased to about 3000 kcal on a "rest" day and increased to 9000 kcal when cycling over a mountain pass. By combining liquid nutrition with normal meals, this cyclist nearly matched daily energy expenditure with energy intake. Unfortunately, the doping scandal involving the U.S. cycling team resulted in the U.S. Anti-Doping Agency and International Cycling Union rescinding seven-time winner Lance Armstrong's consecutive first place finishes for blatant, serial illegal performance-enhancing drug use [www.healio.com/news/endocrinology/20141203/

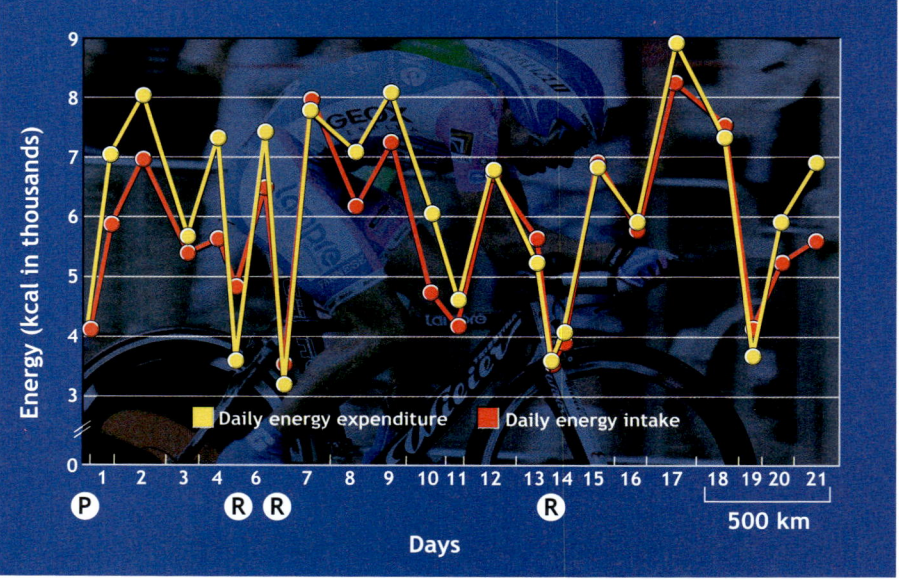

FIGURE 3.10. Daily energy expenditure (*yellow circles*) and energy intake (*red circles*) for a cyclist during the Tour de France. *P*, stage; *R*, rest day.

fyi The Nutrition Rainbow

The Nutrition Rainbow

The more naturally colorful the meal, the more likely it contains abundant cancer-fighting nutrients. The bright colored pigments in fruits and vegetables contain the foods' protective compounds

Colors	Foods	Colorful Protective Substances and Possible Actions
Red	Tomatoes and tomato products, watermelon, guava	Lycopene: antioxidant; cuts prostrate cancer risk
Orange	Carrots, yams, sweet potatoes, mangoes, pumpkins	Beta-carotene: supports immune system; powerful antioxidant
Yellow-orange	Oranges, lemons, grapefruits, papayas, peaches	Vitamin C, flavonoids: inhibit tumor cell growth, detoxify harmful substances
Green	Spinach, kale, collards, and other greens	Folate: builds healthy cells and genetic material
Green-white	Broccoli, Brussels sprouts, cabbage, cauliflower	Indoles, lutein: eliminate excess estrogen and carcinogens
White-green	Garlic, onion, chives, asparagus	Allyl sulfides: destroy cancer cells, reduce cell division, support immune systems
Blue	Blueberries, purple grapes, plums	Anthocyanins: destroy free radicals
Red-purple	Grapes, berries, plums	Resveratrol: may decrease estrogen production
Brown	Whole grains, legumes	Fiber: carcinogen removal

Adapted from: Physicians Committee for Responsible Medicine; www.PCRM.org

to race performance. Energy balance also was studied during a 1000-km/600-mi running race from Sidney to Melbourne, Australia. Greek ultramarathon champion Yiannis Kouros completed the race in 5 days, 5 hr, and 7 min, finishing 24 hr and 40 min ahead of the next competitor. Kouros did not sleep during the first 2 competition days. He covered 463 km/287.8 mi at an average 11.4 km·hr^{-1}/8.5 min·mi^{-1} speed for day 1 and 8.3 km·hr^{-1}/11.6 min·mi^{-1} for day 2. During the remaining days, he took frequent rest periods including periodic breaks for short "naps." Weather ranged from spring to winter conditions (3°C to 8°C/86°F to 46.4°F) and terrain varied.

The near equivalence between Kouros's estimated 55,970 kcal total energy intake and 59,079 kcal total energy expenditure represents energy balance homeostasis to the physical activity extremes. For total energy intake, carbohydrates represented 95.3%, lipids 3%, and proteins 1.7%. Protein intake from food averaged considerably below recommended levels, but Kouros did take protein supplements in tablet form. The unusually large daily energy intake, which ranged from 8600 to 13,770 kcal, came from Greek baklava, cookies, and doughnuts; some chocolates; dried fruit and nuts; various fruit juices; and fresh fruits. Every 30 min after the first 6 hr, Kouros replaced sweets and fruits with a small biscuit soaked in honey or jam. He consumed some roasted chicken on day 4 and drank coffee every morning. He took a 500-mg vitamin C supplement every 12 hr and a protein tablet twice daily.

Kouros's exceptional achievement exemplifies a highly conditioned athlete's exquisite energy balance control during this demanding endurance event. He performed at a pace that averaged 49% of his aerobic capacity during the first 2 competition days and 38% for days 3 through 5. He also finished the competition without muscular injuries or thermoregulatory problems, and his body mass remarkably remained unchanged. He did report severe constipation during the run and frequent urination for several days postrace.

Another case study of a 37-year-old male ultramarathoner further demonstrates the tremendous capacity for prolonged, high daily energy expenditure. The doubly labeled water technique evaluated energy expenditure during a 2-wk 14,500-km/9000-mi run around Australia in 6.5 months (average 70 to 90 km·d^{-1}/43 to 56 mi·d^{-1}) without rest days.[39] Daily energy expenditure over the measurement period averaged 6321 kcal, and daily water turnover equaled 6.1 L. The athlete ran about the same distance each day over the study period as he ran in the entire race period. As such, these data likely represent energy dynamics for the entire run.

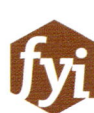

Yiannis Kouros—All-Time Greatest Record-Breaking Ultraendurance Runner

Distance runs			
100 miles	Road	11 hr 46 min 37 s	13.7 km/hr/8.5 mph
1000 km	Track	5 d 16 hr 17 min 0 s	7.3 km/hr/4.6 mph
1000 km	Road	5 d 20 hr 13 min 40 s	7.1 km/hr/4.4 mph
1000 miles	Road	10 d 10 hr 30 min 36 s	6.4 km/hr/4.0 mph
Timed races			
12 hr	Road	162.6 km/101.0 miles	13.5 km/hr/8.5 mph
24 hr	Road	290.2 km/180.3 miles	12.1 km/hr/7.5 mph
24 hr	Track	303.5 km/188.6 miles	12.7 km/hr/7.9 mph
48 hr	Road	433.1 km/269.1 miles	9.0 km/hr/5.6 mph
48 hr	Track	473.5 km/294.2 miles	9.9 km/hr/6.1 mph
6 d	Road	1,028.4 km/639.0 miles	7.2 km/hr/4.4 mph
6 d	Track	1,038.9 km/645.5 miles	7.2 km/hr/4.5 mph

Greek superstar ultraendurance runner Yiannis Kouros (b. 1956) is one of the greatest distance athletes of all time. His running career began in the 1980s, and his athletic achievements include the men's outdoor road world records for 100 to 1000 mi, and road and track records from 12 hr to 6 d duration. In this modern era that features specialization based on training specificity, Kouros's performance accomplishments will remain remarkable for decades to come.

Source:
Adapted from Kouros Y. List of Yiannis Kouros world and course records. 2012. www.yianniskouros.gr/index.php/en/kourosvictories?i=1

Other Extreme Ultraendurance Sports

The **Iditasport ultramarathon** includes choosing one race event from among the following options: run 120 km/75 mi, snowshoe 120 km/75 mi, bicycle 259 km/151 mi, cross-country ski 250 km/155 mi, or snowshoe, ski, and bicycle 250 km/155 mi. Begun in 1983 as a single event (Iditaski), a parallel competition emerged in 1987 with long-distance cycling (Iditabike). In 1991, the two races merged along with foot, snowshoe, and triathlon events. The triathlon was discontinued in 1997, and the lengths for all other races changed to 160 km/99 mi. The competition begins in late February, and the athletes traverse varied terrain, mostly in the wilderness over frozen rivers and lakes; wooded, rolling hills; and packed snow trails. On any given day, racers can experience extremes in weather that range from calm, "balmy" (−1.1°C/30°F) to "harsh" (−40°C/−40°F) with blizzard conditions. During the 48-hr time limit for the event, racers carry a minimum of 15-lb/6.8-kg survival gear; this includes a sleeping bag rated to −28.8°C/20°F, insulated sleeping pad, bivy sack or tent, stove and 8 oz/227 g of fuel with matches or lighter fluid starter, pot to melt snow, insulated water containers to carry 2 qt water, headlamp or flashlight, and minimum 1-day emergency food supply. The supplies, weighing from 6.8 to 13 kg/15 to 30 lb, are carried in a backpack or pulled by sled.

Researchers estimated the total energy and macronutrient requirements for 13 males and 1 female in the 1995 race with 49 entrants (**FIG. 3.11**). The bikers consumed the most total calories (8458 kcal; multiply kcal value by 4.182 to convert to kJ), 74.1% as carbohydrate, 9.4% as protein, and 16.5% as lipid. A comparison study between 1997 and 1998 of Iditasport athletes and their 1995 counterparts showed only small differences in energy and nutrient contents except for higher carbohydrate intake (78.5%) and less lipid (14.5%) and protein (7.3%) for skiers. The authors concluded that even though the event length differed in

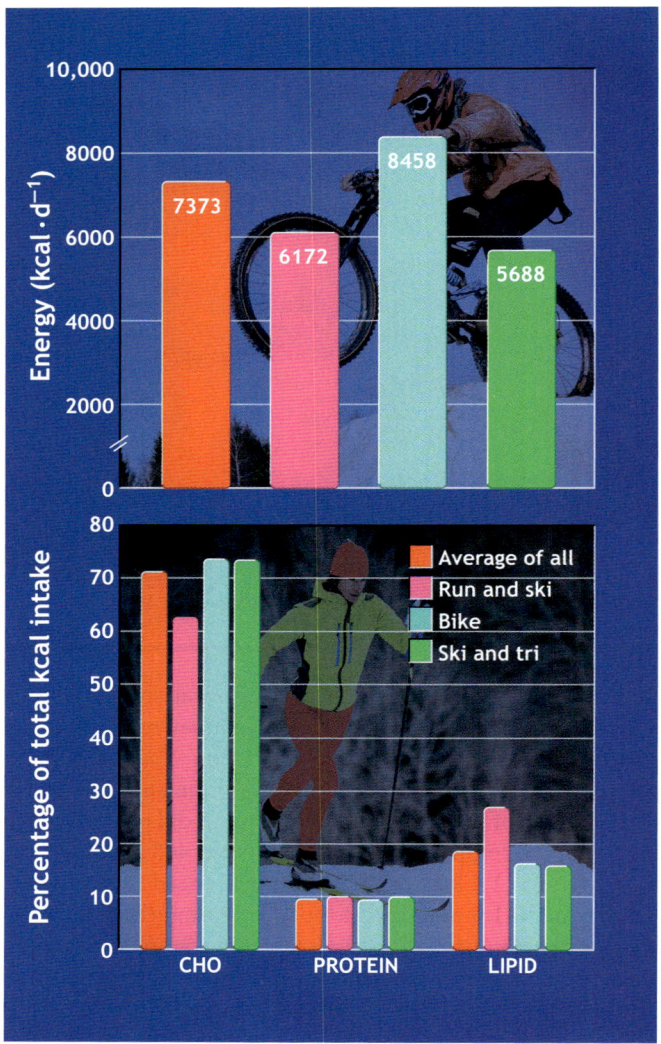

FIGURE 3.11. Energy and macronutrient content of Iditasport competitors' diets.
(Shutterstock: muroPhotographer; michelangeloop)

1994–1996 and 1997–1998, few differences existed in the diet's energy content and its macronutrient percentages among the four competition categories from the two time periods.

High-Risk Sports for Marginal Nutrition

Gymnasts, ballet dancers, ice dancers, and weight-class athletes in boxing, wrestling, rowing, and judo engage in arduous training. The athletes continually strive to maintain a lean, low body mass dictated by either esthetic or mandated weight-class considerations. Energy intake often intentionally falls short of energy expenditure, with relative malnutrition a distinct possibility. Nutritional supplementation for these athletes may prove beneficial as suggested by the data in **FIGURE 3.12** for daily nutrient intake (% RDA) in 97 competitive female gymnasts age 11 to 14 years (mean stature, 152.4 cm/60 in; mean body mass, 43.1 kg/94.8 lb). The percentage RDA on the y-axis (left) reflects only protein, while energy intake, CHO, and lipid reflect "recommended" values. The right-side image shows the percentage of gymnasts consuming less than two thirds of the RDA for vitamins and minerals. Twenty-three percent ($N = 22$) of the gymnasts consumed less than 1500 kcal daily, and more than 40% consumed less than two thirds of the RDA for vitamin E and folic acid, and the minerals iron, magnesium, calcium, and zinc. Clearly, many of the adolescent gymnasts needed to upgrade their diets or consider supplementation to achieve a more favorable nutrition profile.

Eat More and Weigh Less

Physically active individuals generally consume more calories per kilogram body mass than sedentary counterparts. The extra energy for physical activity accounts for the larger caloric intake. Paradoxically, the most active males and females, who eat more on a daily basis, weigh less than those who exercise at a lower total caloric expenditure. Regular physical activity allows a person to "eat more yet weigh less" while maintaining a lower body fat percentage, despite the age-related tendency toward weight gain in middle age.[8] *Physically active persons maintain a lighter and leaner body and a healthier heart disease risk profile, despite increased food intake.* Chapter 30 discusses in more detail regular physical activity's important role for weight control.

Precompetition Meal

Athletes often compete in the morning following an overnight fast. As discussed in Chapter 1, considerable depletion occurs in the body's carbohydrate reserves over an 8- to 12-hr period without eating, even following appropriate dietary recommendations. Consequently, precompetition nutrition takes on considerable importance. *The precompetition meal should provide adequate carbohydrate energy and ensure optimal hydration.* Fasting before competition or training makes no sense physiologically because it rapidly depletes liver and muscle glycogen to impair exercise performance. If a person trains or competes in the afternoon, breakfast becomes the important meal for optimizing glycogen reserves. When training or competing in the late afternoon, lunch becomes the important food source to adequately maintain glycogen stores. Consider three factors when individualizing the precompetition meal plan:

1. Food preference
2. Psychological set
3. Food digestibility

As a general rule on competition day, participants should exclude foods high in lipid and protein because they digest slowly and remain in the digestive tract longer than foods with similar energy content as carbohydrate. Precompetition meal timing also deserves consideration. The increased stress and tension that accompany competition reduce blood flow to the digestive tract to produce depressed intestinal absorption. *A carbohydrate-rich, precompetition meal requires 1 to 4 hr to digest, absorb, and replenish muscle and liver glycogen (high-glycemic carbohydrates digest and absorb more rapidly).*

The meal should accomplish three goals:

1. Contain 150 g/0.33 lb to 300 g/0.66 lb carbohydrate (3 to 5 g · kg body mass^{-1} as either a solid or liquid)

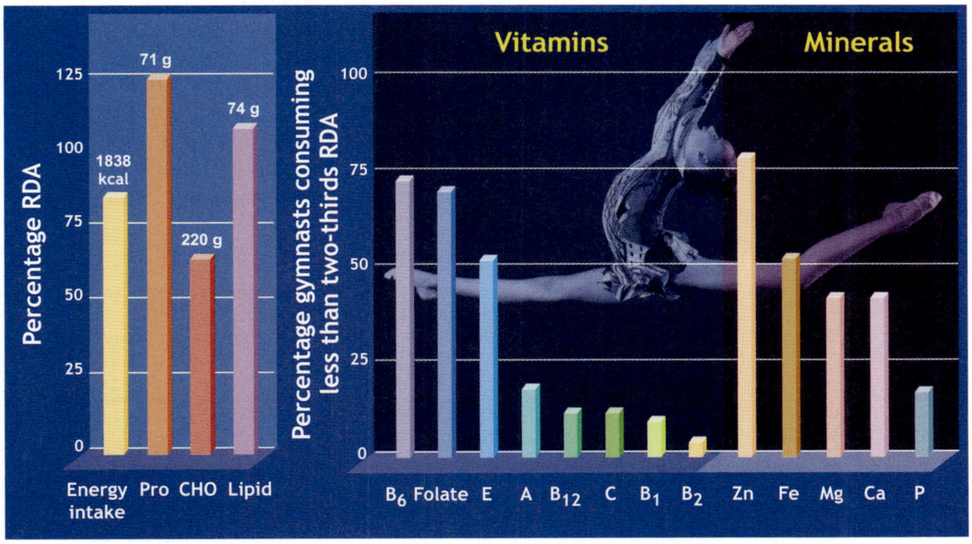

FIGURE 3.12. Average daily nutrient intake for 97 adolescent female gymnasts compared to recommended RDA values.
(Sergey Nivens/Shutterstock)

2. Consumed 1 to 4 hr before exercise for complete digestion and absorption to optimize glycogen stores
3. Contain relatively little lipid and fiber to facilitate gastric emptying and minimize gastrointestinal distress

The benefits of proper precompetition feeding occur only if the athlete maintains a nutritionally sound diet throughout training. Pre-exercise feedings cannot correct existing nutritional deficiencies or inadequate nutrient intake prior to competition. Chapter 23 discusses how endurance athletes can augment precompetition glycogen storage in conjunction with specific exercise/nutritional modifications using "carbohydrate-loading" techniques.

The following five reasons justify modifying and/or abolishing the high-protein precompetition meal with one featuring carbohydrate:

1. Dietary carbohydrates replenish liver and muscle glycogen depletion from the overnight fast.
2. Carbohydrate digestion and absorption occur more rapidly than either protein or lipid, so carbohydrate can provide energy faster and reduce fullness following a meal.
3. A high-protein meal elevates resting metabolism more than a high-carbohydrate meal from its greater energy requirements to digest, absorb, and assimilate protein. The additional thermic effect could strain the body's heat-dissipating mechanisms and impair exercise in hot weather.
4. Protein catabolism for energy facilitates dehydration during physical activity because the amino acid breakdown by-products require water for urinary excretion. One gram of urea excretion coincides with 50 mL of water elimination.
5. Carbohydrate, not protein, represents the main energy nutrient for both short-term anaerobic activity and longer-term intense aerobic activity.

Liquid Meals and Prepackaged Nutrition Bars, Powders, and Drinks

Commercially prepared nutrition bars, powders, and liquid meals offer an alternative approach to precompetition feeding or supplemental feedings during competition. Nutrient supplements also effectively enhance energy and nutrient intake during training, particularly if energy output exceeds energy intake from mismanaged feedings.

Liquid Meals

Liquid meals provide high-carbohydrate content but also contain enough lipid and protein to contribute to satiety. A liquid meal digests rapidly, leaving essentially no intestinal tract residue. Liquid meals prove particularly effective during day-long swimming and track meets or during tennis, soccer, softball, and basketball tournaments. In these outings, the person usually has little time for or interest in food. Liquid meals offer a practical approach to supplementing caloric intake during the high energy output training phase. Athletes can use liquid nutrition to help maintain body weight and as an extra calorie source to gain weight.

Nutrition Bars

Nutrition bars (called "energy bars," "protein bars," and "diet bars") contain a relatively high protein content that ranges between 10 and 30 g per bar. The typical 60-g bar contains 25 g (100 kcal) carbohydrate (equal amounts starch and sugar), 15 g (60 kcal) protein, and 5 g (45 kcal) lipid (3 g or 27 kcal saturated fat), with water as the remaining weight. This represents about 49% of the bar's total 205 calories from carbohydrates, 29% from protein, and 22% from lipid. The bars often include vitamins and minerals at 30 to 50% recommended values, and some contain β-hydroxymethylbutyrate labeled as a dietary supplement rather than as a food.

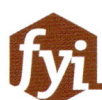 Do Vegetarians Get Adequate Protein?

In 2013, the largest study of its kind compared differences in nutrient profiles between nonvegetarians, semivegetarians, pescovegetarians, ovolactovegetarians, and strict vegetarians (vegans). Subjects included 71,751 participants (mean age 59). Nonvegetarians had the lowest intakes of plant proteins, fiber, β-carotene, and magnesium and the highest intakes of saturated, *trans*, arachidonic, and docosahexaenoic fatty acids compared with those following vegetarian dietary patterns. Vegetarians had the lowest caloric intake, yet their total daily protein intake was within 5% of the nonvegetarian group's intake. All groups exceeded the recommended protein intake, averaging in excess of 70 g · d^{-1}, a value almost twice the recommended value. In a later study, vegetarian athletes (in contrast to nonathlete vegetarians) would require an additional 10 g protein daily to reach a recommended protein intake of 1.2 g · kg · d^{-1}. An additional 22 g protein consumed daily would achieve 1.4 g · kg · d^{-1}, the upper end of the recommended intake range for competitive athletes.

Nina Firsova/Shutterstock

Sources:
Ciuris C, et al. A comparison of dietary protein digestibility, based on DIASSs scoring, in vegetarian and non-vegetarian athletes. *Nutrients*. 2019;11:3016.
Rizzo NS, et al. Nutrient profiles of vegetarian and nonvegetarian dietary patterns. *J Acad Nutr Diet*. 2013;113:1610.

Nutrition bars provide a relatively easy way to consume important nutrients. But these should not totally substitute for normal food intake because they lack plant-based fibers and phytochemicals, with relatively high saturated fatty acid levels. Additionally, these bars, generally sold as dietary supplements, have no independent assessment by the FDA through the 1994 Dietary Supplement Health and Education Act (https://ods.od.nih.gov/About/DSHEA_Wording.aspx) or other federal or state agency to validate the labeling claims for nutrient content and composition—so buyer beware!

High-Protein Bar's Monetary Value

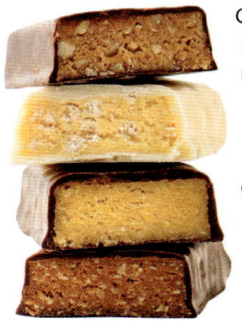

NatalyaBond/Shutterstock

Consider two nutritional bars, one costing $1.00 and the other $1.50. Checking the nutrition label, both bars contain 13 g of protein. Which is the better deal regarding how much protein the bar provides for its cost? Dividing the number of protein grams by the bar's cost provides the cost for each protein gram. For the first bar, $1.00 ÷ 13 g equals 7.7¢ per g protein; for the other bar, the protein cost per g equals 11.5¢. Clearly, the cheaper bar provides more value per unit protein (7.7¢ vs. 11.5¢ per g). The savings can be substantial over several years of purchasing such bars. In consuming the $1.00-bar daily over a 2-year period, how much money will be saved compared with the other, more expensive bar? The answer—not an insignificant $350.00!

Nutrition Powders and Drinks

A high protein content between 10 and 50 g per serving represents a unique aspect of nutritional powders and drinks. They also contain added vitamins, minerals, and other dietary supplement ingredients. The powders come in canisters or packets that mix with water or other liquids premixed in cans. These products often serve as alternatives to nutrition bars; they are marketed as meal replacements, dieting aids, energy boosters, or concentrated protein sources.

The nutrient composition for powders and drinks varies considerably from nutrition bars. Most nutrition bars contain at least 15 g of carbohydrates to provide texture and taste, whereas powders and drinks do not. This accounts for powders' and drinks' relatively high protein content. Nutrition powders and drinks generally contain fewer calories per serving than nutrition bars, but this can vary for a powder depending on the mixing liquid.

The recommended serving for a powder averages about 45 g/1.5 oz, the same amount as a nutrition bar minus its water content. A typical high-protein powder serving contains about 10 g carbohydrate (two thirds as sugar), 30 g protein, and 2 g lipid. This amounts to 178 kcal or 23% calories from carbohydrate, 67% from protein, and 10% from lipid. These powdered nutrient supplements exceed the recommended protein intake percentage and fall below recommended lipid and carbohydrate percentages. A drink typically contains slightly more carbohydrate and less protein than a powder. As with nutrition bars, the FDA and other federal or state agencies make no independent assessment about the validity of labeling claims for ingredients, macronutrient content, and composition.

Energy Beverages and Sports Drinks

Unfortunately, energy beverage consumption correlates positively with high-risk behaviors—increased illicit drug use, sexual risk taking, fighting, failure to use seat belts, taking risks on a dare, smoking, and excessive alcohol abuse.

Sports drinks serve as hydrating agents and a way to replenish electrolytes and carbohydrates, yet their consumption can create undesirable side effects from elevated caffeine levels and other ingredients. The following recommendations apply to the nonathlete consumer and athlete:

Nonathlete:

1. Limit energy beverage consumption to no more than 500 mL or 1 can daily.
2. Do not mix energy beverages with alcohol—this can mask intoxication and is dehydrating.
3. Rehydrate with water or an appropriately formulated sports drink following intense physical activity.
4. Avoid energy beverages if under treatment for hypertension.
5. Consult a physician before using energy beverages if under treatment for a serious medical condition—coronary artery disease, heart failure, or arrhythmia.

Athlete participating in physical activity lasting less than 1 hr:

1. Do not use energy beverages.
2. Do not consume energy beverages during physical activity to avoid dehydration, blood pressure elevation, and lack of equivocal benefits versus water or sports drinks.

Athlete participating in exercise lasting 1 hr or longer:

1. Do not use energy beverages.
2. Sports drinks containing carbohydrates and electrolytes can help avoid dehydration and restore minerals lost through perspiration, and may produce better hydration than water.

Buyer Beware: Energy Beverages Provide More Than Energy!

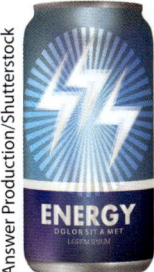

Answer Production/Shutterstock

Consuming energy drinks increases blood pressure and precipitates electrocardiographic abnormalities. Forty healthy volunteers ages 18 to 40 consumed either one of two unmarked 16-oz energy drinks or a placebo within 60 min on 3 separate days. The energy drinks included 304 to 320 mg caffeine with taurine, glucuronolactone, B-vitamins, and other ingredients. Compared to the placebo, consuming either 32-oz energy drink changed the heart's electrical activity (prolonged QTc), a risk factor for heart arrhythmias. The energy drinks also significantly elevated blood pressure.

Sources:
Gutiérrez-Hellín J, Varillas-Delgado D. Energy Drinks and sports performance, cardiovascular risk, and genetic associations; future prospects. *Nutrients.* 2021;13:715.
Veselska ZD, et al. Energy drinks consumption associated with emotional and behavioural problems via lack of sleep and skipped breakfast among adolescents. *Int J Environ Res Public Health.* 2021;18:6055.

Carbohydrate Feedings Prior to, During, and in Recovery from Physical Activity

Intense aerobic activity for 1 hr decreases liver glycogen by about 55%, whereas a 2-hr strenuous workout almost depletes liver and active muscle fiber glycogen content. Even supramaximum, repetitive 1- to 5-min activity bouts interspersed with brief rest intervals—soccer, ice hockey, field hockey, European handball, and tennis—dramatically lower liver and muscle glycogen. The body's glycogen stores' vulnerability during strenuous exercise has focused research on the potential benefits of carbohydrate feedings immediately before and during physical activity.

Prior to Physical Activity

Some researchers argue that consuming rapidly absorbed high-glycemic carbohydrates within 1 hr before physical activity accelerates glycogen depletion to negatively impact endurance performance by two mechanisms:

1. Rapid blood sugar rise triggers an insulin release overshoot. Excess insulin causes a relative hypoglycemia, also called **rebound hypoglycemia** or reactive hypoglycemia. Significant blood sugar reduction impairs central nervous system function during physical activity.
2. A large insulin release facilitates glucose movement into muscle, which disproportionately increases glycogen catabolism during physical activity. Simultaneously, high insulin levels *inhibit* lipolysis, which reduces fatty acid mobilization from adipose tissue. Enhanced carbohydrate breakdown and depressed lipid mobilization contribute to premature glycogen depletion and early fatigue.

Research in the late 1970s showed that drinking a highly concentrated sugar solution before physical activity precipitated early fatigue during endurance activities. When young males and females consumed a 300-mL solution containing 75 g glucose 30 min before cycling, endurance declined by 19% compared to similar trials preceded by 300 mL plain water or a protein, lipid, and carbohydrate liquid meal.[25] Paradoxically, the concentrated sugar drink depleted muscle glycogen reserves prematurely compared with drinking plain water. The researchers hypothesized that the dramatic blood glucose rise within 5 to 10 min following the concentrated pre-event sugar drink caused the pancreas to oversecrete insulin (called accentuated hyperinsulinemia). This triggered rebound hypoglycemia as glucose moved rapidly into muscle.[36,100] Concomitantly, insulin inhibited mobilization and lipid use for energy, referred to as lipolysis suppression.[77] Consequently, intramuscular glycogen catabolized to a greater extent causing early glycogen depletion and fatigue compared with control conditions. Subsequent research has *not* corroborated negative effects of concentrated pre-exercise sugar feedings on endurance.[24,77,86] The discrepancy in research findings has no clear explanation. One way to eliminate any potential for negative pre-exercise simple sugar consumption effects is to ingest them at least 60 min before activity to sufficiently re-establish hormonal balance before activity begins.[32]

The Glycemic Index and Pre-Physical Activity Feedings

The **glycemic index** is a numerical indicator of how carbohydrate-containing foods affect glucose appearance in the systemic circulation. A rise in blood sugar—termed **glycemic response**—is determined after ingesting a food containing 50 g of a digestible carbohydrate (total carbohydrate minus fiber) and comparing it over 2 hr with a carbohydrate "standard," usually white bread or glucose with an assigned 100 value. The GI, first developed in 1980–1981 by nutrition researchers Dr. David Jenkins and colleagues at Toronto University's St. Michael's Hospital (http://stmichaelshospitalresearch.ca/researchers/david-jenkins/), expresses the percentage total area under the blood glucose response curve for 1 g of a specific food compared with glucose. The **glycemic load** refers to the estimate of how much a food will elevate blood glucose where one glycemic load unit approximates eating one gram of glucose. **FIGURE 3.13** displays the general response curve for intestinal glucose absorption (expressed as change in blood glucose, left axis)

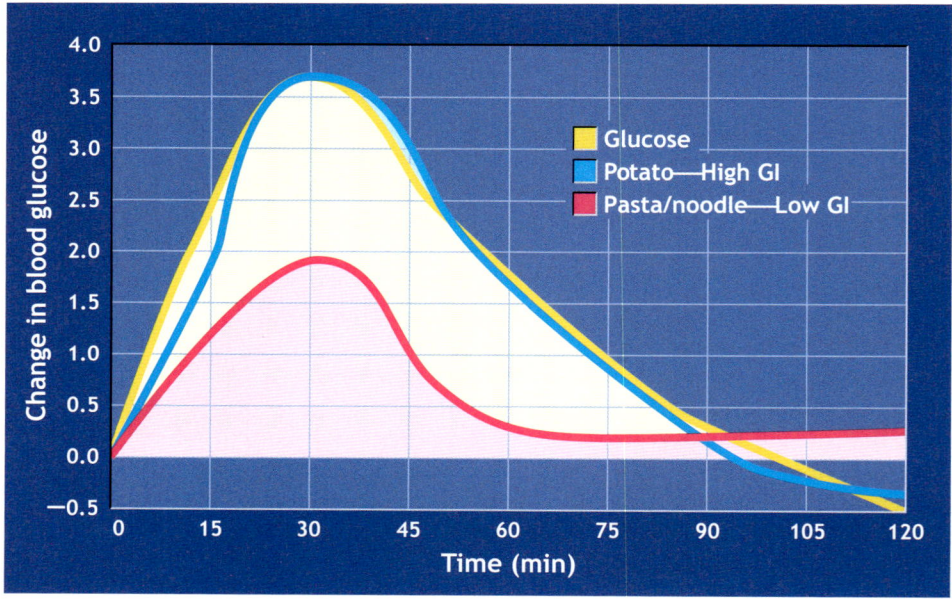

FIGURE 3.13. General response curve of intestinal glucose absorption expressed as change in blood glucose following food feedings with either a low or high glycemic index plotted over a 2-hr time duration.

following feedings with either a low GI (*magenta curve*) or a high GI, such as a potato (*light blue curve*), followed over a 2-hr duration. The low-GI food absorbs at a slower rate, reflected by the more gradual upward sloping for changes in blood glucose, throughout the small intestine's full length to produce a more gradual or blunted blood glucose rise compared with the high-GI food.

By convention, a food with GI of 45 indicates that ingesting a 50-g food portion raises blood glucose concentrations to levels that achieve 45% of that achieved with 50 g of glucose. The GI provides a more useful physiologic concept than just classifying a carbohydrate based on its chemical configuration as a simple or complex sugar or starch, or available or unavailable. The key international listing for GI values—from 2008 but still relevant—contains nearly 2480 entries that represent data from over 205 separate studies and 1879 individual food entries (https://care.diabetesjournals.org/content/31/12/2281).

FIGURE 3.14 lists GI values for common food items categorized as high glycemic (70 or higher), medium glycemic (55 to 69), and low glycemic (55 and under). A food's index rating does not depend simply on its classification as "simple" such as monosaccharides and disaccharides or as "complex" such as starch and fiber carbohydrate. The plant starch in white rice and potatoes has a higher GI than simple sugars, particularly for fructose in apples and peaches. A food's fiber content slows digestion rate, so peas, beans, and other legumes have a

Low glycemic (55 and lower) Slower-release		Medium glycemic (55–69)		High glycemic (70 and higher) Faster-release	
Grapefruit juice	48	Cantaloupe	65	Glucose	100
Carrot juice	43	Papaya	59	Carrots	92
Orange juice	46—53	Raisins	64	Honey	87
Strawberries	40	Corn, sweet	59	Corn flakes	80
Pears	33—42	Shredded wheat cereal	67	White rice	72
Grapes	46—49	Brown rice	66	Potato, instant mashed	80
Plums	24—53	Beets	64	White bread	70
Apples	28—44	Pineapple	66	Pretzels	83
Bananas, underripe/overripe	30—52	Pancakes	67	French baguette	95
Lentils	29	Popcorn	55	Watermelon	72
Peanuts	13	Spaghetti	58	Dates	103
Navy, kidney, butter beans	29—36	Sports drinks, Gatorade	50	Lucozade, glucose sweetened beverage	95
Cherries	23	Buns, hamburger/hot dog	61	Kaiser roll	73
Ice cream, vanilla	38	Crackers, wheat thins/muffins	53—65	Potato, Russet baked without skin	98
Milk, whole/2%/1%/soy/chocolate	27—35	Kellogg's Raisin Bran/Special K	54—61	Maltose	110
Yogurt, low fat with/without fruit	24—40	Jam/jellies	55—63	Jelly beans	80
Chocolate bar, peanut M&Ms/Snickers bar	33—49	Pasta	51—55	Onions	75
Bagel, plain white	33	Quinoa, boiled	53	Rice, jasmine	89
Potato chips	51	Pizza, cheese	60	Tortilla, corn	70
Oatmeal	49	Waffles	67	Quiche	98
		Peas, canned/frozen	52		
		Bread, whole wheat	52		

FIGURE 3.14. Glycemic index for common carbohydrate sources categorized by release speed as high glycemic (70 and higher; faster release), medium glycemic (55–69), or low glycemic (55 and lower; slower release).

low GI. Ingesting lipids and proteins tends to slow food passage into the small intestine, thereby reducing the GI of the meal's accompanying carbohydrate content. The most rapid strategy to replenish glycogen following longer duration physical activity is to consume foods with medium-to-high GIs rather than foods rated low, even when the replenishment meal contains a small amount of lipid and protein.[12,19,46,98,116] Adding liquid protein to the carbohydrate supplement can enhance glycogen's resynthesis magnitude. Consuming fat-free milk after an endurance activity replenishes carbohydrate as effectively as a non-nitrogenous carbohydrate control beverage, with the added postexercise benefit of supporting skeletal muscle and whole-body protein recovery.[50,56] During the first 2 hr of recovery (with muscle glycogen content at its lowest level), consuming a glucose polymer solution with low osmolality restores glycogen faster than an energy-equivalent solution containing high-osmolality monomers.

Two factors help to explain why low-osmolality solutions benefit glycogen replenishment:

1. More rapid gastric emptying and glucose delivery to the small intestine
2. Augmented postexercise-stimulated, non–insulin-dependent glucose uptake by muscle; adding L-arginine to a carbohydrate-containing beverage offers no additional benefit to carbohydrate replenishment

The glycogen requirement in previously active muscle augments glycogen resynthesis post physical activity. Four factors facilitate cellular glucose uptake following physical activity when food becomes available:

1. Hormonal milieu as reflected by elevated insulin.
2. Increased tissue sensitivity to insulin and other transporter proteins; examples include GLUT1 and GLUT4, facilitative monosaccharide transporters that mediate glucose transport activity by passive diffusion
3. Low catecholamine levels
4. Increased glycogen synthase activity (a specific glycogen-storing enzyme)

Pre-Exercise Fructose: Not a Good Alternative

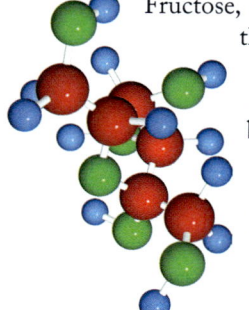
Vasilyev/Shutterstock

Fructose, a six-carbon glucose isomer shown in the inset (same molecular formula but structurally different; see the inset represented as spheres [hydrogen = blue, carbon = red, oxygen = green]) was discovered in 1847 by French industrial "sugar" chemist Augustin-Pierre Dubuffet (1797–1881; also discovered hydrogen peroxide).

The fructose molecule, the sweetest among all naturally occurring carbohydrates—1.73 times more than sucrose—absorbs more slowly from the gut than either glucose or sucrose. Fructose, with a low 19 glycemic index compared with other natural sugars, causes only minimal insulin response with essentially no blood glucose decline. Carbohydrates that degrade quickly during digestion and release glucose rapidly into the bloodstream have a high GI, whereas carbohydrates that degrade more slowly release glucose gradually into the bloodstream and have a low GI. These observations have stimulated debate about the possible benefits of fructose as an immediate pre-exercise exogenous carbohydrate fuel source for prolonged physical activity. From an undesirable standpoint, consuming a high-fructose beverage often produces vomiting and diarrhea, which obviously would negatively impact subsequent exercise performance. Once the small intestine absorbs fructose, it travels to the liver for conversion to glucose, thus limiting its availability for energy production or glycogen conversion. Fructose exists in foods as either a monosaccharide (free fructose) or a unit of the sucrose disaccharide molecule. The small intestine directly absorbs free fructose. When consumed as sucrose, however, fructose digestion occurs only in the small intestine's upper anatomic region. By the time sucrose contacts intestinal membranes, the enzyme sucrase catalyzes its cleavage to produce one unit each of glucose and fructose. Fructose then enters the hepatic portal vein that drains blood from the gastrointestinal tract and spleen for transport to the liver's capillary beds. *The take-home message seems clear—do not substitute exogenous fructose for glucose during prolonged physical activity because less fructose oxidizes when consuming equivalent amounts of both sugars.*

During Physical Activity

Physical and mental performance improves with carbohydrate supplementation *during* physical activity.[11,42,92,99] Adding protein to the carbohydrate-containing beverage in a 4:1 carbohydrate to protein ratio may delay fatigue and reduce muscle damage compared with supplementation during the activity with carbohydrate only.[43,44,72] When a person consumes carbohydrates during endurance activities, the carbohydrate form has little negative effect on hormonal response, metabolism, or endurance performance. The reason is straightforward: Increased levels of sympathetic nervous system hormones (catecholamines epinephrine and norepinephrine) released during physical activity inhibit insulin release. Concurrently, exercise increases muscles' glucose absorption, so any exogenous glucose moves into the cells with a lower insulin requirement.

Ingested carbohydrate provides a readily available energy nutrient for active muscles in intense physical activities. Consuming about 60 g/2.1 oz of liquid or solid carbohydrate hourly benefits intense, long-duration (≥1 hr) aerobic activity and repetitive brief bouts of near-maximum exercise.[13,45,60] The beneficial effect reflects improved muscle function, possibly from the protection of muscle membrane excitability. Supplemental carbohydrate during protracted intermittent exercise to fatigue also facilitates skill performance such as improved stroke quality during the final stages of prolonged tennis play. Supplementation also blunts depression of neuromuscular function with prolonged exercise, possibly as a consequence of its protection of muscle membrane excitability.[82] Ingesting multiple

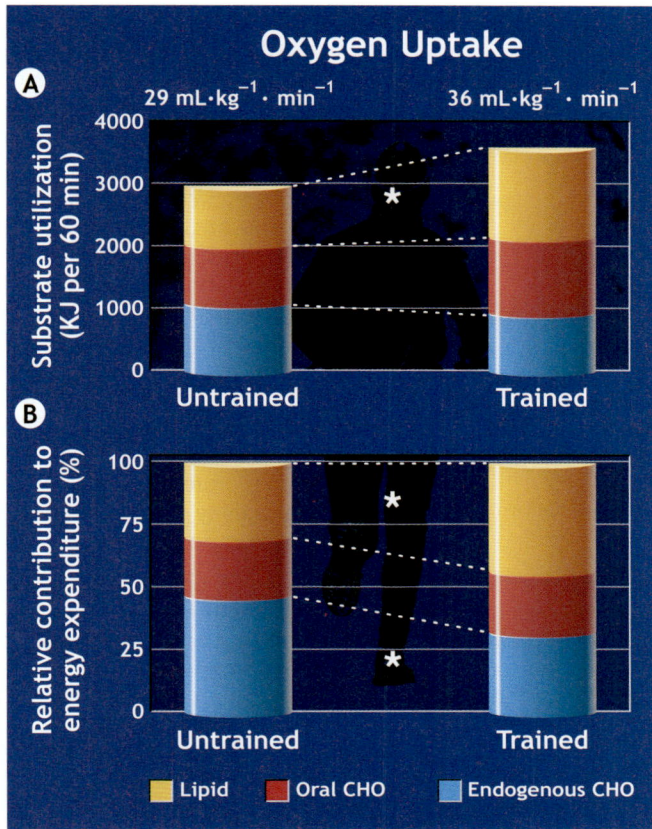

FIGURE 3.15. (A) Absolute (kilojoules per 60 min exercise) and (B) relative substrate contribution (%) to energy expenditure in endurance-trained and untrained men. *Statistically significant difference between trained and untrained men. Multiply by 0.239 to convert kilojoules to kilocalories.

untrained individuals perform at the same relative intensity. Seven trained cyclists and seven untrained subjects exercised for 2 hr at 60% aerobic capacity. At activity onset, each subject consumed 8 mL · kg body mass^{-1} of an 8% naturally labeled [^{13}C]-glucose solution with 2 mL · kg body mass^{-1} of fluid ingested every 20 min thereafter. Total exogenous [^{13}C]-glucose use (3.2 kcal · min^{-1}) was similar in both groups despite a 24% higher absolute oxygen uptake in the trained subjects (36 vs. 29 mL O$_2$ · kg^{-1} · min^{-1}; Fig. 3.15A) and higher total lipid oxidation. About 1.5 to 1.7 g/6.0 to 6.8 kcal · min^{-1} represents the upper limit to oxidize exogenous carbohydrate. The equivalence in exogenous glucose use between trained and untrained subjects displayed in Figure 3.15B occurred even with smaller exogenous and endogenous carbohydrate contributions to the higher total energy expenditure of the trained subjects. Carbohydrates absorbed from the gastrointestinal tract into the circulation likely limit ingested carbohydrate's catabolism rate during exercise independent of training state.

Carbohydrate feedings during physical activity at 60 to 80% aerobic capacity postpone fatigue by 15 to 30 min.[20] **FIGURE 3.16** presents data from a classic 1989 study showing (https://pubmed.ncbi.nlm.nih.gov/2927302/) that a single concentrated carbohydrate feeding about 30 min before

transportable carbohydrates may further enhance endurance performance.[21] Ingesting glucose plus fructose improved timed-trial cycling performance by 8% compared with glucose-only feedings. Combined glucose, fructose, and sucrose mixtures ingested at a high rate (about 1.8 to 2.4 g · min^{-1}) produced 20 to 55% higher exogenous carbohydrate oxidation rates, peaking as high as 1.7 g · min^{-1} with reduced endogenous carbohydrate oxidation, compared with an isocaloric glucose amount.[70]

Exogenous carbohydrate intake during intense physical effort confers three benefits:

1. Spares muscle glycogen in highly active type I, slow-twitch muscle fibers because the ingested glucose powers physical activity.[90,91]
2. Maintains a more optimal blood glucose level, which lowers perceived exertion ratings; elevates plasma insulin; lowers cortisol and growth hormone levels; prevents headache, light-headedness, and nausea; and reduces central nervous system distress and diminished muscular performance.[9,62,63]
3. Blood glucose maintenance supplies muscles with glucose when glycogen reserves run low in prolonged exercise.[17,35]

FIGURE 3.15 shows that training status did *not* alter glucose-oxidizing capacity during exercise when trained and

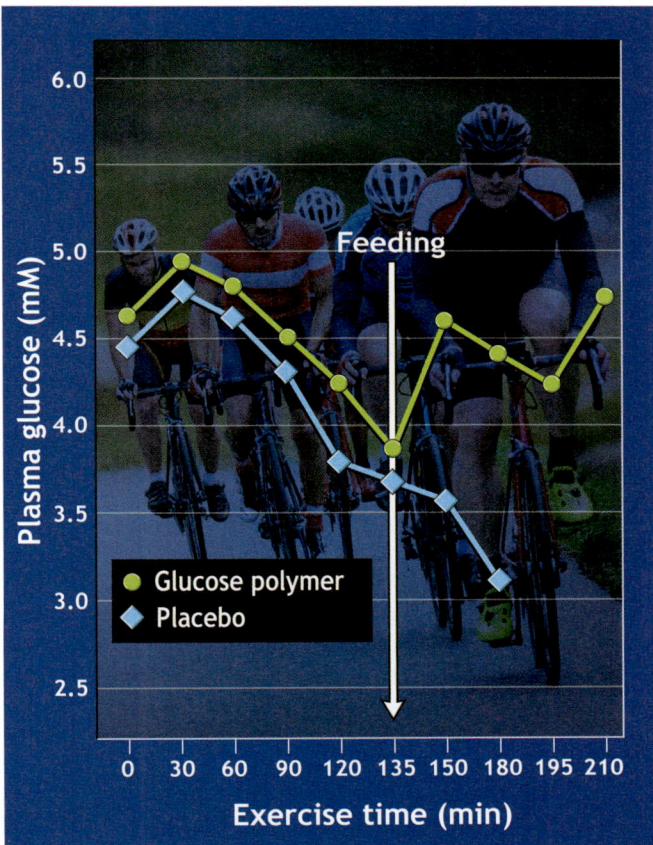

FIGURE 3.16. Average plasma glucose concentration during prolonged intense aerobic exercise when trained cyclists consumed either an artificially sweetened placebo or glucose polymer (3 g · kg^{-1} in a 50% solution).
(Duncan Andison/Shutterstock)

anticipated fatigue about 2 hr into the cycling activity proves as effective as periodic carbohydrate feedings throughout exercise. The single concentrated feeding restores blood glucose level and thereby delays fatigue by increasing carbohydrate availability to resupply this crucial substrate for oxidation by active muscles.

The greatest benefits from carbohydrate feeding emerge during prolonged exercise at about 75% aerobic capacity.[17] Lipid provides the primary energy fuel in light-to-moderate activity below 50% maximum; at this intensity, glycogen reserves do not decrease to a level that limits endurance.[2] Repeated carbohydrate feedings in solid form (43 g sucrose with 400 mL water) at the beginning and at 1, 2, and 3 hr into activity maintain blood glucose and slow glycogen depletion during 4 hr of cycling. Glycogen conservation not only extends endurance but also enhances sprint performance to exhaustion toward the end of exercise.[68,78,84] These findings demonstrate that carbohydrate feeding during prolonged, intense physical activity either conserves muscle glycogen for later use or maintains blood glucose for use as physical activity progresses and muscle glycogen depletes, or both.

The end result produced two effects:

1. Improved endurance at a high steady pace or during intense intermittent physical activity
2. Augmented sprint capacity toward the end of prolonged physical effort

In Recovery from Physical Activity

To speed glycogen replenishment following intense training or competition, consume high-glycemic carbohydrate-rich foods quickly (see next section). Follow these two practical recovery strategies to restore depleted glycogen:

1. Consume high-glycemic foods (57 to 85 g) within 15 min after stropping exercise. This equates to moderate- to high-glycemic carbohydrates every 2 hr for a total of 500 to 700 g (7 to 10 g · kg body mass^{-1}) or until consuming a large high-carbohydrate meal.
2. Eat meals that contain 2.5 g high-glycemic carbohydrate per kg body mass at 2, 4, 6, 8, and 22 hr postexercise to replenish glycogen to levels achieved with a similar protocol but begun immediately following exercise.

For a 70-kg runner, this would amount to little more than 6 oz (2.5 g × 70 ÷ 28.4 g · oz^{-1}). The carbohydrate type consumed makes a difference because all carbohydrates do not digest and absorb at the same rate. Plant starch with high amylose content represents a resistant carbohydrate from its relatively slow hydrolysis rate. By contrast, starch with a relatively high amylopectin content digests and absorbs more rapidly.

High-Glycemic Foods' Possible Role in Obesity

About 25% of the adult population produces excessive insulin with ingestion of rapidly absorbed or high-glycemic carbohydrates. Insulin-resistant individuals who

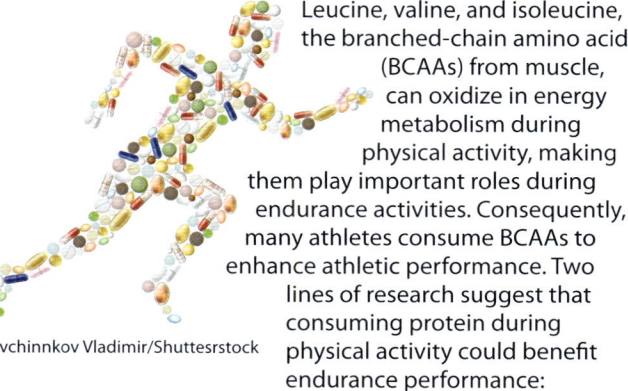

Ingested Protein During Endurance Activity May Delay Fatigue

Ovchinnkov Vladimir/Shuttesrstock

Leucine, valine, and isoleucine, the branched-chain amino acids (BCAAs) from muscle, can oxidize in energy metabolism during physical activity, making them play important roles during endurance activities. Consequently, many athletes consume BCAAs to enhance athletic performance. Two lines of research suggest that consuming protein during physical activity could benefit endurance performance:

1. Increased insulin stimulation: A combined carbohydrate-plus-protein supplement stimulates insulin secretion during physical activity, which in turn conserves muscle and liver glycogen as the activity progresses.
2. Central fatigue suppression: Circulating BCAA levels normally decrease as activity progresses. The essential amino acid tryptophan concurrently unloads from albumin at a high rate into plasma. Ingesting BCAAs during physical activity to maintain plasma concentration should delay serotonin-induced fatigue and subsequently enhance endurance performance.

Sources:

Burke LM, et al. Adaptation to a low carbohydrate high fat diet is rapid but impairs endurance exercise metabolism and performance despite enhanced glycogen availability. *J Physiol*. 2021;599:7710.

Gervasi M, et al. Effects of a commercially available branched-chain amino acid-alanine-carbohydrate-based sports supplement on perceived exertion and performance in high intensity endurance cycling tests. *J Int Soc Sports Nutr*. 2020;17:6.

Guest NS, et al. International society of sports nutrition position stand: caffeine and exercise performance. *J Int Soc Sports Nutr*. 2021;18:1.

Kritikos S, et al. Effect of whey vs. soy protein supplementation on recovery kinetics following speed endurance training in competitive male soccer players: a randomized controlled trial. *J Int Soc Sports Nutr*. 2021;18:23.

require more insulin to regulate blood glucose increase obesity risk by consistently consuming a high-glycemic food diet. These individuals often gain weight because excessive insulin facilitates glucose oxidation rather than fatty acid oxidation; excessive insulin also stimulates lipid storage in adipose tissue.

The insulin surge to a high-glycemic carbohydrate intake "challenge" abnormally decreases blood glucose. This rebound hypoglycemia triggers hunger signals to stimulate overeating. A repetitive scenario of high blood sugar followed by low blood sugar exerts the most profound effect on sedentary obese individuals who exhibit the greatest insulin resistance and exaggerated insulin response to a blood glucose challenge. Low-to-moderate physical activity produces the following three beneficial effects:

1. Improves insulin sensitivity to reduce the insulin requirement for a given glucose uptake
2. Stimulates plasma-derived fatty acid oxidation to decrease liver's fatty acid availability, thereby depressing any increase in plasma very low density lipoprotein (VLDL) cholesterol and triacylglycerol concentration
3. Exerts a potent positive calorie-burning influence for weight control

Foods' Insulin Index

While the GI ranks foods according to the extent they increase blood glucose concentration, it does not consider the concurrent insulin response. In general, insulin secretion largely remains proportional to postprandial (following a meal) glycemia. The stimulus for insulin secretion, however, does not solely depend on carbohydrate. The **insulin index** concept explores the importance of dietary stimulus and the postprandial **insulinemia** of different foods with different glycemic indices. Protein-rich foods or addition of protein to a carbohydrate-rich meal modestly raises insulin secretion in diabetic individuals without increasing blood glucose concentration. Adding lipid to a carbohydrate-rich meal also increases insulin secretion while plasma glucose responses decrease.

The insulin index compares insulin's response to different foods administered as a standard 1000-kJ portion (1 kJ = 0.239 kcal) with 220 mL/7.4 oz of water, using white bread as the reference comparison.

The glycemic index generally predicts the insulin index with some notable exceptions. Brown rice with a 104 GI has a corresponding insulin index score of only 62; a chocolate bar has a 79 GI score with a 122 insulin index. Also, some protein-rich and lipid-rich foods (e.g., eggs, beef, fish, lentils, cheese, cake, and doughnuts) cause as much insulin secretion as some carbohydrate-rich foods.

How Protein Intake During Recovery Impacts Insulin

Consuming an amino acid–protein mixture of whey protein hydrolysate with free leucine and phenylalanine (0.4 g · kg^{-1} · hr^{-1}) in a carbohydrate-containing beverage (0.8 g · kg^{-1} · hr^{-1}) facilitates more muscle glycogen storage without gastrointestinal discomfort than the same concentration in a carbohydrate-only beverage. This advantage relates to the **insulinotropic effect** (increased insulin production and activity) of higher plasma amino acid levels. The benefit of added protein and/or amino acids and associated insulin release on glycogen replenishment is no greater than simply adding additional carbohydrate to the recovery supplement. Well-trained athletes attained glycogen synthesis rates equivalent to a glucose-plus-protein supplement with a 1.2 g · kg^{-1} · hr^{-1} carbohydrate-only intake. Supplements taken at 30-min intervals over a 5-hr recovery period produced maximum glycogen resynthesis. Additional protein or amino acid intake does not increase glycogen synthesis rate.

Optimizing Glycogen Replenishment

Research has addressed the following question: To optimize glycogen replenishment, is it better to consume large meals or more frequent high-glycemic carbohydrate snacks? Studies have compared 24-hr carbohydrate replenishment with two ways to consume an energy-equivalent meal of high-GI carbohydrates:

1. "Gorging" on a single large meal, with its greater incremental glucose and insulin response
2. "Nibbling" on frequent smaller snacks, which produces a more stable glucose and insulin response

These two eating strategies produced *no difference* in the final muscle glycogen level. Accordingly, persons should consume high-glycemic carbohydrates following intense exertion; meal and snack frequency should dovetail with appetite and food availability following physical activity.

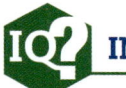 **INTEGRATIVE QUESTION**

Why does glycemic index affect nutritional recommendations for immediate pre-exercise feedings differently than for immediate postexercise feedings?

Cellular Glucose Uptake

Normal blood glucose concentration called **euglycemia** approximates 5 mM, equivalent to 90 mg glucose · dL^{-1} (100 mL) blood. Following a meal, blood glucose can rise above the hyperglycemic level to about 9 mM (162 mg · dL^{-1}). A decrease in blood glucose concentration well below normal to 2.5 mM (<45 mg · dL^{-1}) classifies as hypoglycemia and can occur during starvation or extreme, prolonged physical activity.

Glucose entry into red blood cells, brain cells, and kidney and liver cells depends on the maintenance of a positive glucose concentration gradient across the cell membrane, termed unregulated glucose transport. By contrast, skeletal and heart muscle and adipose tissue require glucose transport via regulated uptake with insulin and GLUT 4, the predominant intracellular glucose transporter protein, as regulating compounds.[58] Active skeletal muscle increases glucose uptake from the blood, independent of insulin's effects. This effect persists into the early postexercise period and helps to replenish glycogen stores.[22] Maintaining adequate blood glucose levels during physical activity and in recovery decreases possible negative effects from a low blood glucose concentration.

INTEGRATIVE QUESTION

Advise an endurance athlete whose pre-event nutrition consists of a fast-food hamburger and high-protein shake consumed 1 hr before competition.

Glucose Feedings, Electrolytes, and Water Uptake

Ingesting fluid before and during exercise minimizes dehydration's detrimental effects on cardiovascular dynamics, temperature regulation, and exercise performance (see Chapter 25). Adding carbohydrate to an **oral rehydration solution** also provides additional glucose energy. Determining the optimal fluid/carbohydrate mixture and volume becomes important to minimize fatigue and prevent dehydration. Concern highlights the dual observations that a large fluid volume intake impairs carbohydrate uptake, whereas a concentrated sugar solution impairs fluid replenishment.

Important Considerations

The rate that the stomach empties affects the small intestine's fluid and nutrient absorption. **FIGURE 3.17** illustrates major factors that influence gastric emptying. Little negative effect on gastric emptying occurs up to 75% maximum exercise intensity, after which emptying rate slows.[54] *A major factor to speed gastric emptying (and compensate for any inhibitory effects of a beverage's carbohydrate contents) involves maintaining a high stomach fluid volume.* Consuming 400 to 600 mL of fluid immediately before physical activity optimizes the beneficial effects of increased stomach volume on fluid and nutrient passage into the small intestine. Then, regularly drinking 150 to 250 mL at 15-min intervals throughout exercise continually replenishes fluid passed into the intestine.[53,61] This protocol produces a $1\text{-L} \cdot \text{hr}^{-1}$ fluid delivery rate, sufficient to meet the fluid needs for most endurance athletes. Moderate hypohydration of up to 4% body mass does not impair gastric emptying rate.[71] Fluid temperature does not exert a major effect during exercise, but highly carbonated beverages retard gastric emptying.[66] Beverages containing alcohol or caffeine induce a diuretic effect, with alcohol most pronounced, making alcoholic beverages inappropriate in a fluid replacement strategy.

Particles in Solution

Gastric emptying slows when ingested fluids contain a high concentration of particles in solution (**osmolality**) or possess high caloric content.[6,71,95] The negative effect of a concentrated sugar solution on gastric emptying diminishes (and plasma volume remains unaltered) when the drink contains a short-chain glucose polymer (**maltodextrin**) rather than simple sugars. Short-chain polymers (3 to 20 glucose units) derived from cornstarch breakdown reduce the particle number in solution. Fewer particles facilitate water movement from the stomach for intestinal absorption. Adding small amounts of glucose and sodium, with glucose the more important factor, to oral rehydration solutions exert little negative effect on gastric emptying.[29,37] Glucose plus sodium facilitates fluid uptake in the intestinal lumen from the rapid, active glucose-sodium cotransport across the intestinal mucosa. Absorption of these particles stimulates water's passive uptake by osmotic action.[30,53] Extra glucose uptake also helps to preserve blood glucose. Additional glucose then spares muscle and liver glycogen and/or maintains blood glucose should glycogen reserves decrease with prolonged activity.

Adding sodium to a fluid helps to maintain plasma sodium concentrations. Extra sodium benefits ultraendurance athletes at risk for hyponatremia from their large sweat-sodium loss coupled with their copious plain water intake (see Chapter 2). Maintaining plasma osmolality by adding sodium to the rehydration beverage also reduces urine output and sustains the sodium-dependent osmotic

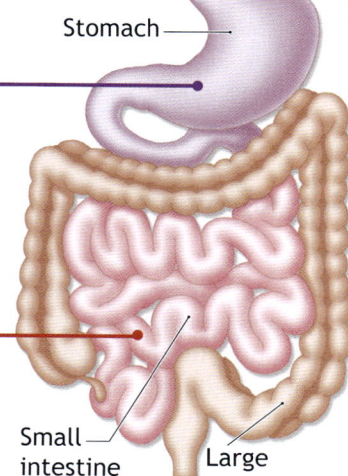

Gastric emptying
- **Volume:** increased gastric volume *increases* emptying rate
- **Caloric content:** increased energy content *decreases* emptying rate
- **Osmolality:** increased solute concentration *decreases* emptying rate
- **Exercise:** intensity exceeding 75% maximum *decreases* emptying rate
- **pH:** marked deviation from 7.0 *decreases* emptying rate
- **Hydration level:** dehydration *decreases* gastric emptying and *increases* gastrointestinal distress risk

Intestinal fluid absorption
- **Carbohydrate:** low to moderate glucose + sodium *increase* fluid absorption
- **Sodium:** low to moderate sodium levels *increase* fluid absorption
- **Osmolality:** hypotonic to isotonic fluids with NaCl and glucose *increase* fluid absorption

FIGURE 3.17. Major factors affecting gastric emptying from the stomach and fluid absorption from the small intestine.

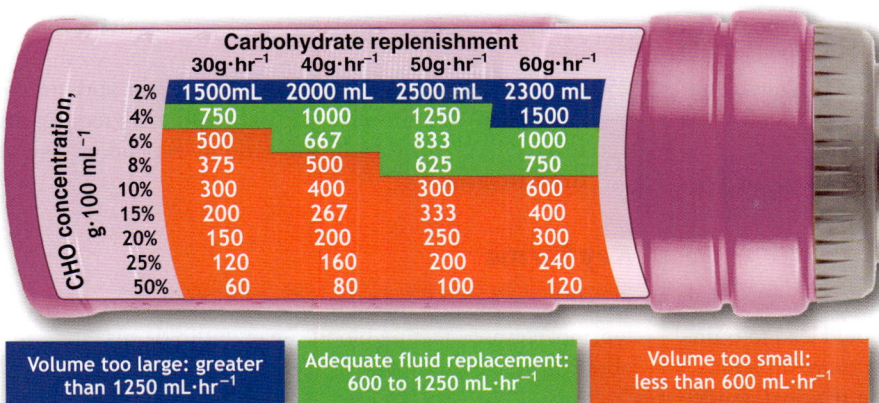

FIGURE 3.18. Fluid volume to ingest hourly to obtain the desired carbohydrate quantity expressed in g · hr.⁻¹
(Fotogroove/Shutterstock)

drive to drink (see Chapter 25). A normal plasma and extracellular fluid osmolality promote continued fluid intake and fluid retention during recovery.

Recommended Oral Rehydration Beverages

A 5 to 8% carbohydrate-electrolyte beverage consumed during exercise in the heat contributes to temperature regulation and fluid balance as effectively as plain water.[33,74] Consuming this solution in recovery from prolonged physical activity in a warm environment also improves endurance capacity for subsequent physical activity. To determine a drink's percentage carbohydrate, divide carbohydrate content (g) by fluid volume (mL) and multiply by 100. For example, 80 g carbohydrate in 1 L (1000 mL)

Three Ways to Replenish Fluid and Carbohydrate During Physical Activity

1. Monitor dehydration rate from changes in body weight; require urination before postexercise body weight measurement for precise determination of the body's total fluid loss. Each pound of weight loss corresponds to 450 mL/15 oz dehydration.
2. Drink fluids at the same rate as their estimated depletion (or at least drink at a rate close to 80% of sweating rate) during prolonged activity that increases cardiovascular stress, metabolic heat load, and dehydration.
3. Achieve carbohydrate (30 to 60 g · hr⁻¹) and fluid requirements by drinking a 4 to 8% carbohydrate beverage each hour (625 to 1250 mL; average 250 mL every 15 min).

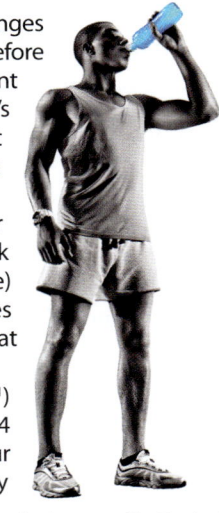

Rocksweeper/Shutterstock

water represents an 8% solution. Effective fluid absorption during prolonged physical activity occurs over a wide osmolality range. Total fluid absorption from carbohydrate-electrolyte beverages with 197 osmolalities (hypotonic), 295 (isotonic), and 414 (hypertonic) mOsm · L H_2O^{-1} did not differ from the absorption rate of a plain water placebo.[31]

FIGURE 3.18 presents a general guideline for fluid intake hourly during exercise for a given carbohydrate replenishment amount. A trade-off exists between how much carbohydrate to consume and its rate of gastric emptying. The stomach still empties up to 1700 mL of water each hour, even when drinking an 8% carbohydrate solution. Approximately 1000 mL (about 1 qt) of fluid consumed each hour probably represents an optimal volume to offset dehydration because larger fluid volumes can lead to cramping, diarrhea, and abdominal discomfort.

Environmental and physical activity conditions interact to influence the rehydration solution's optimal composition. Fluid replenishment is crucial to health and safety when intense aerobic effort performed under high thermal stress lasts 30 to 60 min. Under these conditions, the individual should consume a more dilute carbohydrate-electrolyte solution with 5% carbohydrate. In cooler weather, when dehydration does not pose a problem, a more concentrated 15% carbohydrate beverage suffices. Little difference exists among liquid glucose, sucrose, or starch as the ingested carbohydrate fuel source during physical activity. Fructose is undesirable from its potential to cause gastrointestinal distress. Fructose absorption by the gut does not involve the active cotransport process required for glucose-sodium. This makes fructose absorption relatively slow and promotes less fluid uptake than an equivalent glucose amount. *The optimal carbohydrate replacement rate during intense aerobic exercise ranges from 30 to 60 g/1 to 2 oz hourly.*

Summary

1. A balanced diet with only 1200 kcal provides the athlete and other individuals who train regularly an adequate intake of vitamins, minerals, and proteins.
2. The recommended 0.83 g/0.029 oz · kg⁻¹ body mass intake for protein represents a liberal but adequate intake for nearly all persons and most physical activity levels.
3. A protein intake between 1.2 and 1.8 g · kg⁻¹ body mass should adequately meet the added protein needs during intense exercise training.
4. Athletes generally consume two to four times the protein RDA because their greater caloric intake provides proportionately more protein.
5. No precise recommendations exist for daily lipid and carbohydrate intake.

6. Prudent advice recommends no more than 30% of daily calories from lipids; of this amount, most should be unsaturated fatty acids.
7. For physically active persons, unrefined polysaccharides should provide 60% or more of the daily calories (400 to 600 g).
8. A high-fat diet stimulates adaptive responses to augment lipid catabolism, but consistent exercise or training benefits have not been demonstrated for this dietary modification.
9. Successive hard training days gradually deplete the body's liver and muscle glycogen reserves and could lead to training staleness making continued training more difficult.
10. USDA's revised MyPlate highlights nutritional guidelines for healthy eating. Strategy, emphasizing more plant-based eating from vegetables from all five subgroups, attempts to help Americans become healthier in their battle against the cardiometabolic disorders.
11. Athletes' daily caloric needs in strenuous sports do not consistently exceed 4000 kcal.
12. The precompetition meal should include foods high in carbohydrates and relatively low in lipids and proteins, with 3 hr sufficient time to digest and absorb the meal.
13. Commercially prepared liquid meals offer a well-balanced nutritive value, contribute to fluid needs, absorb rapidly, and leave little residue in the digestive tract.
14. Carbohydrate-containing rehydration solutions consumed in physical activity enhance intense endurance performance by maintaining a desirable blood glucose concentration.
15. Glucose supplied via the blood can spare existing glycogen in active muscles during physical activity and/or serve as reserve blood glucose when muscle glycogen becomes depleted.
16. The glycemic index provides a relative measure of blood glucose increase after consuming a specific carbohydrate food.
17. For rapid carbohydrate replenishment after exercise, individuals should consume 50 to 75 g each hour of moderate- to high-glycemic index carbohydrate-containing foods.
18. Glycogen stores replenish at a rate of 5 to 7% an hour with optimal carbohydrate intake; it takes about 20 hr for full liver and muscle glycogen replenishment following glycogen-depleting exercise.
19. Foods with a low-glycemic index digest and absorb at a relatively slow rate to supply slow-release glucose during prolonged exercise.
20. The insulin index concept explores the important dietary stimulus and postprandial insulinemia for different foods with different glycemic indices.
21. Protein-rich foods and additional protein added to a carbohydrate-rich meal raise insulin secretion in type 2 diabetics without increasing blood glucose concentration.
22. Adding lipid to a carbohydrate-rich meal increases insulin secretion and decreases plasma glucose levels.
23. Drinking 400 to 600 mL fluid immediately before exercise followed by regular 250 mL every 15 min fluid ingestion during exercise optimizes gastric emptying by maintaining a relatively large stomach fluid volume.
24. The ideal 5 to 8% carbohydrate oral rehydration solution maintains fluid balance during physical activity and heat stress.
25. Adding sodium to a fluid stabilizes plasma sodium concentrations to minimize hyponatremia risk, reduce urine production, and sustain the sodium-dependent osmotic drive to drink.

Key Terms

Cardiometabolic disorders: Interrelated risk factors—hypertension, elevated fasting blood sugar, dyslipidemia, abdominal obesity, and elevated triacylglycerols

Dietary Guidelines for Americans: Nutritional advice from healthcare professionals and policymakers to advise Americans about healthful dietary choices

Euglycemia: Normal blood glucose concentration of about 5 mM (90 mg) glucose · dL (100 mL) blood^{-1}

Glycemic index: Relative increase in blood glucose concentration 2 hr after ingesting a food compared with a carbohydrate "standard," usually white bread or glucose with an assigned 100 value

Glycemic load: Estimate of how much a food will elevate blood glucose where one glycemic load unit approximates eating one gram of glucose

Glycemic response: A food or meal's effect on blood glucose level

Healthy Eating Plate: Harvard School of Public Health's plant-based nutrition guide rich in vegetables, whole grains, and healthful lipids and proteins as a MyPlate alternative to lower weight gain and chronic disease risk

Iditasport ultramarathon: Alaskan race competition—run 120 km, snowshoe 120 km, bicycle 259 km, cross-country ski 250 km, or snowshoe, ski, and bicycle 250 km

Insulin index: Elevated blood insulin concentration during 2-hr period after ingesting food

Insulinemia: Excessive insulin release to a rapid rise in blood glucose concentration

Insulinotropic effect: Increase in insulin production and activity

Maltodextrin: Short-chain glucose polymer produced from starch by partial hydrolysis that easily digests and absorbs rapidly

Mediterranean Diet Pyramid: Includes fruits, nuts, vegetables, fish, beans, and grains, with dietary lipid composed mostly of monounsaturated fatty acids with mild ethanol intake

Muscle glycogen: Multibranched polysaccharide molecule that serves as both anaerobic and aerobic energy source in skeletal muscle

MyPlate: Current nutrition guide published by the USDA Center for Nutrition Policy and Promotion featuring a place setting proportionally depicting a desirable intake of five food groups

Oral rehydration solution: Rehydration fluid containing an optimal fluid/carbohydrate/electrolyte mixture and volume to minimize fatigue and deter dehydration

Osmolality: Concentration of all solutes in a given weight of water expressed as units of osmolality (milliosmoles solute per kilogram water) or osmolarity (milliosmoles solute per liter water)

Precompetition meal: Foods selected prior to athletic competition generally consisting of carbohydrate-rich foods that require 1 to 4 hr to fully digest, absorb, and replenish muscle and liver glycogen and liquids to assure adequate hydration

Rebound hypoglycemia: Rapid rise in blood sugar triggers an insulin release overshoot and relative hypoglycemia (also called reactive hypoglycemia)

Tour de France: Annual 21 stage 23-day professional bicycle race primarily held in France but also occasionally passing through nearby countries

References are available online at Lippincott Connect.

Additional References

Ahmed J, et al. Glycemic index and glycemic load values. *Pak J Med Sci.* 2021;37:1246.

Astrup A, et al. Saturated fats and health: a reassessment and proposal for food-based recommendations: JACC state-of-the-art review. *J Am Coll Cardiol.* 2020;76:844.

Burke LM. Ketogenic low-CHO, high-fat diet: the future of elite endurance sport? *J Physiol.* 2021;599:819.

Burke LM, et al. Adaptation to a low carbohydrate high fat diet is rapid but impairs endurance exercise metabolism and performance despite enhanced glycogen availability. *J Physiol.* 2021;599:771.

Chiavaroli L, et al. Effect of low glycaemic index or load dietary patterns on glycaemic control and cardiometabolic risk factors in diabetes: systematic review and meta-analysis of randomised controlled trials. *BMJ.* 2021;374:n1651.

Chrisman M, Diaz Rios LK. Evaluating MyPlate after 8 years: a perspective. *J Nutr Educ Behav.* 2019;51:899.

Elizabeth L, et al. Ultra-processed foods and health outcomes: a narrative review. *Nutrients.* 2020;12:1955.

Gillen JB, et al. Interrupting prolonged sitting with repeated chair stands or short walks reduces postprandial insulinemia in healthy adults. *J Appl Physiol (1985).* 2021;130:104.

Gubert C, et al. Exercise, diet and stress as modulators of gut microbiota: implications for neurodegenerative diseases. *Neurobiol Dis.* 2020;134:104621.

Gürdeniz G, et al. Analysis of the SYSDIET Healthy Nordic Diet randomized trial based on metabolic profiling reveal beneficial effects on glucose metabolism and blood lipids. *Clin Nutr.* 2022;41:441.

Kissock KR, et al. Aligning nutrient profiling with dietary guidelines: modifying the Nutri-Score algorithm to include whole grains. *Eur J Nutr.* 2022;61:541.

Laitinen TT, et al. Dietary fats and atherosclerosis from childhood to adulthood. *Pediatrics.* 2020;145:e20192786.

Martinovic D, et al. Adherence to Mediterranean diet and tendency to orthorexia nervosa in professional athletes. *Nutrients.* 2022;14:237.

Mentella MC, et al. Cancer and Mediterranean diet: a review. *Nutrients.* 2019;11:2059.

Mohr AE, et al. The athletic gut microbiota. *J Int Soc Sports Nutr.* 2020;17:24.

Stierwalt HD, et al. Diet and exercise training influence skeletal muscle long-chain acyl-CoA synthetases. *Med Sci Sports Exerc.* 2020;52:569.

van den Heuvel EGHM, et al. Editorial: food-based dietary guidelines: the relevance of nutrient density and a healthy diet score. *Front Nutr.* 2020;7:576144.

Table 3.1 Research Findings: Dietary Components Associated with Different Health Outcomes

Health Outcomes	All-cause Mortality	CV Disease	Overweight/Obesity	Type 2 Diabetes	Bone Health	Colorectal Cancer	Breast Cancer	Lung Cancer	Neurocognitive Health
Dietary patterns associated with lower risk of disease consistently include the following:									
Fruits	Yes	Yes	Yes	Yes	Yes	Yes	Yes	Yes	Yes
Vegetables	Yes	Yes	Yes	Yes	Yes	Yes	Yes	Yes	Yes
Whole grains/cereal	Yes	Yes	Yes	Yes	Yes	Yes	Yes	Yes	
Legumes	Yes	Yes	Yes (adults)		Yes	Yes	Yes		Yes
Nuts	Yes	Yes			Yes	Yes	Yes	Yes	Yes
Low-fat dairy	Yes	Yes	Yes		Yes	Yes	Yes	Yes	Yes
Fish and/or seafood	Yes	Yes	Yes (adults)	Yes	Yes	Yes	Yes	Yes	Yes
Unsaturated oils	Yes	Yes	Yes (adults)		Yes	Yes	Yes	Yes	Yes
Lean meat	Yes					Yes		Yes	
Poultry	Yes								
Dietary patterns associated with higher disease risk consistently include the following:									
Red meat	Yes	Yes (adults)	Yes (adults)	Yes		Yes			
Processed meat	Yes	Yes	Yes	Yes	Yes	Yes			
High-fat meat								Yes	
High-fat dairy	Yes			Yes					
Animal source foods							Yes		
Saturated fat		Yes (adults)	Yes (adults)			Yes			
Sugar-sweetened beverages/foods	Yes	Yes	Yes	Yes	Yes	Yes			
Refined grains	Yes	Yes	Yes	Yes			Yes		
Potatoes (French fries, regular)			Yes (children)						
Sodium		Yes	Yes (adults)						

An empty box indicates the research did not consistently include that component as part of the in dietary patterns.

Source: Dietary Guidelines Advisory Committee. *Scientific Report of the 2020 Dietary Guidelines Advisory Committee: Advisory Report to the Secretary of Agriculture and the Secretary of Health and Human Services.* Washington, DC: U.S. Department of Agriculture, Agricultural Research Service; 2020.

SECTION 2

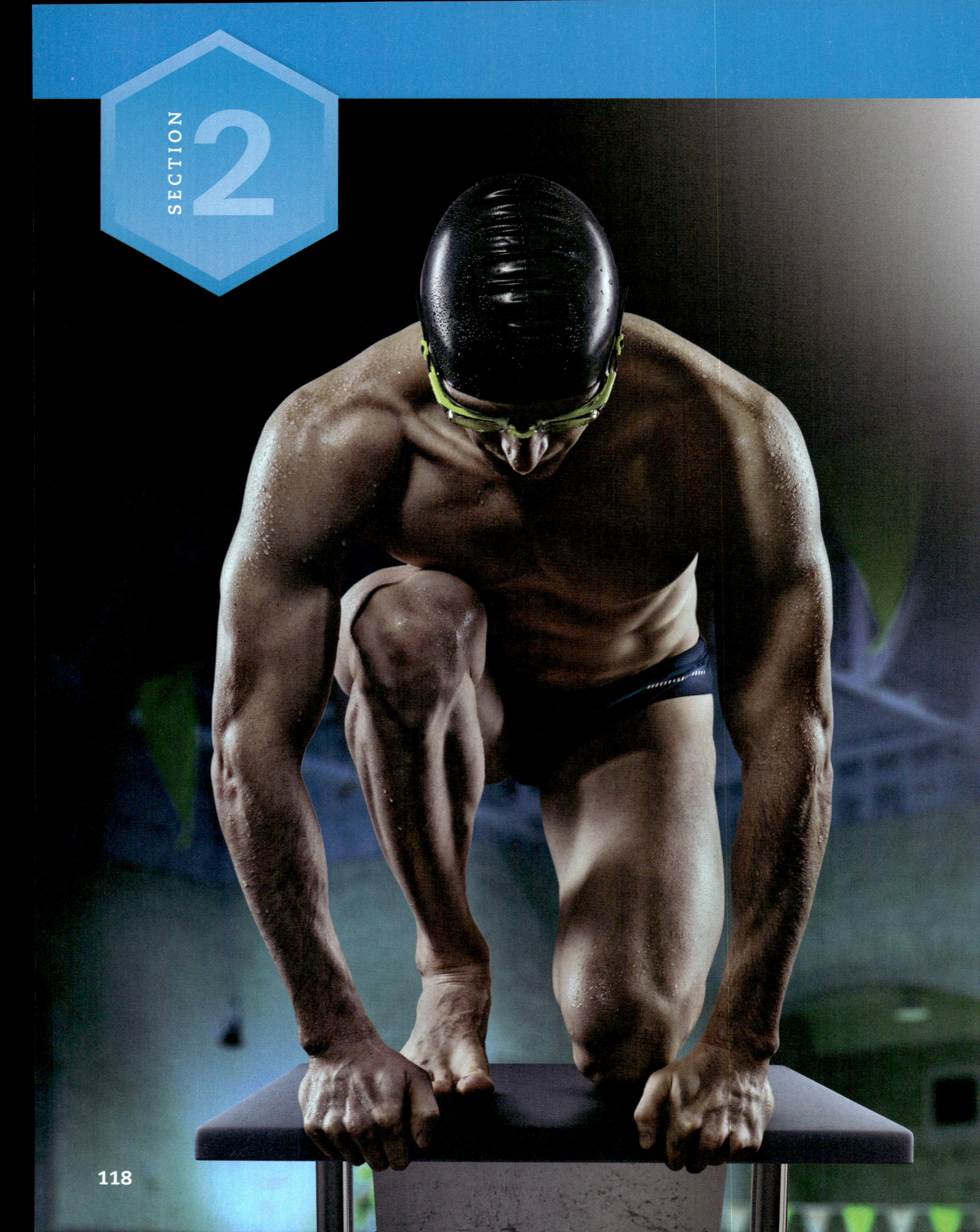

Energy for Physical Activity

OVERVIEW

Biochemical reactions that do not consume oxygen produce rapid energy for brief durations. This anaerobic cellular strategy for rapid energy generation remains crucial to sustain performance during sprint activities and other all-out physical activity bursts. In contrast, longer-duration, less-intense physical activity relies on energy extracted from food through reactions that depend on oxygen. For greatest effectiveness, training key physiologic systems requires understanding about three important factors:

1. How the body generates energy to sustain physical activity
2. How cells deliver energy
3. Physical activity energy requirements

This section describes how cells extract chemical energy bound within food molecules and use it to power all biologic work forms. We highlight food nutrients and energy transfer processes to maintain optimal physiologic function during light, moderate, and strenuous physical activities.

CHAPTER 4: Food's Energy Value

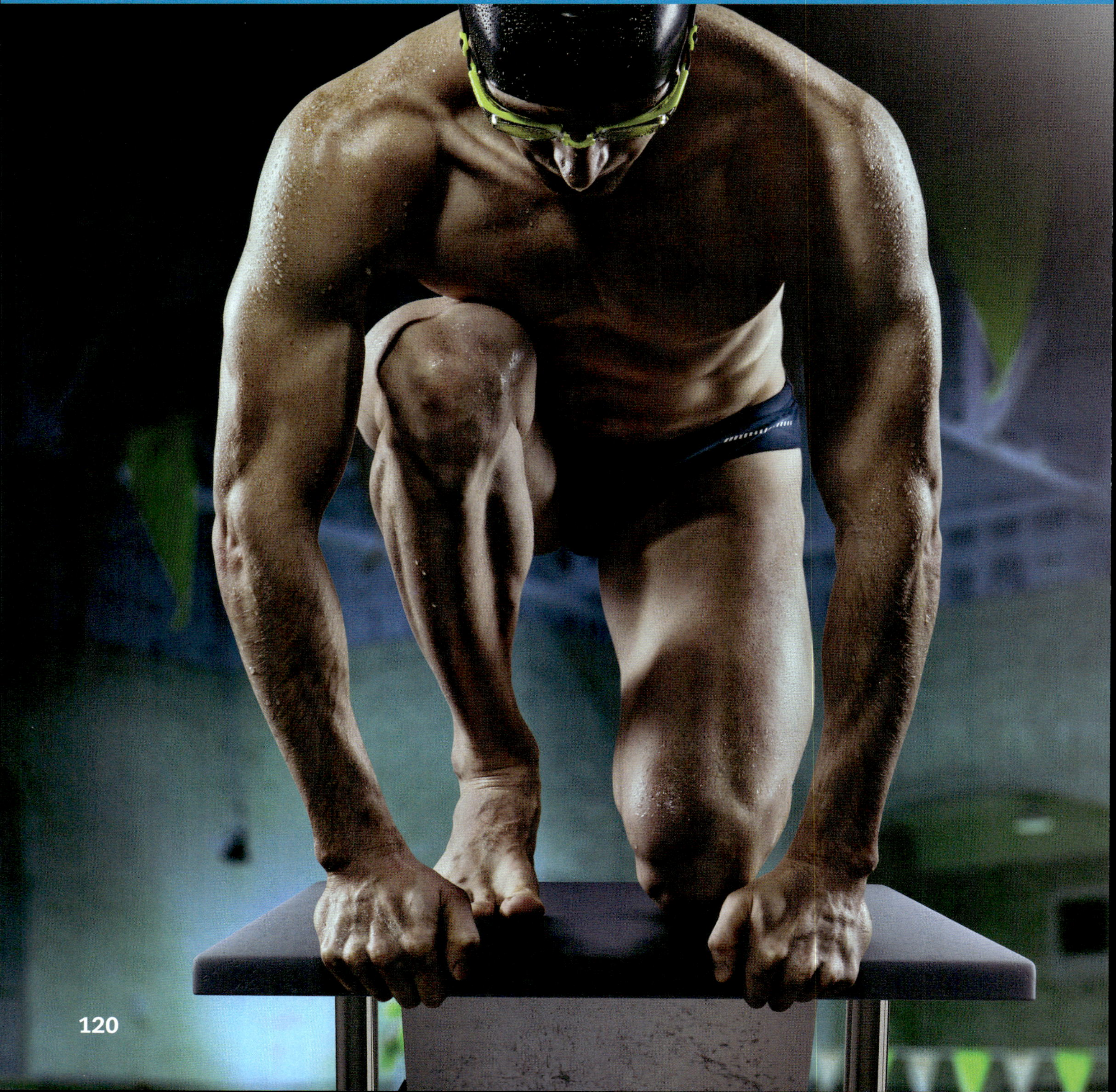

Chapter Objectives

- Describe the primary laboratory method to directly determine a food's macronutrient energy content
- Discuss three factors that influence the difference between a food's *gross* energy value and its *net* physiologic energy value
- Define combustion heat, digestive efficiency, and Atwater general factors to directly determine a food's energy content
- Compute the energy content for a sample breakfast from its macronutrient composition consisting of 8 oz of orange juice, 2 soft-boiled medium-grade eggs, 2 pieces of whole-wheat toast, 1 pat of butter, 1 tbs of strawberry jam (½ fl oz), and ½ medium grapefruit

Ancillaries at-a-Glance

Visit Lippincott Connect to access the following resources.

- References: Chapter 4
- Appendix D: The Metric System and Conversion Constants in Exercise Physiology
- Appendix E: Nutritive Values for Common Foods, Alcoholic and Nonalcoholic Beverages, and Specialty and Fast-Food Items
- Animations: General Digestion, Hydrolysis
- Focus on Research: Obesity-Related Thermogenic Response

All biologic functions require energy. The carbohydrate, lipid, and protein macronutrients contain the energy that ultimately powers biologic work from respiration within the body's cells. This includes the energy expended when muscles contract and relax during any type of physical activity, including racing down a ski trail, riding a giant wave, chewing food and processing it, brushing and flossing one's teeth, surfing the web, and answering an e-mail. In all these examples, creating cellular energy and processing it in the cells' energy factories serve as the common factor to classify both food and physical activity.

Measuring Food's Energy Content

Calorie

For food energy, 1 kilogram calorie (or kilocalorie; abbreviated kcal, from the Latin *calor* meaning "heat") expresses an amount of heat required to raise the temperature of 1 kg/2.2 lb of water (or its equivalent 1 L/0.264 gal) 1°C/1.8°F from 14.5 to 15.5°C/58.1 to 59.9°F at 1 atmosphere of pressure. Note that 1 kilogram calorie equals 1 Calorie (with a capital "c") but 1000 calories (with a lowercase "c"). Technically, 1 calorie (with a lowercase "c") indicates the quantity of heat necessary to raise the temperature of 1 g/0.04 oz (or its equivalent 1 mL/0.03 fl oz) of water 1°C/31.8°F.

French chemist and physicist professor Nicolas Clément-Desormes (1779–1841) was the first to scientifically define the kilogram calorie as an energy unit directly related to heat. He presented his ideas in lectures from 1819 to 1823 at the Conservatoire des Arts et Métiers in Paris, which were subsequently published in the 1824 journal *Le Producteur Philosophique De L'industrie, Des Sciences Et Des Beaux Artsin*.

Calories Versus Kilocalories

The small calorie, or gram calorie (abbreviated cal or c), identifies an amount of energy needed to raise the temperature of 1 g of water by one degree Celsius. The large Calorie— also known as the kilogram calorie, dietary calorie, nutritionist's calorie, or food calorie (abbreviated Cal or kcal)— is the amount of energy required to raise the temperature of one kilogram of water by one degree Celsius. The large Calorie thus equals 1000 small calories or 1 **kilocalorie (kcal)** and is widely used as a unit to represent food energy in the United States, United Kingdom, and other Western countries. The small calorie precisely quantifies the infinitesimally small amount of energy expressed as heat released in the body's billions of chemical reactions per second in the human body.

Bogdan Wankowicz/Shutterstock

For example, if a vegetable and hummus sandwich contains 400 kcal, then releasing the potential energy trapped within this food's chemical structures would increase the temperature of 400 L/106 gal of water 1°C/31.8°F. Different foods and their combinations contain quantitatively dissimilar potential energy values. Consider these two examples:

1. Two thirds of a cup of Ben and Jerry's Boots on the Moooo'n milk chocolate ice cream with fudge and toffee chunks contains about 420 kcal (26 g lipid, 41 g carbohydrate, 2 g fiber, 34 g added sugars, and 6 g protein) and the equivalent heat energy to increase the temperature for 420 L/111 gal of water by 1°C/31.8°F.
2. A Burger King Double Whopper sandwich with cheese but without mayo contains 980 kcal and thus would increase 980 L/259 gal of water by 1°C/31.8°F. For the Double Whopper, this large water quantity represents the equivalent of 490 2-L bottles of Gatorade or 521 12-oz cans of nondiet soda!

Temperature Versus Heat

Distinct differences exist between temperature and heat. **Temperature** reflects a relative, quantitative measure of an object's hotness or coldness on a numerical scale. In essence, temperature relates to the average kinetic energy of a substance's molecules, but it is not energy. **Heat** describes thermal energy and its *transfer* or *exchange* from one object or system to another. Heat, measured in energy units, reflects the energy within a substance. Adding heat to a substance *adds* energy to the substance. To a molecular biologist, physicist, or chemist, the added heat (or energy) reflects an increase in the kinetic energy of the substance's molecules. If that energy changes the state of the substance (e.g., a melting ice cube or ice cream cone), then the added energy breaks the ice molecule's bonds (or the semisolid milk mixture serving as in the cone) instead of changing its kinetic energy. In essence, when a substance *gains* heat, energy transfers to the substance.

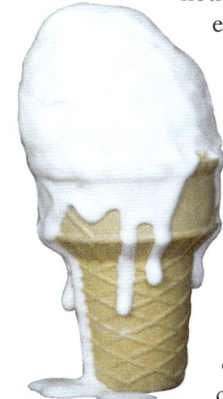
Captured by Nicole/Shutterstock

British Thermal Unit

The **British thermal unit (BTU)** represents a corresponding heat unit using Fahrenheit degrees. Credit for naming this unit belongs to British civil engineer Thomas Tredgold (1788–1829), who in 1824 described the BTU in one of his texts about warming and ventilating public buildings (https://archive.org/details/b21365283). One BTU represents the quantity of heat required to raise the temperature of 1 lb/0.543 kg (weight) of water 1°F/0.56°C from 63 to 64°F/17.2 to 17.7°C. Because heat is equivalent to energy, one BTU unit is convertible to approximately 1055 joules (J; 1.054 to 1.060 kilojoules [kJ]) and about 252 to 253 cal or 0.25 kcal. Interestingly, the BTU measurement unit, although it uses the name "British," is not used as a popular standard heat unit in Britain or the rest of the world. Instead, the International System of Units (see next section) serves as the accepted standard.

In the United States, an engineer might explain that when you burn a match to its end, its **exothermic** combustion reaction gives off heat equal to about one BTU. Living in a cold winter climate and relying on a wood stove as the heat source, the stove's heat-generating capacity rates at 40,000 BTU·h^{-1}. This equates to burning about 40,000 kitchen matches continuously each hour. Similarly, burning other fuels besides wood in the stove can be expressed in BTU. One gallon of gasoline generates 120,476 BTU, while a propane gallon generates about 25% less energy, or 91,333 BTU, and the same quantity of heating oil liberates 138,500 BTU. An exercising human who weighs 70 kg/154 lb would generate on average about 100 kcal during a one-mile walk or run regardless of speed, or the equivalent 400 BTU (1 BTU = 0.25 kcal). To preserve computational sanity, fortunately the kcal unit remains the preferred energy expenditure unit, as do gallons rather than BTU when filling a car's gas tank.

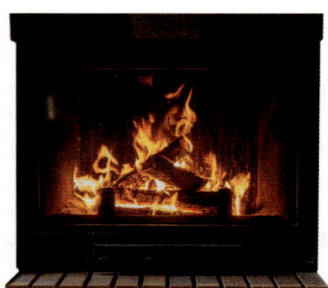
Syda Productions/Shutterstock

International System of Units

The **International System of Units (SI)**, also known as Système International d'Unités, had its origins in the 1790s during the French Revolution (http://physics.nist.gov/cuu/Units/history.html). The system began with just the meter (m) and kilogram (kg) as standards, but since then, the SI has undergone continuous updates and refinements. The 2019 (9th) edition, published by the Bureau International des Poids et Mesures (known in English as the *International Bureau of Weights and Measures*), promotes and explains the SI metric system definitions and calculations (www.bipm.org/documents/20126/41483022/SI-Brochure-9-EN.pdf).

Electrical energy, mechanical energy, and heat energy basically reflect the same state and in isolation are interconvertible from one form into another. The SI energy unit, the, **joule (J)**, and was named to honor the English physicist James Prescott Joule (1818–1889), whose work essentially postulated the **first law of thermodynamics**. This immutable natural law posits that energy in its various states can be changed from one state into another because energy remains fundamentally the same regardless of its state. Joule had studied how vigorous paddlewheel stirring warmed water, relying on earlier waterwheel concepts developed in the ancient Syrian cities for farming, maritime transportation on European waterways, and United States paddlewheel transportation methods. He determined that paddlewheel circular movement added energy to water, raising its water temperature in direct proportion to the work done by the wooden blades. The blades were arranged on the outside rim of a central wheel and formed the driving surface to thrust the "waterwheel" through the water. This was depicted in an 1841 *Magazine of Science* cover about waterwheel propulsion used in 19th century maritime transportation, which began in 1807 in the United States with Robert Fulton's (1765–1815) successful commercial steamboat service between New York City and Albany, NY, and included his design of the first steam warship, used in the War of 1812 to defend New York City. In ancient times, waterwheel engineering served farming and irrigation delivery systems, such as in the ancient Syrian city Hama, the "City of wheels," where waterwheels were in operation about

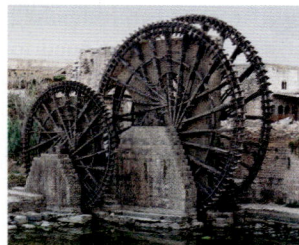
OPIS Zagreb/Shutterstock

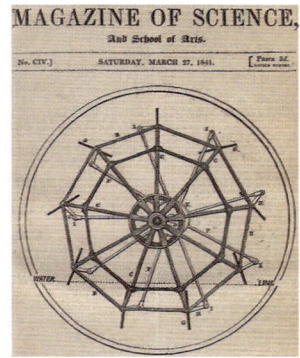

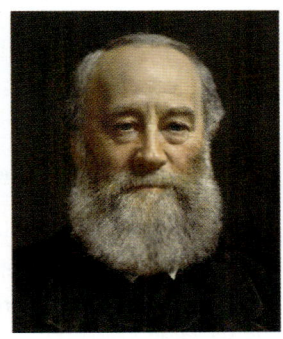
Morphart Creation/Shutterstock

fyi The Seven SI Base Units

The definitions for each of the seven base unit definitions are deduced by using previously defined constants to give their definitions from this consensus document (see www.bipm.org/documents/20126/41483022/SI-Brochure-9-EN.pdf).

Base Quantity		Base Unit	
Name	Symbol	Name	Symbol
Time	t	Second	s
Length	L, x, r	Meter	m
Mass	m	Kilogram	kg
Electric current	I, i	Ampere	A
Thermodynamic temperature	T	Kelvin	K
Amount of substance	n	Mole	mol
Luminous intensity	I_v	Candela	cd

The symbols for quantities are generally single Latin or Greek alphabet letters printed in an italic font. The symbols for the base units are printed in an upright (Roman) font and not italicized.

469 BC (www.waterhistory.org/histories/waterwheels/). Joule's classic and pioneering experiments have continued to impact worldwide thermodynamic science.

Energy Interconversions

One joule represents the work done or energy expended when one Newton (N) of force acts through a 1-m distance along the force direction; in essence 1 J = 1 Newton-meter (Nm). The J, or, more properly in nutritional science, the kilojoule (kJ; equals 1000 J), represents the standard SI unit to express food energy. To convert kcal to kJ, multiply the kcal value by 4.184. The **megajoule (MJ)** equals 1000 kJ; its use avoids unmanageably large numbers. As an example, the kilojoule value for 4 cups (8 oz) of air-popped white kernel popcorn without butter would equal 120 kcal × 4.184 or 502 kJ. Stovetop preparation with minimal vegetable oil adds about 5 to 10 kcal/21 to 42 kJ to the total calorie value. The following conversions apply: 1000 cal = 1 kcal × 4184 J or 0.004184 kJ; 1 BTU = 778 foot-pounds (ft-lb) = 252 cal = 1055 J. Appendix D lists metric system transpositions and conversion constants common to exercise physiology.

Vitaly Korovin/Shutterstock

Lippincott® Connect **Appendix D, available online at on** Lippincott Connect**, provides relationships among metric units and U.S. units, and common expressions for work, energy, and power.**

Food's Gross Energy Value

Food and nutrition laboratories use the **bomb calorimeter** to quantify the total or **gross energy value** for various food macronutrients. The bomb calorimeter (derived from the Latin *calor* = heat, and the Greek *metry* = measure), shown in the inset image and **FIGURE 4.1**, operates on the **direct calorimetry** principle by measuring the heat liberated as the food completely burns in a constant-volume container that serves as the "bomb" to record the equivalent change in its internal energy component or temperature (www.youtube.com/watch?v=VG9YG0VviHc). Burning (oxidizing) foods under high oxygen pressure (about 435 psi) and extreme temperature (sometimes exceeding 954°C/1750°F) identifies the calorie content in every food product sold to consumers.

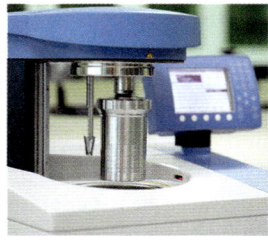
Choksawatdikorn/Shutterstock

Challenges in Determining Food's Gross Energy Value

Fast-food restaurants in the United States and worldwide face the challenge of providing consumers reliable and valid information about their food purchases. For example, the United States in 2020 had the most number of fast-food locations (https://en.wikipedia.org/wiki/List_of_the_largest_fast_food_restaurant_chains). The top five are Subway, 42,600;

Conversion Between Calories and Joules

An energy equivalency exists between 1 kcal of heat and 4.184 J of work. Energy and work unit conversion calculators on the Internet (see for example: www.calculatorsoup.com/calculators/conversions/energy.php) easily perform the calculations among joules (J), kilojoules (kJ), and megajoules (MJ). For example, 10,000 J = 10 kJ = 0.01 MJ. Further interconversions for 10,000 J include 7376 ft-lb, 9478 BTU, and 2.39 kcal. In everyday life, one J equals the energy *required* to lift a small apple with a mass of about 102 g 1 m off a table, and conversely the energy *released* when that same apple falls 1 m to the table. An animal pulling a plow generates the required energy to pull the plow through the fields over a specified time and distance. In human terms, one J equals the energy released in 1 s as heat by an average-size person at rest. In engineering terms, one nanojoule (nJ) equals one billionth of one J, and a microjoule (μJ) equals one millionth of one J.

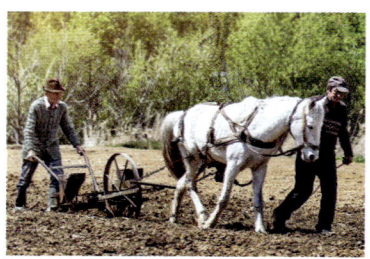
Alexandru Logel/Shutterstock

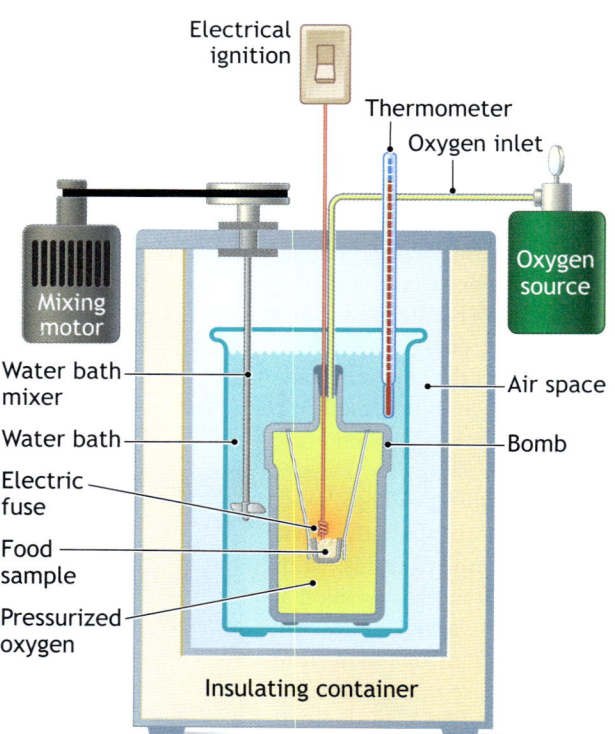

FIGURE 4.1. A bomb calorimeter directly measures a food's energy value.

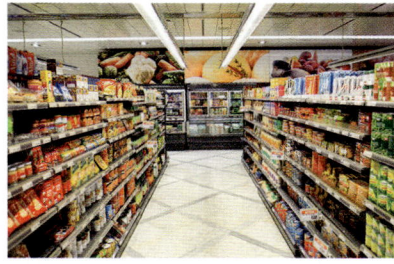
Sorbis/Shutterstock

McDonald's, 38,700; Starbucks, 31,256; KFC, 24,104; and Burger King, 18,838. These are followed by Tim Hortons in Canada (4774), Jollibee in Southeast Asia and the Middle East (4593), and CNHLS in China (4000). The bomb calorimeter provides the experimentally derived basis to establish a given food quantity's energy content. For the more than 40,000 supermarkets in the United States in 2019, approximately 28,112 different foods were sold, with the super warehouse retailers averaging from 40,000 to 50,000 different items—each with its own nutritional label to help consumers make decisions about a food's nutrient composition and caloric content per serving based on bomb calorimeter science.

Bomb Calorimeter Methodology

A bomb calorimeter, shown in Figure 4.1, contains a small, stainless steel insulated chamber filled with oxygen under high pressure and a weighed food sample placed in a small container within the bomb. An electric current ignites an iron or nickel electric fuse within the bomb chamber, making the food sample literally explode and burn. A surrounding water bath absorbs the heat released as the food burns. An insulating water jacket surrounding the bomb prevents heat loss to the outside environment. A sensitive, highly accurate thermometer measures the heat absorbed by the water. For example, the complete combustion for one 20-oz skinless beef hot dog and 1.4-oz bun with mustard and small French fries (68 g/2.4) liberates 512 kcal of heat energy. This is the equivalent heat to change the temperature of 5.12 kg/11.3 lb of water from 0°C/32°F to its boiling point of 100°C/212°F. The Web site www.siamzim.com/pdf/calorimeters/TN_101.pdf provides bomb calorimetry calibration methods, with different calorimeter types and methodologies.

Combustion Heat

Heat liberated by food oxidation in a bomb calorimeter represents the food's **combustion heat** or total energy value. *Burning 1 g pure carbohydrate yields 4.20 kcal, 1 g pure protein releases 5.65 kcal, and 1 g pure lipid yields 9.45 kcal.* Most foods in a daily food regimen contain these three macronutrients in different proportions. In effect, a particular food's caloric content represents the summed heats of combustion for the carbohydrate, lipid, and protein components. In the bomb calorimeter, complete lipid oxidation liberates about 65% more energy per gram than protein oxidation, and 120% more energy than does carbohydrate oxidation.

Consider a real-world example when a typical triacylglycerol molecule with the following chemical composition completely oxidizes in the body's 30 to 40 trillion cells: $C_{55}H_{104}O_6$ + $78 O_2 \rightarrow 55 CO_2 + 52 H_2O$ + Heat (~8084 kcal · mol^{-1}). In this case, the heat per mole generated corresponds to the mass of the oxidized triacylglycerol molecule (6.023×10^{23} carbon, hydrogen, and oxygen particles in the molecule), which ultimately liberates 8804 kcal per mole. In practical terms when humans sleep, for example, all the body's cells continue to liberate heat to maintain every human function at rest. The most observable "heat factor" during sleep is body temperature, which remains stable at about 37°C/98.6°F throughout the sleeping period. *In effect, the recorded body temperature at rest and all physical activities represents the cumulative heat produced during all forms of cellular oxidation or the heat equivalent expressed as body temperature* (see previous section: Temperature versus Heat).

fizkes/Shutterstock

INTEGRATIVE QUESTION

How can the oxygen required to burn food in a calorimeter translate to the number of calories in a meal?

Carbohydrate Combustion Heat

Carbohydrate combustion heat varies depending on the atom's arrangement in the particular carbohydrate molecule. The glucose molecule's combustion heat (sucrose shown in the inset image with conventional atom coding for carbon [gray], oxygen [red], hydrogen [white]) equals 3.74 kcal · g^{-1}, whereas glycogen (4.19 kcal) and starch (4.20 kcal) yield larger values. *The carbohydrate combustion heat for 1 g averages about 4.2 kcal.*

Maryna Olyak/Shutterstock

Lipid Combustion Heat

Lipid combustion heat varies with the triacylglycerol molecule's fatty acid three-dimensional structural composition shown for the derived lipid cholesterol with the same conventional atom coding shown for sucrose. One g of either beef or pork fat yields 9.50 kcal, whereas oxidizing 1 g of butterfat liberates 9.27 kcal. The average caloric value for 1 g of lipid in meat, fish, and eggs equals 9.50 kcal. In dairy products, the calorific equivalent amounts to 9.25 kcal · g^{-1}, and 9.30 kcal in vegetables and fruits. *The average lipid combustion heat equals 9.4 kcal · g^{-1}.*

Maryna Olyak/Shutterstock

Protein Combustion Heat

Two factors impact a food's protein component energy release during combustion:

1. The food's protein type
2. The protein's relative nitrogen content

Common proteins in eggs, meat, corn, and beans (jack, lima, navy, soy) contain approximately 16% nitrogen and have corresponding combustion heats averaging 5.75 kcal·g⁻¹. Proteins in other foods have higher nitrogen content (e.g., most nuts and seeds [18.9%] and whole-kernel wheat, rye, millets, and barley [17.2%]). Whole milk (15.7%) and bran (15.8%) contain a slightly lower nitrogen percentage. The molecular model represents lysozyme protein found in human milk. **Protein combustion heat** averages 5.65 kcal·g⁻¹.

Kateryna Kon/Shutterstock

The average combustion heats for the three macronutrients (carbohydrate, 4.2 kcal·g⁻¹; lipid, 9.4 kcal·g⁻¹; protein, 5.65 kcal·g⁻¹) demonstrate that lipid's complete oxidation in the bomb calorimeter liberates about 65% more energy per gram than protein oxidation and 120% more energy than carbohydrate oxidation. In Chapter 1, we emphasized that lipid molecules contain more hydrogen atoms than either carbohydrate or protein molecules. For example, the common fatty acid palmitic acid with 16 carbon atoms, 32 hydrogen atoms, and 2 oxygen atoms (structural formula $C_{16}H_{32}O_2$) is found naturally in palm and kernel oils, butter, cheese, milk, and meat (https://oil-palmblog.wordpress.com/2014/01/25/1-composition-of-palm-oil/). The hydrogen-to-oxygen atom ratios in fatty acids always exceed the 2:1 carbohydrate ratio. Simply stated, lipid molecules have more hydrogen atoms available for cleavage and subsequent oxidation for energy than carbohydrates and proteins.

Lipid-rich foods have higher energy contents than foods relatively fat-free. One cup of whole milk contains 160 kcal, whereas the same quantity of skim milk contains 56% less or 90 kcal. If a person who normally consumes 0.95 L/1 qt of whole milk daily switches to skim milk, the total calories ingested yearly would decrease by the equivalent calories in 11.3 kg/25 lb of body fat! In 3 y, all other things remaining constant, body fat loss would approximate 34 kg/75 lb. Such a theoretical comparison merits serious consideration because of the almost identical nutritional composition between whole milk and skim milk except for the lipid content. Drinking 226.7 g/8 oz of skim milk rather than whole milk also considerably reduces saturated fatty acid intake (0.4 vs. 5.1 g) and cholesterol intake (0.3 g vs. 33 mg).

In the 1960s and 1970s, parents who wanted to reduce a child's lipid intake (and save money) often switched from whole milk to much cheaper powdered fat-free milk mixed with cold water. The bottom line is that small differences in energy intake (particularly lipid-rich foods) add up over time to potentiate large differences in energy balance. A college-age male (age 20, 79.4 kg/175 lb) who gains *just* 0.45 kg/1 lb yearly would increase his body weight to 99.8 kg/220 lb by age 65! Similarly, a 20-year-old college-age female who weighs 56.7 kg/125 lb would have gained 20.4 kg/45 lb by age 65. Not surprisingly, those gains are almost identical to what occurs in the United States population on a year-by-year basis through age 65, as we discuss in Chapters 28 and 30, which deal with body composition and basic principles about the energetics of weight control and physical activity.

Interchangeable Expressions for Energy, Heat, and Work

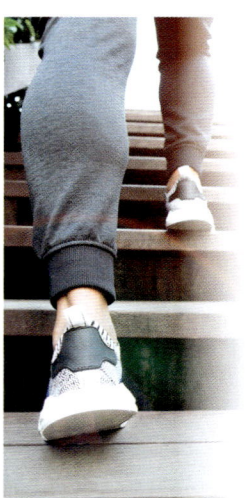

1 ft-lb = 0.13825 kg-m

1 kg-m = 7.233 ft-lb = 9.8066 J

1 kcal = 3.0874 ft-lb = 426.85 kg-m = 4.186 kJ

1 J = 1 Nm

1 kJ = 1000 J = 0.23889 kcal

1 BTU = 778 ft-lb = 252 cal = 1055 J

1 kcal = 1000 cal = 4186 J = 4.184 kJ

1 cal = 4.184 J

BEAUTY STUDIO/Shutterstock

Food's Net Energy Value

Differences exist in a food's energy value when comparing heats of combustion determined by direct calorimetry (gross energy value) to the body's **net energy value**. This pertains particularly to proteins because the body cannot oxidize its nitrogen component. Rather, nitrogen atoms combine with hydrogen to form urea (NH_2CONH_2) for excretion through the skin and in urine. Eliminating hydrogen represents an approximately 19% loss in the protein molecule's stored potential energy. This hydrogen loss reduces protein combustion heat in the body to approximately 4.6 kcal·g^{-1} instead of 5.65 kcal·g^{-1} released during bomb calorimeter oxidation. In contrast, identical physiologic fuel values exist for carbohydrates and lipids (which contain no nitrogen) compared with their respective bomb calorimeter determined heats of combustion.

Limitations of Basing Food's Energy Value on Combustion Heat

The basic assumptions concerning combustion heats for carbohydrates, lipids, and proteins assume that a given food portion digests and absorbs equally with little or no variation within a food's category. Researchers now appreciate that the cell walls of some plants are more difficult to break down than others and that cooking generally disrupts the cell wall's integrity to increase accessibility to the food's energy nutrients compared to the identical food in the raw state where some calories pass unavailable from the body. Some nuts (e.g., walnuts, hazelnuts, almonds, Brazil nuts) resist complete digestion so they too release fewer calories to the body than "expected," computed from their actual macronutrient content. Many different protein types demonstrate a broad range in variability in net energy available to the body owing to their specific requirements for complete digestion, absorption, and assimilation. Food processing also makes the energy in food more readily available than food in the unprocessed state. The standard Atwater model for computing a food's energy content we discuss in the next section appears relatively effective, yet the caloric values in food tables represent *averages*—and averages sometimes fail to account for fluctuations related to the type, form, preparation (raw and whole, raw and pounded, cooked and whole, cooked and pounded), or whether the food is processed or consumed in a more natural unprocessed form. This also applies to individual differences in digestive efficiency among individuals of all ages.

 See the animation "General Digestion" on Lippincott Connect for a demonstration of this process.

Digestibility Coefficients

Digestive efficiency influences the ultimate caloric yield from macronutrients. Numerically defined as the **coefficient of digestibility**, digestive efficiency represents the percentage of food digested and absorbed to serve the body's metabolic needs. In essence, the small intestine's fingerlike projections (villi), shown here, extend the full length into the small intestine's lumen, providing a large surface area to absorb and catabolize the foods consumed as they pass through the digestive passages beginning in the mouth where the food is reduced to smaller units and mixed with fluids, and then through the esophagus into the stomach, and finally through the small and large intestines for excretion. Food remaining unabsorbed in the intestinal tract becomes voided in the feces. Dietary fiber reduces the coefficient of digestibility—a high-fiber meal has less total energy absorbed than a fiber-free meal or highly processed foods with equivalent caloric content. This difference occurs because fiber moves food more rapidly through the small intestine thereby reducing absorption time. Fiber also may cause mechanical erosion of intestinal mucosa, which then becomes resynthesized through energy-requiring processes. **TABLE 4.1** shows factors for digestibility, heats of combustion, and net physiologic energy values for dietary protein, lipid, and carbohydrate.

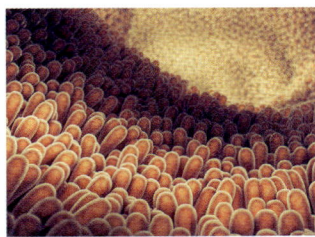
nobeastsofierce/Shutterstock

> **TABLE 4.1** Factors for digestibility, heats of combustion, and net physiologic energy values for dietary protein, lipid, and carbohydrate

The relative macronutrient percentages completely digested and absorbed averages 97% for carbohydrate, 95% for lipid, and 92% for protein. Little difference exists in digestive efficiency between obese and lean persons. Considerable variability nevertheless exists in efficiency percentages for any food within a particular food category. Proteins have highly variable digestive efficiencies; they range from a low of about 78% for high-fiber legumes to a high of 97% for protein from animal sources. Some advocates promote the use of vegetables in weight loss dietary regimens because of plant protein's relatively low digestibility coefficient.

The feces contain food residues remaining unabsorbed in the intestinal tract. Organic chemical bacterial action produces the overall unpleasant fecal odor. These include the aromatic heterocyclic *indole* compound (C_8H_7N produced by the *Escherichia coli* bacteria), *skatole* (white crystalline, foul smelling tryptophan organic compound produced in the digestive tract), *hydrogen sulfide* H_2S (colorless gas with a strong odor of rotten eggs from bacterial organic matter breakdown), and *mercaptans* (pungent smelling organic hydrocarbon components combined with sulfur).

Calculating a Meal's Energy Value

The caloric content of any food can be determined from the Atwater values by knowing its composition and weight. For example, based on laboratory analysis of a standard recipe, one can determine the kcal value for ½ cup (100 g/3.5 oz) of creamed chicken. The macronutrient composition of 1 g creamed chicken contains 0.2 g protein, 0.12 g lipid, and 0.06 g carbohydrate. Using the Atwater net kcal values, 0.2 g of protein contains 0.8 kcal (0.20 × 4.0), 0.12 g of lipid equals 1.08 kcal (0.12 × 9.0), and 0.06 g of carbohydrate yields

0.24 kcal (0.06 × 4.0). The total caloric value of 1 g of creamed chicken thus equals 2.12 kcal (0.80 + 1.08 + 0.24). A 100-g serving for the creamed chicken contains 100 times as much, or 212 kcal. **TABLE 4.2** presents the kcal calculations for 100 g/3/4 cup of vanilla ice cream, including its macronutrient composition.

TABLE 4.2 Method to compute a food's caloric value from its macronutrient composition

If you double the serving size to 1.5 cups, the total calories increase from 217 to 434 kcal. Similar computations can estimate the caloric value for any food serving. Increasing or decreasing portion sizes (or adding lipid-rich sauces or creams or fruits or calorie-rich substitutes) impacts caloric content accordingly.

Computing food caloric values is time consuming and laborious. Various governmental agencies in the United States and abroad have evaluated and compiled nutritive values for thousands of foods. The most comprehensive data bank resources include the U.S. Nutrient Data Bank (USNDB) maintained by the U.S. Department of Agriculture's (USDA; www.usda.gov) Consumer Nutrition Center and a computerized data bank maintained by the Bureau of Nutritional Sciences of Health and Welfare Canada (www.canada.ca/en/health-canada/corporate/about-health-canada/branches-agencies/health-products-food-branch/food-directorate/bureau-nutritional-sciences.html). The USDA Nutrient Database can be viewed at https://fdc.nal.usda.gov; and the Food and Nutrition Information Center, National Agricultural Library, Agricultural Research Service of the USDA can be accessed at www.nal.usda.gov/fnic. Other free excellent resources to quantify food calories can be obtained from the Society for Nutrition Education and Behavior Web site (www.sneb.org).

Lippincott® Connect **Appendix E, available on** Lippincott Connect, presents energy and nutritive values for common foods, including specialty and fast-food items.

Consuming an equal number of calories from diverse foods often requires increasing or decreasing the quantity of a particular food. For example, to consume 100 kcal from each of six common foods—carrots, celery, green peppers, grapefruit, medium-sized eggs, and mayonnaise—one must eat 5 carrots, or 20 stalks of celery, or 6.5 green peppers, or 1 large grapefruit, or 1¼ eggs, but only 1 tablespoon of mayonnaise. Consequently, an average sedentary adult woman would need to consume 420 celery stalks, or 105 carrots, or 136 green peppers, or 26 eggs, yet only 1½ cup of mayonnaise or 227 g/8 oz of salad oil to meet her daily 2100-kcal energy needs. *These examples dramatically illustrate that foods high in lipid content contain considerably more calories than foods low in lipid with correspondingly higher water content.*

Syda Productions/Shutterstock

Atwater General Factors

Atwater general factors were named to honor Wilbur Olin Atwater (1844–1907), the renowned 19th-century chemist who determined the average net energy values for dietary protein, lipid, and carbohydrate. Atwater conducted his research, which pioneered the first human nutrition and energy balance studies, in his laboratory at Wesleyan University at Middleton, Connecticut in the 1890s. Atwater had gained valuable scientific skills in physiological chemistry in Berlin and Leipzig, Germany, where he did postgraduate work with the incomparable chemists Carl von Voit (1831–1908) and Max Rubner (1854–1932), whom we profile in Chapter 1. Atwater conducted human calorimetric study experiments with the physicist Edward Bennet Rosa (1873–1921) and nutritionist Francis Gano Benedict (1870–1957), which included determining the caloric content of various food macronutrients, contributing to a system of dietary standards for the food industry (https://specialcollections.nal.usda.gov/guide-collections/wilbur-olin-atwater-papers). The Atwater general factors provide ingested foods' net metabolizable energy availability to power the body's chemical reactions. The Atwater factors provide reasonable average energy content values in the daily diet. For alcohol, 7 kcal (29.4 kJ) represents each gram (mL) of pure 200 proof alcohol ingested. The efficiency of alcohol's potential energy available to the body equals that of other carbohydrates.

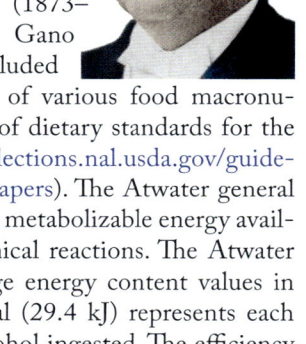

Atwater 4-9-4 kcal Rule

The **Atwater 4-9-4 kilocalorie rule** generally proves useful to quantitatively estimate the intake of food energy. Limitations do exist, particularly when consuming foods that include carbohydrate-bulking agents. For example, polysaccharides obtained from industrial gums, modified starches, and plant cell walls, which contain combinations of cellulose, hemicellulose, and a small amount of lignin, serve as common bulking agents in most prepared foods. These agents may be totally digestible, partially digestible, or indigestible depending on their chemical structure. They pass through the intestinal tract with little breakdown because without naturally occurring enzymes, no hydrolysis occurs; hence, they are of no energy value to the body. Determining digestibility coefficients with bomb calorimetry also plays an essential role in animal husbandry research related to the care and feeding of livestock, because such practices impact products sold in the marketplace. They provide transparency regarding scientific information about an animal's prior overall health status (e.g., caged or free-roaming, organic food sources or pesticides added to feed) and ultimately the consumer's desire to purchase the product.

 See the animation "Hydrolysis" on Lippincott Connect for a demonstration of this process.

By accepting the Atwater 4-9-4 kcal rule, low calorie foods are recommended as the desirable choice to achieve weight loss and maintenance compared to consuming foods higher in lipid content (e.g., 9.0 kcal·g^{-1} for lipid versus only 4 kcal·g^{-1} for protein and carbohydrate). This strategy for weight reduction, known as the energy balance theory (EBT) or the "calories-in, calories-out" rule, posits that body weight decreases only when total calories consumed are less than total calories expended by metabolism and physical activity over a given time period. A recent competing theory, the **mass balance model (MBM)**, favors body weight and body fat loss when total *macronutrient mass intake* (not kcal burned as heat) is less than total *macronutrient mass excretion* via normal oxidative processes than when *macronutrient mass intake* exceeds *macronutrient mass elimination*. In both theories, can celery's low-caloric content qualify as a potential "high-calorie" food to either lose or just stabilize body weight, and therefore, whether overeating celery qualifies as a fattening food as explained in the following example.

Suppose someone consuming 1800 kcal daily decides to eat 1 typical celery stalk (almost 8 kcal) on any given day. How many celery stalks would they need to consume to achieve their total 1800 calorie daily intake? The answer is straight forward—eating 2 normal size celery stalks (about 7 in long) would add about 16 kcal of energy toward the 1800 kcal daily goal. Thus, the person would need to consume 225 celery stalks to achieve the daily maintenance energy goal. Suppose the person now "binged" on succeeding days by eating just 12 additional celery stalks daily equivalent to only about 100 "extra" kcal. This small additional daily energy intake would translate to adding only 1/35th of a kilogram or 0.063 lb to stored body fat each day or 1 kg/2.2 lb of fat gain every 35 days (3500 kcal = 1 kg/2.2 lb body fat). This theoretically improbable, inexact example for daily calorie intake clearly makes the point, that if celery is regularly consumed in excess it too would qualify as a "fattening" food, despite that it clearly represents an excellent low calorie food source high in antioxidant nutrients with more fiber (1.6 g) than protein (<1 g) or sugars per cup! Interestingly, low-calorie versus high-calorie foods may not play the consequential role whether someone succeeds or fails in weight regulation on a particular dietary regimen. The next section describes the new MBM theory that challenges the conventional idea that "calories-in versus calories-out" plays the pivotal role to explain body weight and body fat loss.

MBM: An Alternative Explanation

The energy balance theory (EBT) or "calories-in, calories-out" rule states that body weight decreases only when total calories consumed are less than total calories expended by metabolism and physical activity over a given time period. Without creating an "imbalance," body weight and total fat remain relatively stable because the body's net energy balance ("calories-in equals calories-out") does not favor output over input. This

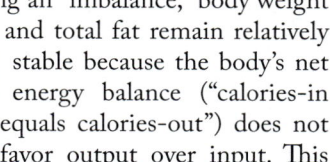
Liudmila P. Sundikova/Shutterstock

means that if energy input equals energy output, there will be little change in body weight and thus essentially little impact on weight loss or body fat reduction. It also follows that different dietary regimens with *identical* energy content (e.g., an isocaloric 1300 kcal high-fat versus low-fat diets) should theoretically produce identical body weight and fat losses independent of the diet's macronutrient composition.

According to MBM theory, in contrast to the EBT theory, the key to weight loss creates an imbalance between the *food mass intake* (not simply *total kcal*) and the corresponding mass elimination equivalent that results from the food oxidation *end-product mass* excretion. Weight gain occurs as the mass of food ingested increases even when its associated calories remain stable at a predetermined maintenance or deficit level to produce weight loss. In the late 1700s, Antoine Lavoisier's experiments (discussed in the History chapter) discovered that for oxidation reactions, the Law of Mass Conservation states that in any oxidation reaction, mass flows from reactants to products and not from calories-in to calories-out. The mass of chemical reactants must equal the mass of the chemical products without mass transfer occurring in the oxidation process as released heat (i.e., calories-out). In the MBM, consuming only 1 g of either protein, lipid, or carbohydrate will increase an individual's body mass by exactly 1 g independent of the nutrient's energy content (i.e., calories-in), independent of its caloric content. For example, if food consumption equals 120 g for the combined macronutrient intake, then 120 g will *add* to the body mass. Accordingly, the oxidation of 1 g of any stored macronutrient will *reduce* body mass by 1 g as the oxidation end-products are eliminated with the source of "burned" calories becoming literally inconsequential.

The MBM theory predicts that in weight reduction interventions with identical energy isocaloric content, the amount of body weight and body fat loss will depend on the diet's macronutrient composition, not the calorie in-and-out. For example, consider a 1300 kcal low-fat diet (LFD) with calories distributed as 20% lipid, 65% carbohydrate, and 15% protein. Using traditional Atwater factors, the nutrient mass intake with this regimen approximates 289 g. In contrast, a similar calculation for a 1300 kcal low-carbohydrate diet (LCD), with calories distributed as 70% lipid, 15% carbohydrate, and 15% protein, reduces the nutrient mass ingestion to 199 g (289 g from the 65% carbohydrate diet minus 90 g

In a Practical Sense

Three Nutrient Timing Phases to Optimize Performance

Findings from sports and exercise nutrition research emphasize not only specific types and nutrient mixtures but also the timing of nutrient intake to enhance exercise performance. Nutrient timing's goal attempts to know when and what to eat to achieve top performance and accelerate subsequent recovery. Nutrient timing can blunt a catabolic state from the effects of glucagon, epinephrine, norepinephrine, and cortisol release, and activate natural muscle-building hormones testosterone, growth hormone, insulin-like growth factor-1, and insulin to speed recovery and maximize muscle growth. Three phases optimize specific nutrient intake:

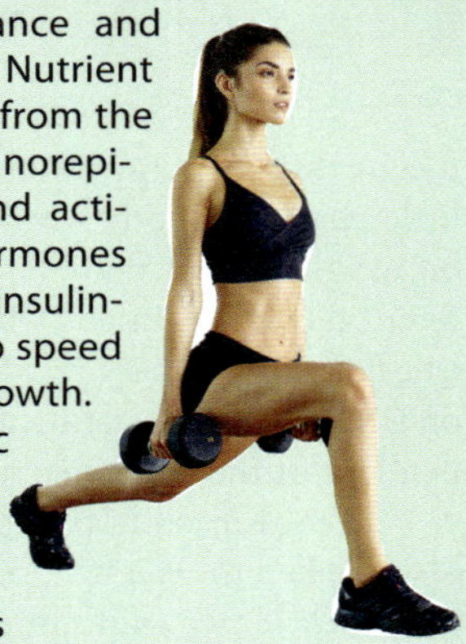

Energy phase: (1) Enhances nutrient intake to spare muscle glycogen and protein, (2) enhances muscular endurance, (3) limits immune system suppression, (4) reduces muscle damage, and (5) facilitates postexercise recovery. Consuming a carbohydrate + protein supplement in the immediate pre-activity period and during physical activity extends endurance; ingested protein promotes protein metabolism reducing demand for muscle's release of amino acids. Carbohydrates consumed during physical activity suppress cortisol release—this blunts the suppressive effects of physical activity on immune system function and reduces the use of branched-chain amino acids generated by protein breakdown for energy. The recommended energy phase supplement profile contains the following nutrients: 20 to 26 g high glycemic carbohydrates (glucose, sucrose, maltodextrin), 5 to 6 g whey protein (rapidly digested, high-quality protein separated from milk in the cheese-making process), 1 g leucine, 30 to 120 mg vitamin C, 20 to 60 IU vitamin E, 100 to 250 mg sodium, 60 to 100 mg potassium, and 60 to 220 mg magnesium.

Anabolic phase: Consists of the 45-min postexercise metabolic window—a period that enhances insulin sensitivity for muscle glycogen replenishment and muscle tissue repair and synthesis. This shift from a catabolic to anabolic state occurs largely by blunting cortisol's catabolic action and increasing insulin's anabolic, muscle-building effects by consuming a standard high-glycemic carbohydrate + protein supplement in liquid form (e.g., whey protein and high-glycemic carbohydrates). In essence, a high-glycemic carbohydrate consumed following physical activity serves as a nutrient activator to stimulate insulin release, which in the presence of amino acids, increases muscle tissue synthesis and decreases protein degradation. The recommended anabolic phase supplement contains the following nutrients: 40 to 50 g of high-glycemic carbohydrates (glucose, sucrose, maltodextrin), 13 to 15 g whey protein, 1 to 2 g leucine, 1 to 2 g glutamine, 60 to 120 mg vitamin C, and 80 to 400 IU vitamin E.

Growth phase: Extends from the end of the anabolic phase to the start of the next workout. This time interlude maximizes insulin sensitivity and maintains an anabolic state to accentuate gains in muscle mass and muscle strength. The rapid segment, which involves the first several hours, helps to maintain increased insulin sensitivity and glucose uptake to maximize glycogen replenishment. It also speeds elimination of metabolic waste by increasing blood flow and stimulates tissue repair and muscle growth. The next sustained 16 to 18 hr segment maintains positive nitrogen balance by consuming a relatively high daily protein intake (between 0.91 and 1.2 g protein per 0.54 kg/1 lb body weight), which fosters sustained but slower muscle tissue synthesis. An adequate carbohydrate intake emphasizes glycogen replenishment, with a recommended growth phase supplement containing 14 g whey protein, 2 g casein, 3 g leucine, 1 g glutamine, and 2 to 4 g high-glycemic carbohydrates.

Sources:
Arent SM, et al. Nutrient timing: a garage door of opportunity? *Nutrients*. 2020;12:1948.
Huecker M, et al. Protein supplementation in sport: source, timing, and intended benefits. *Curr Nutr Rep*. 2019;8:382.
Queiroz JDN, et al. Time-restricted eating and circadian rhythms: the biological clock is ticking. *Crit Rev Food Sci Nutr*. 2021;61:2863.
Rangaraj VR, et al. Association between timing of energy intake and insulin sensitivity: a cross-sectional study. *Nutrients*. 2020;16:12. pii: E503.
Stecker RA, et al. Timing of ergogenic aids and micronutrients on muscle and exercise performance. *J Int Soc Sports Nutr*. 2019;16:37.

---

from the 15% carbohydrate diet). Accordingly, for both isocaloric 1300 kcal diets, the LCD results in *greater* weight loss versus the LFD because the 199 g weight difference in favor of LCD necessarily produces the greatest body weight loss. **FIGURE 4.2** summarizes key points about the MBM—the food mass ingested is based on its macronutrient composition, and the mass of the elimination oxidation products, not total heat (kcal with LCD or LFD), determines the amount and rate of body weight and body fat loss during weight reduction.

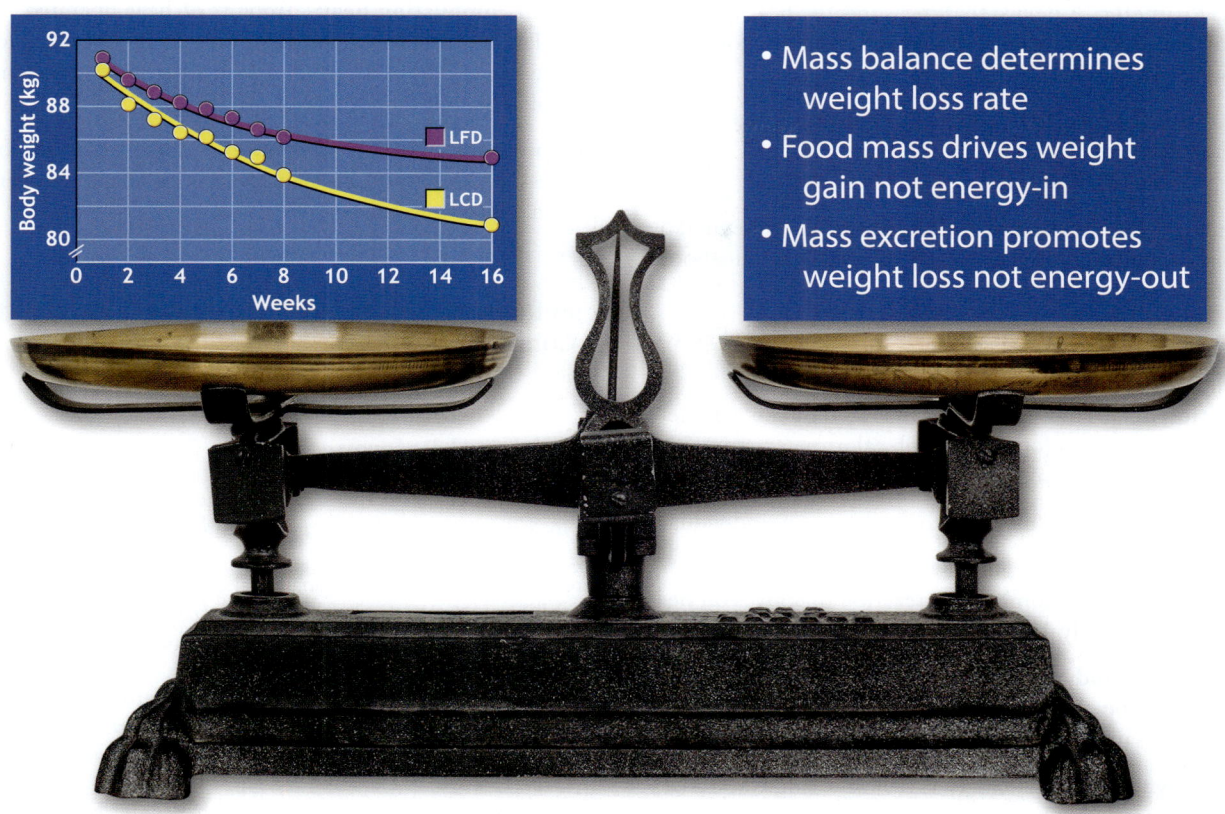

FIGURE 4.2. The new mass balance model predicts successful weight reduction interventions with diets of identical energy content but different macronutrient compositions, as shown on the left scale: a low-fat diet (LFD; *purple line*) versus a high-fat, low-calorie diet (LCD; *yellow line*). The amount and rate of body weight and body fat loss produced by each dietary treatment depend on the diet's macronutrient blend. The LCD favors greater losses because there is less food mass as the energy proportion from lipid increases—a consequence of the higher caloric density of lipids than carbohydrates.
(Image of scales: DJTaylor/Shutterstock)

Summary

1. A calorie or kilocalorie (kcal) represents a food's energy value expressed as heat.
2. Burning food in a bomb calorimeter directly quantifies a food's energy content.
3. A clear distinction exists between temperature and heat. Temperature reflects a relative, quantitative measure or number of an object's hotness or coldness measured on a scale (e.g., 14.5°C/59.9°F).
4. Heat describes thermal energy and its transfer or exchange from one object or system to another.
5. The combustion heat quantifies the amount of heat liberated in a food's complete oxidation.
6. Average gross energy values equal 4.2 kcal·g^{-1} for carbohydrate, 9.4 kcal·g^{-1} for lipid, and 5.65 kcal·g^{-1} for protein.
7. The coefficient of digestibility represents the proportion of food digested and absorbed during the digestive processes.
8. Coefficients of digestibility average 97% for carbohydrates, 95% for lipids, and 92% for proteins.
9. The net energy values equal 4 kcal·g^{-1} for carbohydrate and protein, and 9 kcal·g^{-1} for lipid and provide an accurate estimate about a food's typical net energy value.
10. Atwater calorific values refer to the energy (caloric) content of a meal from the food's carbohydrate, lipid, and protein compositions.
11. Calories represent heat energy regardless of food source (e.g., 500 chocolate chip cookie dough ice cream kcal = 500 raw asparagus kcal = 500 pepperoni and cheese pizza kcal = 500 Hawaiian macadamia nut kcal).
12. The new MBM predicts that for successful weight reduction, low carbohydrate diets (LCD) produce greater body weight and body fat loss than low-fat diets (LFD) of an equivalent caloric value.
13. An LCD is the preferred dietary intervention because there is *less* food mass as the energy proportion from lipid increases—a consequence from lipids high caloric density compared to the carbohydrate or protein macronutrients.

Key Terms

Atwater 4-9-4 kilocalorie rule: The rule establishing that carbohydrates yield 4 kcal·g^{-1}, lipids yield 9 kcal·g^{-1}, and proteins yield 4 kcal·g^{-1}

Atwater general factors: Estimates of the net energy value for a typical food portion consumed equal to 4 kcal·g^{-1} carbohydrate, 9 kcal·g^{-1} lipid, and 4 kcal·g^{-1} protein

Bomb calorimeter: A device that measures the heat liberated as a food burns completely in a constant-volume container, which serves as the "bomb"

British thermal unit (BTU): Amount of heat needed to raise the temperature of 0.45 kg/1 lb of liquid water 1°F from 17.2°C/63°F to 17.7°C/64°F

Carbohydrate combustion heat: Amount of heat liberated by the complete burning or oxidation of carbohydrate in a bomb calorimeter; averages 4.2 kcal·g^{-1}

Coefficient of digestibility: The percentage of food digested and absorbed to serve the body's metabolic needs

Combustion heat: Amount of heat liberated by the complete burning or oxidation of food in a bomb calorimeter, representing food's total energy value

Direct calorimetry: A method to measure an individual's total heat production

Exothermic: A type of combustion reaction that gives off heat equal to approximately 1 BTU (0.25 kcal)

First law of thermodynamics: A physical law that establishes that energy can be changed from one state into another as it remains at the same quantity in its various states

Gross energy value: Total energy value for various food macronutrients determined by bomb calorimetry

Heat: Thermal energy and its transfer or exchange from one object or system to another

International System of Units (SI): A complete international system of units used for scientific measurements containing seven standard quantities (time, length, mass, electric current, thermodynamic temperature, substance amount, luminous intensity) and seven corresponding base units (second, meter, kilogram, ampere, kelvin, mole, candela); also known as Système International d'Unités

Joule (J): A standard unit of heat measurement (1 J = 1 Nm)

Kilocalorie (kcal): A unit of energy equivalent to 1000 calories, representing the energy required to raise the temperature of one liter of water 1°C at sea level

Lipid combustion heat: Amount of heat liberated by the complete burning or oxidation of lipid in a bomb calorimeter; averages 9.4 kcal·g^{-1} with complete oxidation

Mass balance model (MBM): Theoretical model that weight loss occurs by creating an imbalance between the food mass intake and corresponding mass elimination from the excretion of food oxidation end-products, not heat produced by the "calories-in, calories-out" traditional way to explain weight loss

Megajoule (MJ): A unit of heat measurement equal to 1 million J, or 1000 kJ

Net energy value: A measure of energy equal to the coefficient of digestibility times the heat of combustion adjusted for energy loss in urine

Protein combustion heat: Amount of heat liberated by the complete burning or oxidation of protein in a bomb calorimeter; averages 5.65 kcal·g^{-1} based on an average nitrogen content of 16%

Temperature: A relative, quantitative measure of an object's hotness or coldness on a scale to determine the internal energy within a given system

References are available online at Lippincott Connect.

Additional References

Alghannam AF, et al. Regulation of energy substrate metabolism in endurance exercise. *Int J Environ Res Public Health.* 2021;18:4963.

Arencibia-Albite F. Serious analytical inconsistencies challenge the validity of the energy balance theory. *Heliyon.* 2020;6:e04204.

Burke LM. Ketogenic low-CHO, high-fat diet: the future of elite endurance sport? *J Physiol.* 2021;599:819.

Cao J, et al. The effect of a ketogenic low-carbohydrate, high-fat diet on aerobic capacity and exercise performance in endurance athletes: a systematic review and meta-analysis. *Nutrients.* 2021;13:2896.

Coleman JL, et al. Body composition changes in physically active individuals consuming ketogenic diets: a systematic review. *J Int Soc Sports Nutr.* 2021;18:41.

Collins J, et al. UEFA expert group statement on nutrition in elite football. Current evidence to inform practical recommendations and guide future research. *Br J Sports Med.* 2021;55:416.

Devrim-Lanpir A, et al. Efficacy of popular diets applied by endurance athletes on sports performance: beneficial or detrimental? A narrative review. *Nutrients.* 2021;13:491.

Gejl KD, Nybo L. Performance effects of periodized carbohydrate restriction in endurance trained athletes—a systematic review and meta-analysis. *J Int Soc Sports Nutr.* 2021;18:37.

Halsey LG. The mystery of energy compensation. *Physiol Biochem Zool.* 2021;94:380.

Hannon MP, et al. Key Nutritional considerations for youth winter sports athletes to optimize growth, maturation and sporting development. *Front Sports Act Living.* 2021;3:599118.

Holtzman B, Ackerman KE. Recommendations and nutritional considerations for female athletes: health and performance. *Sports Med.* 2021;51:43.

Lee HS, Lee J. Influences of ketogenic diet on body fat percentage, respiratory exchange rate, and total cholesterol in athletes: a systematic review and meta-analysis. *Int J Environ Res Public Health.* 2021;18:2912.

Palacios C, et al. Current calcium fortification experiences: a review. *Ann N Y Acad Sci.* 2021;1484:55.

Ribeiro F, et al. Timing of creatine supplementation around exercise: a real concern? *Nutrients.* 2021;13:2844.

Riviere AJ, et al. Nutrition knowledge of collegiate athletes in the United States and the impact of sports dietitians on related outcomes: a narrative review. *Nutrients.* 2021;13:1772.

Shaw KA, et al. Dietary Supplementation for para-athletes: a systematic review. *Nutrients.* 2021;13:2016.

Sprengell M, et al. Brain more resistant to energy restriction than body: a systematic review. *Front Neurosci.* 2021;15:639617.

Table 4.1 — Factors for Digestibility, Heats of Combustion, and Net Physiologic Energy Values of Protein, Lipid, and Carbohydrate

Food Group	Digestibility (%)	Heat of Combustion (kcal·g⁻¹)	Net Energy (kcal·g⁻¹)
Protein			
Animal food	97	5.65	4.27
Meats, fish	97	5.65	4.27
Eggs	97	5.75	4.37
Dairy products	97	5.65	4.27
Vegetable food	85	5.65	3.74
Cereals	85	5.80	3.87
Legumes	78	5.70	3.47
Vegetables	83	5.00	3.11
Fruits	85	5.20	3.36
Average protein	92	5.65	4.05
Lipid			
Meat and eggs	95	9.50	9.03
Dairy products	95	9.25	8.79
Animal food	95	9.40	8.93
Vegetable food	90	9.30	8.37
Average lipid	95	9.40	8.93
Carbohydrate			
Animal food	98	3.90	3.82
Cereals	98	4.20	4.11
Legumes	97	4.20	4.07
Vegetables	95	4.20	3.99
Fruits	90	4.00	3.60
Sugars	98	3.95	3.87
Vegetable food	97	4.15	4.03
Average carbohydrate	97	4.15	4.03

Note: Net physiologic energy values reflect the coefficient of digestibility multiplied by the heat of combustion adjusted for energy loss in urine.
From Merrill AL, Watt BK. *Energy values of foods: basis and derivation. Agricultural Handbook no. 74.* Washington, DC: USDA; 1973.

Table 4.2 — Method to Compute a Food's Caloric Value from Its Macronutrient Composition

Food: Ice cream (vanilla)
Weight: 3/4 cup = 100 g

	Composition		
	Protein	Lipid	Carbohydrate
Percentage	4	13	21
Total g	4	13	21
In 1 g	0.04	0.13	0.21
Calories per g	0.16	1.17	0.84
	(0.04 × 4.0 kcal)	(0.13 × 9.0 kcal)	(0.21 × 4.0 kcal)

CHAPTER 5
Introduction to Energy Transfer

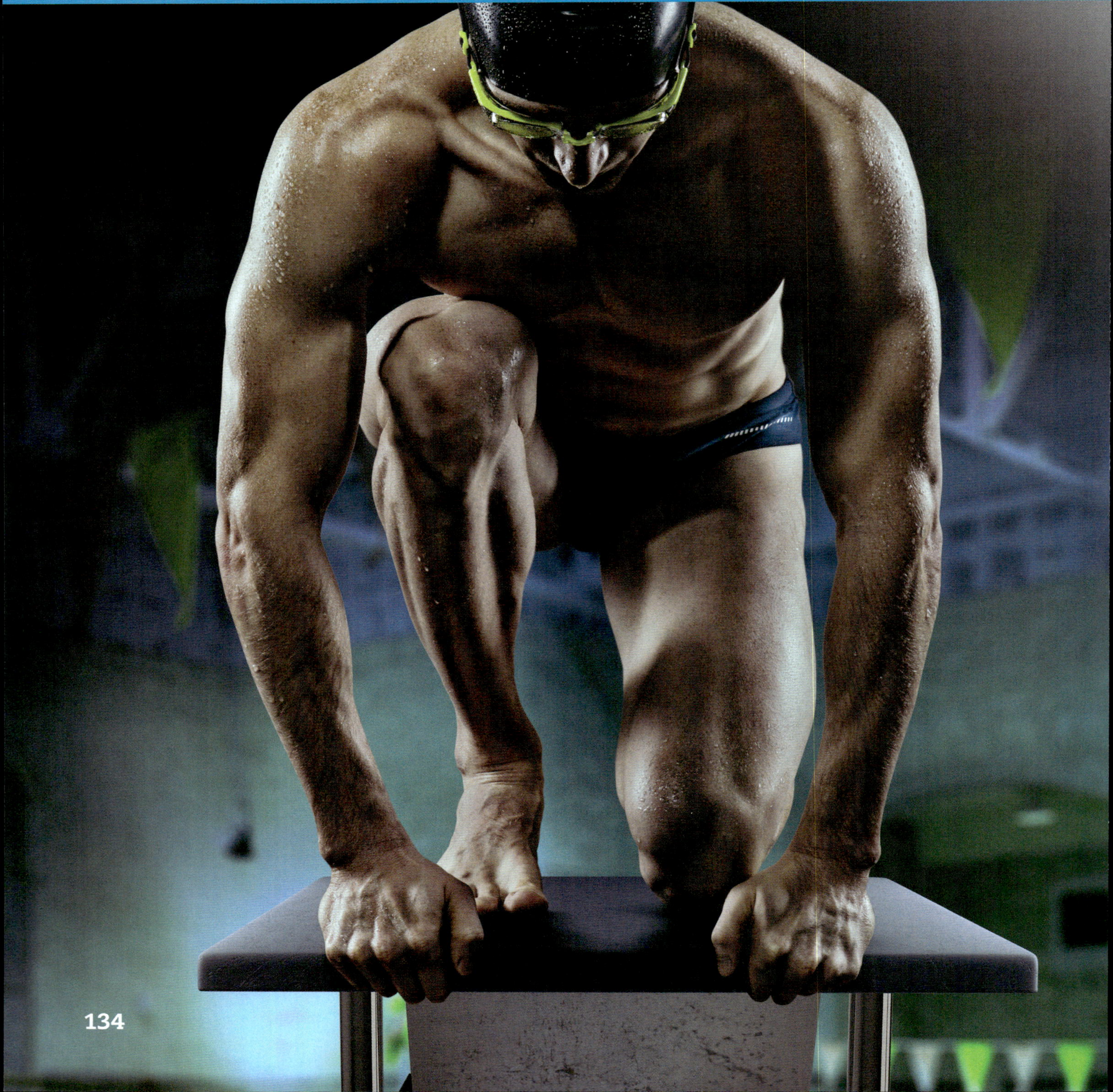

Chapter Objectives

- Explain how the first law of thermodynamics relates to energy balance and work within biologic systems
- Define potential energy and kinetic energy and give two examples for each
- Discuss free energy's role during biologic work
- Give two examples for exergonic and endergonic chemical reactions within the body and their importance
- Explain the second law of thermodynamics and give two practical applications
- Discuss coupled reaction's role in biologic processes
- Differentiate between photosynthesis and respiration and the biologic significance of each
- Identify the three forms of biologic work and give two examples of each form
- Explain how enzymes and coenzymes affect energy metabolism
- Differentiate between hydrolysis and condensation and explain their importance to physiologic function
- Explain the role redox chemical reactions play in energy metabolism

Ancillaries at-a-Glance

Visit Lippincott Connect to access the following resources.

- Reference: Chapter 5
- Animations: Condensation, Hydrolysis
- Focus on Research: Valid Determination for Oxygen Uptake

The capacity to extract energy from food macronutrients and continually transfer it rapidly to skeletal muscle's contractile elements determines one's capacity for prolonged physical activity. Likewise, specific energy-transferring capacities that demand all-out, "explosive" power output for brief durations determine success in weightlifting, sprinting, jumping, and football line play. Muscular activity, as do all forms of biologic work, requires power generated from the direct transfer of chemical energy. *Ingested food's nutrient breakdown provides the energy source for synthesizing chemical fuel that powers all forms of biologic work.*

The sections that follow introduce general concepts about bioenergetics, with application to energy metabolism during all physical activity modes.

Energy: The Capacity for Work

Unlike the physical properties of matter, one cannot define *energy* concretely in terms of size, shape, or mass. Rather, the term *energy* reflects a dynamic state related to *change*, so energy becomes apparent only when change occurs. Within this context, **energy transfer** relates to work performance—as work increases, change occurs proportionally to the energy transferred among molecules, cells, substances, compounds, tissues, and different body systems. From a mechanical perspective, work refers to the product of a given force acting through a given distance (force × distance). In the body, cells more commonly accomplish chemical and electrical work than mechanical work.

Bioenergetics refers to both energy flow and energy exchange within living systems. The first law of thermodynamics, which was verified in the 1850s by German scientists Rudolf Clausius (1822–1888) and Scottish chemist William Thomson (1824–1907; www.wolframscience.com/reference/notes/1019b), described a fundamental principle linked to biologic work. Its basic tenet states that energy can neither be created nor destroyed but transforms from one form to another without being depleted during the transfer process. In essence, this law describes the important **conservation of energy principle** that applies to living and nonliving systems. In the body, chemical energy within macronutrient bonds does not immediately dissipate as heat during energy metabolism; instead, a large portion remains as chemical energy, which the musculoskeletal system configures into mechanical energy and ultimately to heat energy. *The first law of thermodynamics requires that the body does not produce, consume, or use up energy; instead, it transforms it from one state into another as physiologic systems undergo continual change.*

INTEGRATIVE QUESTION

Why is it imprecise to refer to the body's energy "production" when considering the first law of thermodynamics?

Potential and Kinetic Energy

The total energy of the body's physiologic systems includes both potential energy and kinetic energy. **FIGURE 5.1.** illustrates potential energy as positional energy, similar to water cresting over a dam. In the flowing water example, energy change remains proportional to the water's vertical drop—the greater the vertical drop, the greater the potential energy before the drop. A waterwheel inserted into the water flow harnesses some energy to produce useful work. For a falling boulder, all the potential energy transforms to kinetic energy and dissipates to the environment as unusable heat.

Other potential energy examples include bound energy within a battery's internal structure, a dynamite stick, and a macronutrient before releasing its stored energy in metabolism. *The release of potential energy transforms it into kinetic energy of motion.* In some cases, bound energy in one substance directly transfers to other substances to increase their potential energy. This type of energy transfer provides the required energy for the body's chemical work of **biosynthesis**. In this process, specific building-block carbon, hydrogen, oxygen, and nitrogen atoms join other atoms and molecules to synthesize important biologic compounds and tissues. Some newly created compounds provide structure, as, for example, bone or the bilayer lipid-containing plasma membrane that encapsulates all cells. The synthesized high energy compounds **adenosine triphosphate (ATP)** and **phosphocreatine** contribute to every cell's energy requirements.

Energy-Releasing and Energy-Conserving Processes

Exergonic describes any physical or chemical process that releases energy to its surroundings. Such reactions represent "downhill" processes because of a decline in free energy— "useful" energy to support the cell's continuing energy-requiring, life-sustaining processes. Normally, a cell's internal pressure and

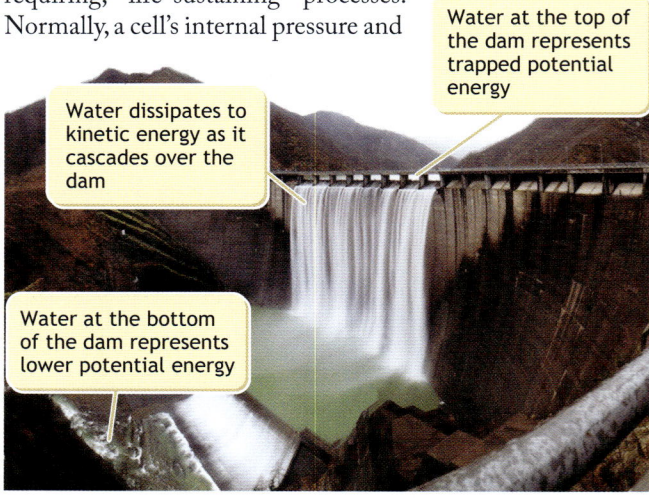

FIGURE 5.1. High-grade potential energy powering work degrades to an unusable kinetic energy form. In the example, water falling over the dam represents potential energy, which dissipates to kinetic heat energy as water crashes below. (Iafoto/Shutterstock.)

volume remain relatively stable, and free energy determines the potential energy within a molecule's chemical bonds. The following relationship describes free energy quantitatively:

$$G = H - TS$$

where G = free energy (denoted by the symbol G to honor American scientist Josiah Willard Gibbs [1839–1903; https://mathshistory.st-andrews.ac.uk/Biographies/Gibbs/], whose theoretical research provided the foundation for biochemical thermodynamics), H = **enthalpy** (thermodynamic measure of the thermal energy change in a reaction), S = randomness from energy unavailability, and T = (temperature °C + 273).

Endergonic chemical reactions store or absorb energy; they represent "uphill" processes and proceed with an increase in free energy for biologic work. An endergonic reaction proceeds because the reaction's product has more energy than the reactant. Exergonic reactions release energy, resulting in less energy in the product than in the reactant. Exergonic chemical processes sometimes link or *couple* with endergonic reactions to transfer some energy to the endergonic process. In the body, coupled reactions conserve in usable form a large portion of the chemical energy stored within a macronutrient, as described in a useful article with accompanying video (www.thoughtco.com/endergonic-vs-exergonic-609258).

FIGURE 5.2 illustrates energy flow in endergonic and exergonic chemical reactions. Free energy change occurs when the reactant molecule's bonds form new product molecules with different bonding. In endergonic reactions, the new product receives the energy. In exergonic reactions, energy release occurs as the reactant's energy "flows downhill." An important equation expresses these changes under constant temperature, pressure, and volume conditions:

$$\Delta G = \Delta H - T\Delta S$$

The symbol Δ (delta) designates change. The change in free energy represents a keystone of chemical reactions. ΔG remains negative in exergonic reactions—the products contain *less* free energy than the reactants, with the energy differential released as heat. For example, the union of hydrogen with oxygen to form water releases 68 kcal·mol⁻¹ (molecular weight in grams) free energy in the following reaction:

$$H_2 + O \rightarrow H_2O - \Delta G\ 68\ \text{kcal} \cdot \text{mol}^{-1}$$

In the reverse endergonic reaction, ΔG stays positive because the product contains *more* free energy than the reactant. Releasing 68 kcal energy per water mole causes water's chemical bonds to split apart, freeing the original hydrogen and oxygen atoms. This "uphill" energy transfer process allows the hydrogen and oxygen atoms with their original energy content to satisfy the basic tenant of the first law of thermodynamics—*the conservation of energy.*

$$H_2 + O \leftarrow H_2O + \Delta G\ 68\ \text{kcal} \cdot \text{mol}^{-1}$$

Cellular energy transfer reactions follow the basic principles illustrated in the Figure 5.1 waterfall example. Carbohydrate, lipid, and protein macronutrients possess considerable potential energy within their chemical bonds. Formation of new products progressively *reduces* the nutrient molecule's original potential energy with a corresponding *increase* in kinetic energy. Enzyme-regulated transfer systems harness or conserve some chemical energy in new compounds for biologic work. In essence, living cells serve as transducers with the capacity to extract and use chemical energy stored within a compound's atomic structure. Conversely, and equally important, cells also bind atoms and molecules together to raise them to a *higher* potential energy level. The transfer of potential energy in any spontaneous process always proceeds in a direction that *decreases* the capacity to perform work.

The tendency for potential energy to degrade to kinetic energy of motion with a lower capacity for work (i.e., increased **entropy**) reflects the second law of thermodynamics, described in the 1850s by scientists Rudolf Clausius and William Thomson. A flashlight battery provides a salient illustration. The electrochemical energy stored within its cells slowly dissipates, even if the battery remains unused. Energy from sunlight provides another illustration—it continually degrades to heat energy when light strikes an object and the surface it interacts with absorbs it. Food and other chemicals also represent excellent potential energy storehouses. This stored energy continually decreases as the compounds decompose through normal oxidative processes. Energy, like water, always runs downhill, so potential energy decreases. Ultimately, all potential energy in a biological system degrades to unusable kinetic form or heat energy.

Energy Interconversions

The total energy in a closed system remains constant, so a decrease in one energy form matches an equivalent increase in another energy form. During energy conversions,

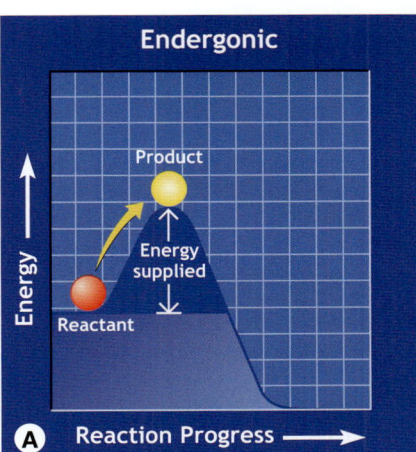
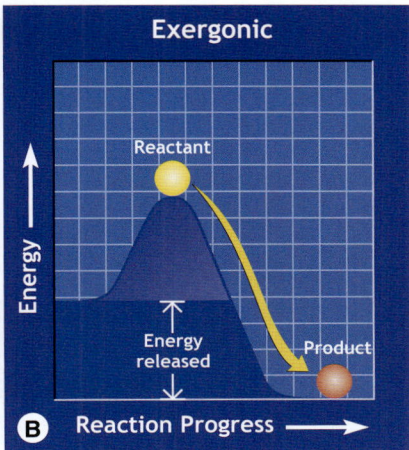

FIGURE 5.2. Energy flow in endergonic (**A**) and exergonic (**B**) chemical reactions.

a loss in potential energy from one source produces a temporary increase in potential energy in another source. This fundamental process in nature allocates tremendous quantities of potential energy for useful purposes. Under the most favorable conditions, however, the net energy flow in the biologic world moves toward entropy, ultimately producing a net potential energy loss. Entropy reflects the continual process of energy change. All chemical and physical processes proceed in a direction in which total randomness or disorder *increases* and the energy available for work *decreases*. In coupled chemical reactions during biosynthesis, one part of a system may decrease in entropy while another part increases. *The second law of thermodynamics can never be circumvented—the entire system always reveals a net entropy increase.*

Six Energy Categories

FIGURE 5.3 shows energy placed into six categories—chemical, mechanical, heat, light, electrical, and nuclear.

Energy Interconversion Examples

Energy interconversions, from one form to another, occur routinely in both the inanimate and animate worlds. In living cells, **photosynthesis** and **respiration** represent key fundamental examples of energy interconversions.

Photosynthesis. In the sun, **nuclear fusion** releases the potential energy stored in the hydrogen atom's nucleus. The penetrating electromagnetic radiation or gamma radiation then converts to radiant energy.

FIGURE 5.4. depicts photosynthesis dynamics, an endergonic process powered by sunlight's energy. The photosynthetic green pigment chlorophyll ($C_{55}H_{70}MgN_4O_6$), contained in large chloroplast organelles within a leaf's cells, traps radiant solar energy to synthesize glucose from carbon dioxide and water, while its by-product oxygen flows to the environment. Plants also convert carbohydrates to lipids and proteins for storage as a future energy reserve and to sustain growth. Animals then ingest plant nutrients to serve their own energy and growth needs. *In essence, solar energy coupled with photosynthesis furnishes animals with food and oxygen.*

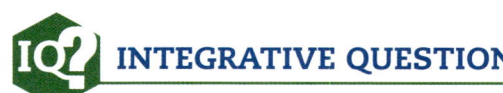

INTEGRATIVE QUESTION

In human bioenergetics, discuss the significance of the statement: "Have you thanked a green plant today?"

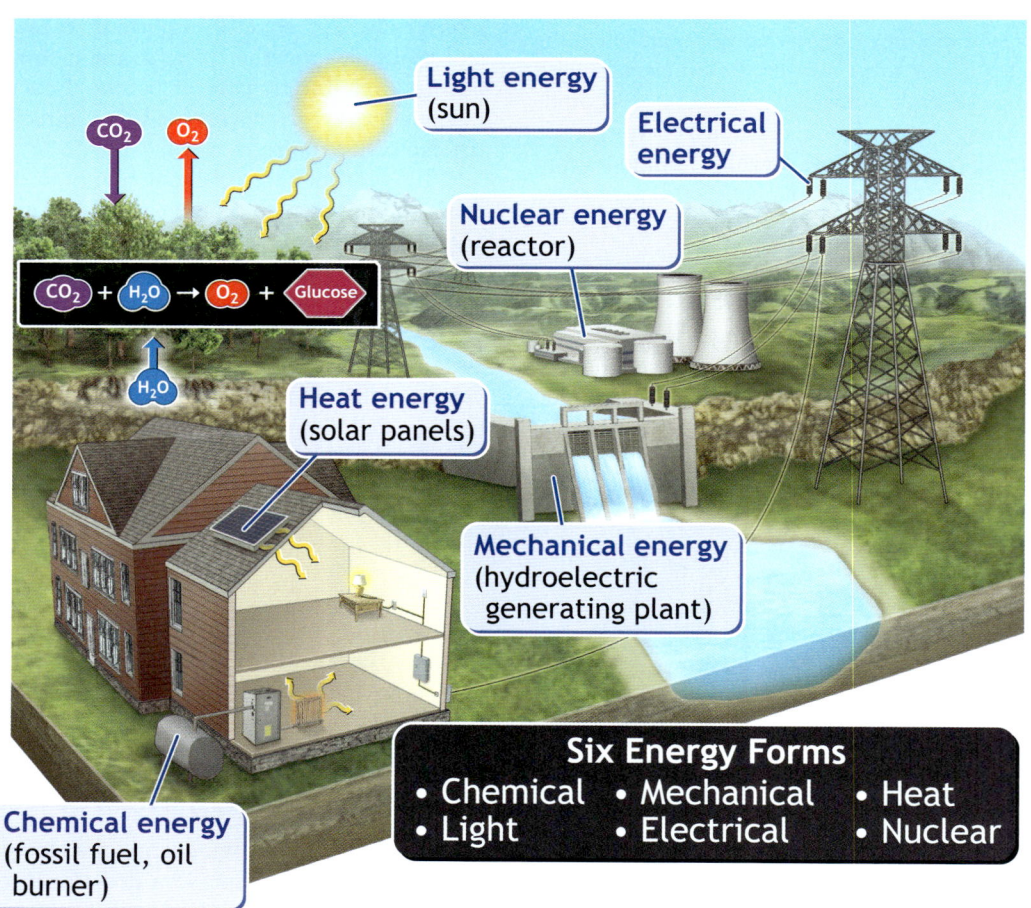

FIGURE 5.3. Interconversions among six energy forms.

Mechanical Work

Mechanical work generated by muscle action and subsequent movement provides an obvious physical example of energy transformation. A muscle fiber's protein filaments directly convert chemical energy into mechanical energy. This does not represent the body's only mechanical work form. In the cell nucleus, contractile elements literally tug at chromosomes to facilitate cell division crucial in inherited characteristics, first discovered in 1902 by German biologist Theodore Boveri (1862–1915) and American geneticist Walter Sutton (1877–1916). "In a Practical Sense" illustrates three common exercise devices to quantify muscular work and power.

Chemical Work

All cells perform chemical work for maintenance and growth. Continuous synthesis of new cellular components occurs as other components degrade. For example, ions can move at extremely rapid rates up and down concentration gradients at speeds up to 10^8 molecules per second across cell membranes to interact with other substances to create new ones, while other specialized transporters move relatively "slowly" at 10^2 to 10^4 molecules per second. Chemical energy transfer occurs most notably from different protein substances during DNA and RNA molecular transformations and in other related molecular substances, which are discussed in Chapter 33.

Muscle tissue hypertrophy that occurs in response to chronic overload in resistance training vividly illustrates chemical work as individual fibers increase their protein contractile content.

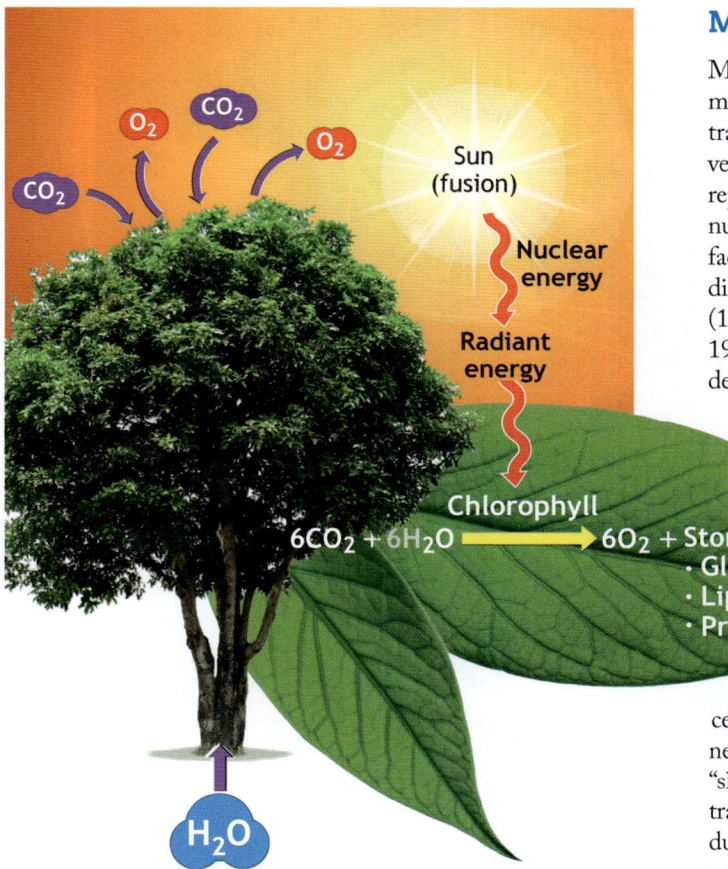

FIGURE 5.4. Endergonic photosynthesis processes in plants, algae, and some bacteria synthesize carbohydrates, lipids, and proteins. A glucose molecule forms when carbon dioxide binds with water with positive, useful free energy change ($+\Delta G$).

Respiration. **FIGURE 5.5** illustrates the exergonic reactions of respiration (reverse of photosynthesis) as the plant's stored energy transfers in the form of ATP for the mechanical work of muscle contraction, chemical work of glycogen, triacylglycerol, and protein synthesis, and transport work that shuttles substances across cell membranes against their concentration gradients. With oxygen, the cells extract the chemical energy stored in the carbohydrate, lipid, and protein molecules. For the glucose molecule ($C_6H_{12}O_6$), respiration releases 689 kcal · mol^{-1} (180 g) oxidized. *Some energy released during* *cellular respiration* *is harnessed in other chemical compounds for use in energy-requiring processes, with the remaining energy flowing as heat to the environment.*

Biologic Work in Humans

Figure 5.5 also illustrates three biologic work categories:

1. **Mechanical work** of active muscles
2. **Chemical work** that synthesizes cellular molecules such as glycogen, triacylglycerol, and protein
3. **Transport work** that concentrates substances such as sodium (Na$^+$) and potassium (K$^+$) ions in the intracellular and extracellular fluids

Transport Work

Concentrating substances in the body's cells progresses much less conspicuously than mechanical or chemical work. Cellular materials normally flow from a high concentration region to a lower concentration region. This passive **diffusion** does not require energy. Under normal physiologic conditions, some chemicals require transport "uphill" from a lower to higher concentration. **Active transport** describes this energy-requiring process. For example, when cells produce ATP in the mitochondria, organelles in the cell membrane pump the ATP up the concentration gradient from a specific cellular *lower* concentration area to a *higher* concentration area. Secretion and reabsorption in the kidney tubules rely on active transport mechanisms, as does neural tissue to establish the proper electrochemical gradients about its plasma membranes. These "quiet" forms of biologic work require a continual expenditure of stored chemical energy.

Enzymes and Coenzymes: Energy Release Rate Alteration

The upper exercise intensity limits ultimately depend on the rate that cells extract, conserve, and transfer chemical energy from food

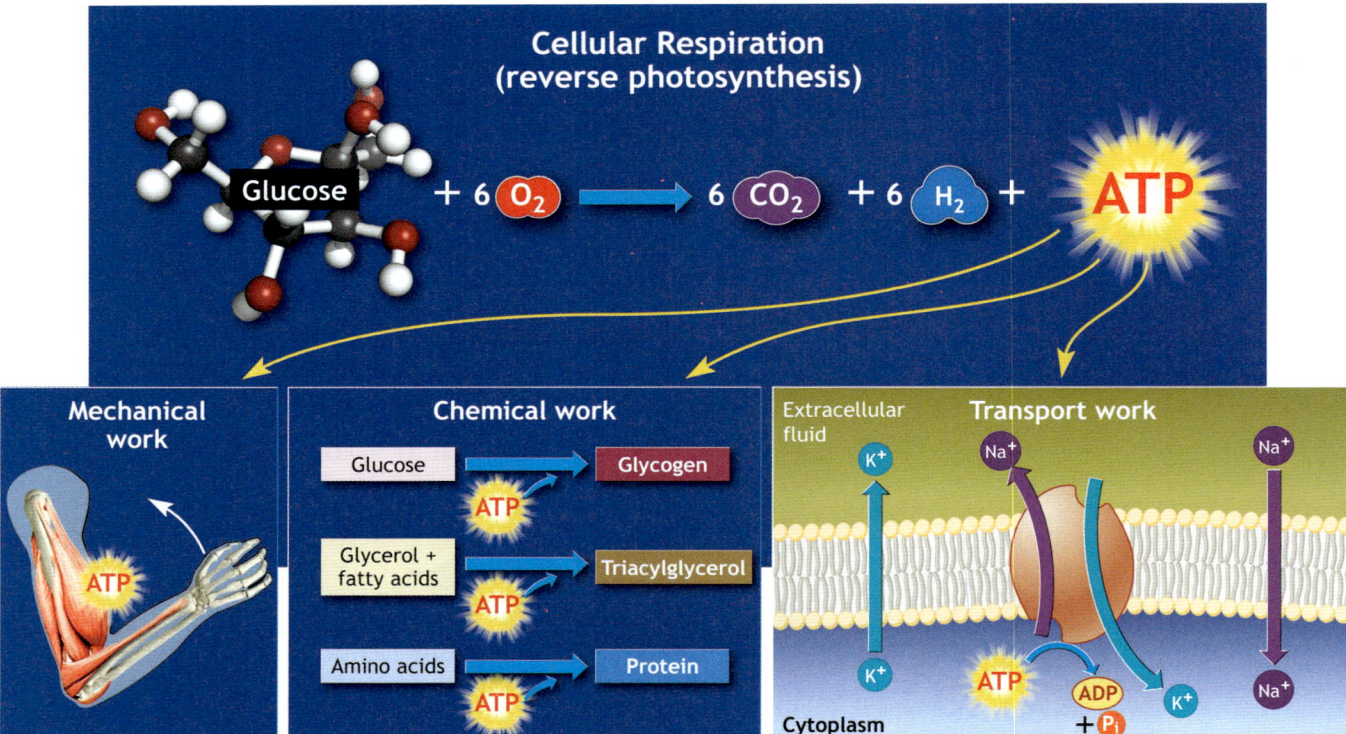

FIGURE 5.5. Exergonic cellular respiration (reverse photosynthesis). Exergonic reactions release potential energy to produce a negative standard free energy change ($-\Delta G$). The top image highlights how cellular respiration harvests food's potential energy to form ATP to power all mechanical, chemical, and transport work forms.
(Shutterstock: StudioMolekuul; Mitar Vidakovic.)

nutrients to the skeletal muscle's contractile filaments. *Sustaining marathon pace at close to 90% aerobic capacity or a sprinter's speed in all-out running directly reflects the body's capacity to transfer chemical energy and transform it into mechanical work.*

Enzymes as Biologic Catalysts

Enzymes, highly specific and large protein catalysts, accelerate forward and reverse chemical reaction rates without being consumed or changed during the reaction. Enzymes only govern reactions that normally take place, but at a much slower rate. In a way, enzymes reduce required **activation energy**—the energy input to initiate a reaction—so the reaction's rate changes. Enzyme action takes place without altering equilibrium constants and total energy released (free energy change or ΔG) in the reaction. **TABLE 5.1** presents the six enzyme classifications.

Table 5.1 Six enzyme classification types, main functions, and the controlling enzymes

Enzymes cannot be readily altered by the reactions they affect. Consequently, enzyme turnover in the body remains slow, and specific enzymes are continually reused. A typical mitochondrion may contain up to 10 billion enzyme molecules, each carrying out millions of operations within milliseconds (1 s equal 1000 ms). During all-out physical activity, enzyme activity increases as energy demands rise about 100 times resting levels. A single cell can contain thousands of different enzymes, each with a specific function that catalyzes a distinct cellular reaction. In the body, for example, glucose breakdown to carbon dioxide and water with the release of energy for use in biologic work shown in the reaction below requires 19 different chemical reactions, each catalyzed by its own specific enzyme.

$$C_6H_{12}O_6 + 6O_2 = 6CO_2 + 6H_2O + \text{Energy}$$
Glucose Oxygen   Carbon   Water   Chemical (40%)
                 Dioxide   Heat (60%)

Many enzymes operate outside the cell—in the bloodstream, digestive mixture, or intestinal fluids.

Enzymes and Reaction Rate Alteration

Enzymes operate along a continuum from exceedingly fast to relatively slow. Consider the enzyme carbonic anhydrase, which catalyzes carbon dioxide (CO_2) hydration to form carbonic acid (H_2CO_2). Its maximum **turnover number**, the number of substrate moles that react to form a product per enzyme mole per unit time, approximates 800,000. In contrast, the turnover number is only two for tryptophan synthetase, which catalyzes the final step in tryptophan synthesis. This essential amino acid required in the diet for normal infant growth and to maintain nitrogen balance in adults was discovered by English Nobel prize biochemist Frederick Gowland Hopkins (1861–1947) in 1901.

In a Practical Sense

Measuring Work on a Treadmill, Cycle Ergometer, and Step Bench

An **ergometer**, an exercise apparatus that quantifies and standardizes movement relating to work and/or power, includes treadmills, cycle and arm-crank ergometers, stair steppers, and rowers.

Work (W) represents application of force (F) through a distance (D):

$$W = F \times D$$

For example, for a body mass of 70 kg and vertical jump score of 0.5 m, work accomplished equals 35 kilogram-meters (70 kg × 0.5 m). The most common work measurement units include kilogram-meters (kg-m), foot-pounds (ft-lb), joules, Newton-meters, and kilocalories (kcal).

Power (P) represents W performed per unit time (T):

$$P = F \times D \div T$$

TREADMILL WORK CALCULATION

Consider the treadmill a moving conveyor belt with a variable angle of incline and speed. Work performed on a treadmill equals the product of the weight (mass) of the person (F) and the vertical distance (vert distance) the person achieves walking or running up the incline. Vert distance equals the sine of the treadmill angle (theta, or θ) multiplied by the distance traveled (D) along the incline (treadmill speed × time):

$$W = \text{body mass (force)} \times \text{vertical distance (D)}$$

ANGLES (°) AND SINE θ FOR DIFFERENT PERCENT AGE GRADES (%)

Angle (°)	Sine θ	Grade (%)
1	0.0175	1.75
2	0.0349	3.49
3	0.0523	5.23
4	0.0698	6.98
5	0.0872	8.72
6	0.1045	10.51
7	0.1219	12.28
8	0.1392	14.05
9	0.1564	15.84
10	0.1736	17.63
15	0.2588	26.80
20	0.3420	36.40

Example

For an angle θ of 8° (measured with an inclinometer or determined by knowing the percent age grade of the treadmill), the sine of angle θ equals 0.1392 (see table). The vert distance D represents treadmill speed multiplied by duration multiplied by sine θ. For example, D on the incline while walking at 5000 m · h^{-1} for 1 h equals 696 m (5000 × 0.1392). If a person weighing 50 kg walks on a treadmill at an incline of 8° (grade approximately 14%) for 60 min at 5000 m · hr^{-1}, work accomplished computes as

$$W = F \times \text{Vert D (Sine } \theta \times D)$$
$$= 50 \text{ kg} \times (0.1395 \times 5000 \text{ m})$$
$$= 34{,}800 \text{ kg-m}$$

The value for power equals 34,800 kg-m ÷ 60 min, or 580 kg-m · min^{-1}.

CYCLE ERGOMETER WORK CALCULATION

Most mechanically braked cycle ergometers contain a flywheel with a belt around it connected by a small spring at one end and an adjustable tension lever at the other end. As the wheel turns, a pendulum balance indicates the resistance against the flywheel. Increasing belt tension increases flywheel friction, which increases resistance to pedaling. The force (flywheel friction) represents braking load in kg or **kilopounds (kp**; kp = force acting on 1-kg mass at the normal acceleration of gravity). The distance traveled equals pedal revolution number multiplied by flywheel circumference.

Example

A person pedaling a bicycle ergometer with a 6-m flywheel circumference at 60 rpm for 1 min covers a distance (D) = 360 m each min (6 m × 60 rpm). If the flywheel's frictional resistance equals 2.5 kg, total work computes as

$$W = F \times D$$
$$= \text{frictional ressitance} \times \text{distance traveled}$$
$$= 2.5 \text{ kg} \times 360 \text{ m}$$
$$= 900 \text{ kg-m}$$

Power generated by the effort equals 900 kg-m in 1 min, or 900 kg-m · min^{-1} (900 kg-m ÷ min).

BENCH STEPPING WORK CALCULATION

Only the vertical (positive) work calculates during bench stepping. Distance (D) computes as bench height times step number; force (F) equals the person's body mass (kg).

Example

If a 70-kg person steps up and down a 0.375-m high bench at 30 steps per min for 10 min, total work computes as

$$W = F \times D$$
$$= \text{body mass, kg} \times (\text{vertical distance [m]}$$
$$\times \text{steps per min} \times 10 \text{ min})$$
$$= 70 \text{ kg} \times (0.375 \text{ m} \times 30 \times 10)$$
$$= 7875 \text{ kg-m}^{-1}$$

Power generated during stepping equals 787 kg-m · min^{-1} (7875 kg-m ÷ 10 min).

Enzymes also act along small regions of substrate, each time working at a different rate than previously. Some enzymes delay initiating their work. The precursor digestive enzyme trypsinogen, manufactured by the pancreas in its inactive form, serves as a good example. Trypsinogen enters the small intestine where enzyme action activates it and changes its molecular configuration so it now becomes the active enzyme trypsin first discovered in 1876 by German chemist Wilhelm Kuhne (1837–1900). This "changed" enzyme breaks down complex proteins into simple amino acids. Without the delay in activity, trypsinogen would literally digest the pancreatic tissue that produced it.

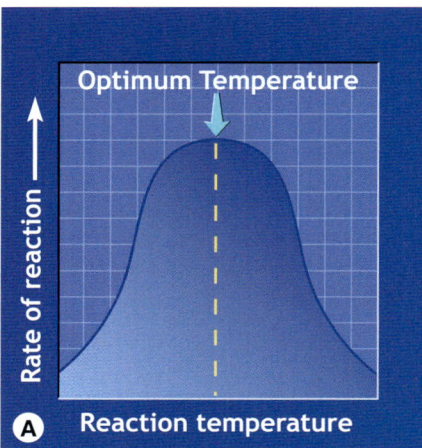 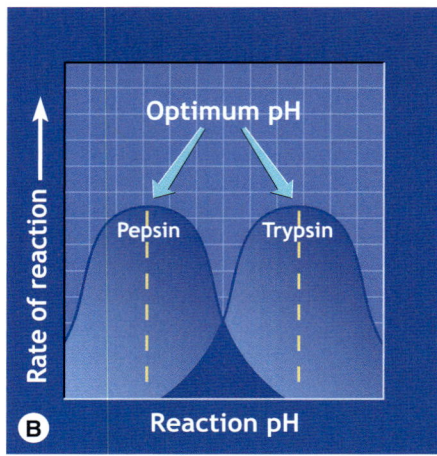

FIGURE 5.6. **(A)** Reaction temperature and **(B)** reaction pH effects on enzyme action turnover rate.

FIGURE 5.6 shows that pH and temperature dramatically alter enzyme activity to change reaction rates. For some enzymes, peak activity requires high acidity, whereas others function optimally on the alkaline side of neutrality. Note that the two enzymes pepsin and trypsin (Fig. 5.6B) exhibit different pH profiles that modify their activity rates and determine optimal function. Pepsin operates optimally at a pH between 2.4 and 2.6, whereas trypsin's optimum range approximates saliva and milk's value of 6.2 to 6.6. This pH effect on enzyme dynamics takes place because changing a fluid's hydrogen ion concentration alters the balance between positively and negatively charged molecular complexes in the enzyme's amino acids. Increases in temperature generally accelerate enzyme reactivity. As temperature rises above 104°F/40°C to 122°F/50°C, the protein enzymes permanently alter their natural qualities (called denaturing), causing their activity to cease.

Enzyme Action

An enzyme's unique three-dimensional globular protein structure defines the interaction with its specific substrate. **FIGURE 5.7** illustrates how this interaction works similarly to a key fitting a lock. The enzyme "turns on" when its active site, usually a groove, cleft, or cavity on the protein's surface, joins in a "perfect fit" with the substrate's active site illustrated in the figure. Upon forming an enzyme-substrate complex, the splitting of chemical bonds forms a new product with new bonds. This immediately frees the enzyme to act on additional substrate. A more contemporary hypothesis considers the "lock-and-key mechanism" more of an "induced fit" because of the required conformational characteristics of enzymes. This is outlined in the three-step sequence for the maltase enzyme as it disassembles or hydrolyzes maltase into its component two glucose building blocks:

Step 1: The enzyme's active site and substrate align for a perfect fit to form an enzyme-substrate complex.
Step 2: The enzyme catalyzes (accelerates) the chemical reaction with the substrate. Note the hydrolysis reaction adds a water molecule.
Step 3: Two glucose molecule end products form, freeing the enzyme to act on additional substrate.

German chemist and 1902 Nobel laureate Emil Fischer (1852–1919; www.nobelprize.org/prizes/chemistry/1902/fischer/biographical/) first proposed the lock-and-key mechanism to describe enzyme-substrate interactions. This process ensures that the correct enzyme "mates" with its specific substrate to perform a specific function. Once the enzyme and substrate join, a *conformational change* in enzyme shape takes place as it molds to the substrate. Even if an enzyme links with a substrate, unless the specific conformational change occurs in the enzyme's shape, it will not interact chemically with the substrate.

The lock-and-key mechanism serves a protective function so only the correct enzyme activates a given substrate. Consider the enzyme hexokinase, which accelerates a chemical reaction by linking with a six-carbon glucose molecule in a process called phosphorylation. When this occurs, a phosphate molecule transfers from ATP to a specific binding site on one of glucose's carbon atoms. Once the two binding sites join to form a glucose-hexokinase complex, the substrate begins its stepwise degradation, controlled by other specific enzymes, to form fewer complex molecules during energy metabolism.

Coenzymes

Some enzymes remain totally dormant unless activated by additional **coenzyme** substances. These nonprotein organic substances facilitate enzyme action by binding the substrate with a specific enzyme. Coenzymes then regenerate to assist in further similar reactions. The metallic ions iron and zinc play coenzyme roles, as do the B vitamins or their derivatives. Oxidation-reduction reactions use the B vitamins riboflavin and niacin, whereas other vitamins serve as transfer agents for groups of compounds in different metabolic processes (see Table 2.1).

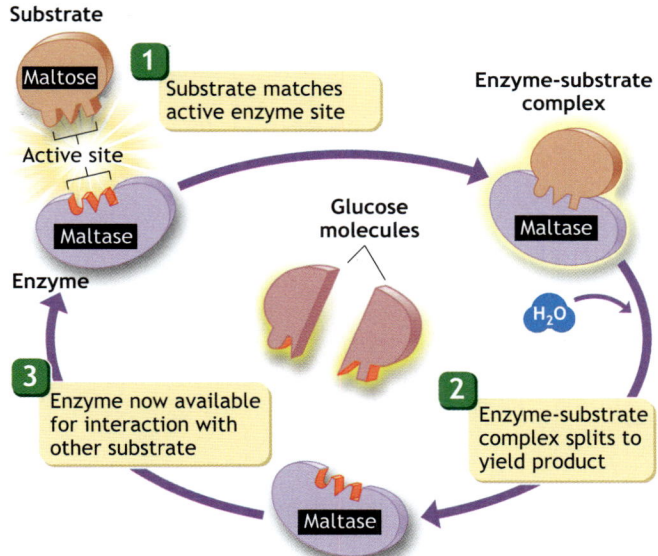

FIGURE 5.7. Sequence of steps in the "lock-and-key mechanism" of an enzyme with its substrate at the "active site." Example illustrates how two monosaccharide glucose molecules form when maltase interacts with its disaccharide substrate maltose.

Vitamins Serve as Coenzymes But Do Not Provide Energy

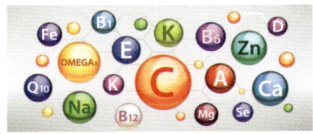
Siberian Art/Shutterstock

Some advertisements for vitamins imply that taking vitamin supplements provides immediate usable energy for exercise. This simply does not occur. Vitamins often serve as coenzymes to "make reactions go," but they contain no chemical energy for biologic work.

A coenzyme requires less specificity in its action than an enzyme because the coenzyme affects different reactions. It acts either as a "cobinder" or temporary carrier of intermediary products in the reaction. For example, the coenzyme **nicotinamide adenine dinucleotide (NAD^+)** forms NADH in transporting hydrogen atoms and electrons released from food fragments during energy metabolism. The electrons then pass to other special transporter molecules in another series of chemical reactions that ultimately deliver the electrons to oxygen.

Enzyme Inhibition

Many substances inhibit enzyme activity to slow a reaction rate. **Competitive inhibitors** closely resemble the enzyme's normal substrate structure. They bind to the enzyme's active site, but the enzyme cannot change them. The inhibitor repetitively occupies the active site and blunts the enzyme's interaction with its substrate. **Noncompetitive inhibitors** do not resemble the enzyme's substrate and do not bind to its active site. Instead, they bind to the enzyme at a site other than the active site. This changes the enzyme's structure and ability to catalyze the reaction because of the presence of the bound inhibitor. Some drugs used in treatment of cancer, depression, and acquired immunodeficiency syndrome act as noncompetitive enzyme inhibitors (as do some poisons, pesticides, antibiotics, and painkillers).

Hydrolysis and Condensation: The Basis for Digestion and Synthesis

In general, hydrolysis reactions digest or degrade complex molecules into simpler subunits; condensation reactions build larger molecules by bonding their subunits.

Hydrolysis Reactions

Hydrolysis catabolizes carbohydrates, lipids, and proteins into simpler forms that the body absorbs and assimilates. This basic decomposition process splits chemical bonds by adding H^+ and OH^- to the reaction by-products. Hydrolytic reactions include starch and disaccharide digestion to monosaccharides, proteins to amino acids, and lipids to their glycerol and fatty acid constituents. Specific enzymes catalyze each breakdown step in the process. For disaccharides, the enzymes are lactase (lactose), sucrase (sucrose), and maltase (maltose). The lipid enzymes called lipases degrade the triacylglycerol molecule by adding water. This cleaves the fatty acids from their glycerol backbone. During protein digestion, protease enzymes accelerate amino acid release when the addition of water splits the peptide linkages. The following represents the general form for all hydrolysis reactions:

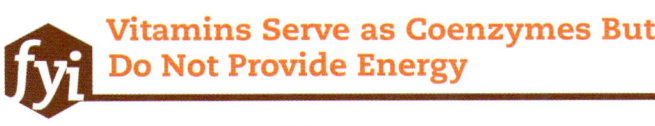

$$AB + HOH \rightarrow A-H + B-OH$$

Water added to the substance AB causes the chemical bond that joins AB to decompose and produce the breakdown products A-H (H refers to a hydrogen atom from water) and B-OH (OH refers to the hydroxyl group from water). **FIGURE 5.8A** illustrates the hydrolysis reaction for the disaccharide sucrose to its end-product molecules glucose and fructose. Note that B reactions show the reverse for the dipeptide hydrolysis reaction, freeing water (H_2O) from the macronutrient glucose and amino acid molecules. This similar degradation process occurs before carbohydrate and lipid macronutrient absorption in the small intestine.

 See the animation "Hydrolysis" at Lippincott Connect to view this process.

Condensation Reactions

Hydrolysis reactions can reverse direction when compound AB synthesizes from A-H and B-OH. One water molecule also forms in this buildup process of **condensation**, also termed *dehydration synthesis*. The nutrients' structural components bind together in condensation reactions to form more complex molecules and compounds. Figure 5.8B shows the condensation reactions for maltose synthesis from two glucose units, and the synthesis of a more complex protein from two amino acid units. In protein synthesis, a hydroxyl group (OH) removed

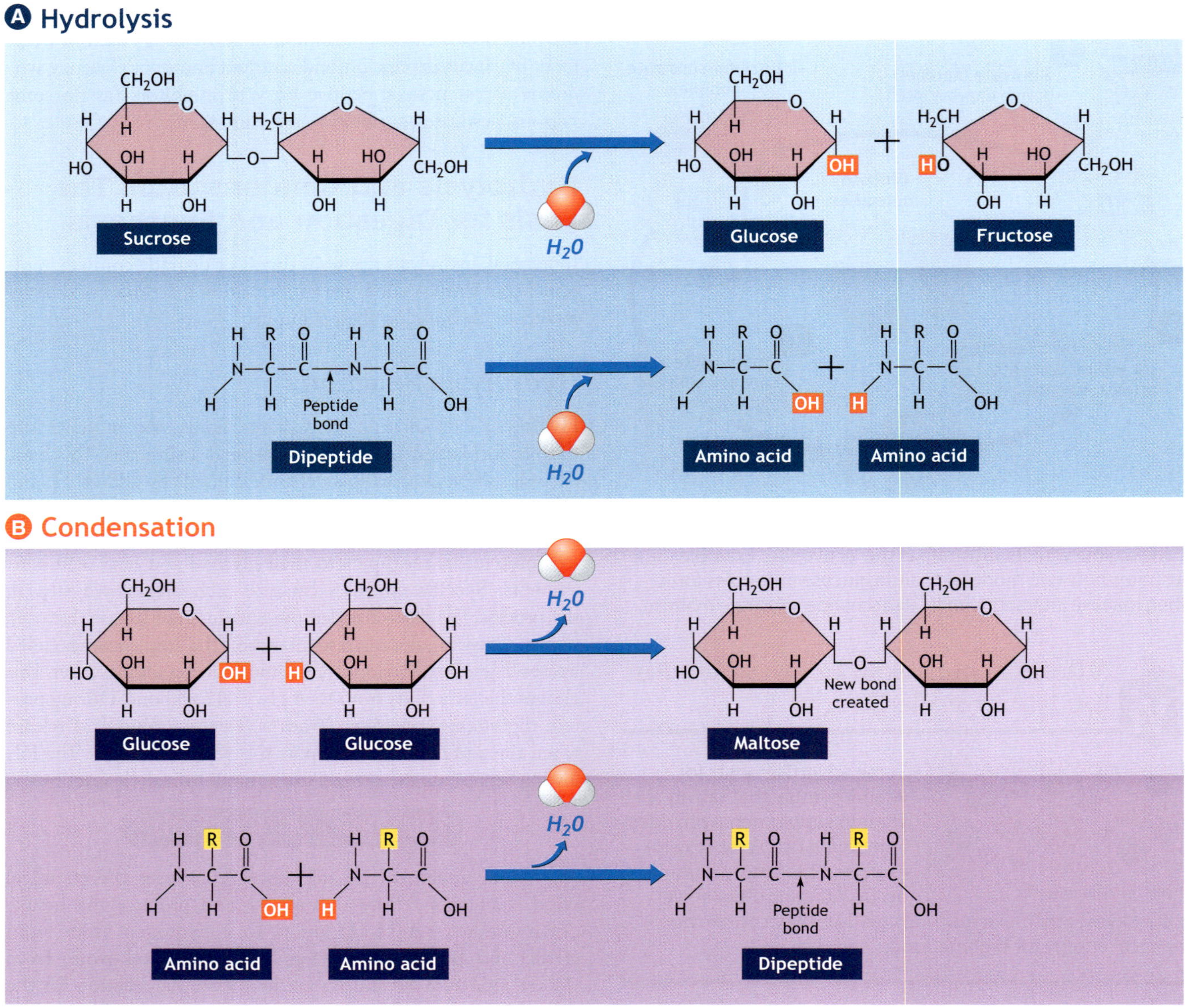

A Hydrolysis

B Condensation

FIGURE 5.8. **(A)** Disaccharide sucrose hydrolysis forms the end-products glucose and fructose molecules, and dipeptide protein hydrolyzes into two amino acid components. **(B)** Condensation chemical reaction synthesizes maltose from two glucose units and creates a protein dipeptide from two amino acid subunits. The symbol *R* in yellow represents the amino acid molecule's remaining atoms and bonds.

from one amino acid and a hydrogen ion (H^+) removed from the other amino acid join to create a water molecule. The term **peptide bond** describes the new protein bond. More complex carbohydrate synthesis from simple sugars also produces water molecules. For lipids, water forms when glycerol and fatty acid components combine to form a triacylglycerol molecule.

 See the animation "Condensation" at Lippincott Connect to view this process.

Oxidation and Reduction Reactions

Thousands of simultaneous chemical reactions involve electron transfer from one substance to another. **Oxidation** reactions *transfer oxygen atoms, hydrogen atoms, or electrons*. An electron *loss* always occurs in oxidation reactions, with a corresponding net valence *gain*. **Reduction** involves a process in which the atoms in an element gain electrons, with a corresponding net decrease in valence.

fyi An Aid to Remember

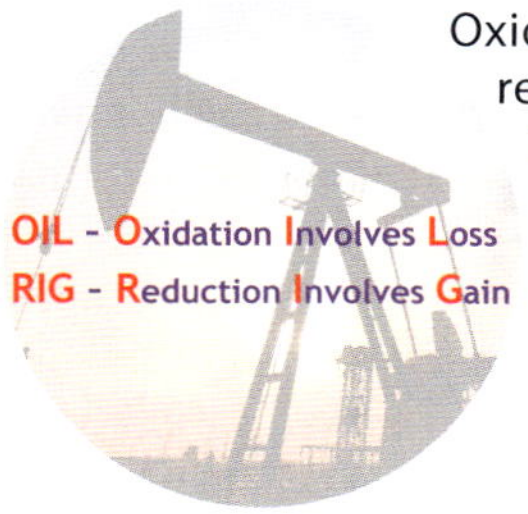

Oxidation involves electron loss and reduction involves electron gain. The mnemonic **OIL RIG** can help you to recall the difference between oxidation and reduction, electron loss, and electron gain.

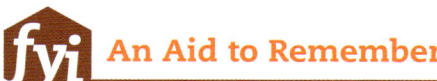

OIL - **O**xidation **I**nvolves **L**oss
RIG - **R**eduction **I**nvolves **G**ain

pan demin/Shutterstock

The term **reducing agent** describes the substance that donates or loses electrons as it oxidizes. The substance reducing or gaining electrons is called the electron acceptor or **oxidizing agent**. Electron transfer requires both oxidizing and reducing agents, and the process of oxidation and reduction are characteristically coupled. Whenever oxidation occurs, the reverse reduction also occurs. That is, when one substance loses electrons, the other substance gains them. The term **redox reaction** describes a coupled oxidation-reduction reaction.

An example redox reaction involves electron transfer within a mitochondrion. Here, special carrier molecules transfer oxidized hydrogen atoms and their removed electrons to oxygen, which becomes reduced. The carbohydrate, lipid, and protein substrates provide a ready source of hydrogen atoms. Dehydrogenase (oxidase) enzymes (see Table 5.1) accelerate the redox reactions. Two hydrogen-accepting dehydrogenase coenzymes are the vitamin B–containing NAD^+ and flavin adenine dinucleotide (FAD). Transferring electrons from NADH to $FADH_2$ harnesses energy in the form of ATP.

Energy release in glucose oxidation occurs when electrons reposition as they move closer to oxygen atoms, their final destination. **FIGURE 5.9** shows the mitochondrion and its intramitochondrial structures, and the inset table summarizes the different chemical events in relation to mitochondrial structures.

IQ2 INTEGRATIVE QUESTION

What biologic benefit comes from the coupling of oxidation and reduction reactions?

The transport of electrons by specific carrier molecules constitutes the respiratory chain. **Electron transport** represents the final common pathway in oxidative (aerobic) metabolism by specific carrier molecules. For each hydrogen atom pair, two electrons flow down the chain and reduce one oxygen atom. The process terminates when oxygen accepts two hydrogens to form water. This coupled redox process constitutes hydrogen oxidation and subsequent oxygen reduction. Chemical energy conserved or "trapped" during cellular oxidation-reduction creates the energy-rich ATP molecule that powers all forms of biologic work.

FIGURE 5.10 illustrates redox (oxidation-reduction) reactions from light to strenuous physical activity. As physical effort intensifies, hydrogen atoms strip away from the carbohydrate substrate faster than their oxidation along the respiratory chain. To continue energy metabolism, a substance other than oxygen must "accept" the nonoxidized excess hydrogens. This occurs when pyruvate, an intermediate molecule formed in carbohydrate catabolism's initial phase, accepts a pair of hydrogens (electrons) to form ionized lactic acid or lactate in the body. More intense activity produces greater excess hydrogen flow to pyruvate and forms lactate, which rises rapidly in blood and active muscles. In recovery, the excess hydrogens in lactate oxidize (electrons removed and passed to NAD^+) to reform a pyruvate molecule, with the enzyme lactate dehydrogenase accelerating this reversal. Chapter 6 more fully discusses oxidation-reduction reactions in human energy metabolism.

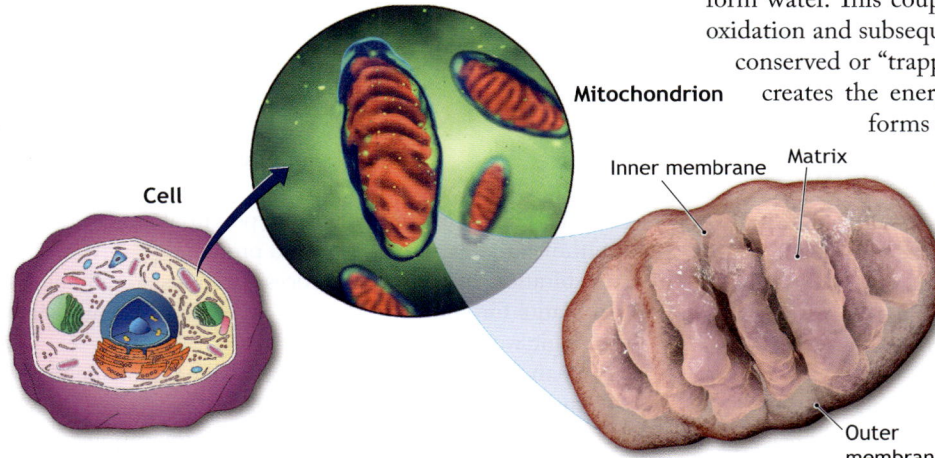

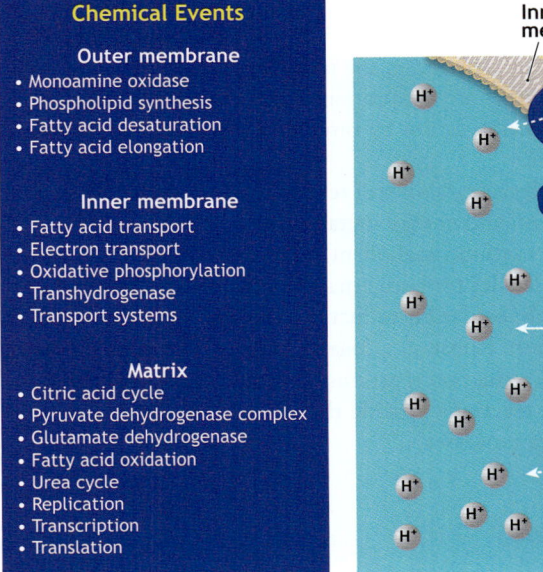

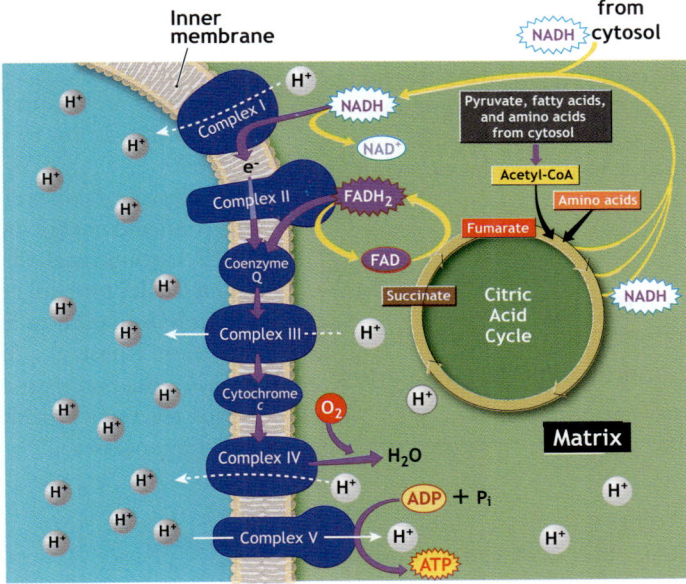

FIGURE 5.9. Primary chemical reactions on the outer and inner mitochondrial membrane and matrix. The table summarizes different chemical events related to mitochondrial structures.
(Shutterstock: Angallen Rogozha; Kateryna Kon; nobeastsofierce.)

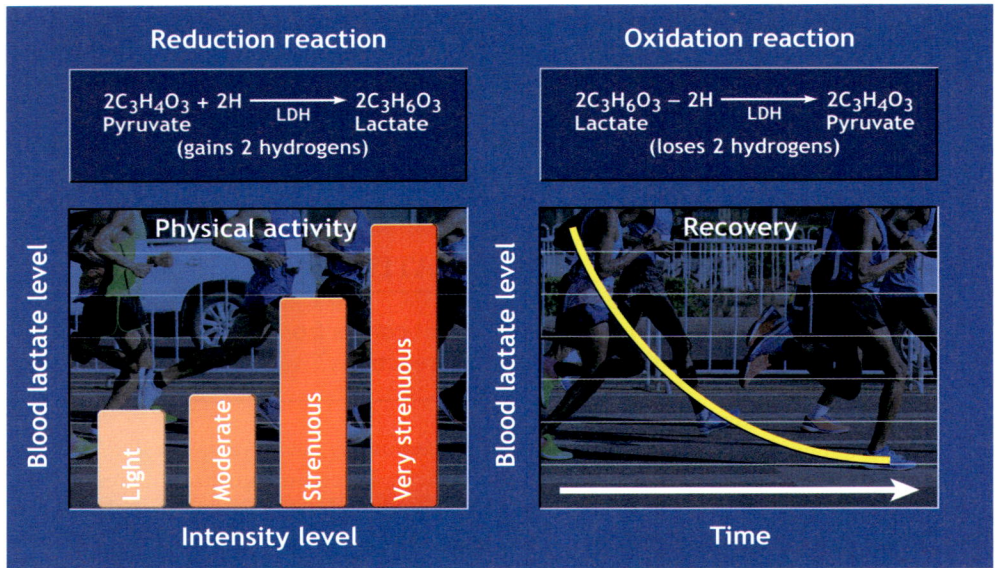

FIGURE 5.10. Redox (oxidation-reduction) reaction. During progressively strenuous physical activity when oxygen supply becomes inadequate, some pyruvate formed in energy metabolism gains two hydrogens (two electrons) and becomes *reduced* to lactate. In recovery with adequate oxygen supply or use, lactate loses two hydrogens (two electrons) and *oxidizes* back to pyruvate.
(Izf/Shutterstock.)

Measuring Human Energy Transfer

Heat gain or loss in a biologic system provides a simplified way to assess energy dynamics in any chemical process. In food catabolism, a human calorimeter (see Fig. 8.1), similar to the bomb calorimeter described in Chapter 4 (see Fig. 4.1), measures the energy change directly as heat released from the chemical reactions and expressed in kilocalories.

Complete food combustion occurs at the expense of molecular oxygen, so any heat generated in these exergonic reactions can be inferred from measurements of oxygen uptake. Such measurements can, therefore, use indirect calorimetry to quantitatively assess the energy expended during rest and diverse physical activities from mountain climbing to playing the guitar to running a mile in the sand, to performing basic tasks during spaceflight. Chapter 8 discusses how direct and indirect calorimetry determine human heat production or energy expenditure.

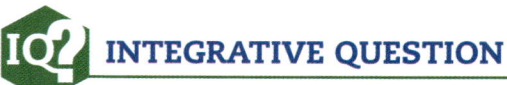 **INTEGRATIVE QUESTION**

How does the second law of thermodynamics relate to the measurement of energy expenditure?

Summary

1. Energy refers to capacity to perform work and may exist in chemical, mechanical, heat, light, nuclear, or electrical forms.
2. Energy exists in either potential or kinetic form.
3. Potential energy refers to energy associated with a substance's structure or position; kinetic energy refers to energy of motion.
4. The six energy categories include chemical, mechanical, heat, light, electrical, and nuclear.
5. Exergonic energy reactions release energy to the immediate surroundings; endergonic energy reactions store, conserve, or increase free energy.
6. All potential energy ultimately degrades into kinetic or heat energy.
7. Living organisms temporarily conserve some potential energy within a new compound's internal structures to power biologic work.
8. Entropy describes potential energy's tendency to degrade to kinetic energy with a lower capacity for work.
9. In the endergonic photosynthetic process, plants transfer the energy of sunlight to the potential energy bound within carbohydrates, lipids, and proteins.
10. Respiration, an exergonic process, releases stored energy in plants for coupling to other chemical compounds for biologic work.
11. Human energy transfer supports three biologic work forms: chemical (cellular biosynthesis), mechanical (muscle contraction), or transport (substance relocation among cells).
12. Enzymes represent highly specific protein catalysts that accelerate chemical reaction rates without being consumed or changed in the reaction.
13. Coenzymes are nonprotein organic substances that facilitate enzyme action by binding a substrate to its specific enzyme.
14. Hydrolysis (catabolism) reactions occur in macronutrient digestion and energy metabolism.
15. Condensation (anabolism) reactions synthesize complex biomolecules for tissue maintenance and growth.
16. Linking oxidation-reduction (redox) reactions enables oxidation (substance loses electrons) to coincide with reverse reduction reactions (substance gains electrons).
17. Redox reactions provide the basis for the body's energy-transfer processes.

Key Terms

Activation energy: Minimum energy required to initiate a chemical reaction; measured in joules per mole (J/mol) or kilocalories per mole (kcal/mol)

Active transport: Molecular movement that requires cellular energy across a membrane from a lower concentration region (against a concentration gradient) into a higher concentration region

Adenosine triphosphate (ATP): Molecular intracellular energy unit or "currency" that transfers its stored energy in complex organic chemical reactions in all life forms

Bioenergetics: Chemical processes involved with making and breaking chemical bonds to produce cellular ATP

Biosynthesis: Multistep, enzyme-catalyzed process that modifies or converts simple compounds into other more complex compounds, or compounds joined to form macromolecules

Cellular respiration: Chemical process that converts macronutrients into useful cellular energy

Competitive inhibitors: Substances that bind an enzyme's active site without enzyme interference

Conservation of energy principle: Principle stating that an isolated system's total energy remains constant regardless of how the system changes

Diffusion: Net molecule or atom passive movement from a higher concentration region (high chemical potential) to a lower concentration region (low chemical potential)

Electron transport: Final common pathway in aerobic (oxidative) metabolism

Endergonic: Physical or chemical process that stores or absorbs energy with increases in free energy for biologic work

Energy: In biological systems, the capacity to perform work (e.g., potential, kinetic, endergonic, exergonic) with energy transfer possible from one object to another object

Energy transfer: Energy relocation from the chemical bonds within a substance to the chemical bonds in another substance

Enthalpy: Sum of a system's internal energy and the product of its pressure and volume

Entropy: Continual energy change process with net potential energy loss

Enzymes: Macromolecular biological catalysts that accelerate chemical reaction rates

Ergometer: Exercise apparatus for measuring the work performed

Exergonic: Physical or chemical process that releases energy to its surroundings

Hydrolysis: Chemical reaction where a water molecule breaks one or more chemical bonds

Kilopound (kp): Force acting on 1-kg mass at gravity's normal acceleration on Earth ($9.80665 \text{ m} \cdot \text{s}^2$)

Kinetic energy: Object's energy based on its motion

Nicotinamide adenine dinucleotide (NAD$^+$): Cofactor in all living cells that transfers electrons from one reaction to another in metabolic redox reactions

Noncompetitive inhibitors: Substances that bind to an enzyme at a location other than its active site

Nuclear fusion: Atomic reaction in which two or more atomic nuclei fuse together to create a larger nucleus with substantial energy release

Oxidation: Process involving electron loss and corresponding net valence increase

Oxidizing agent: Substance that reduces or gains electrons

Phosphocreatine: Phosphorylated creatine molecule that rapidly mobilizes high-energy phosphate reserve in skeletal muscle to regenerate ATP

Photosynthesis: Converts light energy into chemical energy to fuel plant and animal cellular activities

Potential energy: Object's stored energy, determined by its position relative to another object

Power (P): Rate of doing work; $P = F \times D \div T$

Redox reaction: Coupled oxidation-reduction reaction

Reducing agent: Substance that donates or loses electrons during oxidation

Reduction: Process involving electron gain and corresponding net valence decrease

Respiration: All processes in which nutrients convert into useful energy in cells

Turnover number: Moles of substrate react to form a product per mole of substrate

Work (W): Applied force (F) through a distance (D): $W = F \times D$

> References are available online at Lippincott Connect.

Additional References

Denniston K. *General, Organic, and Biochemistry*. 10th ed. New York: McGraw-Hill; 2020.

Dowling L, et al. MicroRNAs in obesity, sarcopenia, and commonalities for sarcopenic obesity: a systematic review. *J Cachexia Sarcopenia Muscle*. 2022. doi:10.1002/jcsm.

Fox S, Rompoiski K. *Human Physiology*. 16th ed. New York: McGraw-Hill; 2022.

Li W, et al. Selective autophagy of intracellular organelles: recent research advances. *Theranostics*. 2021;11:222.

Llurda-Almuzara L, et al. Biceps femoris activation during hamstring strength exercises: a systematic review. *Int J Environ Res Public Health*. 2021;18:8733. doi:10.3390/ijerph18168733.

Mthembu SXH, et al. The potential role of polyphenols in modulating mitochondrial bioenergetics within the skeletal muscle: a systematic review of preclinical models. *Molecules*. 2021;26:2791.

Murphy NE, et al. High-fat ketogenic diets and physical performance: a systematic review. *Adv Nutr*. 2021:223. doi:10.1093/advances/nmaa101.

Nelson EL, Cox MM. *Lehninger Principles of Biochemistry*. 8th ed. New York: MacMillian Learning; 2021.

Ramsey KA, et al. The association of objectively measured physical activity and sedentary behavior with skeletal muscle strength and muscle power in older adults: a systematic review and meta-analysis. *Ageing Res Rev*. 2021;67:101266.

Reginato A, et al. The role of fatty acids in ceramide pathways and their influence on hypothalamic regulation of energy balance: a systematic review. *Int J Mol Sci*. 2021;22:5357. doi:10.3390/ijms22105357.

Sanjaya A, et al. Elaborating the physiological role of yap as a glucose metabolism regulator: a systematic review. *Cell Physiol Biochem*. 2021;55:193.

Sprengell M, et al. Proximal disruption of brain energy supply raises systemic blood glucose: a systematic review. *Front Neurosci*. 2021;15:685031. doi:10.3389/fnins.2021.

Stryer L. *Biochemistry*. 9th ed. Gordonsville, VA: Macmillan Learning; 2019.

Trumpff C, et al. Stress and circulating cell-free mitochondrial DNA: a systematic review of human studies, physiological considerations, and technical recommendations. *Mitochondrion*. 2021;59:225.

Uwamahoro R, et al. Assessment of muscle activity using electrical stimulation and mechanomyography: a systematic review. *Biomed Eng Online*. 2021;20:1.

Višnjić D, et al. AICAr, a widely used AMPK activator with important AMPK-independent effects: a systematic review. *Cells*. 2021;10:1095.

Table 5.1 Six Enzyme Classification Types, Main Functions, and Controlling Enzymes

Name	Action	Control Enzyme
Oxidoreductases	Catalyze oxidation-reduction reactions where the substrate oxidized becomes an hydrogen or electron donor; include dehydrogenases, oxidases, oxygenases, reductases, peroxidases, hydroxylases	Lactate dehydrogenase
Transferases	Catalyze the transfer from the methyl or glycosyl group from one compound (donor) to another compound (acceptor); include kinases, transcarboxylases, transaminases	Hexokinase
Hydrolases	Catalyze reactions that add water; include esterases, phosphatases, peptidases	Lipase
Lyases	Catalyze reactions that cleave C–C, C–O, C–N, and other bonds by hydrolysis or oxidation; differ from other enzymes because two substrates engage in one reaction direction, but only one in the other direction; include synthases, deaminases, decarboxylases	Carbonic anhydrase
Isomerases	Catalyze reactions that rearrange molecular structure and catalyze changes within one molecule (e.g., isomerases, epimerases)	Phosphoglycerate mutase
Ligases	Catalyze bond formation between two substrate molecules with related diphosphate bond hydrolysis in ATP or similar triphosphate	Pyruvate carboxylase

CHAPTER 6
Energy Transfer in the Body

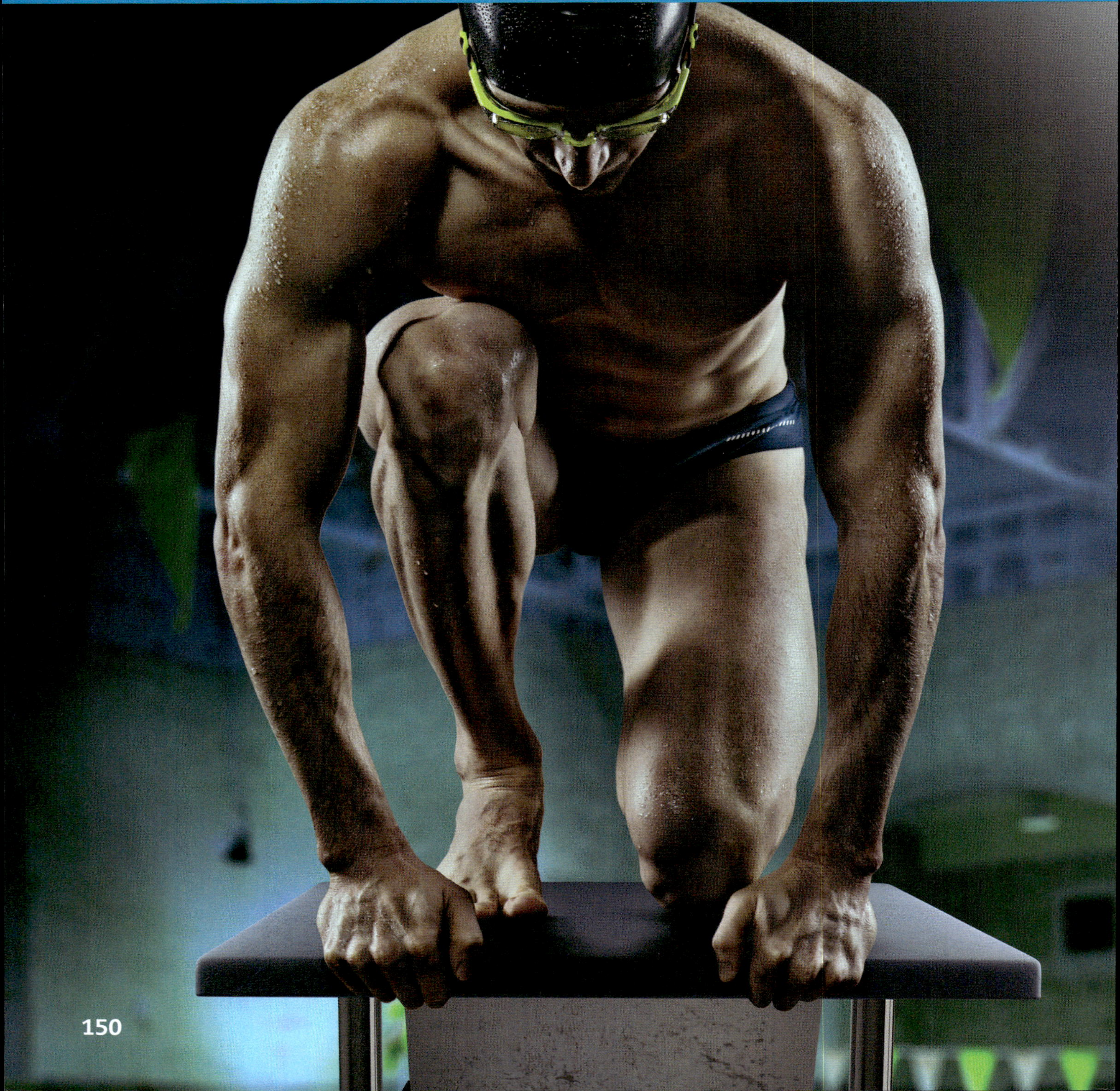

Chapter Objectives

- Discuss how the high-energy phosphates contribute to energizing biologic work
- Quantify the body's adenosine triphosphate (ATP) and phosphocreatine (PCr) reserves and give two examples of physical activity where each energy source predominates
- Outline the steps during electron transport–oxidative phosphorylation
- Explain oxygen's role during energy metabolism
- List three important functions of carbohydrate's role in energy metabolism
- Explain cellular energy release during anaerobic metabolism
- Contrast the energy-conserving efficiencies for aerobic versus anaerobic metabolic processes
- Discuss lactate formation dynamics and accumulation in the blood during increasing exercise intensity
- Describe the role the citric acid cycle plays in energy metabolism
- Outline the general pathways for energy release during macronutrient catabolism
- Contrast the ATP yield from catabolizing a carbohydrate, lipid, and protein molecule
- Discuss the role the Cori cycle plays in energy metabolism during physical activity
- Outline the potential molecular interconversions among carbohydrate, lipid, and protein
- Explain the meaning of this phrase: "Fats burn in a carbohydrate flame"

Ancillaries at-a-Glance

Visit Lippincott Connect to access the following resources.

- References: Chapter 6
- Animations: ATPase, Electron Transfer Chain, Metabolism of Amino Acids, Protein Synthesis, Protein Synthesis Overview, Tricarboxylic Acid Cycle
- Focus on Research: Aerobic Metabolism and Exercise

SECTION 2 • Energy for Physical Activity

Humans require a continual chemical energy supply to sustain their many complex physiologic functions. The energy extracted from food oxidation does not release suddenly at a kindling temperature as occurs when organic materials combust and release heat. The body, unlike a mechanical engine, cannot use heat energy. If the body required only heat energy, body fluids would boil and tissues would burst into flames.

In contrast, human energy dynamics involve transferring energy via chemical bonds. Potential energy within the carbohydrate, lipid, and protein molecules releases stepwise in small quantities by the splitting of chemical bonds. Some energy is conserved when new bonds form during enzymatically controlled reactions within the cell's cytoplasm. Energy lost by one molecule transfers to the chemical structure of other molecules without appearing as heat. This provides for a relatively high energy transformation efficiency.

Biologic work occurs when compounds low in potential energy become "juiced up" from energy transfer via high-energy phosphate bonds. In essence, healthy cells usually receive adequate energy to carry out their numerous functions. The story of how the body maintains its continuous energy supply begins with adenosine triphosphate (ATP) the special free energy carrier molecule.

Part 1 — Phosphate Bond Energy

Adenosine Triphosphate: The Energy Currency

Energy in food does not transfer directly to cells for biologic work. Rather, energy from macronutrient oxidation is harvested and funneled through the energy-rich compound ATP. The potential energy within this nucleotide molecule powers all of a cell's energy-requiring processes. In essence, the energy donor–energy receiver role of ATP represents the cell's two major energy-transforming activities:

1. Extract potential energy from food and conserve it within ATP bonds
2. Extract and transfer the chemical energy in ATP to power biologic work

See the animation "ATPase" on **Lippincott Connect** to view this process.

ATP serves as the ideal energy-transfer agent. It "traps" within its phosphate bonds a large portion of the original food molecule's potential energy. ATP also readily transfers this trapped energy to other compounds to raise them to a higher activation level. The cell contains other high-energy compounds (e.g., phosphoenolpyruvate; 1,3-diphosphoglycerate; phosphocreatine), but ATP remains the most important. **FIGURE 6.1** illustrates how ATP forms from a molecule of adenine and ribose (called **adenosine**) linked to three phosphates (triphosphate), each consisting of phosphorus and oxygen atoms. The bonds that link the two outermost phosphates (symbolized by 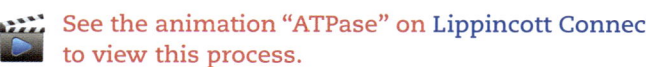) represent high-energy bonds because they release useful energy during hydrolysis. The released energy powers bodily functions including glandular secretion, digestion, tissue synthesis, circulatory function, muscle action, and nerve transmission. In muscle, energy from ATP stimulates specific sites on the contractile elements to activate the molecular motors that power muscle fibers to shorten. A new compound, **adenosine diphosphate (ADP)**, forms when ATP joins with water, catalyzed by the enzyme **adenosine triphosphatase (ATPase)**.

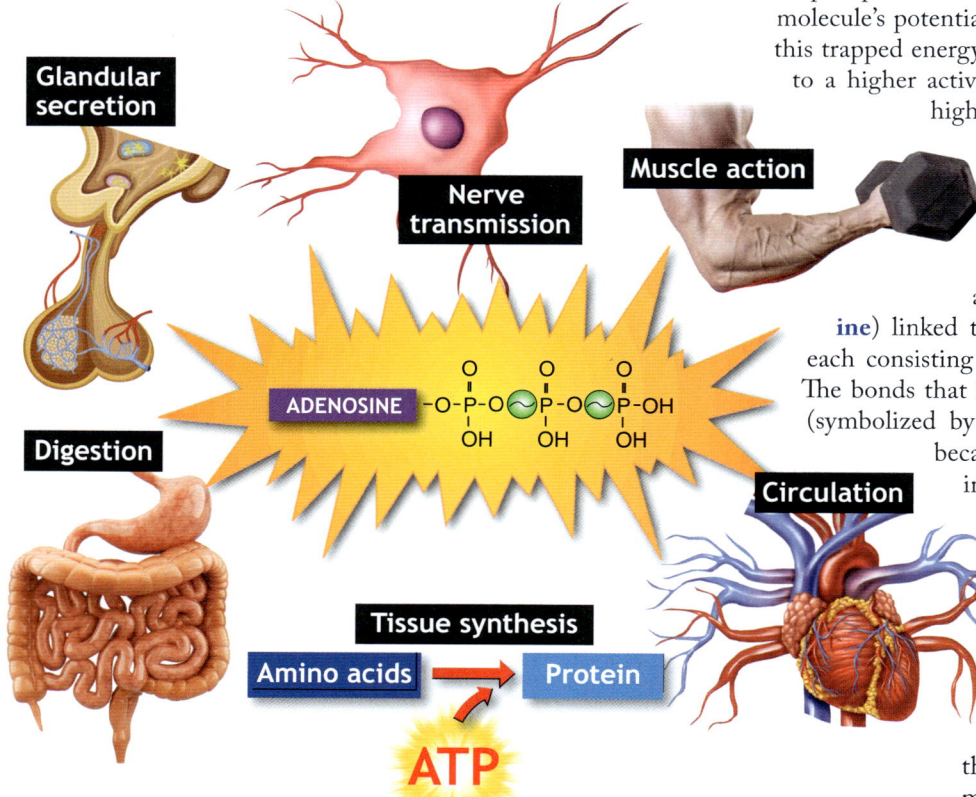

FIGURE 6.1. ATP, the energy currency that powers all biologic work forms. The 🟢 represent high-energy bonds.
(Shutterstock: Mitar Vidakovic; Vecton; BlueRingMedia; cirkoglu; Lightspring; Liya graphics)

This reaction cleaves ATP's outermost phosphate bond to release an inorganic phosphate ion and approximately 7.3 kcal of **free energy** (ΔG; i.e., energy available for work) per mole of ATP hydrolyzed to ADP. The symbol ΔG refers to the standard free energy change measured under laboratory conditions (77°F/25°C; 1 atmosphere pressure; concentrations maintained at 1 molal at pH = 7.0). Standard laboratory conditions are seldom achieved in the body, yet this expression of free energy change makes comparisons possible under different conditions. In the intracellular environment, the free energy value may actually approach 10 kcal · mol^{-1}.

$$ATP + H_2O \xrightarrow{ATPase} ADP + P_i - \Delta G\ 7.3\,kcal \cdot mol^{-1}$$

The free energy liberated in ATP hydrolysis reflects the energy difference between reactant and end product. This reaction generates considerable free energy, making ATP a high-energy phosphate compound. Infrequently, additional energy releases when another phosphate splits from ADP. In some reactions of biosynthesis, ATP donates its two terminal phosphates simultaneously to construct new cellular material. The remaining molecule, **adenosine monophosphate (AMP)**, has a single phosphate group.

The energy liberated during ATP breakdown directly transfers to other energy-requiring molecules. *Energy from ATP hydrolysis powers all biologic work forms; thus, ATP constitutes the cell's "energy currency."*

FIGURE 6.2 illustrates ATP's role as energy currency for the biologic work of macronutrient synthesis in anabolic (endergonic) processes and its subsequent reconstruction from ADP and a phosphate ion (P_i) via stored macronutrients' oxidation in catabolic (exergonic) processes.

ATP splits almost instantly without need for molecular oxygen. This capability to hydrolyze ATP without oxygen (termed **anaerobic**) generates rapid energy transfer. Bodily movements requiring this type of "rapid" energy include sprinting 10 s to catch a bus, lifting an object, swinging a golf club, spiking a volleyball, or performing a pull-up or push-up. In each case, energy metabolism proceeds uninterrupted because the energy required for the activity derives almost exclusively from intramuscular ATP hydrolysis. The body always attempts to maintain a continuous ATP supply through different metabolic pathways; some are located in the cell's cytosol, whereas others operate within the mitochondria (**FIG. 6.3**). For example, the cytosol contains the pathways for ATP production from the anaerobic breakdown of PCr, glucose, glycerol, and the carbon skeletons of some deaminated amino acids. Within the mitochondria, reactive processes harness cellular energy to generate ATP aerobically (see "Cellular Oxidation," later in this chapter)—the citric acid cycle and respiratory chain—featuring fatty acid, pyruvate, and some amino acid catabolic mechanisms.

Cells contain limited ATP and must continually resynthesize it as used. Only under extreme physical activity conditions do ATP levels in skeletal muscle decrease. A limited ATP supply provides a biologically useful mechanism to

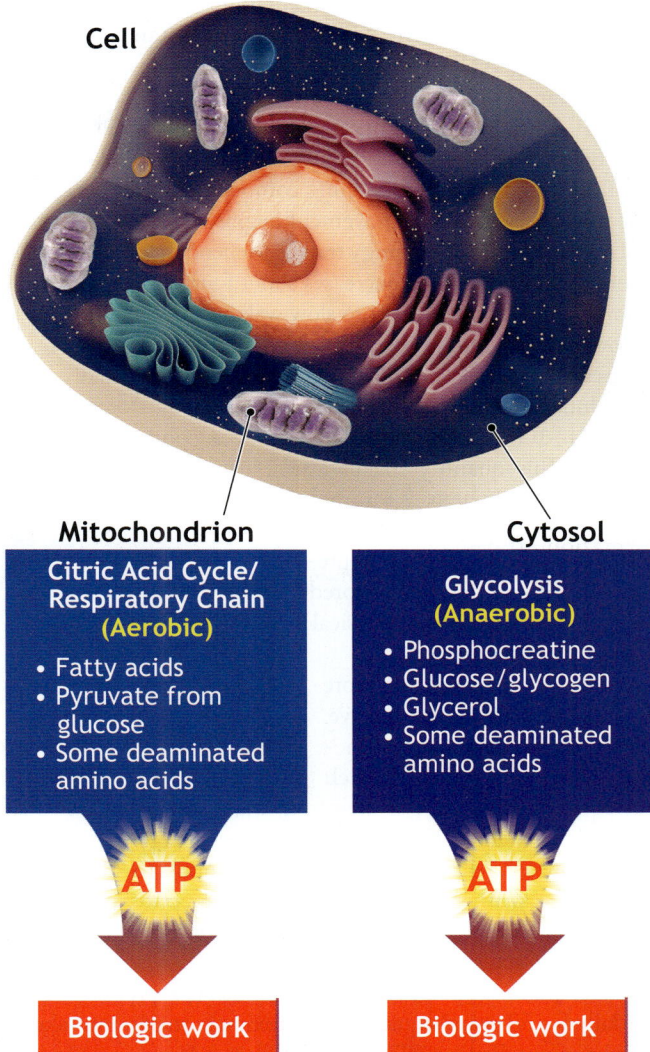

FIGURE 6.3. Different ways to produce ATP. The body maintains a continuous ATP supply through different metabolic pathways in the mitochondrion and cytosol. (Shutterstock: Mitar Vidakovic; Vecton; eranicle;Kateryna Kon)

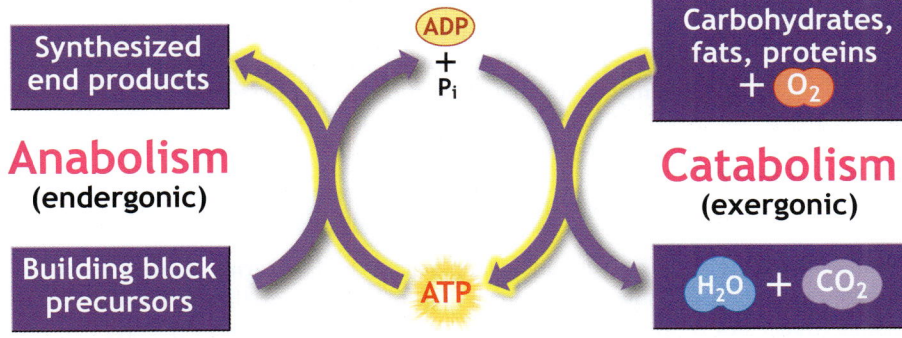

FIGURE 6.2. ATP recycling in macronutrient breakdown (catabolic or exergonic process) and its subsequent reconstruction (anabolic or endergonic process) from ADP and a phosphate ion (P_i).
(Mitar Vidakovic/Shutterstock)

regulate energy metabolism. By maintaining a limited ATP reserve, the relative ATP concentration (and corresponding ADP, P_i, and AMP concentrations) changes rapidly in response to only minimal decreases in ATP. Any increase in energy requirement immediately disrupts the balance between ATP, ADP, and P_i. The imbalance stimulates the breakdown of other stored energy-containing compounds to resynthesize ATP. In this way, when muscular movement begins, it rapidly activates several systems to increase energy transfer depending on movement intensity. Energy transfer increases about fourfold in the transition from sitting in a chair to slow walking. Changing from a slow walk to an all-out sprint almost immediately accelerates active muscles' energy transfer rate about 120-fold!

Under normal resting conditions the body stores only 80 to 100 g (about 3.0 oz) of ATP at any point in time. This quantity makes available each second, approximately 2.4 mmol ATP per kg wet muscle weight, or about 1.44×10^{10} ATP molecules. This represents enough intramuscular stored energy to power all-out physical activity for several seconds.[41]

ATP alone does not represent a significant energy reserve. A sedentary person resynthesizes an amount of ATP each day equal to about 75% of their body mass. For endurance athletes who generate 20 times their resting energy expenditure throughout a 2.5-hr marathon race, this amounts to 80 kg/176.4 lb of ATP resynthesis during the run. To appreciate the tremendous ATP quantity produced over adult portion of a life span (assuming a body weight 80 kg/176.4 lb and a relatively sedentary lifestyle for 50 years after age 20), total ATP production (60 kg daily for 50 years) equals the approximate maximum takeoff weight of two Boeing 787 Dreamliner aircraft.

Phosphocreatine: The Energy Reservoir

To overcome its storage limitation, ATP resynthesis proceeds uninterrupted to continuously supply energy for all of the body's biologic work. Lipid and glycogen represent the major energy sources to maintain as-needed ATP resynthesis. Some energy for ATP resynthesis also comes directly from the anaerobic splitting of a phosphate from phosphocreatine (PCr), another intracellular high-energy phosphate compound. **FIGURE 6.4** schematically illustrates the reversible release and use of phosphate-bond energy in ATP and PCr. The energy liberated from PCr hydrolysis rebonds ADP and P_i to form ATP. The term high-energy phosphates describes these compounds.

The PCr and ATP molecules share a similar characteristic: a large amount of free energy releases when the bond cleaves between the PCr's creatine and phosphate molecules. The double-pointing arrows in Figure 6.4 show the reversible reactions. In other words, phosphate (P) and creatine (Cr) rejoin to form PCr. This also applies to ATP synthesis: ADP plus P re-forms ATP. Because PCr has a larger free energy

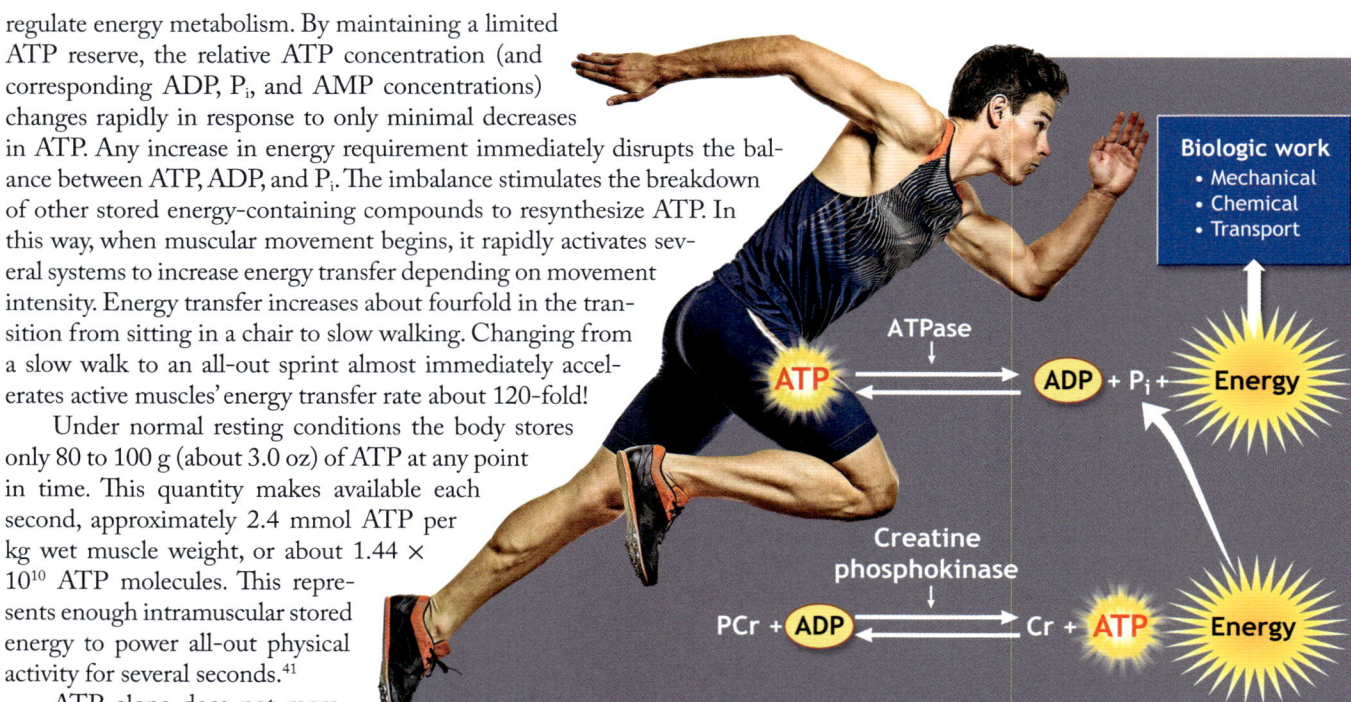

FIGURE 6.4. ATP and PCr provide anaerobic phosphate-bond energy sources. (Mitar Vidakovic/Shutterstock)

of hydrolysis than does ATP, its hydrolysis catalyzed by the **creatine kinase** enzyme (4 to 6% on the outer mitochondrial membrane, 3 to 5% in the sarcomere, and 90% in the cytosol) drives ADP phosphorylation to ATP. Cells store approximately four to six times more PCr than ATP.

Transient increases in ADP within the muscle's contractile unit during exercise shift the creatine kinase reaction toward PCr hydrolysis and ATP production (*the upper reaction in* Fig. 6.4); the reaction does not require oxygen and reaches a maximum energy yield in about 10 s.[39] In this case, PCr serves as a "reservoir" for high-energy phosphate bonds. The rapidity of ADP phosphorylation considerably exceeds energy transfer from stored muscle glycogen because of the high creatine kinase activity rate.[18] If maximal effort continues beyond 10 s, energy for continual ATP resynthesis must originate from less-rapid stored macronutrients' catabolism. Chapter 23 discusses the potential for exogenous creatine supplementation to enhance short-term, explosive exercise performance.

The **adenylate kinase reaction** represents another single-enzyme–mediated reaction for ATP regeneration. The reaction uses two ADP molecules to produce one ATP molecule and AMP as follows:

$$2\ ADP \xrightleftharpoons{\text{adenylate kinase}} ATP + AMP$$

The adenylate kinase and **creatine kinase reactions** (lower reaction in Fig. 6.4) augment the muscle's ability to rapidly increase energy output (increased ATP availability), and also produce the molecular byproducts AMP, P_i, and ADP that activate the initial stages of glycogen and glucose catabolism and the cellular oxidation (respiration) pathways of the mitochondrion.

Cellular Oxidation

Most energy for phosphorylation derives from the oxidation ("biologic burning") of the dietary carbohydrate, lipid, and protein macronutrients. Recall from Chapter 5 that a molecule becomes reduced when it accepts electrons from an electron donor. In turn, the molecule that gives up the electron becomes oxidized. *Oxidation reactions (those that donate electrons) and reduction reactions (those that accept electrons) remain coupled and constitute the biochemical mechanism that underlies energy metabolism.* This process continually provides hydrogen atoms from catabolizing the stored macronutrients. The mitochondria, in essence the cell's "energy factories," contain carrier molecules that remove electrons from hydrogen (oxidation) and eventually pass them to oxygen (reduction).[42] ATP synthesis occurs during oxidation-reduction (redox) reactions.[43]

Electron Transport

FIGURE 6.5 illustrates the general schema for hydrogen oxidation and accompanying electron transport to oxygen.

 See the animation "Electron Transfer Chain" on Lippincott Connect to view this process.

During cellular oxidation, hydrogen atoms are not merely turned loose in intracellular fluids. Rather, substrate-specific **dehydrogenase enzymes** catalyze hydrogen's release from the nutrient substrate. The coenzyme component of the dehydrogenase (usually the niacin-containing nicotinamide adenine dinucleotide [NAD^+]) accepts electron pairs from hydrogen. Although the substrate oxidizes and gives up hydrogens (electrons), NAD^+ gains hydrogen and two electrons and reduces to NADH; the other hydrogen appears as H^+ in the cell fluid. The riboflavin-containing coenzyme **flavin adenine dinucleotide (FAD)** serves as another electron acceptor to oxidize food fragments. Like NAD^+, FAD catalyzes dehydrogenation and accepts electron pairs. Unlike NAD^+, FAD becomes $FADH_2$ by accepting both hydrogens. *NADH and $FADH_2$ provide energy-rich molecules because they carry electrons with high energy-transfer potential.*

The cytochromes, a series of iron-protein electron carriers dispersed on the inner mitochondrial membranes, then pass in "bucket brigade" fashion pairs of electrons carried by NADH and $FADH_2$. The cytochrome's iron portion exists in either its oxidized (ferric, or Fe^{3+}) or reduced (ferrous, or Fe^{2+}) ionic state. By accepting an electron, a specific cytochrome's ferric portion reduces to its ferrous form. In turn, ferrous iron donates its electron to the next cytochrome and so on down the line. *By shuttling between these two iron forms, the cytochromes transfer electrons to ultimately reduce oxygen to form water. NAD^+ and FAD then recycle for subsequent electron transfer.* The NADH generated during glycolysis (see section "Rapid Glycolysis: Anaerobic Energy Release from Glucose") converts back to NAD via hydrogen "shuttling" from NADH across the mitochondrial membrane.

Electron transport by specific carrier molecules constitutes the **respiratory (cytochrome) chain**, the final common pathway where electrons extracted from hydrogen pass to oxygen. For each hydrogen atom pair, two electrons flow down the chain and reduce one oxygen atom to form one water molecule. Passage of electrons down the five-cytochrome chain releases enough energy to rephosphorylate ADP to ATP at three of the sites. At the last site, **cytochrome oxidase (cytochrome aa$_3$)** with strong oxygen affinity, discharges its electron directly to oxygen.

FIGURE 6.6 shows the route for hydrogen oxidation, electron transport, and energy transfer in the respiratory chain that releases free energy in relatively small amounts. In several of the electron transfers, the formation of high-energy phosphate bonds conserves energy. Each electron acceptor in the respiratory chain has a progressively greater affinity for electrons. In biochemical terms, this affinity for electrons represents a substance's reduction potential. Oxygen, the last electron receiver in the transport chain, possesses the largest reduction potential. Mitochondrial oxygen ultimately drives the respiratory chain and other catabolic reactions that require continual availability of NAD^+ and FAD. In oxidation-reduction, much of the chemical energy stored within the hydrogen atom does not dissipate to kinetic energy but instead is conserved within the ATP bonds.

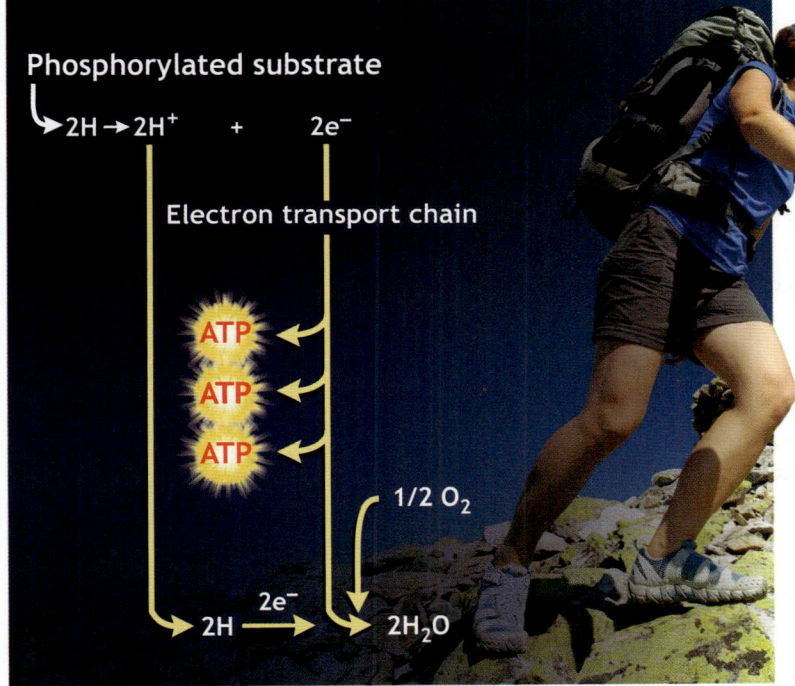

FIGURE 6.5. General schema to remove hydrogen electrons (oxidation) in the electron transport chain.
(Mitar Vidakovic/Shutterstock)

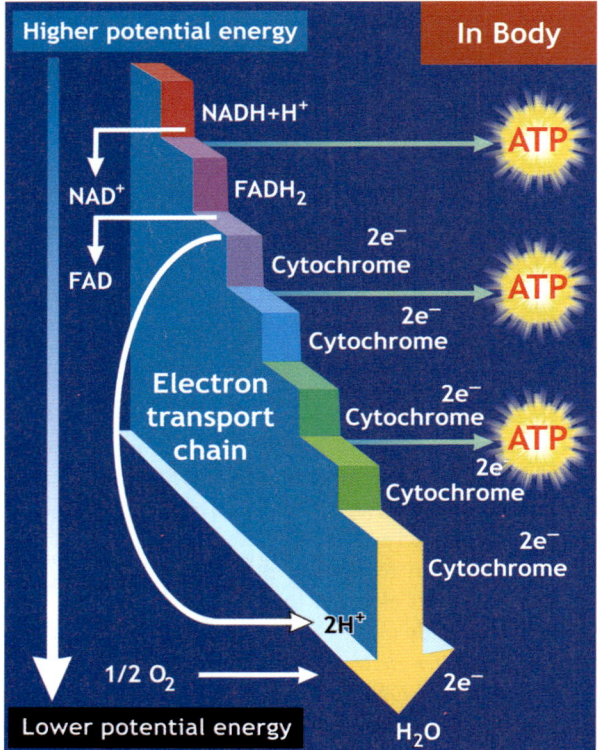

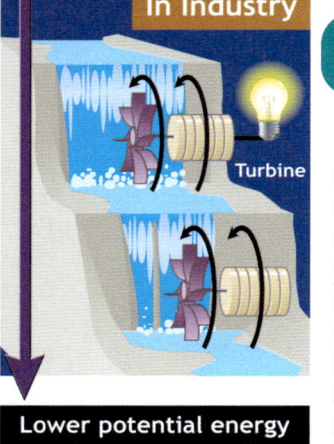

FIGURE 6.6. Examples of harnessing potential energy. The smaller inset figure shows how falling water rotates waterwheels to generate energy trapped by the turbine to turn on a lightbulb. In the body, the electron transport chain removes electrons from hydrogens attached for ultimate delivery to oxygen. In oxidation-reduction much of the chemical energy within hydrogen atoms does not dissipate to kinetic energy, but instead is conserved within ATP.
(Shutterstock: Mitar Vidakovic; yukipon)

Oxidative Phosphorylation

Oxidative phosphorylation synthesizes ATP by transferring electrons from NADH and FADH$_2$ to oxygen. **FIGURE 6.7** illustrates how the energy generated in the electron transport reactions pump protons across the inner mitochondrial membrane into the intermembrane space. The electrochemical gradient generated by a reverse proton flow across the inner membrane (see arrow pointing into the intermembrane space) represents stored potential energy and provides the coupling mechanism that binds ADP and a phosphate ion to synthesize ATP. The mitochondrion's inner membrane remains impermeable to ATP, so the protein enzyme complex ATP/ADP translocase exports the newly synthesized ATP molecule. In turn, ADP and P$_i$ move into the mitochondrion for subsequent synthesis to ATP, referred to as **chemiosmotic coupling**. This represents the cell's primary endergonic means to extract and trap chemical energy within the high-energy phosphates. *More than 90% of ATP synthesis takes place in the respiratory chain by oxidative reactions coupled with phosphorylation.*

Oxidative phosphorylation can be likened to a waterfall divided into several separate cascades by intervening turbines at different heights as illustrated in Figure 6.6. Similarly, electrochemical energy generated during electron transport becomes harnessed and transferred (coupled) to ADP. Energy transfer from NADH to ADP to re-form ATP happens at three distinct electron transport coupling sites. Hydrogen oxidation and subsequent phosphorylation occurs as follows:

$$NADH + H^+ + 3ADP + 3P_i + \tfrac{1}{2}O_2 \rightarrow NAD^+ + H_2O + 3ATP$$

The ratio of phosphate bond formation to oxygen uptake (**P/O ratio**) reflects quantitative ATP production coupling to electron transport. In the preceding equation, note that the P/O ratio equals 3 for each NADH plus H$^+$ oxidized. If FADH$_2$ originally donates hydrogen, only two ATP molecules form for each hydrogen pair oxidized (P/O ratio = 2). This occurs because FADH$_2$ enters the respiratory chain at a lower energy level at a point beyond the first ATP synthesis in Fig. 6.6.

fyi Mitochondrial Oxygen Shuttle

NADH from cell cytoplasm must be converted back to NAD$^+$ to enter the electron transport chain within mitochondria to release its hydrogen electrons for ATP production. By itself, NADH cannot cross the inner mitochondrial membrane, but it can reduce another molecule that can cross the membrane. This transport/shuttle system located within mitochondrial membranes transfers NADH-released hydrogens from the cell cytosol into the electron transport chain. Movement of reducing agents across the membrane is called mitochondrial or hydrogen shuttling. The electron microscopy image shows the mitochondrion membranes as black, with OM = outer membrane and IM = inner membrane, the latter partitioned into the inner boundary membrane (IBM) and cristae membranes (CM).

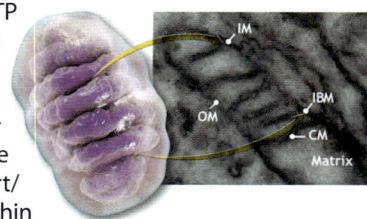
Kateryna Kon/Shutterstock

Sources:
Giacomello M, et al. The cell biology of mitochondrial membrane dynamics. *Nat Rev Mol Cell Biol.* 2020;21:204.
Gupta A, Becker T. Mechanisms and pathways of mitochondrial outer membrane protein biogenesis. *Biochim Biophys Acta Bioenerg.* 2021;1862:148323.
Schlame M. Protein crowding in the inner mitochondrial membrane. *Biochim Biophys Acta Bioenerg.* 2021;1862:148305.

indicates an average number of ATP produced per NADH oxidation with the energy for mitochondrial transport subtracted. When $FADH_2$ donates hydrogen, at one step below the first ATP formation site, then on average only 1.5 molecules of ATP form for each hydrogen pair oxidized.

Electron Transport–Oxidative Phosphorylation Efficiency

Each ATP mole formed from the union of ADP and P_i conserves approximately 7 kcal of energy. Because 2.5 moles ATP regenerate from the total 52 kcal energy released in the oxidation of 1 mole (1-g molecular weight) of NADH, about 18 kcal (7 kcal · mol^{-1} × 2.8) are conserved as chemical energy. This represents a relative 34% efficiency (18 kcal ÷ 52 kcal × 100) to harness chemical energy by electron transport-oxidative phosphorylation, a relatively high efficiency rate considering a steam engine transforms its fuel into useful energy at only about 30% efficiency.

Oxygen's Role in Energy Metabolism

Three prerequisites exist for continual ATP resynthesis during coupled oxidative phosphorylation. Satisfying the following three conditions causes hydrogen and electrons to shuttle uninterrupted down the respiratory chain to oxygen during energy metabolism:

1. Tissue availability for the NADH (or $FADH_2$) reducing agents
2. Oxidizing agent oxygen present in the tissues
3. Sufficient enzyme and mitochondrial concentrations so energy transfer reactions proceed at their appropriate rate

During strenuous physical activity, inadequacy in oxygen delivery (condition 2) or its rate of use (condition 3) creates an imbalance between hydrogen release and its terminal oxidation. In both cases, electron flow down the respiratory chain "backs up" and hydrogens accumulate bound to NAD^+ and FAD. In the section "More About Lactate," in Part 2, we describe how pyruvate temporarily binds excess hydrogens (electrons) to form lactate. Lactate formation allows electron transport–oxidative phosphorylation to provide energy as needed.

Aerobic metabolism refers to energy-generating catabolic reactions where oxygen serves as the final electron acceptor in the respiratory chain to combine with hydrogen to form water. In one sense, the term *aerobic* seems misleading because oxygen does not participate directly in ATP synthesis. On the other hand, oxygen's presence at the "end of the line" largely determines the capacity for aerobic ATP production and the ability to sustain intense endurance activities.

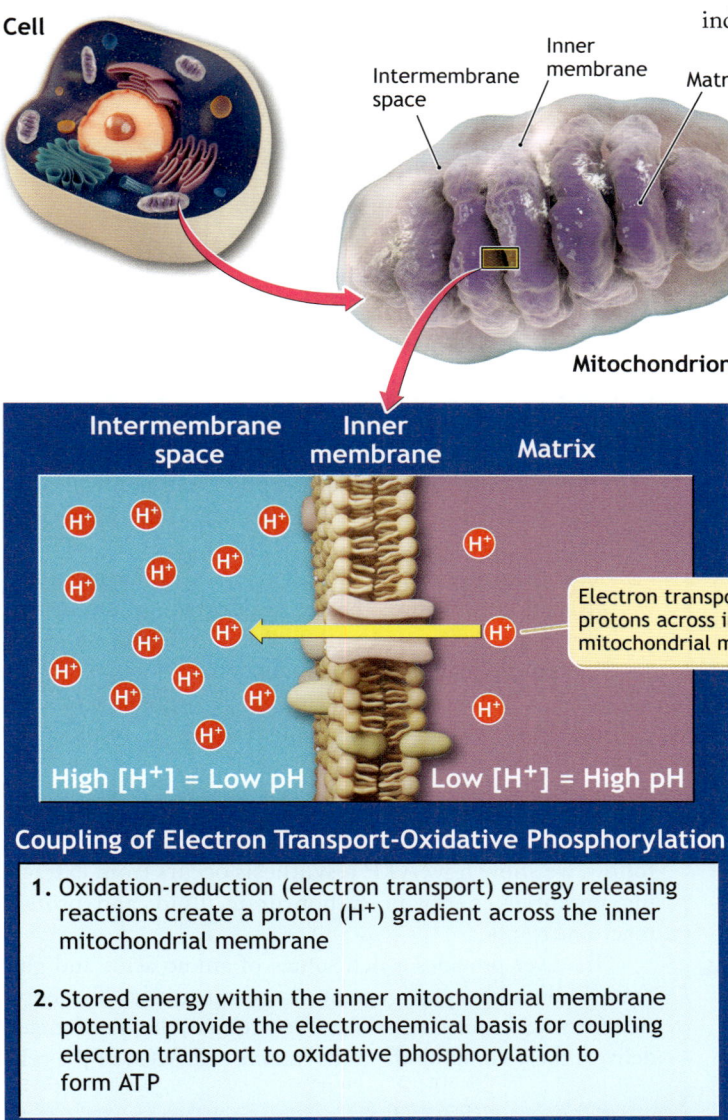

FIGURE 6.7. The mitochondrion is the site for aerobic energy metabolism. Electron transport creates a proton (H^+) gradient across the inner mitochondrial membrane to produce a net proton flow to provide the coupling mechanism to drive ATP resynthesis.
(Shutterstock: eranicle; Kateryna Kon; OSTILL is Franck Camhi; jivacore)

Biochemists have adjusted their accounting transpositions regarding energy conservation in resynthesizing an ATP molecule in aerobic pathways. Energy provided by NADH and $FADH_2$ oxidation resynthesizes ADP to ATP. Additional energy (H^+) is also required to shuttle the NADH from the cell's cytoplasm across the mitochondrial membrane to deliver H^+ to electron transport. This added energy exchange from NADH shuttling across the mitochondrial membrane reduces the net ATP yield for glucose metabolism and changes the overall ATP production efficiency (see the section of "Electron Transport–Oxidative Phosphorylation Efficiency"). The oxidation of one NADH molecule produces on average only 2.5 ATP molecules. This decimal value for ATP does not indicate the formation of one-half an ATP molecule but rather

fyi Newborn Oxygen Uptake

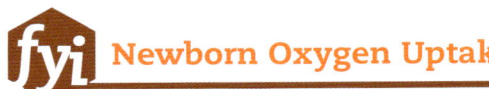

Oxygen uptake during rest is relatively stable when expressed relative to body weight or size for children and adult humans. Less is known regarding a newborn's oxygen uptake immediately upon delivery, particularly differences between those delivered vaginally following normal labor and those delivered by cesarean section before labor begins. Oxygen uptake was determined in twenty healthy women at term (38 to 42 wk), 10 delivered by elective cesarean section and 10 by normal vaginal delivery. Newborn weight was determined and umbilical venous and arterial blood obtained immediately following delivery. Newborn oxygen uptake was calculated as umbilical venous blood flow × the difference in umbilical arterial and venous oxygen content. The mean oxygen uptake in human newborns at term (median gestational age 39 wk) was 6.58 mL · min^{-1} · kg^{-1}. There was no significant difference in oxygen uptake between newborns delivered following uncomplicated normal labor and those delivered by elective cesarean section before labor onset. Human newborns tolerate intermittent uterine blood flow and oxygen supply reductions associated with myometrial contractions during normal labor.

Leptospira/Shutterstock

Source:
Acharya G, et al. Oxygen uptake of the human fetus at term. *Acta Obstet Gynecol Scand.* 2009;88:104.

Summary

1. Energy within the carbohydrate, lipid, and protein molecules does not suddenly release in the body at some kindling temperature.
2. Energy releases slowly in small amounts during complex, enzymatically controlled reactions to promote more efficient energy transfer and conservation.
3. About 40% of the potential energy available from food nutrients' breakdown is conserved within the bonds of the high-energy compound ATP.
4. Splitting the terminal phosphate bond from ATP liberates free energy to power all biologic work, making ATP the body's energy currency despite its limited 3.0-oz supply.
5. PCr interacts with ADP to form ATP to replenish ATP almost instantaneously.
6. Phosphorylation refers to energy transfer via phosphate bonds as ADP with creatine continually recycle into ATP and PCr.
7. Cellular oxidation occurs on the inner mitochondrial membrane linings by transferring electrons from NADH and FADH$_2$ to oxygen.
8. Electron transport–oxidative phosphorylation produces coupled chemical energy transfer to form ATP from ADP plus a phosphate ion.
9. During aerobic ATP resynthesis, oxygen serves as the final electron acceptor in the respiratory chain to combine with hydrogen to form water.

Part 2 Energy Release from Macronutrients

Energy release in macronutrient catabolism serves one crucial purpose—to phosphorylate ADP to reform the energy-rich compound ATP. **FIGURE 6.8** outlines three broad stages that ultimately lead to the release and conservation of energy by the cell for biologic work:

1. *Stage 1* involves digestion, absorption, and assimilation of large food macromolecules into smaller subunits for cellular metabolism.
2. *Stage 2* involves amino acid, glucose, and fatty acid and glycerol units within the cytosol degrading into acetyl-coenzyme A (formed within the mitochondrion), with limited ATP and NADH production.
3. *Stage 3* involves acetyl-coenzyme A degrading to CO_2 and H_2O within the mitochondrion with considerable ATP production.

The specific degradation pathways differ depending on the nutrient substrate catabolized. In the sections that follow, we show how ATP resynthesis occurs from extracting potential energy in carbohydrate, lipid, and protein macronutrients.

The liver provides a rich source of amino acids and glucose, while adipocytes generate large quantities of energy-rich fatty acid molecules. After their release, the bloodstream delivers these compounds to the muscle cell. Most of the cells'

fyi Glycogenolysis Cascade

Epinephrine's action has been termed the **glycogenolysis cascade** because this hormone impacts progressively greater phosphorylase activation to ensure rapid glycogen mobilization in stressful situations. Phosphorylase activity remains at the highest level during intense physical activity when sympathetic activity increases and carbohydrate represents the optimum energy fuel. Sympathetic outflow and subsequent glycogen catabolism decrease considerably during low-to-moderate intensity exercise when the slower fatty acid oxidation rate adequately maintains ATP concentrations in active muscle.

StudioMolekuul/Shutterstock

Source:
Briski KP, et al. Norepinephrine regulation of ventromedial hypothalamic nucleus astrocyte glycogen metabolism. *Int J Mol Sci.* 2021;22759.

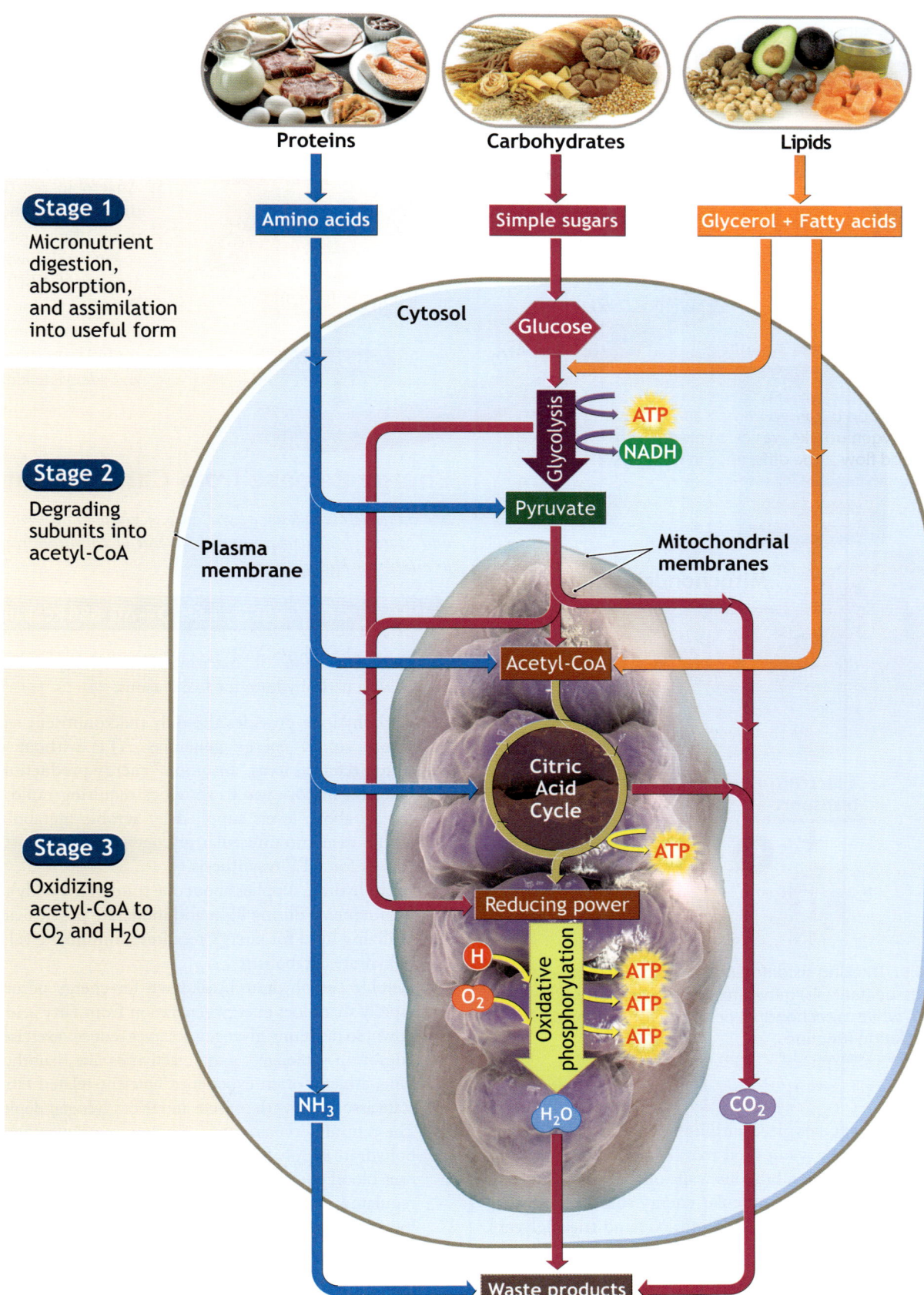

FIGURE 6.8. Three broad stages for protein, carbohydrate, and lipid use during energy metabolism.
(Shutterstock: Mitar Vidakovic; Alexander Prokopenko; Elena Schweitzer; Tina Larsson; Kateryna Kon)

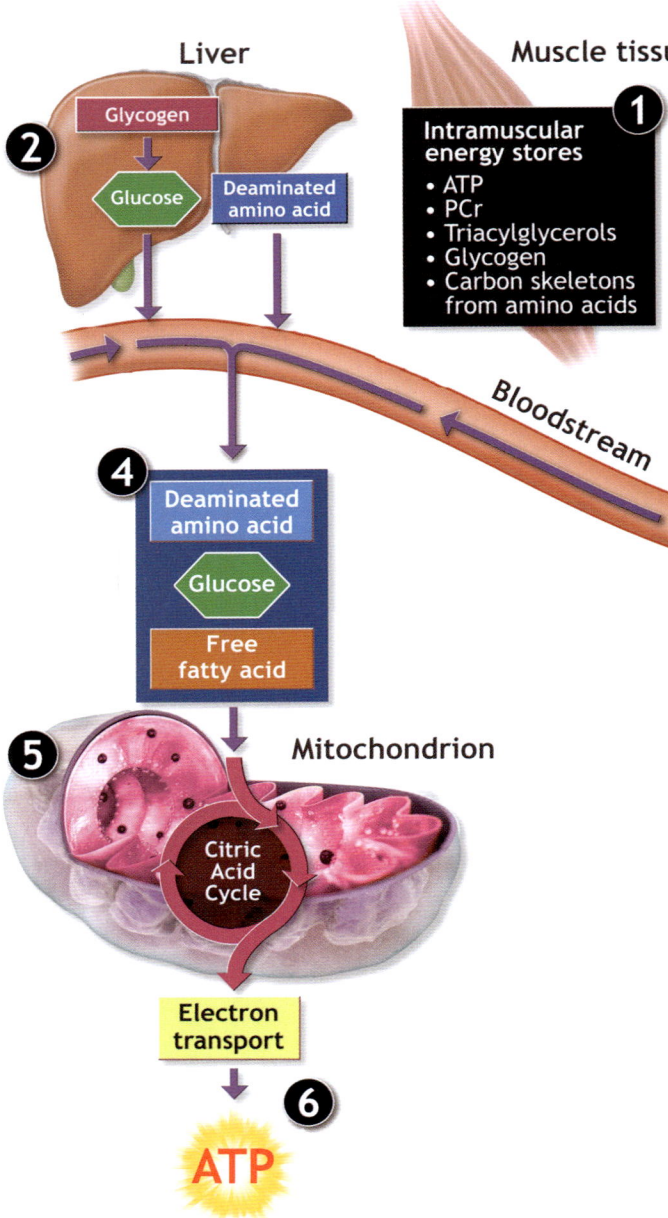

FIGURE 6.9. Tracking six different stages of ATP regeneration. Adipose tissue (fat cells) generates energy-rich fatty acid molecules, while mitochondrial proteins carry out oxidative phosphorylation functions.
(Shutterstock: Mitar Vidakovic; SciePro; Crevis)

energy production takes place within the mitochondria. Mitochondrial proteins carry out their roles in oxidative phosphorylation on the inner membranous walls of this architecturally elegant complex. The intramuscular energy sources consist of the high-energy phosphates ATP and PCr and triacylglycerols, glycogen, and amino acids.

FIGURE 6.9 outlines the following six fuel sources that supply substrate for ATP formation:

1. Triacylglycerol and glycogen molecules stored within muscle cells
2. Blood glucose (derived from liver glycogen)
3. Free fatty acids (derived from triacylglycerols in liver and adipocytes)
4. Intramuscular- and liver-derived carbon skeletons from amino acids
5. Anaerobic reactions in the cytosol in the initial phase of glucose or glycogen breakdown (small amount of ATP)
6. Phosphorylation of ADP by PCr under enzymatic control by creatine kinase and adenylate kinase

Energy Release from Carbohydrate

The complete breakdown of one mole of glucose to carbon dioxide and water yields a maximum 686 kcal of chemical-free energy available for biologic work.

$$C_6H_{12}O_6 + 6O_2 \rightarrow 6CO_2 + 6H_2O - \Delta G\ 686\ kcal \cdot mol^{-1}$$

Our discussion of macronutrient energy metabolism begins with carbohydrate for five reasons:

1. Carbohydrate provides the only macronutrient substrate whose stored energy generates ATP without oxygen (often referred to as "anaerobic" energy production). This takes on importance in activities requiring rapid energy release above levels supplied by aerobic metabolism. In such a case, intramuscular glycogen supplies most of the energy for ATP resynthesis.
2. Carbohydrate supplies about one third of the body's energy requirements during light and moderate physical activity.
3. Utilizing lipid for energy requires a minimal level of carbohydrate catabolism.
4. Aerobic carbohydrate breakdown for energy occurs more rapidly than does energy generation from fatty acid breakdown, so depleting glycogen reserves reduces exercise power output. In prolonged aerobic activities like marathon running, athletes often experience nutrient-related fatigue—a state associated with muscle and liver glycogen depletion.
5. The central nervous system requires an uninterrupted carbohydrate supply to function properly. The brain normally uses blood glucose almost exclusively as its fuel. In poorly regulated diabetes, during starvation, or with prolonged low carbohydrate intake, the brain adapts after about 8 days and metabolizes lipid (ketones) as an alternative fuel.

Complete glucose breakdown conserves only some released energy as ATP. Synthesizing 1 mole of ATP from ADP and a phosphate ion requires 7.3 kcal of energy. Coupling all of the energy from glucose oxidation to phosphorylation could theoretically form 94 ATP moles per glucose mole (686 kcal ÷ 7.3 kcal·mol^{-1} = 94 mol). In the muscle, phosphate bond formation conserves only 34% or about 233 kcal, with the remainder dissipated as heat (see Electron Transport–Oxidative Phosphorylation Efficiency). As such, glucose breakdown regenerates 32 ATP moles (233 kcal ÷ 7.3 kcal·mol^{-1} = 32 mol) with an accompanying 233-kcal free energy gain.

Anaerobic Versus Aerobic Glycolysis

Two forms of carbohydrate breakdown occur in several fermentation reactions collectively termed **glycolysis** ("the dissolution of sugar"), or the Embden-Meyerhof pathway named for its two German chemist discoverers (Otto Meyerhof [1884–1951]; 1922 Nobel Prize in Physiology or Medicine; www.nobelprize.org/nobel_prizes/medicine/laureates/1922/meyerhof-bio.html; and Gustav Embden [1874–1933]). In one form, lactate, formed from pyruvate, becomes the end product. In the other form, pyruvate remains the end product. With pyruvate as the end substrate, carbohydrate catabolism proceeds and couples to further break down in the citric acid cycle with subsequent electron transport production of ATP. Carbohydrate breakdown in this form (sometimes termed *aerobic* [with oxygen] *glycolysis*) is a relatively *slow* process resulting in substantial ATP formation. In contrast, glycolysis that results in lactate formation (referred to as *anaerobic* [without oxygen] *glycolysis*) represents rapid but limited ATP production. The net lactate or pyruvate formation depends more on the relative glycolytic and mitochondrial activities than on molecular oxygen's presence. The relative demand for rapid or slow ATP production determines the form of glycolysis. The glycolytic process itself, from beginning substrate (glucose) to end substrate (lactate or pyruvate), does *not* involve oxygen. *From our perspective, rapid (anaerobic) and slow (aerobic) glycolysis are the appropriate terms to describe glycolysis.*

Glucose degradation occurs in two stages. In stage one, glucose breaks down rapidly into two pyruvate molecules. Energy transfer for phosphorylation occurs without oxygen (rapid glycolysis). In stage two, pyruvate degrades further to carbon dioxide and water. Energy transfers from these reactions require electron transport and accompanying oxidative phosphorylation (**slow glycolysis**).

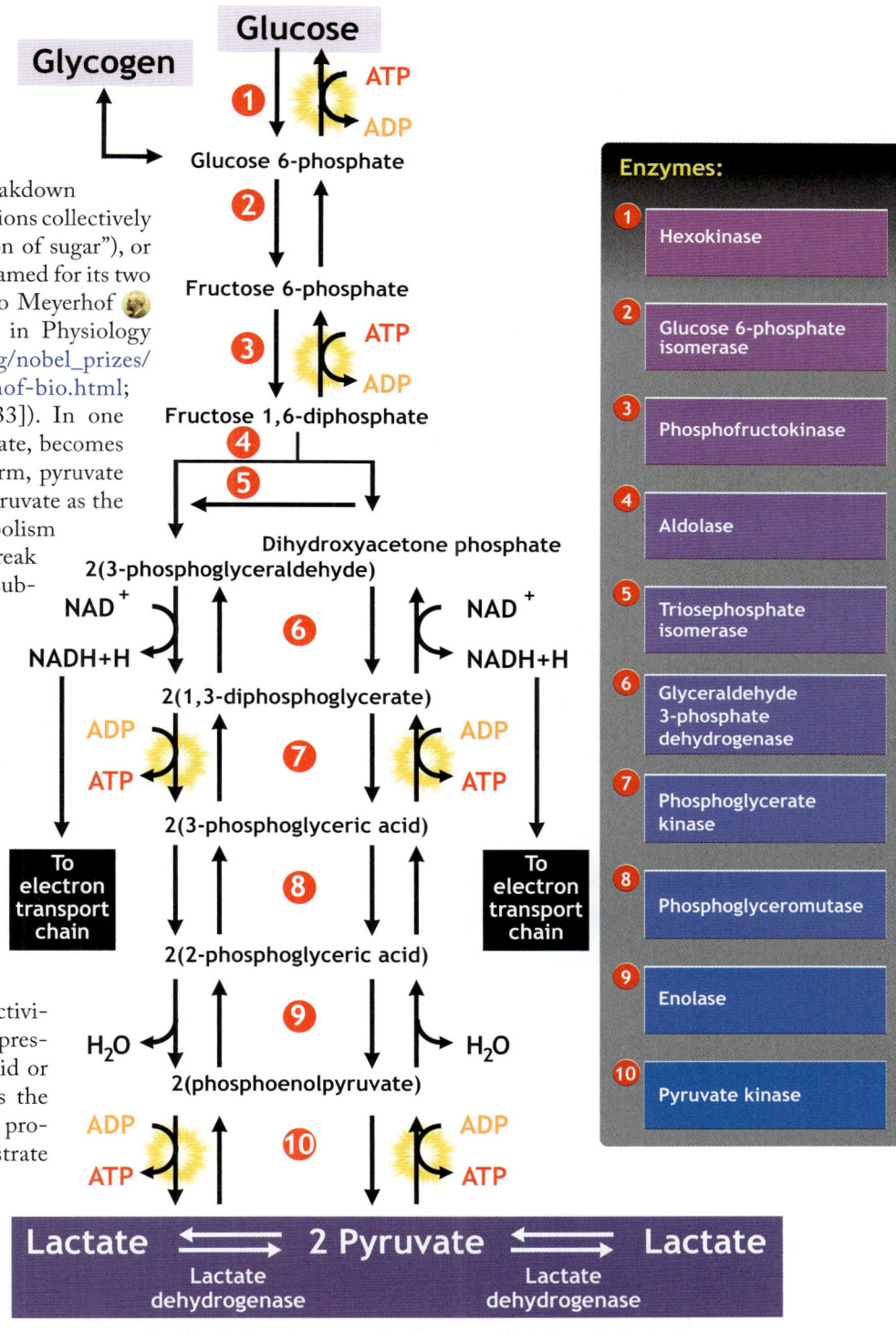

FIGURE 6.10. In glycolysis, 10 enzymatically controlled chemical reactions create two pyruvate molecules from the anaerobic breakdown of glucose. Lactate forms when NADH oxidation does not keep pace with its formation in glycolysis. The insert at the right lists the enzymes that play regulatory roles in the 10 key metabolic reactions.
(Mitar Vidakovic/Shutterstock)

Rapid Glycolysis: Anaerobic Energy Release from Glucose

FIGURE 6.10 illustrates the first stage of glucose degradation in glycolysis, which occurs in the cell's watery medium outside the mitochondrion. Glycolysis represents a more primitive form of rapid energy transfer prevalent in amphibians, reptiles, fish, and marine mammals. In humans, the cells' capacity for glycolysis remains crucial during maximum-effort physical activities for up to about 90s.

In reaction ❶, ATP acts as a phosphate donor to phosphorylate glucose to glucose 6-phosphate. In most tissues, this "traps" the glucose molecule in the cell. With action of the enzyme glycogen synthase, glucose links or polymerizes with other glucose molecules to form a large glycogen molecule (see Fig. 1.3). The liver and kidney cells, however, contain the **phosphatase** enzyme that splits the phosphate from glucose 6-phosphate. This frees glucose from the cell for transport throughout the body. During energy metabolism, glucose 6-phosphate changes to fructose 6-phosphate (reaction ❷). At this stage, energy is not yet released, but some energy incorporates into the original glucose molecule at the expense of one ATP molecule. In a way, consider phosphorylation as "priming the pump" to continue energy metabolism. The fructose 6-phosphate molecule gains an additional phosphate and changes to fructose 1,6-diphosphate under control of **phosphofructokinase (PFK**; reaction ❸). The activity level of this enzyme probably limits the glycolysis rate during maximum-effort activity. Fructose 1,6-diphosphate then splits into two phosphorylated molecules with three carbon chains (*3-phosphoglycerasdehyde*); these further decompose to **pyruvate** in five successive reactions. Fast-twitch (type II) muscle fibers (see Chapter 7) have a high PFK concentration; this makes them ideally suited to generate anaerobic energy from glycolysis.

The Reversal: Metabolism of Glucose to Glycogen and Glycogen to Glucose

The cytoplasm of liver and muscle cells contains glycogen granules and the enzymes for glycogen synthesis (glycogenesis) and glycogen breakdown (glycogenolysis). Under normal conditions following a meal, glucose does not accumulate in the blood. Rather, surplus glucose takes one of three routes—enters the energy metabolic pathways, stores as glycogen, or converts to lipid.

During high cellular activity, available glucose oxidizes by the glycolytic pathway, citric acid cycle, or respiratory chain to form ATP. In contrast, low cellular activity and/or depleted glycogen reserves inactivate key glycolytic enzymes. This causes surplus glucose to form glycogen. Glycogenolysis describes a cleaving process to liberate glucose from the glycogen molecule. The glucose residue then reacts with a phosphate ion to produce glucose 6-phosphate, bypassing step 1 of the glycolytic pathway. When glycogen supplies a glucose molecule for glycolysis, it creates a net gain of three ATPs rather than two during glucose breakdown.

Glycogen Metabolism Regulation

In the liver, glycogen phosphorylase enzymes become inactive following a meal, while glycogen synthase activity increases to facilitate storing of glucose obtained from food. Conversely, between meals when glycogen reserves decrease, liver phosphorylase becomes active (concurrently depressing glycogen synthase activity) to maintain blood glucose stability. Skeletal muscle at rest shows higher synthase activity, whereas physical activity increases phosphorylase activity while concomitantly blunting the synthase enzyme. **Epinephrine**, a sympathetic nervous system hormone, accelerates the rate at which phosphorylase cleaves one glucose component at a time from the glycogen molecule.[7,9]

Substrate-Level Phosphorylation in Glycolysis

Most energy generated in glycolysis does not result in ATP resynthesis but instead dissipates as heat. In reactions ❼ and ❿ in Figure 6.10, the energy released from glucose intermediates stimulates direct phosphate group transfer to four ADP molecules, generating four ATP molecules. *Because two ATP molecules contribute to the initial glucose molecule's phosphorylation, glycolysis generates a net gain of two ATP molecules. This represents a 14.6 kcal · mol^{-1} endergonic conservation without involving molecular oxygen.* Instead, the energy transferred from substrate to ADP by phosphorylation in rapid glycolysis occurs via phosphate bonds in anaerobic **substrate-level phosphorylation** reactions. Energy conservation operates at an efficiency of about 30% during this form of glycolysis.

Rapid glycolysis generates about 5% of the total ATP during the glucose molecule's complete degradation to energy. Activities that rely heavily on ATP generated by rapid glycolysis include sprinting at the end of a mile run, swimming all-out from start to finish in a 50- or a 100-m swim, routines on gymnastics apparatus, and sprint-running up to 200 m.

Glycolysis Regulation

Three factors regulate glycolysis:

1. Four key glycolytic enzyme concentrations: hexokinase, phosphorylase, phosphofructokinase, and pyruvate kinase
2. Levels of the substrate fructose 1,6-disphosphate
3. Oxygen, which in abundance inhibits glycolysis

Glucose delivery to cells also influences its subsequent use in energy metabolism.

Glucose locates in the surrounding extracellular fluid for transport across the cell's plasma membrane. Five proteins, collectively called *facilitative glucose transporters*, mediate this process of **facilitative diffusion**. Muscle fibers and adipocytes contain the insulin-dependent transporter Glu T4 or **GLUT 4**. In response to both insulin's actions and physical activity (independent of insulin's actions), this transporter migrates from vesicles within the cell to the plasma membrane.[33] Its action facilitates glucose transport into the sarcoplasm, where it subsequently catabolizes and forms ATP. Another glucose transporter, GLUT 1, accounts for transporting basal levels of glucose into muscle.

Hydrogen Release in Glycolysis

Glycolytic reactions strip two pairs of hydrogen atoms from the glucose substrate and pass their electrons to NAD⁺ to form NADH (Fig. 6.10, reaction ❻). Normally, if the respiratory chain processed these electrons directly, 2.5 ATP molecules would form for each NADH molecule oxidized (P/O ratio = 2.5). Within heart, kidney, and liver cells, extramitochondrial hydrogen appears as NADH in the mitochondrion termed the **malate-aspartate shuttle**. This produces 2.5 ATP molecules from oxidizing each NADH molecule. The mitochondria in skeletal muscle and brain cells remain impermeable to cytoplasmic NADH formed during glycolysis. Consequently, electrons from extramitochondrial NADH must shuttle indirectly into the mitochondria. This route terminates when electrons pass to FAD to form FADH$_2$ (termed the **glycerol-phosphate shuttle**) at a point below the first formation of ATP. *Thus, 1.5 rather than three ATP molecules form when the respiratory chain oxidizes cytoplasmic NADH (P/O ratio = 1.5).* From two molecules of NADH formed in glycolysis, four ATP molecules generate aerobically by subsequent coupled electron transport–oxidative phosphorylation in skeletal muscle.

More About Lactate

Sufficient oxygen bathes the cells during light-to-moderate levels of energy metabolism. The hydrogens (electrons) stripped from the substrate and carried by NADH oxidize within the mitochondria to form water when they join with oxygen. In a biochemical sense, a "steady state" or more precisely a "steady rate" exists because hydrogen oxidizes at about the same rate it becomes available.

During strenuous physical activity, when energy demands exceed either oxygen supply or its rate of use, the respiratory chain cannot process all of the hydrogen joined to NADH. Continued anaerobic energy release in glycolysis depends on NAD⁺ availability to oxidize 3-phosphoglyceraldehyde (see reaction 6, Fig. 6.10); otherwise the rapid glycolysis rate would "grind to a halt." During rapid glycolysis, NAD⁺ "frees up" or regenerates when "excess" nonoxidized hydrogen pairs combine with pyruvate to form lactate. Lactate formation requires one additional step (catalyzed by **lactate dehydrogenase**) in a reversible reaction shown in **FIGURE 6.11**.

During rest and moderate physical activity, some lactate continually forms in two ways:

1. Energy metabolism of red blood cells (they contain no mitochondria)
2. Limitations posed by enzyme activity in muscle fibers with high glycolytic capacity

Any lactate that forms in one or both of these ways readily oxidizes for energy in neighboring muscle fibers with high oxidative capacity, or in more distant heart and ventilatory muscle tissues. Lactate also serves as an indirect liver glycogen precursor. Consequently, lactate does not *accumulate* because its removal rate equals its production rate. Endurance athletes show an enhanced ability for lactate clearance (or turnover) during exercise.[22,45,46]

As discussed previously, a direct pathway exists for liver glycogen synthesis from dietary carbohydrate. Liver glycogen synthesis also occurs indirectly from converting the 3-carbon precursor lactate to glucose. Erythrocytes and adipocytes also contain glycolytic enzymes, but skeletal muscle possesses the largest quantity so

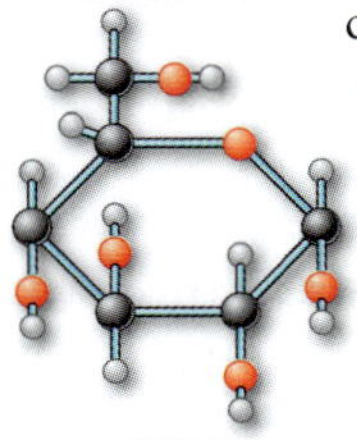

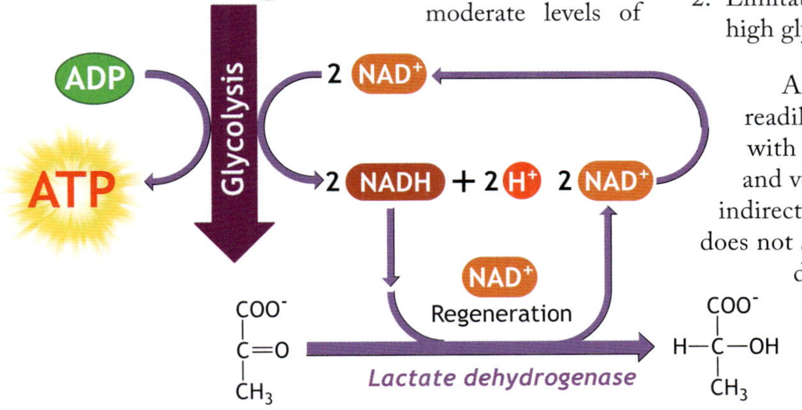

> ### Lactic Acid Versus Lactate
>
> Lactic acid ($C_3H_6O_3$), also known as "milk acid," and lactate are related but technically different molecules. Lactic acid is formed during anaerobic glycolysis that quickly dissociates in the body to release a hydrogen ion (H⁺). The remaining molecule, the acid's conjugate base, binds with a positively charged sodium (Na⁺) or potassium ion (K⁺) to form the acid salt lactate. Under physiological conditions, the majority of lactic acid dissociates and presents as lactate.
>
> StudioMolekuul/Shutterstock

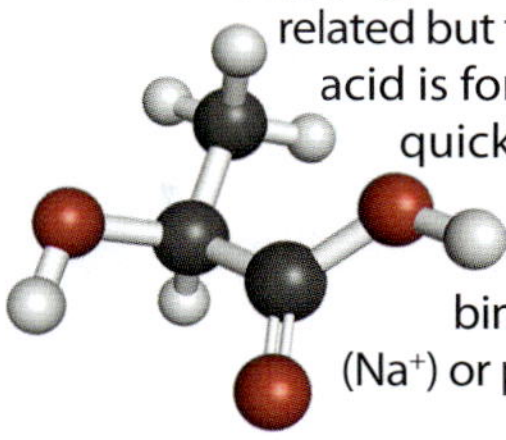

FIGURE 6.11. Lactate forms within muscle when hydrogens from NADH combine temporarily with pyruvate to free up NAD to accept additional hydrogens generated in glycolysis.
(Mitar Vidakovic/Shutterstock)

most lactate-to-glucose conversion occurs in this tissue. This indirect pathway, from lactate-to-liver glycogen synthesis (particularly after eating), is called the **glucose paradox**.[46] Later in this chapter, we discuss the glucose paradox as part of the lactate shuttle to explain how lactate is formed, distributed, and utilized in carbohydrate metabolism.

Temporarily storing hydrogen with pyruvate represents a unique aspect of energy metabolism because it provides a ready "collector" for temporary storage of the rapid glycolysis end product. Once lactate forms in muscle, it can take two different routes:

1. Diffuses into interstitial spaces and blood for buffering and removal from the energy metabolism site
2. Provides gluconeogenic substrate for glycogen synthesis

In this way, rapid glycolysis (with lactic acid production) continues to supply anaerobic energy for ATP resynthesis. This avenue for extra energy production remains temporary because blood and muscle lactate levels increase, and ATP formation fails to keep pace with its rate of use. The end result—fatigue—soon sets in, and physical performance diminishes. Increased intracellular acidity under anaerobic conditions facilitates fatigue by inactivating energy transfer enzymes to impair the muscle's contractile properties.[2,6,17,23]

Lactate: A Valuable "Waste Product". Lactate should not be viewed as a metabolic waste product.[47,48] To the contrary, it serves as a valuable chemical energy source that accumulates with intense physical activity.[12,13] When sufficient oxygen becomes available during recovery, or when pace slows, NAD^+ scavenges hydrogens attached to lactate to form ATP by oxidative processes. The pyruvate molecule's carbon skeletons re-formed from lactate during physical activity (one pyruvate molecule + two hydrogens form a molecule of lactate) become either oxidized for energy or synthesized to glucose (gluconeogenesis) in muscle or in the **Cori cycle** (**FIG. 6.12**). The Cori cycle removes lactate released from active muscles and uses it to replenish glycogen reserves depleted from intense physical activity.[37,46]

 See the animation "Biochemical Reactions of Cori Cycle" on Lippincott Connect to view this process.

During intense physical activity exceeding 80% aerobic capacity with elevated carbohydrate catabolism, glycogen within inactive tissues supplies the active muscle's energy needs. Active glycogen turnover through an exchangeable lactate pool occurs because inactive tissues release lactate into the circulation. This lactate then can serve as a precursor to synthesize carbohydrate in the Cori cycle in

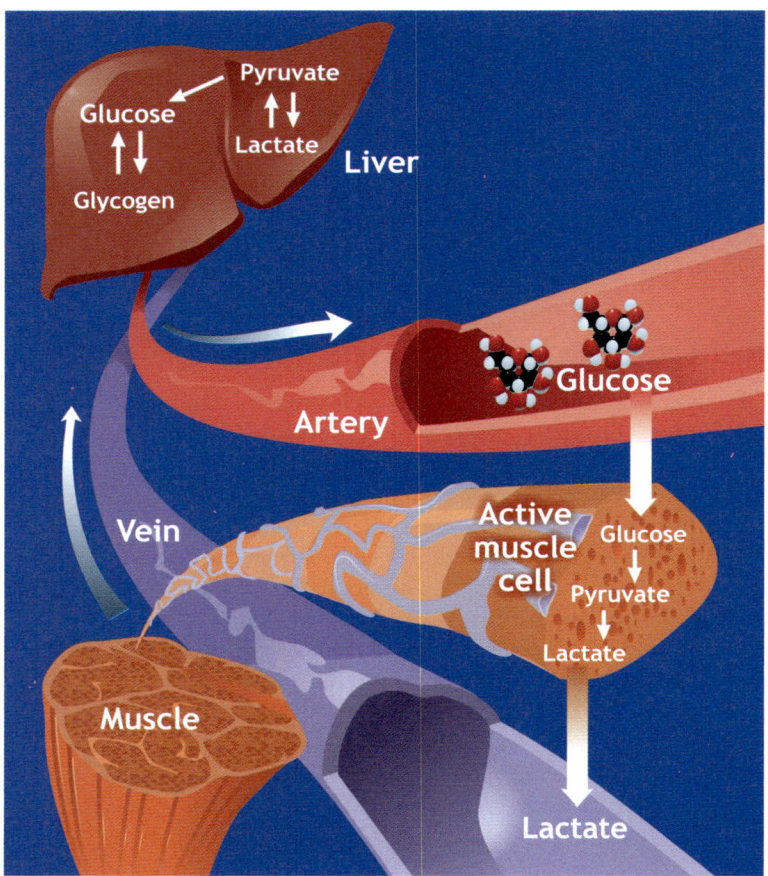

FIGURE 6.12. The Cori cycle biochemical reactions in the liver synthesize glucose from the lactate released from active muscles to stabilize carbohydrate reserves.

the liver and kidneys to support blood glucose levels and the exercise energy requirements.[3,22]

Lactate Shuttle: Blood Lactate as an Energy Source. Isotope tracer studies show that lactate produced in fast-twitch muscle fibers (and other tissues) circulates to other fast-twitch or slow-twitch fibers for conversion to pyruvate. Pyruvate, in turn, converts to acetyl-coenzyme A and enters into the citric acid cycle (see next section) for aerobic energy metabolism. The **lactate shuttling** among cells enables glycogenolysis in one cell to supply other cells with fuel for oxidation. *This makes muscle not only a major lactate producing site but also a primary tissue for lactate removal by oxidation.*[4,13,15,45–48]

Aerobic Energy Release from Glucose

Anaerobic glycolytic reactions release only about 5% of the energy within the original glucose molecule. Extracting the remaining energy continues when pyruvate irreversibly converts to **acetyl-coenzyme A (acetyl-CoA)**, a form of acetic acid. Acetyl-CoA enters the **citric acid cycle** (also termed the Krebs cycle for its discoverer, 1953 Nobel Prize–winning chemist Sir Hans Adolf Krebs, or tricarboxylic acid cycle; www.nobelprize.org/nobel_prizes/medicine/laureates/1953/press.html), the second carbohydrate breakdown stage.

As **FIGURE 6.13** shows within mitochondria, the citric acid cycle degrades the acetyl-CoA substrate to carbon dioxide and hydrogen atoms. The reduced coenzyme carrier molecules transfer hydrogen to the electron transport chain. ATP forms when hydrogen atoms oxidize during electron transport–oxidative phosphorylation.

▶ See the animation "Tricarboxylic Acid Cycle" on **Lippincott Connect** to view this process.

FIGURE 6.14 shows pyruvate preparing to enter the 10-step enzymatically controlled citric acid cycle by joining with coenzyme A (A for acetic acid) to form the 2-carbon compound acetyl-CoA. All values are doubled when computing the net gain of hydrogen and carbon dioxide because two molecules of pyruvate form from one glucose molecule in glycolysis. Enzymes colored purple are key regulatory enzymes. The two released hydrogens transfer their electrons to NAD^+ to form one carbon dioxide molecule as follows:

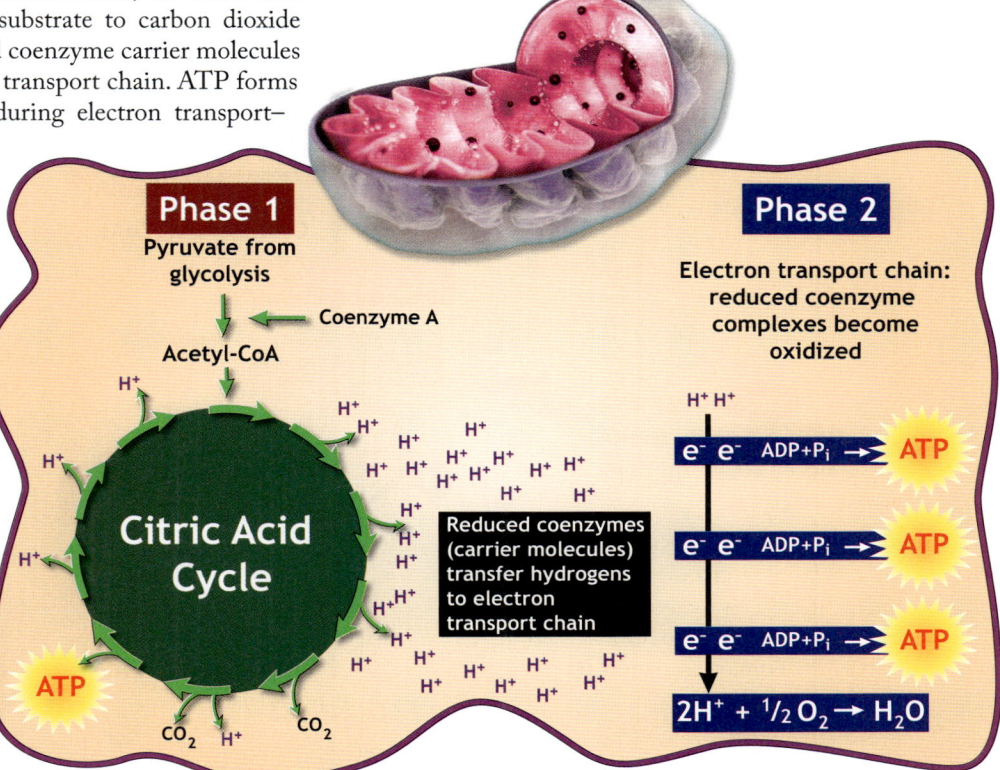

FIGURE 6.13. Aerobic energy metabolism. Phase 1. The citric acid cycle in mitochondria generates hydrogen atoms during acetyl-CoA breakdown. Phase 2. Significant ATP regenerate when hydrogens are oxidized in the electron transport chain.
(Shutterstock: Mitar Vidakovic; Crevis)

$$Pyruvate + NAD^+ + CoA \rightarrow Acetyl\text{-}CoA + CO_2 + NADH^+ + H^+$$

The acetyl portion of acetyl-CoA joins with **oxaloacetate** to form **citrate** (the same 6-carbon citric acid compound found in citrus fruits), which then proceeds through the citric acid cycle. This cycle continues to operate because it retains the original oxaloacetate molecule to join with a new acetyl fragment that enters the cycle. Each acetyl-CoA molecule entering the cycle releases two carbon dioxide molecules and four hydrogen atom pairs. One ATP molecule also regenerates directly by substrate-level phosphorylation from citric acid cycle reactions (reactions 7–8, **FIG. 6.14**). As summarized at the bottom of Figure 6.14, the formation of two acetyl-CoA molecules from two pyruvate molecules created in rapid glycolysis releases four hydrogens, while the citric acid cycle releases 16 hydrogens for a total of 20 hydrogens. *The citric acid cycle's primary function generates energy-rich electrons for passage in the respiratory chain to NAD^+ and FAD forming $NADH + H$ and $FADH_2$, respectively.*

Oxygen does not participate directly in citric acid cycle reactions. The chemical energy within pyruvate transfers to ADP through electron transport–oxidative phosphorylation. With adequate oxygen, including enzymes and substrate, NAD^+ and FAD regenerate, and citric acid cycle metabolism

fyi — Aerobic Metabolism Produces Free Radicals

Passage of electrons along the electron transport chain

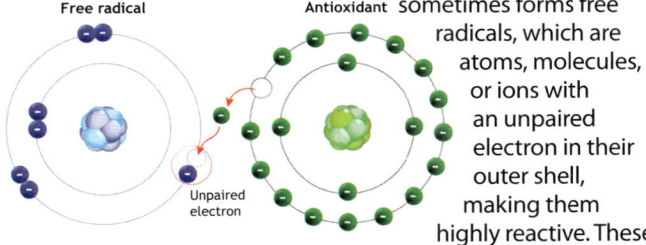

Designua/Shutterstock

sometimes forms free radicals, which are atoms, molecules, or ions with an unpaired electron in their outer shell, making them highly reactive. These reactive free radicals bind quickly to other molecules and promote potential damage to the combining molecule. Free radical formation in muscle, for example, might contribute to muscle fatigue, soreness, or possibly reduced metabolic capacity. Increased interest in monitoring an athlete's oxidative stress status will open future research opportunities linking antioxidant supplement to physical activity.

Sources:
Ruocco C, et al. Essential amino acid formulations to prevent mitochondrial dysfunction and oxidative stress. *Curr Opin Clin Nutr Metab Care*. 2021;24:88.
Taherkhani S, et al. A short overview of changes in inflammatory cytokines and oxidative stress in response to physical activity and antioxidant supplementation. *Antioxidants (Basel)*. 2020;9:886.

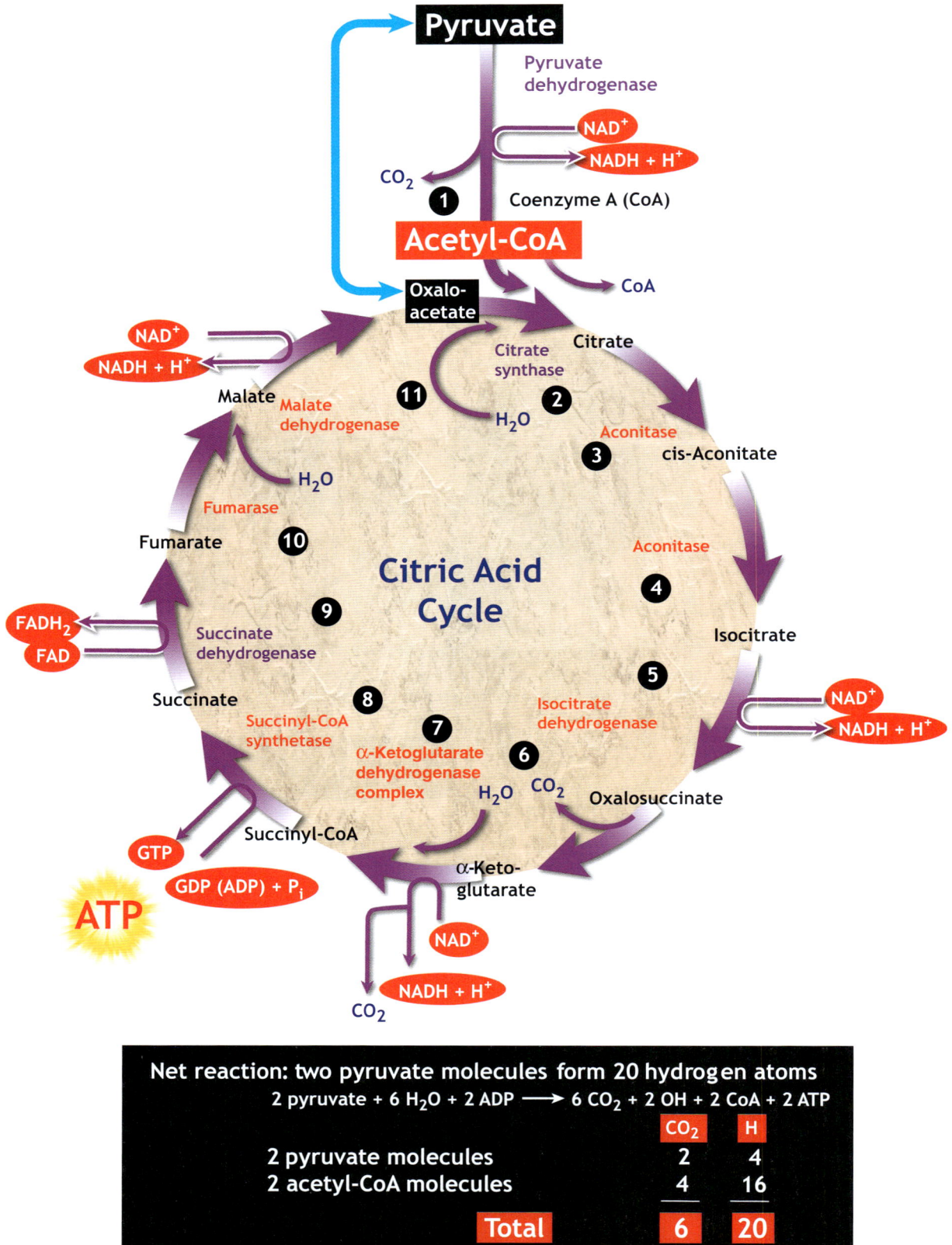

FIGURE 6.14. Flow sheet for releasing hydrogen and carbon dioxide in the mitochondrion during one pyruvate molecule's breakdown.
(Mitar Vidakovic/Shutterstock)

proceeds unimpeded. *The three components in aerobic metabolism include the citric acid cycle, electron transport, and oxidative phosphorylation.*

Total Energy Transfer from Glucose Catabolism

FIGURE 6.15 summarizes the pathways for energy transfer during glucose catabolism in skeletal muscle. Two net ATPs form from substrate-level phosphorylation in glycolysis; similarly, two ATPs emerge from acetyl-CoA degradation in the citric acid cycle. The 24 released hydrogen atoms can be accounted for as follows:

1. Four extramitochondrial hydrogens (two NADH) generated in glycolysis yield five ATPs during oxidative phosphorylation.
2. Four hydrogens (two NADH) released in the mitochondrion when pyruvate degrades to acetyl-CoA yield five ATPs.
3. Two guanosine triphosphates (GTP; a molecule similar to ATP) produced in the citric acid cycle via substrate-level phosphorylation.
4. Twelve of the 16 hydrogens (6 NADH) released in the citric acid cycle to yield 15 ATPs (6 NADH × 2.5 ATP per NADH = 15 ATP).
5. Four hydrogens joined to FAD (two $FADH_2$) in the citric acid cycle to yield three ATPs.

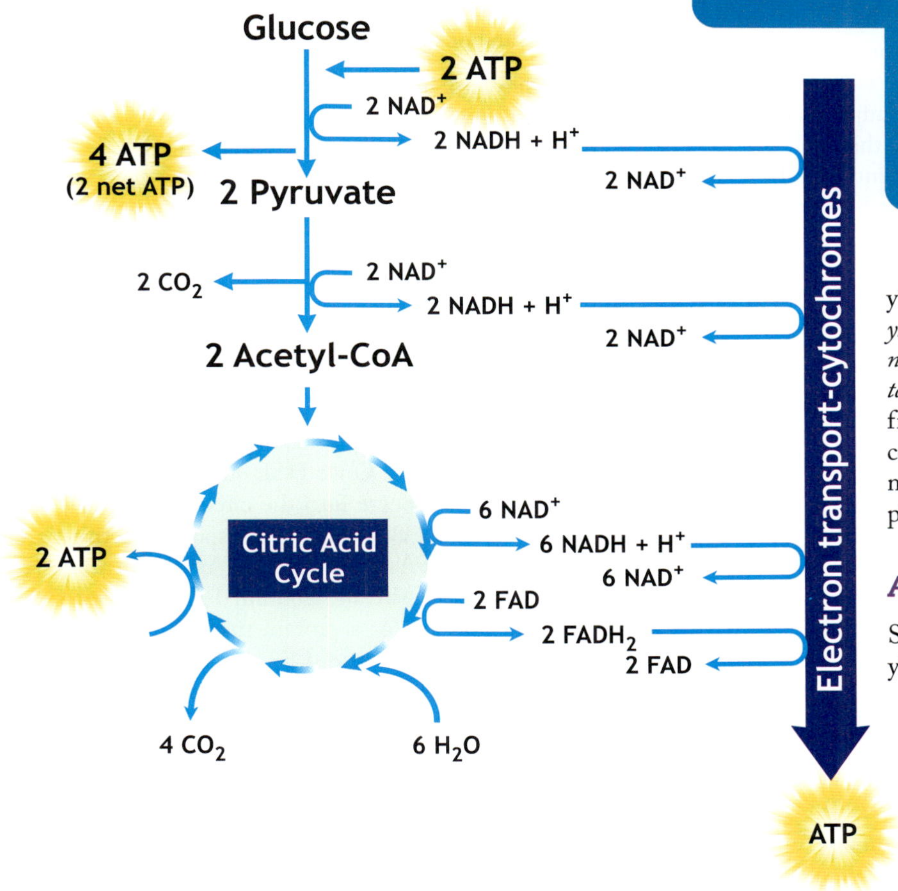

The complete glucose breakdown yields 34 ATPs. *Two ATPs initially phosphorylate glucose making 32 ATP molecules equal the net ATP yield from glucose catabolism in skeletal muscle.* Four ATP molecules form directly from substrate-level phosphorylation (glycolysis and citric acid cycle), whereas 28 ATP molecules regenerate during oxidative phosphorylation.

Adjusted ATP Accounting

Some textbooks quote a 36 to 38 net ATP yield from glucose catabolism. The disparity depends on which shuttle system (the glycerol-phosphate or malate-aspartate) transports NADH + H⁺ into the mitochondrion and the ATP yield per H oxidation used in the computations. One must temper the theoretical values for ATP yield in energy metabolism because only 30 to 32 ATP actually enter the cell's cytoplasm. The differentiation between theoretical versus actual ATP yield can be attributed to the added energy cost to transport ATP out of the mitochondria.[10,49]

Energy Metabolism Regulation

Electron transport and subsequent energy release normally tightly couple to ADP phosphorylation. Without ADP availability for phosphorylation to ATP, electrons generally do not shuttle down the respiratory chain to oxygen. *Metabolites*

Net ATP from glucose metabolism

Source	Reaction	Net ATP
Substrate phosphorylation	Glycolysis	2
2 H_2 (4 H⁺)	Glycolysis	5
2 H_2 (4 H⁺)	Pyruvate → Acetyl-CoA	5
Substrate phosphorylation	Citric acid cycle	2
6 H_2 (12 H⁺)	Citric acid cycle	15
2 H_2 (4 H⁺)	Citric acid cycle	3
	Total:	**32 ATP**

FIGURE 6.15. Pathways for energy transfer during glucose catabolism in skeletal muscle. (Mitar Vidakovic/Shutterstock)

that either inhibit or activate enzymes at key control points in the oxidative pathways modulate glycolysis and citric acid cycle regulatory control.[14,16,28,31,50] Each pathway contains at least one enzyme considered rate limiting because the enzyme controls that pathway's overall reactive speed. *Cellular ADP concentration exerts the greatest effect on the rate-limiting enzymes that control macronutrient energy metabolism.* This makes sense because any increase in ADP signals a need to supply energy to restore depressed ATP levels. Conversely, high cellular ATP levels indicate a relatively low energy requirement. More broadly, ADP concentrations function as a cellular feedback mechanism to maintain relative homeostasis in the energy currency level required for biologic work. Other rate-limiting modulators include cellular levels of phosphate, cyclic AMP, AMP-activated protein kinase (AMPK), calcium, NAD^+, citrate, and pH. More specifically, ATP and NADH serve as enzyme inhibitors, whereas intracellular calcium, ADP, and NAD^+ function as activators. This chemical feedback allows rapid metabolic adjustment to the cells' energy needs. Within the resting cell, the ATP concentration considerably exceeds the ADP concentration by about 500:1. A decrease in the ATP/ADP ratio and intramitochondrial $NADH/NAD^+$ ratio when exercise begins signals a need to increase metabolism. In contrast, a relatively low energy metabolism maintains high ATP/ADP and $NADH/NAD^+$ ratios to depress energy metabolism.[1]

Independent Effects

No single chemical regulator dominates mitochondrial ATP production. *In vitro* and *in vivo* experiments show that changes in these regulators independently alter the oxidative phosphorylation rate. All exert regulatory effects, each contributing differently depending on energy demands, cellular conditions, substrate availability, and specific tissue involvement.[50]

Energy Release from Lipid

Stored lipid represents the body's most plentiful potential energy source. Relative to carbohydrate and protein, stored lipid provides almost unlimited energy. The fuel reserves from lipid in a typical young adult male come from two main sources:

1. Between 60,000 and 100,000 kcal (enough energy to power about 25 to 40 marathon runs) from triacylglycerol in fat cells (adipocytes) distributed throughout the body (see Chapter 28)
2. About 3000 kcal from intramuscular triacylglycerol (12 $mmol \cdot kg\ muscle^{-1}$)

In contrast, carbohydrate energy reserves generally amount to less than 2000 kcal.

Three specific energy sources for lipid catabolism include the following:

1. Triacylglycerols stored directly within the muscle fiber in close proximity to the mitochondria (more in slow-twitch than in fast-twitch muscle fibers)
2. Circulating triacylglycerols in lipoprotein complexes that become hydrolyzed on a tissue's capillary endothelium surface
3. Circulating free fatty acids mobilized from triacylglycerols in adipose tissue

Prior to energy release from lipid, hydrolysis (lipolysis) in the cell's cytosol splits the triacylglycerol molecule into a glycerol molecule and three water-insoluble fatty acid molecules. **Hormone-sensitive lipase** (HSL, activated by cyclic AMP; see section on "Hormonal Effects" in Chapter 20) catalyzes triacylglycerol breakdown as follows:

$$Triacylglycerol + 3H_2O \xrightarrow{lipase} Glycerol + 3\ Fatty\ acids$$

Adipocytes: Lipid Storage and Mobilization Sites

FIGURE 6.16 outlines the dynamics of fatty acid mobilization in adipose tissue and delivery to skeletal muscle. Lipid mobilization and catabolism involve seven discrete processes:

1. Triacylglycerol breakdown to free fatty acids
2. Free fatty acid transport in blood
3. Free fatty acid uptake from blood to muscle
4. Fatty acid preparation for catabolism
5. Activated fatty acid entry into muscle mitochondria
6. Breakdown of fatty acid to acetyl-CoA by β-oxidation with NADH and $FADH_2$ production
7. Coupled oxidation in citric acid cycle and electron transport chain

All cells store some lipid, but adipose tissue supplies the most. Adipocytes specialize in synthesizing and storing triacylglycerols. Triacylglycerol lipid droplets occupy up to 95% of adipocyte cell volume. Once HSL stimulates fatty acids to diffuse from the adipocyte into the circulation, nearly all of them bind to plasma albumin for transport to active tissues as free fatty acids (FFAs).[8,34] Hence, FFAs are not truly "free" entities. At the muscle site, the albumin-FFA complex releases FFAs by diffusion and/or a protein-mediated carrier system across the plasma membrane. FFAs accomplish two results once inside the muscle fiber:

1. Re-esterify to form triacylglycerols
2. Bind with intramuscular proteins and enter the mitochondria for energy metabolism by **carnitine acyltransferase** action on the inner mitochondrial membrane

Carnitine acyltransferase catalyzes an acyl group's transfer to carnitine to form acylcarnitine, a compound that readily crosses the mitochondrial membrane. Medium-chain and short-chain fatty acids do not depend on this enzyme-mediated transport, but diffuse freely into the mitochondria.

The water-soluble glycerol molecule formed during lipolysis diffuses from the adipocyte into the circulation, which allows plasma glycerol levels to reflect triacylglycerol catabolism.[32] Glycerol, when delivered to the liver, serves as a precursor for glucose synthesis. This relatively slow process explains why supplementing with exogenous glycerol (consumed in liquid form) contributes little as an energy substrate or glucose replenisher during exercise.[27]

Adipose tissue's release of FFAs and their subsequent use for energy during light and moderate physical activity increase directly with blood flow through adipose tissue

CHAPTER 6 • Energy Transfer in the Body

(threefold increase not uncommon) and active muscle. FFA catabolism increases principally in slow-twitch muscle fibers whose ample blood supply and large, numerous mitochondria make them ideal for lipid breakdown.

Circulating triacylglycerols carried in lipoprotein complexes also provide an energy source. The lipoprotein lipase (LPL) enzyme synthesized within the cell and localized on surrounding capillary surfaces catalyzes the hydrolysis of these triacylglycerols. LPL also facilitates a cell's fatty acid uptake for energy metabolism or for *re-esterfication* of the triacylglycerols stored within muscle and adipose tissues.[34,51]

Hormonal Effects on Lipid Metabolism

Epinephrine, *norepinephrine*, *glucagon*, and *growth hormone* augment lipase activation and subsequent lipolysis and FFA mobilization from adipose tissue. Plasma concentrations of these lipogenic hormones increase during physical activity to continually supply active muscles with energy-rich substrate. An intracellular mediator, **adenosine 3′,5′-cyclic monophosphate (cyclic AMP)**, activates HSL to regulate lipid breakdown. Various lipid-mobilizing hormones, which themselves do not enter the cell, activate cyclic AMP.[35] Circulating lactate, ketones, and particularly insulin inhibit cyclic AMP activation.[8] Physical training–induced increases in the activity level of skeletal muscle and adipose tissue lipases, including biochemical and vascular adaptations in the muscles themselves, enhance lipid use for energy during moderate physical activity.[19–21,24] Paradoxically, excess body fat decreases FFA availability during physical activity.[25,52] Chapter 20 presents a more detailed evaluation regarding hormone regulation in exercise and training.

Fatty acid molecules' availability regulates both lipid breakdown and synthesis. After a meal, when energy metabolism remains relatively low, digestive processes increase FFA and triacylglycerol delivery to cells to stimulate triacylglycerol synthesis. By contrast, moderate physical activity increases fatty acid use for energy, which reduces their cellular concentration. The decrease in intracellular FFAs stimulates triacylglycerol breakdown into glycerol and fatty acid components. Concurrently, hormonal release triggered by physical activity stimulates adipose tissue lipolysis to further augment FFA delivery to active muscle.

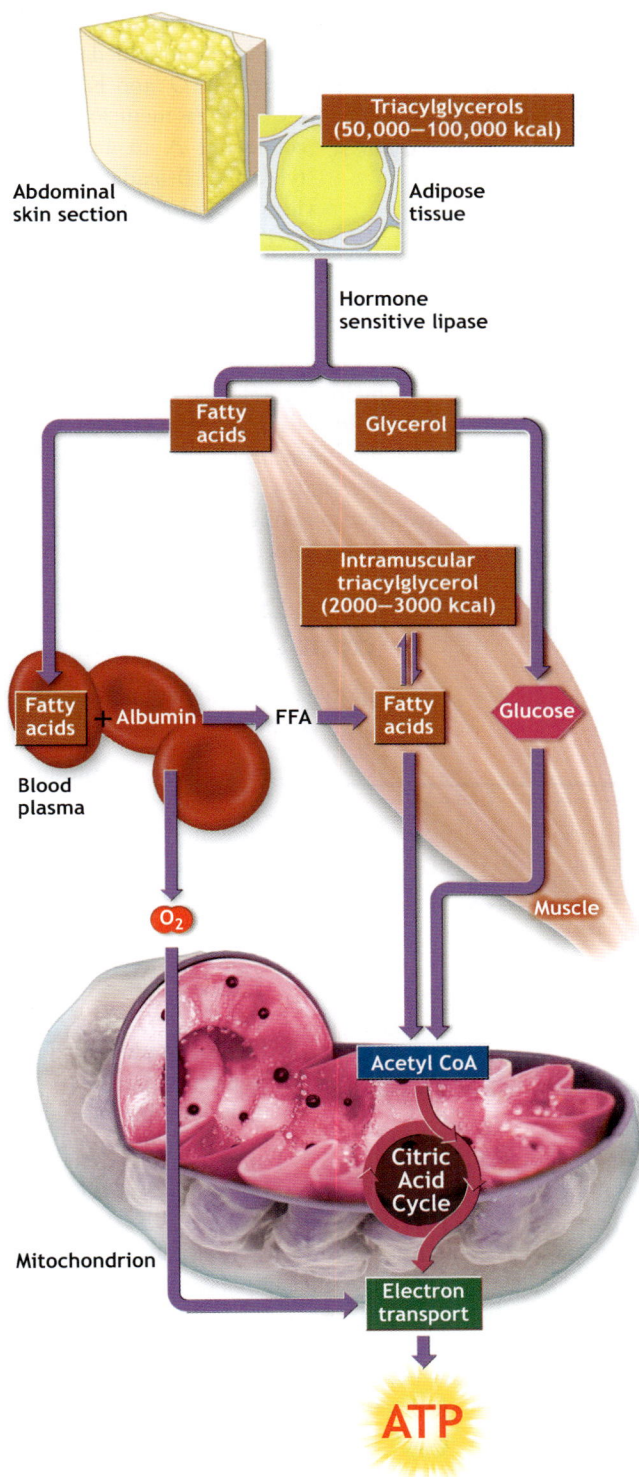

FIGURE 6.16. Dynamics of lipid mobilization and use. Hormone-sensitive lipase stimulates triacylglycerol breakdown into its glycerol and fatty acid components. The blood transports free fatty acids (FFAs) released from adipocytes and bound to plasma albumin. Energy releases when triacylglycerols stored within the muscle fiber also degrade to glycerol and fatty acids.
(Shutterstock: Mitar Vidakovic; Crevis)

 **INTEGRATIVE QUESTION**

If elite marathoners run at an intensity that does not cause appreciable blood lactate accumulation, why do some athletes appear disoriented and fatigued and slow down toward the end of a 26.2-mile competition?

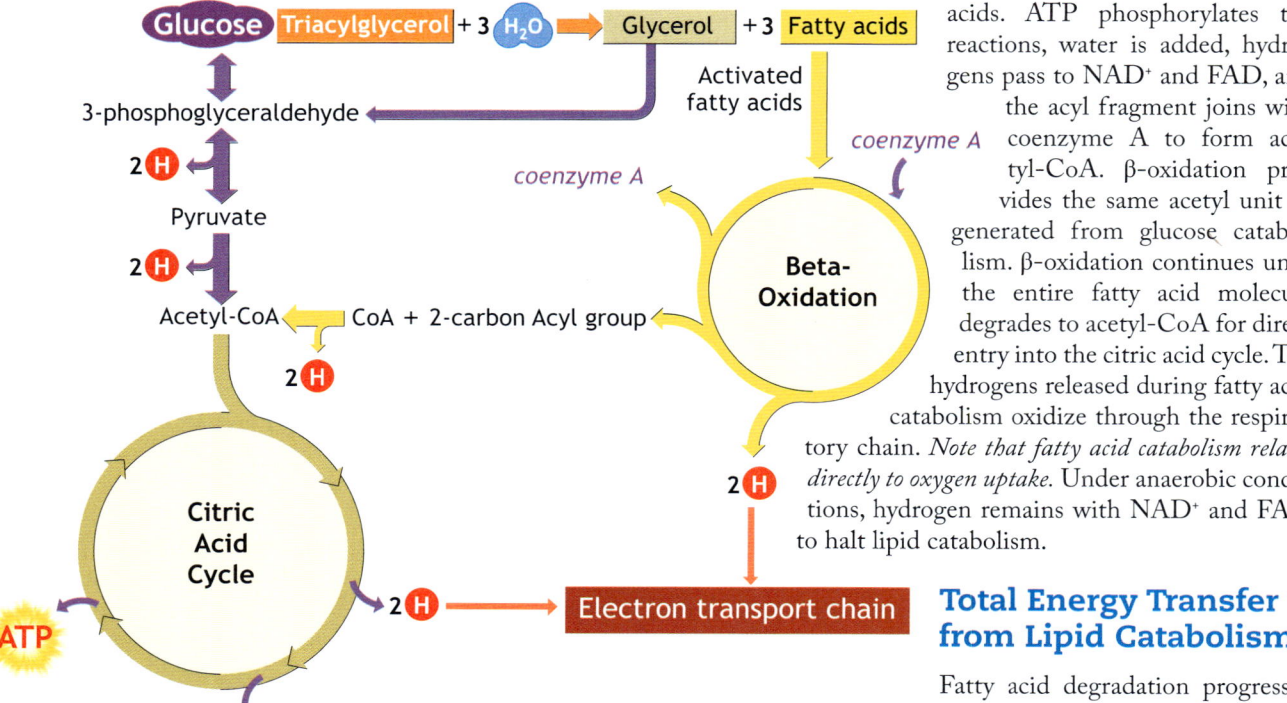

FIGURE 6.17. Pathways for degrading the glycerol and fatty acid components of the triacylglycerol molecule.
(Mitar Vidakovic/Shutterstock)

Glycerol and Fatty Acid Catabolism

FIGURE 6.17 summarizes the pathways for degrading the glycerol and fatty acid fragments of the triacylglycerol molecule.

Glycerol

The anaerobic glycolysis reactions accept glycerol as **3-phosphoglyceraldehyde**, which degrades to pyruvate to form ATP by substrate-level phosphorylation. Hydrogen atoms pass to NAD^+, and the citric acid cycle oxidizes pyruvate. *The complete breakdown of a single glycerol molecule synthesizes 19 ATP molecules.* Glycerol also provides carbon skeletons for glucose synthesis (see "In a Practical Sense"). Glycerol's gluconeogenic role becomes important when glycogen reserves deplete from dietary restriction of carbohydrates, long-term physical activity, or intense training.

Fatty Acids

Fatty acid molecules transform into acetyl-CoA in the mitochondria during **beta (β)-oxidation**. This involves successive splitting of carbon acyl fragments from long chain fatty acids. ATP phosphorylates the reactions, water is added, hydrogens pass to NAD^+ and FAD, and the acyl fragment joins with coenzyme A to form acetyl-CoA. β-oxidation provides the same acetyl unit as generated from glucose catabolism. β-oxidation continues until the entire fatty acid molecule degrades to acetyl-CoA for direct entry into the citric acid cycle. The hydrogens released during fatty acid catabolism oxidize through the respiratory chain. *Note that fatty acid catabolism relates directly to oxygen uptake.* Under anaerobic conditions, hydrogen remains with NAD^+ and FAD to halt lipid catabolism.

Total Energy Transfer from Lipid Catabolism

Fatty acid degradation progresses in three stages:

1. β-oxidation produces NADH and $FADH_2$ by cleaving the fatty acid molecule into 2-carbon acyl fragments.
2. Citric acid cycle degrades acetyl-CoA into carbon dioxide and hydrogen atoms.
3. Hydrogen atoms oxidize by electron transport–oxidative phosphorylation.

For each 18-carbon fatty acid molecule, 147 ADP molecules phosphorylate to ATP during β-oxidation and citric acid cycle metabolism. Each triacylglycerol molecule contains three fatty acid molecules to form 441 ATP molecules from the fatty acid components (3 × 147 ATP). Also, 19 ATP molecules form during glycerol breakdown to generate 460 ATP molecules for each triacylglycerol molecule catabolized. This represents a considerable energy yield compared to the net 32 ATPs formed when skeletal muscle catabolizes a glucose molecule (see Fig. 6.15). Energy conservation efficiency for fatty acid oxidation amounts to about 40%, a value slightly higher than glucoses' approximately 34% oxidation efficiency.[53,54]

Intracellular and extracellular lipid molecules usually supply between 30 and 80% of the energy for biologic work, depending on a person's nutritional status, training level, and physical activity intensity and duration.[38,53] Lipid becomes the *primary* energy fuel for exercise and recovery when intense, long-duration exercise depletes glycogen.[21] Furthermore, enzymatic adaptations occur with prolonged exposure to a high-fat, low-carbohydrate diet because this dietary regimen enhances lipid oxidation capacity in physical activity.[26]

In a Practical Sense

Glucose Synthesis from Triacylglycerol Components

Circulating glucose provides vital fuel for brain and red blood cell functions.[44] Maintaining blood glucose homeostasis remains a challenge in prolonged starvation or intense endurance activity because the limited muscle and liver glycogen reserves deplete rapidly. When this occurs, the central nervous system eventually metabolizes ketone bodies as an energy fuel. The ketones consist of three water-soluble dissolved compounds—acetone, acetoacetic acid, and β-hydroxybutyric acid—produced when fatty acids break down for energy in the liver. Concurrently, muscle protein (amino acids) degrades to gluconeogenic constituents to sustain plasma glucose levels. Excessive muscle protein catabolism eventually produces a muscle-wasting effect. Reliance on protein catabolism, coincident with depleted glycogen, continues because fatty acids from triacylglycerol hydrolysis in muscle and adipose tissue fail to provide gluconeogenic substrates.

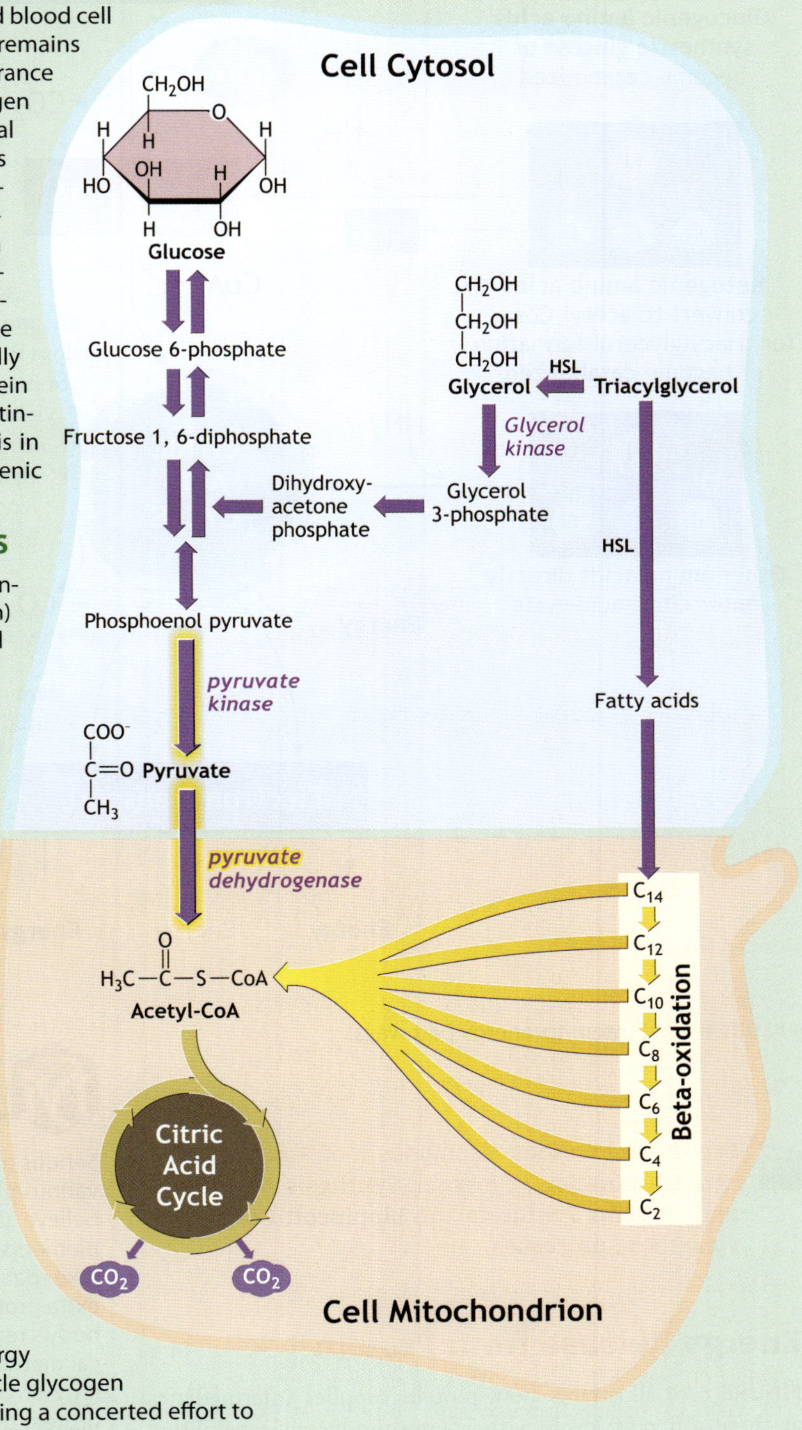

NO GLUCOSE SYNTHESIS FROM FATTY ACIDS

The accompanying figure illustrates why humans cannot convert fatty acids (palmitate in example shown) to glucose from triacylglycerol breakdown. Fatty acid oxidation within the mitochondria produces acetyl-CoA. The pyruvate dehydrogenase and pyruvate kinase reactions proceed irreversibly, so acetyl-CoA cannot simply form pyruvate by carboxylation and synthesize glucose by reversing glycolysis. Instead, the 2-carbon acetyl group formed from acetyl-CoA degrades further when it enters the citric acid cycle. In humans, fatty acid hydrolysis produces no net glucose synthesis.

LIMITED GLUCOSE FROM TRIACYLGLYCEROL-DERIVED GLYCEROL

The figure shows that triacylglycerol hydrolysis via hormone-sensitive lipase (HSL) produces a single 3-carbon glycerol molecule. Unlike fatty acids, the liver can use glycerol for glucose synthesis. After delivering glycerol in the blood to the liver, glycerol kinase phosphorylates it to glycerol 3-phosphate. Further reduction produces dihydroxyacetone phosphate, a substance that provides the carbon skeleton for continuing glucose synthesis. There is a clear "practical application" to sports and exercise nutrition from an understanding about the limited metabolic pathways available for glucose synthesis from the body's triacylglycerol energy depots. Replenishing and maintaining liver and muscle glycogen reserves depend on the physically active person making a concerted effort to regularly consume nutritious, low-to-moderate glycemic foods.

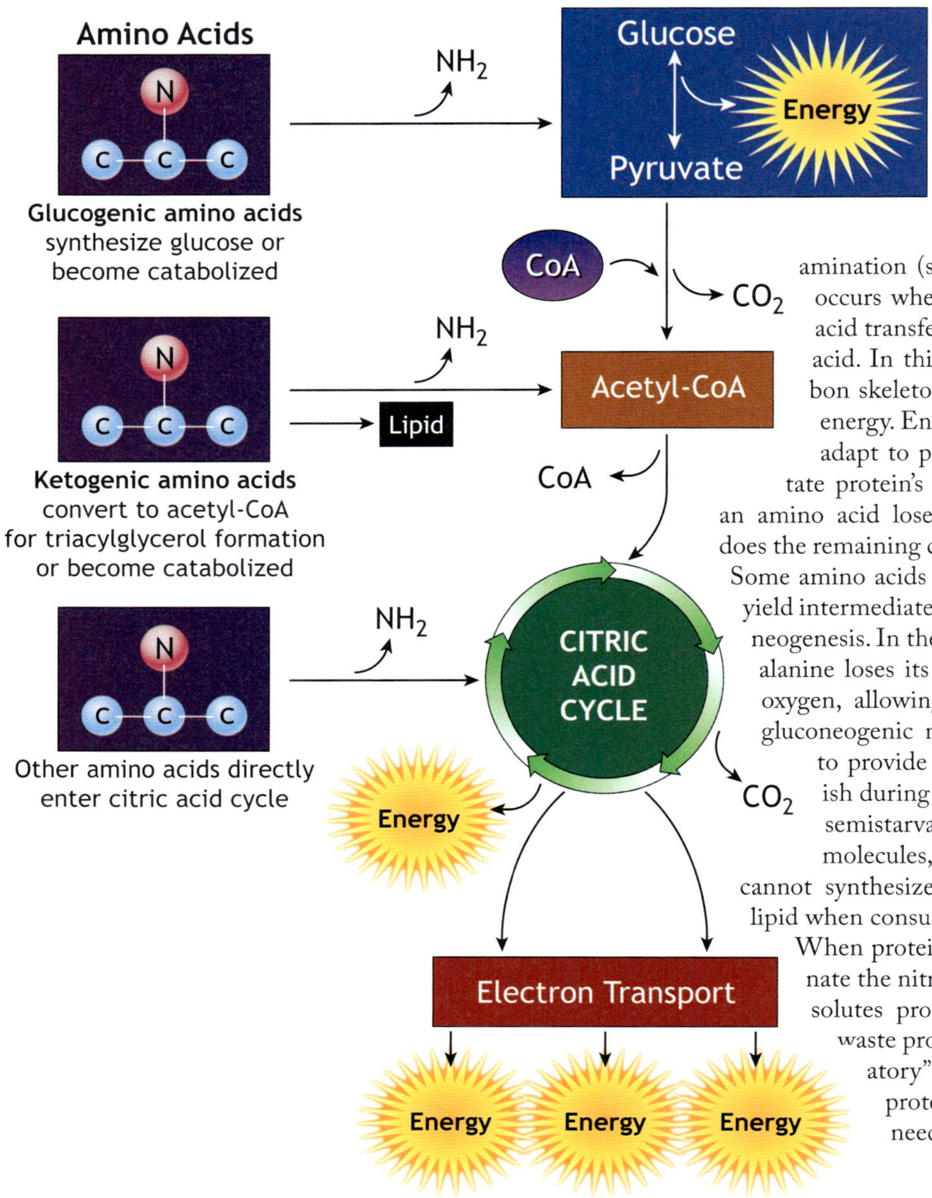

Figure 6.18

FIGURE 6.18. Protein-to-energy pathways.

- **Glucogenic amino acids** synthesize glucose or become catabolized
- **Ketogenic amino acids** convert to acetyl-CoA for triacylglycerol formation or become catabolized
- **Other amino acids** directly enter citric acid cycle

Pathways: Amino Acids → (NH₂ removed) → Glucose ↔ Pyruvate (Energy) → Acetyl-CoA (via CoA, releasing CO_2) → Citric Acid Cycle (releasing CO_2, Energy) → Electron Transport (Energy, Energy, Energy). Ketogenic amino acids feed into Acetyl-CoA and can form Lipid.

requires removing nitrogen from the amino acid molecule, a process known as deamination (refer to Chapter 1). The liver serves as the main deamination site. Skeletal muscle also contains specialized enzymes that remove nitrogen from an amino acid and pass it to other compounds during transamination (see Fig. 1.21). Nitrogen removal usually occurs when an amine group from a donor amino acid transfers to an acceptor acid from a new amino acid. In this way, the muscle directly uses the carbon skeleton by-products of donor amino acids for energy. Enzyme levels for transamination favorably adapt to physical training; this may further facilitate protein's use as an energy substrate. Only when an amino acid loses its nitrogen-containing amine group does the remaining compound contribute to ATP formation. Some amino acids are **glucogenic**; when deaminated, they yield intermediate products for glucose synthesis via gluconeogenesis. In the liver, for example, pyruvate forms when alanine loses its amino group and gains a double-bond oxygen, allowing pyruvate to synthesize glucose. This gluconeogenic method is important to the Cori cycle to provide glucose when glycogen reserves diminish during prolonged physical activity or periods of semistarvation. Similar to lipid and carbohydrate molecules, certain amino acids are **ketogenic**; they cannot synthesize to glucose, but instead synthesize to lipid when consumed in excess.

When protein provides energy, the body must eliminate the nitrogen-containing amine group and other solutes produced from protein breakdown. These waste products leave the body dissolved in "obligatory" fluid (urine). For this reason, excessive protein catabolism increases the body's water needs.

 See the animations "Metabolism of Amino Acids," "Transamination," "Protein Synthesis Overview," and "Protein Synthesis" on **Lippincott Connect** to view these processes.

Energy Release from Protein

FIGURE 6.18 illustrates how protein supplies intermediates at three different levels with energy-producing capabilities. Protein acts as an energy substrate during long-duration, endurance activities. Amino acids first convert to a form that readily enters pathways for energy release. These forms primarily include the branched-chain amino acids—leucine, isoleucine, valine, glutamine, and aspartic acid. This conversion

---

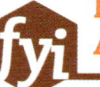 **Excess Dietary Protein Accumulates as Fat**

Serious athletes and others involved in various physical training modes who believe that taking protein supplements builds muscle should take pause and consider that extra protein consumed above the body's requirement (achieved with a typical diet) ends up either catabolized for energy or converted to body fat! The excess protein does **not** contribute to muscle tissue synthesis.

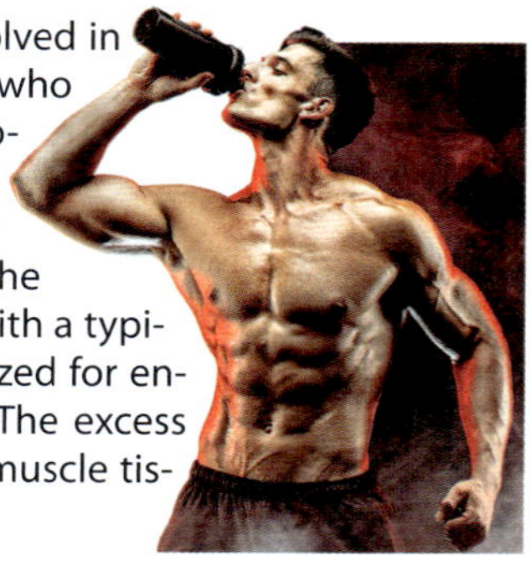

Source:
Remesar X, Alemany M. Dietary energy partition: the central role of glucose. *Int J Mol Sci*. 2020;21:E7729.

Oleksandr Zamuruiev/Shutterstock

The Metabolic Mill: Interrelationships Among Carbohydrate, Lipid, and Protein Metabolism

The "metabolic mill" illustrated in **FIGURE 6.19** depicts the citric acid cycle as the vital link between macronutrient energy and chemical energy in ATP. The citric acid cycle also serves as a metabolic hub to provide intermediates that cross the mitochondrial membrane into the cytosol to synthesize bionutrients for maintenance and growth. For example, excess carbohydrates provide glycerol and acetyl fragments to synthesize triacylglycerol, which can contribute to increased body fatness. Acetyl-CoA functions as the entry point to synthesize cholesterol and hormones. Fatty acids *cannot* contribute to glucose synthesis because the conversion of pyruvate to acetyl-CoA is not reversible (notice the one-way arrow in Figs. 6.17 and 6.19). Many carbon compounds generated in citric acid cycle reactions also provide the organic starting points to synthesize nonessential amino acids.

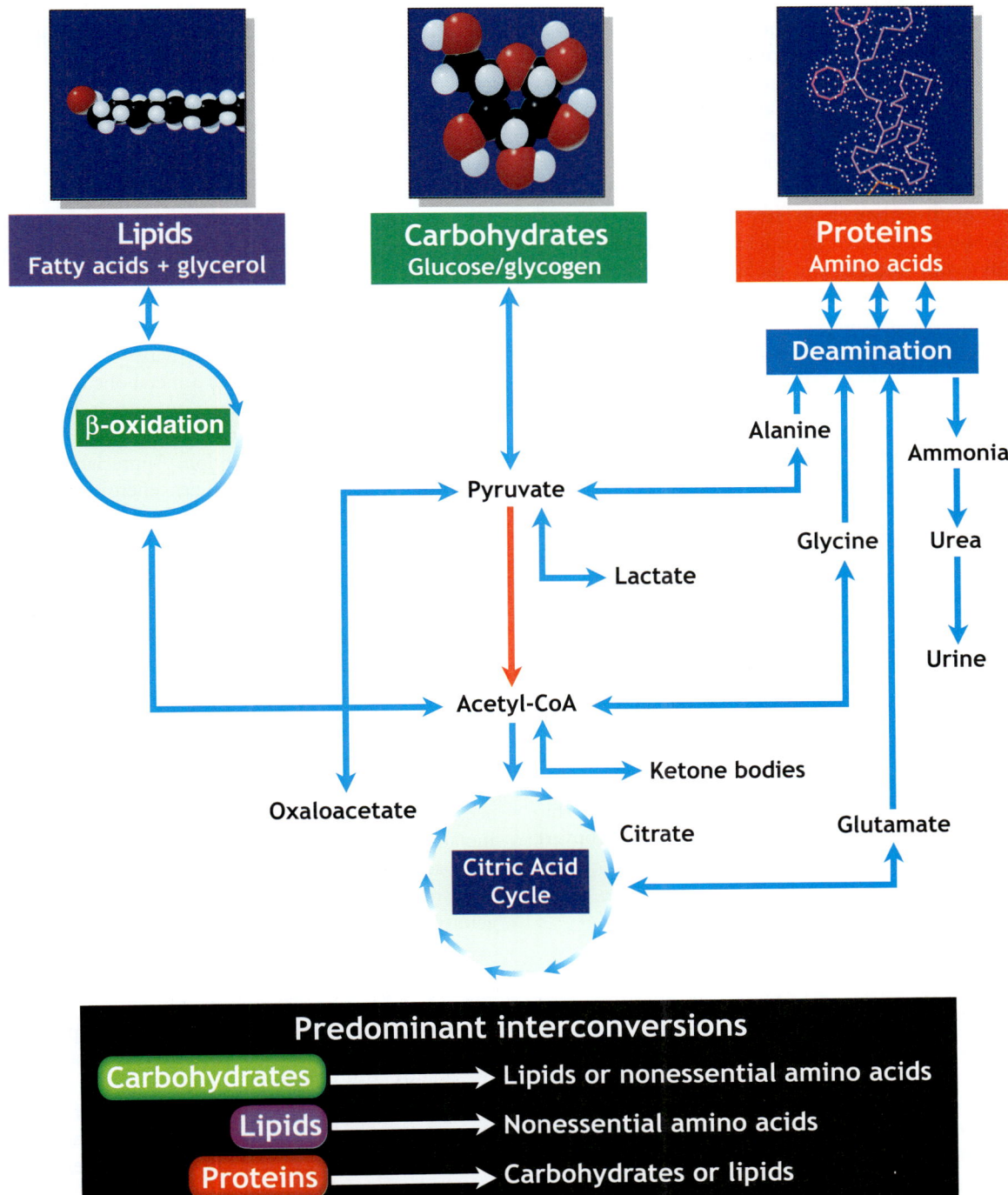

FIGURE 6.19. The "metabolic mill" allows important interconversions for catabolism and anabolism among carbohydrates, lipids, and proteins.

Glucose Conversion to Lipid

Lipogenesis describes lipid formation, mostly in liver cells. It occurs when ingested glucose or protein not used to sustain energy metabolism converts into stored triacylglycerol. For example, when muscle and liver glycogen stores fill (as after a large carbohydrate meal), pancreatic release of insulin causes a 30-fold increase in glucose transport into adipocytes. Insulin initiates the translocation of GLUT 4 transporters from the adipocyte cytosol to the plasma membrane. GLUT 4 facilitates glucose transport into the cytosol for synthesis to triacylglycerols and subsequent storage within the adipocyte. This lipogenesis requires ATP energy working in concert with the B vitamins biotin, niacin, and pantothenic acid.

Lipogenesis begins with carbons from glucose and the carbon skeletons from amino acid molecules that metabolize to acetyl-CoA (see the section "Energy Release from Protein," below). Liver cells bond the acetyl-CoA molecules' acetate parts in a sequential step process to form the 16-carbon saturated fatty acid palmitic acid. This molecule then lengthens to an 18- or 20-carbon chain fatty acid in either the cytosol or mitochondrion. Three fatty acid molecules ultimately join (esterify) with one glycerol molecule produced during glycolysis to yield one triacylglycerol molecule. Triacylglycerol releases into the circulation as a very low-density lipoprotein (VLDL), which cells can use for ATP production or store it in adipocytes along with other lipids from dietary sources.

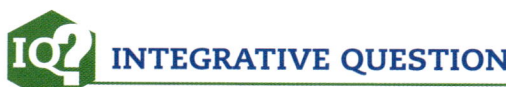

INTEGRATIVE QUESTION

How does cellular ATP vary depending on where a deaminated amino acid enters the catabolic pathways?

Protein Conversion to Lipid

Surplus dietary protein, similar to carbohydrate, readily converts to lipid. After protein's digestion, the circulation transports the amino acids absorbed by the small intestine to the liver. Figure 6.19 illustrates that the carbon skeletons from these amino acids after deamination convert to pyruvate. This six-carbon molecule then enters the mitochondrion to convert to acetyl-CoA for one of two purposes:

1. Catabolism in the citric acid cycle
2. Fatty acid synthesis

Fats Burn in a Carbohydrate Flame

In metabolically active tissues, fatty acid breakdown depends somewhat on continual background levels of carbohydrate catabolism. Recall that acetyl-CoA enters the citric acid cycle by combining with oxaloacetate to form citrate. Oxaloacetate then regenerates from pyruvate during carbohydrate breakdown. This conversion occurs under enzymatic control by pyruvate carboxylase, which adds a carboxyl group to the pyruvate molecule. Fatty acid degradation in the citric acid cycle continues only if sufficient oxaloacetate and other intermediates from carbohydrate breakdown combine with the acetyl-CoA formed during β-oxidation. These intermediates are continually lost or removed from the cycle and require replenishment. Pyruvate formed during glucose catabolism plays an important role in maintaining sufficient oxaloacetate levels (see Figs. 6.14 and 6.18). Low pyruvate levels from inadequate carbohydrate breakdown reduce levels of the citric acid intermediates oxaloacetate and malate. Lipids require these intermediates generated during carbohydrate breakdown for their continual catabolism for energy in the metabolic mill.[5,11,30,36,40] In the sense that carbohydrate acts as a metabolic primer, we can state that "*fats burn in a carbohydrate flame.*"

Lipid's Slower Energy Release

A rate limit exists for fatty acid use by active muscle.[41,55] *The power generated solely by lipid breakdown represents only about one-half that achieved with carbohydrate as the chief aerobic energy source.* Accordingly, depleting muscle glycogen must decrease a muscle's maximum aerobic power output. Just as the hypoglycemic condition coincides with a "central" or neural fatigue, muscle glycogen depletion contributes to "peripheral" or local muscle fatigue during physical activity.[29]

Gluconeogenesis provides a metabolic option to synthesize glucose from noncarbohydrate sources. This process does not replenish or even maintain glycogen stores without adequate carbohydrate consumption. Appreciably reducing carbohydrate availability jeopardizes energy transfer capacity. Glycogen depletion occurs under these five conditions:

1. Prolonged physical activity (e.g., marathon running)
2. Consecutive intense training days
3. Inadequate energy intake (routinely skipping meals)
4. Elimination of dietary carbohydrates (as advocated with high-fat, low-carbohydrate "ketogenic diets")
5. Impaired cellular glucose uptake as in diabetes

Glycogen depletion depresses aerobic exercise intensity, even if adequate fatty acid substrates circulate to muscle. With extreme carbohydrate depletion, the acetate fragments acetoacetate and α-hydroxybutyrate produced in β-oxidation accumulate in extracellular fluids because they cannot enter the citric acid cycle. The liver then converts them to ketone bodies, some of which pass in the urine. If ketosis persists, body fluid acidity can increase to potentially toxic levels.[56–58]

Summary

1. Food macronutrients provide the major potential energy sources to form ATP (when ADP and a phosphate ion rejoin).
2. Complete combustion of one mole of glucose liberates 689 kcal of energy. Of this, the bonds within ATP conserve about 224 kcal (34%), with the remaining energy dissipated as heat.

3. During glycolytic reactions in the cell's cytosol, a net two ATP molecules form during anaerobic substrate-level phosphorylation.
4. Pyruvate converts to acetyl-CoA during the second stage of carbohydrate breakdown in the mitochondrion before progressing through the citric acid cycle.
5. The respiratory chain oxidizes the hydrogen atoms released during glucose breakdown; a portion of the released energy couples with ADP phosphorylation.
6. Complete oxidation of a glucose molecule in skeletal muscle yields 32 ATP molecules.
7. Hydrogen atom oxidation at its formation rate establishes a "steady rate" of aerobic metabolism.
8. During intense physical activity when hydrogen oxidation fails to keep pace with its production, pyruvate temporarily binds hydrogen to form lactate, which briefly allows for the continuation of anaerobic glycolysis.
9. Compounds that either inhibit or activate enzymes at key control points in the oxidative pathways modulate control of glycolysis and the citric acid cycle.
10. Cellular ADP concentration exerts the greatest effect on the rate-limiting enzymes that control energy metabolism.
11. Completely oxidizing a triacylglycerol molecule yields about 460 ATP molecules.
12. Protein can serve as a potentially important energy substrate.
13. After nitrogen removal from an amino acid molecule during deamination, the remaining carbon skeleton enters metabolic pathways to produce ATP aerobically.
14. Numerous interconversions take place among the food nutrients. Fatty acids represent a noteworthy exception because they cannot synthesize to glucose.
15. Lipids require intermediates generated in carbohydrate breakdown for their continual catabolism for energy in the metabolic mill.
16. The power generated solely by lipid breakdown represents only about half that achieved with carbohydrate as the chief aerobic energy source.
17. Muscle glycogen depletion considerably decreases a muscle's maximum aerobic power output.

Key Terms

3-phosphoglyceraldehyde: Intermediate molecule in several central metabolic pathways for energy

Acetyl-coenzyme A (acetyl-CoA): Participates in protein, carbohydrate, and lipid catabolism to deliver the acetyl group to the citric acid cycle to release energy

Adenosine: Purine nucleoside containing adenine attached to a ribose molecule that combines with triphosphate to form adenosine triphosphate (ATP)

Adenosine 3′,5′-cyclic monophosphate (cyclic AMP): Activates hormone-sensitive lipase to regulate lipid catabolism

Adenosine diphosphate (ADP): Sugar backbone attached to adenine and two phosphate groups bonded to the 5-carbon ribose molecule

Adenosine monophosphate (AMP): Nucleotide containing a phosphate group, ribose, and the nucleobase adenine for conversion to ADP and/or ATP

Adenosine triphosphatase (ATPase): Enzyme that catalyzes ATP into ADP and a free phosphate ion or the reverse of that reaction

Adenylate kinase reaction: Single-enzyme–mediated reaction for ATP regeneration: (2 ADP $\xrightarrow{\text{adenylate kinase}}$ ATP + AMP)

Aerobic glycolysis: Cellular respiration component during glucose catabolism

Anaerobic: Related to an absence of free oxygen

Anaerobic glycolysis: Transforms glucose to lactate under conditions of inadequate oxygen availability or utilization

Beta (β)-oxidation: Removing two-carbon units from the carboxyl end of a fatty acid molecule to produce acetyl-CoA

Carnitine acyltransferase: Enzyme that catalyzes transfer of an acyl group to carnitine to form acylcarnitine, which transfers triacylglycerol into mitochondria

Chemiosmotic coupling: Energy producing mechanisms to synthesize ATP via passage of electrons through the electron transport chain

Citrate: Citric acid derivative in the citric acid cycle

Citric acid cycle: Chemical reactions release stored energy through acetyl-CoA oxidation of carbohydrates, lipids, and proteins to form adenosine triphosphate (ATP)

Cori cycle: Lactate produced by anaerobic glycolysis in muscle moves to the liver for glucose conversion and transport to muscle

Creatine kinase: Catalyzes creatine conversion via ATP to create phosphocreatine (PCr) and ADP

Creatine kinase reaction: Single-enzyme–mediated conversion of creatine and adenosine triphosphate (ATP) to form phosphocreatine (PCr) and adenosine diphosphate (ADP)

Cytochrome oxidase (cytochrome aa$_3$): Last enzyme in the electron transport chain, which receives an electron from each of four cytochrome c molecules and transfers them to one dioxygen molecule, converting the molecular oxygen to two molecules of water

Dehydrogenase enzymes: Oxidize substrate by reducing an electron acceptor (e.g., NAD$^+$, FAD)

Epinephrine: Sympathetic nervous system hormone accelerates cleaving of glucose from glycogen

Facilitative diffusion: Passive movement of molecule or ion across a biological membrane via specific transmembrane integral proteins

Flavin adenine dinucleotide (FAD): Reactive coenzyme involved in enzyme-regulated metabolic reactions

Free energy (ΔG): Energy in a physical system with capacity to perform work

Glucogenic: Amino acid converted to glucose through gluconeogenesis

Glucose paradox: Indirect pathway synthesizes liver glycogen from lactate

GLUT 4: Insulin-dependent transporter protein in fat cells and muscle fibers facilitates glucose transport to form ATP

Glycerol-phosphate shuttle: Mechanism regenerates NAD$^+$ from NADH in glycolysis

Glycogenolysis cascade: Progressively greater phosphorylase activation to ensure rapid glycogen mobilization for energy

Glycolysis: Initial metabolic pathway converts the monosaccharide (glucose) into pyruvate and produces ATP; also known as Embden-Meyerhof pathway

Hormone-sensitive lipase: Enzyme that mobilizes stored lipids

Ketogenic: Degraded directly into acetyl-CoA for subsequent lipid synthesis

Lactate dehydrogenase: Catalyzes reversible conversion of lactate to pyruvate and reconversion of NAD$^+$ to NADH

Lactate shuttling: Lactate produced in fast-twitch muscle fibers circulates to other fast-twitch and slow-twitch fibers for conversion to pyruvate and acetyl-CoA in aerobic energy metabolism

Lipogenesis: Lipid formation when ingested glucose or protein not used in energy metabolism converts to triacylglycerol

Malate-aspartate shuttle: Translocates electrons produced in glycolysis for oxidative phosphorylation

Oxaloacetate: Intermediate citric acid cycle product reacts with acetyl-CoA to form citrate in gluconeogenesis

Oxidative phosphorylation: ATP formation by electron transfer from NADH or FADH$_2$ to oxygen

Phosphatase: Enzyme that catalyzes substrate hydrolysis

Phosphofructokinase (PFK): Kinase enzyme that phosphorylates fructose 6-phosphate in glycolysis

P/O ratio: Ratio of phosphate bonds formed to oxygen atoms consumed; reflects ATP coupling to electron transport

Pyruvate: Conjugated pyruvic acid base converts back to glucose via gluconeogenesis, or to fatty acids through acetyl-CoA reactions

Re-esterfication: Fatty acid resynthesis in muscle and adipose tissue

Respiratory (cytochrome) chain: Final common pathway where extracted hydrogen electrons transfer to oxygen

Slow glycolysis: Energy transfers from reactions include anaerobic glycolysis, electron transport, and oxidative phosphorylation

Substrate-level phosphorylation: Energy transferred in rapid (anaerobic) glycolysis via phosphate bond phosphorylation

References are available online at Lippincott Connect.

Additional References

Alberts B, et al. *Essential Cell Biology: An Introduction to the Molecular Biology of the Cell*. 5th ed. New York: W.W. Norton; 2019.

Berg JM, et al. *Biochemistry*. 8th ed. San Francisco: WH Freeman; 2019.

Condon KJ, et al. Genome-wide CRISPR screens reveal multitiered mechanisms through which mTORC1 senses mitochondrial dysfunction. *Proc Natl Acad Sci USA*. 2021;118:e2022120118. doi:10.1073/pnas.2022120118.

Husain A, et al. Approaches to minimize the effects of P-glycoprotein in drug transport: a review. *Drug Dev Res*. 2022. doi:10.1002/ddr.21918.

Janssen JJE, et al. Extracellular flux analyses reveal differences in mitochondrial PBMC metabolism between high-fit and low-fit females. *Am J Physiol Endocrinol Metab*. 2022;322:E141.

Liu S, et al. Effect of Urolithin A Supplementation on muscle endurance and mitochondrial health in older adults: a randomized clinical trial. *JAMA Netw Open*. 2022;5:e2144279.

Marieb EN, Hoehn KN. *Human Anatomy & Physiology*. 11th ed. San Francisco: Pearson; 2019.

Mathews CK, et al. *Biochemistry*. 4th ed. Redwood City: Pearson; 2019.

Oliveira AN, et al. Measurement of protein import capacity of skeletal muscle mitochondria. *J Vis Exp*. 2022. doi:10.3791/63055.

Rubenstein AB, et al. Skeletal muscle transcriptome response to a bout of endurance exercise in physically active and sedentary older adults. *Am J Physiol Endocrinol Metab*. 2022. doi:10.1152/ajpendo.00378.2021.

Schurr A, Passarella S. Aerobic glycolysis: a deOxymoron of (Neuro) Biology. *Metabolites*. 2022;12:72.

Sheng D, Hattori M. Recent progress in the structural biology of P2X receptors. *Proteins*. 2022. doi:10.1002/prot.26302.

Spinelli JB, et al. Fumarate is a terminal electron acceptor in the mammalian electron transport chain. *Science*. 2021;374:1227.

Wen J, et al. Metal-free colorimetric detection of pyrophosphate ions by the peroxidase-like activity of ATP. *Spectrochim Acta A Mol Biomol Spectrosc*. 2022;267:120479.

Xu G, et al. Acute succinate administration increases oxidative phosphorylation and skeletal muscle explosive strength via SUCNR1. *Front Vet Sci*. 20228:808863. doi:10.3389/fvets.2021.808863.

CHAPTER 7: Energy Transfer During Physical Activity

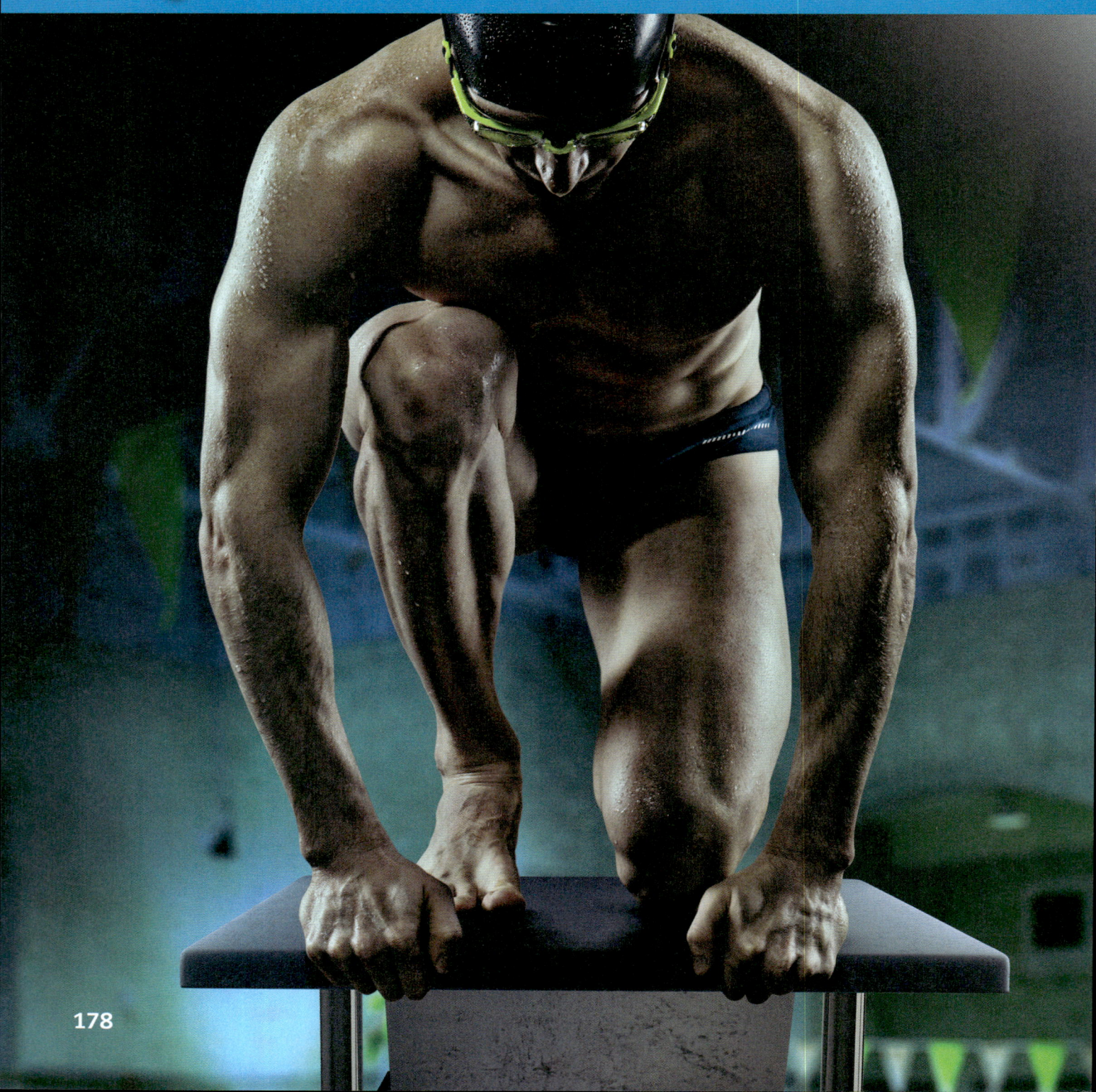

Chapter Objectives

- Identify the three energy transfer systems and outline their irrelative contribution for intensity and duration for specific sport activities
- Discuss the blood lactate threshold concept and indicate differences between sedentary and endurance-trained individuals
- Outline the time course for oxygen uptake during 10 min of moderate-intensity physical activity
- Draw the oxygen uptake curve during progressive physical activity increments to maximum
- Differentiate between type I and type II muscle fibers
- Discuss two differences in postexercise oxygen uptake patterns for moderate and exhaustive physical activity
- Outline two optimal recovery procedures from steady-rate and non–steady-rate physical activity
- Discuss the rationale for intermittent physical activity applied to interval training

Ancillaries at-a-Glance

Visit Lippincott Connect to access the following resources.

- References: Chapter 7
- Focus on Research: A Challenge to Conventional Wisdom

Physical activity provides the greatest demand for energy transfer. In sprint running and swimming, for example, energy output from active muscles exceeds their resting value by 120 times or more. During marathon running, the whole-body energy requirement increases 20 times or more above resting levels. The relative contribution of the body's energy transfer systems differs markedly depending on physical activity intensity, duration, and fitness status.

Immediate Energy: The Adenosine Triphosphate-Phosphocreatine System

Intense, short-duration physical activity, as in a 100-m dash, a 25-m swim, or lifting a heavy weight, requires immediate energy. This energy comes almost exclusively from two intramuscular high-energy phosphate or phosphagen sources—**adenosine triphosphate (ATP)** and phosphocreatine (PCr)—collectively termed **phosphagens**.

Skeletal muscles contain about 3 to 8 mmol of ATP per 1 kg/2.2 lb and four to five times more PCr. This represents between 570 and 690 mmol of high-energy phosphagens for a 70-kg/154-lb person with a 30-kg/66-lb muscle mass. Assuming that 20 kg/44 lb of muscle becomes active during "big-muscle" activity, sufficient stored phosphagen energy will supply the energy to move from standing or sitting to brisk walking for 1 min, running at a marathon pace for 20 to 30 s, or sprint-running for 5 to 8 s. Theoretically, these high-energy compounds should become fully depleted within about 20 to 30 s during all-out physical activity.[8,19] The maximum energy transfer rate from the high-energy phosphates exceeds by four to eight times the maximal energy transfer from aerobic metabolism. For example, in the 100-m dash, in which Usain Bolt of Jamaica set world and Olympic records (world record 9.58 s, August 16, 2009; Olympic record 9.63 s, August 5, 2012), the body cannot maintain maximum speed for the entire run and actually slows down toward the end of the race; the winner is often the one who slows down least. *Thus, the quantity of intramuscular phosphagens substantially influences "all-out" energy for brief durations.* The enzyme 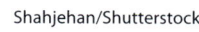 **creatine kinase** triggers PCr hydrolysis to resynthesize ATP to regulate the phosphagen breakdown rate.

Shahjehan/Shutterstock

Short-Term Energy: The Glycolytic (Lactate-Forming) System

Resynthesizing high-energy phosphates proceeds at a rapid rate in intense, short-duration activities. The energy to phosphorylate adenosine diphosphate during such movements comes mainly from stored muscle glycogen breakdown via rapid anaerobic glycolysis with resulting lactate formation (see Chapter 6). With inadequate oxygen supply and/or use, all of the hydrogens formed in rapid glycolysis fail to oxidize, causing pyruvate to convert to lactate in the chemical reaction Pyruvate + 2H → Lactate. This chemical conversion allows for the continuation of rapid ATP formation by anaerobic substrate-level phosphorylation. Recall that this process allows ATP to form rapidly *without* oxygen; rapid anaerobic glycolysis for ATP resynthesis can be considered reserve fuel. It comes into play when a person accelerates during the activity. Examples also include at the start of movement or the last few hundred yards in a mile run or when one goes "all-out" from start to finish during a 440-m run or 100-m swim. *Blood lactate accumulates rapidly during large-muscle, maximal movements lasting between 60 and 180 s.* Decreasing intensity to extend the movement period correspondingly decreases lactate accumulation rate and final blood lactate level.

Lactate Flux

Lactate forms and is used continuously in different cells under fully aerobic conditions. In this way, lactate can be viewed as an important link between glycolytic and aerobic pathways as the product of two processes:

1. Glycolytic metabolic pathways
2. Substrate for mitochondrial respiration

In **FIGURE 7.1A**, lactate, represented in yellow, serves as a go-between among cells, tissues, and organs via glycolytic and oxidative metabolic processes. In Figure 7.1B, a cell-to-cell

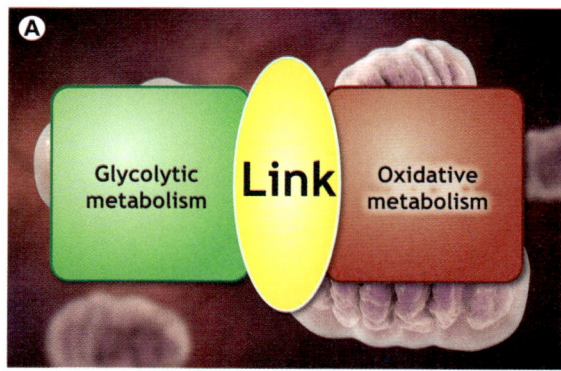

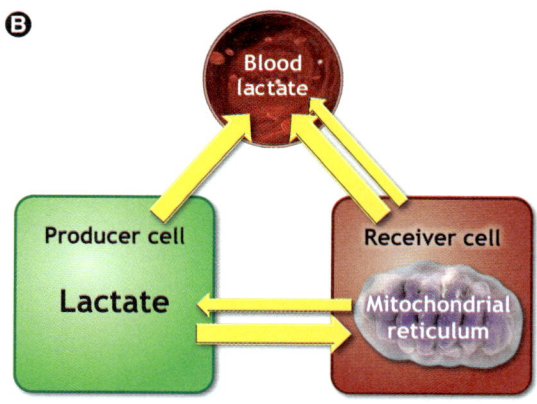

FIGURE 7.1. Generalized contemporary lactate shuttle concept. **(A)** Lactate interfaces between glycolytic and oxidative metabolism. **(B)** Cell-to-cell lactate shuttle within cells and mitochondria.
(Shutterstock: Kateryna Kon; SciePro)

shuttling occurs within the tissue, hence the term "lactate shuttle." In this scenario, lactate concentration is greatest in highly glycolytic cells and lowest in highly oxidative cells, in which lactate becomes a highly oxidizable substrate in the mitochondrion. During continuous submaximal exercise of greater than 10-min duration, blood lactate is greater in consumer "receiving" cells but lower in producer (originating) cells, thus making blood lactate accumulation essentially zero within the whole muscle. According to the **lactate shuttle hypothesis**, the linkage occurs under fully aerobic conditions, with lactate serving not as a metabolic waste product or a fatigue-producing agent but as an important messenger in a complex feedback loop.

At the whole-body level, lactate metabolism is important for at least three reasons, as it serves as a

1. Major energy source
2. Major gluconeogenic precursor
3. Signaling-like lactormone molecule with autocrine, paracrine, and endocrine-mimicking effects

Lactate Accumulation During Physical Activity

Blood lactate does not accumulate at all physical activity levels. **FIGURE 7.2** illustrates the general relationship between oxygen uptake, expressed as a percentage of maximum, and blood lactate during light, moderate, and strenuous activity for endurance athletes and untrained subjects. During light and moderate activity (<50% aerobic capacity), blood lactate formation equals lactate disappearance and oxygen-consuming reactions adequately meet the energy demands. In biochemical terms, energy generated from hydrogen oxidation provides the predominant ATP "fuel" for muscular activity. Any lactate formed in one part of a working muscle becomes oxidized by muscle fibers with high oxidative capacity in the same muscle or less active nearby muscles such as the heart and other tissues.[11,32,37] When lactate oxidation equals its production, blood lactate level remains stable even though increases may occur in exercise intensity and oxygen uptake.

For healthy, untrained persons, blood lactate begins to accumulate and rise in an exponential manner at about 50 to 55% of the maximal capacity for aerobic metabolism. The traditional explanation assumes a relative tissue hypoxia that allows blood lactate to accumulate. When glycolytic metabolism predominates, nicotinamide adenine dinucleotide (NADH) production exceeds the cell's capacity to shuttle its hydrogens (electrons; sometimes referred to as the **hydrogen shuttle**) down the respiratory chain from insufficient oxygen supply or oxygen use at the tissue level. It may even be stimulated by the hormones epinephrine and norepinephrine independent of tissue hypoxia. The imbalance in hydrogen release and subsequent oxidation (more precisely, the cytoplasmic NAD+/NADH ratio) causes pyruvate to accept the excess hydrogens as two hydrogen ions join to the pyruvate molecule. The original pyruvate with two additional hydrogens forms a new molecule—lactic acid (changed to lactate in the body), which begins to accumulate.[33]

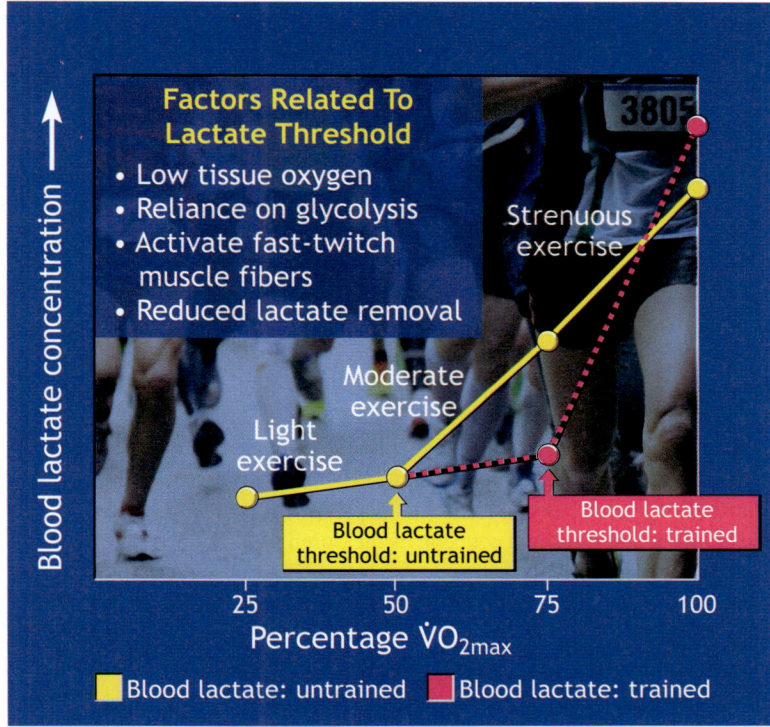

FIGURE 7.2. Blood lactate concentration for trained and untrained subjects at different exercise levels expressed as a $\dot{V}O_{2max}$ percentage. (Mikael Damkier/Shutterstock)

Radioactive tracer studies that label carbon in the glucose molecule advanced the hypothesis to explain lactate buildup in muscle and its subsequent appearance in blood.[10] The research revealed that, while lactate continuously forms in muscle during rest and moderate physical activity, about 70% oxidizes, 20% converts to glucose in muscle and liver, and 10% synthesizes to amino acids with no *net* lactate accumulation (i.e., blood lactate concentration remains stable). *Blood lactate accumulates only when its disappearance by oxidation or substrate conversion does not match its production.*

Aerobic training adaptations allow for high rates of lactate turnover at a given movement intensity, so lactate begins to accumulate at higher intensity levels than those in the untrained state.[44,53] Another explanation for lactate buildup during physical activity includes the tendency for the lactate dehydrogenase (LDH) enzyme in fast-twitch muscle fibers to favor the conversion of pyruvate to lactate. In contrast, LDH levels in slow-twitch fibers favor lactate-to-pyruvate conversion. Recruitment of fast-twitch fibers with increasing exercise intensity thus favors lactate formation, independent of tissue oxygenation.

Lactate production and accumulation accelerate as exercise intensity increases. In such cases, muscle cells can neither meet the additional energy demands aerobically nor oxidize lactate at its formation rate. A similar pattern exists for both untrained subjects and endurance athletes, except the threshold for lactate buildup, termed the **blood lactate threshold**, occurs at a *higher* aerobic capacity percentage in athletes.[21,51,52] Trained endurance athletes perform steady-rate aerobic physical activity at intensities between 80 and

90% of maximum aerobic capacity,[48] and likely relates to three factors[11,14,20,35]:

1. Athlete's specific genetic endowment (e.g., muscle fiber type, muscle blood flow responsiveness)
2. Specific local training adaptations that favor *less* lactate production
3. More rapid lactate removal rate via greater lactate turnover and/or conversion at any physical activity intensity

Endurance training increases capillary density and mitochondrial size and number, as well as the concentration of enzymes and transfer agents in aerobic metabolism,[30,45] a response unimpaired with aging.[15] Training adaptations enhance cellular capacity to generate ATP aerobically through glucose and fatty acid catabolism. Maintaining a low lactate level also conserves glycogen reserves to inhibit muscular fatigue processes and extend the duration of intense aerobic effort.[49] Chapter 14 further develops the blood lactate threshold concept, its measurement, and its relation to endurance performance. In Chapter 21, we discuss how training impacts blood lactate threshold adaptations.

Lactate-Producing Capacity

Producing high blood lactate levels during maximum physical activity increases with specific sprint-power anaerobic training and decreases when training ceases. Sprint-power athletes often achieve 20 to 30% higher blood lactate levels than untrained counterparts during *maximum* short-duration activities. One or more of three mechanisms help to explain this response:

1. Improved motivation with training
2. Increased intramuscular glycogen stores with training, which allow a greater energy contribution via anaerobic glycolysis
3. Training-induced increase in glycolytic-related enzymes, particularly phosphofructokinase, as the 20% increase in glycolytic enzymes falls well below the two- to threefold increase in aerobic enzymes with endurance training

Blood Lactate as an Energy Source

In Chapter 6, we pointed out how blood lactate serves as substrate for gluconeogenesis and as a direct fuel source for active muscle. Isotope tracer studies of muscle metabolism reveal that lactate produced in fast-twitch muscle fibers circulates to other fast-twitch or slow-twitch fibers for conversion to pyruvate. Pyruvate, in turn, converts to acetyl-coenzyme A for entry to the citric acid cycle for aerobic energy metabolism. Lactate shuttling between cells enables **glycogenolysis** in one cell to supply other cells with fuel for oxidation. *This makes muscle not only a major site of lactate production but also a primary tissue for lactate removal via oxidation.*

A muscle oxidizes much of its produced lactate without releasing it into the bloodstream. The liver also accepts muscle-generated lactate from the bloodstream and synthesizes it to glucose through the Cori cycle's gluconeogenic reactions, which are diagrammed in Chapter 6. Glucose derived from lactate takes one of two routes:

1. Returns in the blood to skeletal muscle for energy metabolism
2. Synthesizes to glycogen for storage

These two routes make lactate the anaerobic by-product of intense activity a valuable metabolic substrate, and certainly not an unwanted by-product.

Long-Term Energy: The Aerobic System

Glycolytic reactions produce relatively few ATPs. Accordingly, aerobic metabolism provides nearly all of the energy transfer when physical activity continues beyond several minutes.

Oxygen Uptake During Physical Activity

FIGURE 7.3 shows the time course for oxygen uptake—also referred to as *pulmonary oxygen uptake* because oxygen measurements occur at the lung and not the active muscles—during a slow 10-min run in endurance-trained and untrained individuals. Oxygen uptake rises exponentially during the first minutes of physical activity, called the **oxygen uptake fast component**, to attain a plateau between the third and fourth minutes of the run. The orange and purple regions indicate the oxygen deficit: the quantity of oxygen that would have been consumed had oxygen uptake reached steady rate immediately. If the individual maintains the same running pace, oxygen uptake then remains relatively stable. **Steady rate**, also known as *steady state*, generally describes the oxygen uptake flattening along the curve. It reflects a balance between energy required by the active muscles and ATP production in aerobic metabolism. Within the steady-rate exercise region, coupled redox reactions supply the energy for the activity. Any lactate produced either oxidizes or recon-

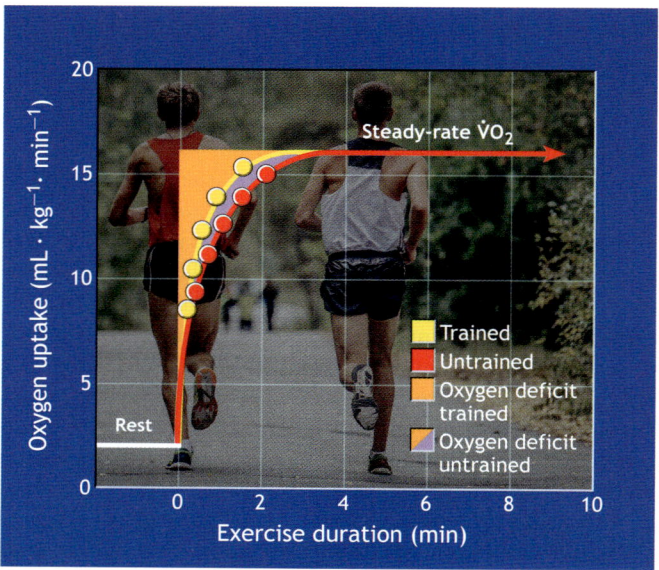

FIGURE 7.3. Oxygen uptake versus time during a continuous jog at a relatively slow pace in endurance trained and untrained individuals.
(sportpoint/Shutterstock)

verts to glucose. *No appreciable blood lactate accumulates under steady-rate aerobic metabolic conditions.*

Once a steady rate of aerobic metabolism occurs, physical activity theoretically could progress indefinitely if the individual wished to continue. This assumes that steady-rate aerobic metabolism singularly determines the capacity to sustain steady-rate activity. Fluid loss and electrolyte depletion during activity often pose limiting factors, especially in hot weather. Maintaining adequate liver glycogen for central nervous system function and muscle glycogen to power physical activity takes on added importance at high intensities of prolonged aerobic effort. Glycogen depletion dramatically reduces exercise capacity.

Individuals have many steady-rate levels of physical activity. For some, the spectrum ranges from computer chores to mowing the lawn. An elite endurance runner, on the other hand, can maintain a steady aerobic metabolic rate throughout a 26.2-mi marathon, averaging slightly less than 5 min/mi, or during a 658-mi ultramarathon, averaging 118 mi/d for slightly over 5 days! Maintaining adequate aerobic metabolism necessitates well-developed functional capacities from diverse physiologic systems that deliver oxygen continuously at a sufficient rate to all active muscles. Two major factors help to explain exceptional endurance accomplishments:

1. Central circulation that functions with high capacity to *deliver* oxygen to active muscles
2. Active muscles that function with high capacity to *use* available oxygen

Oxygen Deficit

At activity onset, the oxygen uptake curve, as shown in Figure 7.3, does not increase instantaneously to steady rate. In the initial, transitional stage of constant-load effort, oxygen uptake remains below a steady-rate level even though the energy requirement remains unchanged throughout the activity. An early lag in oxygen uptake should not be surprising because energy for muscle action comes directly from the immediate anaerobic ATP breakdown. Even with experimentally increased oxygen availability and increased oxygen diffusion gradients at the tissue level, the initial increase in exercise oxygen uptake is always lower than the steady-rate oxygen uptake.[24,25] Due to the intrinsic inertia in cellular metabolic signals and enzyme activation and relative sluggishness in oxygen delivery to the mitochondria, the hydrogens produced in energy metabolism do not immediately oxidize and combine with oxygen.[40,46] Oxygen uptake increases rapidly in subsequent energy transfer reactions under three conditions, in which oxygen combines with the hydrogens liberated in

1. Glycolysis
2. Fatty acid β-oxidation
3. Citric acid cycle reactions

After several minutes of submaximal physical activity, hydrogen production and subsequent oxidation to power ATP production become matched to the exercise-energy requirement. At this stage, oxygen uptake attains a balance indicating a relative steady rate between energy requirement and aerobic energy transfer.

fyi Lactic Acid, Lactate, and pH

Hydrogen ions (H^+) that dissociate from lactic acid present a primary problem to the body's homeostatic mechanisms. At normal pH levels, lactic acid almost immediately and completely dissociates to H^+ and lactate. Few disruptions exist if the amount of free H^+ does not exceed the body's ability to buffer them and maintain pH at a relatively stable level. The pH decreases when excessive lactic acid exceeds the body's immediate buffering capacity. Discomfort and possible performance impairment occur as the blood becomes more acidic.

JeffreyRasmussen/Shutterstock

The **oxygen deficit** *quantitatively expresses the difference between the total oxygen uptake during activity and the total that would be consumed had steady-rate oxygen uptake been achieved at the onset.* The oxygen deficit represents the immediate anaerobic energy transfer from intramuscular high-energy phosphate and rapid glycolytic hydrolysis until steady-rate energy transfer matches the exercise energy requirements. Interestingly, lactate begins to increase in active muscle well before the high-energy phosphates reach their lowest levels. This indicates that rapid glycolysis also contributes anaerobic energy in the initial stages of vigorous physical activity, well before full use of the high-energy phosphates. *Energy for physical activity does not occur from activating different energy systems that "switch on" and "switch off," but rather from smooth blending with overlap from one energy transfer mode to another.*[26,43]

Oxygen uptake kinetics at activity onset do not differ between children and adults.[27] Regardless of age, the endurance-trained person achieves steady rate more rapidly, with a smaller oxygen deficit than sprint-power athletes, cardiac patients, older adults, or untrained individuals.[7,16,31,34] Consequently, a faster aerobic response allows a trained person

fyi Rate-Limiting Enzymes

Energy Pathway	Enzyme	Stimulated by	Inhibited by
ATP/PCr	Creatine kinase	ADP	ATP
Glycolysis	Phosphofructokinase	AMP, ADP, P_i, ↑ pH	ATP, CPr, citrate, ↓ pH
Citric acid cycle	Isocitrate dehydrogenase	ADP, Ca^{++}, NAD^+	ATP, NADH
Electron transport	Cytochrome oxidase	ADP, P_i	ATP

Andrii Vodolazhskyi/Shutterstock

to consume a greater total amount of oxygen to reach steady rate, which makes the anaerobic energy transfer component proportionately smaller. The following three aerobic training adaptations facilitate the rate of aerobic metabolism when activity begins:

1. More rapid increase in muscle bioenergetics
2. Increase in overall cardiac output
3. Disproportionately large regional blood flow to active muscle complemented by cellular adaptations

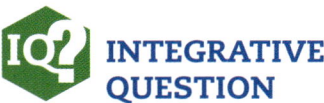

INTEGRATIVE QUESTION

At what physical activity level does the body switch to anaerobic energy metabolism?

FIGURE 7.4. Maximal oxygen uptake ($\dot{V}O_{2max}$) while running up hills of progressively increasing slope occurs in a region designated by the *yellow data points* along the top part of the curve and not a single point in the flattened region.
(Jacob Lund/Shutterstock)

Maximal Oxygen Uptake

FIGURE 7.4 depicts oxygen uptake during constant-speed runs up six progressively steeper "hills." The lime green dots represent measured oxygen uptake values while traversing the treadmill's hills. In the laboratory, increasing treadmill elevation serves as the "hills" metaphor, as does increasing stepping rate on a step bench, progressively increasing resistance to pedaling at a constant rate on a bicycle ergometer, or increasing the rate of water flow as a swimmer tries to maintain a steady pace during a swim flume test. Each successive "hill" imposes a greater energy output that places additional demand for aerobic ATP resynthesis. During the first several hills, oxygen uptake increases rapidly, with each new steady-rate value in direct proportion to exercise intensity. The runner maintains speed up the two last hills, but oxygen uptake fails to increase as rapidly or to the same extent as in the previous hills. Further increases in exercise intensity produce a less-than-expected increase in oxygen uptake. No increase in oxygen uptake occurs during the run up the last hill. *The region in yellow at the top right of the figure where oxygen uptake plateaus or increases only slightly with additional increases in exercise intensity represents the* **maximal oxygen uptake ($\dot{V}O_{2max}$)**, *also called maximal aerobic power, or aerobic capacity*. Energy transfer via anaerobic glycolysis allows more-intense physical activity with additional lactate accumulation, until the runner becomes exhausted and refuses to continue.

The $\dot{V}O_{2max}$ quantitatively expresses a person's capacity for aerobic ATP resynthesis. This makes the $\dot{V}O_{2max}$ an important indicator of how well a person can maintain intense exercise for longer than 4 or 5 min. Attaining a high $\dot{V}O_{2max}$ has important physiologic meanings in addition to its role in sustaining exercise energy metabolism. A high $\dot{V}O_{2max}$ requires integration of the diverse physiologic support systems (pulmonary ventilation, hemoglobin concentration, blood volume and cardiac output, peripheral blood flow, and cellular metabolic capacity), which are illustrated in **FIGURE 7.5**.

ATP Generation: Fast- Versus Slow-Twitch Muscle Fibers

Humans have two distinct muscle fiber types, each generating ATP differently. **Fast-twitch (FT) muscle fibers,**

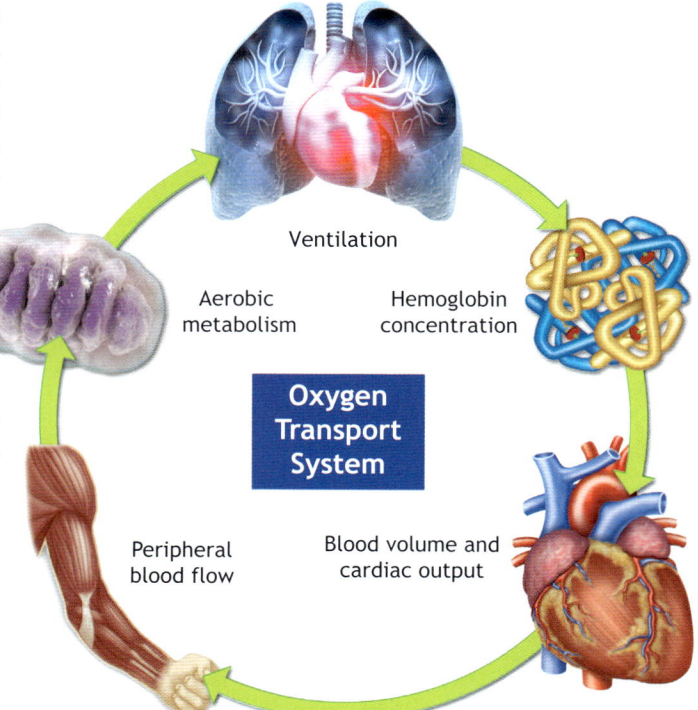

FIGURE 7.5. $\dot{V}O_{2max}$ depends on five components and their functional capacity and integration for oxygen supply, transport, delivery, and use.
(Shutterstock: Kateryna Kon; Explode; ilusmedical; Emre Terim)

also known as type II muscle fibers, are subdivided into type IIa and type IIx fiber types. Each fiber possesses rapid contraction speed and high capacity for anaerobic ATP production via glycolysis. The type IIa fiber also possesses somewhat high aerobic capacity. Type II fibers predominate in change-of-pace and stop-and-go basketball, field hockey, lacrosse, soccer, and ice hockey. They also increase force output when running or cycling up hills at a constant speed or during all-out effort requiring rapid, powerful movements powered by energy from anaerobic metabolism.

The second fiber type, the **slow-twitch (ST) muscle fibers**, also known as type I muscle fibers, generates energy primarily through aerobic pathways. It possesses a slower contraction speed compared with fast-twitch fibers. Capacity to generate ATP aerobically intimately relates to the type I fiber's numerous large mitochondria, which include high enzyme levels that aerobic metabolism requires, particularly for fatty acid catabolism. Slow-twitch muscle fibers primarily sustain continuous activities requiring a steady rate of aerobic energy transfer. Fatigue in prolonged running associates with glycogen depletion in the leg muscles' type I and type IIa muscle fibers.[2,22] Selective glycogen depletion also occurs in the arms of wheelchair-dependent athletes during extended physical activity.[42] More than likely, predominance of slow-twitch muscle fibers contributes to the high blood lactate thresholds in elite endurance athletes.

Athletes who excel in high-power rather than endurance activities usually have a greater number of muscle fibers of the type that supports their sport's energy demands. For example, **FIGURE 7.6** illustrates the muscle-fiber composition of two athletes in sports that rely on distinctly different energy transfer systems favored by specific muscle fiber type predominance. The

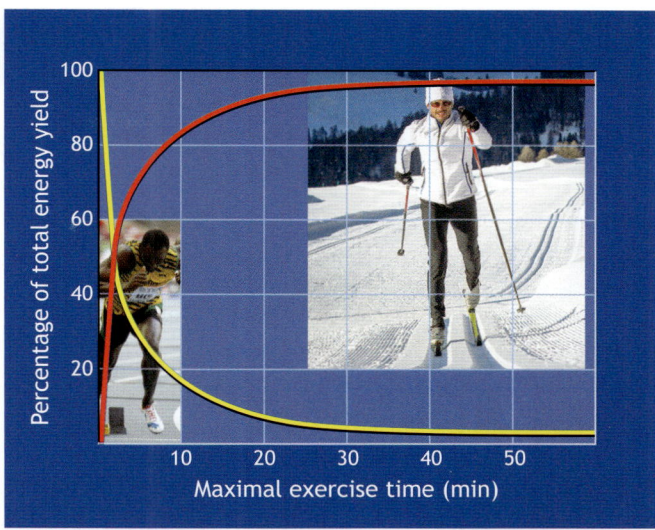

FIGURE 7.7. Relative contribution of aerobic and anaerobic energy metabolism during maximal physical effort of various durations.
(Data from Åstrand P-O, Rodahl K, et al. *Textbook of Work Physiology: Physiological Bases of Exercise*, 4th ed., p. 257. New York: McGraw-Hill, 2003. Shutterstock: michelangeloop; Kaliva)

Duration of maximal exercise									
	Seconds			Minutes					
	10	30	60	2	4	10	30	60	120
Percentage anaerobic	90	80	70	50	35	15	5	2	1
Percentage aerobic	10	20	30	50	65	85	95	98	99

type I fibers stain dark, whereas type II fibers remain unstained. For the 50-m sprint swim champion (*left panel*), type II fibers represent nearly 80% of the total muscle fibers, whereas the endurance cyclist possesses 80% type I fibers. Most sports require relatively slow, sustained muscle actions interspersed with short energy bursts, as in basketball, soccer, lacrosse, and field hockey. Understandably, these activities require an equal percentage and activation of *both* muscle fiber types. This suggests that a muscle's predominant fiber type contributes to success in certain sports or activities. Chapter 18 explores this idea more fully, including other considerations concerning each fiber type's metabolic, contractile, and fatigue characteristics and training effects.

Physical Activity Energy Spectrum

FIGURE 7.7 illustrates the relative contribution from anaerobic and aerobic energy sources related to maximal exercise time, while **TABLE 7.1** shows the major fuel use during various running competitions. For example, a 100-m sprint run corresponds to any all-out physical activity for about 10 s, whereas an 800-m run and 200-m swim last approximately 2 min. All-out 1-min activities include the 400-m run, the 100-m swim, and repeated full-court presses during basketball. In the 1500- to 10,000-m runs, PCr provides the immediate fuel for the first few seconds and, if resynthesized during the run, supplies some additional energy (although minor) in the sprint to the finish, but the major energy is supplied via aerobic reactions.

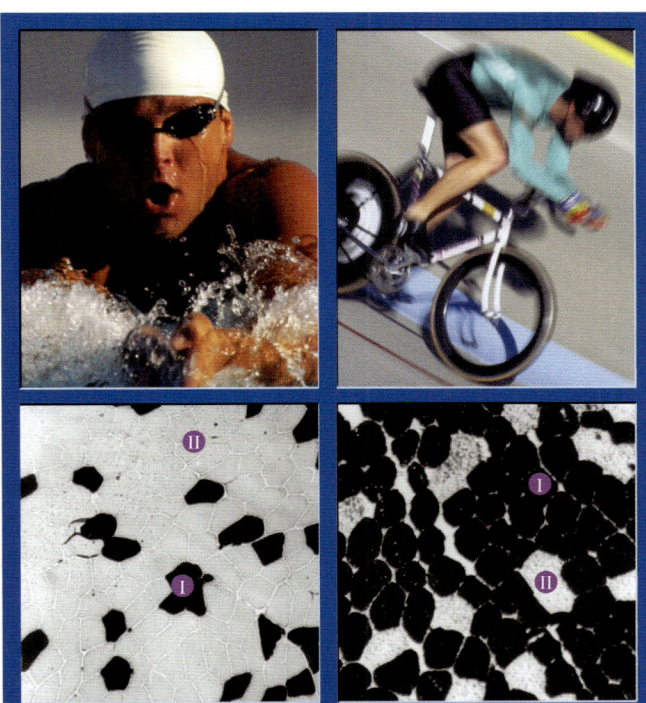

FIGURE 7.6. Differences in muscle-fiber type composition between a sprint swimmer and endurance cyclist.
(Photos and photomicrographs courtesy Dr. R. Billeter, School of Life Sciences, University of Nottingham, Great Britain.)

In a Practical Sense

Interpreting $\dot{V}O_{2max}$: Establishing Cardiovascular Fitness Categories

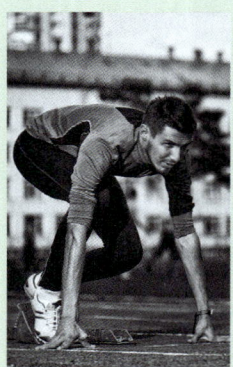
Danil Nevsky/Shutterstock

Cardiovascular fitness reflects the maximal oxygen uptake during each minute of near-maximum exercise assessed in the laboratory and expressed as milliliters oxygen per kilogram body mass per minute ($mL \cdot kg^{-1} \cdot min^{-1}$). Individual values range from about 10 $mL \cdot kg^{-1} \cdot min^{-1}$ in cardiac patients to 80 or 90 $mL \cdot kg^{-1} \cdot min^{-1}$ in world-class runners and cross-country skiers. Male and female distance runners, swimmers, cyclists, and cross-country skiers generally attain $\dot{V}O_{2max}$ values nearly two times greater than those of sedentary persons (see Fig. 11.7 in Chapter 11).

Researchers have measured $\dot{V}O_{2max}$ in thousands of individuals of different ages. The average values and respective ranges for males and females have been applied to establish cardiovascular fitness classification categories. The table presents the five categories from literature data for nonathletes.

Sources:
Hermosilla F, et al. Periodization and programming for individual 400 m medley swimmers. *Int J Environ Res Public Health*. 2021;18:6474.
Wu ZJ, et al. Impact of high-intensity interval training on cardiorespiratory fitness, body composition, physical fitness, and metabolic parameters in older adults: a meta-analysis of randomized controlled trials. *Exp Gerontol*. 2021;150:111345.

CARDIOVASCULAR FITNESS CLASSIFICATION CATEGORIES IN MALES AND FEMALES BASED ON MAXIMUM OXYGEN UPTAKE LEVELS

Gender	Age (y)	$\dot{V}O_{2max}$ ($mL \cdot kg^{-1} \cdot min^{-1}$)				
		Poor	Fair	Average	Good	Excellent
Male	≤29	≤24.9	25–33.9	34–43.9	44–52.9	≥53
	30–39	≤22.9	23–30.9	31–41.9	42–49.9	≥50
	40–49	≤19.9	20–26.9	27–38.9	39–44.9	≥45
	50–59	≤17.9	18–24.9	25–37.9	38–42.9	≥43
	60–69	≤15.9	16–22.9	23–35.9	36–40.9	≥41
Female	≤29	≤23.9	24–30.9	31–38.9	39–48.9	≥49
	30–39	≤19.9	20–27.9	28–36.9	37–44.9	≥45
	40–49	≤16.9	17–24.9	25–34.9	35–41.9	≥42
	50–59	≤14.9	15–21.9	22–33.9	34–39.9	≥40
	60–69	≤12.9	13–20.9	21–32.9	33–36.9	≥37

TABLE 7.1 Estimated percentage contribution from different fuels to ATP generation in various running events for a 70-kg/154-lb male

The energy allocation for physical activity from each energy transfer system progresses along a continuum. At one extreme, the intramuscular high-energy phosphates supply almost all of the energy needs for intense, extremely brief activity. The ATP-PCr and lactic acid systems supply about half the energy for intense activity lasting 2 min, with the remainder supplied by aerobic reactions. To excel under these conditions requires a well-developed anaerobic and aerobic metabolic capacity. Intense intermediate-duration activity performed for 5 to 10 min places greater demand on aerobic energy transfer (e.g., middle-distance running and swimming, or basketball). Long-duration marathon running, distance swimming, cycling, recreational jogging, and trekking require a constant aerobic energy supply with little reliance on anaerobic energy transfer sources.

Understanding the energy demands of diverse activities helps to explain why a world-record holder in the 1-mi run does not necessarily excel in distance running. Conversely, champion-level marathon runners rarely run 1 mi in less than 4 min, yet can complete a 26.2-mi marathon at a 5-min/mi pace, generating almost all the energy for the run from aerobic processes. *The appropriate approach to physical training analyzes* an activity for its specific energy components and then formulates training strategies to ensure optimal adaptations in physiologic and metabolic function. Improved capacity for energy transfer usually translates into improved performance.

INTEGRATIVE QUESTION

If athletes generally perform marathon running under intense but steady-rate aerobic conditions, why do some have reduced capacity to sprint to the finish at the end of the race?

Recovery Oxygen Uptake

Bodily processes do not immediately return to resting levels following physical activity, except in relatively light, short-duration effort when recovery proceeds rapidly and almost unnoticed. In contrast, after running all-out for one-half mile or swimming 200 yards, recovery time to pre-activity levels requires considerable time. How rapidly an individual responds in recovery from light, moderate, and strenuous physical activity depends on specific metabolic and physiologic processes during exercise and in recovery from each type of effort.

FIGURE 7.8 illustrates oxygen uptake during activity and recovery from different movement intensities. Light activity (A), with rapid attainment of steady-rate oxygen uptake, produces a small oxygen deficit. The magnitude of recovery oxygen uptake, coincidently, approximates the size of the oxygen deficit at the beginning of physical activity. Recovery proceeds rapidly. Oxygen uptake decreases by about 50% over each subsequent 30-s period until reaching the preactivity level.

Oxygen uptake, usually expressed as $mL \cdot min^{-1}$, $L \cdot min^{-1}$, or $mL \cdot kg^{-1} \cdot min^{-1}$, during steady-rate and non–steady-rate activity and recovery, plots logarithmically related to time.[6,50] The function increases during exercise or decreases during recovery by a constant fraction for each time unit as oxygen uptake approaches an asymptote or level value. Consider recovery from 10 min of steady-rate exercise at a 2000 $mL \cdot min^{-1}$ oxygen uptake. If recovery oxygen uptake decreased by half over 30 s, then oxygen uptake would equal 1000 $mL \cdot min^{-1}$ at 30 s recovery and 500 $mL \cdot min^{-1}$ at 60 s, with the resting value of 250 $mL \cdot min^{-1}$ achieved in about 90 s.

Moderate-to-intense aerobic exercise shown in Figure 7.8B requires a longer time to achieve steady-rate oxygen uptake and creates a larger oxygen deficit than less-intense effort. Consequently, it takes longer for the recovery oxygen uptake to return to pre-activity, resting levels. The oxygen uptake recovery curve demonstrates an initial rapid decline, similar to recovery from light activity, followed by a more gradual decline to baseline resting levels. In Figure 7.8A and B, the oxygen deficit and recovery oxygen uptake compute by using the steady-rate oxygen uptake to represent the oxygen or energy requirement of the physical activity performed. Figure 7.8C shows that all-out, exhaustive effort does not produce steady-rate oxygen uptake. Such effort demands a larger energy requirement than aerobic processes can supply. Consequently, anaerobic energy transfer increases and blood lactate

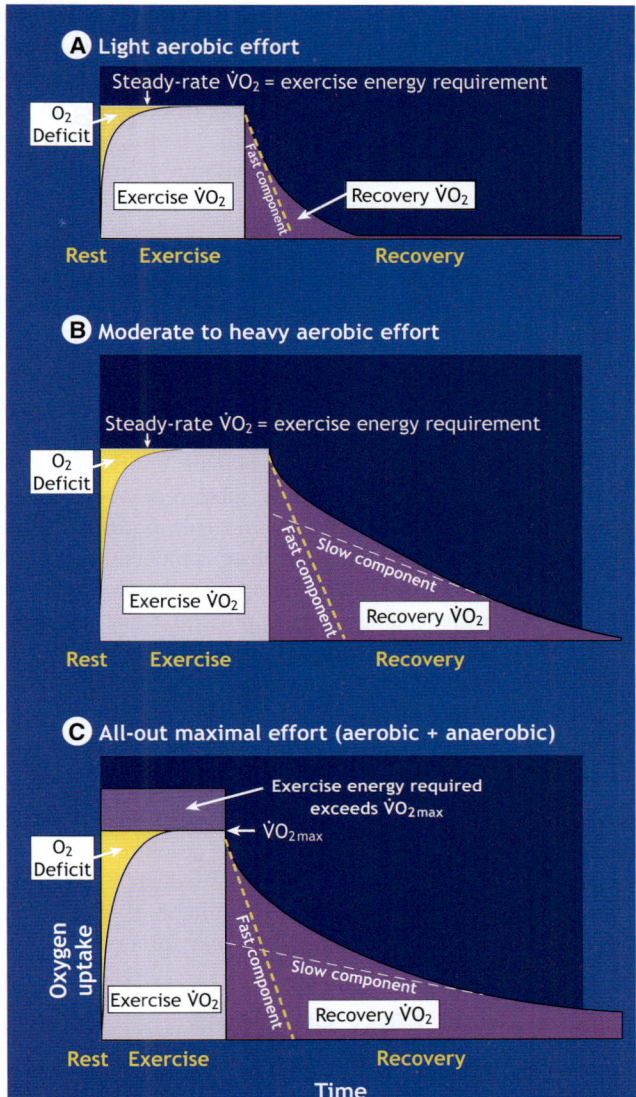

FIGURE 7.8. Oxygen uptake during exercise and recovery from **(A)** light steady-rate effort, **(B)** moderate-to-intense steady-rate effort, and **(C)** exhaustive effort that does not produce a steady rate of aerobic metabolism.

accumulates, with considerable time required to achieve complete recovery. Failure to achieve steady-rate oxygen uptake makes it unfeasible to accurately quantify an oxygen deficit.

Each of the curves in Figure 7.8 shows that oxygen uptake during recovery always exceeds the resting value, independent of activity intensity. In the 1940s–1970s, the excess oxygen uptake had been called oxygen debt or recovery oxygen uptake. Currently, the newer preferred term is **excess postexercise oxygen consumption (EPOC)**; indicated by the *purple* shaded area under each recovery curve. EPOC is computed as total oxygen uptake in recovery minus total oxygen theoretically consumed at rest during recovery. For example, if a total of 5.5 L of oxygen are consumed in recovery until attaining the 0.310 $L \cdot min^{-1}$ resting value, and recovery required 10 min, the recovery oxygen uptake would equal 5.5 L minus 3.1 L (0.310 L × 10 min) or 2.4 L. This suggests that the preceding activity "caused" physiologic alterations during activity *and* during recovery that required an additional 2.4 L oxygen uptake before it returned to pre-exercise levels at rest. These calculations assume that resting oxygen uptake remains unaltered during activity and recovery. As we discuss later in the section on Contemporary Concepts, this assumption is not correct, particularly following more strenuous effort.

Two important characteristics emerge from Figure 7.8 about recovery oxygen uptake:

1. With relatively short-duration, mild aerobic activity with constancy in body temperature and hormonal milieu, about half the total recovery oxygen uptake occurs within 30 s, and complete recovery within 2 to 4 min. The decline in oxygen uptake follows a single-component exponential curve termed the **fast component for recovery oxygen uptake**.
2. Recovery from strenuous activity presents a different situation because three factors increase substantially—blood lactate, body temperature, and thermogenic hormone levels. In addition to the fast recovery phase component, a second recovery phase exists—a **slow component for recovery oxygen uptake**. Depending on prior physical activity intensity and duration, the slow component can take up to 24 hr to return to pre-exercise oxygen uptake levels.[5,23,43] Even with shorter, intermittent "supramaximal" effort (e.g., three 2-min bouts at 108% $\dot{V}O_{2max}$ interspersed with 3-min rest intervals), recovery oxygen uptake remains elevated for 1 hr or longer.[4]

Trained subjects have a faster rate recovery oxygen uptake rate when exercising at either the same absolute or relative intensities compared to untrained individuals.[42] Training adaptations that facilitate rapid achievement of steady-rate oxygen uptake also facilitate a rapid recovery process.

Oxygen Debt: Early Concepts

A precise biochemical explanation for the recovery oxygen uptake remains elusive because no current, comprehensive explanation exists regarding interactions among contributory factors.

In 1922, Nobel laureate Archibald Vivian Hill (www.nobelprize.org/nobel_prizes/medicine/laureates/1922/hill-bio.html) and colleagues first coined the term **oxygen debt**. These pioneer scientists discussed energy metabolism during physical activity and recovery in financial-accounting terms.[28] The body's carbohydrate stores were likened to energy "credits." Expending stored credits during exercise incurred an energy "debt." The greater energy "deficit" or use of available stored energy credits, the larger the energy debt. Hill believed that the recovery oxygen uptake represented the cost to repay the debt—hence the logical descriptive term *oxygen debt*.

Lactate accumulation from the activity's anaerobic component represented the use of glycogen, the stored energy credit. The ensuing oxygen debt served two purposes:

1. Reestablish the original glycogen stores or credits by synthesizing approximately 80% of the lactate back to glycogen in the liver via the Cori cycle
2. Catabolize the remaining lactate through the pyruvate-citric acid cycle pathway, with the new ATP presumably powering glycogen resynthesis from lactate

This early explanation regarding recovery oxygen uptake was subsequently termed the "lactic acid theory of oxygen debt." In 1933, following Hill and colleagues work, researchers at the Harvard Fatigue Laboratory (https://en.wikipedia.org/wiki/Harvard_Fatigue_Laboratory) deduced that the initial recovery oxygen uptake phase stopped before blood lactate could decline.[36] They showed that a physically active individual could incur an almost 3-L oxygen debt without any appreciable blood lactate accumulation. To resolve these findings, they proposed two phases to explain the oxygen debt:

1. **Alactic oxygen debt** (meaning without lactate buildup; also known as alactacid oxygen debt)
2. **Lactic acid oxygen debt** (associated with elevated blood lactate levels; also known as lactacid oxygen debt)

The researchers speculated that these two explanations occurred because the early chemical methodology did not allow them to measure ATP and PCr replenishment or to assess the relationship between blood lactate and glucose and glycogen levels.

Metabolic Dynamics: Contemporary Concepts

The elevated aerobic metabolism in recovery (EPOC) restores the body to its pre-exercise condition. In short-duration, light-to-moderate activity, recovery oxygen uptake generally replenishes the high-energy phosphates depleted by the activity. Recovery from physical activity typically proceeds rapidly within several minutes. In longer-duration intense 60-min or longer aerobic activity, recovery oxygen uptake remains elevated considerably longer.[9] **FIGURE 7.9** illustrates the effect physical activity duration has on recovery oxygen uptake.[40] Eight trained women walked

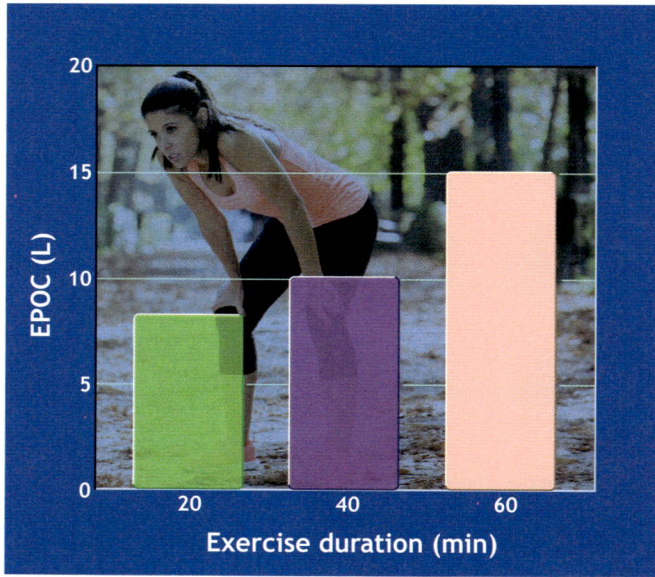

FIGURE 7.9. Total excess postexercise oxygen consumption (EPOC) during a 3-hr recovery from 20, 40, to 60 min of treadmill walking at 70% $\dot{V}O_{2max}$.
(Adapted with permission from Quinn TJ, et al. Postexercise oxygen consumption in trained females: effect of exercise duration. *Med Sci Sports Exerc*. 1994;26:908. Marcos Mesa Sam Wordley/Shutterstock)

Physiological Characteristics for an 83-Year-Old Champion Female Master Runner

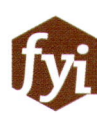

The $\dot{V}O_{2max}$, HR_{max}, maximal knee extensor muscle isometric torque, thigh and triceps surae muscle volumes, and proximal femur region bone mineral density (BMD) were assessed in an 83-year-old champion Mexican female Master runner currently competing in the 90+ age category. The measured 42.3 $mL \cdot kg^{-1} \cdot min^{-1}$ $\dot{V}O_{2max}$ is the highest ever observed for a female older than age 80 and gave her a remarkable physiological age of a 27-year-old! By contrast, her physiological age was closer to her biological age for maximal isometric torque strength (90 years) and HR_{max} (74 years). Her BMD (−1.7 T score) revealed that she had osteopenia but not osteoporosis. This case study revealed that existing specific muscular and skeletal characteristics did not interfere with the remarkable cardiorespiratory fitness and exercise performance in an older female master athlete coupled with her yearly endurance training schedule.

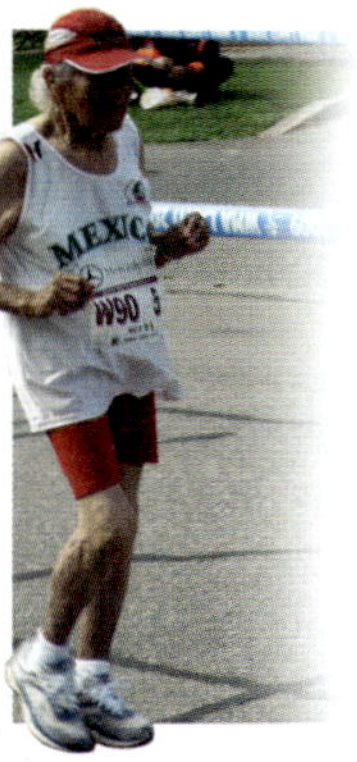

Denis Kuvaev/Shutterstock

Source:
Cattagni T. The physiological characteristics of an 83-year-old champion female master runner. *Int J Sports Physiol Perform*. 2019;14:1.

considerably larger oxygen uptake during recovery (EPOC) than oxygen deficit in prolonged aerobic activity and exhaustive anaerobic effort. Body temperature, for example, rises about 5.4°F/3°C during a long bout of intense aerobic activity and can remain elevated for several hours into recovery. Elevated body temperature directly stimulates metabolism to increase EPOC.

Other factors also impact EPOC. Up to 10% recovery oxygen uptake reloads the blood returning to the lungs from the previously active muscles. An additional 2 to 5% restores oxygen dissolved in bodily fluids and bound to myoglobin within muscle. Ventilation volumes in recovery from intense activity remain 8 to 10 times above the resting requirement, a cost equal to 10% of the EPOC. The heart also works harder and requires a greater oxygen supply during recovery. Tissue repair and redistribution of calcium, potassium, and sodium ions within muscle and other body compartments also demand additional energy. The residual thermogenic effects from epinephrine, norepinephrine, and thyroxine, including the glucocorticoids released during physical activity, elevate metabolism during recovery. *In essence, all of the physiologic systems activated during* physical activity *increase their own particular oxygen need during recovery* (see text boxes in **FIGURE 7.10**). Two factors impact recovery oxygen uptake:

1. Level of anaerobic metabolism during physical activity
2. Respiratory, circulatory, hormonal, ionic, and thermal adjustments that elevate metabolism during recovery

at 70% $\dot{V}O_{2max}$ for 20, 40, or 60 min. Recovery oxygen uptake totaled 8.6 L for the 20-min workout and 9.8 L for the 40-min session. Note the oxygen uptake during the 60-min workout nearly doubled to 15.2 L. The increase in recovery oxygen uptake in each steady-rate walking session failed to relate to lactate accumulation. Rather, disequilibrium in other physiologic functions elevated the recovery metabolism.

During exhaustive physical effort with its large anaerobic component and lactate accumulation, a small EPOC resynthesizes lactate to glycogen. This gluconeogenic mechanism also progresses during physical activity, particularly in trained individuals.[17,35] A significant EPOC component relates to physiologic processes that take place during recovery, in addition to metabolic events during physical activity. Such factors likely account for the

- Normalize thermogenic catecholamine increases
- Normalize elevated core temperature
- Normalize oxygen to myoglobin
- Normalize elevated physiologic functions
- Resynthesize ATP and PCr
- Resynthesize lactate to glycogen (Cori cycle)
- Oxidize lactate in energy metabolism

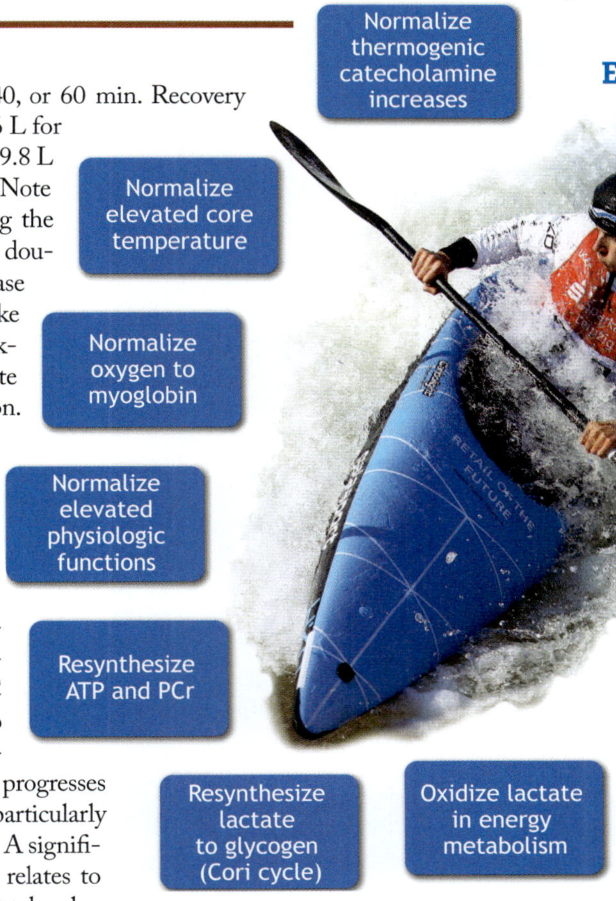

FIGURE 7.10. Factors contributing to EPOC following exhaustive physical activity and their normalization.
(Michele Morrone/Shutterstock)

EPOC Implications for Physical Activity and Recovery

Understanding the EPOC dynamics provides a rational basis to structure exercise intervals and optimize recovery. No appreciable lactate accumulates with either steady-rate aerobic activity or brief 5- to 10-s bouts of all-out effort powered by intramuscular high-energy phosphates. In such cases, recovery progresses rapidly and activity can begin again with only a short, passive recovery rest period.[18] In contrast, prolonged anaerobic effort durations that exceed 2 min produce considerable lactate buildup in active muscles and blood, with subsequent disruption in various physiologic systems, which require considerable time before returning to pre-activity baseline levels. Prolonged recovery between activity intervals would impair performance in basketball, hockey, soccer, tennis, and badminton. An athlete pushed to high levels of anaerobic metabolism may not fully recover during brief time-outs or intermittent intervals of less intense activity.

Procedures to speed recovery generally are either **active recovery** or **passive recovery**. In active recovery, often termed "cooling down" or "tapering off," the individual performs submaximal effort with large muscle groups desiring to prevent muscle cramps and stiffness and facilitate lactate removal and a more rapid and full recovery. With passive recovery, the person usually lies down, presuming that total inactivity reduces the resting energy requirements and thus "frees" oxygen to fuel the recovery process. Modifications have included massage, cold showers, specific body positions, and consuming cold liquids.

Optimal Recovery from Steady-Rate Physical Activity

For most individuals, little lactate accumulates during steady-rate physical activity below 55 to 60% $\dot{V}O_{2max}$. Recovery requires high-energy phosphate resynthesis with oxygen replenishment in the blood, bodily fluids, and muscle myoglobin, with only a small energy cost required to sustain elevated circulation and ventilation. Passive procedures facilitate recovery because any additional activity during recovery would only elevate total metabolism to delay recovery.

Optimal Recovery from Non–Steady-Rate Physical Activity

Blood lactate accumulates when physical activity intensity exceeds the maximum steady-rate level and lactate formation in muscle exceeds its removal rate. With increasing intensity, blood lactate levels rise sharply and the exerciser soon becomes exhausted. The precise mechanisms for exhaustion during anaerobic activity remain unclear, but blood lactate levels still provide an objective indication about a physical activity's relative strenuousness and the adequacy of recovery. Lactate anions induce a fatiguing effect on skeletal muscle independent of reduced pH,[29] so any procedure that accelerates lactate removal probably augments subsequent physical performance.[1]

Performing aerobic activity in recovery accelerates blood lactate removal.[13,21,39,41,47] The optimal recovery activity level ranges between 30 and 45% $\dot{V}O_{2max}$ for cycling and 55 to 60% $\dot{V}O_{2max}$ when recovery involves running.[38] This difference between activity modes reflects more localized muscle involvement in bicycling that lowers the blood lactate accumulation threshold.

FIGURE 7.11 illustrates blood lactate recovery patterns for trained men who performed 6 min of supramaximal exercise on a bicycle ergometer. Active recovery involved continuous cycling at either 35 or 65% $\dot{V}O_{2max}$ for 40 min. The horizontal white line indicates the blood lactate level produced by exercise at 65% $\dot{V}O_{2max}$ without previous exercise. A combined bout of 65% $\dot{V}O_{2max}$ for 7 min followed by 35% $\dot{V}O_{2max}$ for 33 min evaluated whether a higher-intensity exercise interval early in recovery would accelerate lactate removal. Moderate aerobic activity (35% $\dot{V}O_{2max}$, *yellow curve*) better facilitates lactate removal compared with a passive recovery procedure (*aqua*

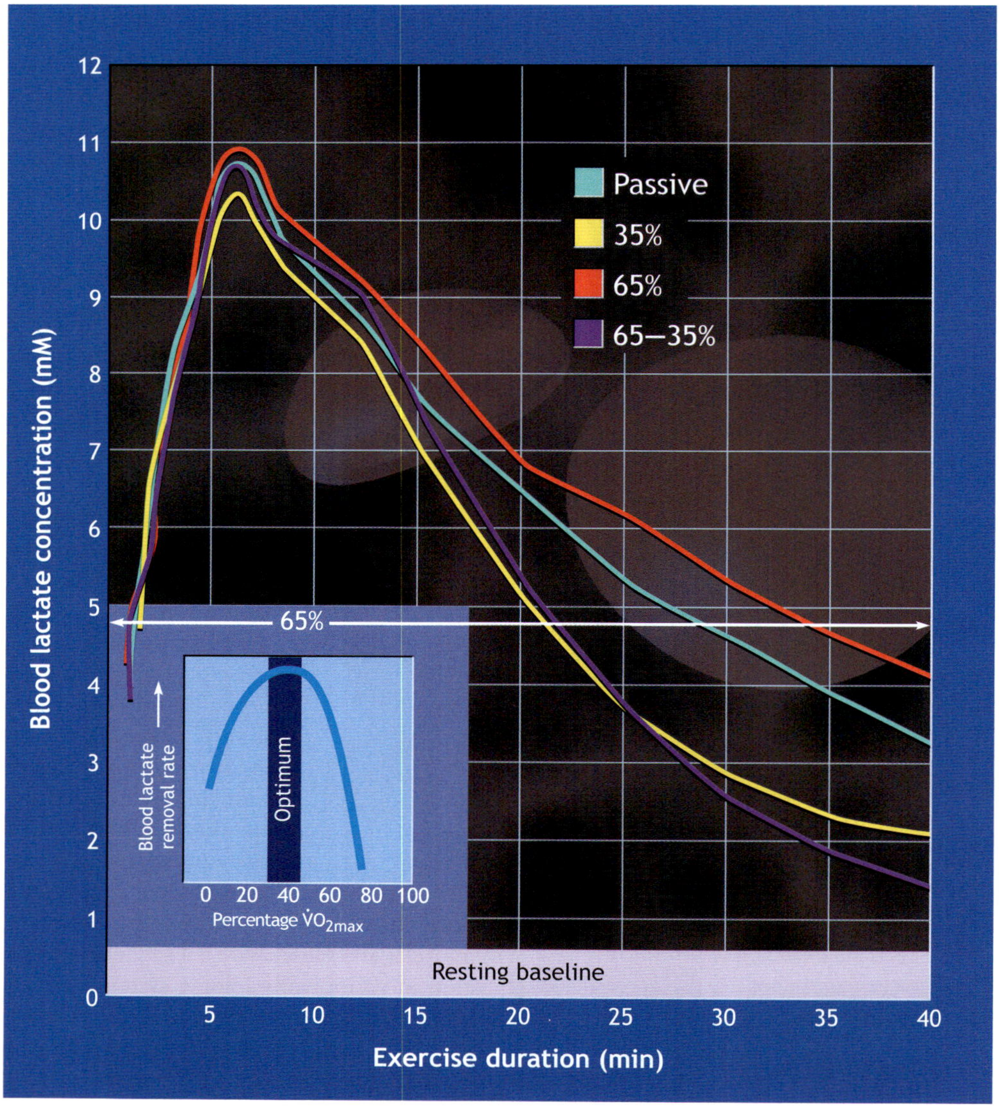

FIGURE 7.11. Blood lactate concentration following maximal exercise using passive recovery and active recoveries at 35%, 65%, and a combination 35 and 65% $\dot{V}O_{2max}$.
(Adapted with permission from Dodd S, et al. Blood lactate disappearance at various intensities of recovery exercise. *J Appl Physiol: Respir Environ Exerc Physiol* 1984;57:1462. jaras72/Shutterstock)

curve). Combining higher-intensity followed by lower-intensity exercise (*purple curve*) had no greater benefit than a single moderate-intensity exercise level. Physical activity during recovery above the lactate threshold (65% $\dot{V}O_{2max}$, *red curve*) offers no advantage and may even prolong recovery by triggering lactate formation and accumulation. The bottom inset curve depicts the generalized relationship between exercise intensity and lactate removal rate and illustrates that optimal recovery exercise intensity probably ranges between 30 and 40% $\dot{V}O_{2max}$.

Facilitated lactate removal with active recovery likely occurs from increased blood perfusion through "lactate-using" liver and heart and inspiratory muscles. These structures serve as net lactate consumers during recovery from intense physical activity.[3,12] Increased blood flow through muscles during active recovery also enhances lactate removal because citric acid cycle metabolism readily oxidizes lactate from muscle tissue.

Intermittent Interval Physical Activity

One approach to performing continuous physical activity that normally produces exhaustion within several minutes requires exercising *intermittently* with pre-established activity spacing and rest intervals. The physical conditioning **interval training** strategy characterizes this approach. This training regimen applies different work-to-rest intervals with supramaximal effort to overload specific energy transfer systems. In all-out movement of up to 8 s, the intramuscular high-energy phosphates predominantly provide the energy with only minimal reliance on the glycolytic pathway. This produces rapid recovery in the alactic or fast component postexercise oxygen uptake, enabling another intense activity to begin following only a brief recovery.

TABLE 7.2 summarizes classic experiments with combined exercise and rest intervals. On one day, the subject ran about 0.8 mi at a speed that would normally exhaust him within 5 min and attained a 5.6 L·min⁻¹ $\dot{V}O_{2max}$. A high blood lactate level confirmed a substantial level of anaerobic metabolism before exhaustion (last table column). On another day, he ran at the same fast speed but intermittently, with 10-s run periods and 5 s of recovery. For 30 min of intermittent running, the time actually running amounted to 20 min and the distance covered equaled 4 mi, compared with less than 5 min and 0.8 mi in the continuous run! This protocol's effectiveness becomes even more impressive considering that blood lactate remained low despite a 5.1 L·min⁻¹ (91% $\dot{V}O_{2max}$) oxygen uptake during the 30-min period. A relative balance existed between the exercise energy requirements and aerobic energy transfer within the active muscles throughout the exercise and rest intervals.

TABLE 7.2 Total distance run, average oxygen uptake, and blood lactate levels during intense intermittent exercise

Manipulating the duration of physical activity and rest intervals effectively overloads a specific energy-transfer system. When the rest interval increased from 5 to 10 s, oxygen uptake averaged 4.4 L·min⁻¹; 15-s exercise and 30-s recovery intervals produced only a 3.6-L oxygen uptake. For each 30-min intermittent running bout, the runner achieved a longer distance and substantially lower blood lactate level than when running continuously at the same intensity. Chapter 21 focuses on applying the basic principles of intermittent physical activity for aerobic and anaerobic training and sports performance.

Summary

1. Physical activity intensity and duration impact ATP production pathways.
2. The intramuscular ATP and PCr (immediate energy system) stores provide energy for short-duration, intense activities (e.g., 100-m "all-out" dash, repetitively lifting heavy weights).
3. For less intense longer duration activities of 1 to 2 min, the anaerobic glycolysis reactions (short-term, lactate-forming energy system) generate most of the energy.
4. The aerobic system (long-term energy system) predominates as physical activity progresses beyond several minutes.
5. Humans possess two distinct muscle fiber types, each with unique metabolic and contractile properties: low glycolytic–high oxidative, slow-twitch fibers (type I) and low oxidative–high glycolytic, fast-twitch fibers (type II). Intermediate fast-twitch type fibers exist with overlapping metabolic characteristics.
6. Understanding the physical activity energy spectrum allows for specific training to improve the capacity of the different energy transfer systems.
7. Steady-rate oxygen uptake represents a balance between active muscles' energy requirements and aerobic ATP resynthesis.
8. Oxygen deficit defines the difference between the exercise oxygen requirement and the oxygen uptake during the activity.
9. $\dot{V}O_{2max}$ quantitatively defines the maximum capacity to resynthesize ATP aerobically. The $\dot{V}O_{2max}$ serves as an important indicator of physiologic functional capacity to sustain intense aerobic activity.
10. Oxygen uptake remains elevated above the resting level following physical activity.
11. Recovery oxygen uptake reflects both the metabolic demands of exercise and the exercise-induced physiologic imbalances in recovery.
12. Moderate physical activity following intense physical activity, referred to as active recovery, facilitates recovery compared with passive procedures.
13. Proper work-to-rest interval spacing provides a way to augment physical activity intensity that normally would prove fatiguing if performed continuously.

Key Terms

Active recovery: Low- to moderate-level physical activity during recovery from previous more intense physical activity

Alactic oxygen debt: Fast component of postexercise oxygen uptake unassociated with lactate buildup; also known as alactacid oxygen debt

Blood lactate threshold: Point or region during increasing exercise intensity when blood lactate concentration increases abruptly

Excess postexercise oxygen consumption (EPOC): Oxygen uptake above a resting level during exercise recovery required to restore body to a resting state; also known as oxygen debt and recovery oxygen uptake

Fast component for recovery oxygen uptake: Rapid increase in the oxygen uptake curve at the start of physical activity

Fast-twitch (FT) muscle fibers: Fast-contracting muscle fibers identified by staining for myosin ATPase activity subdivides into type IIA and type IIx based on unique metabolic and biochemical characteristics; also known as type II muscle fibers

Hydrogen shuttle: Hydrogen's passage from the sarcoplasma into mitochondria via NADH

Interval training: Intermittent training involving multiple brief intense exercise intervals interspersed with brief recovery periods

Lactate shuttle hypothesis: Describes lactate intracellular and intercellular transport

Lactic acid oxygen debt: Oxygen uptake during the slow component postexercise period associated with lactate build-up and subsequent removal; also known as lactacid oxygen debt

Maximal oxygen uptake ($\dot{V}O_{2max}$): Highest oxygen uptake measured during incremental exercise to maximal effort; also known as maximal aerobic power and aerobic capacity

Oxygen debt: Term described as energy "credits" the energy metabolism during recovery from physical activity to reflect excess postexercise oxygen uptake and recovery oxygen uptake

Oxygen deficit: Quantitative difference between total oxygen uptake during an activity and additional oxygen that would have been consumed if a steady-rate aerobic metabolism occurred immediately when exercise begins

Oxygen uptake fast component: Mathematical expression for rapidly declining postexercise oxygen uptake curve during recovery

Passive recovery: Complete inactivity during recovery following physical activity

Phosphagens: ATP and PCr

Slow component for recovery oxygen uptake: Mathematical expression of the slower decline in oxygen uptake during postexercise recovery

Slow-twitch (ST) muscle fibers: Muscle fiber type identified by myosin ATPase activity staining; referred to as type I fibers with high capacity for aerobic metabolism

Steady rate: Relative plateau in exercise oxygen uptake to denote balance between active muscles' energy requirements and aerobic ATP production; also known as steady state

References are available online at Lippincott Connect.

Additional References

AbdelMassih AF, et al. The potential use of lactate blockers for the prevention of COVID-19 worst outcome, insights from exercise immunology. *Med Hypotheses*. 2021;148:110520.

Bräuer EK, Smekal G. VO2 Steady state at and just above maximum lactate steady state intensity. *Int J Sports Med*. 2020;41:574.

Brooks GA, et al. The blood lactate/pyruvate equilibrium affair. *Am J Physiol Endocrinol Metab*. 2022;322:E34. doi:10.1152/ajpendo.00270.2021.

Brooks GA. Role of the heart in lactate shuttling. *Front Nutr*. 2021; 8:663560.

Brooks GA. The tortuous path of lactate shuttle discovery: from cinders and boards to the lab and ICU. *J Sport Health Sci*. 2020;9:446.

Charron J, et al. Physiological responses to repeated running sprint ability tests: a systematic review. *Int J Exerc Sci*. 2020;13:1190.

Christiansen D, et al. The effect of blood-flow-restricted interval training on lactate and H+ dynamics during dynamic exercise in man. *Acta Physiol (Oxf)*. 2021;231(3):e13580.

Dong S, et al. Lactate and myocadiac energy metabolism. *Front Physiol*. 2021;12:715081.

Glancy B, et al. Mitochondrial lactate metabolism: history and implications for exercise and disease. *J Physiol*. 2021;599:863.

Hashimoto T, et al. Effect of exercise on brain health: the potential role of lactate as a myokine. *Metabolites*. 2021;11:813.

Hill DW, et al. Exercise above the maximal lactate steady state does not elicit a $\dot{V}O_2$ slow component that leads to attainment of $\dot{V}O_{2max}$. *Appl Physiol Nutr Metab*. 2021;46:133.

Kabasakalis A, et al. Response of Blood biomarkers to sprint Interval swimming. *Int J Sports Physiol Perform*. 2020:1. doi:10.1123/ijspp.2019-0747.

Keir DA, et al. Identification of non-invasive exercise thresholds: methods, strategies, and an online app. *Sports Med*. 2022;52:237.

Kurtz JA, et al. Taurine in sports and exercise. *J Int Soc Sports Nutr*. 2021;18:39.

Liegnell R, et al. Elevated plasma lactate levels via exogenous lactate infusion do not alter resistance exercise-induced signaling or protein synthesis in human skeletal muscle. *Am J Physiol Endocrinol Metab*. 2020;319:E792.

McCarthy SF, et al. The emerging role of lactate as a mediator of exercise-induced appetite suppression. *Am J Physiol Endocrinol Metab*. 2020;319:E814. doi:10.1152/ajpendo.

Quittmann OJ, et al. Maximal lactate accumulation rate and postexercise lactate kinetics in handcycling and cycling. *Eur J Sport Sci*. 2021;21:539.

Takeda R, et al. Effect of endurance training and PGC-1α overexpression on calculated lactate production volume during exercise based on blood lactate concentration. *Sci Rep*. 2022;12:1635.

Van den Tillaar R, et al. Comparison of a traditional graded exercise protocol with a self-paced 1-km test to assess maximal oxygen consumption. *Int J Sports Physiol Perform*. 2020:1. doi:10.1123/ijspp.2019-0843.

| Table 7.1 | Estimated Percentage Contribution from Different Fuels to ATP Generation in Various Running Events for a 70-kg/154-lb Male |||||

| | Percentage Contribution to ATP Generation |||||
| | | Glycogen || | |
Event	Phosphocreatine	Anaerobic	Aerobic	Blood Glucose (Liver Glycogen)	Triacylglycerol (Fatty Acids)
100 m	50	50	—	—	—
200 m	25	65	10	—	—
400 m	12.5	62.5	25	—	—
800 m	6	50	44	—	—
1500 m	a	25	75	—	—
5000 m	a	12.5	87.5	—	—
10,000 m	a	3	97	—	—
Marathon	—	—	75	5	20
Ultramarathon 80 km/50 mi	—	—	35	5	60
24-h race	—	—	10	2	88
Soccer game	10	70	20	—	—

^aIn such events, phosphocreatine is used for the first few seconds and, if it has been resynthesized during the race, in the sprint to the finish.
ATP, adenosine triphosphate.
Source: Newsholme EA, et al. Physical and mental fatigue: metabolic mechanisms and importance of plasma amino acids. *Br Med Bull.* 1992;48:477.

| Table 7.2 | Total Distance Run, Average Oxygen Uptake, and Blood Lactate Levels During Intense Intermittent Exercise ||||

Exercise-Rest Periods	Total Distance Run (yd)	Average Oxygen Uptake ($L \cdot min^{-1}$)	Blood Lactate ($mg \cdot dL$ $Blood^{-1}$)
4-min continuous	1422	5.6	150
10-s exercise 5-s rest	7294	5.1	44
10-s exercise 10-s rest	5468	4.4	20
15-s exercise 30-s rest	3642	3.6	16

Source: Christenson EH, et al. Intermittent and continuous running. *Acta Physiol Scand.* 1960;60:269.
Photo: wavebreakmedia/Shutterstock

CHAPTER 8

Measuring Energy Expenditure

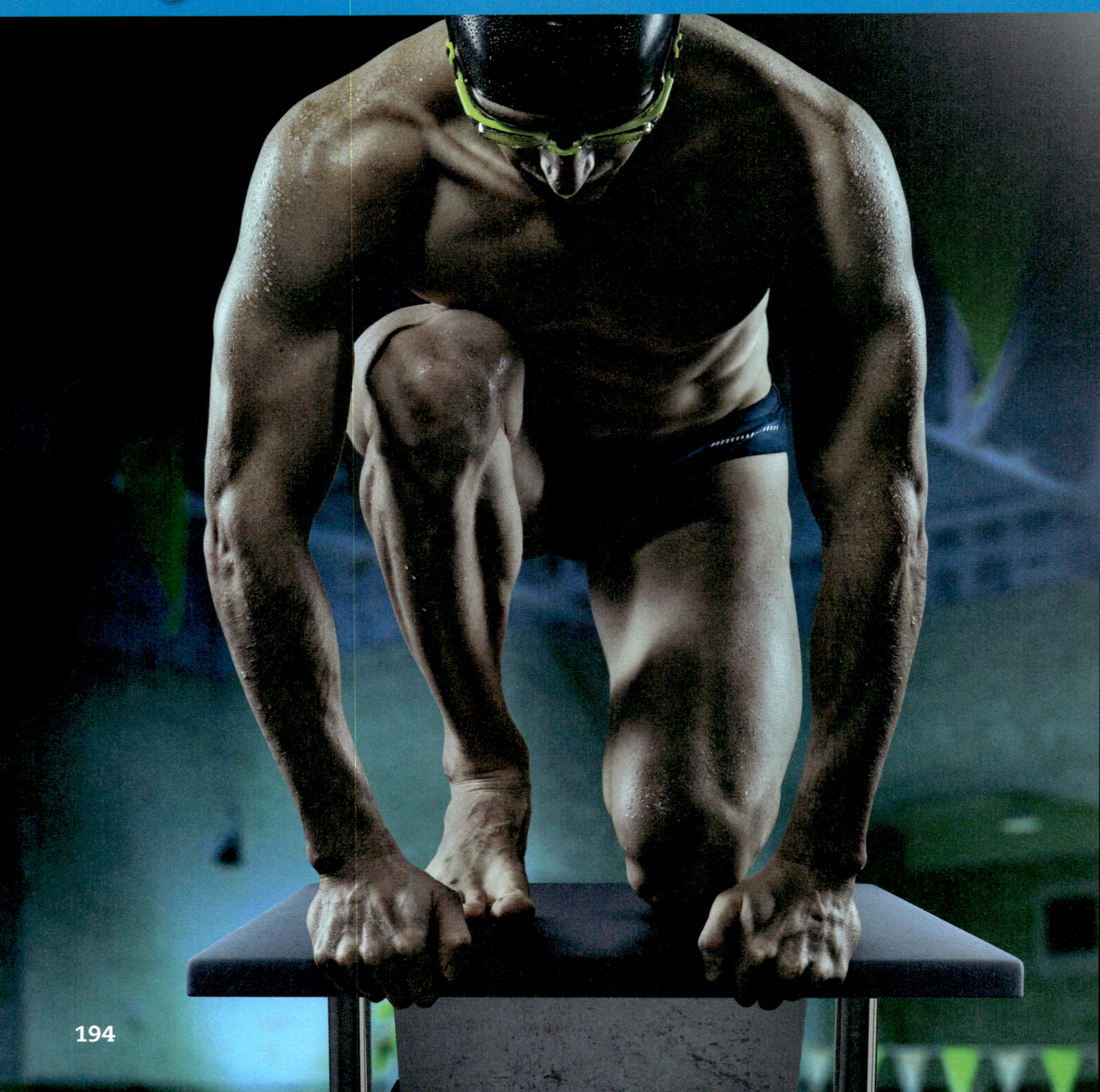

Chapter Objectives

- Explain the differences between direct calorimetry and indirect calorimetry, and closed-circuit spirometry and open-circuit spirometry
- Diagram the closed-circuit spirometry system for oxygen uptake determinations
- Describe portable spirometry, bag technique, and computerized instrumentation systems for open-circuit spirometry
- Explain the micro-Scholander and Haldane methods to chemically analyze expired air samples
- Discuss two advantages and two limitations for doubly labeled water to estimate human energy expenditure
- Define respiratory quotient and respiratory exchange ratio, and explain their differences for quantifying energy release in metabolism and the composition of the food mixture metabolized during rest and physical activity

Ancillaries at-a-Glance

Visit Lippincott Connect to access the following resources.

- References: Chapter 8
- Appendix F: Energy Expenditure in Household, Occupational, Recreational, and Sports Activities
- Appendix G: Standardizing Gas Volumes: Environmental Factors
- Focus on Research: Respiratory Gas Exchange Implies Metabolic Mixture

Measuring the Body's Heat Production

All metabolic processes within the body ultimately result in heat production. Thus, the heat production rate by cells, tissue, and even the whole body operationally defines the energy metabolism rate. The calorie represents the basic heat measurement unit, and the term **calorimetry** defines the measurement of heat transfer. **FIGURE 8.1** illustrates two different approaches, **direct calorimetry** and **indirect calorimetry**, to accurately quantify human energy (heat) transfer.

Direct Calorimetry

Heat represents the ultimate fate for all of the body's metabolic processes. The early experiments of French chemist Antoine Lavoisier (1743–1794) and his contemporaries in the 1770s to 1780s provided the impetus to directly measure energy expenditure during rest and physical activity (http://scienceworld.wolfram.com/biography/Lavoisier.html). The idea, similar to that used with the bomb calorimeter described in Chapter 4 to determine food energy, provided a convenient though elaborate methodology to measure heat production in humans.

In his classic experiment, Lavoisier collaborated with French mathematician Pierre Simon de Laplace (1749–1827; https://mathshistory.st-andrews.ac.uk/Biographies/Laplace/) on problems in respiration chemistry. Their experiments with guinea pigs in 1780 were the first to quantify oxygen uptake and carbon dioxide produced by metabolism using their initial ice calorimeter. Over a 10-hr period, approximately 3 g of carbonic acid were collected from an animal breathing oxygen. In a second experiment, a guinea pig was placed into a wire cage, which in turn was placed into a double-walled container. Ice packed into the outer container's wall maintained a constant chamber temperature. Ice between the cage and the wall of the inner container melted from the animal's body heat, yielding 370 g/13 oz of ice melted over 24 hr. They concluded that the total heat produced by the animal equaled the amount of heat required to melt the ice.

These scientists paved the way for future energy balance studies by initially recognizing that the elements carbon, hydrogen, nitrogen, and oxygen involved in metabolism appeared neither suddenly nor disappeared mysteriously. Rather, they reasoned that these elements reconfigured in a predictable sequence during combustion. Lavoisier supplied the basic truth—*"Only oxygen participates in animal respiration, and the "caloric" liberated during respiration is itself the combustion."*

In the 1890s at Wesleyan University, professors Wilber Olin Atwater (a chemist; 1844–1907; see, e.g., https://academic.oup.com/jn/article-abstract/124/suppl_9/1707S/4730392) and Edward Bennett Rosa (a physicist; 1861–1921; see, e.g., www.nasonline.org/publications/biographical-memoirs/memoir-pdfs/rosa-e-b.pdf) used the first **human calorimeter** of major scientific importance.[1,30] Their pioneering and elegant calorimetric experiments with the **Atwater-Rosa calorimeter** related energy input (food consumption) to energy expenditure, verified the energy conservation law, and validated the indirect calorimetric technique.

The calorimeter, diagramed schematically in **FIGURE 8.2**, included an airtight, thermally insulated chamber in which a subject could live, eat, sleep, and exercise on a bicycle ergometer. A known water volume at a specified temperature circulated through coils at the chamber top. Water absorbed the heat produced and radiated by the person in the calorimeter. Insulation protected the entire chamber, so any change in water temperature related directly to the person's energy metabolism level. For adequate ventilation, the person's exhaled air continually passed from the room through chemicals to remove moisture and absorb carbon dioxide. Oxygen added to the air recirculated through the chamber.

In the calorimeter, a thin copper sheet lined the chamber's interior wall, to which heat exchangers were attached overhead, through which cold water circulated. Water cooled to 35.6°F/2°C moved at a high flow rate, absorbing the heat radiated from the subject during diverse activities. Insulation surrounded the entire chamber, so any changes in water temperature, measured in 0.01°C units with a microscope mounted alongside a thermometer, reflected the subject's energy metabolism. As the subject rested, warmer water flowed more slowly.

In the original bicycle ergometer shown in the schematic, the rear wheel contacted the generator shaft, which powered a light bulb. The rear wheel rotated through the

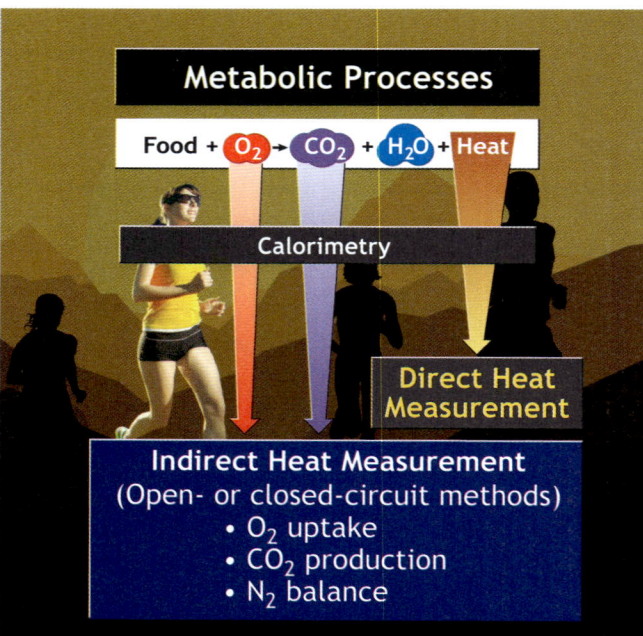

FIGURE 8.1. Measuring the body's heat production rate directly assesses metabolic rate, which also can be estimated indirectly from carbon dioxide and oxygen exchange during food macronutrient breakdown and nitrogen excretion.
(Shutterstock: Kuznetcov_Konstantin; kstudija.)

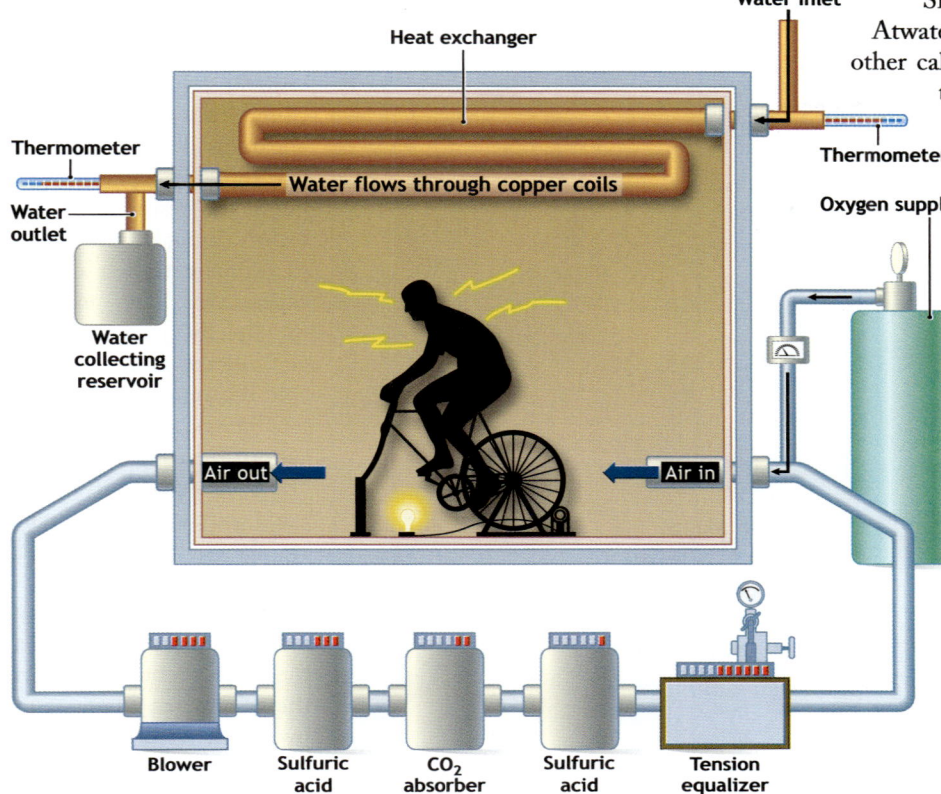

FIGURE 8.2. Early human calorimeter directly measured the body's energy metabolism rate or heat production in an airtight, thermally insulated chamber. Adding an ergometer to their experiments quantified energy expenditure during controlled cycling exercise for preset durations pedaling at different speeds and relative strenuousness.

electromagnetic field to produce an electric current to quantify power output.

Experiments lasted from several hours to 13 days, and some involved cycling performed for 16 hr, with total energy expenditure exceeding 10,000 kcal! A staff of 16, working in teams for 8- to 12-hr shifts, operated the calorimeter.

A modern-day human calorimeter, as shown in **FIGURE 8.3**, contains an air-tight chamber with an oxygen supply sufficient for a person to live and work for extended time periods. The system depicted in the four panels includes an airtight room (14 m³/46 ft³) with two exchange ports, through which food and supplies may be passed between the chamber's inside and outside, sufficient living space for the subject to sleep and do work, a lavatory, and exercise equipment. Oxygen uptake and CO_2 production are continuously monitored while the person "lives" in the chamber by analyzing the differential concentration for the gases between ambient air flowing into and out of the chamber. A known water volume at a specified temperature circulates through coils at the chamber top. The water absorbs the heat produced and radiated by the person in the calorimeter. Insulation surrounds the entire chamber, so any change in water temperature relates directly to the person's energy metabolism. For adequate ventilation, exhaled air continually passes through chemicals to remove moisture and absorb carbon dioxide. Oxygen added to the air recirculates through the chamber.

Since the seminal papers published by Atwater and Rosa in the early 20th century, other calorimetric methods have been designed to infer energy expenditure based on metabolic gas exchange for extended periods in respiration chambers and metabolic and thermal balance with water flow and airflow calorimeters.[5,8,13,19–21] The modern space suit worn by astronauts (shown in the left insert image) during water immersion practice for extravehicular activities (EVAs) in space represents a "suit calorimeter," designed to maintain respiratory gas exchange, thermal balance, and protection from a potentially hostile space environment. These suits played a crucial role in the moon explorations and in EVAs on the International Space Station (www.nasa.gov/mission_pages/station/main/index.html) and will continue to do so in the establishment of a manned Mars outpost within the next several decades.[23] (Note: photo credit—NASA TV.)

Credit: NASA TV

Over the years, various heat-measuring devices have been developed for human use, each based on a different operational principle.

1. An *airflow calorimeter* determines heat production by multiplying temperature change in air that flows through an insulated space by the air's mass and specific heat and by calculating evaporative heat loss.
2. A *water flow calorimeter* operates similarly, except that the change in temperature it measures is in water flowing through coils that constitute part of the environmentally self-contained body suit worn in space missions.
3. *Gradient layer calorimetry* measures body heat flow from the subject through a sheet of insulating materials with appropriate piping and cooler water flowing on the gradient's outside.

Direct heat production measurement in humans has theoretical implications but limited practical applications. Accurate measurements in the calorimeter require considerable time and expense and formidable engineering expertise. Thus, heat-measuring calorimeters are not practical for determining energy release in most sport, occupational, and recreational activities.

Indirect Calorimetry

All energy-releasing reactions in humans ultimately depend on oxygen use. Measuring a person's oxygen uptake during physical activities provides researchers with an indirect yet highly accurate way to estimate energy expenditure. Compared with direct calorimetry, indirect calorimetry remains simpler and much less expensive.

Caloric Transformation for Oxygen

Careful experiments have shown that approximately 4.82 kcal release when a typical mixed diet of carbohydrate, lipid, and protein combusts with 1 L oxygen in a bomb calorimeter. Even with large variations in the metabolic mixture, the caloric value for oxygen varies only slightly, generally within 2 to 4%. Thus, a rounded value of 5.0 kcal · L O_2^{-1} consumed provides an appropriate conversion factor to estimate energy expenditure under steady-rate metabolic conditions. This conversion provides a suitable yardstick to express any aerobic physical activity in energy units (see Appendix F).

Lippincott® Connect — Appendix F, available online at Lippincott Connect, provides energy expenditure in household, occupational, recreational, and sport activities.

Indirect calorimetry yields results comparable to those of direct measurement with the human calorimeter. Closed-circuit spirometry and open-circuit spirometry are the two main types of indirect calorimetry.

IQ? INTEGRATIVE QUESTION

What rationale underlies early experiments that quantified energy metabolism of small animals by measuring the rate ice melted in a container surrounding the animal?

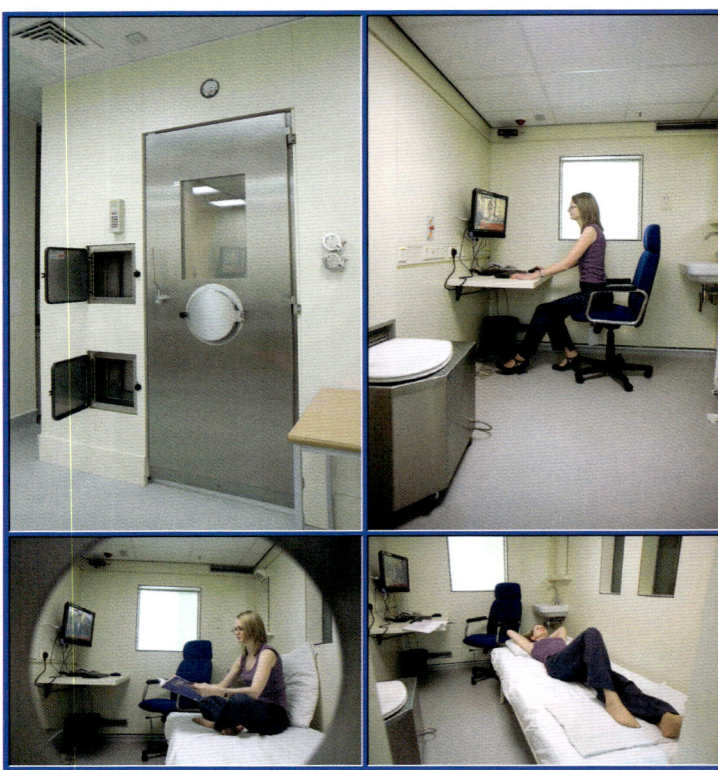

FIGURE 8.3. Example of a modern, whole-body human calorimetry room with sufficient space for a person to live, sleep, and perform routine work tasks.
(Photos courtesy of Dr. Debbie Girdlestone, Sector Lead (Life Sciences), Business Development and Translational Medicine. www2.warwick.ac.uk/services/ris/impact/analyticalguide/wbc)

Closed-Circuit Spirometry

FIGURE 8.4 illustrates the closed-circuit spirometric apparatus developed in the late 1800s and used in hospitals and research laboratories through the 1980s to estimate resting energy expenditure. This method to directly measure oxygen uptake has considerable theoretical importance but limited practical application. The subject breathes 100% oxygen from a prefilled container or spirometer. The equipment is called "closed" because the subject rebreathes only the gas from the spirometer. As the subject rebreathes from the spirometer, a potassium hydroxide (soda lime) canister placed in the breathing circuit absorbs, or "washes," exhaled carbon dioxide. A drum attached to the spirometer revolves at a known speed to measure and record the volume of oxygen removed (i.e., oxygen uptake) based on changes in the system's total volume. The difference between the initial and final oxygen volumes in the calibrated spirometer reflects the oxygen uptake during the measurement interval.

Closed-circuit spirometry measurement during physical activity is challenging. The subject must remain close to the equipment, the apparatus presents considerable resistance to large breathing volumes, and carbon dioxide removal lags behind its production during intense effort. For these reasons, open-circuit spirometry remains the most widely used laboratory procedure to measure oxygen uptake and infer caloric expenditure during human movement.

Open-Circuit Spirometry

The open-circuit method provides a simple way to measure oxygen uptake. A subject inhales ambient air with constant 20.93% oxygen, 0.03% carbon dioxide, 79.04% nitrogen composition, and a negligible quantity of inert gases. The changes in oxygen and carbon dioxide percentages in expired air compared with the percentages in inspired ambient air indirectly reflect the ongoing energy metabolism process. Thus, analyzing two factors—inspired and expired air volume breathed during a specified time and composition of inspired and expired air—provides a practical way to measure oxygen uptake and infer energy expenditure. This chapter's "In a Practical Sense" illustrates the step-by-step procedure to compute the metabolic variables obtained with open-circuit spirometry.

Four common indirect calorimetry procedures measure oxygen uptake during physical activity:

1. Portable spirometry
2. Bag technique
3. Ventilated hood technique
4. Computerized instrumentation

Portable Spirometry

Two German scientists at the Max Plank Institute for Nutritional Research (now called the Max Plank Institute for Metabolism Research; www.sf.mpg.de/en) in the early 1940s perfected a lightweight, portable system first devised by German respiratory physiologist and altitude physiologist and aviation medicine pioneer Nathan Zuntz (1847–1920; www.ncbi.nlm.nih.gov/pubmed/7726784). When the 20th century began, Zuntz determined energy expenditure indirectly during war-related operations (e.g., traveling over different terrain with full battle gear, operating tanks and aircraft, performing physical tasks encountered during combat operations).[15]

Carrying the portable spirometer secured to the upper torso also allowed considerable freedom to move while mountain climbing, downhill skiing, sailing, golfing, and performing many common household activities (Appendix F). Nevertheless, the equipment becomes cumbersome during vigorous activity, and the flow meter underrecords at near-maximum or maximum air volumes with rapid breathing.[17]

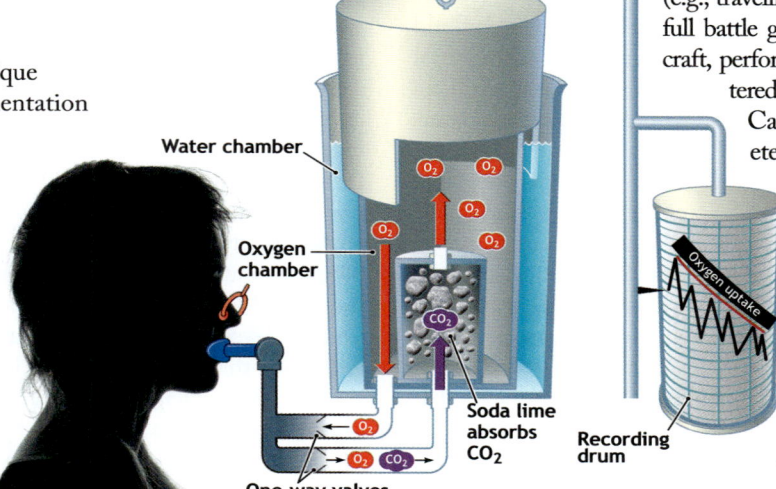

FIGURE 8.4. The closed-circuit spirometry method to estimate resting energy expenditure via oxygen uptake measurement. (fantom_rd/Shutterstock)

 Extravehicular Activity Physiology and Energy Metabolism

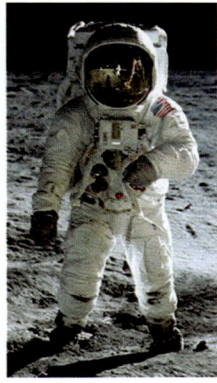

Credit: NASA

Extravehicular activities (EVAs), more commonly known as spacewalks, have been a critical component of space exploration for both the United States and Russia. During EVAs, crewmembers wear life support suits called extravehicular mobility units (EMUs) that offer atmospheric containment, cooling, and thermal insulation and that protect the wearer from solar radiation and micrometeoroids. Crewmembers wore such EMUs when the Apollo lunar module Eagle landed on the moon in July 1969 (www.nasa.gov/stem-ed-resources/sfs-extravehicular-mobility-unit.html). A risk crewmembers face on EVAs is decompression sickness (DCS), which can occur due to a failure to sufficiently eliminate nitrogen from the lungs prior to the EVA and to the pressure within the EMU being much lower than the ambient pressure on the International Space Station (www.nasa.gov/mission_pages/station/main/index.html). DCS can result in joint pain, neurologic and cardiopulmonary complications, and even death. Astronauts can avoid DCS by breathing 100% O_2 before the EVA to displace tissue N_2, which prevents N_2 gas bubble formation. NASA's Human Health and Performance Directorate's EVA Physiology team (www.nasa.gov/feature/eva-physiology) conducts research to develop prebreathe protocols with shorter separation time while reducing or preventing DCS. EVA physiology scientists and engineers develop and test the flight protocols, and support crew training. Astronauts train using individualized exercise prescriptions for the prebreathe protocol prior to training in the neutral buoyancy laboratory pool (www.nasa.gov/image-feature/neutral-buoyancy-laboratory). Scientists and engineers also perform suit and life support system hardware development and testing, including suit ventilation evaluations for carbon dioxide washout, metabolic rate measurement for suited evaluations, and integrated portable life support testing.

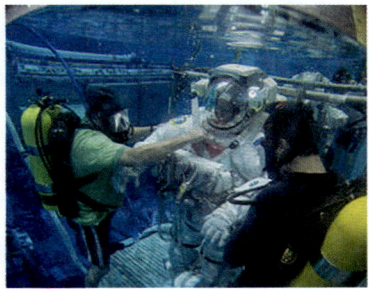

Credit: NASA

Sources:

Belobrajdic B, et al. Planetary extravehicular activity (EVA) risk mitigation strategies for long-duration space missions. *NPJ Microgravity*. 2021;7:16.

de la Cruz RA, et al. Aerospace Decompression Illness. 2021 Nov 29. In: StatPearls [Internet]. Treasure Island (FL): StatPearls Publishing; 2022 Jan; 28846248.

Kluis L, Diaz-Artiles A. Revisiting decompression sickness risk and mobility in the context of the SmartSuit, a hybrid planetary spacesuit. *NPJ Microgravity*. 2021 5;7:46.

Lippincott® Connect Appendix F, available online at Lippincott Connect, lists calorie expenditures for different physical activities, including common household activities.

Different portable systems have been designed, tested, and used in sport, industrial, military, scientific, and commercial applications. Portable systems incorporate the latest advances in miniaturized computer technology to produce results comparable to more fixed, dedicated desktop systems or the traditional Douglas bag system described in the Section "Bag Technique." FIGURE 8.5 shows different commercially available portable metabolic collection systems. The most current miniaturized systems include whole-body multisensor devices worn on the wrist or arm, or a collection system similar to a lightweight headset microphone. In these applications, an integrated computer performs the metabolic calculations based on electronic signals it receives from microdesigned instruments that measure oxygen and carbon dioxide in expired air and respiratory flow dynamics and volumes with a highly sensitive microflowmeter. Microchips store the data for later analyses. More advanced systems also include automated blood pressure, heart rate, and temperature monitors, with preset instructions to regulate speed, duration, and workload (and force output where applicable) for treadmills, bicycle ergometers, steppers, rowers, swim flumes, resistance devices, or other exercise apparatus. Private laboratories investigating caloric expenditure for common activities can have about 30 fully automated systems collect data at the same time throughout the day or for years, to provide invaluable normative data by sex, age, and fitness level (https://fortune.com/2017/09/05/apple-secret-exercise-lab/; www.menshealth.com/technology-gear/a18923364/inside-apples-secret-performance-lab/).[34] In private exercise physiology laboratories in 2017, 13 exercise physiologists and 29 nurses and medics monitored data on a continuous daily basis. Over a 5-year period, the laboratory logged 33,000 sessions with more than 66,000 hours of data collection, involving more than 10,000 participants. Several research studies became integrated into projects sponsored by the National Institutes of Health and published in 2020 for assessing wristwatch-based photoplethysmography to identify cardiac arrhythmias (https://clinicaltrials.gov/ct2/show/NCT03335800).

Bag Technique

FIGURE 8.6 depicts two classic bag techniques to secure expired air volumes. One occurs during stationary cycling (Fig. 8.6A) and involves the subject pedaling a bicycle ergometer wearing headgear attached to a two-way, high-velocity, low-resistance breathing valve. The other occurs during front crawl swimming (Fig. 8.6B) and involves the subject swimming freely while the exercise physiologist walks along the pool edge carrying a pole with electronic instruments, including a heart rate transmitter, with waterproof electrodes attached to the swimmer's chest. In both examples, subjects breathe ambient air through one side of the valve, which is then expelled through the other side into standard rubber meteorological balloons (also routinely used in weather-related research) and then evacuated into a gas meter to measure the total expired air volume. The expired air also can pass into a canvas **Douglas bag** (named for distinguished British respiratory physiologist Claude G. Douglas [1882–1963]; www.douglashistory.co.uk/history/claude_douglas.htm). The meter draws off an aliquot air sample into multiple smaller rubber bags for subsequent O_2 and CO_2 compositional analysis. In experiments in the 1920s using Douglas bags (and then meteorological balloons in exercise physiology laboratories, including the famous Harvard Fatigue laboratory), multiple collection samples were analyzed for O_2 and CO_2, mostly with the chemical Haldane or Scholander methods, which often would require many 8-hr days to analyze the air samples. It was not unusual to collect up to 165 total air samples covering a 15-min rest period, 60-min treadmill run, and 90-min recovery period! An experienced technician could analyze a single air sample by the Haldane method in 5 to 10 min. For the above treadmill experimental protocol, this translates to about 14 to 28 hr to complete the Haldane analyses

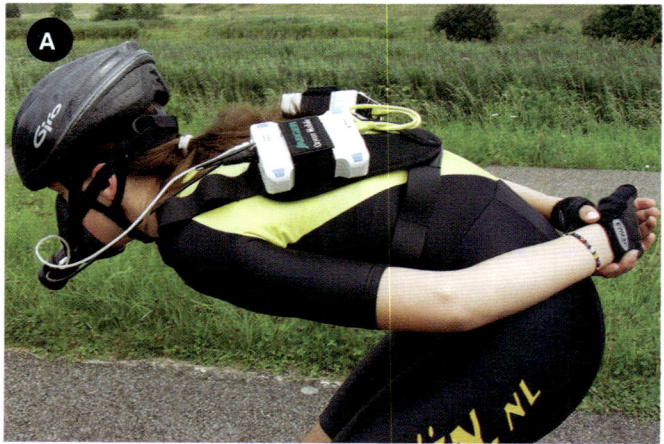

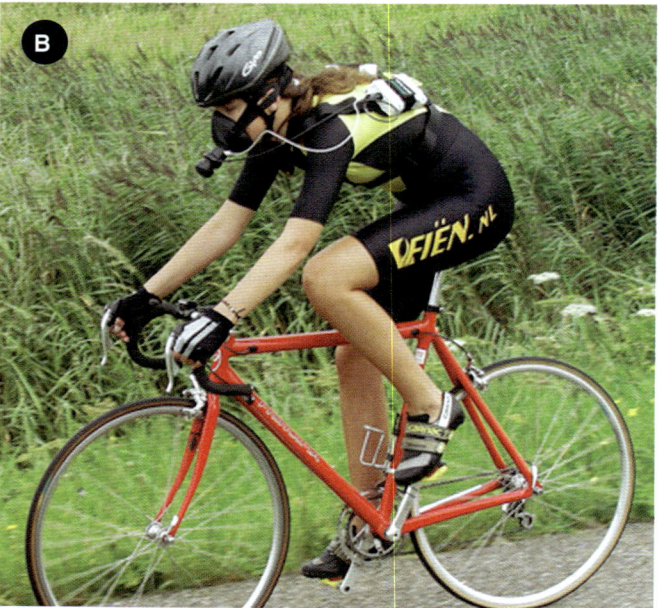

FIGURE 8.5. Examples of metabolic collection system to measure oxygen uptake by the open-circuit method for **(A)** in-line skating and **(B)** cycling.

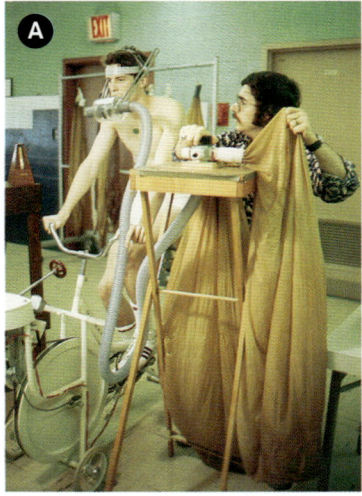 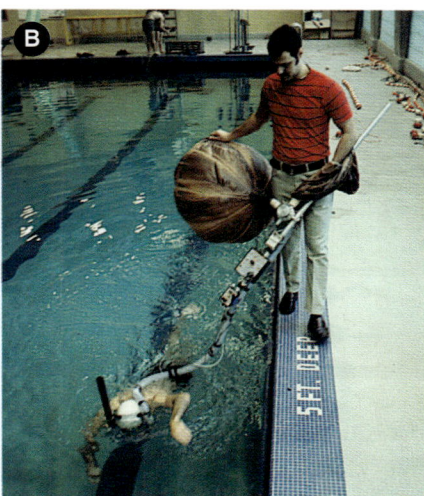

FIGURE 8.6. Oxygen uptake measurement by open-circuit spirometry (bag technique) during stationary cycle ergometer exercise (**A**) and during front-crawl swimming (**B**).
(Images courtesy Fitness Technologies.)

to determine the oxygen uptake during rest, exercise, and recovery (allowing 5 to 10 min per analysis for each of the 165 aliquot samples).

Ventilated Hood Technique

The open **ventilated hood technique** (FIG. 8.7) relies on modifications of open-circuit spirometry. With this method, a flexible cone or tent surrounds the subject's head and shoulders to capture expired gases by airflow pumped through the tent to microprocessor-controlled analyzers to assess oxygen and carbon dioxide concentrations. This method permits continuous monitoring over longer rest periods and sleep durations than tolerated with restrictions imposed by mouthpieces, nose clips, and hoses with typical open-circuit spirometric methods.[35,36]

Computerized Instrumentation

With advances in computer and microprocessor technology, the exercise scientist can rapidly assess metabolic and physiologic exercise responses. A computer interfaces with at least two instruments:

1. System to continuously sample the subject's expired air volume
2. High-speed analyzers to measure the expired air mixture's oxygen and carbon dioxide composition

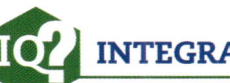

The computer performs metabolic calculations based on electronic signals it receives from the instruments. A printed or graphic display appears throughout the measurement period. FIGURE 8.8 depicts a typical computerized system to assess and monitor metabolic and physiologic responses during physical activity. The flowchart in the figure illustrates the breath-by-breath sequence to compute ventilation volume and oxygen uptake and carbon dioxide produced during the measurement period.

FIGURE 8.7. Open-circuit spirometry assessed with a ventilated hood system.

Computerized systems offer advantages in operation and data analysis speed, and also disadvantages of high equipment cost and delays from system breakdowns.[4,10,32] Regardless of a particular automated system's sophistication, the output data still reflect the measuring device's accuracy. Instrument reliability and validity require careful and frequent calibration that employs established reference or criterion standards.

Metabolic measurements require frequent instrument calibration to validate the accuracy of the air volume breathed and the expired air volume's oxygen and carbon dioxide fractional concentrations. In this regard, most laboratories use established criterion methods to calibrate the measurement instruments.

 **INTEGRATIVE QUESTION**

What is the common energy basis to equate food intake and physical activity?

Before the conversion to electronic and computerized instrumentation, oxygen uptake determinations used either the **micro-Scholander method** or **Haldane gas analysis method**. The Scholander technique,[22] developed by Swedish physician and biologist Per Scholander (1905–1980; www.nasonline.org/publications/biographical-memoirs/memoir-pdfs/scholanderper.pdf), remained the preferred method through the 1980s to validate gas analysis procedures. The Haldane analyzer,[11] also used in early exercise physiology research, was devised by the British physiologist who invented the gas mask used in World War I, John Scott Haldane (1860–1936; www.ncbi.nlm.nih.gov/pmc/articles/PMC4091013/). Both methods involved time-consuming separate analyses for a single experiment, with frequent duplicate measurements to verify results. This partly explains why energy metabolism studies from the early exercise physiology literature (1920s–1950s) often relied on only one or two subjects and took so long to complete. When performed properly with attention to detail, these chemical analyzers produced highly accurate and reliable data and are even used to validate today's high-speed analysis methods.

INTEGRATIVE QUESTION

What is the rationale for measuring only CO_2 production to estimate energy expenditure during steady-rate physical activity?

Direct Versus Indirect Calorimetry

Energy metabolism comparisons with direct and indirect calorimetry provide convincing evidence for the indirect method's validity. Research in the early 19th century compared the two calorimetry methods over 40 days for three men who lived in a calorimeter similar to the one in Figure 8.3. Daily energy expenditure averaged 2723 kcal when measured directly by heat production and 2717 kcal when computed indirectly by closed-circuit oxygen uptake measures. Other experiments with animals and humans, using rest and light and moderate (steady-rate) physical activity, also show close agreement between direct and indirect methods; in most instances, the difference averages less than ±1%. In Atwater and Rosa calorimetry experiments, methodological errors averaged only ±0.2%. This remarkable achievement, using mostly handmade instruments, resulted from the scientists' dedication to precise calibration methods long before electronic instrumentation availability.

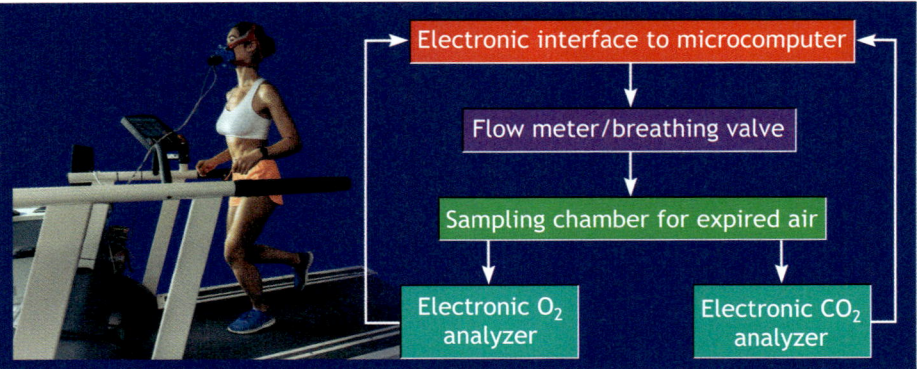

FIGURE 8.8. Systems approach to collect, analyze, and monitor physiologic and metabolic data during physical activity.
(Jacob Lund/Shutterstock)

Doubly Labeled Water Technique

The **doubly labeled water technique** provides an isotope-based method to safely estimate total (average) daily energy expenditure for children and adults in free-living conditions without the normal constraints imposed by laboratory procedures.[7,24,25,27,33] The technique does not furnish sufficient refinement for accurately estimating a person's energy expenditure at any one time but is more applicable to estimate average values over a prescribed time period and also for group energy expenditure estimates. The high technical accuracy for the doubly labeled water method allows for use as a criterion to validate other methods (e.g., physical activity questionnaires and physical activity records) to estimate total daily energy expenditure for groups over prolonged time periods.[3,6,9,17,23,28,37]

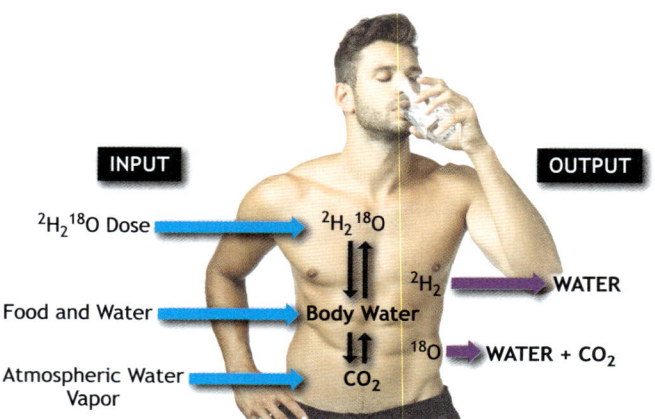

Mix and Match Studio/Shutterstock

The subject consumes water with a known concentration of the heavy, nonradioactive forms of the stable isotopes of hydrogen (^{2}H or deuterium) and oxygen (^{18}O or oxygen-18)—hence the term "doubly labeled water." The isotopes distribute throughout bodily fluids. Labeled hydrogen leaves the body as water (^{2}H$_2$O) in sweat, urine, and pulmonary water vapor, whereas labeled oxygen leaves as both water (H$_2^{18}$O) and carbon dioxide (C^{18}O$_2$) produced during macronutrient oxidation during energy metabolism. Differences between elimination rates for the two isotopes (determined by isotope ratio mass spectrometry) relative to the body's normal background levels estimate total CO$_2$ production during measurement. Oxygen uptake is easily estimated by CO$_2$ production and an assumed or measured respiratory quotient value of 0.85 (see the next section).

Under normal circumstances, urine or saliva analysis before consuming the doubly labeled water serves as control baseline values for ^{18}O and ^{2}H. Ingested isotopes require about 5 hr to distribute throughout the body water. The researchers then measure the enriched urine or saliva sample initially and then every day (or week) thereafter for the study's duration, typically up to 3 wk. The progressive decrease in the sample concentrations between the two isotopes yields the CO$_2$ production rate.[26] Doubly labeled water's accuracy versus directly measured energy expenditure in controlled settings averages between 3 and 5%. This magnitude of error probably increases in field studies mostly among physically active individuals.[31]

The doubly labeled water technique provides an ideal way to assess total energy expenditure of individuals over prolonged periods (e.g., bed rest, climbing Mt. Everest, Tour de France cycling, trekking across Antarctica, military maneuvers, space EVAs, and endurance running and swimming).[2,12,18,29] Drawbacks to the method include the expense for enriched ^{18}O and spectrometric analysis of both isotopes.

Respiratory Quotient

Research in the early 20th century discovered a way to evaluate the food mixture metabolized during rest and steady-rate physical activity from pulmonary gas exchange measures.[16] Inherent chemical differences among carbohydrate, lipid, and protein composition require different oxygen amounts to completely oxidize each molecule's carbon and hydrogen atoms to CO_2 and H_2O end products. Thus, carbon dioxide produced per unit oxygen uptake varies with the substrate type catabolized. The **respiratory quotient (RQ)** describes the ratio to express gas exchange in the lungs as follows:

$$RQ = CO_2 \text{ produced} \div O_2 \text{ consumed}$$

The RQ provides a convenient guide to approximate the nutrient mixture catabolized for energy during rest and aerobic physical activity. Note, that precisely determining the body's heat production by indirect calorimetry requires measuring both RQ and oxygen uptake.

Carbohydrate RQ

The complete oxidation of one glucose molecule requires six oxygen molecules and produces six carbon dioxide and water molecules as follows:

Gas exchange during glucose oxidation produces CO_2 molecules equal in number to O_2 molecules consumed; therefore, the RQ for carbohydrate equals 1.00.

$$C_6H_{12}O_6 + 6\,O_2 \rightarrow 6\,CO_2 + 6\,H_2O$$
$$RQ = 6\,CO_2 \div 6\,O_2$$
$$RQ = 1.00$$

Lipid RQ

Lipid's chemical composition differs from carbohydrate's because lipids contain considerably more hydrogen and carbon atoms than oxygen atoms. Consequently, lipid catabolism requires more oxygen in relation to carbon dioxide production. For example, palmitic acid, a typical fatty acid, oxidizes to carbon dioxide and water, producing 16 carbon dioxide molecules for every 23 oxygen molecules consumed. The following equation summarizes this exchange to compute the RQ:

$$C_{16}H_{12}O_2 + 23\,O_2 \rightarrow 16\,CO_2 + 16\,H_2O$$
$$RQ = 16\,CO_2 \div 23\,O_2$$
$$RQ = 0.696$$

Generally, a 0.70 value represents the RQ for lipid, with values ranging between 0.69 and 0.73 depending on the oxidized fatty acid's carbon-chain length.

Protein RQ

Proteins do not simply oxidize to carbon dioxide and water in energy metabolism. Rather, the liver first deaminates the amino acid molecule, followed by nitrogen excretion with sulfur fragments in urine, sweat, and feces. The remaining keto acid fragment oxidizes to carbon dioxide and water to provide energy for biologic work. To achieve complete combustion, the short-chain keto acids require more oxygen than carbon dioxide produced. The protein albumin oxidizes as follows:

$$C_6H_{112}O_{11}S + 77\,O_2 \rightarrow 63\,CO_2 + 38\,H_2O + SO_3 + 9\,CO(NH_2)_2$$
$$RQ = 63\,CO_2 \div 77\,O_2$$
$$RQ = 0.818$$

The value 0.82 characterizes protein's general RQ value.

Nonprotein RQ

The RQ based on expired air's compositional analysis usually reflects catabolizing a blend of carbohydrates, lipids, and proteins. One can precisely determine each one's contribution to the metabolic mixture. For example, the kidneys excrete approximately 1 g of urinary nitrogen for every 5.6 (current value) to 6.25 g (classic value) protein metabolized for energy.[14] Each gram of nitrogen excreted represents approximately 4.8 L carbon dioxide produced and oxygen uptake of about 6.0 L. Within this framework, the following example illustrates the stepwise procedure to calculate the **nonprotein RQ**—that is, the respiratory exchange portion attributed to combustion of *only* carbohydrate and lipid with protein excluded.

This example considers data from a subject who consumes 4.0 L oxygen and produces 3.4 L carbon dioxide during a 15-min rest period. During this time, the kidneys excrete 0.13 g of nitrogen in urine.

1. Step 1. 4.8 L CO_2 per g protein metabolized × 0.13 g = 0.62 L CO_2 produced in protein catabolism
2. Step 2. 6.0 L O_2 per g protein metabolized × 0.13 g = 0.78 L O_2 consumed in protein catabolism
3. Step 3. Nonprotein CO_2 produced = 3.4 L CO_2 − 0.62 L CO_2 = 2.78 L CO_2
4. Step 4. Nonprotein O_2 consumed = 4.0 L O_2 − 0.78 L O_2 = 3.22 L O_2
5. Step 5. Nonprotein RQ = 2.78 ÷ 3.22 = 0.86

TABLE 8.1 presents the thermal energy equivalents for oxygen uptake for different nonprotein RQ values and the lipid and carbohydrate percentages catabolized for energy. For the 0.86 nonprotein RQ computed in the previous example, each liter of oxygen uptake liberates 4.875 kcal. Also, for this RQ, 54.1% for nonprotein calories come from carbohydrate and 45.9% from lipid. The total 15-min heat production at rest attributable to lipid and carbohydrate catabolism equals 15.70 kcal (4.875 kcal·L^{-1} × 3.22 L O_2). The energy from protein breakdown equals 3.5 kcal (4.5 kcal·L^{-1} × 0.78 L O_2). The total energy from protein combustion and nonprotein macronutrients during the 15-min period equals 19.2 kcal (15.7 kcal nonprotein + 3.5 kcal protein).

TABLE 8.1 Thermal energy equivalents for oxygen of different nonprotein RQ values and percentage lipid and carbohydrate catabolized for energy

If the thermal equivalent for a mixed diet (RQ = 0.82) had been used in the caloric transformation or if RQ had been computed from total respiratory gas exchange and applied to Table 8.1 without considering the protein component, the estimated energy expenditure would be 19.3 kcal (4.825 kcal·L^{-1} × 4.0 L O_2; assuming a mixed diet). This corresponds to only a

In a Practical Sense

Open-Circuit Spirometry to Calculate Oxygen Uptake, Carbon Dioxide Production, and Respiratory Quotient

Inspired air percentage composition remains relatively constant (CO_2 = 0.03%, O_2 = 20.93%, N_2 = 79.04%), so determining a person's oxygen uptake ($\dot{V}O_2$) requires measuring the expired air's amount and composition. Expired air always contains more CO_2 (usually 2.5 to 5.0%), less O_2 (usually 15.0 to 18.5%), and more N_2 (usually 79.04 to 79.60%) than does inspired air.

NITROGEN EXCHANGE: THE HALDANE TRANSFORMATION

Nitrogen is inert in terms of energy metabolism, so any change in its concentration in expired air compared with that in inspired air reflects that the number of oxygen molecules removed from inspired air is not replaced by the same carbon dioxide molecule number produced in metabolism. Thus, the expired air volume ($\dot{V}_{E,STPD}$) is unequal to the inspired air volume ($\dot{V}_{I,STPD}$). For example, if the respiratory quotient is less than 1.00 (i.e., less CO_2 produced in relation to O_2 consumed), with 3 L of air inspired, less than 3 L of air will be expired. In this case, the nitrogen concentration is higher in expired air than in inspired air. This is not because nitrogen has been produced, but rather nitrogen molecules now represent a larger percentage of $\dot{V}_E$ compared with $\dot{V}_I$. $\dot{V}_E$ differs from $\dot{V}_I$ in direct proportion to the change in nitrogen concentration between inspired and expired air volumes. Thus, $\dot{V}_I$ can be determined from $\dot{V}_E$ using the ratio nitrogen expired to nitrogen inspired in an equation known as the Haldane transformation.

$$\dot{V}_{I,STPD} = \dot{V}_{E,STPD} \times \frac{\%N_2E}{\%N_2I} \quad \text{Equation 1}$$

where $\%N_2I$ = 79.04 and $\%N_2E$ = percent nitrogen in expired air computed from gas analysis as $[(100 - (\%O_{2E} + \%CO_{2E})]$.

CALCULATING $\dot{V}O_2$ USING EXPIRED AIR VOLUME

The following examples assume that all ventilation volumes are expressed at standard temperature and pressure and dry (STPD).

Lippincott® Connect Appendix G, available online at Lippincott Connect, explains how to standardize gas volumes to reference conditions (STPD and body temperature, ambient pressure, and gas saturated with water vapor [BTPS]).

The volume of O_2 in inspired air per minute ($\dot{V}O_{2I}$) is determined as follows:

$$\dot{V}O_{2I} = \dot{V}_I \times \%O_{2I} \quad \text{Equation 2}$$

Using the Haldane transformation and substituting Equation 1 for $\dot{V}_I$,

$$\dot{V}O_{2I} = \dot{V}_E \times \frac{\%N_2E}{79.04} \times \%O_{2I} \quad \text{Equation 3}$$

where $\%O_2$ = 20.93%.

The amount or volume of oxygen in expired air ($\dot{V}O_{2E}$) computes as follows:

$$\dot{V}O_{2E} = \dot{V}_E \times \%O_{2E} \quad \text{Equation 4}$$

where $\%O_{2E}$ is the fractional concentration for oxygen in expired air determined by gas analysis (chemical or electronic methods).

The O_2 amount removed from inspired air each minute ($\dot{V}O_2$) is computed as follows:

$$\dot{V}O_2 = \dot{V}_I \times \%O_{2I} - \dot{V}_E \times \%O_{2E} \quad \text{Equation 5}$$

By substitution,

$$\dot{V}O_2 = \left\langle \left[\left(\dot{V}_E \times \frac{\%N_2E}{79.04\%} \right) \times 20.93\% \right] - (\dot{V}_E \times \%O_{2E}) \right\rangle \quad \text{Equation 6}$$

where $\dot{V}O_2$ = oxygen volume consumed per minute, expressed in mL or L, and $\dot{V}_E$ = expired air volume consumed per minute, expressed in mL or L, STPD.

Equation 6 can be simplified to:

$$\dot{V}O_2 = \dot{V}_E \left[\left(\frac{\%N_2E}{79.04\%} \times 20.93\% \right) - \%O_{2E} \right] \quad \text{Equation 7}$$

After dividing 20.93 by 79.04, the final equation becomes:

$$\dot{V}O_2 = \dot{V}_E [(\%N_{2E} \times 0.265) - \%O_{2E}] \quad \text{Equation 8}$$

Equation 8 is the choice equation to calculate $\dot{V}O_2$ when ventilation expired (STPD) is determined.

True O_2

The value obtained within the brackets in Equations 7 and 8 is referred to as the *True O_2* and represents "oxygen extraction," or more precisely, the percentage oxygen uptake for any air volume expired.

CALCULATING $\dot{V}O_2$ USING INSPIRED AIR VOLUME

In situations where only $\dot{V}_I$ is measured, the $\dot{V}_E$ can be calculated from the Haldane transformation:

$$\dot{V}_E = \dot{V}_I \frac{\%N_{2I}}{\%N_{2E}} \quad \text{Equation 9}$$

By substitution in Equation 5, the computational equation becomes:

$$\dot{V}O_2 = \dot{V}_I \left[\%O_{2I} - \left(\frac{\%N_{2I}}{\%N_{2E}} \times \%O_{2E} \right) \right] \quad \text{Equation 10}$$

CALCULATING CARBON DIOXIDE PRODUCTION

The carbon dioxide production per minute ($\dot{V}CO_2$) calculates as follows:

$$\dot{V}CO_2 = \dot{V}_E(\%CO_{2E} - \%CO_{2I}) \quad \text{Equation 11}$$

where $\%CO_{2E}$ = percent carbon dioxide in expired air determined by gas analysis, and $\%CO_2$ = percent carbon dioxide in inspired air, which is essentially constant at 0.03%.

The final equation becomes:

$$\dot{V}CO_{2E} = \dot{V}_E(\%CO_{2E} - 0.03\%) \quad \text{Equation 12}$$

RESPIRATORY QUOTIENT CALCULATION

Calculate the respiratory quotient (RQ) in one of two ways:

$$RQ = \frac{\dot{V}CO_2}{\dot{V}O_2}$$

or \quad Equation 13

$$RQ = \frac{\%CO_{2E} - 0.03\%}{\text{"True"}O_2}$$

Example

Compute $\dot{V}O_2$, $\dot{V}CO_2$, and RQ from the following data:
a. $\dot{V}_{E,STPD}$ = 60.0 L
b. $\%O_{2E}$ = 16.86 or (0.1686)
c. $\%CO_{2E}$ = 3.62 or (0.0362)

$$\dot{V}O_2 = \dot{V}_E[(\%N_{2E} \times 0.265) - \%O_{2E}] \quad \text{Equation 8}$$

$\dot{V}O_2 = 60.0\ [(1.00 - (0.1686 + 0.0362)) \times 0.265 - 0.1686]$
$\dot{V}O_2 = 60.0\ [(0.7952 \times 0.265) - 0.1686]$
$\dot{V}O_2 = 2.527\ L \cdot min^{-1}$

$$\dot{V}CO_{2E} = \dot{V}_E(\%CO_{2E} - 0.03\%) \quad \text{Equation 12}$$

$\dot{V}CO_{2E} = 60.0\ (0.0362 - 0.0003\%)$

$\dot{V}CO_{2E} = 2.154\ L \cdot min^{-1}$

$$RQ = \frac{\dot{V}CO_2}{\dot{V}O_2} \quad \text{Equation 13}$$

$RQ = \frac{2.154}{2.527}$

$RQ = 0.85$

0.5% difference from the value obtained with the more elaborate and time-consuming method requiring urinary nitrogen analysis. *In most cases, the gross metabolic nonprotein RQ calculated from pulmonary gas exchange and applied without urinary and other nitrogen sources introduces only minimal error because protein's contribution to energy metabolism remains small.*

The last two columns in Table 8.1 present conversions for the nonprotein RQ to carbohydrate and lipid grams metabolized per liter oxygen uptake. For the subject with RQ of 0.86, this represents approximately 0.62 g carbohydrate and 0.25 g lipid. For the 3.22 L of oxygen uptake during the 15-min rest period, this represents 2.0 g carbohydrate (3.22 L O_2 × 0.62) and 0.80 g fat (3.22 L O_2 × 0.25) metabolized for energy.

Mixed Diet RQ

The RQ seldom reflects pure carbohydrate or pure lipid oxidation during activities ranging from complete bed rest to mild aerobic walking or slow jogging. Instead, catabolizing a nutrient mixture occurs with an RQ intermediate between 0.70 and 1.00. For most purposes, assume a 0.82 RQ (40% carbohydrate and 60% lipid) and apply the caloric equivalent 4.825 kcal per liter oxygen in the energy transformations. In using 4.825, the maximum error possible in estimating energy expenditure from steady-rate oxygen uptake averages about 4%. When requiring greater precision, compute the actual RQ and refer to Table 8.1 to obtain a more precise caloric transformation and percentage contribution from carbohydrate and lipid to the metabolic mixture.

 **INTEGRATIVE QUESTION**

How did exercise physiologists determine that between 70 and 80% of the energy comes from lipid combustion in the last phases of a marathon run?

Respiratory Exchange Ratio

The RQ assumes the oxygen and carbon dioxide exchange measured at the lungs reflects gas exchange from macronutrient catabolism in the cell. This assumption remains reasonable during rest and steady-rate conditions with little reliance on anaerobic metabolism. Several factors other than food combustion can spuriously alter the oxygen and carbon dioxide exchange in the lungs. When this occurs, the gas exchange ratio no longer reflects only the substrate mixture in energy metabolism. Respiratory physiologists refer to the ratio between carbon dioxide produced to oxygen uptake under such conditions as the **respiratory exchange ratio (RER)**. In this case, the pulmonary oxygen and carbon dioxide exchange no longer reflects a specific food mixture's cellular oxidation. The RER computes exactly the same as the RQ.

Carbon dioxide elimination increases during hyperventilation because breathing increases to disproportionately higher levels compared with metabolic demands (see Chapter 14). Overbreathing decreases the blood's normal carbon dioxide level because this nonmetabolic carbon dioxide "blows off" from the lungs in the expired air without corresponding increases in

In a Practical Sense

The Weir Method to Calculate Energy Expenditure

In 1949, John Brash de Vere Weir (1908–1985), a senior lecturer in physiology from Glasgow University, presented a simple method to estimate caloric expenditure (kcal · min^{-1}) from pulmonary ventilation and expired oxygen percentage measures, accurate to within ±1% of the traditional respiratory quotient (RQ) method.

BASIC EQUATION

Weir showed that the following formula could calculate energy expenditure if total energy production from protein breakdown equaled 12.5% (a reasonable percentage for most people under most conditions):

$$\text{kcal} \cdot \text{min}^{-1} = \dot{V}_{E(STPD)} \times (1.044 - 0.0499 \times \%O_{2E})$$

where $\dot{V}_{E(STPD)}$ represents expired minute ventilation (L · min^{-1}) corrected to standard temperature and pressure and dry (STPD) conditions, and $\%O_{2E}$ represents expired oxygen percentage. The value in parentheses $(1.044 - 0.0499 \times \%O_{2E})$ represents the "Weir factor." The table displays Weir factors for different $\%O_{2E}$ values.

To use the table, locate the $\%O_{2E}$ and corresponding Weir factor. Compute energy expenditure in kcal · min^{-1} by multiplying the Weir factor by $\dot{V}_{E(STPD)}$.

EXAMPLE

A person runs on a treadmill and $\dot{V}_{E(STPD)} = 50$ L · min^{-1} and $\%O_{2E} = 16.0\%$. Compute energy expenditure by the Weir method as follows:

$$\begin{aligned}\text{kcal} \cdot \text{min}^{-1} &= \dot{V}_{E(STPD)} \times (1.044 - [0.0499 \times \%O_{2E}]) \\ &= 50 \times (1.044 - [0.0499 \times 16.0]) \\ &= 50 \times 0.2456 \\ &= 12.3\end{aligned}$$

Weir also derived the following equation to calculate kcal · min^{-1} from RQ and $\dot{V}O_2$ in L · min^{-1}:

$$\text{kcal} \cdot \text{min}^{-1} = ([1.1 \times RQ] + 3.9) \times \dot{V}O_2$$

WEIR FACTORS

$\%O_{2E}$	Weir Factor	$\%O_{2E}$	Weir Factor
14.50	0.3205	17.00	0.1957
14.60	0.3155	17.10	0.1907
14.70	0.3105	17.20	0.1857
14.80	0.3055	17.30	0.1807
14.90	0.3005	17.40	0.1757
15.00	0.2955	17.50	0.1707
15.10	0.2905	17.60	0.1658
15.20	0.2855	17.70	0.1608
15.30	0.2805	17.80	0.1558
15.40	0.2755	17.90	0.1508
15.50	0.2705	18.00	0.1468
15.60	0.2656	18.10	0.1408
15.70	0.2606	18.20	0.1368
15.80	0.2556	18.30	0.1308
15.90	0.2506	18.40	0.1268
16.00	0.2456	18.50	0.1208
16.10	0.2406	18.60	0.1168
16.20	0.2366	18.70	0.1109
16.30	0.2306	18.80	0.1068
16.40	0.2256	18.90	0.1009
16.50	0.2206	19.00	0.0969
16.60	0.2157	19.10	0.0909
16.70	0.2107	19.20	0.0868
16.80	0.2057	19.30	0.0809
16.90	0.2007	19.40	0.0769

Source:
Data from Weir JB. New methods for calculating metabolic rates with special reference to protein metabolism. *J Physiol.* 1949;109:1. If $\%O_{2E}$ does not appear in the table, compute individual Weir factors as $1.044 - 0.0499 \times \%O_{2E}$.

---

oxygen uptake. This raises the RER (usually to above 1.00) to a level that does not reflect macronutrient oxidation.

Exhaustive activity presents another situation in which RER rises above 1.00. Sodium bicarbonate in the blood buffers or neutralizes the lactate generated during anaerobic metabolism to maintain proper acid-base balance. Lactate buffering produces carbonic acid, a weaker acid, as follows:

$$HLa + NaHCO_3 \rightarrow NaLa + H_2CO_3$$

fyi Respiratory Quotient Versus Respiratory Exchange Ratio

The respiratory exchange ratio (RER) expresses the amount of CO_2 produced to the amount of O_2 consumed during various physiologic occurrences on a total body level unrelated to macronutrient combustion (e.g., substrate catabolism, buffering, hyperventilation). By contrast, the RQ represents the ratio between the amount of CO_2 produced to the amount of O_2 consumed under rest and steady-rate exercise conditions. This ratio characterizes the same gas exchange ratio as RER but reflects only cellular level substrate catabolism.

Jacob Lund/Shutterstock

Sources:
Erickson JR, et al. Effects of one versus two doses of a multi-ingredient pre-workout supplement on metabolic factors and perceived exertion during moderate-intensity running in females. *Sports (Basel)*. 2020;8:E52.

Gilbertson NM, et al. Tolerance is linked to postprandial fuel use independent of exercise dose. *Med Sci Sports Exerc*. 2018;50:2058.

In the pulmonary capillaries, carbonic acid degrades to its component carbon dioxide and water molecules. Carbon dioxide readily exits the lungs in the reaction:

$$H_2CO_3 \rightarrow H_2O + CO_2 \rightarrow Lungs$$

The RER increases above 1.00 because buffering adds "extra" nonmetabolic-created carbon dioxide to the expired air above the quantity normally released during energy metabolism. In rare instances, the exchange ratio exceeds 1.00 when a person gains body fat through excessive dietary carbohydrate intake. In this lipogenic situation, carbohydrate-to-lipid conversion liberates oxygen as the excess calories accumulate in adipose tissue. The released oxygen then supplies energy metabolism to reduce the lungs' atmospheric oxygen uptake despite maintaining normal carbon dioxide production.

Relatively low RER values also can occur. Following exhaustive physical activity, the cells and bodily fluids retain carbon dioxide to replenish the sodium bicarbonate that buffered the accumulating lactate. This alkaline reserve replenishment decreases the expired carbon dioxide level without impacting oxygen uptake and may decrease the RER to below 0.70.

Summary

1. Direct calorimetry and indirect calorimetry represent two methods to determine human energy expenditure.
2. Direct calorimetry measures heat production in an insulated calorimeter.
3. Indirect calorimetry infers energy expenditure from oxygen uptake and carbon dioxide production, using either closed-circuit spirometry or open-circuit spirometry.
4. The doubly labeled water technique estimates energy expenditure in free-living conditions without the normal constraints imposed by laboratory procedures.
5. Complete macronutrient oxidation requires a different oxygen uptake quantity for comparable carbon dioxide production.
6. The RQ relates the ratio between carbon dioxide produced to oxygen uptake.
7. The RQ averages 1.00 for carbohydrate, 0.70 for lipid, and 0.82 for protein.
8. For each RQ value, a corresponding caloric value exists per liter oxygen uptake.
9. The RQ-kcal relationship accurately determines energy expenditure for most mild-to-moderate intensity physical activities.
10. The RER reflects carbon dioxide and oxygen pulmonary exchange under differing physiologic and metabolic conditions unrelated to macronutrient combustion.
11. RER does not mirror gas exchange for the macronutrient mixture catabolized.

Key Terms

Atwater-Rosa calorimeter: Human calorimeter to measure energy metabolism designed by research scientists W.O. Atwater and E.B. Rosa in the 1890s

Caloric value for oxygen: Energy release in kcal measured by bomb calorimetry for a given nutrient "exploded" (burned) in 1 L oxygen

Calorimetry: Measures heat transfer (calories) into or out of a system during a chemical reaction or physical process

Closed-circuit spirometry: Uses principles of indirect calorimetry in a closed system to estimate energy expenditure

Direct calorimetry: Directly measures heat as kcal transferred directly from food combustion in a bomb calorimeter or heat produced by a person in a human calorimeter

Doubly labeled water technique: Isotope-based method using ^2H or deuterium and oxygen ^{18}O or oxygen-18 to safely estimate total and average daily energy expenditure of groups of children and adults in free-living conditions without the normal constraints imposed by typical laboratory procedures

Douglas bag: An inflatable canvas bag named for British respiratory physiologist Claude G. Douglas (1882–1963) to collect expired air volume, which is then sampled and measured through a gas meter to determine oxygen uptake

Haldane gas analysis method: Method to chemically measure the composition of relatively small expired air samples

Human calorimeter: Special chamber to directly measure human heat production under diverse living conditions

Indirect calorimetry: Method to calculate heat production by measuring either carbon dioxide production or oxygen uptake for a given duration

Micro-Scholander method: Method to measure oxygen and carbon dioxide concentrations in a microsample of expired air to an accuracy of ±0.015 mL per 100 mL

Nonprotein RQ: Portion of the respiratory exchange attributed to only carbohydrate and lipid combustion *excluding* protein

Open-circuit spirometry: Indirect calorimetry to estimate energy expenditure breathing ambient air (20.93% O_2, 0.03% CO_2, and 79.04% N_2)

Respiratory exchange ratio (RER): Ratio of carbon dioxide produced to oxygen uptake under conditions of non–steady-rate physical activity (computes identically to RQ)

Respiratory quotient (RQ): Ratio of carbon dioxide produced to oxygen uptake for complete macronutrient oxidation measured during steady-rate metabolic conditions (computes as RQ = CO_2 produced ÷ O_2 uptake)

Ventilated hood technique: Flow-dilution-based hood for indirect human calorimetry without a closed-circuit system

References are available online at Lippincott Connect.

Additional References

Bacelis-Rivero AP, et al. Assessment of physical activity in adults: a review of validated questionnaires from a nutritionist's point of view. *Eval Health Prof.* 2020;43:235.

Barclay CJ, Loiselle DS. Historical perspective: heat production and chemical change in muscle. Roger C. Woledge. *Prog Biophys Mol Biol.* 2021;161:3.

Burrows T, et al. A systematic review of the validity of dietary assessment methods in children when compared with the method of doubly labelled water. *Eur J Clin Nutr.* 2020;74:669.

Cano A, et al. Analysis of sex-based differences in energy substrate utilization during moderate-intensity aerobic exercise. *Eur J Appl Physiol.* 2022;122:29.

Cohen P, Kajimura S. The cellular and functional complexity of thermogenic fat. *Nat Rev Mol Cell Biol.* 2021;22:393.

Crawford CK, et al. Prolonged standing reduces fasting plasma triglyceride but does not influence postprandial metabolism compared to prolonged sitting. *PLoS One.* 2020;15:e0228297.

Dominelli PB, Molgat-Seon Y. Sex, gender and the pulmonary physiology of exercise. *Eur Respir Rev.* 2022 31:210074.

O'Driscoll R, et al. Improving energy expenditure estimates from wearable devices: a machine learning approach. *J Sports Sci.* 2020;6:1.

Pisanu S, et al. Validity of accelerometers for the evaluation of energy expenditure in obese and overweight individuals: a systematic review. *J Nutr Metab.* 2020;2020:2327017.

Porter J, et al. Understanding total energy expenditure in people with dementia: a systematic review with directions for future research. *Australas J Ageing.* 2021;40:243.

Ramakrishnan R, et al. Objectively measured physical activity and all-cause mortality: a systematic review and meta-analysis. *Prev Med.* 2021;143:106356.

Sanchez-Delgado G, Ravussin E. Assessment of energy expenditure: are calories measured differently for different diets? *Curr Opin Clin Nutr Metab Care.* 2020;23:312.

Sato H, et al. Energy expenditure and physical activity in COPD by doubly labelled water method and an accelerometer. *ERJ Open Res.* 2021;7:00407.

Stickland MK, et al. How we do it - Using cardiopulmonary exercise testing to understand dyspnea and exercise intolerance in respiratory disease. *Chest.* 2022:S0012-3692(22)00145.

Tatucu-Babet OA, et al. Doubly labelled water for determining total energy expenditure in adult critically ill and acute care hospitalized inpatients: a scoping review. *Clin Nutr.* 2022;41:424.

Van Drunen R, Eckel-Mahan K. Circadian rhythms of the hypothalamus: from function to physiology. *Clocks Sleep.* 2021;3:189.

Zhang L, et al. Butyrate in energy metabolism: there is still more to learn. *Trends Endocrinol Metab.* 2021;32:159.

Table 8.1 — Thermal Energy Equivalents for Oxygen of Different Nonprotein RQ Values and Percentage Lipid and Carbohydrate Catabolized for Energy

Nonprotein RQ	kcal·L O_2^{-1}	% kcal Derived from		g·L O_2^{-1}	
		Carbohydrate	Lipid	Carbohydrate	Lipid
0.707	4.686	0.0	100.0	0.000	0.496
0.71	4.690	1.1	98.9	0.012	0.491
0.72	4.702	4.8	95.2	0.051	0.476
0.73	4.714	8.4	91.6	0.090	0.460
0.74	4.727	12.0	88.0	0.130	0.444
0.75	4.739	15.6	84.4	0.170	0.428
0.76	4.750	19.2	80.8	0.211	0.412
0.77	4.764	22.8	77.2	0.250	0.396
0.78	4.776	26.3	73.7	0.290	0.380
0.79	4.788	29.9	70.1	0.330	0.363
0.80	4.801	33.4	66.6	0.371	0.347
0.81	4.813	36.9	63.1	0.413	0.330
0.82	4.825	40.3	59.7	0.454	0.313
0.83	4.838	43.8	56.2	0.496	0.297
0.84	4.850	47.2	52.8	0.537	0.280
0.85	4.862	50.7	49.3	0.579	0.263
0.86	4.875	54.1	45.9	0.621	0.247
0.87	4.887	57.5	42.5	0.663	0.230
0.88	4.899	60.8	39.2	0.705	0.213
0.89	4.911	64.2	35.8	0.749	0.195
0.90	4.924	67.5	32.5	0.791	0.178
0.91	4.936	70.8	29.2	0.834	0.160
0.92	4.948	74.1	25.9	0.877	0.143
0.93	4.961	77.4	22.6	0.921	0.125
0.94	4.973	80.7	19.3	0.964	0.108
0.95	4.985	84.0	16.0	1.008	0.090
0.96	4.998	87.2	12.8	1.052	0.072
0.97	5.010	90.4	9.6	1.097	0.054
0.98	5.022	93.6	6.4	1.142	0.036
0.99	5.035	96.8	3.2	1.186	0.018
1.00	5.047	100.0	0	1.231	0.000

RQ, respiratory quotient.
Source: From Zuntz N. Ueber die Bedeutung der verschiedenen Nährstoffe als Erzeuger der Muskelkraft. *Arch Gesamte Physiol.* 1901;LXXXIII:557; *Pflugers Arch Physiol.* 1901;83:557.

CHAPTER 9

Energy Expenditure During Rest and Physical Activity

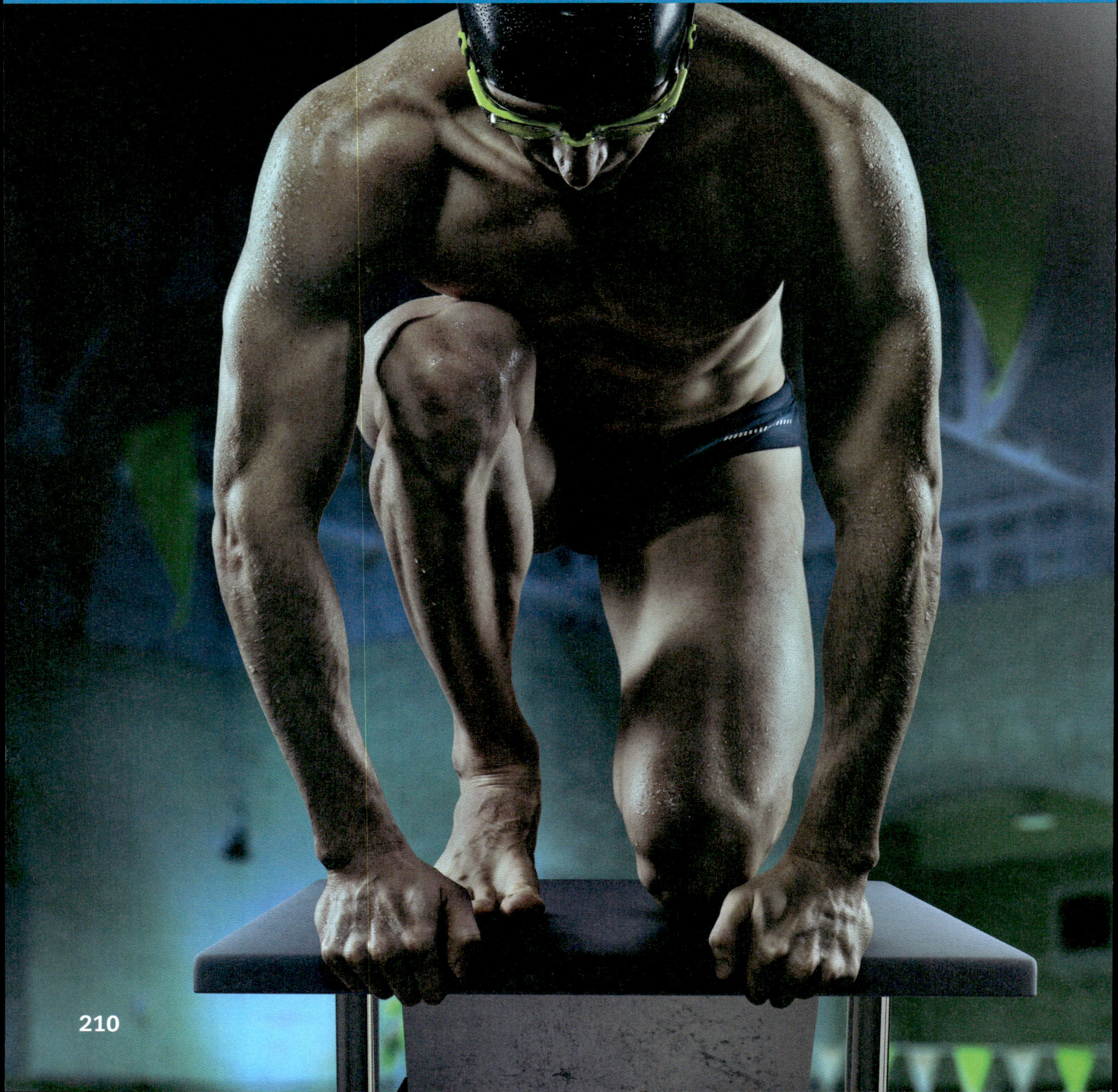

Chapter Objectives

- Define basal metabolic rate and list three factors that affect it
- Discuss three factors that affect total daily energy expenditure
- Outline two classification systems to rate physical activity's relative strenuousness
- Explain body weight's role in determining the energy cost for diverse physical activities
- Discuss two advantages and limitations in estimating physical activity energy expenditure from heart rate

Ancillaries at-a-Glance

Visit Lippincott Connect to access these resources.

- References: Chapter 9
- Appendix F: Energy Expenditure in Household, Occupational, Recreational, and Sports Activities
- Focus on Research: Factors that Affect Recovery Oxygen Uptake

Metabolism involves all of the chemical reactions of the body's biomolecules that contribute to **anabolism** and **catabolism**. The figure below illustrates the following three general factors that impact **total daily energy expenditure (TDEE)**. Combined, these three components constitute the energy requirements for nongrowing individuals.

1. Thermogenic effect of feeding
2. Thermic effect of physical activity
3. Resting metabolic rate

Part 1 — Energy Expenditure at Rest

Basal and Resting Metabolic Rate

Each individual requires a minimum energy level to sustain vital functions in the waking state, a level known as **basal metabolic rate (BMR)**. This energy requirement reflects the sum total of the body's many avenues to produce heat. Measuring oxygen uptake under stringent laboratory conditions indirectly determines the BMR. For example, the person must remain in the postabsorptive (fasting) state, not consuming any food, for the 12 to 18 hr preceding measurement to avoid metabolic increases from digestion, absorption, and assimilation of ingested nutrients. To reduce other calorigenic influences, the person cannot perform any physical activity for a minimum of 2 hr prior to the assessment. In the laboratory, the person rests supine for about 30 min in a comfortable, thermoneutral environment prior to measuring oxygen uptake for a 10-min minimum. Oxygen uptake values for BMR usually range between 160 and 290 $mL \cdot min^{-1}$ (0.8 to 1.43 $kcal \cdot min^{-1}$) depending on gender, age, overall body size (stature and body mass), fat-free body mass (FFM), and health/fitness status.

BMR establishes the energy baseline required to develop prudent weight control strategies through food restriction, regular physical activity, or their combination. Basal values measured under controlled laboratory conditions vary only slightly below values for **resting metabolic rate (RMR)** measured 3 to 4 hr following a light meal without prior physical activity. RMR and BMR often are used interchangeably, yet subtle differences exist. For example, BMR is always slightly lower than RMR depending on body size, muscle mass, age, health/fitness level, hormonal status, and body temperature. When measured under standardized conditions, both BMR and RMR show high reproducibility and stability.[8]

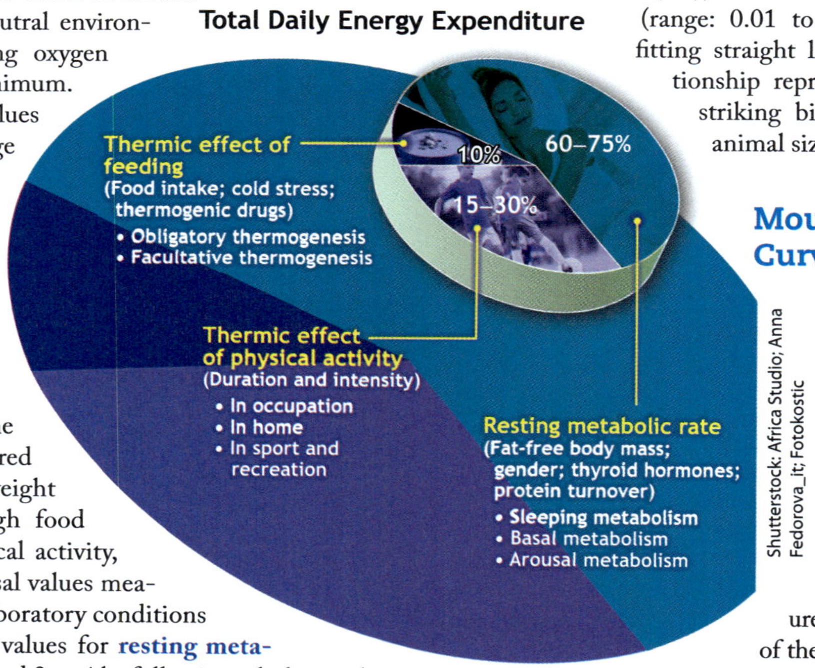

Essentially, BMR and RMR both refer to metabolic processes of the active cell mass required to sustain normal regulatory balance and body functions during basal or the less stringent resting state. For the typical person, RMR accounts for between 60 and 75% of TDEE, whereas thermic effects from food account for approximately 10%, and physical activity for 15 to 30%.

Metabolic Size Concept

Experiments in the late 1800s determined that a person's body size related to basal and resting metabolism in a predictable way. Careful experiments validated that these variables varied in proportion to body surface area (BSA). Experiments determined the total energy metabolism of a dog and man for 24 hr. The heat generated by the larger man exceeded the dog's energy metabolism by about 200%. The researchers deduced that expressing heat production in relation to either the man's BSA or dog's BSA reduced their metabolic difference to only about 10%. This important observation provided the basis to express basal (and resting) metabolic rate relative to BSA expressed as square meters per hour ($kcal \cdot m^{-2} \cdot hr^{-1}$). The "*surface area law*" describes the fundamental relationship between the body's heat production and its overall body size. **FIGURE 9.1** illustrates a logarithmic plot for body mass (range: 0.01 to 10,000 kg) versus metabolic rate expressed in watts (W), where 1 W = 0.01433 $kcal \cdot m^{-2}$ (range: 0.01 to 10,000 W). The best-fitting straight line describing this relationship represents one of the more striking biologic concepts relating animal size to metabolism.

Mouse-to-Elephant Curve

Numerous experiments have confirmed the "mouse-to-elephant curve" for metabolic rate using body mass to the 0.75 power displayed in Figure 9.1, whereas metabolic rate relates to BSA to the 0.67 power. The schematic inset figure compares the body size of the world's tallest man (2.89 m/9 ft 5¾ in) and woman (2.48 m/8 ft 1¾ in) with the world's largest land mammal (*Baluchitherium*, rhinoceros predecessor), whose body mass approximated 30 tons at 5.26 m/17 ft 3 in. Comparisons between a

---

Total Daily Energy Expenditure

- Thermic effect of feeding (Food intake; cold stress; thermogenic drugs)
  - Obligatory thermogenesis
  - Facultative thermogenesis — 10%
- Thermic effect of physical activity (Duration and intensity)
  - In occupation
  - In home
  - In sport and recreation — 15–30%
- Resting metabolic rate (Fat-free body mass; gender; thyroid hormones; protein turnover)
  - Sleeping metabolism
  - Basal metabolism
  - Arousal metabolism — 60–75%

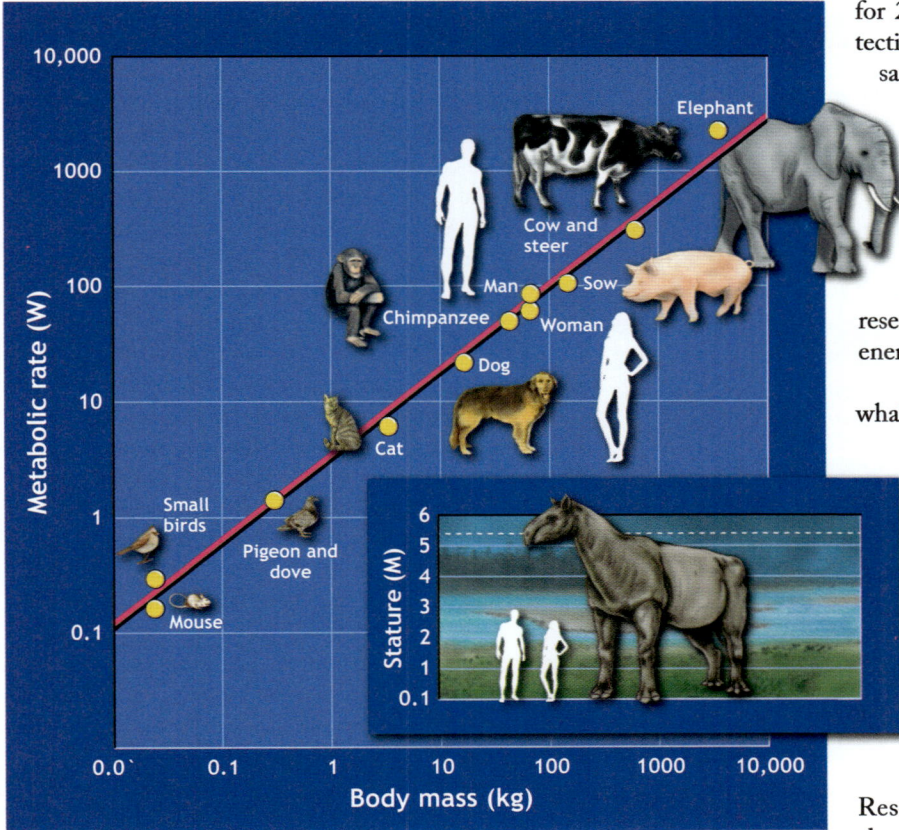

FIGURE 9.1. Metabolic rate expressed in watts from mouse to elephant differing substantially in overall body size (including body volume) and body shape.
(Shutterstock: Evgeniya Chertova; vladmark)

micro-organism (amoeba: mass, 0.1 mg) and 100-ton blue whale (*Balaenoptera musculus*)—or the smallest Gabon dwarf shrew specimen discovered in the Philippines, that weighed 1.4 g and one tenth the size for a small mouse or one millionth the size for an elephant—illustrate the importance that appropriate scaling procedures have when relating oxygen uptake, heart size, and blood volume to body mass.

Marine Mammal Biology—Exercise Physiology

In the emerging field of marine mammal biology–exercise physiology, researchers study the impact of climate change on aquatic animal "exercise physiology" and their ecosystem behaviors. The methodology and equipment to determine respiratory flow rates and resting metabolism are essentially the same equipment found in most exercise physiology laboratories (e.g., pneumotachometer, fast-response breath-by-breath O_2 and CO_2 analyzers, and miniaturized computer data acquisition and respiratory gas sampling systems). Large capture/release bottlenose dolphins (*Tursiops truncatus*) and counterpart aquatic-center–housed dolphins are assessed for metabolic responses in water for 15 to 20 min and on land for 20- to 60-min periods with adequate protection to sustain normal functions during gas sampling procedures. The results for RMR fit nicely on the inset figure's purple line of best fit in Figure 9.1. For example, RMR for a 150-kg/331-lb dolphin averaged 3.9 mL $O_2 \cdot kg^{-1} \cdot min^{-1}$, and the metabolic rate while active ranged from 11.7 to 23.4 mL $O_2 \cdot kg^{-1} \cdot min^{-1}$. The marine studies indicated that RMR represents about 30 to 40% of a dolphin's daily energy requirement.

In more difficult metabolic studies of killer whales, their estimated field metabolic rate (FMR) ranged from 35,048 to 228,216 kcal $\cdot day^{-1}$ for males (465 to 4434 kg/1025 to 9775 lb) and from 35,048 to 184,444 kcal $\cdot day^{-1}$ for females (465 to 3338 kg/1025 to 7359 lb). Contrast this level of energy output with typical TDEE in adult human males and females of about 2000 to 3000 kcal.

Metabolic Size Concept

Research in the 1920s provided solid evidence that the surface area law did not apply universally to all temperature-regulating species or homeotherms. To more fully describe the relationship between metabolic heat production and body size, a newer concept, *metabolic size*, related BMR to body mass raised to the 0.75 power (body mass, $kg^{0.75}$). BMR, often expressed relative to body mass,$^{0.75}$ holds true for humans, mammals, and birds, which differ considerably in size and shape.

Allometric Scaling

Chapter 22 discusses allometric scaling as an alternative mathematical procedure to establish a scientifically defensible relationship between a body-size variable (e.g., stature, body mass, lean body mass, FFM) and other variables, such as muscular strength or aerobic capacity. This allometric "correction" attempts to statistically correct comparisons among individuals or groups that exhibit large differences in body size and avoid simply using a standard ratio by dividing oxygen uptake by a body-size variable, such as body mass.

Further research showed that indexing BMR or RMR to lean body mass (nonadipose tissue) or FFM (nonlipid mass) accounts for gender differences in resting energy metabolism. For an individual or same-sex group, BSA provides as good an index for RMR as does FFM because of the strong within-sex association between BSA and FFM.

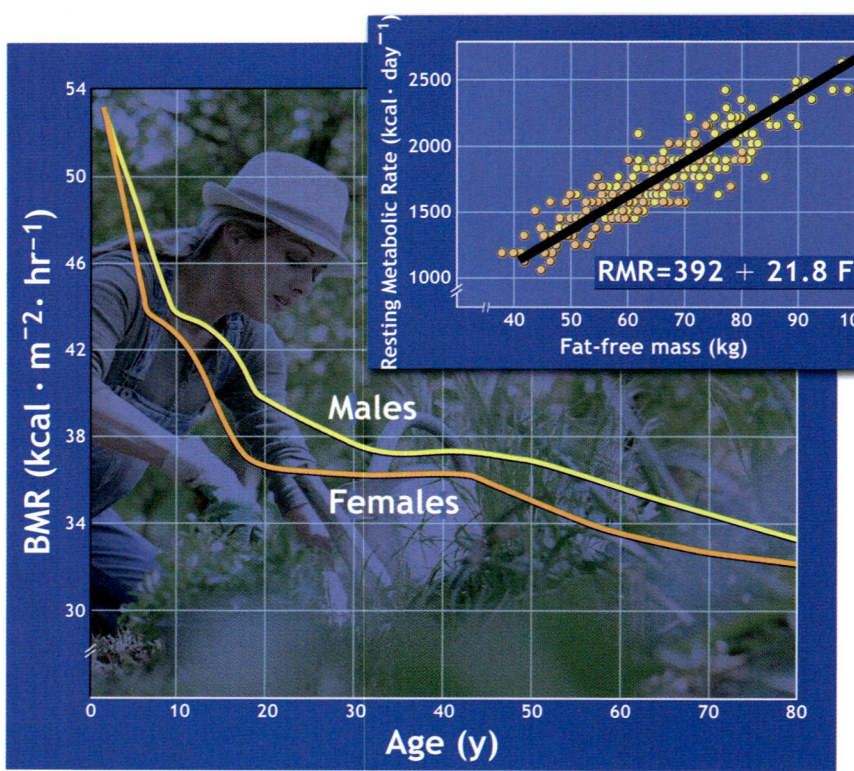

FIGURE 9.2. Basal metabolic rate (BMR) as a function of age and sex.
(goodluz/Shutterstock)

Metabolic Rate: Age and Sex Comparisons

FIGURE 9.2 presents BMR data for males and females of different ages and body weights expressed relative to BSA as $kcal \cdot m^{-2} \cdot hr^{-1}$. An individual's BMR or RMR estimated from the curves generally falls within ±10% of the value obtained during laboratory measurements. The inset figure illustrates the positive "best-fit" relationship between FFM and daily RMR for males (yellow data) and females (orange data). Females exhibit an average 5 to 10% lower rate than do same-age males. This does not necessarily reflect true "gender differences" in metabolic rates of specific tissues. Rather, it results largely because females possess a larger ratio of body fat to FFM than do similar-size males (i.e., fat tissue has lower metabolic activity than muscle). Changes in body composition with aging, either a decrease in FFM or increase in body fat during adulthood, help explain the 2 to 3% per decade BMR reduction observed for adults.[2,7,22] Reduced metabolic activity in lean tissue components also progresses with increasing age,[19] helping to contribute to the age-related increase in body fat, particularly in the trunk/abdominal regions (see Chapter 30).

Physical Activity Effects

Similar BMR measures occur when comparing young and middle-aged endurance-trained men, who exhibited no group difference in FFM.[16] Resting metabolism increased by 8% when 50- to 65-year-old men increased their FFM with resistance training.[23] An 8-wk aerobic training program for older individuals also produced a 10% increase in resting metabolism without any changes in FFM.[20] Apparently, regular physical activity, in addition to body composition, influences factors that increase RMR. *Regular endurance and resistance exercise offsets any decrease in resting metabolism with aging.* For athletes, an added bonus occurs because maintaining FFM during weight reduction counters any potential negative effects of weight loss on physical performance.

Each curve in Figure 9.2 can accurately estimate the average RMR in males (yellow) and females (orange) beginning at about the age of 10 years. For example, for individuals between ages 20 and 40, the BMR averages about 38 $kcal \cdot m^{-2} \cdot hr^{-1}$ for males and 35 $kcal \cdot m^{-2} \cdot hr^{-1}$ for females. To estimate hourly metabolic rate, multiply BMR from the appropriate curve by the calculated BSA (see next section).

Determining BSA

Accurate BSA assessment can pose a considerable challenge. Experiments by German, French, and Japanese scientists in the late 1800s and early 1900s provided data to determine BSA by a simple prediction using only body mass (kg) and stature (cm). In a classic study published 106 years ago,[29] researchers clothed eight males and two females in tight, whole-body underwear and applied melted paraffin and paper strips over their bodies. After removing the treated cloth, it was cut into flat pieces that, when combined, provided a precise measure of the total surface area (length × width). The close relationship between stature, body mass, and BSA culminated in the following empirical formula to predict BSA:

$$BSA, m^2 = 0.20247 \times Stature^{0.725} \times Body\ mass^{0.425}$$

Stature is height in meters (inches × 0.254 converts to meters), and body mass is weight in kilograms (pounds ÷ 2.205 converts to kilograms).

Example: BSA computations for a man 1.778 m/70 in tall who weighs 75 kg/165.3 lb:

$$\begin{aligned} BSA &= 0.20247 \times 1.778^{0.725} \times 75^{0.425} \\ &= 0.20247 \times 1.51775 \times 6.2647 \\ &= 1.925\ m^2 \end{aligned}$$

Using the nomogram in **FIGURE 9.3** to determine BSA produces results similar to the BSA empirical formula. To determine surface area from the nomogram, locate stature on scale I and body mass on scale II. Connect these two points with a straightedge; the intersection on scale III gives the surface area in square meters (m²). Repeat the procedure twice to verify the numbers. For example, if stature equals 185 cm and body mass equals 75 kg, surface area from scale III on the nomogram equals 1.98 m².

BMR Normalcy

It is possible to compare a person's actual BMR by indirect calorimetry to the average or standard BMR for the same age and sex. **FIGURE 9.4** presents standard metabolic rates for different-aged males and females. Use directly determined BMR and then use Figure 9.4 to determine the standard metabolic rate. Compute the percentage difference between actual and standard to determine BMR "normalcy." Any value within ±10% of the standard represents a normal BMR. The following formula computes the deviation expressed as a percentage:

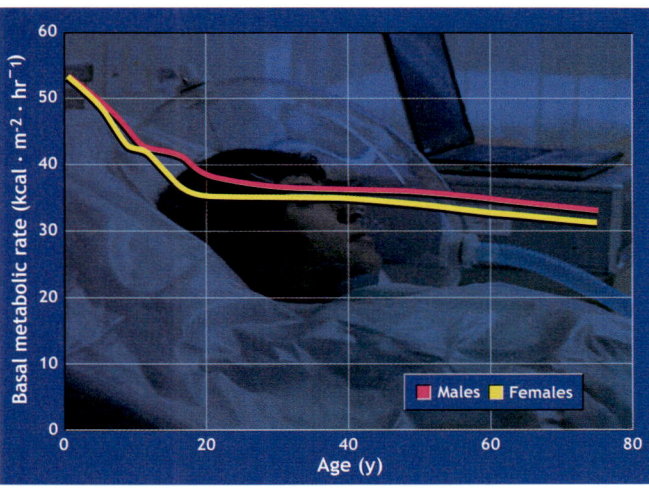

FIGURE 9.4. Standard basal metabolic rates.

$$\Delta BMR = (\text{measured BMR} - \text{standard BMR}) \times 100 \div \text{standard BMR}$$

For example, the measured BMR for a 20-year-old female is 36.5, whereas the standard metabolic rate from Figure 9.4 is 35.3. Thus, this person's BMR falls 3.4% above the standard BMR and is considered within normal range.

$$\Delta BMR = (\text{measured BMR} - \text{standard BMR}) \times 100 \div \text{standard BMR}$$
$$\Delta BMR = (36.5 - 35.3) \times 100 \div 35.3$$
$$\Delta BMR = +3.4\%$$

INTEGRATIVE QUESTION

Why should middle-aged men and women try to maintain or even increase muscle mass for weight control?

Estimating Resting Daily Energy Expenditure

To estimate a person's **resting daily energy expenditure (RDEE)**, multiply his or her BMR value by BSA. For example, for a 50-year-old woman with an estimated BMR of 35.0 kcal · m⁻² · hr⁻¹ (see Fig. 9.4) and with a BSA of 1.40 m², the

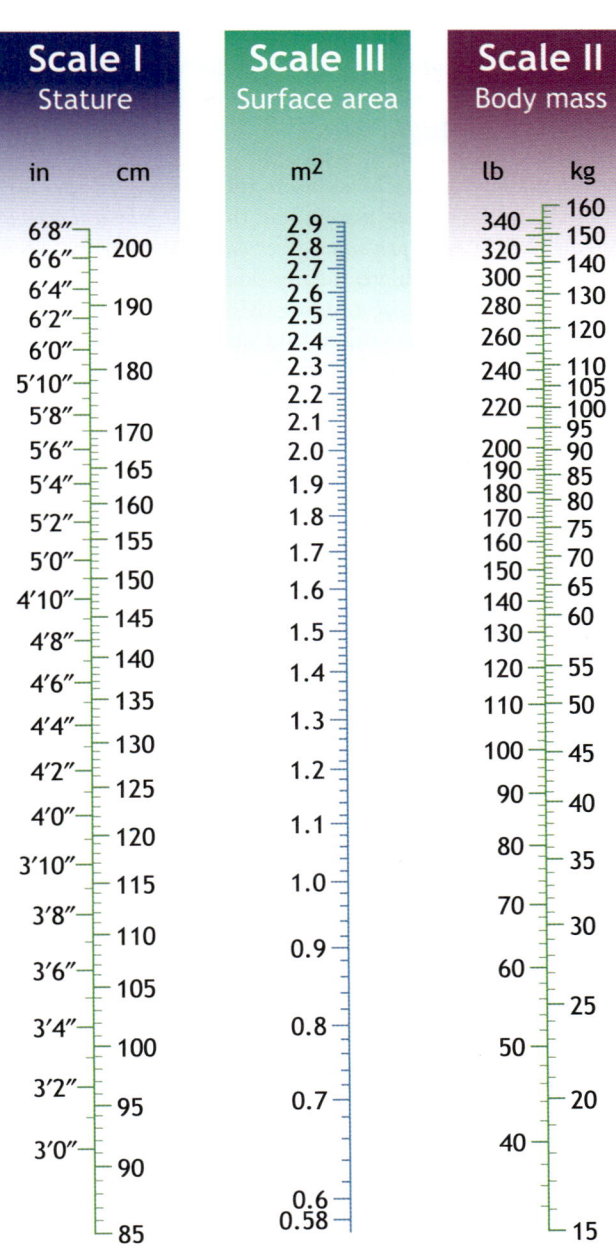

FIGURE 9.3. Nomogram to estimate body surface area from stature and body mass.

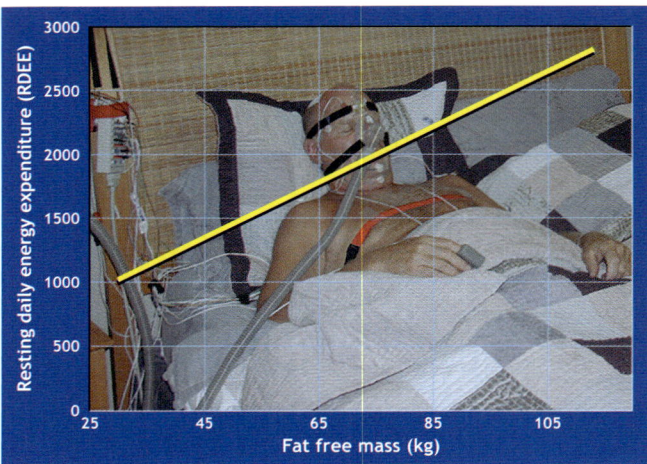

FIGURE 9.5. Resting daily energy expenditure (RDEE; kcal · 24 hr⁻¹) based on fat-free body mass (FFM). (Data from V. Katch. Exercise Physiology Laboratory, University of Michigan. Prediction equation for RDEE derived as the weighted mean constants for males and females from the world literature. To convert kcal to kJ, multiply by 4.18; to convert kcal to MJ, multiply by 0.0042. Image courtesy F. Katch.

hourly energy expenditure equals 49.0 kcal · hr⁻¹ (35.0 kcal × 1.40 m²). On a daily basis, this amounts to a RDEE of 1140 kcal (47.5 kcal · hr⁻¹ × 24 hr).

FIGURE 9.5 provides a prediction of RDEE from FFM estimated from several indirect procedures described in Chapter 28. The data in the table were computed from the following generalized equation, applicable to males and females over a wide body weight range:

$$\text{RDEE (kcal} \cdot 24 \text{ hr}^{-1}) = 370 + 21.6 \times \text{FFM, kg}$$

A male who weighs 90.9 kg at 21% body fat has an estimated FFM of 71.7 kg. Rounding to 72 kg translates to a 1925-kcal or 8047-kJ (8.08-MJ) RDEE.

The table below presents estimates of absolute and relative energy needs, expressed as oxygen uptake in mL · min⁻¹ for various organs and tissues in adults at rest.

Estimates of Absolute and Relative Energy Needs for Various Organs and Tissues in Adults at Rest

Organ	$\dot{V}O_2$ (mL · min⁻¹)	Percentage RMR
Liver	67	27
Brain	47	19
Heart	17	7
Kidneys	26	10
Skeletal muscle	45	18
Remainder	48	19
Total	**250**	**100**

RMR, resting metabolic rate; $\dot{V}O_2$, oxygen uptake.

The brain and skeletal muscles consume about the same total oxygen quantity even though the brain weighs only 1.6 kg (2.3% of body mass), whereas muscle constitutes almost 50% body mass. For children, brain metabolism represents nearly 50% of total resting energy expenditure. This similarity in metabolism does not transfer to maximal exercise because the energy generated by active muscle increases nearly 100 times, whereas brain's total energy requirement increases only marginally.

Five Factors That Affect TDEE

The following five key factors affect TDEE:

1. Physical activity
2. Diet-induced thermogenesis
3. Food's calorigenic effect on exercise metabolism
4. Climate
5. Pregnancy

Physical Activity

Physical activity generally accounts for between 15 and 30% of TDEE. As we discuss throughout this text, *physical activity exerts by far the most profound effect on human energy expenditure*. World-class athletes nearly double their TDEE with 3 or 4 hr of daily intense training. Most persons can sustain metabolic rates 10 times the resting value in continuous "big-muscle" activities such as fast walking, running, uphill hiking, bicycling, and swimming.

Diet-Induced Thermogenesis

Food consumption generally increases energy metabolism. **Diet-induced thermogenesis (DIT**; sometimes referred to as thermic effect of food) consists of two components. **Obligatory thermogenesis** (formerly called specific dynamic action) results from energy required to digest, absorb, and assimilate food nutrients. **Facultative thermogenesis** relates to sympathetic nervous system activation and its stimulating influence on metabolic rate.

The influential German nutritional physiologist Max Rubner (1854–1932; www.mri.bund.de/en/about-us/max-rubner/) in 1891 used indirect calorimetry to experiment with DIT. His research established a 24-hr, 742 kcal energy expenditure for a fasting dog.[13] Rubner then fed the dog 2 kg (1926 kcal) of meat. Food consumption increased the dog's daily energy expenditure to 1046 kcal. Rubner attributed the 304-kcal (41%) increase to the "glands chemical work metabolizing absorbed nutrients" or the "work of digestion." The increased metabolism represented 16% of the dog's total energy ingested. Numerous subsequent experiments showed that the following five factors differentially affected DIT magnitude:

1. Meal size
2. Macronutrient composition
3. Time since prior meal
4. Nutritional status
5. Health status

Regular Physical Activity in Older Adults Positively Impacts Brain Structure and Function

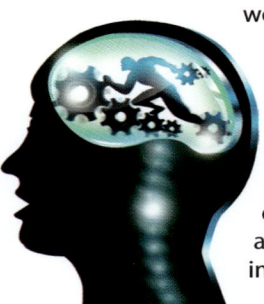

Crystal Eye Studio/Shutterstock

By 2050, the projected number of adults older than age 60 will rise to more than two billion, reaching 21% of the world's population. Regular physical activity has emerged as a low-cost, nonpharmacological treatment to slow the age-related cognitive decline progression that includes loss in information processing speed, loss of memory and executive function, brain atrophy, and decreased brain function in the prefrontal and temporal cortices and hippocampus. Systematic exercise training improves cognitive functioning in community-dwelling healthy older adults. A meta-analyses review identified 24 randomized control trial empirical studies that assessed relationships among specific exercise training characteristics—frequency, intensity, time, type, volume, and progression—and brain structure and function judged by magnetic resonance imaging (MRI) and functional MRI techniques. Most studies reported that the following exercise variables positively affect brain function: vigorous intensity aerobic ($\geq$45 min · d^{-1}) and/or resistance exercise (70 to 90% of maximum heart rate) and increased exercise duration and frequency ($\geq$3 d · wk^{-1}). Data on exercise volume and exercise training progression were unremarkable. Despite a wealth of evidence demonstrating that exercise interventions benefit functional brain outcomes, the dose-response relationship was not straightforward and requires further, insightful research strategies.

Source:
Belcher BR, et al. The roles of physical activity, exercise, and fitness in promoting resilience during adolescence: effects on mental well-being and brain development. *Biol Psychiatry Cogn Neurosci Neuroimaging*. 2021;6:2256.

Food's thermic effect generally reaches maximum within 1 hr following a meal. Considerable variability exists among individuals. DIT magnitude usually varies between 10 and 30% depending on food quantity and type consumed. A pure protein meal, for example, would elicit a thermic effect nearly 25% of the meal's total caloric value. This large thermic effect results largely from activation of digestive processes. It also includes extra energy required by the liver to assimilate and synthesize protein and/or deaminate amino acids for conversion to glucose or triacylglycerols.

Overweight individuals often have a blunted thermic response to eating that contributes to excess body fat accumulation.[24,25] DIT's magnitude also may be lower in endurance-trained individuals than untrained counterparts.[11,21,27] Any "training effect" probably reflects a calorie-sparing adaptation to conserve energy and glycogen during increased physical activity. Energy conservation in any form seems counterproductive to the goal of increasing energy output as a weight control strategy. For the physically active person, however, DIT represents only a small portion of TDEE compared with energy expenditure through regular physical activity.

Food's Calorigenic Effect on Exercise Metabolism

DIT has been compared for resting and exercising subjects after consuming meals of identical macronutrient composition and caloric content. In one study, six men performed moderate physical activity on a bicycle ergometer before breakfast on one day; then on separate days, they performed exercise for 30 min after a breakfast containing 350, 1000, or 3000 kcal.[3] Three results emerged:

1. Breakfast increased resting metabolism by 10%.
2. Variations in the meal's caloric value exerted no influence on the thermic effect.
3. Performing physical activity following a 1000- or 3000-kcal meal produced a larger energy expenditure than exercise without prior food.

Food's calorigenic effect on energy metabolism during physical activity nearly doubled the food's resting thermic effect. Apparently, physical activity increases DIT. This agrees with previous findings in which the thermic response to a 1000-kcal meal averaged 28% of the basal requirement at rest, yet increased to 56% when subjects exercised following a meal.[17] The DIT for carbohydrate and protein exceeded that for lipid. As with rest, some obese men and women exhibit a depressed DIT when they exercise after eating. For most individuals, however, it seems reasonable to encourage moderate physical activity following a meal to increase a diet-induced caloric expenditure.

Climate

Environmental factors influence RMR, as the resting metabolism for people living and working in a tropical climate averages 5 to 20% higher than that for counterparts living in more temperate areas. Physical activity performed in hot weather also imposes a small additional metabolic load. It causes an oxygen uptake of about 5% higher than that in a thermoneutral environment, probably from the thermogenic effect of an elevated core temperature *per se*. This would include additional energy required for greater sweat gland activity and enhanced circulatory dynamics related to performing work in the heat.

Cold environments generally increase energy metabolism during rest and physical activity, depending largely on

In a Practical Sense

Harris-Benedict Equations to Estimate Basal Metabolic Rate from Body Mass, Stature, and Age

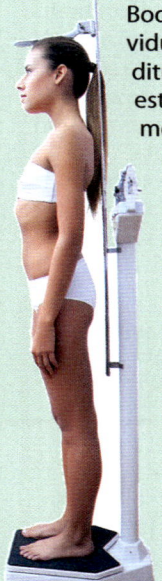

Ambrophoto/Shutterstock

Body mass, stature, and age contribute to individual differences in resting daily energy expenditure (RDEE), making it possible to accurately estimate RDEE using these variables. The original method first published in 1919 by Drs. Jay Arthur Harris and Francis G. Benedict (www.ncbi.nlm.nih.gov/pmc/articles/PMC1091498/) used closed-circuit spirometry to carefully measure oxygen uptake in individuals who varied widely in body size and age. Their original study measured 136 males, 103 females, and 94 newborns. Subsequent revisions have updated the original Harris-Benedict equation to slightly improve prediction accuracy, but the original formula still remains the most-used method in clinical practice, applied calorimetry, and hospital settings. The authors correctly surmised their approach could also be applied in future studies when comparing athletes and nonathletes, and in individuals with disease.

ORIGINAL HARRIS-BENEDICT EQUATIONS FOR PREDICTING BASAL METABOLIC RATE

Women

$$RDEE\ (kcal \cdot 24\ hr^{-1}) = 9.563 \times BM + 1.8496 \times HT - 4.6756 \times age + 655.0955$$

where BM = body mass in kg; HT = stature in cm; and age = years.

Men

$$RDEE\ (kcal \cdot 24\ hr^{-1}) = 13.7516 \times BM + 5.0033 \times HT - 6.7550 \times age + 66.4730$$

where BM = body mass in kg; HT = stature in cm; and age = years.

Example: Woman

Data: Body mass = 62.7 kg; stature = 172.5 cm; age = 22.4 years

$$RDEE\ (kcal \cdot 24\ hr^{-1}) = 9.563 \times BM + 1.8496 \times HT - 4.6756 \times age + 655.0955$$

$$RDEE\ (kcal \cdot 24\ hr^{-1}) = 9.563 \times 62.7 + 1.8496 \times 172.5 - 4.6756 \times 22.4 + 655.0955$$

$$RDEE\ (kcal \cdot 24\ hr^{-1}) = 599.600 + 319.056 - 104.7334 + 655.0955$$

$$RDEE\ (kcal \cdot 24\ hr^{-1}) = 1469$$

Example: Man

Data: Body mass, 80 kg; Stature, 189.0 cm; Age, 30 years

$$RDEE\ (kcal \cdot 24\ hr^{-1}) = 13.7516 \times BM + 5.0033 \times HT - 6.7550 \times age + 66.4730$$

$$RDEE\ (kcal \cdot 24\ hr^{-1}) = 13.7516 \times 80 + 5.0033 \times 189.0 - 6.7550 \times 30 + 66.4730$$

$$RDEE\ (kcal \cdot 24\ hr^{-1}) = 1100.128 + 945.623 - 202.65 + 66.473$$

$$RDEE\ (kcal \cdot 24\ hr^{-1}) = 1910$$

REVISED HARRIS-BENEDICT EQUATION

In 1984, the original Harris-Benedict equations were revised using new data. In comparisons with actual energy expenditure, the revised equations were slightly more accurate, particularly when applied to the obese.

Women

$$RDEE\ (kcal \cdot 24\ hr^{-1}) = 9.247 \times BM + 3.098 \times HT - 4.330 \times age + 447.593$$

where BM = body mass in kg; HT = stature in cm; and age = years.

Men

$$RDEE\ (kcal \cdot 24\ hr^{-1}) = 13.397 \times BM + 4.799 \times HT - 5.677 \times age + 88.362$$

where BM = body mass in kg; HT = stature in cm; and age = years.

Sources:
Harris JA, Benedict FG. *A Biometric Study of Basal Metabolism in Man.* Publ. No. 279. Washington, DC: Carnegie Institute; 1919.
Roza AM, Shizgal HM. The Harris Benedict equation reevaluated: resting energy requirements and the body cell mass. *Amer J Clin Nutr* 1984;40:168.
Müller B, et al. Calculating the basal metabolic rate and severe and morbid obesity. *Praxis* (Bern 1994). 2001;90:1955. [Article in German].

In a Practical Sense

Predicting Maximum Oxygen Uptake During Pregnancy from Submaximum Exercise Heart Rate and Oxygen Uptake

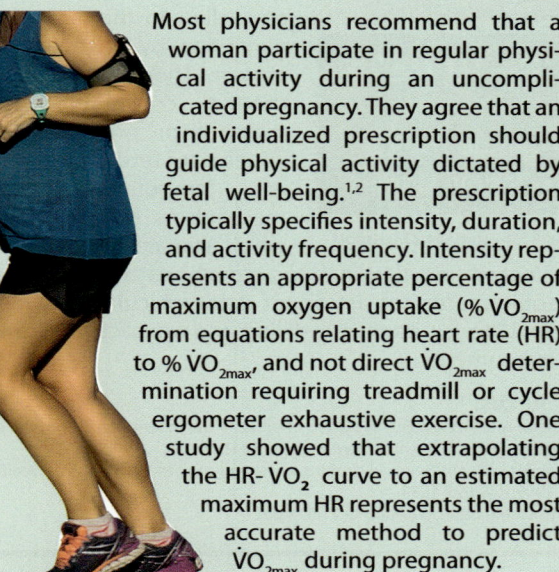

CHURN/Shutterstock

Most physicians recommend that a woman participate in regular physical activity during an uncomplicated pregnancy. They agree that an individualized prescription should guide physical activity dictated by fetal well-being.[1,2] The prescription typically specifies intensity, duration, and activity frequency. Intensity represents an appropriate percentage of maximum oxygen uptake (% $\dot{V}O_{2max}$) from equations relating heart rate (HR) to % $\dot{V}O_{2max}$, and not direct $\dot{V}O_{2max}$ determination requiring treadmill or cycle ergometer exhaustive exercise. One study showed that extrapolating the HR-$\dot{V}O_2$ curve to an estimated maximum HR represents the most accurate method to predict $\dot{V}O_{2max}$ during pregnancy.

PREDICTING $\dot{V}O_{2max}$ FROM SUBMAXIMUM EXERCISE

Predicting $\dot{V}O_{2max}$ during pregnancy involves a three-stage, submaximum cycle ergometer test. The $\dot{V}O_2$ and HR, measured toward the end of the final exercise stage, predict $\dot{V}O_{2max}$ via regression analyses.

SUBMAXIMUM CYCLE ERGOMETER TEST

Procedure: Subject rests for 10 min and then performs a continuous three-stage, 6-min/stage cycle ergometer test as follows:

1. *Stage 1:* 0 watts (W; unloaded cycling)
2. *Stage 2:* 30 W (184 kg-m · min^{-1})
3. *Stage 3:* 60 W (367 kg-m · min^{-1})

PREDICTION EQUATIONS

Measure $\dot{V}O_2$ (L · min^{-1}) and HR (b · min^{-1}) for each of the last 3 min during the final exercise stage. Average the three HR values to predict % $\dot{V}O_{2max}$ as follows:

$$\text{Predicted \% } \dot{V}O_{2max} = 0.634 \times \text{HR (b·min}^{-1}) - 30.79$$

Use the predicted $\dot{V}O_{2max}$ and measured $\dot{V}O_2$ (L · min^{-1}) during the last exercise stage to predict $\dot{V}O_{2max}$ (L · min^{-1}) in the following equation:

$$\text{Predicted } \dot{V}O_{2max} = \dot{V}O_2 \div \text{predicted \% } \dot{V}O_{2max} \times 100$$

EXAMPLE

A woman 20 wk pregnant weighing 70.4 kg performs the three-stage cycle ergometer test. Final-stage HR equals 155 b · min^{-1} and $\dot{V}O_2$ equals 1.80 L · min^{-1}.

$$\text{Predicted \% } \dot{V}O_{2max} = (0.634 \times \text{HR [b·min}^{-1}]) - 30.79$$
$$= 67.5\%$$

$$\text{Predicted } \dot{V}O_{2max} = \dot{V}O_2 \div \text{predicted \% } \dot{V}O_{2max} \times 100$$
$$= 1.80 \div 67.5 \times 100$$
$$= 2.67 \text{ L·min}^{-1} \text{ (2670 mL·min}^{-1})$$
$$= 2670 \text{ mL·min}^{-1} \div 70.4 \text{ kg}$$
$$= 37.9 \text{ mL·kg}^{-1}\text{·min}^{-1}$$

Sources:
Goli P, et al, Kelishadi R. Intergenerational influence of paternal physical activity on the offspring's brain: a systematic review and meta-analysis. *Int J Dev Neurosci.* 2021;81:10.
Haakstad LAH, et al. Pregnancy and advanced maternal age. The associations between regular exercise and maternal and newborn health variables. *Acta Obstet Gynecol Scand.* 2020;99:240.
Sady SP, et al. Prediction of $\dot{V}O_{2max}$ during cycle exercise in pregnant women. *J Appl Physiol.* 1988;65:657.

---

the individual's body fat content and clothing's effectiveness to retain body heat. Metabolic rate increases in extreme cold water up to fivefold at rest because shivering generates additional body heat in an attempt to maintain a stable core temperature.[26]

Pregnancy

One area of interest concerns the degree that pregnancy affects the metabolic cost and physiologic strain imposed by physical activity.[4] One investigation studied 13 women from the 6th month to 6 wk after gestation.[9] Physiologic measures taken every 4 wk included heart rate and oxygen uptake during bicycle and treadmill exercise. Heart rate and oxygen uptake during weight-bearing walking at constant speed on a level grade increased progressively during the measurement period but remained unchanged during bicycle riding at a constant intensity. The added energy cost to weight-bearing locomotion during walking, jogging, and stair climbing during pregnancy results *primarily* from the additional weight transported, with a relatively small contribution from the developing fetus *per se*. Chapter 21 fully discusses the physiologic and metabolic impact of physical activity on the mother and fetus during pregnancy.

Origin of the Term MET

In the early 1900s, researchers began to study varied exercise protocol effectiveness on human physiologic responses to hot and cold environmental stressors. Wearing efficient clothing to withstand extreme environmental stressors remains the basic need in cold environments. One concern was how to balance thermal clothing qualities with metabolic heat production at rest and during increasing exercise intensities. One strategy defined clothing's thermal characteristics to provide optimal protection from the cold to maintain a stable thermal equilibrium or central core body temperature. Seventy years ago, three environmental physiologists—Drs. A. Pharo Gagge (1908–1993) from Yale University (John B. Pierce Foundation Laboratory; http://jbpierce.org/research/), Alan Burton from the University of Toronto, and H.C. Bazett, MD from the University of Pennsylvania—first proposed a practical measurement system to describe heat exchange applicable to persons of varying body sizes and shapes. The researchers were first to coin the term *MET* to indicate a heat unit to represent a thermal metabolic heat constant to maintain body temperature. One **metabolic equivalent (MET)** to maintain body heat varied depending on body size. In this system, 1 MET serves as the baseline equivalent to the heat (or energy) generated by an average person at rest. Their empirically derived thermal constants for energy metabolism provided the early impetus for future experimentation in temperature regulation mechanisms and clothing design, which ultimately produced thermally balanced suits designed to accommodate the clothing design requirements for astronaut extravehicular activities, polar expeditions, underwater diving, and work activities in industrial environments.

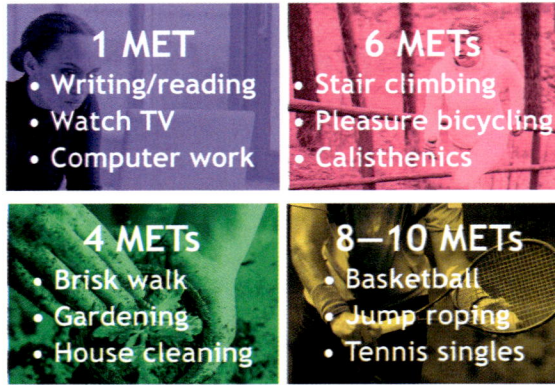

Shutterstock: Jacob Lund; Kaspars Grinvalds; Shyntartanya; Maxisport

Sources:
Gagge AP, et al. A practical system of units for the description of the heat exchange of man with his environment. *Science.* 1941;94:428.
Holmér I. Recent trends in clothing physiology. *Scand J Work Environ Health.* 1989;15(Suppl 1):58.
https://oig.nasa.gov/docs/IG-21-025.pdf.

Summary

1. TDEE equals the sum of resting metabolism, thermogenic effects of food and environmental influences, and energy generated in physical activity.
2. The BMR represents the minimum energy required to maintain vital functions in the waking state measured under controlled laboratory conditions. The BMR averages only slightly lower than the RMR and relates closely to BSA.
3. RMR and BMR both decrease with age from variations in FFM. The RMR for males generally exceeds values for females of similar body size. One can accurately predict RMR from FFM in males and females who vary considerably in body size.
4. Different organs expend energy in differing amounts during rest and physical activity. At rest, muscle contributes about 20% to the body's total energy expenditure. During all-out sustained physical effort, active muscles can increase their expenditure to more than 100 times above rest, which accounts for nearly 85% of the total energy expenditure.
5. Five major factors affect exercise metabolism: physical activity, DIT, food's calorigenic effect, climate, and pregnancy, with physical activity exerting the greatest effect.

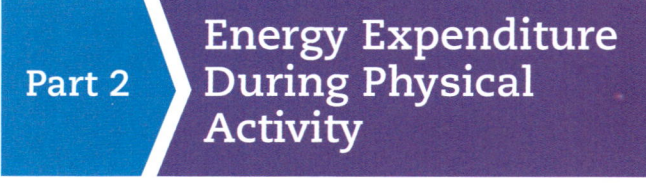

Part 2 — Energy Expenditure During Physical Activity

Energy Expenditure Classification for Physical Activities

Most individuals have performed physical activity they would classify as "exceedingly difficult." This might include walking up a long flight of stairs, shoveling snow for 60 min, sprinting a long block to catch a bus, digging a deep trench, skiing or snowshoeing through a blizzard, or hiking up steep terrain. *Two important factors, exercise intensity and duration, impact the relative strenuousness* of a particular *task*. One person might expend considerable energy running at maximum steady-rate pace (e.g., 80% $\dot{V}O_{2max}$) and complete the distance in a little more than 2 hr. Another equally fit runner might select a slower, more comfortable pace (e.g., 55% $\dot{V}O_{2max}$) and complete the run in 3 hr. In this example, the intensity of effort distinguishes the task's physical demands. In another example, two persons of equal fitness may run at the same speed, but one person runs for twice as long as the other. In this case, exercise duration becomes key to classify strenuousness.

Several classification systems differ in how they categorize physical activity exertion levels from light to maximum. One system recommends intensity classification by the ratio of the activity's energy requirement to the resting energy requirement.[1] This system, called the **physical activity ratio (PAR)**, classifies three activity levels:

1. *Light work* elicits an oxygen uptake (i.e., energy expenditure) up to three times the resting requirement.
2. *Heavy work* encompasses physical activity requiring six to eight times resting metabolism.
3. *Maximal work* includes tasks requiring energy expenditure increases from nine times or more above resting metabolism.

As a frame of reference, most industrial jobs and household tasks require *less* than three times resting energy expenditure. These work classifications rated in multiples of resting metabolism average slightly lower for women because of their generally lower aerobic capacity. Work classification based on the PAR model rates occupational task strenuousness at a lower level than typical general exercise classifications. This is because the time devoted to occupational and industrial tasks typically extends for much longer durations than routine exercise training; they often require smaller muscle mass involvement performed under stressful environmental conditions and physical constraints.

Converting METs to Calories

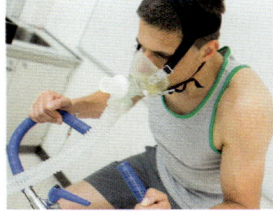
wavebreakmedia/Shutterstock

Conversion from MET to kcal · min^{-1} requires body weight with the following conversion: **1 MET = 1.0 kcal · kg^{-1} · h^{-1}**. For example, if a person weighing 70 kg bicycles at 10 mph (listed as a 10-MET activity), the corresponding kcal expenditure value = 11.7 kcal · min^{-1}:

10.0 METs = 10.0 kcal·kg^{-1}·hr^{-1} × 70 kg ÷ 60 min
= 700 kcal ÷ 60 min
= 11.7 kcal·min^{-1}

The MET

TABLE 9.1 presents a five-level classification system based on the energy expressed in kcal required by untrained males and females who perform different physical activities including a broad range of occupational tasks.[6] The early energy expenditure experiments showed that 5-kcal energy output approximated 1 L oxygen uptake, thus enabling transposition of these calorie values into liters of oxygen uptake per minute (L · min^{-1}) or milliliters of oxygen per kilogram of body mass per minute (mL · kg^{-1} · min^{-1}) or METs, a *multiple of RMR*. One MET is equivalent to 250 mL · min^{-1} resting oxygen uptake for an average-sized man and 200 mL · min^{-1} for an average-sized woman. Hence, physical activity performed at a 2-MET level requires twice the resting metabolism or about 500 mL · min^{-1}, and 3 METs equal three times rest, and so on. For a different but usually more accurate classification that considers variations in body size, one should express the MET as oxygen uptake per unit body mass: *1 MET equals 3.5 mL · kg^{-1} · min^{-1}; 2 METs equal 7.0 · mL · kg^{-1} · min^{-1}, 3 METs equal 10.5 mL · kg^{-1} · min^{-1}, while 10 METs would equal 35.0 mL · kg^{-1} · min^{-1}.*

> **TABLE 9.1** Five-level physical activity classification based on energy expenditure

TABLE 9.2 presents a classification system to characterize leisure-time physical activity intensity in absolute (METs) and relative ($\%\dot{V}O_{2max}$) intensity by age categories. To account for the general aging effect on aerobic capacity, the categories for activity intensity in METs adjust lower with increasing age.

> **TABLE 9.2** Leisure-time physical activity energy expenditure expressed in Metabolic equivalents and percentage maximum oxygen uptake

Average Daily Energy Expenditure Rates

TABLE 9.3 presents averages for daily energy expenditure for males and females living in the United States for ages ranging from 15 to 50+ years. The average male aged 15 to 50 years expends about 2900 kcal daily, whereas the average female expends about 24% less, or 2200 kcal daily. On average, most individuals spend nearly 75% of their day in activities that require only light energy expenditure (e.g., 8 hr sleeping/lying down, 6 hr sitting and standing, 2 hr walking, 2 hr recreational activities). For most individuals, energy expenditure rarely rises substantially above the resting level, with walking the most common physical activity. The term *Homo-sedentarius* all too appropriately describes most of the world's population! This compelling descriptor reinforces that physical *inactivity* in highly mechanized societies has become the equivalent of a medical disease despite the admonitions of scientists, physicians, educators, and governmental agencies to cure this condition or at least reverse the trend. The Centers for Disease Control and Prevention (www.cdc.gov) estimates that physical inactivity and poor eating habits in the United States account for about 360,000 deaths yearly, and probably more in the 2020 decade. Such estimates are unavailable for other industrialized countries.

> **TABLE 9.3** Daily energy expenditure by gender and age

Energy Cost of Household, Industrial, and Recreational Activities

Appendix F lists energy expenditure expressed by body mass (kcal · kg^{-1}) for common household activities, selected industrial tasks, and popular recreational and sports activities. These data highlight the large variation in energy expenditure for diverse physical activities as lawn bowling and kite flying. The caloric values also represent averages, with values for an individual varying considerably depending on skill, pace, and fitness level.

Lippincott® Connect Appendix F, available on Lippincott Connect, provides examples of energy expenditure in household, occupational, recreational, and sports activities.

The values listed in the column for body mass represent the activity's caloric expenditure for 1 min. This equals the gross energy value because it includes the energy expenditure of rest for an equivalent 1-min interval (see Chapter 10). To estimate total expenditure for an activity, multiply the caloric value in the table by minutes of participation. For example, if a 70-kg man spends 30 min vacuuming (carpet sweeping), the total energy expenditure for this household task would equal 102 kcal (3.4 kcal × 30 min). The same individual would expend approximately 690 kcal during a 50-min judo workout, but only 90 kcal while sitting quietly watching television for 2 hr. Golf (without a cart) requires about 6.0 kcal each minute or 360 kcal · hr^{-1}. The same person expends 708 kcal · hr^{-1} swimming backstroke. Viewed somewhat differently, 25 min of swimming backstroke requires about the same calorie expenditure as playing golf for 1 hr. Increasing the pace of either the swim or golf game proportionally increases the energy expenditure.

Photo courtesy V. Katch

Body Mass Influence

Increases in body mass raise the energy expenditure during physical activity (see Appendix F), particularly in **weight-bearing activity** such as walking and running. **FIGURE 9.6** demonstrates that energy cost of walking increases proportionately to body mass (i.e., larger body mass requires greater energy expenditure). For persons with the same body mass, surprisingly few practical variations are evident in oxygen uptake, allowing body mass to accurately predict the energy expended in walking.

The influence of body mass on energy metabolism during weight-bearing activity occurs whether the person gains weight naturally as body fat or FFM, or as a short-term added

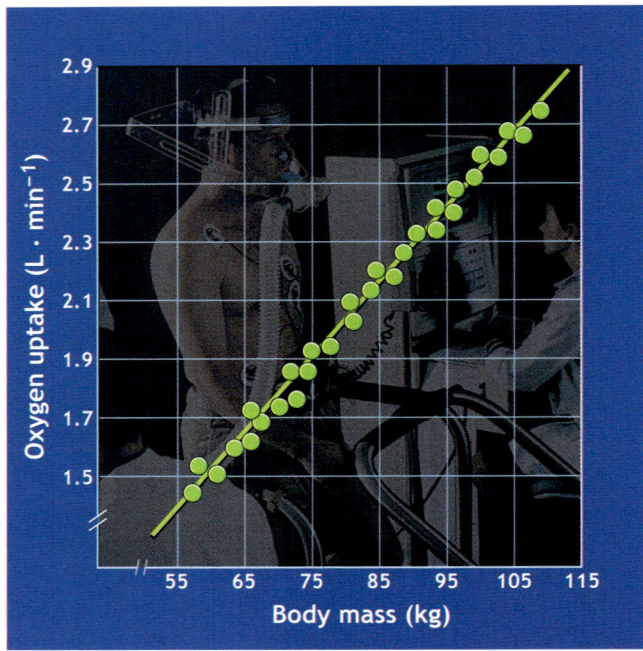

FIGURE 9.6. Relationship between body mass and oxygen uptake measured during submaximal, brisk treadmill walking.

load from sports equipment or a weighted torso vest.[5,28] With **weight-supported activity** (e.g., stationary cycling or elliptical exercise), the body mass influence on energy cost decreases considerably. It averages only about 5% higher in stationary cycling among heavy people because of extra energy required to lift the heavier lower limbs.[10,12] The body weight effect during stationary cycling slightly lowers energy cost values for females compared with males. For overweight persons, non–weight-supported physical activity for weight loss generates additional caloric expenditure from transporting a heavier body weight.

Appendix F shows that the energy expended for cross-country running ranges between 8.2 kcal · min^{-1} for a 50-kg person and 16.0 kcal · min^{-1} for a person who weighs 98 kg. Expressing the energy requirement by body mass as kcal · kg^{-1} · min^{-1} attempts to eliminate this variation. In this case, energy cost averages about 0.164 kcal · kg^{-1} · min^{-1}. Expressing energy cost per kilogram of body mass (kcal · kg^{-1} · min^{-1}) reduces differences among individuals independent of age, race, and sex. Nevertheless, a heavier person still expends more *total* calories than a lighter person for an equivalent exercise because the activity mainly requires transporting body mass—and this requires proportionately greater energy output.

Heart Rate to Estimate Energy Expenditure

For each person, heart rate and oxygen uptake relate linearly during exercise up to about 80% maximum intensity. This intrinsic relationship allows for heart rate to estimate oxygen uptake and thus energy expenditure during most steady-rate aerobic activities. This approach has proven useful when oxygen uptake could not be measured during the desired activity.

FIGURE 9.7 presents data for two members of a women's basketball team during a laboratory treadmill running test. For each woman, heart rate increased linearly with oxygen uptake—a proportionate increase in heart rate (HR) accompanied each increase in oxygen uptake ($\dot{V}O_2$). Both HR-$\dot{V}O_2$ lines display linearity, but the same heart rate does not correspond to the same oxygen uptake for both women because each has a different rate of change or slope. Heart rate for subject B increases less than does that for subject A for each increase in oxygen uptake (see Chapters 11, 17, 21). For the current discussion, exercise heart rate estimates exercise oxygen uptake with reasonable accuracy. For player A, a 140 b · min^{-1} heart rate corresponds to a 1.08 L · min^{-1} oxygen uptake, whereas the same heart rate for player B corresponds to a 1.60 L · min^{-1} oxygen uptake. Heart rate by radiotelemetry during basketball competition was then applied to each player's HR-$\dot{V}O_2$ line to estimate energy expenditure under game conditions.[15]

Heart rate to estimate energy expenditure appears practical but has limited research or "real-life" applications because it has been validated for only a few general, large muscle activities. One major problem concerns the similarity between the laboratory test to establish the HR-$\dot{V}O_2$ line and specific activities to which it applies. For example, the following seven factors other than oxygen uptake influence exercise heart rate response:

1. Environmental temperature
2. Emotions
3. Previous food intake
4. Body position
5. Muscle groups exercised
6. Continuous or discontinuous (stop-and-go) activity
7. Static or dynamic muscle actions

In aerobic dance, for example, heart rate while dancing at a specific oxygen uptake exceeds the heart rate at the same oxygen uptake during treadmill walking or running.[18] Consistently higher heart rates occur in upper-body physical activity; they also are higher when muscles act statically in straining-type movements than in dynamic movements at any submaximal oxygen uptake. Applying heart rate during upper-body or static-type activity to a HR-$\dot{V}O_2$ line developed during lower-body dynamic running or cycling overpredicts the measured oxygen uptake.[14]

INTEGRATIVE QUESTION

A high-tech computer company asks you to validate a wrist-mounted device to measure energy expenditure. The person exhales one breath onto the top of the device while moving. The device's electronic components and microprocessor analyze expired air to compute oxygen uptake and energy expenditure. What are the steps to establish the instrument's validity?

Summary

1. Different classification systems rate physical activity strenuousness.
2. The ratio of the activity energy cost to the resting energy requirement, oxygen uptake expressed in mL · kg^{-1} · min^{-1}, and METs the strenuousness of physical activity.
3. TDEE for those ages 19 to 50 years averages 2900 kcal for males and 2200 kcal for females.
4. Variations in physical activity make the largest contribution to disparities among individuals in TDEE.
5. Daily energy expenditure provides a framework to classify different occupations. Within any classification, energy expended during leisure-time recreational pursuits contributes additional variability.
6. Heavier individuals expend more total energy than lighter counterparts in weight-bearing walking, climbing, and running activities than in weight-supported activities (stationary cycling, elliptical exercise).
7. For most physical activities, heart rate offers only limited practical benefit to predict oxygen uptake and caloric expenditure.

Key Terms

Anabolism: Synthesizing complex molecules in living organisms from simpler ones with energy storage; requires energy

Basal metabolic rate (BMR): Energy expenditure rate at rest in a thermoneutral environment in the postabsorptive state expressed in kilocalories per meter squared per hour (kcal · m^{-2} · hr^{-1})

Catabolism: Complex molecule's breakdown with energy release

Diet-induced thermogenesis (DIT): Increased metabolism from energy-requiring processes to digest, absorb, and assimilate food nutrients; also known as food's thermic effect

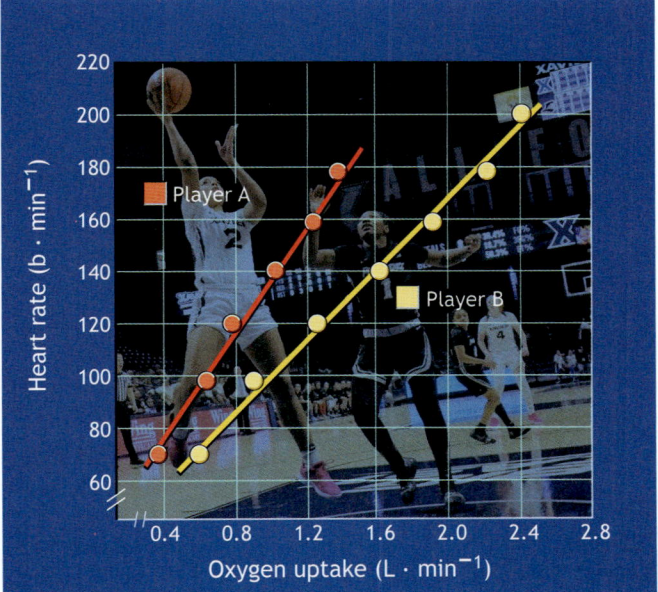

FIGURE 9.7. Linear relationship between heart rate and oxygen uptake for two female collegiate basketball players of different aerobic fitness levels. Measurements made during a graded exercise test on a motor-driven treadmill.
(Jason Whitman/Shutterstock)

Facultative thermogenesis: Sympathetic nervous system activation by food ingestion stimulating the metabolic rate

Metabolic equivalent (MET): Unit to express activity intensity relative to resting energy expenditure where 1 MET = adult's average seated resting VO_2 or energy expenditure, about 250 mL $O_2 \cdot min^{-1}$, 3.5 mL $O_2 \cdot kg^{-1} min^{-1}$, 1 kcal $\cdot kg^{-1} \cdot hr^{-1}$, or 0.017 kcal $\cdot kg^{-1} \cdot min^{-1}$ (1 kcal $\cdot kg^{-1} \cdot hr^{-1} \div 60$ min = 0.017)

Metabolic size: An Animal's basal metabolic rate proportional to the animal's body surface area raised to the 0.75 power (body mass, $kg^{0.75}$)

Obligatory thermogenesis: Energy required to digest, absorb, and assimilate food nutrients formerly known as specific dynamic action

Physical activity ratio (PAR): System to rate physical activity's "strenuousness" expressed in resting metabolism multiples for light, heavy, and maximum work

Resting daily energy expenditure (RDEE): Energy expenditure for 24 hr during resting conditions expressed in kcal

Resting metabolic rate (RMR): Energy expenditure measured 3 to 4 hr following a light meal without physical activity

Total daily energy expenditure (TDEE): Total calories expended in 24 hr

Weight-bearing activity: Any activity that relies on body weight to support movement (walking, jogging, running, climbing)

Weight-supported activity: Any activity that supports body weight during external movement (cycling, swimming)

References are available online at Lippincott Connect.

Additional References

Abou Ghayda R, et al. Body mass index and mortality in patients with cardiovascular disease: an umbrella review of meta-analyses. *Eur Rev Med Pharmacol Sci.* 2021;25:273.

Bartke A, et al. Energy metabolism and aging. *World J Mens Health.* 2021;39:222.

Bendavid I, et al. The centenary of the Harris-Benedict equations: how to assess energy requirements best? Recommendations from the ESPEN expert group. *Clin Nutr.* 2021;40:690.

Bi X, Forde CG, Goh AT, Henry CJ. Basal metabolic rate and body composition predict habitual food and macronutrient intakes: gender differences. *Nutrients.* 2019;11.

Bosy-Westphal A, et al. What is the impact of energy expenditure on energy intake? *Nutrients.* 2021;13:3508

Calcagno M, et al. The thermic effect of food. A review. *J Am Coll Nutr.* 2019;38:547.

Chae SA, et al. Prenatal exercise in fetal development: a placental perspective. *FEBS J.* 2021;doi: 10.1111/febs.16173.

Clark NW, et al. The acute effects of thermogenic fitness drink formulas containing 140 mg and 100 mg of caffeine on energy expenditure and fat metabolism at rest and during exercise. *J Int Soc Sports Nutr.* 2020;17:10.

de Paula T, et al. Acute effect of aerobic and strength exercise on heart rate variability and baroreflex sensitivity in men with autonomic dysfunction. *J Strength Cond Res.* 2019;33:2743.

Ehrenwald M, et al. Exercise capacity and body mass index—important predictors of change in resting heart rate. *BMC Cardiovasc Disord.* 2019;19:307.

Frischhut C, et al. Effects of a heat and moisture exchanger on respiratory function and symptoms post-cold air exercise. *Scand J Med Sci Sports.* 2020;30:591.

Goldbogen JA, Madsen PT. The largest of August Krogh animals: physiology and biomechanics of the blue whale revisited. *Comp Biochem Physiol A Mol Integr Physiol.* 2021;254:110894.

Gür F, Can Gür G. Is exercise a useful intervention in the treatment of alcohol use disorder? Systematic review and meta-analysis. *Am J Health Promot.* 2020;34(5):520.

Heine M, et al. Developing a complex understanding of physical activity in cardiometabolic disease from low-to-middle-income countries-a qualitative systematic review with meta-synthesis. *Int J Environ Res Public Health.* 2021;18:11977.

Jesus F, et al. Are predictive equations a valid method of assessing the resting metabolic rate of overweight or obese former athletes? *Eur J Sport Sci.* 2020;7:1.

Li H, Wang C, et al. Skeletal muscle non-shivering thermogenesis as an attractive strategy to combat obesity. *Life Sci.* 2021;269:119024.

Lim H, et al. Operationalization of intersectionality in physical activity and sport research: a systematic scoping review. *SSM Popul Health.* 2021;14:100808.

Lytle JR, et al. Predicting energy expenditure of an acute resistance exercise bout in men and women. *Med Sci Sports Exerc.* 2019;51:1532.

McNab BK. What determines the basal rate of metabolism? *J Exp Biol.* 2019;222(Pt 15).

Oh SK, et al. Association between basal metabolic rate and handgrip strength in older Koreans. *Int J Environ Res Public Health.* 2019;16:22.

Okabe K, Uchiyama S. Intracellular thermometry uncovers spontaneous thermogenesis and associated thermal signaling. *Commun Biol.* 2021;4:1377.

Podrekar N, et al. Effects of cycle and treadmill desks on energy expenditure and cardiometabolic parameters in sedentary workers: review and meta-analysis. *Int J Occup Saf Ergon.* 2021;27:728.

Ramakrishnan R, et al. Objectively measured physical activity and all cause mortality: a systematic review and meta-analysis. *Prev Med.* 2021;143:106356.

Tabuchi C, Sul HS. Signaling pathways regulating thermogenesis. *Front Endocrinol (Lausanne).* 2021;12:595020.

Table 9.1 Five-Level Physical Activity Classification Based on Energy Expenditure

Level	Energy Expenditure			
	kcal·min^{-1}	L·min^{-1}	mL·kg^{-1}·min^{-1}	METs
Males				
Light	2.0–4.9	0.40–0.99	6.1–15.2	1.6–3.9
Moderate	5.0–7.4	1.00–1.49	15.3–22.9	4.0–5.9
Heavy	7.5–9.9	1.50–1.99	23.0–30.6	6.0–7.9
Very heavy	10.0–12.4	2.00–2.49	30.7–38.3	8.0–9.9
Unduly heavy	≥12.5	≥2.50	≥38.4	≥10.0
Females				
Light	1.5–3.4	0.30–0.69	5.4–12.5	1.2–2.7
Moderate	3.5–5.4	0.70–1.09	12.6–19.8	2.8–4.3
Heavy	5.5–7.4	1.10–1.49	19.9–27.1	4.4–5.9
Very heavy	7.5–9.4	1.50–1.89	27.2–34.4	6.0–7.5
Unduly heavy	≥9.5	≥1.90	≥34.5	≥7.6

MET, metabolic equivalent.
Note: L·min^{-1} based on 5 kcal per liter of oxygen; mL·kg^{-1}·min^{-1} based on 65-kg male and 55-kg female; 1 MET equals the average resting oxygen uptake (250 mL·min^{-1} for males, 200 mL·min^{-1} for females).

Table 9.2 Leisure-Time Physical Activity Energy Expenditure Expressed in Metabolic Equivalents and Percentage Maximum Oxygen Uptake

Categorization	Relative Intensity (%$\dot{V}O_{2max}$)	Absolute Intensity (METs)			
		Young	Middle-Aged	Old	Very Old
Rest	<10	1.0	1.0	1.0	1.0
Light	<35	<4.5	<3.5	<2.5	<1.5
Fairly light	<50	<6.5	<5.0	<3.5	<2.0
Moderate	<70	<9.0	<7.0	<5.0	<2.8
Heavy	<70	>9.0	>7.0	>5.0	>2.8
Maximal	100	13.0	10.0	7.0	4.0

%$\dot{V}O_{2max}$, percent maximum oxygen uptake; MET, metabolic equivalent.
Source: Reprinted with permission from Bouchard C, Shephard RJ. Physical activity, fitness, and health: the model and key concepts. In: Bouchard C, et al., eds. *Physical Activity, Fitness, and Health: International Proceedings and Consensus Statement*. Champaign, IL: Human Kinetics, 1994: 77.

Table 9.3 Daily Energy Expenditure by Gender and Age

Gender	Age (yr)	Energy Expenditure (kcal)
Male	15–18	3000
	19–24	2900
	25–50	2900
	>51	2300
Female	15–18	2200
	19–24	2200
	25–50	2200
	>50	1900

Data from Food and Nutrition Board, National Research Council. *Recommended Dietary Allowances, Revised*. Washington, DC: National Academy of Sciences; 1989.

CHAPTER 10
Energy Expenditure During Walking, Jogging, Running, and Swimming

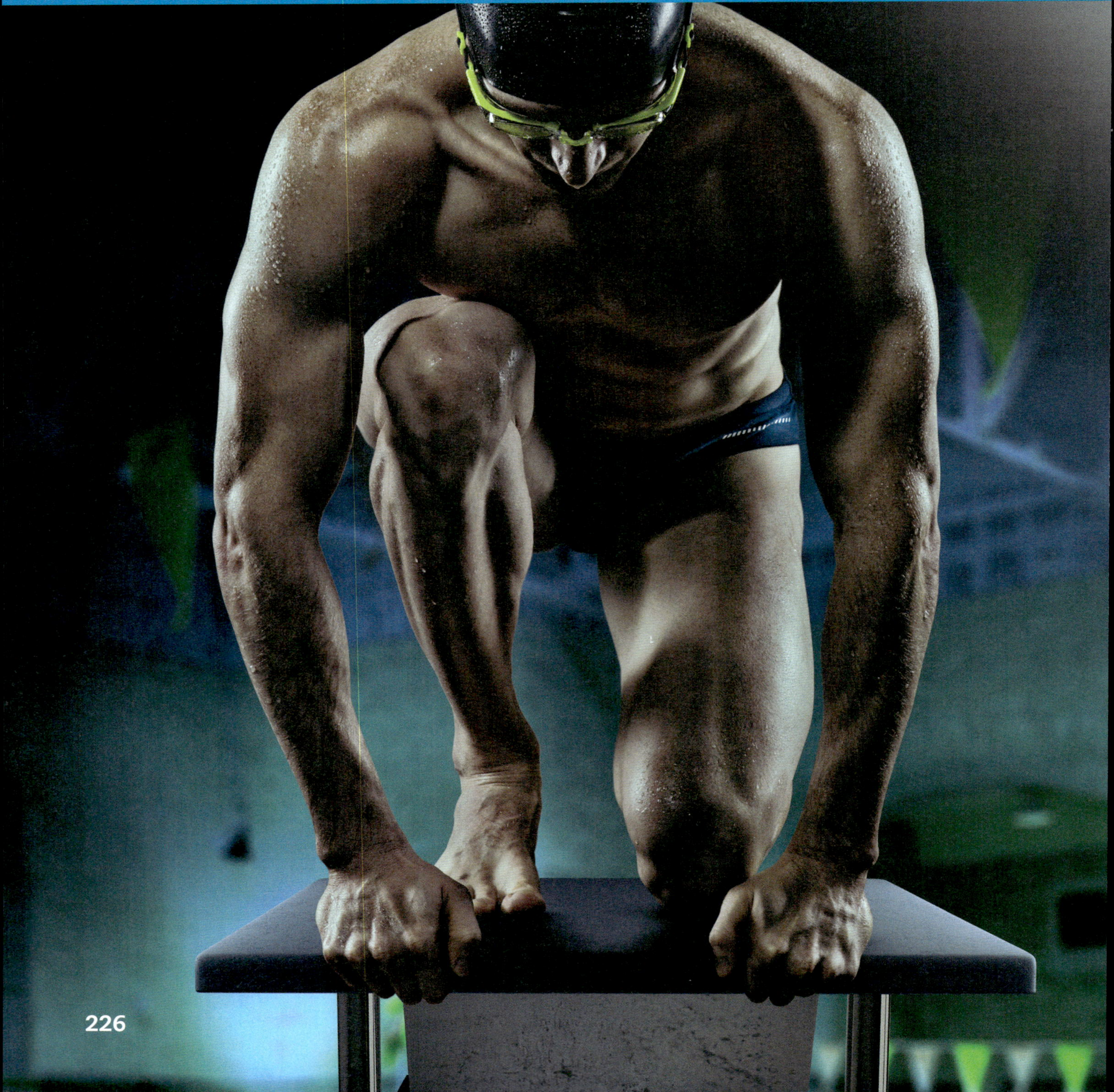

Chapter Objectives

- Differentiate between gross and net energy expenditure
- Explain movement economy
- Explain mechanical efficiency
- Describe differences in running economy between trained and untrained children and adults
- Graph the relationship between walking velocity and energy expenditure up to maximum values
- Discuss influences of body weight, activity surface, and footwear on energy expenditure during walking and running
- List two advantages and two disadvantages of ankle and handheld weights to increase energy expenditure during walking and running
- Graph the relationship between running velocity and energy expenditure
- Explain the association between running velocity and energy expenditure per unit distance traveled
- For running versus competitive racewalking, explain the interactions among stride length, stride frequency, and linear velocity
- Quantify how a drafting strategy influences energy expenditure during running, swimming, and bicycling
- Identify three factors contributing to lower swimming exercise economy compared with running economy

Ancillaries at-a-Glance

Visit Lippincott Connect to access these resources.

- References: Chapter 10
- Focus on Research: It Costs More Energy to Move More

Walking, running, and swimming take on special significance for their important roles played in weight control, physical conditioning, and health maintenance and rehabilitation.

Human Movement Efficiency and Economy

Three factors largely determine success in aerobic endurance performance:

1. Aerobic capacity ($\dot{V}O_{2max}$)
2. Ability to sustain effort at a large $\dot{V}O_{2max}$ percentage
3. Efficiency of energy use termed **movement economy**

Exercise physiologists consider a high $\dot{V}O_{2max}$ a prerequisite for endurance success. Among elite long-distance runners with nearly identical aerobic capacities, other factors often explain competitive success. For example, a performance edge would clearly exist for an athlete able to run at a higher $\dot{V}O_{2max}$ percentage (i.e., higher blood lactate threshold) than competitors. Similarly, the runner who maintains a given pace with relatively low-energy expenditure or greater movement economy maintains a competitive advantage.

Human Movement Efficiency

The energy expenditure related to external work represents a fraction of the total energy utilized when an individual engages in physical activity—the remainder appears as heat. **Mechanical efficiency (ME)** indicates the percentage of the total chemical energy expended (denominator) that contributes to the **external work output** (numerator). Within this context:

> **ME (%) = Work Output ÷ Energy Expended × 100**

Force, acting through a vertical distance (F × D), usually records as foot-pounds (ft-lb) or kilogram-meters (kg-m) and represents external work output accomplished. External work output during cycle ergometry, stair climbing, and bench stepping requires lifting the body mass vertically. In contrast to horizontal walking or running, work output cannot be computed because no external work occurs. Reciprocal leg and arm movements negate each other, and the body achieves no net gain in vertical distance. If a person walks or runs up a grade, the work component depends on body mass and vertical distance or lift achieved during the activity interval (see Chapter 5, "*In A Practical Sense: Measuring Work on a Treadmill, Cycle Ergometer, and Step Bench*"). Work output converts to kilocalories using these standard conversions:

> **1 kcal = 426.8 kg-m**
> **1 kcal = 3087.4 ft-lb**
> **1 kcal = 1.5593 × 10⁻³ hp·h⁻¹**
> **1 kcal = 0.01433 kcal·min⁻¹**
> **1 watt = 6.12 kg·m·min⁻¹**

Steady-rate oxygen uptake during physical activity represents the energy input in the efficiency equation (denominator). To obtain common units, oxygen uptake converts to energy units (1.0 L O_2 = 5.0 kcal; see Table 8.1 for precise calorific transformations based on the nonprotein respiratory quotient [RQ]).

Three terms, gross, net, and delta, express efficiency. Each expression exhibits a particular advantage. Each calculation method assumes a submaximal steady-rate condition and requires that work output and energy expenditure be expressed in the same units—typically kilocalories. Applying the different calculation methods to the same activity modality yields varying results for ME that range from 8 to 25% using gross calculations, 10 to 30% using net calculations, and 24 to 35% using delta calculations.

Gross Mechanical Efficiency

Gross mechanical efficiency, the most frequently calculated efficiency measure, applies when requiring a specific work rate and speed, or in nutritional studies that express energy expenditure over extended durations. Gross efficiency computations use the total oxygen uptake during the activity.

As an example, suppose a 15-min ride on a stationary bicycle generates 13,300 kg-m of work or 31.2 kcal (13,300 kg-m ÷ 426.8 kcal per kg-m). The oxygen uptake to perform the work totals 25 L at an RQ of 0.88, which indicates that each liter of oxygen uptake generated an energy equivalent of 4.9 kcal (see Table 8.1). Thus, the activity required 122.5 kcal (25 L × 4.9 kcal). ME (%) computes as follows:

> **Gross ME (%) = Work Output ÷ Energy Expended × 100**
> **= 31.2 kcal ÷ 122.5 kcal × 100**
> **= 25.5%**

As with all machines, the human body's efficiency to produce mechanical work falls considerably below 100%. The energy required to overcome internal and external friction becomes the biggest factor affecting ME. Overcoming friction represents essentially wasted energy because it accomplishes no external work; consequently, work input *always* exceeds work output. Human locomotion ME in most walking, running, and cycling activities ranges between 20 and 30%.

Net Mechanical Efficiency

Net mechanical efficiency involves subtracting the resting energy expenditure from the total energy expended during activity. This calculation indicates the work efficiency *per se*, unaffected by the energy expended to sustain the body at rest. Net ME calculates as follows:

> **Net ME (%) = Work Output ÷ Energy Expended Above Rest × 100**

Resting energy output is determined for the same time duration as the work output.

In the previous example for gross ME, if resting oxygen uptake equaled 250 mL·min⁻¹ (0.25 L·min⁻¹) and RQ equaled 0.91 (4.936 kcal·L O_2^{-1}; 0.250 L·min⁻¹ × 4.936 = 1.234 kcal·min⁻¹), then net ME computes as:

$$\text{Net ME (\%)} = 31.2 \div 122.5 \text{ kcal} - (1.234 \text{ kcal·min}^{-1} \times 15 \text{ min}) \times 100 = 30\%$$

Delta Efficiency

Delta efficiency calculates as the *relative* energy cost to perform an additional work increment; that is, the ratio of the difference between *work output* at two work output levels to the *difference* in *energy expenditure* determined for the two exercise levels.

$$\Delta \text{ Efficiency} = \frac{\text{Difference in work output between two exercise levels}}{\text{Difference in energy expended between two exercise levels}} \times 100$$

As an example, suppose an individual cycles at 100 watts for 5 min (100 W = 1.433 kcal·min⁻¹) at a steady-rate oxygen uptake of 1.70 L·min⁻¹ at an RQ of 0.83 (4.838 kcal·L O_2^{-1}). This corresponds to an energy expenditure of 8.23 kcal·min⁻¹. The person then cycles another 5 min at 200 watts (200 W = 2.866 kcal·min⁻¹) at a steady-rate oxygen uptake of 2.80 L·min⁻¹ with RQ of 0.90 (4.924 kcal·L O_2^{-1}). This results in 13.8 kcal·min⁻¹ energy expenditure. Delta efficiency computes as:

$$\Delta \text{ Efficiency} = 2866 \text{ kcal·min}^{-1} - 1.433 \text{ kcal·min}^{-1} \div 13.79 \text{ kcal·min}^{-1} - 8.23 \text{ kcal·min}^{-1} \times 100$$
$$= -1.433 \text{ kcal·min}^{-1} \div 5.56 \text{ kcal·min}^{-1} \times 100$$
$$= 25.8\%$$

Use the delta efficiency method when assessing treadmill activity efficiency because it is impossible to determine work output accurately during horizontal movement.

Factors Influencing Exercise Efficiency

Seven factors influence exercise efficiency:

1. **Work rate**: Efficiency generally decreases as work rate increases from a curvilinear rather than linear relation between energy expenditure and work rate. As work rate increases, total energy expenditure increases disproportionately to work output, resulting in a lowered ME.
2. **Movement speed:** Every individual has an optimum movement speed for any given physical activity. Generally, the optimum movement speed increases as power output increases (i.e., higher power outputs require greater movement speed to create optimum efficiency). Any deviation from the optimal movement speed decreases efficiency. Low efficiencies at slow speeds most likely result from inertia (i.e., increased energy expended to overcome internal starting and stopping). Declines in efficiency at high speeds can result from increases in muscular friction, with resulting increases in internal work and energy expenditure.
3. **Extrinsic factors**: Improvements in equipment design have increased efficiency in many physical activities. For example, lighter and softer running shoes with different insole cushioning properties permit running at a given speed with lower energy expenditure, which increases movement efficiency. Changes in clothing have produced a similar effect (e.g., lighter, more absorbent fabrics and more hydrodynamic full-body swimsuits).
4. **Muscle fiber composition**: Activation of slow-twitch muscle fibers produces greater efficiency than the same work accomplished by fast-twitch fibers. Slow-twitch fibers require less adenosine triphosphate per unit work than fast-twitch fibers.[21,22,45] Consequently, individuals with a higher slow-twitch fiber percentage exhibit increased ME.
5. **Fitness level:** More fit individuals perform a given task at a higher efficiency from decreased energy expenditure for the non–exercise-related functions of temperature regulation, increased circulation, and waste product removal.
6. **Body composition:** Overweight individuals perform weight-bearing walking and running activities at a lower efficiency from the increased energy cost to transport extra poundage.
7. **Technique:** Improved technique produces fewer extraneous body movements and lower energy expenditure and hence higher efficiencies. The golf swing serves as a prime example. Millions of men and women expend considerable "energy" trying to direct ball flight where they want it to go—mostly with less than ideal execution. In contrast, tour players give the impression they expend little "energy" to coordinate movement patterns of their feet, legs, hips, shoulders, and arms to strike the ball on a preplanned trajectory toward a target in a precise, sequenced, and coordinated manner that appears "effortless."

Changes in Efficiency During a Competitive Season Relate to Training Volume and Intensity

Cyclists who spend the most time training at or above their lactate threshold increase gross efficiency cycling compared to their preseason and postseason values. The increase in gross efficiency averages a modest 1%, yet this can make a difference in winning or losing and the posting of a rider's best times.

OSTILL is Franck Camhi/Shutterstock

Source:
Carlsson M, et al. Gross and delta efficiencies during uphill running and cycling among elite triathletes. *Eur J Appl Physiol*. 2020;120:961.

Human Movement Economy

The exercise economy concept encompasses the relation between energy input and energy output. The energy to perform a particular task relative to performance quality represents an important concern. In a sense, many of us assess economy by visually comparing the ease of movement among highly trained athletes. It does not require a trained eye to discriminate how "easy" elite swimmers, skiers, golfers, dancers, gymnasts, and platform divers perform compared to less proficient counterparts who seem to expend considerable "wasted energy" to essentially performing the same tasks. A world-class swimmer glides through the water with the greatest of ease, as do ballet dancers who leap, twist, and turn with grace and power. Anyone who has learned a new sport experiences the difficulties encountered in executing the most basic movement patterns, which with proper practice over thousands of hours became automatic and indeed appear "effortless."

Physical Activity Oxygen Uptake; A Reflection of Movement Economy

A common method to assess differences in movement economy among individuals evaluates the steady-rate oxygen uptake during the activity at a set power output or movement speed. This approach only applies to steady-rate physical activity that mirrors oxygen uptake with energy expenditure. *At a given submaximal running, cycling, or swimming speed, an individual with greater movement economy consumes less oxygen.* Economy takes on importance during longer duration activities in which aerobic capacity and the task's oxygen requirements largely determine success.[32,52,61] *All else being equal, any training adjustment that improves economy of effort directly translates to improved performance.*[83,84]

FIGURE 10.1 relates running economy to endurance performance in elite athletes with comparable $\dot{V}O_{2\,max}$ values. As depicted in the figure, athletes with greater running economies (i.e., lower oxygen uptake at the same running pace) achieve better performance.

No single biomechanical factor accounts for individual differences in running economy. Significant variation in economy at a particular running speed occurs even among trained runners, and not to measurement error or inconsistency.[46,79] In general, improved running economy results from years of arduous training with particular attention to training specific running *movement* patterns. Short-term training that emphasizes only "proper running techniques" (e.g., synchronized arm movements and body alignment) probably does not improve running economy. Distance runners who lack an economical stride-length pattern benefit from a short-term program involving audiovisual feedback that focuses on optimizing stride length.[13,60]

fyi Running Economy Improves with Age

Running economy improves steadily from age 10 to age 18. This partly explains young children's relatively poor performance in distance running and their progressive improvements throughout adolescence. Improved endurance occurs even though aerobic capacity relative to body mass (mL $O_2 \cdot kg^{-1} \cdot min^{-1}$) remains constant during this time.

Source:
Mendonca GV, et al. Running economy in recreational male and female runners with similar levels of cardiovascular fitness. *J Appl Physiol (1985).* 2020;129(3):508.

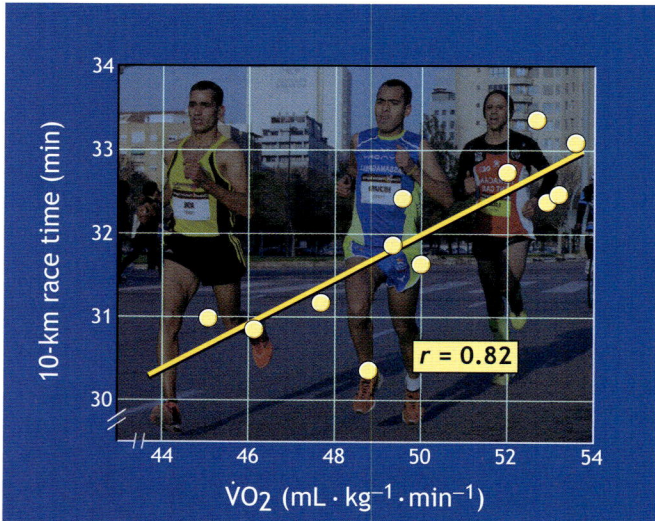

FIGURE 10.1. Relationship between submaximal oxygen uptake running at 268 m · min⁻¹ and 10-km race time in elite male runners of comparable aerobic capacity.
(Adapted with permission from Morgan DW, Craib M. Physiological aspects of running economy. *Med Sci Sports Exerc.* 1992;24:456. Background photo: Rob Wilson/Shutterstock)

Walking Energy Expenditure

For most individuals, walking represents their major daily physical activity. **FIGURE 10.2** displays the combined research from five countries on energy expenditure in men walking at speeds from 1.5 to 9.5 km · hr⁻¹/0.9 to 5.9 mph. The yellow line represents average values from various studies reported in the literature. The relationship between walking speed and oxygen uptake remains approximately linear between 3.0 and 5.0 km · hr⁻¹/1.9 and 3.1 mph; as walking economy decreases at faster speeds, the relationship curves upward with a disproportionate increase in energy expenditure with increasing speed. This explains why per unit distance traveled, faster, less efficient walking speeds require more total calories expended per unit distance traveled.

Body Mass Influence

An equation based on the combined data in Figure 10.2 and additional studies,[1,30] accurately predicts energy expenditure for horizontal walking at speeds between 3.2 and 6.4 km · hr⁻¹/2.0 and 4.0 mph for males and females who differ in body weight.

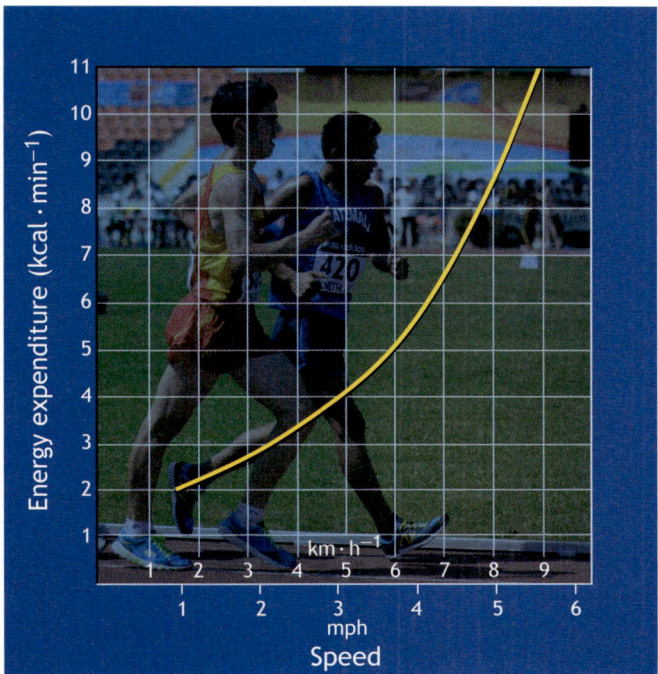

FIGURE 10.2. Energy expenditure walking on a level surface at different speeds.
(Background photo: StockphotoVideo/Shutterstock)

The values listed in **TABLE 10.1** achieve accuracy to within ±15% of measured energy expenditure. On a daily basis, the error in estimating walking energy expended from body weight generally ranges from 50 to 100 kcal, assuming the person walks 2 hr daily. The predictions become less accurate when extrapolations are made for light (<36 kg/79 lb) and heavy (>91 kg/201 lb) individuals.

TABLE 10.1 Energy expenditure (kcal · min⁻¹) prediction from level walking speed and body mass

Terrain and Walking Surface

TABLE 10.2 summarizes how different terrains and surfaces influence energy expenditure for walking. Similar movement economies exist for level walking on a grass track or paved surface. In contrast, walking in sand requires almost twice the energy expenditure compared to walking on a hard surface because of sand's hindering effects on the forward movement of the foot and added force required by calf muscles to compensate for foot slippage. Walking in soft snow triples energy expenditure compared with similar walking on a treadmill.[82] A brisk walk or jog along a beach or in freshly fallen snow provides an excellent way to "burn" additional calories or improve physiologic fitness.[80]

TABLE 10.2 Different terrain effects on energy expenditure walking at 5.6 km · hr–1/3.2 mph and 5.6 km · hr–1/3.5 mph

Individuals generate about the same energy expenditure walking on a firm, level surface or walking on a treadmill at an equivalent speed and distance.[72] Energy expenditure determined from laboratory studies provide confidence in translating human energy expenditure data to "real-life" situations.

Grade

Walking downhill on a mountain hike or golf course provides welcome relief compared with uphill walking. Downhill walking or running represents a form of **negative work** as the body's center of mass moves in a downward vertical direction with each step cycle. At the same speed and elevation, it requires less energy to perform eccentric muscle actions (negative work) than the concentric actions involved in positive work.

FIGURE 10.3 illustrates the net oxygen uptake for both level and negative-grade walking at constant speeds from 6.3 to 5.4 km · hr⁻¹/3.9 to 3.35 mph. Percent grade reflects the vertical distance moved downward per unit horizontal distance traversed. Compared with walking on level ground, progressive negative-grade walking decreases oxygen uptake down to a −9% grade for speeds of 5.4 km · hr⁻¹/3.35 mph. Energy expenditure begins to increase at more severe negative grades. The additional energy expenditure to resist or "brake" the body from gravity's pull while trying to achieve a proper and safe walking rhythm increases the oxygen uptake for walking down steeper grades.

Footwear and Other Distal Leg Loads

It requires considerably more energy to carry weight on the feet or ankles than to carry the same weight on the torso.[12] A weight equal to 1.4% body mass placed on the ankles increases energy expenditure walking an average 8%, or nearly six times more than with the same weight on the torso.[39] Wearing boots

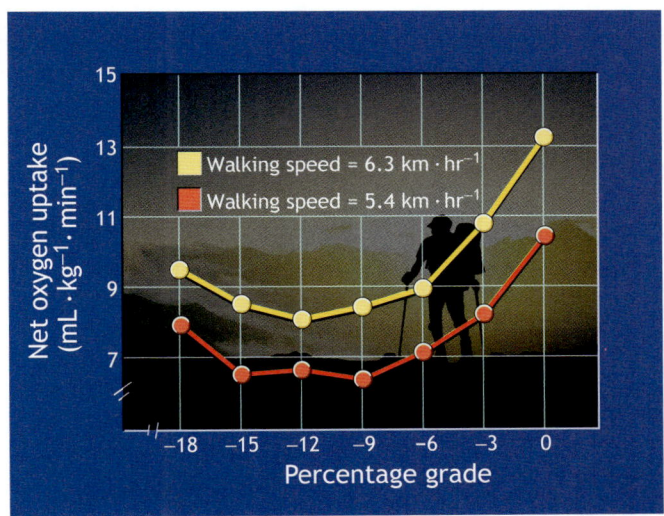

FIGURE 10.3. Net oxygen uptake (0% grade) and downhill walking at grades between −3 and −18% and speeds between 5.4 and 6.3 km · hr⁻¹.
(Adapted with permission from Wanta DM, et al. Metabolic response to graded downhill walking. *Med Sci Sports Exerc.* 1993;25:159. biletskiyevgeniy.com/ Shutterstock)

disproportionately increases the walking and running energy expenditure compared with energy expenditure wearing lighter running shoes. Adding only an additional 100 g/3.5 oz to each shoe increases oxygen uptake during moderate running by 1%. Running barefoot offers no metabolic advantage over running in lightweight, cushioned shoes.[33] In designing running shoes, hiking and climbing boots, and work boots for mining, forestry, fire-fighting, and the military, small changes in shoe weight produce meaningful changes in movement economy and hence total energy expenditure.[36] Minimally shod runners show 2.4 to 3.3% greater running economy than traditionally shod runners after accounting for shoe weight and stride frequency.[66] Greater elastic energy storage and release in the lower extremity during minimal-shoe running helps to explain this difference. The cushioning properties and longitudinal bending stiffness of the shoe also impact walking and running economy. A more flexible and softer-soled running shoe reduced oxygen uptake with increased running economy at a moderate speed by −2.4% compared with a similar shoe with a firmer cushioning system, although the softer-soled shoes weighed an additional 31 g/1.1 oz.[34,64,77]

Walking

Ankle weights increase energy expenditure during walking to values usually observed for running.[54] The effect benefits individuals who use only walking as a low-impact training modality yet require greater energy expenditures than normal walking. Handheld weights, walking poles that simulate arm action in cross-country skiing, power belts worn around the waist with resistance cords with handles for arm action, weighted vests, and swinging the arms in upper-body exercise increase walking's energy expenditure.[29,71,73,91]

Handheld weights and walking poles may disproportionately increase exercise systolic blood pressure most likely from the pressure-elevating effects of upper-body exercise (see Chapter 15, "Upper Body Physical Activity") and increased intramuscular tension from gripping. An amplified blood pressure response contraindicates using handheld weights for individuals with existing hypertension or coronary heart disease.

Running

Considering the relatively small increase in energy expenditure with hand or ankle weights in running, it seems more practical to simply increase unweighted running speed or distance. This reduces injury potential from the added impact force imparted by the weights and eliminates any discomfort from carrying them. For individuals with orthopedic limitations, in-line skating offers a less-stressful alternative for an equivalent aerobic demand.[48,53]

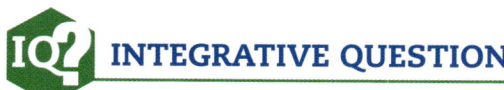

INTEGRATIVE QUESTION

Discuss recommendations for mode-specific aerobic physical activities to train individuals with knee osteoarthritis?

Competition Walking

For Olympic-caliber walkers, walking speed during competition averaged 13.0 km·hr^{-1} (ranging from 11.5 to 14.8 km·hr^{-1}/7.1 to 9.2 mph) over distances from 1.6 to 50 km/1.0 to 31.1 mi. This represents a relatively fast speed. The world record for the 20-km/12.6-mi walk for men is 1:16:436 (Yusuke Suzuki, Japan, March 2015) and for women is 1:23:39 (Elena Lashmanova, Russia, June 2018), which equal speeds of 15.74 km·hr^{-1}/9.78 mph for men and 16 km·hr^{-1}/9.94 mph for women! **FIGURE 10.4** illustrates that the break point in locomotion economy between walking and running ranges between 8.0 and 9.0 km·hr^{-1}/4.97 and 5.59 mph. These data, plus biomechanical evidence, indicate about the same crossover speed—when running becomes more economical than walking—for conventional and competitive walking styles (**FIG. 10.5**). The preferred 7.2 km·hr^{-1}/4.5 mph (nonrunners) and 7.4 km·hr^{-1}/4.6 mph (runners) transition speed is slower than the energetically optimal speed, and these speeds remain independent of training state or aerobic capacity.[75] Treadmill walking at competition speeds produced only slightly lower oxygen uptakes for racewalkers than their highest oxygen uptakes during treadmill running. A linear relationship exists between oxygen uptake and walking at speeds above 8 km·hr^{-1}/5.0 mph, but the slope of the line is *twice* as steep compared to running at the same speeds (athletes walked at velocities of nearly 16 km·hr^{-1}/9.9 mph). *The economy of walking faster than 8 km·hr^{-1} equaled only half the economy running at the same speeds.* Attaining a similar $\dot{V}O_{2\,max}$ during racewalking and running by elite competitors further supports the model for aerobic training specificity—$\dot{V}O_{2\,max}$ in untrained subjects during walking generally remains 5 to 15% below running values.[35,51]

Competition walkers achieve high yet uneconomical movement rates unattainable with a conventional walking style, with a unique modified walking technique that constrains

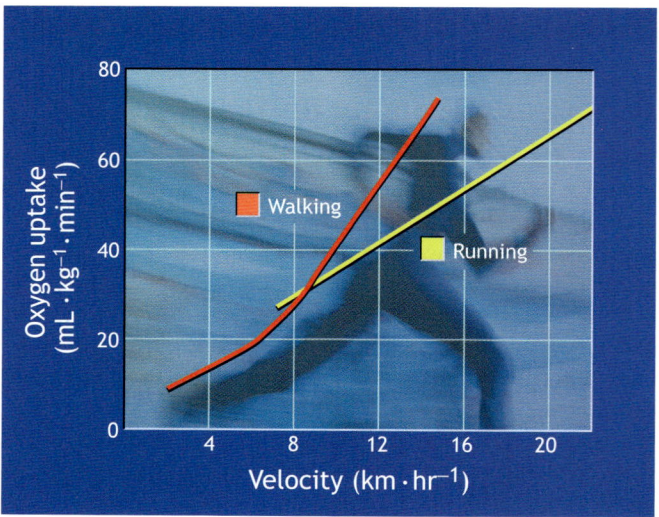

FIGURE 10.4. Relationship between oxygen uptake and horizontal velocity for walking and running in competition walkers.
(Adapted with permission from Menier DR, Pugh LGCE. The relation of oxygen intake and velocity of walking and running in competition walkers. *J Physiol*. 1968;197:717.)

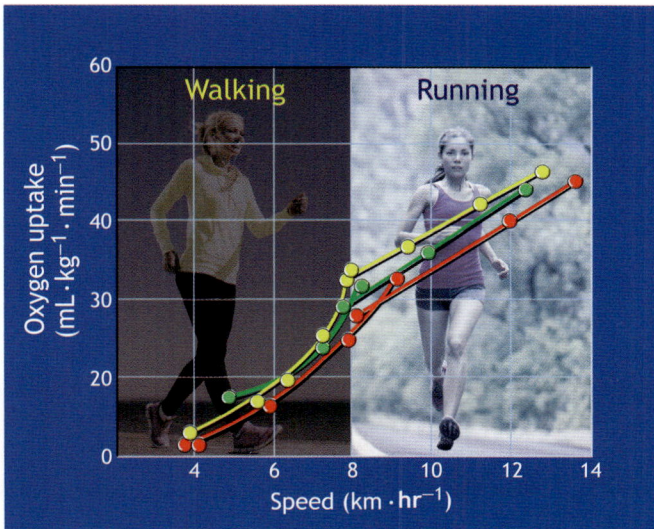

FIGURE 10.5. Relationship between oxygen uptake and horizontal walking and running speed in women and men. Different colored lines represent values from various research studies.
(Adapted with permission from Falls HB, Humphrey LD. Energy cost of running and walking in young women. *Med Sci Sports*. 1976;8:9. Shutterstock background photos: Syda Productions (left), Maridav (right).)

the athlete to certain movement patterns regardless of walking speed (www.youtube.com/watch?v=W1sxFgTUbWo). The athlete must maintain this gait despite progressive decreases in walking economy as duration progresses and fatigue increases.[10,11] Among elite racewalkers, variations in walking economy contribute more to successful performance than do economy variations in competitive runners.[35]

Running Energy Expenditure

Biomechanical factors that determine running energy expenditure related to velocity among mammals include magnitude and rate of muscular force generation to counteract gravity and to operate the spring-like properties of the muscle-tendon system.[43] Energy expenditure for running has been quantified during the actual activity and on a treadmill while precisely controlling speed and grade. The terms *jogging* and *running* reflect qualitative assessments related to speed and strenuousness. At identical submaximal speeds, an endurance athlete runs at a lower $\dot{V}O_{2max}$ percentage than an untrained person, yet both maintain nearly similar oxygen uptake rates. The demarcation between a jog and a run relates more to the participant's fitness level: *A jog for one person represents a run for another.*

 Speed, Pace Times, and Target Distance Conversions

The table provides useful conversions for different speeds, paces, and distances.

MPH	km/hr	min/mi	min/km	3 mi	5 km	8 km	10 km	Half marathon	Marathon
3.0	4.8	0:20:00	0:12:26	1:00:00	1:02:08	1:39:25	2:04:16	4:22:13	8:44:26
4.0	6.4	0:15:00	0:09:19	0:45:00	0:46:36	1:14:34	1:33:12	3:16:40	6:33:20
5.0	8.0	0:12:00	0:09:19	0:36:00	0:37:17	0:59:39	1:14:34	2:37:20	5:14:40
6.0	9.7	0:10:00	0:06:13	0:30:00	0:31:04	0:49:43	0:02:08	2:11:07	4:22:13
7.0	11.3	0:08:34	0:05:20	0:25:43	0:26:38	0:42:36	0:53:16	1:52:23	3:44:46
8.0	12.9	0:07:30	0:04:40	0:22:30	0:23:18	0:37:17	0:46:36	1:38:20	3:16:40
9.0	14.5	0:06:40	0:04:09	0:20:00	0:20:43	0:33:08	0:41:25	1:27:24	2:54:49
10.0	61.1	0:06:00	0:03:44	0:18:00	0:18:38	0:29:50	0:37:17	1:18:40	2:37:20
11.0	17.7	0:05:27	0:03:23	0:16:22	0:16:57	0:27:07	0:33:54	1:11:31	2:23:02
12.0	19.3	0:05:00	0:03:06	0:15:00	0:15:32	0:24:51	0:31:04	1:05:33	2:11:07

David Acosta Allely/Shutterstock

Independent of fitness, it becomes more economical from an energy expenditure standpoint to discontinue walking and begin running at speeds above about 8 km·hr^{-1}/4.97 mph. Figure 10.5 illustrates the relationship between oxygen uptake and horizontal walking and running for males and females at speeds between 4 and 14 km·hr^{-1}/2.5 and 8.7 mph. For data depicted in green and yellow, the lines relating oxygen uptake and speed intersect at an 8.0 km·hr^{-1}/4.97 mph running speed; the breakpoint in competition walkers locomotion economy shown in red occurs at about 8.7 km·hr^{-1}/5.4 mph.

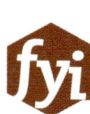

Elite Runners Run More Economically Even at a Young Age

At a particular speed, elite endurance runners run at a lower oxygen uptake than less trained or less successful similar-age counterparts. This holds for 8- to 11-yr-old cross-country runners and adult marathoners. Elite distance athletes as a group run with 5 to 10% greater economy than well-trained middle-distance runners.

Economy of Running Fast or Slow

The data for running in Figure 10.5 illustrate an important principle about running speed and energy expenditure. *The linear relationship between oxygen uptake and running speed indicates an equivalency in total energy requirement for running a given distance (at steady rate), which is nearly the same regardless of speed throughout a broad running speed range.* Simply stated, running a mile at 10 mph requires about twice the energy each min as running a mile at 5 mph; at the faster speed, completing the mile requires 6 min, but running at the slower speed takes about twice as long or 12 min. The *net* energy expenditure (minus resting value) to traverse a mile remains nearly the same.[74] Equivalent energy expenditure per mile regardless of running speed occurs for horizontal running and for running at a specific grade that ranges from −45 to +15%.[24,49] *During horizontal running, the net energy expenditure per kilogram body mass per km traveled averages 1 kcal or 1 kcal·kg^{-1}·km^{-1}.* The net energy expenditure running 1 km/0.62 mi for individuals who weigh 78 kg/172 lb averages 78 kcal, independent of running speed. Expressed as oxygen uptake (5 kcal = 1 L O_2), this amounts to 15.6 L oxygen uptake per km (78 kcal·km^{-1} ÷ 5 kcal). Comparing the net energy expenditure for locomotion per unit distance traveled for walking and running indicates greater energy expenditure when running a distance.[6]

Net Energy Expenditure

TABLE 10.3 presents *net energy expenditure* during running for 1 hr at various speeds—expressed in km per hr, mi per hr, and min required to complete 1 mi at a given speed. Bolded values indicate net calories expended running 1 mi for a given body mass. Recall that energy requirement for each mile remains fairly constant regardless of running speed. *A person who weighs 62 kg/137 lb requires approximately 2600 kcal (net) to run a 26.2-mi marathon regardless of whether the run takes just over 2, 3, or 4 hr!*

> **TABLE 10.3** Net energy expenditure during horizontal running per hour related to velocity and body mass

Table 10.3 also reveals that energy expenditure per mi increases proportionately with body mass. A 102-kg/225-lb person who runs 5 mi/d at a comfortable pace expends 163 kcal for each mi completed, or 815 kcal for 8.1 km/5 mi. The influence of body mass on an activity's energy expenditure supports weight-bearing physical activity as an additional caloric "stressor" for persons who desire to increase daily energy expenditure. Increasing or decreasing the speed within a broad steady-rate pacing range simply alters the 8.1 km/5 mi run duration; it has little effect on total energy (kcal) expended!

TABLE 10.4 summarizes data from energy expenditure studies using horizontal and grade walking and running on a firm surface. The energy requirement represents MET multiples (1 MET = 3.5 mL O_2·kg^{-1}·min^{-1}).

> **TABLE 10.4** Energy requirements (METs) for horizontal and grade walking and running on a solid surface

Stride Length, Stride Frequency, and Speed

Running

Three ways to increase running speed:

1. Increase steps per minute (*stride frequency*)
2. Increase distance between steps (*stride length*)
3. Increase *both* length and stride frequency

The third option may seem obvious, but several experiments provide objective data concerning this alternative. Research in 1944 evaluated the stride pattern for a Danish champion in 5- and 10-km running events.[8] At a running speed of 9.3 km·hr^{-1}/5.78 mph, this athlete's stride frequency equaled 160 per min, with a corresponding 97 cm/3.66 in stride length. When running speed increased 91% to 17.8 km·hr^{-1}/11.1 mph, stride frequency increased only

In a Practical Sense

Predicting Energy Expenditure for Treadmill Walking and Running

A linear relationship exists between oxygen uptake (energy expenditure) and walking speeds between 3.0 and 5.0 km·hr^{-1}/1.9 and 3.1 mph, and running speeds faster than 8.0 km·hr^{-1}/5 to 10 mph; see Figure 10.5. Adding the resting oxygen uptake to the oxygen requirements for the horizontal and vertical walk or run components allows for estimating total (gross) exercise oxygen uptake ($\dot{V}O_2$) and energy expenditure. Recall that a metabolic equivalent (MET) is a unit of measure used to express activity intensity relative to resting energy expenditure.

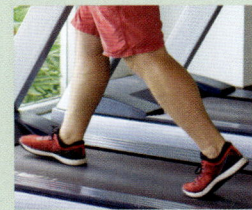
Den4is/Shutterstock

BASIC EQUATION

$\dot{V}O_2$ (mL·kg^{-1}·min^{-1}) = Resting component (1 MET [3.5 mL O_2·kg^{-1}·min^{-1}]) + Horizontal component (speed [m·min^{-1}] × oxygen uptake of horizontal movement) + Vertical component (percentage grade × speed [m·min^{-1}] × oxygen uptake of vertical movement).

[To convert mph to m·min^{-1}, multiply by 26.82; to convert m·min^{-1} to mph, multiply by 0.03728.]

Walking

Oxygen uptake for the horizontal movement component equals 0.1 mL·kg^{-1}·min^{-1}, and 1.8 mL·kg^{-1}·min^{-1} for the vertical component.

Running

Oxygen uptake for the horizontal movement component equals 0.2 mL·kg^{-1}·min^{-1}, and 0.9 mL·kg^{-1}·min^{-1} for the vertical component.

PREDICTING TREADMILL WALKING ENERGY EXPENDITURE

Problem

A 55-kg person walks on a treadmill at 2.8 mph (2.8 × 26.82 = 75 m·min^{-1}) up a 4% grade. Calculate (1) $\dot{V}O_2$ (mL·kg^{-1}·min^{-1}), (2) METs, and (3) energy expenditure (kcal·min^{-1}).

[Note: Express % grade as a decimal value (i.e., 4% grade = 0.04)]

Solution

1. $\dot{V}O_2$ = Resting $\dot{V}O_2$ (mL·kg^{-1}·min^{-1})
   + [speed (m·min^{-1}) × 0.1 mL·kg^{-1}·min^{-1}]
   + [%grade × speed (m·min^{-1})
   × 1.8 mL·kg^{-1}·min^{-1}]
   = 3.5 + (75 × 0.1) + (0.04 × 75 × 1.8)
   = 3.5 + 7.5 + 5.4
   = 16.4 mL·kg^{-1}·min^{-1}

2. METs = $\dot{V}O_2$ (mL·kg^{-1}·min^{-1})
   ÷ 3.5 mL·kg^{-1}·min^{-1}
   = 16.44 ÷ 3.5
   = 4.7

3. kcal·min^{-1} = $\dot{V}O_2$ (mL·kg^{-1}·min^{-1})
   × Body mass (kg) × 5.05 kcal·LO_2^{-1}
   = 16.4 mL·kg^{-1}·min^{-1}
   × 55 kg × 5.05 kcal·L^{-1}
   = 0.902 L·min^{-1} × 5.05 kcal·L^{-1}
   = 4.6

PREDICTING TREADMILL RUNNING ENERGY EXPENDITURE

Problem

A 55-kg person runs on a treadmill at 5.4 mph (5.4 × 26.82 = 145 m·min^{-1}) at a 6% grade. Calculate (1) $\dot{V}O_2$ in mL·kg^{-1}·min^{-1}, (2) METs, and (3) energy expenditure (kcal·min^{-1}).

Solution

1. $\dot{V}O_2$ = Resting $\dot{V}O_2$ (mL·kg^{-1}·min^{-1})
   + [speed (m·min^{-1}) × 0.2 mL·kg^{-1}·min^{-1}]
   + [%grade × speed (m·min^{-1})
   × 0.9 mL·kg^{-1}·min^{-1}]
   = 3.5 + (145 × 0.2) + (0.06 × 145 × 0.9)
   = 3.5 + 29.0 + 7.83
   = 40.33 mL·kg^{-1}·min^{-1}

2. METs = $\dot{V}O_2$ (mL·kg^{-1}·min^{-1})
   ÷ 3.5 mL·kg^{-1}·min^{-1}
   = 40.33 ÷ 3.5
   = 11.5

3. kcal·min^{-1} = $\dot{V}O_2$ (mL·kg^{-1}·min^{-1})
   × Body mass (kg) × 5.05 kcal·LO_2^{-1}
   = 40.33 mL·kg^{-1}·min^{-1}
   × 55 kg × 5.05 kcal·L^{-1}
   = 2.22 L·min^{-1} × 5.05 kcal·L^{-1}
   = 11.2

Adapted with permission from *ACSM Guidelines for Exercise Testing and Prescription*. 10th ed. Baltimore: Lippincott Williams & Wilkins; 2017.

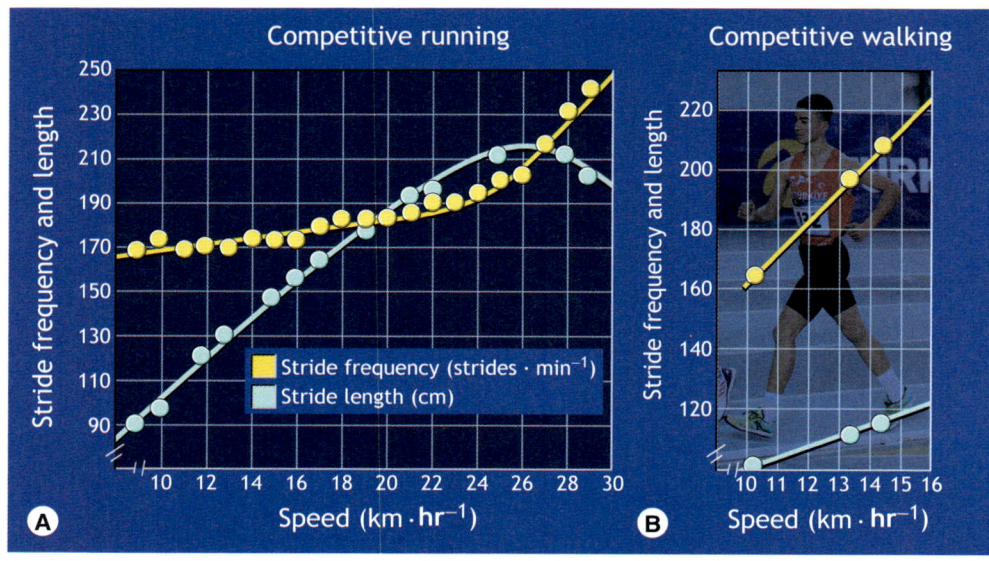

FIGURE 10.6. **(A)** Stride frequency and stride length as a function of running speed. **(B)** Data for an Olympic walker during racewalking.
(Adapted with permission from Hogberg P. Length of stride, stride frequency, flight period and maximum distance between the feet during running with different speeds. *Arbeitsphysiologie* 1952;14:431. Background photo: EvrenKalinbacak/Shutterstock)

10% to 176 per min, whereas stride length increased 83%, to 168 cm/66.1 in. **FIGURE 10.6A** displays the interaction between stride frequency and stride length as running speed increases. Doubling speed from 10 to 20 km · hr^{-1} increases stride length by 85%, whereas stride frequency increases only about 9%. Running at speeds above 23 km · hr^{-1} occurs mainly by increasing stride frequency. *As a general rule, running speed increases mainly by lengthening stride: Stride frequency becomes important at faster speeds.* Relying on increasing length in the "stroke" cycle, not frequency, to achieve rapid speeds in endurance performance also occurs among top-flight kayakers, rowers, cross-country skiers, and speed skaters.

Competition Walking

A competitive walker does not increase speed the same way as a runner. Figure 10.6B illustrates the stride length–stride frequency relationship for an Olympic 10-km medal winner who walked at speeds from 10 to 14.4 km · hr^{-1}/6.2 to 8.95 mph. When walking speed increased within this range, stride frequency increased 27% and stride length increased 13%. Faster speeds produced an even greater increase in stride frequency. Unlike running, where the body essentially "glides" through the air, competitive racewalking requires that the back foot remain on the ground until the front foot makes contact. Thus, lengthening stride becomes difficult and ineffectual to increase speed. Involving trunk and arm musculature to move the leg forward rapidly requires additional energy expenditure; this explains the poorer economy for walking than running at speeds above 8 or 9 km · hr^{-1}/5.0 or 5.6 mph (see Fig. 10.4).

Optimum Stride Length

Each person runs at a constant speed with an optimum stride length and stride frequency combination. This optimum depends largely on the person's mechanics or running "style" and cannot be determined from body measurements.[16] Nevertheless, energy expenditure increases more for overstriding than understriding. **FIGURE 10.7** relates oxygen uptake to different stride lengths altered by a subject running at the relatively fast 14 km · hr^{-1}/8.7 mph speed.

For this runner, a 135 cm/53.1 in stride length produced the lowest 3.35 L · min^{-1} oxygen uptake. When stride length decreased to 118 cm/46.5 in, oxygen uptake increased 8%; lengthening the distance between steps to 153 cm/60.23 in increased oxygen uptake by 12%. The inset graph shows a similar pattern for oxygen uptake when running speed increased to 16 km · hr^{-1}/9.9 mph and stride lengths varied between 135 and 169 cm/53 and 66.5 in. Decreasing this runner's stride length from the optimum 149 to 135 cm/58.6 to 53.1 in increased oxygen uptake by 4.1%; lengthening the stride to 169 cm/66.5 in increased aerobic energy expenditure nearly 13%. As one might expect, stride length selected by the subject (marked in the figure by the *solid orange circle*) produced the most economical stride length (lowest $\dot{V}O_2$). Lengthening the stride above the optimum produced a larger increase in oxygen uptake than a shorter-than-optimum length. Urging a runner who shows early fatigue signs to "lengthen your stride" to maintain speed actually proves counterproductive in running economy and subsequent performance.

Well-trained runners have "learned" through experience to run at the stride length they are accustomed to. In keeping with the concept that the body attempts to achieve a level requiring minimum effort, a self-selected stride length and frequency generally produce the most economical running performance. This reflects an individual's unique body size, limb segment inertia, and anatomic development.[15,55,56] *No "best" style characterizes elite runners.* For the competitive runner, any minor improvement in running economy generally improves race performance.

Running Economy: Children and Adults, Trained and Untrained

Children are less economical runners than adults; they require 20 to 30% more oxygen per unit body mass to run at a given speed.[2,42,63] Adult models to predict energy expenditure during weight-bearing locomotion fail to account for the increased and changing energy expenditures in children and adolescents.[37,62]

FIGURE 10.8 illustrates the relationship between 60 to 200 m · min^{-1}/2 and 8 mph walking and running speeds in male and female adolescent volunteers and oxygen uptake. The white line represents the best-fit curve for walking; the yellow line represents the best-fit line for running. Despite higher oxygen uptake and energy expenditure values during walking

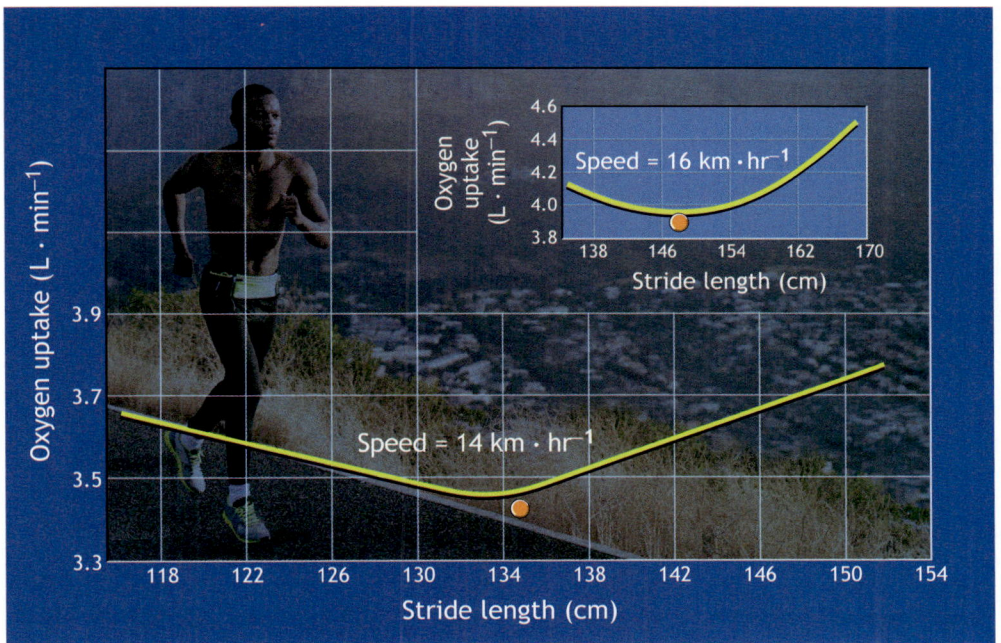

FIGURE 10.7. Oxygen uptake while running at 14 km · hr^{-1} affected by different stride lengths. The inset graph plots oxygen uptake at a faster speed of 16 km · hr^{-1}.
(Adapted with permission from Hogberg P. Length of stride, stride frequency, flight period and maximum distance between the feet during running with different speeds. *Arbeitsphysiologie* 1952;14:431. Background photo: WAYHOME studio/Shutterstock)

and running for adolescents than adults (see Fig. 10.5), the curves for both groups remain remarkably similar in shape.

Differences exist in energy expenditure among children and adolescents in weight-bearing physical activities. This has been attributed to a larger surface area-to-body mass ratio, greater stride frequencies, and shorter stride lengths, and to differences in anthropometric variables and mechanics that reduce movement economy.[31,76] Movement economy in weight-bearing activity also improves in obese adolescents and adults following weight loss.[27,67]

FIGURE 10.9 illustrates that running economy (lower steady rate $\dot{V}O_2$ at a given running speed) improves steadily during ages 10 through 18. Poorer running economy among young children partly explains their poorer performance in distance running compared with adults and their progressive performance improvement through adolescence. Aerobic capacity (mL $O_2 \cdot kg^{-1} \cdot min^{-1}$) remains relatively unchanged throughout this period. Consequently, improvement in a weight-bearing 1-mi walk-run fitness test during the growth years does not necessarily imply concomitant improvement in $\dot{V}O_{2\,max}$.[23]

Elite adolescent and adult endurance runners generally have lower oxygen uptake scores when running at a particular speed than less trained or less successful age-matched counterparts.[40,51] For trained runners, economy values and biomechanical characteristics during running remain fairly stable from day to day, even during intense running, with probably no difference between genders.[25,58,59]

Air Resistance

Anyone who has run into a headwind knows it requires greater effort ("energy") to maintain a given pace than running in calm

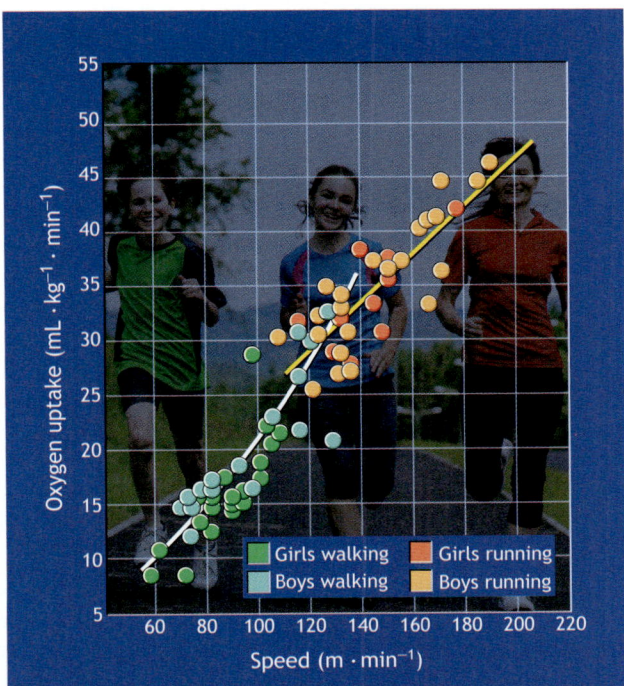

FIGURE 10.8. Relationship among walking speed and running speed and oxygen uptake for adolescent boys (N = 47) and girls (N = 35).
(Adapted with permission from Walker JL, et al. The energy cost of horizontal walking and running in adolescents. *Med Sci Sports Exerc*. 1999;31:311. Background photo: Jacek Chabraszewski/Shutterstock)

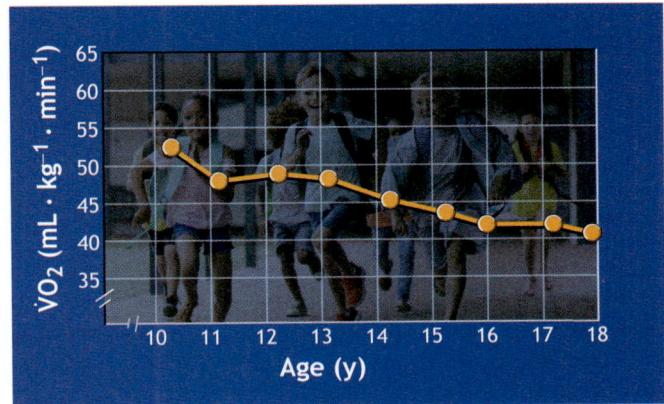

FIGURE 10.9. Age effects during childhood and adolescence on submaximal oxygen uptake during running at 202 m · min^{-1}.
(Adapted with permission from Daniels J, et al. Differences and changes in among runners 10 to 18 years of age. *Med Sci Sports*. 1978;10:200. Background photo: wavebreakmedia/Shutterstock)

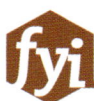

Edward Payson Weston: Walker Extraordinaire

Born in 1839, when life span averaged 40 years, Edward Payson Weston (1839–1929) in his prime would walk 50 to 100 mi a day. In 1861, he walked 453 mi from Boston to Washington, DC, in 10 days and 10 hr to attend Lincoln's inauguration on March 4. The new 16th president Abraham Lincoln gave Weston a congratulatory handshake, which inspired Weston to compete in many professional "pedestrian" competitions. These included 6 days ultramarathon races before huge crowds in New York City's Madison Square Garden and in London's Agricultural Hall. At age 71, Weston was first to walk across America from Los Angeles to New York City, covering approximately 5794 km/3600 mi in 88 days, averaging 66 km/41 mi daily. In his mid-80s, Weston still walked the equivalent of a marathon distance daily! Other notable achievements included walking 161 km/100 mi from Philadelphia to New York in less than 24 hr. At age 68, he repeated his 1867 Maine-to-Chicago walk, beating his prior time by over 24 hr. In 1909, Weston walked for 100 consecutive days, covering 6437 km/4000 mi from New York City to San Francisco following many routes not on the standard trail of that era. Weston, a professional racewalker extraordinaire and early American champion for vigorous exercise, died in 1929 at age 90, in a fate of irony being struck by a New York City taxicab that crushed his legs.

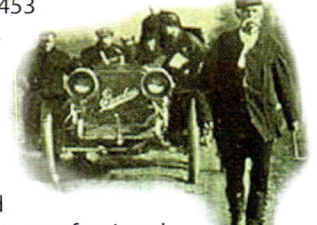

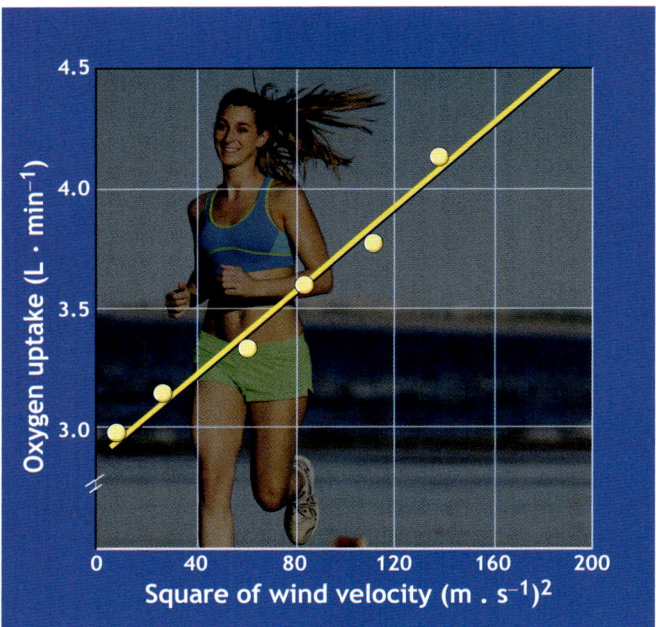

FIGURE 10.10. Oxygen uptake as a function of the square of the wind velocity while running at 15.9 km · hr^{-1} against various headwinds.
(Adapted with permission from Pugh LGCE. Oxygen intake and treadmill running with observations on the effect of air resistance. *J Physiol*. 1970;207:823.)

air or with a strong wind at one's back. Air resistance effects on energy expenditure running vary with three factors:

1. Air density
2. Runner's projected surface area
3. Wind velocity squared

Overcoming air resistance requires 3 to 9% of the total energy expenditure running in calm air depending on running speed.[69] Running into a headwind creates an additional energy "expense." **FIGURE 10.10** shows that oxygen uptake while running at 15.9 km · hr^{-1}/9.9 mph in calm conditions averaged 2.92 L · min^{-1}. This increased 5.5% to 3.09 L · min^{-1} against a 16-km · hr^{-1}/9.9 mph headwind, and further to 4.1 L · min^{-1} when running against the strongest wind (66 km · hr^{-1}/41 mph)—an additional 41% energy expenditure to maintain running velocity.

Some have argued that running with a tailwind counterbalances the negative effects of running into a headwind. This does not occur because the energy expenditure running through a headwind exceeds the reduced oxygen uptake with an equivalent wind velocity at one's back. Wind tunnel tests show that clothing modification or even trimming one's hair improves aerodynamics and reduces air resistance effects up to 6%. The reduced magnitude translates into improved running performance, particularly for elite athletes. Wind velocity has less effect on energy expenditure at higher altitudes than at sea level from the lower air density at higher elevations. Moderate altitude lowers oxygen uptake during competitive ice skating at a given speed compared with sea level.[3] An altitude effect also applies to energy expenditure running, cross-country skiing, and cycling.

Drafting: Beneficial Outcomes

The negative air resistance and headwind effects on energy expenditure running confirm the goal of running in an aerodynamically desirable position directly behind a competitor. This technique, called **drafting**, shelters the person taking advantage of it. Running 1 m/3.3 ft behind another runner at 21.6 km · hr^{-1}/13.4 mph decreases total energy expenditure by about 7%.[68] Drafting's beneficial effect also impacts cross-country skiing, short-track speed skating, and bicycling.[7,28,48,78] Bicycling at 40 km · hr^{-1} on a calm day requires about 90% of the total exercise power simply to overcome air resistance. At this speed, energy expenditure decreases 26 to 38% when a competitor closely follows another cyclist.[44]

For elite speed skaters, drafting within 1 m/3.3 ft behind the leader during controlled-pace 4-min skating trials lowers exercise heart rate and blood lactate concentration.[78] Reduced physical stress with drafting should theoretically give the competitor an additional energy reserve for the crucial sprint to the finish. When triathletes draft during the cycling leg in a sprint-distance triathlon (0.75-km/0.47-mi swim, 20-km/12.4-mi bike, 5-km/3.1-mi run), oxygen uptake, heart rate, and blood lactate concentrations remain lower than when the athletes cycle at the same speed without drafting.[38] These physiologic benefits translate into improved subsequent performance. Maximal running speed after biking with drafting translates to faster running performance than without prior drafting.

More modern equipment also plays a role. For elite cyclists, helmets now weigh under 170 g/6 oz—less than a full soda can. Helmet shape reduces drag by directing air over the head and past the rider's back when leaning forward; adding dimples to the jersey reduces the drag, and microfiber polyester garments suck moisture away from the body to facilitate a cooler and drier ride. These economy-enhancing and thermal-optimizing modifications to equipment surely benefit world class–level performance.[20]

Treadmill Versus Track Running

The treadmill provides the primary exercise mode to evaluate running physiology. One might question this procedure's validity to determine energy metabolism during running and relating it to competitive track performance. For example, does the energy required to run at a given treadmill speed equal that required to run on a track in calm weather? To answer this question, eight distance runners ran on a treadmill and track at three submaximal speeds (180 m·min^{-1}/6.7 mph, 210 m·min^{-1}/ 7.8 mph, and 260 m·min^{-1}/9.7 mph) under calm air conditions. Graded running tests determined possible differences between treadmill and track running on maximal oxygen uptake. **TABLE 10.5** summarizes the results for one submaximal speed and one maximal run test while running on the treadmill or on the track.

TABLE 10.5 No differences in metabolic responses during submaximal and maximal running on a treadmill and track

From a practical standpoint, there were no measurable differences in the energy required in submaximal running up to 286 m·min^{-1}/10.7 mph on the treadmill and track, or between $\dot{V}O_{2max}$ in both activity modes. The possibility exists that at faster speeds achieved by elite endurance runners, the impact of air resistance on a calm day increases oxygen uptake in track running compared with "stationary" treadmill running at the same fast speed. This occurs in activities requiring the athlete to move at high velocities in cycling[5] and speed skating, where the retarding effects of air resistance become considerable.

Marathon Running

The current men's fastest marathon ever run is 1:59:40 by the Kenyan, Eliud Kipchoge on October 12, 2019 in Vienna, Austria. This was the first time that a runner finished a marathon in under 2 hr. This race was part of the INEOS 1:59 Challenge and not included in any sanctioned race and thus does not count as a world record. Kipchoge carved 2 min from his own 2 hr:01 min:39 s world record set at the Berlin Marathon in 2018. His speed averaged nearly four and a half min per mile, which represents an extraordinary achievement in human running capacity. Not only does this blistering pace require a steady-rate oxygen uptake that exceeds the aerobic capacity of most male college students, it also demands that the marathoner sustain 80 to 90% $\dot{V}O_{2max}$ for over 2 hr.

Researchers measured two distance runners during a marathon to assess min-by-min and total energy expenditure.[50] They determined oxygen uptake every 3 mi using open-circuit spirometry (see Chapter 8). Marathon times were 2 hr: 36 min:34 s ($\dot{V}O_{2max}$ = 70.5 mL·kg^{-1}·min^{-1}) and 2 hr: 39 min:28 s ($\dot{V}O_{2max}$ = 73.9 mL·kg^{-1}·min^{-1}). The first runner maintained an average 16.2 km·hr^{-1}/10.0 mph speed that required an oxygen uptake equal to 80% $\dot{V}O_{2max}$. For the second runner, who averaged a "slower" 16.0 km·hr^{-1}/9.94 mph speed, the aerobic component averaged 78.3% of maximum. For both runners, the total energy required to run the marathon ranged between 2300 and 2400 kcal.

Swimming

Swimming differs in several important aspects from walking or running. One obvious difference entails energy expenditure to maintain buoyancy while simultaneously generating horizontal arm and leg movement by using either in combination or separately. Other differences include requirements to overcome **drag forces** that impede a swimmer's forward movement. The drag depends on the fluid medium and the swimmer's size, shape, and velocity. These four factors contribute to a ME in front-crawl swimming that ranges between only 5 and 9.5%.[88] *A considerably lower ME makes the energy expenditure during swimming a given distance average about four times more than the energy expenditure running the same distance.*

Measurement Methods

Subjects can hold their breath for short swims of 22.9 m/25 yd at different velocities. Net oxygen uptake during a 20- to 40-min recovery estimates energy expenditure. For longer swims, including 12- to 14-hr endurance events, energy expenditure is determined from oxygen uptake measured with open-circuit spirometry during the swim. **FIGURE 10.11A** and **B** shows the first attempts to measure oxygen uptake for a swimmer in 1919 by pioneering Swedish researcher-physicians Göran Liljestrand and Nils Stenström.[47] The swimmer used a snorkel-type mouthpiece connected to a flexible hose while the investigators rowed alongside the swimmer. Expired air was collected in canisters and taken back to the laboratory for analysis. **FIGURE 10.11C** illustrates the oxygen uptake measurement conducted in a swimming pool where the researcher walks alongside the swimmer and carries portable gas-collection equipment.[41]

In an alternate maximum capacity swimming test, the subject remains stationary while attached or tethered to a cable and pulley system by a belt worn around the waist. Periodic increases in the weight stack attached to the cable force the swimmer to exert greater effort to maintain a constant body position. In a flume or "swimming treadmill," water circulates at velocities

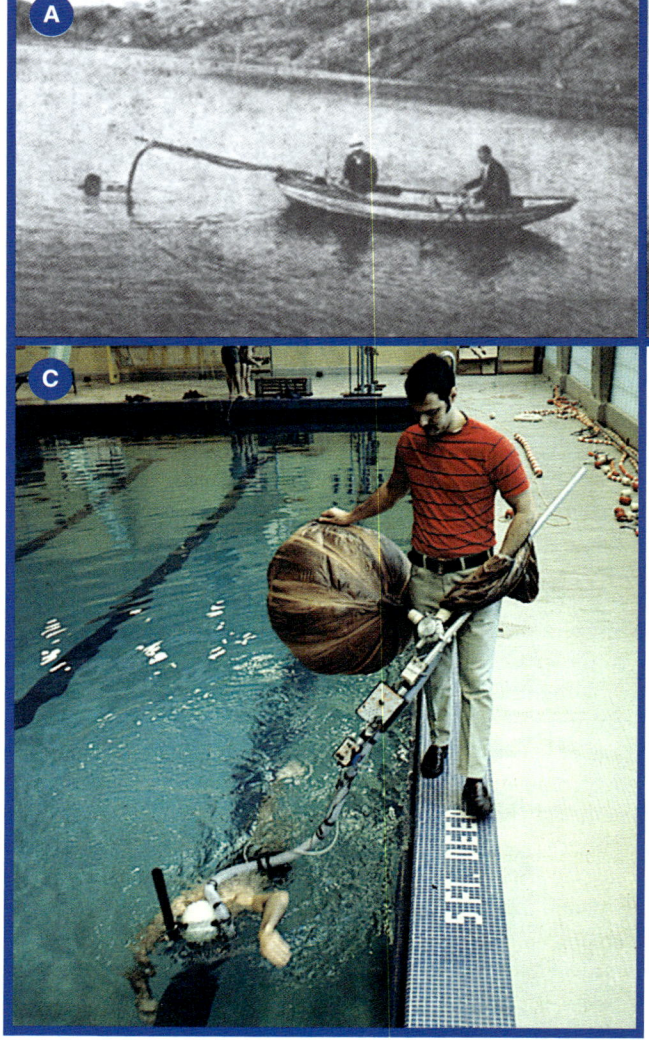

FIGURE 10.11. (A, B) First recorded open-circuit oxygen uptake spirometry measurements in 1919 during swimming and in (C) updated technique where the investigator walks alongside the swimmer to collect expired air for later laboratory analyses for oxygen uptake.
(A and B reprinted with permission from Liljestrand G, Stenström N. Studien über die physiologie des schwimmens. *Scand Arch Physiol.* 1920;39:1.)

swimming at slow velocities, but its influence increases at faster swimming speeds.

2. **Skin friction drag**—produced as water slides over the skin surface. Even at fast swimming velocities, the quantitative skin friction drag contribution to the total drag component remains small. Research supports the common practice of "shaving down" to reduce skin friction drag and thereby decrease energy expenditure.[81]

3. **Viscous pressure drag**—caused by the pressure differential created in front of and behind the swimmer, which substantially counters propulsive efforts at slow velocities. Viscous pressure drag forms adjacent to the swimmer from separation of a thin sheet of water or boundary layer. Its effect decreases for highly skilled swimmers who master streamline stroke mechanics. Such enhanced techniques reduce the separation region by moving it closer to the water's trailing edge, similar to an oar slicing through water with the blade parallel rather than perpendicular to water flow.

Drag force increases with increasing swimming speed. Generally, drag force averages 2 to 2.5 times more during swimming than passive towing.[86] Variations in swimsuit designs tend to reduce overall drag when compared to conventional suits, with positive effects noted for suits that cover the body from the shoulder to either the ankle or knee and for those that cover only the lower body.[17,57] Wet suits worn by triathletes during swimming reduce body drag by about 14%, thus lowering oxygen uptake at a given speed.[87,89] Improved swimming economy largely explains triathletes' faster swim times when varying from a slow swimming speed to near-record pace for a freestyle sprint. Aerobic capacity measurements using tethered, free, or flume swimming produce essentially identical values.[9] Any of these measurement modes objectively assess metabolic and physiologic dynamics and capacities during swimming.

Energy Expenditure and Drag

Total drag force encountered by a swimmer includes three components:

1. **Wave drag**—caused by waves that build up in front of and form hollows behind the swimmer moving through the water. This drag component does not significantly impact

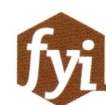 **Exercise Economy and Muscle Fiber Type**

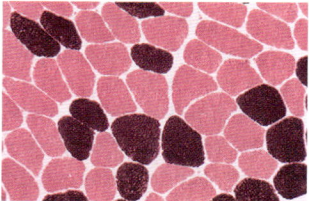

Muscle fiber type impacts the economy of cycling effort. During submaximum cycling, trained cyclists varied up to 15% in cycling economy from differences in muscle fiber types within the active muscles. Cyclists who exhibit the most economical cycling pattern possessed a greater slow-twitch (type I) percentage in their leg muscles. Type I fibers probably act with greater mechanical efficiency than the faster-acting type II fibers.

Sources:
Spiliopoulou P, et al. Effect of concurrent power training and high-intensity interval cycling on muscle morphology and performance. *J Strength Cond Res.* 2021;35(9):2464.
Methenitis S, et al. Muscle fiber composition, jumping performance, and rate of force development adaptations induced by different power training volumes in females. *Appl Physiol Nutr Metab.* 2020;45:996.

wearing wet suits. As in running, cross-country skiing, and cycling, drafting in swimming by following up to 50 cm/20 in behind a lead swimmer's toes reduces drag force, metabolic cost (by 11 to 38%), and physiologic demand[4,19] and improves economy in a subsequent cycling session.[26] This effect enables an endurance triathlete or ocean racer to conserve energy toward the end of competition. Triathletes swimming 400 m/437 yd swam the total distance 3% faster in a drafting position with lower blood lactate and stroke rate compared to swimming in the lead position.[18] Performance changes coincided with large reductions in passive drag force in the drafting position, while faster and leaner swimmers showed the greatest drag force reduction and performance improvement.

Kayaking's energy demands largely reflect the resistance provided by the water to the craft's forward movement. Consequently, drafting or "wash riding" behind a competitor reduces the energy requirements of paddling between 18 and 32%.[65] The assist to forward movement provided by the wash generated by the lead boat improves kayaking economy. This effect decreases resistance and water pressure that impacts boat movement.

Energy Expenditure, Swimming Velocity, and Skill

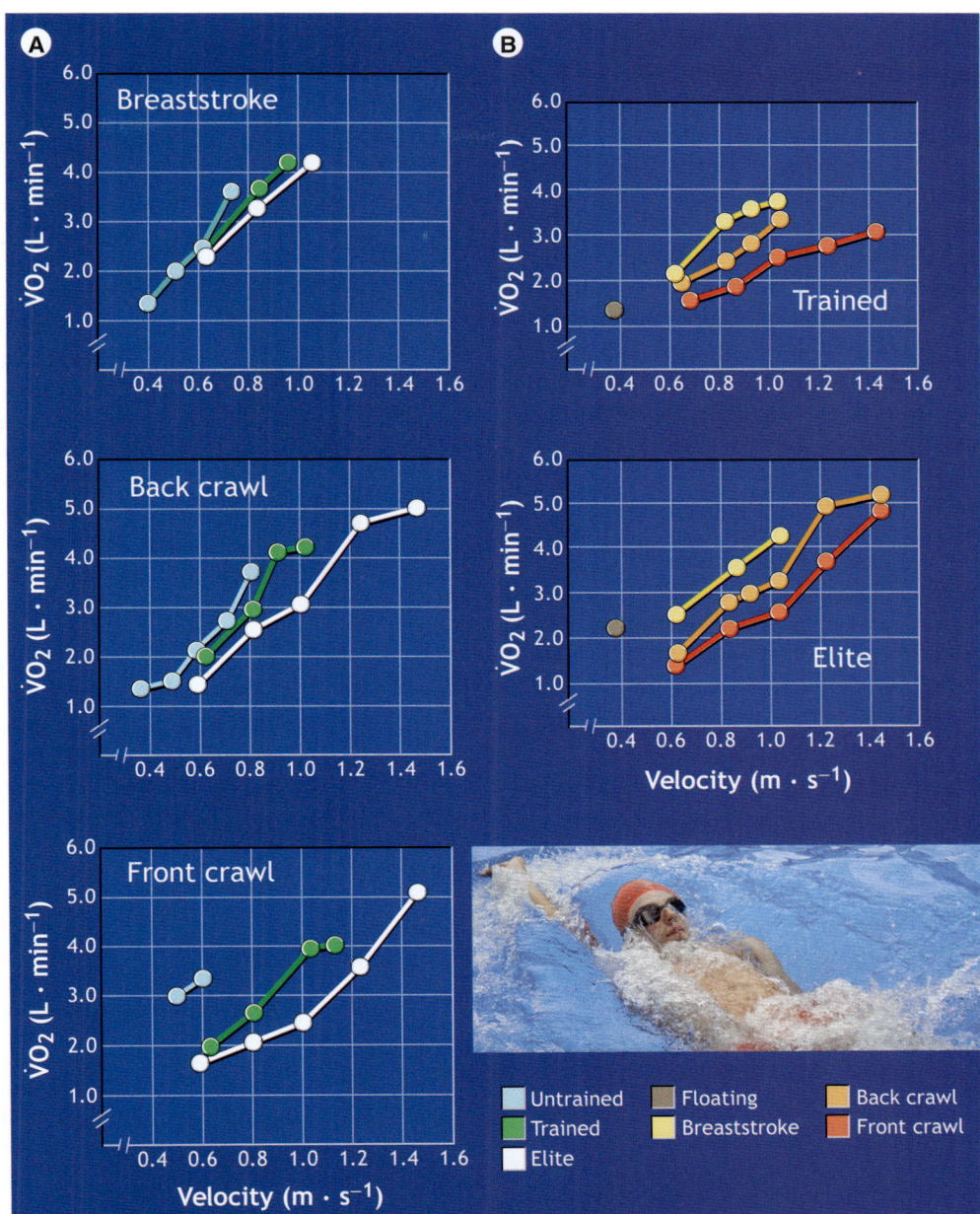

FIGURE 10.12. **(A)** Oxygen uptake related to swimming velocity for the breaststroke, front crawl, and back crawl in subjects at three skill levels. **(B)** Oxygen uptake for two trained swimmers during three competitive strokes.
(Adapted with permission from Holmér I. Oxygen uptake during swimming in man. *J Appl Physiol*. 1972;33:502. Photo: Albert Garrido/Shutterstock.)

Elite swimmers swim a particular stroke at a given velocity with greater economy than less trained or recreational swimmers. Highly skilled swimmers use more of the energy they generate per stroke to overcome drag forces, so they cover a greater distance per stroke than less skilled swimmers who in effect "waste" considerable energy in moving the water during the swim. **FIGURE 10.12A** compares three swimming ability levels for oxygen uptake and velocity in the breaststroke, back crawl, and front crawl. One subject, a recreational swimmer, did not participate in swim training; the trained subject, a top Swedish swimmer, swam on a daily basis; the elite swimmer was a European champion. Except during the breaststroke, the elite swimmer had a lower oxygen uptake at a given speed than trained and untrained swimmers. Figure 10.12B illustrates that the breaststroke for the trained swimmers required greater oxygen uptake at any speed, followed by the backstroke, with the front crawl being the least "expensive" among the three strokes. The marked accelerations and decelerations within each stroke cycle cause the energy expended for the butterfly and breaststroke to nearly double compared to front and back crawl at the same speeds.[85] At comparable speeds sustained aerobically, the energy expenditure in surface swimming with fins averaged about 40% lower than swimming without them.[90]

Water Temperature Effects

Relatively, cold water places the swimmer under thermal stress and elicits different metabolic and cardiovascular adjustments than swimming in warmer water. These responses primarily maintain a stable core temperature by compensating for considerable heat loss, particularly at water temperatures below 25°C/77°F. Body heat loss occurs most readily in lean swimmers who lack the insulatory benefits from subcutaneous fat.

FIGURE 10.13 illustrates oxygen uptake during breaststroke swimming at 18°C/64.4°F, 26°C/78.8°F, and 33°C/91.4°F. Cold water produced the highest oxygen uptakes at all swimming speeds. The body begins to shiver in cold water to regulate core temperature, which accounts for the higher energy expenditure when swimming in colder water temperatures. For individuals with an average body fat percentage, optimal water temperature for competitive swimming ranges between 28°C/82°F and 30°C/86°F. Within this range, metabolic heat generated during this exercise mode readily transfers to the water. Nonetheless, the heat flow gradient from the body is not large enough to stimulate shivering (which would increase energy metabolism) or reduce core temperature.

Buoyancy: Men Versus Women

Women at all ages possess a higher body fat percentage than men. Fat readily floats and muscle and bone sink in water, allowing a female to gain a hydrodynamic lift and expend less energy to stay afloat than a male.[92] More than likely, gender differences in percentage body fat and thus body **buoyancy** partially explain a female's greater swimming economy. For example, females swim a given distance at about 30% lower total energy expenditure than males.[93,94] Expressed another way, females achieve higher swimming velocities than males at the same energy expenditure.

Females also present with a greater peripheral body fat distribution. This causes their legs and arms to float relatively high in water, making them swim more streamlined. In contrast, males leaner legs tend to swing down and float lower in the water.[14] Lowering the legs to a deeper position increases body drag and reduces swimming economy. Enhanced flotation and the females' smaller body size, which also reduces drag, contribute to gender difference in swimming economy.[85,86] Females potential hydrodynamic benefits become evident during longer distance ocean swims because swimming economy and body insulation contribute to success. For example, the female record to swim the 21-mi/33.8-km English Channel from England to France equals 7 hr 25 min 15 s (Yvetta Hlavacova; Czech Republic, 2006). For males, the record (Trent Grimsey; Australia, 2012) equals 6 hr 55 min, only a 6.8% difference (www.dover.uk.com/channel-swimming/records). The first female to successfully cross the Channel in 1926 swam 35% faster than the first male to complete the swim 50 years earlier.

Some Trained Women Actually Swim Faster Than Some Trained Men!

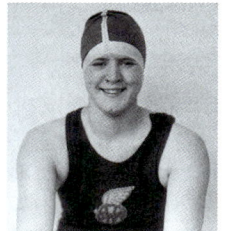

In several instances, women actually swim faster than men (www.bbc.com/news/world-49284389). For example, American Gertrude Ederle (1905–2003; www.britannica.com/biography/Gertrude-Ederle; www.bbc.co.uk/newsround/49483420) achieved a milestone by becoming the first woman without a life vest to swim the English Channel on August 6, 1926, in 14 hr 31 min. Her time was faster by more than 2 hr than British steamship Captain Matthew Webb (1848–1883), the first man to complete the swim without a vest 51 years earlier in 1875 in 21 hr 45 min. Muscle fiber type, body fat and its distribution, buoyancy, and insulation are all factors that could account for the considerable success of women in long-distance ocean swimming.

Endurance Swimmers

Distance swimming in ocean water poses a severe metabolic and physiologic challenge. A study of nine English Channel swimmers included measurements taken under race conditions in a saltwater pool at swimming speeds that ranged from

FIGURE 10.13. Energy expenditure related to swimming velocity for the breaststroke at three water temperatures. (Adapted with permission from Nadel ER, et al. Energy exchanges of swimming man. J Appl Physiol. 1974;36:465. Background photo: Erich Sacco/Shutterstock)

2.6 to 4.9 km·hr⁻¹/1.6 to 3.04 mph.⁷⁰ During the race, competitors maintained a constant stroke rate and pace until the last few hours, when fatigue set in. From detailed observations in one male swimmer, the average 2.85 km·hr⁻¹/1.77 mph speed during a 12-hr swim required an average 1.7 L·min⁻¹ oxygen uptake or an equivalent 8.5 kcal·min⁻¹ energy expenditure. The gross caloric expenditure for the 12-hr swim approximated 6120 kcal (8.5 kcal × 60 min × 12 h). The net energy expenditure to swim the English Channel, assuming a 1.2 kcal·min⁻¹ (0.260 L O_2·min⁻¹) resting energy expenditure, exceeds 5200 kcal or approximately twice the calories of running a marathon.

INTEGRATIVE QUESTION

Does swim training improve swimming economy more than run training improves running economy? Why or why not?

Summary

1. Total or gross energy expenditure includes the resting energy requirement.
2. Net energy expenditure represents activity energy expenditure excluding the resting value.
3. Movement economy refers to the oxygen uptake during steady-rate exercise.
4. Mechanical efficiency evaluates the relationship between work accomplished and energy expended doing the work.
5. Walking, running, and cycling produce MEs between 20 and 25%.
6. Efficiencies decrease below 20% for activities with considerable resistance to movement (drag).
7. A linear relationship exists between walking speed and oxygen uptake at normal walking speeds. Walking on sand requires about twice the energy as walking on firm surfaces.
8. A proportionately larger energy expenditure exists for heavier persons during weight-bearing physical activities.
9. Running becomes more economical than walking at speeds that exceed 8 km·hr⁻¹/5.0 mph.
10. Handheld and ankle weights can increase walking energy expenditure to values similar to running.
11. Net energy expenditure running a given distance at steady-rate oxygen uptake remains about the same regardless of running speed.
12. Net energy expenditure during horizontal running approximates 1 kcal·kg⁻¹·km⁻¹.
13. Shortening running stride and increasing stride frequency to maintain a constant running speed requires less energy than lengthening stride and reducing frequency.
14. An individual subconsciously "selects" an optimal stride length and frequency combination to achieve minimum effort.
15. Energy expended to overcome air resistance running in calm air includes 3 to 9% of the total energy expended.
16. Children generally require more oxygen to transport their body mass while running than do adults.
17. Running a given distance or speed on a treadmill requires similar energy output as running on a track under identical environmental conditions.
18. About four times more energy is expended to swim a set distance than to run the same distance.
19. Elite swimmers expend fewer calories to swim a given stroke at any velocity than less skilled counterparts.
20. Significant gender differences exist in body drag, ME, and net oxygen uptake during swimming.
21. Females swim a given distance at approximately 30% lower energy expenditure than males.
22. The net energy expenditure to swim the English Channel exceeds 5200 kcal or approximately twice the calories to complete a marathon run.

Key Terms

Buoyancy: Upward force exerted by a fluid that opposes an immersed object's weight

Delta efficiency: Difference in work output between two exercise levels ÷ difference in energy expended between two exercise levels × 100

Drafting: Technique to follow directly behind a competitor to counter the negative effects on energy cost imposed by air, oncoming headwind, or water resistance

Drag forces: Forces that slow down a swimmer's movement in the water

External work output: Force acting through a vertical distance (F × D), usually recorded as foot-pounds (ft-lb) or kilogram-meters (kg-m) and expressed in kcal units (1 kcal = 3087 ft-lb, or 426.4 kg-m in a perfect machine without loss in efficiency)

Gross mechanical efficiency: Total chemical energy percentage expended that contributes to external work, with the remainder lost as heat; includes energy expended during rest

Mechanical efficiency (ME): Chemical energy expended as a percentage (denominator) that contributes to external work output (numerator); Work output ÷ Energy expended × 100

Movement economy: Energy to perform a steady-rate submaximal task, measured as $\dot{V}O_2$ in mL·kg⁻¹·min⁻¹

Negative work: Work that occurs when the body's center of mass moves in a downward vertical direction with each step cycle, (downhill walking or running)

Net mechanical efficiency: Total oxygen uptake excluding resting value converted to kilocalories minus resting oxygen uptake (kcal) for the equivalent physical activity time period

Skin friction drag: Force against a swimmer produced as water slides over the skin surface

Viscous pressure drag: Force against a swimmer caused by the pressure differential created in front of and behind the swimmer to substantially counter propulsive efforts at slow swim velocities

Wave drag: Force against a swimmer caused by waves that build up in front of and form hollows behind the swimmer at slow swim velocities

> References are available online at Lippincott Connect.

Additional References

Baek S, Ha Y. Estimation of energy expenditure of Nordic walking: a crossover trial. *BMC Sports Sci Med Rehabil.* 2021;13:14.

Bohm S, et al. Enthalpy efficiency of the soleus muscle contributes to improvements in running economy. *Proc Biol Sci.* 2021;288:20202784.

Bohm S, et al. Muscle-specific economy of force generation and efficiency of work production during human running. *Elife.* 2021;10:e67182.

Büchel D, et al. Exploring intensity-dependent modulations in EEG resting-state network efficiency induced by exercise. *Eur J Appl Physiol.* 2021;121:2423.

Charles JP, et al. Foot anatomy, walking energetics, and the evolution of human bipedalism. *J Hum Evol.* 2021;156:103014.

Gemmell BJ, et al. The most efficient metazoan swimmer creates a 'virtual wall' to enhance performance. *Proc Biol Sci.* 2021;288:20202494.

Gupta S, Raja K. Energy Expenditure Index as a measure of efficiency of walking on outdoor uneven surface in individuals with cerebral palsy. *Disabil Rehabil.* 2021;43:568.

Hamidi Rad M, et al. A novel macro–micro approach for swimming analysis in main swimming techniques using IMU sensors. *Front Bioeng Biotechnol.* 2021;8:597738.

Lazzari CD, et al. Virtual cycling effort is dependent on power update rate. *Eur J Sport Sci.* 2020;20:831.

Li S, et al. Comparison of energy expenditure and substrate metabolism during overground and motorized treadmill running in Chinese middle-aged women. *Sci Rep.* 2020;10:1815.

Liu F, et al. Association between walking energetics and fragmented physical activity in mid- to late-life. *J Gerontol A Biol Sci Med Sci.* 2021;76:e281.

Miao J, et al. Enhancing swimming performance by optimizing structure of helical swimmers. *Sensors (Basel).* 2021;21:494.

Post AK, et al. Multigenerational performance development of male and female top-elite swimmers-A global study of the 100-m freestyle event. *Scand J Med Sci Sports.* 2020;30:564.

Sasada S, et al. Arm cycling increases the short-latency reflex from ankle dorsiflexor afferents to knee extensor muscles. *J Neurophysiol.* 2021;125:110.

Slater L, et al. Improving gait efficiency to increase movement and physical activity - The impact of abnormal gait patterns and strategies to correct. *Prog Cardiovasc Dis.* 2021;64:83.

Yuan J, et al. Cognitive measures during walking with and without lower-limb prosthesis: protocol for a scoping review. *BMJ Open.* 2021;11:e039975.

Zamparo P, et al. The energy cost of swimming and its determinants. *Eur J Appl Physiol.* 2020;120:41.

Table 10.1 Energy Expenditure (kcal · min^{-1}) Prediction from Level Walking Speed and Body Mass

Walking Speed		Body Mass						
mph	km · hr^{-1}	36 kg/ 80 lb	45 kg/ 100 lb	54 kg/ 120 lb	64 kg/ 140 lb	73 kg/ 160 lb	82 kg/ 180 lb	91 kg/ 200 lb
2.0	3.22	1.9	2.2	2.6	2.9	3.2	3.5	3.8
2.5	4.02	2.3	2.7	3.1	3.5	3.8	4.2	4.5
3.0	4.83	2.7	3.1	3.6	4.0	4.4	4.8	5.3
3.5	5.63	3.1	3.6	4.2	4.6	5.0	5.4	6.1
4.0	6.44	3.5	4.1	4.7	5.2	5.8	6.4	7.0

Note: How to use the table: A 54-kg/120 lb person who walks at 3.0 mph (4.83 km · hr^{-1}) expends 3.6 kcal · min^{-1} or 216 kcal in a 60-min walk (3.6 × 60).
Data from Passmore R, Durnin JVGA. Human energy expenditure. *Physiol Rev.* 1955;35:801.

Table 10.2 Different Terrain Effects on Energy Expenditure Walking at 5.6 km·hr⁻¹/3.2 mph and 5.6 km·hr⁻¹/3.5 mph

Terrain	Correction Factor
Paved road (similar to grass track)	0.0
Plowed field	1.5
Hard snow	1.6
Sand dune	1.8

Note: The correction factor is a multiple for energy expenditure walking on a paved road or grass track. For example, the walking energy expenditure in a plowed field equals 1.5 times that walking on a paved road. Divide by 1.6 to convert to mph.
First entry: Data from Passmore R, Durnin JVGA. Human energy expenditure. *Physiol Rev*. 1955;35:801.
Last three entries: Data from Givoni B, Goldman RF. Predicting metabolic energy cost. *J Appl Physiol*. 1971;30:429.

Table 10.3 Net Energy Expenditure During Horizontal Running Per Hour Related to Velocity and Body Mass[a]

Body Mass (kg)	(lb)	km·hr⁻¹ / min·mi⁻¹ / kcal·mi⁻¹[b]	8 / 4.97 / 12:00	9 / 5.60 / 10:43	10 / 6.20 / 9:41	11 / 6.84 / 8:46	12 / 7.46 / 8:02	13 / 8.08 / 7:26	14 / 8.70 / 6:54	15 / 9.32 / 6:26	16 / 9.94 / 6:02
50	110	**80**	400	450	500	550	600	650	700	750	800
54	119	**86**	432	486	540	594	648	702	756	810	864
58	128	**93**	464	522	580	638	696	754	812	870	928
62	137	**99**	496	558	620	682	744	806	868	930	992
66	146	**106**	528	594	660	726	792	858	924	990	1056
70	154	**112**	560	630	700	770	840	910	980	1050	1120
74	163	**118**	592	666	740	814	888	962	1036	1110	1184
78	172	**125**	624	702	780	858	936	1014	1092	1170	1248
82	181	**131**	656	738	820	902	984	1066	1148	1230	1312
86	190	**138**	688	774	860	946	1032	1118	1204	1290	1376
90	199	**144**	720	810	900	990	1080	1170	1260	1350	1440
94	207	**150**	752	846	940	1034	1128	1222	1316	1410	1504
98	216	**157**	784	882	980	1078	1176	1274	1372	1470	1568
102	225	**163**	816	918	1020	1122	1224	1326	1428	1530	1632
106	234	**170**	848	954	1060	1166	1272	1378	1484	1590	1696

[a]Interpret the table as follows: For a 50-kg/110 lb person, the net energy expenditure for running 1 hr at 8 km·hr⁻¹ or 4.97 mph equals 400 kcal; this speed represents a 12-min per mi pace. Thus, 5 mi would be run in 1 hr and 400 kcal would be expended. Increasing the pace to 12 km·hr⁻¹ expends 600 kcal during the 1-hr training run. The values in **boldface type** are *net* calories expended to run 1 mi for a given body mass independent of running speed.
[b]Running speeds are expressed as kilometers per hour (Km·hr⁻¹, miles per hour (mph), and minutes required to complete each mile (min per mile).

Table 10.4 Energy Requirements (METs) for Horizontal and Grade Walking and Running on a Solid Surface

		\multicolumn{6}{c}{Horizontal and Grade Walking}					
% Grade	mph	1.7	2.0	2.5	3.0	3.4	3.75
	m · min⁻¹	45.6	53.7	67.0	80.5	91.2	100.5
0		2.3	2.5	2.9	3.3	3.6	3.9
2.5		2.9	3.2	3.8	4.3	4.8	5.2
5.0		3.5	3.9	4.6	5.4	5.9	6.5
7.5		4.1	4.6	5.5	6.4	7.1	7.8
10.0		4.6	5.3	6.3	7.4	8.3	9.1
12.5		5.2	6.0	7.2	8.5	9.5	10.4
15.0		5.8	6.6	8.1	9.5	10.6	11.7
17.5		6.4	7.3	8.9	10.5	11.8	12.9
20.0		7.0	8.0	9.8	11.6	13.0	14.2
22.5		7.6	8.7	10.6	12.6	14.2	15.5
25.0		8.2	9.4	11.5	13.6	15.3	16.8

		\multicolumn{7}{c}{Horizontal and Grade Jogging/Running}						
% Grade	mph	5	6	7	7.5	8	9	10
	m · min⁻¹	134	161	188	201	215	241	268
0		8.6	10.2	11.7	12.5	13.3	14.8	16.3
2.5		10.3	12.3	14.1	15.1	16.1	17.9	19.7
5.0		12.0	14.3	16.5	17.7	18.8		
7.5		13.9	16.4	18.9				
10.0		15.5	18.5					

Adapted with permission from *ACSM Guidelines for Exercise Testing and Prescription*. 10th ed. Baltimore: Lippincott Williams & Wilkins; 2017.

Table 10.5 No Differences in Metabolic Responses During Submaximal and Maximal Running on a Treadmill and Track

Measurement	Treadmill	Track	Difference
Submaximum Exercise			
Oxygen uptake, mL · kg⁻¹ · min⁻¹	42.2	42.7	0.5
Respiratory exchange ratio	0.89	0.87	−0.02
Running speed, m · min⁻¹	213.7	216.8	3.1
Maximum Exercise			
Oxygen uptake, L · min⁻¹	4.40	4.44	0.04
mL · kg⁻¹ · min⁻¹	66.9	66.3	−0.6
Ventilation, L · min⁻¹, BTPS	142.5	146.5	4.0
Respiratory exchange ratio	1.15	1.11	0.04

BTPS = body temperature (37°C), ambient pressure, and gas saturated with water vapor.
Data from McMiken DF, Daniels JT. Aerobic requirements and maximum aerobic power in treadmill and track running. *Med Sci Sports*. 1976;8:14.

CHAPTER 11
Individual Differences and Measuring Energy Capacities

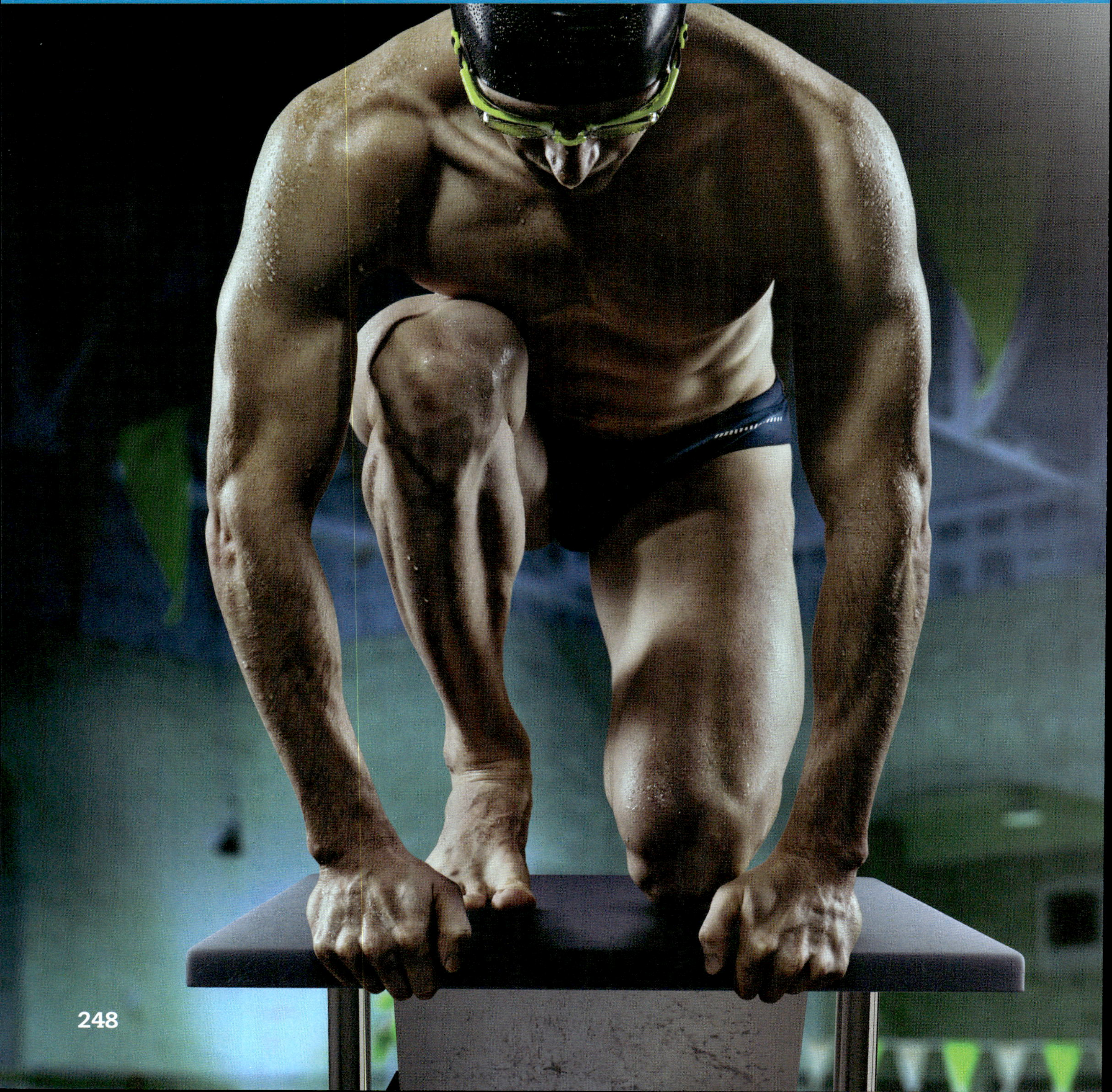

Chapter Objectives

- Explain specificity and generality applied to physical performance and physiologic functions
- Outline the anaerobic-to-aerobic exercise energy transfer continuum
- Describe two practical "field tests" to measure the immediate energy system's power output capacity
- Describe a common test to assess the short-term energy system's power output capacity
- Explain how motivation, buffering, and physical training impact the glycolytic energy pathway
- Define maximum oxygen uptake ($\dot{V}O_{2max}$) and its physiologic significance
- Differentiate between $\dot{V}O_{2max}$ and peak oxygen uptake
- Define graded exercise test and list two criteria to indicate achieving a "true" $\dot{V}O_{2max}$
- Outline three common treadmill protocols to assess $\dot{V}O_{2max}$
- Explain how activity mode, heredity, training state, gender, body composition, and age affect $\dot{V}O_{2max}$
- Describe a walking field test to predict $\dot{V}O_{2max}$
- List three valid assumptive requirements to predict $\dot{V}O_{2max}$ from submaximal exercise heart rate

Ancillaries at-a-Glance

Visit Lippincott Connect to access the following resources.

- References: Chapter 11
- Focus on Research: An important Measure of Cardiorespiratory Functional Capacity

Metabolic Capacity and Exercise Performance: Specificity Versus Generality

The body draws useful energy from different metabolic pathways, yet considerable variability exists among individuals in the capacity of each energy transfer type. Individual variability serves as a cornerstone for the concept of **individual differences** in metabolic capacity. A large $\dot{V}O_{2max}$ during running, for example, does not necessarily ensure a similarly large $\dot{V}O_{2max}$ when using the different muscle groups required in swimming and rowing. That some individuals with exceptional aerobic power in one activity possess above-average aerobic power in other activities illustrates the **generality principle** of metabolic functions.

The nonoverlapped areas in **FIGURE 11.1** represent metabolic function specificity among the body's three energy systems, while the three overlapped portions represent generality. In the broadest sense, specificity indicates a low likelihood for an individual to excel in each of a particular sport's sprint, middle-distance, and long-distance competitions. In a narrow definition of metabolic and physiologic specificity, most individuals do not possess an equally high-energy-generating capacity for aerobic activities as different as running (lower body) and swimming or arm-crank (upper body) exercises.

Based on the **specificity concept**, training to achieve a high aerobic power or $\dot{V}O_{2max}$ contributes little to one's capacity to generate energy anaerobically, and vice versa. A high specificity component also exists for physical training effects on neuromuscular movement patterning. The terms "speed," "power," and "endurance" must be applied precisely within the specific movement patterns and specific metabolic and physiologic requirements of the activity.

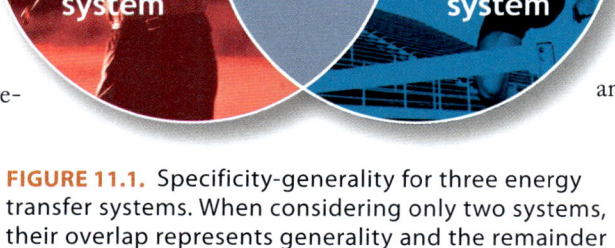

FIGURE 11.1. Specificity-generality for three energy transfer systems. When considering only two systems, their overlap represents generality and the remainder specificity.

This chapter assesses the three energy transfer systems discussed in Chapters 6 and 7, with emphasis on individual differences, specificity, and appropriate measurement.

IQ? INTEGRATIVE QUESTION

Why should a triathlete train in each of the sport's three events?

Overview: Exercise Energy Transfer Capacity

The immediate and short-term energy systems predominantly power by anaerobic processes all-out movements for up to 2 min. A greater reliance on anaerobic energy exists for fast, short-duration movements or under increasing resistance to movement at a given speed.

FIGURE 11.2 illustrates the relative activation of the anaerobic and aerobic energy transfer systems for different durations of all-out effort. When movement begins at either fast or slow speed, intramuscular high-energy phosphates adenosine triphosphate (ATP) and phosphocreatine (PCr) provide immediate energy to power muscle action. After the first few seconds, the glycolytic pathway generates an increasingly greater total energy percentage required for continuous ATP resynthesis. Continued activity places progressively greater demands on the long-term aerobic system. All physical activities and sports lend themselves to classification based on an immediate-to-glycolytic-to-aerobic continuum. Some activities rely predominantly on a single energy transfer system, whereas most require activating more than one energy system depending on activity intensity and duration. Performing at higher intensity but shorter duration markedly increases demand on anaerobic energy transfer. The fact that specific metabolic requirements in intense activities vary with the duration of effort and because of the highly specific nature of one's metabolic capacity (see nonoverlapped areas in Fig. 11.1) largely explain why athletes have difficulty becoming proficient in multiple events such as sprint, middle-distance, endurance, and ultraendurance running.

Anaerobic Function Physiologic and Performance Tests

Two general approaches assess anaerobic power and capacity for both the immediate and short-term energy systems' response to physical activity:

1. Physiologic tests that measure changes in ATP and PCr levels metabolized or lactate produced from a preponderance of anaerobic metabolism
2. Performance tests that quantify external work performed or power generated during short-duration, intense activity that demands high levels of anaerobic energy transfer

Both approaches assume that short-duration, intense activity could not occur without a high anaerobic energy

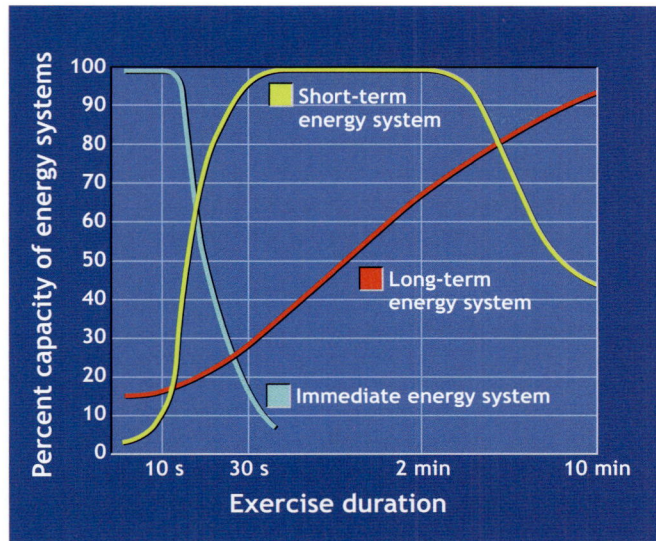

FIGURE 11.2. Three systems of energy transfer and percentage total capacity during all-out physical activity for different durations.

transfer level; thus, measuring work or power indirectly can gauge or predict anaerobic energy utilization.

Anaerobic Energy Transfer: The Immediate and Short-Term Energy Systems

Performance Tests to Assess the Immediate Energy System

Football, weightlifting, and other short-duration, maximal-effort activities that require rapid energy release rely nearly exclusively on energy supplied from the intramuscular high-energy phosphates. Performance tests that maximally activate the **ATP-PCr energy system** serve as practical field tests to evaluate the capacity for "immediate" energy transfer. Two assumptions underlie performance test scores to infer the high-energy phosphate's power-generating capacity:

1. All ATP at maximal power output regenerates via ATP-PCr hydrolysis
2. Adequate ATP and PCr exist to support maximal effort for about 6-s duration

The term *power test* generally describes these brief maximal power output measurements. Power in this context refers to the time-rate to accomplish work as follows:

$$P = (F \times D) \div T$$

where **F** equals *force* generated, **D** equals *distance* the force moves, and **T** represents exercise *time* or duration. Power is expressed in **watts**: 1 watt equals 0.73756 ft-lb · s^{-1}, 0.01433 kcal · min^{-1}, 1.341 × 10^{-3} hp (or 0.0013 hp), or 6.12 kg-m · min^{-1}.

Stair-Sprinting Power Tests

FIGURE 11.3 illustrates a practical way to assess high-energy phosphate power output by recording the time required to run up a staircase, three steps at a time, as fast as possible. External work accomplished includes the total vertical distance traversed up the stairs, usually 1.05 m for six stairs. For example, when a 65-kg/143-lb woman traverses six steps in 0.52 s, power computes as follows:

$$\text{Power} = (65 \text{ kg} \times 1.05) \div 0.52 \text{ s}$$
$$= 131.3 \text{ kg-m} \cdot \text{s}^{-1} \text{ (1288 watts)}$$

Based on the equation, body mass influences power calculations in stair-sprinting tests because a heavier person who achieves the same speed as a lighter counterpart would achieve a higher power score. This implies that the heavier person possesses a more highly developed immediate energy system. Unfortunately, no direct evidence justifies this conclusion; athletes, coaches, and trainers must use care interpreting differences in stair-sprinting power scores and inferring individual differences in ATP-PCr energy transfer capacity among individuals who differ in body weight. *The test should be used in one of two ways:*

1. With individuals of similar body mass (within about 2 kg/4.5 lb)
2. With the same individuals before and after specific training designed to develop leg power output from the immediate energy system (assuming no change in body mass)

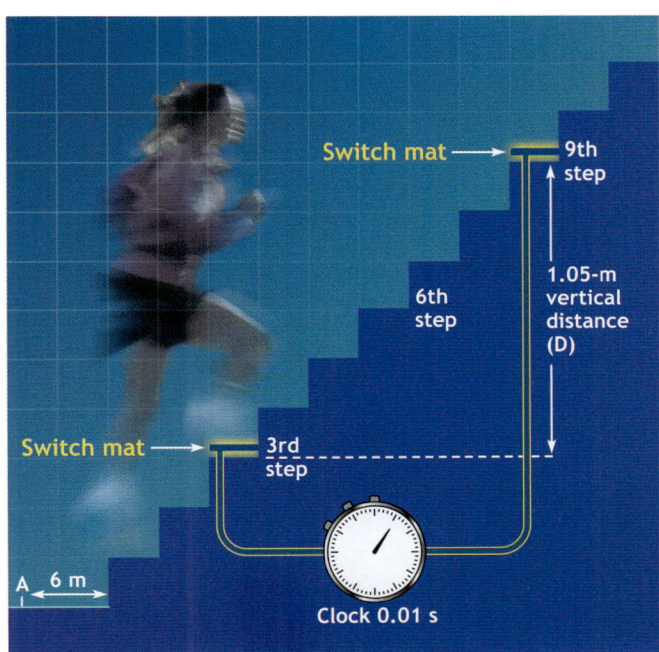

FIGURE 11.3. Stair-sprinting power test. The subject begins at point A (lower left) and runs as fast as possible up a flight of stairs, taking three steps at a time. Electric switch mats placed on the steps record the time needed to cover the distance between stairs 3 and 9 to the nearest 0.01 s. Power output equals the product of the subject's body mass (F) and vertical distance covered (D), divided by the time (T).

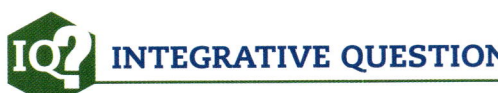

INTEGRATIVE QUESTION

Considering training specificity, how would you test the immediate energy system power output capacity for volleyball players, swimmers, and soccer players?

Jumping-Power Tests

The popular vertical jump-and-reach test or a standing broad jump often appear in physical fitness test batteries to measure immediate energy power output. The vertical jump score reflects the difference between a person's standing reach and maximal vertical jump-and-touch height (see In a Practical Sense: Predicting Power with a Vertical Jump Test). The broad jump score consists of the horizontal distance traversed in a leap from a semi-crouched position. Both tests purport to measure leg power, but they probably fail to achieve this goal. For example, jump tests generate power to propel the body from the crouched position only while the feet maintain contact with the surface. *This extremely brief muscle activation period probably does not adequately evaluate a person's maximal ATP/PCr energy transfer capacity.* Also, we are aware of no data to show a relationship between jump test scores and actual ATP-PCr levels or depletion patterns in the primary muscles activated during the jump.

Other Power Performance Tests

Figure 11.2 suggests that any all-out 6- to 8-s physical effort probably reflects a person's capacity for immediate power performance from high-energy phosphates in the specific muscles activated. Other possible tests include sprint running or cycling, brief shuttle runs, and localized movements produced by arm-cranking or leg movements.

In a Practical Sense

Predicting Power with a Vertical Jump Test

Peak anaerobic power output for brief duration underlies success in many sport activities. The vertical jump test has become a widely used measure to express "explosive" or peak anaerobic power.

VERTICAL JUMP TEST

The vertical jump measures the highest distance jumped from a semi-crouched position with this specific protocol:

1. Establish standing reach height. The individual stands with the shoulder adjacent to a wall with the feet flat on the floor or before reaching up as high as possible to touch the wall with the longest finger. Measure the distance (in cm) from the wall mark to the floor.
2. Bend the knees to roughly a 90° angle, and place both arms back in a winged position.
3. Thrust forward and upward, touching as high as possible on the wall; no foot or leg movement is permitted before jumping.
4. Perform three trials of the jump test, and use the highest score to represent the individual's "best" vertical jump height.
5. Compute the vertical jump height as the difference between the standing reach height and the vertical jump height in centimeters.

ANAEROBIC POWER OUTPUT EQUATION

The following equation applies to males and females for predicting peak anaerobic power output from the immediate energy system in watts (PAP_W) from vertical jump height in cm (VJ_{cm}) and body weight in kg (BW_{kg}).

$$PAP_W = (60.7 \times VJ_{cm}) + (45.3 \times BW_{kg}) - 2055$$

Example

A 21-year-old man weighing 78 kg records a vertical jump height of 43 cm (standing reach height = 185 cm; vertical jump height = 228 cm); predict peak anaerobic power output in watts.

$$PAP_W = (60.7 \times VJ_{cm}) + (45.3 \times BW_{kg}) - 2055$$
$$PAP_W = (60.7 \times 43\ cm) + (45.3 \times 78\ kg) - 2055 = 4088.5\ W$$

Applicability to Males and Females

For comparison purposes, average peak power output measured with this protocol averages 4620.2 W (SD = ±822.5 W) for males and 2993.7 W (SD = ±542.9 W) for females.

Sources:
Ferland PM, et al. Validation of the alpine skiing 90 seconds box jump field test and prediction of power output. *J Sports Med Phys Fitness.* 2021;61:3803.
Mohammadian M, Saet al. The relationship between vertical stiffness during bilateral and unilateral hopping tests performed with different strategies and vertical jump performances. *Eur J Sport Sci.* 2021:18.
Parmar A, et al. Concurrent validity of the portable gFlight system compared to a force plate to measure jump performance variables. *Physiol Meas.* 2021;42:015003.

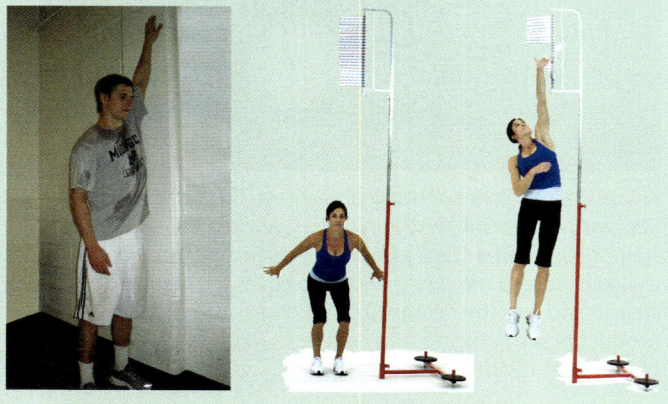

Interrelationships Among Power Performance Tests

If the various power tests measure the same "general" metabolic capacity, then individuals who perform best on one test should rank correspondingly high on a second or third different test.

Unfortunately, this does not usually occur to any great extent. Although some individuals who score well on one power performance test tend to score well on another test, a poor relationship generally exists.[88] The unnumbered table below represents data from 31 male college-age students from one of our laboratories shows the interrelationship, expressed statistically as a correlation coefficient, between several tests purported to measure immediate energy power output. The relationship ranges from poor to good, depending on the test. The fairly strong relationship between stair-sprinting power test scores and 40-yard dash scores ($r = -0.88$) indicates that one can obtain almost the same information on short-term power performance through sprint running on a track as the more elaborate procedures required in the stair sprint.

Variable	Jump and Reach	Stair-Sprinting
40-yard dash	−0.48	−0.88
Jump and reach	—	−0.31

Data from the Applied Physiology Laboratory, University of Michigan (N = 31 males).
Note: Negative correlations mean faster times (lower scores) associate with higher jumps or greater power outputs.

Several factors explain relatively low relationships among the other power test scores. First, human exercise performance remains highly task specific. This means that the best sprint runner does not necessarily rank as the best sprint swimmer, sprint cyclist, "stair sprinter," or "arm cranker." While it is true that identical metabolic reactions generate energy to power each performance, these reactions occur within the specific muscles activated by exercise. Each specific test also requires different neuromuscular and skill components that introduce variability and specificity into test scores.

Power tests offer an excellent way for self-testing and motivation and serve as a modality to train the immediate energy system. For example, football coaches use the 40-yard dash for power training and to evaluate "football speed." Forty-yard dash test scores may provide relevant information concerning "speed" in football, even though no data exist to quantify how a 40-yard sprint in a straight line relates to all of the complex skills and movements involved in game performance or as a valid way to gauge overall football ability. A shorter 20-yd run test with multiple changes in direction would probably provide a more appropriate, task-specific football performance measure.

Physiologic Tests to Assess the Immediate Energy System

Several physiologic and biochemical measures assess the **immediate energy system's** energy-generating capacity:

1. Size of the intramuscular ATP-PCr pool
2. Depletion rates of ATP and PCr in all-out, short-duration activity

ATP and PCr depletion rates provide the most direct estimate and correlate highly (≥0.80) with physical performance assessments of the immediate energy system. For example, one experiment determined muscle PCr depletion at different 100-m sprint intervals based on the muscle biopsy technique.[35] Compared with resting values (22 mmol · kg wet weight^{-1}), PCr decreased by 60% during the first 40 m (<6 s) and only another 20% for the sprint's remainder. It remains nearly impossible with current technology to obtain precise biochemical data during all-out brief duration efforts. Researchers must rely on the "face validity" from various specific performance measures as satisfactory markers to assess capacity for ATP-PCr energy transfer during intense physical activity.

Anaerobic Energy Transfer: The Short-Term Glycolytic (Lactate-Forming) Energy System

Performance Tests to Assess the Short-Term Energy System

Figure 11.2 illustrates that when all-out physical effort continues for longer than a few seconds, the **short-term glycolytic energy system** generates increasingly more energy for ATP resynthesis. This does not mean that aerobic metabolism is unimportant at this stage of activity or that oxygen-consuming reactions have not "switched on." To the contrary, the aerobic energy transfer contribution increases early in physical activity.[84] During short-duration maximal effort, the energy requirement greatly exceeds energy generated by hydrogen oxidation in the respiratory chain. Consequently, glycolytic ATP production predominates, with lactate accumulation in active muscle and ultimately in the blood.

Unlike tests for $\dot{V}O_{2max}$, no specific criteria exist to indicate that a person has attained maximal glycolytic effort. More than likely, self-motivation and the testing environment influence such performance tests.[105] Performance test scores show good reproducibility from day to day, particularly under standardized conditions.[4,52,64] *Performances that activate the short-term energy system require maximal effort for up to 3 min.* All-out runs, stationary cycling, shuttle runs, and repetitive weightlifting at a certain percentage of maximal capacity have assessed anaerobic power. The influence of age, gender, skill, motivation, and body size creates difficulty selecting a suitable criterion test or developing appropriate norms to evaluate anaerobic power. Above-normal intramuscular glycogen levels do not affect test performance or final blood lactate accumulation level.[92] Based on the exercise specificity principle, one should *not* use a test that requires maximally activating the leg musculature to assess short-term anaerobic capacity for an upper body rowing or swimming activity. *The performance test must closely resemble the activity that requires energy capacity assessment*. In most cases, the activity itself should serve as the performance test.

Katch and Wingate Tests

In 1973, the **Katch test** (all-out, short-duration stationary cycling) estimated the anaerobic energy systems' power capacity.[43] Further experiments created a stationary bicycle test with frictional resistance against the flywheel preset at a high load (6 kg/13 lb for males; 5 kg/11 lb for females). Subjects turned as many revolutions as possible in 40 s while pedal rate was continuously recorded. Peak cycling power expressed in watts represented the subject's anaerobic power, whereas total work accomplished indicated anaerobic capacity expressed in joules. The popular **Wingate test** involves a 30-s supramaximal effort on either an arm-crank or leg-cycle ergometer.[4,107] Body mass determines resistance to pedaling (originally set to 0.075 kg per kg body mass but now can exceed 0.12 kg for athletes) with resistance applied within 3 s after overcoming the initial inertia and the ergometer's unloaded frictional resistance. **Peak power** represents the highest mechanical power generated during any 3 to 5 s in the test sequence, with **relative power** representing peak power divided by body mass. **Anaerobic fatigue** represents the percentage decline in power output during the test, and **anaerobic capacity** represents the total work accomplished over the 30-s exercise period. The **fatigue rate** corresponds to the decline in power relative to the peak value. The Katch and Wingate tests assume that peak power output reflects the high-energy phosphate's energy-generating capacity, while average power reflects glycolytic capacity.

fyi Power Versus Capacity

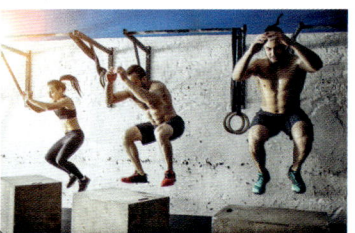
UfaBizPhoto/Shutterstock

The terms *power* and *capacity* refer to distinct measurements, particularly in anaerobic test procedures. Originally, the idea was to create measures of anaerobic performance similar to aerobic performance to reflect power. Some authors incorrectly used the term *capacity* to infer total work (joules) but instead used power scores (joules · s⁻¹ = watts) to represent this entity. To represent anaerobic power in this context, the term *capacity* must be a power score (much like $\dot{V}O_{2max}$) and not a work score; thus, watt represents the correct unit to express capacity. The joule is used to compute total anaerobic work.

In a Practical Sense: The Wingate Cycle Ergometer Test to Assess Anaerobic Power and Capacity provides the procedures to determine anaerobic power and capacity using the Wingate cycle ergometer test. **TABLE 11.1** presents normative standards for average and peak power outputs in young, physically active males and females during the test.

Table 11.1 Wingate test percentile norms for average power and peak power for physically active young adult men and women

Performance scores, blood lactate concentrations, and peak heart rates show high test-retest reproducibility and moderate validity compared with other anaerobic capacity criteria.[67,102] Elite volleyball and ice hockey players have achieved some of the highest Wingate power scores.

FIGURE 11.4A and B presents each of the three energy system's relative contribution during three different

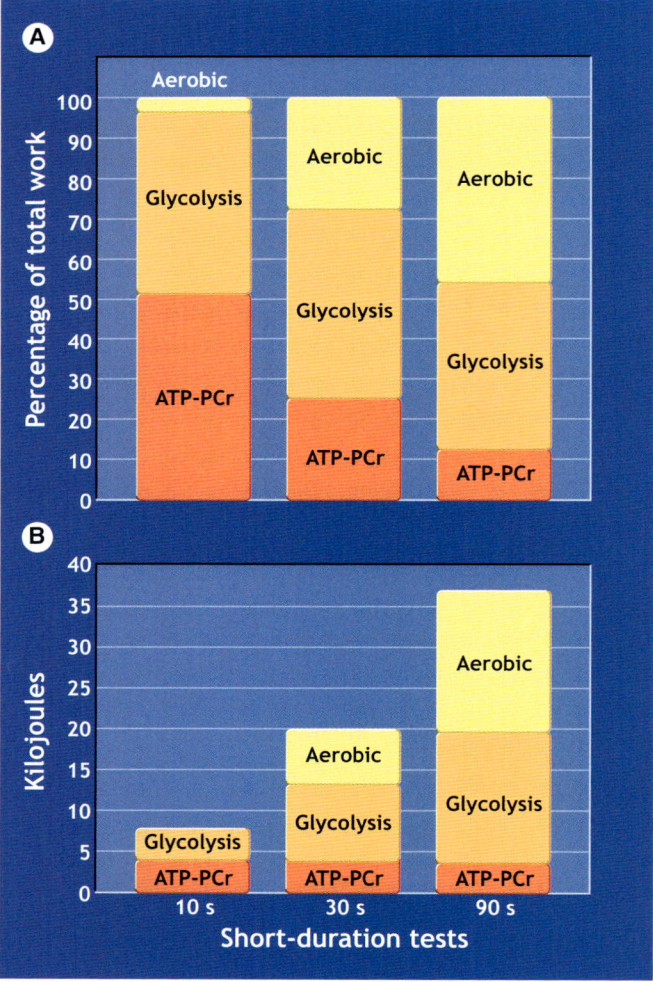

FIGURE 11.4. Relative contribution of each energy system to total work accomplished in three short-duration exercise tests. **(A)** Percentage of total work output. **(B)** Total kilojoules of energy. Test results based on Katch test protocol (see section Performance Tests to Assess the Short-Term Energy System). ATP-PCr, adenosine triphosphate-phosphocreatine energy system.
(Data from Applied Physiology Laboratory, University of Michigan, Ann Arbor, MI.)

In a Practical Sense

The Wingate Cycle Ergometer Test to Assess Anaerobic Power and Capacity

The Wingate cycle ergometer test represents the most popular test to assess anaerobic capacity. Developed at the Wingate Institute in Israel in the 1970s, its scores can reliably determine peak anaerobic power and anaerobic fatigue.

THE TEST

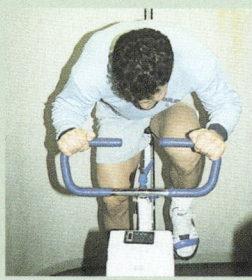

A mechanically braked bicycle ergometer serves as the testing device. After warming up (3 to 5 min), the subject begins pedaling as fast as possible, without resistance. Within 3 s, a fixed resistance is applied to the flywheel; the subject continues to pedal "all out" for 30 s. An electrical or mechanical counter continuously records flywheel revolutions in 5-s intervals. Total work during the 30 s computes in joules and power computes as joules · s^{-1}, or watts.

RESISTANCE

Flywheel resistance equals 0.075 kg per kg body mass. For a 70-kg person, the flywheel resistance would equal 5.25 kg (70 kg × 0.075). Resistance often increases to 0.10 kg per kg body mass or higher (up to 0.12 kg) when testing power- and sprint-type athletes. The Wingate test was originally designed using the Swedish Monarch cycle ergometer (https://sport-medical.monarkexercise.se/astrands-konditionstest-pa-cykel/). The unit of resistance was the former standard Swedish unit of force called the *kilopond*. Measurement of the kilopond (kp) was a cleverly engineered system composed of a basket containing a weight representing the braking force applied to the flywheel, equal to the weight of the basket and its contents. The standard corresponded to the weight of a 1-kg mass; hence, 1 kp has come to represent 1 kg. The proper unit of force when using the Monarch bike should be kp-m · min^{-1}, not kg-m · min^{-1}. When Sweden joined the European Union, they switched to the SI unit of force using the Newton (N). One kilopond corresponds to the force exerted by Earth's gravity (9.80665 m · s^{-2} on 1 kg of mass; thus, one kilogram-force equals 9.80665 Newtons (N)).

TEST SCORES

1. **Peak power (PP) output**—The highest power output, observed during the first 5-s exercise interval, indicates the energy-generating capacity of the immediate energy system (intramuscular high-energy phosphates ATP and PCr). PP, expressed in watts (1 W = 6.12 kp-m · min^{-1}), computes as Force in Newtons (kp resistance × acceleration due to gravity) × Distance (number of revolutions × distance per revolution) ÷ Time in minutes (5 s = 0.0833 min).
2. **Relative peak power (RPP) output**—Peak power output (W) relative to body mass: PP ÷ Body mass (kg).
3. **Anaerobic fatigue (AF)**—Percentage declines in power output during the test; AF is thought to represent the total capacity to produce ATP via the immediate and short-term energy systems. AF computes as (Highest 5-s PP − Lowest 5-s PP) ÷ Highest 5-s PP × 100.
4. **Anaerobic work (AW)**—Total work accomplished in watts for duration of the test (30 s).

EXAMPLE

A male weighing 73.3 kg performs the Wingate test on a Monark cycle ergometer (6.0 m traveled per pedal revolution) with an applied resistance (force) of 5.5 kp (73.3-kg body mass × 0.075 = 5.497, rounded to 5.5 kg); pedal revolutions for each 5-s interval equal 12, 10, 8, 7, 6, and 5 (48 total revolutions in 30 s).

CALCULATIONS

1. **Peak power output**
   PP = Force × Distance ÷ Time
   = (5.5 kp × 9.8 m · s^{-2}) × (12 rev × 6 m · rev^{-1}) ÷ 5 s
   = 776.8 kg · m^{-2} · s^{-3}
   = 776.8 N · m · s^{-2}
   = 776.8 W

2. **Relative peak power output**
   RPP = PP ÷ Body mass, kg
   = 776.8 W ÷ 73.3 kg
   = 10.6 W · kg^{-1}

3. **Anaerobic fatigue**
   AF = (Highest PP − Lowest PP) ÷ Highest PP × 100
   Highest PP = Force × Distance ÷ Time = 5.5 kp × 9.8 m · s^{-2}
   × (12 rev × 6 m) ÷ 0.0833 min
   = 4753.9 kp-m · min^{-1}, or 776.8 W
   Lowest PP = Force × Distance ÷ Time = 5.5 kp × 9.8 m · s^{-2}
   × (5 rev × 6 m) ÷ 0.0833 min
   = 1980.8 kp-m · min^{-1}, or 323.7 W
   AF = 776.8 W − 323.7 W ÷ 776.8 W
   = 58.3%

4. **Anaerobic work**
   AW = Force × Total Distance (in 30 s)
   = (5.5 kg × 9.8 m · s^{-2}) × [(12 rev + 10 rev + 8 rev + 7 rev + 6 rev + 5 rev) × 6 m]
   = 15,523 joules, or 15.5 kJ

short-duration cycle ergometer tests of anaerobic power. The lower figure in B gives estimated kilojoules for total energy. The upper figure presents the percentage contribution for each system's total work accomplished. Note the progressive change in the percentage contribution from each energy system with increasing duration of effort.

Age Differences. The reason for children's poor performance compared with adolescents and young adults on the Wingate test remains unclear. Possible explanations include child's relatively lower intramuscular glycogen concentrations, poorer motivation, and a slower glycogen hydrolysis rate during physical activity.

Gender Differences. Large gender differences exist in anaerobic power when comparing test scores on an absolute basis.[22,78] These observations, as with most physiologic and performance tests are explained by gender differences in factors that affect absolute anaerobic power output—body mass, active muscle mass, and fat-free body mass (FFM). Expressing power output capacity relative to a body mass or body composition component should minimize gender differences in anaerobic capacity. This adjustment should offer insight into whether gender truly impacts a muscle's capacity to generate energy anaerobically.

Gender differences in body composition, physique, muscular strength, or neuromuscular factors do *not* fully explain a female's lower anaerobic performance.[53,68] For a given fat-free leg volume, the peak oxygen deficit (a measure of anaerobic power[3,58] during supramaximal cycling) remained higher in males than in females.[103] These differences averaged about 20%, even when adjusting for the estimated gender difference in active muscle mass. Similar gender differences in anaerobic performance exist for children and adolescents.[66,78] The gender effect among adolescents remains apparent for the lower body musculature even when considering gender differences in body composition.[68] Males' greater relative muscle area and fast-twitch fiber type's metabolic capacity and larger catecholamine response to physical activity may help to explain their larger anaerobic performance.

Available evidence indicates an inherent biologic gender difference in glycolytic exercise power/capacity. Physical testing that focuses on this fitness component would inflate observed performance differences between males and females. Even adjusting the performance score to body size or body composition does not eliminate this difference. In occupational settings, the justifiable concern when using all-out anaerobic physical effort to predict job performance relates to the potential to exacerbate gender differences in performance scores and magnify any adverse impact on females. Female maximal anaerobic performance remains unaffected by variations in menstrual cycle phase.[30]

The Fastest Creatures in the Sky, Land, and Water

In the Sky
The *peregrine falcon* is considered the fastest creature in the sky. It can fly horizontally at speeds up to 55 mph and dive downward at over 280 mph.

On Land

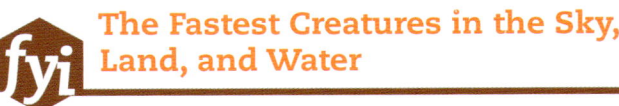

The *cheetah* achieves speeds up to 75 to 80 mph with only one foot touching the ground at a time and reaches maximum speed in about 3 s.

Stu Porter/Shutterstock

In the Sea
The Indo-Pacific *sailfish* with an average 4-year life span measures about 170.2 cm/5′7″ to 335.3 cm/11 ft in length and weighs 54 kg/119 lb to 100 kg/220 lb; it has been measured at a top speed of 109 kmh/68 mph.

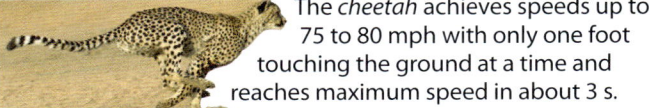

niceregionpics/Shutterstock

Maximally Accumulated Oxygen Deficit Test

The **maximally accumulated oxygen deficit (MAOD)** provides another indirect attempt to measure anaerobic metabolic capacity.[58,59,81,100] MAOD determination relies on an extrapolation procedure using the linear exercise intensity–oxygen uptake relationship established from several submaximal treadmill exercise levels. From these data, a regression line predicts the individual's supramaximal oxygen uptake, usually set at 125% of the subject's directly measured $\dot{V}O_{2max}$. MAOD represents the difference between the predicted supramaximal oxygen uptake from the exercise intensity–oxygen uptake relationship and oxygen uptake measured during a 2- to 3-min all-out treadmill run to fatigue. It correlates positively with the Wingate test, sprint-running, and stair-climbing anaerobic performance test scores and demonstrates independence from aerobic energy estimates. It also differentiates between aerobically and anaerobically trained individuals and remains unchanged with varying durations of intense physical effort.

Physiologic Tests to Assess the Short-Term Energy System

Blood Lactate Levels

Considerable blood lactate accumulates from glycolytic energy pathway activation during maximal short-duration activity; thus, blood lactate levels should reflect this energy system's level of activation and capacity.

FIGURE 11.5 presents data from 10 college men who performed 10 all-out different duration exercise on a bicycle ergometer on different days. Subjects included men involved in physical conditioning programs and varsity athletics. Unaware of test duration, the men were urged to turn as many revolutions as possible on the ergometer. Venous blood lactate was measured

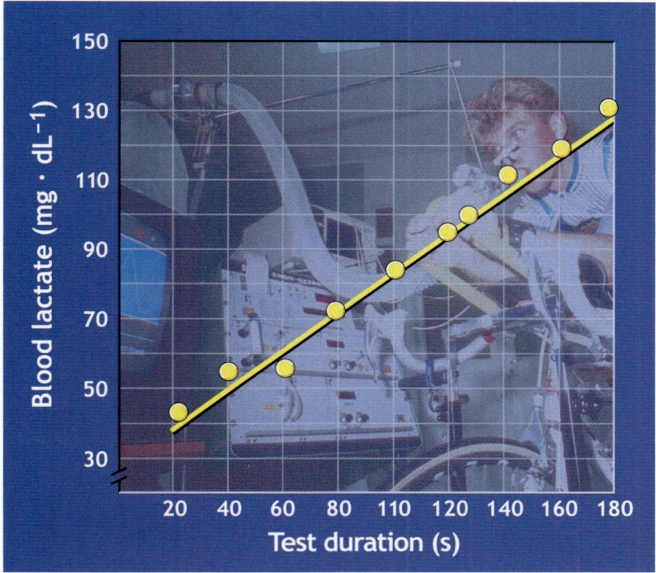

FIGURE 11.5. Pedaling a stationary bicycle ergometer at each subject's highest possible power output increases blood lactate in direct proportion to test duration for up to 3 min. Each value represents the average of 10 subjects.
(Data from the Applied Physiology Laboratory, University of Michigan.)

before and immediately following each test and throughout recovery. The plotted points represent the average peak blood lactate values at the end of cycling for each test. Blood lactate levels increased linearly with test duration and total work output. The highest blood lactates occurred at the end of 3 min, averaging about 130 mg in each 100 mL blood (approximately 16 mmol).

Physiologists have traditionally interpreted any "excess" lactate appearance in muscle and blood following exercise to indicate contributions from anaerobic metabolism to the total exercise energy requirement. Muscle or venous blood measurements routinely verified steady-rate exercise or glycolytic activity magnitude consequent to non–steady-rate exercise. This view now appears overly simplified in light of research showing lactate's role as a metabolic intermediate rather than a metabolic "dead end" whose only fate involves reconversion to pyruvate. We now know that lactate serves as an important substrate in energy-storing and energy-generating pathways in different tissues. Lactate measured during or following physical activity does not necessarily reflect absolute anaerobic energy transfer levels via glycolysis.[12,19,31,32] With increasing intensity, including near-maximal and supramaximal levels, greater lactate production reflects increasing ATP resynthesis from anaerobic pathways.[85] Anaerobic glycolysis and PCr degradation provide about 70% of the total energy yield for 30 s of maximal effort, with aerobic pathways generating the remaining energy (see Fig. 11.4).

 INTEGRATIVE QUESTION

Why do females score poorly when using absolute scores for "average power" and "peak power" on the Wingate leg-cycle ergometer test?

Glycogen Depletion

Glycogen depletion patterns reveal glycolytic contributions to physical activity because glycogen stored in specific muscles activated by the activity powers the short-term energy system. **FIGURE 11.6** illustrates the close connection between glycogen depletion rate in the quadriceps femoris muscle during cycling and exercise intensity.

During prolonged but relatively light activity (31% $\dot{V}O_{2max}$), a considerable muscle glycogen reserve remains even after 180 min. Relatively large fatty acid quantities provide fuel for exercise at this intensity, with only minimal reliance on stored glycogen. The two intense supramaximal workloads (120 and 150% $\dot{V}O_{2max}$) produced the most rapid and pronounced glycogen depletion. This outcome makes sense from a metabolic standpoint: *Glycogen provides the most rapid ATP phosphorylation of the three macronutrients, and glycogen serves as the only stored macronutrient that resynthesizes ATP anaerobically.*

Changes in total muscle glycogen, like those illustrated in Figure 11.6, do not necessarily indicate precise glycogen catabolism in specific fibers within active muscle. Depending on intensity, glycogen depletion progresses selectively in either fast- or slow-twitch muscle fibers. Fast-twitch fibers provide most of the power requirements for intense effort (e.g., repeated 1-min sprints on a bicycle ergometer at an extreme load). The glycogen content of these fibers almost totally depletes from the activity's anaerobic nature. In contrast,

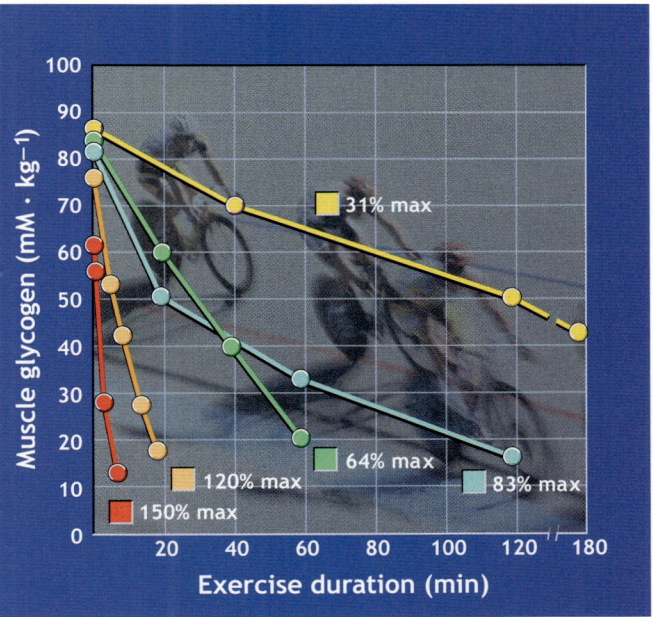

FIGURE 11.6. Glycogen depletion from the vastus lateralis of the quadriceps femoris muscles during bicycle exercise of different intensities and durations. Exercise at 31% of maximum oxygen uptake ($\dot{V}O_{2max}$; the lightest workload) caused some depletion of muscle glycogen, but the most rapid depletion occurred during exercise between 83 and 150% of $\dot{V}O_{2max}$.
(Adapted with permission from Gollnick PD. Selective glycogen depletion pattern in human muscle fibers after exercise of varying intensity and at varying pedaling rates. J Physiol. 1974;241:45.)

during moderately intense but more prolonged aerobic exercise, slow-twitch muscle fibers become glycogen depleted first. Specificity in glycogen use and depletion by specific fiber types makes it difficult to evaluate the anaerobic involvement of distinct fibers from changes in a muscle's total glycogen content before and after exercise.

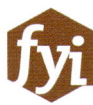

Marathon Records Difficult to Repeat

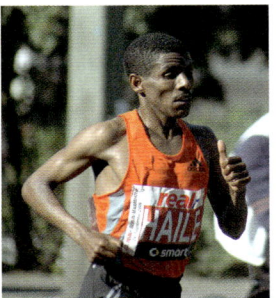

360b/Shutterstock

Only five men and eight women have been able to follow one marathon world record with another. James Peters set four marathon records between 1952 and 1954, while Abebe Bikila, Derek Clayton, Khalid Khannouchi, and most recently Haile Gebrselassie shown in the image each set two world records back-to-back. On the women's side, Greta Weitz set four consecutive world records from 1978 to 1983 (the last stood for only one day!), while Chantal Langlace, Jacqueline Hansen, Christa Vahlensieck, Joyce Smith, Tegla Loroupe, and most recently Paula Radcliffe each broke the marathon record twice. Perhaps, the most famous of all of the world records were the races of Abebe Bikila, the barefoot Ethiopian, who set world records 4 years apart while winning Olympic Marathons in 1960 (Rome, barefoot) and 1964 (Tokyo, wearing shoes).

Individual Differences in Short-Term Energy Transfer Capacity

Three factors contribute to differences among individuals in capacity to generate short-term anaerobic energy:

1. Previous training effects
2. Capacity to buffer acid metabolites
3. Motivation

Training Effects

Many factors relate to differences in anaerobic metabolism between sprint-trained athletes and untrained subjects. Swedish researchers in a classic 1971 experiment determined that trained subjects always exhibit higher muscle lactic acid, blood lactate, and greater muscle glycogen depletion levels following short-term maximal bicycle ergometer exercise compared to untrained counterparts. Significant reductions occurred in the intramuscular high-energy phosphates with essentially no differences observed between groups.[39]

Buffering of Acid Metabolites

Buffering capacity refers to how well different substances resist increases in free hydrogen ion concentration by binding free protons to prevent decreases in pH. When anaerobic energy transfer predominates, lactate accumulates and muscle and blood acidity increase to negatively affect the intracellular environment and the active muscles' contractile capacity. Anaerobic training might enhance short-term energy capacity by improving the body's alkaline reserve for buffering. Such a training adaptation would theoretically enable greater lactate production through more effective buffering. This reasoning seems appealing, yet athletes have only a slightly larger alkaline reserve than sedentary counterparts. Additionally, no appreciable change in alkaline reserve occurs following intense physical training. *Exercise training most likely confers a buffering capability within the range expected for healthy untrained individuals.* Chapter 23 discusses the potential ergogenic effect of pre–exercise-induced alkalosis.

Motivation

Individuals with a higher "pain tolerance," "toughness," or ability to "push" beyond discomforting fatigue accomplish more work anaerobically. This coincides with higher blood lactate concentrations and greater glycogen depletion. Motivational factors prove difficult to quantify, yet undoubtedly play an integral role in achieving superior performance at most competition levels.

Aerobic Energy Transfer: The Long-Term Energy System

FIGURE 11.7 illustrates that male and female athletes who excel in endurance sports have a superior capacity for aerobic energy transfer. The $\dot{V}O_{2max}$ for elite cross-country skiers, distance runners, swimmers, bicyclists, and skaters exceeds values for sedentary men and women by almost twofold. This does not mean that $\dot{V}O_{2max}$ provides the sole endurance performance determinant. Other factors at the local tissue level include improved capillary density, enzyme concentration, mitochondrial size and number, and muscle fiber type. These intrinsic qualities strongly influence a muscle's capacity to sustain high aerobic activity levels.[36] The $\dot{V}O_{2max}$ does provide important information about the capacity of the long-term energy system. This conveys important physiologic meaning because attaining a high $\dot{V}O_{2max}$ requires integration of high levels of pulmonary, cardiovascular, and neuromuscular function (see Fig. 7.5). *Integration of these factors makes* the $\dot{V}O_{2max}$ *a fundamental measure of physiologic functional capacity for physical activity.*

Physiologic Tests to Assess the Long-Term Energy System

Over the past 80 years, considerable research has perfected methodology to assess the $\dot{V}O_{2max}$. Normative standards exist related to age, gender, state of training, and body size and composition.

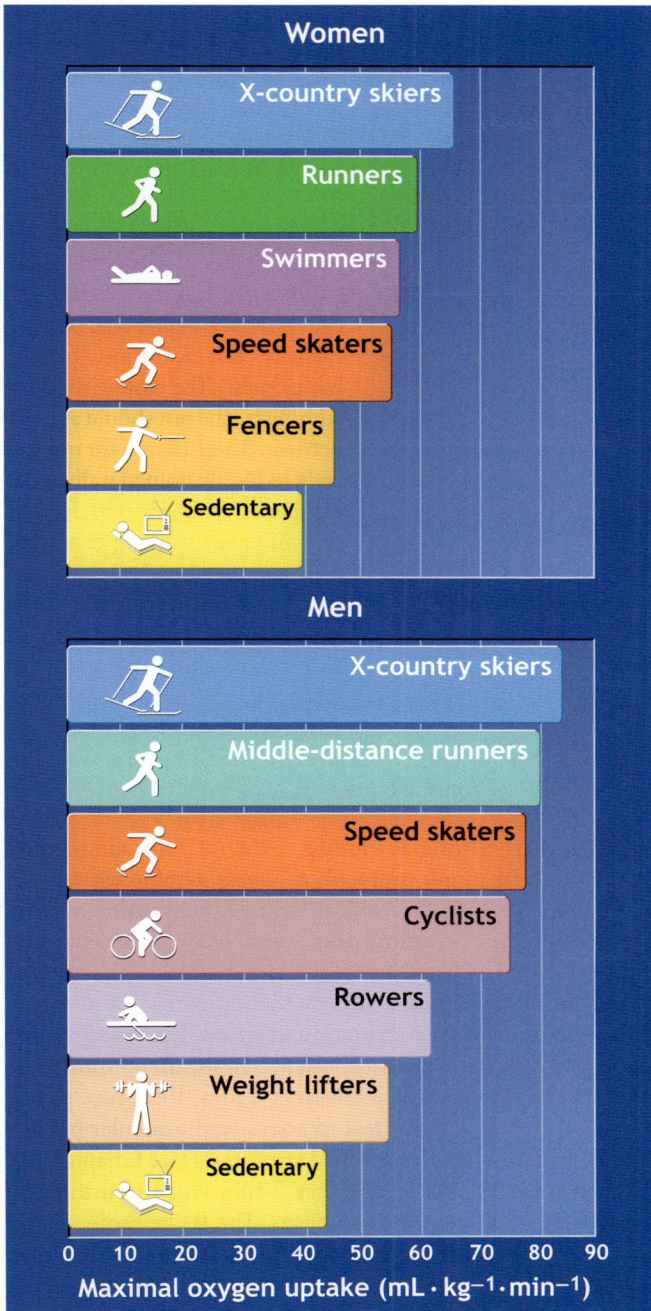

FIGURE 11.7. Maximal oxygen uptake of male and female Olympic-caliber athletes in different sport categories compared with healthy sedentary subjects.
(Adapted with permission from Saltin B, Åstrand PO. Maximal oxygen consumption in athletes. *J Appl Physiol.* 1967;23:353. ©The American Physiological Society (APS). All rights reserved)

$\dot{V}O_{2max}$ Criteria

The plot in **FIGURE 11.8** relates oxygen uptake and exercise intensity during progressive increases in treadmill effort. The test terminated when the subject could not complete the full duration of a particular interval. The highest oxygen uptake (average of 18 subjects) occurred before subjects achieved their maximal effort level. *A leveling-off or peaking-over in oxygen uptake with increasing exercise intensity generally provides assurance that a person has reached maximum aerobic metabolism (i.e., achieved "true" $\dot{V}O_{2max}$).* Agreement on a precise standard for the criterion remains controversial.[21,37,83] Less stringent criteria, besides failure for oxygen uptake to increase in graded exercise, also establish $\dot{V}O_{2max}$ attainment. Oxygen uptake that fails to increase by the value expected from previous observations with the specific test protocol often serves as an appropriate criterion.[1,37,87]

Oxygen uptake at progressively higher exercise intensity levels does not readily plateau, particularly among children,[76] except during treadmill running. The term **peak oxygen uptake** ($\dot{V}O_{2peak}$) applies when leveling-off does not occur or maximal performance appears limited by local muscular factors rather than central circulatory dynamics. $\dot{V}O_{2peak}$ *generally refers to the highest oxygen uptake value measured during a graded exercise test.* The highest oxygen uptake value often occurs during the last minute of the activity. Secondary criteria that objectify $\dot{V}O_{2peak}$ include attaining the age-predicted maximum heart rate or a respiratory exchange ratio (R) that exceeds 1.15. Some researchers posit that to accept an oxygen uptake value as near maximum, blood lactate should attain 70 or 80 mg · dL^{-1} of blood (8 to 10 mmol) or higher.[21]

Tests to Assess $\dot{V}O_{2max}$

Different tests can activate the body's large muscle groups to determine $\dot{V}O_{2max}$, provided exercise intensity and duration maximize aerobic energy transfer. Usual activity modes include treadmill running or walking, bench stepping, and stationary cycling. In accord with exercise test and training specificity, other testing modes employ free, tethered, and flume swimming[6,48]; swim-bench ergometry[29]; in-line skating[97]; roller skiing[77]; simulated arm-leg climbing[11]; rowing[15]; ice skating[24]; and arm-crank and wheelchair exercise.[80,91,93] These performance tests remain substantially unaffected by a subject's general strength level, movement speed, body size, and skill, except for specialized tests that measure aerobic capacity in sport-specific activities.

The $\dot{V}O_{2max}$ test may require a single, continuous 3- to 5-min supramaximal effort. The test, however, usually includes progressive increments in **graded exercise** (effort) until the subject will no longer continue despite strong verbal encouragement. Some researchers term this end point "exhaustion." In reality, the person terminates the test—a decision often influenced by motivational factors that do not necessarily reflect true physiologic strain. Bringing the subject to the point of acceptable criteria for either $\dot{V}O_{2max}$ or $\dot{V}O_{2peak}$ often requires considerable urging and prodding.[96] Practical experience indicates that attaining a plateau in oxygen uptake during a graded exercise test in well-trained athletes also requires a high level of anaerobic energy output. This poses some difficulty for untrained males and females and elderly persons who normally do not perform strenuous physical activity with its associated discomforts and potential health concerns.

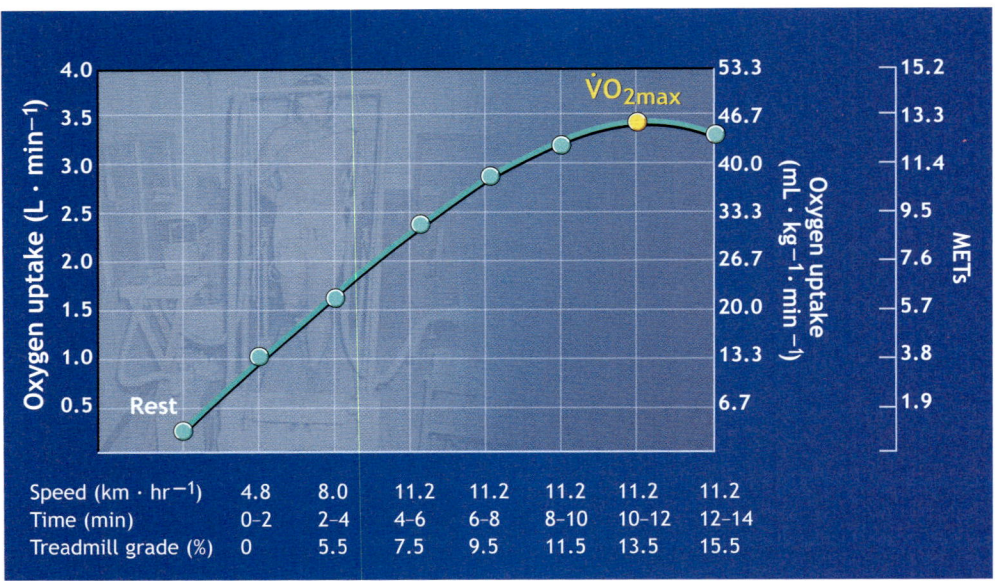

FIGURE 11.8. Peaking-over in oxygen uptake with increasing treadmill exercise intensity in 18 sedentary males. The region where oxygen uptake fails to increase the expected amount or even decreases slightly with increasing intensity represents the maximum oxygen uptake ($\dot{V}O_{2max}$). METs, metabolic equivalents.
(Data from V. Katch from the Applied Physiology Laboratory, University of Michigan, Ann Arbor, MI.)

 INTEGRATIVE QUESTION

How does $\dot{V}O_{2max}$ provide important insights about the functional capacity of different physiologic systems?

Test Comparisons. There are two popular maximum oxygen uptake test protocols:

1. *Continuous*—progressively increasing exercise increments without interspersed recovery or rest intervals
2. *Discontinuous*—progressively increasing exercise increments interspersed with pre-set recovery intervals

Both test protocols yield similar $\dot{V}O_{2max}$ values.[21] The data in **TABLE 11.2** reveal a systematic comparison of $\dot{V}O_{2max}$ scores from six common continuous and discontinuous treadmill and bicycle protocols.

TABLE 11.2 Average maximum oxygen uptake during continuous and discontinuous tests on the treadmill and bicycle ergometer

Only an 8 mL difference in $\dot{V}O_{2max}$ occurred between the continuous and discontinuous bicycle tests, but $\dot{V}O_{2max}$ during cycling averaged 6.4 to 11.2% below treadmill values. The largest difference among the three run tests equaled only 1.2%. In contrast, the walking test elicited $\dot{V}O_{2max}$ scores nearly 7% higher than stationary bicycle ergometer values but 5% lower than the three running tests.

Subjects commonly complained that intense local discomfort in the thigh muscles during both continuous and discontinuous bicycle tests limited their ability to achieve a true maximal effort. They often experienced discomfort in the lower back and calf muscles during treadmill walking at treadmill elevations beyond a 12% incline. Running tests rarely produced local discomfort; subjects complained more of general fatigue usually categorized as feeling "winded." For administrative ease, the continuous treadmill run provides a practical aerobic capacity test for most healthy individuals. The total time to administer the test should average between 8 and 10 min for moderately to highly trained individuals compared with 65 min for the discontinuous running test. Subjects tolerate the continuous test and prefer the shorter test duration.[106] Achievement of $\dot{V}O_{2max}$ also occurs with a continuous protocol that increases intensity progressively in 15-s intervals.[23] Total test time for either bicycle or treadmill exercise with this approach averages only about 5 min.

Common Treadmill Protocols. **FIGURE 11.9** summarizes six common treadmill protocols to assess aerobic capacity in normal individuals and cardiac patients. Manipulation of exercise duration and treadmill speed and grade share common features. The Naughton protocol **(A)** includes 3-min exercise periods of increasing intensity alternating with 3 min of rest. Exercise periods vary in % grade and speed. The Åstrand protocol **(B)** involves a constant speed at 5 mph; after 3 min at 0% grade, the grade increases 2½% every 2 min. The Bruce protocol **(C)**, the most popular test to assess cardiovascular parameters during physician-monitored stress tests (see Chapter 32), changes grade and/or speed every 3 min while omitting the 0 and 5% grades for healthy subjects. The Balke protocol **(D)** involves 1 min at 0% grade and 1 min at 2% grade, the grade increases 1% per minute thereafter while speed is maintained at 3.3 mph. The Ellestad protocol **(E)** includes an initial grade of 10% and later a grade of 15%, while speed increases every 2 or 3 min. Finally, with the Harbor protocol **(F)**, often referred to as a *ramp test*, after 3 min of walking at a comfortable speed, the grade increases at a constant preselected amount each minute: 1%, 2%, 3%, or 4%, so that the subject achieves $\dot{V}O_{2max}$ in approximately 10 min. This relatively quick procedure—well tolerated by both healthy subjects and cardiac patients—elicits a linear increase in oxygen uptake up to maximum.[13,18,71,99]

 **INTEGRATIVE QUESTION**

Why should training experiments objectively demonstrate attainment of a true $\dot{V}O_{2max}$ in both pre- and post-test measures, and how could this goal be verified?

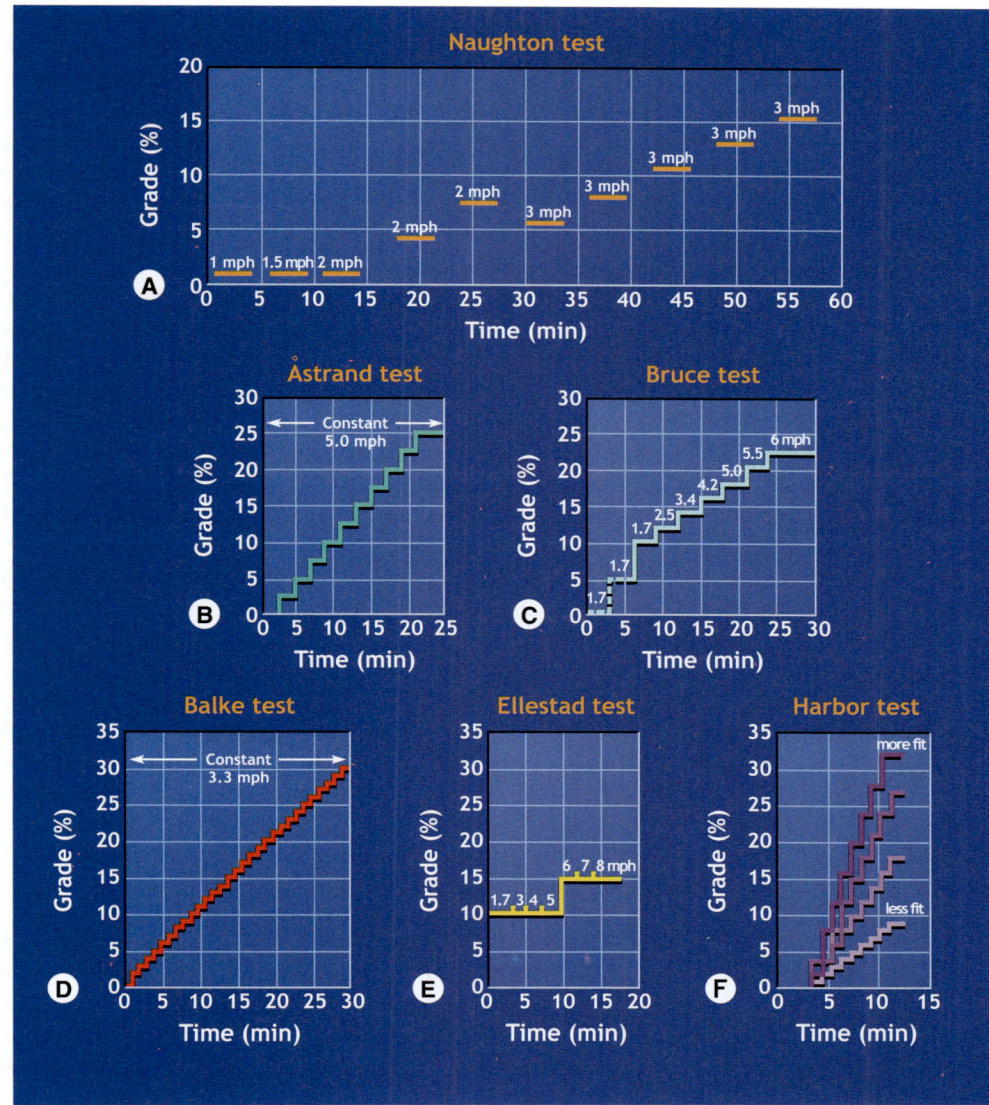

FIGURE 11.9. Six commonly used treadmill protocols to assess maximum oxygen uptake. (Adapted from Wasserman K, Sietsema KE et al. *Wasserman & Whipp's Principles of Exercise Testing and Interpretation.* 6th ed., Fig. 5.4, p. 130. Philadelphia: Wolters Kluwer, 2021.)

Factors That Affect $\dot{V}O_{2max}$

The six most important factors that influence the maximum oxygen uptake score include the following:

1. Activity mode
2. Heredity
3. Training state
4. Gender
5. Body size and composition
6. Age

Activity Mode. *Variations in $\dot{V}O_{2max}$ with different physical activity modes generally reflect variations in the activated muscle mass. Treadmill exercise usually produces the highest values among diverse activity modes.* Bench stepping produces $\dot{V}O_{2max}$ scores similar to treadmill values and higher than values on the cycle ergometer.[40] During arm-crank exercise, aerobic capacity averages only about 70% of the treadmill score.[91] For skilled but untrained swimmers, the $\dot{V}O_{2max}$ during swimming usually averages about 80% of treadmill values.[48,56] A definite test specificity exists for swimmers because trained collegiate swimmers achieve $\dot{V}O_{2max}$ values swimming only 11% below treadmill values.[54] Some elite swimmers even equal or exceed their treadmill scores during swim tests.[48] Similarly, distinct exercise specificity exists for competitive race-walkers who achieve similar $\dot{V}O_{2max}$ values during treadmill walking and treadmill running.[60] When competitive cyclists pedal at the rapid frequencies of competition, they too achieve $\dot{V}O_{2max}$ values equivalent to treadmill $\dot{V}O_{2max}$ scores.[33,86]

Treadmill exercise proves highly desirable to determine $\dot{V}O_{2max}$ in healthy subjects in the laboratory because it is easy to regulate effort intensity. Compared with other exercise modes, the treadmill allows subjects to more readily meet one or more $\dot{V}O_{2max}$ associated criteria or $\dot{V}O_{2max}$. In field experiments outside the laboratory setting, bench stepping and cycle ergometry remain suitable alternatives.

Heredity. The interaction between inherited factors (DNA sequence variation; see Section 8, "A Look to the Future") and physical activity enhances understanding about individual variations in training responsiveness and anticipated health-related benefits of regular physical activity.[7,34,63,75] Frequent questions concern the relative contribution of natural endowment (genotype) to physiologic function, daily physical activity level, neuromuscular coordination, and physical performance (phenotype).[10,27,47,62,65,74,79,104] For example, to what extent does heredity determine the extremely high aerobic capacities for the endurance athletes listed in Figure 11.7? Do exceptionally high functional capacity levels simply reflect intensive training effects? How does familial aggregation affect skeletal muscle capillary density and enzyme activity and their response to training?

In general, most physical fitness characteristics demonstrate high heritability. Early research focused on 15 identical twin pairs (homozygous; same heredity from a single fertilized ovum) and 15 fraternal twin pairs (dizygous;

like ordinary siblings, derived from two separate fertilized ovum) raised in the same city and with parents of similar socioeconomic backgrounds. Heredity alone accounted for up to 93% the observed $\dot{V}O_{2max}$ differences. Short-term glycolytic energy system capacity revealed an 81% genetic component, while an 86% genetic determination emerged for maximum heart rate.[45] In larger groups of brothers, fraternal twins, and identical twins, there was a smaller inherited factor effect for aerobic capacity and endurance performance.[8,9] **FIGURE 11.10** presents data for $\dot{V}O_{2max}$ in identical twin and fraternal twin brothers. Lesser variation in aerobic capacity between brother pairs emerges for identical twins (yellow circles) with identical genetic constitutions. Chapters 21 and 33 discuss the potential contribution of genetic makeup to aerobic training improvements.

Researchers estimate the genetic effect at about 20 to 30% for $\dot{V}O_{2max}$, 50% for maximum heart rate, and 70% for physical working capacity.[7,8,70] Combining the estimated genetics and familial environment effects raises the upper genetic determination limit to about 50% for $\dot{V}O_{2max}$ when adjusted for age, gender, and body mass and/or body composition.[9] Identical twins have similar muscle fiber type composition, whereas fiber type varies widely between fraternal twins and brothers.[46] Genetic factors account for between 15 and 40% of the variation in muscular strength.[69,90] Current thinking maintains that inherited factors substantially contribute to many physiologic functions, daily physical activity level, training responsiveness, superior physical accomplishments, and specific health-related physical fitness components.[26,47,73,75,94]

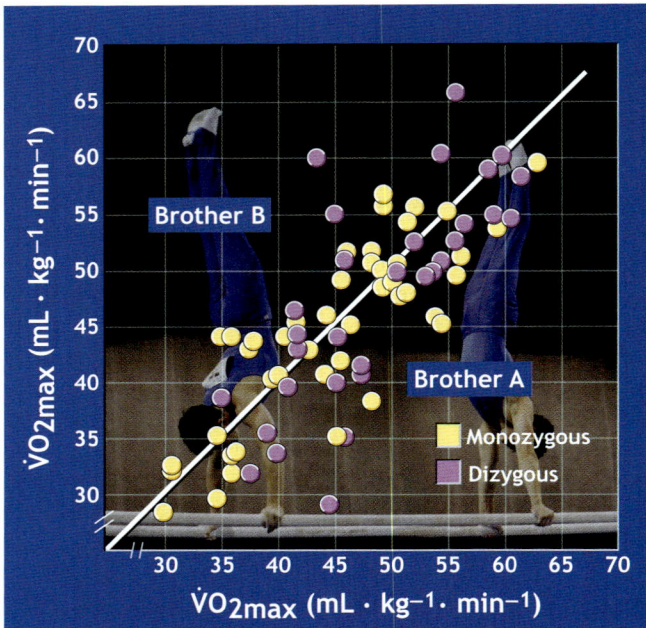

FIGURE 11.10. Maximum oxygen uptake ($\dot{V}O_{2max}$) for monozygotic (identical) and dizygotic (fraternal) twin brothers.
(From Bouchard C, et al. Aerobic performance in brothers, dizygotic and monozygotic twins. Med Sci Sports Exerc. 1986;18:639.)

Training State. Aerobic training contributes substantially to the $\dot{V}O_{2max}$, which normally varies between 5 and 20% for a person depending on their fitness at the time of testing. Chapter 21 discusses how training influences aerobic capacity.

Gender. *Females typically achieve $\dot{V}O_{2max}$ scores 15 to 30% below male values.*[82,95] Among trained endurance athletes, the gender difference ranges between 15 and 20%.[5] These differences are considerably larger for $\dot{V}O_{2max}$ expressed in absolute units ($L \cdot min^{-1}$) rather than expressed relative to body mass ($mL \cdot kg^{-1} \cdot min^{-1}$).[101] Among world-class cross-country skiers, for example, females achieved 43% lower absolute $\dot{V}O_{2max}$ value compared to males (6.54 vs. 3.75 $L \cdot min^{-1}$), which became 15% lower when expressed relative to body mass (83.8 vs. 71.2 $mL \cdot kg^{-1} \cdot min^{-1}$).

Differences in body composition (discussed below) and hemoglobin concentration usually explain $\dot{V}O_{2max}$ gender differences. Untrained young adult women generally average about 25% body fat, whereas men average 15%. The average male generates more total aerobic energy simply because he possesses more muscle mass and has less fat than the average female. Trained athletes have lower fat percentages than average individuals, yet trained females still possess more body fat than trained male counterparts. Perhaps because of higher testosterone levels, males also have a 10 to 14% greater hemoglobin (Hb) concentration than females throughout the life span, although the absolute Hb declines for both groups over time. This difference in the blood's oxygen-carrying capacity enables men to circulate more oxygen during physical activity, which increases their aerobic capacities above females.

Factors other than lower body fat and higher Hb concentrations may help to explain male-female aerobic capacity differences. For example, normal physical activity levels differ between average males and females. One could argue that social constraints reduce the female's opportunities at all ages to participate in extracurricular athletic activities and recreational pursuits. Among prepubertal children, boys engage in more daily physical activity than girls of the same age. Despite these fitness-inhibiting factors, the physically active female's aerobic capacity generally exceeds values for the sedentary male. For female cross-country skiers, their $\dot{V}O_{2max}$ exceeds untrained males by 40%.[5]

Body Size and Composition. Variations in body mass explain nearly 70% of the difference in absolute $\dot{V}O_{2max}$ scores among individuals. This limits interpretations about physical performance achievements or absolute oxygen uptake when comparing individuals who vary in body size or composition. The body size impact on aerobic capacity has led to the practice of expressing oxygen uptake related to surface area, body mass, FFM, or even limb volume. The table on the next page illustrates different ways to express $\dot{V}O_2$; it reveals a 43% gender difference in $\dot{V}O_{2max}$ when expressed in absolute terms as $L \cdot min^{-1}$ for an untrained male and female who differ considerably in body composition.

Variable	Female	Male	% Diff (Female – Male)
$\dot{V}O_{2max}$, L · min^{-1}	2.00	3.50	−43
$\dot{V}O_{2max}$, mL · kg^{-1} · min^{-1}	40.0	50.0	−20
$\dot{V}O_{2max}$, mL · kg FFM^{-1} · min^{-1}	53.3	58.8	−9
Body mass, kg	50	70	−29
Percentage body fat	25	15	+67
FFM, kg	37.5	59.5	−37

Diff, difference; FFM, fat-free body mass; $\dot{V}O_{2max}$, maximum oxygen uptake.

When expressed in relative terms per unit body mass as mL · kg^{-1} · min^{-1}, the $\dot{V}O_{2max}$ for females remains about 20% lower than for the males. Expressing aerobic capacity by FFM reduces between-subject difference even more (by 29%). Adjusting for muscle mass variation activated in physical activity provides additional information to explain interindividual variation in $\dot{V}O_{2max}$. For example, adjusting oxygen uptake values obtained during maximal arm-cranking for variations in estimated arm and shoulder size completely eliminates gender differences in $\dot{V}O_{2max}$.[98] Expressing oxygen uptake per unit appendicular skeletal muscle mass often negates the difference in $\dot{V}O_{2max}$ between similarly trained males and females.[14] The size of the contracting muscle mass activated in an activity largely explains the gender differences in aerobic capacity.

Age. Age does not spare its impact on maximum oxygen uptake.[41,51,57,72] Available data provide insight into the possible aging effects on physiologic function, although one can draw only limited inferences from cross-sectional studies of different age group. **FIGURE 11.11** summarizes trends in children and adults' aerobic capacity between ages 10 to 60 years.

Absolute $\dot{V}O_{2max}$ in (L · min^{-1}) for boys and girls remains similar until about age 12. Then, at age 14, $\dot{V}O_{2max}$ for boys averages 25% higher than for girls, and by age 16, the difference exceeds 50%. The difference generally relates to the combined effects from greater muscle mass in boys and their greater daily physical activity levels. The relative $\dot{V}O_{2max}$ (mL · kg^{-1} · min^{-1}) for boys remains steady at about 52 mL · kg^{-1} · min^{-1} from ages 6 to 16; for girls, the relative $\dot{V}O_{2max}$ slopes downward beginning at about age 6 to 8 years, achieving about 40 mL · kg^{-1} · min^{-1} at age 16 (32% below same age males). The greater body fat accumulation in adolescent females partially accounts for the lower values because females must transport this extra fat, which does not enhance capacity for aerobic metabolism. $\dot{V}O_{2max}$ declines steadily at about 1% yearly for both men and women after age 25, so at age 55, it averages approximately 27% below values reported for 20-year-olds (Fig. 11.11). $\dot{V}O_{2max}$ declines at an accelerated rate among the elderly.[25] For eight women about age 80 years, $\dot{V}O_{2max}$ averaged 13.4 mL · kg^{-1} · min^{-1}, or about 3.7 metabolic equivalents (METs).[26] Despite this apparent aging effect, strong evidence indicates that a person's habitual physical activity level exerts far greater influence on aerobic capacity than chronological age *per se*.[61] Chapter 31 continues the discussion about age-related influences on physiologic function.

Performance and Prediction Tests to Assess the Long-Term Energy System

Direct $\dot{V}O_{2max}$ measurement requires an extensive laboratory, specialized equipment, and considerable subject effort and motivation. Consequently, laboratory tests remain impractical to assess large groups of untrained individuals. Medically, strenuous

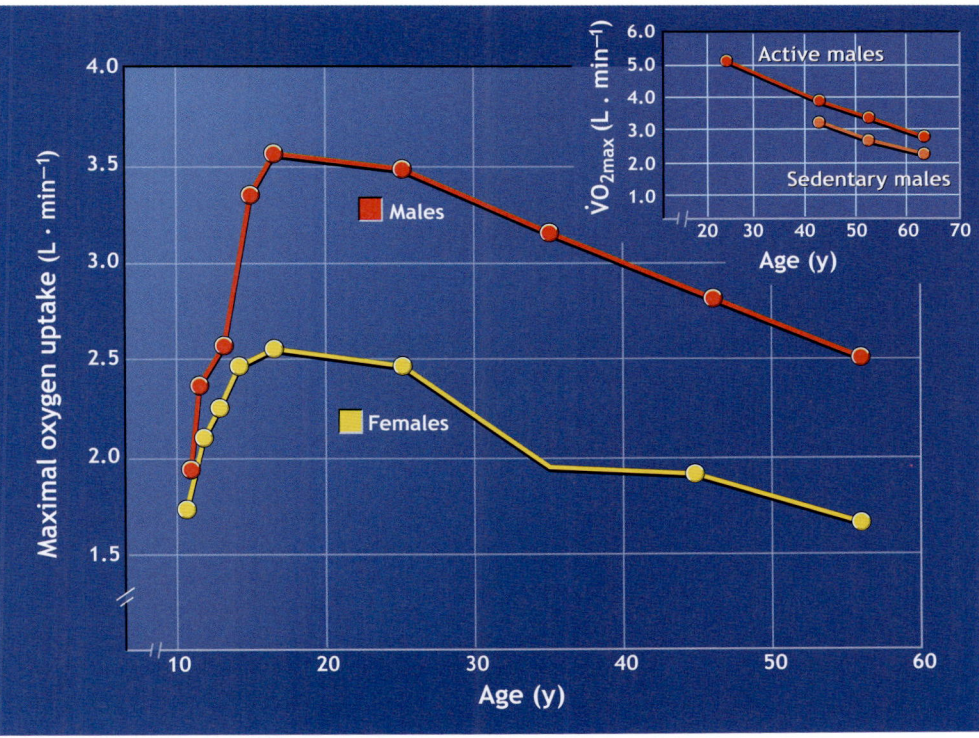

FIGURE 11.11. Maximal oxygen uptake ($\dot{V}O_{2max}$) related to age in males and females between ages 10 and 60 y.
(Adapted with permission from Hermansen L. Individual differences. In: Larson LA, ed. *Fitness, Health, and Work Capacity: International Standards for Assessment*. New York: Macmillan; 1974. Inset graph redrawn from table data of Åstrand PO, Rodahl KR. *Textbook of Work Physiology*. New York: McGraw-Hill; 1970.)

exertion could prove risky to older adults (greater than age 50) who do not receive proper medical clearance and appropriate supervision, particularly if they have underlying conditions, which include overweight/obesity, diabetes, hypertension, and have a chronic history of cigarette smoking. These considerations increase the importance of substituting submaximal exercise testing to *predict* $\dot{V}O_{2max}$ from performance during walking and running or from heart rate during or immediately postexercise.

A Word of Caution About Predictions

All predictions contain error referred to as the **standard error of estimate (SEE)**. Errors are estimates expressed in the predicted variables measurement units (e.g., kg, mL, min, s) or their percentage. For example, suppose the $\dot{V}O_{2max}$ (mL·kg^{-1}·min^{-1}) predicted from time on a walking test equals 55 mL·kg^{-1}·min^{-1}, with SEE ±10 mL·kg^{-1}·min^{-1}. This means that the actual $\dot{V}O_{2max}$ probably (68% confidence) lies within ±10 mL·kg^{-1}·min^{-1} or between 45 and 65 mL·kg^{-1}·min^{-1} of the predicted value! This represents a relatively large potential error (±18% of the absolute value). Standard errors within ±3 to 5% compared to a criterion measurement would be more desirable.

Some predictions associate with relatively small errors (SEE = 3–5%) and others with larger errors as in the previous example. Obviously, a larger error translates to a less useful predicted score because the likely true score encompasses such a large range for possible values. Without knowing the SEE magnitude, it becomes problematic to judge a predicted score's usefulness based singularly on a correlation coefficient.

Walking Tests

Walking tests can predict $\dot{V}O_{2max}$ with reasonable accuracy, which means a prediction within about ±3–5% had the criterion test been performed on a treadmill in the laboratory. The following equation accurately predicts $\dot{V}O_{2max}$ in L·min^{-1} from walking speed, heart rate, body weight, age, and gender in men and women[44]:

$$\dot{V}O_{2max} = 6.9652 + (0.0091 \times Wt) - (0.0257 \times Age) \\ + (0.5955 \times Gender) - (0.224 \times T1) \\ - (0.0115 \times HR1\text{–}4)$$

where Wt is body weight in pounds; Age = years; Gender = 0 for females and 1 for males; T1 is time for the 1-mile track walk, expressed as min and hundredths of a min; and HR1–4 is heart rate in beats per min measured immediately following the last quarter-mile.

The following equation predicts $\dot{V}O_{2max}$ in mL·kg^{-1}·min^{-1} using the same variables with an SEE equal to ±0.335 L·min^{-1} or ±4.4 mL·kg^{-1}·min^{-1}.

$$\dot{V}O_{2max} = 132.853 - (0.0769 \times Wt) - (0.3877 \times Age) \\ + (6.315 \times Gender) - (3.2649 \times T1) \\ - (0.1565 \times HR1\text{–}4)$$

The multiple correlation is $r = 0.92$ for predicting $\dot{V}O_{2max}$ from 1-mi walking performance for both prediction equations with low SEE reported means that about 68% of the people tested have an actual $\dot{V}O_{2max}$ within ±0.335 L·min^{-1} (±4.4 mL·kg^{-1}·min^{-1}) of the predicted value. The group ranged in age from 30 to 69 years, which means that the predictive method applies to a large segment of an adult population.

The following data for a 30-year-old female illustrate the prediction method:

$$\text{Body weight} = 155.5 \text{ lb} \\ T1 = 13.56 \\ HR_{1\text{–}4} = 145 \text{ b·min}^{-1}$$

Substituting in the equation to predict $\dot{V}O_{2max}$ in mL·kg^{-1}·min^{-1}:

$$\dot{V}O_{2max} = 132.853 - (0.0769 \times 155.5) \\ - (0.3877 \times 30.0) + (6.315 \times 0) \\ - (3.2649 \times 13.56) - (0.1565 \times 145)$$

$$\dot{V}O_{2max} = 132.853 - (11.96) - (11.63) + (0) \\ - (44.27) - (22.69)$$

$$\dot{V}O_{2max} = 42.3 \text{ mL·kg}^{-1}\text{·min}^{-1}$$

Endurance Runs

As with walking tests, runs of various durations or distances evaluate aerobic fitness. Test use reasonably assumes that a person's ability to maintain a high, steady-rate oxygen uptake largely determines the distance run over at least 5-min duration. This ability depends on the maximum capacity to generate energy aerobically (i.e., $\dot{V}O_{2max}$). This rationale provided the framework for a field performance test devised in 1959 to evaluate aerobic fitness of military personnel.[2] The test required subjects to run as far as possible in 15 min. A 1968 study by Cooper shortened run time to 12 min.[16]

In his original 12-min test validation study, Cooper reported a strong association between $\dot{V}O_{2max}$ in Air Force personnel and distances run-walked in 12 min. The correlation coefficient was $r = 0.90$ between 12-min run-walk distance and $\dot{V}O_{2max}$ (mL·kg^{-1}·min^{-1}) in 47 men who varied considerably in age (17 to 54 years), body mass (52 to 123 kg), and $\dot{V}O_{2max}$ (31 to 59 mL·kg^{-1}·min^{-1}). Other researchers reported the same correlation for 9 ninth-grade boys.[20] Subsequent studies have failed to demonstrate as strong a correlation between "Cooper 12-min run scores" and aerobic capacity. For example, one study measured 11- to 14-year-old boys and reported a correlation of $r = 0.65$.[49] For a group of 26 female athletes, the correlation was $r = 0.70$ between run-walk scores and $\dot{V}O_{2max}$[50] and $r = 0.67$ for 36 untrained college women.[42]

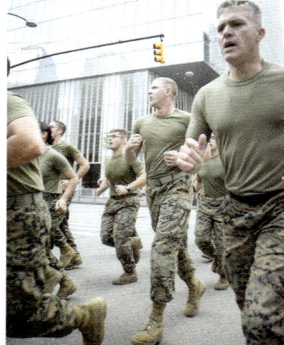

Glynnis Jones/Shutterstock

Most importantly, a simple correlation between run-walk scores and $\dot{V}O_{2max}$ does not consider the interacting but confounding age and body mass effects. These variables themselves relate to both run-walk times and $\dot{V}O_{2max}$ scores. When restricting these original data for females to the same age range as subjects in the preceding study for 36 untrained women, the computed correlation coefficient decreased dramatically from $r = 0.90$ to $r = 0.59$. This decrease changes the test result interpretations. In one case, $r = 0.90$ indicates a strong relationship exists between run test scores and $\dot{V}O_{2max}$, without age or weight exerting as large an influence. On the other hand, a correlation of $r = 0.59$ simply indicates the walk-run test has a relatively low predictive power—there simply is little chance the walk-run test would reveal much about the person's "true" $\dot{V}O_{2max}$ score.

One must, therefore, view $\dot{V}O_{2max}$ predictions based on running performance with caution. The need to establish a consistent motivation level and effective pacing during running becomes critical with inexperienced subjects. Some individuals achieve an optimal pace throughout the run while some may run too fast early and be forced to slow down or even stop before completing the test. Other individuals may begin too slowly and continue this way, so that their final performance scores reflect inappropriate pacing or poor motivation rather than poor physiologic capacity. The $\dot{V}O_{2max}$ does not singularly determine endurance running performance. Body mass and fatness levels, running economy, and aerobic capacity percentage sustained without blood lactate buildup also contribute to successful running. Generally, the SEE of predicting $\dot{V}O_{2max}$ from run-walk performance averages about ±8 to ±10% of the predicted value. At best, an 8 to 10% predictive spread compared to a "true" $\dot{V}O_{2max}$ score measured in the laboratory is generally of too great a magnitude for use other than general fitness screening.

Limitations for Use with Children

Maximum 1-mile run or walk times serve only limited use for $\dot{V}O_{2max}$ prediction in growing children because the age-related exercise performance improvements in youth relate poorly to aerobic capacity changes.[17] The largest contributions to test score improvement in children as they grow older result from increased $\dot{V}O_{2max}$ percentage sustained during the activity (i.e., increased blood lactate threshold) and improved running economy. Both factors contribute substantially to faster times independent of $\dot{V}O_{2max}$ improvements.

Predictions Based on Heart Rate

Tests to predict $\dot{V}O_{2max}$ use exercise or postexercise heart rate during a standardized submaximal effort performed on a bicycle ergometer, treadmill, or step test. These tests apply the essentially linear relationship between heart rate (HR) and oxygen uptake ($\dot{V}O_2$) during increasing light to relatively intense aerobic exercise. The slope of the line describing the HR-$\dot{V}O_2$ relationship (i.e., rate of heart rate increase) reflects cardiovascular response and aerobic fitness capacity. The $\dot{V}O_{2max}$ is estimated by drawing a best-fit straight line through several submaximal points that relate heart rate and oxygen uptake (or exercise intensity); the **HR-$\dot{V}O_2$ line** is then extended to an assumed maximum heart rate for the subject's age.

FIGURE 11.12 illustrates the extrapolation procedure for an untrained and an endurance-trained college student. Four submaximal measures during graded exercise provided the data points to construct the HR-$\dot{V}O_2$ line. Each person's HR-$\dot{V}O_2$ line tends toward linearity, although the slope of the line often differs considerably. A person with relatively high aerobic fitness performs more intense effort at about 160 b · min^{-1} heart rate (i.e., achieves higher $\dot{V}O_2$) than a less-fit person. Heart rate increases linearly with exercise intensity ($\dot{V}O_2$), so the person with the smallest heart rate increase tends to achieve the highest exercise capacity and highest $\dot{V}O_{2max}$. Extrapolating the HR-$\dot{V}O_2$ line to 195 b · min^{-1}—the assumed maximum heart rate for college age individuals—predicted the two students $\dot{V}O_{2max}$ as shown in Figure 11.12.

Four assumptions impact the $\dot{V}O_{2max}$ prediction accuracy from submaximal exercise heart rate:

1. *Linearity of heart rate-oxygen uptake or exercise intensity relationship.* This assumption generally holds, particularly during light to moderate physical activity. In some subjects, the HR-$\dot{V}O_2$ line curves or asymptotes at more intense workloads in a direction indicating a larger than expected oxygen uptake increase per unit increase in heart

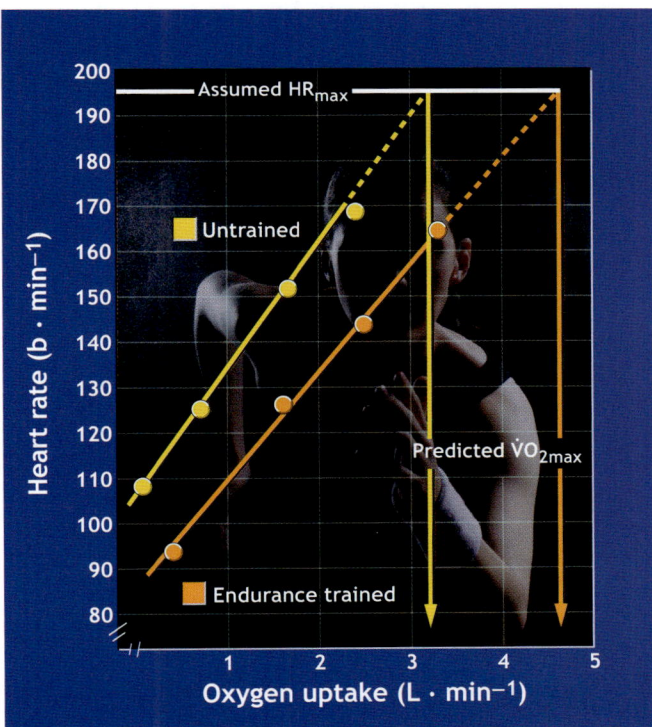

FIGURE 11.12. Extrapolating the linear relationship between submaximal heart rate and oxygen uptake up to an assumed maximal heart rate (HR$_{max}$) in graded exercise by an untrained subject and endurance-trained subject. $\dot{V}O_{2max}$, maximum oxygen uptake.

rate. Oxygen uptake increases more than predicted by linearly extrapolating the HR-$\dot{V}O_2$ line, thereby underestimating these subjects' $\dot{V}O_{2max}$.

2. *Similar maximum heart rates for all subjects.* One standard deviation from the average maximum heart rate for individuals of the same age equals ±10 b·min^{-1}. Extrapolating the HR-$\dot{V}O_2$ line of a young adult to 195 b·min^{-1}, for example, overestimates the person's $\dot{V}O_{2max}$ with a 185 b·min^{-1} actual maximum heart rate. The opposite occurs for a subject with an actual 205 b·min^{-1} maximum heart rate. Maximum heart rate also decreases with age. Failure to consider an age effect (i.e., extrapolating to an average 195 b·min^{-1} heart rate for 25-year-olds) consistently overestimates $\dot{V}O_{2max}$ in older subjects. Chapter 31 discusses the aging effect on maximum heart rate.

3. *Assumed constant economy and mechanical efficiency during activity.* Variations in exercise economy contribute to $\dot{V}O_{2max}$ prediction errors with tests that estimate submaximal oxygen uptake from the external workload (rather than measuring $\dot{V}O_2$ directly). More specifically, underestimating $\dot{V}O_{2max}$ would occur for a subject with poor exercise economy whose submaximal oxygen uptake increases more than assumed based on estimates from exercise intensity. This occurs from the elevated heart rate from the added uneconomical movement's oxygen cost. Variation in walking or cycling economy among individuals usually does not exceed 6%; for bench stepping, the variation can equal about 10%, a value unrelated to age, leg length, aerobic fitness, or percentage body fat.[89] Seemingly, small modifications in test procedures profoundly affect exercise economy. Allowing individuals to support themselves with the treadmill handrails reduces the exercise oxygen cost by as much as 30%.[108]

4. *Day-to-day heart rate variation.* Under standardized conditions, the day-to-day variation in heart rate averages about 5 b·min^{-1} during submaximal exercise.

Considering these four limitations, $\dot{V}O_{2max}$ predicted from submaximal heart rate would generally fall within ±10 to ±20% of a person's actual value assessed in the laboratory. This accuracy level remains *unacceptable* for research purposes, yet the prediction tests can "sort-of" screen and classify individuals for aerobic fitness in a gymnasium or health-club setting. The run-walk test has been used to estimate aerobic capacity during pregnancy (see In a Practical Sense, Chapter 9).

The Step Test

"Prediction equations" applied to step test results can estimate $\dot{V}O_{2max}$ with reasonable accuracy. In one of our laboratories, we devised a 3-min step test to evaluate heart rate responses in thousands of college men and women.[55] Gymnasium bleacher steps 16¼ in/41.3 cm high were used to test approximately 60 students at the same time (30 students stepping, 30 students acting as recorders with each stepper). Subjects performed each stepping cycle to a four-step cadence, "up-up-down-down." The women performed 22 complete step-ups per min, regulated by a metronome set at 88 b·min^{-1}. Males tended to be "fitter" for step-up exercise than females, so their cadence was 24 step-ups per min or 96 b·min^{-1} on the metronome. The step test began after a brief demonstration and practice period. After stepping, students remained standing while pulse rate was measured for 15 s, 5 to 20 s into recovery. Recovery heart rate was converted to beats per min (15 s HR × 4).

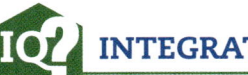

INTEGRATIVE QUESTION

Why do $\dot{V}O_{2max}$ values measured directly in the laboratory not always agree with those predicted with a 12-min run?

Based on the linear relationship between heart rate and oxygen uptake during submaximal effort, one would expect a person with a low step test heart rate (i.e., farther from maximum) to experience less stress than someone the same age who performed identical exercise with a relatively higher heart rate. In other words, a lower heart rate during a standard exercise corresponds to a higher $\dot{V}O_{2max}$. To determine step test validity to estimate aerobic capacity, we then measured the $\dot{V}O_{2max}$ for a group of untrained, young adult men and women who also performed the step test. **FIGURE 11.13** illustrates the relationship between $\dot{V}O_{2max}$ and female's step test scores. The results clearly indicated that step test heart rate provided useful information about $\dot{V}O_{2max}$. Females with a high recovery heart rate tended to have a lower $\dot{V}O_{2max}$, whereas a faster recovery (lower heart rate) related to a relatively higher $\dot{V}O_{2max}$. The following equations predict $\dot{V}O_{2max}$ (mL·kg^{-1}·min^{-1}) from step test pulse rate (ST$_{pulse}$) for similar young adult male and female groups:

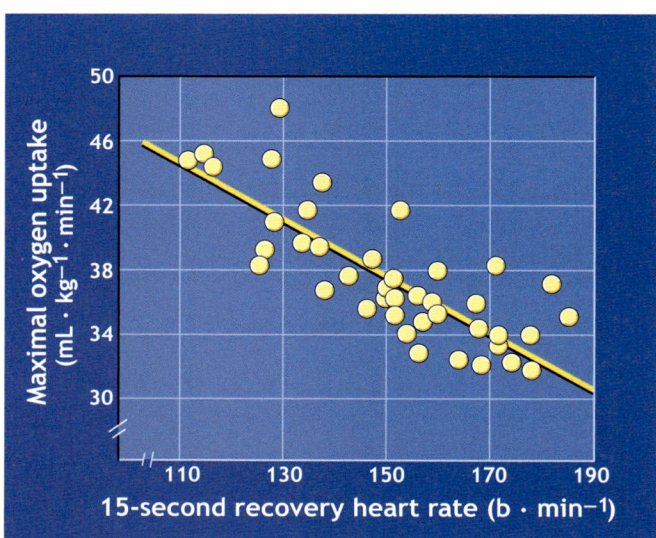

FIGURE 11.13. Scattergram and line of "best fit" that relates step test heart rate scores and maximal oxygen uptake in untrained college females.

Males:

$$\dot{V}O_{2max} = 111.33 - (0.42 \times ST_{pulse}\,[b \cdot min^{-1}])$$

Females:

$$\dot{V}O_{2max} = 65.81 - (0.1847 \times ST_{pulse}\,[b \cdot min^{-1}])$$

For example, an untrained college-age male with a 152 b · min^{-1} step test recovery pulse rate has a 47.5 mL · kg^{-1} · min^{-1} (111.33 − [0.42 × 152]) predicted $\dot{V}O_{2max}$. For predictive accuracy, one can be 95% confident that the predicted $\dot{V}O_{2max}$ falls within ±16% of the person's "true" $\dot{V}O_{2max}$.

A Novel Approach to Prediction from Nonexercise Data

A unique approach to $\dot{V}O_{2max}$ prediction for quick screening of large groups of individuals requires specific nonexercise data obtained via a questionnaire.[28,38]

TABLE 11.3 Input information on level of physical activity and perceived functional capacity for predicting $\dot{V}O_{2max}$ from nonexercise data

The SEE for a predicted score from the method described below equals ±3.44 mL O$_2$ · kg^{-1} · min^{-1}.

The following example shows how to predict $\dot{V}O_{2max}$ using the data from **TABLE 11.3**.

Input Data:

1. **Sex**—(female = 0; male = 1).
2. **Body mass index** (**BMI; kg · m^{-2}**)—Self-reported body mass (kg) and stature (m) to compute BMI as follows:

$$BMI = Body\ mass\ (kg) \div Stature\ (m^2)$$

3. **Physical activity rating** (**PA-R**)—A point value between 0 and 10 represents overall physical activity level for the previous 6 months (Table 11.3A).
4. **Perceived functional ability** (**PFA**)—Point value sum between 0 and 13 for questions about current perceived functional ability level to maintain a continuous pace on an indoor track for 1 mi and perceived pace to cover 3 mi without becoming breathless or overly fatigued (Table 11.3B).

Equation

$$\dot{V}O_{2max}(mL \cdot kg^{-1} \cdot min^{-1}) = 44.895 + (7.042 \times Sex)$$
$$- (0.823 \times BMI)$$
$$+ (0.738 \times PFA)$$
$$+ (0.688 \times PA\text{-}R)$$

Example

1. Sex, female
2. BMI = 22.66 (self-reported body mass 61.7 kg/136 lb; self-reported height 1.65 m/5 ft 5 in; BMI = 61.7 ÷ (1.65 × 1.65) = 22.66
3. PA-R score = 5 (self-reported from Table 11.3A)
4. PFA score = 15 (sum of 7 scored on first question set and 8 on the second set; see Table 11.3B)

Computation

$$\dot{V}O_{2max}(mL \cdot kg^{-1} \cdot min^{-1}) = 44.895 + (7.042 \times Sex)$$
$$- (0.823 \times BMI)$$
$$+ (0.738 \times PFA)$$
$$+ (0.688 \times PA\text{-}R)$$
$$= 44.895 + (7.042 \times 0)$$
$$- (0.823 \times 22.66)$$
$$+ (0.738 \times 15) + (0.688 \times 5)$$
$$= 44.895 - 18.65 + 11.07$$
$$+ 3.77$$
$$= 41.1\ mL \cdot kg^{-1} \cdot min^{-1}$$

Summary

1. The individual differences and exercise specificity concepts provide an important underlying framework to understand anaerobic and aerobic power capacities.
2. Precise anaerobic and aerobic energy transfer contributions depend largely on effort intensity and duration.
3. Energy transfer during strength and power-sprint activities primarily involves the immediate and short-term (anaerobic) energy systems.
4. The long-term (aerobic) energy system becomes progressively more active during activity lasting longer than 2 min.
5. Physiologic measurements and performance tests can assess each energy transfer system's capacity.
6. The stair-sprinting test assesses the intramuscular high-energy phosphates (ATP and PCr) energy-generating power capacity.
7. The 30-s Wingate test evaluates peak power and average power output capacity from the glycolytic pathway.
8. The maximal accumulated oxygen deficit (MAOD) correlates positively with other anaerobic performance tests; it demonstrates independence from aerobic energy sources to differentiate aerobically from anaerobically trained individuals.
9. Training status, acid-base regulation, and motivation contribute to individual differences in the immediate and short-term anaerobic energy systems.
10. Maximum oxygen uptake ($\dot{V}O_{2max}$) provides important, reproducible information about the long-term energy system's power capacity and the physiologic support systems' functional capacity.
11. Heredity, training mode, age, gender, and body composition uniquely contribute to an individual's $\dot{V}O_{2max}$.
12. Expressing $\dot{V}O_{2max}$ as a ratio, which includes body size or composition (e.g., mL · kg^{-1} · min^{-1} or mL · kg FFM^{-1} · min^{-1}), reduces $\dot{V}O_{2max}$ sex differences.

13. $\dot{V}O_{2max}$ prediction tests from submaximal physiologic and performance data often prove useful for placing individuals into different fitness classifications.
14. Tests to predict $\dot{V}O_{2max}$ from submaximal physiologic and performance data rely on the validity of four assumptions: HR-$\dot{V}O_2$ relationship linearity, constancy in maximum heart rate, relatively constant and typical exercise economy, and minimal day-to-day variation in exercise heart rate.
15. Field testing methods provide useful information about cardiovascular-aerobic function for groups, but should be undertaken with caution for individual $\dot{V}O_{2max}$ predictions.
16. Nonexercise data to predict $\dot{V}O_{2max}$ are useful to classify and screen individuals for physical activity programs participation.

Key Terms

Anaerobic capacity: Total mechanical work in a given time period during short-duration maximal effort

Anaerobic fatigue: Percentage decline in power output during short-duration maximal effort

ATP-PCr energy system: Energy system from catabolizing adenosine triphosphate (ATP) and phosphocreatine (PCr) energy reserves known as the immediate energy system

Fatigue rate: Decline in power output rate relative to peak power output

Generality principle: Individuals with a high $\dot{V}O_{2max}$ in one physical activity mode to also possess above-average aerobic capacity in other diverse big muscle activities

Graded exercise: Laboratory exercise test that involves progressive increases in effort intensity

HR-$\dot{V}O_2$ line: Best-fit straight line through several submaximal points that relate heart rate (HR) and oxygen uptake ($\dot{V}O_2$ or exercise intensity)

Immediate energy system: Energy system catabolizes adenosine triphosphate (ATP) and phosphocreatine (PCr) energy reserves

Individual differences: True differences among individuals on test variables distinguished from trial-to-trial differences within an individual

Katch test: "All-out" stationary short-duration (40-s) cycling test (frictional resistance = 6 kg/13 lb for males and 5 kg/11 lb for females) to estimate the anaerobic energy system's power output capacity

Maximally accumulated oxygen deficit (MAOD): Extrapolation procedure calculates the difference between predicted supramaximal oxygen uptake from the exercise intensity-oxygen uptake relationship and oxygen uptake measured during a 2- to 3-min all-out treadmill run to fatigue

Peak oxygen uptake ($\dot{V}O_{2peak}$): Highest measured oxygen uptake value during a test when the accepted maximum oxygen uptake criteria are not met, or when local arm or leg muscle fatigue rather than central circulatory dynamics limits test performance

Peak power: Highest mechanical power output, measured in watts, generated during a short-duration maximal physical effort

Relative peak power (RPP) output: Peak power output (in watts) relative to body mass: PP ÷ body mass (kg)

Relative power: Peak power output divided by body weight

Short-term glycolytic energy system: Energy system from glucose breakdown in glycolysis, which refers to rapid glycolytic ATP production and lactate formation known as the lactate-producing energy system

Specificity concept: Individuals with a high score in one exercise form do not necessarily score high in another exercise form

Standard error of estimate (SEE): Degree of prediction errors for a given data set, expressed in the same units as the actual score, with two thirds of the data points falling within a ±1SEE and about 95% within ±2SEE

Watts: A unit of power in the International System of Units; 1 W = 1 kg · m² · s⁻³/0.73756 ft-lb · s⁻¹or 6.12 kg-m · min⁻¹

Wingate test: Assess anaerobic energy system's power output capacity using "all-out" supramaximal effort on stationary cycling for 30 s with resistance set at 0.075 kg per kg body weight

References are available online at Lippincott Connect.

Additional References

Andrade VL, et al. Determination of maximum accumulated oxygen deficit using backward extrapolation. *Int J Sports Med*. 2021;42:161.

Cheng AJ, et al. Intramuscular mechanisms of overtraining. *Redox Biol*. 2020;35:101480.

De Oliveira Tavares VD, et al. Reliability and convergent validity of self-reported physical activity questionnaires for people with mental disorders: a systematic review and meta-analysis. *J Phys Act Health*. 2020;1:7.

Dzik KP, et al. Single bout of exercise triggers the increase of vitamin D blood concentration in adolescent trained boys: a pilot study. *Sci Rep*. 2022;12:1825.

Gil-Cabrera J, et al. Traditional versus optimum power load training in professional cyclists: a randomized controlled trial. *Int J Sports Physiol Perform*. 2021;16:496.

Jamnick NA, et al. An examination and critique of current methods to determine exercise intensity. *Sports Med*. 2020;50:1729.

Jordan AC, et al. Promoting a pro-oxidant state in skeletal muscle: potential dietary, environmental, and exercise interventions for enhancing endurance-training adaptations. *Free Radic Biol Med*. 2021;176:189.

Kaufmann S, et al. The metabolic relevance of type of locomotion in anaerobic testing: Bosco continuous jumping test versus Wingate anaerobic test of the same duration. *Int J Sports Physiol Perform*. 2021:1.doi:10.1123/ijspp.2020-0669.

Kim MC, Ahn Y. The value of exercise stress test in patients with stable ischemic heart disease. *J Korean Med Sci.* 2020;35:e21.

Knaier R, et al. Diurnal variation in maximum endurance and maximum strength performance: a systematic review and meta-analysis. *Med Sci Sports Exerc.* 2022;54:169.

Muriel X, et al. Physical demands and performance indicators in male professional cyclists during a grand tour: Worldtour versus Proteam category. *Int J Sports Physiol Perform.* 2022;17:22.

Nowak AM, et al. Application of the arm-cranking 30-second Wingate Anaerobic Test (the WAnT) to assess power in amputee football players. *Acta Bioeng Biomech.* 2021;23:13.

Özbay S, Ulupınar S. Strength-power tests are more effective when performed after exhaustive exercise in discrimination between top-elite and elite wrestlers. *J Strength Cond Res.* 2022;36:448.

Poole DC, et al. The anaerobic threshold: 50+ years of controversy. *J Physiol.* 2021;599:737.

Possamai LT, et al. Similar maximal oxygen uptake assessment from a step cycling incremental test and verification tests on the same or different day. *Appl Physiol Nutr Metab.* 2020;45:357.

Quittmann OJ, et al. Maximal lactate accumulation rate and postexercise lactate kinetics in handcycling and cycling. *Eur J Sport Sci.* 2020;12:1.

Ravindrakumar A, et al. Daily variation in performance measures related to anaerobic power and capacity: a systematic review. *Chronobiol Int.* 2022:1.doi:10.1080/07420528.2021.1994585.

Yoshimura M, et al. Effects of artificial CO_2-rich cold-water immersion on repeated-cycling work efficiency. *Res Sports Med.* 2022;30:215..

Table 11.1 Wingate Percentile Norms for Average Power and Peak Power for Physically Active Young Adult Men and Women

| | Male | | Female | | Male | | Female | |
| | Avg Power Watts | Avg Power Watts · kg BM^{-1} | Avg Power Watts | Avg Power Watts · kg BM^{-1} | Peak Power Watts | Peak Power Watts · kg BM^{-1} | Peak Power Watts | Peak Power Watts · kg BM^{-1} |
% Rank								
90	662	8.24	470	7.31	822	10.89	560	9.02
80	618	8.01	419	6.95	777	10.39	527	8.83
70	600	7.91	410	6.77	757	10.20	505	8.53
60	577	7.59	391	6.59	721	9.80	480	8.14
50	565	7.44	381	6.39	689	9.22	449	7.65
40	548	7.14	367	6.15	671	8.92	432	6.96
30	530	7.00	353	6.03	656	8.53	399	6.86
20	496	6.59	336	5.71	618	8.24	376	6.57
10	471	5.98	306	5.25	570	7.06	353	5.98

Note: Avg, average; Watts · kg BM^{-1}, watts per kg body mass.

Adapted from Maud PJ, Schultz BB. Norms for the Wingate anaerobic test with comparisons in another similar test. *Res Q Exerc Sport.* 1989;60:144. Use with permission of the Society of Health and Physical Educators, www.shapeamerica.org.

Table 11.2 Average Maximum Oxygen Uptake During Continuous and Discontinuous Tests on the Treadmill and Bicycle Ergometer

| | Bike | | Treadmill | | | |
Variable	Discont.	Cont.	Discont. Run-Walk	Cont. Walk	Discont. Run	Cont. Run
$\dot{V}O_{2max}$, mL · min^{-1}	3691 ± 453	3683 ± 448	4145 ± 401	3944 ± 395	4157 ± 445	4109 ± 424
$\dot{V}O_{2max}$, mL · kg^{-1} · min^{-1}	50.0 ± 6.9	49.9 ± 7.0	56.6 ± 7.3	53.7 ± 7.6	56.6 ± 7.6	55.5 ± 6.8

Note: Values are means ± standard deviations. Cont., continuous; Discont., discontinuous; $\dot{V}O_{2max}$, maximum oxygen uptake.

Adapted with permission from McArdle WD, et al. Comparison of continuous and discontinuous treadmill and bicycle tests for max Vo2. *Med Sci Sports.* 1973;5:156.

Table 11.3 Input Information on Level of Physical Activity and Perceived Functional Capacity for Predicting $\dot{V}O_{2max}$ from Nonexercise Data

A. Physical Activity Rating (PA-R)

Select the number that best describes your overall level of physical activity for the previous 6 months:

Points	Exertion Level	Miles/wk Run	Time/wk Spent	Description of Activity
0	Inactive	—	—	Avoid walking or exertion (e.g., always use elevator, drive rather than walk)
1	Light	—	—	Walk for pleasure, routinely use stairs, occasionally exercise with heavy breathing/perspiration
2	Moderate	—	10–60 min	Golf, horseback riding, calisthenics, table tennis, bowling, weightlifting, yard work, cleaning house, walking for exercise
3	Moderate	—	>1 hr	See activities listed for 2 points
4	Vigorous	<1	<30 min	Running or comparable activity: lap swimming, cycling, rowing, aerobics, skipping rope, running in place, soccer, basketball, tennis, racquetball, handball
5	Vigorous	1 to <5	30 to <60 min	Running or comparable activity (see 4 points)
6	Vigorous	5 to <10	1 to <3 hr	Running or comparable activity (see 4 points)
7	Vigorous	10 to <15	3 to <6 hr	Running or comparable activity (see 4 points)
8	Vigorous	15 to <20	6 to <7 hr	Running or comparable activity (see 4 points)
9	Vigorous	20–25	7–8 hr	Running or comparable activity (see 4 points)
10	Vigorous	>25	>8 hr	Running or comparable activity (see 4 points)

B. Perceived Functional Ability (PFA) Questions

Suppose you exercise continuously on an indoor track for 1 mile. Which exercise pace is right for you—not too easy or not too hard? Circle the appropriate number from 1 to 13.

How fast could you cover a distance of 3 miles and NOT become breathless or overly fatigued? Be realistic. Circle the appropriate number from 1 to 13.

Points	Activity	Pace (min/mi)	Points	Activity	Pace (min/mi)
1	Walking	Slow (18 min/mi)	1	Walking	Slow (18 min/mi)
2			2		
3	Walking	Medium (16 min/mi)	3	Walking	Medium (16 min/mi)
4			4		
5	Walking	Fast (14 min/mi)	5	Walking	Fast (14 min/mi)
6			6		
7	Jogging	Slow (12 min/mi)	7	Jogging	Slow (12 min/mi)
8			8		
9	Jogging	Medium (10 min/mi)	9	Jogging	Medium (10 min/mi)
10			10		
11	Jogging	Fast (8 min/mi)	11	Jogging	Fast (8 min/mi)
12			12		
13	Running	Fast (≤7 min/mi)	13	Running	Fast (≤7 min/mi)

Adapted with permission from George JD, et al. Non-exercise $\dot{V}O_{2max}$ estimation for physically active college students. *Med Sci Sports Exerc.* 1997;29:415.

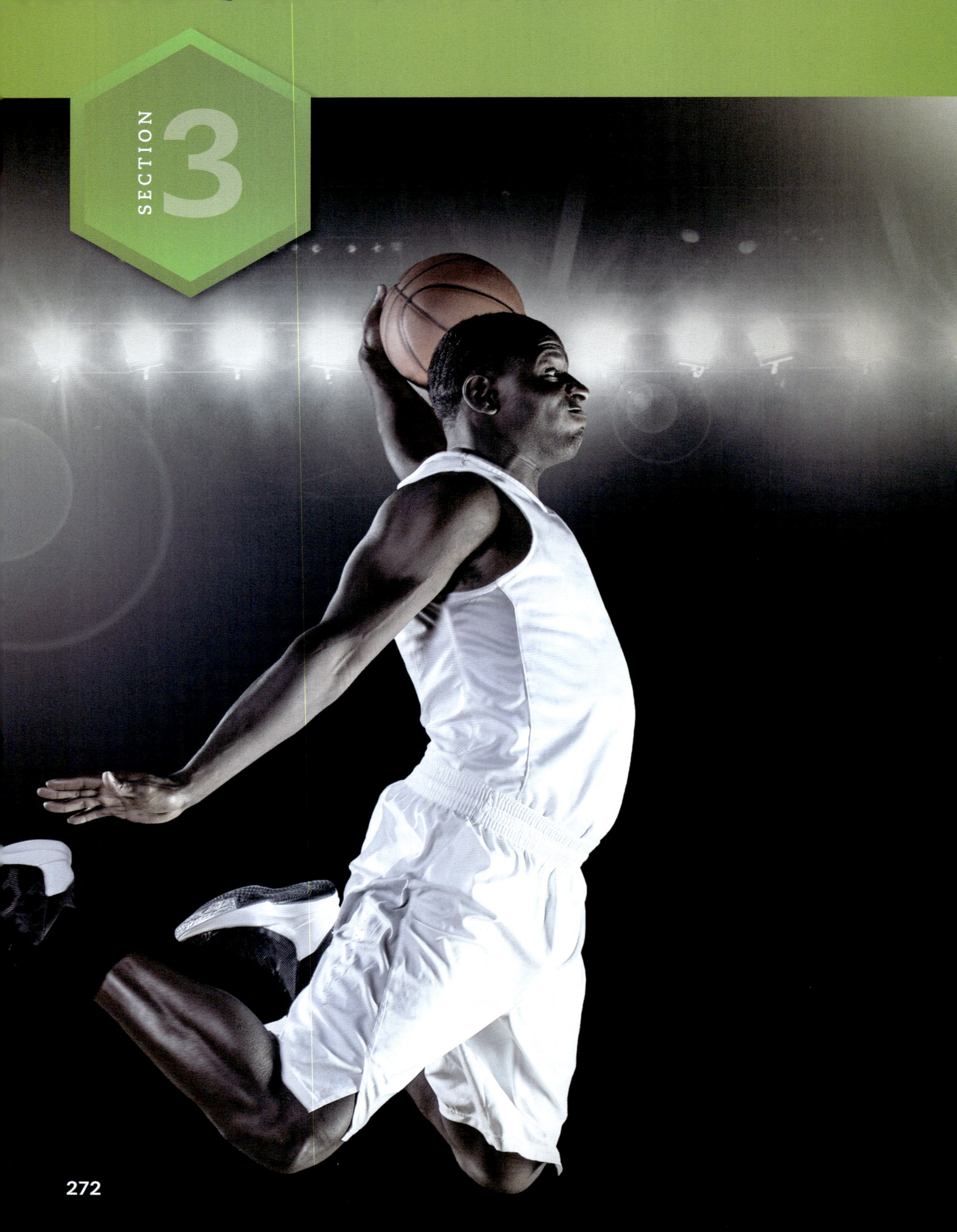

SECTION 3

Aerobic Energy Delivery and Use

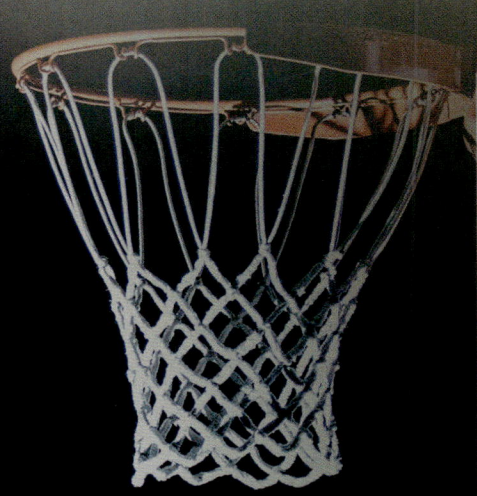

Overview

Many sports, recreational, and occupational activities depend on a moderately intense and sustained energy release. Carbohydrate, lipid, and protein breakdown through aerobic processes provide energy for activities powered by phosphorylating adenosine diphosphate to the energy-rich cellular currency adenosine triphosphate (ATP). Two factors influence how well individuals keep up a high steady-rate (aerobic) physical activity level with negligible fatigue:

1. **Capacity and integration for physiologic support systems for oxygen delivery**
2. **Capacity for specific muscle fibers activated during physical activity to create ATP aerobically**

Individual differences in aerobic capacity depend on the contributions from ventilatory, circulatory, muscular, and endocrine systems described in this section. Experimental evidence about the energy requirements and corresponding physiologic adjustments to exercise provides a solid basis to formulate effective physical activity training programs.

CHAPTER 12
Pulmonary Structure and Function

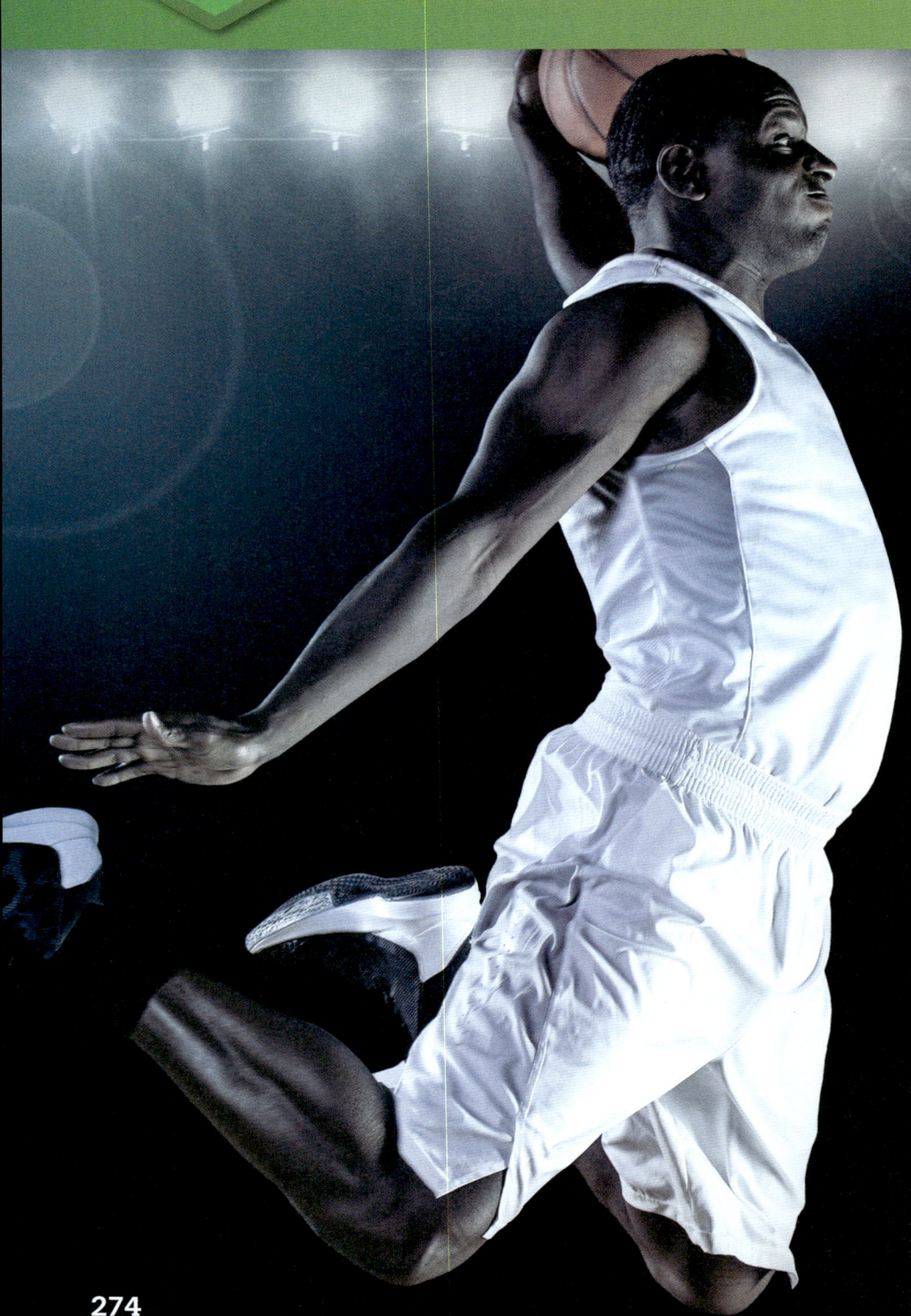

Chapter Objectives

- Diagram the ventilatory system, labeling the glottis, trachea, bronchi, bronchioles, and alveoli
- Describe the ventilatory system's conducting, transitional, and respiratory zones
- Discuss the mechanical and muscular aspects of inspiration and expiration during rest and physical activity
- Define and quantify static and dynamic lung function measures and how they relate to physical performance
- Define minute ventilation, alveolar ventilation, ventilation-perfusion ratio, and anatomic and physiologic dead space
- Discuss how breathing rate and tidal volume relate to minute ventilation and alveolar minute ventilation at rest and during physical activity
- Discuss factors that account for variations in the ventilation-perfusion ratio among healthy individuals and those with pulmonary limitations, and how this ratio varies in different lung areas
- Explain the four phases of the Valsalva maneuver and its physiologic consequences
- Describe how cold-weather exercise affects respiratory system function

Ancillaries at-a-Glance

Visit Lippincott Connect to access the following resources:

- References: Chapter 12
- Animations: Accessory Muscles of Respiration, Asthma, Perform a Pulmonary Function Test, Pulmonary Ventilation, The Respiratory System
- Focus on Research: Physiologic Control of Pulmonary Ventilation

If oxygen supply to muscle depended only on diffusion through the skin surface, one could not sustain the 0.2- to 0.4-L·min⁻¹ basal oxygen requirement, let alone the 4- to 5-L·min⁻¹ oxygen uptake and carbon dioxide elimination required to run at a world-class, sub–5-min·mi⁻¹ marathon pace. The body's compact and efficient **ventilatory system** meets the requirements for gas exchange. This system, depicted in **FIGURE 12.1**, regulates the body's "external" pulmonary environment to effectively aerate body fluids.

Ventilation Anatomy

Pulmonary ventilation describes moving ambient air and exchanging it for air in the lungs. Air entering the nose and mouth flows into the ventilatory system's conductive portions to adjust to body temperature and become filtered and humidified as it travels through the **trachea**. The inspired air then passes into two **bronchi**, the airway passages that serve as primary conduits into each lung. The bronchi further subdivide into numerous **bronchioles**, which conduct inspired air through a winding, narrow route until eventually mixing it with existing air in the alveolar ducts. Microscopic **alveoli**, hollow terminal capillary-rich cavities that are spherical outcroppings of the respiratory bronchioles, completely envelop these ducts.

Pulmonary Respiration Versus Cellular Respiration: A Conflict in Terms?

Physiologists use the term *respiration* in two different yet inexorably linked contexts. *Cellular respiration* defines metabolic processes that occur within the cell that generate energy via oxygen use and carbon dioxide production. **Pulmonary respiration** defines lung ventilation with resulting uptake of oxygen and carbon dioxide elimination to maintain blood-gas homeostasis.

RAJ CREATIONZS/ Shutterstock

The Lungs

The lungs provide the **gas exchange surface** that separates blood from the surrounding alveolar gaseous environment. Oxygen transfers from alveolar air into alveolar capillary blood. Simultaneously, the blood's carbon dioxide flows into the alveolar chambers, where it comes in contact with ambient air separated only by a thin cellular barrier.

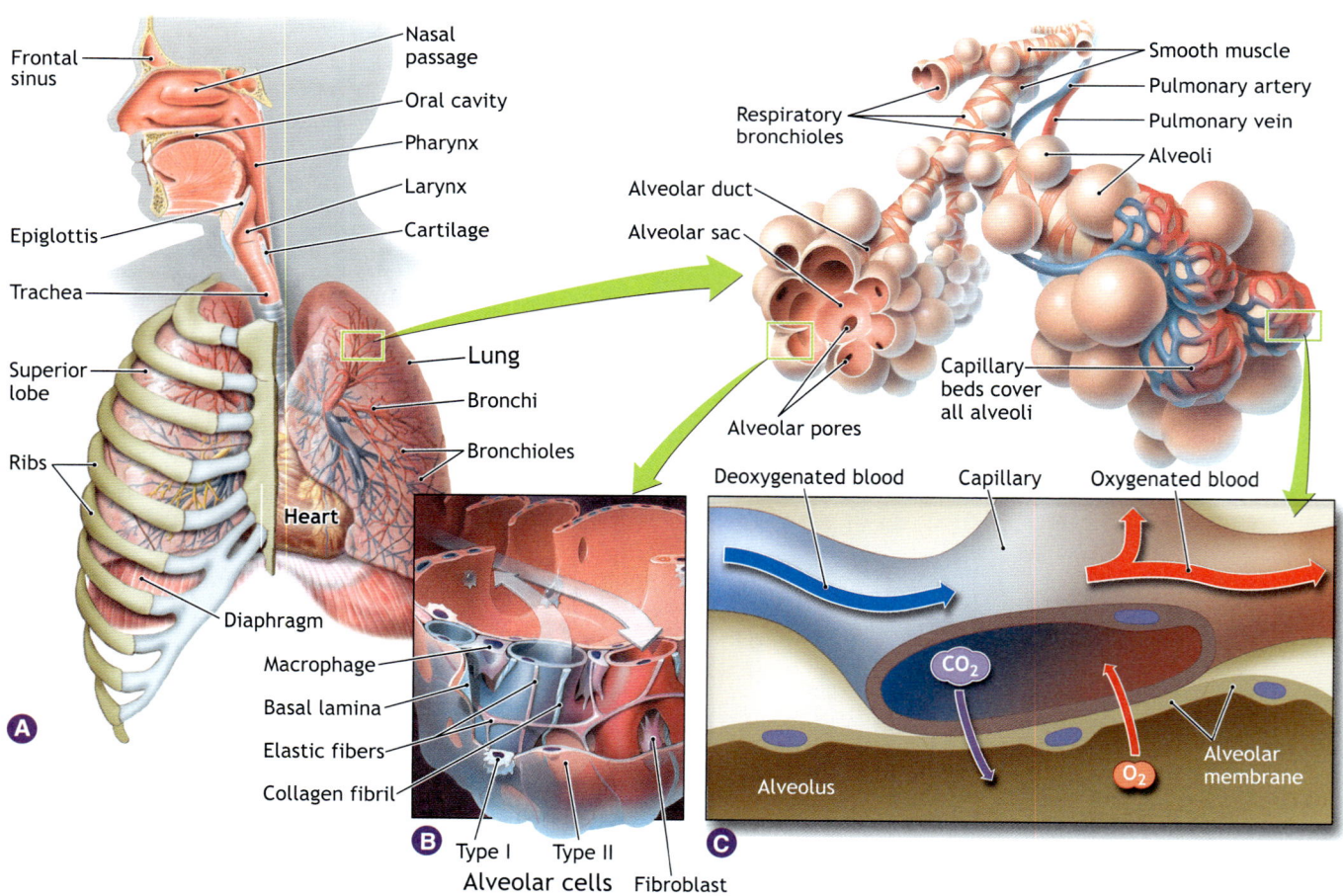

FIGURE 12.1. **(A)** Major pulmonary structures within the thoracic cavity including the respiratory tree's terminal branches. **(B)** Lung tissue slice showing individual alveolus including type I cells that form the alveolar wall, type II cells secrete pulmonary surfactant, and macrophages that destroy foreign substances including bacteria. **(C)** Alveolus gas exchange function.

The paired lungs weigh about 2.3 kg for an average-size adult, with volume ranging between 4 and 6 L—about the air volume in a standard basketball. The lungs have about 10% solid tissue, with the remainder filled by air and blood. They provide an exceptionally large surface for gas exchange. If spread out onto a basketball court, the total lung tissue would cover an area 50 to 140 m² (depending on body mass and stature), a value 20 to 65 times larger than the body's external surface.

Within the chest cavity, the highly vascularized, moist lung tissue includes 1500 miles of airways and 600 miles of capillaries. The capillaries represent the body's smallest blood vessels, shrouded by a thin cell membrane to allow a single file of red blood cells to pass through its 5 to 10 μm diameter. The lung membranes fold over onto themselves to provide a considerable interface to aerate blood. At rest, a single red blood cell remains in a pulmonary capillary for only about 0.5 to 1.0 s as it traverses two to three individual alveoli. During any 1 s of maximal effort, no more than 1 pint of blood flows within the delicate mesh network of lung tissue blood vessels.

Common Symbols in Pulmonary Physiology

The following table shows the most common symbols related to pulmonary ventilation, external respiration, and internal respiration.

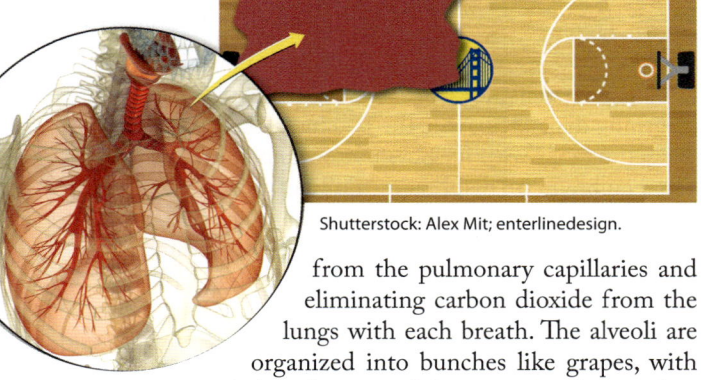

Shutterstock: Alex Mit; enterlinedesign.

Pulmonary Ventilation	External Respiration	Internal Respiration
$\dot{V}_E$ = Minute ventilation	$\dot{V}_A$ = Alveolar minute ventilation	a-$\bar{v}O_{2\,diff}$ = O_2 quantity in arteries minus amount carried in veins
V_d = Dead space	P_AO_2 = Alveoli O_2 partial pressure	PaO_2 = Arterial blood O_2 partial pressure
V_T = Tidal volume	PaO_2 = Arterial blood O_2 partial pressure	$PaCO_2$ = Arterial blood CO_2 partial pressure
F = Breathing frequency	(A-a)$PO_{2\,diff}$ = Oxygen or PO_2 pressure gradient between alveoli and arteries	$PvCO_2$ = Venous blood CO_2 partial pressure
V_d/V_T = Ratio dead space to tidal volume	$SaO_{2\%}$ = Arterial blood %O_2 saturation	$SvO_{2\%}$ = Venous blood O_2 % saturation
	P_ACO_2 = Alveoli CO_2 partial pressure	PvO_2 = Venous blood O_2 partial pressure

The Alveoli

The lungs, on average, contain about 600 million alveoli (from Latin alveolus, meaning "*little cavity*"), ranging from 270 to 790 million, depending on a person's size. These microscopic, balloonlike structures are responsible for capturing oxygen from the pulmonary capillaries and eliminating carbon dioxide from the lungs with each breath. The alveoli are organized into bunches like grapes, with each bunch grouped into an alveolar sac (see Fig. 12.4). The diameter of each alveolus (singular for alveoli) averages about 0.2 mm/0.008 in. Alveolar number closely relates to total lung volume, with larger lungs having more alveoli and taller people having larger lungs.

These elastic, thin-walled membranous alveolar sacs composed of simple squamous epithelial cells provide the vital surface for gas exchange between lung tissue and blood. Alveolar tissue receives the largest blood supply of any body organ. Millions of capillaries and alveoli lie side by side; air moves along one side and blood along the other. Gases diffuse across the extremely thin alveolar and capillary cell barrier (approximately 0.3 μm); the diffusion distance remains relatively constant throughout varying physical activity intensity levels. Integrity of the thin pulmonary blood-gas barrier remains constant during sustained effort. The surface remains as thin as possible to accelerate rapid gas exchange without compromising structural integrity. In elite endurance athletes, alveolar mechanical stress from a large ventilation and accompanying pulmonary blood flow in near-maximal exercise can impair the blood-gas barrier's permeability. For these individuals, an increased permeability is reflected by elevated red blood cell concentrations, total protein, and leukotriene B_4 (a potent chemotactic agent that initiates, coordinates, and amplifies the inflammatory response) in bronchoalveolar lavage fluid with maximal exertion.[22,23,46]

Small **pores of Kohn** within each alveolus evenly disperse surfactant (see the section "Surfactant" below) over the respiratory membranes to reduce surface tension for easier alveolar inflation. The pores also provide for collateral gas interchange for uniform air distribution between adjacent alveoli. Mixing in this manner sustains indirect ventilation of alveoli damaged or blocked due to lung disease (see Chapter 32).[49,50]

Each minute at rest, approximately 250 mL of oxygen leaves the alveoli and enters the blood, and 200 mL of carbon dioxide diffuses in the opposite direction. When endurance athletes perform intense exercise, nearly 25 times this quantity of oxygen and carbon dioxide transfers across the alveolar-capillary membrane. In healthy individuals, pulmonary ventilation during rest and physical activity maintains a constant and favorable oxygen and carbon dioxide concentration in the alveolar chambers to ensure complete gaseous exchange before the blood exits the lungs for transport throughout the body.

See the animation "The Respiratory System" on Lippincott Connect to view this process.

Ventilation Mechanics

FIGURE 12.2 illustrates the physical principle that underlies breathing dynamics. Note the two lung-shaped balloons suspended in a jar with its glass bottom replaced by a thin rubber membrane or diaphragm. Pulling the membrane down increases jar volume, whereas the membrane's recoil following release after this action decreases jar volume, causing the air to rush out. Similarly, during inspiration in humans, the chest cavity increases in size because the ribs rise and the diaphragm descends, causing air to flow into the lungs. Inhalation increases the anteroposterior (A-P) and vertical rib-cage diameters. Approximately 70% of lung expansion results from A-P enlargement and 30% from diaphragmatic descent. In addition to diaphragmatic action, the external intercostal muscles become active and the internal intercostal muscles relax during inhalation. During expiration, the ribs swing down and the diaphragm returns to a relaxed position. This reduces thoracic cavity volume, and air rushes out. In the jar analogy, moving the jar's rubber bottom causes air to enter and exit the two balloons, simulating diaphragmatic action. Movement of the bucket handle simulates rib action. The diaphragm, external intercostals, sternocleidomastoids, scapular elevators, anterior serrati, and spinal erector muscles compose the inspiratory muscles that elevate and enlarge the thorax; expiratory muscles (rectus abdominis, internal intercostals, posterior inferior serrati muscles) depress the thorax and reduce its size. Deep-breathing exercise increases the power and efficiency of the intercostal muscles and diaphragm and is used as a therapeutic strategy for patients with asthma.[63]

FIGURE 12.3 illustrates the ventilatory system, subdivided into two parts:

1. **Conducting zones** 1–16, *shown in blue at the right*, which include the trachea and terminal bronchioles
2. **Transitional and respiratory zones** 17–23, *shown in brown at the right*, which comprise the bronchioles, alveolar ducts, and alveoli

The conducting zone structures contain no alveoli, so the term **anatomic dead space** describes this volume, which is usually about 150 mL. It represents the inhaled air portion that remains in the conducting airways following inhalation and does not participate in gas exchange. The respiratory zone represents the gas exchange site. It occupies about 2.5 to 3.0 L and

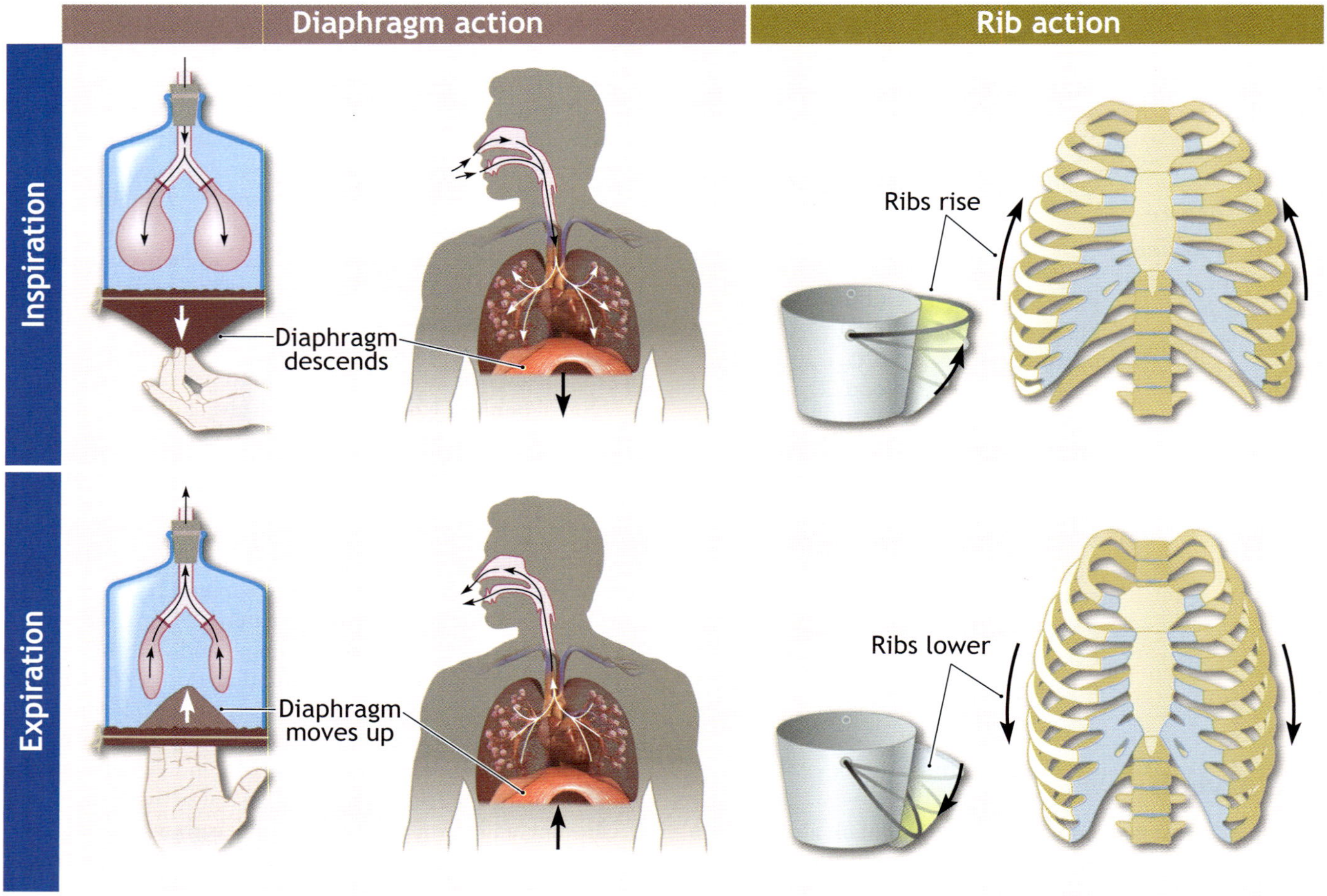

FIGURE 12.2. Breathing mechanics involving diaphragm and rib action. (Lungs image: sciencepics/Shutterstock)

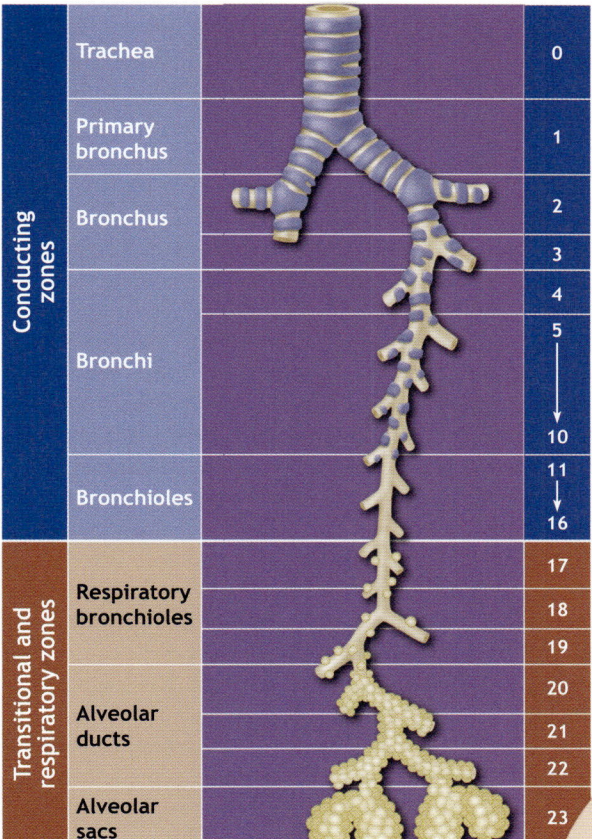

FIGURE 12.3. Separation of human lung tissue into discrete conduction zones 1 through 16 and transitional and respiratory zones 17 through 23. The alveolar sacs provide the vital surface for gas exchange between lung tissue and blood. (Alveoli image: first vector trend/Shutterstock)

constitutes the largest portion of the total lung volume. Air moving into the lungs literally flows down the trachea to the terminal bronchi, much like water flowing through a hose. As air reaches the smaller air passages in the transitional zone, the tremendous increase in surface area slows airflow into the alveoli.

The ventilatory conducting zone functions also include the following:

1. Air transport
2. Humidification
3. Warming
4. Particle filtration
5. Vocalization
6. Immunoglobulin secretion

The four respiratory zone functions encompass the following:

1. Surfactant production (in the alveolar endothelium)
2. Molecule activation and inactivation (in the capillary endothelium)
3. Blood clotting regulation
4. Endocrine function

FIGURE 12.4 depicts the relationship between the lung's airway generation and total cross-sectional area for various lung segment zones. Airway cross section increases and velocity slows as air moves through the conducting zone to the terminal bronchioles. At this stage, diffusion governs gas movement and distribution. In the alveoli, gas pressures rapidly equilibrate on each side of the alveolar-capillary membrane. **Fick law of diffusion** (derived in 1845 by German physiologist Adolf Gaston Eugen Fick [1852–1937], contact lens inventor and first to devise a technique to measure cardiac output [see Chapter 17]) regulates gas diffusion across a fluid membrane.[51] This two-part law states that a gas diffuses through a sheet of tissue at a rate (1) proportional to the tissue area, a diffusion constant, and the pressure differential of the gas on each side of the membrane and (2) inversely proportional to tissue thickness. Because carbon dioxide is more soluble than oxygen, it requires a much smaller pressure differential for an equivalent volume of gas movement.

Inspiratory and Expiratory Dynamics

The lungs do not merely remain suspended in the chest cavity as the balloons do in Figure 12.2. Instead, they adhere to the double-walled pleural sacs that line both the thoracic wall and the exterior lung surface. The pressure differential between the air in the lungs and the lung–chest wall interface causes them to adhere to the chest wall and follow the breathing movements. Any change in thoracic cavity volume correspondingly alters lung volume.

Inspiration

The **diaphragm**, an upward-curving, dome-shaped striated musculofibrous tissue sheet that separates the thoracic and abdominal cavities, serves the same purpose as the jar's lower rubber membrane (see Fig. 12.2). This primary ventilatory muscle—whose mitochondrial volume density, muscle fiber oxidative capacity, and aerobic capacity exceed by up to fourfold those of most other skeletal muscles[33]—creates an airtight separation between the abdominal and thoracic cavities. The diaphragm contains openings for the esophagus, blood vessels, and nerves. This separating membrane possesses high oxidative potential and the greatest capacity of all of the ventilatory muscles for shortening and volume displacement.[13,34]

During **inspiration**, the diaphragm muscle contracts, flattens, and moves downward toward the abdominal cavity by as much as 10 cm. Chest cavity elongation and enlargement increase the air volume in the lungs, causing **intrapulmonic pressure** to decrease to slightly below atmospheric pressure. The lungs inflate as the nose and mouth literally suck air inward, with the degree of filling dependent on inspiratory movements. Maximum inspiratory muscle activation produces pressures that range from −80 to +140 mm Hg. Inspiration ends when thoracic cavity expansion ceases. This causes intrapulmonic pressure to equal ambient atmospheric pressure.

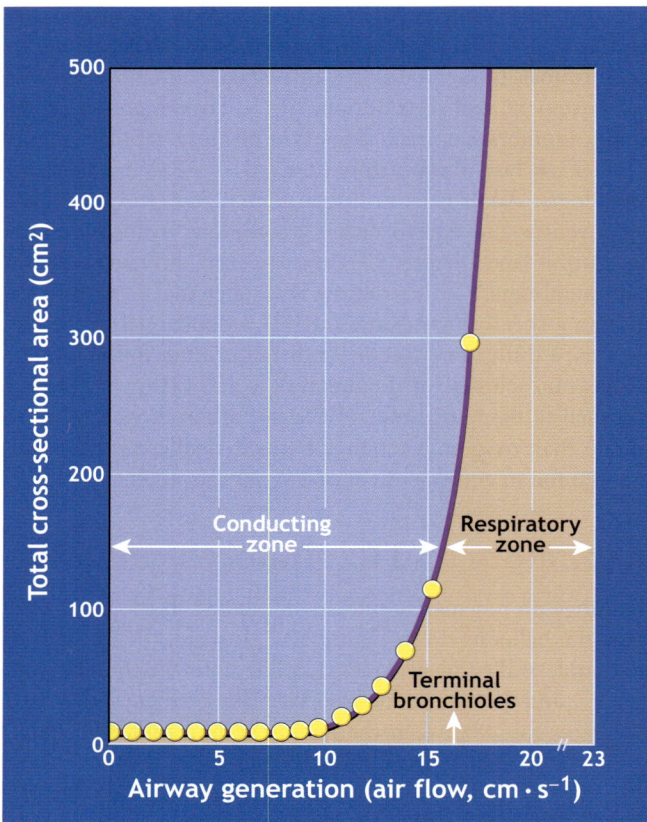

FIGURE 12.4. Lung airflow generation related to total cross-sectional lung tissue area.

During physical activity, the highly efficient movements of the diaphragm, rib cage (ribs and sternum), and abdominal muscles synchronize to contribute to inspiration and expiration.[2,25] During inspiration, the **scaleni and external intercostal muscles** between the ribs contract, causing the ribs to rotate and lift up and away from the body. This action corresponds to lifting the handle up and away from the bucket (see Fig. 12.2, *upper right*). Inspiratory action increases during physical activity when the diaphragm descends, the ribs swing upward, and the sternum thrusts outward to increase the lateral and A-P diameters of the thorax.

fyi — Common Body Position After Intense Running Facilitates Breathing

Athletes often bend forward from the waist to facilitate breathing following sustained physical effort. This body position serves two purposes:

1. Promotes blood flow to the heart
2. Minimizes gravity's antagonistic effects on the usual upward trajectory of inspiratory movements

Martin Novak/Shutterstock

Expiration

Expiration during rest and light physical activity represents a passive process of air movement from the lungs and results from two factors:

1. Stretched lung tissue's natural recoil
2. Inspiratory muscle relaxation

The sternum and ribs swing down, and the diaphragm rises toward the thoracic cavity. These movements decrease chest cavity volume and compress alveolar gas so air moves from the respiratory tract to the atmosphere. Expiration ends when the expiratory muscles' compressive force ceases and intrapulmonic pressure decreases to atmospheric pressure. During strenuous activity, **internal intercostal and abdominal muscles** act powerfully on the ribs and abdominal cavity to reduce thoracic dimensions.[14] This makes exhalation rapid and more extensive.

No major differences exist in ventilatory mechanics between males and females of different ages. At rest in the supine position, most persons breathe diaphragmatically ("abdominal breathers"), whereas in the upright position, rib and sternum actions become more apparent. Rib-cage movement dictates the rapid alterations in thoracic volume in strenuous exertion. Distinct biochemical differences among muscles that compose the respiratory pump provide evidence that the rib musculature acts more rapidly than the diaphragm and abdominal muscles.[35] The position of the head and back that distance runners naturally adopt—forward lean from the waist, neck flexed, and head extended forward with mandible parallel to the ground—favors pulmonary ventilation during intense activity.

Surfactant

Pressures vary continually within the alveolar and pleural spaces throughout the ventilatory cycle. Resistance to normal lung cavity and alveoli expansion progressively increases during inspiration due to **surface tension**, primarily in the alveoli. Surface tension relates to a resisting force created at the liquid surface in contact with a gas, a structure, or another liquid. In the alveoli, surface tension results from the attractive forces between the liquid molecules that line these structures. The tension or force created causes the liquid to assume a shape that presents the smallest surface area to the surrounding medium. The greater the surface tension surrounding a spherical alveolus, the greater the force required to overcome pressure within the sphere and cause it to enlarge or inflate. **Surfactant** (contraction of "surface active agent," or, literally, a wetting agent) consists of a lipoprotein mixture of phospholipids, proteins, and calcium ions produced by alveolar epithelial cells. The main component of surfactant, the phospholipid dipalmitoylphosphatidylcholine, reduces surface tension. It mixes with the fluid that encircles the alveolar chambers. Its action interrupts the surrounding water layer, reducing the alveolar membrane's surface tension to increase overall lung compliance, which reduces the energy required for alveolar inflation and deflation.[48] Without surfactant, small alveoli would collapse (called *atelectasis*) from high collapsing pressures, which would make it more difficult for them to remain open. The opposite effect occurs in alveoli with larger radii and thus lower collapsing pressure.

Lung Volumes and Capacities

FIGURE 12.5 illustrates eight lung volume measurements and average values for males and females. The individual rebreathes through a water-sealed, volume-displacement recording spirometer, similar to the one described in Chapter 8 (Fig. 8.4), for measuring oxygen uptake by closed-circuit spirometry. As with many anatomic and physiologic measures, lung volumes vary with age, gender, and body size and composition, but particularly stature.[52] It is common practice to compare measured values with established standards that consider these factors.

 See the animation "Perform a Pulmonary Function Test" on Lippincott Connect to view this process.

Static Lung Volumes

The spirometer bell falls and rises during inhalation and exhalation to record ventilatory volume and breathing rate. **Tidal volume (TV)** describes air volume moved during either the inspiratory or expiratory phase of each breathing cycle. Under resting conditions, TV usually ranges from 0.4 to 1.0 L of air per breath. After recording several TV trials, the subject inspires as deeply as possible following a normal inspiration. The additional 2.5- to 3.5-L volume above inspired tidal air represents the reserve ability for inhalation referred to as **inspiratory reserve volume (IRV)**, which in the example in Figure 12.5 attained 3.0 L. After a normal exhalation, the subject continues to exhale and forces as much air as possible from the lungs. This additional **expiratory reserve volume (ERV)** ranges from 1.0 to 1.5 L for an average-size man. During physical activity, encroachment on IRV and ERV, particularly IRV, considerably increases TV.

The total air volume voluntarily moved in one breath, from full inspiration to maximum expiration, represents the vital capacity (VC) or more precisely, **forced vital capacity (FVC)**. FVC includes TV plus IRV and ERV. FVC usually ranges from 4 to 5 L in healthy young males and 3 to 4 L in healthy young females. In total, 6- to 7-L values are common in tall individuals, and unusually large FVC values of close to 8 L have been published for world-class athletes.[3,47] These athletes' large lung volumes generally reflect genetic influences and body size characteristics, because exercise training does not appreciably change static lung volumes.

The **residual lung volume (RLV)** represents the air volume remaining in

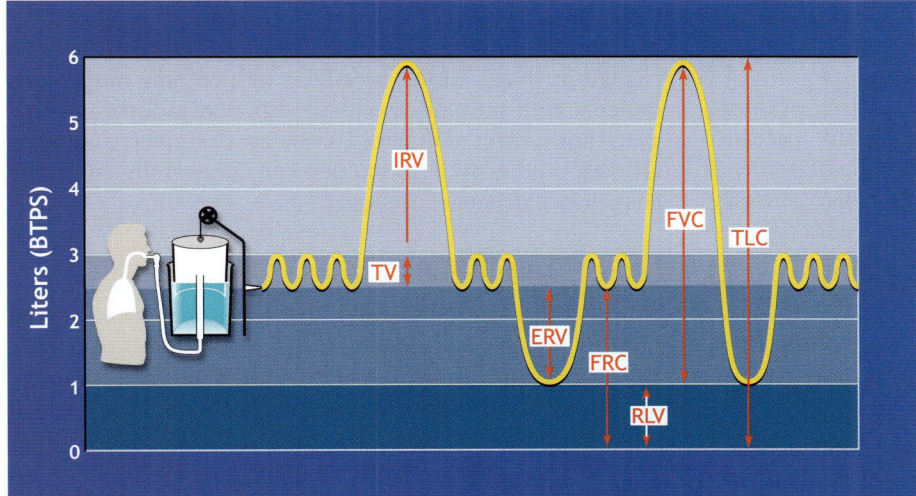

Lung volume/capacity	Definition	Average values (mL) Men	Women
Tidal Volume (TV)	Volume inspired or expired per breath	600	500
Inspiratory Reserve Volume (IRV)	Maximum inspiration at end of tidal inspiration	3000	1900
Expiratory Reserve Volume (ERV)	Maximum expiration at end of tidal expiration	1200	800
Total Lung Capacity (TLC)	Volume in lungs after maximum inspiration	6000	4200
Residual Lung Volume (RLV)	Volume in lungs after maximum expiration	1200	1000
Forced Vital Capacity (FVC)	Maximum volume expired after maximum inspiration	4800	3200
Inspiratory Capacity (IC)	Maximum volume inspired following tidal expiration	3600	2400
Functional Residual Capacity (FRC)	Volume in lungs after tidal expiration	2400	1800

RLV prediction equations in normal weight and overweight males and females*

Normal-weight males and females	R	SEE
RLV = 0.0275 AGE + 0.0189 HT − 2.6139	0.70	0.405

Overweight males and females	R	SEE
RLV = 0.0277 AGE + 0.0048 WT + 0.0138 HT − 2.3967	0.65	0.404

R, multiple correlation coefficient; Age (y); HT, height (cm); WT, weight (kg); SEE, standard error of estimate.

*From Miller WC, et al. Derivation of prediction equations for RV in overweight men and women. *Med Sci Sports Exerc*. 1998;30:322.

FIGURE 12.5. Static lung volume measurements.

the lungs following a maximum forceful exhalation. This volume averages 0.8 to 1.2 L for college-age, healthy females and 0.9 to 1.4 L for college-age, healthy males. RLV for apparently healthy professional football players ranges from 0.96 to 2.46 L.[45] RLV increases with age, whereas IRV and ERV decrease proportionally. A decline in the elasticity of lung tissue components with aging probably decreases breathing reserve and concomitantly increases RLV. Alterations in pulmonary function may not entirely reflect an aging phenomenon because regular aerobic training diminishes the typical age-related decline in static and dynamic lung functions.[16] The RLV allows for an uninterrupted gas exchange between the blood and alveoli to prevent fluctuations in blood gases during different breathing cycle phases including deep breathing. RLV plus FVC constitutes **total lung capacity**.

The RLV temporarily increases from a bout of either short-term or prolonged physical activity. In one study, RLV increased during recovery from a maximal treadmill test by 21% after 5 min, 17% after 15 min, and 12% after 30 min.[5] RLV generally reverts to its original value within 24 hr. Two possible factors help to explain RLV increases with physical activity:

1. Closure of small peripheral airways
2. Increased thoracic blood volume

The added blood volume does not alter the lungs' mechanical properties, but it does displace a portion of their air contents, thus preventing complete exhalation (reduced FVC).[8] Any temporary RLV increase would affect subsequent body volume computations by hydrostatic weighing for body composition studies (see Chapter 28). When RLV measurement is impractical, prediction equations based on the relation between RLV and age, stature, gender, and body mass provide reasonably accurate estimates for normal-weight and overweight males and females (see RLV prediction equations at bottom of Fig. 12.5).

Dynamic Lung Volumes

Pulmonary ventilation depends on how well one sustains high airflow levels rather than how quickly one moves air in a single breath. Dynamic ventilation depends on two factors:

1. Maximum lung "stroke volume" (FVC)
2. Moving air volume quickly (breathing rate)

Airflow velocity depends on respiratory passage resistance to smooth airflow and the "stiffness" imposed by mechanical properties of the chest and lung tissue to a change in shape during breathing termed *lung compliance*. Patients with lung disease rarely experience distress symptoms until their ventilatory capacity decreases. Individuals with mild airway obstruction can successfully engage in competitive distance running.[29]

FEV-to-FVC Ratio

Some individuals with severe lung disease achieve near-normal FVC values if measured with no time limit for this maneuver. For this reason, clinicians prefer a "dynamic" lung function measurement called **forced expiratory volume (FEV)**, which is usually measured over 1 s **(FEV$_{1.0}$)**. FEV$_{1.0}$ divided by FVC (FEV$_{1.0}$ ÷ FVC) indicates pulmonary airflow capacity. It reflects pulmonary expiratory power and overall resistance to air movement upstream in the lungs. Healthy individuals normally expel about 85% of the VC in 1 s. Severe obstructive lung disease (emphysema or bronchial asthma)—with accompanying reduced airway caliber and loss of lung-tissue elastic recoil—considerably reduces FEV$_{1.0}$/FVC, often to values less than 45% of VC (e.g., the middle panel in **FIG. 12.6** shows 42%).[28,42] The demarcation point for airway obstruction during dynamic spirometry represents an FEV$_{1.0}$/FVC of 70% or less. Figure 12.6 presents pulmonary function test results for FEV$_{1.0}$ and FVC in individuals with normal lung function (*left*), those with obstructive lung disease (*middle*; chronic inflammatory disease that obstructs airflow from the lungs [e.g., emphysema, chronic bronchitis]), and those with restrictive lung disease (*right*; restricted lung expansion that decreases lung volume [stiffness in

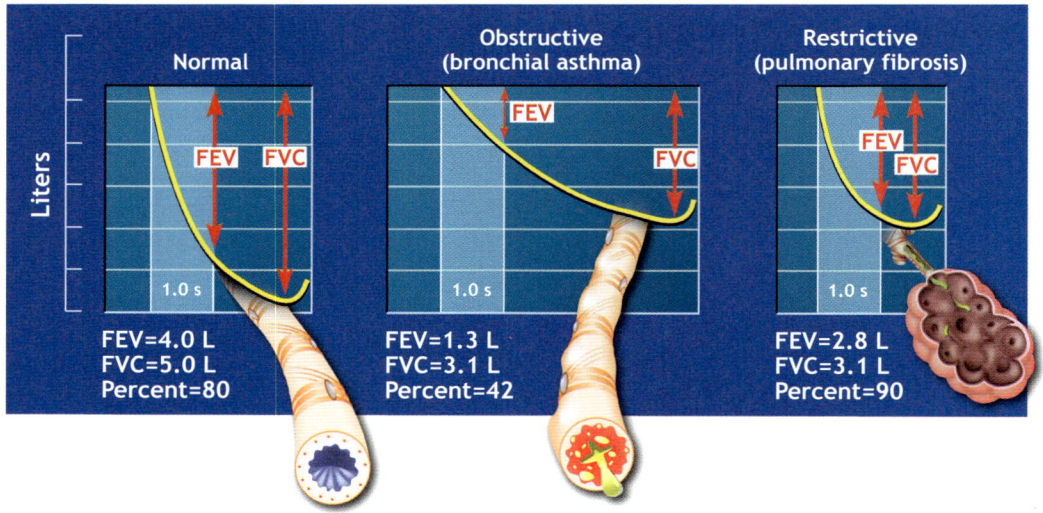

FIGURE 12.6. Example spirometric tracings during standard pulmonary function tests for FEV$_{1.0}$ and FVC in individuals with normal dynamic lung function (*left*) and in patients with either obstructive lung disease (*middle*; e.g., bronchial asthma or emphysema with irreversibly damaged alveolar sacs) and/or restrictive lung disease (*right*; restricted lung expansion that decreases lung volume [lung stiffness making it difficult to inflate lungs]).
(Shutterstock: Designua; ilusmedical.)

lungs themselves making it difficult to fully inflate lungs to produce adequate ventilation and/or oxygenation]). Clinicians also compute other values generated in the forced spirometry maneuver (e.g., mid-50% or instantaneous flows at 25, 50, or 75% FVC) to assess airflow dynamics in the pulmonary tract's small airway passages.[44]

 See the animation "Asthma" on Lippincott Connect to view how this condition impacts pulmonary function.

Maximum Voluntary Ventilation

The **maximum voluntary ventilation (MVV)** evaluates ventilatory capacity with rapid and deep breathing for 15 s. The 15-s volume, extrapolated to the volume the subject would achieve if continued for 1 min, represents MVV and typically ranges from 35 to 40 times the $FEV_{1.0}$.[45] MVV also averages 25% higher than ventilation during maximal exercise because exercise does not maximally stress how a healthy person breathes. MVV ranges from 140 to 180 L·min^{-1} for healthy, college-age males and 80 to 120 L·min^{-1} for healthy, college-age females. MVV in male members from the United States Nordic Ski Team averaged 192 L·min^{-1}; the individual high was 239 L·min^{-1}.[17] Conversely, patients with chronic obstructive pulmonary disease (e.g., emphysema) achieve only about 40% of the MVV considered normal for age and body size.

 **INTEGRATIVE QUESTION**

How does regular resistance and aerobic training affect the typical aging decline in lung function?

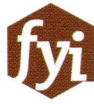 **Response of Ventilatory Muscles to Training**

Specific ventilatory muscle training, generalized resistance training, or simply increasing daily physical activity level improves ventilatory muscle strength and endurance and increases both inspiratory muscle function and maximal voluntary ventilation (MVV).[1,37,42,53,54,61] Ventilatory muscle training in patients with chronic obstructive pulmonary disease (COPD) enhances exercise capacity and reduces physiologic strain.[9,39,55,56] Progressive desensitization to the feeling of breathlessness and greater self-control of respiratory symptoms represent important benefits of ventilatory muscle training and regular physical activity for patients with COPD.[57,62]

SciePro/Shutterstock

Effect of Gender Differences on Exercise Performance

Adult females consistently have reduced lung size, static and dynamic lung function measures, airway diameters, and diffusion surface than males even when accounting for differences in stature. This disparity produces expiratory flow limitations, greater respiratory muscle work, and relatively greater use of ventilatory reserve compared with males during maximum physical effort. This is particularly true for highly trained females compared with trained males and less-fit females.[31] A relatively smaller lung volume plus a high expiratory flow rate requirement in trained females during intense activity places considerable demand on the maximum flow-volume envelope of the airways (i.e., mechanical constraints of TV and pulmonary minute ventilation). This adversely affects the ability of highly fit females to maintain alveolar-to-arterial oxygen exchange, which could compromise arterial oxygen saturation and aerobic capacity to a greater degree than in males.[19,20]

Lung Function, Aerobic Fitness, and Physical Performance

Unlike the other aerobic system components, regular endurance activity does not stimulate large increases in the pulmonary system's functional capacity. Dynamic lung function tests indicate the severity of COPD but provide little information about aerobic fitness or performance when values fall within the normal range. For example, no difference emerges when comparing the average FVC for prepubescent and Olympic wrestlers, middle-distance athletes, and untrained, healthy subjects.[36,38] Professional American football players averaged only 94% of predicted FVC; the defensive backs achieved only 83% of predicted "normal" values for body size (see "In a Practical Sense"). Somewhat surprisingly, similar values emerged for static and dynamic lung function in accomplished marathon runners and other endurance-trained athletes compared with untrained controls of similar body size.[16,27,30] Nevertheless, some research has reported higher dynamic lung function measures in endurance athletes when compared with power athletes or a sedentary control group.[58]

Swimming and scuba diving may stimulate larger-than-normal static lung volumes. These sports strengthen the inspiratory muscles, which must work against the additional resistance from the water mass that compresses the thorax. Enhanced ventilatory muscle strength and power explain the relatively large FVC in scuba divers and competitive swimmers.[6,10,11] Little relationship exists among different lung volumes and capacities and various track performances, including distance running in teenage boys and girls, even after adjusting for body size differences.[12] For marathon runners versus sedentary subjects of similar body size, no difference existed for lung function values (**TABLE 12.1**).[24,29] For healthy, untrained individuals, no relationship exists between maximal oxygen uptake and FVC or MVV (adjusted for body size). Fatigue from strenuous physical activity frequently relates to feeling "out of breath," or "winded," yet normal capacity for pulmonary ventilation for most individuals does not limit maximal aerobic performance. The larger-than-normal lung volumes and breathing capacities in some athletes probably reflect genetic endowment.

> **TABLE 12.1** Anthropometric data, pulmonary function, and resting minute ventilation in 20 marathon runners and healthy controls

Pulmonary Ventilation

One can view pulmonary ventilation from two perspectives:

1. Air volume moved into or out the ventilatory tract each minute (minute ventilation)
2. Air volume that ventilates only the alveolar chambers each minute (alveolar minute ventilation)

 See the animation "Pulmonary Ventilation" on Lippincott Connect to view this process.

Minute Ventilation

The normal breathing rate during quiet breathing at rest in a thermoneutral environment averages 12 breaths $\cdot$ min^{-1}, and TV averages 0.5 L of air per breath. Consequently, the air volume breathed each minute, referred to as **minute ventilation**, equals 6 L.

$$\begin{aligned}\text{Minute Ventilation } (V_E) &= \text{Breathing rate} \times \text{TV} \\ &= 12 \times 0.5\,\text{L} \\ &= 6\,\text{L}\cdot\text{min}^{-1}\end{aligned}$$

An increase in either the rate or depth of breathing or both increases minute ventilation. During strenuous physical activity, healthy young adults readily increase breathing rate to 35 to 45 breaths $\cdot$ min^{-1}. Some elite endurance athletes breathe as rapidly as 60 to 70 times $\cdot$ min^{-1} during maximal effort. TVs in the 2.0-L range and higher commonly occur in most adults during physical activity. Such increases in breathing rate and TV increase minute ventilation to 100 L or more (about 17 to 20 times resting value). In male endurance athletes, ventilation may increase to 160 L $\cdot$ min^{-1} during maximal effort. Minute ventilation volumes of 200 L, with a high of 208 L in an American football player, have been observed during bicycle exercise.[47] Even with such large minute ventilations, TVs for trained and untrained individuals rarely exceed 60% of VC.

Alveolar Minute Ventilation

Some air in each breath does not enter the alveoli to participate in gaseous exchange with the blood. The term anatomic dead space describes this air volume that fills the upper airway structures (mouth, nasal passages, nasopharynx, larynx, trachea, and other nondiffusible conducting passages). The anatomic dead space generally ranges from 150 to 200 mL in healthy individuals (about 30% resting TV). The dead space composition remains almost identical to ambient air except for its full saturation with water vapor.

The dead-space volume permits about 350 mL of the 500 mL resting inspired TV to enter into and mix with existing alveolar air. This does not mean that only 350 mL of air enters and leaves the alveoli with each breath. Instead, if TV equals 500 mL, then 500 mL of air enters the alveoli, but only 350 mL is fresh air, or about one-seventh of the total alveolar air. Such relatively small and seemingly inefficient **alveolar minute ventilation**—inspired air portion reaching the alveoli and participating in gas exchange—prevents drastic changes in alveolar air composition to ensure consistency in arterial blood gases throughout the breathing cycle.

TABLE 12.2 indicates that minute ventilation does not always reflect alveolar ventilation. The first example of shallow breathing shows that one can reduce TV to 150 mL, yet still maintain a 6-L minute ventilation by increasing breathing rate to 40 breaths $\cdot$ min^{-1}. The same 6-L minute volume occurs from decreasing breathing rate to 12 breaths $\cdot$ min^{-1} and increasing TV to 500 mL. By contrast, doubling TV and halving breathing rate, as in the deep-breathing example, also produce a 6-L minute ventilation. Each of these ventilatory adjustments drastically affects alveolar ventilation. In the shallow-breathing example, dead-space air represents the only air volume moved without any alveolar ventilation. In the other examples, deeper breathing causes a larger portion from each breath to enter into and mix with alveolar air. Alveolar ventilation determines the gaseous concentrations at the alveolar-capillary membrane.

> **TABLE 12.2** Tidal volume, breathing rate, and total and alveolar minute ventilation

Dead Space Versus TV

The preceding examples for alveolar ventilation represent oversimplifications because they assumed a constant dead space despite changes in TV. Actually, anatomic dead space increases as TV becomes larger; it often doubles during deep breathing due to some respiratory passages stretching with a fuller inspiration. Importantly, any increase in dead space still represents proportionately less volume than the accompanying TV increase. Consequently, deeper breathing provides more effective alveolar ventilation than similar minute ventilation achieved through increased breathing rate.

Ventilation-Perfusion Ratio

Adequate gas exchange between alveoli and blood requires effective matching of alveolar ventilation to the blood perfusing the pulmonary capillaries. It normally requires approximately 4.2 L of air to ventilate the alveoli each minute at rest, with an average of 5.0 L of blood flowing through the pulmonary capillaries. In this case, the **ventilation-perfusion ratio** (alveolar ventilation ÷ pulmonary blood flow) equals 0.84 (4.2 ÷ 5.0). This ratio means that 0.84 L of alveolar ventilation matches

In a Practical Sense

Predicting Pulmonary Function Variables in Young and Older Males and Females

Pulmonary function variables do not directly relate to physical fitness measures in healthy individuals. Instead, their measurement often forms part of a standard medical/health/fitness examination, particularly for at-risk individuals with limited pulmonary function (e.g., chronic cigarette smokers, those with asthma). Measuring pulmonary dimensions and lung functions with a water-filled spirometer (see Fig. 12.5) or electronic spirometer provides the framework to assess pulmonary dynamics during rest and physical activity. Proper pulmonary function evaluation requires comparison with "expected" values (norms) from the clinical literature.

EQUATIONS

Pulmonary function scores associate closely with stature (ST) and age (A), enabling these two variables to predict an individual's expected normal lung function values as in the examples for Kevin: A, 22 y; ST, 165.1 cm/65 in; and Erika: A, 22 y; ST, 182.9 cm/72 in.

EXAMPLES

Female

1. *Forced vital capacity (FVC)*

$$FVC(L) = (0.0414 \times ST[cm]) - (0.0232 \times A[y]) - 2.20$$
$$= 6.835 - 0.5104 - 2.20$$
$$= 4.12\ L$$

2. *Forced expiratory volume in 1 s ($FEV_{1.0}$)*

$$FEV_{1.0}(L) = (0.0268 \times ST[cm]) - (0.0251 \times A[y]) - 0.38$$
$$= 4.425 - 0.5522 - 0.38$$
$$= 3.49\ L$$

3. *Percentage forced vital capacity in 1 s ($FEV_{1.0}/FVC$)*

$$FEV_{1.0}/FVC(\%) = (-0.2145 \times ST[cm]) - (0.1523 \times A[y]) + 124.5$$
$$= -35.41 - 3.35 + 124.5$$
$$= 85.7\%$$

4. *Maximum voluntary ventilation (MVV)*

$$MVV\ (L \cdot min^{-1}) = 40 \times FEV_{1.0}$$
$$= 40 \times 3.49\ (from\ \#2)$$
$$= 139.6\ L \cdot min^{-1}$$

Male

1. *Forced vital capacity (FVC)*

$$FVC\ (L) = (0.0774 \times ST[cm] - (0.0212 \times A[y]) - 7.75)$$
$$= 14.156 - 0.4664 - 7.75$$
$$= 5.49\ L$$

2. *Forced expiratory volume in 1 s ($FEV_{1.0}$)*

$$FEV_{1.0}(L) = (0.0566 \times ST[cm]) - (0.0233 \times A[y]) - 0.491$$
$$= 10.35 - 0.5126 - 4.91$$
$$= 4.93\ L$$

3. *Percentage forced vital capacity in 1 s ($FEV_{1.0}/FVC$)*

$$FEV_{1.0}/FVC(\%) = (-0.1314 \times ST[cm]) - (0.1490 \times A[y]) + 110.2$$
$$= -24.03 - 3.35 + 110.2$$
$$= 82.8\%$$

4. *Maximum voluntary ventilation (MVV)*

$$MVV(L \cdot min^{-1}) = 40 \times FEV_{1.0}$$
$$= 40 \times 4.93\ L\ (from\ \#2)$$
$$= 197.2\ L \cdot min^{-1}$$

EQUATIONS TO PREDICT PULMONARY FUNCTION VARIABLES IN YOUNG AND OLDER MALES AND FEMALES

Variable	Male		Female	
	<25 y	>25 y	<25 y	>25 y
$FVC\ (L) =$	$(0.0774 \times ST) - (0.0212 \times A) - 7.75$	$(0.065 \times ST) + (0.029 \times A) - 5.459$	$(0.0414 \times ST) - (0.0232 \times A) - 2.20$	$(0.037 \times ST) + (0.092 \times A) - 3.469$
$FEV_{1.0}\ (L) =$	$(0.0566 \times ST) - (0.0233 \times A) - 0.491$	$(0.052 \times ST) + (0.027 \times A) - 4.203$	$(0.0268 \times ST) - (0.0251 \times A) - 0.38$	$(0.027 \times ST) - (0.021 \times A) - 0.794$
$FEV_{1.0}/FVC\ (\%) =$	$(-0.1314 \times ST) - (0.1490 \times A) + 110.2$	$103.64 - (0.87 \times ST) - (0.14 \times A)$	$(-0.2145 \times ST) - (0.1523 \times A) + 124.5$	$107.38 - (0.111 \times ST) - (0.109 \times A)$
$MVV(L \cdot min^{-1}) =$	$40 \times FEV_{1.0}$	$(1.15 \times H) - (1.27 \times A) + 14$	$40 \times FEV_{1.0}$	$(0.55 \times ST) - (0.72 \times A) + 50$

A, age, y; $FEV_{1.0}$, forced expiratory volume in 1 s; $FEV_{1.0}/FVC$, percentage of forced vital capacity expired in 1 s; FVC, forced vital capacity; MVV, maximum voluntary ventilation; ST, stature (height), cm.

Sources:
Myers J, Nieman D. *ACSM's Resources for Clinical Exercise Physiology*. 2nd ed. Baltimore: Wolters Kluwer Health; 2009.

West JB, Luks AM. *West's Respiratory Physiology. The Essentials*. 11th ed. Baltimore: Wolters Kluwer Health; 2020.

each liter of pulmonary blood flow. In light activity, the ventilation-perfusion ratio remains at approximately 0.8. By contrast, intense physical activity produces a disproportionate increase in alveolar ventilation. In healthy individuals, the ventilation-perfusion ratio may exceed 5.0; in most instances, this response guarantees adequate venous blood aeration. This mismatching of alveolar ventilation to perfusion (blood flow) accounts for many gas exchange problems occurring in pulmonary disease and possibly during intense physical activity among highly trained endurance athletes. The ventilation-perfusion ratio varies depending on the lung region (zone) due to gravitational effects and the positions of the lung's base (lower region) below the heart and its apex (upper region) above the heart (see FYI, "Bronchopulmonary Segments").[4]

Blood flow through the lungs is greatest at the base and least at its apex. This results in a ventilation-perfusion ratio of less than 1.0 at the base (indicative of overperfusion or underventilation) and greater than 1.0 at the apex (indicative of underperfusion or overventilation). In essence, abnormally large ventilation-perfusion ratios waste pulmonary ventilation in overventilating alveoli that cannot use the oxygen while providing inadequate oxygen for alveoli in need. Despite these regional variations in ventilation related to blood flow, ventilation-perfusion ratios that exceed 0.50 sufficiently meet most gas exchange requirements at rest.

Physiologic Dead Space

Sometimes alveoli may not function adequately due to two factors that can impair gas exchange:

1. Blood underperfusion
2. Inadequate ventilation relative to alveolar surface area

The term **physiologic dead space** describes the alveolar volume fraction with a ventilation-perfusion ratio that

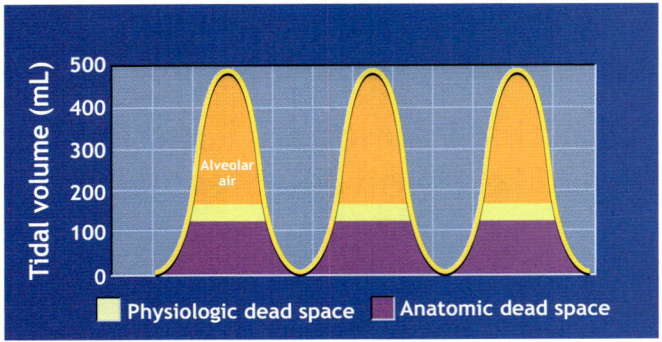

FIGURE 12.7. Tidal volume (TV) distribution in a healthy subject at rest. TV includes about 350 mL ambient air that mixes with alveolar air, 150 mL ambient air that remains in the larger air passages (anatomic dead space), and a small air portion distributed to either poorly ventilated or poorly perfused alveoli (physiologic dead space).

approaches zero. **FIGURE 12.7** shows the negligible physiologic dead space in the healthy lung shown by the yellow horizontal bar. In certain pathologic situations, physiologic dead space increases to 50% TV, as with inadequate perfusion from hemorrhage or pulmonary circulation blockage by an embolism or inadequate ventilation in emphysema, asthma, and pulmonary fibrosis. An increased physiologic dead space from decreased functional alveolar surface in emphysema produces extreme ventilation even at low physical activity intensities. Many patients cannot achieve maximal circulatory capacity because of ventilatory muscle fatigue from excessive breathing. Adequate gas exchange becomes impossible when lung dead space exceeds 60% of total lung volume.

Breathing Rate Versus TV

Increasing the breathing rate and depth increases alveolar ventilation in physical activity. In moderate activity, well-trained athletes maintain alveolar ventilation by increasing TV with only a small increase in breathing rate.[15] As breathing becomes deeper during activity, alveolar ventilation increases from 70% of the total minute ventilation at rest to more than 85% of the exercise ventilation. **FIGURE 12.8** shows that encroachment on the IRV, with a smaller decrease in the end expiratory level, increases exercise TV. With more intense activity, the increase in TV plateaus at approximately 60% VC; minute ventilation increases further through nonconscious increases in breathing rate. Each person develops a breathing "style" in which breathing rate and TV blend to provide efficient alveolar ventilation. Conscious breathing manipulation usually disturbs the exquisitely regulated physiologic adjustments to physical activity. Attempts to modify

Typical Pulmonary Ventilation Values During Rest and Moderate and Intense Physical Activity

Condition	Breathing rate (breaths · min⁻¹)	Tidal volume (L · breath⁻¹)	Pulmonary ventilation (L · min⁻¹)
Rest	12	0.5	560
Moderate exercise	30	2.5	75
Intense exercise	50	3.0	150

Shutterstock: Stokkete; dwphotos; anatoliy_gleb

fyi Bronchopulmonary Segments

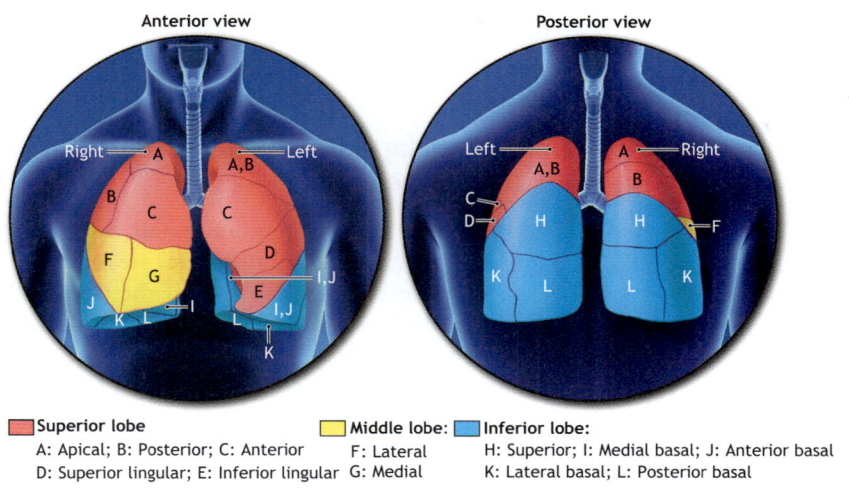

Anterior view / Posterior view

- Superior lobe — A: Apical; B: Posterior; C: Anterior; D: Superior lingular; E: Inferior lingular
- Middle lobe: F: Lateral; G: Medial
- Inferior lobe: H: Superior; I: Medial basal; J: Anterior basal; K: Lateral basal; L: Posterior basal

sciencepics/Shutterstock

INTEGRATIVE QUESTION

How can a person increase breathing volume at rest without disrupting normal alveolar ventilation?

Dyspnea

Dyspnea refers to inordinate shortness of breath or subjective distress in breathing. Breathing incapacity characterized by shortness of breath or "air hunger" also occurs during physical activity, particularly in novice exercisers. The disorder usually accompanies elevated arterial carbon dioxide and H^+ concentrations. Both conditions excite the inspiratory center to increase breathing rate and depth. Failure to adequately regulate arterial carbon dioxide and H^+ concentrations most likely relates to low aerobic fitness levels and a poorly conditioned ventilatory musculature.

breathing during running or other general physical activities offer no benefit to exercise performance. During rest and all exertion levels, a healthy person should breathe in the manner that seems most natural.

Variations from Normal Breathing Patterns

Breathing patterns during physical activity generally progress in an effective and highly economical manner, yet some pulmonary responses can adversely affect performance and/or physiologic balance.

Hyperventilation

Hyperventilation refers to an increase in pulmonary ventilation that exceeds the metabolic needs for oxygen uptake and carbon dioxide elimination. This "overbreathing" quickly lowers normal alveolar carbon dioxide concentration and causes excess carbon dioxide to leave bodily fluids via the expired air. An accompanying decrease in hydrogen ion (H^+) concentration increases plasma pH. Hyperventilating for several seconds generally produces lightheadedness; prolonged hyperventilation leads to unconsciousness from excessive carbon dioxide unloading.

Valsalva Maneuver

The expiratory muscles, besides their normal role in pulmonary ventilation, provide for the coughing and sneezing ventilatory maneuvers. They also contribute to stabilizing the abdominal and chest cavities during heavy lifting. In quiet breathing, intrapulmonic pressure decreases only about 3 mm Hg during inspiration and rises a similar amount above atmospheric pressure in exhalation (**FIG. 12.9A**).

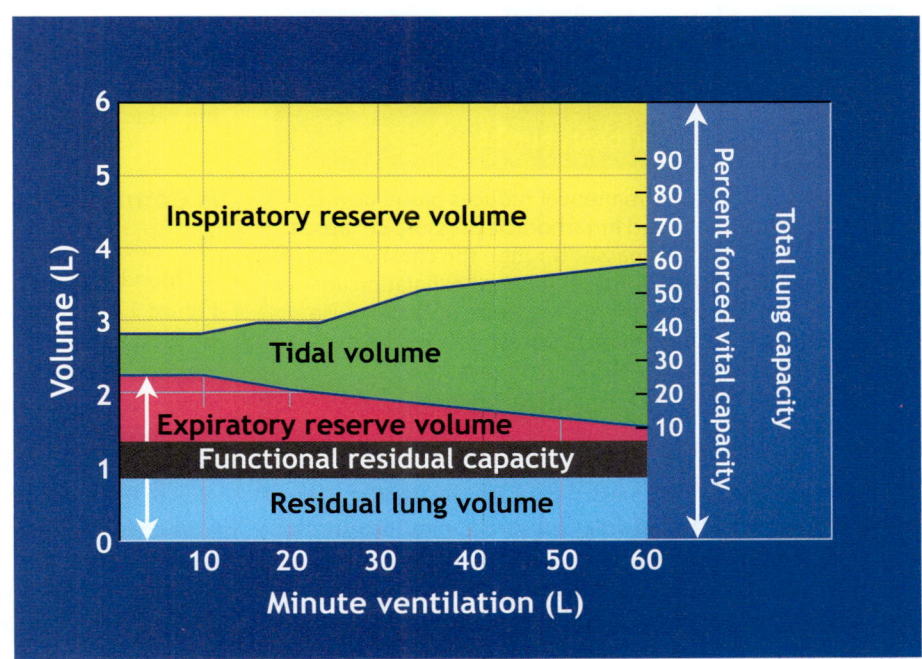

FIGURE 12.8 Tidal volume and pulmonary air subdivisions during rest and physical activity.

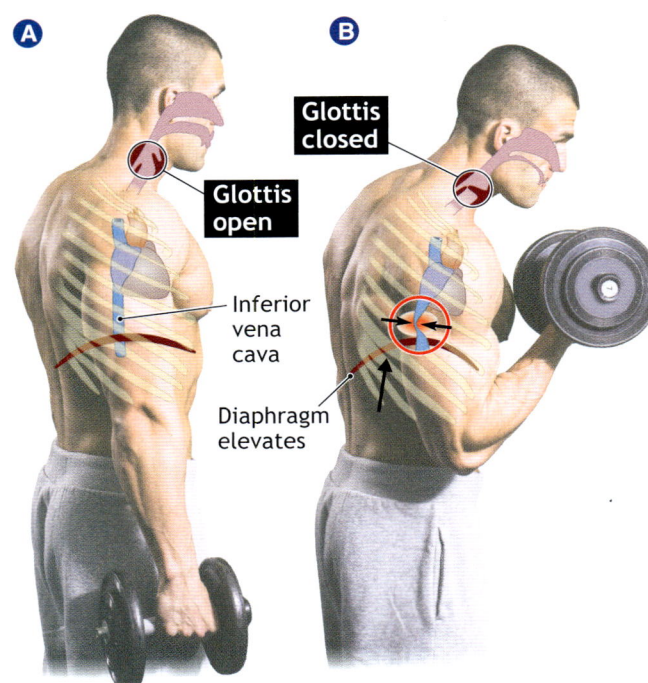

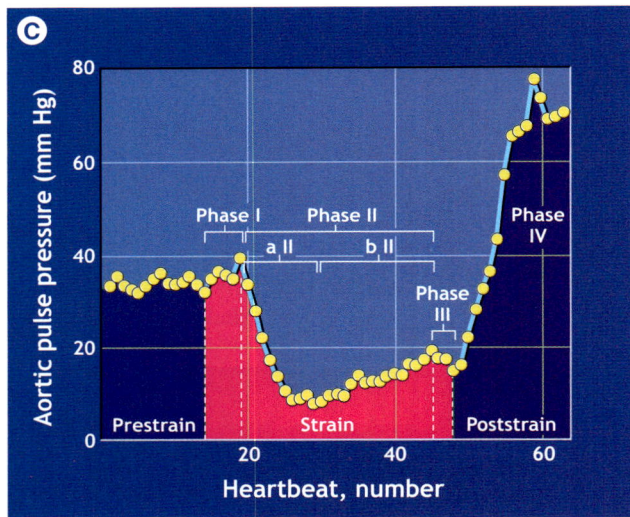

FIGURE 12.9 The Valsalva maneuver reduces blood flow to the heart because increased intrathoracic pressure collapses the inferior vena cava that passes through the chest cavity. **(A)** Normal breathing. **(B)** Straining with forced exhalation against a closed glottis. **(C)** Typical normal response of aortic pulse pressure (systolic pressure minus diastolic pressure) with a Valsalva maneuver during calibrated muscle strain.
(Alexander Lukatskiy/Shutterstock.)

Closing the glottis (narrowest part in the throat region for air to pass into the trachea) following a full inspiration while maximally activating the expiratory muscles creates compressive forces that increase intrathoracic pressure more than 150 mm Hg above atmospheric pressure (Fig. 12.9B). Pressures increase to even higher levels within the abdominal cavity during a maximal exhalation against a closed glottis.[18,59,60]

Forced exhalation against a closed glottis, termed the **Valsalva maneuver**, occurs commonly in weightlifting and other activities that require rapid, maximum force application for a brief duration. This maneuver stabilizes the abdominal and thoracic cavities to enhance muscle action.

Physiologic Consequences When Performing the Valsalva Maneuver

A prolonged Valsalva maneuver produces an acute drop in blood pressure. Increased intrathoracic pressure during a Valsalva maneuver transmits through the thin walls of veins that pass through the thoracic region. Because venous blood remains under relatively low pressure, thoracic veins collapse, which reduces blood flow to the heart. Reduced venous return sharply lowers the heart's stroke volume, triggering a fall in blood pressure below the resting level.[7,26] Performing a prolonged Valsalva maneuver during static, straining-type exercise as in Figure 12.9B dramatically reduces venous return and arterial blood pressure. These effects diminish the brain's blood supply, often producing dizziness, "spots before the eyes," or fainting. Once the glottis reopens and intrathoracic pressure normalizes, blood flow re-establishes with an "overshoot" in arterial blood pressure.[41,43]

Figure 12.9C illustrates a typical four-phase blood pressure response, heartbeat by heartbeat, during a Valsalva maneuver in a healthy subject. Aortic pulse pressure increases slightly as the Valsalva maneuver begins in Phase I from an elevated intrathoracic pressure effect, which expels blood from the left ventricle into the aorta. A biphasic response occurs at the Valsalva maneuver onset within six heartbeats. This reduces aortic pulse pressure in Phase IIa followed by a relatively small gradual rise in Phase IIb and secondary Phase III decrease during the continued Valsalva strain. When the maneuver ceases in Phase IV, blood pressure rises rapidly and overshoots the resting value.

A Common Misconception

The Valsalva maneuver does not cause the large increases in blood pressure during heavy resistance exercises. In Figure 12.9, we showed that a prolonged Valsalva maneuver dramatically reduces blood pressure. Confusion arises because a Valsalva maneuver of insufficient duration to lower blood pressure usually accompanies straining muscular efforts common during isometric and dynamic resistance exercise. These activities, with or without the Valsalva maneuver, greatly increase resistance to blood flow in active muscle with a resulting rise in systolic blood pressure.[21] For example, intramuscular fluid pressure increases linearly at all isometric force levels up to maximum.[40] Increased peripheral vascular resistance increases the arterial blood pressure and the heart's workload throughout exercise. These responses pose a potential danger to individuals with cardiovascular disease; they form the basis for advising cardiac patients to refrain from heavy resistance exercise and training with such exercise. By contrast, performing rhythmic muscular activity, including moderate weightlifting, promotes a steadier blood flow and only modest increase in blood pressure and work of the heart. Chapter 15 more fully discusses the blood pressure response to different activity modes.

INTEGRATIVE QUESTION

After completing a maximum-lift standing press, a person exclaims, "I feel slightly dizzy and see spots before my eyes." What is a plausible physiologic explanation for this response?

The Respiratory Tract During Cold-Weather Physical Activity

Cold ambient air normally does not damage the respiratory passages. Even in extremely cold weather, incoming air generally warms to between 26.5°C/79.7°F and 32.2°C/89.9°F by the time it reaches the bronchi. Nonetheless, values as low as 20°C/68°F can occur in the bronchi when breathing cold, dry air.[32] Airway warming of inspired air greatly increases the air's capacity to hold moisture, which produces considerable water loss from respiratory passages. In cold weather, the respiratory tract loses considerable water and heat, most notably during strenuous activities with large ventilatory volumes. Fluid loss from the airways often contributes to overall dehydration, dry mouth, burning sensation in the throat, and generalized respiratory passage irritation. Wearing a scarf or cellulose mask-type "balaclava" that covers the nose and mouth traps the water in exhaled air and subsequently warms and moistens the next incoming breath, an effect that reduces respiratory discomfort.

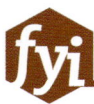

Ventilatory Distress with Cold Weather Exercise

Physical activity in cold weather can dry the throat and trigger coughing during recovery. The response becomes more prevalent during cold weather when the respiratory tract loses considerable water. Postexercise coughing relates directly to overall respiratory water loss (not respiratory heat loss) associated with larger ventilatory volumes breathed during exercise. The condition intensifies not only in exercise but also when encountering sudden changes in temperature, particularly for those who suffer from chronic obstructive lung diseases (www.ncbi.nlm.nih.gov/pmc/articles/PMC6031196/).

Fotoupro/Shutterstock

Summary

1. The lungs provide a large surface between the body's internal fluid environment and the gaseous external environment.
2. No more than 1 pint of blood flows in the pulmonary capillaries during any 1 s of physical activity.
3. Normal pulmonary ventilation regulation maintains favorable alveolar oxygen and carbon dioxide concentrations to ensure adequate aeration of blood flowing through the lungs.
4. Fick's diffusion law governs gas movement across a fluid membrane.
5. Surfactant consists of a lipoprotein mixture secreted within lung tissue that reduces surface tension between the alveolar membrane and surrounding tissues.
6. Pulmonary airflow depends on small pressure differentials between ambient air and air within the lungs.
7. Lung volumes vary with age, gender, and body size (particularly stature) and should only be evaluated in the context of established norms for these variables.
8. The RLV represents air remaining in the lungs following maximal exhalation; it allows for uninterrupted gas exchange during the breathing cycle.
9. FEV and MVV dynamically measure the ability to sustain a high airflow level.
10. Lung function measures serve as excellent screening tests to detect lung disease.
11. Static and dynamic lung function assessments that fall within the normal range poorly predict aerobic fitness and exercise performance.
12. Breathing rate and TV determine pulmonary minute ventilation.
13. Minute ventilation averages 6 $L \cdot min^{-1}$ at rest and can increase to 200 $L \cdot min^{-1}$ during maximal effort.
14. Alveolar ventilation reflects the minute ventilation portion that enters the alveoli for gaseous exchange with the blood.
15. The ventilation-perfusion ratio reflects the association between alveolar minute ventilation and pulmonary blood flow.
16. At rest, an alveolar ventilation of 0.8 L matches each liter of pulmonary blood flow.
17. During intense physical activity, alveolar ventilation increases disproportionately to pulmonary blood flow to increase the ventilation-perfusion ratio to 5.0.
18. TV increases during physical activity by encroachment into IRV and ERV.
19. During intense exercise, TV plateaus at approximately 60% of VC; minute ventilation increases further by an increase in breathing rate.
20. Hyperventilation refers to increased pulmonary ventilation that exceeds metabolic gas exchange needs.
21. A Valsalva maneuver describes a forced exhalation against a closed glottis, which causes large pressure increases within the thoracic and abdominal cavities that compress the thoracic veins and reduce venous return to the heart.
22. The straining muscular effort that typically accompanies the Valsalva maneuver temporarily elevates blood pressure and adds to the heart's workload.

23. Individuals with heart and vascular disease should refrain from heavy weightlifting and sustained isometric muscle actions because of their adverse effect on the heart's workload.
24. Breathing cold ambient air normally does not damage the respiratory passages.

Key Terms

Alveolar minute ventilation: Inspired air participating in alveolar gas exchange

Alveoli: Hollow terminal spherical capillary-rich cavities at the end of respiratory bronchioles where gas exchange occurs

Anatomic dead space: Inhaled air volume that fills the nondiffusible conducting portions of the upper respiratory tract, which lack alveoli and therefore do not participate in gas exchange

Bronchi: Primary airway conduits into each lung

Bronchioles: Smaller airway ducts branching off of the bronchi that conduct inspired air through a winding, narrow route to mix with existing air in alveolar ducts

Conducting zone: Area in the upper airway that includes the trachea and terminal bronchioles and that lacks alveoli for gas exchange

Diaphragm: Large, dome-shaped sheet of striated musculofibrous tissue that separates the thoracic and abdominal cavities

Dyspnea: Inordinate shortness of breath or subjective breathing distress

Expiratory reserve volume (ERV): Maximum air volume expelled from the lungs after normal exhalation

$FEV_{1.0}$: Forced expiratory volume measured over 1 s

Fick's law of diffusion: States that a gas or solute moves passively from a higher to lower concentration across a concentration gradient

Forced expiratory volume (FEV): Air volume moved from maximum inspiration to maximum expiration with no imposed time limit

Forced vital capacity (FVC): Total air volume voluntarily moved in one breath from full inspiration to full expiration

Gas exchange surface: Lung area separating blood from the surrounding alveolar gaseous environment

Hyperventilation: Pulmonary ventilation that exceeds the oxygen uptake and carbon dioxide elimination needs of metabolism

Inspiration: Process of taking air into the lungs, in which the diaphragm muscle contracts, flattens, and moves downward toward the abdominal cavity to create the pressure differential for air inflow

Inspiratory reserve volume (IRV): Additional 2.5- to 3.5-L volume above inspired tidal air that represents the reserve ability for inhalation

Internal intercostal and abdominal muscles: Muscles that act powerfully on the ribs and abdominal cavity to reduce thoracic dimensions to make exhalation rapid and more extensive

Intrapulmonic pressure: Pressure within the lungs that varies between inspiration (lower than atmospheric) and expiration (higher than atmospheric)

Lung compliance: "Stiffness" imposed by the mechanical properties of the chest and lung tissue to a change in shape during breathing

Maximum voluntary ventilation (MVV): Maximum air volume moved with deep and rapid breathing, usually for a 15-s period

Minute ventilation: Air volume breathed each minute

Physiologic dead space: Alveolar volume with a ventilation-perfusion ratio approaching zero

Pores of Kohn: Small holes within adjacent alveoli for collateral ventilation

Pulmonary respiration: Lung ventilation with resulting uptake of oxygen and elimination of carbon dioxide to maintain blood-gas homeostasis

Pulmonary ventilation: Moving and exchanging ambient air with air in lungs

Residual lung volume (RLV): Air volume remaining in the lungs after exhaling as deeply and forcibly as possible

Scaleni and external intercostal muscles: Inspiratory muscles that act on the ribs, causing them to rotate and lift up and away from the body to increase thoracic dimensions, causing air inflow

Surface tension: Resisting force created at the surface of a liquid in contact with a gas, a structure, or another liquid

Surfactant: Wetting agent produced by alveolar epithelial cells to reduce surface tension for easier lung inflation

Tidal volume (TV): Air volume moved during either the inspiratory or expiratory phase of each breathing cycle

Total lung capacity: Residual lung volume plus forced vital capacity

Trachea: Ventilatory system portion in which inspired air adjusts to body temperature and is filtered and almost completely humidified

Transitional and respiratory zones: Area comprising the bronchioles, alveolar ducts, and alveoli

Valsalva maneuver: Forced exhalation against a closed glottis causing considerable increase in intrathoracic pressure

Ventilation-perfusion ratio: Alveolar ventilation ÷ pulmonary blood flow

Ventilatory system: Specific organs and structures responsible for oxygen and carbon dioxide exchange

References are available online at Lippincott Connect.

Additional References

Behnia M, et al. Alterations in central hemodynamic in patients with COPD after acute high intensity exercise. *Pulmonology*. 2020;1:S2531-0437(20)30140-9.

Elliott L, Loomis D. Respiratory effects of road pollution in recreational cyclists: a pilot study. *Arch Environ Occup Health*. 2020;1-9.

Fritz C, et al. Inspiratory muscle training did not improve exercise capacity and lung function in adult patients with Fontan circulation: a randomized controlled trial. *Int J Cardiol*. 2020;27:S0167-5273(20)33416-1.

Heiden GI, et al. Mechanisms of exercise limitation and prevalence of pulmonary hypertension in pulmonary Langerhans cell histiocytosis. *Chest*. 2020;158:2440.

Mendes LPS, et al. Validity and responsiveness of the Glittre-ADL test without a backpack in people with chronic obstructive pulmonary disease. *COPD*. 2020;17:392.

Moawd SA, et al. Inspiratory muscle training in obstructive sleep apnea associating diabetic peripheral neuropathy: a randomized control study. *Biomed Res Int*. 2020;2020:5036585.

Sovová M, et al. Is population's cardiorespiratory fitness really declining? *Cent Eur J Public Health*. 2020;28:120.

Tanner EA, et al. Optimized curcumin, pomegranate extract, and methylsulfonylmethane reduce acute, systemic inflammatory response to a half-marathon race. *Altern Ther Health Med*. 2020;AT6137.

Volianitis S, et al. The physiology of rowing with perspective on training and health. *Eur J Appl Physiol*. 2020;120:1943.

Table 12.1 Anthropometric Data, Pulmonary Function, and Resting Minute Ventilation in 20 Marathon Runners and Healthy Controls

Measure	Runners	Controls	Difference
Anthropometric			
Age, y	27.8	27.4	0.4
Stature, cm	175.8	176.7	0.9
Surface area, m²	1.82	1.89	0.07
Pulmonary Function			
FVC, L	5.13	5.34	0.21
TLC, L	6.91	7.13	0.22
$FEV_{1.0}$, L	4.32	4.47	0.15
$FEV_{1.0}$/FVC, %	84.3	83.8	0.5
MVV, L · min^{-1}	179.8	176.0	3.8
Resting Ventilation			
$\dot{V}_I$, L · min^{-1}	11.9	11.9	0.9
Breathing rate, breaths · min^{-1}	10.9	11.1	0.2
Tidal volume, L	1.16	1.06	0.10

Note: All differences (last column) are not statistically significant.

Table 12.2 Tidal Volume, Breathing Rate, and Total and Alveolar Minute Ventilation

Condition	Tidal Volume (mL)	× Breathing Rate (min) =	Total Min $\dot{V}_E$ (mL · min^{-1})	− Dead Space Min $\dot{V}_E$ (mL · min^{-1}) =	Alveolar Min $\dot{V}_E$ (mL · min^{-1})
Shallow breathing	150	40	6000	(150 mL × 40)	0
Normal breathing	500	12	6000	(150 mL × 12)	4200
Deep breathing	1000	6	6000	(150 mL × 6)	5100

$\dot{V}_E$ = expired volume

CHAPTER 13
Gas Exchange and Transport

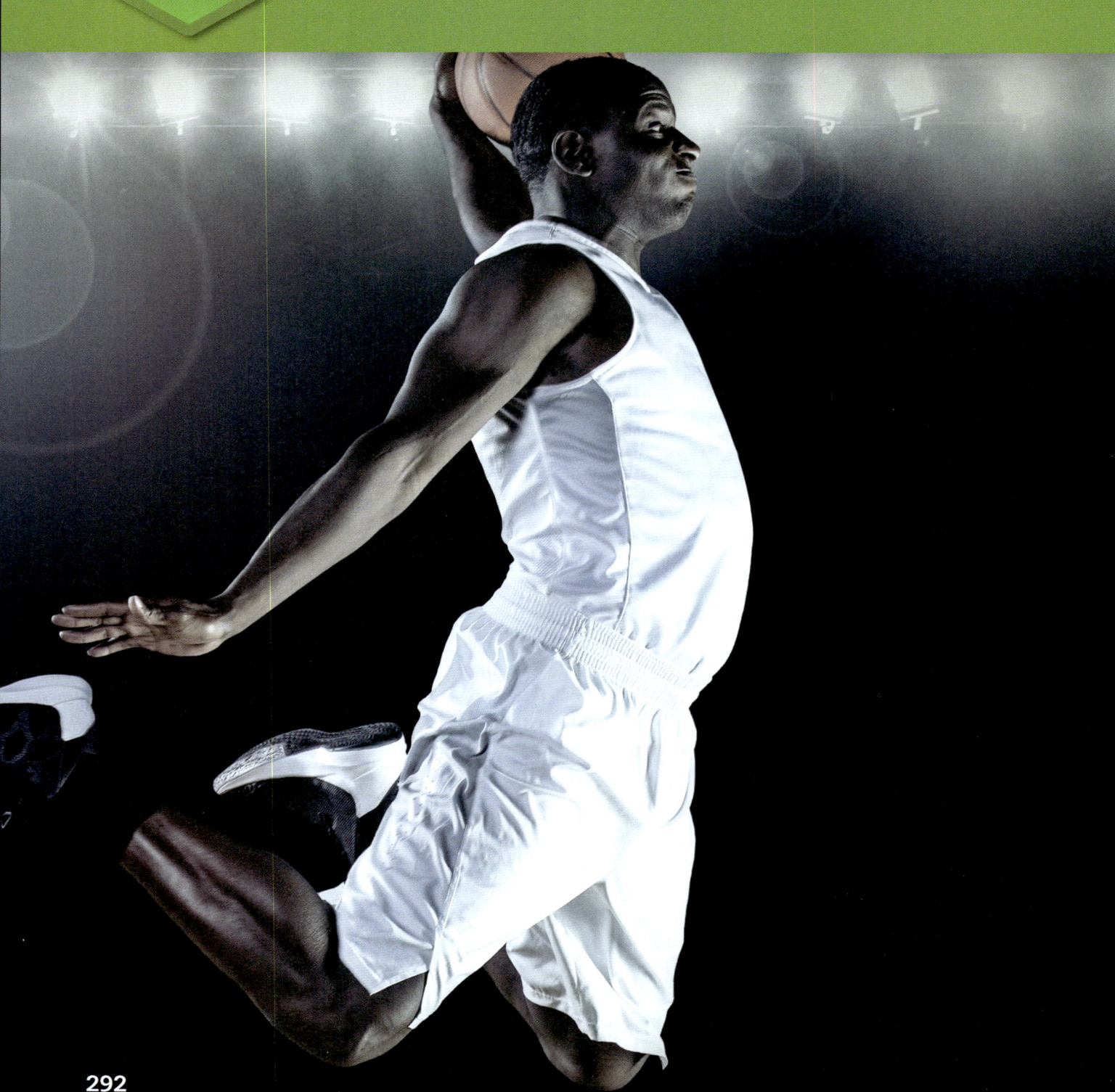

Chapter Objectives

- List the partial pressures of respired gases in the alveoli, arterial blood, active muscles, and mixed-venous blood during rest and maximal physical activity
- Explain how Henry's law impacts pulmonary gas exchange
- Discuss the role partial pressure plays in metabolic gas loading and unloading in the lungs and tissues
- Quantify oxygen transport in arterial plasma and combined with hemoglobin under sea-level ambient conditions
- Discuss the physiologic advantage of oxyhemoglobin's S-shaped dissociation curve
- Describe myoglobin's role in oxygen delivery to capillaries and red blood cells during physical exertion
- Describe factors that produce the "Bohr effect" and their major beneficial effect in physical activity
- Explain myoglobin's role during intense physical activity
- Describe three ways carbon dioxide is transported in blood

Ancillaries at-a-Glance

Visit Lippincott Connect to access the following resources.

- References: Chapter 13
- Animations: Gas Exchange in Alveoli, Oxygen Transport
- Focus on Research: Muscle: A Remarkably Adaptable Tissue

The body's oxygen supply in ambient air depends on two factors:

1. Gas concentration
2. Gas pressure

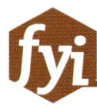
Weather Changes and Barometric Pressure

At sea level, the pressure of air's gas molecules raises a mercury column to an average height of 760 mm/29.9 in. Barometric readings vary with changing weather conditions and decrease predictably as altitude increases. As an example of the influence of changing weather conditions, consider the barometric pressure in Ann Arbor, Michigan (48109), area recorded at the local municipal airport near the University of Michigan Stadium on March 3, 2020 at 3:00 PM—barometric pressure 29.47 in at 3.9°C/39°F and 66% relative humidity. Only 30 min later at the same temperature but slightly elevated humidity (69%), barometric pressure decreased slightly to 29.40 in. By 6:45 PM, when temperature decreased to −3.9°C/25°F, barometric pressure had declined further to 29.16 in (https://weather.com/maps/currentusweather).

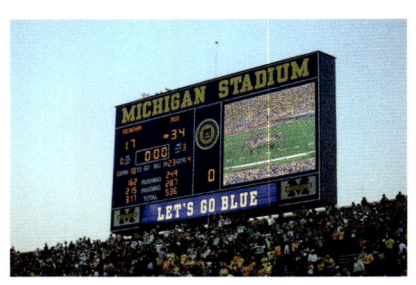
Susan Montgomery/Shutterstock

Ambient air's composition remains relatively constant at 20.93% oxygen; 79.04% nitrogen, including inert gases in small quantities that behave physiologically like nitrogen; 0.03% carbon dioxide; and usually small water vapor quantities. The gas molecules move at relatively high speeds and exert a pressure against any contacted surface. At sea level, the pressure of air molecules raises a column of mercury in a barometer to a height of 760 mm/29.9 in or the equivalent of 1 torr. The **torr**—named for Italian physicist and mathematician Evangelista Torricelli (1608–1647), who invented the barometer in 1644—is not an SI unit but an expression for gas pressure. *One torr equals the pressure necessary to raise a 1-mm mercury column 1 mm high at 0°C/32°F against the standard acceleration of gravity at 45° north latitude (980.6 cm · s^{-2}).* One standard atmosphere equals 760 torr. The barometric reading varies with changing weather conditions and becomes lower with increasing altitude (see Chapter 24).

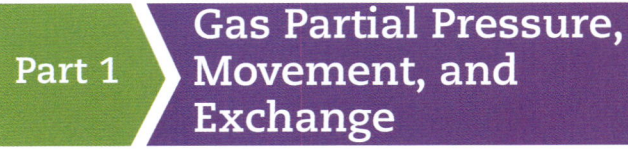

Part 1 — Gas Partial Pressure, Movement, and Exchange

Respired Gas Concentrations and Partial Pressures

Each specific gas molecule in a mixture of different gas molecules exerts an individual **partial pressure**. Collectively, the mixture's total pressure equals the sum of the partial pressures for all individual gases in the mixture. This principle, known as **Dalton law**, honors the British chemist and physicist John Dalton who also developed the atomic matter theory (1766–1844; www.famousscientists.org/john-dalton). Partial pressure computes as follows:

> Partial pressure = Percentage concentration of specific gas
> × Total pressure of gas mixture

Mercury Instead of Water

During the last 3 months of his life, Galileo (1564–1642; http://inventors.about.com/od/gstartinventors/a/Galileo_Galilei.htm) suggested to Torricelli that he include mercury in his ongoing vacuum experiments. Two years later, Torricelli filled a 4-foot-long glass tube with mercury, 13.6 times heavier than water, reducing dramatically the need for an extremely long water-filled tube that was taller than his house; he inverted the tube into a dish to create a sustained vacuum. He observed that the mercury did not flow, leaving the air above the mercury undisturbed in a vacuum. Thus, Torricelli became the first scientist to discover the barometer's basic principle—changes in atmospheric pressure could be measured by changes in the height of mercury in a tube. He also deduced that day-to-day changes in atmospheric pressure (clear, cloudy, rainy, stormy) affected the atmospheric pressure, in effect paving the way for modern weather forecasting. Vice Admiral Robert Fitzroy (1805–1865), captain on Charles Darwin's exploration ship HMS Beagle, began the first published daily weather forecasting in London in 1860 that detailed air pressure's rise and fall.

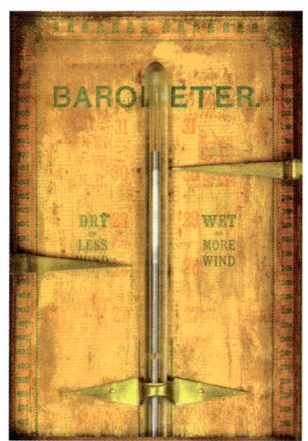
Martin Bergsma/Shutterstock

Ambient Air Composition at Sea Level (760 mm Hg)

Gas	Percentage	Ambient Partial Pressure (mm Hg)	Gas Volume (mL · L⁻¹)
Oxygen	20.93	159	209.3
Carbon dioxide	0.03	0.2	0.4
Nitrogen	79.04	600	790.3

Note: Nitrogen includes 0.93% argon and other rare trace gases

Vibrant Image Studio/Shutterstock

Ambient Air

The partial pressure of oxygen equals 20.93% of the total 760 mm Hg pressure exerted by air or 159 mm Hg (20.93 ÷ 100 × 760 mm Hg). Carbon dioxide exerts only 0.23 mm Hg pressure (0.03 ÷ 100 × 760 mm Hg), whereas nitrogen molecules exert a pressure that raises the mercury in a manometer about 600 mm (79.04 ÷ 100 × 760 mm Hg). The letter *P* placed before the gas symbol denotes partial pressure. The partial pressures at sea level for the principal ambient air components average as follows:

- Oxygen (P_{O_2}) = 159 mm Hg
- Carbon dioxide (P_{CO_2}) = 0.2 mm Hg
- Nitrogen (P_{N_2}) = 600 mm Hg

Tracheal Air

Air completely saturates with water vapor as it enters the nasal cavities and mouth and passes down the respiratory tract. The vapor dilutes the inspired air mixture somewhat. At a body temperature of 37°C/98.6°F, the water molecule pressure in humidified air equals 47 mm Hg; this leaves 713 mm Hg (760 − 47 mm Hg) as the total pressure exerted by the inspired dry air molecules. Consequently, the effective P_{O_2} in tracheal air decreases by about 10 mm Hg from its ambient air value of 159 to 149 mm Hg [0.2093 × (760 − 47 mm Hg)]. Carbon dioxide's negligible contribution to inspired air means that humidification exerts little effect on inspired P_{CO_2}.

Alveolar Air

The composition of alveolar air differs considerably from that of the incoming breath of moist ambient air because carbon dioxide continually enters the alveoli from the blood. In contrast, oxygen flows from the lungs into the blood for transport throughout the body. The inset table shows that alveolar air, in contrast to ambient air, contains on average 14.5% oxygen, 5.5% carbon dioxide, and 80.0% nitrogen.

After subtracting the vapor pressure from moist alveolar gas, the average alveolar partial pressure becomes 103 mm Hg [0.145 × (760 − 47 mm Hg)] for P_{O_2} and 39 mm Hg [0.055 × (760 − 47 mm Hg)] for P_{CO_2}. These values represent average pressures exerted by oxygen and carbon dioxide molecules against the alveolar side of the alveolar-capillary membrane. They do not remain physiologic constants; rather, they vary somewhat with the ventilatory cycle phase and the adequacy of ventilation in various lung regions. Recall that a relatively large air volume remains in the lungs after each normal exhalation. This functional residual capacity serves as a damper, so each incoming breath exerts only a small effect on alveolar air composition. This explains why alveolar gas partial pressures remain relatively stable.

Alveolar Air Composition at Sea Level (37°C/98.6°F)

Gas	Percentage	Partial Pressure (mm Hg)	Gas Volume (mL · L⁻¹)
Oxygen	14.5	103	145
Carbon dioxide	5.5	39	55
Nitrogen	80.0	571	800
Water vapor		47	

Vibrant Image Studio/Shutterstock

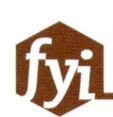

Approximate Solubility Coefficients of Gases in Physiologic Fluids

Gas	Water	Plasma	Blood	Quantity Dissolved (per dL blood)
Oxygen	2.39	2.14	2.26	0.3 mL
Carbon dioxide	56.7	51.5	57.03	3.0 mL
Nitrogen	1.23	1.18	1.30	0.8 mL

Olga Hmelevskaya/Shutterstock

Gas Movement in Air and Fluids

In accordance with **Henry's law** (named for decorated English chemist and physician William Henry [1774–1836]; https://peoplepill.com/people/william-henry/), the mass of a gas that dissolves in a fluid at a given temperature varies directly with the gas pressure over the liquid (if no chemical reaction takes place between the gas and liquid). Two factors govern gas diffusion rate into a fluid:

1. **Pressure differential** between the gas above the fluid and the gas dissolved in the fluid
2. Gas **solubility** in the fluid

Impaired Alveolar Gas Transfer Can Compromise Survival

Two factors can impair gas transfer capacity at the alveolar-capillary membrane: (1) a layer of accumulated environmental pollutants (e.g., secondhand cigarette smoke, solid and liquid particles and gases from combusting fossil fuels in the air, power plant emissions) that "thickens" the alveolar membrane and (2) reduced alveolar effective surface area from respiratory diseases (e.g., viral or bacterial pneumonia, emphysema). Each factor extends the time before alveolar-capillary gases equilibrate and, in severe disease, can totally overwhelm the inflammatory response and lead to acute respiratory disease syndrome. When this occurs from the novel coronavirus SARS-CoV-2, the virus invades the deeper, more numerous alveolar receptors of angiotensin-converting enzyme 2, causing surrounding healthy cells to die. As the condition worsens, individuals must rely on external ventilator support to replace normal ventilatory function. The mechanical ventilator (respirator) assumes the role of the the ventilatory muscles in the breathing process when they fail to provide on their own sufficient oxygen to sustain life. The image shows a three-dimensional schematic of a coronavirus molecule (COVID-19), depicted in red and yellow oblong shapes, embedded in an alveoli cluster in a former collegiate athlete. A normal, noninfected lung has from 270 to 800 million alveoli.

Kateryna Kon/Shutterstock

Sources:
De Sousa RAL, et al. Physical exercise effects on the brain during COVID-19 pandemic: links between mental and cardiovascular health. *Neurol Sci*. 2021;42:1325.
Mihalick VL, et al. Cardiopulmonary exercise testing during the COVID-19 pandemic. *Prog Cardiovasc Dis*. 2021;67:353.
Vancini RL, et al. Physical exercise and COVID-19 pandemic in PubMed: two months of dynamics and one year of original scientific production. *Sports Med Health Sci*. 2021;3:80.

Pressure Differential

FIGURE 13.1 illustrates the concept of gas pressure differential. In this example, oxygen molecules continually bombard the water surface in three chambers. The water depicted in chamber A initially contains no oxygen (P = 0 mm Hg), but then many oxygen molecules enter the water and dissolve in it. Dissolved gas molecules also move randomly, allowing for some oxygen molecules to exit the fluid. In chamber B, oxygen still shows a *net* movement into the fluid from the gaseous state. In chamber C, the numbers of molecules entering and leaving the fluid eventually equalize. This means that the gas pressures equilibrate without net oxygen diffusion into or out of the water. Conversely, if the pressure of dissolved oxygen molecules exceeds the free gas air pressure, oxygen leaves the fluid until it attains a new pressure equilibrium. *In humans, the pressure difference between alveolar and pulmonary blood gases creates the driving force for gas diffusion across the pulmonary membrane.*

Solubility: Dissolving Power of a Gas

For two different gases at identical pressure differentials, each gas solubility value (expressed in milliliters of gas per 100 mL [dL] of fluid) determines how many gas molecules move into or out of a fluid. Oxygen, carbon dioxide, and nitrogen have different solubility coefficients in whole blood. Carbon dioxide dissolves most readily, with a solubility coefficient of 57.03 mL/dL of fluid at 760 mm Hg and 37°C/98.6°F. Oxygen, with a solubility coefficient of 2.26 mL, remains relatively insoluble. Nitrogen is least soluble, with a coefficient of 1.30 mL.

The amount of gas dissolved in a fluid computes as follows:

> **Quantity of gas (mL·dL^{-1}) = Solubility coefficient × (Gas partial pressure ÷ Total barometric pressure)**

For example, the quantity of oxygen dissolved in 1 dL of arterial whole blood (Po_2 = 100 mm Hg) at sea level (760 mm Hg) computes as:

> **Quantity of gas = 2.26 × (100 ÷ 760) = 0.3 mL·dL^{-1}**

For each pressure unit that favors diffusion, approximately 25 times more carbon dioxide than oxygen moves into or out of a fluid. Viewed another way, equal amounts of oxygen and carbon dioxide enter or leave a fluid under considerably different pressure gradients for each gas—precisely what occurs in the body.

At rest, dissolved oxygen contributes about 4% to the total oxygen uptake by the body each minute. In maximal physical activity, it provides less than 2% of the total requirement. Even if one increases arterial

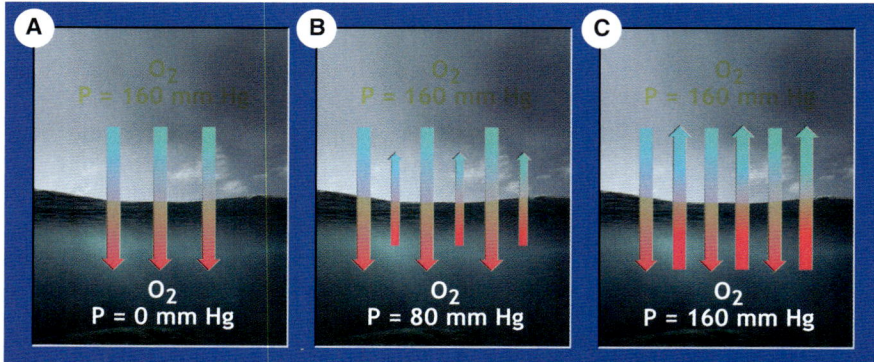

FIGURE 13.1. **(A)** Oxygen enters the water. **(B)** Dissolved oxygen halfway to equilibrium with gaseous oxygen. **(C)** Equilibrium between oxygen in air and oxygen dissolved in water.
(rangizzz/Shutterstock)

Po$_2$ by breathing 100% oxygen (ambient Po$_2$ = 760 mm Hg), dissolved oxygen (1.5 to 2.0 mL·dL blood^{-1}) still supplies only 40% of the total oxygen at rest and about 10% in maximal exertion. The physiologic significance of the solubility of oxygen and carbon dioxide comes not from its role as a transport medium, but in determining the partial pressures for these gases. In the lungs and tissues, partial pressure plays a central role in loading and unloading oxygen and carbon dioxide.

Gas Exchange in the Lungs and Tissues

Gas exchange between the lungs and blood and gas movement at the tissue level continue passively by diffusion, depending on pressure gradients. **FIGURE 13.2** illustrates pressure gradients that favor gas transfer in different body regions at rest.

See the animation "Oxygen Transport" on Lippincott Connect to view this process.

Gas Exchange in the Lungs

Figure 13.2A shows that, at rest, the 100-mm Hg pressure of oxygen molecules in the alveoli exceeds by about 60-mm Hg the 40 mm Hg pressure of oxygen in blood that enters the pulmonary capillaries. Consequently, oxygen travels from higher to lower pressure as it dissolves and diffuses through the alveolar membranes into the blood. In contrast, carbon dioxide exists under slightly greater pressure in returning venous blood than in the alveoli. This causes net carbon dioxide diffusion from the blood into the lungs. Despite the relatively small 6 mm Hg pressure gradient for carbon dioxide diffusion (compared with the 60 mm Hg diffusion gradient for oxygen), carbon dioxide transfer occurs rapidly due to its high plasma

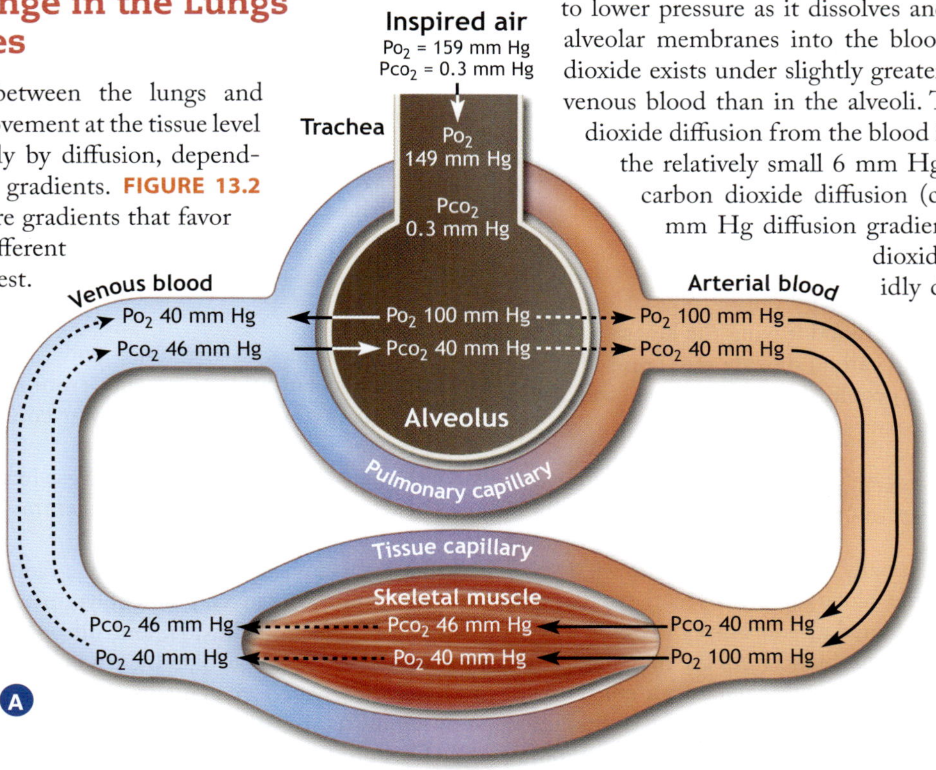

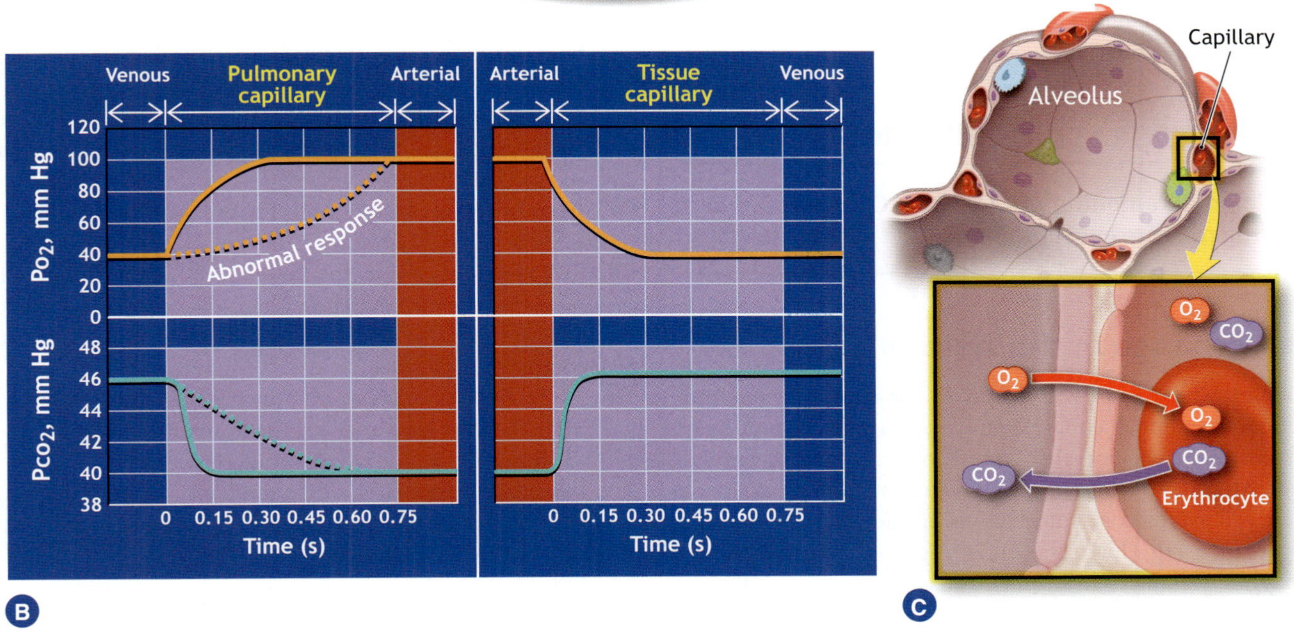

FIGURE 13.2. **(A)** Gas transfer pressure gradients at rest, showing the partial pressure of oxygen (Po$_2$) and partial pressure of carbon dioxide (Pco$_2$) for ambient, tracheal, and alveolar air and gas pressures in venous and arterial blood and muscle tissue. **(B)** Time required for gas exchange. **(C)** Gas exchange (diffusion) between a pulmonary capillary and its adjacent alveolus. (Aldona Griskeviciene/Shutterstock)

solubility. Nitrogen remains essentially unchanged in alveolar-capillary gas, neither used nor produced in metabolic reactions.

Gas exchange occurs so rapidly in the healthy lung that alveolar gas-blood gas equilibrium takes place in about 0.25 s, or within one third of the blood's transit time through the lungs (Fig. 13.2B). At rest, blood remains in the pulmonary and tissue capillaries for about 0.75 s. Pulmonary disease (dashed line) impairs the rate of gas transfer across the alveolar-capillary membrane, thus prolonging the time for gas equilibration. Blood's transit time through the pulmonary capillaries during maximal exercise decreases to about 0.4 s, but this still remains adequate for complete aeration in the healthy lung. Even in intense activity, a red blood cell's velocity through a pulmonary capillary generally does not exceed by more than 50% its velocity at rest. With increasing exercise intensity, the pulmonary capillaries increase the blood volume within them by about three times the resting value.[7] Accommodating a larger blood volume helps to maintain a relatively slow pulmonary blood flow velocity during physical activity. With complete aeration, the blood leaving the lungs contains oxygen at 100 mm Hg and carbon dioxide at 40 mm Hg, on average. For most healthy people, these values vary little during vigorous physical activity.

  See the animation "Gas Exchange in Alveoli" on Lippincott Connect to view this process.

Arterial blood P_{O_2} usually remains slightly lower than alveolar P_{O_2} because some blood in the alveolar capillaries passes through poorly ventilated alveoli. Also, the blood leaving the lungs mixes with venous blood from the bronchial and cardiac circulations. The term *venous admixture* defines this small quantity of poorly oxygenated blood. Venous admixture reduces the arterial P_{O_2} slightly below the value in pulmonary end-capillary blood and only exerts a small influence in healthy individuals.

 INTEGRATIVE QUESTION

Why do small amounts of CO_2 and CO impurities in a breathing mixture exert profound physiologic effects?

Gas Exchange in the Tissues

In tissues, where energy metabolism consumes oxygen and produces an almost equal amount of carbon dioxide, gas pressures differ considerably from those recorded in arterial blood. At rest, the P_{O_2} in the fluid immediately outside a muscle cell averages 40 mm Hg and intracellular P_{CO_2} averages 46 mm Hg (Fig. 13.2A). In vigorous physical activity, oxygen pressure within muscle tissue falls toward 0 mm Hg, whereas carbon dioxide pressure approaches 90 mm Hg. Pressure differences between gases in plasma and tissues establish diffusion gradients. Oxygen leaves the blood and diffuses *toward* cells, whereas carbon dioxide flows *from*

cells into the blood. Blood then passes into venules and veins (venous circuit) for return to the heart and delivery to the lungs. Diffusion occurs rapidly as blood enters the dense pulmonary capillary network. The body does not attempt to eliminate all carbon dioxide. Rather, each liter of blood leaving the lungs, assuming a P_{CO_2} of 40 mm Hg, contains about 50 mL of carbon dioxide. As discussed in Chapter 14, this small "background level" of carbon dioxide provides the chemical basis for ventilatory control through its stimulating effect on the brainstem's pons and medullary centers. The term respiratory center describes these neural tissue collections for ventilatory control. In this sense, alveolar ventilation couples tightly to metabolic demands to keep alveolar gas composition remarkably constant. Stability in alveolar gas concentrations persists even during strenuous activity that increases oxygen uptake and carbon dioxide output to 25 times those of resting values.

Summary

1. Gas molecules in the lungs and tissues diffuse along their concentration gradients from a higher concentration (higher pressure) to lower concentration (lower pressure).
2. The partial pressure for a specific gas in a mixture of gases varies directly with the gas concentration and the mixture's total pressure.
3. Henry's law states that pressure gradient and solubility determine how much gas dissolves in a fluid.
4. Oxygen, carbon dioxide, and nitrogen exhibit different solubilities in whole blood. Carbon dioxide dissolves most readily, whereas oxygen and nitrogen show relatively low solubility.
5. Carbon dioxide solubility in plasma is 25 times that of oxygen, allowing carbon dioxide to move into and out of body fluids down a relatively small diffusion (pressure) gradient.
6. Maintaining a constant alveolar gas composition during rest and physical activity reflects fine adjustments in pulmonary ventilation.
7. Alveolar ventilation maintains P_{O_2} at about 100 mm Hg and P_{CO_2} at 40 mm Hg.
8. Oxygen diffuses into the blood and carbon dioxide diffuses into the lungs because venous blood contains oxygen at lower pressure and carbon dioxide at higher pressure compared with alveolar gas.
9. Alveolar-blood gas exchange at rest achieves equilibrium in the healthy lung at about the midpoint of blood's transit through the pulmonary capillaries.
10. In intense exertion, blood flow velocity through the lungs generally does not compromise full oxygen loading and carbon dioxide unloading.
11. Diffusion gradients favor oxygen movement from the capillaries to the tissues and carbon dioxide from the tissues to the blood.
12. During physical activity, oxygen and carbon dioxide diffuse rapidly as their pressure gradients widen.

Part 2: Oxygen Transport in Blood

The blood carries oxygen in two ways:

1. In physical solution, dissolved in blood's fluid component
2. In loose combination with hemoglobin, the iron-protein molecule within the red blood cell

Oxygen Transport in Physical Solution

Within bodily fluids, oxygen's relative insolubility in water keeps its concentration low. At a 100 mm Hg alveolar P_{O_2}, only about 0.3 mL of gaseous oxygen dissolves in each deciliter of blood (0.003 mL for each additional 1 mm Hg increase in P_{O_2}). This equals 3 mL of oxygen per liter of blood. The blood volume of a 70-kg person averages about 5 L; thus, 15 mL of oxygen dissolves in the blood's fluid portion (3 mL per L × 5). This small amount of oxygen would sustain life for about 4 s. Viewed from a different perspective, if oxygen in physical solution in blood provided the body's sole oxygen source, about 80 L of blood would need to circulate each minute to supply the resting oxygen requirements—a blood flow about twice the maximum ever recorded!

As with carbon dioxide, the small oxygen quantity transported in physical solution serves several important functions. Dissolved oxygen's random movement establishes the P_{O_2} in blood and tissue fluids. The pressure of oxygen in solution helps to regulate breathing, particularly at higher altitudes, when ambient P_{O_2} decreases considerably. It also determines oxygen loading of hemoglobin in the lungs and subsequent release in tissues.

Oxygen Transport in Hemoglobin

Metallic compounds exist in the blood of many animal species to augment its oxygen-carrying capacity. **FIGURE 13.3A** illustrates the iron-containing globular protein pigment **hemoglobin (Hb)**, which is carried within each of the more than 25 trillion human red blood cells. The incomparable French physiologist Claude Bernard (see Introduction: A View From the Past) described Hb's role in the blood. Derived from the words *heme* and *globin*, the term describes each Hb subunit as a bulbous protein with an embedded heme group containing one iron atom acting as an oxygen "magnet" (Fig. 13.3B). In mammals, a single Hb molecule contains four heme subunits. With a normal Hb concentration, the blood carries 65 to 70 times more oxygen than normally dissolves in plasma. Thus, the approximately 280 million Hb molecules temporarily "capture" and transport about 197 mL of oxygen in each liter of blood. Each of the four iron atoms embedded within the Hb molecule's structure loosely binds with one oxygen molecule in the following reversible reaction:

$$Hb_4 + 4O_2 \leftrightarrow Hb_4O_8$$

The reaction requires no enzymes; it proceeds without a change in the valence of Fe^{2+}, as occurs in the more permanent oxidation process. *The P_{O_2} dissolved in physical solution controls Hb's oxygenation to oxyhemoglobin.*

Hb's Oxygen-Carrying Capacity

For males, each deciliter of blood contains about 15 g of Hb. The value decreases 5 to 10% for females (14 g·dL^{-1}). This gender difference partly explains the lower aerobic capacity of females relative to males, even when considering differences in body mass and body fat. Males have larger Hb concentrations from testosterone's stimulating effect on red blood cell production.[13,28]

Each of the four iron atoms in the Hb molecule combines loosely with 1.34 mL of oxygen. Thus, if one knows blood's Hb content, its oxygen-carrying capacity computes as follows:

Blood's oxygen capacity (mL·dL blood^{-1})		Hemoglobin (g·dL blood^{-1})		Oxygen capacity of hemoglobin
20 mL O_2	=	15	×	1.34 mL·g^{-1}

 See the animation "Asthma" on Lippincott Connect for a demonstration of asthma's effects on the pulmonary system.

Anemia's Effects on Oxygen Transport

Iron insufficiency prevalent among endurance athletes occurs with greater-than-normal frequency in women engaged in

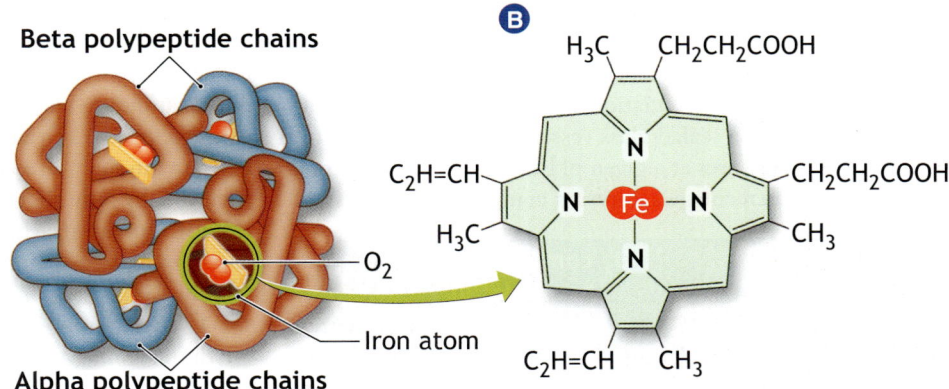

FIGURE 13.3. (A) The hemoglobin molecule consists of the protein globin and four subunit polypeptide chains. (B) Each polypeptide contains a single heme group with its single iron atom acting as an oxygen "magnet."

intense training.[2,6] The blood's capacity to transport oxygen changes only slightly with normal variations in Hb content. In contrast, a significant decrease in the iron content of red blood cells reduces the blood's oxygen-carrying capacity. Iron deficiency anemia diminishes an individual's capacity to sustain even mildly intense aerobic activity.[3,11,26,27]

TABLE 13.1 presents data from 29 iron-deficient anemic males and females with low Hb levels. They formed two groups; one received intramuscular iron injections over an 80-day period, whereas the placebo group received similar intramuscular injections of colored saline solution. A third group with normal Hb levels served as controls. The researchers tested all groups during exercise prior to the experiment and after 80 days of either iron therapy or placebo treatment. The results clearly show that the anemic group given iron supplements improved in exercise response compared with non-supplemented counterparts. Peak heart rate while stepping for 5 min declined from 155 to 113 b·min^{-1} for males and from 152 to 123 b·min^{-1} for females. This translates into an average of 15% more oxygen delivered per heartbeat.

TABLE 13.1 Hemoglobin and peak exercise heart rate in normal and anemic subjects prior to and following supplemental iron treatment

PO_2 and Hb Saturation

The term *cooperative binding* describes a union between oxygen and Hb. Binding of an oxygen molecule to an iron atom in one of four globin chains (Fig. 13.3) progressively facilitates subsequent molecule binding. The cooperative binding phenomenon explains Hb's sigmoid, or S-shaped, oxygen saturation curve.

FIGURE 13.4A illustrates the **oxyhemoglobin dissociation curve**, showing Hb's saturation with oxygen at various PO_2 values, including alveolar-capillary gas at sea level (PO_2, 100 mm Hg). The right ordinate gives the oxygen amount carried in each deciliter of normal blood at a particular plasma PO_2 value. The term **volume percent (vol%)** describes blood's oxygen content. In this regard, vol% refers to milliliters of oxygen extracted from a deciliter sample from either whole blood (with plasma) or packed red blood cells (without plasma) measured in a vacuum.

Physical chemists establish the oxygen content and percentage saturation in dissociation curves by exposing about 200 mL of blood in a sealed glass vessel called a tonometer to various oxygen pressures at a given pH in a constant temperature water bath. Percentage saturation computes as follows:

$$\text{Percentage saturation} = \frac{O_2 \text{ combined with hemoglobin}}{O_2 \text{ capacity of hemoglobin}} \times 100$$

If an individual's Hb oxygen-carrying capacity in whole blood equals 20 vol%, yet only 12 vol% oxygen actually combines with Hb, then percentage saturation computes as:

$$\text{Percentage saturation} = 12 \text{ vol\%} \div 20 \text{ vol\%} \times 100 = 60\%$$

For 100% saturation, the oxygen combined with Hb equals its oxygen-carrying capacity.

Figure 13.4B depicts the **oxygen transport cascade** for oxygen partial pressure as oxygen moves from ambient air at sea level to the mitochondria embedded within maximally active muscle fibers. The shiny purple background image shows a close-up mitochondrial structure integral in processing the complex but highly energetic reactions within the muscle's submicroscopic structures.

PO_2 in the Lungs

In the discussion of Hb, the assumption has been that Hb fully saturates with oxygen when exposed to alveolar gas. This does not occur because at the average alveolar PO_2 at sea level (100 mm Hg), Hb achieves only 98% oxygen saturation. The right ordinate in Figure 13.4A shows that at the PO_2 of 100 mm Hg, the Hb in each deciliter of blood leaving the lungs carries about 19.7 mL of oxygen. The two yellow lines indicate the Hb percentage saturation (solid line) and myoglobin (dashed line) in relation to oxygen pressure. The right ordinate shows the oxygen amount carried in each deciliter of blood under normal conditions. The two inset curves within the figure illustrate the temperature and acidity effects in altering Hb's affinity for oxygen (Bohr effect). The black inset box presents oxyhemoglobin saturation and arterial blood's oxygen-carrying capacity for different PO_2 values with a Hb concentration of 14 g·dL^{-1} blood at pH 7.40. The white horizontal line at the top of the graph indicates percentage Hb saturation at the average alveolar PO_2 at sea level of 100 mm Hg. Clearly, any additional increase in alveolar PO_2 contributes little to how much more oxygen can combine with Hb. In addition to the oxygen bound to Hb, the plasma for each deciliter of arterial blood contains 0.3 mL of oxygen in solution. In healthy individuals who breathe ambient air at sea level, each deciliter of blood leaving the lungs carries approximately 20.0 mL of oxygen: 19.7 mL bound to Hb and 0.3 mL dissolved in plasma.

Figure 13.4 also reveals that Hb saturation with oxygen changes little until oxygen pressure declines to about 60 mm Hg. This flat upper portion of the oxyhemoglobin dissociation curve provides a safety margin to ensure adequate arterial blood saturation with oxygen despite considerable fluctuations in ambient PO_2.[24] Even if alveolar PO_2 decreases to 75 mm Hg, as occurs in lung disease or at higher altitudes, Hb saturation decreases by only about 6%. At an alveolar PO_2 of 60 mm Hg, Hb still remains nearly 90% saturated with oxygen! Below this pressure, oxygen quantity combined with Hb declines more rapidly.

On television, one frequently views competitive athletes on the sidelines breathing a concentrated oxygen gas mixture during and even following strenuous sea-level physical activity. This makes no sense from an oxygen transport perspective. The oxyhemoglobin dissociation curve shows little or no potential for increased Hb loading from additional

PO_2	Percentage saturation	Arterial O_2 content ($mL \cdot L^{-1}$)
10	13.3	24.9
20	35.5	66.6
30	58.0	108.8
40	73.9	138.6
44	78.4	147.1
48	82.0	153.8
52	84.9	159.3
56	87.3	163.8
60	89.3	167.5
64	90.9	170.5
68	92.2	173.0
76	94.1	176.5
80	94.9	178.0
90	96.3	180.7
100	97.2	182.4

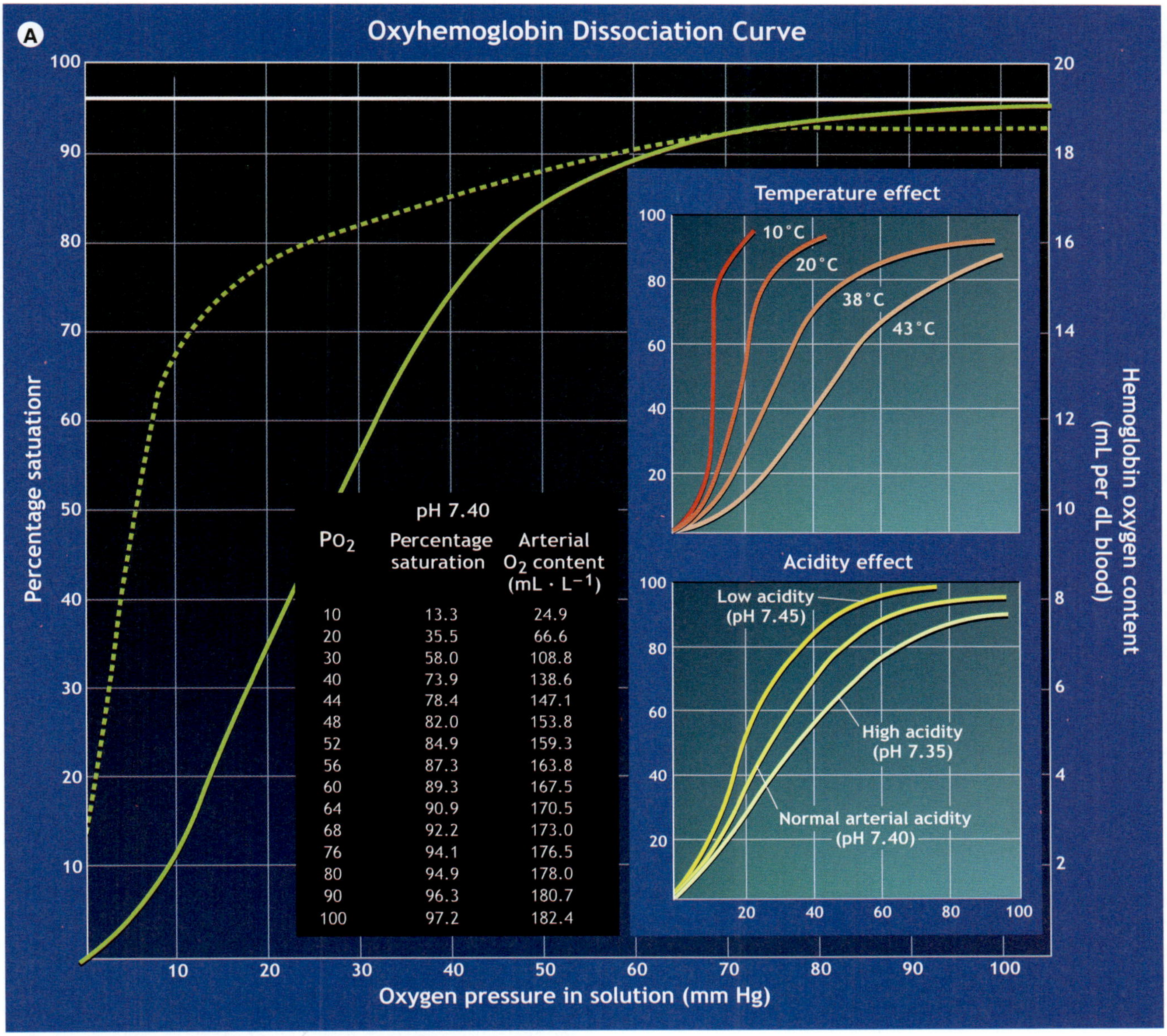

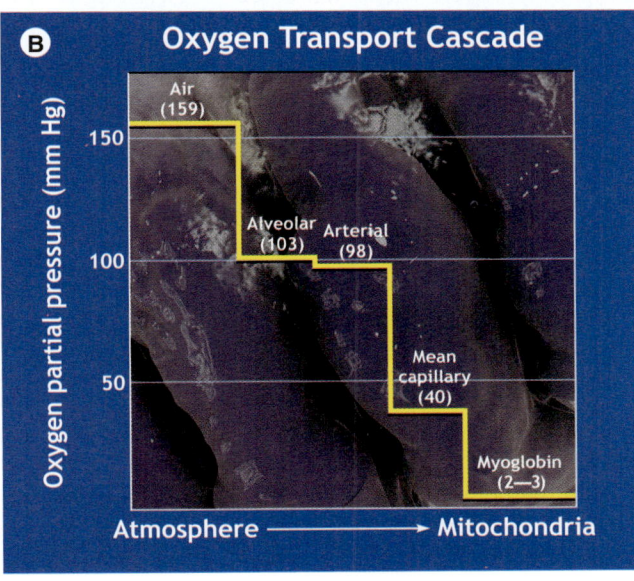

FIGURE 13.4. **(A)** Oxyhemoglobin dissociation curve. **(B)** The oxygen transport cascade characterizes partial pressures as oxygen moves from ambient air at sea level to the mitochondria in maximally active muscle tissue.
(Kateryna Kon/Shutterstock)

In a Practical Sense

Exercise-Induced Asthma

Asthma, a chronic obstructive pulmonary disease, affects more than 25 million individuals in the United States (7.7% of adults, 8.4% of children). Asthma has been increasing in prevalence since the early 1980s in all age, sex, and racial groups and represents the most common chronic children's disease (www.aafa.org/asthma-facts/).

This public health problem does not impact just high-income countries but occurs in all countries regardless of economic development. Unfortunately, most asthma-related deaths occur in low- and lower-middle-income economies (http://data.worldbank.org/about/country-and-lending-groups#MENA).

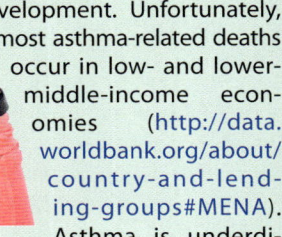
Lopolo/Shutterstock

Asthma is underdiagnosed and undertreated and often restricts individuals' activities for a lifetime.

A high fitness level does not confer immunity from asthma. Pulmonary airway hyperirritability usually manifests by coughing, wheezing, and shortness of breath, all characteristic of the asthmatic condition.[4,5,10,19]

With physical activity, catecholamines released from the sympathetic nervous system produce a relaxation effect on smooth muscle that lines pulmonary airways. Everyone experiences initial bronchodilation with physical activity. For people with asthma, in contrast, bronchospasm and exertion cause mucous secretion following normal bronchodilation. An acute airway obstruction episode often occurs 10 min following physical activity, and recovery usually occurs spontaneously within 30 to 90 min. One means to diagnose exercise-induced asthma (EIA) uses progressive treadmill or bicycle ergometer increments of exercise. During a 10- to 20-min recovery following each activity bout, spirometric testing assesses pulmonary airflow capacity (forced expiratory volume in 1 s divided by forced vital capacity). A 15% reduction in pre-exercise values confirms the EIA diagnosis.

SENSITIVITY TO THERMAL GRADIENTS

An attractive theory to explain EIA relates to the rate and magnitude for pulmonary heat exchange alterations as ventilation increases with activity. As the incoming breath of air moves down the pulmonary pathways, air warms and humidifies as heat and water transfer from the respiratory tract. This "air conditioning" effect both cools and dries the respiratory mucosa, allowing for an abrupt airway rewarming during recovery. The thermal gradient from cooling and subsequent rewarming and water loss from mucosal tissue stimulates proinflammatory chemical mediators that cause bronchospasm.

ENVIRONMENT MAKES A DIFFERENCE

Physical activity in a humid environment diminishes the EIA response regardless of ambient air temperature. Inhaling ambient air fully saturated with water vapor in physically active patients often abolishes the bronchospastic response. This also explains why people with asthma tolerate walking or jogging on a warm, humid day or swimming in an indoor pool, yet outdoor winter sports usually trigger an asthmatic attack. People with asthma should perform 15- to 30-min continuous warm-up activity because it initiates a "refractory period" that minimizes the bronchoconstrictive response severity during subsequent more intense physical activity.

Medications offer considerable relief from bronchoconstriction. Exercise training cannot "cure" the asthmatic condition, but it does increase airway reserve to reduce breathing work during all physical activity modes.

EVEN PHYSICALLY FIT ATHLETES CAN HAVE ASTHMA

Champion athletes are not immune from asthma. One of the most famous examples, 1984 Olympic marathon champion Joan Benoit Samuelson (1957–), experienced breathing problems during races in 1991 that led to the discovery of her asthmatic condition (https://en.wikipedia.org/wiki/Joan_Benoit). Despite experiencing breathing difficulties during the 1991 New York Marathon, she finished with a time of 2 hr 33 min 40 s!

Sources:
Goossens J, et al. How to detect young athletes at risk of exercise-induced bronchoconstriction? *Paediatr Respir Rev*. 2021:S1526-0542(21)00095-6.
Satia I, et al. Exercise-induced bronchoconstriction and bronchodilation: investigating the effects of age, sex, airflow limitation and FEV1. *Eur Respir J*. 2021;58:2004026.
Tikkakoski AP, et al. Outdoor pollen concentration is not associated with exercise-induced bronchoconstriction in children. *Pediatr Pulmonol*. 2021. doi: 10.1002/ppul.25782.
Zeiger JS, Weiler JM. Special Considerations and perspectives for exercise-induced bronchoconstriction (EIB) in Olympic and other elite athletes. *J Allergy Clin Immunol Pract*. 2020;S2213-2198(20)30099-4.

---

oxygen pressure inhaled at sea level or at relatively low altitude. The next time you see an American professional football player breathing from a mask connected to an oxygen tank, you will know this procedure has little merit, and no hope at all for "supercharging" the lungs with additional oxygen for subsequent performance or recovery! We explore breathing hyperoxic gas mixtures and exercise performance more fully in Chapter 23.

The sigmoid, solid lime green line in Figure 13.4A represents the oxyhemoglobin dissociation curve under resting physiologic conditions at a 7.4 arterial pH and 37°C/98.6°F tissue temperature. The two *inset curves* depict other important characteristics of Hb's affinity for oxygen. Any increase in plasma acidity (including carbon dioxide concentration) or temperature causes the dissociation curve to shift downward and to the right. Note the range of temperature from 10°C to 40°C/50°F to 109.4°F and acidity from pH 7.45 to 7.35, a fairly narrow range, considering that normal arterial acidity is pH 7.40. These important characteristics are called the **Bohr effect**, to honor its 1891 discoverer, Danish physiologist Christian Bohr (1855–1911; father of Nobel physicist Niels Bohr [1885–1962]). The salient features reveal that hydrogen ions and carbon dioxide alter Hb's molecular structure to decrease its oxygen-binding affinity. The reduced Hb effectiveness to hold oxygen occurs particularly in the P_{O_2} range of 20 to 50 mm Hg. The Bohr effect remains evident during intense exertion as more oxygen releases to tissues due to increases in the following three factors:

1. Metabolic heat
2. Carbon dioxide
3. Acidity from blood lactate accumulation

At normal alveolar P_{O_2}, the Bohr effect exerts almost no effect on pulmonary capillary blood (even during maximal exertion), so Hb binds fully with oxygen as blood flows through the lungs.

FIGURE 13.5 shows the percentage composition for centrifuged whole blood for red blood cells (termed **hematocrit**) and plasma, including representative values for the oxygen amount carried in each component for an untrained person in a pretraining experiment and following 4 days of aerobic training. Note that the increase in plasma volume (hemodilution) early in training decreases red blood cell concentration toward borderline anemia. Oxygen transport capacity does not decrease with training because the total erythrocyte mass of blood remains constant or increases slightly.[25]

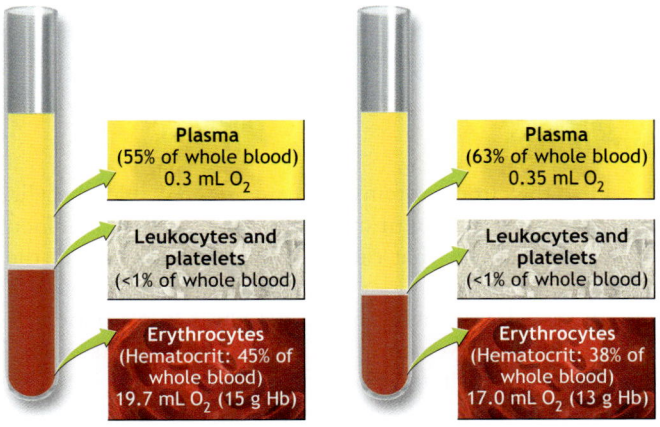

FIGURE 13.5. **(A)** Major components of centrifuged whole blood, including oxygen carried in each deciliter of blood in an untrained individual. **(B)** Changes in whole-blood constituents following aerobic exercise training for 4 days.
(Shutterstock: Monika Wisniewska; Anna Kireieva)

INTEGRATIVE QUESTION

How would you explain the "bottom line" to a coach who requires football players to breathe from an oxygen tank during time-outs or rest breaks to speed recovery?

P_{O_2} in the Tissues

At rest, the P_{O_2} in the cell fluids averages 40 mm Hg. This makes dissolved oxygen from the plasma diffuse across the capillary membrane through the tissue fluids into the cells. This reduces plasma P_{O_2} below the P_{O_2} in the red blood cell, causing Hb to lower its oxygen saturation level. The released oxygen ($HbO_2 \rightarrow Hb + O_2$) moves from blood cells through the capillary membrane into tissues.

At the 40-mm Hg tissue-capillary P_{O_2} at rest, Hb holds about 70% of its original oxygen (see Fig. 13.4). Thus, when blood leaves the tissues and returns to the heart, it carries about 15 mL of oxygen in each deciliter of blood, releasing 5 mL of oxygen to the tissues.

Arteriovenous Oxygen Difference

The **arterio-mixed venous oxygen difference ($a-\bar{v}O_2$ diff)** describes the difference between the oxygen content of arterial blood and that of mixed venous blood. The $a-\bar{v}O_2$ diff in blood at rest normally averages 4 to 5 mL of oxygen per deciliter of blood. The remaining oxygen quantity still attached to Hb provides an "automatic" reserve for cells to immediately obtain oxygen should metabolic demands suddenly increase, whether sprinting for a bus or starting a marathon run. Tissue P_{O_2} decreases as the cell's oxygen use increases in physical activity. This causes Hb to immediately release a larger oxygen amount. During intense activity when extracellular P_{O_2} decreases to nearly 15 mm Hg, only about 5 mL of oxygen remains bound to Hb. This makes the $a-\bar{v}O_2$ diff increase to 15 mL oxygen per 100 mL (**FIG. 13.6A AND B**). When active muscle P_{O_2} falls to 2 or 3 mm Hg during exhaustive exercise, the blood perfusing these tissues gives up virtually all its oxygen (**FIG. 13.6C**).[20] Oxygen release from Hb can occur without any increase in blood flow to local tissues. The oxygen amount released to muscle increases almost three times above that supplied at rest—just from more complete unloading of Hb as blood flows through the active muscles. *An active muscle's uncompromising capacity to use available oxygen in its large blood flow supports the position that oxygen supply (blood flow), not muscle oxygen use, limits aerobic capacity.*[17,21,23]

Red Blood Cell 2,3-Diphosphoglycerate

A red blood cell derives its energy solely from the anaerobic glycolysis reactions because they contain no mitochondria; this establishes the normal plasma lactate levels at rest. Red blood cells produce the compound **2,3-diphosphoglycerate (2,3-DPG**, also referred to as 2,3-biphosphoglycerate [2,3-BPG]) during glycolysis. This compound binds loosely with

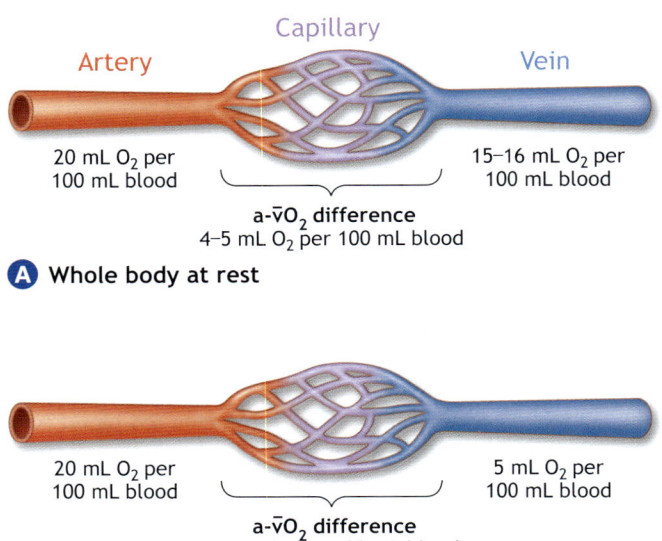

Myoglobin and Muscle Oxygen Storage

Myoglobin, an iron-containing globular protein in skeletal and cardiac muscle fibers with some 240 times greater affinity for oxygen than Hb, provides for intramuscular oxygen storage. Sir John C. Kendrew (1917–1997; 1962 Nobel Prize in Chemistry; www.nobelprize.org/nobel_prizes/chemistry/laureates/1962/) revealed myoglobin's structural details using x-ray crystallography in his studies of the structure of globular proteins. The molecule contains a peptide backbone embedded with the heme group and its metallic Fe^{2+}. Reddish muscle fibers have a high respiratory pigment concentration, whereas myoglobin-deficient fibers appear pale or white.[14] Myoglobin resembles Hb because it also combines reversibly with oxygen, but each molecule contains one iron atom while Hb contains four. Myoglobin adds additional oxygen to the muscle in the following chemical reaction:

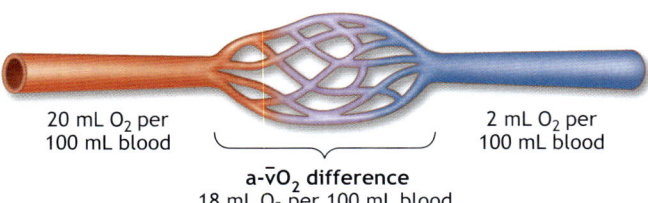

Oxygen Released at Low Pressures

Myoglobin facilitates oxygen transfer to the mitochondria when movement begins and during intense effort when cellular P_{O_2} declines rapidly and dramatically. The dissociation curve for myoglobin (Fig. 13.4; *dashed lime green line*) does not form an S-shaped line comparable to Hb but instead plots as a rectangular hyperbola (i.e., perpendicular asymptotes). Compared with the oxygen saturation curve for Hb, the curve for myoglobin shows that it binds more readily and retains oxygen at low oxygen pressures. During rest and moderate physical activity, myoglobin maintains high oxygen saturation. For example, at a 40-mm Hg P_{O_2}, myoglobin retains 95% of its oxygen. The greatest oxygen quantity releases from MbO_2 when tissue P_{O_2} declines below 5 mm Hg.[18] Myoglobin's oxygen-binding affinity, unlike Hb, is unaffected by acidity, carbon dioxide, and temperature so it does not exhibit a Bohr effect. Chapter 21 discusses the effects of aerobic training on muscles' myoglobin content.

FIGURE 13.6. **(A)** Average values for whole-body arteriovenous oxygen difference in skeletal muscle during rest, **(B)** intense aerobic exercise, and **(C)** active skeletal muscle during intense aerobic exercise.

the Hb molecule subunits, reducing its affinity for oxygen. This causes greater oxygen release to the tissues for a given P_{O_2} decrease.[8]

Increased red blood cell 2,3-DPG levels occur in individuals with cardiopulmonary disorders and those who live at high altitudes. This compensatory adjustment facilitates oxygen release to cells. During strenuous activity, 2,3-DPG also aids in oxygen transfer to muscles.[12] Conflicting results emerge in comparison of 2,3-DPG levels in trained and untrained subjects.[1,9,16] One study reported higher resting 2,3-DPG levels in two athletic groups than in untrained subjects.[22] This metabolic intermediate level increased by 15% for middle-distance runners following short-duration maximal effort. In contrast, prolonged steady-rate exercise in endurance athletes produced a small decrease in 2,3-DPG. These data support the proposition that increases in 2,3-DPG concentration with intense physical activity and training reflect an adaptive response to augment oxygen delivery to more metabolically active tissues. More than likely, the different effects of different activities on erythrocyte 2,3-DPG level reflect the specific metabolic demands of each activity. Females have more red blood cell 2,3-DPG than males of similar fitness status and physical activity level. This gender difference might compensate for lower Hb levels in females.[15]

Summary

1. Hb, the iron-protein pigment in red blood cells, increases the amount of oxygen carried in whole blood about 65 times that carried in physical solution in the plasma.
2. The small amount of oxygen dissolved in plasma exerts molecular movement that establishes oxygen's partial pressure (P_{O_2}) in the blood.
3. Plasma P_{O_2} determines Hb's loading at the lungs (oxygenation) and its unloading at the tissues (deoxygenation).
4. The blood's oxygen transport capacity varies only slightly with normal variations in Hb content.
5. Iron deficiency anemia lowers Hb concentration, thus decreasing the blood's oxygen-carrying capacity and impairing aerobic exercise performance.

6. Hb saturation changes little until P_{O_2} declines below 60 mm Hg.
7. The oxygen quantity bound to Hb falls sharply as oxygen moves from capillary blood to the tissues when metabolic demands increase.
8. Arterial blood releases about 25% of its total oxygen content to the tissues at rest, with the remaining 75% returning "unused" to the heart in venous blood.
9. The difference in oxygen content of arterial and venous blood under resting conditions indicates an automatic oxygen reserve exists should metabolism increase suddenly.
10. The Bohr effect reflects alterations in Hb's molecular structure from increased acidity, temperature, carbon dioxide concentration, and red blood cell 2,3-DPG that reduce its effectiveness to hold oxygen.
11. The iron-protein pigment myoglobin in skeletal and cardiac muscle provides an "extra" oxygen store to release oxygen at low P_{O_2}.
12. During intense physical activity, myoglobin facilitates oxygen transfer to the mitochondria when intracellular P_{O_2} in active skeletal muscle decreases dramatically.

Part 3 — Carbon Dioxide Transport in Blood

Once carbon dioxide forms in the cell, diffusion and subsequent transport in venous blood provides the only means for its "escape" through the lungs. The blood carries carbon dioxide in three ways:

1. In physical solution in plasma (a small amount)
2. As plasma bicarbonate
3. Combined with Hb within the red blood cell

FIGURE 13.7 illustrates the three ways for transporting carbon dioxide from the tissues to the lungs as explained in the following sections.

Carbon Dioxide Transport in Physical Solution

Approximately 5% carbon dioxide formed during energy metabolism moves into physical solution in the plasma as free carbon dioxide. The random movement for this small quantity of dissolved carbon dioxide molecules establishes the blood P_{CO_2}.

Carbon Dioxide Transport as Bicarbonate

Carbon dioxide in solution slowly combines with water to form carbonic acid in the following reversible reaction:

$$CO_2 + H_2O \longleftrightarrow H_2CO_3$$

Little carbon dioxide transport would occur as carbonic acid without carbonic anhydrase, a zinc-containing enzyme within the red blood cell. One mole of this catalyst tremendously accelerates the union between a carbon dioxide mole with water to a rate about 800,000 times per second (about 5000 times faster than without enzymatic action). The reaction attains equilibrium as the red blood cell moves through the tissue's capillary.

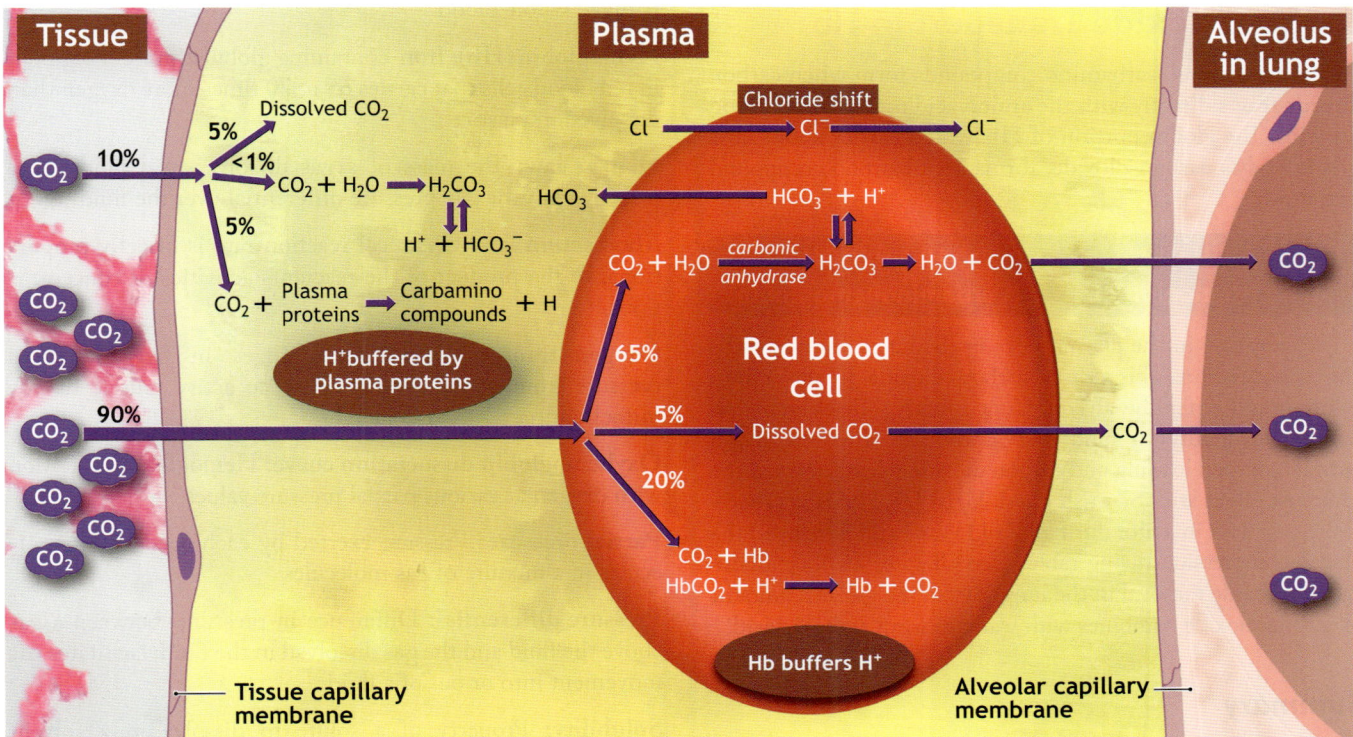

FIGURE 13.7. Carbon dioxide transports in the plasma and red blood cells as dissolved CO_2, bicarbonate, and carbamino compounds. (Choksawatdikorn/Shutterstock)

Once carbonic acid forms in the tissues, most ionizes into hydrogen ions (H⁺) and bicarbonate ions (HCO_3^-) as follows:

In Tissues

$$CO_2 + H_2O \xrightarrow{\text{carbonic anhydrase}} H_2CO_3 \rightarrow H^+ + HCO_3^-$$

Buffering of the H⁺ by Hb's protein component maintains blood pH within relatively narrow limits (see "Acid-Base Regulation," Chapter 14). The HCO_3^- remains soluble so it diffuses from the red blood cell into plasma. There it exchanges for a chloride ion (Cl⁻) that moves into the blood cell to maintain ionic equilibrium. This phenomenon, termed *chloride shift* shown at the top of the red blood cell, increases erythrocytes' Cl⁻ content in venous blood more than in arterial red blood cells, particularly during exercise.

Sixty to eighty percent of total carbon dioxide exists as plasma bicarbonate. Bicarbonate forms in accordance with the *mass action law*; carbonic acid formation accelerates as tissue Pco_2 increases. Plasma Pco_2 lowers as carbon dioxide leaves the blood via the lungs. This disturbs the equilibrium between carbonic acid and bicarbonate ion formation. The H⁺ and HCO_3^- recombine to form carbonic acid. In turn, carbon dioxide and water reform and carbon dioxide exits through the lungs as follows:

In Lungs

$$H^+ + HCO_3^- \rightarrow H_2CO_3 \xrightarrow{\text{carbonic anhydrase}} CO_2 + H_2O$$

The Cl⁻ moves from the red blood cell back into the plasma because plasma HCO_3^- decreases in the pulmonary capillaries.

Carbon Dioxide Transport in Hb

At the tissue level, carbamino compounds form when carbon dioxide reacts directly with the amino acid molecules of blood proteins. The globin portion of Hb, which carries about 20% of the body's carbon dioxide, forms a carbamino compound as follows:

$$CO_2 + \underset{\text{(Hemoglobin)}}{HbNH} \rightarrow \underset{\text{(Carbaminohemoglobin)}}{HbNHCOOH}$$

A decrease in the plasma Pco_2 in the lungs reverses carbamino formation. This causes carbon dioxide to move into solution and enter the alveoli. Concurrently, Hb oxygenation reduces its ability to bind carbon dioxide. The interaction between oxygen loading and carbon dioxide release, termed the **Haldane effect** after Scottish physiologist J. S. Haldane (1860–1936; gas mask inventor during World War I and developed the first decompression diving tables [see Chapter 26]), facilitates carbon dioxide removal in the lung. By far, the greatest amount of carbon dioxide combines with water to form carbonic acid.

Summary

1. About 5% carbon dioxide travels in the plasma as free carbon dioxide in physical solution.
2. Dissolved carbon dioxide establishes the blood's Pco_2, which modulates important physiologic functions.
3. The major quantity of carbon dioxide (80%) transports in chemical combination with water to form bicarbonate as follows:

$$CO_2 + H_2O \longrightarrow H_2CO_3 \longrightarrow H^+ + HCO_3^-$$

In the lungs, the reaction reverses and carbon dioxide exits the blood into the alveoli.
4. About 20% carbon dioxide combines with blood proteins and Hb to form carbamino compounds.

Key Terms

2,3-Diphosphoglycerate (2,3-DPG): Chemical produced by red blood cells during glycolysis to facilitate oxygen release by decreasing oxygen affinity for hemoglobin.

Arterio-mixed venous oxygen difference (a-v̇O₂ diff): Difference between arterial blood's oxygen content and the content of mixed venous blood

Bohr effect: Hydrogen ions and carbon dioxide alter hemoglobin's molecular structure to decrease its oxygen-binding affinity, mostly oxygen partial pressure between 20 and 50 mm Hg

Cooperative binding: Binding an oxygen molecule to the iron atom in one of hemoglobin four globin chains progressively facilitates binding oxygen molecules

Dalton's law: A gas mixture's total pressure equals the sum of the partial pressures of the individual gases in the mixture

Hematocrit: Red blood cell percentage composition in centrifuged whole blood

Hemoglobin (Hb): Iron-containing globular protein pigment in red blood cells that carries 65 to 70 times more oxygen than dissolved in plasma

Henry's law: The mass of a gas dissolves in a fluid varies directly with the gas' pressure differential over the fluid

Mass action law: Chemical reaction rate is directly proportional to the product of the reactants activities or concentrations.

Oxygen transport cascade: Changes in oxygen partial pressure from sea level ambient air to active muscle tissue's mitochondria

Oxyhemoglobin dissociation curve: Hemoglobin saturation with oxygen at various partial pressure values

Partial pressure: Pressure exerted by each specific gas molecules in a mixture of gas molecules

Pressure differential: Difference in pressures between a gas above the fluid and the gas dissolved in the fluid; facilitates gas movement into or out of a fluid

Solubility: Property of a solute to dissolve in a solvent depending on the solute and solvents temperature, pressure, and additional chemicals in the solvent

Torr: Pressure to raise a 1-mm column of mercury 1 mm high at 0°C/32°F

Venous admixture: Small amount of blood in alveolar capillaries that passes through poorly ventilated alveoli plus the blood leaving the lungs that mixes with venous blood from the bronchial and cardiac circulations

Volume percent (vol%): Blood's oxygen content in milliliters oxygen extracted from a deciliter sample of whole blood (with plasma) or packed red blood cells (without plasma)

> References are available online at Lippincott Connect.

Additional References

Böning D, Schmidt WF. Role of haemoglobin oxygen affinity for oxygen uptake during exercise. *J Physiol.* 2020;598:3531.

Dobbe L, et al. Cardiogenic pulmonary edema. *Am J Med Sci.* 2019;358:389.

Dominelli PB, Molgat-Seon Y. Sex, gender and the pulmonary physiology of exercise. *Eur Respir Rev.* 2022;31:210074.

Harper J, et al. How does hormone transition in transgender women change body composition, muscle strength and haemoglobin? Systematic review with a focus on the implications for sport participation. *Br J Sports Med.* 2021;55:865.

Klain A, et al. Exercise-induced bronchoconstriction in children. *Front Med (Lausanne).* 2022;8:814976.

Lagiou O, et al. Exercise limitation in children and adolescents with mild-to-moderate asthma. *J Asthma Allergy.* 2022;15:89.

Lundgren KM, et al. Blood volume, hemoglobin mass, and peak oxygen uptake in older adults: the Generation 100 study. *Front Sports Act Living.* 2021;3:638139.

Marinus N, et al. The impact of different types of exercise training on peripheral blood brain-derived neurotrophic factor concentrations in older adults: a meta-analysis. *J Sports Med.* 2019;49:1529.

Rhibi F, et al. Increase interval training intensity improves plasma volume variations and aerobic performances in response to intermittent exercise. *Physiol Behav.* 2019;199:137.

Singh I, et al. Persistent exertional intolerance after COVID-19: insights from invasive cardiopulmonary exercise testing. *Chest.* 2022;161:54.

Stickland MK, et al. How we do it - Using cardiopulmonary exercise testing to understand dyspnea and exercise intolerance in respiratory disease. *Chest.* 2022:S0012-3692(22)001453.

Webb KL, et al. Influence of high hemoglobin-oxygen affinity on humans during hypoxia. *Front Physiol.* 2022. 12:763933.

Weng X, et al. Intermittent hypoxia exposure helps to restore the reduced hemoglobin concentration during intense exercise training in trained swimmers. *Front Physiol.* 2021;12:736108.

Zouhal H, et al. The effects of exercise training on plasma volume variations: a systematic review. *Int J Sports Med.* 2021. doi:10.1055/a-1667-6624.

Zubac D, et al. No differences in splenic emptying during on-transient supine cycling between aerobically trained and untrained participants. *Eur J Appl Physiol.* 2022: doi:10.1007/s00421-021-04843-w.

Zysman M, et al. Women's COPD. *Front Med (Lausanne).* 2022;8:600107.

Table 13.1 Hemoglobin and Peak Exercise Heart Rate in Normal and Anemic Subjects Prior to and Following Supplemental Iron Treatment

Subjects	Hb (g·dL^{-1})	HR (b·min^{-1})
Normal		
Men	14.3	119
Women	13.9	142
Iron-Deficient Males		
Pretreatment	7.1	155
Posttreatment	14.0	113
Iron-Deficient Females		
Pretreatment	7.7	152
Posttreatment	12.4	123
Iron-Deficient Males		
Preplacebo	7.7	146
Postplacebo	7.4	137
Iron-Deficient Females		
Preplacebo	8.1	154
Postplacebo	8.4	144

b, beats; Hb, hemoglobin; HR, heart rate.

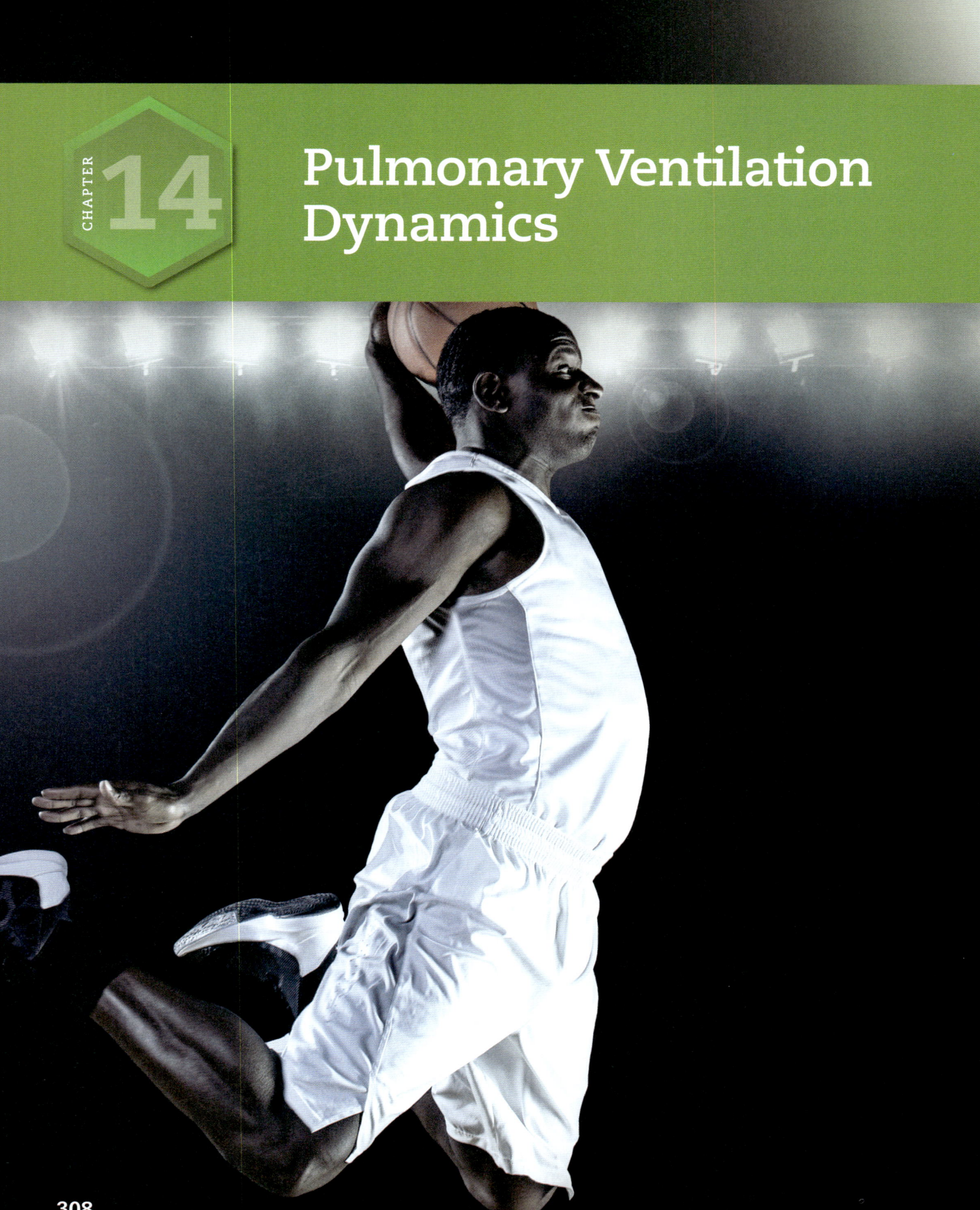

CHAPTER 14
Pulmonary Ventilation Dynamics

Chapter Objectives

- Describe how the hypothalamic neural command center controls pulmonary ventilation
- Explain how major chemical and nonchemical factors regulate pulmonary ventilation during rest and physical activity
- Describe how hyperventilation extends breath-holding time but also poses a danger in sport diving
- Outline the dynamic phases of minute ventilation at the onset, early phase, and late stage of moderate physical activity and recovery
- Graph relationships among pulmonary ventilation, blood lactate, and oxygen uptake during incremental exercise, indicating the point of onset of blood lactate accumulation (OBLA)
- Explain two reasons for the increase in ventilatory equivalent during the transition from steady-rate to non–steady-rate activity
- Give the rationale for substituting the blood lactate threshold or OBLA for maximum oxygen uptake to predict endurance performance
- Quantify the energy cost of breathing during rest and strenuous exertion in health and pulmonary disease
- Describe acute cigarette smoking effects on heart rate and energy cost of breathing during physical activity
- Outline endurance training adaptations in pulmonary ventilation during submaximal and maximal physical activity
- Discuss pros and cons to the argument that pulmonary ventilation represents the "weak link" in oxygen supply during intense physical activity
- Summarize how chemical and physiologic buffer systems regulate acid-base quality of body fluids during rest and physical activity

Ancillaries at-a-Glance

Visit Lippincott Connect to access these resources.

- References: Chapter 14
- Animation: Renal Function
- Focus on Research: Detecting the Onset of Anaerobic Metabolism

Part 1: Pulmonary Ventilation

Ventilatory Control

Complex neural, humoral, and chemoreceptor mechanisms exquisitely adjust breathing rate and depth to the body's metabolic needs. Intricate neural circuits relay information from higher brain centers, lungs, and other sensors throughout the body to coordinate ventilatory control.[5,60] The gaseous and chemical states of the blood that bathes the medulla and aortic and carotid artery chemoreceptors also mediate alveolar ventilation. In healthy individuals, these control mechanisms maintain relatively constant alveolar and arterial gas pressures over a broad exercise intensity range. **FIGURE 14.1** illustrates the key input factors for the respiratory center's (medullary) control of pulmonary ventilation.

Neural Factors

The inherent activity of inspiratory neurons with cell bodies located in the medial portion of the **medulla** governs the normal respiratory cycle. These neurons activate the diaphragm and intercostal muscles to cause the lungs to inflate. The inspiratory neurons cease firing from self-limitations and inhibitory influence of expiratory neurons in the medulla. Inhibitory and excitatory signals throughout the body influence the medullary neurons' normal rhythm. For example, lung inflation stimulates stretch receptors mainly in the bronchioles. These receptors act through afferent fibers to inhibit inspiration and stimulate expiration. Exhalation occurs as the inspiratory muscles relax, allowing for the passive recoil of stretched lung tissue and raised ribs. This passive phase relies on synchronous activation of expiratory neurons and associated muscles that facilitate expiration. As expiration proceeds, the inspiratory center becomes progressively less inhibited and once again becomes active.

The inherent respiratory center activity alone cannot account for the smooth ventilatory adjustment patterns to metabolic demands. The inspiratory cycle duration and intensity respond to the neural center in the hypothalamus that integrates input from descending neurons in the higher locomotor areas of the cerebral hemisphere, the pons, and other brain regions. During physical activity, ventilatory adjustments occur through ascending neural signals from mechanical and/or chemical changes within active muscles and its vasculature to provide peripheral feedback control from the cerebellum to the respiratory center.

Humoral Factors

At rest, the blood's chemical state exerts the greatest control over pulmonary ventilation. Variations in arterial P_{O_2}, P_{CO_2}, pH, and temperature activate sensitive

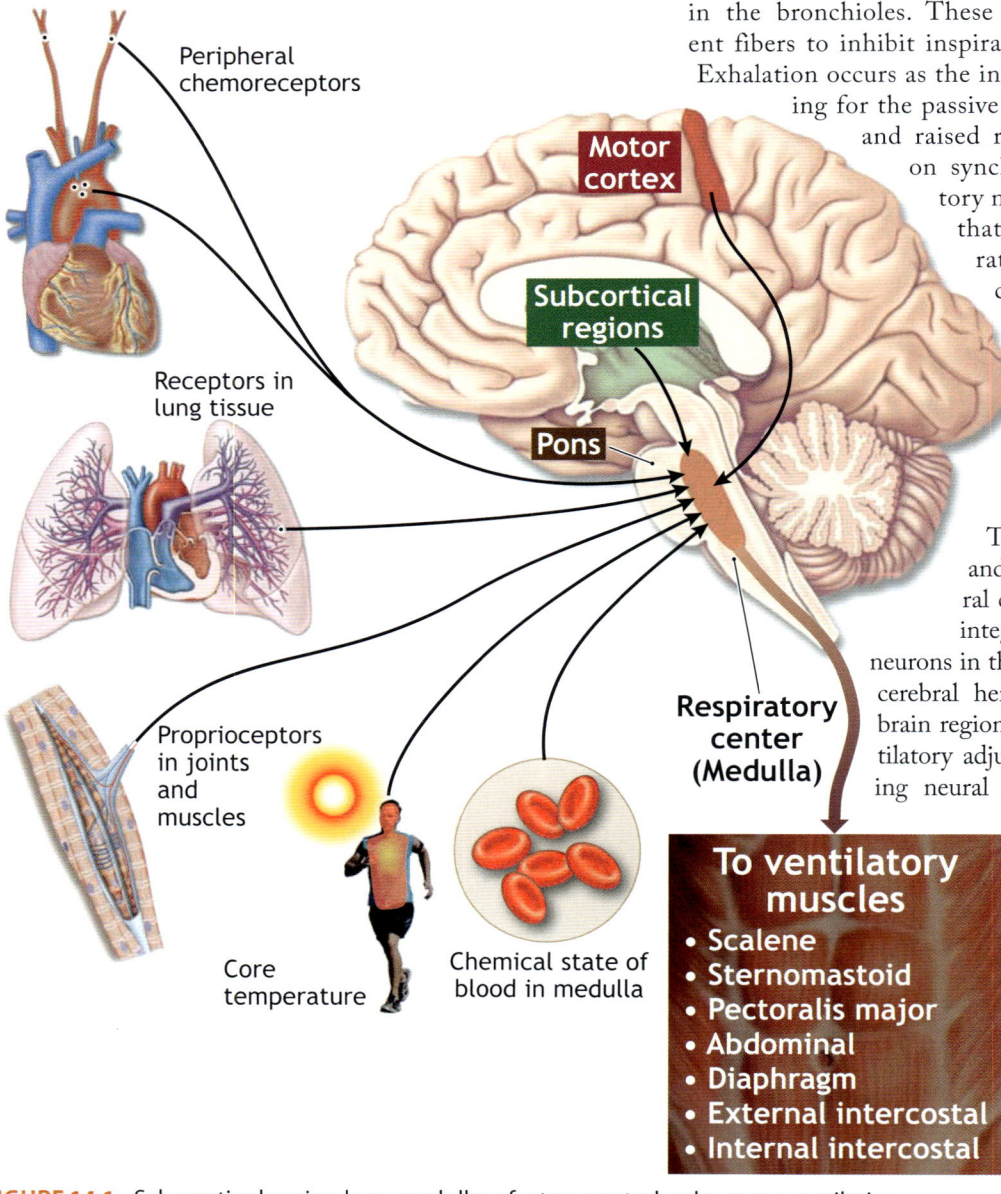

FIGURE 14.1. Schematic showing how medullary factors control pulmonary ventilation. (Brain illustration adapted from Bear MF, et al. *Neuroscience: Exploring the Brain*. 3rd Ed. Baltimore: Lippincott Williams & Wilkins, 2007: 207. Lung illustration adapted with permission from Moore KL, et al. *Clinically Oriented Anatomy*. 8th Ed. Baltimore: Wolters Kluwer, 2018: 336. Fig. 4.37. Abdomen illustration: BigBlueStudio/Shutterstock)

neural units in the medulla and arterial system to adjust ventilation and maintain arterial blood chemistry within narrow limits.

Plasma P_{O_2} and Peripheral Chemoreceptors

Inhaling a gas mixture with 80% oxygen greatly increases alveolar P_{O_2} and reduces minute ventilation by 20%. Conversely, ventilation increases if inspired oxygen concentration decreases below ambient levels, particularly if alveolar P_{O_2} falls below 60 mm Hg. Hemoglobin saturation at this P_{O_2} begins to decrease considerably (see Fig. 13.2).

Sensitivity to reduced oxygen pressure does not reside in the respiratory center. Rather, peripheral **chemoreceptors** serve as the primary detection sites for arterial hypoxia to reflexly initiate a ventilatory response. **FIGURE 14.2** shows these tiny specialized neurons located in the aortic arch and carotid artery branching along the neck's right and left sides. Strategic carotid body positioning monitors arterial blood just before it perfuses the brain. The peripheral chemoreceptors defend against arterial hypoxia in pulmonary disease and ascent to high altitude. The chemoreceptors also help to regulate exercise hyperpnea through the increased arterial carbon dioxide and H^+ concentrations' stimulating effects. These receptors *alone* protect the organism against reduced oxygen pressure in inspired air.

Peripheral chemoreceptor afferents also stimulate ventilation in physical activity, even though reductions in arterial P_{O_2} do not normally occur.[46,49] The stimulating exercise effects on carotid afferent chemoreceptor discharge mainly come from increases in temperature, acidity, and carbon dioxide and potassium concentrations.[20,66]

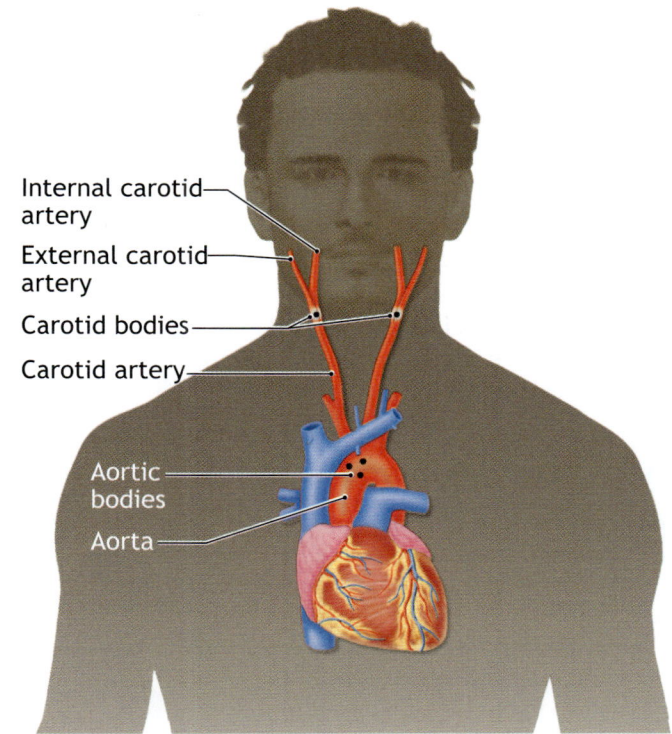

FIGURE 14.2. The aortic arch and carotid artery bifurcations contain cell bodies sensitive to reduced P_{O_2} and increased P_{CO_2} and H^+ concentrations in arterial blood.

Plasma P_{CO_2} and H^+ Concentration

At rest, carbon dioxide pressure in arterial plasma provides the most important respiratory stimulus. Small increases in P_{CO_2} in inspired air trigger large increases in minute ventilation. For example, the resting ventilation nearly doubles by

---

 Overbreathing Before Entering the Underwater Environment Can Kill You

The term "overbreathing" (hyperventilating) commonly describes a voluntary, above-normal increase in alveolar ventilation to reduce arterial CO_2 and increase breath-hold time while underwater. Young people often perform overbreathing before competitions over who can swim the farthest underwater in a pool without coming up for air (or remaining submerged as long as possible at the pool bottom). While the maneuver can increase the time of an underwater breathhold and distance covered, it considerably decreases the normal arterial blood CO_2 level—the stimulus to breathe. Even slight blood chemistry alterations can end in death from such competitions. The seven bulleted items describe the mechanisms involved in this technique and its potential for deadly outcomes:

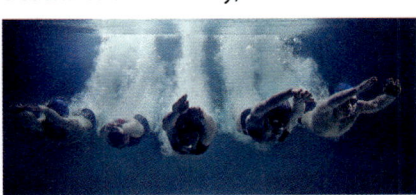
S.Pytel/Shutterstock

- Hyperventilation (rapid deep breathing) before prolonged underwater swimming is a dangerous practice that may end in drowning.
- Hyperventilation does not increase the amount of oxygen in the blood; rather, it lowers the blood's carbon dioxide to abnormal levels.
- Abnormally low CO_2 poses risks because arterial blood carbon dioxide governs the drive to breathe.
- When the underwater swimmer finally does take a breath instinctively, water rushes in, beginning the drowning process.
- Prolonged underwater swimming should be discouraged as an adjunct to swim training or as a competitive play tool.
- Aggressive hyperventilation should be avoided before any long underwater swim because it elevates risk from Shallow Water Blackout and possible death.
- Swimmers should not be permitted to swim underwater past the 15-m/50-ft mark. Such underwater distance guidelines are incorporated into the U.S. Swimming Rules to minimize Shallow Water Blackout incidence.

increasing inspired P_{CO_2} to just 1.7 mm Hg (0.2% CO_2 in inspired air).

Molecular carbon dioxide *per se* does not mediate ventilatory responses to arterial P_{CO_2}. Instead, plasma acidity, which varies directly with the blood's carbon dioxide content, exerts considerable command over minute ventilation. A fall in blood pH signals acidosis and usually reflects carbon dioxide retention and subsequent carbonic acid formation. Blood pH also can decrease from lactate accumulation in strenuous physical activity or fatty acid (ketone) accumulation in diabetes. Independent of cause, as arterial pH declines and hydrogen ions accumulate, inspiratory activity increases to eliminate carbon dioxide and reduce arterial carbonic acid levels (see Chapter 13).

Hyperventilation and Breath Holding

Following a normal exhalation and then immediately holding one's breath, it takes approximately 40 s before the urge to breathe increases enough to initiate inspiration. The stimulus to breathe comes primarily from increased arterial P_{CO_2} and H^+ concentration, not decreased P_{O_2} in the breath-holding condition. The break point for breath holding corresponds to an increase in arterial P_{CO_2} to approximately 50 mm Hg.

If one consciously increases ventilation above normal level (hyperventilation) before breath holding, alveolar air composition becomes more like ambient air. Alveolar P_{CO_2} decreases from its normal 40 mm Hg value to a low of 15 mm Hg. This creates a considerable diffusion gradient for carbon dioxide runoff into the alveoli from venous blood that enters the pulmonary capillaries. Consequently, a larger than normal carbon dioxide quantity leaves the blood and arterial P_{CO_2} decreases. Hyperventilation extends breath-holding duration until arterial P_{CO_2} and/or H^+ concentration rises to levels that again stimulate the urge to breathe.

WAYHOME studio/Shutterstock

Ventilatory Regulation During Physical Activity

Chemical Control

Neither chemical stimulation nor any other single mechanism entirely accounts for the increase in ventilation (**hyperpnea**) during physical activity. For example, the classic resting ventilation feedback control via oxygen- and carbon dioxide–mediated mechanisms does not adequately explain exercise hyperpnea. Inducing maximum changes in plasma acidity and inspired P_{O_2} and P_{CO_2} does not increase minute ventilation to values seen during vigorous exertion.

FIGURE 14.3 illustrates relationships among oxygen uptake during graded exercise and venous and alveolar P_{CO_2} and alveolar P_{O_2}. As intensity increases, alveolar (arterial) P_{O_2} does not decrease to an extent that increases ventilation through chemoreceptor stimulation.[21] The large ventilatory volumes during intense physical activity cause alveolar P_{O_2} to rise *above* the average 100-mm Hg resting value. Any increase in alveolar P_{O_2} during physical activity hastens blood oxygenation in alveolar capillaries. Despite increased metabolism with physical activity, alveolar P_{O_2} and P_{CO_2} remain near resting levels. Increases in mixed-venous P_{CO_2} result from increased carbon dioxide production in metabolism. Pulmonary ventilation during light and moderate activity closely couples with metabolism proportional to oxygen uptake and carbon dioxide production. Under these conditions, alveolar (and arterial) P_{CO_2} generally averages 40 mm Hg. During strenuous activity with its relatively large anaerobic component (lactate accumulation), increased carbon dioxide and subsequent H^+ concentrations provide an additional ventilatory stimulus. The resulting hyperventilation *reduces* alveolar and arterial P_{CO_2}, sometimes to as low as 25 mm Hg. Any reduction in arterial P_{CO_2} decreases the ventilatory drive from carbon dioxide during physical activity.

Nonchemical Control

The rapid ventilatory response at movement onset and cessation suggests that input other than changes in arterial P_{CO_2} and H^+ concentration mediate these exercise hyperpnea phases.

Neurogenic Factors

Neurogenic factors for ventilatory control during physical activity include cortical and peripheral influences.

- *Cortical influence*: Neural outflow from motor cortex regions and cortical activation in activity anticipation stimulate respiratory neurons in the medulla to initiate the abrupt increase in exercise ventilation.

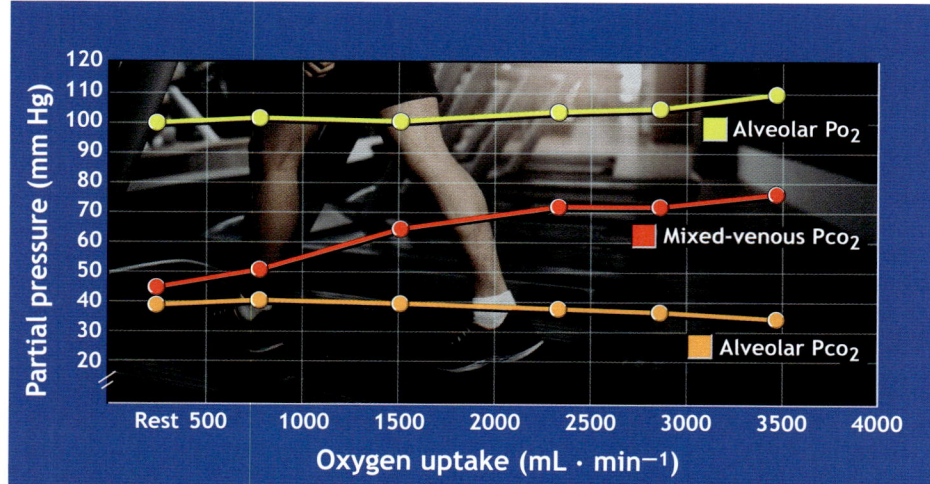

FIGURE 14.3. Values for partial pressure of oxygen (P_{O_2}) in alveolar blood entering the lungs and of carbon dioxide (P_{CO_2}) in mixed-venous and alveolar blood, related to oxygen uptake during graded exercise.
(Data courtesy of the Laboratory of Applied Physiology, Queens College. Ivan Kurmyshov/Shutterstock.)

- *Peripheral influence*: Sensory input from joints, tendons, and muscles influences ventilatory adjustments throughout physical activity. Experiments involving passive limb movements, electrical muscle stimulation, and voluntary movements with the muscle's blood flow occluded support the contribution from local mechanoreceptors and chemoreceptors to a reflex exercise hyperpnea.

Temperature Influence

Except for extreme hyperthermia, an increase in body temperature exerts little effect on ventilatory regulation during physical activity. In most conditions, the rise in ventilation at activity onset and its decline during recovery occur too quickly to reflect control from core temperature changes.

Integrated Regulation
During Physical Activity

The combined and perhaps simultaneous effects of several chemical and neural stimuli initiate and modulate exercise alveolar ventilation. **FIGURE 14.4** shows the three dynamic minute ventilation phases during moderate physical activity and recovery.

In **phase I ventilation** as physical activity begins, neurogenic stimuli from the cerebral cortex (**central command**), combined with feedback from the active limbs, stimulate the medulla to increase ventilation abruptly to about 20 L · min^{-1}. Cortical and locomotor peripheral input continue throughout the activity period.

After a short plateau (approximately 20 s), minute ventilation then rises exponentially in **phase II ventilation** to achieve a steady level related to the metabolic gas exchange demands. Central command input, including factors intrinsic to respiratory control system neurons, regulates this exercise ventilation phase. Continued respiratory neuron activity in the medulla causes short-term potentiation that augments their responsiveness to the same continuing stimulation. This brings minute ventilation to a new, higher level. In all likelihood, input from peripheral chemoreceptors in the carotid bodies also contributes to regulation during phase II ventilation.[66]

The final phase III ventilation control involves fine-tuning steady-state ventilation through peripheral sensory feedback mechanisms. Central and reflex stimuli from the main byproducts of increased muscle metabolism—carbon dioxide and H$^+$ concentration—modulate alveolar gas pressures in this phase. These factors stimulate chemoreceptor group IV unmyelinated neurons that communicate with central nervous system regions to regulate cardiorespiratory function.[48] An additional stimulus to increase ventilation in strenuous activity occurs from the lactate anion itself, apart from lactic acidosis.[24] Reflexes related to pulmonary blood flow and mechanical lung and respiratory muscle movements also provide regulatory input during physical activity.

During Recovery

The abrupt decline in ventilation when physical activity ceases reflects removal of both central command drive and sensory input from previously active muscles. Two factors help to explain the slower recovery phase:

1. Gradual diminution from short-term respiratory center potentiation
2. Reestablishment of the body's normal metabolic, thermal, and chemical functions

Summary

1. Inherent neuronal activity in the medulla regulates the normal respiratory cycle.
2. Input from higher brain centers, the lungs, and other sensors throughout the body interact with medullary neural output to regulate ventilation.
3. Chemical factors that act directly on the respiratory center or modify its activity through peripheral chemoreceptors control alveolar ventilation at rest.
4. Arterial Pco_2 and H$^+$ concentration are the most important regulatory factors of ventilation.
5. Hyperventilation lowers arterial Pco_2 and H$^+$ concentration to prolong breath-holding time until carbon dioxide and acidity levels increase to stimulate breathing.
6. Anticipatory cortical activation and motor cortex outflow when movement begins, peripheral chemoreceptor and mechanoreceptor sensory input, and increased body temperature are nonchemical factors to augment ventilatory adjustments to physical activity.
7. The ventilatory response to physical activity occurs in three phases.
8. In phase I, cortical stimulus plus feedback from active limbs cause the abrupt increase in ventilation as activity begins.
9. Phase II ventilation rises exponentially to reach a steady level related to the activity's metabolic demands.
10. Phase III ventilation involves fine-tuning steady-state ventilation through peripheral sensory feedback mechanisms.

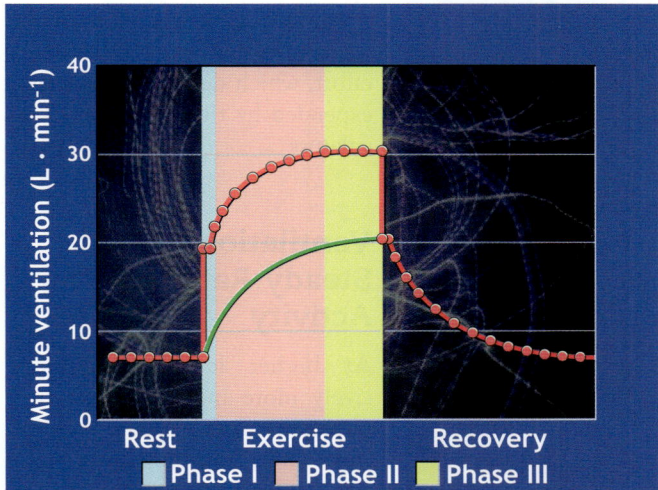

FIGURE 14.4. Phases I to III of pulmonary ventilation, showing dynamics during exercise hyperpnea. The *lower green curve* depicts only the contribution from central neuronal short-term potentiation and rising arterial H$^+$ concentration to the total respiratory response.
(Dmitry Moldavanov/Shutterstock)

Part 2: Pulmonary Ventilation During Physical Activity

Ventilation and Energy Demands During Physical Activity

Physical activity affects oxygen uptake and carbon dioxide production more than any other physiologic stress. With physical activity, oxygen diffuses from the alveoli into the venous blood as it returns to the lungs, while about the same carbon dioxide quantity moves from the blood into the alveoli. Concurrently, increased alveolar ventilation maintains proper gas concentrations to facilitate rapid gas exchange.

Ventilation in Steady-Rate Physical Activity

FIGURE 14.5 relates oxygen uptake and minute ventilation during increasing exertion levels up to maximum oxygen uptake ($\dot{V}O_{2max}$) shown as the final orange point along the curve. During light-to-moderate activity, ventilation increases *linearly* with oxygen uptake and carbon dioxide production, averaging between 20 and 25 L of air for each liter oxygen uptake. Ventilation, in this case, increases mainly through increases in tidal volume; at higher intensities, breathing frequency takes on a more important role. Such ventilatory adjustments provide complete blood aeration because alveolar P_{O_2} and P_{CO_2} remain near resting levels. Transit time for blood in the pulmonary capillaries remains long enough for complete lung-blood gas equilibration (see Fig. 13.2 in Chapter 13). Note that the lower dashed white line, from about 2.3 L · min^{-1} extending to about 3.3 L · min^{-1}, extrapolates the linear relationship between $\dot{V}_E$ and $\dot{V}O_2$ during submaximal effort.

The lactate threshold (not necessarily the threshold for anaerobic metabolism) represents the highest exercise intensity (oxygen uptake) not associated with elevated blood lactate concentration. It occurs at a point where the $\dot{V}_E$-$\dot{V}O_2$ relationship deviates from linearity, indicated as the *point of ventilatory threshold*. Onset of blood lactate accumulation represents the point of lactate increase just above a 4.0-mM baseline. *Respiratory compensation* represents a further disproportionate ventilation increase indicated by the deviation from the *upper dashed white line* to counter the plasma pH decrease in intense physical activity.

The term **ventilatory equivalent**, symbolized $\dot{V}_E/\dot{V}O_2$, describes the ratio of minute ventilation to oxygen uptake. Healthy young adults usually maintain this ratio at 25 (i.e., 25 L air breathed per liter O_2 uptake) during submaximal physical activity up to approximately 55% $\dot{V}O_{2max}$. Higher ventilatory equivalents occur in children, with values averaging 32 L air breathed per liter O_2 uptake. Activity mode also affects the ventilatory equivalent. Prone swimming, for example, generates lower $\dot{V}_E/\dot{V}O_2$ ratios than running at all energy expenditure levels. Swimming's restrictive nature on breathing lowers the ventilatory equivalent; this could constrain adequate gas exchange at maximal swimming velocities and partly explain the lower $\dot{V}O_{2max}$ during swimming than during running, even among moderately trained swimmers. Pulmonary ventilation dynamics are highly adaptive to regular physical activity. Aerobic training performed for several weeks reduces the ventilatory equivalent during submaximal effort, which decreases the energy expended by the ventilatory musculature

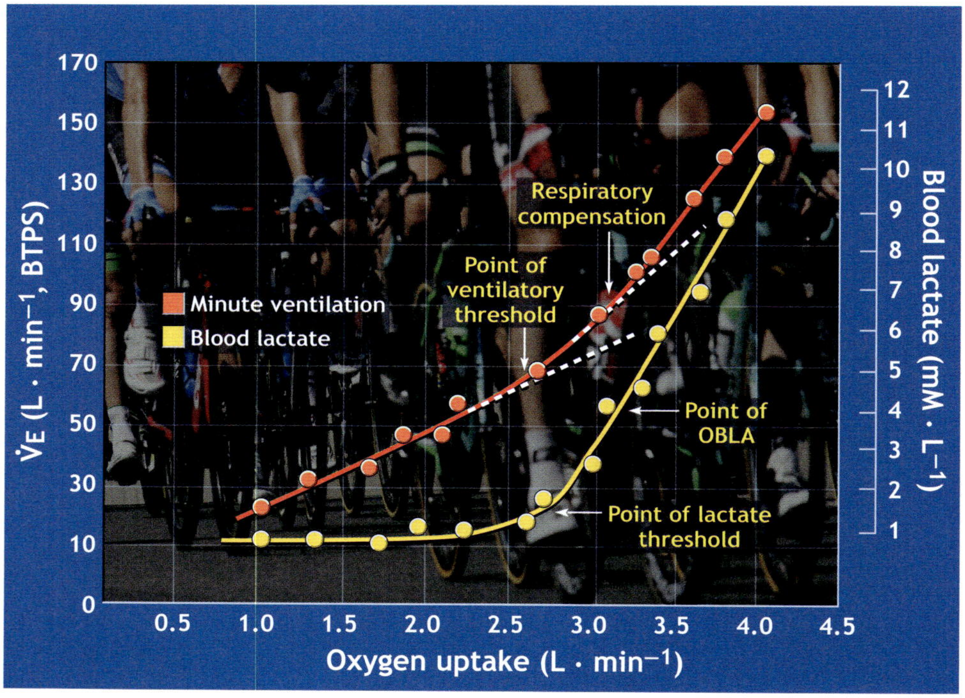

Ventilation in Non–Steady-Rate Physical Activity

At higher levels of progressively more intense submaximal physical effort, minute ventilation shifts sharply upward and increases disproportionately to oxygen uptake. In this case, the ventilatory equivalent can attain 35 or 40 L air breathed per liter oxygen uptake.

FIGURE 14.5. Pulmonary ventilation, blood lactate concentration, and oxygen uptake during graded exercise to maximum. BTPS, body temperature (37°C), ambient pressure and gas saturated with water vapor; OBLA, onset of blood lactate accumulation. (ChiccoDodiFC/Shutterstock)

Ventilatory Threshold

The term **ventilatory threshold (Tvent)** describes the point where pulmonary ventilation increases disproportionately relative to increases in oxygen uptake (i.e., a precipitous increase in the $\dot{V}_E/\dot{V}O_2$ ratio during graded exercise; see Fig. 14.5, *dashed white line* and "In a Practical Sense," later in this chapter). At this point, pulmonary ventilation no longer links tightly to oxygen demand at the cellular level. In fact, the "excess" ventilation comes directly from carbon dioxide's release from the buffering of lactic acid that begins to accumulate from increased glycolysis. Sodium bicarbonate in the blood buffers almost all the lactic acid generated in anaerobic metabolism to sodium lactate in the following reaction:

$$\text{Lactic acid} + \text{NaHCO}_3 \rightarrow \text{Na Lactate} + \text{H}_2\text{CO}_3$$
$$\updownarrow$$
$$\text{H}_2\text{O} + \text{CO}_2$$

The excess carbon dioxide released in the buffering reaction stimulates pulmonary ventilation that disproportionately increases the $\dot{V}_E/\dot{V}O_2$ ratio. Additional carbon dioxide exhaled from acid buffering causes the respiratory exchange ratio (R; $\dot{V}CO_2/\dot{V}O_2$) to exceed 1.00. Traditionally, researchers believed that the disproportionate increase in $\dot{V}_E$ and R increase exceeding 1.00 indicated active muscles' oxygen demands exceeded mitochondrial oxygen supply with an increase in anaerobic energy transfer. Tvent indicated the *threshold* for anaerobiosis, and the researchers termed it **anaerobic threshold (AT)** to denote increased reliance on anaerobic processes. Attempts to validate a linkage between ventilatory changes and glycolytic events at the cellular level have proven elusive.

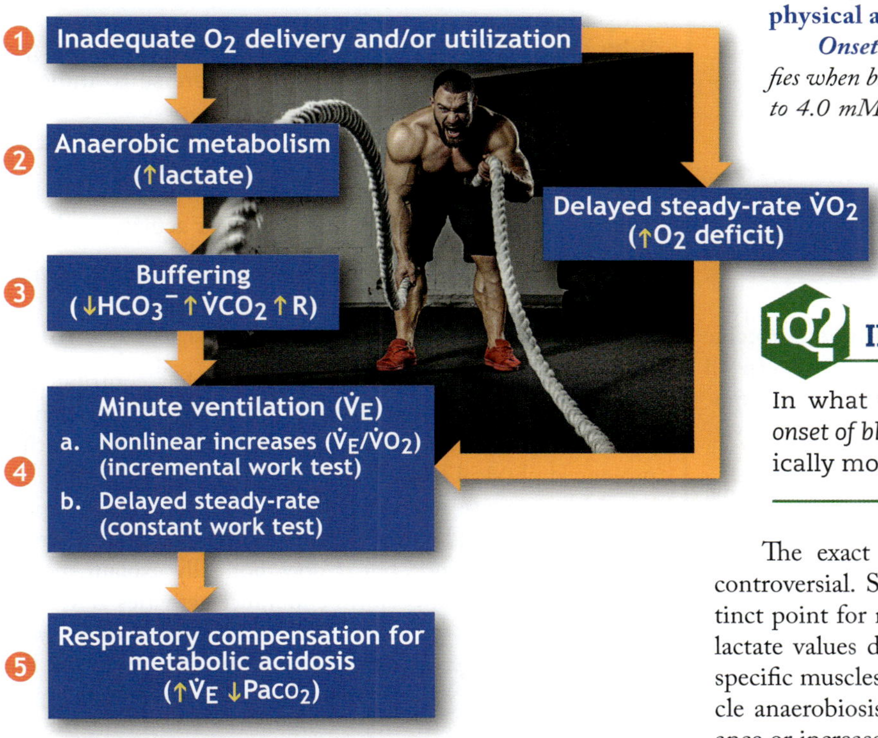

Onset of Blood Lactate Accumulation

During steady-rate physical activity, aerobic metabolism matches active muscles' energy requirements. Little or no blood lactate accumulates because any lactate production equals lactate disappearance. *The term **lactate threshold** describes the highest oxygen uptake or exercise intensity achieved with less than a 1.0 mM increase in blood lactate concentration above the pre-exercise level.*[63] By convention, blood lactate concentration is usually expressed in millimoles (mM) per liter whole blood or as mg per deciliter whole blood, also termed volume percent (vol%); 1.0 mM equals 9.0 vol%. **FIGURE 14.6** outlines possible underlying factors related to lactate threshold detection based on pulmonary gas exchange dynamics during progressively more intense **physical activity**.

Onset of blood lactate accumulation (OBLA) signifies when blood lactate concentration systematically increases to 4.0 mM.[12,53,63] Some researchers often use the terms *lactate threshold* and *OBLA* interchangeably, although each represents an operationally different precise reference point for exercise intensity and blood lactate levels.

INTEGRATIVE QUESTION

In what ways do the terms *lactate threshold* and *onset of blood lactate accumulation* become biochemically more precise than *anaerobic threshold*?

The exact triggering mechanism for OBLA remains controversial. Some researchers assume it represents a distinct point for muscle anaerobiosis onset even though blood lactate values do not always reflect lactate concentration in specific muscles. Lactate can accumulate not only from muscle anaerobiosis but also from decreased total lactate clearance or increased lactate production in specific muscle fibers. Four factors signal a threshold for lactate appearance:

1. Imbalance between glycolysis rate and mitochondrial respiration
2. Decreased redox potential (increased NADH relative to NAD$^+$)
3. Lower blood oxygen content
4. Lower blood flow to skeletal muscle

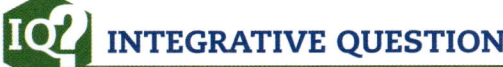

FIGURE 14.6 Underlying factors related to lactate threshold detection from pulmonary gas exchange dynamics during progressively more intense exercise. Paco$_2$, arterial partial pressure of carbon dioxide; R, respiratory exchange ratio ($\dot{V}CO_2/\dot{V}O_2$); $\dot{V}CO_2$, carbon dioxide exhaled; $\dot{V}_E$, minute ventilation (expired); $\dot{V}_E/\dot{V}O_2$, ventilatory equivalent (ratio of minute ventilation [expired] to oxygen uptake); $\dot{V}O_2$, oxygen uptake.

(sutulastock/Shutterstock)

Flowchart content:
1. Inadequate O$_2$ delivery and/or utilization
2. Anaerobic metabolism (↑lactate)
3. Buffering (↓HCO$_3^-$ ↑$\dot{V}CO_2$ ↑R)
   — Delayed steady-rate $\dot{V}O_2$ (↑O$_2$ deficit)
4. Minute ventilation ($\dot{V}_E$)
   a. Nonlinear increases ($\dot{V}_E/\dot{V}O_2$) (incremental work test)
   b. Delayed steady-rate (constant work test)
5. Respiratory compensation for metabolic acidosis (↑$\dot{V}_E$ ↓Paco$_2$)

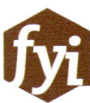

Lactate Threshold: Production Versus Clearance

Early experiments linked lactate appearance in the blood to signal the onset of anaerobic conditions within active muscle, a term called *anaerobic threshold*. Subsequent research using radioactive-labeled carbohydrate indicated that lactate's appearance in venous blood indicates an imbalance between lactate production and lactate clearance within the muscle rather than signaling

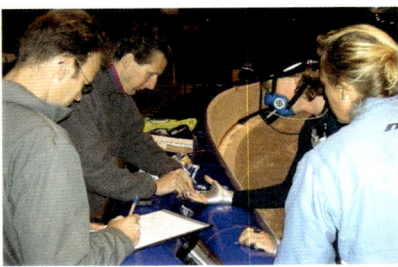

Photo courtesy Professor Stephen Seiler, Faculty of Health and Sport Sciences, University of Agder, Kristiansand, Norway.

onset of anaerobic conditions. This is because fast-twitch fibers that produce lactate "shuttle" the lactate to the muscle's slow-twitch oxidative fibers as aerobic energy substrate. The active muscles take up any released lactate in venous blood, as do the heart and brain, lactate-using organs that catabolize lactate as an aerobic energy substrate. The inset image shows Norwegian exercise physiology researchers obtaining finger-prick blood samples for lactate determination in Olympic level speed skaters during normal high-intensity oval track training.

Sources:
Iannetta D, et al. A "step-ramp-step" protocol to identify the maximal metabolic steady state. *Med Sci Sports Exerc.* 2020;52:2011.
Lee MJ, et al. Order of same-day concurrent training influences some indices of power development, but not strength, lean mass, or aerobic fitness in healthy, moderately-active men after 9 weeks of training. *PLoS One.* 2020;15:e0233134.
Snarr RL, et al. Comparison of lactate and electromyographical thresholds after an exercise bout. *J Strength Cond Res.* 2019;33:3322.

Caution should temper interpretations of the specific metabolic significance and cause regarding OBLA. In all likelihood, it probably does signify initiation for the exponential accumulation of lactate in active muscle during physical activity.[29,32]

Blood lactate accumulation is reflected by plasma changes in pH, bicarbonate and H^+ concentrations, and carbon dioxide production from buffering, to provide an indirect OBLA assessment.[2,33,34,61] Changes in these measures do indeed relate to OBLA, but they probably cannot serve independently to establish muscles' anaerobic metabolism onset. However, they do provide practical information about exercise performance. "In a Practical Sense," in this chapter, illustrates several common methods to indicate an imbalance between lactate formation and its clearance during physical activity.

OBLA Specificity. Task specificity characterizes OBLA, as do other physiologic functions related to exercise performance. Differences in OBLA relative to oxygen uptake levels emerge in comparing bicycle, treadmill, and arm-crank exercise.[67] Variations in muscle mass activated in each activity help to explain these differences. At a particular intensity or submaximal oxygen uptake, a higher metabolic rate per unit active muscle mass exists for arm-crank and bicycle exercise than treadmill walking or running. OBLA therefore occurs at a lower level ($\dot{V}O_2$) during bicycling and arm-crank exercise. *Different activity modes cannot interchangeably define the point of OBLA during graded exercise testing. Each must be determined during its own exercise mode.*

Some Independence Between OBLA and $\dot{V}O_{2max}$. Blood lactate in trained individuals accumulates at higher submaximum oxygen uptakes and at higher $\dot{V}O_{2max}$ percentages compared to untrained individuals. For children and adults, endurance training often improves the exercise intensity at OBLA *without* concomitant increases in $\dot{V}O_{2max}$,[4,15,35,40] suggesting that different factors influence OBLA and $\dot{V}O_{2max}$. Muscle fiber type, capillary density, mitochondrial size and number, and enzyme concentrations play major roles in establishing the percentage of aerobic capacity sustainable without lactate accumulation.[11,30,62] In contrast, the cardiovascular system's functional capacity for oxygen transport and the total muscle mass activated during physical activity determine the $\dot{V}O_{2max}$.

INTEGRATIVE QUESTION

Why can one measure pulmonary ventilation and gas exchange dynamics during graded exercise to indicate lactate buildup at the cellular level?

OBLA and Endurance Performance. Two important factors influence endurance performance in specific activity modes:

1. Maximum capacity to transport and consume oxygen ($\dot{V}O_{2max}$)
2. Maximum level for steady-rate physical activity (OBLA)

FIGURE 14.7 identifies 11 variables that contribute to oxygen transport and use. These factors ultimately determine the maximum exercise intensity a person can maintain during prolonged physical effort such as running.

Most exercise physiologists use $\dot{V}O_{2max}$ to gauge capacity to sustain endurance activity. This measure generally relates to performance, but it does not fully explain success because one does not perform endurance activities at $\dot{V}O_{2max}$. *The physical activity intensity at OBLA consistently and strongly predicts endurance performance of males and females.*[6,13,44,55] For race-walkers, race-walking velocity at OBLA accurately predicted 20-km times to within 0.6% of the actual time.[23] Similar results occurred in elite cyclists. Cycling power output at lactate threshold showed a strong relationship ($r = 0.93$) to average absolute power output maintained during a 1-hr ride in the laboratory.[14] The laboratory measurement accurately predicted performance in a 40-km road race. Improved endurance performance with training more closely relates to training-induced improvement in the physical activity level at OBLA than $\dot{V}O_{2max}$ changes.[68]

sustain a relatively higher percentage of maximal exercise capacity (i.e., superior fatigue resistance) from considerably higher oxidative enzyme profiles (citrate synthase and 3-hydroxyacyl-CoA dehydrogenase) and lower plasma lactate concentrations during sustained submaximal effort.[52] Greater running economy also probably contributes to superior endurance performance of elite African runners.[65] African runners perform better in high ambient temperatures than Caucasians due partly to their smaller size. This size "benefit" (larger surface-to-mass ratio) augments capacity to more readily transfer metabolic heat to the environment compared to the heavier Caucasian runners.[41]

Unbelievable Human Capacity for Marathon Running

On October 12, 2019 in Vienna, Austria, Olympic Champion and world record holder Kenya's Eliud Kipchoge (age 36 years, weight 52 kg/115 lb, height 1.67 m/5'6") became the first person to shatter the sub–2-hr marathon barrier, a milestone few believed could be reached for decades if at all, yet it will not count in the record books. Rotating teams of 36 runners paced him in alternating groups helped by a pace car guided by a laser beam projecting the ideal road position—one reason it is not record setting—Kipchoge smashed the 2-hr barrier by 20 s finishing the race in 1 hr:59 min:40.2 s! He currently holds the official world record marathon time of 2:01:39 (Berlin, 2018). Not to be outdone, the following day female Kenyan counterpart Brigid Kosgei (age 27 years in 2021, no weight or height data available) won the 2019 Chicago Marathon in 2:14:04. This broke the woman's world record of 2:15:25 in the event held for over 16 years by Paula Radcliffe, which had stood as one of the most "unbreakable" running records.

photocosmos1/Shutterstock

Dave Smith 1965/Shutterstock

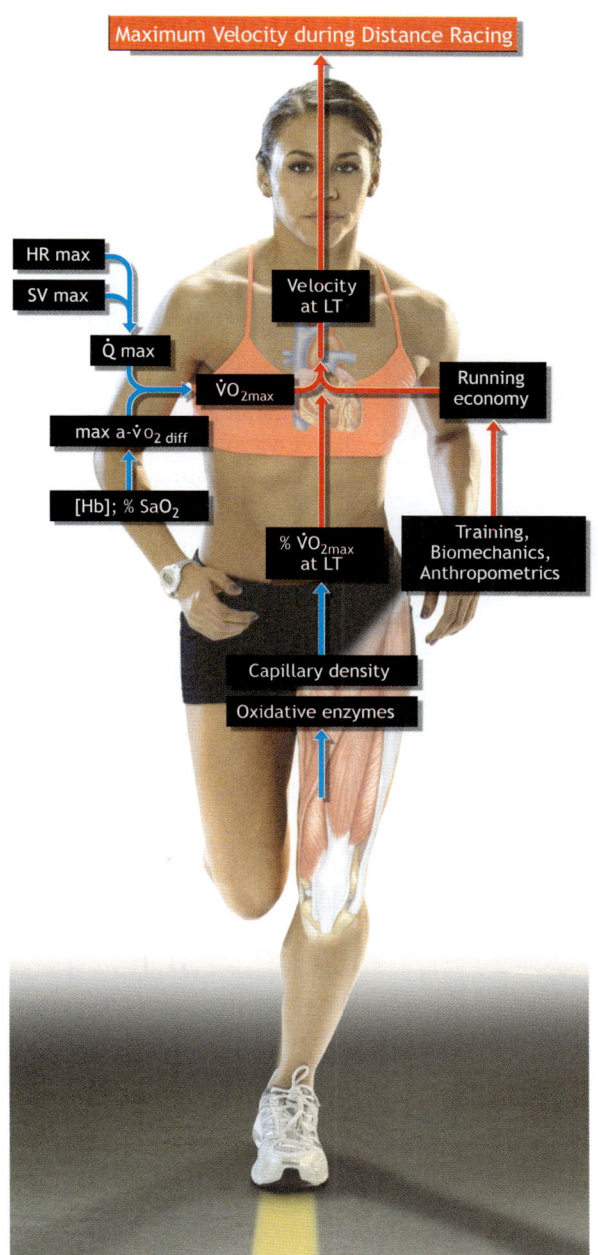

FIGURE 14.7. Major variables related to maximum oxygen uptake, blood lactate onset, and maximum running velocity during endurance exercise races. a-$\dot{V}O_2$ diff, arterial-mixed-venous oxygen difference; Hb, hemoglobin; HR, heart rate; LT, lactate threshold; max, maximum; $\dot{Q}$, perfusion; Sao_2, arterial oxygen saturation; SV, stroke volume; $\dot{V}O_{2max}$, maximum oxygen uptake.
(Gino Santa Maria/Shutterstock)

Racial Differences. The overwhelming dominance of African athletes in competitive endurance running between 3000 and 10,000 m has stimulated research into possible racial differences in resistance to fatigue, blood lactate accumulation, temperature regulation, and intramuscular oxidative enzyme capacity.[58] African and South African endurance runners consistently show greater resistance to fatigue at the same percentage of peak treadmill running velocity than Caucasian counterparts despite similar values for $\dot{V}O_{2max}$ and peak treadmill velocity.[10,64,65] African athletes

Oxygen Cost of Breathing

FIGURE 14.8 displays the oxygen cost of breathing during graded exercise up to maximum. Figure 14.8A indicates the effects of increasing minute ventilation on the oxygen cost of breathing expressed as a percentage of total exercise oxygen uptake. Figure 14.8B illustrates the influence of increasing minute ventilation on oxygen cost per liter air breathed per minute. The oxygen requirement of breathing remains relatively small at rest and during light to moderate activity with no differences observed between nonobese women and men.[39] For ventilations up to about 100 L · min^{-1}, oxygen cost averaged between 1.5 and 2.0 mL · L^{-1} air breathed each minute. This represented from 3 to 5% of the total oxygen uptake in moderate activity and 8 to 11% for minute ventilations at $\dot{V}O_{2max}$ values typical for most individuals. Among highly trained endurance athletes with 150 L · min⁻¹ and higher maximum minute ventilations, the cost associated with physical activity hyperpnea can exceed 15% of the total oxygen uptake.[9] At this level, the inspiratory muscles operate at 40 to 60% maximum capacity to generate force.[1] The blood flow rate to these muscles may equal flow to the limb locomotor muscles.[18]

Up to 15% of the total blood flow sustains the respiratory muscles' metabolic demands during maximal effort.[25,27] Evidence from healthy, fit individuals indicates a "competition" for blood flow and oxygen between respiratory and locomotor muscles during intense activity. For example, altering respiratory muscle work during maximal physical effort to increase breathing's energy cost vasoconstricts the locomotor muscles. Redirecting cardiac output to the respiratory musculature compromises perfusion to active, nonrespiratory muscles. This reduced the total $\dot{V}O_{2max}$ percentage used by the active locomotor muscles. Conversely, easing breathing effort during maximal exercise with an assist ventilator elicited a corresponding increase in oxygen uptake (greater % $\dot{V}O_{2max}$) for the active leg musculature.

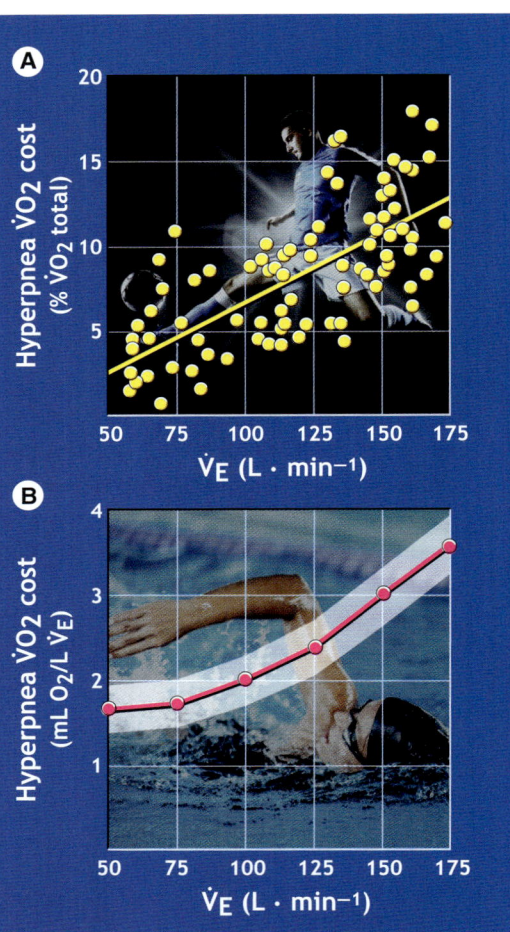

FIGURE 14.8. Oxygen cost of breathing during physical activity up to maximum. **(A)** Increasing minute ventilation ($\dot{V}_E$) effects expressed as a percentage for total exercise oxygen uptake ($\dot{V}O_2$). **(B)** Increasing minute ventilation effects on the oxygen cost per liter air breathed per minute.
(Shutterstock: Alex Kravtsov; Microgen)

Respiratory Disease

During light to moderate physical activity, the healthy person rarely senses the effort to breathe. In respiratory disease, breathing becomes an exhaustive effort in itself.[69,70,72] In chronic obstructive pulmonary disease (COPD), the added expiratory resistance can triple the normal breathing cost at rest; during light physical activity, ventilatory cost may reach 10 mL oxygen for each liter air breathed. In severe pulmonary disease, breathing cost easily attains 40% of the total oxygen uptake. Competition between locomotor and respiratory muscles for oxygen and blood flow limits the amount of oxygen available to the active, nonrespiratory muscle mass.[26] In COPD, the increased breathing cost severely limits the individuals exercise capacity with this debilitating condition. Regular physical activity or specific ventilatory muscle training can, however, improve exercise capacity, reduce dyspnea, decrease ventilatory equivalents for oxygen, improve respiratory and peripheral muscle function, and enhance psychological state.[8,16,47,54,71,73] Chapter 32 more fully discusses regular physical activity's role in rehabilitating COPD patients.

Cigarette Smoking

Airway resistance at rest increases up to threefold in both chronic smokers and nonsmokers following 15 puffs on a cigarette during a 5-min period.[43] The added resistance to breathing lasts 35 min on average and probably exerts only a minor effect during light activity when breathing cost remains small. The residual smoking effect could prove detrimental during vigorous activity from the additional oxygen cost to move larger air volumes. Increased peripheral airway resistance with smoking comes mainly from two sources:

1. Vagal reflex—possibly triggered from sensory stimulation by minute particles in cigarette smoke
2. Parasympathetic ganglia stimulation by nicotine

Researchers determined the oxygen cost of breathing in six habitual smokers immediately after smoking two cigarettes and 1 day after tobacco abstinence. The subjects ran on a treadmill at a speed and grade requiring 80% $\dot{V}O_{2max}$. Two methods increased ventilation during the "smoking" and "nonsmoking" runs:

1. Subjects voluntarily hyperventilated during the run (voluntary HV)
2. Induced hyperventilation by increasing alveolar P_{CO_2} by breathing through a large-diameter tube that increased anatomic dead space by 1400 mL (dead space HV)

The oxygen cost associated with "extra" breathing equaled the difference between normal oxygen uptake and uptake in the hyperventilation experiments.

TABLE 14.1 shows the oxygen cost of breathing decreased between 13 and 79% with smoking abstinence. Breathing's energy requirement during physical activity averaged 14% of the total oxygen uptake after smoking, but only 9% in the nonsmoking trials for the heaviest smokers. Also, heart rate averaged 5 to 7% lower during physical activity following cigarette abstinence for 1 day. All subjects reported feeling better when they exercised in the nonsmoking condition. These findings indicate a substantial reversal for increased breathing cost with only 1 day of

TABLE 14.1 Hyperventilation's oxygen cost during "smoking" and "nonsmoking" exercise at approximately 80% of maximum oxygen uptake

In a Practical Sense

Determining the Lactate Threshold

Conceptually, the lactate threshold (LT) represents an exercise level (power output, $\dot{V}O_2$, or energy expenditure) where tissue hypoxia triggers an imbalance between lactate formation and its clearance, with a resulting increase in blood lactate concentration. The following terms refer to the same LT phenomenon: *expiratory compensation threshold, anaerobic threshold, onset of blood lactate accumulation, optimal ventilatory efficiency, aerobic-anaerobic threshold, onset of plasma lactate accumulation, individual anaerobic threshold,* and *point of metabolic acidosis.*

LT measurement serves three important functions:

1. Provides a sensitive indicator of aerobic training status
2. Predicts endurance performance with greater accuracy than $\dot{V}O_{2max}$
3. Establishes training intensity to the active muscles' aerobic metabolic dynamics

One of three major variables indicate LT:

- Fixed blood lactate concentration
- Ventilatory threshold
- Blood lactate-exercise $\dot{V}O_2$ response

FIXED BLOOD LACTATE CONCENTRATION

During low-intensity, steady-rate exercise, blood lactate concentration does not increase beyond normal resting variation. As intensity increases, blood lactate exceeds normal variation. Exercise intensity (or $\dot{V}O_2$) associated with a fixed blood lactate concentration that exceeds normal resting variation denotes LT (often coincides with 2.5-mM value). A 4.0-mM lactate value indicates onset for blood lactate accumulation (OBLA). The top figure illustrates LT and OBLA from fixed blood lactate concentrations during incremental, 4-min exercise stages on a cycle ergometer. Interpolation from a visual power output ($\dot{V}O_2$) plot versus blood lactate determines the exercise level associated with a fixed blood lactate concentration.

The decision regarding stage duration, number of stages, and interval between stages becomes important. Stages 4 min or longer provide better predictability than shorter ones. For top figure (**A**), LT occurred at a 205 W power output; 225 W predicted the OBLA fixed blood lactate concentration.

VENTILATORY THRESHOLD

Pulmonary minute ventilation ($\dot{V}_E$) during physical activity increases disproportionately to oxygen uptake coinciding when blood lactate begins to accumulate. The ventilatory threshold (Tvent) predicts LT from the graded exercise $\dot{V}_E$ response.

The test involves a ramp test of 1- or 2- min increments with continuous measurement of $\dot{V}_E$ (breath-by-breath or every 10, 20, or 30 s) to the point of fatigue (usually within 8 to 12 min). The point of nonlinear increase in $\dot{V}_E$ versus $\dot{V}O_2$ represents Tvent, expressed as a specific $\dot{V}O_2$ value rather than as running speed or power output common with the fixed blood lactate concentration method. The middle figure (**B**) shows the relationship between $\dot{V}_E$ and $\dot{V}O_2$ during incremental exercise; Tvent occurs at an exercise $\dot{V}O_2$ of 3.04 L·min^{-1}. It is common to express the $\dot{V}O_2$ at LT as a percentage of $\dot{V}O_{2max}$ (71% in this example).

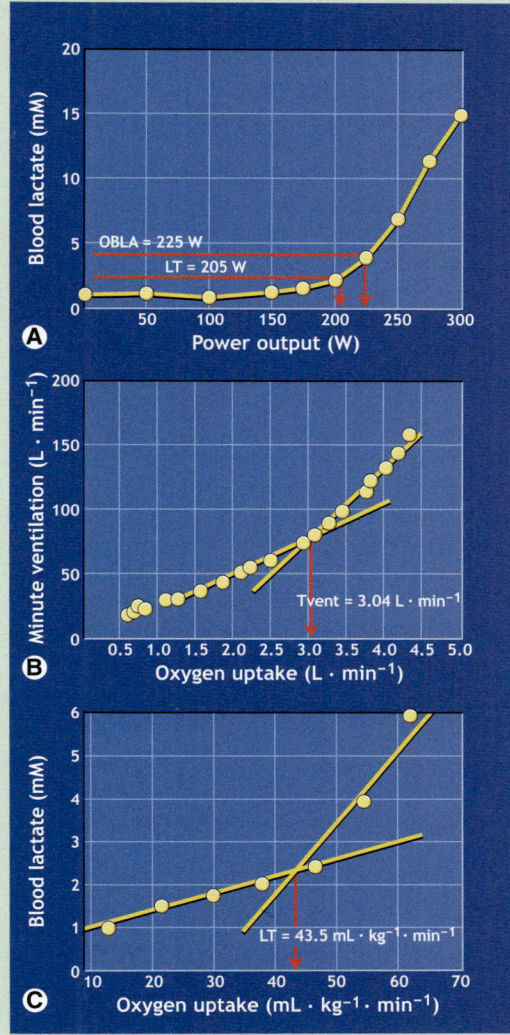

(**A**) Fixed blood lactate concentration method to determine LT and onset of blood lactate accumulation (OBLA). This example shows LT at a fixed blood lactate of 2.5 mM and OBLA at a fixed blood lactate of 4.0 mM. (**B**) Determination of LT from the relationship between pulmonary minute $\dot{V}_E$ and $\dot{V}O_2$ during incremental exercise. (**C**) Determination of LT from the relationship between blood lactate concentration and $\dot{V}O_2$ during incremental exercise.

BLOOD LACTATE-EXERCISE RESPONSE

This protocol plots blood lactate concentration versus either $\dot{V}O_2$ or exercise intensity in a manner similar to determination of fixed blood lactate concentration. The person exercises for 3- or 4-min increments on a bicycle ergometer or treadmill. With treadmill exercise, blood is sampled for lactate determination during a brief pause at the end of each stage or without pause when using stationary cycling. The bottom figure plots blood lactate versus oxygen uptake throughout the test. A best-fitting straight line depicts the linear portion of the curve; a second line describes the upward-trending curve after it "breaks" from linearity. The intersection of the two lines represents LT.

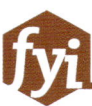

Cigarette Smoking Blunts Exercise Heart Rate Response

A paradox exists between cigarette smokers maximal exercise capacity and their submaximal heart rate response to exercise. Otherwise healthy chronic smokers exhibit significantly less endurance during graded exercise to maximum than nonsmokers.[28,36] Despite their poorer performance in maximal testing (i.e., shorter time to fatigue), the smokers spent more time to attain a 130 b·min^{-1} heart rate during a graded exercise test. This result indicates a relatively *higher* fitness level (i.e., more exercise accomplished before reaching a submaximal heart rate value). An altered sensitivity in autonomic neural control from cigarette smoking may inhibit smokers' submaximal effort heart rate response.[37] Public health policy must consider smoking status when evaluating fitness standards based on submaximal heart rate responses step test or heart rate prediction tests. Failure to account for cigarette smoking inflates an individual's fitness status because smoker's lower submaximal heart rate response erroneously implies higher aerobic capacity.

R-Type/Shutterstock

Sources:
Jackson SE, et al. Combined health risks of cigarette smoking and low levels of physical activity: a prospective cohort study in England with 12-year follow-up. *BMJ Open.* 2019;9:e032852.
Mandraffino G, et al. Abnormal left ventricular global strain during exercise-test in young healthy smokers. *Sci Rep.* 2020;10:5700.

---

smoking abstinence in chronic smokers. *From a practical standpoint, an athlete who cannot eliminate smoking completely should at least abstain the day before a competition.* Additional research complements these findings; a 7-day smoking abstinence period by young men reduced submaximal exercise heart rate and enhanced time to exhaustion during graded treadmill testing.[28]

 INTEGRATIVE QUESTION

What is the biochemical rationale for measuring oxygen uptake and carbon dioxide production during graded exercise to indicate the onset of lactate buildup (metabolic anaerobiosis) at the cellular level?

Does Ventilation Limit Aerobic Power and Endurance Performance?

Aerobic training produces considerably less adaptation in pulmonary structure and function than in cardiovascular and neuromuscular adaptations.[17,19]

With inadequate breathing during graded exercise, the relationship between pulmonary ventilation and oxygen uptake would curve in a direction opposite to that indicated in Figure 14.5 (i.e., decreased ventilatory equivalent). This common response in COPD patients indicates a *failure* of ventilation to keep pace with oxygen uptake.[3] During strenuous effort, healthy individuals overbreathe at higher oxygen uptake levels. The hyperventilation response generally decreases alveolar P_{CO_2} (see Fig. 14.3) and slightly increases alveolar P_{O_2}. Physical activity conditions that trigger hyperventilation-induced reductions in arterial carbon dioxide restrict cerebral blood flow, which may compromise oxygen delivery to active brain areas and contribute to central fatigue.[45] Even during maximal activity, a considerable **breathing reserve** exists because minute ventilation at $\dot{V}O_{2max}$ equals only 60 to 85% of a healthy person's maximum voluntary ventilation (MVV). Most individuals have a 20 to 40% MVV reserve during intense physical activity. *Pulmonary function does not form a "weak link" in the oxygen transport system of healthy individuals with average to moderately large aerobic capacities.*

For endurance athletes, the pulmonary system lags behind their exceptional cardiovascular and aerobic muscular adaptations to training.[59] The potential for inequality in alveolar ventilation relative to pulmonary capillary blood flow (i.e., impaired ventilation-perfusion ratio) during intense activity may compromise arterial saturation and oxygen transport capacity—a condition termed **exercise-induced arterial hypoxemia (EIH)**.[31,38,42,50] EIH among trained individuals remains variable. It sometimes occurs at physical activity levels as low as 40% $\dot{V}O_{2max}$ at sea level and mild to moderate altitudes.[7,22,51] When highly trained endurance athletes exercised near $\dot{V}O_{2max}$ (>65 mL·kg^{-1}·min^{-1}; **FIG. 14.9**), pressure differentials

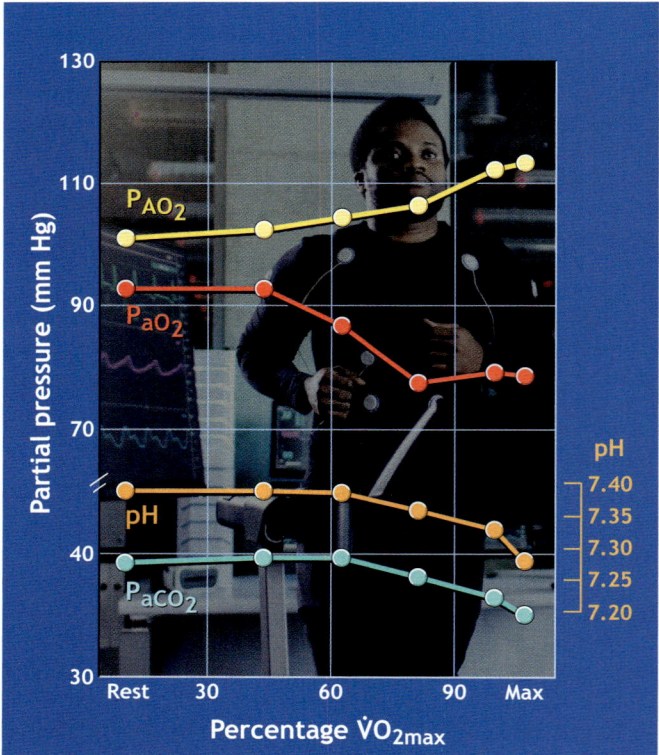

FIGURE 14.9. Average blood gas pressures (partial pressures of oxygen [P_{aO_2}] and carbon dioxide [P_{aCO_2}]), acid-base status (pH), and difference between alveolar (P_{AO_2}) and arterial (P_{aO_2}) oxygen partial pressure in eight male athletes during graded exercise to maximum oxygen uptake ($\dot{V}O_{2max}$).
(Gorodenkoff/Shutterstock)

between alveolar and arterial oxygen widened to more than 30 mm Hg. This caused arterial oxygen saturation to fall below 90% with a corresponding arterial Po₂ below 75 mm Hg. For some elite endurance athletes, arterial desaturation becomes more apparent as exercise duration progresses. Alterations in pulmonary structure at the alveolar-capillary interface do not produce EIH, although intrapulmonary shunt vessel recruitment during physical activity may contribute to impaired pulmonary gas exchange.[56,57]

Three functionally based causes for arterial desaturation include:

1. Inequality in ventilation-perfusion ratio within the lungs or specific lung regions
2. Blood shunting between venous and arterial circulations, thus bypassing diffusion areas
3. Failure to achieve end-capillary equilibrium between alveolar oxygen pressure and oxygen's pressure in blood perfusing pulmonary capillaries

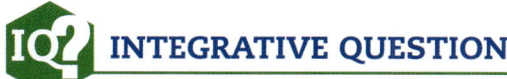

INTEGRATIVE QUESTION

Why does pulmonary ventilation not limit aerobic exercise performance for most healthy persons?

Summary

1. In light-to-moderate physical activity, pulmonary ventilation increases linearly with oxygen uptake so the ventilatory equivalent ($\dot{V}_E/\dot{V}O_2$) averages 20 to 25 L of air breathed per liter of oxygen intake.
2. In non–steady-rate physical activity, ventilation increases disproportionately with increases in oxygen uptake, with ventilatory equivalents exceeding 35 L.
3. A disproportionately sharp rise in minute ventilation during incremental exercise provides a "bloodless" way to estimate the onset of blood lactate accumulation (OBLA).
4. OBLA provides a submaximal aerobic fitness measure that relates to the beginning of anaerobiosis in the active musculature.
5. OBLA occurs without significant metabolic acidosis or severe cardiovascular strain.
6. The oxygen cost of breathing for healthy individuals remains relatively small throughout the submaximal effort range.
7. For individuals with respiratory disease, the breathing effort becomes excessive, often producing inadequate alveolar ventilation.
8. Cigarette smoking causes airway resistance to rise considerably and increase breathing cost, adversely impacting endurance performance.
9. Exercise training generally reduces the ventilatory equivalent in submaximal activity, which "conserves" oxygen during a particular task.
10. For individuals of average aerobic fitness, maximal physical activity does not tax pulmonary ventilation to a point that limits optimal alveolar gas exchange and arterial oxygen saturation.
11. Pulmonary function improvements for the endurance athlete can lag behind their exceptional adaptations in cardiovascular and muscle function, thereby compromising blood aeration during maximal effort.

Part 3 — Acid-base Regulation

Buffering

Acids and bases (and salts) dissociate in water to form electrolytes, which can substantially alter the properties of the solution in which they dissolve. **Acids** dissociate in solution and releases H⁺, whereas **bases** accept H⁺ to form hydroxide ions (OH⁻). The term **buffering** designates reactions that minimize changes in H⁺ concentration, while **buffers** refer to chemical and physiologic mechanisms that impede such changes. Every strong base dissociates to produce a high OH⁻ concentration. In contrast, weak bases release only limited OH⁻ or absorb only a few H⁺. The body's buffering systems function efficiently, with different systems operating at different rates. The chemical buffers adjust pH within milliseconds, while physiologic buffers operate with a longer time requirement. For example, it may take minutes for respiratory tract mechanisms to adjust and become evident so as to alter the blood pH upward by exhaling above-normal CO₂ from the body.

The term **pH** refers to the inverse of a solution's H⁺ concentration or the acidity or alkalinity (basicity) of a liquid solution. Specifically, pH refers to the concentration of protons or H⁺. Acid solutions have more H⁺ than OH⁻ at a pH below 7.0, and vice versa for basic solutions whose pH exceeds 7.0. Chemically pure (distilled) water, considered neutral, has equal H⁺ and OH⁻ and thus a pH of 7.0.

In 1909, Danish chemist Sören Sörensen (1868–1939; http://protomag.com/assets/soren-sorensen-pioneer-ph) designed the pH scale displayed in **FIGURE 14.10**. Sörensen achieved considerable notoriety for his work in amino acid synthesis and enzyme reactions at Carlsberg Laboratory in Copenhagen, Denmark (www.carlsbergfondet.dk/en/About-the-Foundation/The-Carlsberg-Foundation/The-Carlsberg-family/The-Carlsberg-Laboratory-). The pH scale ranges from between 1.0 and 14.0, with an inverse relation existing between pH and H⁺ concentration (strictly defined as $-\log_{10} c$, where c is the hydrogen ion concentration in moles per liter). The pH logarithmic scale means a one-unit change in pH produces a 10-fold change in H⁺ concentration. A solution with pH 4 is 10 times more acidic than a solution with pH 5. For another example, lemon juice and gastric juice (pH = 2.0) have 1000 times the H⁺ concentration compared to black coffee (pH = 5.0), whereas hydrochloric acid (pH = 1.0) has approximately 1 million times the blood's H⁺ concentration at pH 7.4. Values for blood pH rarely fall below pH 6.9, even during the most strenuous physical activity, while pH values within active muscle cytoplasm are lower. A digital pH meter can accurately determine pH for any

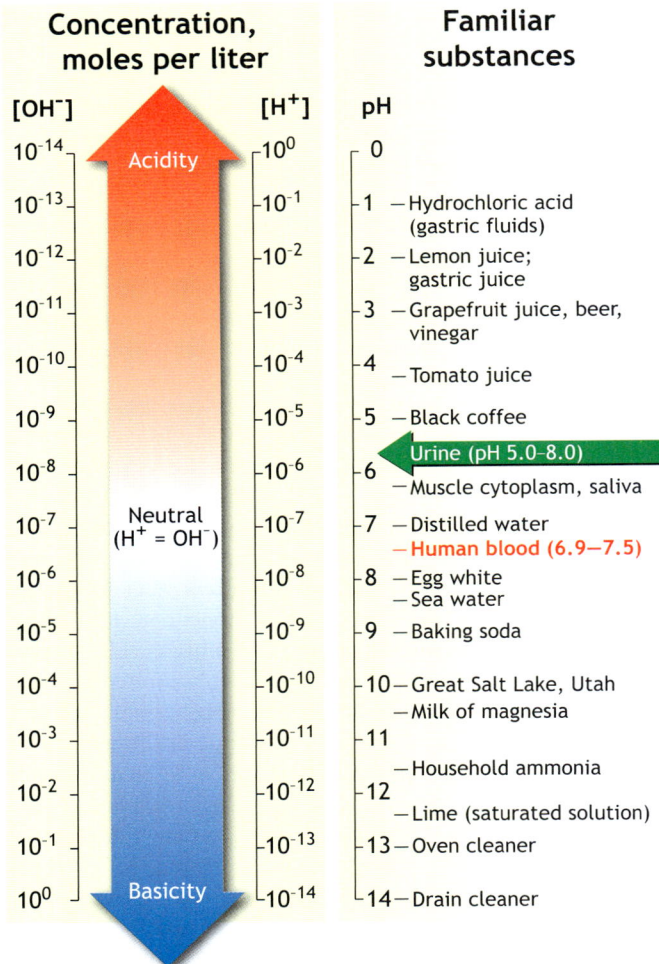

FIGURE 14.10. The pH scale represents a liquid solution's acidity and alkalinity (basicity). Blood pH normally stabilizes at the slightly alkaline pH of 7.4.

Chemical Buffers

The chemical buffering system consists of a weak acid and salt of that acid. Bicarbonate buffer, for example, contains the weak acid carbonic acid and its salt, sodium bicarbonate. Carbonic acid forms when bicarbonate binds H^+. When H^+ concentration remains elevated, the reaction produces the weak acid because excess H^+ ions bind in accord with the general reaction:

$$H^+ + \text{Buffer} \rightarrow H\text{-Buffer}$$

In contrast, when H^+ concentration decreases—as during hyperventilation, when plasma carbonic acid declines because carbon dioxide leaves the blood and exits through the lungs—the buffering reaction moves in the opposite direction and releases H^+:

$$H^+ + \text{Buffer} \leftarrow H\text{-Buffer}$$

Most carbon dioxide generated during energy metabolism reacts with water to form the relatively weak carbonic acid that dissociates into H^+ and HCO_3^-. Likewise, the stronger lactic acid reacts with sodium bicarbonate to form sodium lactate and carbonic acid; in turn, carbonic acid dissociates and increases extracellular fluid H^+ concentration. The organic fatty acids dissociate and liberate H^+, as do sulfuric and phosphoric acids generated during protein catabolism. Bicarbonate, phosphate, and protein chemical buffers provide the rapid first line of defense to maintain consistency in the acid-base character of the internal environment.

Bicarbonate Buffer

The bicarbonate buffer system consists of carbonic acid and sodium bicarbonate in solution. During buffering, hydrochloric acid (a strong acid) converts to the much weaker carbonic acid by combining with sodium bicarbonate in the following reaction:

$$HCl + NaHCO_3 \rightarrow NaCl + H_2CO_3 \leftrightarrow H^+ + HCO_3^-$$

Hydrochloric acid buffering produces only a slightly reduced pH. Sodium bicarbonate in plasma exerts a strong buffering action on lactic acid to form sodium lactate and carbonic acid. Any additional increase in H^+ concentration from carbonic acid dissociation causes the reaction to move in the opposite direction to release carbon dioxide into solution as follows:

For acidosis:

$$H_2O + CO_2 \leftarrow H_2CO_3 \leftarrow H^+ + HCO_3^-$$

An increase in plasma carbon dioxide or H^+ concentration immediately stimulates ventilation to eliminate "excess" carbon dioxide.

substance. The example shows a urine sample with pH 6.32. When expressed in ionic terms, hydrogen ion concentration at each pH value represents 10 times the next pH. For instance, a pH value 4 corresponds to 10^{-4} M or 0.0001 M proton concentration, whereas a pH value 5 denotes a 10^{-5} M or 0.00001 M proton concentration.

Bodily fluid pH ranges between 1.0 for digestive hydrochloric acid to a slightly basic pH between 7.35 and 7.45 for arterial and venous blood and most other bodily fluids. A decrease in H^+ concentration (increased pH or **alkalosis**) produces an increase in pH above the normal 7.4 average. Conversely, acidosis refers to increased H^+ concentration (decreased pH). The acid-base bodily fluid characteristics fluctuate within narrow limits because metabolism remains highly sensitive to H^+ concentrations in the reacting medium. Three mechanisms regulate the pH of internal processes because fluctuations—either too acidic or too basic—often precipitate life-threatening disorders:

1. Chemical buffers
2. Pulmonary ventilation
3. Renal function

Conversely, a decrease in plasma H^+ concentration inhibits the ventilatory drive and retains carbon dioxide to combine with water to increase acidity (carbonic acid) and normalize pH.

For alkalosis:

$$H_2O + CO_2 \rightarrow H_2CO_3 \rightarrow H^+ + HCO_3^-$$

Phosphate Buffer

Phosphoric acid and sodium phosphate comprise the **phosphate buffering system**. These chemicals act similarly to the bicarbonate buffers. Phosphate buffer exerts an important effect to regulate acid-base balance in the kidney tubules and intracellular fluids where phosphate concentration remains high.

Protein Buffer

Venous blood buffers the H^+ released from dissociating the relatively weak carbonic acid (produced from $H_2O + CO_2$). *By far, hemoglobin provides the most important H^+ acceptor for this buffering function.* Hemoglobin is almost six times more potent in regulating acidity than the other plasma proteins. Hemoglobin's oxygen release to cells makes hemoglobin a weaker acid, thereby increasing its affinity to bind H^+. The H^+ generated when carbonic acid forms in the red blood cell (erythrocyte) readily combines with deoxygenated hemoglobin (Hb^-) in the reaction:

$$H^+ + Hb^- \text{ (Protein)} \rightarrow HHb$$

Intracellular tissue proteins also regulate plasma pH. Some amino acids possess free acidic radicals. When dissociated, they form OH^-, which readily reacts with H^+ to form water.

Chemical Buffering's Relative Power

The table below lists the relative power of the blood's chemical buffers compared with those of blood only and blood and interstitial fluids combined. As a frame of reference, the bicarbonate system's buffering power has the value 1.00.

Chemical buffering power		
Chemical buffer	Blood	Blood and interstitial fluids
Bicarbonate	1.0	1.0
Phosphorate	0.3	0.3
Proteins (excluding Hb)	1.4	0.8
Hemoglobin (Hb)	5.3	1.5

thinkhubstudio/Shutterstock

Physiologic Buffers

The pulmonary and renal systems provide the second line of defense against disruptions in acid-base regulation. Their buffering function occurs only when changes in pH have already occurred.

Ventilatory Buffer

When extracellular fluids and plasma gain free H^+, it directly stimulates the respiratory center to immediately increase alveolar ventilation. This rapid adjustment reduces alveolar P_{CO_2} and causes carbon dioxide removal from the blood for exit in expired air. Reduced plasma carbon dioxide levels accelerate H^+ and HCO_3^- recombination, lowering free H^+ concentration in plasma to provide a **ventilatory buffer** effect. For example, doubling alveolar ventilation by hyperventilation at rest increases blood alkalinity and pH by 0.23 units, from 7.40 to 7.63. Conversely, reducing normal alveolar ventilation (hypoventilation) by one-half increases blood acidity by approximately 0.23 pH units. The ventilatory buffering potential equals twice the combined effect of all the body's chemical buffers.

Renal Buffer

Chemical buffers only temporarily affect excess acid buildup. H^+ excretion by the kidneys (**renal buffer**), although relatively slow, provides an important longer-term defense to maintain the body's buffer reserve (**alkaline reserve**). To this end, the kidneys stand as the final sentinels, guarding against the potentially lethal consequences of abnormal pH alterations. The renal tubules regulate acidity through complex chemical reactions that secrete ammonia and H^+ into the urine and then reabsorb alkali, chloride, and bicarbonate.

 See the animation "Renal Function" on **Lippincott Connect** to view this process.

Intense Physical Activity Effects

Increased H^+ concentration from carbon dioxide production and lactate formation during strenuous physical activity makes pH regulation progressively more difficult. Acid-base regulation becomes exceedingly difficult during repeated, brief all-out effort that elevates blood lactate values to 30 mM (270 mg lactate $\cdot$ dL blood^{-1}) or higher.[29] **FIGURE 14.11** illustrates the inverse linear relationship between blood lactate concentration and blood pH. Blood lactate concentration in these experiments varied between 0.8 mM at rest (pH 7.43) and 32.1 mM during exhaustive exercise (pH 6.8). In active muscle, pH reaches even lower values than in blood, declining to 6.4 or lower at exhaustion.

Clearly, humans *temporarily* tolerate pronounced disturbances in acid-base balance during maximal physical effort. A plasma pH below 7.00 does not occur without consequences,

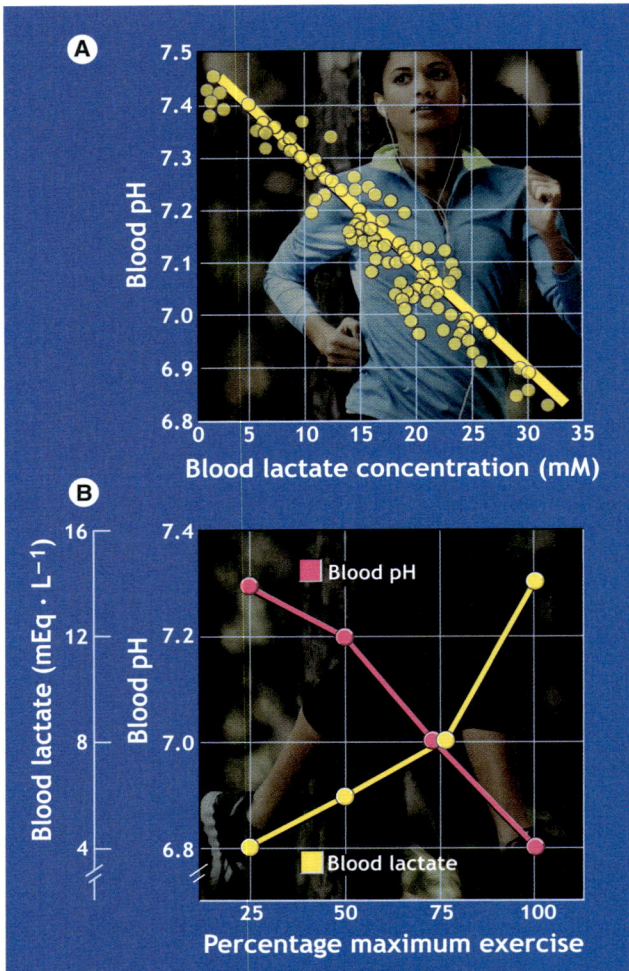

FIGURE 14.11. **(A)** Relationship between blood pH and blood lactate concentration during rest and increasing intensity short-duration exercise up to maximum. **(B)** Blood pH and blood lactate concentration expressed as a percentage of maximum. Decreases in blood pH accompany increases in blood lactate concentration.
(Daxiao Productions/Shutterstock)

This level of acidosis produces nausea, headache, and dizziness, in addition to discomfort and pain that ranges from mild to debilitating within active muscles.

Summary

1. The chemical and physiologic buffer systems normally regulate bodily fluid acid-base quality within narrow limits.
2. The bicarbonate, phosphate, and protein chemical buffers provide the rapid first-line defense in acid-base regulation.
3. Chemical buffers consist of a weak acid and that acid's salt, converting a strong acid to a weaker acid and neutral salt.
4. The lungs and kidneys help to regulate pH.
5. Changes in alveolar ventilation rapidly alter free H^+ concentration in extracellular fluids.
6. The renal tubules act as the body's final defense by secreting H^+ into the urine and reabsorbing bicarbonate.
7. Intense anaerobic exercise increases buffering demand to make pH regulation progressively more challenging.

Key Terms

Acids: Dissociate in solution and release hydrogen ions (H^+)

Alkaline reserve: Sum total of the basic ions (mainly bicarbonate) of blood and other body fluids, which acting as buffers, maintain the blood's normal pH

Alkalosis: Decrease in H^+ concentration increases pH above 7.4

Anaerobic threshold (AT): The abrupt increase in ventilatory equivalent caused by nonmetabolic carbon dioxide production from lactate buffering; believed by some to be a noninvasive measure to signal the body's shift to anaerobic metabolism

Bases: Accept hydrogen ions (H^+) to form hydroxide ions (OH^-)

Breathing reserve: Difference between maximal voluntary ventilation (MVV) and ventilation measured during a maximal exercise test; equals 20 to 40% MVV

Central command: Central nervous system influences on ventilatory and circulatory dynamics

Chemoreceptors: Specialized nerve cells that respond to chemical stimuli

Exercise-induced arterial hypoxemia (EIH): Alveolar ventilation inequality relative to pulmonary capillary blood flow (i.e., impaired ventilation-perfusion ratio) during intense activity; compromised arterial saturation and oxygen transport capacity

Hyperpnea: Increased breathing rate and/or depth

Lactate threshold: Highest oxygen uptake or exercise intensity level achieved with less than a 1.0-mM increase in blood lactate concentration above pre-exercise levels

Medulla: Hindbrain portion that controls autonomic functions (e.g., breathing, digestion, heart and blood vessel dynamics, swallowing, sneezing)

Onset of blood lactate accumulation (OBLA): Exercise intensity at which blood lactate concentration equals 4.0 mM

pH: A measure of acidity or alkalinity expressed as H^+ concentration equal to $-\log_{10}c$, where c = hydrogen ion concentration in moles per liter

Phase I ventilation: Neurogenic stimuli from the cerebral cortex and feedback from the active limbs stimulate the medulla to abruptly increase ventilation

Phase II ventilation: Minute ventilation rises exponentially to achieve a steady level related to metabolic gas exchange demands

Phosphate buffering system: Phosphoric acid and sodium phosphate impact kidney tubule and intracellular fluid acid-base balance

Renal buffer: The regulation of acidity through complex chemical reactions that secrete ammonia and H^+ into the urine and then reabsorb alkali, chloride, and bicarbonate

Ventilatory buffer: Increased free H^+ in extracellular fluid and plasma increases alveolar ventilation, which reduces the level of blood CO_2

Ventilatory equivalent: Ratio of minute ventilation to oxygen uptake ($\dot{V}_E/\dot{V}O_2$)

Ventilatory threshold (Tvent): Point where pulmonary ventilation increases disproportionately relative to increases in oxygen uptake

References are available online at Lippincott Connect.

Additional References

Driver S, et al. Effects of wearing a cloth face mask on performance, physiological and perceptual responses during a graded treadmill running exercise test. *Br J Sports Med.* 2022;56:107.

Freire APCF, et al. Resistance training using different elastic components offers similar gains on muscle strength to weight machine equipment in Individuals with COPD: a randomized controlled trial. *Physiother Theory Pract.* 2022;38:14.

Jones AM, et al. Physiological demands of running at 2-hour marathon race pace. *J Appl Physiol* (1985). 2021;130:369.

Koreny M, et al. Patterns of physical activity progression in patients with COPD. *Arch Bronconeumol (Engl Ed).* 2021;57:214.

Ktenidis CK, et al. Priming exercise increases Wingate cycling peak power output. *Eur J Sport Sci.* 2021;21:705.

Leary BK, et al. Differences in joint power distribution in high and low lactate threshold cyclists. *Eur J Appl Physiol.* 2021;121:231.

Morris NR, et al. Exercise & Sports Science Australia (ESSA) position statement on exercise and chronic obstructive pulmonary disease. *J Sci Med Sport.* 2021;24:52.

Oguz S, et al. Walking training augments the effects of expiratory muscle training in Parkinson's disease. *Acta Neurol Scand.* 2022;145:79.

Poffé C, et al. Bicarbonate unlocks the ergogenic action of ketone monoester intake in endurance exercise. *Med Sci Sports Exerc.* 2021;53:431.

Poole DC, et al. The anaerobic threshold: 50+ years of controversy. *J Physiol.* 2021;599:737.

Snarr RL, et al. Validity of wearable electromyographical compression shorts to predict lactate threshold during incremental exercise in healthy subjects. *J Strength Cond Res.* 2021;35:702.

Støa EM, et al. Factors influencing running velocity at lactate threshold in male and female runners at different levels of performance. *Front Physiol.* 2020;11:585267.

Tanji F, Nabekura Y. Oxygen uptake and respiratory exchange ratio relative to the lactate threshold running in well-trained distance runners. *J Sports Med Phys Fitness.* 2019;59:895.

Zanforlini BM, et al. Clinical trial on the effects of oral magnesium supplementation in stable-phase COPD patients. *Aging Clin Exp Res.* 2022;34:167.

Table 14.1 Hyperventilation's Oxygen Cost During "Smoking" and "Nonsmoking" Exercise at Approximately 80% of Maximum Oxygen Uptake

	Smoking				Nonsmoking			
	Voluntary HV		Dead Space HV		Voluntary HV		Dead Space HV	
Subject	$\dot{V}_E$ (L·min^{-1})	O_2 Cost (mL·L^{-1})	$\dot{V}_E$ (L·min^{-1})	O_2 Cost (mL·L^{-1})	$\dot{V}_E$ (L·min^{-1})	O_2 Cost (mL·L^{-1})	$\dot{V}_E$ (L·min^{-1})	O_2 Cost (mL·L^{-1})
1	26.4	15.1	18.9	12.7	22.7	11.4	23.0	6.5
2	39.0	10.3	28.1	5.9	42.6	11.3	41.3	4.8
3	22.8	7.9	27.2	7.0	23.8	7.2	22.8	5.7
4	36.3	5.0	28.7	5.6	44.7	3.8	18.6	−1.6
5	52.7	13.5	26.7	12.4	75.2	6.1	22.8	5.7
6	22.4	8.5	27.3	1.1	23.2	3.4	30.1	3.0
Average	32.6	10.1	26.2	7.4	38.7	7.2	26.5	4.0

HV, hyperventilation; $\dot{V}_E$, minute ventilation (expired).

Note: The "negative" $\dot{V}_E$ cost for this subject (last column) implies that the added dead space reduces the normal exercise $\dot{V}_E$ cost.

CHAPTER 15
The Cardiovascular System

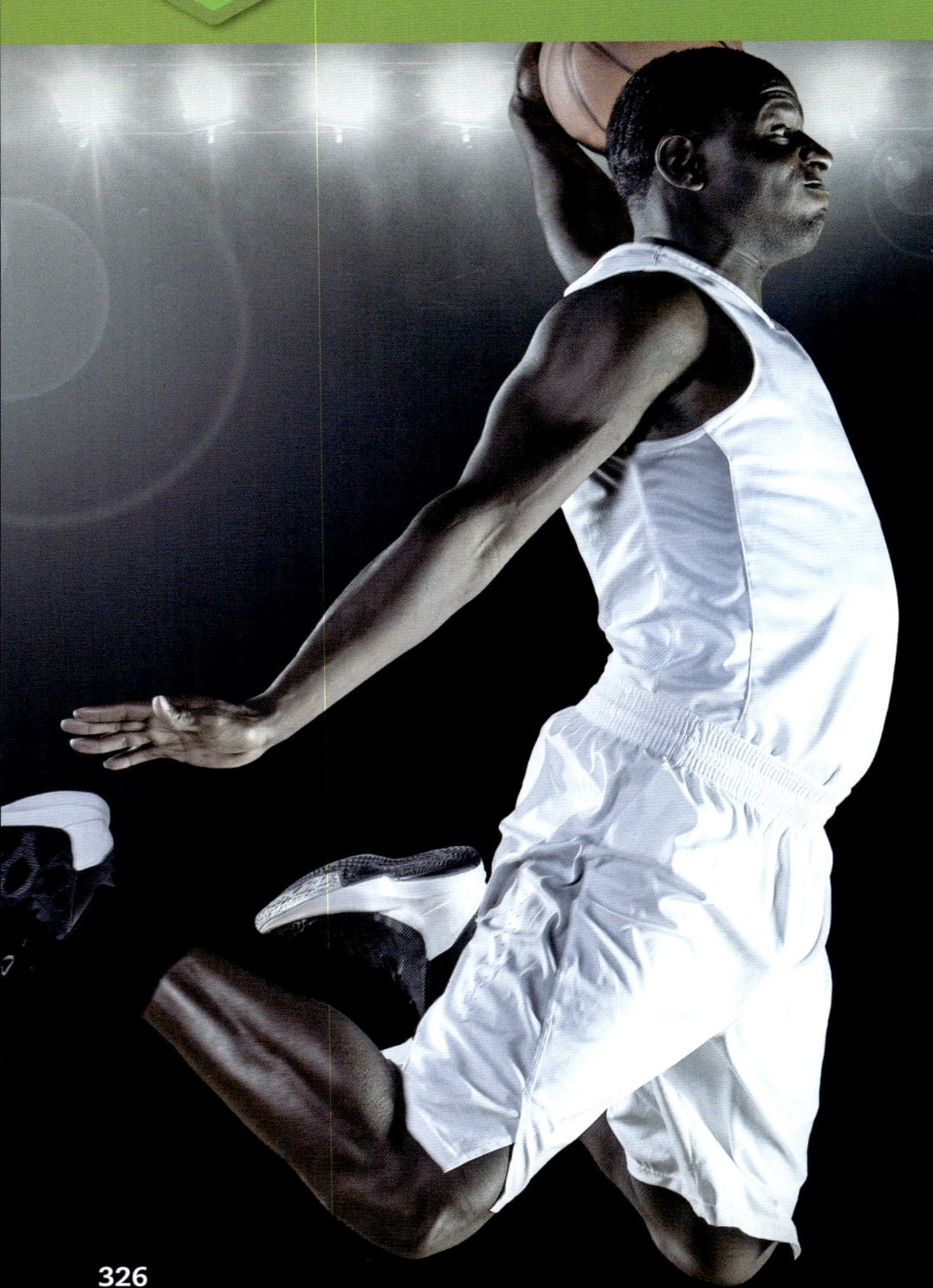

Chapter Objectives

- List four important cardiovascular system functions
- Describe the interactions among cardiac output, total peripheral resistance, and arterial blood pressure
- Explain the venous system's role as an active blood reservoir
- Outline the structural differences among various blood vessel types
- Explain how to measure blood pressure with auscultation
- List typical systolic and diastolic blood pressures at rest and during moderate and intense aerobic physical activity
- Explain the time course for the blood pressure response during resistance exercise and upper body exercise
- Explain why a "hypotensive response" might occur in recovery from physical activity
- Diagram the coronary circulation's major vessels
- Describe myocardial blood flow patterns, oxygen uptake, and substrate use during rest and various physical exertion intensities
- Explain the rate-pressure product and its meaning in clinical exercise physiology

Ancillaries at-a-Glance

Visit Lippincott Connect to access the following resources.

- References: Chapter 15
- Appendix H: Links for Supplemental Animations and Videos
- Animations: Blood Circulation, Cardiac Cycle, Hypertension, Measuring Blood Pressure, Myocardial Blood Flow
- Focus on Research: Required Exercise Intensity to Improve Fitness

The early "physiologists" during Galen's time, almost 2000 years ago (see Introduction: A View From the Past), proposed that the **cardiovascular system** integrates the body as a unit. For contemporary exercise physiologists, an important cardiovascular function entails how well this highly integrated system supplies active muscles with a continuous nutrient and oxygen stream to sustain high energy transfer levels while removing metabolic byproducts from the tissues' active energy release sites.

Chapters 15, 16, and 17 explore circulation dynamics, particularly its oxygen delivery role during physical activity. The maximum level for aerobic energy transfer during activity depends on oxygen transport and delivery, and most importantly, how muscles continuously generate adenosine triphosphate (ATP) aerobically, whether for relatively brief durations, as in most physical activities, or for demanding ultra-endurance events under challenging environmental conditions.

Cardiovascular System Components

The cardiovascular system has four main components:

1. A pump to provide continuous linkage with the other three components
2. A high-pressure distribution circuit
3. Exchange vessels
4. A low-pressure collection and return circuit

If an average-sized adult's 60,900 km/100,000 miles of blood vessels were stretched end to end, they would encircle the Earth about 2.4 times. Over a typical 72-year life span (26,300 days carrying about 1800 gallons daily at rest plus movement), that vast vessel transportation network will move more than 47.3 million gallons of blood! **FIGURE 15.1** schematically shows the cardiovascular system (A) and its major arteries that comprise the adult systemic circulation (B). The red shading depicts oxygen-rich arterial blood, whereas the blue shading denotes deoxygenated venous blood. The situation reverses in the pulmonary circuit; oxygenated blood returns to the heart in the right and left pulmonary veins. The inset table at the top left shows the absolute and percentage distribution for total blood volume in the pulmonary and systemic vascular circuits for a typical adult male at rest. The systemic circulation's small arteries, veins, and capillaries contain approximately 75% of total blood volume, whereas the heart contains only 7%. Note that in the systemic circulation, the small veins account for 46%, the largest blood volume at any one time, compared with 6% in the largest arteries and 18% in veins.

 See the animation "Blood Circulation" on **Lippincott Connect** to view this process.

The Heart

The **heart** provides the impetus for blood flow. Situated in the chest cavity's midcenter, about two thirds of its mass lies to the left of the body's midline. The four-chambered muscular organ weighs 11 oz for an average-sized adult male and 9 oz for an average-sized adult female and pumps about 70 mL/2.4 oz per beat. For a person who rates average in fitness status, the maximum blood output from the heart in 1 min exceeds the fluid output from a household faucet turned wide open.

FIGURE 15.2 summarizes general functional and structural characteristics and activation mode for the body's three muscle types—skeletal, cardiac, and smooth. The heart muscle or **myocardium** represents a homogenous striated muscle form similar to the slow-twitch fibers in skeletal muscle with high capillary density and numerous mitochondria. In contrast to skeletal muscle, the multinucleated, individual cells or fibers interconnect in latticework fashion via **intercalated discs**. The stimulation (depolarization) in one cell spreads the action potential through the myocardium to *all* cells allowing the heart to function as a unit.

 See the animation "Cardiac Cycle" on **Lippincott Connect** to view this process.

FIGURE 15.3 shows heart and lung anatomy during a cardiac cycle. Part **(A)** indicates the heart, its great vessels, and the one-way blood flow indicated by red and blue arrows through valves during the cardiac cycle. Part **(B)** shows how the aortic and pulmonary valves snap closed in diastole; shortly thereafter, the mitral and tricuspid valves open and blood flows into the ventricular cavities. Initiation of systole and ventricular emptying **(C)** closes the tricuspid and **mitral valves**, while the aortic and pulmonary valves open. When viewing the structural details in the figure, note that the right lung is shown on the left side and vice versa for the left lung. This is because when locating the structures, it is always done from the person's viewpoint. Thus, the right lung appears on the left and the left lung on the right because this corresponds to the person's anatomical position while standing and facing forward.

Functionally, one can view the heart as two separate pumps. The hollow chambers on the heart's right side (right heart) perform two crucial functions:

1. Receive blood returning from throughout the body
2. Pump blood to the lungs for aeration through the **pulmonary circulation**

The heart's chambers on the left side (referred to as the left heart) also perform two critical functions:

1. Receive oxygenated blood from the lungs
2. Pump blood into the thick-walled, muscular aorta for distribution throughout the body in the **systemic circulation**

A thick, solid muscular wall or interventricular septum separates the heart's left and right sides. The **atrioventricular valves** within the heart provide one-way blood flow from the right atrium to the right ventricle and from the left atrium to the left ventricle through the **mitral** or **bicuspid valve**. The **semilunar valves**, located in the arterial wall just outside the heart, prevent blood from flowing back into the heart between contractions. The relatively thin-walled, saclike atrial chambers serve as primer or "booster" pumps to receive and store blood during ventricular contraction. Approximately 70% of the blood returning to the atria flows directly into the ventricles before atrial contraction. The simultaneous atrial contractions then force the remaining blood into their respective ventricles directly below. Almost immediately after atrial contraction, the ventricles contract and propel blood into the arterial system.

As ventricular pressure builds, the atrioventricular valves snap closed. All heart valves remain closed for 0.02 to 0.06 s. This brief interval of rising ventricular tension, when heart volume and muscle fiber

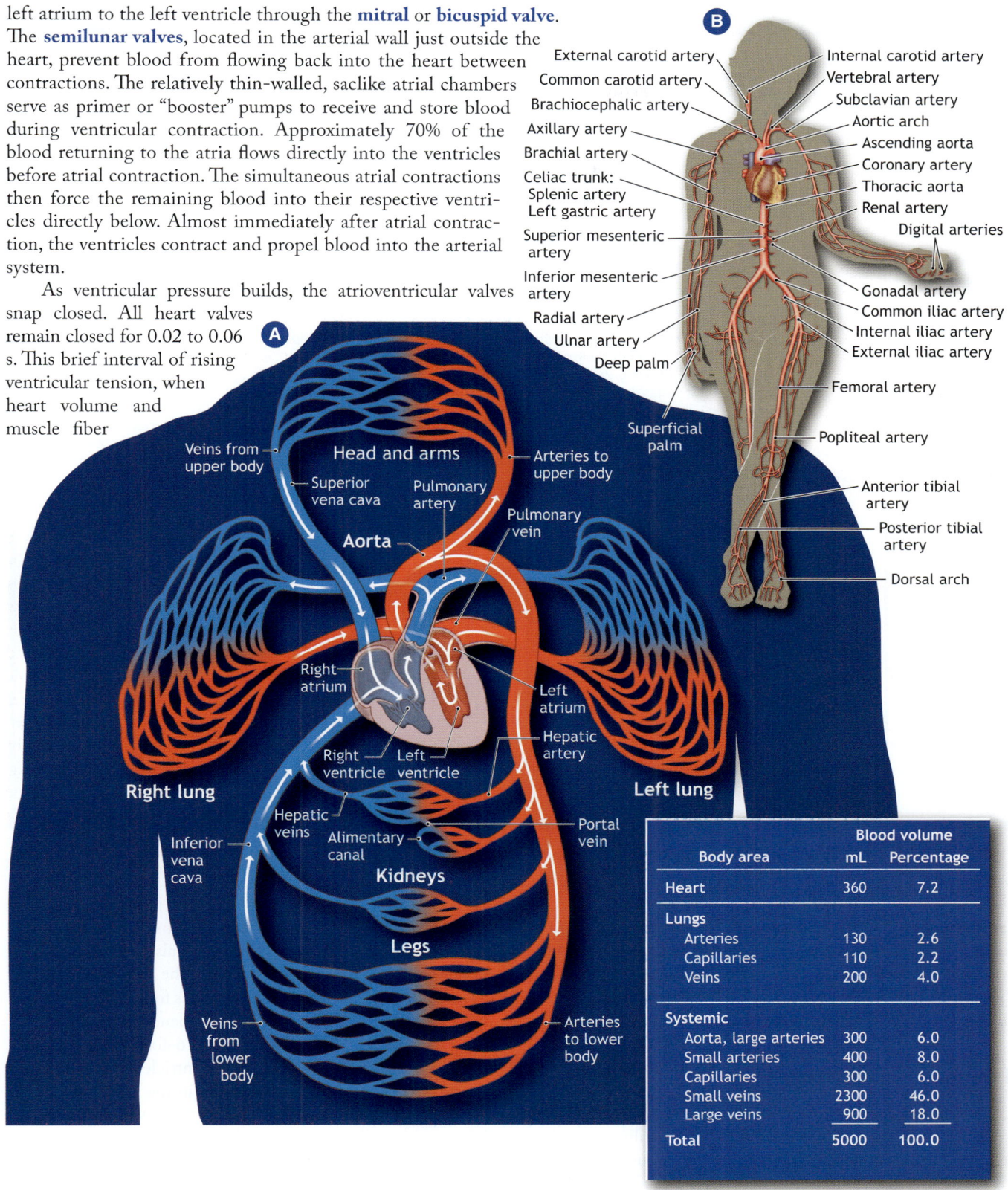

FIGURE 15.1. Cardiovascular system demonstrating the heart **(A)** and pulmonary and systemic **(B)** vascular circuits, and absolute and percentage distribution for total resting blood volume.

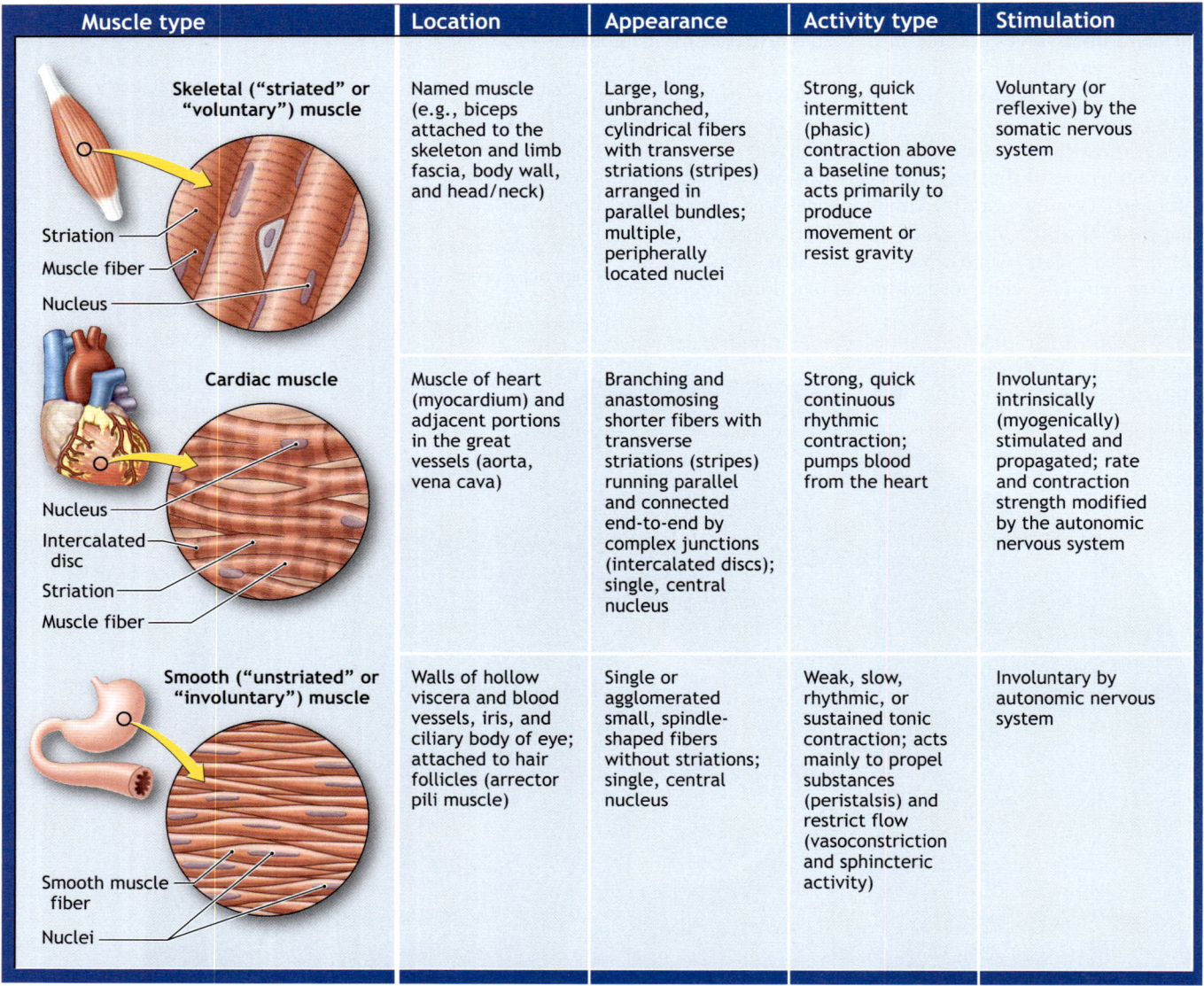

FIGURE 15.2. Functional and structural characteristics and activation mode for skeletal, cardiac, and smooth muscle.

length remain unchanged, represents the heart's **isovolumetric contraction period**. The heart ejects blood when ventricular pressure exceeds arterial pressure. With each contraction, the spiral and circular cardiac muscle band arrangement literally "wrings out" blood from the ventricles.

The Arterial System

The arteries compose the high-pressure tubing that propels oxygen-rich blood to the tissues. **FIGURE 15.4** illustrates that arteries shown on the right have connective tissue and smooth muscle layers. No gaseous exchange takes place between arterial blood and surrounding tissues because of the thickness of these vessels. As illustrated, a single endothelial cell layer lines each vessel. Fibrous tissue wrapped in several smooth muscle layers surrounds the arterial walls. A single muscle cell layer surrounds the arterioles, whereas capillaries have only one endothelial cell layer, often less than 1 micron (μm) thick, with a 300 to 1200 μm^2 flat surface area. In the venule, fibrous tissue encases the endothelial cells; veins also possess a smooth muscle layer. The inset table displays the average values for vessel diameter and corresponding values for blood flow velocity. A vessel's resistance (R) to flow depends on its radius (r). Decreasing vessel r by half increases R 16-fold (see inset table).

Blood pumped from the left ventricle into the highly muscular, yet elastic **aorta**, distributes in the body through an intricate but highly efficient arterial network with smaller arterial branches called **arterioles**. Arterial walls contain circular smooth muscle layers that either constrict or relax to regulate peripheral blood flow. These "resistance vessels" dramatically alter their internal diameter to rapidly adjust blood flow through the vascular circuit. This redistribution function takes on added importance during physical activity because blood rapidly diverts to active muscles from areas that temporarily compromise their blood supply as in the splanchnic (visceral) and cutaneous tissues.[50,58] The inset table lists average values for

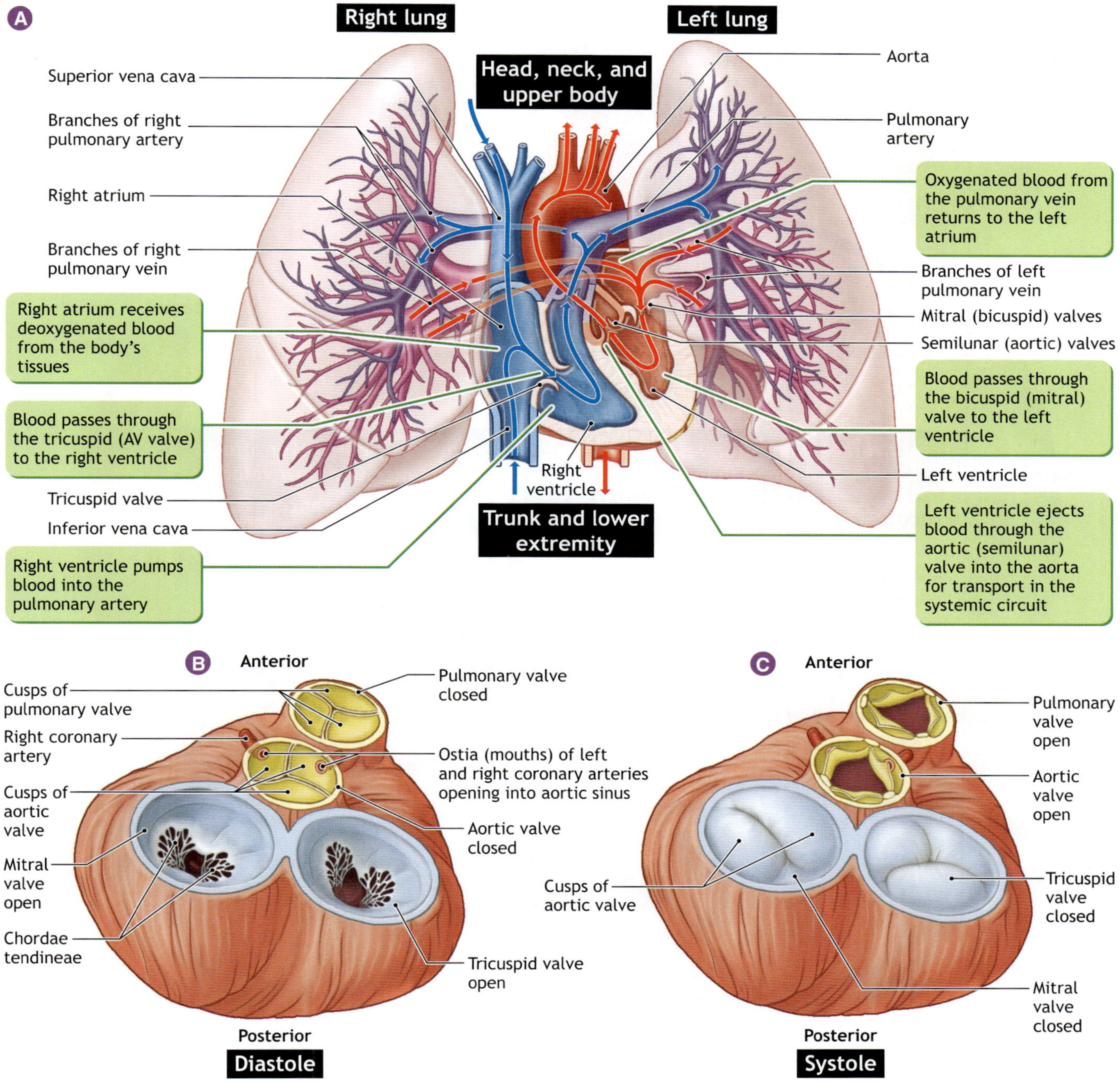

FIGURE 15.3. **(A)** Heart and lung anatomy and blood flow direction. **(B)** Aortic and pulmonary valve function in diastole. **(C)** Tricuspid and mitral valve function in systole.

blood vessel diameter and corresponding blood flow velocities. Note that blood flowing through capillaries moves slowly (0.05 to 0.1 cm·s^{-1}) compared with any main arteries or veins.

INTEGRATIVE QUESTION

What advantage does a "closed" circulatory system provide to the physically active individual?

Blood Pressure

Each left ventricle contraction forces blood to surge through the aorta. Peripheral vessels do not permit blood to "run off" into the arterial system as rapidly as it ejects from the heart. Thus, the distensible aorta "stores" some blood, which creates pressure within the entire arterial system, causing a pressure wave to travel down the aorta to remote arterial tree branches. The characteristic "pulse" in superficial arteries occurs from the stretch and subsequent arterial wall recoil

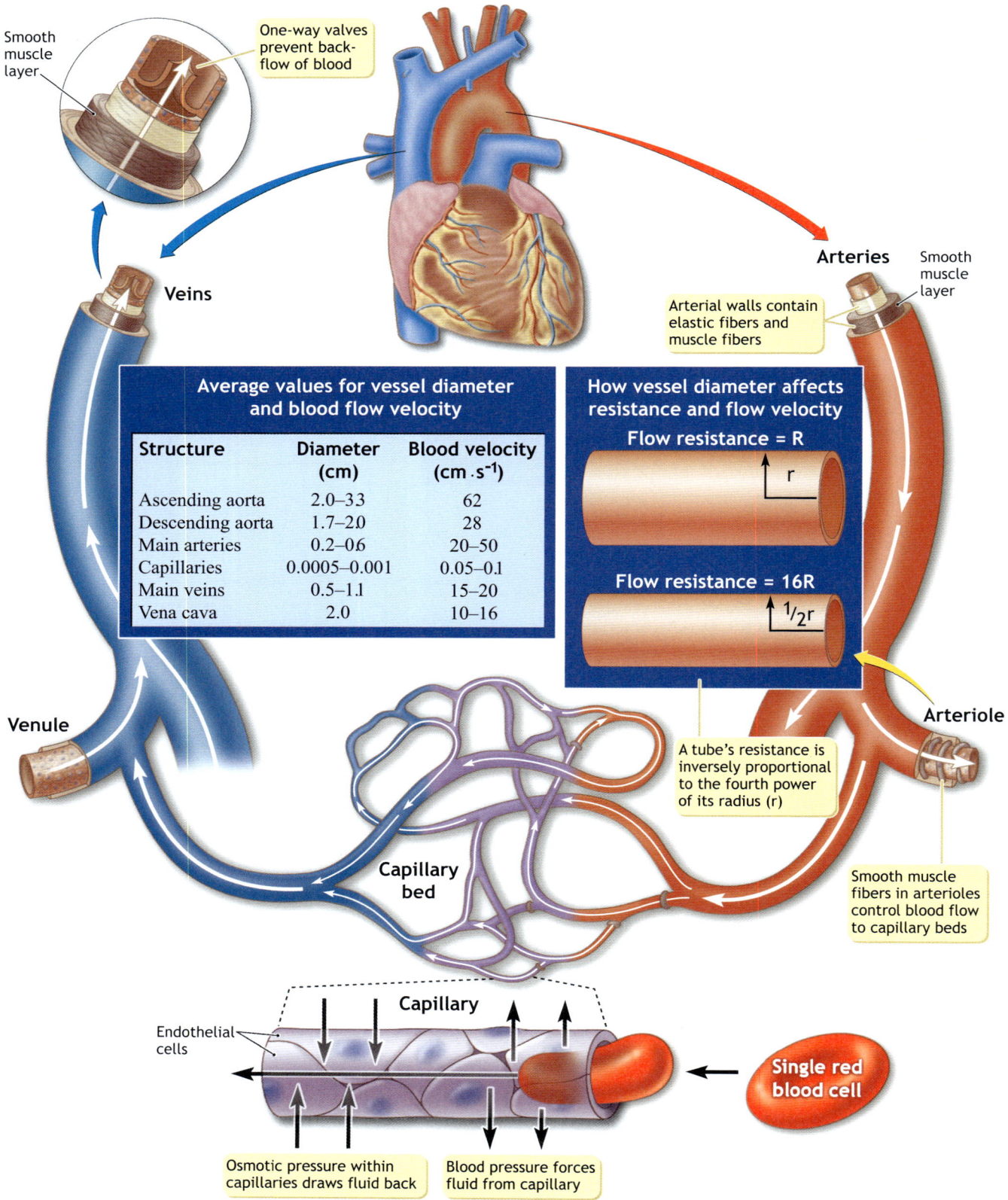

FIGURE 15.4. Blood flow direction and blood vessel wall structure for arteries, capillaries, and veins. Blood surges through the arterial system from the heart's left side moving through the capillaries, returning to the heart in the venous circulation.

Pulse Rate Versus Heart Rate

Each definition defines the differences. Heart rate (HR) describes cardiac muscle contraction and relaxation rate, more specifically the left ventricle rate during the cardiac cycle. Pulse rate (PR), measured by arterial palpation, describes arterial expansion and relaxation rate as blood moves through the vessel during measurement. In healthy individuals, HR and PR are similar. Individuals with heart conditions, where the heart does not efficiently pump enough blood with each contraction to initiate a palpable pulse, may have a PR lower than the actual measured HR.

---

during a cardiac cycle. In healthy individuals, identical values occur for pulse rate and heart rate. In essence, arterial blood pressure reflects the combined effects of arterial blood flow each minute (i.e., cardiac output) and resistance to that flow in the peripheral vasculature. The relationship can be characterized as:

> Blood pressure = Cardiac output × Total peripheral resistance

Systolic Blood Pressure. At rest in normotensive individuals, the highest pressure generated by the heart averages 120 mm Hg during left ventricular contraction, termed *systole*. The brachial artery at the right atrium level usually serves as the reference measurement point. **Systolic blood pressure** (SBP) estimates the heart's work and the force that blood exerts against the arterial walls during ventricular systole. During the heart's relaxation phase, when aortic valves close, the natural elastic arterial system recoil maintains a continuous head of pressure. This provides a steady blood flow into the periphery until the next surge of blood.

Diastolic Blood Pressure. During the cardiac cycle's relaxation phase, termed *diastole*, arterial blood pressure decreases to 60 to 80 mm Hg. **Diastolic blood pressure** indicates peripheral resistance or the ease blood flows from arterioles into capillaries. With high peripheral resistance, pressure within the arteries after systole does not rapidly dissipate. Instead, it remains elevated for a larger portion of time in the cardiac cycle. In a Practical Sense: Blood Pressure Measurement explains the method of **auscultation** to measure blood pressure.

Mean Arterial Pressure. SBP typically averages 120 mm Hg, and the diastolic pressure equals 80 mm Hg in young, healthy adults at rest. The average or **mean arterial pressure (MAP)** is slightly lower than the arithmetic average of systolic and diastolic pressure because the heart remains in diastole longer than in systole. MAP averages 93 mm Hg at rest; this represents the average force exerted by the blood against the arterial walls during a cardiac cycle. MAP computes as (with BP standing for blood pressure):

> MAP = Diastolic BP + [0.333(Systolic BP − Diastolic BP)]

For a person with an 89 mm Hg diastolic blood pressure and 127 mm Hg systolic pressure, MAP equals 89 + [0.333 (127 − 89)], or 102 mm Hg.

Cardiac Output and Total Peripheral Resistance

The hemodynamic equation that relates blood pressure to cardiac output and total peripheral resistance rearranges to illustrate factors that determine either cardiac output or total peripheral resistance:

> Cardiac output = MAP ÷ Total peripheral resistance

> Total peripheral resistance = MAP ÷ Cardiac output

MAP (computed from systolic and diastolic blood pressures) and cardiac output estimate the change in total resistance to blood flow in the transition from rest to physical movement. Suppose SBP at rest equals 120 mm Hg, diastolic pressure equals 80 mm Hg (MAP = 93.3 mm Hg), and cardiac output averages 5.0 L·min^{-1}. Substituting these values in the formula for total peripheral resistance yields 18.7 mm Hg·L^{-1} blood flow (93.3 mm Hg ÷ 5.0 L·min^{-1}). Resistance to peripheral blood flow *decreases* dramatically during strenuous physical activity, when systolic pressure increases considerably more than diastolic pressure and cardiac output increases six

Mean Arterial Pressure: Pulmonary Versus Systemic Circulation

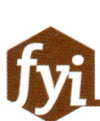

Significant differences exist in blood pressure and vascular resistance in the lung's blood vessels compared to vessels in the systemic circulation. For example, the mean arterial blood pressure in the pulmonary artery averages about 15 mm Hg, whereas the pressure in the large systemic arteries averages about 95 mm Hg. With equivalent blood flow in both circulations, vascular resistance is lower in the pulmonary circuit. This accounts for the difference in blood vessel structure. Pulmonary arterial vessels are relatively thin walled with little smooth muscle compared with their thicker, more muscular systemic counterparts.

or seven times the resting value in an elite endurance athlete. For example, if cardiac output equals 35.0 L·min⁻¹ and MAP equals 130 mm Hg (systolic = 210 mm Hg; diastolic = 90 mm Hg), then resistance to blood flow in the systemic circulation averages 3.71 mm Hg·L⁻¹·min⁻¹, or five times *less* than the resting value.

The Capillaries

The arterioles branch and form smaller and less muscular vessels 10 to 20 microns (μm) in diameter called **metarterioles**. These vessels end in microscopically small capillary vessels, the smallest in the body, which generally contain 6% of the total blood volume. In skeletal muscle, with its widely varying oxygen requirements, each metarteriole interfaces with 8 to 10 capillaries. The capillary diameter ranges between 7 and 10 μm (approximately 1/100th mm). Figure 15.4 illustrates that the capillary wall usually contains a compressed single endothelial cell layer. Some capillaries are so narrow that only one blood cell at a time can squeeze through its 3 to 4 μm diameter. In many instances, the extensive capillary proliferation causes their walls to abut surrounding cell membranes. Capillary density varies throughout the body, depending on a particular tissue's location and function. Capillary density in human skeletal muscle averages between 2000 and 3000 capillaries per square millimeter. Capillary density is considerably greater in heart muscle where no cell lies farther than 0.008 mm/0.0003 in from its nearest capillary.

The **precapillary sphincter**, a smooth muscle ring encircling the vessel at its origin, controls capillary diameter. Sphincter constriction and relaxation provide an important local means to regulate blood flow within a specific tissue to meet its metabolic requirements. Chapter 16 discusses specific factors that autoregulate local blood supply.

 See the animation "Measuring Blood Pressure" on Lippincott Connect to view this process.

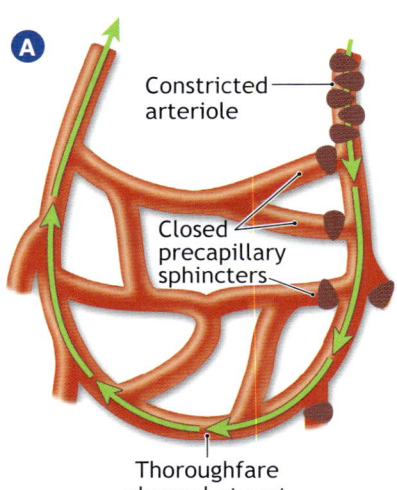

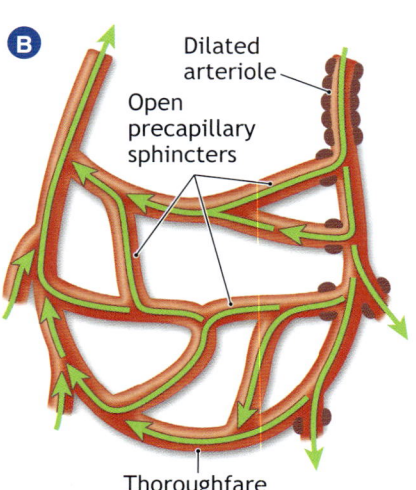

FIGURE 15.5. Capillary blood flow during rest **(A)** and exercise **(B)**, with the pulsatile blood flow pattern from rest, during exercise, and in recovery.

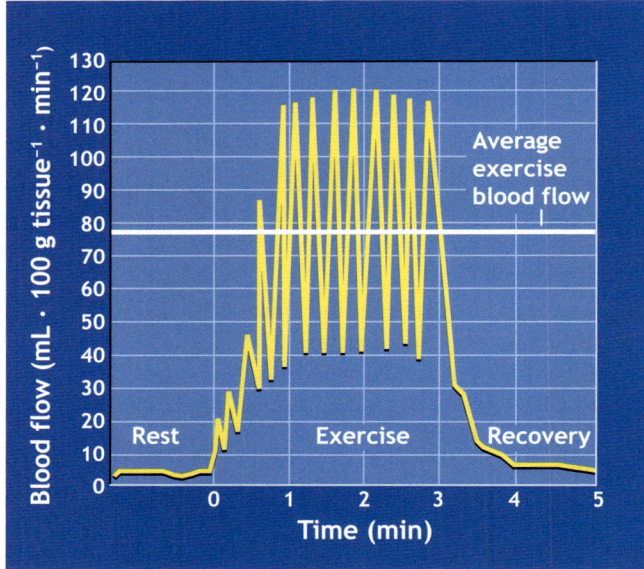

FIGURE 15.5 depicts a generalized view for capillary blood flow dynamics within muscle during rest **(A)** and physical activity **(B)**. In this example for resting gastrocnemius muscle, blood flow each minute averages 5 mL for every 100 g of muscle tissue. Fewer capillaries function at rest than are available. For a muscle that weighs 600 g, approximately 30 mL blood flows through it at rest each minute. During physical activity at any intensity level, from slow walking to sprint running, blood flow increases rapidly to meet metabolic demands as previously dormant or "unused" capillaries open to accommodate the increased flow of blood. Capillary diameter, red blood cell size, and blood viscosity all affect capillary blood flow. The dark red knobs in the figure indicate the closing or opening of dormant capillaries. The right graphic shows that blood flows in a pulsatile pattern under all conditions. During activity, blood flow to active muscles increases rapidly as previously "unused" capillaries dilate. Two factors trigger precapillary sphincter relaxation to open more capillaries and thus increase total blood flow:

1. Driving force from increased local blood pressure plus intrinsic neural control
2. Local metabolites (e.g., lactate, H⁺, CO₂) produced in physical activity

In a Practical Sense

Blood Pressure Measurement

DEFINITIONS

Blood pressure represents the force exerted by blood against the arterial walls during a cardiac cycle. Systolic blood pressure (SBP), the higher of the two pressure measurements, occurs during ventricular contraction (systole) as the heart propels 70 to 100 mL of blood into the aorta. Following systole, the ventricles relax (diastole), the arteries recoil, and arterial pressure continually declines as blood flows into the periphery and the heart refills with blood. The lowest pressure attained during ventricular relaxation represents diastolic blood pressure. **Pulse pressure** refers to the difference between systolic and diastolic pressures. Moderately high blood pressure, 130/80 mm Hg, rather than 140/90 mm Hg, which previously defined this condition, should initially be treated with lifestyle changes and in some patients with medication based on the American College of Cardiology and American Heart Association guidelines (www.ahajournals.org/doi/full/10.1161/HCQ.0000000000000057). Refer to Chapter 32 for a more complete discussion of current hypertension classification stages.

PROCEDURES

The auscultation blood pressure method (listening to sounds; first described in 1902 by Russian vascular surgeon Nikolai S. Korotkoff, 1874–1920; see www.ahajournals.org/doi/full/10.1161/01.cir.94.2.116) follows this typical measurement sequence seated in a quiet room after resting quietly for 3 to 5 min:

1. Locate the brachial artery at the inner upper arm side, approximately 1 in above the elbow bend.
2. Take the cuff's free end and secure it snugly (but not tightly) around the upper arm using an appropriately sized cuff depending on the size of the person (child, adult, or overweight/obese person). Verify the cuff aligns with the brachial artery.
3. Place the stethoscope bell below the antecubital space over the brachial artery, with the connecting tube, inflation bulb, and pressure gauge from the cuff exiting toward the arm.
4. Before inflating the cuff, verify the air-release switch remains closed (knob turns clockwise).
5. Inflate the cuff with quick, even pumps to about 160 to 200 mm Hg.
6. Gradually release cuff pressure about 3 to 5 mm·s^{-1} by slowly opening the air-release knob (counterclockwise turn) and record the pressure reading when you hear the first sound. Turbulence from the sudden blood rush produces the sound as the formerly closed artery briefly opens during the highest pressure in the cardiac cycle. The first sound represents SBP.
7. Continue to reduce cuff pressure, noting when the sound "muffles" (fourth phase diastolic pressure) and when the sound disappears (fifth phase diastolic pressure), which clinicians record as diastolic blood pressure.
8. If the measured pressure exceeds 140/90 mm Hg, allow a 10-min quiet rest and repeat the procedure one or two more times, using the average to represent the most representative blood pressure on that date and time (www.nhlbi.nih.gov/guidelines/hypertension/express.pdf).

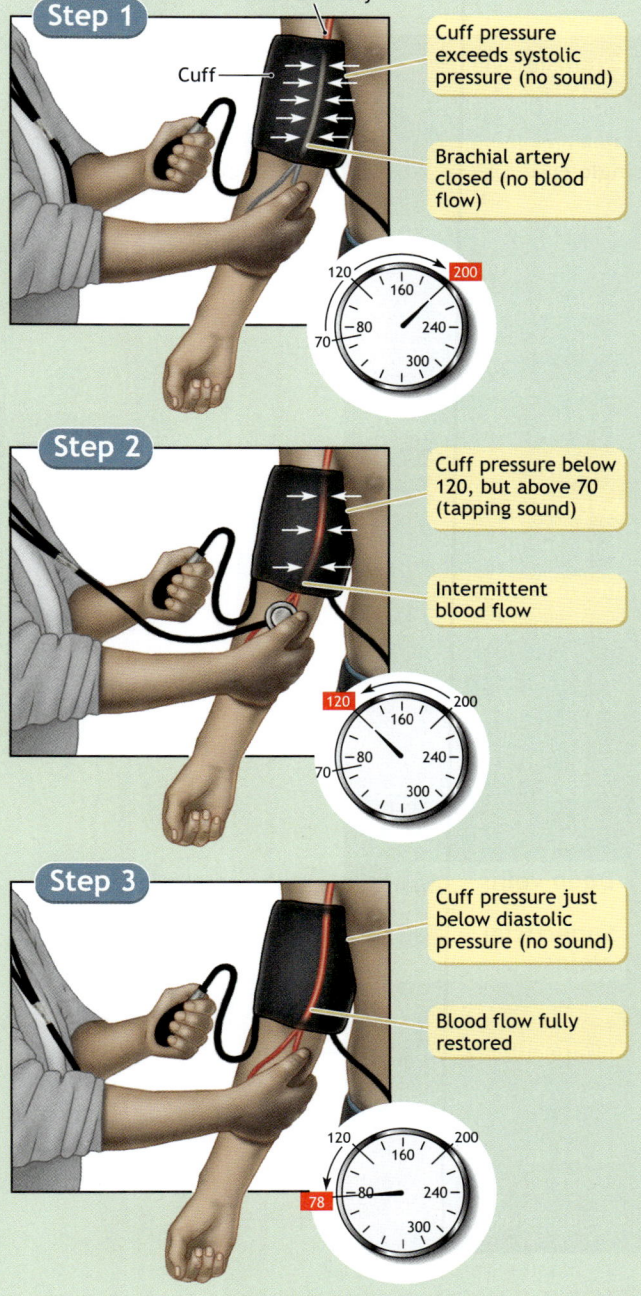

Blood flow in active muscle increases almost linearly with exercise intensity and reaches peak values at maximal exertion from the combined small increase in perfusion pressure with massive vasodilatation.[6] During strenuous activity, sustained local blood flow increases 15 to 20 times the resting value. Blood flow to gastrocnemius muscle tissue averages about 80 mL per 100 g·min^{-1}. Capillary microcirculation branching increases its cross-sectional area to about 800 times the 1-in.- diameter aorta. Blood flow velocity relates inversely to the vasculature's cross section as follows:

$$\text{Velocity, cm·s}^{-1} = \text{Volume flow, cm}^3\text{·s}^{-1} \div \text{Cross-sectional area, cm}^2$$

Velocity progressively decreases as blood moves toward and enters the capillaries. It takes approximately 1.5 s for a single blood cell to pass through an average-sized capillary. The total capillary wall surface area exceeds by 100 times an average adult's external body surface. A huge surface area with a slow blood flow rate of approximately 0.5 to 1.0 mm·s^{-1} provides an effective exchange mechanism between the blood and neighboring tissues.

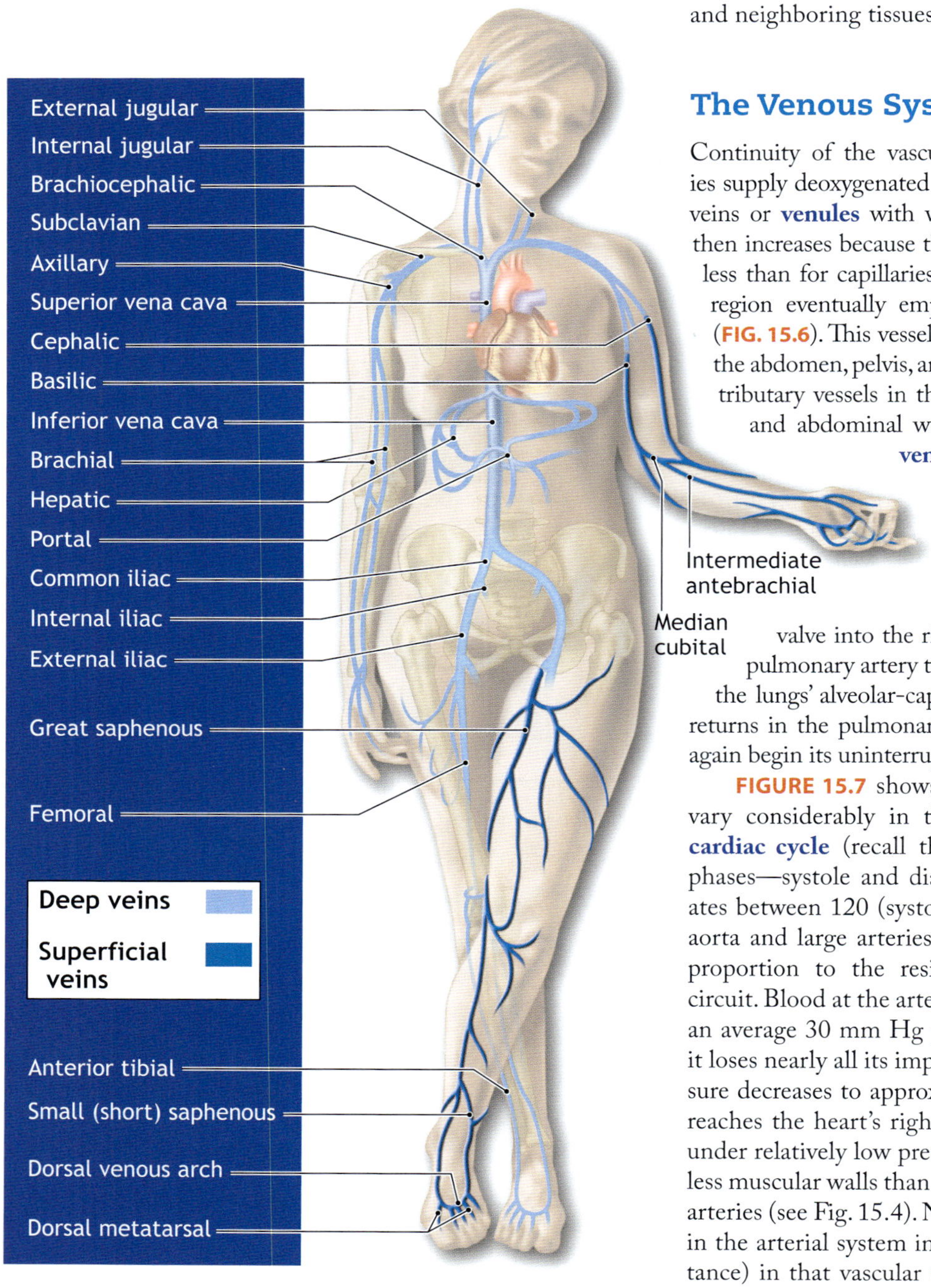

The Venous System

Continuity of the vascular system progresses as the capillaries supply deoxygenated blood at almost a trickle into the small veins or **venules** with which they merge. Blood flow velocity then increases because the venous system cross-sectional area is less than for capillaries. The smaller veins in the body's lower region eventually empty into the large **inferior vena cava** (**FIG. 15.6**). This vessel returns blood to the right atrium from the abdomen, pelvis, and lower extremities. Venous blood from tributary vessels in the head, neck, shoulder regions, thorax, and abdominal wall flows into the 7-cm-long **superior vena cava** to join the inferior vena cava at heart level. The mixture of blood that drains the upper and lower body, called **mixed venous blood**, then enters the right atrium. From there it flows downward through the tricuspid valve into the right ventricle for pumping through the pulmonary artery to the lungs. Gas exchange takes place in the lungs' alveolar-capillary network; oxygenated blood then returns in the pulmonary veins to the heart's left side to once again begin its uninterrupted passage throughout the body.

FIGURE 15.7 shows how blood pressure and blood flow vary considerably in the systemic circulation. During the **cardiac cycle** (recall that cardiac activity divides into two phases—systole and diastole), resting blood pressure fluctuates between 120 (systolic) and 80 (diastolic) mm Hg in the aorta and large arteries. The pressure then declines in direct proportion to the resistance encountered in the vascular circuit. Blood at the arteriole-capillary end, for example, exerts an average 30 mm Hg pressure. As blood enters the venules, it loses nearly all its impetus for forward movement. The pressure decreases to approximately 0 mm Hg by the time blood reaches the heart's right atrium. The venous system operates under relatively low pressure, so veins need much thinner and less muscular walls than the thicker-walled and less distensible arteries (see Fig. 15.4). Note in Figure 15.7 that blood pressure in the arterial system inversely relates to the total area (resistance) in that vascular tree section. For example, when total vascular area approaches 5000 cm^2, blood flow velocity reaches its lowest level.

FIGURE 15.6. Major superficial (*dark blue*) and deep (*light blue*) veins distribution.

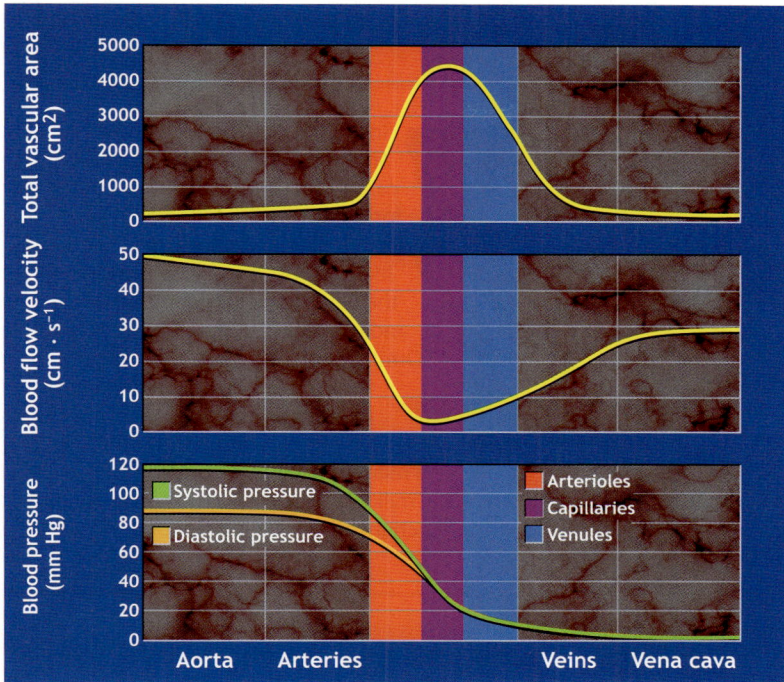

FIGURE 15.7. Resting blood flow and blood pressure in the systemic circulation.
(piyaphong/Shutterstock)

a person would faint from reduced venous return and resulting diminished brain blood flow every time they stood up.

Active Vasculature?

Contemporary exercise physiologists have debated the venous system's role as an active vasculature to mobilize blood volume.[48] At rest, the systemic venous vessels normally contain about 65% of the body's total blood volume, making the veins **capacitance vessels** that serve as blood reservoirs. This has led to speculation about the veins' role as an **active blood reservoir** to either retard or facilitate blood delivery to the systemic circulation. The current prevailing opinion maintains that the major contribution to blood mobilization in physical activity occurs by active muscle pump action and passive effect from arterial vasoconstriction, not visceral venoconstriction, which reduces downstream venous pressure.

Venous Return

The low blood pressure in the venous system poses a problem that a unique structural characteristic of veins partly resolves. **FIGURE 15.8.** shows that thin, membranous, flaplike **valves** spaced at short intervals within veins allow blood to flow in only one direction toward the heart. Valves situated in the veins prevent blood flowing backward (**A**), but this does not hinder the normal one-way blood flow shown in (**B**). Blood moves through veins (**C**) by the nearby active muscle acting as a force to propel blood forward (called muscle pump action), or in (**D**) by contraction of smooth muscle bands within the wall of the veins. This scenario now seems logical, but in 1759 when William Harvey in England first proposed the idea to his colleagues during a medical lecture and demonstration (see, e.g., www.nndb.com/people/269/000085014/), he was vilified for daring to contradict prior medical dogma of almost 2000 years since the physician Galen (129 to c. 200 AD), an early but influential medical practitioner, posited that blood simply "sloshed" back and forth through the heart and blood vessels (see section titled William Harvey in the Introduction).

The low pressure in the venous circuit means that the smallest muscular contractions, or even minor pressure changes within the thoracic cavity with breathing (**respiratory pump**), readily compress the veins.[22] The alternate vein compression and relaxation, including one-way valve action, provides a "milking" or wringing action that propels blood back to the heart. Without valves, blood would stagnate as it sometimes does in extremity veins. Without this protective mechanism,

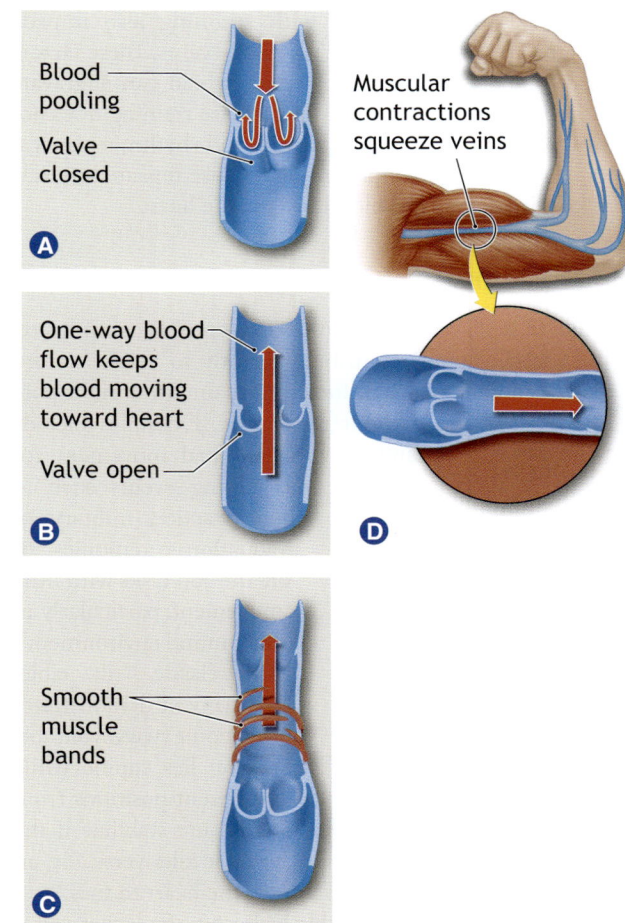

FIGURE 15.8. The valves in veins ensures that blood flows on its one-way return to the heart to prevent blood pooling and facilitate venous return to the heart.

Varicose Veins

Sometimes the valves within a vein fail to maintain their one-way blood flow, a defective condition termed *varicose veins*. This condition usually occurs in lower extremity surface veins. Accordingly, blood gathers in them as they become excessively distended and painful, which impairs the affected area's circulation. In severe cases, the venous wall becomes inflamed and progressively deteriorates—a condition called *phlebitis*. This necessitates vessel removal either surgically or nonsurgically by injecting solutions that irritate the vessel's surface membranes in a process termed *sclerotherapy*. This procedure and laser ablation (also known as photoablation, which removes material from a surface by laser beam irradiation) cause the vein to collapse, fuse, and eventually shrivel up; eventually some blood flow reroutes to the deeper veins.

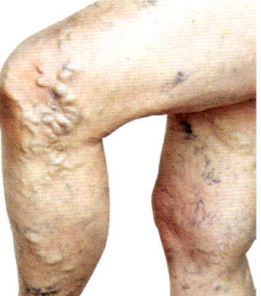
nixki/Shutterstock

Individuals with varicose veins should avoid static, straining resistance-type activities. During sustained, nonrhythmic muscle actions, the muscle and ventilatory "pumps" contribute little to venous return. Increased intrathoracic and abdominal pressures (Valsalva maneuver) with straining also impede venous return by literally squeezing on the veins. These factors act to pool blood in lower body veins, which can aggravate an existing varicose vein condition. Exercise training does not prevent varicose veins; however, regular and rhythmic physical activity can minimize complications because repeated muscle actions continually propel blood toward the heart.

Venous Pooling

Rhythmic muscular activity with vascular tree compression (i.e., the muscle pump) contributes greatly to venous return that many people faint when forced to maintain upright posture without movement. Examples include standing with minimal movement for long periods during events such as choir practice, military or graduation ceremonies, or on-the-job tasks with little movement, particularly in hot, humid environments. The classic "tilt table" experiment demonstrates this point (www.youtube.com/watch?v=5H5FZTAic7c). The person lies supine while secured on a "tilt table" that pivots to different positions from the horizontal. Heart rate and blood pressure stabilize if the person remains horizontal. When the table tilts vertically, an uninterrupted blood column exists from the heart to toes.

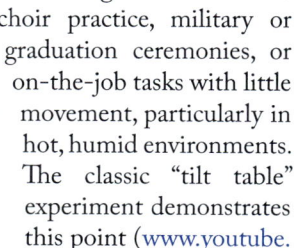

This creates an 80 to 100 mm Hg hydrostatic force that causes blood to pool in the lower extremities. Fluid backs up in the capillary bed and seeps into the surrounding tissues causing swelling or *edema*. Reduced venous return reduces both cardiac output and arterial blood pressure. Simultaneously, heart rate accelerates and blood mobilizes from the splanchnic region by upstream vasoconstriction causing passive mobilization from downstream veins. Some active venoconstriction to counter venous pooling effects also may occur. Forcing the person to maintain the upright position induces fainting from insufficient cerebral blood supply (i.e., reduced cardiac output). Tilting the person either horizontally or head down immediately restores circulation and consciousness. In Chapter 27, we discuss a tilt table experiment applied in experimental microgravity research to induce symptoms and corresponding responses to weightlessness when test subjects remain in a 6° tilt-down position for weeks at a time.

The pressurized suits worn by supersonic aircraft test pilots, as well as special support stockings for individuals with varicose veins or poor venous return from swollen ankles in the upright position, reduce the hydrostatic blood shifts to lower extremity veins in the upright position. A swimming pool provides a similar supportive effect in upright activity because the water's external support facilitates venous return.

External Compression Facilitates Venous Return

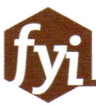

In sedentary older individuals and those with compromised cardiovascular function who drive long distances or take frequent airline flights, wearing full-length leg "support" stockings compresses the veins to minimize blood pooling and prevent blood clot formation. During surgical operations and for 3 to 4 days into recovery, mechanical pneumatic cuffs worn around the lower limbs alternately compress and relax lower limb musculature to mechanically provide a "milking" action to prevent blood pooling and reduce the chances for a blood clot or deep vein thrombosis in those limbs.

sportpoint/Shutterstock

INTEGRATIVE QUESTION

The ancient Romans executed individuals by securing their arms and legs to a cross mounted in the vertical position. What are the physiologic responses that cause death under these circumstances?

Hypertension

Systolic pressure at rest can exceed 300 mm Hg in individuals whose arteries exhibit the following two characteristics:

1. "Hardening" with fatty materials deposited within their walls or the vessel's connective tissue layer has thickened
2. Excessive resistance to peripheral blood flow due to neural hyperactivity or kidney malfunction

Diastolic pressure also can exceed 100 mm Hg under the above two conditions. Abnormally high blood pressure, termed **hypertension**, chronically strains the cardiovascular system, and, left untreated, eventually damages arterial vessels and lead to arteriosclerosis, heart disease, stroke, and kidney failure.[29]

 See the animation "Hypertension" on Lippincott Connect to view this process.

FIGURE 15.9 shows the percentages in the U.S. population with hypertension (systolic pressure >130 mm Hg; diastolic pressure >80 mm Hg) and its increased prevalence with age. Hypertensive risk increases with age, with lifetime risk exceeding 80%. More than three quarters of those older than age 70 have hypertension.[8] An elevated SBP provides a more reliable and accurate way to predict hypertension risk and need for treatment than diastolic blood pressure, particularly during middle age.[32,46]

Prevalence

As America continues to become more overweight and accumulate excess fat, hypertension rate also has been increasing to alarmingly high levels. Hypertensive Americans have increased to about 108 million from 50 million 20 years ago.[64]

Current estimates place nearly 50% of the current adult U.S. population in the hypertensive category.[64] An estimated 1.13 billion people have hypertension, yet fewer than 1 in 5 can control it (www.cdc.gov/bloodpressure/facts.htm). Relatively high hypertension prevalence exists among African Americans who exhibit a higher hypertension and ischemic stroke risk than Caucasians (see Fig. 15.9). Their predisposition for hypertension reflects reduced sensitivity to nitric oxide's vasodilating action[7,18,49] (see Chapter 16, Nitric Oxide Autoregulates Tissue Blood Flow). Projections show that by 2030, hypertension prevalence will increase 10 to 15% from 2019 estimates. An individual on hypertension medication still classifies as hypertensive, even if blood pressure remains within the normal range.

fyi Active Recovery "Cool-Down"

The interaction between muscular contractions and blood flow through the venous system provides a sound rationale to continue walking or jogging at a slow pace following strenuous physical activity. Moderate activity in recovery or "cooling down" facilitates blood flow through the vascular circuit, including myocardial blood vessels. Active recovery also facilitates lactate removal from the blood.

Tyler Olson/Shutterstock

Continuing mild physical activity for 3 to 5 min may blunt potential deleterious effects on cardiac function from elevated epinephrine and norepinephrine catecholamines, glucocorticoids, and aldosterone release during the activity.[9,10,65]

Uncorrected hypertension often leads to congestive heart failure, kidney disease, myocardial infarction, or stroke. In contrast, reducing blood pressure effectively prevents stroke and other vascular events including heart failure, even among the elderly.[4] Lowering SBP 2 mm Hg reduces deaths from stroke by 6% and heart disease by 4%. In general, lowering high blood pressure also may reduce dementia progression and cognitive impairment, which are more prevalent in those with hypertension.[44]

Treatment Strategies

Preventing a chronic rise in blood pressure serves a crucial function. Even when elevated blood pressure normalizes through lifestyle changes or medication, the disease risk remains higher than if the person had never become hypertensive. Blood pressure should be checked periodically because it often progresses unnoticed for years. Effective prevention strategies include substantially increasing regular physical activity to at least 1 hr daily and modest weight loss (especially in the overweight and obese), stress management, smoking cessation, reduced sodium and alcohol consumption, increased dietary nitrate, and adequate calcium and magnesium intake.[1,2,27,41,57,60,62]

A diet containing potassium-rich foods is also an important component as

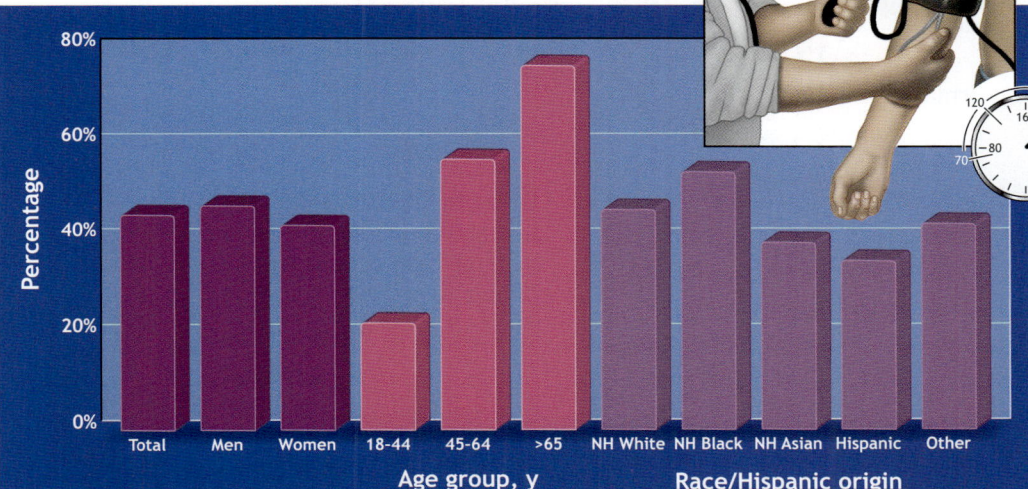

FIGURE 15.9. Hypertension prevalence among U.S. adults ages 18 and older considering criteria from the American College of Cardiology and American Heart Association's (ACC/AHA) 2017 Hypertension Clinical Practice Guideline by Sex, Age and Race/Hispanic Origin. NH = non-Hispanic.
(Data source: National Center for Health Statistics, Centers for Disease Control and Examination Survey. NHANES, 2013–2016.)

In a Practical Sense

Hypertension Effects on Tissues and Organs

Effects in blood vessels
Damage to the interior arterial wall thickens it, thus reducing the space for transporting blood.

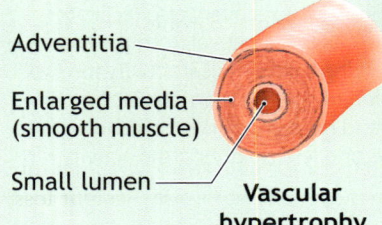

Vascular hypertrophy / Normal blood vessel

The arterial wall may dilate or bulge (aneurysm) and burst, causing blood loss, tissue damage, and death.

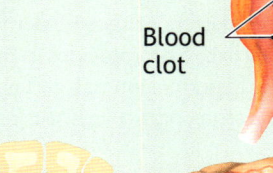

Blood clot

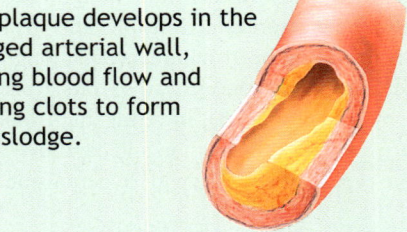

Atherosclerosis

Fatty plaque develops in the damaged arterial wall, clogging blood flow and allowing clots to form and dislodge.

Effects in brain
Blood clots can impair blood flow and cause strokes (and hemorrhage) from aneurysms that burst from increasing pressure.

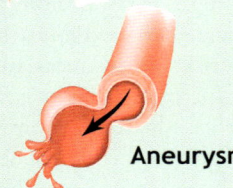

Blood clot / Aneurysm

Blood flow in heart
The right side of the heart receives blood from the body and delivers this deoxygenated blood to the lungs. The left side of the heart receives oxygen-rich blood from the lungs and pumps it to all body organs and tissues.

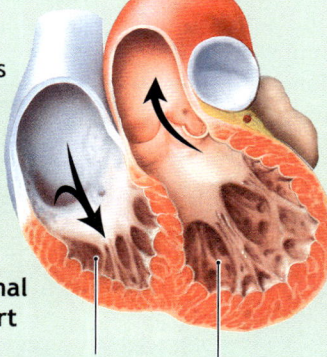

Normal heart — Right ventricle, Left ventricle, Aorta

Effects in eye
Development of abnormal retinal vasculature.

Effects in heart
The left heart must pump more forcefully against a higher pressure from increased arterial resistance (increased preload), causing the left ventricle to enlarge and fail to effectively respond to the increased pressure.

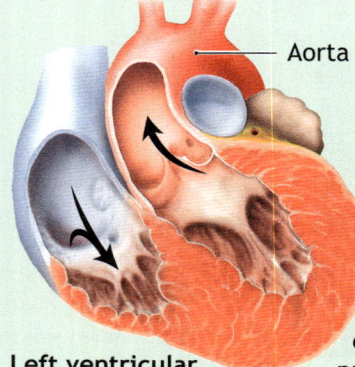

Left ventricular hypertrophy

Effects in kidneys
Damage to kidneys may cause hypertension from their failure to properly regulate salt and water balance.

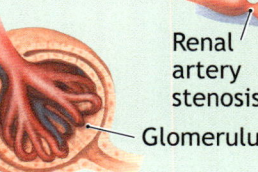

Renal artery stenosis / Glomerulus

fyi Crucifixion Physiology

In the ancient world until about the 4th century CE, the ultimate punishment for the ruling Persians, Carthaginians, and Romans was executing traitors, convicts, and those convicted for civil and capital crimes. The victims were secured to a patibulum (crossbar) with rope or nails that punctured the ends around the extremities to keep the body from falling from the stipes (upright post). Death occurred mainly from blood pooling in the thorax or lower extremities from the prolonged vertical head up or head down suspension position. This produced hypovolemic shock, with accompanying pulmonary edema and asphyxia (suffocation from oxygen deprivation).[12] Asphyxia was not the only mechanism to hasten death—others included pulmonary embolism (blood clot in the lungs) and cardiac rupture from hanging upside down, suspension trauma, and shock. Some have argued that traumatic shock complicated by trauma-induced coagulopathy was a major contributing factor in the execution, not simply excruciating torture as a rapid means to hasten death.

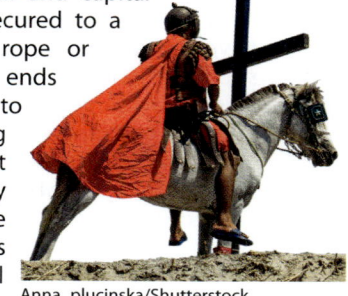
Anna_plucinska/Shutterstock

Sources:
Bordes S, et al. The clinical anatomy of crucifixion. *Clin Anat*. 2020;33:12.
Bergeron JW. The crucifixion of Jesus: review of hypothesized mechanisms of death and implications of shock and trauma-induced coagulopathy. *J Forensic Leg Med*. 2012;19:113.
Habermas G, et al. Medical views on the death by crucifixion of Jesus Christ. *Proc (Bayl Univ Med Cent)*. 2021;34:748.
Retief FP, Cilliers L. The history and pathology of crucifixion. *S Afr Med J*. 2003;93:938.

---

a nonpharmacologic approach to blood pressure control. Regular aerobic physical activity lowers systolic and diastolic blood pressure, while vigorous activity produces a greater lowering effect on diastolic pressure than more moderate physical activity.[52] Low cardiorespiratory fitness remains a significant hypertension risk predictor, whereas body weight emerges as a predictor only for persons in the overweight range.[45]

In addition to modifying lifestyle, hypertension treatment uses medication to reduce extracellular fluid volume and/or peripheral resistance to blood flow. Lowering the odds for having to take hypertension medication relates to both an increase in physical activity level and physical fitness level.[61] A prudent diet, weight control, and regular, moderate physical activity should precede pharmacologic treatment for **stage 1 hypertension** (130 to 139 mm Hg systolic or 80 to 89 mm Hg diastolic) and **stage 2 hypertension** (systolic at ≥140 mm Hg or diastolic at least 90 mm Hg). This is because of possible harmful effects of drug therapy on other coronary artery disease risk factors. The classification *hypertensive crisis* applies to a SBP greater than 180 mm Hg and/or diastolic pressure greater than 120 mm Hg (see In a Practical Sense: Hypertensive Crisis—When to Call 911!).

Lifestyle Choices

1. Every 20-lb weight loss reduces SBP 5 to 20 mm Hg.
2. Eating a lower fat diet rich in vegetables, fruits, and legumes (e.g., DASH diet, see Chapter 3) reduces SBP 8 to 14 mm Hg.
3. Increase aerobic physical activity to 30 min · d^{-1} reduces SBP 4 to 9 mm Hg.
4. Limit sodium intake to ≤1500 mg · d^{-1} reduces SBP 2 to 8 mm Hg.
5. Limit alcohol intake to ≤1 drink · d^{-1} lowers SBP 2 to 4 mm Hg.

Chapter 32 discusses the role of regular aerobic activity and resistance training to treat moderate hypertension.

Pharmacologic Treatment

It may be necessary to seek pharmacologic treatment if an initial 6- to 12-month treatment regimen with diet, weight loss, reduced alcohol intake, and regular physical activity proves ineffective to treat hypertension.

Eleven blood pressure medication categories are used to treat hypertension:

- **Thiazide diuretics:** Referred to as "water pills" act on the kidneys to eliminate sodium and water to reduce blood volume and hence blood pressure
- **Angiotensin-converting enzyme (ACE) inhibitors:** Inhibit the ACE enzyme, which constricts arterial blood vessels and stimulates the adrenal cortex to release aldosterone, to cause the kidneys to retain sodium and salt; also dilates blood vessels to reduce blood pressure
- **Angiotensin II receptor blockers:** Relax blood vessels by blocking the natural chemical that narrows blood vessels
- **Calcium channel blockers:** Relax blood vessels and slow the heart rate
- **Alpha-blockers:** Reduce nerve impulses to blood vessels to minimize natural chemical effects that narrow the vessels
- **Alpha-beta blockers:** Slow the heart to reduce blood pumped through the vascular circuit
- **Beta-blockers:** Reduce the heart's workload and dilate blood vessels, causing the heart to beat slowly with less force
- **Aldosterone antagonists:** Reduce salt and fluid retention, which contribute to elevated blood pressure
- **Renin inhibitors:** Blunt kidneys' renin production to lower blood pressure
- **Vasodilators:** Act on muscle component of arterial wall to prevent tightening and narrowing
- **Central-acting agents:** Prevent brain from signaling the nervous system to increase heart rate and narrow blood vessel diameter

Blood Pressure Response to Physical Activity

The blood pressure response to physical activity varies with the activity mode.

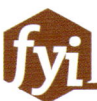

Record Blood Pressure in Both Arms

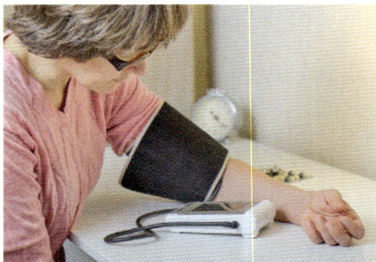
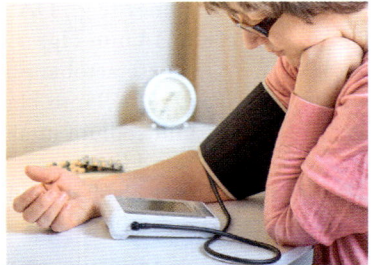

Rudolfovich/Shutterstock (both images)

It may be a good idea to obtain systolic blood pressure (SBP) in both arms because a difference in readings acts as an independent heart disease risk factor. About 4400 healthy individuals (56% female) aged 40 and older from the Framingham Heart Study were followed over an average 13 years. During this period, 598 participants suffered a first heart attack, stroke, or other cardiovascular complication. In those individuals, more than 25% had a 10 mm Hg or greater between-arm difference in SBP that increased cardiac event risk by nearly 40%. The increased risk remained independent for age, cholesterol level, body mass index, hypertension, or other known cardiovascular risk factors. Studies have linked subclavian artery stenosis, which supplies blood to the upper arm, to the differences in interarm blood pressure. In this regard, a systolic interarm blood pressure difference that exceeds 15 mm Hg may serve as an upper limit cutoff to indicate significant valvular disease risk and subsequent death.

Sources:
Clark CE, et al. Association of a difference in systolic blood pressure between arms with vascular disease and mortality: a systematic review and meta-analysis. *Lancet.* 2012;379:905.
Sato K, et al. Association of physical activity with a systolic blood pressure difference between arms in older people. *Geriatr Gerontol Int.* 2018;18:95.
Visaria A, et al. Leg and arm adiposity is inversely associated with diastolic hypertension in young and middle-aged United States adults. *Clin Hypertens.* 2022;28:3.

Resistance Exercise

Straining muscle actions, particularly the concentric (shortening) and/or static phase muscle actions, mechanically compress peripheral arterial vessels supplying the active muscles. Arterial vascular compression dramatically increases total peripheral resistance and reduces muscle perfusion. Muscle blood flow decreases in proportion to the percentage of maximum force capacity exerted. In an attempt to restore muscle blood flow, substantial increases occur in sympathetic nervous system activity, cardiac output, and MAP. The hypertensive response magnitude relates directly to effort intensity and muscle mass activated.[16,24,39] Young and older healthy adults have similar short-term hemodynamic responses to resistance-type activities.[36,37] In resistance-trained individuals, the elevated blood pressure response is considerably reduced.

1. In one of the textbook authors' laboratories, blood pressure was measured in normotensive subjects directly with a pressure transducer connected to a catheter inserted into the femoral artery. Measurements were made during three exercise modes: (1) isometric bench press performed at 25, 50, 75, and 100% of maximal voluntary contraction (MVC); (2) free-weight bench press performed at 25 and 50% isometric MVC; and (3) hydraulic resistance bench press exercise performed "all out" for 20 s at slow and fast speeds. The results, displayed in **TABLE 15.1**, show clearly that the three exercise modes substantially increased arterial blood pressure and the heart's corresponding workload (see Rate-Pressure Product, below).

TABLE 15.1 Peak systolic and diastolic blood pressure during dynamic arm and leg exercise at similar percentages of aerobic capacity

Other studies show that movements that activate a large muscle mass and require relatively great muscle strain dramatically increase blood pressure responses.[14,30,35,40] The exacerbated blood pressure response results from two combined effects:

1. Greater cardiovascular center stimulation by active motor cortex areas
2. Large peripheral feedback from the contracting muscle mass to the cardiovascular center

The acute cardiovascular strain with heavy-resistance exercise could prove harmful to individuals with heart and vascular

Skin's Emergency Mechanism

The skin has an emergency "back-up" to guard against compromised blood supply, achieved by a structural element called an **arteriovenous anastomosis (AVA)**. This mechanism provides a natural direct or indirect communication link between two blood vessels via collateral channels to ensure blood flow continues to an area with reduced or blocked blood supply. The AVAs currently exist in the body; while other vessels can develop under "stress" from compromised blood supply conditions to support the body's response to coronary artery disease.

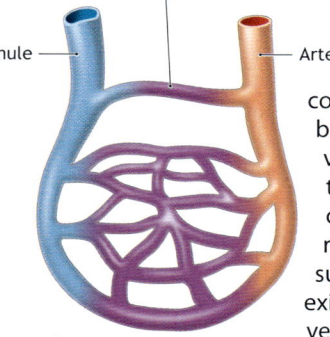

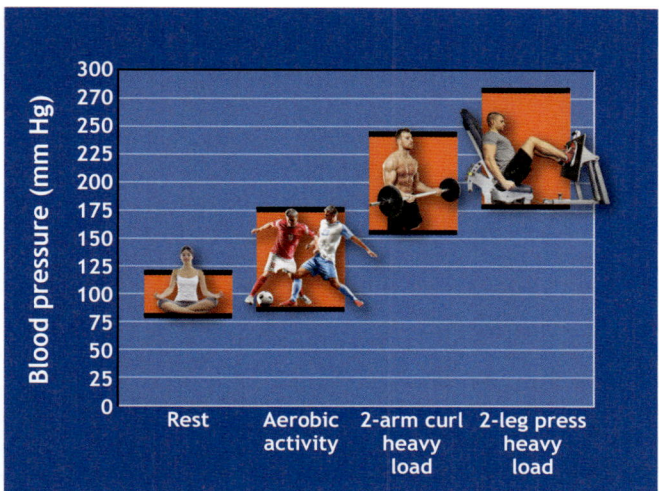

FIGURE 15.10. Heavy-resistance exercise magnifies the exercise blood pressure response (higher with legs than arms) compared with rest and recreational aerobic activities. Bar height indicates the approximate pulse pressure (difference between systolic and diastolic pressures).
(Shutterstock: Josep Suria; Syda Productions; Eugene Onischenko; Slatan)

disease, particularly individuals unfamiliar in this activity mode. **FIGURE 15.10** presents generalized responses for blood pressure during rhythmic aerobic activity and resistance exercises that activate either a relatively small or relatively large muscle mass. Note that intraocular pressure increases considerably during resistance exercise, which increases the risk for eye damage. Breath holding during the lift further magnifies the effect.[55,56]

Steady-Rate Physical Activity

During rhythmic muscular activity (e.g., jogging, swimming, bicycling, soccer, hiking), vasodilation in the active muscles reduces total peripheral resistance to enhance blood flow through a large portion of the peripheral vasculature. Alternate muscle contraction and relaxation also provide an effective force to propel blood through the vascular circuit for its return to the heart. Increased blood flow in the first few minutes during rhythmic, steady-rate activities rapidly increases systolic pressure. Blood pressure then levels off at 140 to 160 mm Hg for healthy men and women. As activity continues, systolic pressure gradually declines because the arterioles in the active muscles continue to dilate, further reducing peripheral resistance to blood flow. Diastolic blood pressure remains relatively unchanged throughout the activity period.

Graded Exercise

FIGURE 15.11 illustrates the general pattern for systolic and diastolic blood pressures during continuous, graded treadmill walking and running. After an initial rapid rise from the resting level, SBP increases linearly with exercise intensity, while diastolic pressure remains stable or decreases slightly at higher activity levels. Healthy sedentary and endurance-trained males and females demonstrate similar blood pressure responses. During maximum exertion by trained individuals with high aerobic capacity, SBP may increase to 200 mm Hg or higher, despite reduced total peripheral resistance.[39] This blood pressure level most likely reflects the heart's large cardiac output.

Upper Body Physical Activity

Physical activity with the arms produces considerably higher systolic and diastolic blood pressures and consequently greater cardiovascular strain than leg activity performed at a given maximum oxygen uptake percentage in each activity (**TABLE 15.2**).[42,53]

TABLE 15.2 Systolic and diastolic blood pressure at similar percentages of maximum oxygen uptake in dynamic arm and leg exercise

This occurs because the smaller arm muscle mass and vasculature offer greater resistance to blood flow than the larger leg mass and blood supply. Individuals with cardiovascular dysfunction should activate relatively large muscle groups (walking, bicycling, and running) in contrast to movements that engage a limited muscle mass in different activity types from shoveling, overhead hammering, and arm-crank exercise.[15,38] Chapter 17 focuses on the cardiovascular adjustments to upper body physical activity.

Recovery from Physical Activity

Upon completing a single submaximal physical activity bout, blood pressure temporarily falls below pre-exercise levels for normotensive and hypertensive individuals from an

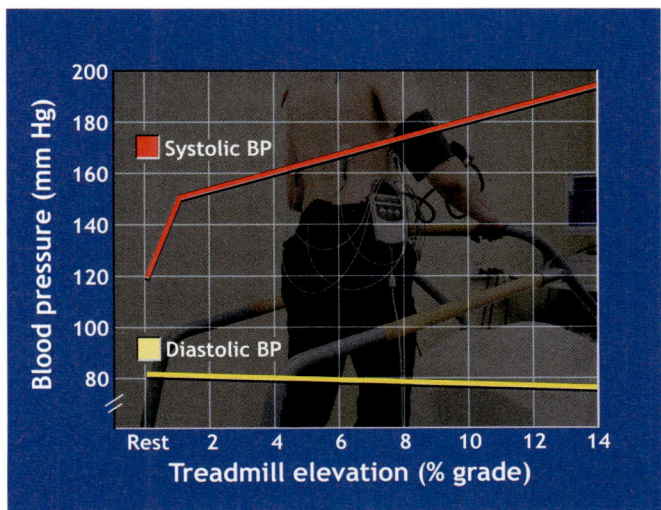

FIGURE 15.11. Generalized, systolic progressive increase and slight decrease in diastolic blood pressure responses during a continuous, maximum treadmill stress test.
(Pavel L Photo and Video/Shutterstock)

In a Practical Sense

Hypertensive Crisis: When to Call 911!

The American Heart Association recognizes five blood pressure categories:

1. **Normal:** Blood pressure normal range (≤120/80 mm Hg).
2. **Elevated:** Readings consistently range from 120 to 129 systolic and ≤80 mm Hg diastolic. Consistently elevated blood pressure requires medical supervision.
3. **Hypertension Stage 1:** Blood pressure consistently ranges ≥130 to 139 systolic or 80 to 89 mm Hg diastolic. Initial intervention includes lifestyle modifications.
4. **Hypertension Stage 2:** Blood pressure consistently ≥140/90 mm Hg or higher. Physicians usually prescribe a combination of blood pressure medications with lifestyle changes.
5. **Hypertensive Crisis:** Blood pressure rises quickly and consistently throughout the day with readings ≥180/120.

Blood Pressure Categories

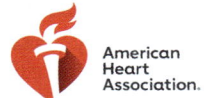

BLOOD PRESSURE CATEGORY	SYSTOLIC mm Hg (upper number)		DIASTOLIC mm Hg (lower number)
NORMAL	LESS THAN 120	and	LESS THAN 80
ELEVATED	120-129	and	LESS THAN 80
HIGH BLOOD PRESSURE (HYPERTENSION) STAGE 1	130-139	or	80-89
HIGH BLOOD PRESSURE (HYPERTENSION) STAGE 2	140 OR HIGHER	or	90 OR HIGHER
HYPERTENSIVE CRISIS (consult your doctor immediately)	HIGHER THAN 180	and/or	HIGHER THAN 120

heart.org/bplevels

Reprinted with permission https://www.heart.org/-/media/files/health-topics/high-blood-pressure/hbp-rainbow-chart-english.pdf © American Heart Association, Inc.

Uncontrolled high blood pressure consequences can include:

- Stroke
- Loss of consciousness
- Memory loss
- Heart attack
- Damage to eyes and kidneys
- Failed kidney function
- Aortic dissection
- Angina (unstable chest pain)
- Pulmonary edema (fluid backup in lungs)
- Eclampsia (persistent high blood pressure in pregnancy)
- Severe headache
- Shortness of breath
- Nosebleeds
- Severe anxiety

Two types of hypertensive crises require immediate attention as early detection enhances treatment effects:

- **Hypertensive urgency:** Blood pressure exceeds 180/120 mm Hg *without* symptoms of associated target organ damage (e.g., chest pain, shortness of breath, back pain, numbness/weakness, vision change, difficulty speaking); may require hospitalization
- **Hypertensive emergency:** Blood pressure exceeds 180/120 mm Hg *with* symptoms of associated target organ damage; DIAL 911!

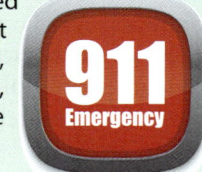

VectorDiploma/Shutterstock

unexplained peripheral vasodilation.[23,26,28,31,33] The **hypotensive response** to activity can last up to 12 hr. It occurs in response to either low- or moderate-intensity aerobic activity or resistance exercise.[34,42] One explanation posits that considerable blood remains pooled in the visceral organs and/or skeletal muscle vascular beds during recovery.[11] The venous pooling effect reduces central blood volume, which in turn decreases atrial filling pressure and systemic arterial blood pressure lowers. A prolonged increase in splanchnic, renal, or cutaneous blood flow in recovery plays only a limited contributory role to the postexercise hypotensive response.[43,59] Postexercise reductions in blood pressure further support moderate physical activity as a nonpharmacologic method to treat hypertension. Prolonged reductions in postexercise blood pressure justify recommending multiple physical activity periods interspersed throughout the day.[5]

Heart's Blood Supply

None of the blood passing through the heart's chambers directly supplies nutrients to the myocardium *per se* because no direct circulatory channels penetrate the chambers into the tissues. Instead, the heart muscle maintains its own intricate circulatory network. As **FIGURE 15.12** shows, the heart has evolved its own visible, crownlike vascular network called the **coronary circulation**.

The right and left coronary arteries emerge from the ascending aorta's upper part. Their openings form just above the semilunar valves at a point where oxygenated blood leaves the left ventricle. These arteries then curl around the heart's surface. The right coronary artery supplies predominantly the right atrium and right ventricle. The greatest blood volume flows in the left coronary artery to the left atrium and left ventricle and small sections of the right ventricle. These vessels divide and eventually form a dense capillary network within the myocardium. Blood leaves the tissues of the left ventricle through the **coronary sinus**; blood from the right ventricle exits via the **anterior cardiac veins**, which empty directly into the right atrium. The circular figure illustrates an obstructed coronary vessel that ultimately leads to tissue death or necrosis. Impaired coronary blood flow and/or arterial blockage and its resulting effects are discussed more fully in the section Impaired Blood Supply, below.

Each systole's driving force pushes some blood into the coronary arteries. The normal 200 to 250 mL · min^{-1} blood flowing within the myocardium at rest represents only about 5% of the heart's total output capacity.

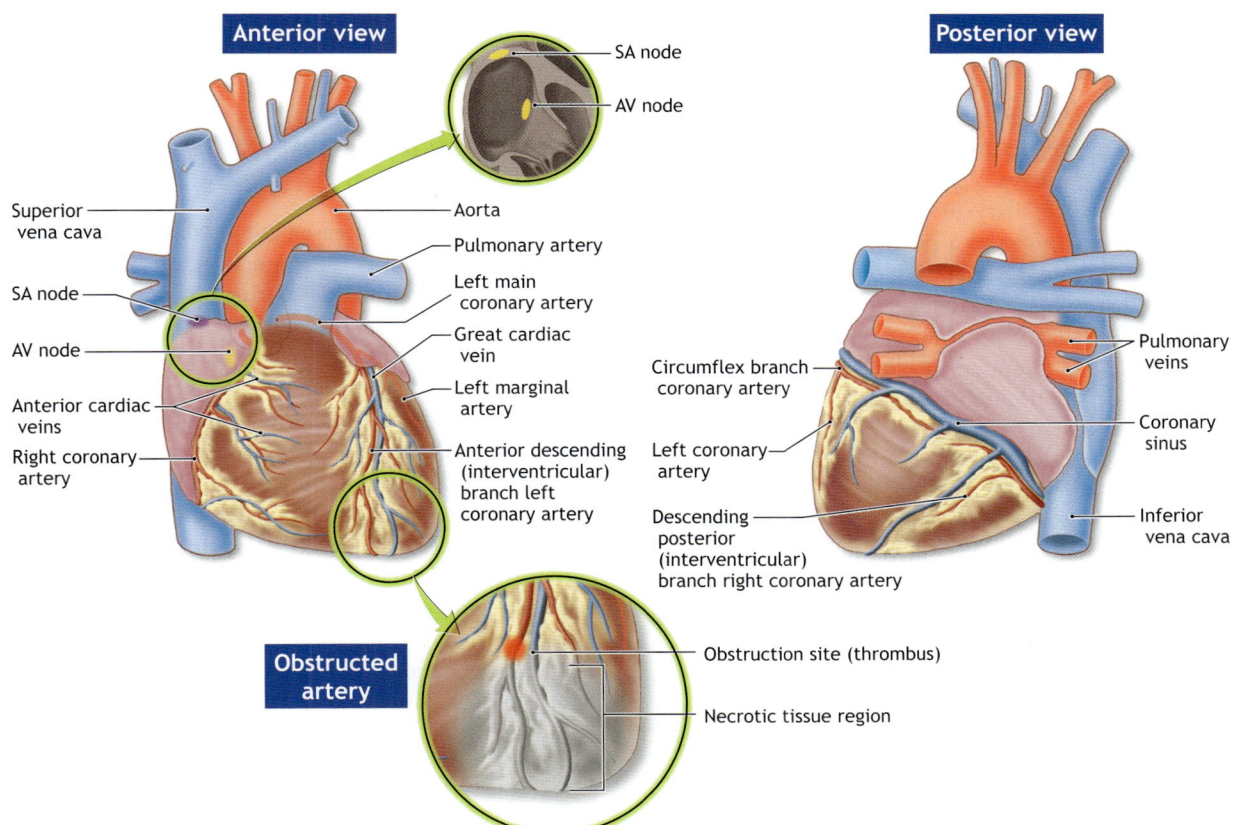

FIGURE 15.12. Coronary circulation anterior and posterior views including sinoatrial (SA) and atrioventricular (AV) nodes (*upper inset*). Arteries are shaded *red* and veins *blue*, except the pulmonary circulation colors reverse. The *lower inset* illustrates a myocardial infarction from an obstructed coronary vessel.

Myocardial Oxygen Supply and Use

At rest, the myocardium requires considerable oxygen relative to its blood flow; it extracts about 70 to 80% of oxygen from the blood in the coronary vessels. The myocardial oxygen extraction magnitude differs considerably from most other tissues, which use only about one fourth of the available blood's oxygen at rest. Consequently, a proportionate increase in coronary blood flow during physical activity essentially provides the sole mechanism to increase myocardial oxygen supply. During vigorous physical effort, coronary blood flow increases by as much as four times above the resting level. In general, coronary blood flow matches myocardial oxygen needs from increases in heart rate during physical activity. Coronary vessels dilate during exercise from the combined feedforward mechanisms (mediated by sympathetic-adrenoceptor vasodilation) and feedback control possibly from vascular-stimulating adenine nucleotides released from erythrocytes.[19,20,54] Arterial blood pressure also facilitates coronary blood flow. Increased aortic pressure during physical activity forces a proportionately greater blood volume into the coronary circulation. The blood's ebb and flow in the coronary vessels consistently fluctuates with each cardiac cycle phase. On average, about 2.5 times more blood flows in the coronary vessels during diastole than systole.

 See the animation "Myocardial Blood Flow" on Lippincott Connect to view this process.

Impaired Blood Supply

The myocardium depends on an adequate oxygen supply because, unlike skeletal muscle, it has limited anaerobic energy-generating capacity.[63] Extensive vascular perfusion supplies at least one capillary to each of the heart's muscle fibers. Tissue hypoxia provides a potent stimulus to myocardial blood flow. Impaired coronary blood flow usually produces severe and crushing chest pains termed **angina pectoris** (from Latin angere "to strangle" and pectus "chest"— translated as strangling feeling in the chest; www.hopkinsmedicine.org/health/conditions-and-diseases/angina-pectoris).

More pronounced pain occurs during physical activity because the heart's energy requirements increase considerably. A blood clot or **thrombus** lodged in a coronary vessel usually impairs normal heart function (**FIG. 15.13**). This "heart attack" or more specifically **myocardial infarction**, may be mild, or more severe with partial or complete blockage of multiple vessels, severely damaging the myocardium and requiring interventional surgical repair and rehabilitation. Fortunately, the various forms of exercise stress testing provide an effective way to evaluate myocardial blood flow and the extent of any vascular disease. Chapters 31 and 32 provide details about coronary heart disease, exercise stress testing, and the role regular physical activity plays in preventative and rehabilitative medicine.

FIGURE 15.13. **(A)** Plaque. **(B)** Thrombus.
(Adapted with permission from Moore KL, et al. *Clinically Oriented Anatomy*. 8th ed., Fig BI.9 [p. 42]. Baltimore: Wolters Kluwer, 2018; based on Willis MC. *Medical Terminology: The Language of Health Care*. Baltimore: Lippincott Williams & Wilkins; 1995.)

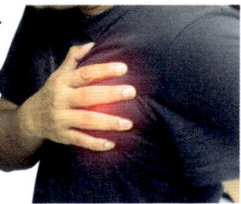
Monster e/Shutterstock

Rate-Pressure Product to Estimate Myocardial Work

Myocardial workload (and resulting oxygen uptake) uses the product of peak SBP, measured at the brachial artery, and heart rate (HR). This relative index termed the double product or **rate-pressure product (RPP)** relates closely to directly measured myocardial oxygen uptake and coronary blood flow in healthy subjects over a wide exercise intensity range, and computes as follows:

$$RPP = SBP \times HR$$

Changes in heart rate and blood pressure contribute equally to changes in RPP. Typical values for RPP range from 6000 at rest (HR = 50 b·min^{-1}; SBP = 120 mm Hg) to 40,000 (HR = 200 b·min^{-1}; SBP = 200 mm Hg) or above, depending on activity intensity and mode. Resistance training and upper body physical activity produce substantially higher heart rate and blood pressure responses, hence higher RPPs than rhythmic movements involving the lower body. Added myocardial work poses an unnecessary risk for coronary heart disease patients with compromised myocardial oxygen supply.

RPP, Physical Activity, and the Heart Disease Patient

Research with heart disease patients shows a physiologic correlation between RPP and angina pectoris onset and electrocardiographic abnormalities during physical activity. The RPP thus provides an objective yardstick to evaluate cardiac performance in clinical, surgical, or exercise interventions. The well-documented lowering of exercise heart rate and SBP (with lower RPP and myocardial oxygen requirement) helps to explain cardiac patients' improved exercise capacity before abnormal cardiac symptoms emerge following training. Prolonged, intense aerobic training also allows cardiac patients to achieve a higher exercise RPP.[13,21] In nine patients followed over a 7-year training period, RPP increased by 11.5% before ischemic symptoms appeared during graded exercise testing.[47] These findings provide indirect evidence for improved myocardial oxygenation from greater coronary vascularization or reduced obstruction from the training adaptation.

 **INTEGRATIVE QUESTION**

Explain why a training-induced increase in the rate-pressure product before a patient experiences angina or electrocardiographic abnormalities implies enhanced myocardial oxygenation.

Lippincott® Connect   Appendix H, available on Lippincott Connect, provides supplemental animations and videos on heart function, dysfunction, and treatment.

Myocardial Metabolism

The myocardium relies almost exclusively on energy released in aerobic reactions, which explains why myocardial tissues have a threefold higher oxidative capacity than skeletal muscle. The heart muscle is always "on" from birth to death, so its functional efficiency through evolutionary adaptation also must operate at a high level. The muscle fibers contain the greatest mitochondrial concentration than any other tissue; they demonstrate exceptional capacity for long-chain fatty acid catabolism as a primary means for ATP resynthesis.

FIGURE 15.14 shows specific myocardium substrate use on a percentage basis during rest and, moderate and intense physical activity. Glucose, fatty acids, and lactate formed from glycolysis provide the energy to sustain myocardial function.[3,25] At rest, these three substrates contribute to ATP resynthesis, with the most energy from free fatty acid breakdown (green bar: 60 to 70%).[17,51] Following a meal, glucose becomes the preferred energy substrate. In essence, the heart uses for energy whatever substrate it "sees" on a physiologic level. During intense physical activity when lactate efflux from active skeletal muscle into the blood increases dramatically, the heart derives its major energy by oxidizing circulating lactate. In more moderate activity, equal lipid and carbohydrate amounts provide the preferred energy fuel. In prolonged submaximal ultra-endurance hikes, swims, cycles, and runs, not illustrated, myocardial free fatty acids metabolism generates almost 80% of the total energy requirement to sustain the activity. Similar myocardial metabolism patterns exist for trained and untrained individuals. An endurance-trained person relies on greater myocardial lipid catabolism during submaximal physical activity. This response, similar to trained skeletal muscle's metabolic profile, illustrates another example of the carbohydrate-sparing influence of aerobic training.

Summary

1. Striated myocardial muscle fibers interconnect to make portions of the heart contract in a unified manner.
2. The heart functions as two separate pumps—one to receive blood from the body and pump it to the lungs for aeration (pulmonary circulation) and the other to receive oxygenated blood from the lungs to pump it throughout the systemic circulation.
3. Pressure changes created during the cardiac cycle act on heart valves to provide one-way blood flow in the vascular circuit.
4. The blood surge with ventricular contraction and subsequent runoff in relaxation creates pressure changes within arterial vessels.
5. Ventricular contraction generates systolic blood pressure, the highest pressure during the cardiac cycle.
6. Diastolic pressure represents the lowest pressure preceding the next ventricular contraction.
7. Dense capillary networks provide a large surface for chemical exchange between blood and the surrounding tissues.
8. Minute-diameter blood vessels possess autoregulatory capacity to regulate blood flow precisely to the tissue's changing metabolic activity.
9. The venous tree contains the largest portion of central blood volume at rest, but venoconstriction increases (venous tone) probably contribute little to blood redistribution in physical activity.
10. Vein compression and relaxation from skeletal muscle action ("muscle pump") impart considerable energy to facilitate venous return and justifies active recovery following vigorous effort.
11. Hypertension imposes a chronic cardiovascular stress that can damage arterial vessels and lead to arteriosclerosis, heart disease, stroke, and kidney failure.
12. One in every three individuals experiences chronic, abnormally high blood pressure sometime during their lifetime.
13. Systolic blood pressure increases in proportion to oxygen uptake and blood flow during graded exercise, whereas diastolic pressure remains relatively unchanged or decreases slightly.
14. At the same relative and absolute exercise levels, upper body exercise produces a greater rise in systolic pressure than leg exercise.
15. Blood pressure decreases below the pre-exercise level following physical activity and may remain lower for up to 12 hr.
16. Peak systolic and diastolic blood pressures mirror a hypertensive state during isometric, free-weight, and hydraulic resistance exercise.
17. Intense resistance exercises pose a risk to individuals with hypertension or heart disease.

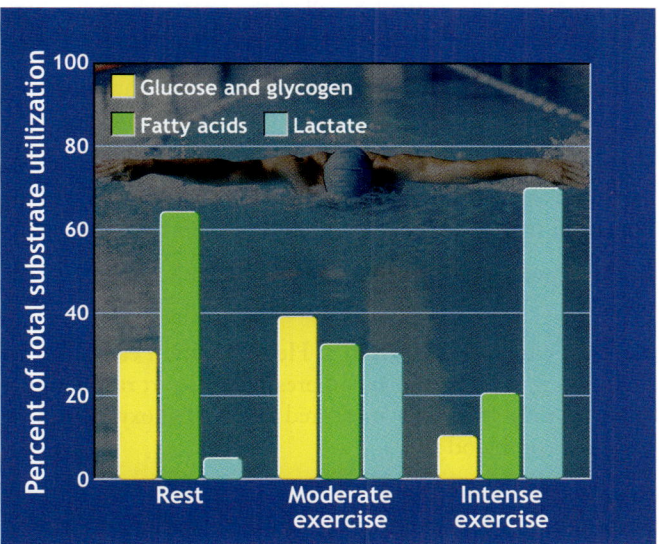

FIGURE 15.14. Generalized myocardial substrate patterns at rest and during moderate and intense exercise.
(Sergey Mironov/Shutterstock)

18. At rest, the myocardium extracts approximately 80% of the oxygen flowing through the coronary arteries.
19. An increase in coronary blood flow primarily provides the myocardial oxygen needs in physical activity.
20. Coronary blood flow impairment initiates chest pains (angina), and a blocked coronary artery can cause irreversible damage to the heart muscle (myocardial infarction).
21. The rate pressure product (heart rate × SBP) estimates myocardial workload.
22. Glucose, fatty acids, and circulating lactate metabolism provide the energy to maintain myocardial function.
23. Myocardial macronutrient energy metabolism varies with physical activity severity, duration, and training status.

Key Terms

Active blood reservoir: Retarding or facilitating blood delivery to the systemic circulation

Angina pectoris: Chest pain from impaired coronary blood flow

Anterior cardiac veins: Three or four small vessels located on the anterior surface of the right ventricle that drain blood from the right ventricle directly into the right atrium

Aorta: Largest artery, originating from the left ventricle and extending down to the abdomen, where it splits into two smaller arteries; distribute oxygenated blood throughout the body

Arterioles: Small-diameter blood vessels that extend and branch out from an artery into the capillary structures

Arteriovenous anastomosis (AVA): Natural direct or indirect communication link between two blood vessels via collateral channels to ensure blood flow to an area with reduced or blocked blood supply

Atrioventricular valves: Valves that provide one-way blood flow from the right atrium to the right ventricle

Auscultation: Assesses circulatory, respiratory, and gastrointestinal system sounds using a stethoscope

Capacitance vessels: Systemic venous vessels containing about 65% of blood's total volume

Cardiovascular system: The body system that comprises the heart and blood vessels and is responsible for transporting oxygen, nutrients, hormones, and cellular waste products throughout the body

Coronary circulation: An extensive crownlike network of blood vessels that wrap around the outside of the heart and provide blood supply to its muscular walls

Coronary sinus: A large vessel that collects blood exiting the heart's left ventricle through veins

Diastole: The relaxation phase of the cardiac cycle

Diastolic blood pressure: The cardiac cycle's lowest pressure, indicating peripheral resistance as blood flows from arterioles into capillaries

Edema: Abnormal interstitial fluid accumulation beneath the skin and within body cavities

Heart: Four-chambered muscular organ pumps blood throughout the body for oxygen and nutrient release to tissues and metabolic waste removal

Hypertension: High blood pressure defined as blood pressure exceeding 130 systolic and 80 diastolic mm Hg

Hypotensive response: Temporary decrease in blood pressure to below pre-exercise levels during submaximal physical activity in normotensive and hypertensive individuals

Inferior vena cava: Body's largest vein that returns blood to the right atrium from the abdomen, pelvis, and lower extremities

Intercalated discs: Interconnected, multinucleated, individual myocardial cells that, when depolarized, spread the action potential through the myocardium so the heart functions as a unit

Isovolumetric contraction period: Rising ventricular tension when heart volume and muscle fiber length remain unchanged

Mean arterial pressure (MAP): Time-weighted blood pressure average over the cardiac cycle that roughly equals diastolic pressure plus one third the difference between systolic and diastolic pressures

Metarterioles: Arterioles that branch and form smaller and less muscular vessels 10 to 20 microns in diameter

Mitral valve: Allows one-way blood flow from the left atrium to left ventricle; also known as the bicuspid valve

Mixed venous blood: Mixture of venous blood that drains from the upper and lower body

Myocardial infarction: Sudden cessation of or decrease in myocardial blood flow that damages the heart muscle; commonly known as a heart attack

Myocardium: The muscular wall of the heart, which has high capillary density and rich mitochondrial content

Precapillary sphincter: Smooth muscle ring that encircles the capillary at its origin to control capillary diameter

Pulmonary circulation: The network of blood vessels that carry deoxygenated blood away from the right ventricle to the lungs and return oxygenated blood to the left atrium

Pulse pressure: Difference between systolic and diastolic pressures

Rate-pressure product (RPP): Heart function calculated by multiplying peak systolic blood pressure by heart rate and that relates closely to directly measured myocardial oxygen uptake and coronary blood flow

Respiratory pump: Physiological mechanism by which small alterations in intrathoracic pressure during the breathing cycle compress veins to create a "milking action" to propel blood to the heart

Semilunar valves: Arterial wall valves outside the heart that prevent blood from flowing back into the heart between contraction cycles

Stage 1 hypertension: Condition in which blood pressure is chronically between 130 and 139 mm Hg systolic or 80 and 89 mm Hg diastolic

Stage 2 hypertension: Condition in which systolic blood pressure is chronically at least 140 mm Hg or diastolic pressure at least 90 mm Hg

Superior vena cava: Large vein that collects venous blood from the head, neck, shoulder regions, thorax, and abdominal wall tributary vessels and joins the inferior vena cava at heart level

Systemic circulation: Circulatory system component that carries oxygenated blood away from the heart and deoxygenated blood back to the heart

Systolic blood pressure (SBP): Force blood exerts against arterial walls during ventricular contraction

Thrombus: A blood clot representing a final blood coagulation product

Valves: Thin, membranous, flaplike structures spaced at short intervals within veins to allow blood to flow in only one direction toward the heart

Varicose veins: Defective valves within lower extremity superficial veins fail to maintain one-way blood flow, causing blood to stagnate and distend the vessel

Venules: Smallest venous blood vessels composed of an endothelial cell tube enclosed in a variable amount of elastic and collagenous tissue

References are available online at Lippincott Connect.

Additional References

Baffour-Awuah B, et al. Safety, efficacy and delivery of isometric resistance training as an adjunct therapy for blood pressure control: a modified Delphi study. *Hypertens Res.* 2022;45:483.

Bolin LP, et al. A pilot study investigating the relationship between heart rate variability and blood pressure in young adults at risk for cardiovascular disease. *Clin Hypertens.* 2022;28:2.

Chen YH, et al. The impact of synchronous telehealth services with a digital platform on day-by-day home blood pressure variability in patients with cardiovascular diseases: retrospective cohort study. *J Med Internet Res.* 2022;24:e22957.

Decaux A, et al. Blood pressure and cardiac autonomic adaptations to isometric exercise training: a randomized sham-controlled study. *Physiol Rep.* 2022;10:e15112.

Dupuy A, et al. Post-exercise heart rate recovery and parasympathetic reactivation are comparable between prepubertal boys and well-trained adult male endurance athletes. *Eur J Appl Physiol.* 2022;122:345.

Hottenrott L, et al. Performance and recovery of well-trained younger and older athletes during different HITT protocols. *Sports (Basel).* 2022;10:9.

Lea JWD, et al. Convergent validity of ratings of perceived exertion during resistance exercise in healthy participants: a systematic review and meta-analysis. *Sports Med Open.* 2022;8:2.

Lee YK, et al. Blood pressure complexity discriminates pathological beat-to-beat variability as a marker of vascular aging. *J Am Heart Assoc.* 2022;11:e022865.

Manoel FA, et al. Novel track field test to determine Vpeak, relationship with treadmill test and 10-km running performance in trained endurance runners. *PLoS One.* 2022;17:e0260338.

Matzka M, et al. Retrospective analysis of training intensity distribution based on race pace versus physiological benchmarks in highly trained sprint kayakers. *Sports Med Open.* 2022;8:1.

Songsorn P, et al. The effect of whole-body high-intensity interval training on heart rate variability in insufficiently active adults. *J Exerc Sci Fit.* 2022;20:48.

Wang KM, Chang TI. Blood Pressure variability: not to be discounted. *Am J Hypertens.* 2022;35:118.

Weber T, et al. International academic 24-hour ambulatory aortic blood pressure consortium. Twenty-four-hour central (aortic) systolic blood pressure: reference values and dipping patterns in untreated individuals. *Hypertension.* 2022;79:251.

Whitaker AA, et al. Cerebrovascular response to an acute bout of low-volume high-intensity interval exercise and recovery in young healthy adults. *J Appl Physiol* (1985). 2022;132:236.

Zhang RM, et al. Immunity and hypertension. *Acta Physiol (Oxf).* 2021;231:e13487..

Table 15.1 Peak Systolic and Diastolic Blood Pressure During Dynamic Arm and Leg Exercise at Similar Percentages of Aerobic Capacity

Condition	Isometric Bench Press[a] (% MVC)				Free-Weight Bench Press[b] (% MVC)		Hydraulic Bench Press[c]	
	25	50	75	100	25	50	Slow	Fast
Peak systolic, mm Hg	172	179	200	225	169	232	237	245
Peak diastolic, mm Hg	106	116	135	156	104	154	101	160

Values are average for seven subjects.
[a]Open glottis (no Valsalva maneuver); average for two trials; contraction time, 2 to 3 s; arm position similar to that of bench press exercise, with hands slightly above chest.
[b]Weight lifted either 25 or 50% of previously determined maximum isometric action.
[c]Hydra-Fitness precision hydraulic chest-press apparatus dial setting 3 (slow) and 5 (fast) for 20 s repeated maximum actions.
MVC, maximum voluntary contraction.

Data from Freedson PF, et al. Intra-arterial blood pressure during free weight and hydraulic resistive exercise. *Med Sci Sports Exerc.* 1984;16:131 and unpublished data from the Human Performance Laboratory, Department of Exercise Science, University of Massachusetts, Amherst.

Table 15.2 Systolic and Diastolic Blood Pressure During Dynamic Arm and Leg Exercise at Similar Percentages of Maximum Oxygen Uptake

Percentage of $\dot{V}O_{2max}$	Systolic Pressure (mm Hg)		Diastolic Pressure (mm Hg)	
	Arms	Legs	Arms	Legs
25	150	132	90	70
40	165	138	93	71
50	175	144	96	73
75	205	160	103	75

$\dot{V}O_{2max}$, maximum oxygen uptake.
From Åstrand PO, et al. Intraarterial blood pressure during exercise with different muscle groups. *J Appl Physiol.* 1965;20:253. ©The American Physiological Society (APS). All rights reserved.

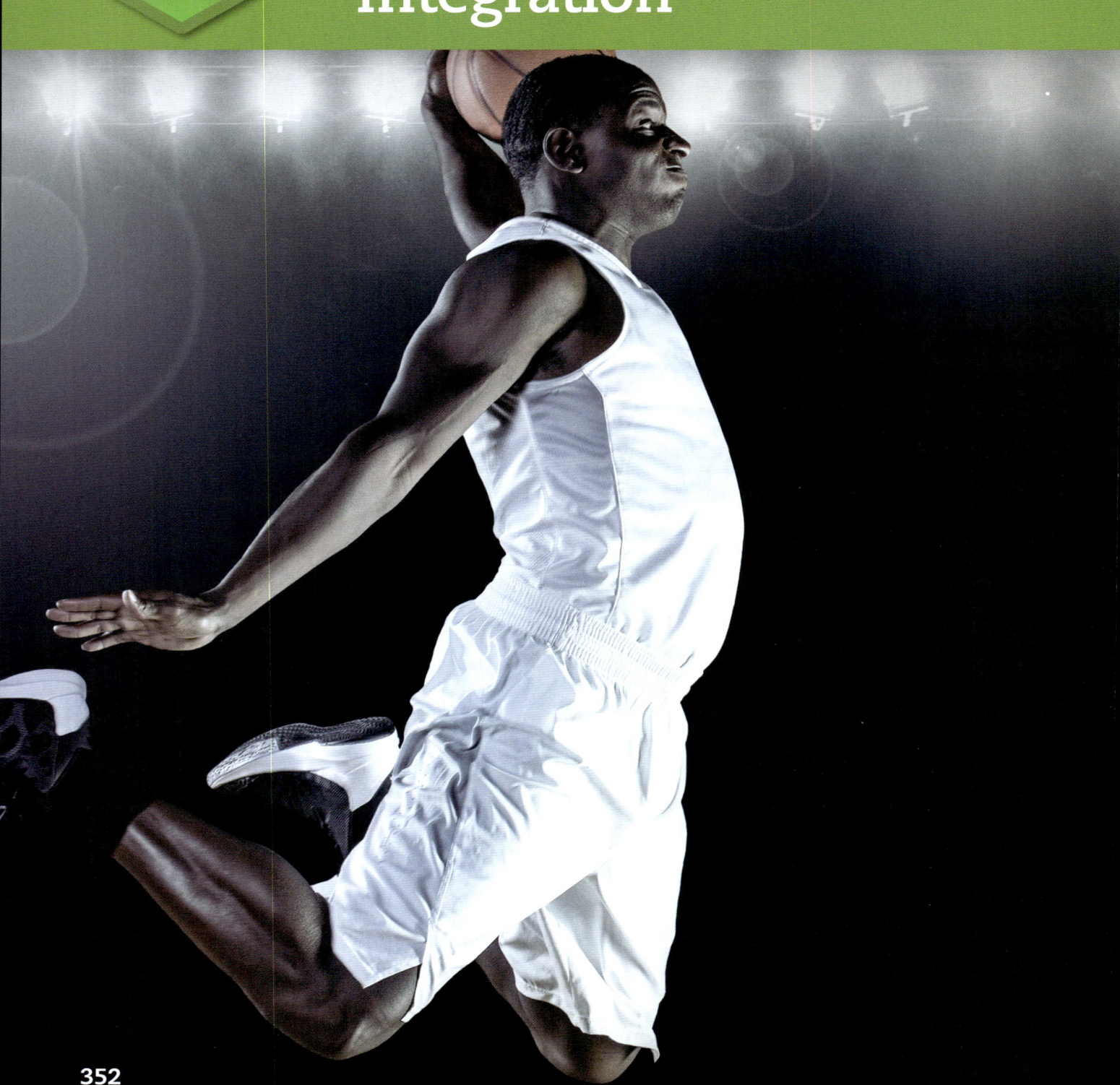

CHAPTER 16
Cardiovascular Regulation and Integration

Chapter Objectives

- Explain how intrinsic and extrinsic factors regulate heart rate during rest and physical activity
- Draw a normal electrocardiogram tracing and identify and describe its major components
- Describe how local metabolic factors regulate blood flow during rest and physical activity
- Explain central command's role in cardiovascular regulation during physical activity
- Describe aerobic training's effects on neural regulation of heart rate
- Outline chemoreceptor, mechanoreceptor, and metaboreflex contributions to cardiovascular regulation during physical activity
- List two physical factors that affect vasculature blood flow
- Describe how each component of Poiseuille's law affects blood flow
- Summarize blood flow dynamics to different tissues at exercise onset and as exercise duration and intensity progress
- Describe the proposed mechanisms for nitric oxide's local blood flow regulation
- Outline the heart transplant patient's cardiovascular response to physical activity

Ancillaries at-a-Glance

Visit Lippincott Connect to access the following resources.

- References: Chapter 16
- Animations: Cardiac Cycle, Perform a Basic 12-Lead Electrocardiogram, Renal Function
- Focus on Research: Age-Related Changes in Exercise-Induced Cardiovascular Function

Throughout the day, while a person is awake or asleep, complex mechanisms continually interact to dynamically balance systemic blood pressure and blood flow to different tissues. Neurochemical factors regulate heart rate and internal blood vessel diameter. Finely regulated cardiovascular responses provide rapid control of heart function and proper blood flow distribution throughout the body. At rest, the skin receives approximately 5% of the 5 L of blood pumped by the heart each minute. By contrast, during physical activity in a hot, humid environment, up to 20% of total blood flow diverts to the body's surface for one major purpose—to dissipate heat. Blood "shunting" and blood pressure control can occur only within a closed vascular system. This dynamic allows a near-immediate increase and blood flow redistribution to meet changing metabolic and physiologic needs and environmental challenges in conditions of cold, heat, submersion in water, high altitude, and zero gravity.

Intrinsic Heart Rate Regulation

Unlike other tissues, cardiac muscle maintains its own rhythm. If left to its inherent rhythmicity, the heart would beat steadily at about 100 b·min^{-1}. Situated within the right atrium's posterior wall lies a small (3 mm wide and 1 cm long) specialized muscle tissue mass called the **sinoatrial (SA) node**. This node spontaneously depolarizes and repolarizes to provide the innate stimulus for heart action. For this reason, the term *pacemaker* describes the SA node. **FIGURE 16.1A** shows the normal route for impulse transmission within the myocardium.

The Heart's Electrical Activity

Electrochemical rhythms originating at the SA node spread across the atria to another small tissue knot situated close to the tricuspid valve known as the **atrioventricular (AV) node**. Figure 16.1B illustrates the time sequence for the propagation of an electrical impulse from the SA node throughout the myocardium.

An approximate 0.10-s delay occurs after the electrical impulse spreads through the atria to allow them to contract and propel blood into the ventricles below. The AV node gives rise to the 1-cm-long **atrioventricular (AV) bundle**, also called the bundle of His, named after Swiss-born anatomist and cardiologist Wilhelm His, Jr. (1863–1934; http://circ.ahajournals.org/content/113/23/2775.full), who in 1893 first described this tissue. Later in his career, His advanced the idea that the heart's individual cells produced the heartbeat.

The AV bundle transmits the impulse rapidly through the ventricles over specialized conducting fibers referred to as the **Purkinje system** (named for Czech [Bohemian] anatomist/physiologist/biologist Jan Evangelista von Purkinje [1787–1869; http://circ.ahajournals.org/content/113/23/2775.full; www.ncbi.nlm.nih.gov/pmc/articles/PMC5832080/]). These fibers form distinct bundle branches that penetrate the right and left ventricles. Purkinje system fibers transmit impulses about six times faster than do normal ventricular muscle fibers. Conducting impulses into the ventricles stimulates each ventricular cell to allow a unified and simultaneous subsequent contraction of both ventricles. The transmission of the cardiac impulse flows as follows:

> SA node → Atria → AV node → AV bundle (Purkinje fibers) → Ventricles

 See the animation "Cardiac Cycle" at on **Lippincott Connect** to view this process.

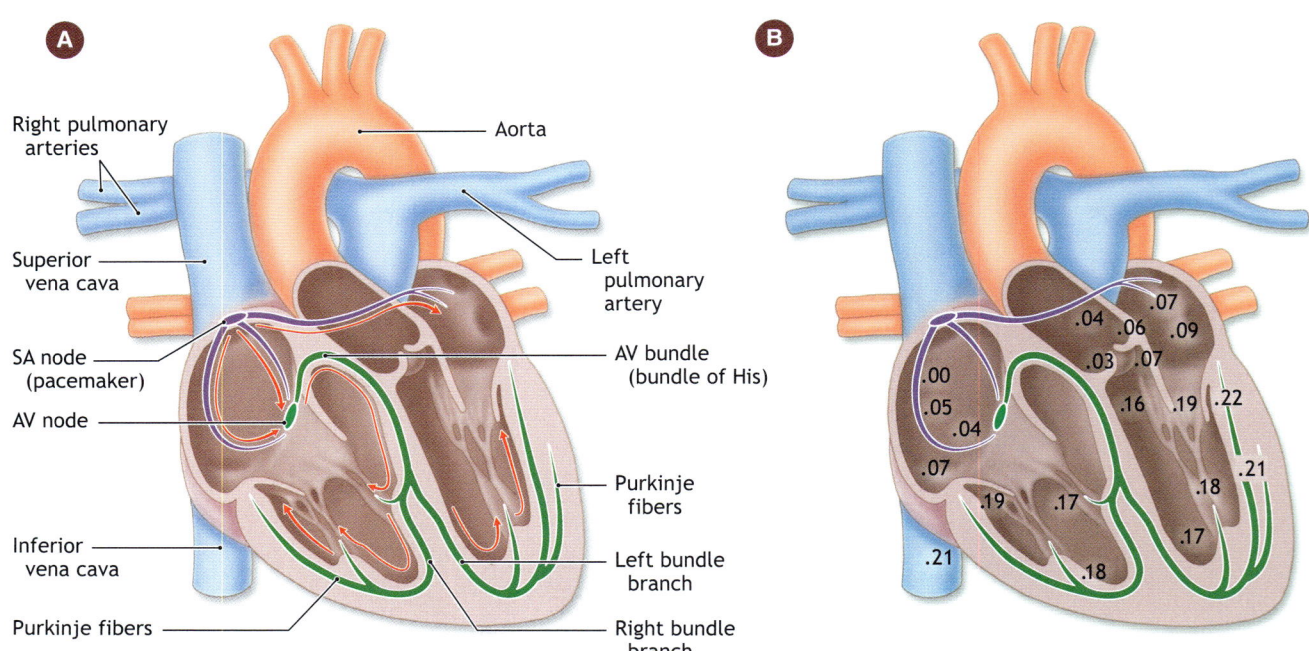

FIGURE 16.1. **(A)** The *red arrows* denote the normal route for excitation and cardiac impulse conduction. The impulse originates at the sinoatrial (SA) node, travels to the atrioventricular (AV) node, and then spreads throughout the ventricular mass. **(B)** Time sequence (in seconds) for electrical impulse transmission from the SA node throughout the myocardium.

In a Practical Sense

Electrode Placement for Bipolar and 12-Lead Electrocardiogram Recordings

Recording the heart's electrical activity began in 1841 when Italian physicist Carlo Matteuci (1811–1868) documented biologist Luigi Galvani's (1737–1798; www.corrosion-doctors.org/Biographies/GalvaniBio.htm) observations about frog muscles' electrical properties. Seven years later, following considerable experiments also with frogs, world-renowned German electrophysiologist Emil Dubois-Reymond (1818–1868; www.informationphilosopher.com/solutions/philosophers/bois-reymond/) described the experimental setups, instruments, and frog preparations to explain the electrical transmission properties through biologic tissues. In 1890, British physiologists Sir William Maddock Bayliss (1860–1924) and Ernest Henry Starling (1866–1927) of University College, London, connected the terminals from a capillary electrometer to the subject's right hand and skin over the heart's apex. This produced a pattern that showed a "triphasic variation accompanying, rather than preceding, each beat of the heart."

The electrocardiogram (ECG) represents a composite record detailing the heart's electrical events during a cardiac cycle. These events provide a way to monitor heart rate during different physical activities and exercise stress testing. A valid ECG tracing requires proper electrode placement. The term *ECG lead* indicates the specific electrode placement pair on the body for transmitting the electrical signal to a recorder or other output device. The record showing electrical differences across different ECG leads creates a composite electrical "picture" regarding myocardial activity.

SKIN PREPARATION

Proper skin preparation reduces extraneous electrical "noise" (interference and skeletal muscle artifact). Abrading the skin with fine sandpaper or commercially available pads and alcohol removes surface epidermis and oil; when done properly, the skin should appear red, slightly irritated, dry, and clean.

BIPOLAR (THREE-ELECTRODE) CONFIGURATION

The typical electrode placement for a three-lead bipolar configuration provides less sensitivity for diagnostic testing but proves useful for routine ECG monitoring in functional exercise testing and radiotelemetry during physical activity. The ground (*green* or *black*) electrode attaches over the sternum; the positive (*red*) electrode attaches on the left side of the chest in the V_5 position (level of fifth intercostal space adjacent to midaxillary line); and the positive (*white*) electrode attaches on the right side of the chest just below the nipple at the fifth intercostal space level. Placement for the positive electrode can be altered to optimize the recording (e.g., third and fourth intercostal spaces, anterior portion of the right shoulder, or near the clavicle). Correct electrode placement can be remembered as follows: *white to right, green to ground, red to left*.

MODIFIED 12-LEAD (10-ELECTRODE TORSO-MOUNTED) CONFIGURATION FOR EXERCISE STRESS TESTING

The standard 12-lead ECG consists of three limb leads, three augmented unipolar leads, and six chest leads. For improved exercise ECG recordings, electrodes mounted on the torso (abdominal level) replace the conventional ankle (leg) and wrist electrodes. This "torso-mounted limb lead system" reduces electrical artifact introduced by limb movement during physical activity.

ELECTRODE POSITIONING FOR THE MODIFIED 10-ELECTRODE, TORSO-MOUNTED SYSTEM

1. RL (right leg): just above right iliac crest on midaxillary line
2. LL (left leg): just above left iliac crest on midaxillary line
3. RA (right arm): just below right clavicle medial to deltoid muscle
4. LA (left arm): just below left clavicle medial to deltoid muscle
5. V_1: on right sternal border in fourth intercostal space
6. V_2: on left sternal border in fourth intercostal space
7. V_3: at midpoint of a straight line between V_2 and V_4
8. V_4: on midclavicular line in fifth intercostal space
9. V_5: on anterior axillary line and horizontal to V_4
10. V_6: on midaxillary line and horizontal to V_4 and V_5

Source:
Phibbs B, Buckels L. Comparative yields of ECG leads in multistage stress testing. *Am Heart J*. 1985;90:275.

Electrocardiogram

Similar to all nerve and muscle tissue, the myocardial cell's or fiber's outer surface maintains a more positive electrical charge than the inside surface. Upon stimulation prior to contraction, polarity reverses and the inside of the myocardial cell becomes more positive than its outside. During the cardiac cycle's diastolic phase, the membranes repolarize to re-establish the normal resting membrane potential.

The myocardium's electrical activity creates an electrical field throughout the body. The salty bodily fluids provide an excellent conducting medium, so electrodes placed on the skin's surface readily detect voltage changes from the electrical sequence of events before and during each cardiac cycle. **FIGURE 16.2A** outlines the conduction pathway for the electrical impulse as it spreads throughout the myocardium to produce the heart muscle's rhythmic contraction and dilation. Figure 16.2B graphically displays the heart's normal electrical activity cycle as recorded by an **electrocardiogram (ECG**; see also, In a Practical Sense: Electrode Placement for Bipolar and 12-Lead Electrocardiogram Recordings). The important electrical deflection patterns are referred to as P, QRS, and T waves, including the P-R and Q-T intervals and the S-T segment.

The **P wave** represents atria depolarization. It lasts approximately 0.15 s and heralds atrial contraction. The relatively large **QRS complex** follows the P wave; it signals electrical changes from ventricular depolarization. At this point, the ventricles contract. Atrial repolarization follows the P wave; it produces a wave so small that the large QRS complex usually obscures it. The **T wave** represents ventricular repolarization that occurs during ventricular diastole. The heart's relatively long 0.20- to 0.30-s depolarization period prevents initiation of the next myocardial impulse (and subsequent contraction). This rest or brief time-out **refractory period** allows sufficient time for ventricular filling between beats.

---

fyi | Behind the Scenes in Electrophysiology with Einthoven's First Tracings of the Heart's Electrical Activity

Electrocardiogram (ECG) sometimes appears abbreviated as EKG. The "K" comes from the German spelling for *electrocardiograph*. In 1895, Dutch physiologist (PhD) and physician (MD) at Leiden University, Holland, Wilhelm Einthoven (1860–1927) received the 1924 Nobel Prize in Physiology or Medicine for pioneering work in electrophysiology for discovering the ECG mechanism obtained from the first tracings of the heart's electrical activity. His early invention relied on a string galvanometer with a thin silver-coated quartz filament placed in a magnetic field, inducing an electrical current to the filament and causing it to move. A light shining on the string produced a shadow on a photographic paper roll rotating at a preset speed. The original machine required water to cool the powerful electromagnets, requiring five people to operate the 270-kg/595-lb machine. The tracing formed a continuous record to represent the heart's electrical activity. To capture the signal, two electrodes were attached to both hands, with another electrode on a hand and foot immersed in a salt-water solution. This three-electrode system calculated the heart's axis, considering it a vector inside an equilateral triangle. In essence, the equilateral triangle with limb leads considered the limbs an extension of the electrodes. The heart's electrical potentials were deduced from the simultaneous configuration from the limb-lead contacts. On March 22, 1905, Einthoven transmitted the first ECG (telecardiogram) a distance of about a mile over a telephone cable from the hospital to his laboratory. This novel approach led to transmitting clinical ECG recordings from patients with heart disease in the hospital to Einthoven's laboratory for interpretation. According to historical reports (Moukabary, 2007), Einthoven's early scientific recording methodology was a precursor to the field now known as vectorcardiography. A normal ECG recording looks like the one in this video clip (see: www.youtube.com/watch?v=RYZ4daFwMa8). Moukabary noted that Einthoven's personal interests included topics that would become relevant to sports medicine a century later and decades before his Nobel Prize achievement in a totally different field:

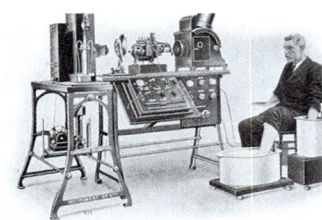

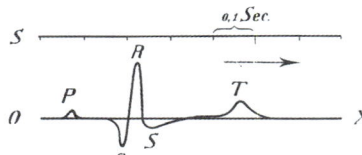

> Einthoven was a great believer in physical education. As a student he urged his fellows "not to let the body perish." He was President of the Gymnastics and Fencing Union, and one of the founders of the Utrecht Student Rowing Club. After suffering from a sports-related elbow fracture he wrote his paper about the functions of the shoulder and elbow joints.

Sources:

Barold SS. Willem Einthoven and the birth of clinical electrocardiography a hundred years ago. *Card Electrophysiol Rev*. 2003;7:99.

Moukabary T. Willem Einthoven (1860–1927): father of electrocardiography. *Card J*. 2007;14:316.

Nobel lectures, physiology or medicine 1922–1941. Amsterdam: Elsevier Publishing Company; 1965. Available at: http://nobelprize.org/nobel_prizes/medicine/laureates/1924/einthoven-bio.html

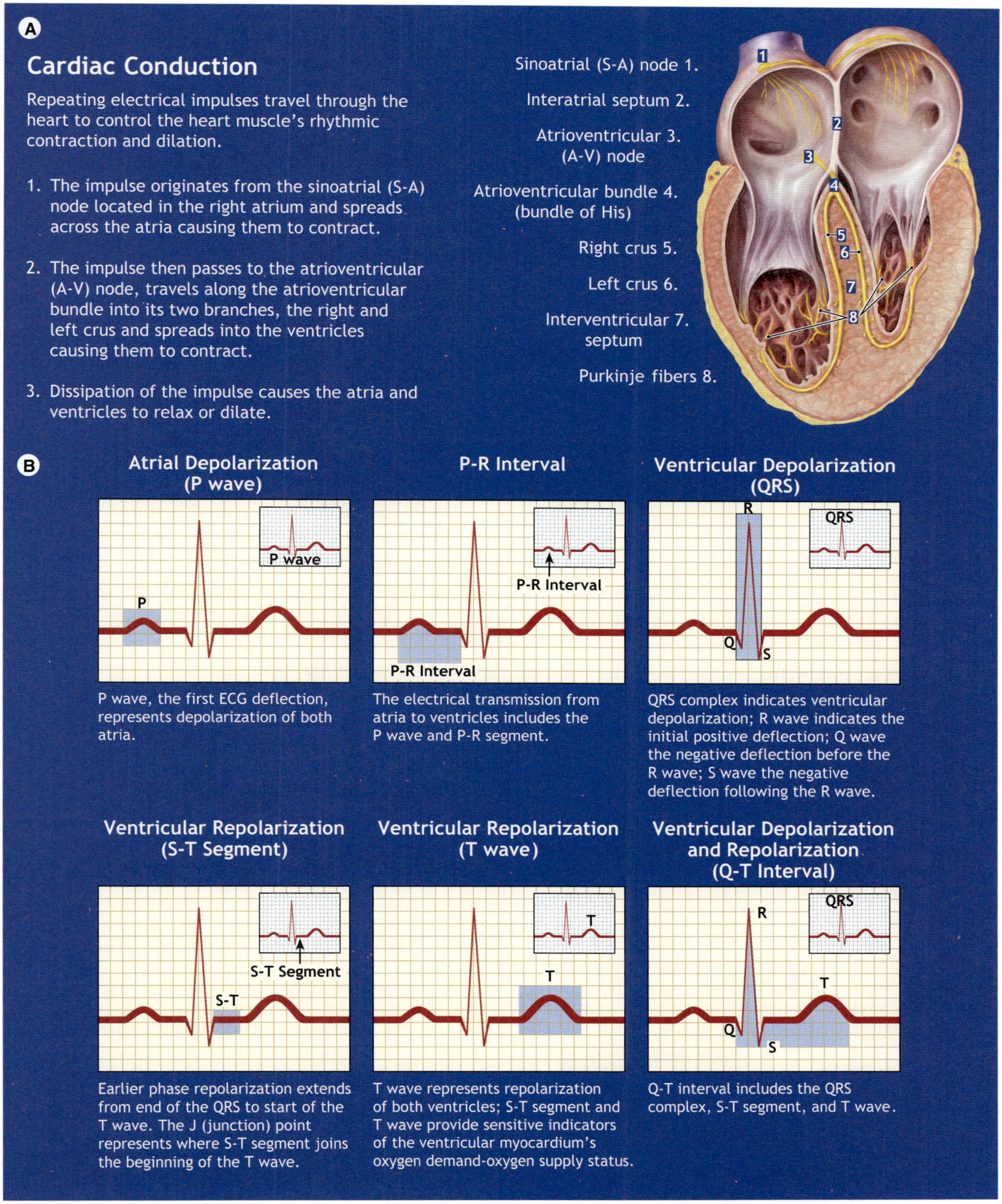

CHAPTER 16 • Cardiovascular Regulation and Integration

A

Cardiac Conduction

Repeating electrical impulses travel through the heart to control the heart muscle's rhythmic contraction and dilation.

1. The impulse originates from the sinoatrial (S-A) node located in the right atrium and spreads across the atria causing them to contract.

2. The impulse then passes to the atrioventricular (A-V) node, travels along the atrioventricular bundle into its two branches, the right and left crus and spreads into the ventricles causing them to contract.

3. Dissipation of the impulse causes the atria and ventricles to relax or dilate.

Sinoatrial (S-A) node 1.
Interatrial septum 2.
Atrioventricular 3.
(A-V) node
Atrioventricular bundle 4.
(bundle of His)
Right crus 5.
Left crus 6.
Interventricular 7.
septum
Purkinje fibers 8.

B

Atrial Depolarization (P wave)
P wave, the first ECG deflection, represents depolarization of both atria.

P-R Interval
The electrical transmission from atria to ventricles includes the P wave and P-R segment.

Ventricular Depolarization (QRS)
QRS complex indicates ventricular depolarization; R wave indicates the initial positive deflection; Q wave the negative deflection before the R wave; S wave the negative deflection following the R wave.

Ventricular Repolarization (S-T Segment)
Earlier phase repolarization extends from end of the QRS to start of the T wave. The J (junction) point represents where S-T segment joins the beginning of the T wave.

Ventricular Repolarization (T wave)
T wave represents repolarization of both ventricles; S-T segment and T wave provide sensitive indicators of the ventricular myocardium's oxygen demand-oxygen supply status.

Ventricular Depolarization and Repolarization (Q-T Interval)
Q-T interval includes the QRS complex, S-T segment, and T wave.

FIGURE 16.2. **(A)** Normal electrical impulse transmission through the myocardium. **(B)** Different normal electrocardiogram (ECG) phases from atrial depolarization (*upper left*) to ventricular repolarization (*lower middle*).
(Part A adapted with permission from Anatomical Chart Company.)

In a Practical Sense

Assessing Heart Rate by Auscultation and Palpation

The cardiac cycle rate (i.e., heart rate) provides a fundamental tool to establish physical activity intensity and assess training changes. Four laboratory methods reliably measure heart rate: (1) sound (auscultation), (2) touch (palpation), (3) heart rate monitor, and (4) electrocardiogram recorder.

HEART RATE BY AUSCULTATION

The method uses a stethoscope to amplify sound waves, bringing the listener's ear closer to the heart sound source.

1. Point the stethoscope ear tips forward, inserting them directly into each ear canal.
2. Gently tap the stethoscope diaphragm to verify you can hear the sound.
3. Position the stethoscope just below the subject's left breast at the pectoralis major muscle over the third intercostal space to the left of the sternum.
4. Place the stethoscope diaphragm firmly against the subject's skin, not on top of clothing.

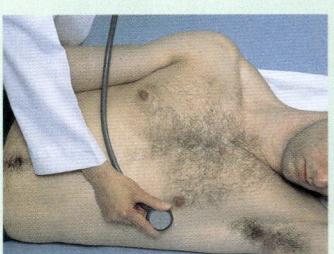

Reprinted with permission from Bickley LS. *Bates' Guide to Physical Examination and History Taking*. 13th Ed. Philadelphia: Lippincott Williams & Wilkins, 2021: 554.

HEART RATE BY PALPATION

1. The pulse wave generated by blood pumping through the arteries is mostly measured with a finger or hand over the radial or carotid arteries.
2. Use the middle and index finger tips; do not use the thumb because it has its own pulse.
3. Press lightly to avoid obstructing blood flow.
4. An apical beat (vibration pulse) generated by the left ventricle hitting the chest wall near the left fifth rib becomes prominent immediately following physical activity. To palpate an apical beat, position the entire hand over the left side at heart level.

Locations for Palpation

1. Temporal artery: At the temple around the hairline
2. Carotid artery: Just lateral to the larynx (do not apply excessive pressure at this site because it may trigger a reflex that slows heart rate)
3. Radial artery: Anterolateral aspect at the wrist directly in line with the base of the thumb
4. Brachial artery: Anteromedial aspect of the arm below the biceps brachii belly, 2 to 3 cm/1 in above the antecubital fossa

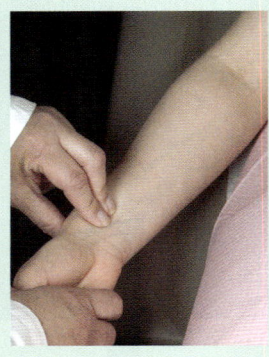 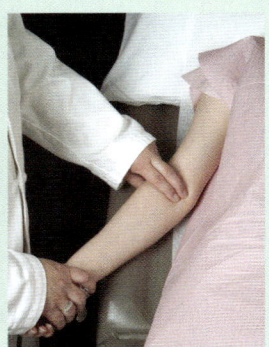

Counting Heart Rate (HR)

Record the HR as a rate per minute (e.g., 150 b·min^{-1}). Two common approaches include the timed heart rate and 30-beat heart rate methods.

Timed Heart Rate Method

This method counts pulse number if counts are taken for 6, 10, or 15 s. If palpating the pulse for 6 s, multiply by 10 to express as a per-min rate; for a 10-s palpation, multiply by 6; and if palpating for 15 s, multiply the pulse count by 4.

Thirty-Beat Heart Rate Method

This method counts time in seconds for 30 pulse beats to occur. Count the first beat as "zero" and simultaneously begin to record the time to count 30-pulse beats. Use the computational formula to compute HR in beats per min (bpm):

$$HR\ (bpm) = 30\ b \div Time\ (s) \times 60\ s \div 1\ min$$

For example, if 30 beats (b) occur in 20 s:

$$\begin{aligned}HR\ (bpm) &= 30\ b \div Time\ (s) \times 60\ s \div 1\ min \\ &= 30\ b \div 20\ s \times 60\ s \div 1\ min \\ &= 1.5 \times 60 \\ &= 90\ bpm\end{aligned}$$

The table on the next page presents a conversion chart to compute HR rounded to the nearest whole number. Find the time for recording 30 beats and corresponding HR (bpm).

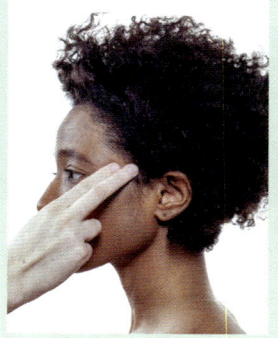 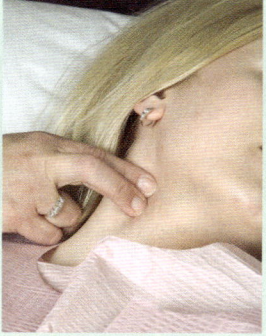

Reprinted with permission from Agur AMR, Dalley AF. *Moore's Essential Clinical Anatomy*. 6th Ed. Baltimore: Wolters Kluwer Health, 2020: 526. Fig. 8.18B.

CONVERSION CHART FOR 30-BEAT HEART RATE METHOD

Time for 30 Beats, s	HR, BPM	Time for 30 Beats, s	HR, BPM	Time for 30 Beats, s	HR, BPM
8	225	21	86	34	53
9	200	22	82	35	51
10	180	23	78	36	50
11	164	24	75	37	49
12	150	25	72	38	47
13	138	26	69	39	46
14	129	27	67	40	45
15	120	28	64	41	44
16	113	29	62	42	43
17	106	30	60	43	42
18	100	31	58	44	41
19	95	32	56	45	40
20	90	33	55		

BPM, beats per minute; HR, heart rate.

Regular physical activity induces structural and electrical cardiac adaptations reflected in the resting 12-lead ECG, which can cause an athlete's ECG recording to differ considerably from that of a sedentary person of similar age, gender, and ethnicity. This raises issues for preparticipation ECG athlete screening in whom false-positive findings are commonplace when comparing standard ECG values derived from sedentary populations.[61]

The Electrocardiogram Objectively Monitors Heart Rate During Physical Activity

Radiotelemetry transmits the electrocardiogram (ECG) from electrodes to a small, lightweight receiver worn on the body while engaging in different physical activity modes (e.g., football, weight lifting, basketball, ice hockey, dancing, swimming, track and field, soccer, baseball, and even extravehicular space flight missions). The latest smartwatches also can transmit heart function from wrist watches and stand-alone electrode-type pads affixed to the back of a phone for transmitting heart rate, heart rate variability, and heart abnormalities (with results uploaded from the phone to a physician or hospital). Watches that detect heart function have been validated with excellent results against heart monitors that record ECG for 24 hr continuously in or outside of clinical settings. Remote cardiac function sensing also detects contraindications to exercise from prior myocardial infarction, ischemic S-T segment changes, conduction defects, and abnormal left ventricular enlargement (see Chapter 31).

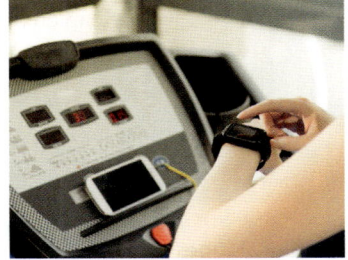

PR Image Factory/Shutterstock

Sources:
De Silva K, et al. A smartwatch to identify atrial fibrillation. *N Engl J Med*. 2020;382:974.
Lahdenoja O, et al. Detection via accelerometer and gyroscope of a smartphone. *IEEE J Biomed Health Inform*. 2018;22:108.
Narasimha D, et al. Validation of a smartphone-based event recorder for arrhythmia detection. *Pacing Clin Electrophysiol*. 2018;41:487.

See the animation "Perform a Basic 12-Lead Electrocardiogram" on **Lippincott Connect** to view this process.

Extrinsic Regulation of Heart Rate and Circulation

Changes in heart rate occur rapidly through nerves that directly supply the myocardium and chemical "messengers" that circulate in blood. These **extrinsic controls** of cardiac function accelerate the heart in anticipation before physical activity begins and then rapidly adjust to physical effort intensity. Extrinsic regulation can decrease heart rate to 25 to 30 b · min^{-1} under normal ambulatory conditions in highly trained endurance athletes and can increase it to 200 b · min^{-1} in maximal exertion in trained and untrained persons.[5]

FIGURE 16.3 illustrates neural mechanisms for cardiovascular regulation before and during activity. Input from the brain and peripheral nervous system continually bombards the cardiovascular control center in the **ventrolateral medulla**. This center regulates the heart's blood output and blood's preferential distribution to all body tissues. The lower box describes the neural activation and response mechanisms during the pre-exercise "anticipatory" and exercise phases.

Heart Rate Variability

Heart rate variability refers to variation in time intervals between heartbeats, usually measured as variation in the R-R time intervals on an electrocardiogram tracing for a particular time period (see blue inset and Fig. 16.2).

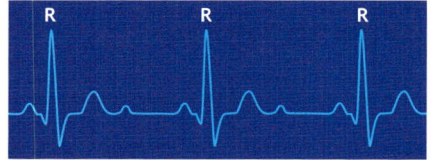
Sofiia Balitckaia/Shutterstock

Wide variation in time intervals generally reflects a "healthy" balance between sympathetic and parasympathetic input to the myocardium, while little variation may reflect dysfunctional autonomic input. *Low* heart rate variability relates to increased risk for heart failure, myocardial infarction, sudden cardiac death, and clinical depression. On the positive side, regular physical activity promotes *increases* in heart rate variability.

Sources:
Binkley PF. Promise of a new role for heart rate variability in the clinical management of patients with heart failure. *JACC Heart Fail*. 2017;5:432.
Emery CF, et al. Sex and family history of cardiovascular disease influence heart rate variability during stress among healthy adults. *J Psychosom Res*. 2018;110:54.
Facioli TP, et al. Study of heart rate recovery and cardiovascular autonomic modulation in healthy participants after submaximal exercise. *Sci Rep*. 2021;11:3620.

 INTEGRATIVE QUESTION

What is the physiologic rationale for biofeedback and relaxation techniques to treat hypertension and stress-related disorders?

 Exercise Pressor Reflex

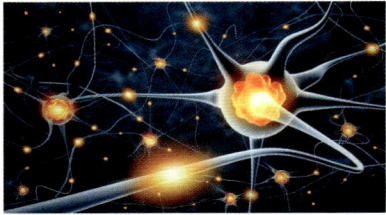
adike/Shutterstock

This neurological reflex, from the French "presser" meaning "to exert pressure" or "to squeeze," contributes to the autonomic, cardiovascular, and ventilatory adjustments to physical activity. The reflex, stimulated by thin fiber sensory muscle afferents (group III and IV afferents) by two complementary receptors, responds to either mechanical distortion or from contracting skeletal muscle's metabolic by-products. Neural signals from active muscle provide peripheral feedback to activate cardiovascular control centers in the brainstem (medulla oblongata) to adjust heart rate and blood pressure via sympathetic activation and parasympathetic withdrawal. The muscle-sensing mechanoreceptor organs are sensitive to and responsive to stretch or pressure while the chemoreceptors monitor the chemical state of the blood perfusing them. These muscle sensors provide central command to continually assess active muscle's mechanical and chemical state. Progressively increasing physical activity intensity activates the exercise pressor reflex. Receptor activation provides reflex-mediated arteriole constriction by increasing blood pressure to maintain perfusion within the muscle's intricate architecture.

Poiseuille's Law of Fluid Flow

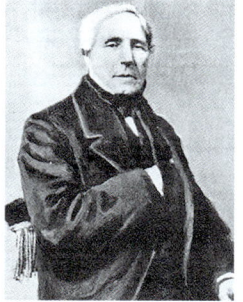

In 1838, French physician and physiologist Jean Louis Poiseuille (1797–1869; http://mahi.ucsd.edu/guy/sio224/stokes-part2.pdf) derived an equation, later named **Poiseuille's law** to honor him. The *poise* represents a standard unit to express resistance to flow. Poiseuille's law expresses the general relationship among pressure differential, vessel radius, vessel length, and fluid viscosity and fluid flow through rigid cylindrical tubes as follows:

$$\text{Flow} = \text{Pressure gradient} \times \text{Vessel radius}^4 \div \text{Vessel length} \times \text{Fluid viscosity}$$

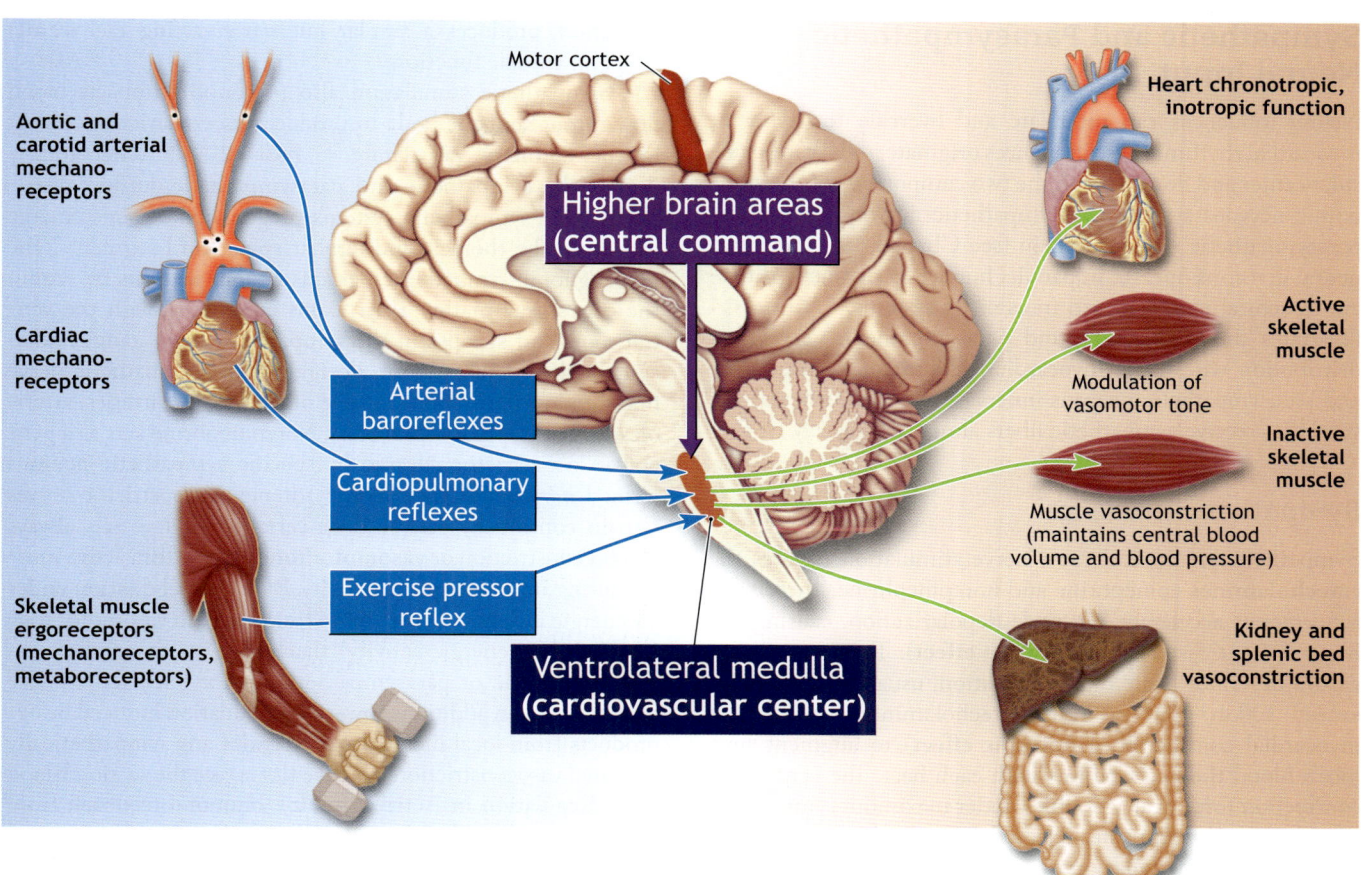

FIGURE 16.3. Cardiovascular system neural regulation in physical activity. ADP, adenosine diphosphate.
(Adapted with permission from Mitchell JH, Raven PB. Cardiovascular adaptation to physical activity. In: Bouchard C, et al., eds. *Physical Activity, Fitness, and Health.: International Proceedings and Consensus Statement* (p. 289) Champaign: Human Kinetics; 1994.)

Sympathetic and Parasympathetic Neural Input

Neural influences can modulate and override the inherent myocardial rhythm. These influences originate in the cardiovascular center and flow through the two components of the autonomic nervous system: the sympathetic nervous system and parasympathetic nervous system (see Chapter 19). These two neural divisions operate in parallel but act by distinctly different structural pathways and transmitter systems. **FIGURE 16.4** illustrates the sympathetic and parasympathetic nerve fiber distribution within the myocardium. Numerous sympathetic and parasympathetic neurons innervate the atria, whereas the ventricles receive sympathetic fibers almost exclusively.

Sympathetic Influence

Sympathetic cardioaccelerator nerve stimulation releases the **catecholamines** epinephrine and norepinephrine. These neurohormones accelerate SA node depolarization, causing the heart to beat faster (**chronotropic effect**). The term **tachycardia** describes heart rate acceleration, usually to rates that exceed 100 b·min^{-1} at rest. Catecholamines also increase myocardial contractility (**inotropic effect**) to augment how much blood the heart pumps with each beat. The ventricular contraction force nearly doubles under maximum sympathetic stimulation. Epinephrine, released into the blood from the adrenal glands' medullary portion during general sympathetic activation, produces a similar but *slower*-acting tachycardia effect on cardiac function.

Sympathetic stimulation also profoundly impacts blood flow throughout the body to produce vasoconstriction, except in the coronary vasculature.[7,53] **FIGURE 16.5** schematically depicts the sympathetic and parasympathetic outflow distribution. The sympathetic system's preganglionic axons emerge *only* from the thoracic and lumbar spinal cord segments. The preganglionic sympathetic nervous system neurons lie within the cord's gray matter. Their axons emerge through the ventral roots and synapse in the sympathetic chain ganglia adjacent to the spinal column. Postganglionic sympathetic nerve fibers end in the smooth muscle of the smaller arteries, arterioles, and precapillary sphincters. Norepinephrine acts as a general vasoconstrictor released by specific sympathetic neurons termed *adrenergic fibers*. Some adrenergic constrictor nerves remain continually active. Thus, certain blood vessels always exhibit constriction or **vasomotor tone** even within active muscle during intense physical activity. Blood vessel dilation under adrenergic influence occurs more from reduced vasomotor tone (decreased adrenergic activity) than from increased cholinergic sympathetic or parasympathetic dilator fiber activity (see next section). In addition, powerful vasodilation induced by by-products from local metabolism overrides any sympathetically activated vasoconstriction in active tissue (see the section Blood Flow Regulation in Active Muscle). Humoral feedback from metabolites released to the circulation from active muscles contributes to heart rate acceleration during physical activity.[31]

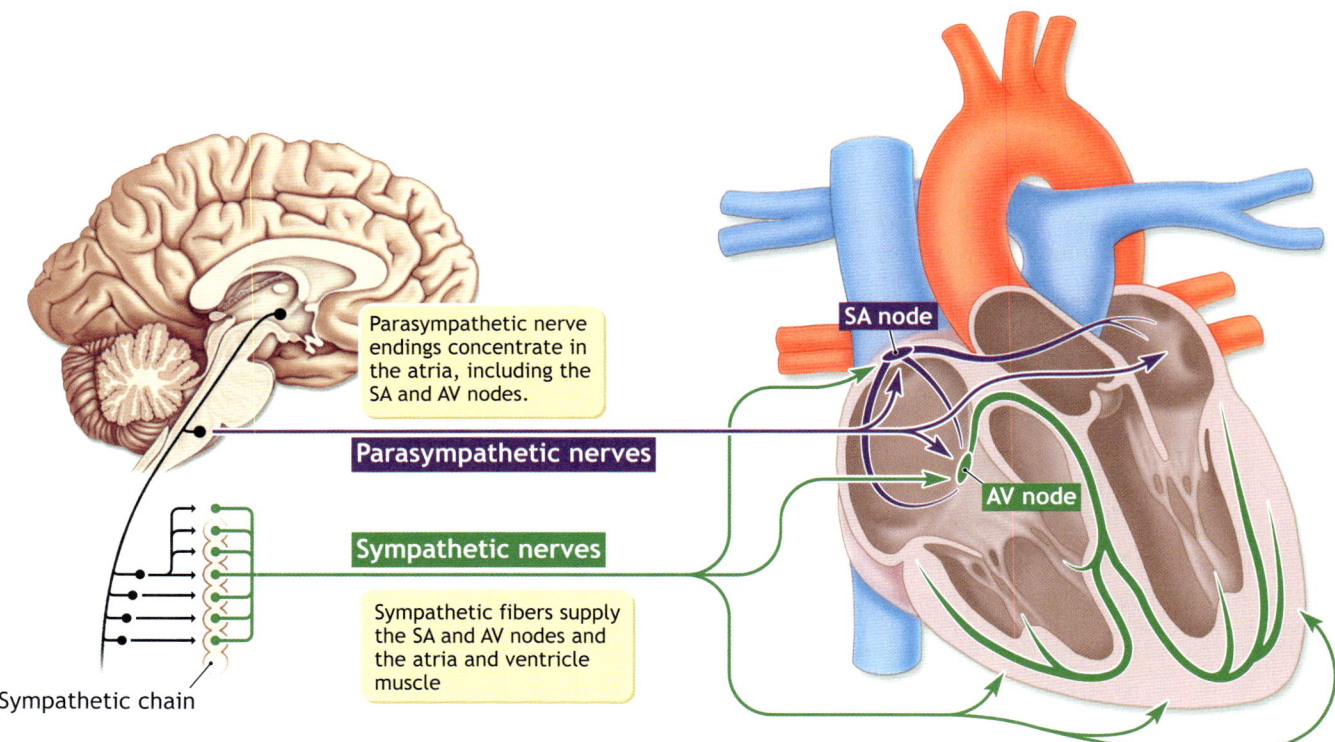

FIGURE 16.4. Myocardium sympathetic and parasympathetic nerve fiber distribution. Sympathetic nerve fiber endings secrete epinephrine. Sympathetic fibers supply the sinoatrial (SA) and atrioventricular (AV) nodes and atria and ventricle muscle. Parasympathetic nerve endings secrete acetylcholine. These fibers and the SA and AV nodes concentrate in the atria.

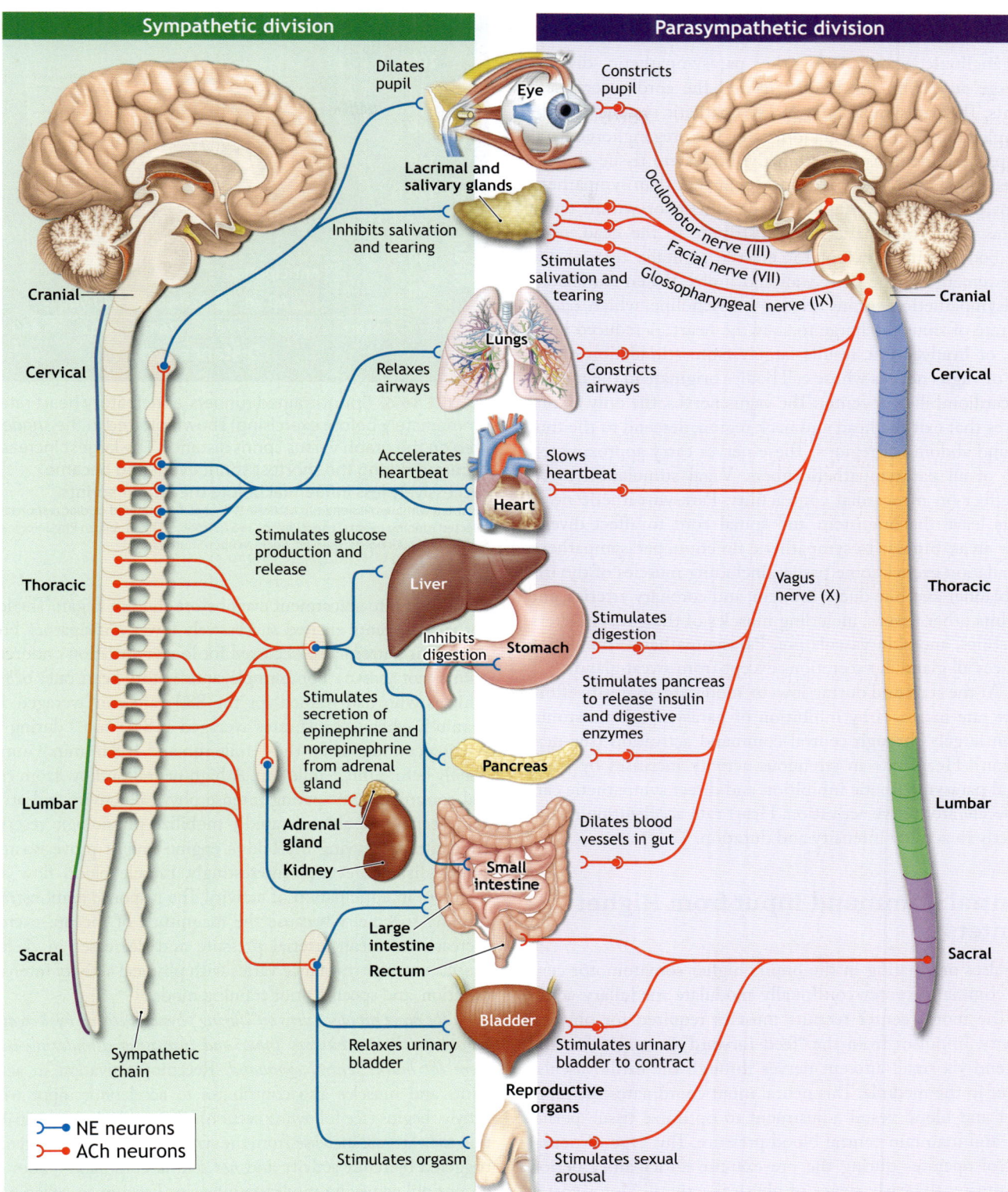

FIGURE 16.5. Chemical, anatomic, and functional organization of the sympathetic and parasympathetic divisions of the autonomic nervous system. The preganglionic input of both divisions use acetylcholine (ACh; *red*) as the neurotransmitter for preganglionic neurons. The parasympathetic division also uses ACh for postganglionic neurons, to innervate visceral organs and sweat glands, but the sympathetic division uses norepinephrine (NE; *blue*) for postganglionic neurons. Preganglionic sympathetic fibers innervate the adrenal medulla with NE release. In general, sympathetic stimulation produces catabolic effects to prepare the body to "fight" or "flee," while parasympathetic stimulation produces anabolic responses to promote normal function and conserve energy.
(Adapted with permission from Bear MF, et al. *Neuroscience: Exploring the Brain*. Baltimore: Lippincott Williams & Wilkins; 2006.)

Parasympathetic Influence

Preganglionic axons from the parasympathetic division emerge *only* from the brainstem and the cord's sacral segments. The parasympathetic and sympathetic systems thereby complement each other anatomically. The preganglionic parasympathetic neurons lie within the brainstem tissue and the lower spinal cord. Their axons travel farther than sympathetic axons because their ganglia lie adjacent to or within target organs. Parasympathetic fibers distribute to the head, neck, and body cavities (except for erectile genitalia tissues) and never emerge in the body wall and limbs. When stimulated, parasympathetic neurons release acetylcholine, which *retards* the rate of sinus discharge to slow the heart. A reduced heart rate, or **bradycardia**, results largely from stimulation of the pair of **vagus nerves** whose cell bodies originate in the medulla's cardioinhibitory center. The vagus nerves, the only cranial nerves that exit the head and neck region, descend to the thorax and abdominal regions. These nerves carry approximately 80% of all parasympathetic fibers. Vagal stimulation exerts no effect on myocardial contractility. Parasympathetic nerve fibers leave the brainstem and spinal cord to affect diverse body areas. Similar to sympathetic function, parasympathetic stimulation excites some tissues, including muscles of the iris, gallbladder and bile ducts, bronchi, and coronary arteries, and inhibits other tissues, including muscles of the gut sphincters, intestines, and skin vasculature. Parasympathetic stimulation induces all glandular secretions except from sweat glands.

At the start and during low-to-moderate–intensity effort, heart rate increases by inhibition of parasympathetic stimulation largely through central command activation (see next section). Heart rate in strenuous activity increases by additional parasympathetic inhibition and direct sympathetic cardioaccelerator nerve activation. Heart rate acceleration relates directly to activity intensity and duration.

Central Command Input from Higher Centers

Impulses originating in the brain's higher somatomotor central command center continually modulate medullary activity. The motor center recruits muscles required for physical activity. Impulses from the "feed-forward" central command descend via small afferent nerves through the cardiovascular center in the medulla. This neural input coordinates the rapid heart and blood vessel adjustment to optimize tissue perfusion and maintain central blood pressure. This type of neural control operates during the pre-exercise anticipatory period and during the early stages of physical activity. Motor cortex medullary stimulation increases with the size of the muscle mass activated in physical activity. *Central command provides the greatest control over exercise heart rate.*[26,38,59]

FIGURE 16.6 shows central command's influence on heart rate when movement begins. Radiotelemetry continuously monitored trained sprint runners' resting heart rate, at the starting commands, and during 60-, 220-, and 440-yard races. Heart rate averaged 148 b·min^{-1} at the starting commands while anticipating the 60-yard sprint; this represented 74% of the run's

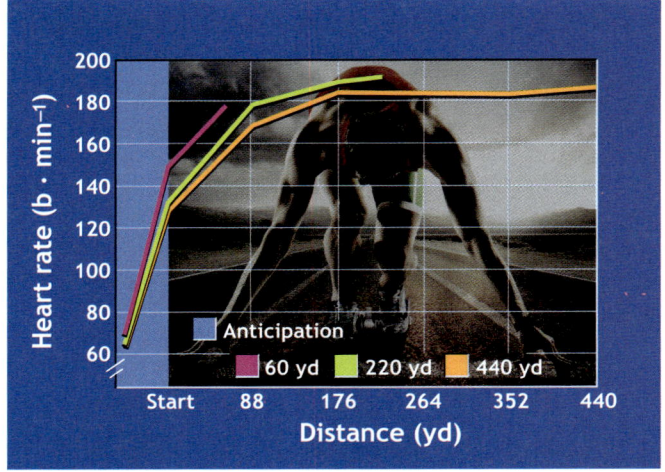

FIGURE 16.6. Sprint-trained runners' anticipatory heart rate (immediately before exercising) shown plotted in the *shaded area* on the graph versus sprint distance. The largest increase occurred during the shortest sprint event and became successively less influential before the longer sprints.
(Adapted with permission from McArdle WD, et al. Telemetered cardiac response to selected running events. *J Appl Physiol*. 1967;23:566. ©The American Physiological Society (APS). All rights reserved. Rocksweeper/Shutterstock)

total heart rate adjustment even before the run began. The longer sprint events elicited successively lower anticipatory heart rates. This pattern also occurred for longer-duration endurance events (not shown). For example, anticipatory heart rates of four athletes who had trained for the 880-yard run averaged 122 b·min^{-1}, whereas heart rates averaged 118 b·min^{-1} during the starting commands for the 1-mile run and 108 b·min^{-1} immediately before the 2-mile run. A high neural outflow from central command anticipating intense physical activity and at the start seems desirable to rapidly mobilize physiologic reserves. By contrast, "revving the body's engine" might prove wasteful before distance events. Interestingly, muscle blood flow also increases in anticipation of activity. The response demonstrates training specificity because the magnitude of the pre-exercise increases in mean arterial pressure and decreases in skeletal muscle vascular resistance varies with physical activity intensity, duration, and specific prior training mode.[13]

The heart rapidly "turns on" during physical activity by decreasing parasympathetic inhibitory input and increasing stimulating input from the brain's central command. Receptor activation in active joints and muscles also contributes to accelerator input when activity begins (see following section). The much slower contribution to heart rate increase from the sympathetic nervous system—triggered by reflex activity and *not* central command—does not occur until achieving moderate intensity. Even in so-called non-sprint events, heart rate reaches 180 b·min^{-1} within 30 s of 1- and 2-mile runs. Further heart rate increases progress gradually with several plateaus during the run. Almost identical results occur for heart rate measured by telemetry during competitive swimming events except for lower maximum heart rates during swimming.

Central command involvement in cardiovascular regulation also explains how variations in emotional state affect cardiovascular response. Such neural input creates difficulty obtaining "true" resting values for heart rate and blood pressure.

Peripheral Input

The cardiovascular center receives reflex sensory input (feedback) from peripheral receptors in blood vessels, joints, and muscles. Chemoreceptors and **mechanoreceptors** within muscle and its vasculature monitor the muscle's chemical and physical state. Afferent impulses from these receptors—slow-conducting, thin-fiber group III and IV afferents from pacinian corpuscles, and unencapsulated nerve-ending receptors—provide rapid feedback. This input modifies either vagal (parasympathetic) or sympathetic outflow to initiate appropriate cardiovascular and respiratory responses to various physical activity intensities.[18,20,24,48] Activating chemically sensitive afferents within the muscle's interstitial space helps to regulate sympathetic neural activation during submaximal effort.[66] Metabolites produced primarily during the concentric muscular activity phase stimulate this **metaboreflex**.[10,65] Three mechanisms continually assess physical activity intensity and the activated muscle mass:

1. Reflex neural input from mechanical deformation of type III afferents within active muscles
2. Type IV afferent chemical stimulation within active muscles (referred to as the **exercise pressor reflex**)
3. Feed-forward outflow from the central command motor areas

Specific mechanoreceptor feedback governs how the central nervous system regulates blood flow and blood pressure during dynamic physical activity.[52] The aortic arch and carotid sinus contain pressure-sensitive baroreceptors, while cardiopulmonary mechanoreceptors assess mechanical activity in the left ventricle, right atrium, and large veins. These receptors function as negative feedback controllers to accomplish the following two functions[45,60,67]:

1. Inhibit sympathetic outflow from the cardiovascular center
2. Blunt an inordinate rise in arterial blood pressure

As blood pressure increases, arterial vessel stretching activates baroreceptors to slow the heart reflexively and dilate the peripheral vasculature. This *decreases* blood pressure toward more normal levels. During physical activity, blood pressure remains effectively regulated but at a higher level. This probably occurs from an arterial baroreflex feedback mechanism override and an upward resetting of its threshold and/or sensitivity (i.e., reduced baroreflex gain), partly from central command activation.[36,46] The baroreceptors more than likely serve as a brake, curtailing abnormally high blood pressure levels during activity. Regular physical activity improves cardiac baroreflex function and beneficially affects blood pressure regulation without negatively affecting cerebral autoregulation of blood flow. This positive effect is maintained into older age in individuals who exercise regularly.[1]

Carotid Artery Palpation Can Depress Heart Rate

External pressure against the carotid artery sometimes slows the heart rate due to direct baroreceptor stimulation at the carotid artery's bifurcation. The potential for bradycardia from **carotid artery palpation** is important to exercise specialists because this location is routinely used to determine heart rate during physical activity. Consistently low heart rate estimation with carotid artery palpation in susceptible individuals would push the person to a higher activity level—certainly an undesirable effect for cardiac patients.

Research in the late 1970s suggested that carotid artery palpation slowed postexercise heart rate and occasionally produced electrocardiographic abnormalities.[57] Subsequent reports indicated rather convincingly for healthy adults and cardiac patients that carotid artery palpation caused little or no heart rate alteration during rest or physical activity and recovery.[41,50] Vascular disease can, nevertheless, negatively impact carotid sinus sensitivity and produce falsely low heart rate values. An excellent substitute location uses pulse rate measured at the radial artery (thumb side of wrist) or temporal artery at the side of the head at the temple; firmly palpating these vessels does not alter heart rate.

Local Factors

Energy metabolism by-products provide a within-muscle autoregulatory mechanism to boost perfusion during physical activity. We discuss local circulatory control in the following sections.

Blood Redistribution

If fully dilated, the body's blood vessels could hold approximately 20 L of blood, four times more than the actual average total 5-L blood volume. Thus, maintaining blood flow and blood pressure during physical activity requires a finely regulated balance between vascular dilation and vascular constriction. *Vasculature constriction or dilation provides for rapid blood redistribution to meet current metabolic requirements, while also optimizing blood pressure throughout the vascular circuit.*

How Physical Factors Impact Blood Flow

Blood flows through the vascular circuit generally following the physical laws of hydrodynamics applied to rigid, cylindrical vessels. Two factors control blood flow volume in any vessel:

1. *Directly* to the pressure gradient between the vessel's two ends, *not* the absolute pressure within the vessel
2. *Inversely* to the resistance encountered to fluid flow

Friction between the blood and internal vascular wall creates resistance or force to impede blood flow governed by three factors:

1. Blood thickness (viscosity)
2. Conducting tube length
3. Blood vessel radius (most crucial factor)

In the body, transport vessel length remains constant, while blood viscosity under most conditions varies only slightly. The conducting tube's radius affects blood flow the most because resistance to flow changes with the vessel's radius raised to the fourth power. For example, halving a vessel's radius decreases flow 16-fold. Conversely, doubling the radius increases volume 16-fold. The pressure differential within the vascular circuit remains relatively constant, so even a small change in vessel radius dramatically alters blood flow. *Constriction and dilation of smaller arterial blood vessels serve as the crucial physiologic mechanism to regulate regional blood flow.*

Exercise Effects

Any increase in energy expenditure requires rapid blood flow adjustments throughout the cardiovascular system. For example, nerves and local metabolites act on smooth muscle arteriole walls to alter their internal diameter almost instantaneously to meet the blood flow demands from increased metabolism. Visceral vasoconstriction and muscle pump action divert a large blood flow into the central circulation.

At movement onset, the active muscles' vascular component increases by local arteriole dilation. These small-supply arteries to skeletal muscle normally possess well-developed flow-mediated and myogenic regulatory mechanisms. They require little modification through training to adequately supply the blood flow requirements in vigorous physical activity.[27] Concurrently, other vessels to tissues that can temporarily compromise their blood supply constrict, or "shut down." Two examples include the splanchnic and renal areas. Here, blood flow decreases in proportion to relative activity intensity (i.e., percent maximum oxygen uptake [$\dot{V}O_{2max}$]). Blood flow shifts from the abdominal viscera to active muscles even during relatively light exertion (HR ≤ 90 b · min^{-1}).[42] Two factors contribute to reduced blood flow to nonactive tissues[33,34,37]:

1. Increased sympathetic nervous system outflow (central and peripheral mechanisms)
2. Local chemicals that directly stimulate vasoconstriction or enhance the effects of other vasoconstrictors

The kidneys vividly illustrate regional blood flow adjustment and bodily fluid conservation via sympathetic vasoconstriction. Renal blood flow at rest normally averages 1100 mL · min^{-1} (20% of total cardiac output), among the highest blood flow to any organ as either a percentage of cardiac output or indexed to organ weight. During maximal exercise effort, renal blood flow decreases to 250 mL · min^{-1} (1% total cardiac output). A large but temporary blood flow reduction also occurs in the liver, pancreas, and gastrointestinal tract.[48,62]

 See the animation "Renal Function" on Lippincott Connect to view this process.

Blood Flow Regulation in Active Muscle

Skeletal muscle blood flow closely couples to metabolic demands, whether at rest or in maximal exercise. Regulation occurs from the interaction of neural vasoconstrictor activity and locally derived vasoactive substances within active tissues' vascular endothelium and red blood cells.[12,15,49,58]

At rest, for every 30 to 40 capillaries in muscle tissue only one remains open. Opening dormant capillaries during physical activity serves three important functions:

1. Increases total muscle blood flow
2. Delivers a large blood volume with only minimal increases in blood flow velocity
3. Increases the effective surface for gas and nutrient exchange between blood and muscle fibers

Vasodilation occurs from local factors related to tissue metabolism that act directly on the smooth muscle bands of small arterioles and precapillary sphincters. This rapid response adjusts precisely to the muscle's force output and metabolic needs. Decreased tissue oxygen supply serves as a potent local stimulus for vasodilation in skeletal and cardiac muscle. Additionally, local increases in blood flow, temperature, carbon dioxide, acidity, adenosine, magnesium and potassium ions, and nitric oxide production by endothelial cells lining the blood vessels trigger the discharge of relaxing factors that enhance regional blood flow.[14,19,32] The venous system also may increase local blood flow by "assessing" increases in the active muscle's metabolic needs and releasing vasodilatory factors from venular endothelial cells that diffuse to and dilate the adjacent arteriole.[21] The **autoregulatory mechanisms** for blood flow make sense physiologically because they reflect elevated tissue metabolism and increased oxygen need. Local regulation provides such strong control that it maintains adequate regional blood flow even in patients in whom the nerves to blood vessels have been surgically removed. Local metabolite stimulation of chemoreceptors also provides peripheral neural reflex input for medullary control of the heart and vasculature.

Nitric Oxide Autoregulates Tissue Blood Flow. **Nitric oxide (NO)** is an important signaling molecule that dilates blood vessels and decreases vascular resistance, thereby increasing blood flow. Most living organisms naturally produce the NO vascular gatekeeper from the nonessential amino acid L-arginine. Stimuli from diverse signal chemicals (including neurotransmitters) and sheering stress and vessel stretch from increased blood flow through the vessel lumen provoke NO synthesis and release by the vascular endothelium. Formerly termed *endothelium-derived relaxing factor* by 1998 Nobel Prize in Physiology or Medicine corecipient **Robert F. Furchgott** (1916–2009; for discovering NO's role as a signaling molecule in the cardiovascular system; www.nobelprize.org/prizes/medicine/1998/furchgott/biographical/), NO rapidly spreads through underlying cell membranes to smooth muscle cells within the arterial wall. Here, it binds with and activates *guanylyl cyclase*, an enzyme important in cellular communication and signal transduction. This initiates a series of reactions that attenuate sympathetic vasoconstriction and induce arterial smooth muscle relaxation to increase blood flow in neighboring blood vessels. NO exerts its potent vasodilator effect on skeletal muscle (including the diaphragm), sponge like vascular tissues, skin, and myocardial tissue (**FIG. 16.7**).[4,8,22,23,54]

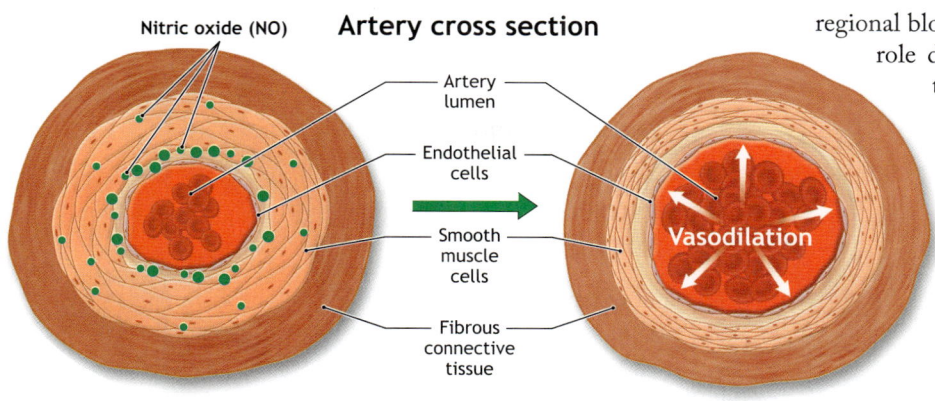

FIGURE 16.7. Mechanism for nitric oxide regulation of local tissue blood flow.

Additional NO Functions

NO regulates an array of physiologic processes affecting skeletal muscle functions. Nitrates in the diet increase NO bioavailability. Dietary nitrate supplementation may increase exercise economy and muscular performance, particularly for type II fast-twitch muscle fibers under low oxygen tensions to promote nitrite's reduction to NO to improve local blood flow, resistance to fatigue, and fiber contractility. Such responses benefit type II muscle fibers in intense, intermittent physical activities; mediate olfaction; enhance immune response regulation; and act as an interneuron to inhibit blood clot formation. NO also contributes to cutaneous active vasodilation with heat stress and dilates coronary vasculature as an early adaptation to moderate exercise training.[28,29,55,57,63]

NO vascular wall receptors contribute to blood pressure regulation in response to central cardiovascular stimulation during emotionally stressful situations including physical activity. Racial differences in resting blood pressure relate to a lower sensitivity to NO's dilating action in Blacks than in Whites.[9] In coronary artery disease, the endothelium produces less NO. Reduced NO bioavailability explains the potent life-saving nitroglycerin treatment, which releases NO gas to reverse chest discomfort or pain called **angina pectoris** from inadequate oxygen delivery from coronary vessel disease.

Hormonal Factors

Sympathetic nerves terminate in the adrenal glands' medullary portion. With sympathetic activation, this glandular tissue secretes large epinephrine quantities and a smaller norepinephrine amount into blood. These hormonal chemical messengers induce a generalized constrictor response, except in blood vessels of the heart and skeletal muscles. Hormonal regional blood flow control plays a relatively minor role during physical activity compared with the more local, rapid, and potent sympathetic neural drive.

Integrative Responses During Physical Activity

The neural command center above the medullary region initiates cardiovascular changes immediately before and at movement onset. Heart rate and myocardial contractility increase from feed-forward input from this center, which also suppresses parasympathetic activation. Concurrently, predictable alterations in regional blood flow occur in proportion to activity severity. Modulation of vascular dilation and constriction optimizes blood flow to areas in need while maintaining blood pressure throughout the arterial system. As activity continues, reflex feedback to the medulla from peripheral mechanical and chemical receptors in active tissue appraises tissue metabolism and circulatory needs. Local metabolic factors act directly to dilate resistance vessels in active muscles. Vasodilation reduces peripheral resistance for greater blood flow in these areas. Arterial blood flow through active muscles progresses in pulsatile oscillations that favor enhanced flow during eccentric (lengthening) muscle actions and/or recovery concentric (shortening) actions.[47] Centrally mediated constrictor adjustments also occur in inactive tissues' vasculature, including skin, kidneys, the splanchnic region, and inactive muscle. Constrictor action maintains adequate perfusion pressure within active muscle while simultaneously increasing blood supply to meet metabolic demands.

Venous Return from Light-to-Maximal–Intensity Physical Activity

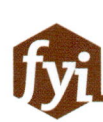

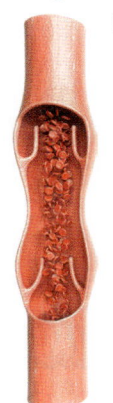

Factors affecting venous return are as important as those regulating arterial blood flow. When exercise movement begins, muscle and ventilatory pump actions in conjunction with visceral vasoconstriction immediately help to return blood to the right ventricle. These acute responses facilitate venous return as cardiac output increases to balance venous return with the heart's output. In upright activity, gravity impedes blood returning from the extremities, thus making autoregulated venous blood flow adjustments an important physiologic response as exercise progresses from light to maximal intensity.

Crevis/Shutterstock

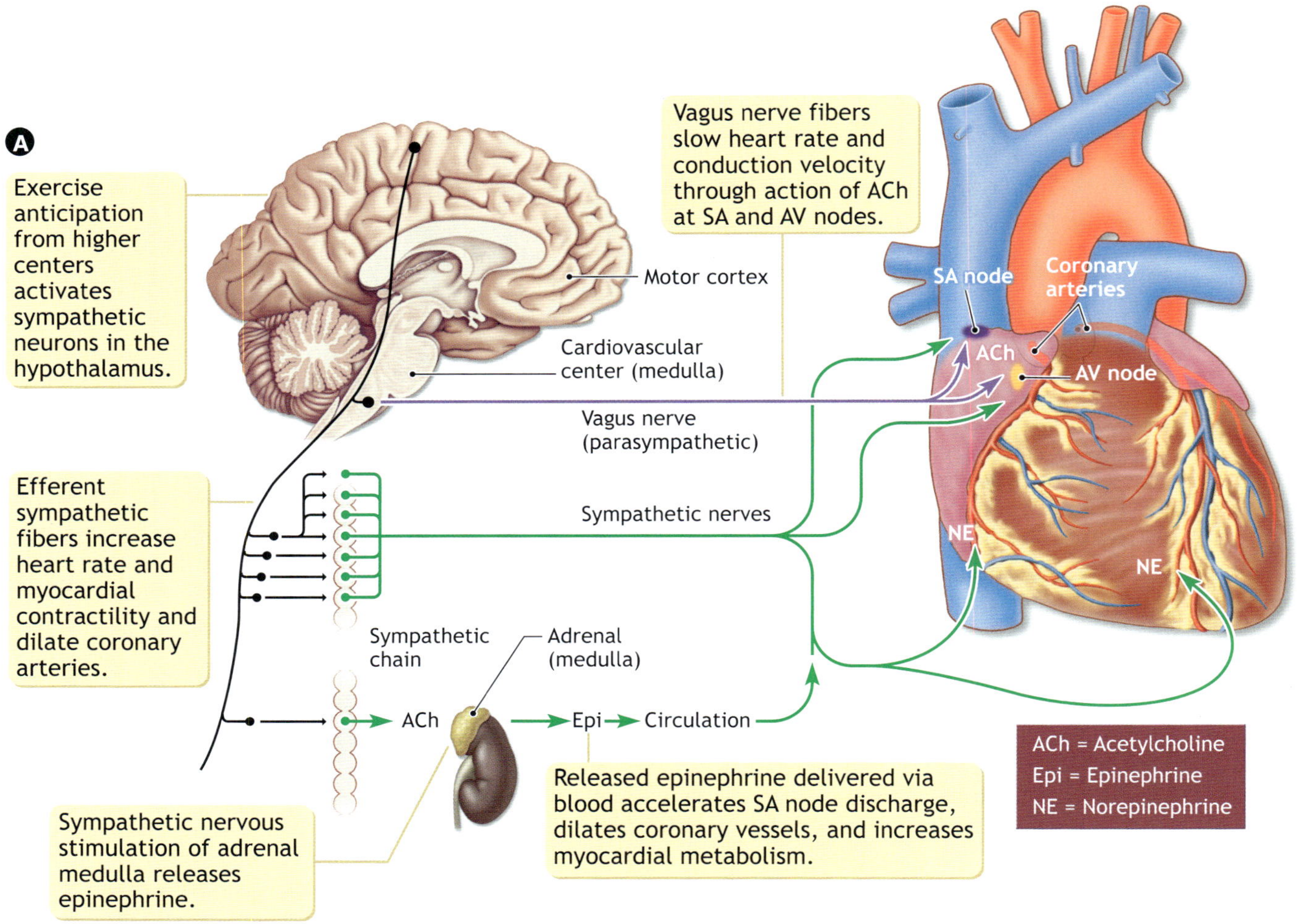

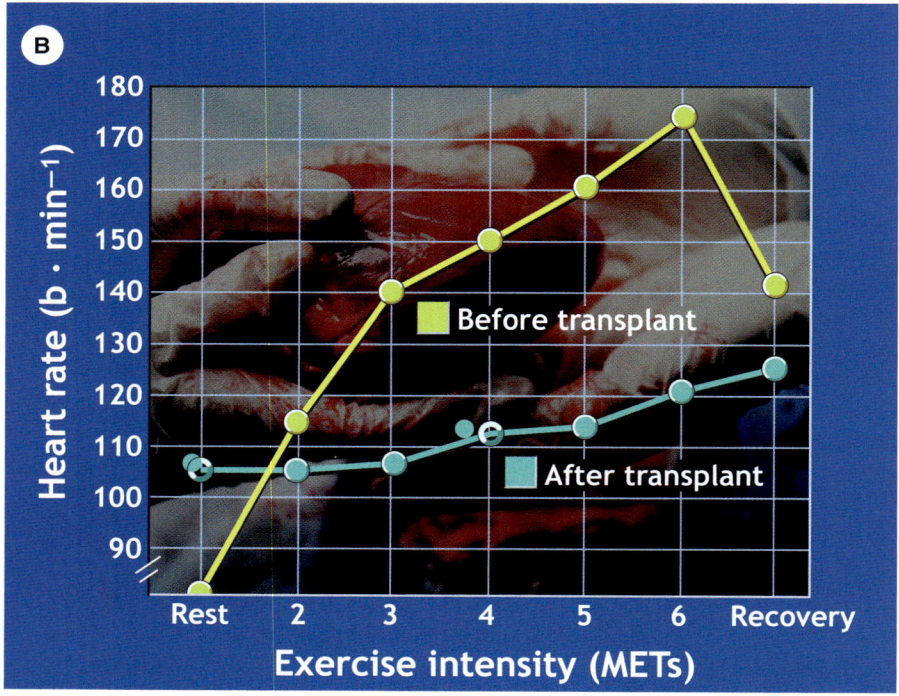

FIGURE 16.8. (A) Normal heart rate (HR) regulation. Heart transplantation produces cardiac denervation by removing myocardium vagal and sympathetic efferent stimulation. Epinephrine from the adrenal medulla regulates exercise HR.
(B) The patient's HR response during graded exercise before and after cardiac transplantation elevates resting HR and delays and depresses HR response after transplantation. AV, atrioventricular; b, beat; MET, metabolic equivalent; SA, sinoatrial.

(Part B adapted with permission from Squires RW. Exercise training after cardiac transplantation. *Med Sci Sports Exerc.* 1991;23:686. Africa Studio/Shutterstock)

Physical Activity After Cardiac Transplantation

Patients with left ventricular dysfunction—ejection fraction less than 20% referred to as *end-stage heart disease*—show poor long-term prognosis. For them, cardiac transplantation becomes their last hope to survive. According to 2019 data from the United Network for Organ Sharing (https://unos.org), 36,529 heart transplantations (HTXs) took place in the United States, more than ever before, in newborns, children, the elderly (70 to 75 years), and oldest old or super-old (above age 90 years; https://onlinelibrary.wiley.com/doi/full/10.1111/ggi.13118). Success with HTX during the past decade has paved the way for multiple-organ transplants—heart-lung, heart-kidney, and heart-liver. The 1-year survival for HTX patients averages close to 90% (www.uptodate.com/contents/heart-transplantation-beyond-the-basics).

Cardiac transplantation, also called **orthotopic transplantation**, illustrates the importance of extrinsic neural control for governing heart rate in physical activity. The procedure removes donor and recipient hearts by transection at the midatrial level—preserving the recipient's pulmonary venous connections to the left atrium's posterior wall—with further aortic transection just above the semilunar valves. Transplantation eliminates the myocardium's neural innervation, while hormonal feedback from circulating catecholamines largely from the adrenal medulla remains intact (**FIG. 16.8A**).

Improved Transplant Function but Altered Circulatory Dynamics

Following successful HTX, patients generally report more favorable quality of life, and approximately 50% return to work. In general, a transplant patient demonstrates prolonged oxygen uptake kinetics, impaired exercise capacity, and diminished physiologic and hemodynamic function that rarely exceeds 45 to 70% of normal.[2,6,17,39,56] This does not necessarily represent the rule for younger, previously active patients who adhere to rehabilitation.[43] In general, HTX recipients can perform relatively intense training and often achieve performance values similar to moderately trained healthy individuals.[11,25,40,44]

FIGURE 16.9A, B, AND C illustrates peak oxygen uptake ($\dot{V}O_{2peak}$) for 140 patients evaluated prior to transplantation and up to 9 years after the procedure. HTX produced an average 50% improvement in $\dot{V}O_{2peak}$ (A) from 14.2 mL · kg^{-1} · min^{-1} before to 21.4 mL · kg^{-1} · min^{-1} 11.2 months after surgery. The patients maintained improved aerobic capacity up to 9 years postsurgery (B). The younger patients below age 40 (includes pediatric patients) exhibited the greatest physiologic improvements following HTX. For both pediatric and adult transplant recipients, increased peripheral oxygen extraction (widened arterio–mixed venous oxygen difference) provides the compensatory mechanism for improved functional capacity.[64]

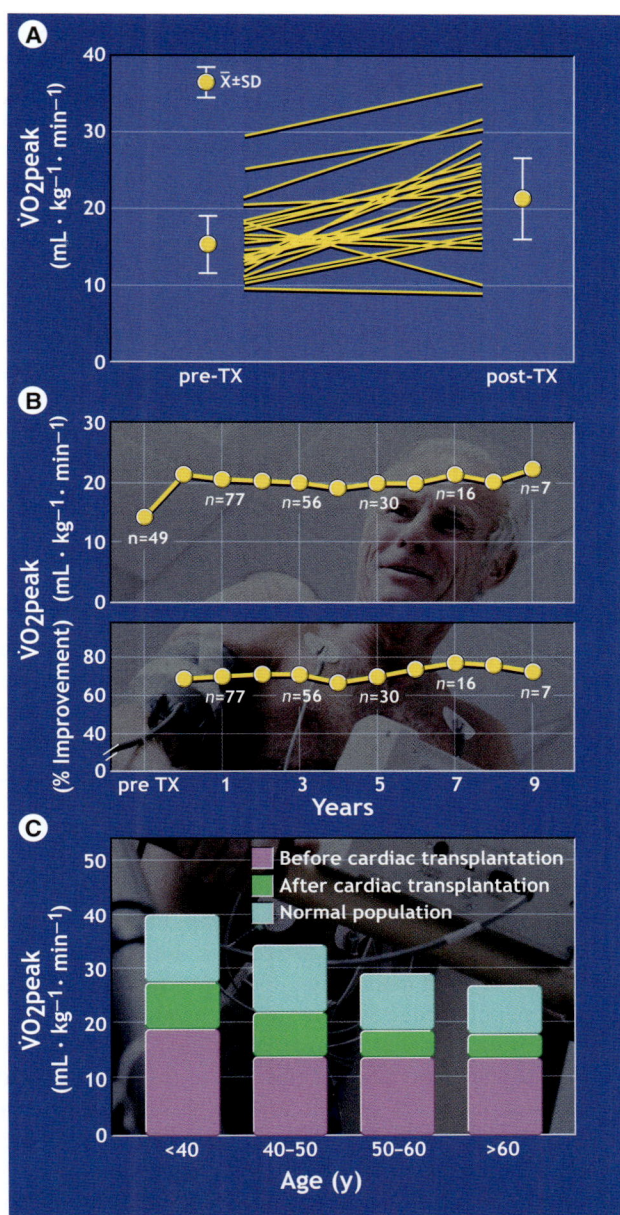

FIGURE 16.9. Heart transplantation (TX) long-term effects on aerobic functional capacity. **(A)** Peak oxygen uptake ($\dot{V}O_{2peak}$) before and 11.2 months after TX in 43 patients who underwent testing at both intervals. Post-TX average significantly surpassed pre-TX. **(B)** Significant percentage improvements in $\dot{V}O_{2peak}$ occurred beginning as early as 6 months post-TX and remained improved for up to 9 years. **(C)** Impact of age on improvement in 43 patients tested before and one year post-TX. SD, standard deviation; x, arithmetic mean.
(Adapted with permission from Osada N, et al. Long-term cardiopulmonary exercise performance after heart transplantation. *Am J Cardiol.* 1997;79:451. Monkey Business Images/Shutterstock)

Sluggish Circulatory Response

The short-term exercise response for the transplant recipient classifies as *abnormal*. These patients demonstrate limited cardiac output and oxygen uptake during exertion, with accompanying reduced left ventricular ejection capacity. Figure 16.8B shows that circulatory sluggishness results from the denervated heart's inability to accelerate significantly with increasing physical demands, often accelerating by only 20 to 40 b·min^{-1} with relatively strenuous effort.[3,16,35] The exercise response of the denervated transplanted heart does improve over the 12-month postsurgery period, but the adaptations exert no meaningful effect on submaximal or peak oxygen uptake.

In healthy individuals, stroke volume increases up to about 50% $\dot{V}O_{2max}$ and then plateaus; further increases in cardiac output come mainly from increases in heart rate. Transplant patients, by contrast, have no stroke volume plateau during graded exercise; instead, stroke volume progressively increases by the Frank-Starling mechanism (i.e., progressive increases in cardiac filling) throughout the exercise range. Chapter 32 discusses regular training's effects for HTX patients.

 INTEGRATIVE QUESTION

How is it that task-specific, regular aerobic physical activity not only trains the cardiovascular system but also "trains" the neuromuscular system to facilitate physiologic adjustments specific to the activity mode?

Summary

1. The cardiovascular system provides rapid heart rate regulation and effective blood distribution through the vascular circuit (while maintaining blood pressure) in response to overall metabolic and physiologic needs.
2. The cardiac rhythm originates at the SA node. The impulse then travels across the atria to the AV node and, after a brief delay, spreads across the large ventricular mass. This conduction pattern initiates atrial and ventricular contractions to provide impetus for blood flow.
3. The ECG records the heart's electrical events during the cardiac cycle. The ECG detects various heart function abnormalities during rest and increasing exercise intensities.
4. Epinephrine and norepinephrine accelerate heart rate and increase myocardial contractility, while acetylcholine acts through the vagus nerve to slow heart rate.
5. The heart "turns on" in the transition from rest to physical activity from increased sympathetic and decreased parasympathetic activity integrated with central command input.
6. Cortical influence in anticipation before and during the initial stage of physical activity governs a substantial part of the heart rate adjustment to the activity.
7. Reflex sensory input from peripheral receptors in blood vessels, joints, and muscles provides the cardiovascular center with continual feedback about active muscles' physical and chemical state.
8. Neural and hormonal extrinsic factors modify the heart's inherent rhythm.
9. Heart rate accelerates rapidly in anticipation of exercise and can attain 200 b·min^{-1} in maximum effort.
10. Carotid artery palpation accurately accesses heart rate during and immediately after exercise in healthy individuals.
11. Nerves, hormones, and local metabolic factors act on the smooth muscle bands in blood vessels to alter the vessels' internal diameter and regulate blood flow to metabolic demands.
12. Blood flow changes with the vessels' radius raised to the fourth power in accord with Poiseuille's law.
13. NO, an extraordinarily important and potent endothelium-derived relaxing factor, facilitates blood vessel dilation and decreases vascular resistance.
14. The kidneys and splanchnic regions dramatically compromise their blood flow in physical activity to augment blood delivery to the active muscles and maintain systemic blood pressure.
15. Patients who successfully undergo orthotopic transplantation have a depressed cardiovascular response to exercise; the denervated heart cannot accelerate rapidly enough to meet the increased physical activity demands.

Key Terms

Adrenergic fibers: Specific sympathetic neurons that release norepinephrine; act as a general vasoconstrictor

Atrioventricular (AV) bundle: Myocardial cells that serve as part of the heart's electrical conduction system; transmits the electrical impulses from right atrium to ventricles; also known as bundle of His

Atrioventricular node (AV node): Electrochemical rhythms originating at the SA node spread across the atria to this small knot of tissue situated close to the tricuspid valve; electrically connects atria and ventricles

Autoregulatory mechanisms: Tendency for maintenance of blood flow to an organ despite changes in arterial pressure in the artery supplying it

Bradycardia: Slower than normal heart rate; usually below 60 beats per minute at rest

Carotid artery palpation: Arterial location at side of neck routinely used to determine heart rate during rest and physical activity

Catecholamines: Adrenal gland amine compounds like dopamine, norepinephrine, and epinephrine that function as neurotransmitters and hormones within the body

Chronotropic effect: Factors that affect the heart's rate of beating

Electrocardiogram (ECG): Normal cycle of the heart's electrical activity

Exercise pressor reflex: Neural signals from active muscle provide peripheral feedback to activate cardiovascular control centers in the brainstem that increase heart rate and blood pressure via sympathetic activation and parasympathetic withdrawal

Extrinsic controls: Neuronal, humoral, reflex, and chemical mechanisms during exercise that regulate heart rate, myocardial contractility, and vascular smooth muscle; maintain cardiac output, blood flow distribution, and arterial blood pressure

Furchgott, Robert F. (1916–2009): Noble Prize in Physiology or Medicine for discovering nitric oxide as a signaling molecule in the cardiovascular system

Inotropic effect: Alterations that affect the force or energy of contractions

Mechanoreceptors: Sensory structures within muscle and its vasculature that monitor physical state: respond to mechanical pressure or distortion

Metaboreflex: Reflex triggered by metaboreceptors during physical activity to increase blood flow and ventilation

Nitric oxide (NO): Signaling molecule that dilates blood vessels and decreases vascular resistance; attenuates sympathetic vasoconstriction and induces arterial smooth muscle relaxation to increase blood flow

Orthotopic transplantation: Transplantation of organ or tissue from a donor into its normal position in the recipient's body

P wave: Represents depolarization of the atria; lasts approximately 0.15 s and heralds atrial contraction

Parasympathetic nervous system: Autonomic nervous system component that slows heart rate, increases intestinal and glandular activity, and relaxes sphincter muscles

Poiseuille's law: Homogeneous fluid volume passing through a tube is directly proportional to pressure differential between its ends and to the fourth power of its internal radius, and inversely proportional to its length and fluid viscosity

Purkinje system: Specialized fibers that transmit electrical impulse from atrioventricular node to ventricles causing them to contract

QRS complex: ECG that follows the P wave by signaling signals electrical changes from ventricular depolarization

Refractory period: Inability of heart to generate a contraction; period during and following an action potential when an excitable membrane cannot be re-excited

Sinoatrial (SA) node: Specialized tissue situated within the posterior wall of the right atrium that spontaneously depolarizes and repolarizes to provide innate stimulus for heart action; also called pacemaker

T wave: ECG portion representing ventricular repolarization that occurs during ventricular diastole

Tachycardia: Describes heart rate acceleration, usually to rates that exceed 100 b · min-1 at rest

Vagus nerve: Tenth cranial nerve that interfaces with parasympathetic control of heart, lungs, and digestive tract

Vasomotor tone: Adrenergic constrictor nerves that remain continually active; causes smooth muscle bands of certain blood vessels to always exhibit a relative state of constriction

Ventrolateral medulla: Cardiovascular control center that regulates heart's output of blood and blood's preferential distribution to body's tissues; receives input from the brain and peripheral nervous system

> References are available online at Lippincott Connect.

Additional References

Calbet JAL, et al. An integrative approach to the regulation of mitochondrial respiration during exercise: focus on high intensity exercise. *Redox Biol*. 2020;35:101478.

Cheng MY, et al. Relationship between cognitive emotion regulation strategies and coronary heart disease: an empirical examination of heart rate variability and coronary stenosis. *Psychol Health*. 2022;37:230.

Christiansen D, Bishop DJ. Aerobic-interval exercise with blood flow restriction potentiates early markers of metabolic health in man. *Acta Physiol (Oxf)*. 2022;234:e13769.

d'Unienville NMA, et al. Heart-rate acceleration is linearly related to anaerobic exercise performance. *Int J Sports Physiol Perform*. 2022;17:78.

Deus LA, et al. Metabolic and hormonal responses to chronic blood-flow restricted resistance training in chronic kidney disease: a randomized trial. *Appl Physiol Nutr Metab*. 2022;47:183.

Dupuy A, et al. Post-exercise heart rate recovery and parasympathetic reactivation are comparable between prepubertal boys and well-trained adult male endurance athletes. *Eur J Appl Physiol*. 2022;122:345.

Guo QN, et al. Nicotine ingestion reduces heart rate variability in young healthy adults. *Biomed Res Int*. 2022;2022:4286621.

Hebisz RG, et al. Heart rate variability after sprint interval training in cyclists and implications for assessing physical fatigue. *J Strength Cond Res*. 2022;36:558.

Joyce W, Wang T. Regulation of heart rate in vertebrates during hypoxia: a comparative overview. *Acta Physiol (Oxf)*. 2022:e13779.

Koep JL, et al. Autonomic control of cerebral blood flow: fundamental comparisons between peripheral and cerebrovascular circulations in humans. *J Physiol*. 2022;600:15.

Liu KY, et al. Heart rate variability in relation to cognition and behavior in neurodegenerative diseases: a systematic review and meta-analysis. *Ageing Res Rev*. 2022;73:101539.

Ng HL, et al. Effects of a taped filter mask on peak power, perceived breathlessness, heart rate, blood lactate and oxygen saturation during a graded exercise test in young healthy adults: a randomized controlled trial. *BMC Sports Sci Med Rehabil*. 2022;14:19.

Papa A, et al. Adrenergic regulation of calcium channels in the heart. *Annu Rev Physiol*. 2022;84:285.

Shanks J, et al. Reverse re-modelling chronic heart failure by reinstating heart rate variability. *Basic Res Cardiol*. 2022;117:4.

Skow RJ, et al. Prenatal exercise and cardiovascular health (PEACH) study: impact of acute and chronic exercise on cerebrovascular hemodynamics and dynamic cerebral autoregulation. *J Appl Physiol (1985)*. 2022;132:247.

Washio T, et al. Site-specific different dynamic cerebral autoregulation and cerebrovascular response to carbon dioxide in posterior cerebral circulation during isometric exercise in healthy young men. *Auton Neurosci*. 2022;238:102943.

Yu TY, et al. Delayed heart rate recovery after exercise predicts development of metabolic syndrome: a retrospective cohort study. *J Diabetes Investig*. 2022;13:167.

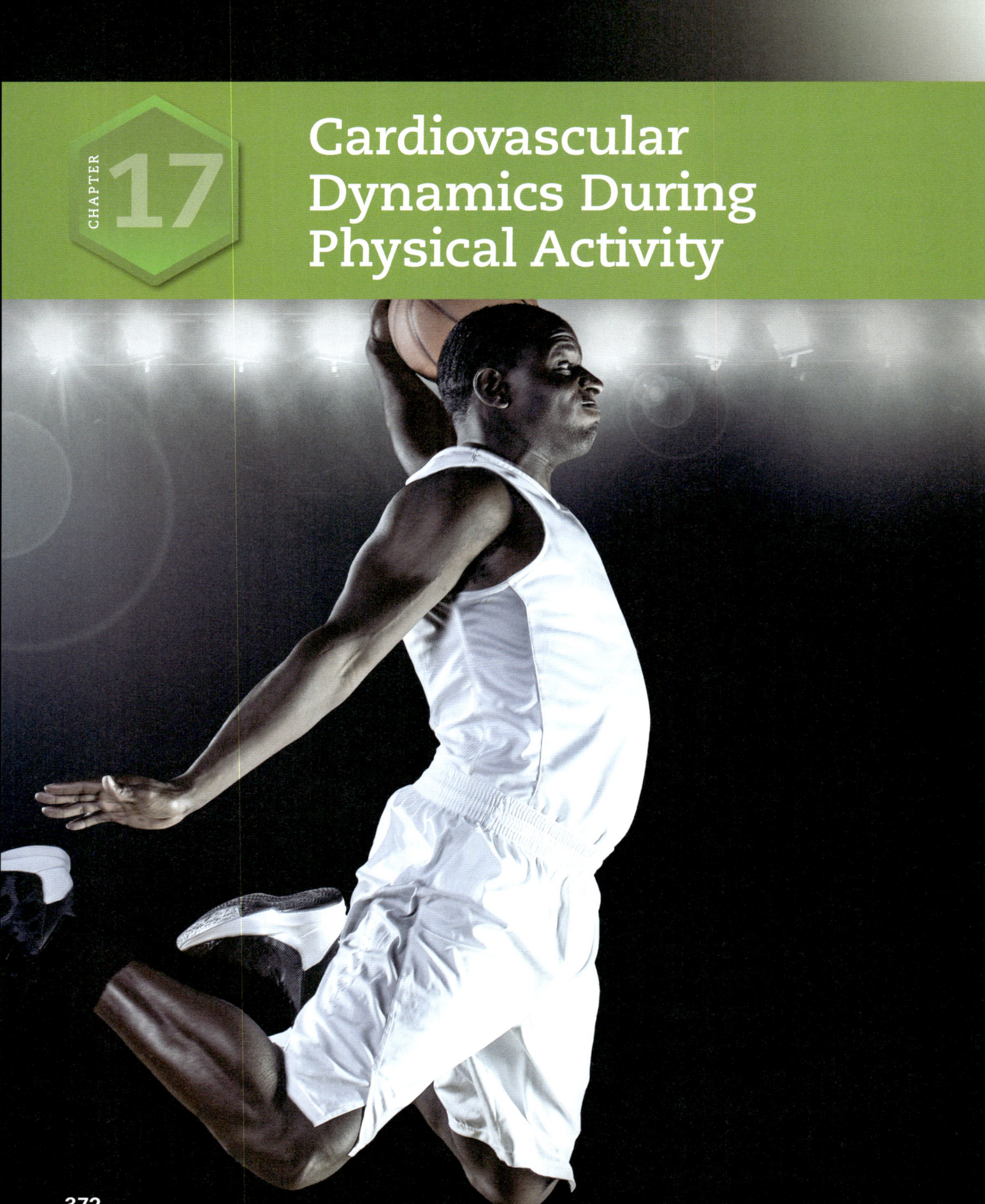

Cardiovascular Dynamics During Physical Activity

CHAPTER 17

Chapter Objectives

- Discuss one advantage and one disadvantage of the direct Fick, indicator dilution, and CO_2 rebreathing cardiac output methods
- Compare cardiac output during rest and maximum effort for an endurance-trained athlete and sedentary nonathlete
- Explain how each Fick equation component influences maximum oxygen uptake ($\dot{V}O_{2max}$)
- Discuss two physiologic mechanisms that influence exercise stroke volume
- Contrast cardiac output component changes from rest to maximum effort for sedentary and endurance-trained individuals
- Explain how the Frank-Starling mechanism impacts cardiac output during different physical activity modes
- Discuss two proposed mechanisms to explain cardiovascular drift
- List the main cardiac output distribution percentages to major body tissues during rest and intense aerobic activity
- Describe how maximum cardiac output and $\dot{V}O_{2max}$ relate among individuals who vary in aerobic fitness
- List three factors responsible for expanding the arterio-mixed venous oxygen difference during graded exercise
- Contrast cardiovascular and metabolic dynamics for upper-body versus lower-body graded exercise

Ancillaries at-a-Glance

Visit Lippincott Connect to access the following resources.

- References: Chapter 17
- Animations: Blood Flow, Myocardial Blood Flow
- Focus on Research: Consequences of Stopping Endurance Exercise Training

Cardiac output ($\dot{Q}$, *meaning quantity*) *refers to how much blood the heart pumps in 1 min.* The maximum value reflects the cardiovascular system's functional capacity. The heart's output, as with any pump, depends on its rate of pumping (**heart rate [HR]**) and how much blood it ejects with each stroke (**stroke volume [SV]**).

$$\text{Cardiac output} = \text{HR} \times \text{SV}$$

 See the animation "Blood Flow" on Lippincott Connect to view this process.

Measuring Cardiac Output

Output from a hose, pump, or faucet can be determined by opening the valve and collecting and measuring the fluid volume ejected over a given time. This is not an acceptable method for application to humans. To more fully understand cardiac output dynamics, we describe three common cardiac output measurement methods to assess the cardiac output of the closed circulatory system in humans:

1. Direct Fick
2. Indicator dilution
3. CO_2 rebreathing

Direct Fick Method

Two factors determine how much fluid a pump circulates within a closed circuit:

1. Change in substance concentration between the pump's outflow and inflow ports
2. Total quantity of that substance taken up or given off in a given time

For cardiovascular dynamics, calculating cardiac output requires knowledge about two variables:

1. Average difference between the oxygen content of arterial blood and the oxygen content of mixed venous blood (a-$\bar{v}O_2$ diff)
2. Oxygen uptake during 1 min ($\dot{V}O_2$)

The important question then becomes how much blood circulates during 1 min to account for the observed oxygen uptake given the observed a-$\bar{v}O_2$ diff?

The **Fick equation**, published in 1870 by German mathematician/physiologist/physicist Adolph Gaston Fick (1829–1901; first to devise a technique to measure cardiac output; see Introduction: A View From the Past), expresses the relationships among cardiac output, oxygen uptake, and a-$\bar{v}O_2$ diff. These variables could not be determined in humans until cardiac catheterization became a standard in clinical medical practice (and later in some contemporary exercise physiology research laboratories).

$$\text{Cardiac output (mL·min}^{-1}\text{)} = \frac{\dot{V}O_2 \text{ mL·min}^{-1}}{\text{a-}\bar{v}O_2 \text{ difference (mL per 100 mL blood)}} \times 100$$

FIGURE 17.1 illustrates use of the Fick principle to determine cardiac output. In this example, 250 mL oxygen is consumed during 1 min at rest, with a-$\bar{v}O_2$ diff averaging 5 mL oxygen per 100 mL (deciliter [dL]) of blood. Substituting these values into the Fick equation yields cardiac output:

$$\text{Cardiac output (mL·min}^{-1}\text{)} = \frac{250 \text{ mL } O_2}{5 \text{ mL } O_2} \times 100 = 5000 \text{ mL blood}$$

Seemingly straightforward in principle, the Fick method requires complex methodology usually performed in a hospital.[18,45,46] Measuring oxygen uptake involves open-circuit spirometry methods (see Chapter 8). Quantifying the a-$\bar{v}O_2$ diff remains more difficult. A representative arterial blood sample can come from any convenient systemic femoral, radial, or brachial artery. These arteries are easily located, but puncturing the artery with a needle confers risk, and sampling mixed-venous blood presents additional difficulties because the blood in each vein only reflects the metabolic activity of the specific area it drains. *An accurate measure of the average oxygen content of all venous blood requires sampling from an anatomic "mixing chamber" (e.g., right atrium, right ventricle, or, most accurately, the pulmonary artery).* Such sampling requires threading a small flexible catheter through the antecubital vein in the arm into the superior vena cava, which drains into the right heart. Arterial and mixed venous blood are then sampled simultaneously while measuring oxygen uptake.

Research about cardiovascular dynamics applies the direct Fick method under different experimental conditions. The method generally serves as the criterion standard to validate other cardiac output measurement techniques. The *invasive* Fick procedure can alter normal cardiovascular dynamics during measurement that may not reflect the person's usual cardiovascular response pattern.

Indicator Dilution Method

The **indicator dilution method** involves venous and arterial needle punctures but does not require cardiac catheterization. Injecting a known inert dye (e.g., indocyanine green) into a large vein is measured in blood from its concentration curve assessed by light absorption. The indicator material remains in the vascular stream usually bound to plasma proteins or red blood cells. It then mixes in the blood as the blood travels to the lungs and returns to the heart before emptying into the systemic circuit. A photosensitive device continually assesses arterial blood samples for dye concentration. The area under the dilution-concentration curve obtained from repetitive sampling reflects the indicator material's average concentration in blood leaving the heart. Cardiac output computes from the dilution of a known quantity of dye in the unknown blood quantity:

$$\text{Cardiac output} = \frac{\text{Quantity of dye injected}}{\text{Average dye concentration in blood for duration of curve} \times \text{Duration of curve}}$$

CO₂ Rebreathing Method

Cardiac output is determined by substituting CO_2 values for O_2 values in the Fick equation.[8,35] The same open-circuit spirometric method to determine oxygen uptake in the typical Fick technique determines CO_2 production in the rebreathing method. Using a rapid CO_2 gas analyzer, and making reasonable assumptions about gas exchange, provides valid mixed venous and arterial CO_2 level estimates. This noninvasive or "bloodless" technique requires breath-by-breath CO_2 analysis, commonly measured in most exercise physiology laboratories. Values for CO_2 production and mixed venous and arterial CO_2 concentrations, derived from expired CO_2 obtained during different time periods, provide the input data to compute cardiac output by the Fick principle as follows:

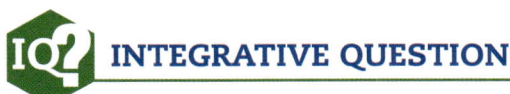

$$\text{Cardiac output (mL·min}^{-1}) = \frac{\dot{V}CO_2}{\bar{v}\text{-a}CO_2 \text{ difference}} \times 100$$

The CO_2 rebreathing method offers obvious advantages over the direct Fick and indicator dilution methods, particularly during physical activity. *It does not require blood sampling or intense medical supervision and only minimally interferes with the subject during movement.* One limitation of CO_2 rebreathing requires that subjects exercise under steady-rate aerobic metabolism. This restricts the method's use during the transition from rest to exercise and maximum and "supra-maximum" activities.

IQ? INTEGRATIVE QUESTION

In what way does the Fick equation fully explain the physiologic components that determine $\dot{V}O_{2max}$?

Cardiac Output at Rest

An individual's cardiac output can vary considerably during rest. Influencing factors include emotional conditions that alter cortical outflow (central command) to the cardioaccelerator nerves that modulate arterial resistance vessels. Each minute, the left ventricle pumps the entire 5-L blood volume (5.0 L·min⁻¹) for a typical 70-kg/154-lb untrained or trained male. Resting cardiac output for the typical 56-kg/124-lb female averages nearly 4.0 L·min⁻¹.

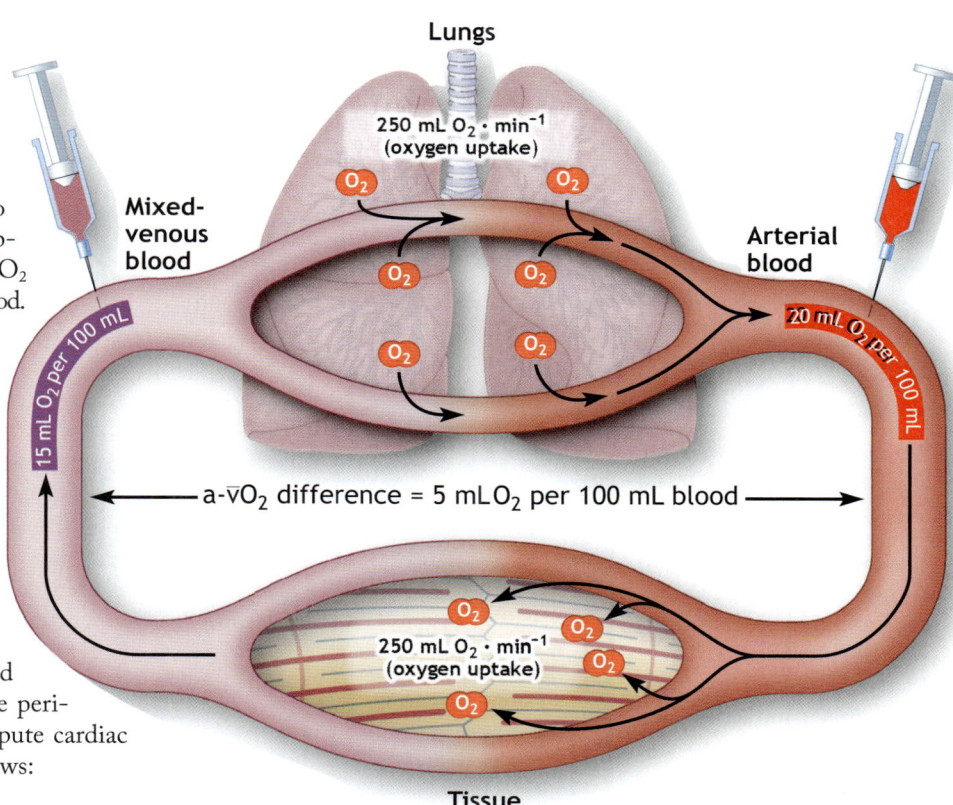

FIGURE 17.1. The Fick principle to measure cardiac output per minute ($\dot{Q}$). a-$\bar{v}O_2$ diff, difference between the oxygen content of arterial blood and mixed-venous blood; $\dot{V}O_2$, oxygen uptake.

Untrained Individuals

For the typical sedentary person at rest, HR averages 70 b·min⁻¹ to sustain a 5-L cardiac output. Substituting this HR value in the cardiac output equation (SV = $\dot{Q}$ ÷ HR), the heart's calculated SV equals 0.0714 L or 71.4 mL. SV and cardiac output for females average about 25% below values for males; in females, the SV at rest averages 50 to 60 mL. This "sex difference" generally relates to the average woman's smaller body size.

Endurance Athletes

Endurance training brings the heart's sinus node under greater acetylcholine influence, the parasympathetic hormone that slows HR. At the same time, resting sympathetic activity decreases. This longer-term training adaptation partially explains many elite endurance athletes' low resting HRs. Relatively brief training periods exert only a minimal lowering effect on resting HR.[1,39]

HRs in healthy endurance athletes generally average 50 b·min⁻¹ at rest, although HRs below 30 b·min⁻¹ have been reported, but infrequently. The endurance athlete's 5 L·min⁻¹ resting cardiac output circulates with a relatively large 100 mL SV. The following summarizes average values for cardiac output, HR, and SV for endurance-trained and untrained men at rest:

> **Rest**
> **Cardiac output = Heart rate × Stroke volume**
> Untrained: 5000 mL·min⁻¹ = 70 b·min⁻¹ × 71 mL
> Trained: 5000 mL·min⁻¹ = 50 b·min⁻¹ × 100 mL

Two factors help to explain the large SV and low HR for endurance-trained athletes:

1. Increased vagal (parasympathetic) tone and decreased sympathetic drive, both of which slow the heart
2. Increased blood volume, myocardial contractility, and compliance (ability to distend in response to pressure; reduced left ventricular cardiac stiffness), all of which augment the heart's SV

Cardiac Output During Physical Activity

Systemic blood flow increases directly with physical activity intensity. Cardiac output increases rapidly during the transition from rest to steady-rate physical activity. Subsequently, cardiac output rises gradually until it plateaus when blood flow meets the exercise metabolic requirements.

In sedentary, college-age men, cardiac output during maximum exertion increased four times above rest to 20 to 22 L·min⁻¹. Maximum HR averaged 195 b·min⁻¹. Consequently, SV generally ranged between 103 and 113 mL (20,000 mL·min⁻¹ ÷ 195 b·min⁻¹ = 103 mL·b⁻¹; 22,000 mL·min⁻¹ ÷ 195 b·min⁻¹ = 113 mL). In contrast, world-class endurance athletes achieve maximum cardiac outputs of 35 to 40 L·min⁻¹. This high value assumes greater significance when one considers that the trained person generally achieves a slightly lower maximum HR than a similar age sedentary person. *The endurance athlete achieves a large maximum cardiac output solely through an enhanced SV.* For example, cardiac output of an Olympic medal winner in cross-country skiing increased to 40 L·min⁻¹ in all-out effort (almost eight times above rest), where SV was 210 mL. This nearly doubled the maximum blood volume pumped per beat by a sedentary counterpart. For an illustrative comparison with nonhuman "athletes," thoroughbred racehorses achieve extraordinarily large cardiac outputs (600 L·min⁻¹) that accompany a $\dot{V}O_{2max}$ ranging between 120 to 150 mL·kg⁻¹·min⁻¹.[7,24]

The equation that follows summarizes average cardiac output, HR, and SV values for endurance-trained and untrained men during maximum physical activity:

> **Cardiac output = Heart rate × Stroke volume**
> Untrained: 22,000 mL·min⁻¹ = 195 b·min⁻¹ × 113 mL
> Trained: 35,000 mL·min⁻¹ = 195 b·min⁻¹ × 179 mL

The following data reveal SV's importance in differentiating among people with high and low $\dot{V}O_{2max}$.

These data were obtained from three groups: athletes (high $\dot{V}O_{2max}$), healthy but sedentary men (normal $\dot{V}O_{2max}$), and men with mitral stenosis (low $\dot{V}O_{2max}$), a narrowing of the orifice of the heart's mitral valve that restricts blood flow. The differences in $\dot{V}O_{2max}$ among groups closely relate to differences in maximum SV. Patients with mitral stenosis had an aerobic capacity and maximum SV half that of sedentary subjects. The relationship also was apparent in comparisons between healthy subjects. The athletes $\dot{V}O_{2max}$ averaged 62.5% larger than the sedentary group. This paralleled a 60% larger SV. The maximum HRs among all groups were similar, making the differences in cardiac output (and $\dot{V}O_{2max}$) almost entirely due to differences in maximum SV.

$\dot{V}O_{2max}$, HR_{max}, SV_{max}, and $\dot{Q}_{max}$ Values in Three Groups with Very Low, Normal, and High $\dot{V}O_{2max}$

	Very Low $\dot{V}O_{2max}$	Normal $\dot{V}O_{2max}$	High $\dot{V}O_{2max}$
$\dot{V}O_{2max}$ (L·min⁻¹)	1.6	3.2	5.2
HR_{max} (b·min⁻¹)	190	200	190
SV_{max} (mL)	50	100	160
$\dot{Q}_{max}$ (L·min⁻¹)	9.5	20.0	30.4

Pavel L Photo and Video/Shutterstock

Enhancing SV: Diastolic Filling Versus Systolic Emptying

Three physiologic mechanisms can increase the heart's SV during physical activity.[9,14,36]

1. Enhanced cardiac filling in diastole followed by a more forceful systolic contraction (Frank-Starling mechanism)
2. Neurohormonal influence that provides for normal ventricular filling in diastole with subsequent forceful systolic ejection with more complete emptying
3. Training adaptations that expand blood volume and reduce peripheral tissue resistance to blood flow

Enhanced Diastolic Filling

Any factor that increases venous return or slows the heart produces greater ventricular filling or **preload** during diastole. An increase in end-diastolic volume stretches myocardial fibers to initiate a powerful ejection stroke during contraction. This ejects the normal SV plus any additional blood that entered the ventricles in diastole and stretched the myocardium.

Ejection fraction refers to the volume of blood ejected from the heart with each heartbeat in relation to the amount initially contained within the left ventricle. This measure of left ventricular pumping efficiency is calculated by dividing SV by **end-diastolic volume**.

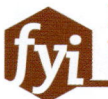 Ejection Fraction Evaluates Ventricular Function

Clinicians use left ventricular ejection fraction (LVEF) as a measure of the heart's pumping ability and subsequent prognosis for cardiovascular health. Individuals with a significantly reduced LVEF generally have poor medical outcomes. Healthy individuals have ejection fractions ranging between 50 and 65% (55 to 73% = normal). Poor left ventricular function often accompanies reduced LVEF, often in the low 40% range or lower (https://www.heart.org/en/health-topics/heart-failure/diagnosing-heart-failure/ejection-fraction-heart-failure-measurement). Physicians determine LVEF by the blood fraction pumped from the left ventricle relative to its end-diastolic volume. For example, if the ventricular end-diastolic volume equals 110 mL, and stroke volume equals 70 mL, LVEF computes as 70 mL ÷ 110 or 0.64 (64%). This translates to mean that with each heartbeat, the left ventricle ejects 64% of its total blood volume before the next beat.

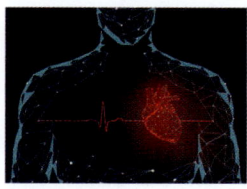
dennistelnovv/Shutterstock

Sources:
Magri D, et al. Cardiovascular death risk in recovered mid-range ejection fraction heart failure: insights from cardiopulmonary exercise test. *J Card Fail.* 2020;26:932. S1071-9164(20)30031-2.

Patriki D, et al. A Prospective pilot study to identify a myocarditis cohort who may safely resume sports activities 3 months after diagnosis. *J Cardiovasc Transl Res.* 2020. doi:10.1007/s12265-020-09983-6.

Two researchers, German physiologist Otto Frank (1865–1944; investigated the heart's isometric and isotonic contractile behavior) and British physiologist Ernest Henry Starling (1866–1927; first to use the term *hormone*), described the relationship between contractile force and the resting length of the heart's muscle fibers. This fundamental phenomenon, the **Frank-Starling law of the heart** (also known as *Starling's law* or the *Frank-Starling mechanism*) states: *Within physiological limits, muscle contraction force relates proportionally to the muscle fiber's initial length.* The principle operates during the cardiac cycle and applies to all heart chambers. For years, physiologists taught that the Frank-Starling mechanism provided the *modus operandi* for *all* SV increases during physical activity. They posited that venous return in exercise facilitated greater cardiac filling. This preload stretched the ventricles in diastole (greater filling) to produce a more forceful ejection stroke.[19,21,47] More than likely, this response pattern for SV operates during the transition from rest to activity or as a person moves from an upright to recumbent position. Enhanced diastolic filling also occurs in swimming as the body's horizontal position optimizes venous return.[48] A more optimal sarcomere myofilament arrangement as the muscle fiber stretches enhances its contractility.

The data in **TABLE 17.1** illustrate the effect of body position on circulatory dynamics. The horizontal position produces the largest and most stable cardiac output and SV. SV remains near maximum in this position at rest and increases only slightly during physical activity as discussed previously. In contrast, in the upright body position, gravity counters blood flow return to the heart (decreased preload) to diminish SV and cardiac output. During upright activity of increasing intensity, SV approaches maximum SV in the supine position.

TABLE 17.1 Body position's effect on cardiovascular dynamics

Greater Systolic Emptying

In most upright physical activity modes, the heart does not fill to increase cardiac volume to the extent it does in the recumbent position. The progressive SV increase in graded upright physical activity in children and adults results from the *combined* effect of enhanced diastolic filling and a more complete emptying during systole.[5,12,23,33] Greater systolic ejection occurs despite increased resistance to blood flow in the arterial circuit from exercise-induced systolic blood pressure elevation known as **afterload**.

Enhanced systolic ejection, with or without increased end-diastolic volume, occurs because the ventricles always contain a **functional residual blood volume**. At rest in the upright position, approximately 40% or 50 to 70 mL of the total end-diastolic blood volume remains in the left ventricle following systole. In physical activity, catecholamine release enhances myocardial contractile force to augment stroke power and facilitate systolic emptying.

Endurance training likely increases left ventricle compliance so as to more readily accept blood in the cardiac cycle's diastolic phase.[9,43] Whether endurance training enhances the myocardium's innate contractile state remains unclear.[10,24] If this adaptation occurs, it too would contribute to a larger SV effect.

Reduced SV and Increased HR During Prolonged Physical Activity: Cardiovascular Drift

Submaximum physical activity performed for more than 15 min in the heat, accompanied by increased core temperature, produces progressive water loss through sweating and a fluid shift from plasma to tissues. The core temperature rise also redistributes blood to the periphery for body cooling. Concurrently, the progressive decrease in plasma volume lowers central venous cardiac filling pressure (preload) to reduce SV. A reduced SV progressively increases HR as activity progresses to maintain a nearly constant cardiac output and body temperature.[8]

The term **cardiovascular drift** describes the gradual time-dependent "drift" in several cardiovascular responses, most notably a decreased SV with concomitant increased HR during prolonged steady-rate physical activity, particularly when outside temperatures exceed 38°C/100°F.[15,49,50]

At high ambient temperatures, a person must exercise at lower intensity than if cardiovascular drift dynamics did not occur.[3,11,41] Decrements in $\dot{V}O_{2max}$ accompany the increased HR and reduced SV with cardiovascular drift, which reduces performance as evidenced by a decreased maximum power output.[42]

One explanation for cardiovascular drift suggests the effects of a progressive increase in cutaneous blood flow (CBF) as core temperature rises in prolonged physical activity. Blood redistribution to the periphery for heat dissipation increases the skin's venous volume, ultimately reducing ventricular filling pressure and SV. **FIGURE 17.2** provides evidence for an alternative explanation for the SV decline during cardiovascular drift in prolonged submaximum physical activity. Seven physically active men cycled for 60 min in a thermoneutral environment while measured for SV (top), HR (middle), and CBF (lower). In one exercise trial, the men received a placebo; at the onset of exercise in the other trial, they received a small β_1-adrenoceptor blocker (atenolol, yellow) dose to prevent the HR increase or cardiovascular drift that normally occurs after cycling for 15 min. Fifteen minutes into activity, HR and SV remained similar during control (green) and β_1-adrenoceptor blockade conditions. From 15 to 55 min during the control trial, a 13% decrease in SV accompanied an 11% HR increase, while CBF showed no increase when cycling from 20 to 60 min. In contrast, from minutes 15 to 55 under blockade conditions when atenolol prevented a HR increase, SV failed to decline compared with control conditions despite similar CBF levels in both trials. Cardiac output remained stable at about 16 L·min^{-1} under both conditions. These observations confirm that a decline in SV results from increased HR and not increased CBF as body temperature rises during prolonged physical activity in a thermoneutral environment.[2] The progressive increases in HR with cardiovascular drift likely decreases end-diastolic volume (i.e., less ventricular filling time) to reduce the heart's SV.

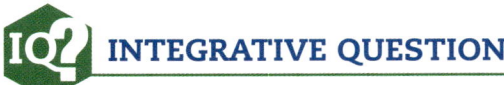 **INTEGRATIVE QUESTION**

Increasing the bloods hemoglobin concentration increases $\dot{V}O_{2max}$ during maximum physical activity at sea level. When this effect occurs, which Fick equation component limits $\dot{V}O_{2max}$?

Cardiac Output Distribution

Blood generally flows to tissues in proportion to their metabolic demands. Thus, blood flow to kidneys, skin, and splanchnic areas generally decreases with skeletal muscles' increased metabolic demands.

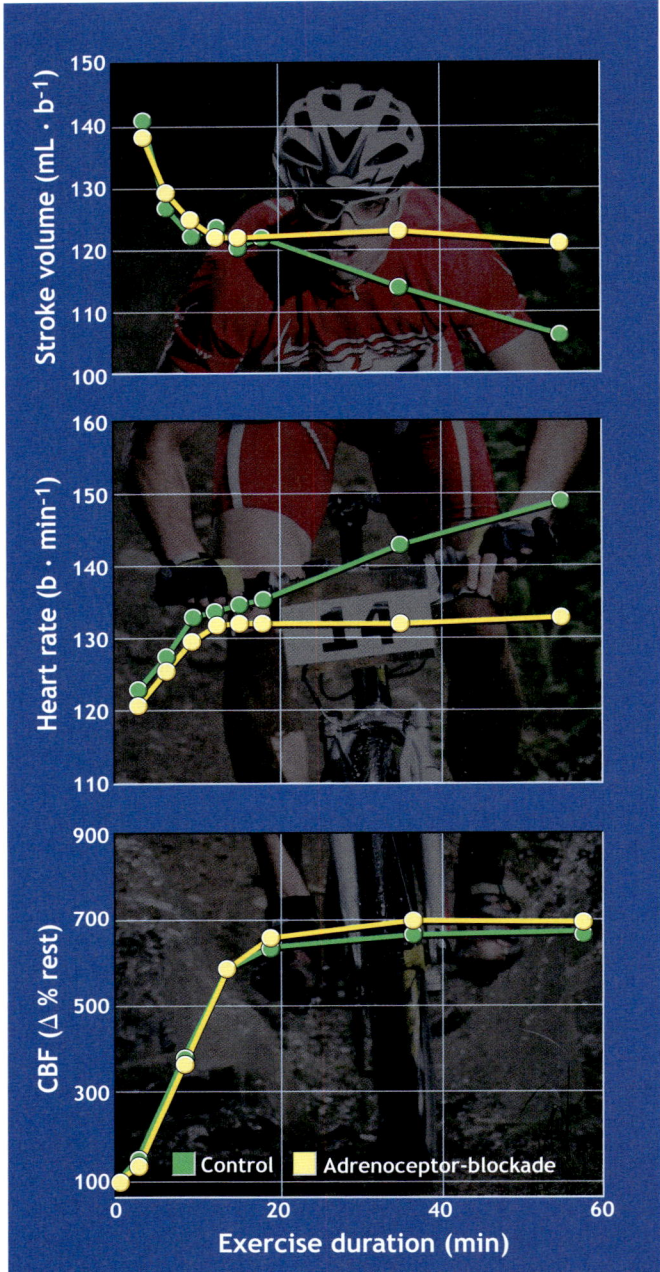

FIGURE 17.2. Stroke volume, heart rate, and cutaneous blood flow (CBF) during exercise for 60 min under β_1-adrenoceptor blockade (*yellow*) and control treatments (*green*).
(Adapted with permission from Fritzsche RG, et al. Stroke volume decline during prolonged exercise is influenced by the increase in heart rate. *J Appl Physiol*. 1999;86:799. ©The American Physiological Society (APS). All rights reserved. forest badger/Shutterstock)

Blood Flow Distribution at Rest

At rest in a thermoneutral environment, the typical 5-L (5000 mL) cardiac output generally distributes in the proportions displayed in **FIGURE 17.3A** pie chart. Muscle tissue requires approximately one fifth of the cardiac output (20%), while the digestive tract, liver, spleen, brain, and kidneys receive the illustrated portions of the remaining distribution.

Blood Flow Redistribution During Physical Activity

Figure 17.3B illustrates the percentage cardiac output distribution for an endurance athlete during intense physical activity. *Environmental stress, fatigue level, and physical activity mode and intensity affect regional blood flow, but the major cardiac output portion diverts to active muscles.* At rest, approximately 4 to 7 mL of blood flows each minute to every 100 g of muscle. In graded exercise, the flow increases steadily with active muscle receiving between 50 and 75 mL per 100 $g^{-1} \cdot min^{-1}$ in maximum exertion.[28,29]

Blood flow *within* active muscle is highly regulated. The greatest quantity of blood diverts to the oxidative portions of the muscle at the expense of those areas with high glycolytic capacity.[4,16] Peak blood flow in a small portion of an active quadriceps muscle can attain values as high as 300 to 400 mL $\cdot$ 100 $g^{-1} \cdot min^{-1}$.[26] During "big muscle" running and cycling at maximum intensity, muscle blood flow accounts for 80 to 85% of total cardiac output.[30]

Blood flow to muscle also increases disproportionately relative to its flow to other tissues. For trained individuals, blood redistribution—from one organ to another by vasoconstriction in one and vasodilation in the other—begins in the anticipatory period just prior to movement.[4] Two factors, hormonal vascular regulation and local metabolic conditions, cause blood to route through active muscles from areas that can temporarily compromise blood flow.[20] Blood redistribution among specific tissues occurs primarily during intense physical activity. For example, blood flow to the skin, the primary heat-exchange organ, increases during light and moderate activity with a rise in core temperature.[3,13,44] In near-maximum effort, the skin restricts its blood flow, redirecting it to active muscle even in hot environments.[27]

At rest, the kidneys and organs in the abdominal cavity (splanchnic tissues or visceral organs) require only 10 to 25% of oxygen in their normal blood supply. These tissues can tolerate a considerably reduced blood flow before oxygen demand exceeds supply and compromises function.[22] Renal blood flow decreases by up to four fifths its normal resting blood supply. Increased oxygen extraction from the available blood supply generally maintains tissue oxygen despite reduced blood flow. In intense effort, the visceral organs can sustain a substantially reduced blood supply for more than 1 hr. Redistributing 2 to 3 L of blood away from these tissues "frees" up to 600 mL oxygen each minute to active tissues. Sustained, reduced blood flow to the liver and kidneys may contribute to fatigue in prolonged submaximum effort. Regular aerobic training diminishes the typical vasoconstrictor response to splanchnic and renal tissues during prolonged exercise[20,34] thus contributing to improved endurance capacity.

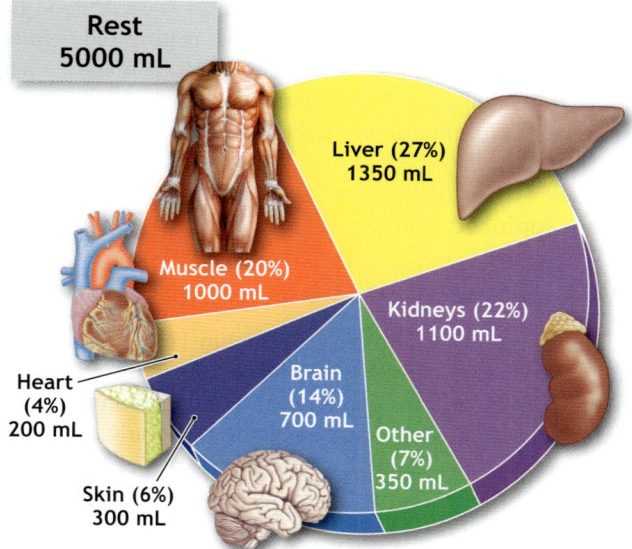

A Cardiac output distribution during rest

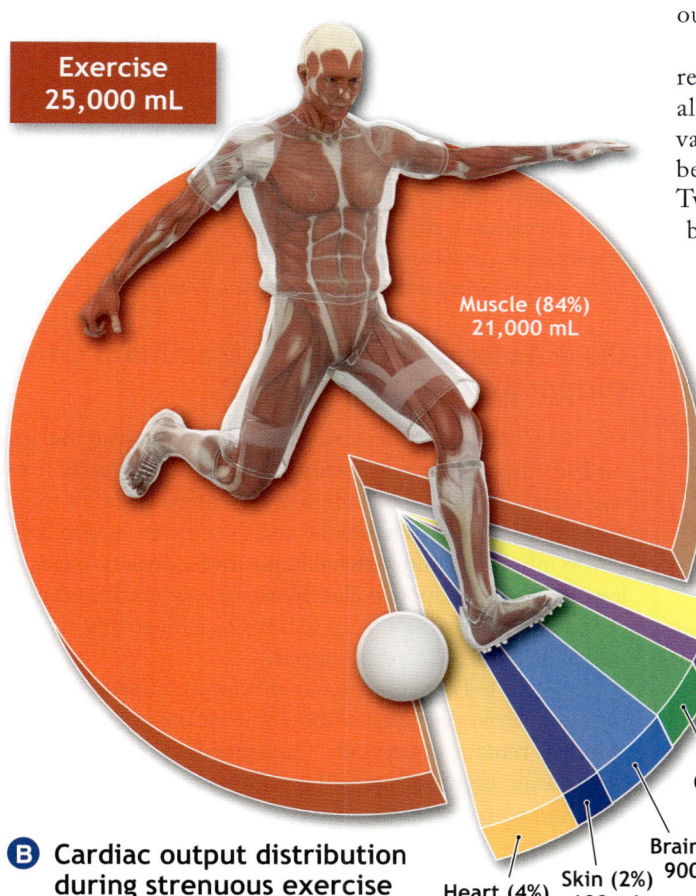

B Cardiac output distribution during strenuous exercise

FIGURE 17.3. Relative cardiac output distribution during **(A)** rest and **(B)** strenuous endurance exercise. The numbers in parentheses indicate total cardiac output percentage. The large absolute muscle tissue mass at rest receives about the same blood quantity as the much smaller kidneys. In strenuous physical activity such as soccer or stop-and-go endurance activities, the active musculature receives the greatest total cardiac output percentage up to 84%.
(Shutterstock: adike; CLIPAREA I Custom media)

Blood Flow to the Heart and Brain

Blood supply to the heart and brain cannot be compromised. At rest, the myocardium normally uses approximately 75% of the oxygen in the blood flowing through the coronary circulation. With such a limited reserve margin, increased coronary blood flow must supply the increased myocardial oxygen needed with exertion. A four- to fivefold increase in coronary circulation accompanies a similar increase in myocardial work during exercise, amounting to a blood flow of about 1 L · min^{-1} during maximum effort. Cerebral blood flow also increases during physical activity by approximately 25 to 30% compared with the resting flow.[37]

The Brain's Blood Flow

Three factors determine cerebral blood flow (CBF)—blood viscosity, blood vessel dilation, and net cerebral perfusion pressure determined by systemic blood pressure. Medically, CBF relates to the net pressure required to drive blood through the aorta into the cranial compartment. The intracranial pressure (ICP) refers to the pressure inside the brain and cerebrospinal fluid (CSF). ICP pressure at rest while lying supine averages between 7 and 15 mm Hg. Increases in ICP can be caused by a tumor mass, bleeding into the brain, or brain swelling (edema) from fluids entering the brain area from trauma (e.g., repeated blows to the head from football, boxing, head butts in soccer, and unplanned sports accidents). The enhanced color image shows an axial cross-sectional computed tomography scan from a patient indicating a large epidural hemorrhage and blood clot in the left cerebral hemisphere with cerebral edema. CBF in an adult at rest typically averages 750 mL · min^{-1} or between 15 and 17% of the cardiac output. This translates to blood flow averaging about 52 mL blood per 100 g tissue^{-1} · min^{-1}. Normally, brain blood flow always meets its metabolic demands. If it does not, excessive blood flow (*hyperemia*) to the area can raise intracranial pressure and damage surrounding tissues. Too little flow (*ischemia*; blood flow below 18 to 20 mL · 100 g tissue^{-1} · min^{-1}) also can cause brain tissue damage (necrosis), and death occurs when blood flow falls below 8 to 10 mL · 100 g tissue^{-1} · min^{-1}. Brain swelling is a serious medical emergency.

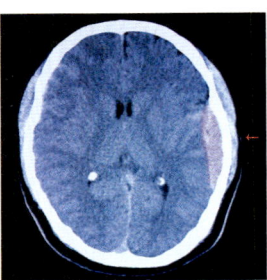

Tomatheart/Shutterstock

Cardiac Output and Oxygen Transport

Rest

Arterial blood carries about 200 mL of oxygen per liter in a person with a normal hemoglobin level (see Chapter 13). If resting cardiac output each minute equals 5 L, potentially 1000 mL of oxygen becomes available to the body (5 L blood × 200 mL O$_2$). Resting oxygen uptake typically averages 250 to 300 mL · min^{-1}, with about 750 mL oxygen returning unused to the heart. This does not reflect wasted blood flow. Rather, extra oxygen circulating above resting requirements represents oxygen in reserve—a relative safety margin when a tissue's metabolism increases dramatically when transitioning from rest to maximum physical effort.

 See the animation "Myocardial Blood Flow" on **Lippincott Connect** to view this process.

Physical Activity

A healthy, young adult with a maximum HR of 200 b · min^{-1} and 80 mL (0.08 L) SV generates a maximum 16 L · min^{-1} (200 × 0.08 L) cardiac output. Even during maximum activity, hemoglobin saturation with oxygen remains nearly complete, so each liter of arterial blood carries about 200 mL of oxygen. Consequently, 3200 mL of oxygen circulates each minute via a 16-L cardiac output (16 L × 200 mL O$_2$ · L^{-1}). Even if the tissues could extract all the oxygen from blood as it traveled throughout the body, the $\dot{V}O_{2max}$ could not exceed 3200 mL. This represents a purely theoretical value because brain and skin tissue's oxygen demands do not increase markedly with increased physical activity, yet they still require a substantial blood supply.

Based on the preceding example, increasing the heart's SV from 80 to 200 mL, while maintaining the maximum HR at 200 b · min^{-1}, dramatically increases maximum cardiac output to 40 L · min^{-1}. This represents a 2.5-fold increase in oxygen circulated during each minute (from 3200 to 8000 mL). *An increase in maximum cardiac output clearly produces a proportionate increase in capacity to circulate oxygen and profoundly impacts $\dot{V}O_{2max}$.*

Close Association Between Maximum Cardiac Output and $\dot{V}O_{2max}$

FIGURE 17.4 depicts the close relationship between maximum cardiac output and the capacity to achieve a high aerobic exercise metabolism. $\dot{V}O_{2max}$ values represent averages for the sedentary person (yellow symbols) and the elite endurance athlete (red symbols). An unmistakable positive association exists—a low $\dot{V}O_{2max}$ corresponds closely with a low maximum cardiac output, whereas a high 5- or 6-L $\dot{V}O_{2max}$ invariably accompanies a 30- to 40-L cardiac output.

A 5- to 6-L increase in blood flow accompanies each 1-L increase in oxygen uptake above the resting value; this relationship remains essentially unchanged over a broad range of dynamic exercise intensities. *High $\dot{V}O_{2max}$ and cardiac output levels represent distinguishing characteristics for preadolescent and adult endurance athletes.* An almost proportionate increase in maximum cardiac output accompanies increases in $\dot{V}O_{2max}$ with endurance training (Chapter 21).

 **INTEGRATIVE QUESTION**

How do factors that influence the a-$\bar{v}O_2$ diff in maximum physical activity account for the specificity of $\dot{V}O_{2max}$ improvement with different aerobic training modes?

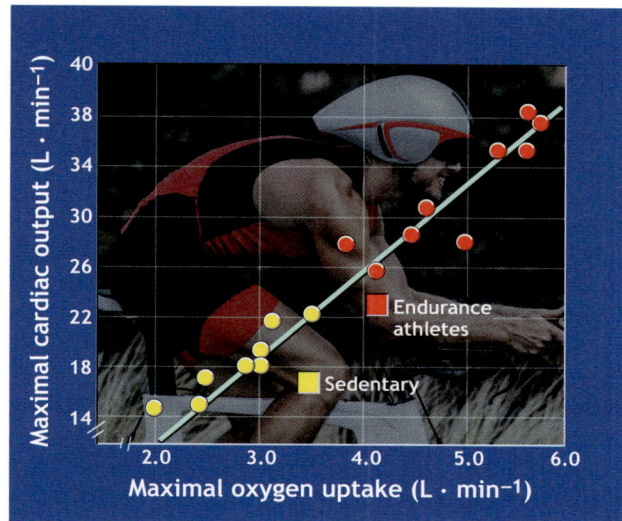

FIGURE 17.4. Relationship between maximal cardiac output and maximal oxygen uptake ($\dot{V}O_{2max}$) in endurance-trained and untrained individuals. Maximal cardiac output relates to $\dot{V}O_{2max}$ in an approximate 6:1 ratio.
(Maridav/Shutterstock)

Cardiac Output Differences Among Men, Women, and Children

Cardiac output and oxygen uptake remain linearly related during graded exercise for boys and girls and males and females. Teenage and adult females generally exercise at any *submaximum* oxygen uptake level with a 5 to 10% larger cardiac output than males.[25] The 10% *lower* hemoglobin concentration in females compared to males explains the apparent sex differences in submaximum cardiac output. A proportionate increase in submaximum cardiac output compensates for the relatively minor decrease in blood's oxygen-carrying capacity.

Higher HRs in children compared to adults during submaximum treadmill and cycle ergometer exercise do not fully compensate for their smaller SV. This produces a smaller cardiac output for children at a given submaximum oxygen uptake.[32,38] Consequently, the a-$\bar{v}O_2$ diff expands to meet oxygen requirements. The biologic significance of this difference in central circulatory function between children and adults remains unclear. Comparison of cardiac responses for SV, aortic peak blood flow velocity, and systolic ejection time between prepubertal children and adults do not reveal any age-related exercise impairment.[31]

Oxygen Extraction: The a-$\bar{v}O_2$ Diff

If blood flow were the only component to increase tissue oxygen supply, then increasing cardiac output from 5 L · min^{-1} at rest to 100 L · min^{-1} during maximum exertion would achieve an endurance athlete's 20-fold oxygen uptake increase. Fortunately, strenuous activity does not require this large cardiac output. Instead, hemoglobin releases a considerable quantity of its "reserve" oxygen from blood that perfuses active tissues. Oxygen uptake during physical activity increases by two mechanisms:

1. Increased cardiac output
2. Expanded a-$\bar{v}O_2$ diff

Rearranging the Fick equation summarizes the important relationship among cardiac output, a-$\bar{v}O_2$ diff, and $\dot{V}O_2$:

$$\dot{V}O_2 = \dot{Q} \times \text{a-}\bar{v}O_2 \text{ difference}$$

Resting a-$\bar{v}O_2$ Diff

Resting metabolism consumes about 5 mL of oxygen from the 20 mL oxygen in each deciliter of arterial blood (50 mL · L^{-1}) that passes through the tissue capillaries. This represents an a-$\bar{v}O_2$ diff of 5 mL of oxygen per deciliter of blood that perfuses the tissue capillary beds. Consequently, 15 mL or 75% of oxygen availability still remains bound to hemoglobin.

a-$\bar{v}O_2$ Diff During Physical Activity

FIGURE 17.5 shows the progressively expanding a-$\bar{v}O_2$ diff from rest to maximum effort in physically active men. A similar pattern emerges for women, except for arterial oxygen content, which averages 5 to 10% lower from their lower hemoglobin concentrations. The figure shows arterial and mixed-venous blood values for different oxygen uptakes. Arterial blood's oxygen content varies little from its 20 mL · dL^{-1} resting value throughout the full exercise intensity range. In contrast, mixed-venous oxygen content varies between 12 and 15 mL · dL^{-1} during rest to a low 2 to 4 mL · dL^{-1} during maximum exertion. The difference between arterial and mixed-venous blood oxygen content at any discrete time (i.e., the a-$\bar{v}O_2$ diff) represents oxygen extraction from circulating arterial blood.

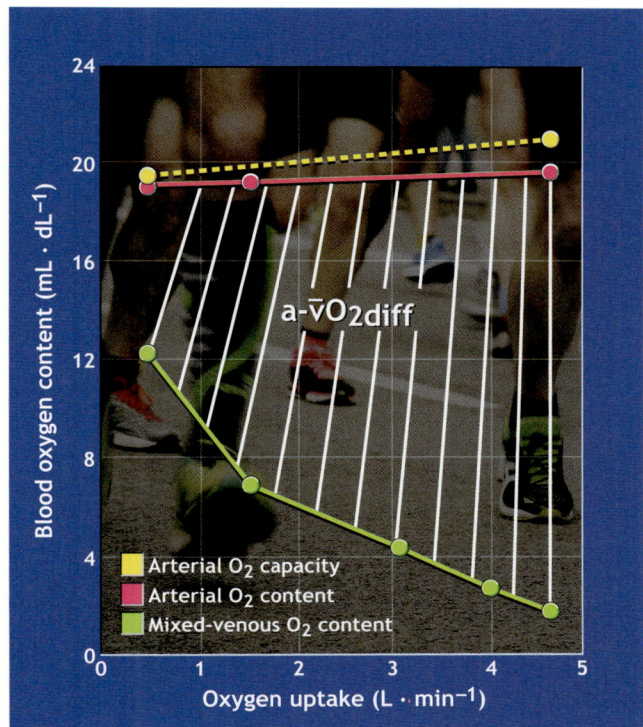

FIGURE 17.5. Changes in the difference between the oxygen content of arterial blood and mixed-venous blood (a-$\bar{v}O_2$ diff) from rest to maximum exercise in physically active males.
(Maxisport/Shutterstock)

Progressive expansion of the a-$\bar{v}O_2$ diff to at least three times the resting value results from a reduced venous oxygen content, which in maximum effort approaches 20 mL · dL^{-1} in active muscle. In this case, essentially all oxygen has been extracted. The oxygen content of a true mixed-venous sample from the pulmonary artery rarely falls below 2 to 4 mL · dL^{-1} because blood returning from active tissues mixes with oxygen-rich venous blood from metabolically less active regions.

Figure 17.5 also shows that capacity for each arterial blood deciliter to carry oxygen (*dashed yellow line*) increases during physical activity from an increase in red blood cell concentration (hemoconcentration) controlled by two mechanisms that direct fluid from plasma into the interstitial space:

1. Increases in capillary hydrostatic pressure as blood pressure rises
2. Metabolic by-products of exercise metabolism that osmotically draw fluid into tissue spaces from the plasma

Factors That Affect the a-$\bar{v}O_2$ Diff During Physical Activity

During physical activity, central and peripheral factors interact to increase oxygen extraction in active tissues. For example, diverting a larger portion of the cardiac output to active musculature during physical effort expands the a-$\bar{v}O_2$ diff in maximum effort. Regular training in a specific exercise mode redirects central circulation to increase its outflow to the active musculature in accord with the specificity of training principle.

When the microcirculation increases in skeletal muscles with training it also increases this tissue's oxygen extraction capacity. Muscle biopsies from the quadriceps femoris revealed a relatively large capillary to muscle fiber ratio in individuals exhibiting a large a-$\bar{v}O_2$ diff. This large ratio reflects a positive endurance training adaptation; it enlarges the interface for both nutrient exchange and metabolic gas exchange during physical activity. Individual muscle cells' increased ability to generate energy aerobically with training represents another important factor in achieving a large oxygen extraction to achieve a large a-$\bar{v}O_2$ diff. Increasing mitochondrial size and number with training augments aerobic enzyme activity and enhances a muscle's metabolic capacity to produce ATP aerobically.[40] These local training adaptations translate to an increased oxygen extraction capacity at the local level.

 INTEGRATIVE QUESTION

What is the physiologic rationale to support the relative importance of central circulatory factors (cardiac output) and peripheral factors in active muscle mass (a-$\bar{v}O_2$ diff) in limiting $\dot{V}O_{2max}$?

Cardiovascular Adjustments to Upper-Body Exercise

Upper-body physical activity creates different metabolic and cardiorespiratory responses than does lower-body physical activity, which requires predominantly leg musculature activation.[51,52]

Maximum Oxygen Uptake

The highest oxygen uptake during arm physical activity averages 20 to 30% lower compared to leg physical activity. Similarly, arm exercise produces lower maximum HR and pulmonary ventilation values. These differences can largely be explained by the arm's relatively smaller muscle mass.

Submaximum Oxygen Uptake

Submaximum physical activity reverses the typical oxygen uptake pattern during maximum effort when comparing upper- and lower-body exercise. The dashed pink line in **FIGURE 17.6** represents oxygen uptake values during arm cycling, which are higher than those for leg cycling at all submaximum power outputs, a difference that increases somewhat as exercise intensity increases. Two factors produce the additional oxygen cost between arm and leg cycling at the higher exercise intensities:

1. Lower mechanical efficiency in upper-body exercise to support an increased energy requirement from static muscle actions that do not contribute to external work
2. Increased energy requirement from additional muscle recruitment to stabilize the torso in upper-body exercise

Physiologic Response

Submaximum oxygen uptake (or percentage $\dot{V}O_{2max}$) or power output at any intensity level with upper-body exercise provides greater physiologic strain than lower-body exercise. Specifically, submaximum arm exercise produces higher HRs, pulmonary ventilations, and perceptions of effort than comparable leg exercise at similar power outputs. This also applies to blood pressure response in arm versus leg exercise (see Chapter 15).

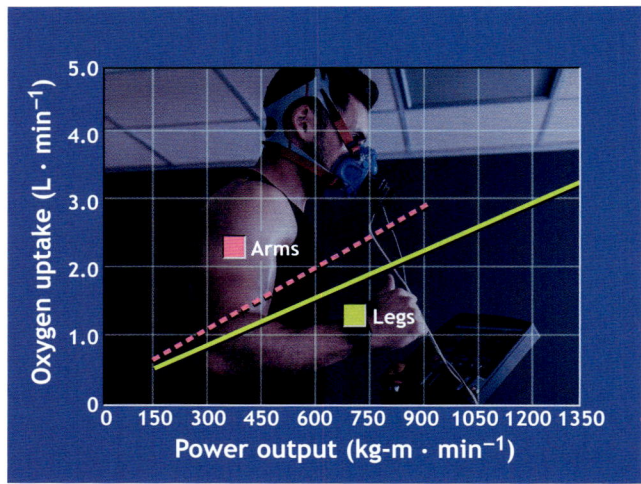

FIGURE 17.6. Arm exercise requires greater oxygen uptake than leg exercise at any submaximum power output throughout the comparison range (data for men and women combined). The largest differences occur during intense exertion.
(Jacob Lund/Shutterstock. Data from Laboratory of Applied Physiology, Queens College, Flushing, NY)

In a Practical Sense

Predicting Maximum Oxygen Uptake Using Walking and Swimming Tests

The 1-mile walk and the 12-min swim provide reliable and valid tests to predict maximum oxygen uptake ($\dot{V}O_{2max}$). The tests are effective for mass testing in schools and with recreational swimmers. We do not recommend these tests for unconditioned beginners, for males over age 40 and females over age 50 without physician clearance, or for symptomatic individuals with known disease or coronary heart disease risk factors. *The swim test assumes relatively high-level swimming skill.*

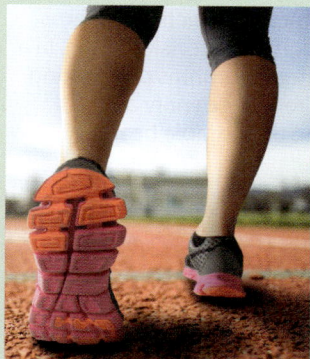
Damon Shaff/Shutterstock

1-MILE WALK TEST

1. Record *gender* and *body weight* (nearest lb)
2. Testing site: a school track (each lap measures ¼ mile) or premeasured 1-mile course
3. Warm up for about 3 min (easy stretching, mild calisthenics, and jogging in place)
4. Walk 1-mile distance as fast as possible without breaking into a jog or faster. On a track, use the inside lane
5. Record run time in min:s and convert to the nearest hundredth minute (e.g., if the time = 13 min 30 s, then time converts to the nearest hundredth minute by dividing sec by 60—thus, the time records as 13.50 min)
6. Immediately after crossing the 1-mile mark, record the 15-s heart rate (HR; use radial or carotid pulse) and convert to b · min⁻¹ by multiplying by 4
7. Predict $\dot{V}O_{2max}$ using the following example:

Where:

gender = 0 for women, and 1 for men

BM = body mass (lb) in walking shoes

T = time to walk 1 mile (converted to nearest hundredth min)

HR = immediate postexercise HR (b·min⁻¹)

Example calculations include the following:
Male (body weight = 160 lb; time to complete 1-mile walk = 13.50 min; HR = 124 b · min⁻¹ [15 s HR = 41])

$\dot{V}O_{2max}$ (mL·kg⁻¹·min⁻¹) = 88.768 + 8.892 (gender) − 0.0957 (B Mlb) − 1.4537 (T) − 0.1194 (HR)

$\dot{V}O_{2max}$ (mL·kg⁻¹·min⁻¹) = 88.768 + 8.892 (1) − 0.0957 (160) − 1.4537 (13.5) − 0.1194 (124)

$\dot{V}O_{2max}$ (mL·kg⁻¹·min⁻¹) = 47.92

12-MINUTE SWIM TEST

Individuals swim as far as possible in 12 min, with distance measured in yards. *Differences in skill level, swim conditioning, and body composition greatly affect oxygen uptake (exercise economy), thus making $\dot{V}O_{2max}$ predictions less valid than those based on walking and running, which have a smaller variation in movement economy.*

1. Warm up for about 3 min with easy stretching and mild calisthenics followed by several laps of easy swimming
2. Swim as many laps as possible in 12 min; paced swimming is preferred to fast and slow effort intervals
3. Determine total distance swam in yards; if the test ends in the middle of the pool, estimate distance; find swim fitness and $\dot{V}O_{2max}$ prediction in the table below

12-MINUTE SWIM TEST FITNESS CATEGORIES (AGE 18 TO 29 YEARS)

Distance (yd)	Fitness Category	Estimated $\dot{V}O_{2max}$ (mL · kg⁻¹ · min⁻¹)	
		Males	Females
>700	Excellent	>52.5	>41.0
500–700	Good	46.5–52.4	37.0–40.0
400–500	Average	42.5–46.4	33.0–36.9
200–400	Fair	36.5–42.4	29.0–32.9
<200	Poor	33.0–36.4	23.6–28.9

$\dot{V}O_{2max}$, maximum oxygen uptake.

Source:
Kline GM, et al. Estimation of from a one mile track walk, gender, age, and body weight. *Med Sci Sports Exerc.* 1987;19:25.

Supercomputers Help to Detect Heart Disease and Sudden Death Risk

Sudden cardiac arrest kills someone in the United States every 5 s. Worldwide, 26 million people succumb to heart rhythm abnormalities, with 50% dying suddenly. Researchers at John Hopkins (www.supercomputingonline.com/latest/59750-john-hopkins-researcher-winslow-builds-new-supercomputer-model-sheds-light-on-biological-events-leading-to-sudden-cardiac-death) have studied these abnormalities to help explain possible factors behind this silent but deadly killer. The image from their supercomputer model shows color bursts depicting propagating calcium waves. Each cell is identical but exhibits a distinct calcium pattern from random ion channel gating. The simulations include the heart's gross anatomy and cellular ultrastructural details. These advanced computational techniques recreate real-world underlying pathologic problems, including scenarios to simulate various antiarrhythmic drug effects on heart cells and surrounding tissues. This novel approach addresses the important issue about genetic disease susceptibility. Adding a supercomputer's speed and capacity to tap into the latest world literature facilitates discovery of interactions between specific gene and possible factors contributing to sudden cardiac arrest. The ultimate plan will prescribe life-saving targeted medications combined with 3D scanning and clinical assessment about the heart's electrical conduction patterns from polygenic assessment known as genetic risk scoring. In a broad sense, sophisticated computer algorithms pinpointing cutting-edge trends will someday reliably identify an individual's predisposition to future undesirable health maladies.

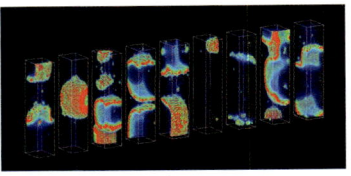

PLOS Computational Biology/Mark A. Walker

Sources:
Maragatham G, Devi S. LSTM Model for prediction of heart failure in big data. *J Med Syst.* 2019;43:111.
Walker MA, et al. Estimating the probabilities of rare arrhythmic events in multiscale computational models of cardiac cells and tissue. *PLoS Comput Biol.* 2017;13:e1005783.

Two factors explain the elevated HR response in submaximum arm exercise:

1. Greater feed-forward stimulation from the brain's central command to the medullary control center
2. Increased feedback stimulation to the medulla from peripheral receptors in active tissue

Upper-body physical activities place a greater force per unit muscle (strain), greater percentage of maximum capacity, and more metabolic by-products on the relatively smaller upper-body musculature for any submaximum exercise level. Added strain augments peripheral feedback to the medulla, which increases HR and blood pressure. A smaller total muscle mass activated in maximum arm movements reduces input to the medullary cardiovascular control center from the motor cortex, with less peripheral feedback from the smaller upper-body muscle mass. This may account for a lower maximum HR in upper-body compared to lower-body activities.

Implications

A standard submaximum exercise load (power output or oxygen uptake) with the upper body produces greater metabolic and physiologic strain than leg exercise. For this reason, exercise prescriptions based on running and bicycling do not apply to arm exercise. Low statistical correlations exist between $\dot{V}O_{2max}$ in arm versus leg exercise, so one should not expect to accurately predict aerobic capacity for arm exercise based on a test that uses the legs and vice versa.[6,17] This lack of strong association between criterion fitness measures from two different activities validates the fundamental specificity principle applied to aerobic fitness and just about every other major fitness component (e.g., strength, power, endurance, speed, flexibility).

Summary

1. Cardiac output reflects the cardiovascular system's functional capacity.
2. HR and SV determine the heart's output capacity expressed as cardiac output = HR × SV.
3. Cardiac output increases proportionally with effort intensity, starting from approximately 5 L·min^{-1} at rest to a maximum 20 to 25 L·min^{-1} in untrained, college-age males and 35 to 40 L·min^{-1} in elite male endurance athletes.
4. The endurance athletes' large SV explains difference in maximum cardiac output compared with untrained persons.
5. SV increases during upright physical activity from the interaction between greater ventricular filling during diastole and more complete emptying during systole.
6. Sympathetic hormones augment systolic ejection by increasing stroke power during systole.
7. Muscles and organs receive blood flow in proportion to their metabolic activity.
8. Cardiac output diverts to active muscles during physical activity because kidneys and splanchnic regions temporarily compromise blood supply to redistribute blood to the active muscles.
9. Maximum cardiac output and maximum a-$\bar{v}O_2$ diff determine $\dot{V}O_{2max}$.
10. A large cardiac output differentiates endurance athletes from untrained counterparts.
11. Arm physical activity generates a 25% lower $\dot{V}O_{2max}$ than leg physical activity.
12. Any submaximum oxygen uptake level (% $\dot{V}O_{2max}$ or power output) with upper-body physical activity provides greater physiologic strain compared with lower-body physical activity.

13. The poor association between $\dot{V}O_{2max}$ in arm versus leg physical activity validates the fundamental specificity principle applied to aerobic fitness and other major fitness components.

Key Terms

Afterload: Left ventricular wall pressure during systole

Cardiac output: Blood volume pumped by the heart each minute

Cardiovascular drift: Gradual "drift" in cardiovascular responses during high ambient temperatures and prolonged steady-rate exercise

Ejection fraction: Fraction of blood pumped from the left ventricle in relation to its end-diastolic volume.

End-diastolic volume: The volume of blood in the ventricle prior to the heart's contraction phase

Fick equation: Equation that expresses the relationships among cardiac output, oxygen uptake, and arterio-mixed venous oxygen difference

Frank-Starling law of the heart: Left ventricle stroke volume increases as left ventricular volume increases due to the myocyte stretch causing a more forceful contraction in systole

Functional residual blood volume: The amount of blood remaining in the ventricles following systole (about 50 to 70 mL)

Heart rate (HR): Heart beats per unit time

Indicator dilution method: Cardiac output measured by adding an indicator substance at a known concentration and constant rate and remeasuring its downstream concentration

Preload: Any factor that increases venous return or slows the heart to produce greater ventricular filling during the cardiac cycle's diastolic phase

Stroke volume (SV): The volume of blood ejected by the left ventricle with each contraction

> References are available online at Lippincott Connect.

Additional References

Abonie US, et al. Effects of 7-week resistance training on handcycle performance in able-bodied males. *Int J Sports Med.* 2022;43:46.

Andersson EP, et al. Physiological responses and cycle characteristics during double-poling versus diagonal-stride roller-skiing in junior cross-country skiers. *Eur J Appl Physiol.* 2021;121:2229.

Billat VL, et al. Pacing strategy affects the sub-elite marathoner's cardiac drift and performance. *Front Psychol.* 2020;10:3026.

Chang KW, et al. The effect of walking backward on a treadmill on balance, speed of walking and cardiopulmonary fitness for patients with chronic stroke: a pilot study. *Int J Environ Res Public Health.* 2021;18:2376.

Christiansen D, Bishop DJ. Aerobic-interval exercise with blood flow restriction potentiates early markers of metabolic health in man. *Acta Physiol (Oxf).* 2022;234:e13769.

Crisafulli A, et al. Editorial: cardiovascular adjustments and adaptations to exercise: from the athlete to the patient. *Front Physiol.* 2020;11:187.

Hammoudi N, et al. Altered cardiac reserve is a determinant of exercise intolerance in sickle cell anaemia patients. *Eur J Clin Invest.* 2022;52:e13664.

Ivanova YM, et al. The influence of a moderate temperature drift on thermal physiology and perception. *Physiol Behav.* 2021;229:113257.

Jørgensen AN, et al. Effects of blood-flow restricted resistance training on mechanical muscle function and thigh lean mass in sIBM patients. *Scand J Med Sci Sports.* 2022;32:359.

Maturana FM, et al. Individual cardiovascular responsiveness to work-matched exercise within the moderate- and severe-intensity domains. *Eur J Appl Physiol.* 2021;121:2039.

Mueller S, et al.; OptimEx-Clin Study Group. Effect of high-intensity interval training, moderate continuous training, or guideline-based physical activity advice on peak oxygen consumption in patients with heart failure with preserved ejection fraction: a randomized clinical trial. *JAMA.* 2021;325:542.

Park HY, et al. Metabolic, cardiac, and hemorheological responses to submaximal exercise under light and moderate hypobaric hypoxia in healthy men. *Biology (Basel).* 2022;11:144.

Reljic D, et al. Effects of very low volume high intensity versus moderate intensity interval training in obese metabolic syndrome patients: a randomized controlled study. *Sci Rep.* 2021;11:2836.

Stadheim HK, et al. Caffeine increases exercise performance, maximal oxygen uptake, and oxygen deficit in elite male endurance athletes. *Med Sci Sports Exerc.* 2021;53:2264.

Swift HT, et al. Acute cardiac autonomic and haemodynamic responses to leg and arm isometric exercise. *Eur J Appl Physiol.* 2022. doi:10.1007/s00421-022-04894-7.

Van Ryckeghem L, et al. Impact of continuous vs. interval training on oxygen extraction and cardiac function during exercise in type 2 diabetes mellitus. *Eur J Appl Physiol.* 2022. doi:10.1007/s00421-022-04884-9.

Table 17.1 Body Position Effects on Cardiac Output, Oxygen Uptake, Stroke Volume, and Heart Rate at Rest and During Strenuous Exercise in Well-Trained Athletes

Variable	Rest		Moderate Exercise		Strenuous Exercise	
	Supine	Upright	Supine	Upright	Supine	Upright
Cardiac output, $L \cdot min^{-1}$	9.2	6.6	19.0	16.9	26.3	24.5
Stroke volume, mL	141	103	163	149	164	155
Heart rate, $beats \cdot min^{-1}$	65	64	115	112	160	159
Oxygen uptake, $mL \cdot min^{-1}$	345	384	1769	1864	3364	3387

Data from Bevegard S, et al. Circulatory studies in well-trained athletes at rest and during heavy exercise, with special reference to stroke volume and the influence of body position. *Acta Physiol Scand*. 1963;57:26. Adapted with permission from McArdle WD, et al. *Exercise Physiology: Nutrition, Energy, and Human Performance*. 8th ed. Baltimore: Wolters Kluwer Health; 2015.

CHAPTER 18
Skeletal Muscle Structure and Function

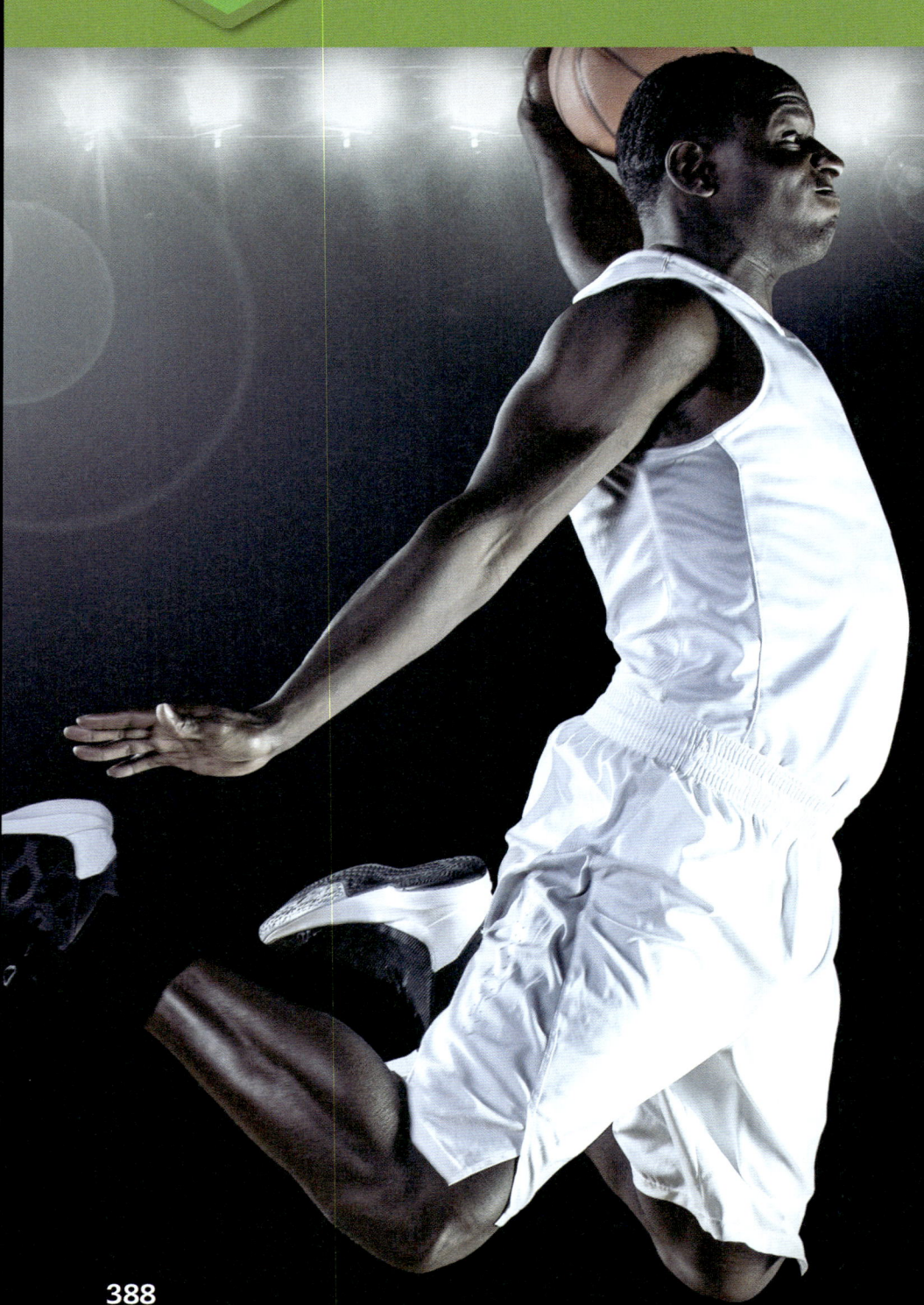

Chapter Objectives

- Outline five levels corresponding to the gross structural organization of skeletal muscle
- List four major skeletal muscle protein constituents and their functions
- Draw and label the structures that, under the light microscope at low magnification, characterize a skeletal muscle fiber's striated appearance
- Describe different individual muscle fiber arrangements along skeletal muscle's long axis and explain the biomechanical advantage of each
- Draw and label a skeletal muscle fiber's ultrastructural components
- Summarize the sliding filament model's salient muscle contraction features
- Outline the key chemical and mechanical events in skeletal muscle excitation-contraction coupling and relaxation
- Discuss two triad and two transverse tubule system functions
- Contrast slow-twitch and fast-twitch (including subdivisions) muscle fiber characteristics
- Outline muscle fiber type distribution patterns among different elite athlete groups
- Discuss how specific exercise training modifies muscle fibers and fiber types
- Explain why mitophagy represents an important mechanism in normal muscle physiology

Ancillaries at-a-Glance

Visit Lippincott Connect to access the following resources.

- References: Chapter 18
- Appendix H: Links for Supplemental Animations and Videos
- Animations: Muscle Contraction Type, Sliding Filament Theory
- Focus on Research: A Tissue Responsive to Regular Exercise

Scientists interested in a muscle's internal structures could not reveal their intimate details until compound microscopes provided basic clues in the 1600s by Dutch spectacles maker Zacharias Jansen (1580–1638; https://micro.magnet.fsu.edu/optics/timeline/people/janssen.html) and Italian observational astronomer, physicist, and mathematician Galileo Galilei (1564–1642; www.thoughtco.com/galileo-galilei-biography-1991864). These observations were soon made easier by Dutch microscopist Antonie van Leeuwenhoek (1632–1723; www.ucmp.berkeley.edu/history/leeuwenhoek.html), who described tiny cells in pond water droplets using his newly perfected microscope. Unlike the earlier Dutch microscopes, which magnified objects only six to nine times, van Leeuwenhoek's microscope included a single glass lens mounted in a flat brass plate that magnified structures up to 200 times—a game-changing scientific advance for the times. The lens was held up to the eye, with the object placed on the movable pin head resting on the lens's other side. This design breakthrough spawned more complex and powerful tools to explore a muscle's inner structural details and other human and animal tissues.

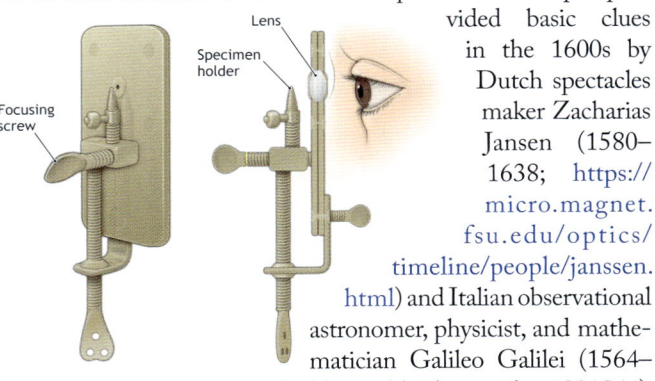

During the next century, thin muscle tissue slices observed under more powerful microscopes showed faint light and dark areas along the tissue's length. We now know that the light and dark areas represent alternating **sarcomere** bands comprising thin and thicker filament substructures that "slide" past each other to alter fiber length and generate force. Hungarian biochemist Albert Szent-Györgyi 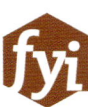 (1893–1986), 1938 Nobel Prize winner in Physiology or Medicine, discovered the vitamin C and fumaric acid combustion reactions (www.nobelprize.org/nobel_prizes/medicine/laureates/1937/szent-gyorgyi-bio.html) and the fundamental muscle contraction processes involving the proteins actin and myosin and their complex architecture and function. His crucial experiments invigorated scientists devoted to basic skeletal muscle research for decades to come.

Szegedi Tudományegyetem

The following sections present skeletal muscle's architectural organization, focusing on gross and microscopic structures. We also highlight the chemical and mechanical events in muscle action and relaxation assessed with the highly sophisticated scanning electron microscope profiled later in this chapter (https://serc.carleton.edu/research_education/geochemsheets/techniques/SEM.html) and muscle fiber differences among untrained individuals and elite athletes in different sports.

 View the animation "Muscle Contraction Type" on Lippincott Connect to view this process.

Muscle Contraction Versus Muscle Action

During the previous half-century, the term *muscle contraction* commonly referred to processes involving muscular tension during muscle shortening. Three striated muscle actions generate tension.

1. Muscle shortens (concentric action)
2. Muscle lengthens (eccentric action)
3. Muscle remains the same length (static action)

In this text, muscle *contraction* and muscle *action* essentially refer to the same event, and we use both interchangeably, although *muscle action* may be preferable. In the image on the left, holding both dumbells without movement at slightly below hip height denotes a static muscle action (no muscle movement); slowly moving both dumbells simultaneously up to chest level in the right image by contracting the biceps characterizes a shortening or concentric muscle action, and slowly lowering the bar back to the original, static position represents an eccentric or lengthening muscle action.

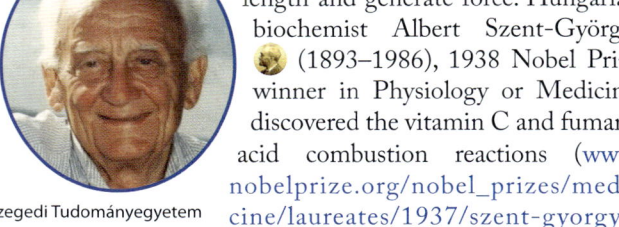

Makatserchyk/Shutterstock

Skeletal Muscle Gross Structure

Humans possess three muscle types—cardiac, smooth, and skeletal—each exhibiting distinct functional and anatomical characteristics. Cardiac muscle resides only in the heart; it possesses the greatest number of mitochondria (2000 to 5000 per cell, compared with only 50 to 200 per cell for **striated** skeletal muscle fibers).

Cardiac cells share several common features with skeletal muscle as both appear striated (striped) viewed under low microscopic magnification, and both contract and shorten similarly. Skeletal muscles also contain fibrous connective tissue wrappings.

Smooth muscle lacks a striated appearance but shares cardiac muscle's nonconscious regulation under autonomic nervous system control. Skeletal muscle operates under *voluntary* control, as in lifting a 25-lb kettlebell overhead or smashing a golf ball 250 yds down the fairway. In the two-handed kettlebell lift, the individual controls three factors:

1. Movement velocity
2. Arm movement range
3. Completed repetitions

In this kettlebell lift, the individual controls all arm, leg, and torso movement sequences in lifting the kettlebell from the ground, through the legs, and with a swinging motion without rotation, thrusts the

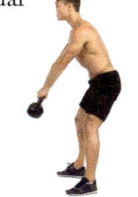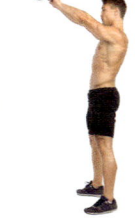

studioloco/Shutterstock

kettlebell to above shoulder height, in a single upward but coordinated movement sequence before returning to the beginning position.

A different situation exists for cardiac and smooth muscle tissue because any muscle activity mostly occurs *involuntarily*. This means a general conscious absence for how fast the heart beats, how fast food moves through the digestive system, or how the body's blood vessels, if stretched end to end to wrap around the Earth about 2.5 times (60,000 miles), could continue to regularly constrict and expand while altering their internal diameter, and thus control blood flow throughout the day, every day until death.

FIGURE 18.1 illustrates cross-sectional details for the body's approximately 600-plus skeletal muscle structures and a tendon's arrangement with its connective tissue wrappings. The endomysium **(A)** covers individual fibers, the perimysium surrounds fibers called fasciculi, and the epimysium wraps the entire muscle in a connective tissue sheath. An endotendon encloses a fiber bundle, and an epitendon sheath, known as a fascicle, surrounds

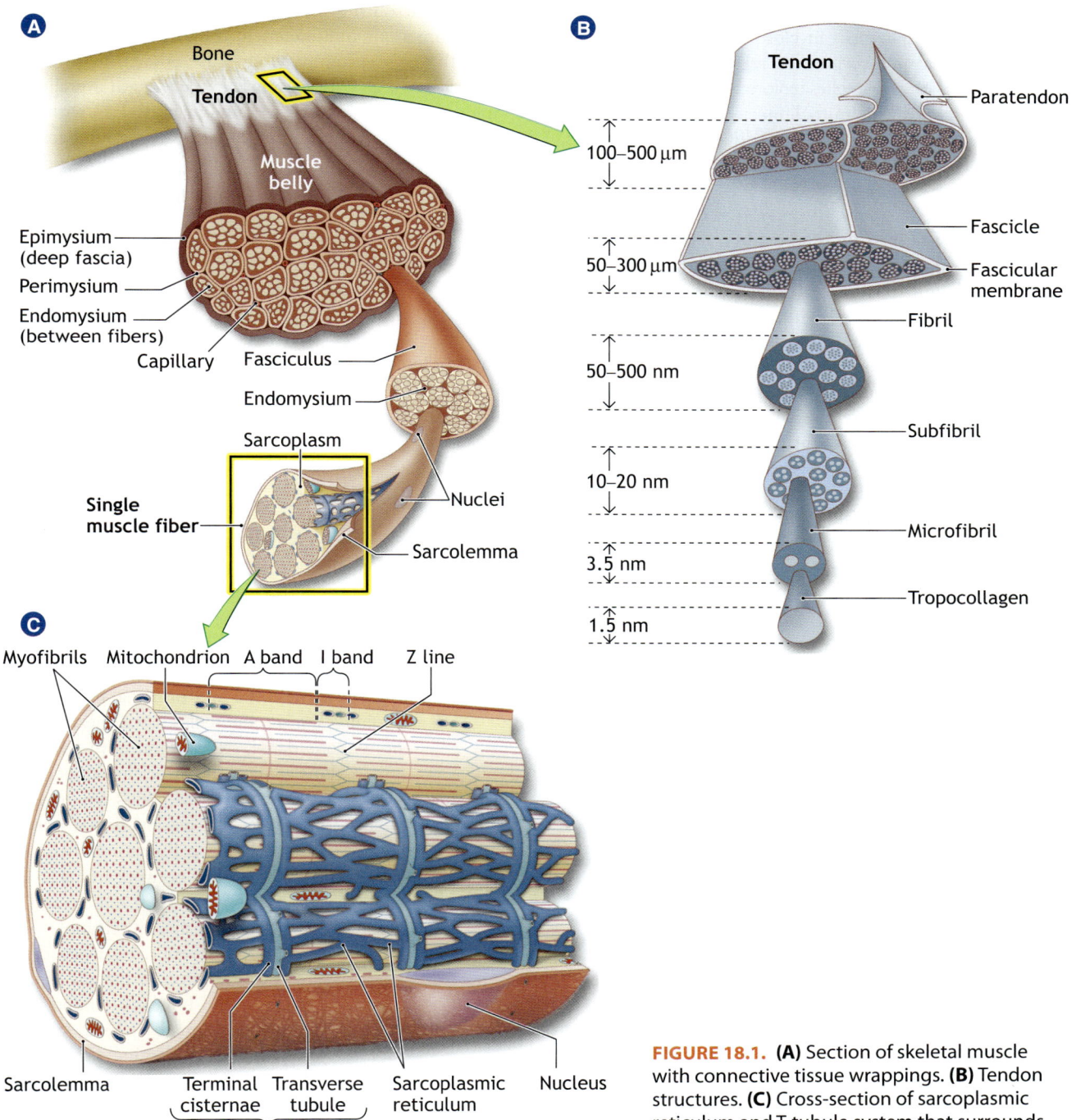

FIGURE 18.1. **(A)** Section of skeletal muscle with connective tissue wrappings. **(B)** Tendon structures. **(C)** Cross-section of sarcoplasmic reticulum and T-tubule system that surrounds the myofibrils.

endotendon groups. Proceeding down in **(A)** illustrates that a single muscle fiber has thousands of cylindrical smaller cells called **muscle fibers**. The **sarcolemma**, a thin, elastic membrane, covers each striated muscle fiber's surface. Details about tendon structure **(B)** illustrate that the microfibril forms from five parallel tropocollagen molecules that unite to form fibrils and then **collagen** fibers. The **fascicles** merge into a tendon that becomes surrounded by its own paratendon sheath. An endotendon encloses the fiber bundle, and an epitendon sheath, called a fascicle, surrounds endotendon groups. The fascicles combine into a tendon that becomes surrounded by its own sheath, the paratendon (μm = 10^{-6} m; nm = 10^{-9} m). The sarcoplasmic reticulum and **transverse (T)-tubule system** cross section in **(C)** surround the **myofibrils**, which remain in close contact with the cell's mitochondrial "energy factories," the relatively tightly packed, oblong mitochondria organelles colored light blue (https://micro.magnet.fsu.edu/cells/mitochondria/mitochondria.html; www.youtube.com/watch?v=RrS2uROUjK4).

Mitophagy

Considerable research from many physiology laboratories worldwide has contributed to a basic understanding about the mitochondrion's important role in energy metabolism. One aspect focuses on how normal mitochondrial functions, when they become defective, could negatively impact cardiovascular physiology and life-threatening diseases. Fortunately, the important roles mitochondrial fission and fusion processes play to protect mitochondria's regulatory role in cellular respiration.[61,62,63] These protective mechanisms, termed **mitophagy**, preserves nondefective mitochondria to carry out their many roles by removing defective or damaged mitochondria as they switch from a normal to abnormal state following cellular damage from a stressor (such as starvation) or a genetic malfunction. The general **autophagy** process removes damaged mitochondria when double-membraned, spherical vesicle phagophores surround the damaged mitochondria (and other cellular substances) and fuses with lysosomes for mitochondrial degradation as shown in the four stage process:

1. **Stage 1**. The phagophore cup-shaped membrane structure precursor (with lipid and protein constituents) begins to isolate the cytosolic proteins (mitochondria) and other organelles
2. **Stage 2**. The phagophore completely engulfs the protein structures ("closes the cup"), and now functions as an autophagosome
3. **Stage 3**. Lysosomes (containing degradative enzymes and hydrolytic enzymes or hydrolases) fuse with the autophagosome to become an autolysosome
4. **Stage 4**. The degradation process concludes

This cellular adaptive process provides an excellent example about the body's intracellular degradation protective system to maintain internal homeostasis. The term **apoptosis** describes the general process relating to normal cell death.

Lippincott® Connect   Appendix H, available online at **Lippincott Connect**, lists supplemental skeletal muscle animations and videos.

The long, slender, multinucleated muscle fibers lie parallel to each other, with the forceful action directed along the fiber's long axis. Their number probably becomes largely fixed in fetal development during months 3 to 6. Individual fiber length varies from a few millimeters in the eye muscles to nearly 30 cm in the large antigravity leg muscles (with width achieving 0.15 mm). Cylindrical muscle fiber length averages 3 cm (ranging between 1 and 4 cm among muscles), with typical fiber diameters about 10 to 100 μm. The unnumbered table compares skeletal muscle microscopic structure width and length dimensions.

Structure	Length	Width
Fiber	1–4 cm	10–100 μm
Myofibril	1–4 cm	10–100 μm
Actin filament	1 μm	20 Å
Myosin filament	1.5 μm	115 Å

Designua/Shutterstock

Organization

As detailed in Figure 18.1 and **FIGURE 18.2**, the **endomysium**, the deepest and smallest muscle connective tissue component, wraps each muscle fiber and separates it from neighboring fibers. Another connective tissue layer, the **perimysium**, surrounds up to 150 fibers called a fasciculus. A fibrous connective tissue fascia, the **epimysium**, surrounds the entire muscle. This protective, fibrous sheath tapers at its distal and proximal ends, blending into and joining the intramuscular tissue sheaths to form the tendon's dense, strong connective tissue. **Tendons** connect the muscle's both ends to the **periosteum**, the bone's outermost covering. The tendon tissues intermesh with the collagenous fibers within bone. This network forms a powerful link between muscle and bone that remains inseparable except during severe stress when the tendon can sever or literally pull away from the bone. A tendon attachment to a long bone's end initiates an adaptation by enlarging at that end to create a more stable union. Depending on bone size, the term *tubercle*, *tuberosity*, or *trochanter* describes this overgrowth, which functions as attachment points for the particular tendon-muscle complex.

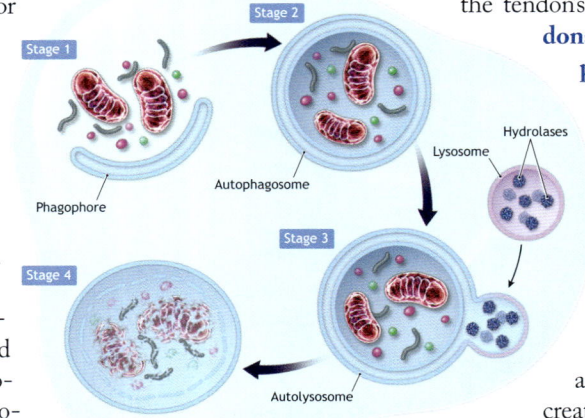
RAJ CREATIONZS/Shutterstock

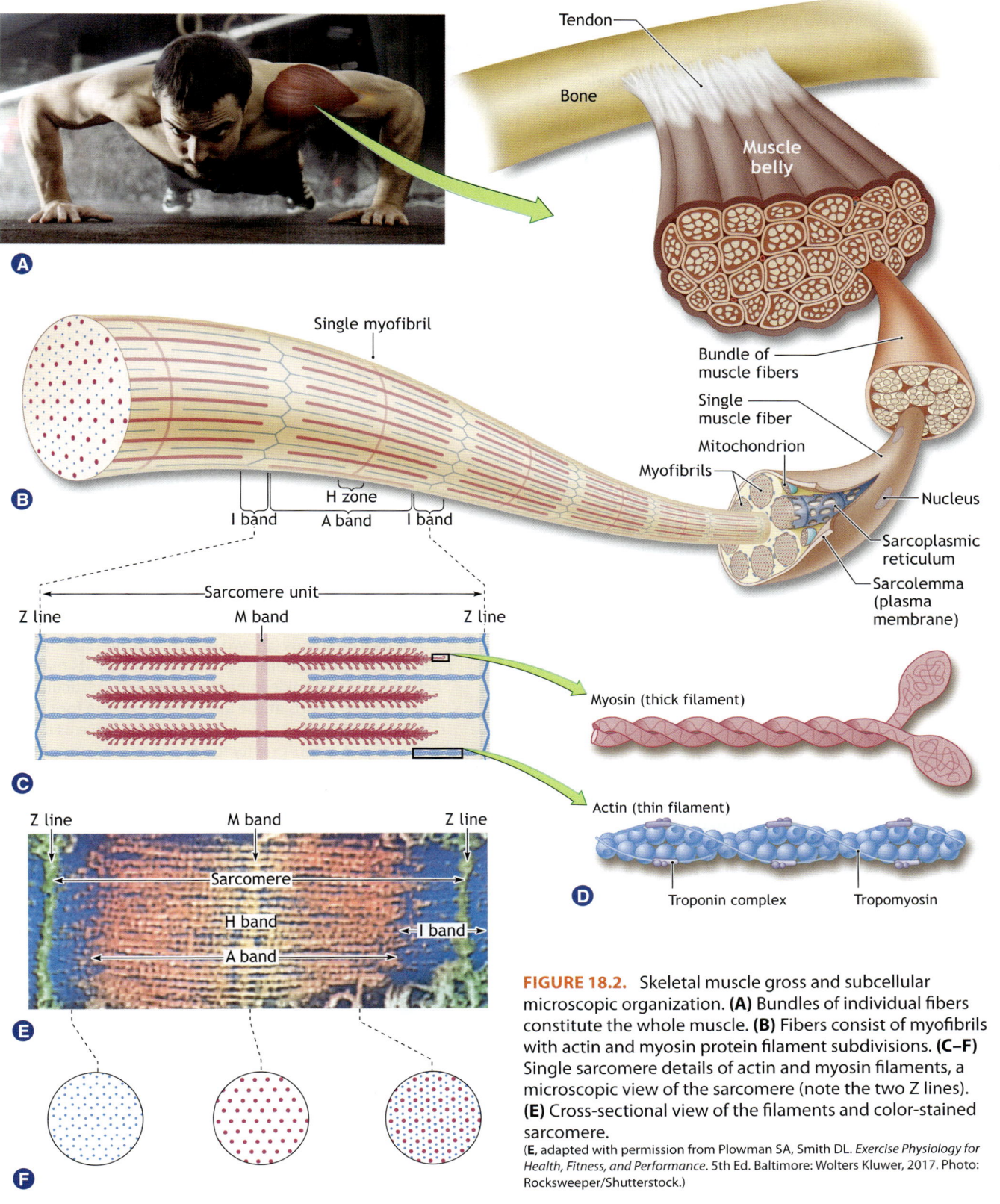

FIGURE 18.2. Skeletal muscle gross and subcellular microscopic organization. **(A)** Bundles of individual fibers constitute the whole muscle. **(B)** Fibers consist of myofibrils with actin and myosin protein filament subdivisions. **(C–F)** Single sarcomere details of actin and myosin filaments, a microscopic view of the sarcomere (note the two Z lines). **(E)** Cross-sectional view of the filaments and color-stained sarcomere.

(**E**, adapted with permission from Plowman SA, Smith DL. *Exercise Physiology for Health, Fitness, and Performance.* 5th Ed. Baltimore: Wolters Kluwer, 2017. Photo: Rocksweeper/Shutterstock.)

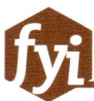

Interesting Facts About Muscles

External Eye Muscles: During wakefulness, eye muscles constantly move to readjust the eye's many positions. The eye blinks more than 100,000 times daily. When the head moves, the external muscles adjust eye position to maintain a steady fixation point. In 1 hr of continuous reading of this textbook, your eye muscles would make about 10,000 coordinated movements to maintain focus, and unfortunately, these muscles easily fatigue. Frequently changing head position and focusing on different objects helps to dissipate eye muscle fatigue.

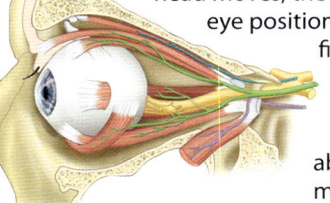

Gluteus Maximus: The gluteus maximus muscle (from the Latin *musculus gluteus maximus*), the body's largest and most powerful antigravity muscle, functions primarily to stabilize an erect posture by extending the hips. Without this muscle's almost continuous contraction state, the body would literally "fold up" like an accordion and collapse in a heap to the ground, unable to structurally support the torso, arms, and head weight.

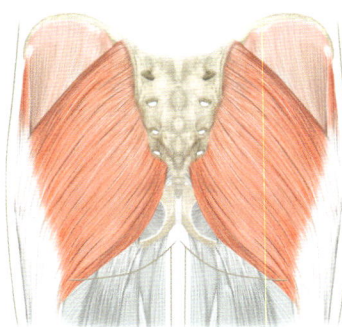

Cardiac Muscle: The heart represents the body's hardest working muscle. It pumps blood at an amount equal to 9450 L/2500 gallons daily, with an average 72 beats a min at rest, and close to 200+ beats a min during maximal exercise. Under essentially resting conditions, during a typical lifetime, the heart beats nonstop over 3 billion times! Even just doubling the resting heart rate during moderate physical activity for 30- to 60-min periods daily during adulthood would add many millions of additional gallons pumped.

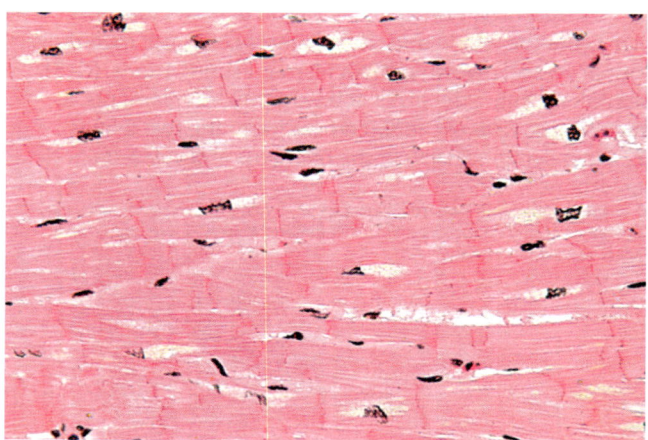

Masseter: One of the jaw muscles involved in chewing, the masseter called a masticatory muscle, represents the body's strongest muscle relative to its relatively small size in the jaw. The masseter connects to the mandible (lower jawbone) and cheekbone. When all the jaw muscles work symbiotically in chewing a piece of steak, for example, the teeth can close with a force of about 25 kg on the incisors or almost four times that on the molars.

Electromyography (EMG) coupled with bite force transducers assesses chewing forces between and among upper and lower teeth, with techniques similar to determining dynamic muscular forces generated during physical activities.

Soleus: The soleus (shown in red) is located below and under the gastrocnemius muscle in the calf. Its major action performs ankle joint plantarflexion, particularly when the leg bends at the knee to extend the foot downward. It contracts with considerable force as it continually counters gravity to keep the body upright during ambulation (e.g., walking, running, hiking). The soleus muscle forms the Achilles tendon when it inserts into the gastrocnemius.

SciePro/Shutterstock

Tongue: The tongue consists of eight striated muscles. Its four *intrinsic* muscles act to change tongue shape and do not attach to any bone. The four *extrinsic* muscles anchored to bone change tongue position. Once food enters the mouth, these muscles work to mix the food into smaller-size pieces. The tongue also contorts itself to form letters and sounds during speech. The tongue seldom "sleeps;" even during the different sleep transition cycles, it provides propulsive forces to maintain salivary flow down the throat. The first real-time MRI video from a German research lab shows the way the mouth and pharynx, along with the lips, tongue, and larynx (voice box), coordinate their movement patterns to form vowels and consonants during speech (www.ncbi.nlm.nih.gov/pmc/articles/PMC2754124/).

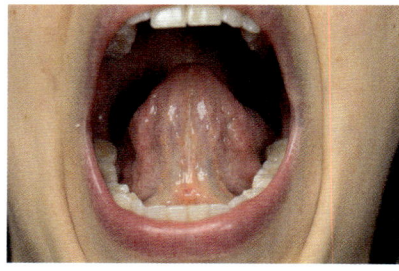

sruilk/Shutterstock

Tendon Structure and Trauma

Tendinitis or tendon inflammation occurs most frequently from trauma at or around the knee's patellar tendon (common in basketball and volleyball athletes), Achilles ankle region (common in high impact lunging and jumping activities), or the stabilizing rotator cuff shoulder region muscle attachments (common in high-velocity baseball pitching, shot put, or discuss throwing). Injuries to these regions usually take 4 months or more to heal, particularly in persons in their mid-40s and older. Tendinitis also can occur from overuse and from putting limbs through extreme movements that exceed the joint's normal motion range. In less severe tendon trauma, common therapies include **nonsteroidal anti-inflammatory drugs (NSAIDs**; www.medicinenet.com/nonsteroidal_antiinflammatory_drugs/article.htm#what_are_nsaids_and_how_do_they_work), immobilization, ice, and rest, with disciplined, gradual return to normal physical activity.

The force generated by a contracting muscle transmits directly from the connective tissue harness to the tendons, which then pull on the bone at the attachment point. The forces exerted on the tendinous attachments under muscular exertion range from 20 to 50 N (197 to 492 kg) per cm^2 cross-sectional area—forces often larger than the muscle fibers themselves can tolerate. The muscle's **origin** refers to the location where the tendon joins a relatively stable skeletal part, generally the proximal or the lever system's fixed end nearest the body's midline. The most distal muscle attachment to the moving bone represents the **insertion** location. The tendon's dry mass includes about 70% collagen, the body's most abundant structural protein. The unnumbered image shows a three-dimensionally rendered collagen model with its linked amino acid structures. The molecule contains triple-helices (two identical chains and one differing slightly in chemical composition and with high hydroxyproline content) plentiful in ligaments, skin, fibrous tendons, corneas, blood vessels, digestive tract, intervertebral discs, and the dentin in teeth.

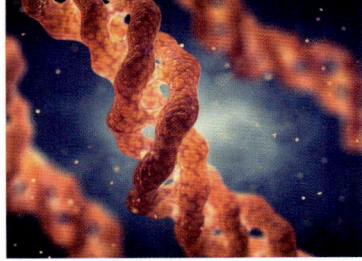
nobeastsofierce/Shutterstock

Membranes

The sarcolemma, a thin, elastic membrane that encloses the muscle fiber's cellular contents, lies beneath the endomysium and surrounds each fiber. It contains a plasma membrane (plasmalemma) and a basement membrane. The plasma membrane, a bilayer lipid structure, conducts an electrochemical **depolarization** wave over the muscle fiber's surface (see Chapter 19). The plasmalemma also insulates one fiber from another during depolarization. Basement membrane proteins and collagen fibril strands fuse with the collagenous fibers in the tendon's outer covering. Between the basement and plasma membranes lie myogenic stem **satellite cells**, the normally quiescent **myoblasts** that function in regenerative cellular growth to provide possible adaptations from exercise training and in recovery from injury.[18,39,52] Satellite cell nuclei incorporated into existing muscle fibers seems a likely explanation for exercise-induced muscle fiber hypertrophy.[22]

The fiber's aqueous **sarcoplasm** contains enzymes, lipid and glycogen particles, nuclei (approximately 250 per mm fiber length) that contain the genes, mitochondria, and other highly specialized organelles. Figure 18.1C details the **sarcoplasmic reticulum**, an extensive longitudinal latticelike tubular channel and vesicle network akin to an interconnected network similar to common roads along a freeway interchange. This specialized system provides for the cell's structural integrity. It allows the depolarization wave to spread rapidly from the fiber's outer surface to its inner environment through the T-tubule system to initiate muscle action. The sarcoplasmic reticulum that surrounds each myofibril contains biologic "pumps" that take up Ca^{2+} from the fiber's sarcoplasm. This produces a calcium concentration gradient between the sarcoplasmic reticulum (higher [Ca^{2+}]) and the sarcoplasm surrounding the filaments (lower [Ca^{2+}]).

Muscle Composition

The total skeletal muscle mass contains approximately 75% water, while protein constitutes 20%. The remaining 5% contains many substance types—including salts; high-energy phosphates; urea; lactate; the minerals calcium, magnesium, and phosphorus; enzymes; sodium, potassium, and chloride ions; amino acids; lipids; and carbohydrates. The most abundant muscle proteins include titin, the largest protein in the body, has 27,000 amino acids (accounts for about 10% muscle mass), myosin (approximately 60% muscle protein), actin, and tropomyosin. For every 100 g muscle tissue, about 700 mg includes the oxygen-binding, conjugated protein myoglobin structurally similar to the hemoglobin subunit that reversibly binds to oxygen (https://jeb.biologists.org/content/207/20/3441).

Aldona Griskeviciene/Shutterstock

Blood Supply

Arteries and veins that lie parallel to individual muscle fibers provide a rich vascular supply. These vessels divide into numerous arterioles, capillaries, and venules to form a diffuse network in and around the endomysium. Extensive blood vessel branching ensures each muscle fiber an adequate oxygenated blood supply from the arterial system and rapid carbon dioxide removal in the venous circulation. During vigorous physical activity in an elite endurance athlete, the muscle's oxygen uptake increases nearly 70 times to approximately 11 mL per 100 g·min^{-1} or a total

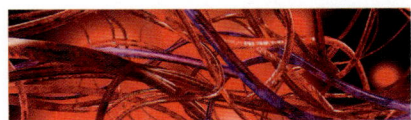
ustas7777777/Shutterstock

3400 mL · min⁻¹ muscle uptake. The local vascular bed illustrated in the unnumbered image delivers blood in large quantities through active tissues to meet oxygen demands. Blood flow distribution fluctuates in rhythmic running, swimming, cycling, climbing, and other similar large muscle activities.

Flow decreases during the muscle's contraction phase and increases during relaxation to provide an auxiliary "milking action" that moves blood through the muscles and propels it via the venous system back to the heart. The rapid dilation for previously dormant capillaries complements the pulsatile blood flow. Between 200 and 500 capillaries deliver blood to each square millimeter of active muscle cross section, with up to four capillaries directly contacting each fiber. In endurance athletes, five to seven capillaries surround each fiber; this positive adaptation ensures greater local blood flow to targeted musculature with adequate tissue oxygenation when needed.

Physical activities that require "straining" (i.e., exerting force against an almost immovable object as in shoveling wet snow) present a different contrasting event for muscle blood flow. When a muscle generates about 60% force-generating capacity for several seconds, elevated intramuscular pressure occludes local blood flow during the contraction. With a sustained high-force contraction, the intramuscular high-energy phosphates and glycolytic anaerobic reactions provide muscular effort's main energy supply.

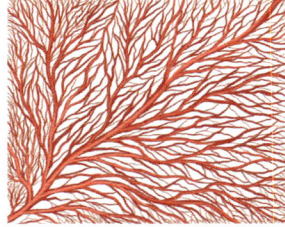
Artemida-psy/Shutterstock

The increased capillary-to-muscle fiber ratio of trained muscles helps to explain improved capacity with endurance exercise.[2,6] An enhanced microcirculation expedites heat removal and metabolic by-products from active tissues, in addition to facilitating oxygen, nutrient, and hormone transfer to these tissues.

With electron microscopy, accelerated electrons rather than light hit an object's surface and reflect from it to turn the scattered electrons into a high-resolution image about 0.1 nm or a magnification exceeding 500,000 times that for a light microscope (see Chapter 33). The resulting image reveals that total capillary number per square millimeter muscle tissue averages about 40% higher in endurance-trained athletes than untrained counterparts. This almost equals the 41% difference in $\dot{V}O_{2max}$ between the two groups. A positive association also exists between $\dot{V}O_{2max}$ and the average muscle capillary number.[42] Enhanced capillary vascularization proves beneficial during activities that require sustained, high-level steady-rate aerobic metabolism. The unnumbered false color micrograph shows capillary endothelium (brown-red),

Jose Luis Calvo/Shutterstock

meninx connective tissue (green), basal lamina (pink), glia limitans astrocytes (yellow-green), and myelinated nerve fiber endings (blue-purple).

Vascular stretch and shear stress on vessel walls from increased blood flow during exercise stimulate capillary development with intense aerobic training.[31]

Skeletal Muscle Ultrastructure

Electron microscopy, x-ray diffraction, histochemical staining, helium-neon laser diffraction, *in vitro* motility assays, and optical tweezer technologies (see Chapter 33) reveal skeletal muscle's ultrastructural details. Figure 18.2A–F illustrates different gross and subcellular organization levels within a skeletal muscle fiber. The whole muscle contains individual fiber bundles (**A**), while each fiber contains myofibrils with actin and myosin protein filament subdivisions (**B**). Insets **C–F** detail a single sarcomere with its actin and myosin filaments, a microscopic sarcomere view (note the two Z lines), a cross-sectional filament view, and a color-stained sarcomere.

A single multinucleated muscle fiber contains smaller functional units that lie parallel to the fiber's long axis. These myofibrils, approximately 1 μm (1 μm = 1/1000 mm) in diameter, contain even smaller subunits called **myofilaments** that lie parallel to the myofibril's long axis. The threadlike myofilaments chiefly exist as ordered assemblages for approximately 85% actin and myosin proteins in the myofibrillar complex. Twelve to fifteen other proteins either serve a structural function or affect protein filament interaction during muscle action. Seven examples with amounts ranging from about 7% to less than 1% include the following:

1. Tropomyosin, located along the actin filaments (5%)
2. Troponin (which contains troponin-1, T, C), located in the actin filaments (3%)
3. α-Actinin, distributed in the Z-band region (7%)
4. β-Actinin, found in the actin filaments (1%)
5. M protein, identified in the M-line regions within the sarcomere (<1%)
6. C protein, which contributes to the sarcomere's structural integrity (<1%)
7. Dystrophin, a rod-shaped protein connecting the actin filaments to dystroglycan, a sarcolemmal transmembrane protein (5%) that creates the dystrophin-dystroglycan complex[59]

INTEGRATIVE QUESTION

What are the advantages of diversity in muscle fiber arrangement?

The Sarcomere

At low magnification, alternating light and dark bands along the skeletal muscle fiber's length impart a characteristic striated appearance. **FIGURE 18.3A** illustrates the myofibrils' cross-striation patterning. The *I band* represents the lighter

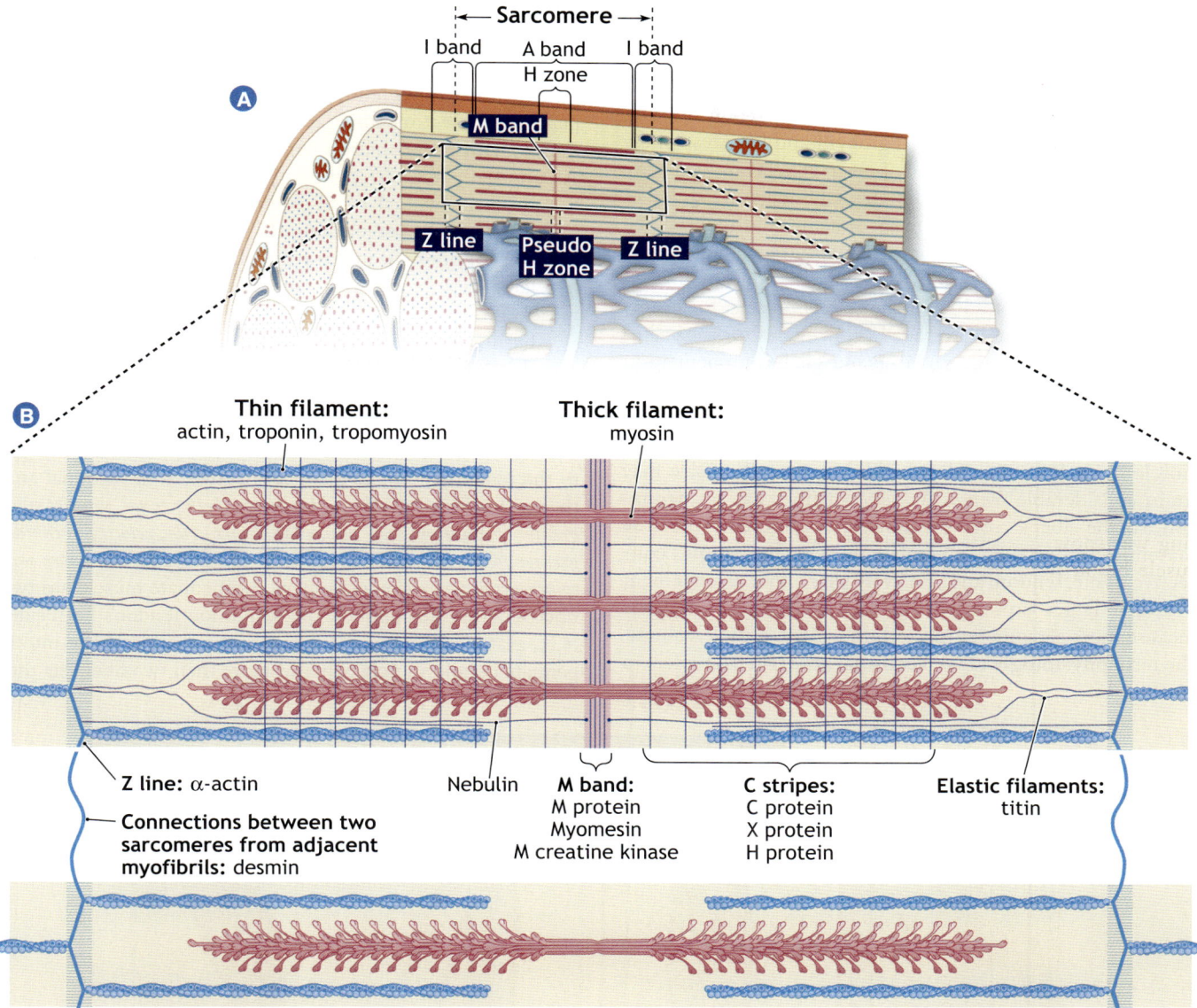

FIGURE 18.3. (A) Myofibril cross-striation pattern. The Z line bounds a sarcomere at both ends. **(B)** Detailed sarcomere view including the proteins listed in **TABLE 18.1**.

blue area, and the *A band* represents the darker reddish area. The *Z line* bisects the I band and adheres to the sarcolemma; it provides stability to the entire structure. Optical properties denote the specific bands. When polarized light passes through the I band, it moves at the same velocity in all directions (isotropic). Light passing through the A band does not scatter equally (anisotropic). The letter *Z* indicates "between" (from German, *zwischenscheibe*), the letter *M* (*mittelscheibe*) denotes "middle," and the letter *H* (*hellerscheibe*) denotes "a clear disk or zone."

The basic repeating units between a sarcomere's two Z lines comprise the muscle fiber's functional unit. The actin and bipolar myosin filaments within the sarcomere contribute primarily to muscle contractile mechanics. Sarcomeres lie in series, and their filaments exhibit a parallel configuration within a given fiber. At rest, each sarcomere averages 2.5 μm in length. A myofibril 15 mm long contains about 6000 sarcomeres joined end to end. The sarcomere's length largely determines a muscle's functional properties.

The relative positioning for the thin actin and thicker myosin protein creates an interdigitating two filament overlap. The A band center contains the *H zone*, a lower optical density area because this region contains no actin filaments. The *M band* bisects the H zone's central region to delineate its center. The M-band protein structures support the myosin filament arrangement. Figure 18.3B shows a sarcomere's detailed view, and **TABLE 18.1** shows 12 sarcomere structural proteins and their proposed functions.

TABLE 18.1 Twelve sarcomere proteins and their functions

Muscle Fiber Alignment

A muscle's long axis determines the individual fiber arrangement from an imaginary line drawn through the origin and insertion, or the fiber angle relative to the force-generating axis. Differences in sarcomere alignment and length strongly affect a muscle's force- and power-generating capacity (**FIG. 18.4**). **Fusiform** or spindle-shaped fibers run parallel to the muscle's long axis (e.g., biceps brachii) and taper at the tendinous attachment. In contrast, **pennate** or fan-shaped fibers' fasciculi (fiber bundles) lie at an oblique pennation angle that varies up to 30°. In the soleus muscle, for example, the pennation angle averages 25°, whereas for the vastus medialis, it equals 5°; the sartorius muscle has no pennation angle. Pennation characteristics directly impact sarcomere number per cross-sectional muscle area. No fibers run the full muscle length. In essence, pennation allows individual muscle fibers to remain *short*, while the overall muscle may attain considerable *length*. A fusiform fiber has no pennation, so the fiber's cross-sectional area represents the true anatomic cross section. In pennate muscle, the complex connective tissue, tendon, and relatively short fiber arrangement creates a larger cross-sectional area than fusiform fibers because more sarcomeres "pack" into a given muscle volume. The term **physiologic cross-sectional area (PCSA)** refers to total cross-sectional areas for all fibers within a particular muscle. Pennation *per se* allows packing many fibers into a smaller cross-sectional area enabling considerable muscle power generation. Figure 18.4B illustrates the fiber-packing pennation effect on force-generating capacity in a fusiform muscle with no pennation angle (ø = 0°) and when ø = 30°. An unusually large 30° pennation angle results in only a 13% loss in an individual fiber's force capacity, creating a huge increase in total fiber-packing ability. From pennation angle geometry, it does not necessarily follow that muscle mass *per se* relates to an equivalent tension output among different muscle groups.[33,45]

Fusiform muscle fibers run parallel to a muscle's long axis. In this case, fiber length equals muscle length, and a fiber's force generation transmits directly to the tendon. *This arrangement facilitates rapid muscle shortening.* A unipennate fiber arrangement, where muscle fibers lie at an oblique angle to the tendon, produces a larger effective cross-sectional area than in fusiform muscle. *Other factors being equal, muscles with greater pennation, yet slower in contractile velocity, generate greater force and power than fusiform muscles because more sarcomeres contribute to muscle action.* A bipennate muscle has two fiber sets that lie obliquely on a common tendon's both sides (e.g., gastrocnemius and rectus femoris muscles). The multipennate deltoid muscle contains more than two fiber sets that

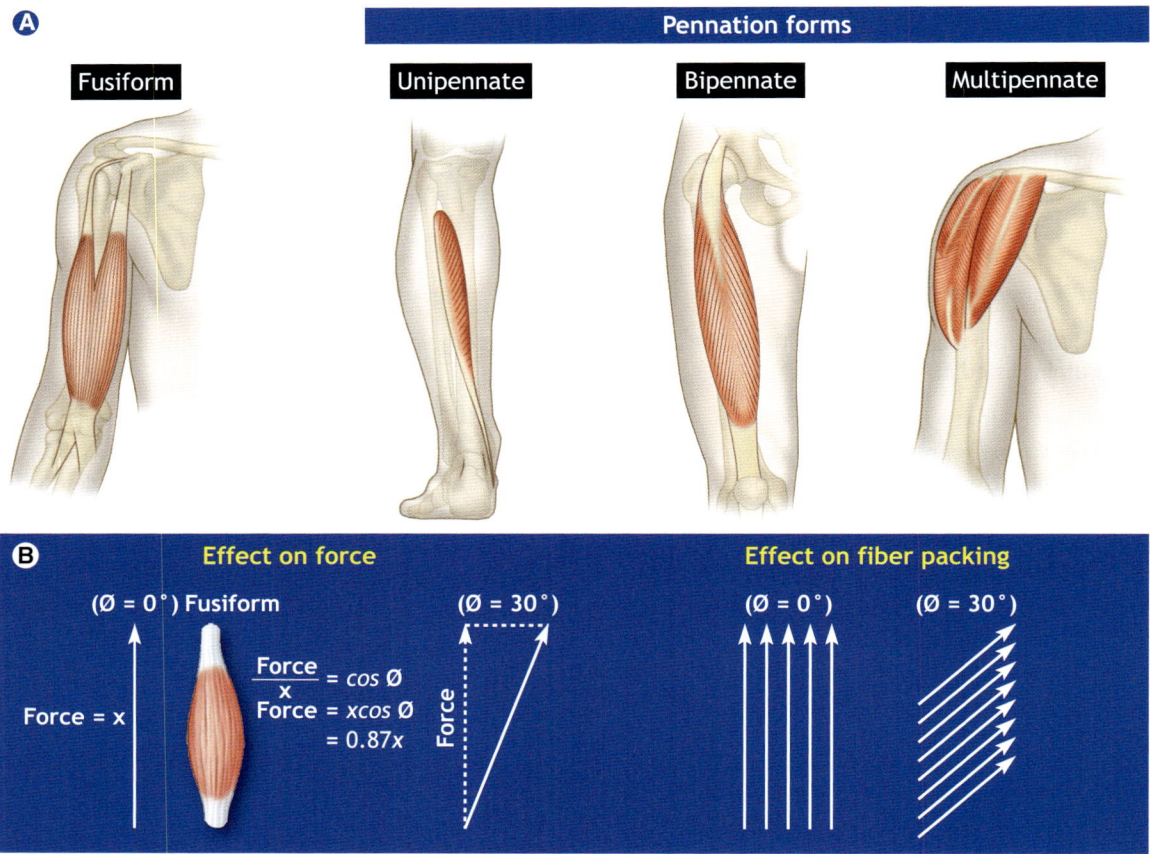

FIGURE 18.4. (A) Various fiber arrangement forms in human skeletal muscle. (B) Force development in a fusiform muscle with no angle of pennation and when angle of pennation equals 30°.
(B, adapted with permission from Lieber RL. *Skeletal Muscle Structure, Function, and Plasticity: The Physiological Basis of Rehabilitation.* 3rd ed. Baltimore: Lippincott Williams & Wilkins; 2009:31.)

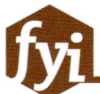

Subcellular Systems and Muscle Function

Skeletal muscle function depends on efficient coordination patterns established among subcellular systems. According to researchers in the Muscle Physiology Laboratory in the Department of Bioengineering and Orthopaedic Surgery at the University of California, San Diego (http://muscle.ucsd.edu/index.shtml), a subset of tightly regulated genes encodes these protein-mediated systems. Even slightly altering system regulation can lead to disease, injury, and dysfunction. For example, nine biologic networks, critical to "normal" muscle function, begin by expressing proteins required to optimize neuromuscular junction function to initiate the muscle cell's action potential. That signal, transmitted to dedicated proteins involved in excitation-contraction coupling, enables Ca^{2+} release to activate contractile proteins to support actin and myosin **crossbridge cycling** (see videos, Muscle contraction—crossbridge cycle animation: www.youtube.com/watch?v=sZuy356qkPM). Cytoskeletal proteins transmitted through the sarcolemma produce forces generated by crossbridge action to support the muscle extracellular matrix. Energy metabolism regulation requires "turning on" target-specific proteins that ultimately control muscle action. Inflammation, a common response to muscle injury, can alter many pathways within muscle. Muscle also possesses multiple pathways to regulate changes in its mass through diminished size (*atrophy*) or enhanced size (*hypertrophy*). Different isoforms associated with "fast" muscle fibers and corresponding isoforms in "slow" muscle fibers perform highly targeted functions.

Naeblys/Shutterstock

The different networks represent critical biological systems that impact skeletal muscle function. Analogous to a modern computer network, combining high-throughput systems analysis with advanced networking software can potentially unravel the tremendous number of yet undiscovered interrelationships among deep neural network systems to predict skeletal muscle force production.

Sources:
Kakurina GV, et al. Relationship between the mRNA expression levels of calpains 1/2 and proteins involved in cytoskeleton remodeling. *Acta Naturae*. 2020;12:110.
Murphy S, et al. Proteomic profiling of giant skeletal muscle proteins. *Expert Rev Proteomics*. 2019;16:241.
Paul DM, et al. In situ cryo-electron tomography reveals filamentous actin within the microtubule lumen. *J Cell Biol*. 2020;219:e201911154.
Rane L, et al. Deep learning for musculoskeletal force prediction. *Ann Biomed Eng*. 2019;47:778.

Lengthened Sarcomeres in Patients with Cerebral Palsy

Patients with cerebral palsy (CP) often exhibit wrist contractures—muscles so highly shortened that the wrist gets "stuck" in the flexed position. Functional genomics research confirms that muscle spasticity has neural origins, yet spastic muscles remain intrinsically abnormal. Muscle fiber size and fiber type distribution are abnormal in cerebral palsy patients, suggesting altered myosin heavy chain expression. Unfortunately, the muscle changes from spasticity are poorly understood. New procedures would be needed to restore muscle length to normal or to permit fibers to shorten to more favorable lengths for active and passive force generation.

Researchers at the Muscle Physiology Laboratory at the University of California, San Diego, were surprised to discover that CP patients had *lengthened* sarcomeres in the cramped flexor carpi ulnaris (FCU) wrist flexors compared to patients without CP. Average sarcomere length measured from 6 CP patients was significantly longer by 31% ($p < .001$) than in 12 patients without CP. This finding displayed at right, using the sophisticated laser diffraction method (see Fig. 18.12), is unprecedented in the literature for any mammalian species including subhuman primates. The researchers hope to unravel unexpected (and as yet unexplained) muscle adaptations to hopefully develop new treatment procedures to return sarcomere-fiber and muscle length to a more effective range.

Lieber and Friden (2019) argue that changes in extracellular matrix collagen amount and arrangement also increase muscle stiffness. Structural light and electron microscopy studies demonstrate that large collagen bundles, referred to as perimysial

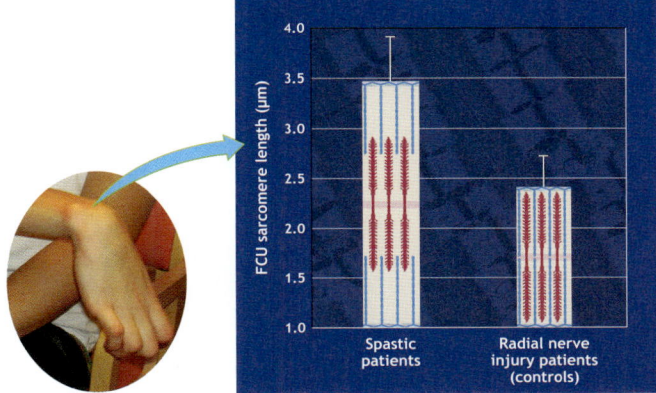

Inset photo of flexed hand courtesy of RL Lieber.

cables, may induce increased stiffness in regulated cell types within the extracellular matrix. Muscle satellite cell degradation may relate to sarcomere and extracellular matrix changes. Discovery of underlying mechanism(s) may lead to effective nonsurgical treatments to positively improve muscle contracture mechanics.

Sources:
Katz RT, Rymer WZ. Spastic hypertonia: mechanisms and measurement. *Arch Phys Med Rehab*. 1989;70:144.
Lieber RL, Fridén J. Muscle contracture and passive mechanics in cerebral palsy. *J Appl Physiol (1985)*. 2019;126:1492.
Smith LR, et al. Contribution of extracellular matrix components to the stiffness of skeletal muscle contractures in patients with cerebral palsy. *Connect Tissue Res*. 2019;1–12.

converge at different angles and insert directly into tendons at both their ends. Pennate muscles differ from fusiform fibers in three ways:

1. Generally contain shorter fibers
2. Possess more individual fibers
3. Exhibit less range of motion

Complex Fusiform Arrangement

The **complex parallel muscle**, also called *series-fibered muscle*, features individual fibers running parallel to the muscle's line of pull. Unlike simple fusiform arrangements where a fiber runs the entire muscle length, the complex parallel arrangement features muscle fibers that terminate in the muscle's mid-belly and taper to interact with the connective tissue matrix or adjacent muscle fibers. This arrangement enables parallel packing in relatively short fibers within a long muscle (e.g., the 50-cm-long sartorius). This structural specialization with diverse intrafascicular terminations also creates lateral tension—either through connective tissue into the tendon or through adjacent and series fibers into connective tissue—at strategic points along the fiber's surface.

Fiber Length-Muscle Length Ratio

The ratio between individual fiber length to a muscle's total length typically varies between 0.2 and 0.6. This means that individual fibers in the longest upper and lower limb muscles remain shorter than the muscle's overall length. **FIGURE 18.5A** illustrates four lower limb muscles and their architectural properties and velocity and force-generating capacities. On average, quadriceps muscle fibers maintain pennation angles that average 4.6°, a PCSA approximately 21.7 cm², with a fiber length that averages about 68 mm. This contrasts with the biceps femoris (hamstring) muscle, with relatively long fibers

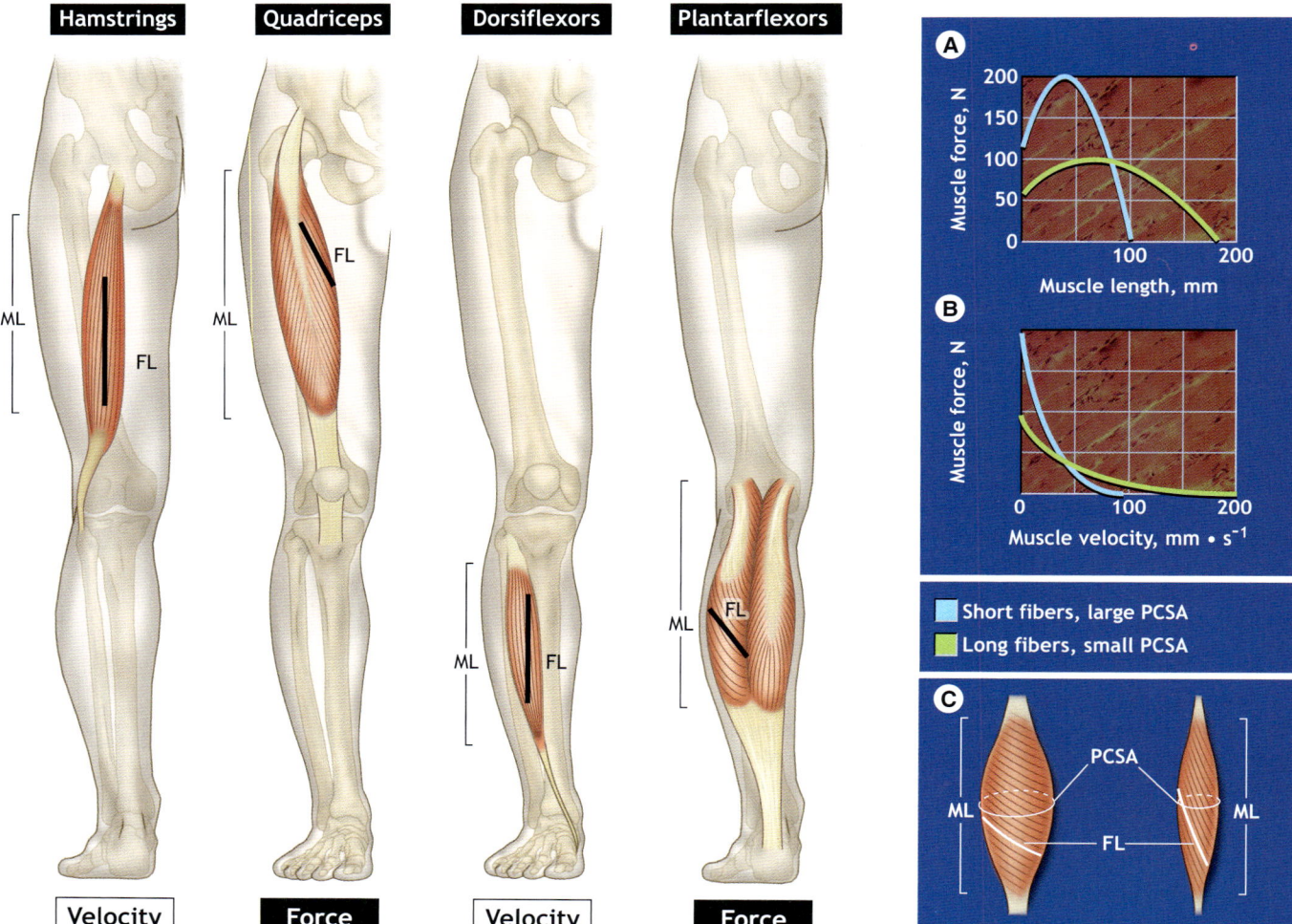

FIGURE 18.5. **Left:** Muscle architectural properties in the lower limb for velocity and force. The quadriceps and plantarflexors exhibit high force production from their low fiber length-to-muscle length (FL:ML) ratios and relatively large physiologic cross-sectional areas (PCSA). **Right:** The muscle force-muscle length curve in **(A)** shows the fusiform muscle with a longer working range and lower maximum force output than the pennate muscle. The curves in **(B)** show that fusiform muscles with longer fibers exhibit higher contractile velocity but lower maximum force output. In **(C)**, a greater PCSA produces substantially more quadriceps and plantarflex or force output.
(Drawings at left modified with permission from Lieber RL. *Skeletal Muscle Structure, Function, and Plasticity: The Physiological Basis of Rehabilitation*. 3rd Ed. Baltimore: Lippincott Williams & Wilkins, 2009: 34. Photo: Arkadiusz Wos/Shutterstock.)

(111 mm) and an intermediate PCSA (11.7 cm²). Quadriceps muscles exhibit approximately 50% greater force capacity than hamstrings, whose architectural quality allows rapid shortening. These design differences suggest susceptibility to hamstring tears as often occurs in sprint running, when an abrupt force output *imbalance* occurs during maximal activation for quadriceps and hamstrings. The imbalance may partly occur from a functional deficit between the hamstrings and quadriceps strength ratio (H:Q), which predisposes individuals to recurrent hamstring injuries and discomfort.[10] The H:Q typically computes by dividing the maximal knee flexor (hamstring) moment by the maximal knee extensor (quadriceps) moment.[1] The right to left sides H:Q peak torque ratios are more similar among female collegiate basketball players (48 to 67%), than collegiate volleyball players (56 to 70%), with significantly greater deficits in volleyball players at 60°, 180°, and 300° · s⁻¹ assessed isokinetically.[50,55,57] Prior studies with male and female collegiate athletes reported that the H:Q increased as velocity increased but without significant right to left limb differences between men's and women's volleyball, men's and woman's soccer, and women's basketball and softball.

The typical H:Q ratio approaches 50 to 80% averaged through the full knee ROM, with a higher ratio at faster movement speeds.[58] If H:Q ratios exceed those expected for a particular sport during preseason screening, trainers and physical therapists can introduce targeted H:Q muscle training at specific, preset velocities and movement patterns to reduce H:Q deficits in routine functional rehabilitation assessments. In essence, the dorsiflexors and hamstrings exhibit lower force capacity because individual sarcomeres lengthen less with a given change in muscle length distributed over more sarcomeres. In Figure 18.5C, a greater PCSA produces a greater force output for quadriceps and plantarflexors.[8,14,34]

At the collegiate and professional levels, the medical team often considers how much symmetry occurs between right and left side limbs in deciding if and when an athlete returns to practice or game participation. Right and left limb muscle symmetry plays a more decisive factor than simply H:Q strength deficits or maximal strength scores, particularly following anterior cruciate ligament reconstruction surgery.[56]

Figure 18.5A and B show generalized muscle force-muscle length and muscle force-muscle velocity relationships for fusiform and pennate muscles with the same contractile protein amount and identical muscle fiber type. In this hypothetical example, the muscle force-muscle length curve for fusiform muscle shows a longer working range and lower maximum force output because longer individual fibers have smaller PCSA (Fig. 18.5C). The opposite occurs for pennate muscle with shorter fibers and larger PCSA—these fibers generate about double the fusiform muscle force. For the muscle force-muscle velocity curve, the fusiform muscle with longer fibers exhibits higher contractile velocity but lower force-output capacity.

Actin-Myosin Orientation

Myosin filaments by the thousands lie packed along the muscle fiber's actin filament line. **FIGURE 18.6A** illustrates a sarcomere's resting length actin-myosin orientation. Figure 18.6B shows

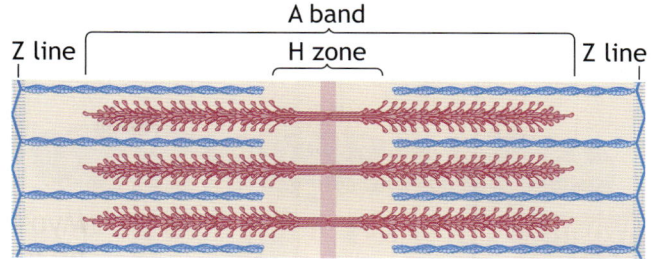

A Resting sarcomere

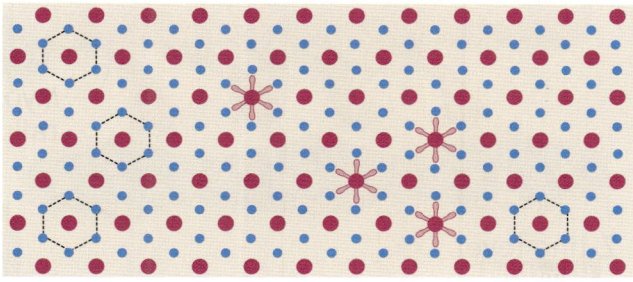

B Crosssection of myofibrils

FIGURE 18.6. (**A**) Ultrastructure of actin-myosin orientation within a resting sarcomere. (**B**) Electron micrographic view through myofibril cross sections in a single muscle fiber. Note the smaller actin and larger myosin filaments' hexagonal orientation, including crossbridges that extend from a thick to thin filament.

the myosin and actin filament hexagonal arrangement. Myosin filaments contain molecule bundles with polypeptide tails and globular heads. Actin filaments have two twisted monomer chains bound by tropomyosin polypeptide chains. Six relatively thin actin filaments, each about 50 Å in diameter and 1 µm long, encircle the thicker myosin filament (150 Å in diameter and 1.5 µm long). This represents an extremely impressive substructural configuration. For example, a myofibril 1 µm in diameter contains approximately 450 thick filaments in the sarcomere's center and 900 thin filaments at each end. A muscle fiber 100 µm in diameter and 1 cm long contains approximately 8000 myofibrils; on average, each myofibril contains 4500 sarcomeres. In a single fiber, this arrangement adds up to approximately 16 billion thick filaments and 64 billion thin filaments!

FIGURE 18.7 illustrates contractile filament component spatial orientation. Projections or "**crossbridges**" spiral around the myosin filament in the actin and myosin filament overlap regions. The crossbridges repeat at approximately 450 Å intervals along the filament. Globular "lollipoplike" myosin heads extend perpendicularly to latch onto the thinner double-twisted actin strands to create structural and functional links between myofilaments. A unique feature about myosin's two heads concerns their opposite orientation at the thick filament ends. ATP hydrolysis activates the two heads, placing them optimally to bind actin's active sites, pulling the sarcomere's thin filaments and Z lines toward the middle. The globular myosin heads contain myosin ATPase, which frees ATP energy for subsequent muscle action.

Tropomyosin and troponin, two other important actin helical structure constituents, regulate the make-and-break

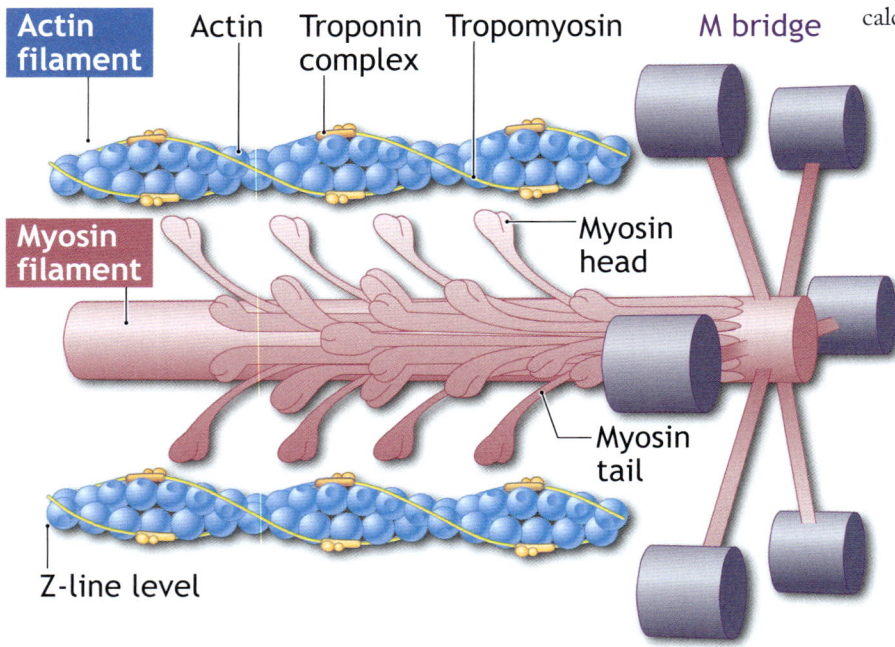

FIGURE 18.7. Thick and thin protein filament details showing tropomyosin and the troponin complex and M bridge. The perpendicularly oriented M bridges interconnect in a hexagonal pattern with adjacent myosin filaments.

calcium ion (Ca^{2+}) affinity, an important mineral that plays a crucial role in muscle action and fatigue.[29] For example, Ca^{2+} and troponin trigger myofibrils to interact and slide past each other. During muscle fiber stimulation, troponin molecules undergo a conformational change that "tugs" on tropomyosin protein strands. Tropomyosin then moves deeper into the groove between two actin strands, "uncovering" actin's active sites so muscle action proceeds. Muscle fatigue relates to considerable Ca^{2+} concentration reductions in the transverse tubules during intense exercise, in addition to intrinsic alterations in the contractile apparatus and sarcoplasmic reticulum function.[7,51]

The M band includes transversely and longitudinally oriented proteins that maintain myosin filament orientation within a sarcomere. Note in Figure 18.7 that the pink, perpendicularly oriented M bridges interconnect in a hexagonal pattern with six adjacent myosin filaments. Exciting areas for investigating muscle biochemistry, physiology, and mechanics involve studying cytoskeletal proteins and structures that serve as an intermediate intracellular filament system.[36] Understanding cytoskeleton characteristics, its diverse proteins, and myofibrillar lattice structure contributes basic knowledge about processes in muscle injury, repair, and overload.

contacts between myofilaments during muscle action. Tropomyosin distributes along the actin filament's length in a groove formed by the double helix. Tropomyosin inhibits actin and myosin interaction (coupling) and prevents their permanent bonding. Troponin and its three-subunit proteins embedded at fairly regular intervals along the actin strands exhibit a high

The intracellular cytoskeleton exhibits three characteristics:

1. Provides structural integrity in the inactive muscle cell
2. Allows for lateral force transmission to adjacent sarcomeres through interaction with actomyosin during muscle action
3. Connects to the cell's surface membrane

Intracellular Cytoskeletal Tubule Systems

FIGURE 18.8 shows a muscle fiber's complex tubular system. Each tubule channel's lateral end terminates in a saclike vesicle that stores Ca^{2+}. Another tubule network—the transverse T-tubule system runs perpendicular to the myofibril. T-tubules lie between the most lateral part in two sarcoplasmic channels; these vesicle structures touch the T-tubule. The term **triad** describes this repeating two vesicles and T-tubule pattern in each Z-line region. Each sarcomere contains two triads, with the pattern repeated regularly along the myofibril's length.

The T-tubules pass through the fiber and open externally from inside the muscle cell. The triad and T-tubule system function

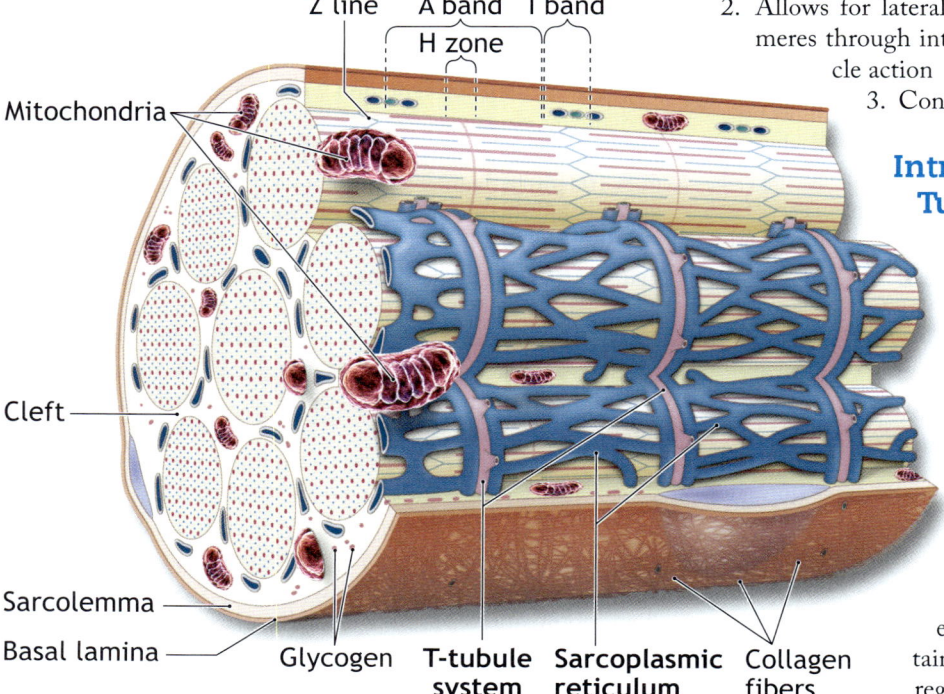

FIGURE 18.8. A muscle fiber's complex "highway" transportation tubule system (*pink* structures) and sarcoplasmic reticulum (*dark blue* structures).
(Mitochondria image: RAJ CREATIONZS/Shutterstock.)

as a microtransportation network by spreading the action potential (*depolarization wave*) *from the fiber's outer membrane inward to deeper cell regions*. Action potential propagation stimulates Ca^{2+} release from the triad sacs, which diffuses a short distance to "activate" the actin filaments. Muscle action begins when myosin filament crossbridges momentarily attach to the actin filament's active sites. When electrical excitation ceases, cytoplasmic Ca^{2+} concentration decreases to relax the muscle. To some extent, propagating an action potential depends on maintaining continued steep Na^+ and K^+ gradients across the sarcolemma. For these electrolytes, decreased chemical gradient, including reduced Na^+/K^+ pump activity, severely impacts muscle fiber excitability and consequent active muscle contractile performance.[35]

Chemical and Mechanical Events During Muscle Action and Relaxation

Electron microscopy, x-ray diffraction, and biochemical methods have unraveled basic information and testable hypotheses concerning chemical and mechanical events during muscle activation and relaxation. Proposed over seven decades ago to explain molecular movements that underlie muscle action, the **sliding filament model** validates the ever-expanding details about muscle ultrastructure and function.[21]

See the animation "Sliding Filament Theory" on **Lippincott Connect** to view this process.

Muscle Action Mechanics: The Sliding Filament Model

The muscle contraction sliding filament model proposed in the early 1950s by two unrelated British biologists with the same last name, had worked independently in the same research area (www.youtube.com/watch?v=sZuy356qkPM). The first, Hugh Esmor Huxley (1924–2013), and the second, Sir Andrew Fielding Huxley (1917–2012; 1963 Nobel Prize in Physiology or Medicine co-winner for insights into ionic mechanisms involved in excitation and inhibition in the peripheral and central nerve cell membrane). A video lecture by Dr. Hugh Huxley provides salient details about his and others' research contributions to the muscle contraction sliding filament model.

Lippincott® Connect Appendix H, available online at **Lippincott Connect**, lists supplemental animations and videos on this subject.

In 1957, A. Huxley extended the theory to include specifics about crossbridge behaviors.[22,23]

The theory proposes a muscle shortens or lengthens because thick and thin filaments slide past each other without changing length. The myosin crossbridges cyclically attach, rotate, and detach from the actin filaments with energy from ATP hydrolysis and provide the molecular motor to drive fiber shortening.[13,40] This produces a major conformational change in relative size within the sarcomere's zones and bands and produces a force

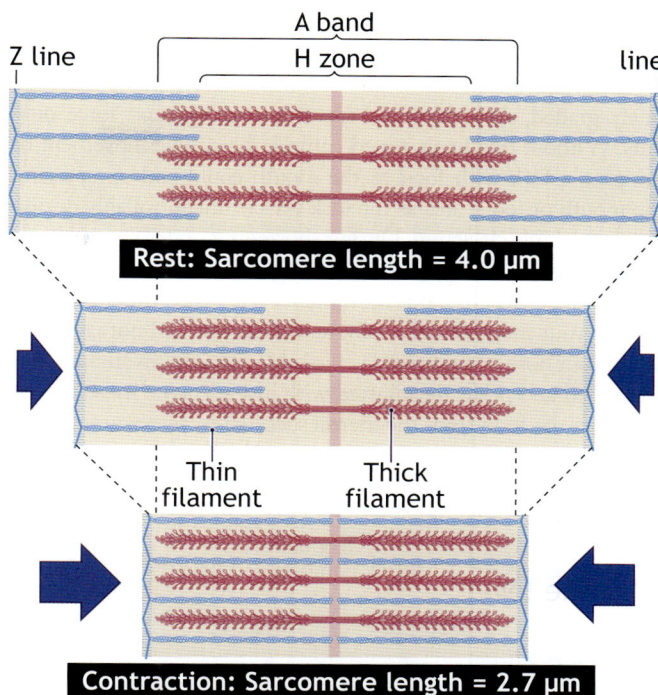

FIGURE 18.9. Structural rearrangement of actin and myosin filaments at rest (4.0 μm sarcomere length) and during muscle shortening (contracted 2.7 μm sarcomere length).

at the Z bands. **FIGURE 18.9** shows that thin actin filaments move past the myosin myofilaments by translating over them by a preset amount and into the A-band region during shortening (2.7 μm) and then move out during the lengthening or relaxation phase (4.0 μm).[4,5] The major structural rearrangement during shortening occurs in the I-band region. This band decreases as the Z bands pull toward each sarcomere's center. No change occurs in the A band width, while the H zone can disappear when the actin filaments make contact at the sarcomere center. A static or isometric muscle action generates force, but the fiber's length remains *unchanged*, keeping the relative I and A bands spacing constant. In this case, the same molecular groups interact continuously. The A band widens in an eccentric action as the fiber lengthens during force generation.

Lippincott® Connect Appendix H provides links to multimedia video animations about muscle action processes available online at **Lippincott Connect**. These videos, produced by students for students, complement our written presentation of muscle action dynamics.

Crossbridge Mechanical Action

Myosin plays both an enzymatic and structural role in muscle action.[50] The myosin crossbridge globular head, which contains actin-activated ATPase in its actin-binding site, generates the mechanical power stroke for actin and myosin filaments to discretely glide past each other. The cyclic, oscillating to-and-fro crossbridge motion powered by ATP hydrolysis move like oars *knifing* through water (**FIG. 18.10**). But unlike oars, crossbridges do not all move synchronously. If they did, muscle action would produce continuous uneven and jerky actions rather than finely graded, smoothly modulated movements and force outputs. Without this finely tuned control, the simple movement of bringing a fork with food to the mouth could end up spearing the mouth or tooth area as the fork wavers uncontrollably during the desired muscle action. During shortening under normal, controlled muscle actions, each crossbridge undergoes repeated but independent asynchronous movement cycles. Next time your food reaches your mouth successfully, remember you did not jab yourself in your nose or eye because crossbridge action was smooth and controlled and perfectly adjusted with just adequate muscle force to deliver the food from the utensil successfully into your mouth!

At any one time, approximately half the crossbridges, which exhibit contractile properties, make contact with actin filaments to form the protein complex actomyosin. The remaining crossbridges move through other positions in their particular vibrating cycle. Figure 18.10 shows each crossbridge action contributes only a small longitudinal displacement to the filament's full sliding action. The process resembles a person's movement in rope climbing. The arms and legs represent the crossbridges. Climbing progresses by first reaching with the arms; then grabbing, pulling, and breaking contact while the legs extend; and then repeating this procedure throughout the climb as the person traverses from one point to the next point and so on along the climb.

In vitro motility assay (www.umass.edu/musclebiophy/techniques%20-%20in%20vitro%20motility%20assay.html) quantifies actin and myosin molecule action.[11,29]

Careful experimentation has determined that myosin elicits a 1 to 10 piconewton (pN; 10^{-2} N) force, in which myosin movement ranges from 1 to 20 nanometers (nm; 10^{-9} m) over a 5-ms interval. Four elegant research tools determine the actomyosin complex's chemical and mechanical properties.

Actomyosin Research Tools

1. *Microneedles.* A glass needle placed in contact with myosin molecules and an actin filament records molecular mechanical movements.[53] Researchers then deduce the forces produced by the myosin heads as they slide along the actin strand.[24]

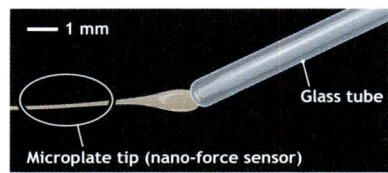

2. *Optical tweezers.* This technique interfaces powerful laser technology with a microscope to isolate individual molecules and measure molecular movement, one molecule at a time (https://blocklab.stanford.edu/optical_tweezers.html).[12]

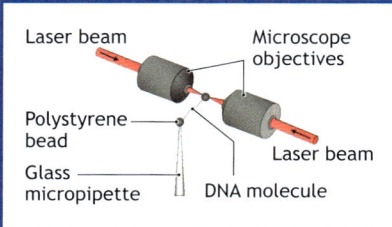

3. *Atomic force microscope* (AFM). The displacement and forces from a probe (with actin and myosin molecules attached; www.nanoscience.com/techniques/atomic-force-microscopy/) interfaced with a specialized microscope yields quantitative data about actin-myosin interaction.[27] German physicist Gerd Binnig (1947–) and Swiss physicist Heinrich Rohrer (1933–2013) shared the 1986 Nobel Prize in Physics for developing the scanning tunneling microscope (www.nobelprize.org/uploads/2018/06/rohrer-lecture.pdf), the precursor to the AFM developed in 1989 by Stanford University researchers (https://microscopy.stanford.edu/atomic-force-microscope).

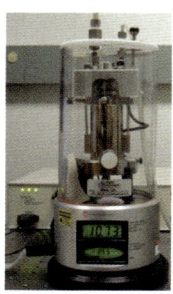

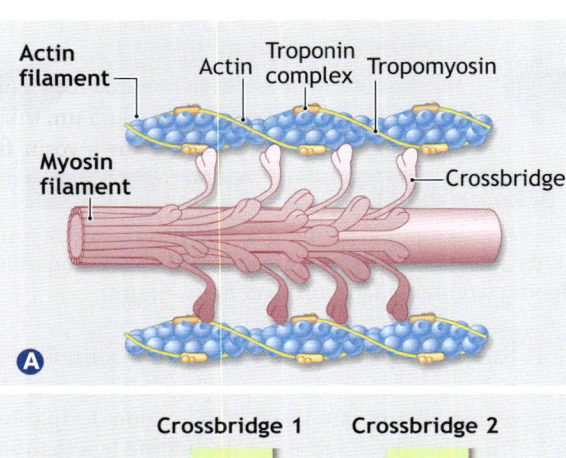
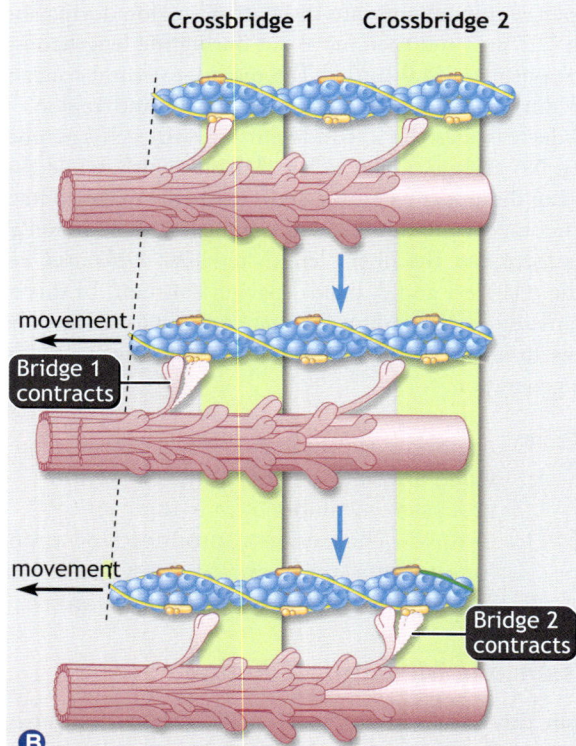

FIGURE 18.10. **(A)** Relative actin and myosin filaments positioning during crossbridge oscillation. **(B)** Each crossbridge action contributes a small movement displacement. For clarity, we show only one actin strand.

4. *Fluorescent probes.* Microscopy with the ability to monitor a cell's physiologic state through high chemical sensitivity fluorescent-labeled probes. 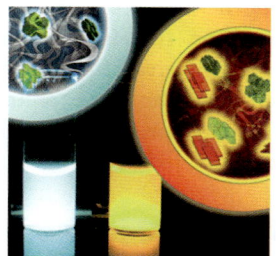 Light-emitting probes quantify molecular binding kinetics and the release between myosin and actin and how ATP liberates useful energy in its degradation.[15] The technique reveals how actin rotates slightly as it moves along myosin and how the myosin heads function during their power stroke.[43]

IQ? INTEGRATIVE QUESTION

How does the term *molecular motor* describe how myofilament crossbridges contribute to muscle fiber action?

Sarcomere Length: Isometric Tension Curve in an Isolated Fiber

FIGURE 18.11 displays interactions between actin and myosin during isometric tension development in an isolated skeletal muscle preparation. Optimal sarcomere length (i.e., the one with the greatest interaction between actin and myosin filaments) occurs between 2.0 and 2.25 μm (*light blue vertical band*). Tension output for optimal sarcomere length decreases steadily as sarcomere length increases beyond the optimal length. Note the actin and myosin filament overlap at various tension-length curve regions and how tension output varies at different sarcomere lengths. Thin filament thickness equals 1.0 μm; thick filament thickness equals 1.6 μm.

In the early 1960s, British and Swedish researchers developed the length-tension curve with sophisticated mechanical experiments by electrically stimulating a single frog muscle fiber 8 mm long and 75 μm in diameter and plotting maximum tension output at selected muscle sarcomere lengths.[17] Sarcomere length along the horizontal axis ranged from 1.6 μm at maximum actin filament overlap (approximately 70% maximum tension) to 3.6 μm when fully relaxed. Note that the upward tension curve occurred at a sarcomere length between 2.0 and 2.25 μm; this length for maximal tension represents the maximum region for actin and myosin filament interaction. Interestingly, the 0.2-μm difference at this part along the curve equals precisely the width in the region where no change takes place in actin-myosin interaction. The curve shifts downward when the sarcomere stretches beyond 2.2 μm, indicating peak tension decline. This decline occurs from reduced overlap between actin and myosin filaments; less overlap produces less crossbridge interaction with concomitant diminished active tension development. Fibers fail to develop tension at the maximum stretch point 3.65 μm (maximum actin filament length, 2.0 μm; maximum myosin filament length, 1.65 μm). Crossbridge interaction cannot take place at sarcomere lengths of 3.65 μm and above.

Sarcomere Length: Isometric Tension Curve in Human Muscle Fibers In Vivo

An elegant technical procedure determines the range over which sarcomeres in intact human muscle operate along their length-tension curve. **FIGURE 18.12** demonstrates sarcomere action during different wrist position angles in patients who undergo surgery to correct chronic lateral epicondylitis or "tennis elbow." The researchers compared length-tension characteristics in an animal preparation (Fig. 18.11) compared to human muscle *in vivo*.

Figure 18.12 (*top right*) depicts the intraoperative helium-neon laser to quantify sarcomere length (and view of the illumination prism) during the surgery. The laser, positioned beneath the extensor carpi radialis brevis (ECRB) muscle's lateral end, quantified sarcomere lengths at three different wrist positions: (1) full flexion to increase sarcomere length, (2) neutral, and (3) full extension to decrease sarcomere length.

The top left in Figure 18.12 shows the laser-generated red diffraction pattern to compute sarcomere length. Biopsy specimens from the same muscle verified the laser determinations. An electron

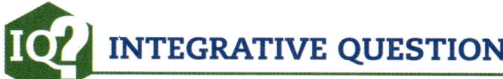

FIGURE 18.11. Relationship between tension and sarcomere length in skeletal muscle during an isometric muscle action.

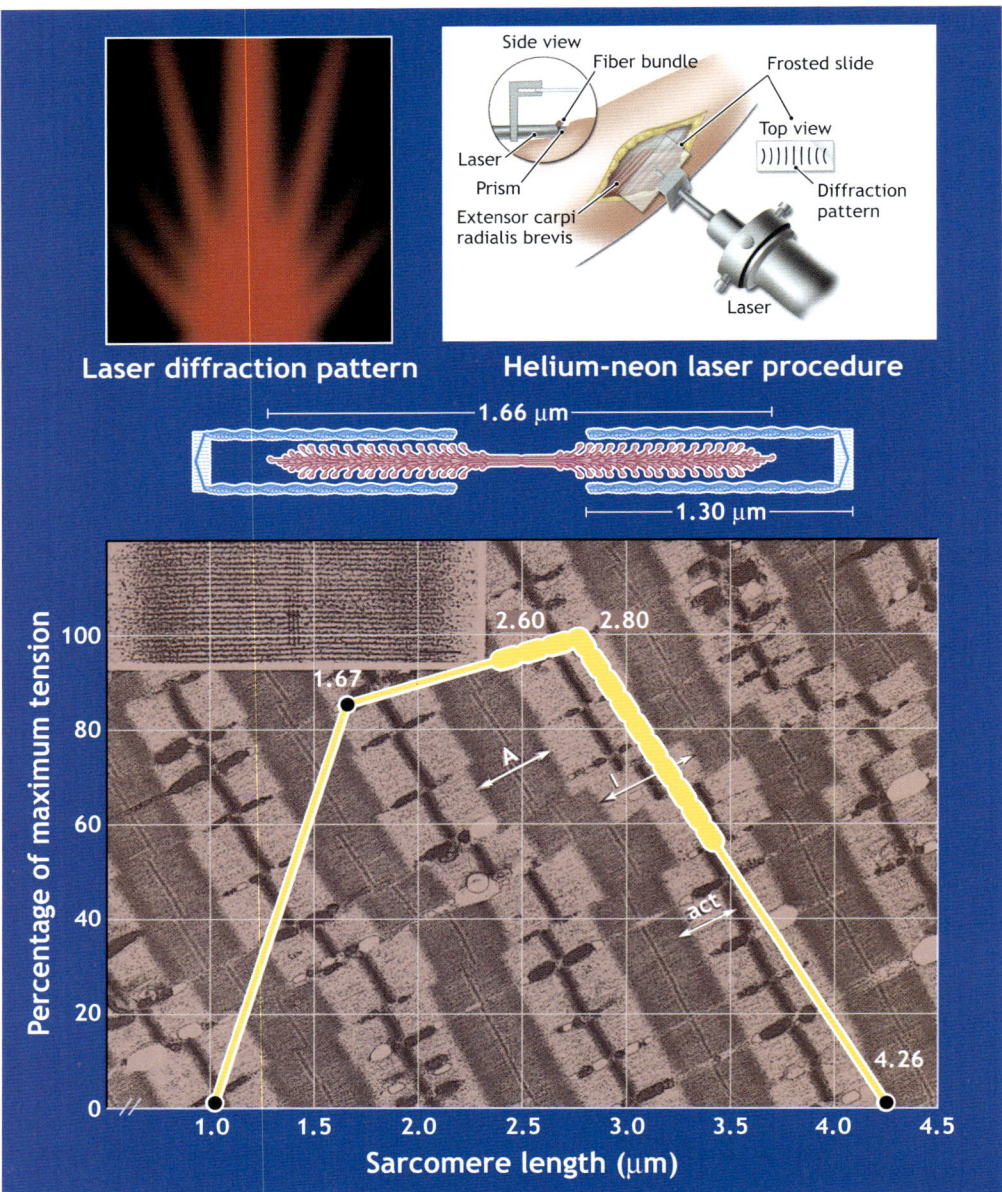

FIGURE 18.12. Changes in the length-tension curve for sarcomeres *in vivo* during human wrist flexion and extension. The electron micrograph depicted behind the length-tension curve shows the actin and myosin filaments and the A and I bands from extensor carpi radialis brevis muscle biopsy samples to verify sarcomere lengths.
(The laser diffraction pattern, electron micrograph, and related images courtesy Dr. Richard L Lieber, Professor of Physical Medicine and Rehabilitation, McCormick School of Engineering and Physiology, Northwestern Feinberg School of Medicine. Evanston, IL.)

length change during wrist flexion (causing sarcomere length increase) and wrist extension (causing sarcomere length decrease). The numbers over the curve represent the inflection points based on measured filament lengths.

Linkage Among Actin, Myosin, and ATP

The interaction and movement for the protein filaments during muscle action require that myosin crossbridges continually undergo oscillatory movements by combining, detaching, and recombining with new sites along the actin strands or the same sites in a static action. When ATP molecules join the actomyosin complex, the myosin crossbridges detach from the actin filament. The myosin crossbridges in this chemical reaction then return to their original state ready to bind to a new active actin site. Actomyosin dissociation occurs as follows:

Actomyosin + ATP → Actin + Myosin-ATP

Energy from ATP hydrolysis transduces into mechanical force when ADP and inorganic phosphate end products form. One reacting site on the myosin crossbridge globular head binds to an actin reactive site. The other myosin active site serves as the actin-activated enzyme **myofibrillar adenosine triphosphatase (myosin ATPase)**. This enzyme hydrolyzes (splits) ATP into ADP and inorganic phosphate (P_i) to yield energy for muscle action. The ATP splitting rate remains relatively slow when myosin and actin continue apart; when they join, myosin ATPase reaction rates increase substantially. Energy released from ATP splitting activates crossbridges, causing them to oscillate. Energy transfer produces a conformational change in myosin's globular head, so it interacts with the appropriate actin molecule. The actin filament slides forward from conformational change at multiple contact points between myosin and actin.

micrograph displayed behind the length-tension curve shows the actin and myosin filaments and A and I bands from a muscle biopsy sample. In this experiment, actin filament length equaled 1.30 μm, while the myosin filaments were 1.66 μm long. The thicker yellow portion for the plateau and downward curve shows the ECRB sarcomere operating range during passive (2.6 to 3.4 μm) and active (2.44 to 3.33 μm) muscle actions.

These data objectify the intrinsic relation between sarcomere length and muscle fiber force capacity (length-tension curve) measured *in vivo* in human muscle. The thickened yellow hypothetical length-tension curve represents sarcomere

Just prior to muscle action, the elongated, pear-shaped, flexible myosin head literally bends around the energy-carrying ATP molecule and cocks like a spring. The myosin then interacts with the adjacent actin filament, splits a phosphate from ATP, and releases its stored mechanical energy as it straightens. This forces the sliding motion that generates muscle tension. Actin and myosin filaments slide past each other at speeds up to 15 μm·s^{-1}.[3]

Excitation-Contraction Coupling

Excitation-contraction coupling represents the physiologic mechanism where an electrical discharge at the muscle initiates chemical events at the cell surface to release intracellular Ca^{2+} and ultimately produce muscle action.

Intracellular Ca^{2+} regulates a muscle fiber's contractile and metabolic activity. Ca^{2+} concentration within a nonactive muscle fiber remains relatively low compared with the extracellular fluid that bathes the cells. Muscle fiber stimulation causes an immediate, small increase in intracellular Ca^{2+}, which precedes contractile activity. Cellular Ca^{2+} increases when the action potential at the transverse tubules causes Ca^{2+} release from the sarcoplasmic reticulum's lateral sacs. Troponin's inhibitory action, which prevents actin-myosin interaction, rapidly dissipates when Ca^{2+} binds with this and other proteins in the actin filaments. In a sense, the muscle "turns on" for action.

Actin + Myosin ATPase → Actomyosin + ATPase

Joining active sites on actin and myosin activates myosin ATPase to split ATP. The energy generated causes myosin crossbridge movement to produce muscle tension.

Actomyosin ATP → Actomyosin + ADP + Pi + Energy

Crossbridges uncouple from actin when ATP binds to the myosin crossbridge. Coupling and uncoupling continue when Ca^{2+} concentration remains high enough to inhibit the troponin-tropomyosin system. When neural stimulation ceases, Ca^{2+} moves back into the sarcoplasmic reticulum's lateral sacs. This restores the troponin-tropomyosin inhibitory action, and actin and myosin stay apart provided ATP concentration remains adequate. In **rigor mortis** (Latin *rigor* "stiffness" + *mortis* "of death"), muscles (and joints) stiffen and become rigid and locked into place about 2 to 6 hr after death and lasts several days. This happens because muscle cells no longer contain ATP—without ATP, myosin crossbridges and actin remain attached and do not separate. In essence, myosin molecules adhere to actin filaments causing muscle rigidity.

The average human muscle fiber ranges in size from 10 to 100 μm, with about 60 μm a more typical size based on sophisticated MRI multi-echo diffusion tensor imaging.

FIGURE 18.13 illustrates the interaction among actin and myosin filaments, Ca^{2+}, and ATP in both a relaxed and shortened muscle fiber. In the relaxed state, troponin and tropomyosin interact with actin, preventing the myosin crossbridge from coupling to actin. During muscle action, the crossbridge couples with actin from Ca^{2+} binding with troponin-tropomyosin.

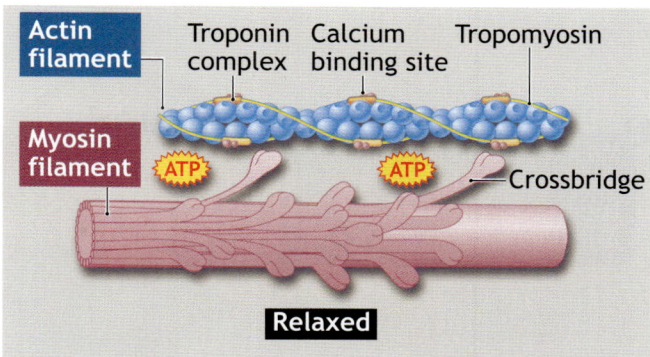
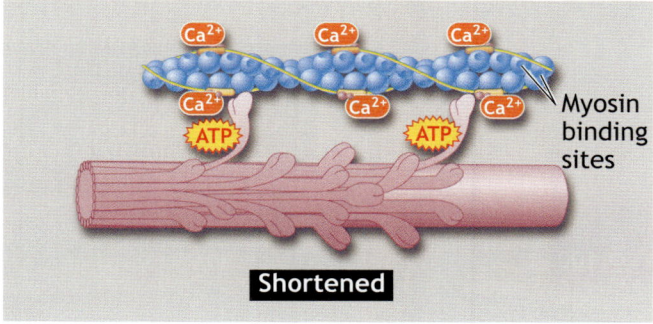

FIGURE 18.13. Interaction among actin-myosin filaments, Ca^{2+}, and adenosine triphosphate (ATP) in relaxed (*upper*) and shortened (*lower*) muscle.

In isolated muscle preparations, stimulation produces a threefold faster rise in Ca^{2+} concentration and accompanying increase in the action potential in type II (fast-twitch) muscle fibers compared with type I (slow-twitch) muscle fibers. Such differences reflect faster Ca^{2+} transport through the sarcoplasmic reticulum and ultimately to the contractile proteins in type II fibers. During excitation-contraction coupling, electrochemical events occur within the cell membrane at the excitation site. The common pathway to precisely target the chemical signal to the contractile proteins largely depends on **ion channel regulators**. Prior to myofilament activation, these microstructures serve as selective "gates" or "sensors" to modulate ion passage between intracellular and extracellular fluids.

Relaxation

When muscle stimulation ceases, Ca^{2+} flow stops, and troponin frees up to inhibit actin-myosin interaction. Recovery involves pumping Ca^{2+} into the sarcoplasmic reticulum where it concentrates in lateral vesicles. Calcium retrieval from the troponin-tropomyosin protein complex "turns off" the actin filament active sites. Muscle relaxation occurs when actin and myosin filaments return to their original states. Deactivation serves two purposes:

1. Prevents any mechanical link between myosin crossbridges and actin filaments
2. Inhibits myosin ATPase activity to curtail ATP splitting

Nine Key Steps in Muscle Action Events

FIGURE 18.14 summarizes nine key steps in muscle activation, contraction, and relaxation. The neurotransmitter **acetylcholine (ACh)**, released from saclike vesicles within

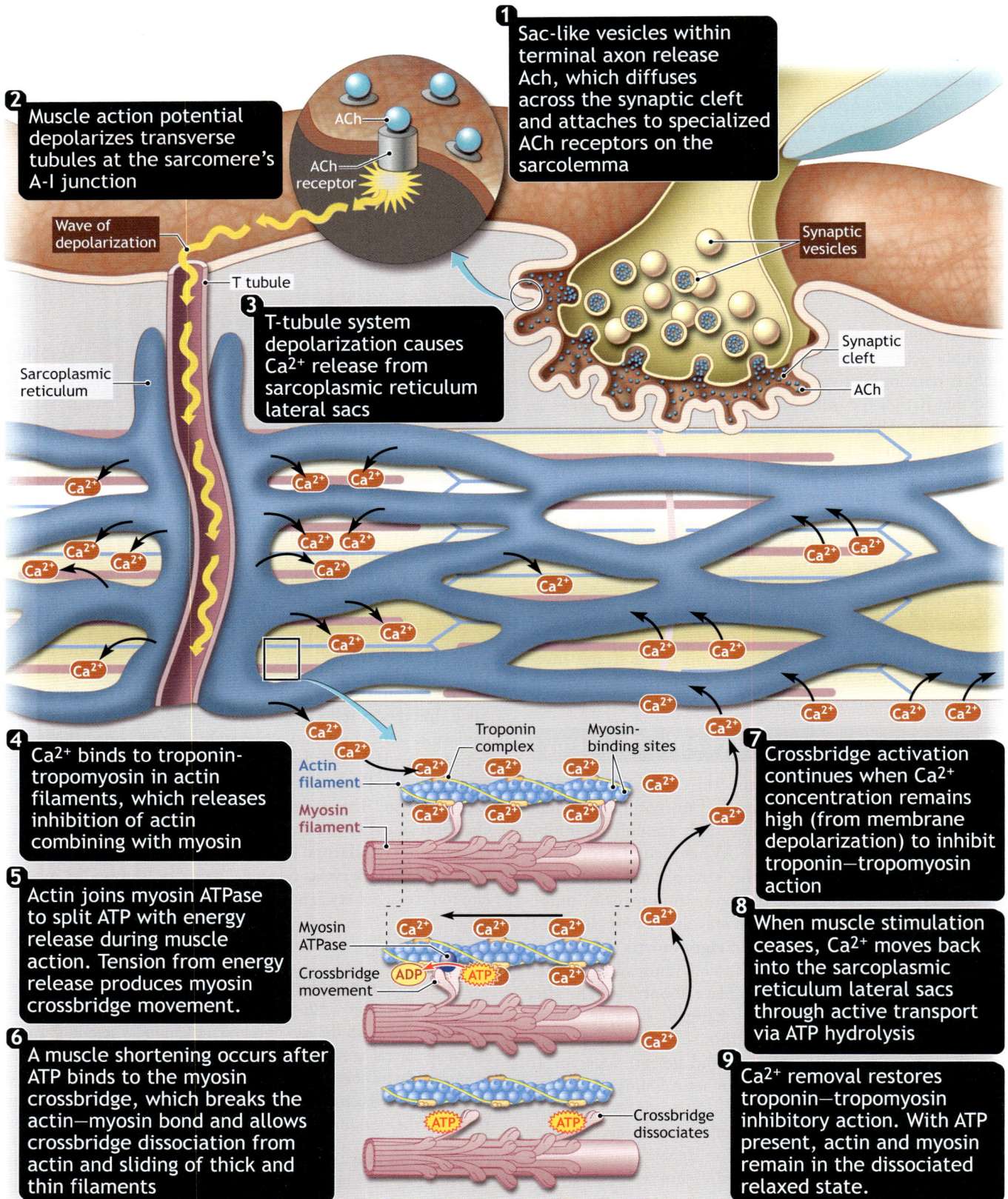

FIGURE 18.14. Nine main events in muscle contraction and relaxation. Numbers correspond to the nine-step sequence outlined under "Nine Key Steps in Muscle Action Events." ACh, acetylcholine; ADP, adenosine diphosphate; ATP, adenosine triphosphate; ATPase, adenosine triphosphatase; T-tubule, transverse tubule.

the terminal axon, initiates transmission at the myoneural junction. Here, the electrochemical signal "jumps" across the 0.05-μm cleft between neuron and muscle fiber. The electrical impulse, traveling at a 1 m·s^{-1} or faster velocity, spreads through the fiber's architecturally elegant tubule system to the myofibril's inner contractile "machinery."

The nine-step sequence begins with the motor nerve's initiating an action potential. A depolarizing impulse then propagates throughout the entire fiber surface (sarcolemma). The nine steps are listed in Figure 18.14.

Lippincott® Connect Appendix H, available online at Lippincott Connect, provides supplemental animations and videos on this subject.

Muscle Fiber Type

Skeletal muscle does not simply contain homogeneous fibers with similar metabolic and contractile properties. Muscle fiber type varies both from muscle to muscle and person to person. Italian physician Stefano Lorenzini made the first distinction between "red" and "white" muscle fibers (myofibers) in 1678 in the electric ray torpedo fish, reaffirmed about 200 years later in 1873 by French histologist Louis-Antoine Ranvier (see Chapter 19).

Skeletal muscle contains two main fiber types that differ in three ways:

1. Primary mechanism to produce ATP
2. Motor neuron innervation type
3. Myosin heavy chain type expressed

A common technique to establish the specific muscle fiber type assesses myosin molecule's heavy chain that exists in three different **isoforms** based on muscle biopsy procedures (see next section). The assessment evaluates a fiber's differential sensitivity to altered enzyme myosin ATPase pH (represents myosin phenotype).[28,30,37,38] This enzyme's different characteristics determine ATP hydrolysis rapidity in the myosin heavy chain region and sarcomere shortening velocity. More specifically, acid pH inactivates the specific myosin ATPase activity in fast-twitch fibers but remains fairly stable at an alkaline pH, the fibers staining *dark* for this enzyme. In contrast, specific myosin ATPase activity for slow-twitch fibers remains high at an acid pH but inactivates in an alkaline milieu, with these fibers staining *light* for myosin ATPase. **TABLE 18.2** lists different classification schemes for skeletal fiber types on the basis of morphology, histochemistry, biochemistry, function, and contractility.

TABLE 18.2 Skeletal muscle fiber classifications

Muscle Biopsy

FIGURE 18.15 illustrates serial cross sections from muscle biopsies obtained from the human vastus lateralis (**A** and **B**), with identification for type I and type IIA, B, and C fibers.

The latter represents a former rare and undifferentiated subtype that may contribute to reinnervation and motor unit transformation. The **muscle biopsy** procedure, originally developed by French neurologist Guillaume-Benjamin-Amand de Boulogne (1806–1875) in the mid-1800s pioneered better understanding about muscular atrophy and paralysis caused by nervous system disorders. In addition to pursuing experiments in electrophysiology, Duchenne described severe muscle weakness in young boys, a disease later identified by a genetic malfunction for the *dystrophin* protein required to maintain normal muscle function resulting in progressive muscle degeneration and weakness (www.mda.org/disease/duchenne-muscular-dystrophy). Unfortunately, the prevalence rate for muscular dystrophy in Europe and the United States now slightly exceeds 6 per 100,000 mostly boys. Duchenne also was first to take muscle tissue biopsies by inventing a needle (literally an "histological harpoon") to extract diseased muscle tissue samples to better understand the disease later named to honor him.

Fast forward to the early 1960s, when two Swedish scientists, Jonas Bergstrom and Eric Hultman at the Karolinska Institute in Sweden (see Introduction: A View From the Past), pioneered a surgical technique first reported by Bergström[60] to excise small muscle tissue snippets primarily from lower leg (quadriceps femoris and vastus lateralis) to identify muscle fiber type functional characteristics during exercise and response to training. The technique called percutaneous muscle biopsy involves inserting a needle similar to that invented by Duchenne into an incision in the muscle belly to extract fibers for subsequent analysis. An excellent video from a modern exercise physiology laboratory shows the step-by-step Bergström methods for muscle biopsy (www.mda.org/disease/duchenne-muscular-dystrophy). The procedure typically takes 15 to 20 min. The procedure has been applied to uncover biochemical alterations from experimental protocols (e.g., dietary manipulation effects and gene expression functions), to training experiments in recreational persons and elite athletes representing both sexes and differing ages on muscle architecture.[64–66] These studies revealed that for male and female World and National caliber athletes, years competing in weight lifting determined fast-twitch fiber percentage more than sex, particularly for type IIa fibers (67% males and 71% females). The extreme fast-twitch myofiber abundance likely explains how these elite weightlifters generate extraordinary force rapidly. The researchers concluded that high fidelity measurement techniques should explore specific fiber type distribution, their size, and contractile properties in elite athlete groups in diverse sports, and body size and composition ideally across several competitive years. The authors posit that future research may ultimately validate genetically based algorithms to personalize success with resistance training methods.

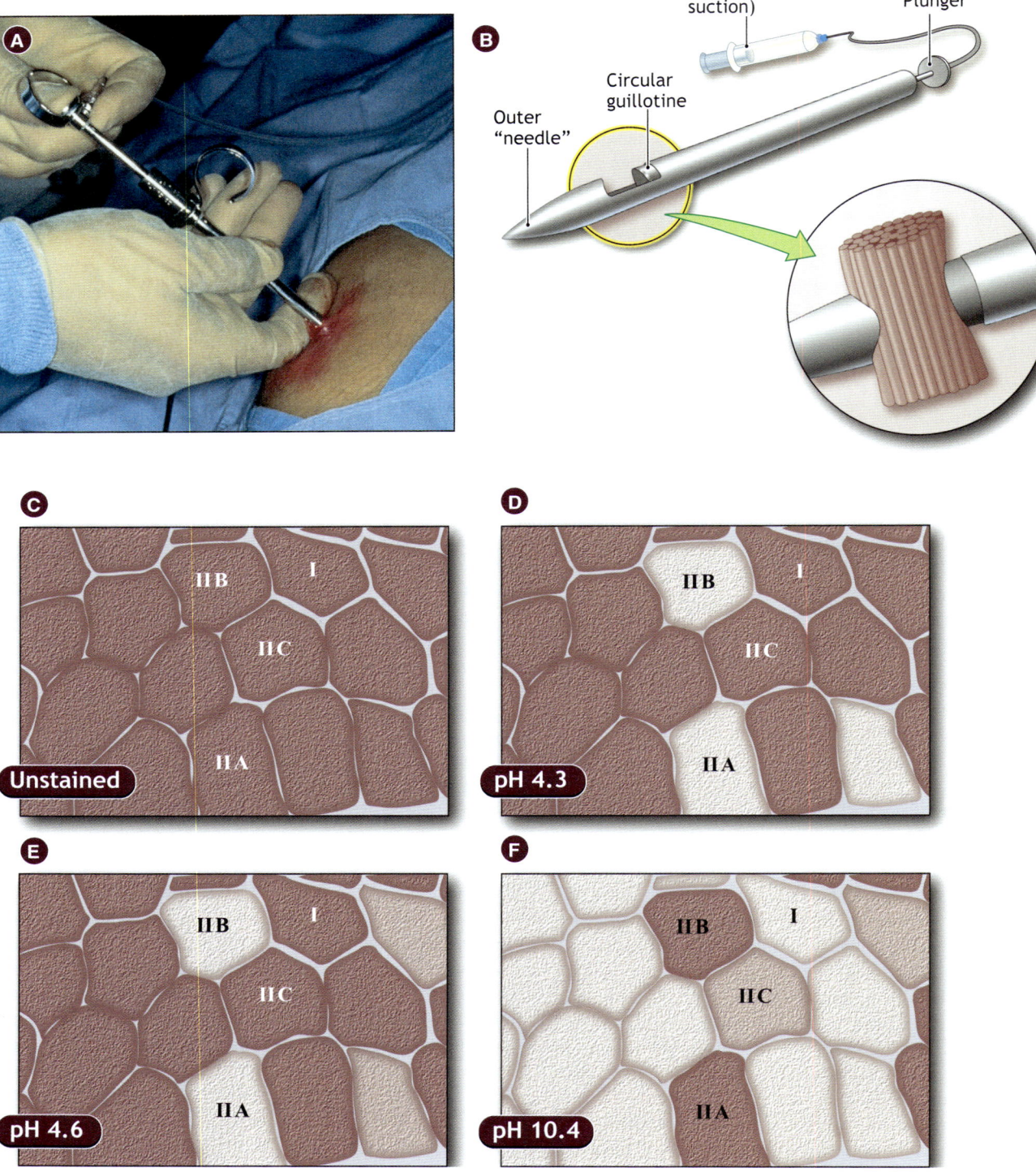

FIGURE 18.15. Serial cross sections obtained by muscle biopsy of human vastus lateralis muscle **(A and B)** with identification of type I and type IIA, B, and C fiber subdivisions. **(C)** Thick unstained section (40 to 50 μm) in which all fibers appear similar. Three other panels indicate some fibers stained for myosin-ATPase activity at a preincubation pH of 4.3 (highly acidic; **D**), 4.6 (intermediate acidity; **E**), and 10.4 (alkaline; **F**).
(**A**, reprinted with permission from Plowman SA, Smith DL. *Exercise Physiology for Health, Fitness, and Performance*. 5th ed. Baltimore: Lippincott Williams & Wilkins; 2017.)

Fast-Twitch Fibers (Type II)

Fast-twitch muscle fibers exhibit four important characteristics:

1. High electrochemical action potential transmission
2. High myosin ATPase activity
3. Rapid sarcoplasmic reticulum Ca^{2+} release and uptake
4. High crossbridge turnover rate

These four factors determine this fiber's rapid energy generation for quick, powerful muscle actions. The fast-twitch fiber's intrinsic shortening speed and tension development ranges three to five times faster than slow-twitch fibers (see following section). Fast-twitch fibers rely on a well-developed, short-term glycolytic energy transfer system. *Fast-twitch fiber activation predominates in anaerobic-type sprint activities and other forceful muscle actions that rely almost entirely on anaerobic energy metabolism.*[3,16,26] Activating fast-twitch fibers plays an important role in the stop-and-go or change-of-pace basketball, soccer, water polo, lacrosse, or field hockey. Such activities demand rapid energy that only anaerobic pathways generate. "In a Practical Sense" describes a popular jumping test, believed to reflect the immediate lower body power output from the anaerobic substrates ATP and PCr.

Type II fibers distribute in three primary subtypes: type IIa, type IIx, and type IIb. Human skeletal muscle contains type I, type IIa, and type IIx fibers (previously referred to as type IIb) and a new type IIb subtype.[46] Type IIa, IIx, and IIb fibers are also present in mammalian rodents and cats.

The **type IIa fiber** exhibits fast shortening speed and well-developed energy transfer capacity from aerobic (high level aerobic enzyme succinic dehydrogenase, or SDH) and anaerobic (high level anaerobic enzyme phosphofructokinase, or PFK) sources. These fibers represent the **fast oxidative-glycolytic (FOG)** fiber type. The **type IIb fiber** possesses the greatest anaerobic potential and most rapid shortening velocity; it represents the "true" fast glycolytic (FG) fiber. A **type IIx fiber** falls midway between type IIa and type IIb counterparts in physiologic and metabolic characteristics.

Slow-Twitch Fibers (Type I)

The aerobic energy transfer system generates considerable energy for ATP resynthesis in predominantly slow-twitch (type I) muscle fibers. Four distinguishing slow-twitch fiber characteristics include the following:

1. Low myosin ATPase activity
2. Slow calcium handling ability and shortening speed
3. Less glycolytic capacity than fast-twitch fibers
4. Large and numerous mitochondria

Slow-twitch fibers receive their characteristic red pigmentation from a rich mitochondrial supply, iron-containing cytochromes, and high myoglobin levels. A high mitochondrial enzyme concentration links closely to a slow-twitch fiber's enhanced aerobic metabolic machinery. *These characteristics make slow-twitch fibers highly fatigue resistant and ideally suited for prolonged aerobic physical activity.* The fibers have been labeled **slow oxidative (SO)**, to describe their slow shortening speed and reliance on oxidative metabolism. Compared to fast-twitch fibers that fatigue readily, longer-duration activities selectively recruit the less fatigable SO fibers, or, more precisely SO motor units.[25]

Muscle glycogen depletion patterns indicate that prolonged, intense aerobic activity demands almost exclusive reliance on slow-twitch muscle fibers. Even after exercising continuously for 12 hr, the limited glycogen remaining in active muscle exists mostly in the relatively "unused" fast-twitch fibers. Differences in oxidative capacity between the two fiber types also determine blood flow through muscle, with slow-twitch fibers receiving the largest quantity.[31]

Exercise physiologists classify slow-twitch fibers as **type I muscle fibers** and fast-twitch fibers (and proposed subdivisions) as **type II muscle fibers**. *Slow and fast muscle fiber types together engage during near-maximum aerobic and anaerobic middle-distance running or swimming or basketball, field hockey, or soccer, which combine both high aerobic and anaerobic efficient energy transfer levels.*

INTEGRATIVE QUESTION

What is a compelling argument for and against muscle fiber typing in children to "guide" them to future sports success?

Genes that Define Skeletal Muscle Phenotype

At least three independent chemical signaling pathways regulate skeletal muscle fiber types in adult animals and most likely humans:

1. Pathways involved with the Ras/mitogen-activated protein kinase (MAPK)
2. Calcineurin, calcium/calmodulin-dependent protein kinase IV
3. Peroxisome proliferator g coactivator 1 (PGC-1α), a coactivator that promotes mitochondrial biogenesis, mitochondrial fatty acid oxidation, and hepatic gluconeogenesis

The PGC-1α provides a direct link between external physiologic stimuli and mitochondrial biogenesis modulation and primarily regulates muscle fiber type determination. This pathway may also act to regulate blood pressure and cellular cholesterol balance and play a role in obesity development. The Ras/MAPK signaling pathway links motor neurons and signaling systems and couples excitation and transcription regulation to promote nerve-dependent muscle regeneration induction.

Mice with an activated PGC-1α form display an "endurance" phenotype, accompanied with a coordinated increase in oxidative enzymes and mitochondrial biogenesis and increased proportion relating to slow-twitch muscle fibers. **Functional genomics research** attempts to

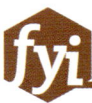

Muscle Fiber Training Specificity

Why do some highly trained athletes who switch to a sport requiring different muscle groups feel essentially untrained for the new activity? The answer is fairly straightforward— only the specific fibers activated in specific exercise training adapt metabolically and physiologically to the particular training regimen. Known as the exercise training specificity principle, swimmers or canoeists should not expect to transfer upper-body "fitness" training to a running sport without training the specific muscles involved in running. This training principle, amply validated over half a century or more from exercise physiology and human performance laboratories worldwide, serves as a bedrock principle that specific muscle fibers activated in training probably will not transfer their functional adaptations, if any, to a dissimilar activity with the expected same physiological and concomitant performance outcomes. In short, specific exercise training with specific muscular movement patterns produces highly specific muscular and performance adaptations.

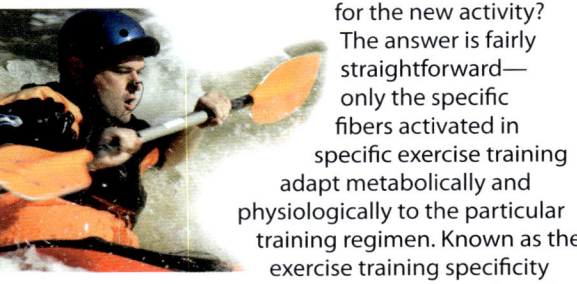
pjmorley/Shutterstock

Sources:
Angleri V, et al. Resistance training variable manipulations are less relevant than intrinsic biology in affecting muscle fiber hypertrophy. *Scand J Med Sci Sports*. 2022. doi:10.1111/sms.14134.
Gergley TJ, et al. Specificity of arm training on aerobic power during swimming and running. *Med Sci Sports Exerc*. 1984;16:34.
Hester GM, et al. Microbiopsy sampling for examining age-related differences in skeletal muscle fiber morphology and composition. *Front Physiol*. 2022;12:756626.
Magel JR, et al. Metabolic and cardiovascular adjustment to arm training. *J Appl Physiol Respir Environ Exerc Physiol*. 1978;45:7.
McArdle WD, et al. Specificity of run training on $\dot{V}O_2$max and heart rate changes during running and swimming. *Med Sci Sports*. 1978;10:16.

---

understanding gene function and other genome characteristics (www.ornl.gov/sci/techresources/Human_Genome/research/function.shtml). These pathways include a signaling network to control skeletal muscle fiber type transformation and metabolic profiles that protect against insulin resistance and obesity.

Other pathways also influence adult muscle characteristics. For example, physical force generated within a muscle fiber may release the serum response transcription factor (SRF) from the structural muscle protein titin first reported in 1976 in chicken skeletal muscle leading to increased muscle growth.[69] Titin acts as a "governor" to control the relative actin and myosin protein positioning, probably by calcium binding upon activation,[19] and regulates contracting muscle's "springiness."[41,44] Titin also plays an important role in muscle force regulation, particularly for eccentric or active lengthening muscle actions.[20,32,54]

Other factors related to **circadian rhythm** (physical, mental, and behavioral changes that follow a daily, mostly repetitive internal 24-hr cycle in humans, plants, animals, fungi, and bacteria) control also contribute to a better understanding about functional genomics research now covered in many undergraduate and graduate kinesiology courses. This new research paradigm centers on feedback loops to control the "molecular clock" components involving transcriptional and translation genetic processes[67,68] (see Chapter 33). This emerging field opens up new interdisciplinary research opportunities in functional genomics related to human movement linked to muscle gene expression.

Fiber Type Differences Among Athletic Groups

Interesting observations concern muscle fiber type and how specific training regimens impact fiber composition and metabolic capacity. Men, women, and children on average possess

Factors in Skeletal Muscle Mass Decline with Aging

Differences in leg muscle cross-sectional area (MCSA) between younger men (age 23) and elderly men (age 71) reflect mainly muscle fiber size differences, not muscle fiber number. The cross-section image shows a 100× microscopic view from a young man's biopsied quadriceps muscle. Quadriceps MCSA and type I and II muscle fiber size were initially measured in 25 healthy young and 26 older men.

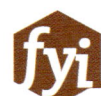
ggw/Shutterstock

Older subjects performed resistance training for 6 months, followed by retesting. Pretraining differences in quadriceps MCSA were compared with differences in type I and II muscle fiber size.

Quadriceps MCSA was substantially smaller in older versus younger men (68 vs. 80 cm). Type II muscle fiber size was smaller in elderly compared to young counterparts by 29%, with only a tendency for smaller type I muscle fibers. Type II muscle fiber size fully explained between group MCSA quadriceps differences. Resistance training for 6 months in the elderly increased type II muscle fiber size by 24%, explaining 100% of the quadriceps MCSA increase from 68 to 74 cm.

These findings reveal that reduced muscle mass with aging results from decreased type II muscle fiber size that is unlikely accompanied by substantial muscle fiber loss. In aging skeletal muscle, mitophagy reflects poorly functional mitochondria accumulation, which moderate-intensity exercise partially can mitigate. The expected yearly skeletal muscle mass declined less in Japanese males ($n = 292$) and females ($n = 363$) who had larger total daily protein intake than individuals with a lower protein intake.

Sources:
Drake JC. Unclogging the garbage disposal: how exercise may improve mitochondria in ageing skeletal muscle. *J Physiol*. 2018;596:3449.
Nilwik R, et al. The decline in skeletal muscle mass with aging is mainly attributed to a reduction in type II muscle fiber size. *Exp Gerontol*. 2013;48:492.
Otsuka R, et al. Protein intake per day and at each daily meal and skeletal muscle mass declines among older community dwellers in Japan. *Public Health Nutr*. 2020;23:1090.

45 to 55% slow-twitch fibers in their arm and leg muscles. The fast-twitch fibers probably distribute equally between type IIa and type IIb subdivisions. No gender differences exist in fiber distribution, yet large inter-individual variation remains prevalent. Generally, the trend in one's muscle fiber type distribution remains consistent among the body's major muscle groups. Muscle fiber distribution patterns generally occur among highly proficient athletes.[47] Successful endurance athletes in a particular sport possess predominantly slow-twitch fibers in the primary muscles activated in their sport, as for example, shoulder muscles in distance swimmers and quadriceps, hamstrings, and gluteal muscles in distance runners. In contrast, elite sprint 100- to 400-m track athletes have predominately fast-twitch fibers, as do male and female elite-caliber weightlifters.

FIGURE 18.16 illustrates fiber type distribution for top Nordic competitors in different sports. Athletic groups with the highest aerobic and endurance capacities (e.g., distance runners and cross-country skiers) possess the highest slow-twitch fiber percentage, often 90 to 95% in the leg's gastrocnemius muscle. Weightlifters, ice hockey players, and sprinters have more fast-twitch fibers with concomitantly lower aerobic capacities. Men and women who perform in middle-distance events display approximately equal fiber type percentages. The same distribution also occurs in the world's top power athletes—throwers, jumpers, and high jumpers.[9]

The relatively clear-cut distinctions between exercise performance and muscle fiber composition pertain mainly to elite athletes with prominence in a distinct sport category (e.g., track and field, and within that category, examples include discus, javelin, high jump, pole vault, 5000-m steeple chase).

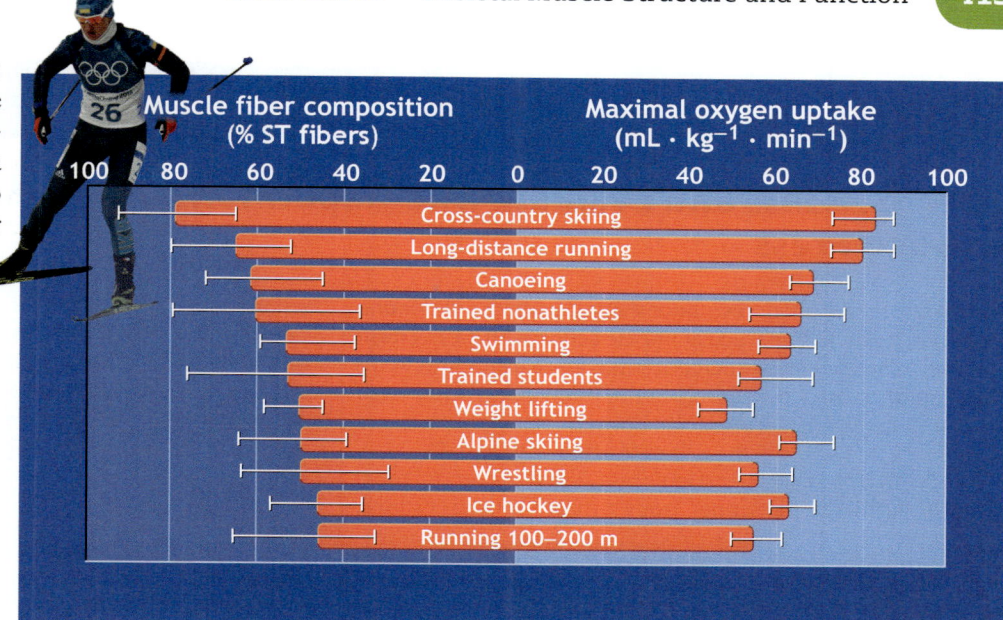

FIGURE 18.16. Muscle fiber composition (% slow-twitch [ST] fibers, *left side*) and maximal oxygen uptake (*right side*) in athletes representing different sports. Data for cross-country skiing features an Olympic competition skier—that sport group has the largest ST fiber percentage and corresponding largest maximal oxygen uptake. The *outer white bars* denote the range.
(Reprinted with permission from Bergh U, et al. Maximal oxygen uptake and muscle fiber types in trained and untrained humans. *Med Sci Sports*. 1978;10:151. Photo: Leonard Zhukovsky/Shutterstock.)

Even among these subgroups, muscle fiber composition does not solely determine performance success because success reflects blending many physiologic, psychological, biochemical, neurologic, and biomechanical "support systems," not simply a particular muscle fiber type.

Endurance athletes have relatively normal-sized muscle fibers, with a tendency toward slow-twitch fiber enlargement. Conversely, weightlifters and other power athletes show more enlarged fiber types, particularly fast-twitch fibers. These may exceed by 45% of those similarly aged endurance athletes or sedentary persons.[48,49] Strength and power training enlarges the fiber's contractile apparatus—specifically the actin and myosin filaments—and total glycogen content. *Larger muscle fibers in male athletes with a larger total muscle mass characterize the principal gender differences in muscle morphology.* Chapter 22 discusses the potential for exercise training to alter skeletal muscles' metabolic and fiber type characteristics and overall muscle size.

In a Practical Sense

How to Assess and Evaluate One-Repetition Maximum for Bench Press and Leg Press

The maximum weight or resistance that a person can lift for one repetition (1-RM) for a particular muscle action with proper form assesses maximum eccentric/concentric muscle strength. A trial-and-error approach determines the 1-RM value. After each successful single lift (rest 2 to 3 min between attempts), increase weight by 2.3 to 4.5 kg/5 to 10 lb until achieving the 1-RM.

The 1-RM bench press and leg press assess maximum muscular strength for the upper body's major muscle groups, while the leg press assesses maximum strength for the lower body's main muscle groups. Dividing the 1-RM weight score (lb or kg) by body weight (lb or kg) assesses relative muscular strength and typically is used to compare groups or individuals between ages 20 to 60 years. The table below presents the relative 1-RM strength ratings for males and females of different ages.

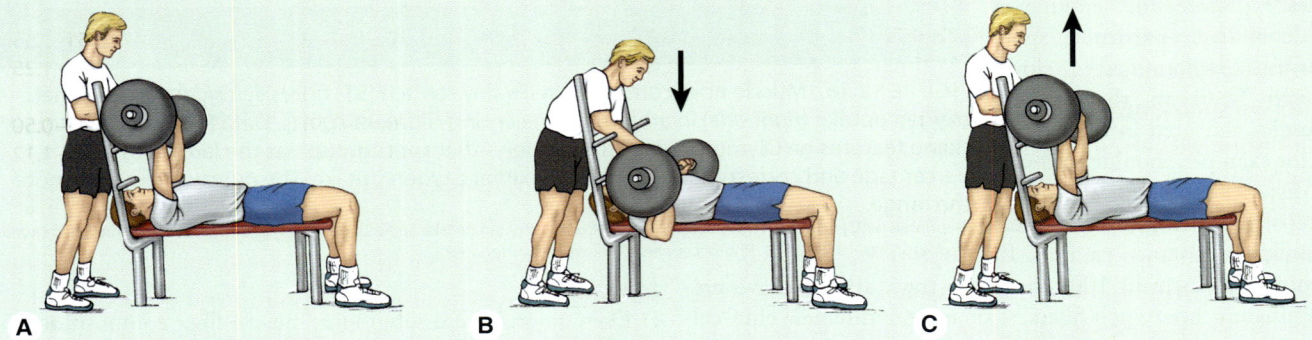

(A) Starting point (standing reach height), **(B)** just prior to jumping, **(C)** final point in determining vertical jump height.

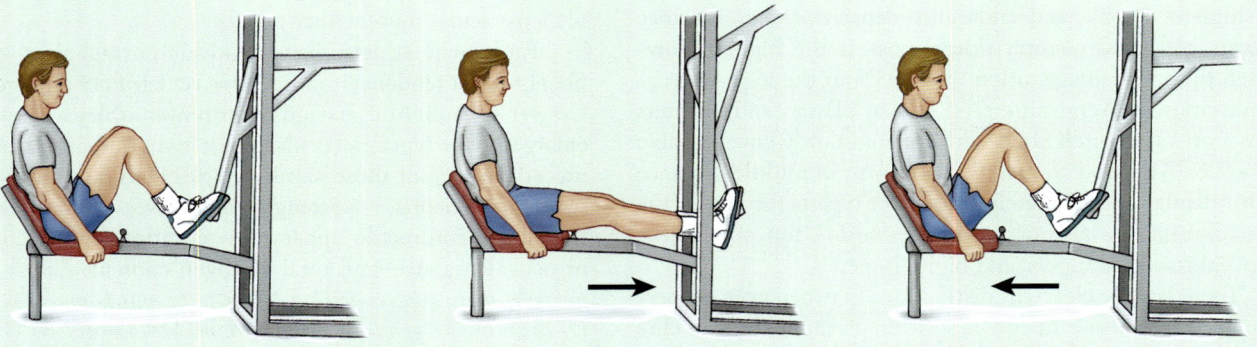

REFERENCE 1-RM BENCH PRESS AND LEG PRESS RELATIVE TO BODY WEIGHT (SCORE = 1-RM, LB ÷ BODY WEIGHT, LB)

	Age, y			
Rating	20–29	30–39	40–49	50–59
Men				
Excellent				
Bench press	>1.26	>1.08	>0.97	>0.86
Leg press	>2.08	>1.88	>1.76	>1.66
Good				
Bench press	1.17–1.25	1.01–1.07	0.91–0.96	0.81–0.85
Leg press	2.00–2.07	1.80–1.87	1.70–1.75	1.60–1.65
Average				
Bench press	0.97–1.16	0.86–1.00	0.78–0.90	0.70–0.80
Leg press	1.83–1.99	1.63–1.79	1.56–1.69	1.46–1.59

Rating	Age, y			
	20–29	30–39	40–49	50–59
Fair				
Bench press	0.88–0.96	0.79–0.85	0.72–0.77	0.65–0.69
Leg press	1.65–1.82	1.55–1.62	1.50–1.55	1.40–1.45
Poor				
Bench press	<0.87	<0.78	<0.71	<0.60
Leg press	<1.64	<1.54	<1.49	<1.39
Women				
Excellent				
Bench press	>0.78	>0.66	>0.61	>0.54
Leg press	>1.63	>1.42	>1.32	>1.26
Good				
Bench press	0.72–0.77	0.62–0.65	0.57–0.60	0.51–0.53
Leg press	1.54–1.62	1.35–1.41	1.26–1.31	1.13–1.25
Average				
Bench press	0.59–0.71	0.53–0.61	0.48–0.56	0.43–0.50
Leg press	1.35–1.53	1.20–1.34	1.12–1.25	0.99–1.12
Fair				
Bench press	0.53–0.58	0.49–0.52	0.44–0.47	0.40–0.42
Leg press	1.25–1.34	1.13–1.19	1.06–1.11	0.86–0.98
Poor				
Bench press	<0.52	<0.48	<0.43	<0.39
Leg press	<1.25	<1.12	<1.05	<0.85

Summary

1. Connective tissue wrappings that encase skeletal muscle blend into and join the tendinous attachment to bone.
2. Muscles act on bony levers to transform ATP's chemical energy into mechanical energy defined by motion.
3. A skeletal muscle fiber by weight contains 75% water, 20% protein, and the remainder inorganic salts, enzymes, pigments, lipids, and carbohydrates.
4. The active muscle's oxygen uptake during vigorous physical activity increases up to 70 times the resting level.
5. The sarcomere represents the muscle fiber's functional unit.
6. Sarcomeres contain the contractile proteins actin and myosin. An average muscle fiber contains 4500 sarcomeres and 16 billion thick (myosin) and 64 billion thin (actin) filaments.
7. Myosin projections or crossbridges serve as structural links between the thick and thin contractile filaments.
8. During muscle action, tropomyosin and troponin regulate the make-and-break contacts between the filaments.
9. Tropomyosin inhibits actin and myosin interaction.
10. Troponin plus Ca^{2+} trigger myofibrils to interact and discreetly slide past each other.
11. The triad and T-tubule system function as a microtransportation network to spread the action potential from the fiber's outer membrane inward to deeper cell regions.
12. During a muscle action, Ca^{2+} activates actin so the myosin crossbridges attach to the actin filaments active sites, while decreased Ca^{2+} concentration produces muscle relaxation.
13. The sliding filament model proposes that a muscle shortens or lengthens because protein filaments slide do not alter their length but just slide past each other.
14. A muscle action links electrochemical and mechanical events by an excitation-contraction coupling mechanism.
15. Three muscle fiber types comprise fast-twitch (FT) fibers that generate energy anaerobically for quick powerful actions, slow-twitch (ST) fibers shorten relatively slowly and generate energy predominantly by aerobic metabolism, and FOG fibers that fall intermediate between the slow-twitch and fast-twitch fiber characteristics.
16. Three independent signaling pathways regulate animal and human skeletal muscle fiber phenotypes; Ras/mitogen-activated protein kinase (MAPK), calcineurin, calcium/calmodulin-dependent protein kinase IV, and peroxisome proliferator g coactivator 1 (PGC-1 α).
17. Genetic factors help to explain intervariability and intravariability in muscle fiber type among individuals.
18. Mitophagy allows the normal adaptive cellular process to selectively target and recognize damaged mitochondria by specific adaptors and receptors to provide for their orderly elimination.

Key Terms

Acetylcholine (ACh): Neurotransmitter released by motoneurons to bind to receptors at the myoneural junction

Apoptosis: Normal cell death process following preprogrammed "death signal instructions" from enzyme proteases called caspases

Autophagy: Biochemical process removes damaged mitochondria (and other cellular substances) when double-membraned, spherical vesicle phagophores surround the damaged mitochondria and fuse with lysosomes to degrade them

Circadian rhythm: Physical, mental, and behavioral changes that follow a daily, mostly repetitive internal 24-hr cycle in humans, plants, animals, fungi, and bacteria

Collagen: Body's most abundant structural protein, consisting of amino acids bound together to form triple helices of elongated fibrils in fibrous tendons, ligaments, skin, corneas, blood vessels, gut, intervertebral discs, and the teeth's dentin

Complex parallel muscle: Muscle type features individual fibers running parallel to the muscle's line of pull

Crossbridge cycling: Conformational change in the filament's myosin head, causing it to glide past the thin actin filament

Crossbridges: Projections spiral around the myosin filament in the actin and myosin filament overlap regions, repeating at intervals of approximately 450 Å along the filament

Depolarization: Process by which a cell's internal charge becomes less negative (more positive) as sodium ions (Na^+) outside the cell membrane migrate into the cell

Endomysium: Smallest connective tissue component in muscle, wrapped around each muscle fiber separating it from neighboring fibers

Epimysium: Fibrous elastic connective tissue sheath that wraps around the entire muscle

Excitation-contraction coupling: Physiologic mechanism that triggers a muscle action from an electrical discharge that releases intracellular Ca^{2+} from chemical events occurring at the cell surface

Fascicles: Groups of muscle fibers

Fast oxidative-glycolytic (FOG): Muscle fiber type with fast contraction speed and well-developed energy transfer capacity from aerobic and anaerobic sources; also known as type IIa muscle fiber

Functional genomics research: Field of study uses genomic data to investigate gene transcription, translation, and different protein interactions

Fusiform: Spindle-shaped; a type of muscle fiber arrangement in which the fibers run parallel to the muscle's long axis (e.g., biceps brachii) and taper at the tendinous attachment

Insertion: Muscle's attachment point to the freely moving bone during a muscle action

Ion channel regulators: Common microstructure pathways (selective "gates" or "sensors") to precisely target the chemical signal to the contractile proteins for modulating ion passage between intracellular and extracellular fluids

Isoforms: Proteins with almost identical functions as other proteins but encoded by a different gene with small sequence differences

Mitophagy: Normal adaptive cellular process that selectively targets and recognizes damaged mitochondria by specific adaptors and receptors to provide for their orderly degradation and elimination

Muscle biopsy: Surgical procedure in which small muscle tissue samples are excised to identify muscle fiber type and nutrient dynamics in exercise and training experiments

Muscle fibers: Thousands of cylindrical cells joined together within a skeletal muscle whose action produces movement

Myoblasts: Primordial muscle cells with potential to develop into muscle fibers

Myofibrillar adenosine triphosphatase (myosin ATPase): Enzyme that hydrolyzes (splits) ATP into ADP and inorganic phosphate (P_i) to yield energy for muscle action

Myofibrils: Thin longitudinal fibrils in skeletal and cardiac muscle fibers consisting of numerous regularly overlapped ultramicroscopic thick and thin myofilaments

Myofilaments: Ultramicroscopic thick (myosin) and thin (actin) filamentous proteins in striated muscle lie parallel to a myofibril's long axis

Nonsteroidal anti-inflammatory drugs (NSAIDs): Drugs that reduce pain, inflammation, and fever; examples include aspirin (Celebrex), ibuprofen (Motrin, Advil), and naproxen (Aleve)

Origin: Muscle's proximal attachment to bone

Pennate: Muscle fiber arrangement in which the fibers are fan-shaped bundles organized at an oblique angle that vary up to 30° and generate considerable muscular power

Perimysium: Connective tissue sheath surrounding a bundle of 10 to more than 100 muscle fibers

Periosteum: Outermost layer of bone, consisting of dense vascular connective tissue except at joint surfaces

Physiologic cross-sectional area (PCSA): Total cross-sectional areas of all fibers within a particular muscle

Rigor mortis: Muscles and joints become rigid and locked into place soon after death because muscle cells no longer contain the ATP required to interact with actin and myosin to produce crossbridge activity

Sarcolemma: Thin, transparent elastic membrane that covers each skeletal muscle fiber's surface to enclose its cellular contents, consisting of a plasma membrane (plasmalemma) and a basement membrane

Sarcomere: Structural unit of a myofibril in striated muscle with basic repeating units between two Z lines

Sarcoplasm: Aqueous cytoplasm in a muscle fiber, containing enzymes, lipid and glycogen particles, and nuclei (approximately 250 per mm of fiber length), which contain the genes, mitochondria, and other specialized organelles

Sarcoplasmic reticulum: Extensive longitudinal latticelike network of tubular channels and vesicle transverse tubules that provides a cell's structural integrity and allows a depolarization wave to spread rapidly from the fiber's outer surface to its inner environment to initiate muscle action

Satellite cells: Stem cells from muscle tissue (myogenic) that lie between the muscle fiber's basement and plasma membranes

Sliding filament model: Theoretical model of muscle contraction in which the muscle shortens or lengthens because thick and thin filaments slide past each other without changing length to produce a conformational change in relative size within the sarcomere's zones and bands to generate force at the Z bands

Slow oxidative (SO): Muscle fiber type with relatively slow shortening speed and reliance on energy release from oxidative metabolism

Striated: Striped, in reference to the characteristic striations in skeletal muscle fibers from regular overlapping of thick and thin myofilaments

Tendinitis: Tendon inflammation caused by overuse or undue stress from poor movement mechanics

Tendons: Fibrous collagenous tissues that attach muscle to bone (outermost periosteum covering)

Transverse (T)-tubule system: Tubule system conduct impulses from the cell surface into the sarcoplasmic reticulum, the cell's longitudinal latticelike tubular channel and vesicle network

Triad: Repeating pattern of two vesicles and a transverse tubule in each sarcomere Z line region

Type I muscle fibers: Slow-twitch muscle fibers

Type II muscle fibers: Fast-twitch muscle fibers

Type IIa fiber: Muscle fiber type exhibits fast shortening speed and well-integrated energy transfer from aerobic (high succinic dehydrogenase level) and anaerobic (high phosphofructokinase level) sources

Type IIb fiber: Muscle fiber type possesses the greatest anaerobic potential and most rapid shortening velocity

Type IIx fiber: Muscle fiber type intermediate between its type IIa and type IIb counterparts in physiologic and metabolic characteristics

> References are available online at Lippincott Connect.

Additional References

Abou Sawan S, et al. Satellite cell and myonuclear accretion is related to training-induced skeletal muscle fiber hypertrophy in young males and females. *J Appl Physiol (1985)*. 2021;131:871.

Angleri V, et al. Resistance training variable manipulations are less relevant than intrinsic biology in affecting muscle fiber hypertrophy. *Scand J Med Sci Sports*. 2022. doi:10.1111/sms.14134.

Besson T, et al. Sex differences in endurance running. *Sports Med*. 2022. doi:10.1007/s40279-022-01651-w.

Bhat N, et al. Dyrk1b promotes autophagy during skeletal muscle differentiation by upregulating 4e-bp1. *Cell Signal*. 2022;90:110186.

Binder-Markey BI, et al. Intramuscular Anatomy drives collagen content variation within and between muscles. *Front Physiol*. 2020;11:293.

Bjerring AW, et al. From talented child to elite athlete: the development of cardiac morphology and function in a cohort of endurance athletes from age 12 to 18. *Eur J Prev Cardiol*. 2020;2047487320921317.

Brigatto FA, et al. High resistance-training volume enhances muscle thickness in resistance-trained men. *J Strength Cond Res*. 2022;36:22.

Brooks GA. Lactate as a fulcrum of metabolism. *Redox Biol*. 2020;35:101454.

Burke LM. Ketogenic low CHO, high fat diet: the future of elite endurance sport? *J Physiol*. 2021;599:819.

Chen X, et al. Effect of dietary L-theanine supplementation on skeletal muscle fiber type transformation in vivo. *J Nutr Biochem*. 2022;99:108859.

De Gasperi R, et al. Numb is required for optimal contraction of skeletal muscle. *J Cachexia Sarcopenia Muscle*. 2022;13:454.

Deshmukh AS, et al. Deep muscle-proteomic analysis of freeze-dried human muscle biopsies reveals fiber type-specific adaptations to exercise training. *Nat Commun*. 2021;12:304.

Fukutani A, et al. Evidence for muscle cell-based mechanisms of enhanced performance in stretch-shortening cycle in skeletal muscle. *Front Physiol*. 2021;11:609553.

Grimby-Ekman A, et al. Pain intensity and pressure pain thresholds after a light dynamic physical load in patients with chronic neck/shoulder pain. *BMC Musculoskelet Disord*. 2020;21:266.

Han S, et al. Filamin C regulates skeletal muscle atrophy by stabilizing dishevelled-2 to inhibit autophagy and mitophagy. *Mol Ther Nucleic Acids*. 2021;27:147.

Harvey NR, et al. Genetic variants associated with exercise performance in both moderately trained and highly trained individuals. *Mol Genet Genomics*. 2020;295:515.

He N, Ye H. Exercise and hyperlipidemia. *Adv Exp Med Biol*. 2020;1228:79.

Hedman K, et al. Limitations of electrocardiography for detecting left ventricular hypertrophy or concentric remodeling in athletes. *Am J Med*. 2020;133:123.

Hennis PJ, et al. Aerobic capacity and skeletal muscle characteristics in glycogen storage disease IIIa: an observational study. *Orphanet J Rare Dis*. 2022;17:28.

Hessel AL, et al. Non-cross bridge viscoelastic elements contribute to muscle force and work during stretch-shortening cycles: evidence from whole muscles and permeabilized fibers. *Front Physiol* 2021;12:648019.

Hester GM, et al. Microbiopsy sampling for examining age-related differences in skeletal muscle fiber morphology and composition. *Front Physiol*. 2022;12:756626.

Hirono T, et al. Relationship between muscle swelling and hypertrophy induced by resistance training. *J Strength Cond Res*. 2022;36:359.

Kilroe SP, et al. Short-term muscle disuse induces a rapid and sustained decline in daily myofibrillar protein synthesis rates. *Am J Physiol Endocrinol Metab*. 2020;318:E117.

Koay YC, et al. Effect of chronic exercise in healthy young male adults: a metabolomic analysis. *Cardiovasc Res*. 2021;117:613.

Kramer A. An overview of the beneficial effects of exercise on health and performance. *Adv Exp Med Biol*. 2020;1228:3.

Kuhtz-Buschbeck JP, et al. The origin of the heartbeat and theories of muscle contraction. Physiological concepts and conflicts in the 19th century. *Prog Biophys Mol Biol*. 2021;159:3.

Lasevicius T, et al. Muscle failure promotes greater muscle hypertrophy in low-load but not in high-load resistance training. *J Strength Cond Res*. 2022;36:346.

Ma W, et al. Myofibril orientation as a metric for characterizing heart disease. *Biophys J*. 2022;121:565.

Martin-Smith R. High intensity interval training (HIIT) improves cardiorespiratory fitness (CRF) in healthy, overweight and obese adolescents: a systematic review and meta-analysis of controlled studies. *Int J Environ Res Public Health*. 2020;17:2955.

McMillin SL, et al. Skeletal muscle wasting: the estrogen side of sexual dimorphism. *Am J Physiol Cell Physiol*. 2022;322:C24.

Melville Z, et al. High-resolution structure of the membrane-embedded skeletal muscle ryanodine receptor. *Structure*. 2022;30:172.

Minari ALA, Thomatieli-Santos RV. From skeletal muscle damage and regeneration to the hypertrophy induced by exercise: what is the role of different macrophage subsets? *Am J Physiol Regul Integr Comp Physiol*. 2022;322:R41.

Mito T, et al. Mosaic dysfunction of mitophagy in mitochondrial muscle disease. *Cell Metab*. 2022;34:197.

Plotkin DL, et al. Muscle fiber type transitions with exercise training: shifting perspectives. *Sports (Basel)*. 2021;9:127.

Quint JP, et al. Nanoengineered myogenic scaffolds for skeletal muscle tissue engineering. *Nanoscale*. 2022;14:797.

Sapp RM, et al. Changes in circulating microRNA and arterial stiffness following high-intensity interval and moderate intensity continuous exercise. *Physiol Rep*. 2020;8:e14431.

Scalzo RL, et al. Single-leg exercise training augments in vivo skeletal muscle oxidative flux and vascular content and function in adults with type 2 diabetes. *J Physiol*. 2022;600:963.

Skelly LE, et al. Human skeletal muscle fiber type-specific responses to sprint interval and moderate-intensity continuous exercise: acute and training-induced changes. *J Appl Physiol (1985)*. 2021;130:1001.

Vann CG, et al. Skeletal muscle protein composition adaptations to 10 weeks of high-load resistance training in previously-trained males. *Front Physiol*. 2020;11:259.

Wahwah N, et al. Subpopulation-specific differences in skeletal muscle mitochondria in humans with obesity: insights from studies employing acute nutritional and exercise stimuli. *Am J Physiol Endocrinol Metab*. 2020;318:E538.

Wang L, et al. The regulatory role of dietary factors in skeletal muscle development, regeneration and function. *Crit Rev Food Sci Nutr*. 2022;62:764.

Wehrstein M, et al. Eccentric overload during resistance exercise: a stimulus for enhanced satellite cell activation. *Med Sci Sports Exerc*. 2022;54(3):388.

Yutaka Igarashi Y, et al. Running to lower resting blood pressure: a systematic review and meta-analysis. *Sports Med*. 2020;50:531.

Table 18.1 Twelve Proteins Associated with a Muscle Fiber's Sarcomere and Proposed Functions

Structure	Protein	Function
Thin filament	Actin	Main protein interacts with myosin during excitation-contraction coupling
	Tropomyosin	Transduces conformational change in the troponin complex to actin
	Troponin	Binds Ca^{2+} and represents a "switch" transforming Ca^{2+} signal into a molecular signal to induce crossbridge cycling
	Nebulin	Adjacent to actin and believed to control actin monomer number joined to each other in a thin filament
Thick filament	Myosin	Splits ATP and responsible for the "myosin head power stroke"
C stripes	C protein	Holds myosin thick filaments in a regular array; holds adjacent thick filament H protein at an even distance during force generation; may control myosin molecule's thick filament number
M line	M protein	Holds thick filaments in a regular array
	Myomesin	Provides a strong anchoring point for the titin protein
	M-CK	Located proximal to the myosin heads and provides ATP from PCr
Z line	α-Actinin	Holds the thin filaments in place spatially
	Desmin	Forms the connection between adjacent Z lines among myofibrils to maintain the sarcomere's striated appearance; can exhibit fiber-type shift from fast to slow isoforms of myosin heavy chain and significantly decreased insulin sensitivity
Elastic filament	Titin	Keeps thick filaments centered between two Z lines during muscle action and controls myosin molecule number in the thick filament

ATP, adenosine triphosphate; CK, creatine kinase; PCr, phosphocreatine.

Table 18.2 Skeletal Muscle Fiber Type Classification and Functions

Fiber Type	Type I Fibers	Type IIa Fibers	Type IIx Fibers	Type IIb Fibers
Contraction time	Slow	Moderately fast	Fast	Very fast
Motor neuron size	Small	Medium	Large	Very large
Fatigue resistance	High	Fairly high	Intermediate	Low
Activity	Aerobic	Long-term An	Short-term An	short-term An
Useful duration	Hours	<30 min	<5 min	<1 min
Force production	Low	Medium	High	Very high
Mitochondrial density	High	High	Medium	Low
Capillary density	High	Intermediate	Low	Low
Oxidative capacity	High	High	Intermediate	Low
Glycolytic capacity	Low	High	High	High
Major storage fuel	Trig	PCr, glycogen	PCr, glycogen	PCr, glycogen
Myosin heavy chains	MYH7	MYH2	MYH1	MYH4

An, anaerobic; PCr, phosphocreatine; Trig, triacylglycerol.

CHAPTER 19
Neural Control and Human Movement

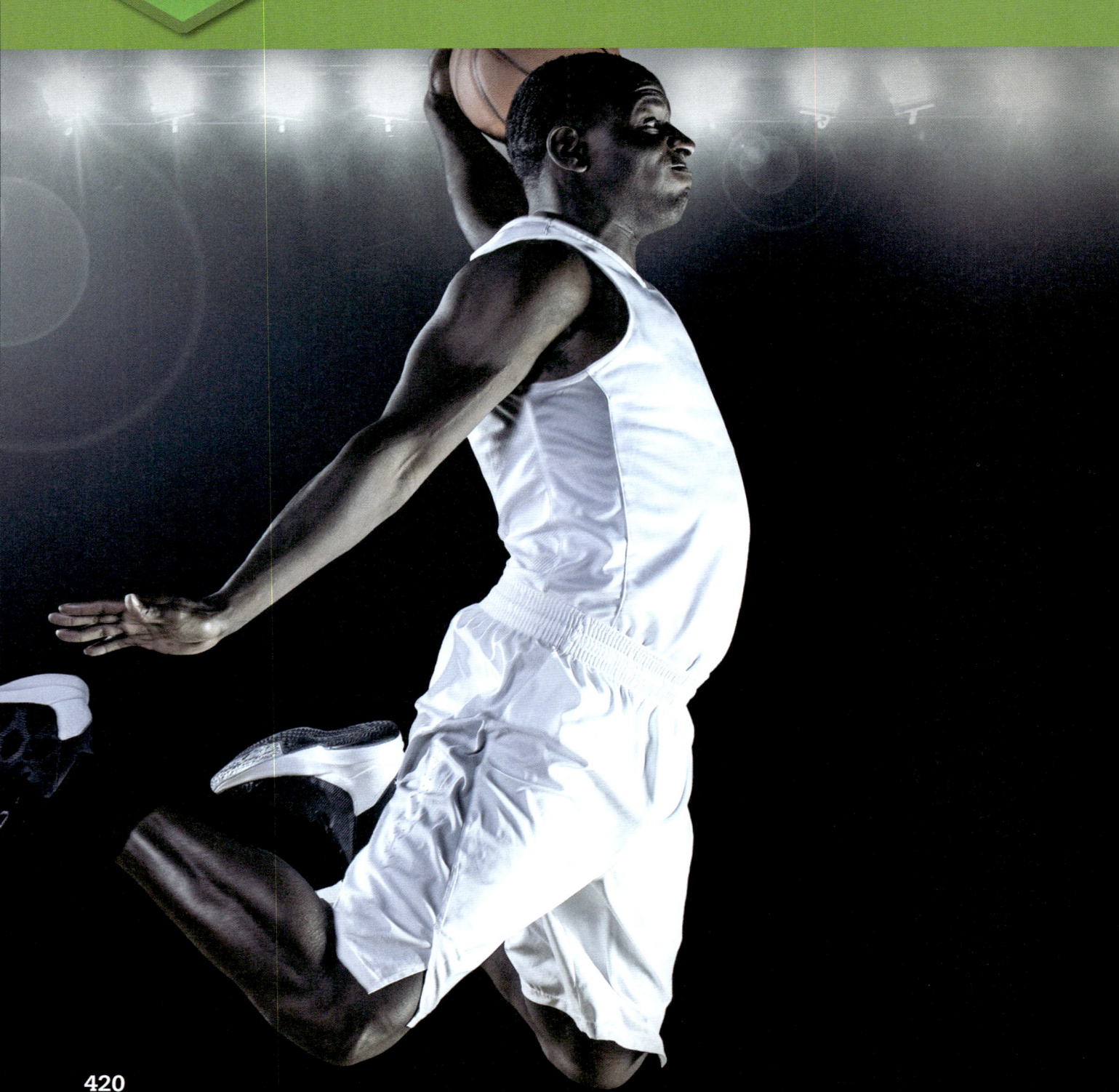

Chapter Objectives

- Draw the brain's major structural components, including the four lobes in the cerebral cortex
- Discuss specific pyramidal and extrapyramidal tract functions
- Diagram the anterior motor neuron and discuss its role in human movement
- Draw and label the basic reflex arc components
- Define the terms motor unit, neuromuscular junction, and autonomic nervous system
- Summarize events in motor unit excitation prior to muscle action
- Outline motor unit facilitation and inhibition and their contribution to exercise performance and responsiveness to resistance training
- Discuss variations in twitch characteristics, resistance to fatigue, and tension development in the different motor unit categories
- Describe two mechanisms that adjust muscle action forces along the continuum from slight to maximum
- Define fatigue and discuss three factors that act and interact to induce neuromuscular fatigue
- Describe proprioceptor functions in joints, muscles, and tendons

Ancillaries at-a-Glance

Visit Lippincott Connect to access the following resources.

- References: Chapter 19
- Appendix H: Links for Supplemental Animations and Videos
- Animations: Action Potential, Flipping the Membrane Potential, Muscle Contraction, Nerve Synapse, Proprioceptors, Saltatory Conduction
- Focus on Research: Muscular Fatigue—A Complex Phenomenon

Effective force application during complex learned movements in a tennis serve, shot put, golf swing, and back somersault off a diving board requires precise, coordinated neuromuscular patterns and movements—not simply the activated region's muscular strength. The intricate sophisticated neural circuitry in the brain, spinal cord, and periphery functions in a manner somewhat similar to the most advanced "cloud" computer network. Sensory inputs from all of the body's systems automatically synchronize for near-instantaneous processing by central neural control mechanisms in response to changing internal and external stimuli. The input must be properly organized, routed, and transmitted in fractions of nanoseconds with high efficiency to the effector organs, the skeletal muscles, to create intended purposeful movements.[27]

Similarities exist between the most advanced supercomputer and the brain's approximately 100 billion nerve cells and their coordinated interconnections to multiple target tissues. Each brain cell "fires" about 200 times per second and connects with a 1000 or more other neurons—a feat unmatched by any other living organism or artificially created entity (www.neuwritewest.org/blog/4541). Not surprisingly, the integrative and organizational human nervous system complexity far exceeds the awe-inspiring processing capacity for all of the public, private, and hybrid "cloud" servers worldwide!

This chapter describes human movement neural control for the following topics:

1. Structural organization of the neuromotor system, with emphasis on the central and peripheral nervous systems
2. Neuromuscular transmission
3. Sensory input for muscular activity
4. Motor unit type, function, and activation

Neuromotor System Organization

Two major subdivisions make up the human nervous system:

1. **Central nervous system (CNS)**: Brain and spinal cord
2. **Peripheral nervous system (PNS)**: Nerves that transmit information to and from the CNS, which include 12 cranial nerves and 31 spinal nerve pairs (8 cervical, 12 thoracic, 5 lumbar, 5 sacral, 1 coccygeal), with each pair connecting to a specific body region

FIGURE 19.1 presents an overview for the two major subdivisions, including their functions in motor control.

CNS: The Brain

Over many thousands of years, the human brain remains remarkably complex yet retains selective growth in different anatomic areas. Comparatively, human brain size exceeds that for most, but not all, mammals. Cortex evolution, particularly the frontal and temporal lobes, coincides with unique spoken and written language functions, reasoning, and abstract thinking. Such differentiation frames the hypothesis that larger, more complex brains allow greater neural circuitry within the cortex and hence increased intellectual and higher center functioning.

For decades, conventional wisdom maintained that brain cell number remained fixed at birth, unlike the cells in other organ systems that continually renew throughout life. Neurobiologists and the science community in general now believe that brain cells, spinal neurons, and neural circuits continually form throughout life but not at the same rate or amount, when unneeded or low functioning synapses develop in neural tissues. From birth through late adolescence, the brain adds billions of new cells, literally constructing and reconstructing new circuits from these newly formed cells.[14,34] Following adolescence, neuronal plasticity adds and forms new circuits but does not stop even with somewhat slower transmission rates, even into older age. Regular physical activity helps to maintain and develop optimal neural circuitry at the appropriate life stages in aging.

FIGURE 19.2A illustrates the brain's six main areas:

1. Medulla oblongata
2. Pons
3. Midbrain
4. Cerebellum
5. Diencephalon
6. Telencephalon

Figure 19.2B shows a superior view of the brain. The longitudinal fissure or groove runs down the midline and separates the brain's right and left sides or **hemispheres**. Below the fissure, a large tract of nerve fibers (**corpus callosum**, not shown) connects the right and left hemispheres. The brain's outer portion, the **cerebral cortex** or **gray matter** (gray because nerve fibers lack a white myelin coating), consists of a series of folded convolutions. Figure 19.2C depicts the four lobes of the cerebral cortex (occipital, parietal, temporal, and frontal) and sensory and motor areas and cerebellum (sometimes known as "little brain"). As a reference, the body has roughly 10 million sensory **afferent neurons**, 50 billion central neurons, and 500,000 motor **efferent neurons**. This represents a ratio of about 20 to 1 between sensory and motor circuits.

The **cerebellum** contains about 50% of the brain's total neurons, yet only 10% the cranial volume involved in four crucial functions:

1. Balance and posture
2. Coordinating voluntary movements
3. Motor learning (coordinating and fine-tuning motor programs for "recall" to make precise muscle movements)
4. Cognition (language)

Traumatic Brain Injury

Four tough membranes (**meninges**), which contain a jellylike cushioning substance, surround and protect the brain and spinal cord from injury by external forces, such as may occur in **sports-related traumatic brain injury (srTBI)**. Epidemiological studies in the United States estimate that 1 to 2 million new cases of srTBI are reported annually, with many more never coming to the attention of health professionals. Approximately 30 to 37% of student athletes at the high school and

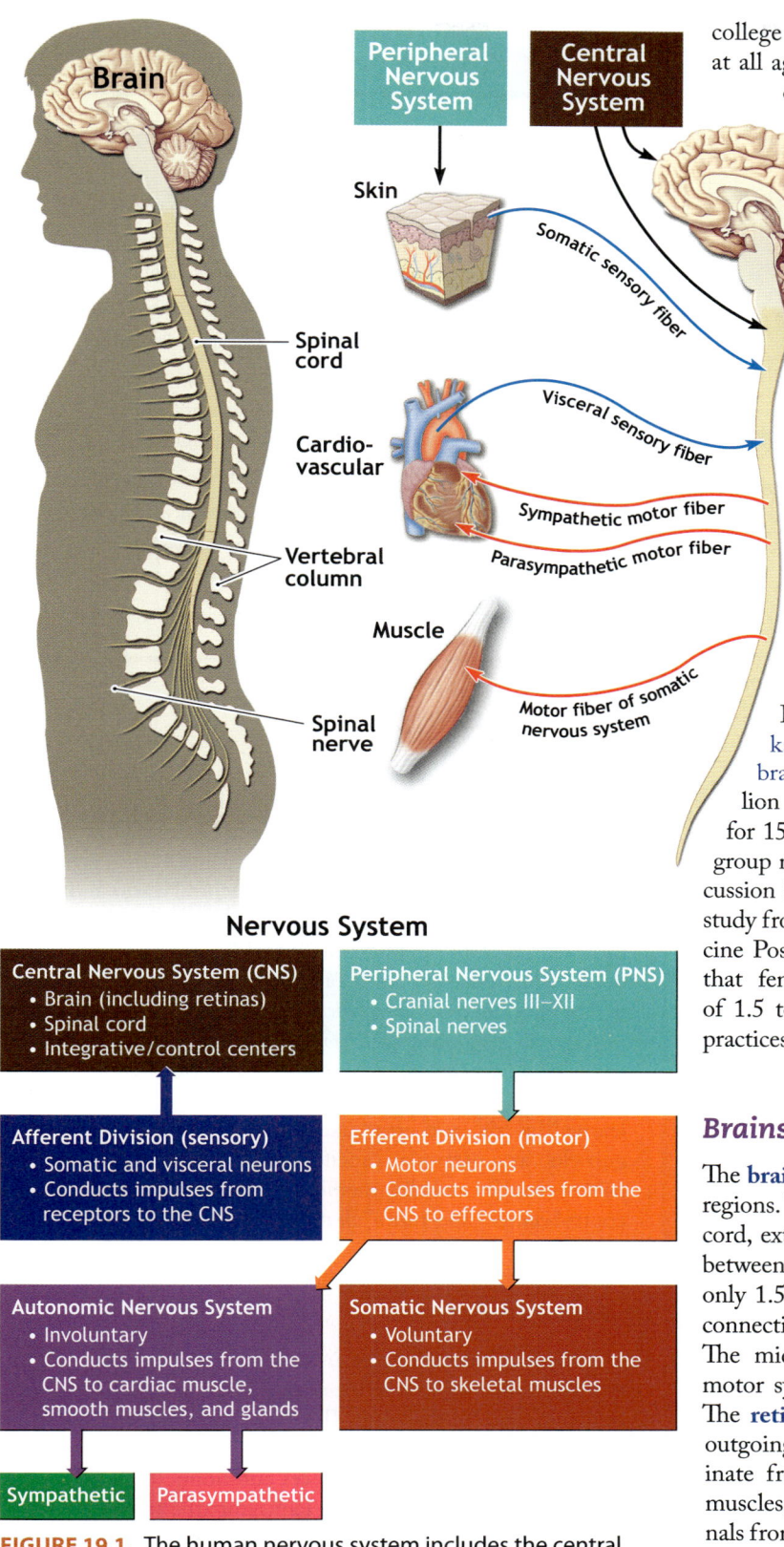

FIGURE 19.1. The human nervous system includes the central nervous system (CNS; brain and retinas, spinal cord, and integrating and control centers) and peripheral nervous system (PNS; cranial nerves and spinal cord). The PNS subdivides into afferent (sensory) and efferent (motor) divisions. The efferent division includes the somatic nervous system and autonomic nervous system (sympathetic and parasympathetic categories.)

college level have suffered a mild brain injury, and in sports at all ages and competitive levels; approximately 300,000 cases have been classified as mild-to-moderate severity **concussions**.[43–45] Intracranial injuries also can occur from a bump, blow, or jolt to the head in vehicle accidents, violent physical confrontations, slips and falls, and military combat.[40–42]

TBI injury type may also result from a simple blow to the head to a penetrating brain injury. In the United States, older adolescents (ages 15 to 19 year) and older adults (ages 65+) are most likely to sustain a TBI in the frontal and temporal brain regions. Mild TBI (mTBI) (also known as **brain concussion**) had been initially considered a benign event; research confirms many adverse neuropsychological outcomes in civilians (e.g., athletes who play contact sports) and military personnel. Unfortunately, moderate-to-severe TBI remains a primary cause related to injury-induced death and disability with an annual incidence rate approaching 500 in 100,000.[46] Researchers at the Korey Stringer Institute at the University of Connecticut (https://ksi.uconn.edu/emergency-conditions/traumatic-brain-injury/#) estimate that about 1.6 to 3.8 million sports-related TBIs occur every year, accounting for 15% of all high school sport-related trauma. The age group most vulnerable for sustaining a sports-related concussion is between ages 9 and 22 for team sports. A 2019 study from the American Medical Society for Sports Medicine Position Statement on Concussion in Sport reported that females have higher concussion rate susceptibility of 1.5 to 1.8 greater than males during competition and practices.

Brainstem

The **brainstem** consists of the medulla, pons, and midbrain regions. The medulla, located immediately above the spinal cord, extends into the pons and serves as a neural bridge between the cerebellum's two hemispheres. The **midbrain**, only 1.5 cm long, attaches to the cerebellum and forms a connection between the **pons** and cerebral hemispheres. The midbrain contains tissues from the extrapyramidal motor system, specifically the red nucleus and substantia. The **reticular formation** integrates various incoming and outgoing signals that flow through it. These signals originate from "stretching" specialized sensors in joints and muscles, from pain receptors in the skin, and as visual signals from the eye and auditory ear impulses. Once activated, the reticular system produces either inhibitory or facilitatory effects on other neurons. The twelve cranial nerve pairs innervate predominantly the head region and were originally named and numbered by the physician Galen about 1800 years ago (see Introduction: A View from the Past).

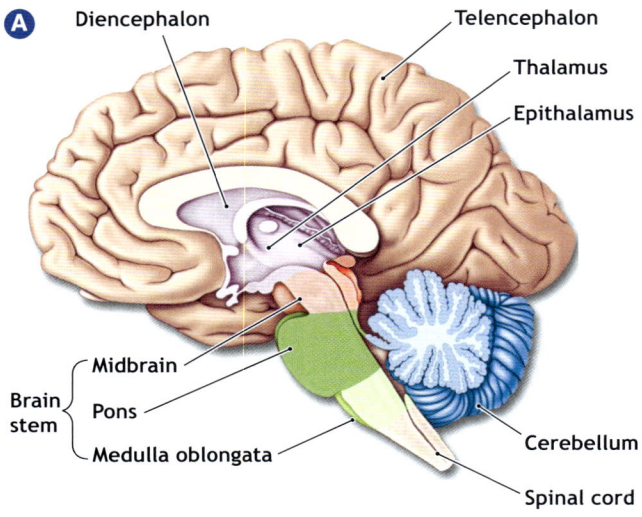

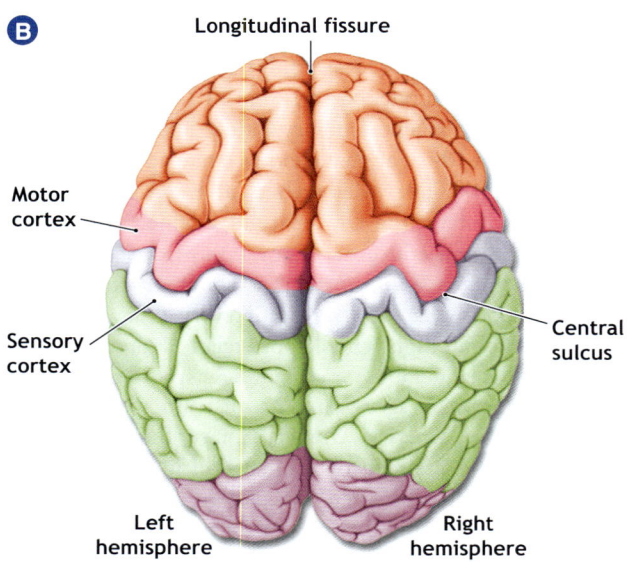

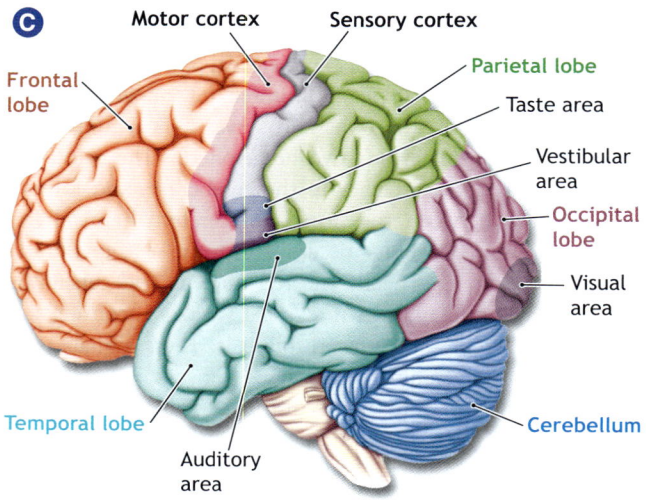

FIGURE 19.2. **(A)** Brain and brainstem medial side view. **(B)** Superior view. **(C)** Four cerebral cortex lobes.

Mnemonic to Remember the 12 Cranial Nerves

On **O**ld **O**lympus' **T**owering **T**op **A** **F**riendly **V**iking **G**rew **V**ines **A**nd **H**ops

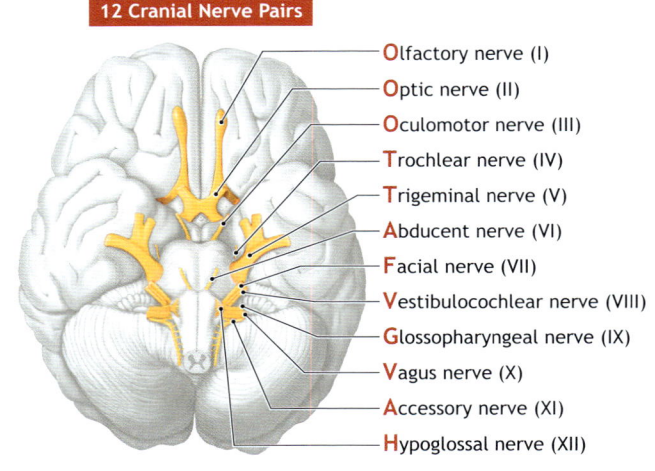

12 Cranial Nerve Pairs
- **O**lfactory nerve (I)
- **O**ptic nerve (II)
- **O**culomotor nerve (III)
- **T**rochlear nerve (IV)
- **T**rigeminal nerve (V)
- **A**bducent nerve (VI)
- **F**acial nerve (VII)
- **V**estibulocochlear nerve (VIII)
- **G**lossopharyngeal nerve (IX)
- **V**agus nerve (X)
- **A**ccessory nerve (XI)
- **H**ypoglossal nerve (XII)

Cerebellum

The cerebellum contains two peach-sized folded tissue mounds with lateral hemispheres and a central vermis. It functions with intricate feedback circuits to monitor and coordinate other brain and spinal cord areas involved in motor control. The cerebellum receives motor output signals from the central command center in the cortex. This specialized brain tissue also obtains sensory information from peripheral receptors located in muscles, tendons, joints, and skin and from visual, auditory, and vestibular end organs. *The cerebellum functions as the major comparing, evaluating, and integrating center for postural adjustments, locomotion, equilibrium maintenance, perceptions about body movement speed, and other reflex-related movement functions.* Movement tasks first learned by trial and error, like riding a bicycle or swinging a golf club at a particular cadence, remain coded as coordinated *patterns* in the cerebellar memory banks. In essence, this motor control center "fine-tunes" all muscular activity forms.[29,37]

Diencephalon

The **diencephalon**, located immediately above the midbrain, contains four major structures—thalamus, hypothalamus, epithalamus, and subthalamus. The hypothalamus, situated below the thalamus, regulates metabolic rate and body temperature. The hypothalamus also influences autonomic nervous system activity (see "Sympathetic and Parasympathetic Nervous Systems"); it receives regulatory input from the thalamus and limbic brain system and responds to diverse hormone effects (see Chapter 20). Changes in arterial blood pressure and blood gas tensions influence hypothalamic activity via peripheral receptors located in the aortic arch and carotid arteries.

Telencephalon

The telencephalon contains the two hemispheres in the cerebral cortex, including the corpus striatum and medulla. The cerebral cortex contains approximately 40% of the brain's total weight. It divides into four lobes: frontal, temporal, parietal, and occipital. Neurons in the cortex provide specialized sensory and motor functions. Beneath each cerebral hemisphere and in close association with the thalamus lie the basal ganglia, which play an important role in controlling motor movement patterns.

Limbic System

In 1878, French anatomist, surgeon, neurologist, and anthropologist Paul Pierre Broca (1824–1880) described areas on the cerebrum's medial surface distinctly different from the surrounding cortex (www.whonamedit.com/doctor.cfm/1982.html). Using the Latin word for "border" (*limbus*), Broca named the area the **limbic lobe** because its structures formed a ring or border around the brainstem and corpus callosum on the temporal lobe's medial surface.[3,38] Broca also discovered the brain's speech center, now known as Broca area, or the third circumvolution of the frontal lobe. Broca should be credited as the founder of modern brain surgery and many other breakthrough findings including the brain's contribution to speech production[39] (www.neuroscientificallychallenged.com/blog/history-of-neuroscience-paul-broca).

CNS: The Spinal Cord

FIGURE 19.3 illustrates the **spinal cord**, about 45 cm in length and 1 cm in diameter, encased by 33 vertebrae (7 cervical, 12 thoracic, 5 lumbar, 5 sacral, and 4 coccygeal). The bony vertebral column encases and protects the spinal cord, which attaches to the brainstem. The spinal cord provides the major conduit for the two-way information transmission from the skin, joints, and muscles to the brain. It provides for communication throughout the body via PNS spinal nerves. These nerves exit the cord through small openings or notches between the vertebrae. Each spinal nerve connects to the spinal cord by the dorsal root and ventral root branches. **TABLE 19.1** lists common names that describe spinal cord neurons and axons.

When viewed in cross section, the spinal cord shows an H-shaped gray matter core (**FIG. 19.4**). The **ventral horn** (anterior) and **dorsal horn** (posterior) describe the limbs depicted by the core. The spinal cord core contains principally three neuron types: **motor neurons**, **sensory neurons**, and **interneurons**. The motor neurons (efferent) run through the ventral horn to supply the extrafusal and intrafusal skeletal muscle fibers (see in a later section). Sensory (afferent) nerve fibers enter the spinal cord from the periphery via the dorsal horn. The white matter, containing the ascending and descending nerve tracts, surrounds the gray matter within the cord.

TABLE 19.1 Common names describing spinal cord neurons and axons

The spinal cord's unique anatomical design allows extreme vertebral movement without affecting spinal nerve function. Twenty-four fibrocartilage **intervertebral disks** separate adjacent vertebrae and, under normal circumstances, provide cushioning and act as a shock absorber protective mechanism. Unfortunately, a disk can bulge into the space occupied by that segment's spinal nerve, compressing it and causing pain. **FIGURE 19.5** shows a normal lumbar disk (A), a **herniated disk** (B), and a removed disk (C). In the latter, a portion of the nucleus pulposus consisting of gel-like structures moves out of its normal enclosure to impinge on a spinal nerve, compressing it and causing referred or radiating pain "downstream" in areas the nerve innervates (e.g., lower back, buttocks, back of the leg [sciatica], and heel into the foot). This cascade of events can disrupt motor control. If the condition persists with significant muscle weakness (e.g., inability to raise and lower the body vertically off the ball of one foot, or numbness in the leg and foot area), surgical repair or removal of the offending herniated disk may be needed to relieve the pressure and pain, although it is not a foolproof solution.

Ascending Nerve Tracts

Ascending nerve tracts in the spinal cord forward sensory information for processing from peripheral receptors to the brain. Three neurons typically form the sensory pathway. The dorsal root ganglion contains the first neuron's cell body whose axon relays information into the spinal cord. The second neuron cell body lies within the spinal cord itself; its axon passes up the cord to the thalamus, which contains the third neuron's cell body. The third neuron axon traverses to the central command center in the cerebral cortex.

Peripheral sensory nerve endings serve as specialized receptors to detect conscious and subconscious sensory information. The "conscious" receptors show sensitivity to kinesthesia (detecting body position, weight, or movement of muscles, tendons, and joints) and proprioception (sensing the relative position of body parts and their effort applied in movement), temperature, and light, sound, smell, taste, touch, and pain sensations.[35] Receptors also monitor subconscious changes in the body's internal environment; these include chemoreceptors that respond to changes in blood gas tension (P_{O_2}, P_{CO_2}) and pH, and **baroreceptors** that react almost instantaneously to any change in arterial blood pressure. The term *mechanoreceptors* refers to sensory receptors sensitive to mechanical stimuli related to touch, pressure, stretch, and motion.

Descending Nerve Tracts

Axons from the brain move downward through the spinal cord along two major pathways, displayed in Figure 19.5. The **pyramidal (lateral) tract** activates skeletal musculature in voluntary movements under direct cortical control. The other pathway, the **extrapyramidal (ventromedial) tract**, controls posture and muscle tone via the brainstem.

Pyramidal (Lateral) Tract. Neurons in the pyramidal tract including the corticospinal and rubrospinal tracts transmit

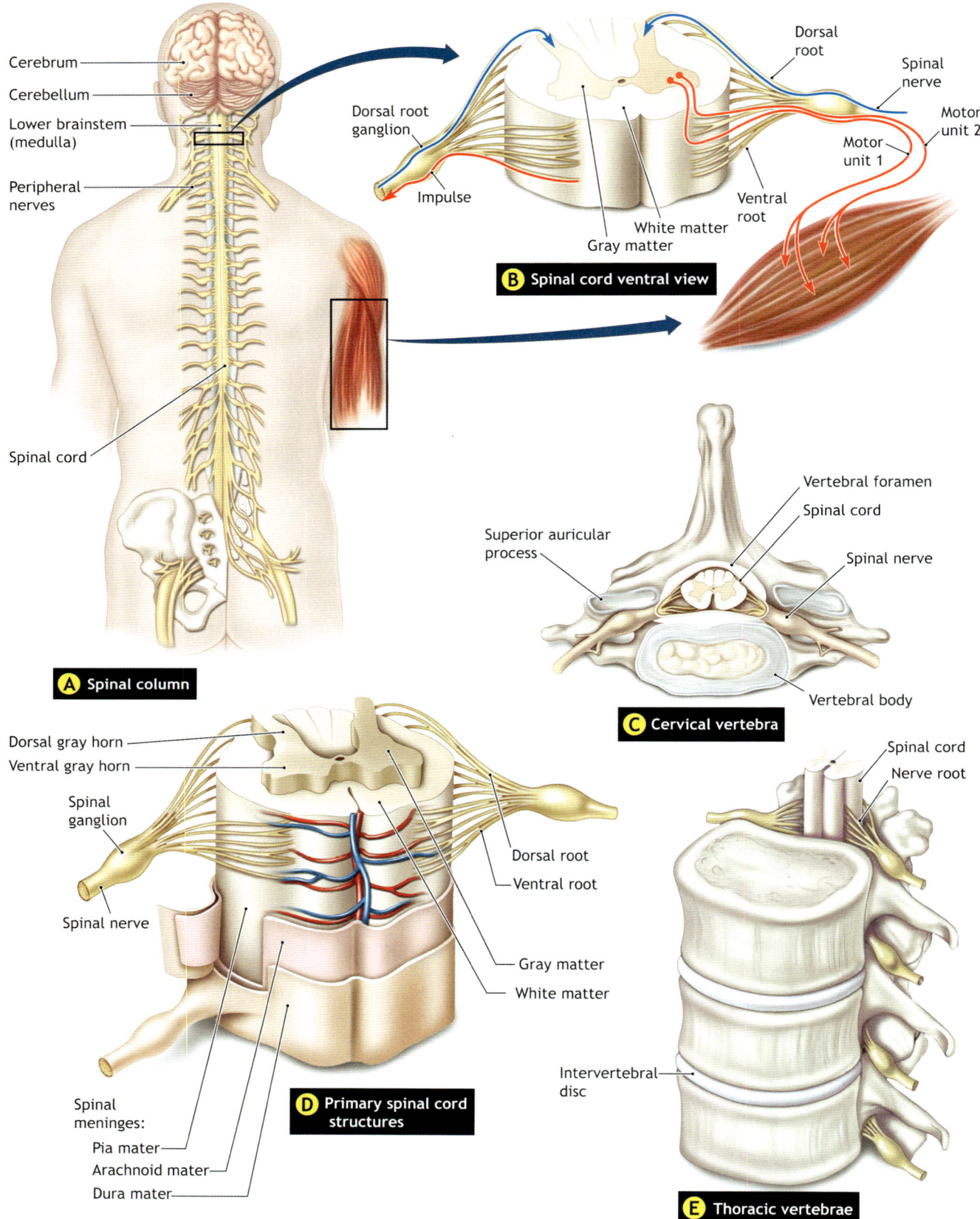

FIGURE 19.3. Human central nervous system anatomy. **(A)** Spinal cord with peripheral nerves. **(B)** Spinal cord ventral view illustrates dorsal and ventral root neural pathways and nerve impulse direction. **(C)** Cross section through one cervical vertebra. **(D)** Primary spinal cord structures. **(E)** Enlarged view among three thoracic vertebrae.

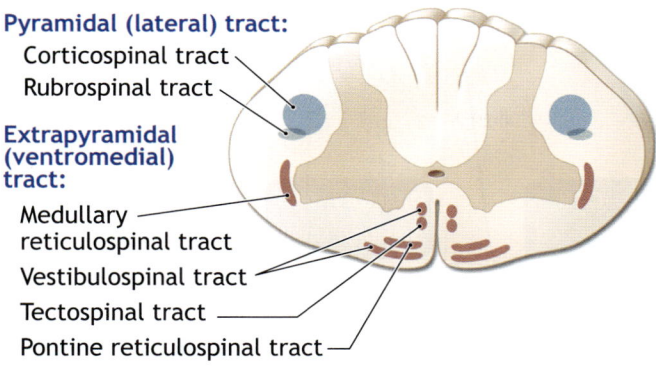

FIGURE 19.4. Brain's descending spinal cord tracts. (Reprinted with permission from Bear MF, et al. *Neuroscience: Exploring the Brain*. 4th ed., p. 486. Wolters Kluwer, 2016.)

impulses downward through the spinal cord. These nerves excite the **alpha (α) motoneurons** that modulate skeletal muscles' fine and gross properties during all purposeful movements. The corticospinal tract, the longest and one of the largest CNS tracts, has two thirds of its axons originating from the brain's frontal lobe, collectively called the **motor cortex**.

Extrapyramidal (Ventromedial) Tract. The extrapyramidal neurons (reticulospinal, vestibulospinal, and tectospinal tracts) originate in the brainstem and connect at all spinal cord levels. They control posture and provide a continual background level related to neuromuscular tone.

Reticular Formation

The reticular formation provides an extensive and intricate neural network through the brainstem core that integrates the spinal cord, cerebral cortex, basal ganglia, and cerebellum. It receives and then processes continuous input from sensory sources. Once activated, it either inhibits or facilitates other neurons. For example, the reticular formation helps to control posture by regulating neuron sensitivity to the antigravity muscles along the body's midline that maintain upright posture and keep the body from collapsing to the floor (soleus, leg extensors, gluteus maximus, quadriceps femoris, neck and back muscles). Peripheral sensory neuron excitation arouses the reticular nerve cells to excite the cerebral cortex and send signals back to the reticular system to maintain appropriate cortical arousal and wakefulness. The reticular formation exerts a powerful regulating influence on cardiovascular and pulmonary functions.

Peripheral Nervous System

The PNS contains 31 pairs of spinal nerves and 12 pairs of cranial nerves. **FIGURE 19.6** shows the distribution for the 12 cranial nerve pairs numbered I through XII. Cranial nerves I and II serve visual and olfactory functions and are part of the CNS. Cranial nerves emerge through foramina or fissures in the skull or cranium. Cranial nerves, as do their spinal counterparts, contain fibers that transmit sensory and/or motor information. Their neurons innervate muscles or glands or transmit impulses from sensory areas into the brain. The spinal nerves consist of 8 cervical nerve pairs, 12 thoracic nerve pairs, 5 lumbar nerve pairs, 5 sacral nerve pairs, and 1 coccygeal nerve pair. A specific letter and number identifies these nerves (e.g., C1, first nerve from the cervical region; T4, fourth nerve in the thoracic region). The exact location for the spinal nerves has been traced using sophisticated surface and needle techniques to map the tissues they innervate (www.sciencedaily.com/releases/2013/03/130323152444.htm). This is fortuitous because an injury to a spinal cord–specific area produces predictable neurologic damage.[21]

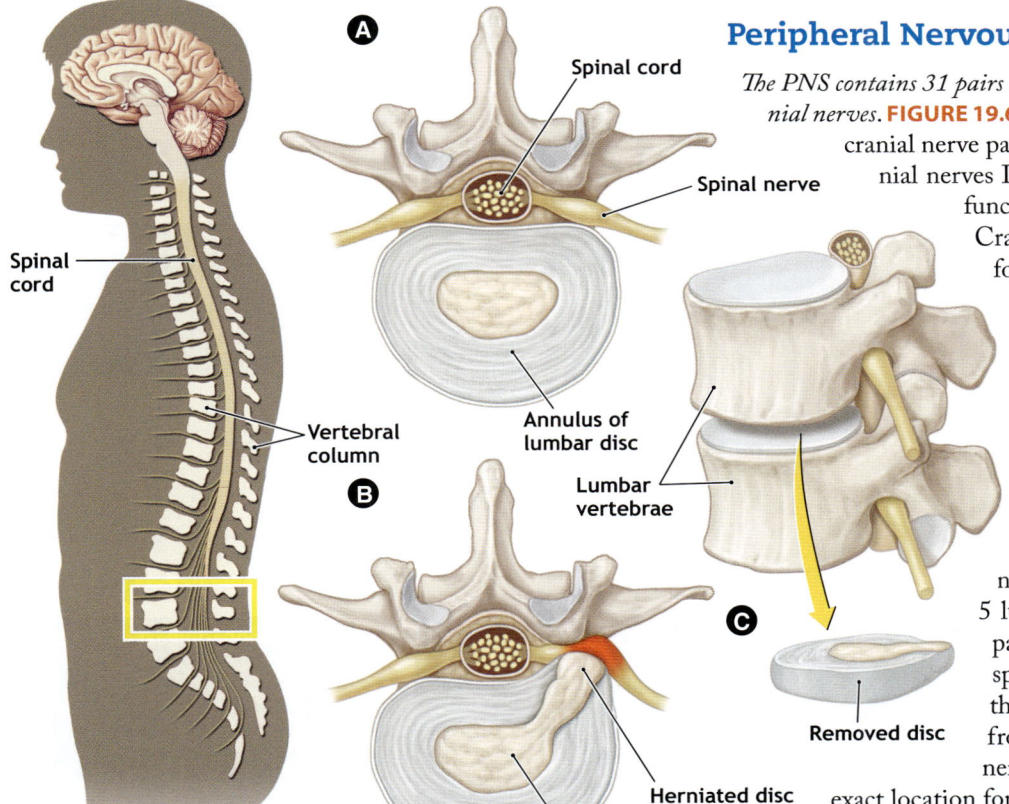

FIGURE 19.5. **(A)** Normal lumbar disk. **(B)** Herniated disk impinging on a spinal nerve. **(C)** Surgically removed disk.

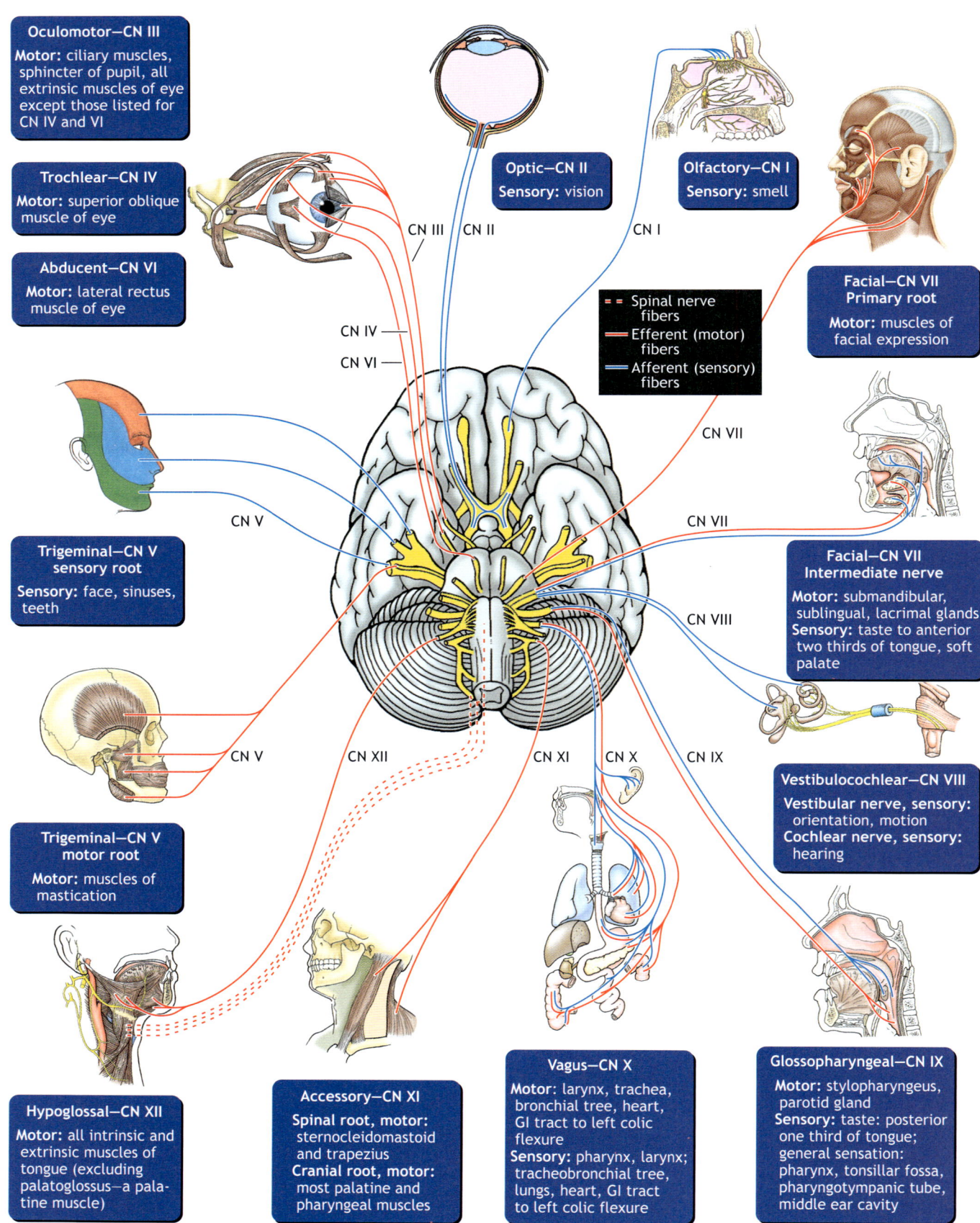

FIGURE 19.6. Distribution for the 12 cranial nerves (CN).
(From Moore KL et al., eds. *Clinically Oriented Anatomy*. 8th ed, Fig. 10.4, p. 1065. Wolters Kluwer, 2018.)

The PNS includes afferent neurons that relay sensory information from receptors in the periphery *toward* the CNS and efferent neurons that transmit information away from the brain to peripheral tissues. Two efferent neuron types include somatic and autonomic nerves.

Somatic and Autonomic Nervous Systems

Somatic nerve fibers, also called *motor neurons* or *motoneurons*, innervate skeletal muscle. Their firing above a threshold level always produces an excitatory response that activates muscle. The autonomic nerves, also called *visceral, involuntary*, or *vegetative nerves*, activate cardiac muscle, sweat and salivary glands, some endocrine glands, and smooth muscle cells, also called *involuntary muscle*, in the intestines and blood vessel walls. Autonomic activity produces either an excitatory or inhibitory effect depending on the specific neurons activated.

Heart and viscera tissues display considerable autonomic excitability, yet conscious control also affects these tissues. For example, individuals who practice yoga or meditation often control heart rate and blood flow "on command" when they assume a particular body pose or breathing sequence. Such conscious autonomic system control has some application as an alternative medical treatment (e.g., gastrointestinal disturbances, hypertension) and to enhance sports performance (e.g., slow heart rate to increase steadiness in target shooting competitions). Competitors in archery and biathlon control cardiovascular activity and respiratory movements to temporarily halt the normal breathing cycle and slow heart rate during the crucial "steadiness" performance phase. The athlete triggers this maneuver immediately prior to releasing the bowstring or pulling the trigger to fire the rifle.

Diego Barbieri/Shutterstock

Sympathetic and Parasympathetic Nervous Systems

The **autonomic nervous system** subdivides into **sympathetic** and **parasympathetic** components. Based on anatomic and physiologic differences, these neurons operate in parallel but use structurally distinct pathways and differ in their transmitter systems. Figure 16.5 in Chapter 16 illustrates that axon's sympathetic division emerges only from the middle third of the spinal cord in the thoracic and lumbar segments; in contrast, preganglionic parasympathetic division axons emerge only from the brainstem and lowest sacral spinal cord segments. The two systems operate independently in some functions and interact cooperatively in others.

Sympathetic fiber distribution, while displaying some overlap with parasympathetic fibers, supplies the heart, smooth muscle, sweat glands, and viscera. Parasympathetic nervous system fibers leave the brainstem and sacral spinal cord segments to supply the thorax, abdomen, and pelvic regions.

Regions in the medulla, pons, and diencephalon control the autonomic nervous system. Fibers that originate in the lower brainstem medullary region control blood pressure, heart rate, and pulmonary ventilation, whereas upper hypothalamic nerve fibers regulate body temperature.

The Reflex Arc

FIGURE 19.7 diagrams the neural arrangement for a typical **reflex arc** in one of the 31 spinal cord segments. Note that the darker shaded or gray matter contains the neuron cell bodies; longitudinal columns of nerve fibers make up the white matter. Stimulating a single α-motor neuron activates up to 3000 muscle fibers. The motor neuron and the fibers it innervates collectively constitute the motor unit. The figure shows only one side for the spinal nerve complex. Afferent neurons that enter the spinal cord through the dorsal (sensory) root transmit sensory input from peripheral receptors. These neurons interconnect or **synapse** in the cord through interneurons that relay information to different cord levels. The impulse then passes over motor sensory pathways via anterior motor neurons to the effector organ—the muscles.

An example for a simple reflex occurs when one suddenly but unexpectedly touches a hot object as shown in Figure 19.7. Pain receptors located in the skin for the fingers touching the hot object transmit sensory information over afferent fibers to the spinal cord. This activates efferent motor fibers to elicit an appropriate muscle response by immediately jerking the hand away. Concurrently, the signal transmits through interneuron activity up the cord to sensory areas in the brain, the area that actually "perceives" the pain. These various operational levels for sensory input, processing, and motor output, including the reflex action just described, cause the hand to move quickly away from the hot object even before the outward perception indicating pain.

Reflex actions in the spinal cord and other subconscious CNS areas control many muscle functions. Literally hundreds and sometimes thousands of hours practicing a particular motor task "grooves" the neuromuscular movements to become automatic, no longer requiring conscious control. Unfortunately, improper practice also can automate a task to produce less-than-optimal neuromuscular actions.

 See the animation "Nerve Synapse" on **Lippincott Connect** to view this process.

Most individuals who practice the golf swing, for example, do so by reinforcing poor habits. It starts with the grip and the first 6 inches during the takeaway in the backswing. Setting up in the stance with an improper grip followed by rapidly cocking the wrists as the backswing begins simply fuels a recipe for disaster. Instead of pounding one ball after another on the range—often hours on end—both aspiring and advanced golfers should purposely practice correct swing movement patterns and sequences, hopefully under the watchful eye from a proficient coach or teacher.

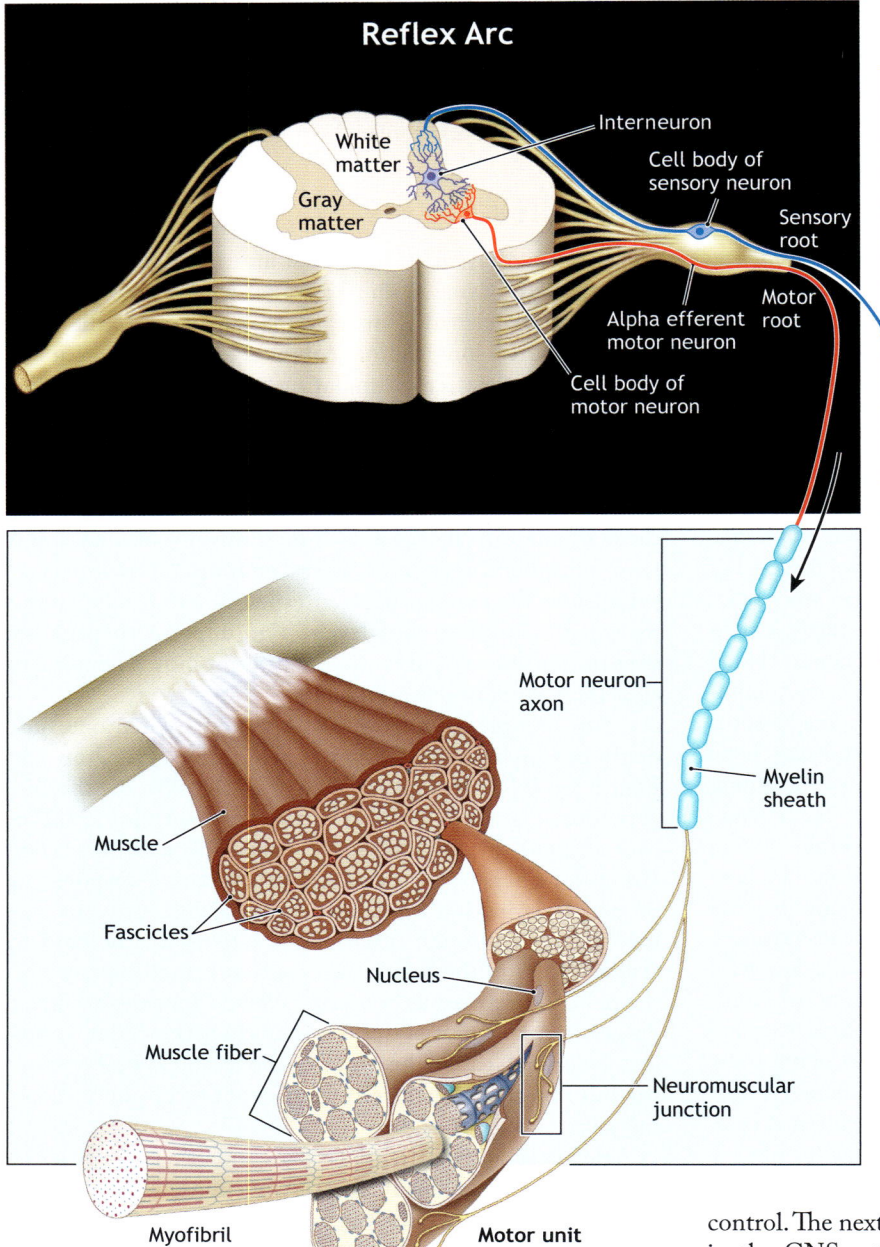

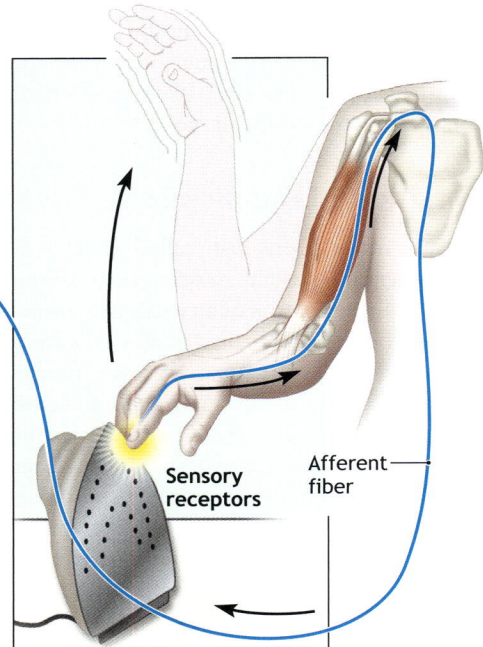

FIGURE 19.7. Reflex arc showing afferent and efferent neurons and interneuron in a spinal cord segment.

Nerve Supply to Muscle

One nerve innervates at least one of the body's approximately 250 million muscle fibers. The typical individual possesses about 420,000 motor neurons; a single nerve usually supplies many individual muscle fibers. *The number of muscle fibers per motor neuron generally relates to a muscle's particular movement function.* Delicate and precise eye muscle work, for example, requires that a neuron control fewer than 10 muscle fibers. For less complex large muscle group movements, a motor neuron may innervate as many as 2000 or 3000 fibers. During any muscular activity, the spinal cord represents the major processing and distribution center for motor control. The next sections examine how information processed in the CNS activates the muscles to trigger an appropriate motor response.

Motor Unit Anatomy

The **motor unit** *makes up the functional movement unit; this anatomic unit includes the anterior motor neuron and the specific muscle fibers it innervates.* The individual and combined motor unit actions produce specific muscle actions. Each muscle fiber generally receives input from only one neuron, yet a motor neuron may innervate many muscle fibers because the axon's terminal end forms numerous branches. The **motor neuron pool** describes the α motor neurons that innervate a single muscle (e.g., triceps or biceps; **FIG. 19.8**). Different motor points exist within the muscle to allow neural stimulation throughout the muscle's length.[26] Some motor units contain up to 1000 or more muscle fibers, whereas motor

The adage "practice makes perfect" should be amended to this five-word mnemonic—"*perfect* practice produces *perfect* performance." If one practices an incorrect movement pattern, no matter how simple or complex the movement, that movement pattern becomes "learned" and "grooved"—in essence, perfecting poor mechanics and grooving improper movement sequencing to produce just the opposite of the desired movement outcome—imperfectly practiced imperfect movement patterns produce predictably imperfect poor performance!

units of the larynx, fingers, or eyeball contain relatively few. For example, the first dorsal interosseous finger muscle contains 120 motor units that control 41,000 fibers; the medial gastrocnemius (calf) muscle contains 580 motor units and 1,030,000 muscle fibers. The ratio between muscle fibers to motor unit averages 340 for the finger muscle and about 1800 for the gastrocnemius muscle. Individual differences in muscle fiber–motor unit ratios probably contribute significantly to variation in sport skill performance and probably help to explain outstanding versus average athletic performance in many individual sport category.

See the animation "Muscle Contraction" on Lippincott Connect to view this process.

Anterior Motor Neuron

The anterior motor neuron illustrated in **FIGURE 19.9** consists of a **cell body**, **axon**, and **dendrites**. Its unique biologic design allows for transmitting an electrochemical impulse from the spinal cord to the muscle. The cell body houses the neuron's control center—the structures involved in genetic code replication and transmission. The spinal cord's gray matter contains the motor neuron's cell body. The axon extends from the cord to deliver the impulse to the muscle; dendrites consist of short neural branches that receive impulses through numerous connections and conduct them toward the cell body. *Nerve cells conduct impulses in one direction only—down the axon away from the original stimulation point.*

The **myelin sheath**, a bilayer lipoprotein membrane that wraps around the axon over most of its length, encases larger nerve fibers. This sheath mostly acts as an electrical insulator that envelops the axon akin to plastic coating surrounding copper electrical wires. A specialized **Schwann cell** covers the bare axon and then spirals around it, sometimes up to 100 times in the largest fibers. A thinner outermost membrane, the **neurilemma**, covers the myelin sheath. The **nodes of Ranvier** named for Paris physician and histologist Louis Antoine Ranvier (1835–1922; www.whonamedit.com/doctor.cfm/3133.html), who also discovered the myelin sheath, interrupt the Schwann cells and myelin every 1 or 2 mm along the axon's length. Whereas myelin insulates the axon to ion flow, the Ranvier nodes permit axon depolarization. This alternating myelin sheath and Ranvier node sequence at about 1-mm intervals allows impulses to "jump" from node to node, called *saltatory conduction* (from the Latin *saltare*, meaning to hop or leap), as the electrical current travels toward the terminal branches at the **motor endplate**. This type of conduction causes faster transmission velocities in myelinated fibers compared to unmyelinated fibers. *Conduction speed in a nerve fiber increases in direct proportion to a fiber's diameter and thickness of its myelin sheath.* Large, myelinated neurons conduct impulses at speeds that exceed 100 m·s^{-1}/224 mph—about 3 times faster than it takes a small Piper Cub airplane to travel one mile, or about half as fast as it takes a commercial airliner to travel one mile!

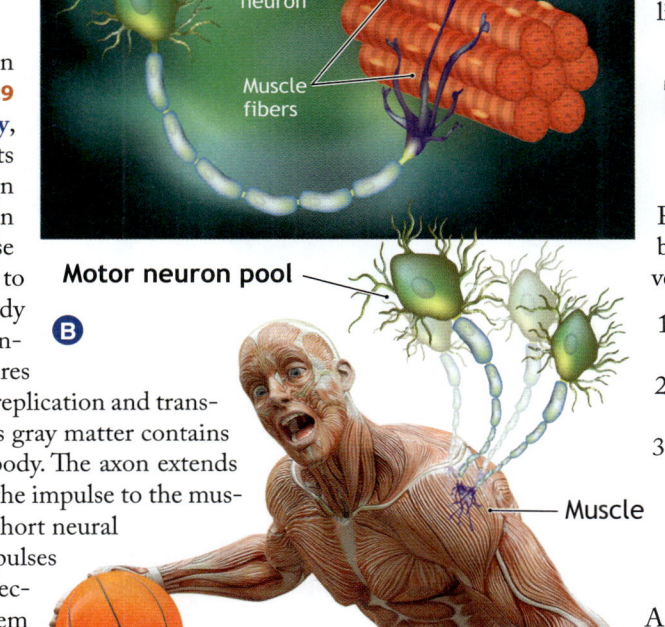

FIGURE 19.8. **(A)** The motor unit represents an α-motor neuron and the fibers it innervates. **(B)** Motor neuron pool represents all the α-motor neurons that innervate one muscle. (Shutterstock: Sakurra; DM7)

See the animation "Saltatory Conduction" on Lippincott Connect to view this process.

Four different nerve fiber groups exist based on size and thus transmission velocity:

1. A-alpha (A-α): 13 to 20 mm; 80 to 120 m·s^{-1}
2. A-beta (A-β): 6 to 12 mm; 35 to 75 m·s^{-1}
3. A-delta (A-δ): 1 to 5 mm; 5 to 35 m·s^{-1}
4. C nerve: 0.2 to 1.5 mm; 0.5 to 2.0 m·s^{-1}

Myelin insulation covers the A-α, A-β, and A-δ nerve fibers, whereas C nerve fibers remain unmyelinated. Nerve fiber thickness dictates neural transmission speed within the fiber—the thickest A-α fibers have the fastest transmission speed, while the smallest C fibers have the slowest transmission speed. These relatively tiny fibers relay information related to pain, temperature, and itch. To give some perspective about transmission speed, impulses in C nerve fibers travel about 2.2 mph, slower than most people walk at about 2.4 mph. In contrast, the A-δ fibers conduct action potentials at a winning Olympic Gold medal 100-m dash velocity in under 10 s, while the A-β fibers that relay information related to touch travel at speeds close to that achieved by the fastest NASCAR and Formula 1 race cars at 200 to 250 mph. As discussed in the section on proprioception, the γ-efferent fibers connect with special stretch sensors in skeletal muscle that detect minute changes in muscle fiber length.

Lippincott® Connect Appendix H, available on Lippincott Connect, provides a list of supplemental animations and videos on this subject.

All muscle action ultimately depends on three primary input sources to α motor neurons (motor units):

1. Dorsal root ganglion cells with axons that innervate specialized muscle spindle sensory units embedded within the muscle
2. Motor neurons in the brain, primarily in the cerebral cortex's precentral gyrus
3. Excitatory and inhibitory spinal cord interneurons

Neuromuscular Junction (Motor Endplate)

The **neuromuscular junction (NMJ)** or motor endplate represents the interface between the myelinated motor neuron's terminal end and the muscle fiber (**FIG. 19.10**). It transmits the nerve impulse to initiate muscle action. Each skeletal muscle fiber usually contains one NMJ.

Five common NMJ characteristics[5]:

1. Schwann cells
2. Neuron's terminal section contains the neurotransmitter acetylcholine (ACh)
3. Basement membrane lines the synaptic space
4. Membrane across from the synaptic space (the postsynaptic membrane) contains ACh receptors
5. Connector microtubules at the postsynaptic membrane transmit the electrical signal within the muscle fiber

The axon's terminal portion below the myelin sheath forms several smaller axon branches whose endings become the **presynaptic terminals**. This region possesses approximately 50 to 70 ACh-containing vesicles per square μm (micrometer, one millionth of a meter). They lie close to but do not come in contact with the muscle fiber's sarcolemma. The invaginated postsynaptic membrane region, also called the *synaptic gutter*, has numerous infoldings that increase the membrane's surface area. The **synaptic cleft** between the synaptic gutter and the axon's presynaptic terminal serves as the region for neural impulse transmission between the nerve and muscle fiber.

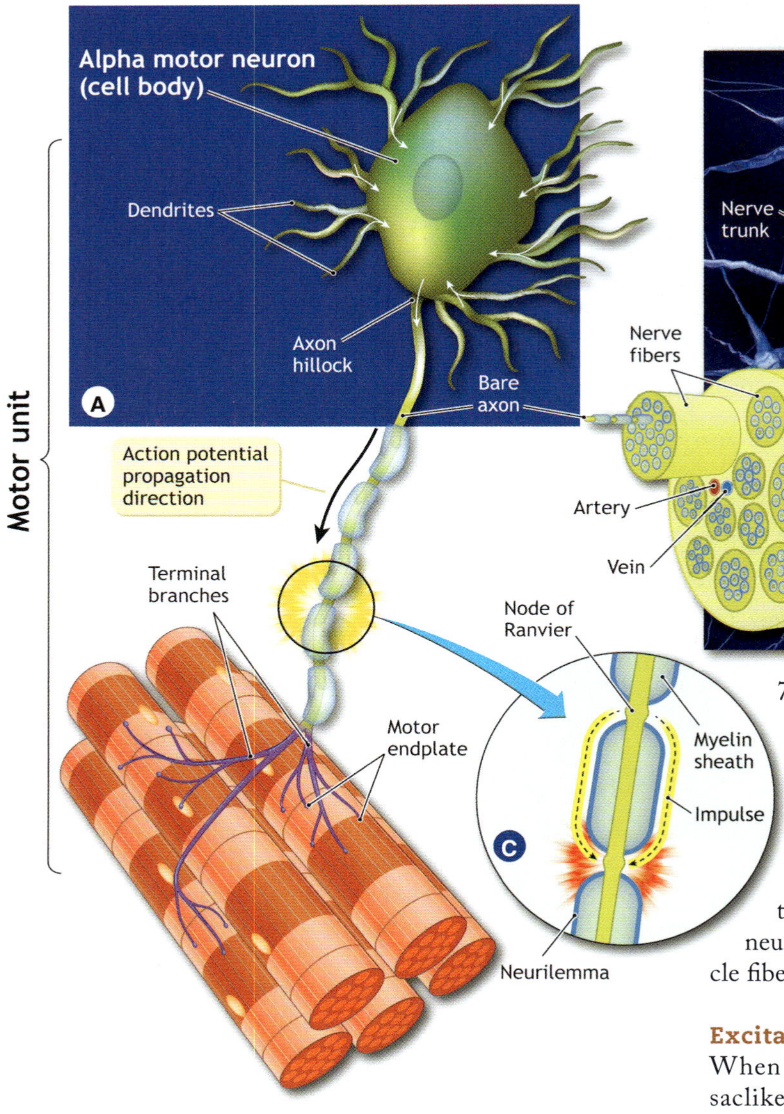

Excitation. *Excitation normally occurs only at the NMJ.* When an impulse arrives at the NMJ, ACh releases from saclike vesicles in the terminal axons into the synaptic cleft. ACh, which changes a basically electrical neural impulse into a chemical stimulus, then combines with a transmitter-receptor complex in the postsynaptic membrane. The resulting change in the postsynaptic membrane's electrical properties elicits an **endplate potential** that spreads from the motor endplate to the muscle's

FIGURE 19.9. **(A)** Anterior α-motor neuron. **(B)** Nerve trunk containing numerous individual nerve fibers including a bare axon. **(C)** Ranvier node on the bare axon, allows impulses to jump from one node to another as the electrical current travels toward the motor endplate's terminal branches. (Shutterstock: Lightspring; Sakurra)

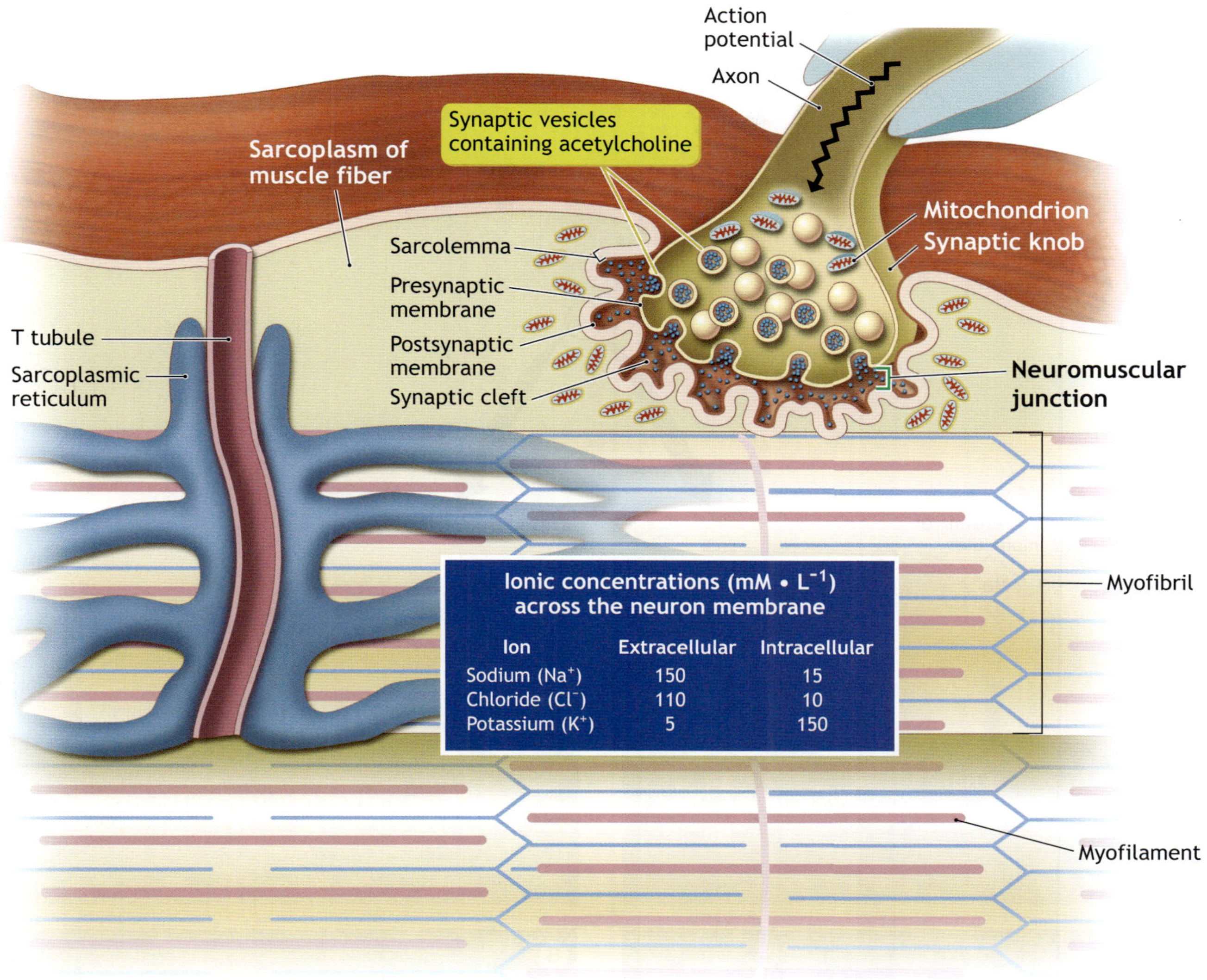

Ionic concentrations (mM • L^{-1}) across the neuron membrane

Ion	Extracellular	Intracellular
Sodium (Na^+)	150	15
Chloride (Cl^-)	110	10
Potassium (K^+)	5	150

FIGURE 19.10. Neuromuscular junction's microanatomy showing the presynaptic and postsynaptic contact areas between the motor neuron and the muscle fiber it innervates. **Inset table** shows representative values for ionic extracellular and intracellular concentrations for Na^+, Cl^-, and K^+ across the motor neuron membrane.

extrajunctional sarcolemma. This causes a depolarization wave (**action potential**) to travel the muscle fiber's length, enter the T-tubule system, and spread to the inner muscle fiber's structures to initiate muscle contraction excitation.

See the animations "Action Potential" and "Flipping the Membrane Potential" on Lippincott Connect to view this process.

The enzyme **cholinesterase**, concentrated at the junctional fold's borders at the synaptic cleft, degrades ACh within 5 ms of its release from the synaptic vesicles. ACh hydrolysis by cholinesterase allows rapid postsynaptic membrane repolarization. The axon resynthesizes cholinesterase end products (composed of acetic acid and choline) to ACh so the entire process continues when another neural impulse arrives.

Facilitation. ACh release from synaptic vesicles excites the postsynaptic membrane belonging to its connecting neuron. This changes membrane permeability so sodium ions diffuse into the stimulated neuron. An action potential occurs if the *change* in transmembrane microvoltage (extracellular sodium influx and/or intracellular potassium efflux) reaches the threshold for excitation. The term ***excitatory postsynaptic potential*** (**EPSP**; www.ncbi.nlm.nih.gov/books/NBK11117/) describes this change in membrane potential at the junction between two neurons (**FIG. 19.11A**). An arriving subthreshold EPSP does *not* cause a neuron to discharge. Rather, positive charges flow into the cell, lower its **resting membrane potential** to temporarily increase its likelihood to "fire." The neuron fires when many subthreshold excitatory impulses arrive in rapid succession and the resting membrane potential lowers to about 50 mV. An impulse arriving in the presynaptic terminal (*top inset A*) causes neurotransmitter release. The molecules bind to

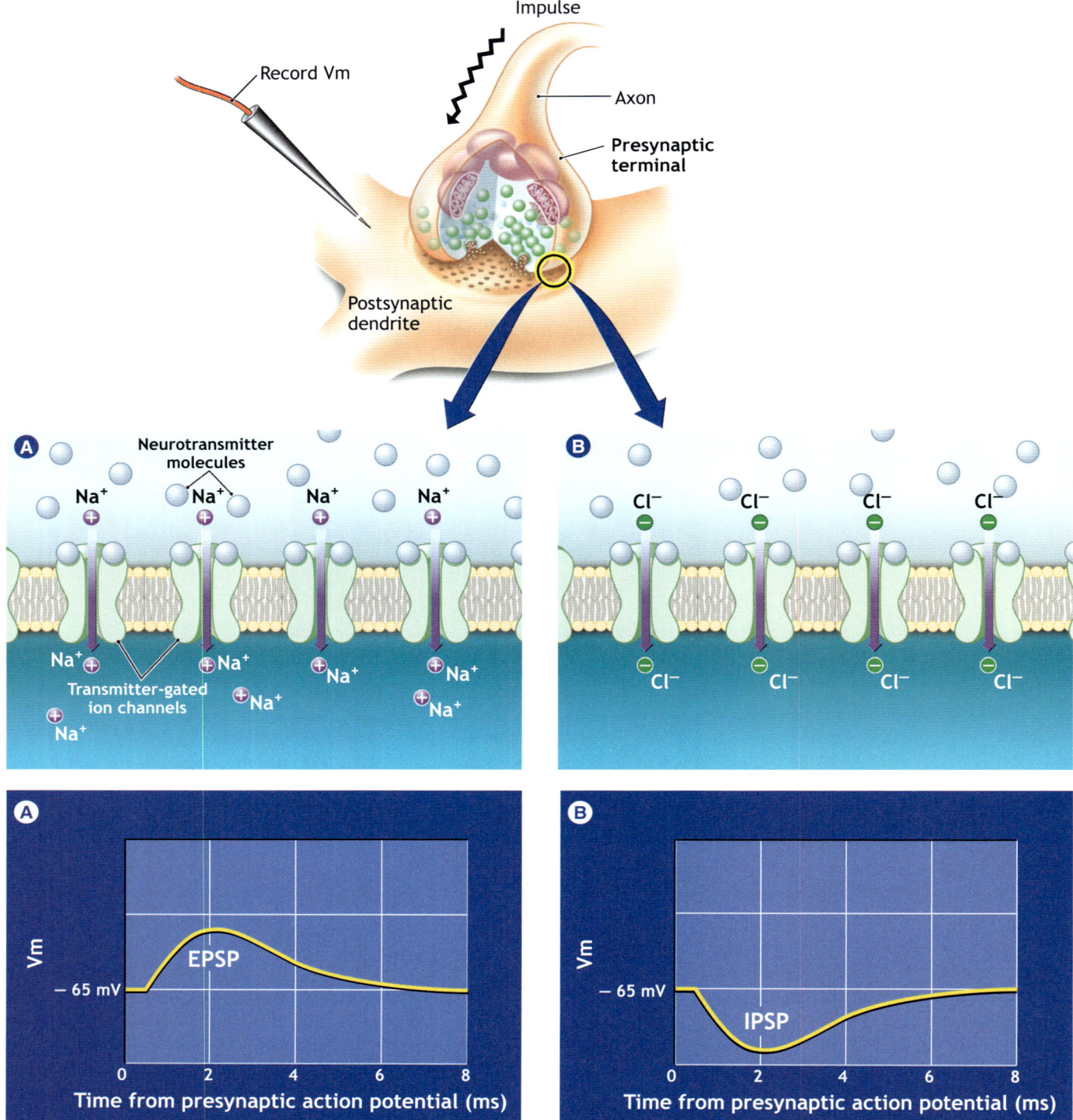

FIGURE 19.11. **(A)** Generating an excitatory postsynaptic potential (EPSP). **(B)** Generation of an inhibitory postsynaptic potential (IPSP). (Reprinted with permission from Bear MF, et al. *Neuroscience: Exploring the Brain*. 4th ed., pp. 128-129. Wolters Kluwer, 2016.)

transmitter-gated ion channels in the postsynaptic membrane. The membrane becomes hyperpolarized when Na⁺ enters the postsynaptic cell through the open channels. The EPSP represents the resulting microvoltage (mV) change in membrane potential recorded by a microelectrode in the cell. An impulse arriving in the presynaptic terminal (*top inset B*) causes neurotransmitter release. The molecules bind to transmitter-gated ion channels in the postsynaptic membrane. The membrane hyperpolarizes if Cl⁻ enters the postsynaptic cell through the open channels. The IPSP represents the resulting change in mV recorded by a microelectrode placed into the muscle cell after piercing the skin under a topical anesthetic. **Temporal summation** describes repeated subthreshold stimulations. Simultaneous surrounding presynaptic terminal stimulation in the same neuron produces **spatial summation**, causing the muscle fiber to fire. This can induce an additive action potential effect from "summing" the individual effects.

See the animation "Nerve Synapse" on Lippincott Connect to view this process.

Neural facilitation known as *disinhibition* impacts the neurons within the CNS rather than electrochemical events at the NMJ because the NMJ does not release inhibitory neurotransmitters. Three mechanisms produce neuronal facilitation:

1. Decreased motor neuron sensitivity to inhibitory neurotransmitters
2. Reduced inhibitory neurotransmitter substance transported to the motor neuron
3. Combined effect of both mechanisms

Neural facilitation exerts an important influence under special, complex movement conditions. A basic principle of strength and power performance is that it requires disinhibiting and maximally activating all motor neurons synchronously during the movement sequences.[14,16,24] *Enhanced facilitation (disinhibition) leads to full muscle group activation during an all-out effort and largely accounts for the rapid and highly specific strength increases in the early strength training phases.*[9,10,25,28,36] Chapter 22 discusses the potential for augmenting maximum strength performance through CNS facilitation with intense concentration or "psyching."

 INTEGRATIVE QUESTION

What are some neuromuscular factors that help explain performance differences among volleyball athletes who devote equal practice time spiking the volleyball over the net?

Inhibition. An **inhibitory postsynaptic potential (IPSP)** temporarily hyperpolarizes the synaptic membrane caused by the flow of negatively charged ions into the postsynaptic cell.

Some presynaptic terminals produce inhibitory impulses. The inhibitory transmitter substance increases the postsynaptic membrane's permeability to potassium and chloride ion efflux, increasing the cell's resting membrane potential to create an IPSP (FIG. 19.11B). The IPSP hyperpolarizes the postsynaptic membrane from the negatively charged ion flow into the postsynaptic cell. The IPSP signal propagates along the dendritic channel and sums with other signal inputs at the axon hillock site. A large IPSP prevents initiating an action potential when a motor neuron receives both excitatory and inhibitory stimulation (https://study.com/academy/lesson/inhibitory-postsynaptic-potential-definition-examples.html). For example, one usually can override or inhibit the reflex to pull the hand away when removing a splinter by steadying the hand to facilitate this unpleasant but necessary task.

The precise neurochemical that provokes an IPSP remains unknown, although gamma (g)-aminobutyric acid (GABA) and the amino acid glycine exert inhibitory effects. Neural inhibition has protective functions and reduces unwanted stimuli input to achieve athletic goals at all skill levels—to execute a smooth, purposeful movement response on demand in the right sequence and tempo.

Transcranial Magnetic Stimulation to Improve Athletic Performance

Developing the brain's complex motor pattern systems in sport holds the key to athletic success—learning how to coordinate then perfect multiple movement patterns simultaneously. An isolated movement is somewhat "delayed" before another movement occurs because a refractory period (delay) exists between at least two movement sequences. The millisecond brief delay following the first movement reflects a central processing limitation at the brain-muscle response stage. As task complexity increases, the brain's processing center must coordinate how to deal with multiple refractory periods efficiently to avoid uncoordinated "jerky" movement sequences. Swinging a baseball bat to hit a 90-mph/144.8-kph to 100-mph/160.9-kph fastball requires coordinating multiple brain strategies to not only anticipate the fast-moving pitch's trajectory but also to coordinate multiple, sequenced movement patterns and refractory periods simultaneously before initiating the swing. Repetitive, purposeful practice swinging at variable speed pitches eventually produces a smooth swing without jerky or hesitant movements. The nerve-to-muscle signaling pattern in complex movements fires involuntarily at the proper time and sequence by fine-tuning or solidifying the brain's specific nerves to multiple muscle pathways. In effect, the normally fast refractory periods among novice athletes reduce to fractional milliseconds in highly skilled athletes. How is this accomplished?

Oligodendrocytes (OL), highly specialized, complex neural cells, consist of a 20% lipid-protein mixture and 80% phospholipid complex. The main OL functions in the CNS are to produce the myelin protective sheath surrounding the axon fiber and to accelerate impulse transmission along the axon (Schwann cells serve the same PNS function). Single OL can spread out its processes to 50 different axons, wrapping approximately 1-μm myelin around individual axons. Practicing both simple and complex motor tasks stimulates OL cells to lay down more myelin, which allows athletes to perform skills faster and more smoothly. To help the athlete better perfect motor skill development, noninvasive transcranial magnetic stimulation or TMS methodology places a magnetic coil above a specific brain region to target a pulsed magnetic field via electromagnetic induction about 2 cm/0.79 in to 3 cm/1.18 in into brain tissues. This procedure may allow the novice to high-performance athlete to facilitate learning complex movement patterns by accelerating the development rate of the brain that develops the myelinated nerve pathways. Combining TMS directed at the brain's motor cortex and

Motor Unit Functional Characteristics

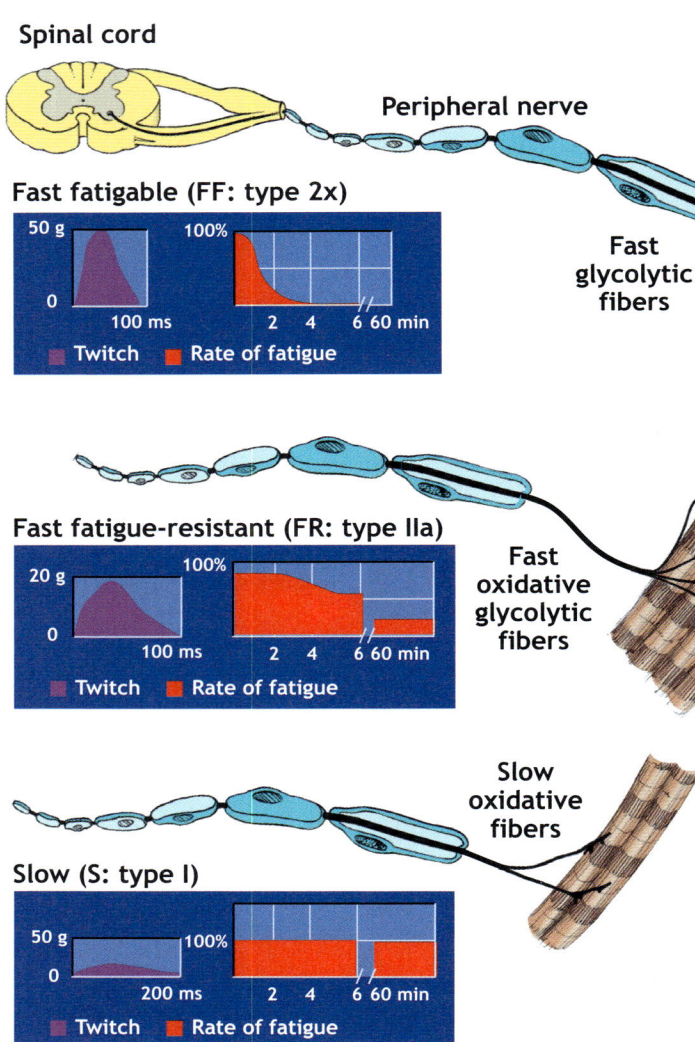

A motor unit contains only one specific muscle fiber type (type I or type II) or a subdivision of the type II fiber with the same metabolic profile. **TABLE 19.2** classifies motor units based on physiologic and mechanical properties and type of muscle fiber each innervates:

1. Twitch characteristics
2. Tension characteristics
3. Force gradation
4. Fatigue resistance

TABLE 19.2 Motor units and muscle fiber types

Twitch Characteristics

Early experiments in muscle/nerve physiology revealed that motor units developed high, low, or intermediate tension in response to a single electrical stimulus. Motor units with low force capacity exhibited a slow shortening time and time to peak force and remained fatigue resistant, but units with higher force capacity shortened rapidly but fatigued earlier. **FIGURE 19.12** illustrates the major characteristics for the three common motor unit categories:

1. Fast twitch, high force, and fast fatigue (type IIx)
2. Fast twitch, moderate force, and fatigue resistant (type IIa)
3. Slow twitch, low force, and fatigue resistant (type I)

Large motor neurons with fast conduction velocities innervate two major fast-twitch muscle fiber subdivisions. These motor units generally contain between 300 and 500 muscle fibers. The fast-fatigable (FF-type IIx) and fast–fatigue-resistant (FR-type IIa) units reach greater peak tension and develop it faster than slow-twitch (S-type I) motor units and receive innervation from smaller motor neurons with slow conduction velocities. The slower contracting units exhibit more fatigue resistance than the fast-twitch units and maintain force output for prolonged time periods. Specific training modifies the unique metabolic characteristics for each specific muscle fiber type. *With prolonged aerobic training, fast-twitch muscle fibers become almost as fatigue resistant as the slow-twitch fibers* (refer to Chapter 22).

Motor neurons themselves have a trophic (stimulating) effect on the muscle fibers they innervate to modulate the fibers' properties and adaptive response to stimuli.[8] Surgically innervating fast-twitch muscle fibers with the neuron from a slow-twitch motor unit eventually alters the fast-contracting fibers' twitch characteristics. Additionally, long-term low-frequency stimulation to intact fast-twitch motor units converts the muscle fibers to the slow-twitch type.[14,22,33] This neurotrophic effect indicates that the myoneural junction takes

FIGURE 19.12. Speed, force, and fatigue characteristics for three motor unit types. "Phasic" motor neurons fire rapidly with short bursts; "tonic" motor neurons fire slowly but continuously.

practicing highly specific movements in the correct sequence thousands of times may allow athletes in the future to enhance performance more efficiently. Brain training with TMS offers a nonpharmacologic ergogenic approach to the athletic training and sports performance world (in addition to its therapeutic role associated with depressive behaviors; www.mayoclinic.org/tests-procedures/transcranial-magnetic-stimulation/multimedia/transcranial-magnetic-stimulation/img-20006838). Ironically, some optimistic coaches and trainers have called the TMS theoretical approach "brain doping" (www.nature.com/articles/nature.2016.19534).

INTEGRATIVE QUESTION

How do drugs that mimic neurotransmitters impact physiological responses and subsequent athletic performance?

on much greater significance than serving just as the site of muscle fiber depolarization. It indicates a remarkable skeletal muscle plasticity that can be altered through long-term use.

Tension Characteristics

A stimulus strong enough to trigger an action potential in the motor neuron activates all the accompanying muscle fibers in the motor unit to contract synchronously. A motor unit does not exert a force gradation—either the impulse elicits an action or it does not. After the neuron fires and the impulse reaches the NMJ, all fibers in the motor unit react simultaneously. This **"all-or-none law"** action was first described by physiologist Henry Pickering Bowditch in 1871 (see Introduction: A View From the Past) who had stated, *"An induction shock produces a contraction or fails to do so according to its strength; if it does so at all, it produces the greatest contraction that can be produced by any strength of stimulus in the condition of the muscle at the time."* The Bowditch discovery has sustained an important biological principle relating to how skeletal and cardiac muscle normally function, which also applies to nerve functioning.

Force Gradation

Graded muscle action forces vary from trivial to maximum by two mechanisms:

1. Increased motor unit recruitment *number*
2. Increased motor unit discharge *frequency*

A muscle generates considerable force when activated by all its motor units. Repetitive stimuli that reach a muscle before it relaxes also increase the total tension. Blending motor unit recruitment and modifying their firing rate permits optimal neural discharge patterns to allow many graded muscle actions. These range from the eye surgeon's delicate touch to repair a torn retina, to the maximum effort in throwing a baseball from deep center field on a straight line to throw out a runner charging home plate.

Low-force muscle actions activate only a few motor units; a higher force requirement progressively enlists more motor units. **Motor unit recruitment** describes adding motor units to increase muscle force. As muscle force requirements increase, progressively larger axons recruit the required motor neurons. This exemplifies the **size principle**—an anatomic basis to orderly recruit specific motor units to produce a smooth muscle action.

All the motor units in a muscle do not fire at the same time (**FIG. 19.13**). If they did, it would be virtually impossible to control muscle force output. Consider the tremendous force and speed gradations muscles generate. When lifting a barbell, for example, some muscles move the limb at a particular speed at a set rate of tension development. One can lift a 3-lb light weight at many speeds. But as weight increases, say to 25 lb and then to 75 lb, the speed options decrease accordingly. When lifting a 6 to 7 g/0.21 to 2.5 oz no. 2 writing pencil, the hand muscles generate just enough force in the fingers to lift the pencil regardless of how fast or slowly the arm moves. When attempting to lift the heaviest weight possible,

fyi Sports Science and Baseball Pitching Speed

Brocreative/Shutterstock

In the 1980s, major and minor league baseball began using radar guns to track pitching speed. From 1997 to 2010, only eight pitchers had thrown 102 mph or higher; one pitch was clocked at 103 mph in 1995 and one at 104.8 mph by Detroit Tigers pitcher Joel Zumaya in 2010. That record was shattered later in the same year when a left-handed pitcher for the Cincinnati Reds, Aroldis Chapman, was clocked at 105 mph. Why is baseball pitching speed included in a chapter dealing with the nervous system? The simple answer, it focuses attention to the tremendous complexity in neural patterns involving millions of "information bits" stored in the nervous system required to activate precise motor patterns over many neural pathways to throw the ball with exquisite muscular control that governs speed, rotation, and direction. Once the pitcher decides on what pitch to throw (e.g., curve, fastball, changeup), the appropriate neural signals activate and transmit the required muscle actions along the body's chain starting at the ankles; moving to the legs, hips, shoulders, and arms; and ending fractions of a second later when the ball releases from the hand and fingers. All these must occur simultaneously with just the right force applied, from the fingers gripping the ball to the hips and shoulders opening and rotating during the motion leading to ball release. Other coordinated minor movements also occur in the proper sequence and timing pattern. The pitcher remains upright while falling forward, maintaining good balance despite unleashing a maximal effort that ultimately gets the arm to release the ball at just the right angle so it flies at maximal velocity from release on the way to the plate. High-speed sports analysis systems have documented important elements in successful muscle action sequences in athletes with exceptional motor skills in all sports from archery to more than 189 martial arts styles (e.g., Japanese martial arts Karate to the Samurai Bajutsu; https://blackbeltwiki.com/martial-arts-styles)!

Sources:
Escamilla RF, et al. Biomechanical comparisons among fastball, slider, curveball, and changeup pitch types and between balls and strikes in professional baseball pitchers. *Am J Sports Med*. 2017;45:3358.
Scarborough DM, et al. Kinematic sequence classification and the relationship to pitching limb torques. *Med Sci Sports Exerc*. 2021;53:351.

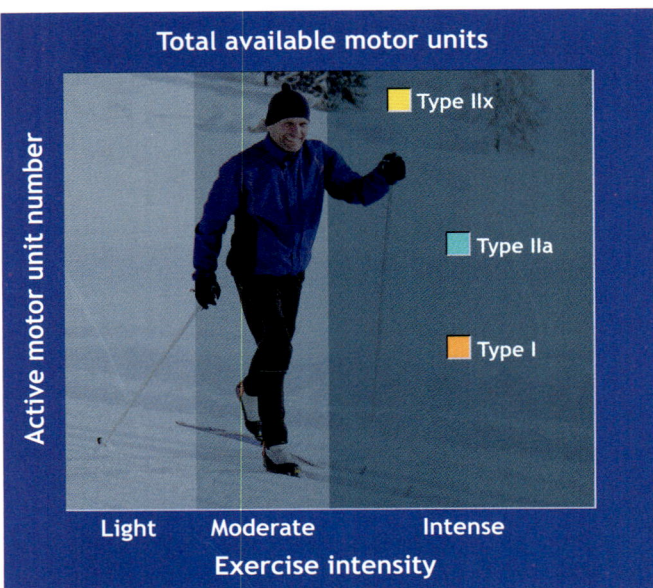

FIGURE 19.13. Slow-twitch (type I) and fast-twitch (type IIa and type IIx) muscle fiber (motor unit) recruitment and physical activity intensity. More intense activity progressively recruits more fast-twitch fibers.
(alenacepl/Shutterstock)

all the available motor units require activation. *From a neural control standpoint, the selective recruitment and firing pattern for the fast-twitch and slow-twitch motor units that control shoulder, arm, hand, and finger movements, and perhaps other stabilizing regions, provide the mechanism to produce the desired coordinated movement response pattern.*

In accord with the *size principle*, slow-twitch motor units with lower activation thresholds are selectively recruited during light to moderate effort. Activating slow-twitch units occurs during sustained slow jogging, cycling, or swimming, or lifting a relatively light weight slowly. More rapid, powerful movements progressively activate fast-twitch fatigue-resistant (type IIa) units up through the fast-twitch fatigable (type IIx) units at peak force. As a runner or cyclist reaches a hill during a distance race, selected fast-twitch units activate to maintain a fairly constant pace over varying terrain. Large single muscles with broad origins and/or insertions (e.g., deltoids) contain smaller, independently controlled "muscles within muscles" that activate depending on the segment's movement plane and intended motion. These movement patterns allow the CNS considerable flexibility to fine-tune skeletal muscle activity to meet the immediate demands imposed by the motor task.[30]

The overall control behind motor unit firing patterns represents a major distinguishing factor that separates skilled from unskilled performers in mainly one-person sport events (e.g., track and field, swimming, tennis) and outstanding performers acting as a team in different athletic groups (e.g., basketball, baseball, soccer).[6] Weightlifters generally exhibit a *synchronous* motor unit firing pattern (i.e., many motor units recruited simultaneously during a lift), whereas the firing pattern for endurance athletes is more *asynchronous* as some motor units fire while others are in various recovery states. Synchronous firing in fast-twitch motor units allows the weightlifter to mobilize forces quickly for the desired lift. In contrast, the asynchronous firing in predominantly slow-twitch, fatigue-resistant units for the endurance ski racer serves as a built-in recuperative period so performance can continue with minimal fatigue. If this were not the case, the endurance athlete could not sustain high-level muscle force output for relatively long durations, as motor units must share the burden employing multiple movements and intensities during their performance.

 INTEGRATIVE QUESTION

How does knowledge regarding neuromuscular exercise physiology help enhance an athlete's (1) strength and power and (2) sports skill performance?

Fatigue Resistance

Fatigue represents a decline in muscle tension or force-output capacity with repeated stimulation or decline throughout a given time period. This also includes one's perceptual alterations about the increased difficulty to achieve a desired submaximum or maximum activity outcome. Many interrelated complex factors lead to motor unit fatigue, each including specific demands unique to the activity that produce it.[1,13,15,17,18]

Voluntary muscle actions depend on four main components relating to nervous system hierarchy:

1. CNS
2. PNS
3. Neuromuscular junction
4. Muscle fiber

Fatigue occurs from disruption in the connection between the CNS and muscle fiber regardless of the reason as illustrated by four examples:

1. Exercise-induced alterations that alter the psychic or perceptual state to disrupt physical ability from changing concentrations in serotonin, 5-hydroxytryptamine (5-HT), dopamine, and ACh concentrations in different brain regions,[4,19] including ammonia and the cytokines secreted by immune cells.
2. Reduced glycogen content of active muscle fibers relates to fatigue during prolonged intense activity.[2,7] This "nutrient fatigue" occurs even with sufficient oxygen available to generate energy through aerobic pathways. Depleted phosphocreatine (PCr) and decline in the total adenine nucleotide pool (ATP + ADP + AMP) accompany the fatigue state in prolonged submaximum effort.[2]
3. Diminished oxygen and increased blood and muscle lactate levels relate to muscle fatigue in short-term, maximum exertion. The dramatic $[H^+]$ increase in active muscle

dramatically disrupts the intracellular environment.[12,23] Alterations in contractile function in anaerobic physical activity also relate to these six factors:

a. PCr depletion
b. Changes in myosin ATPase
c. Impaired glycolytic energy transfer capacity from reduced concentration in phosphorylase and phosphofructokinase
d. Disturbed T-tubule system function to transmit the impulse throughout the cell
e. Ionic imbalances.[11] Down-regulation occurs in the muscle Na^+, K^+, and Ca^{+2} release, distribution, and uptake, which alters myofilament activity and impairs muscular performance,[16] despite nerve impulses continuing to bombard the muscle fiber.

4. Fatigue can occur at the NMJ when an action potential fails to pass from the motor neuron to the muscle fiber, but this "neural fatigue" mechanism remains unknown.

As overall muscle function declines during prolonged submaximum effort, additional motor-unit recruitment maintains the required force outputs to maintain a relatively unvarying performance level. During all-out exercise requiring activating all of the motor units, a decrease occurs in neural activity accompanying fatigue assessed by the electromyogram (EMG; www.hopkinsmedicine.org/health/treatment-tests-and-therapies/electromyography-emg). Reduced neural activity supports the conclusion that failed neural or myoneural transmission produces fatigue in maximum effort.

Proprioceptors: Specialized Receptors in Muscles, Tendons, and Joints

Muscles and tendons contain highly specialized sensory receptors sensitive to three factors—stretch, tension, and pressure. These terminal end organs known as **proprioceptors** almost instantaneously relay information about muscular dynamics and limb movement to the CNS conscious and subconscious brain areas. Proprioception allows for continual monitoring about any limb movements and their movement patterns involved in subsequent motor behavior.[20]

Muscle Spindles

The **muscle spindles**, named for their similar shape to the spindle on a spinning wheel, provide mechanosensory information about changes in two muscle fiber characteristics—fiber length and fiber tension. Both primarily respond to any stretch within the muscle. Through reflex response, the spindles initiate a stronger muscle action to counteract the stretch.

 See the animation "Proprioceptors" on **Lippincott Connect** to view this process.

Structural Organization

FIGURE 19.14 displays a fusiform muscle spindle aligned in parallel to regular muscle fibers or **extrafusal fibers**. When the muscle stretches so do the spindles. The number of spindles within a muscle varies depending on the muscle group. On a relative basis, muscles involved in complex movements contain more spindles per gram muscle than muscles that perform gross movement patterns. The spindle, covered by a connective tissue sheath, contains two specialized muscle fiber types called **intrafusal fibers**. One type, the fairly large **nuclear bag fiber**, contains numerous nuclei packed centrally through its diameter. Each spindle usually contains two nuclear bag fibers. The other type, the **nuclear chain fiber**, contains many nuclei along its length. These fibers attach to the longer nuclear bag fiber's surface. Each spindle usually contains four to five chain fibers. The intrafusal fibers contain actin and myosin filaments and exhibit shortening capability.

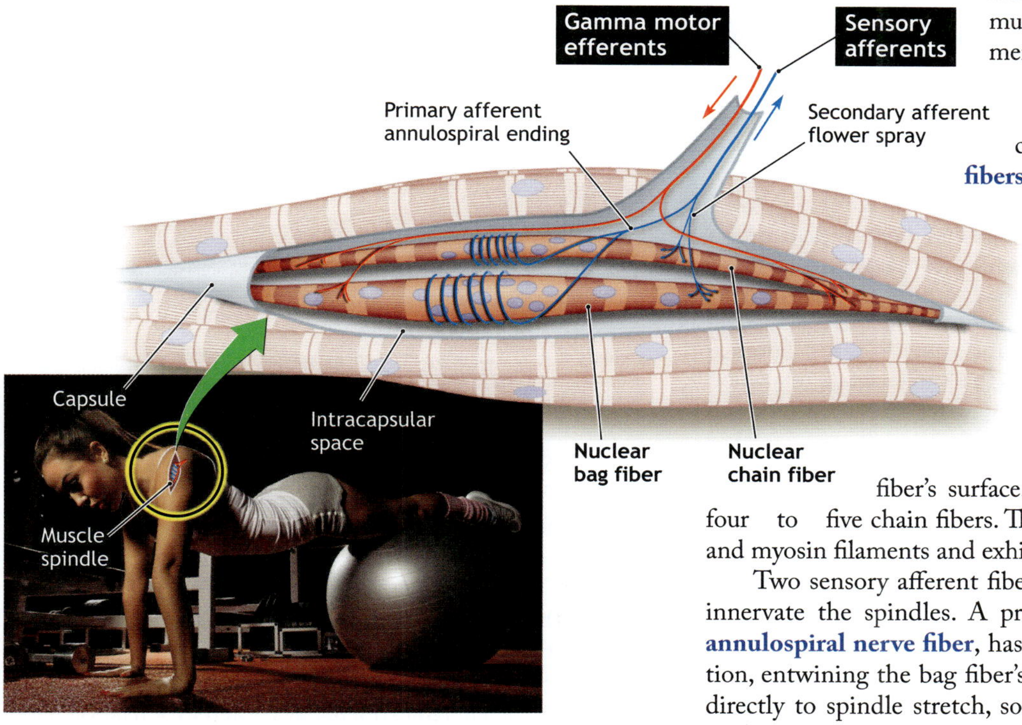

Two sensory afferent fibers and one motor efferent fiber innervate the spindles. A primary afferent nerve fiber, the **annulospiral nerve fiber**, has rings set in a spiral configuration, entwining the bag fiber's midregion. This fiber responds directly to spindle stretch, so its firing frequency (discharge rate) increases in proportion to the stretch. A second group of smaller sensory nerve fibers, the **flower-spray endings**, makes connections mainly on the chain fibers but also attaches to

FIGURE 19.14. Muscle spindle's structural organization with an enlarged spindle's equatorial region view.
(Wallenrock/Shutterstock)

In a Practical Sense

Proprioceptive Neuromuscular Facilitation Stretching

The four static stretching techniques are as follows:

1. Passive: relaxation of all voluntary and reflex muscular resistance followed by passive assistance from another person or device during voluntary movement.
2. Active assistive: involves assistance from another person as the segment moves through its normal range of motion (ROM).
3. Active: a muscle or joint actively moves through its ROM.
4. Proprioceptive neuromuscular facilitation (PNF): inverse stretch reflex induces relaxation in a muscle prior to it being stretched, allowing for increased stretch.

PNF STRETCHING TECHNIQUES

PNF stretching increases ROM by augmenting prior muscle relaxation through spinal reflex mechanisms using these techniques:

1. Contract-relax stretch (hold-relax stretch). Involves a prior isometric action of the muscle group to be stretched followed by a slow, static stretch (relaxation phase).
2. Contract-relax-contract stretch (hold-relax-contract stretch), also referred to as the contract-relax with agonist contraction (CRAC) technique. Involves an isometric action of the muscle group to be stretched; the relax stretching phase is accompanied by a submaximal action of the opposing (agonist) muscle group.

Both PNF techniques use reciprocal inhibition, the isometric action of antagonist muscle group being stretched to induce a reflex facilitation and agonist contraction. Reciprocal inhibition that suppresses contractile activity in the antagonist muscle during the slow static stretch phase allows for greater antagonist stretch.

PERFORMING PNF STRETCHES

1. Stretch the target muscle group by moving the joint to the end of its ROM (**FIG. A**).
2. Isometrically contract the prestretched muscle group against an immovable resistance (e.g., partner) for 5 to 6 s.
3. Relax the contracted muscle group as the partner stretches the muscle group to a new, increased ROM (**FIG. B**). With CRAC, the opposing muscle group (agonist) contracts submaximally for 5 to 6 s to facilitate relaxation and produce further stretching of the muscle group.

PNF Example: To stretch the hamstring and lower back muscles, the individual sits on the floor with the arms extended forward along the side of the legs (Fig. A). The person contracts the lower back muscle isometrically as the partner offers resistance to horizontal extension. After the isometric action, the partner stretches the hamstrings to a new increased ROM (Fig. B).

GUIDELINES FOR PROPER PNF STRETCHING

1. Determine the appropriate posture or position to ensure proper position and alignment.
2. Emphasize proper breathing. Inhale through the nose and exhale during the stretch through pursed lips with the eyes closed 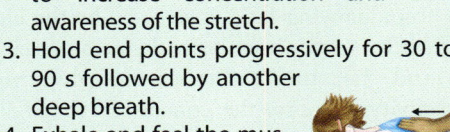 to increase concentration and awareness of the stretch.
3. Hold end points progressively for 30 to 90 s followed by another deep breath.
4. Exhale and feel the muscle being stretched and relaxed to achieve further ROM.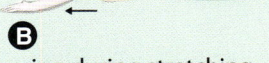
5. Do not bounce or spring during stretching.
6. Do not force a stretch during breath-holding.
7. Increasing stretching range during exhalation encourages full-body relaxation.
8. Slowly reposition from the stretch posture and allow the muscles to recover to their natural resting length.

Sources:
Kay AD, Blazevich AJ. Effect of acute static stretch on maximal muscle performance: a systematic review. *Med Sci Sports Exerc.* 2015;44:154.
Peck E, et al. The effects of stretching on performance. *Curr Sports Med Rep.* 2014;13:179.
Wanderley D, et al. Contract-relax technique compared to static stretching in treating migraine in women: a randomized pilot trial. *J Bodyw Mov Ther.* 2020;24:43.

---

the bag fibers. These endings show less sensitivity to stretch than annulospiral fibers. Activating the annulospiral and flower-spray sensors relays impulses through the dorsal root into the cord to produce reflex motor neuron activation to the stretched muscle. This causes the muscle to act more forcefully and shorten, reducing the stretch stimulus from the spindles.

The third spindle nerve fiber type, the thin **gamma (γ)-efferent fiber**, innervates the contractile, intrafusal fiber striated ends and serves a motor function. Higher centers in the brain activate these fibers to maintain optimal spindle sensitivity at all muscle lengths. Stimulating the γ-efferents activates the intrafusal fibers to regulate their length and sensitivity for any muscle length. This mechanism prepares the spindle for other lengthening actions, even when the muscle remains shortened. Adjustments in γ-efferent activation allow the spindle to continuously monitor the length of muscles that contain them.

CHAPTER 19 • Neural Control and Human Movement 441

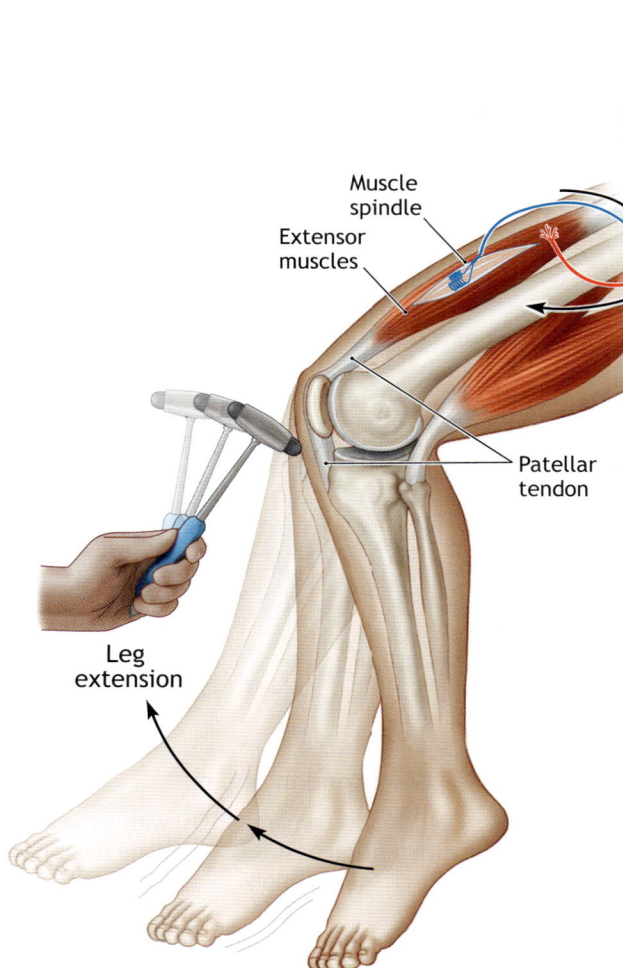

FIGURE 19.15. Activating the patella tendon stretch reflex using percussion with the reflex hammer to stimulate the muscle spindles' afferents and Golgi tendon organs.

2. Afferent nerve fiber that carries the sensory impulse from the spindle to the spinal cord
3. Efferent spinal cord motor neuron that activates the stretched muscle fibers

FIGURE 19.15 illustrates the patellar tendon stretch reflex (also called the *knee-jerk reflex*), the simplest autonomic reflex arc that involves only one synapse called a *monosynaptic synapse*. The spindles lie parallel to the extrafusal fibers so they stretch when these fibers elongate as the hammer strikes the patellar tendon. The spindle's sensory receptors fire when its intrafusal fibers stretch. This immediately directs impulses through the dorsal root into the spinal cord to activate anterior motor neurons. The gray matter contains neuron cell bodies; the white matter carries longitudinal nerve fiber columns. Stimulating a single α-motor neuron affects up to 3000 muscle fibers. The reflex also activates interneurons within the cord to facilitate the appropriate motor response. For example, excitatory impulses activate synergistic muscles that support the desired movement, while inhibitory impulses flow to motor units that normally counter the movement.[31] In this way, the stretch reflex acts as a self-regulating, compensating mechanism. This salient feature allows the muscle to adjust automatically to differences in load and length without requiring immediate information processing through higher CNS centers.

Stretch Reflex

The muscle spindle detects, responds to, and modulates changes in the extrafusal muscle fiber's length. This provides an important regulatory function for movement and posture regulation. Postural muscles continuously receive neural input to sustain their readiness to respond to conscious voluntary movements. These muscles require continual subconscious activity to adjust to gravity's pull downward while standing in an upright postural position. Without this monitoring and feedback mechanism, the body would literally collapse into a heap on the ground from any tension in neck muscles, spinal muscles, hip flexors, abdominal muscles, and large leg musculature. To this end, the stretch reflex provides a fundamental controlling mechanism in all human movements during exercise and in all resting and sleeping activities.

The stretch reflex has three main components:

1. Muscle spindle that responds to stretch

Golgi Tendon Organs

In contrast to muscle spindles that lie parallel to extrafusal muscle fibers, the **Golgi tendon organs (GTOs)**—first identified in 1898 by Italian physician Camillo Golgi (1843–1926; www.nobelprize.org/prizes/medicine/1906/golgi/biographical/) and named in his honor—connect up to 25 extrafusal fibers near the tendon-muscle junction. These fine-tuned sensory receptors detect differences in tension generated by active muscle rather than muscle length. **FIGURE 19.16** shows that the GTOs respond as a feedback monitor to discharge impulses under either of two conditions:

1. Tension created in the muscle when it shortens
2. Tension when the muscle stretches passively

When stimulated by excessive tension, the GTO receptors transmit signals to the spinal cord to elicit *reflex inhibition* in the muscles they supply. This happens from the overriding inhibitory spinal interneuron influence on the particular muscle motor neurons. The GTOs serve as a *protective* sensory mechanism, much like a "governor" mechanism that sets the speed limit for motorized go-carts—no matter how "hard" you depress the gas pedal, the car only travels at a predetermined top speed. Another way to think about GTOs is to consider them law enforcement officers—attempting to thwart hostile actions before any harm occurs to anyone! Excessive change in muscle tension increases the GTO sensor's discharge to depress motor neuron activity and reduce force output. GTO receptors remain relatively inactive and exert little influence if muscle action produces little tension.[32] Ultimately, the GTOs protect the muscle and surrounding connective tissue harness from injury when a sudden, unaccustomed movement occurs, or when a muscle is pushed to its limit as in trying to lift a heavy object without the prerequisite strength to execute the movement safely.

Pacinian Corpuscles

Pacinian corpuscles are small, ellipsoidal bodies located close to the GTOs and embedded in a single, unmyelinated nerve fiber. These sensitive sensory receptors respond to quick movement and deep pressure. Deformation or compression by a mechanical force to the onionlike capsule transmits pressure to the sensory nerve ending within its core to change

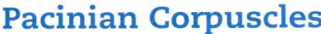

FIGURE 19.16. Golgi tendon organs (GTOs) within the muscle respond to excessive tension or stretch to initiate reflex inhibition in the muscles they supply.

the sensory nerve ending's electric potential. If this generator potential achieves sufficient magnitude, a sensory signal propagates down the myelinated axon that leaves the corpuscle and enters the spinal cord.

Pacinian corpuscles act as fast-adapting mechanical sensors; they discharge a few impulses at a steady stimulus onset and then remain electrically silent or discharge an additional volley when the stimulus ceases. Pacinian corpuscles detect *changes* in movement or pressure rather than how much movement or pressure occurred.

Summary

1. Neural control mechanisms located in the CNS regulate human movement.
2. Skeletal muscles respond to internal and external stimuli where sensory input is automatically coded, routed, organized, and transmitted to the skeletal muscles.
3. Neural tissue tracts descend from the brain to influence spinal cord neurons. Extrapyramidal tract neurons control posture and provide a continual background level of neuromuscular tone, while pyramidal tract neurons stimulate discrete muscular movements.
4. The cerebellum fine-tunes muscle activity by functioning as the major comparing, evaluating, and integrating center.

fyi Intricate Spinal Nerve Cells Photographed in 1878

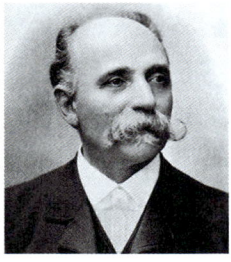 In 1878, Camillo Golgi (1843–1926), an Italian neurohistochemist, discovered the minute tendon organs that now bear his name using a silver nitrate stain described in his masterpiece text, *On the Fine Anatomy of the Nervous System*. Golgi received the Nobel Prize in Physiology or Medicine in 1906 with Santiago Ramón y Cajal (1852–1934; www.nobelprize.org/uploads/2018/06/golgi-lecture.pdf) for insightful contributions about nervous system structures. Golgi's greatest contributions were his creative staining method involving individual nerve and cell structures using a weak solution of silver nitrate, which he named "the black reaction." This invaluable but laborious process at that time traced the outlines of intricate cell spinal cord neuron image he photographed about 150 years ago.

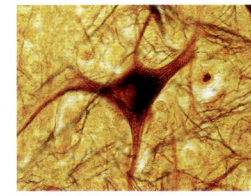

5. The spinal cord and other subconscious CNS areas control many muscle functions.
6. The reflex arc provides the basic mechanism to process "automatic" muscle actions.
7. The motor unit makes up movement's functional unit.
8. Muscle fiber number in a motor unit depends on a muscle's movement function. Intricate movement patterns require a small fiber-to-neuron ratio, where a single neuron can innervate 1000 muscle fibers for gross movements.
9. The anterior motor neuron contains the cell body, axon, and dendrites and transmits electrochemical nerve impulses from the spinal cord to the muscle.
10. The dendrites receive impulses and conduct them toward the cell body; the axon transmits the impulse one way along the axon to the muscle.
11. The neuromuscular junction (NMJ) establishes the interface between the motor neuron and muscle fiber.
12. Acetylcholine (ACh) release at the NMJ provides the chemical stimulus to activate muscle fiber firing.
13. Excitatory and inhibitory impulses continually bombard the synaptic junctions between neurons, altering a neuron's excitation threshold by increasing or decreasing its tendency to fire.
14. During all-out power movements, neural facilitation (disinhibition) proves beneficial because it maximally activates a muscle's motor units.
15. Motor units classify into three types depending on speed of muscle action, force generated, and fatigability: (a) fast twitch, high force, fast fatigue; (b) fast twitch, moderate force, fatigue resistant; and (c) slow twitch, low force, fatigue resistant.
16. Muscle force gradation progresses through interacting factors to regulate the number and type of motor units recruited and their discharge frequency.
17. Low-intensity physical activity recruits slow-twitch motor units, followed by fast-twitch unit activation when requiring more powerful forces.
18. Alterations in motor unit recruitment and firing pattern help to explain the rapid strength improvement during the early resistance training stages.
19. Sensitive sensory receptors in muscles, tendons, and joints relay information about muscle dynamics and limb movement to specific CNS areas to provide important sensory feedback during physical activity.
20. Golgi tendon organ sensory receptors respond to quick movement and deep pressure, while pacinian corpuscles detect changes in movement or pressure.

Key Terms

Action potential: Electrical potential change between the inside and outside of the stimulated nerve or muscle fibers during nerve impulse transmission.

Afferent neurons: Transmit sensory input from peripheral receptors.

All-or-none law: Muscle cells always contract to the fullest extent once the neuron fires and the impulse reaches the neuromuscular junction.

Alpha (α) motor neuron: Large brainstem and spinal cord motor neurons, which innervate extrafusal skeletal muscle fibers to directly initiate their contraction.

Annulospiral nerve fiber: Primary afferent nerve fiber with rings set in a spiral configuration entwining the bag fiber's midregion.

Autonomic nervous system: Subdivides into sympathetic and parasympathetic components.

Axon: Portion of neuron extending from the spinal cord to transmit an impulse to the muscle fibers it innervates.

Baroreceptors: Receptors that react almost instantaneously to any change in arterial blood pressure.

Brain concussion: Mild traumatic brain injury (mTBI).

Brainstem: Includes the medulla, pons, and midbrain regions.

Cell body: Neural area located within the spinal cord's gray matter.

Cerebellum: Composed of two hemispheres located at the base of the brain just above the brainstem, which receives information from the sensory system, spinal cord, and other brain areas to regulate motor movements.

Cerebral cortex: Brain's neural tissue covering the surface of each cerebral hemisphere (occipital, parietal, temporal, and frontal) with folded convolutions.

Cholinesterase: Enzyme that degrades acetylcholine within 5 ms of its release from synaptic vesicles, which immediately repolarizes the postsynaptic membrane to receive another stimulus.

Concussion: Most common form of traumatic brain injury resulting from external trauma to the head as occurs in contact sports, vehicle accidents, violence, slips and falls, and military combat.

Corpus callosum: Large tract of nerve tissue that connects the brain's right and left hemispheres.

Dendrites: Short neural branches that receive impulses through spinal cord connections and conduct them to the cell body.

Diencephalon: Located immediately above the midbrain containing the thalamus, hypothalamus, epithalamus, and subthalamus.

Dorsal horn: Longitudinal gray matter subdivision in the lateral half of the spinal cord that receives terminals from some afferent fibers of the spinal nerves' dorsal roots.

Efferent neurons: Transmit information away from the brain to peripheral tissues.

Endplate potential: Change in the postsynaptic membrane's electrical properties that spreads from the motor endplate to the muscle's extrajunctional sarcolemma.

Excitatory postsynaptic potential (EPSP): Describes the change in membrane potential at the junction between two neurons.

Extrafusal fibers: Standard muscle fibers that, when innervated by alpha motor neurons, generate tension to allow skeletal movement.

Extrapyramidal (ventromedial) tract: Neurons that control posture and muscle tone via the brainstem.

Flower-spray endings: Smaller sensory nerve fibers make connections mainly on the chain fibers and attaches to the bag fibers.

Gamma (γ)-efferent fiber: Third spindle nerve fiber type innervates the contractile, striated intrafusal fiber ends and serves a motor function.

Golgi tendon organs (GTOs): Tiny sensory receptors located near the tendon's junction to the muscle that primarily detect differences in muscle tension rather than length.

Gray matter: Thin outer layer of the brain's neural tissue; appears grey because nerve fibers lack a white myelin coating.

Hemispheres: Longitudinal fissure or groove down the brain's midline, which separates the brain's right and left sides.

Herniated disk: When a gel-like nucleus pulposus structure moves from its normal enclosure to impinge on a spinal nerve, which causes pain in the neck region, trunk, lower back, or leg and foot.

Inhibitory postsynaptic potential (IPSP): Increase in the cell's resting membrane potential making it more difficult to fire.

Interneuron: Nerve that distributes or relays information to various brain and spinal cord levels to convey information between a motor and sensory neuron.

Intervertebral disks: Separate adjacent vertebrae designed to provide cushioning and act as a shock absorber protective mechanism.

Intrafusal fibers: Skeletal muscle fibers that serve as proprioceptors to detect the amount and rate of change in muscle length.

Limbic lobe: Arc-shaped region of cortex on the medial surface of each cerebral hemisphere of the mammalian brain, consisting of parts of the frontal, parietal, and temporal lobes.

Meninges: Four tough membranes that surround the brain and spinal cord.

Midbrain: Attaches to the cerebellum and forms a connection between the pons and cerebral hemispheres; contains the red nucleus and substantia tissues from the extrapyramidal motor system.

Motor cortex: Corticospinal tract region contains axons originating from the brain's frontal lobe.

Motor endplate: Interface between the myelinated motor neuron's terminal end and the muscle fiber.

Motor neuron pool: Describes the α motor neurons that innervate a single muscle.

Motor neurons: Conduct impulses outward from the brain or spinal cord.

Motor unit: Skeletal muscle fibers and their corresponding, innervating anterior (alpha) motor neuron; transmits the neural impulse to initiate muscle action.

Motor unit recruitment: Process of adding motor units to increase muscle force.

Muscle spindle: Provide mechanosensory information about changes in muscle fiber length and tension.

Myelin sheath: Lipid-rich tissue cover, either long in length or large in diameter; surrounds the axon and acts as an electrical insulator to speed neural conduction along the fiber.

Neurilemma: Myelin sheath that surrounds a nerve axon.

Neuromuscular junction (NMJ): Interface between the end of a myelinated motor neuron and the muscle fiber it innervates to transmit the neural impulse to initiate muscle action.

Nodes of Ranvier: Neural tissue that interrupts the Schwann cells and myelin every 1 or 2 mm along an axon's length.

Nuclear bag fiber: One of two specialized muscle fiber types contains numerous nuclei packed centrally through its diameter.

Nuclear chain fiber: One of two specialized muscle fiber types containing numerous nuclei packed centrally through its diameter and attaching to the longer nuclear bag fiber's surface.

Oligodendrocytes (OL): Highly specialized, complex neural cells, consisting of a 20% fatty protein mixture and 80% phospholipid complex.

Parasympathetic: One of the two divisions of the autonomic nervous system; activation inhibits excitation except for vagal parasympathetic excitation of gastrointestinal motility and tone and pancreatic insulin secretion.

Pons: Region in the medulla controls the autonomic nervous system.

Presynaptic terminal: Distal terminations of an axon's smaller branches, which lie close to the muscle fiber's plasma membrane.

Proprioceptor: Specialized sensory receptors sensitive to stretch, tension, and pressure in muscles, joints, and tendons.

Pyramidal (lateral) tract: Neurons that activate skeletal musculature in voluntary movements under direct cortical control.

Reflex arc: A neural pathway that controls a reflex with a sensory nerve and a motor nerve connected by a synapse.

Resting membrane potential: Minimum 65 mV electrical potential (outside vs. inside the cell).

Reticular formation: Section in the midbrain that integrates incoming and outgoing signals that flow through it.

Schwann cells: PNS specialized cells encasing the bare axon and spiraling around it.

Sensory neurons: Conduct impulses from sensory receptors toward the CNS.

Size principle: Motor neurons with progressively larger axons become recruited as muscle force increases.

Spatial summation: Simultaneous repetitive stimulation of different presynaptic terminals on the same neuron.

Spinal cord: Nervous tissue cord extending from the brain lengthwise along the back in the spinal canal, which carries impulses to and from the brain to the cranial nerves, serving as a center to initiate and coordinate reflex action.

Sports-related traumatic brain injury (srTBI): External force injures the brain while engaged in a sports-related activity.

Sympathetic: One of the autonomic nervous system's two divisions; serves to accelerate heart rate, constrict blood vessels, and raise blood pressure via the fight or flight response.

Synapse: Junction between the presynaptic end of one nerve cell that interfaces with the postsynaptic membrane of another nerve cell to excite, inhibit, or modulate neural activity.

Synaptic cleft: Space between the synaptic gutter and an axon's presynaptic terminal; region where neural impulse transmission occurs.

Telencephalon: Contains the two hemispheres in the cerebral cortex—corpus striatum and medulla.

Temporal summation: Arrival of many rapid, successive subthreshold excitatory impulses to fire a neuron.

Ventral horn: One of two spinal nerve roots that passes ventrally from the spinal cord and that consists of motor fibers.

References are available online at Lippincott Connect.

Additional References

Ackerley R, et al. Passive proprioceptive training alters the sensitivity of muscle spindles to imposed movements. *eNeuro*. 2022;9:ENEURO.0249-21.2021.

Aimo A, et al. Function in health and disease. *Eur J Heart Fail*. 2021;23:1458.

Alix-Fages C, et al. The role of the neural stimulus in regulating skeletal muscle hypertrophy. *Eur J Appl Physiol*. 2022. doi:10.1007/s00421-022-04906-6.

Andrews SC, et al. Motor cortex plasticity response to acute cardiorespiratory exercise and intermittent theta-burst stimulation is attenuated in premanifest and early Huntington's disease. *Sci Rep*. 2022;12:1104.

Brady M, et al. What is the evidence on natural recovery over the year following sports-related and non-sports-related mild traumatic brain injury: a scoping review. *Front Neurol*. 2022;12:756700.

Brett BL, et al. The association between persistent white-matter abnormalities and repeat injury after sport-related concussion. *Front Neurol*. 2020;10:1345.

Calvert GHM, Carson RG. Neural mechanisms mediating cross education: With additional considerations for the ageing brain. *Neurosci Biobehav Rev*. 2022;132:260.

Çelik MS, et al. Effectiveness of proprioceptive neuromuscular facilitation and myofascial release techniques in patients with subacromial impingement syndrome. *Somatosens Mot Res*. 2022;7:1.

Chen YS, et al. Acute effects of kinesiology taping stretch tensions on soleus and gastrocnemius h-reflex modulations. *Int J Environ Res Public Health*. 2021;18:4411.

de Lima LL, et al. Analysis of mechanoreceptors and free nerve endings of the transverse carpal ligament. *Hand (NY)*. 2022:15589447211066974.

Del Vecchio A, et al. Lack of increased rate of force development after strength training is explained by specific neural, not muscular, motor unit adaptations. *J Appl Physiol (1985)*. 2022;132:84.

Dhote VV, et al. Sports-related brain injury and neurodegeneration in athletes. *Curr Mol Pharmacol*. 2022;15:51.

Di Virgilio TG, et al. The reliability of transcranial magnetic stimulation-derived corticomotor inhibition as a brain health evaluation tool in soccer players. *Sports Med Open*. 2022;8:7.

Didehbani N, et al. Mild cognitive impairment in retired professional football players with a history of mild traumatic brain injury: a pilot investigation. *Cogn Behav Neurol*. 2020;33:208.

Dobson N. The effect of low-load resistance training on skeletal muscle hypertrophy in trained men: a critically appraised topic. *J Sport Rehabil*. 2022;31:99.

Donnelly CR, et al. How do sensory neurons sense danger signals? *Trends Neurosci*. 2020;43:822.

Gao P, et al. The effects of proprioceptive neuromuscular facilitation in treating chronic low back pain: a systematic review and meta-analysis. *J Back Musculoskelet Rehabil*. 2022;35:21.

Godoy DA, Rabinstein AA. How to manage traumatic brain injury without invasive monitoring? *Curr Opin Crit Care*. 2022. doi:10.1097/MCC.0000000000000914.

Hand BJ, et al. Motor cortex plasticity and visuomotor skill learning in upper and lower limbs of endurance-trained cyclists. *Eur J Appl Physiol*. 2022;122:169.

Jobanputra RD, et al. Modelling the effects of age-related morphological and mechanical skin changes on the stimulation of tactile mechanoreceptors *J Mech Behav Biomed Mater*. 2020;112:104073.

Johansson ME, et al. Aerobic exercise alters brain function and structure in Parkinson's disease: a randomized controlled trial. *Ann Neurol*. 2022;91:203.

Kalra S, et al. An update on pathophysiology and treatment of sports-mediated brain injury. *Environ Sci Pollut Res Int*. 2022. doi:10.1007/s11356-021-18391-5.

Kashyap P, et al. Normalized brain tissue-level evaluation of volumetric changes of youth athletes participating in collision sports. *Neurotrauma Rep*. 2022;3:576.

Kim M, Heo G, Kim SY. Neural signalling of gut mechanosensation in ingestive and digestive processes. *Nat Rev Neurosci*. 2022. doi:10.1038/s41583-021-00544-7.

Le TM, et al. Functional neural network configuration in late childhood varies by age and cognitive state. *Dev Cogn Neurosci*. 2020;45:100862.

Lota KS, et al. Rotational head acceleration and traumatic brain injury in combat sports: a systematic review. *Br Med Bull*. 2022: doi:10.1093/bmb/ldac002.

Maas H, et al. Detection of epimuscular myofascial forces by Golgi tendon organs. *Exp Brain Res*. 2022;240:147.

Machek SB, et al. Myosin heavy chain composition, creatine analogues, and the relationship of muscle creatine content and fast-twitch proportion to Wilks coefficient in powerlifters. *J Strength Cond Res*. 2020;34:3022.

Marillier M, et al. The exercising brain: an overlooked factor limiting the tolerance to physical exertion in major cardiorespiratory diseases? *Front Hum Neurosci*. 2022;15:789053.

Matsuo H, et al. The effect of static stretching duration on muscle blood volume and oxygenation. *J Strength Cond Res*. 2022;36:379.

Matsuo T, et al. Neural mechanism by which physical fatigue sensation suppresses physical performance: a magnetoencephalography study. *Exp Brain Res*. 2022;240:237.

Mendonca GV, et al. Sex differences in soleus muscle H-reflex and V-wave excitability. *Exp Physiol*. 2020. doi:10.1113/EP088820.

Michalik P, et al. The influence of menstrual cycle on the efficiency of stretching. *Adv Clin Exp Med*. 2022. doi:10.17219/acem/140163.

Mingorance JA, et al. A comparison of the effect of two types of whole body vibration platforms on fibromyalgia. A randomized controlled trial. *Int J Environ Res Public Health*. 2021;18:3007.

Nemade DP, Cottrill N, Payne M. Prevalence and duration of post-concussive headaches in a pediatric sports clinic: a cross-sectional study. *Neurology*. 2022;98:S7.

Norbury R, et al. The effect of elevated muscle pain on neuromuscular fatigue during exercise. *Eur J Appl Physiol*. 2022;122:113.

Papadopoulos P, et al. The role of the rhythm step on pro-agility test performance in Division I football players. *Res Q Exerc Sport*. 2021;92:529.

Sarmento AO, et al. Effect of exercise training on cardiovascular autonomic and muscular function in subclinical Chagas cardiomyopathy: a randomized controlled trial. *Clin Auton Res*. 2020. doi:10.1007/s10286-020-00721-1.

Tomalka A, et al. Power amplification increases with contraction velocity during stretch-shortening cycles of skinned muscle fibers. *Front Physiol*. 2021;12:644981.

Visser K, et al. Blood-based biomarkers of inflammation in mild traumatic brain injury: a systematic review. *Neurosci Biobehav Rev*. 2022;132:154.

Wilke J, Groneberg DA. Neurocognitive function and musculoskeletal injury risk in sports: a systematic review. *J Sci Med Sport*. 2022;25:41.

Yuan C, et al. Potential cross-talk between muscle and tendon in Duchenne muscular dystrophy. *Connect Tissue Res*. 2020;62:40.

Table 19.1 Common Names Describing Spinal Cord Neurons and Axons

Name	Description/Example
Neurons	
Gray matter	Generic term for a collection of neuronal cell bodies in the CNS (neurons appear gray in a freshly dissected brain).
Cortex	Collection of neurons forming a thin sheet, usually at the brain's surface; example: cerebral cortex, the sheet of neurons found just under the surface of the cerebrum.
Nucleus	Distinguishable mass of neurons, usually deep in the brain (not to be confused with the nucleus of a cell); example: lateral geniculate nucleus, a cell group in the brainstem relaying information from the eye to the cerebral cortex.
Substantia	Related neurons deep within the brain, but with less distinct borders than those of nuclei; example: substantia nigra, a brainstem cell group involved in voluntary movement control.
Locus (plural—loci)	Small, well-defined group of cells; example: locus coeruleus, a brainstem group of cells involved in control of wakefulness and behavioral arousal.
Ganglion (plural—ganglia)	From the Greek term for "knot"; collection of neurons in the peripheral nervous system; example: dorsal root ganglia, which contain the cell bodies of sensory axons entering the spinal cord in the dorsal roots; only one cell grouping in the CNS, the basal ganglia, goes by this name; the basal ganglia that lie deep within the cerebrum control movement.
Axons	
Nerve	A bundle of axons in the peripheral nervous system; the optic nerve is the only collection of CNS axons termed nerve.
White matter	Generic term for a collection of CNS axons (neurons appear white in a freshly dissected brain).
Tract	Collection of CNS axons having a common site of origin and a common destination; example: corticospinal tract that originates in the cerebral cortex and ends in the spinal cord.
Bundle	Collection of axons running together but not necessarily having the same origin and destination; example: medial forebrain bundle that connects the brainstem with the cerebral cortex.
Capsule	Collection of axons that connect the cerebrum with the brainstem; example: internal capsule that connects the brainstem with the cerebral cortex.
Commissure	Any collection of axons that connect one side of the brain to the other side.
Lemniscus	A tract that meanders through the brain in ribbonlike fashion; example: medial lemniscus that brings tactile information from the spinal cord through the brainstem.

CNS, central nervous system.
Reprinted with permission from Bear MF, et al. *Neuroscience: Exploring the Brain*. 4th ed. Baltimore: Wolters Kluwer, 2016: 192.

Table 19.2 Characteristics and Correspondence Among Motor Units and Three Muscle Fiber Types

Motor Unit Designation	Force Production	Contraction Speed	Fatigue Resistance	Sag[a]	Muscle Fiber Type in the Motor Unit
Fast fatigable (FF—type IIx)	High	Fast	Low	Yes	Fast glycolytic (FG)
Fast—fatigue-resistant (FR—type IIa)	Moderate	Fast	Moderate	Yes	Fast oxidative glycolytic (FOG)
Slow (S—type I)	Low	Slow	High	No	Slow oxidative (SO)

[a]Under repetitive stimuli, some motor units respond smoothly with a systematic increase in tension, while others first increase tension and then decrease or "sag" in response to the same tetanic stimulus. These sag characteristics can classify the different motor units. Only the slow motor units do not exhibit sag. This probably relates more to their diminished force-generating capabilities than fatigue characteristics.
Adapted with permission from Lieber RL. *Skeletal Muscle Structure, Function, and Plasticity: The Physiologic Basis of Rehabilitation*. 3rd ed. Baltimore: Lippincott Williams & Wilkins; 2009: 79. Tables 2.8 & 2.9.

CHAPTER 20
The Endocrine System: Organization and Acute and Chronic Responses to Physical Activity

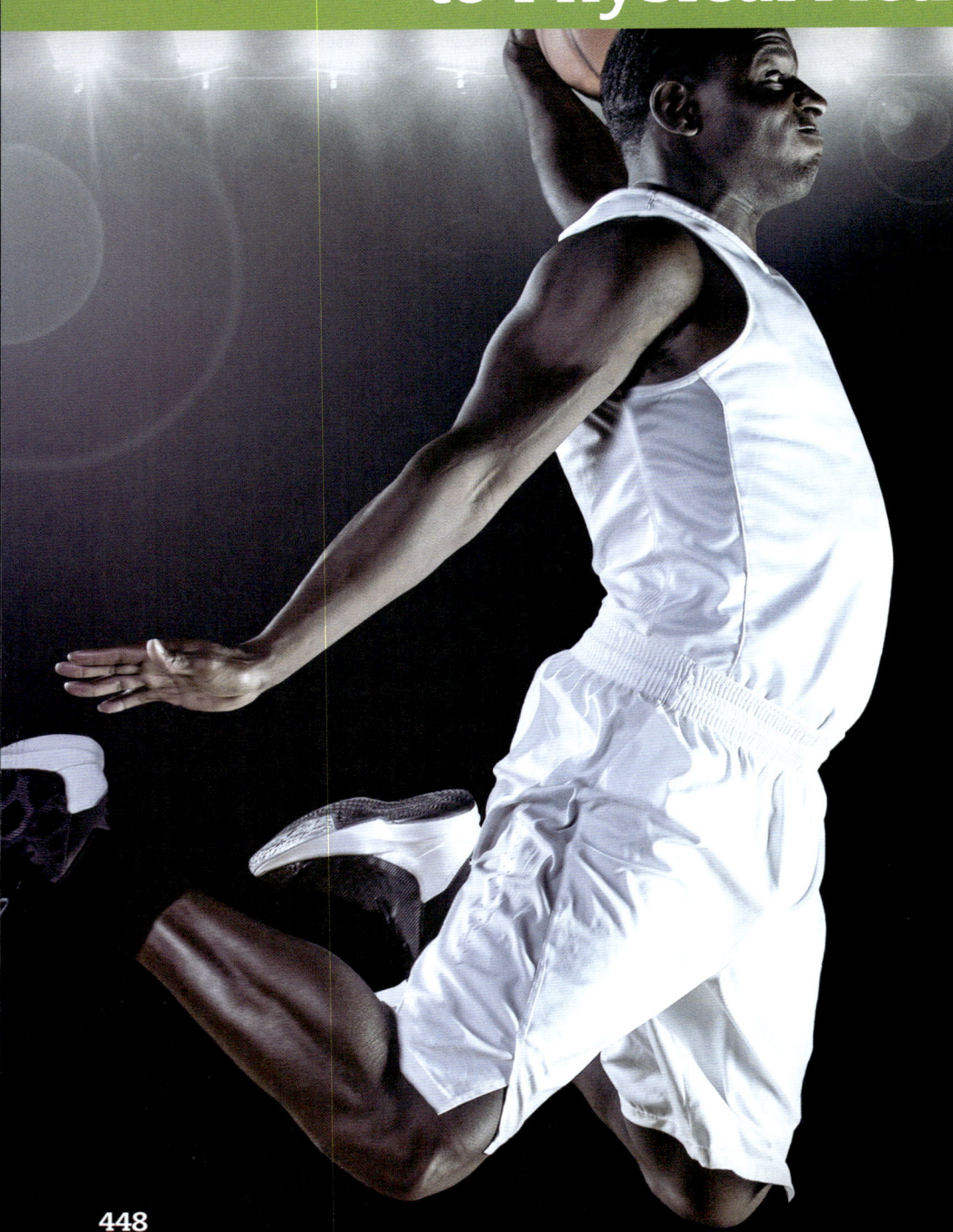

Chapter Objectives

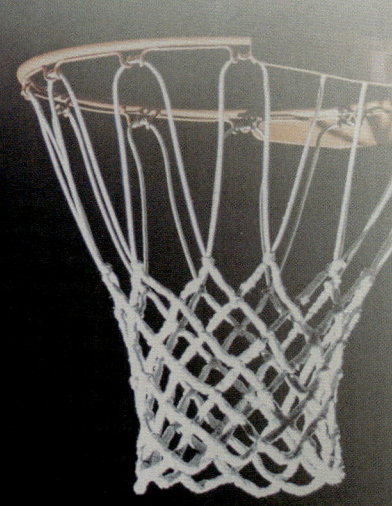

- Draw the body's major endocrine gland locations
- List the sequence of events to show how hormones affect specific "target cell" functions
- Explain how hormones affect enzyme activity and enzyme-mediated membrane transport
- Describe the hormonal, humoral, and neural stimulation influences on endocrine gland activity
- List the anterior and posterior pituitary gland hormones, their functions, and how both acute and chronic physical activity affect their release
- List the thyroid gland hormones, their functions, and how both acute and chronic physical activity affect their release
- List the adrenal medulla and adrenal cortex hormones, their functions, and how both acute and chronic physical activity affect their release
- Define type 1 and type 2 diabetes mellitus, their symptoms, and each disorder's effects
- List three risk factors for type 2 diabetes and two regular physical activity benefits to prevent and treat this disease
- Outline how exercise training affects endocrine functions
- Describe three resistance training effects on testosterone and growth hormone release
- Characterize the opioid peptide functions, their response to physical activity, and possible role in the "exercise high"

Ancillaries at-a-Glance

Visit Lippincott Connect to access the following resources.

- References: Chapter 20
- Animations: Diabetes, Endocrine Gland Stimulation, Hormonal Control, Immune Response, Insulin Functions
- Focus on Research: Training Intensity Affects Growth Hormone Release

The endocrine system integrates and regulates bodily functions to stabilize the body's internal environment. **Hormones** produced by endocrine glands affect all expressions of human function; they activate enzyme systems, alter cell membrane permeability, trigger muscular contraction and relaxation, stimulate protein and lipid synthesis, initiate cellular secretion, and determine how the body responds to physical and psychological stressors. This chapter provides a general overview about the endocrine system, its functions during rest and physical activity, and responses to acute exercise and training.

Endocrine System Overview

Small compared with other body organs, the combined weight for the endocrine organs averages 0.5 kg/1.1 lb. **FIGURE 20.1** illustrates the six major endocrine organ locations—pineal, pituitary, thyroid, parathyroid, thymus, and **adrenal glands**. Several other organs contain discrete endocrine tissue areas that also produce hormones. These include the pancreas, gonads (ovaries and testes), hypothalamus, and adipose (fat) tissues (not shown). The hypothalamus also serves as a major nervous system organ and functions as a neuroendocrine organ. Clusters of hormone-producing cells also form in the walls of the small intestine, stomach, kidneys, and myocytes in the heart's atria, yet these organs exert little influence on total hormone production.

Endocrine System Organization

The **endocrine system** (endocrine means "hormone secreting") has a host organ (gland), minute chemical messenger (hormone), and a target or receptor organ. Glands classify as either endocrine or exocrine; some glands serve both functions. The ancient Chinese and Arab physicians observed bodily dysfunctions related to specialized "glands," but the written evidence relating to such disorders began in Egypt 3000 years before the Christian era with the *Smith papyrus*, the oldest medical text in existence (www.annclinlabsci.org/content/40/4/386.full). Housed in a vault in the library of the New York Academy of Medicine in New York City, the Smith papyrus details 48 medical case reports written on 15 feet of papyrus organized according to symptoms, diagnosis, treatment, and prognosis (www.sciencedirect.com/science/article/pii/S0741521414008659). An app, *Turning the Pages*, allows users to virtually turn the pages of rare medical books from the U.S. National Library of Medicine collections. Centuries later, beginning in the Renaissance Period, many careful investigative studies and human surgeries began to unravel these structures and their functions, known formally as endocrine glands.

Endocrine glands possess no ducts, referred to as *ductless glands*, and secrete substances directly into extracellular spaces around the gland. **FIGURE 20.2** shows that secreted hormones diffuse into blood for transport throughout the body to bind with specific tissue receptors to fulfill their intercellular communication functions. **Exocrine glands** contain secretory ducts that carry substances directly to a specific compartment or surface. Exocrine gland examples include sweat glands and upper digestive tract glands. The nervous system controls almost all exocrine gland functions.

 See the animation "Endocrine Gland Stimulation" on **Lippincott Connect** for a demonstration of endocrine gland functions.

Hormone Types

Hormones, chemical substances synthesized by specific host glands, enter the bloodstream for transport throughout the body. Hormones generally fit into one of two categories:

1. **Steroid**-derived hormones
2. **Amine**- and polypeptide-derived hormones synthesized from amino acids

In contrast to steroid hormones, amine and peptide hormones are soluble in blood plasma. This allows easy uptake at target sites. The term *half-life* describes the time required to reduce a hormone's blood concentration by one half. For example, epinephrine's half-life is slightly less than 3 min, while most orally consumed anabolic hormones (e.g., testosterone) have a half-life of approximately 3.5 hr. A hormone's half-life gives a good indication of how long its effects persist. **TABLE 20.1** compares the storage, synthesis, release mechanism, transport medium, receptor location and receptor-ligand binding, and target organ response for the peptide, steroid, and amine hormones.

The Term *Hormone* Enters the English Lexicon

The term *hormone* (from the Greek *hormao*, meaning "to excite" or "rapid motion toward") entered the English lexicon in 1905 when renowned British physiologists William Bayliss (1860–1924) and Ernest Starling (1866–1927) discovered *secretin*, a compound from the intestine that functioned as an active chemical messenger. At the time it was known that the pancreas secreted digestive juices in response to how food's breakdown products (chyme) passed into the duodenum. Bayliss and Starling discovered that by cutting all the nerves to the pancreas in experimental animals, the hormone released by this gland was not governed by the nervous system. Instead, they determined that secretin, a substance secreted by the intestinal linings, stimulated the pancreas. This early discovery about the first "chemical messengers" circulating in the blood, subsequently called "hormones," foreshadowed the new but important birth of endocrinology into the medical sciences.

Andrea Danti/Shutterstock

Sources:
Chey WY, Chang TM. Secretin: historical perspective and current status. *Pancreas*. 2014;43:162.
Laurila S, et al. Novel effects of the gastrointestinal hormone secretin on cardiac metabolism and renal function. *Am J Physiol Endocrinol Metab*. 2022;322:E54.
Wabitsch M. Gastrointestinal hormones induced the birth of endocrinology. *Endocr Dev*. 2017;32:1.

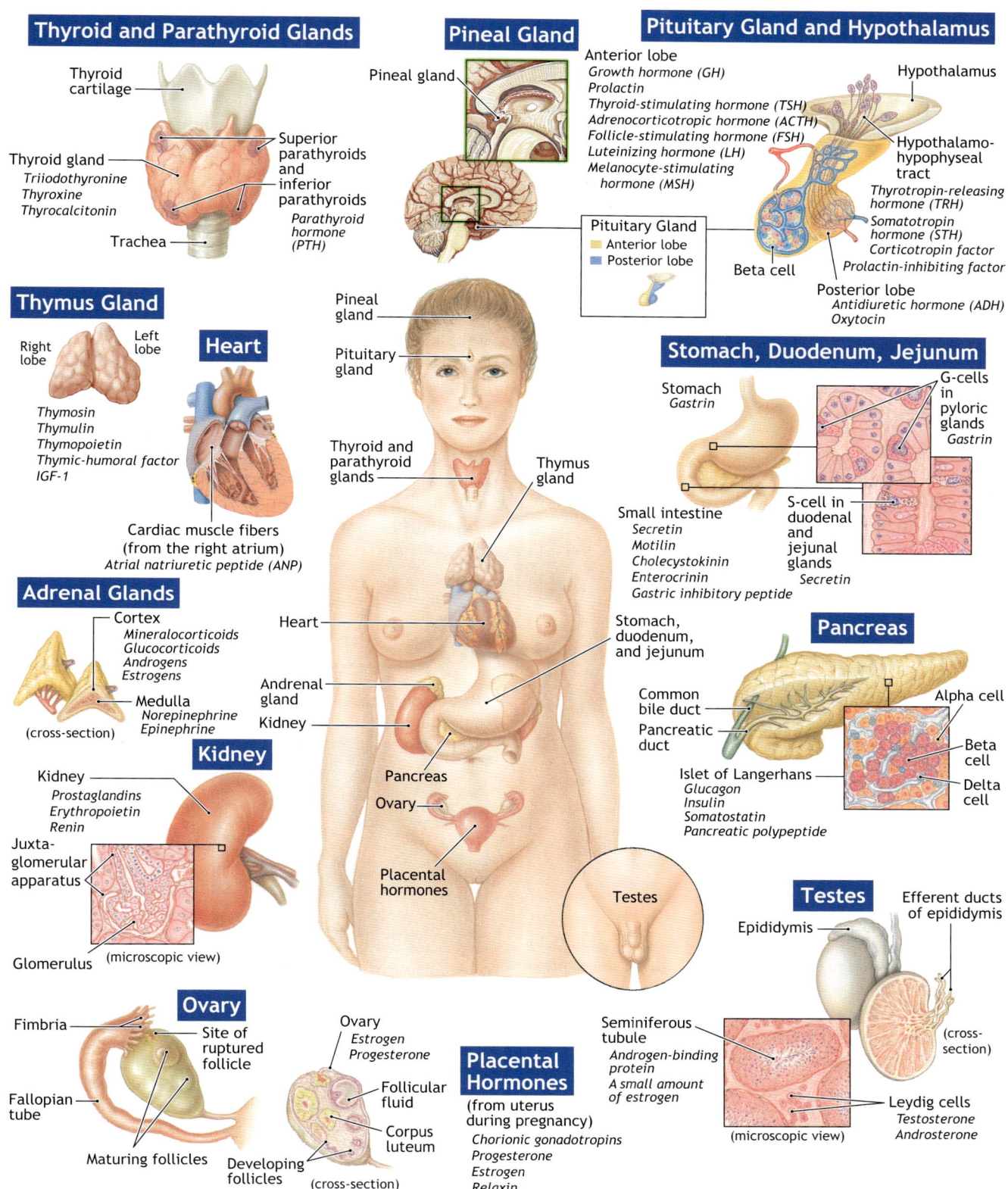

FIGURE 20.1. Hormones produced by endocrine system glands.
(Adapted with permission from Anatomical Chart Co. The Endocrine System. Copyright 2000 Anatomic Chart Company.)

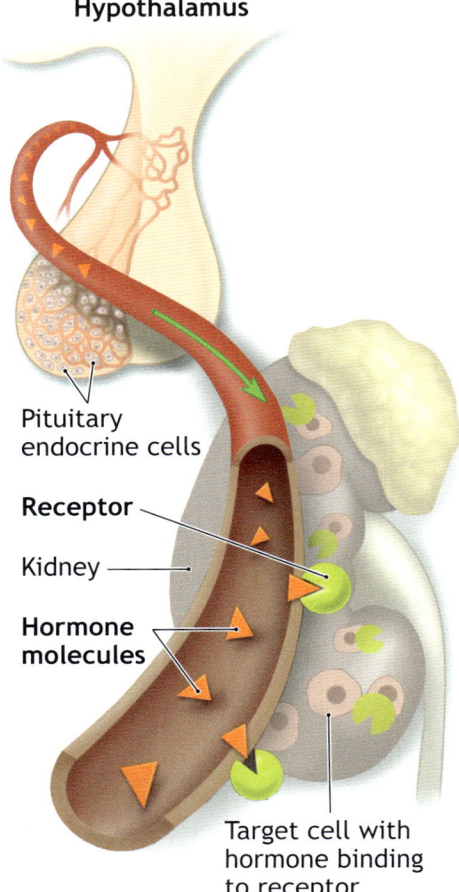

FIGURE 20.2. Endocrine gland hormones travel in the bloodstream to exert their influence on body tissues.

TABLE 20.1 Storage, synthesis, release, transport medium, receptor-ligand binding, and target organ response for peptide, steroid, and amine hormones

TABLE 20.2 lists eight different hormones produced by organs other than the major endocrine glands. Of these, prostaglandins constitute a third chemical hormone class; they represent biologically active lipids in the plasma membrane of nearly all cells. Erythropoietin, a glycoprotein, stimulates the bone marrow's red blood cell production.

TABLE 20.2 Hormones produced by organs other than the major endocrine organs

Most hormones circulate in the blood as messengers that affect tissues a distance from the specific gland. Other hormones (e.g., prostaglandins and the gastrointestinal hormone gastrin) exert local effects in their synthesis region.

 See the animation "Hormonal Control" on Lippincott Connect for a demonstration of hormone activity.

Hormone-Target Cell Specificity

Hormones alter cellular reactions in specific "target cells" in four ways:

1. Modify intracellular protein synthesis rate by stimulating nuclear DNA
2. Change enzyme activity rate
3. Alter plasma membrane transport via a second-messenger system
4. Induce secretory activity

A target cell's response to a hormone depends largely on specific protein receptors that bind the hormone in a complementary way. Target cell receptors occur either on the plasma membrane (up to 10,000 receptors per cell) or in the cell's interior as occurs for fat-soluble steroid hormones that pass through the plasma membrane. Hormone receptors exist in specific local areas or more diffusely throughout the body. For example, adrenal cortex cells contain receptors for adrenocorticotropic hormone (ACTH). In contrast, all cells contain receptors for thyroxine, the principal hormone that stimulates an increase in cellular metabolism.

Must Hormones Be Transported to Distant Targets?

Physiologists have begun to question whether a chemical molecule must be transported to a distant target to classify as a hormone. For example, the different hypothalamic-regulating hormones, the trophic chemical messengers that include releasing and release-inhibiting chemicals, and the different "growth factors" seem to lack widespread distribution in the circulation.

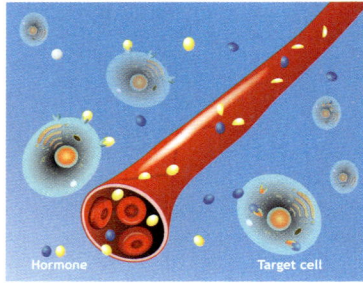

Designua/Shutterstock

Nevertheless, they meet the other qualifications for hormone classification. In fact, one hormone secretion can trigger the release of another hormone with a different function. For example, luteinizing hormone acts on Leydig cells in testes to stimulate testosterone production; adrenocorticotropic hormone floods the inner zone of the adrenal cortex (zona fasciculata) to stimulate cortisol production; thyroid-stimulating hormone stimulates thyroid gland tissue to release triiodothyronine and thyroxine. These examples provide rather convincing evidence that hormone classifications need not rest on meeting the criterion of "transport in the blood."

Source:
Kraemer WJ, et al. Growth hormone(s), testosterone, insulin-like growth factors, and cortisol: roles and integration for cellular development and growth with exercise. *Front Endocrinol (Lausanne).* 2020;11:33.

Hormone-Receptor Binding

Hormone-receptor binding represents the first step to initiate hormone action. A target cell's activation by a hormone depends on three factors:

1. Hormone concentration in the blood
2. Hormone's target cell receptor number
3. Sensitivity or strength of the union between the hormone and receptor

Consider cell hormone receptors as dynamic structures that continually adjust to physiologic demands. **Up-regulation** describes the state whereby target cells form more receptors in response to increasing hormone levels to increase the hormone's effect. In contrast, prolonged exposure to high hormone concentrations desensitizes target cells to blunt hormonal stimulation. Such **down-regulation** also involves a loss of receptors to prevent target cells from overresponding to chronically high hormone levels to decrease a particular hormone's effect.

3′5′-Cyclic Adenosine Monophosphate: The Intracellular Messenger

The binding of a hormone with its specific receptor in the plasma membrane alters the target cell's permeability to a particular chemical (e.g., insulin's effect on cellular glucose uptake) or modifies the target cell's ability to manufacture primarily intracellular proteins. Such actions ultimately affect cellular function. **FIGURE 20.3** shows a schematic for a nonsteroid hormone (displayed as a triangle) as it binds to its receptor and penetrates the intracellular space through the bilayer plasma membrane. The binding hormone acts as first messenger to react with the enzyme **adenylate cyclase** in the plasma membrane to form the compound 3′5′-cyclic adenosine monophosphate (cyclic AMP) from an original ATP molecule.[226] Cyclic AMP then acts as a ubiquitous second messenger to activate a specific protein kinase, which then activates a target enzyme to alter cellular response.

Three factors establish the reaction sequence set into motion by cyclic AMP:

1. Type of target cell
2. Specific enzymes contained in the target cell
3. Specific hormone that acts as first messenger

In thyroid cells, for example, cyclic AMP promotes thyroxine synthesis from the binding of thyroid-stimulating hormone (TSH). In bone and muscle, cyclic AMP produced by growth-hormone binding activates anabolic reactions to synthesize amino acids into tissue proteins.

Hormone Effects on Enzymes

Major hormone actions include altering enzyme activity and enzyme-mediated membrane transport. A hormone increases enzyme activity in one of three ways:

1. Stimulates enzyme production
2. Combines with the enzyme to alter its shape and ability to act, a chemical process known as **allosteric modulation**, and increases or decreases the enzyme's catalytic effectiveness
3. Activates inactive enzyme forms to increase the total active enzyme amount

Hormones either facilitate or inhibit cellular substance uptake. **Insulin**, for example, facilitates glucose transport into the cell by combining with extracellular glucose and a glucose carrier within the plasma membrane. Epinephrine, in contrast, inhibits insulin release to slow cellular glucose uptake.

Hormone action can exert potent although often indirect secondary effects. Insulin release, for example, increases glucose uptake by muscle fibers (primary effect), which in turn increases muscle glycogen synthesis (secondary effect). This insulin effect on glucose uptake and glycogen synthesis maintains fuel homeostasis during physical activity. In insulin-deficient individuals, depressed glucose metabolism impairs exercise performance. Inadequate cellular glucose uptake from chronic insulin deficiency abnormally increases blood glucose

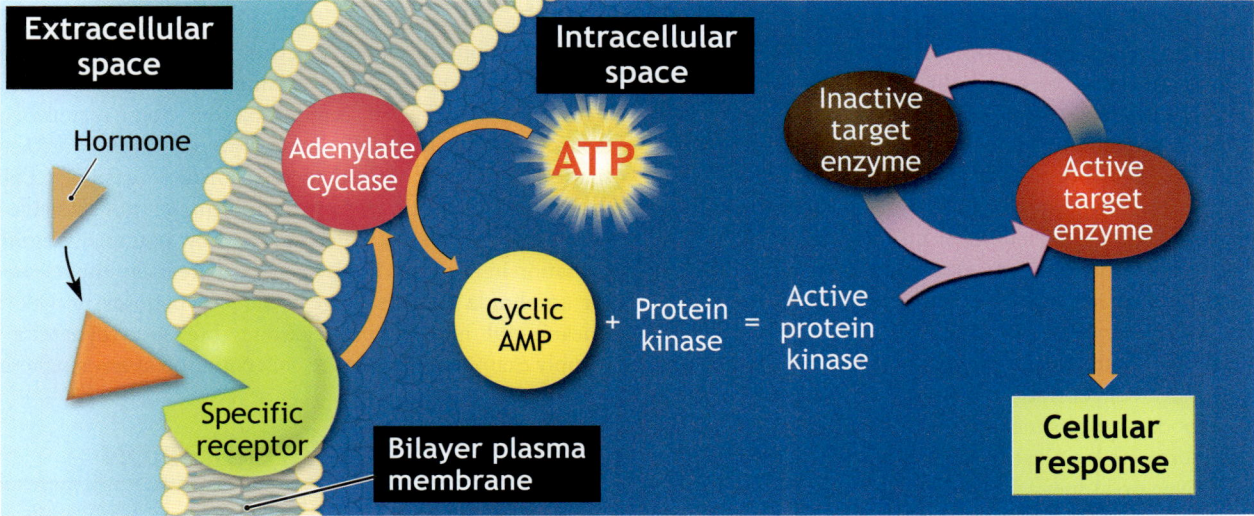

FIGURE 20.3. Nonsteroid hormone action.
(Mitar Vidakovic/Shutterstock)

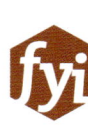

Caffeine Stimulates Lipolysis Through 3'5'-Cyclic Adenosine Monophosphate

Caffeine affects these three key cellular functions:

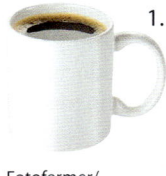

Fotofermer/Shutterstock

1. Increases 3'5'-cyclic adenosine monophosphate (cyclic-AMP) activity in fat cells
2. Increased cyclic-AMP activates hormone-sensitive lipase to promote lipolysis and release fatty acids into the plasma
3. Increased plasma free fatty acid levels stimulate lipid oxidation to conserve liver and muscle glycogen

Source:
Faudone G, Arifi S, Merk D. The medicinal chemistry of caffeine. *J Med Chem*. 2021;64:7156.

---

concentrations.[8] In the extreme, glucose spills into the urine. We discuss insulin insufficiency and/or insulin resistance in more detail later in this chapter.

Factors That Determine Hormone Levels

Hormone secretion rarely occurs at a constant rate. As with nervous system activity, hormone secretion usually adjusts rapidly to meet changing bodily demands. For this reason, all protein hormones secrete in a pulsatile manner as explained in the next section. Four factors determine a particular hormone's plasma concentration:

1. Quantity synthesized in the host gland
2. Catabolism or secretion rate into the blood
3. Quantity of transport proteins present for some hormones
4. Plasma volume changes

Hormone secretion rate depends on the magnitude of chemical stimulatory or inhibitory input from more than one source. Insulin secretion from the pancreas, for example, responds directly to plasma changes in glucose and amino acids, norepinephrine (from sympathetic neurons) and circulating epinephrine, and acetylcholine released from parasympathetic neurons. Each of these chemical messengers supplies inhibitory or excitatory input that determines whether insulin secretion increases or decreases. Over an extended time, which differs for each hormone, their synthesis tends to equal hormone release. For a relatively short duration, hormone release can exceed its synthesis. The term **secreted amount** describes a hormone's plasma concentration. In reality, this represents the sum for hormone synthesis and release by the host gland and its uptake by receptor tissues and removal by liver and kidneys.

Hormone concentration depends on its secretion rate into the blood and/or its metabolism rate causing it to become inactive. Hormone inactivation takes place at or near receptors or in the liver or kidneys. Because blood flow to splanchnic and renal areas decreases during physical activity (blood redistributes to active muscle), hormone inactivation rate decreases and plasma hormone concentration rises.

Changes in plasma volume also alter hormone concentrations independent of the host organ's secretion rate. For example, decreased plasma volume during prolonged hot-weather activity concurrently increases plasma hormone concentration, even without changing the hormone's absolute amount.

FIGURE 20.4 shows how three factors—hormonal, humoral, and neural—stimulate pituitary, pancreas, and adrenal endocrine gland activity.

1. **Hormonal stimulation.** Hormones influence other hormone secretions. For example, release-inhibiting hormones produced by the hypothalamus regulate most anterior pituitary hormone secretions. Anterior pituitary hormones, in turn, stimulate other endocrine organs to release their hormones into the bloodstream. The increased blood hormone levels produced by the final target gland provide feedback to *inhibit* anterior pituitary hormone release and ultimately their own release.

2. **Humoral stimulation.** Changing ion and nutrient levels transported in blood, bile, and other body fluids stimulate hormone release. The term *humoral stimuli* describe these chemicals to distinguish them from bloodborne hormonal stimuli, which also are fluid-borne chemicals. An increase in blood sugar concentration, for example, which acts as the humoral agent, prompts the pancreas to release the hormone insulin. Insulin promotes glucose entry into cells, causing blood sugar levels to decline, ending the humoral stimulus for insulin release.

3. **Neural stimulation.** Neural activity affects hormone release. For example, sympathetic neural adrenal medulla activation during stress releases epinephrine and norepinephrine. The nervous system can override normal endocrine control to maintain homeostasis. Insulin action normally maintains blood sugar levels between 80 and 120 mg per 100 mL or 1 dL. During physical activity, activating the hypothalamus and sympathetic nervous system blunts insulin release to slow a further decrease in blood sugar to ensure sufficient carbohydrate to fuel neural tissue and active muscle.

Hormone Release Patterns

Most hormones respond to peripheral stimuli on an as-needed basis. Others release at regular intervals during a 24-hr cycle referred to as a diurnal secretion pattern. Some secretory cycles span several weeks while others follow daily cycles.[202,203] Cycling patterns are not confined to one hormone category. Pulsatile hormone release patterns reveal information not available from a single blood sample, which fails to show potentially significant variation in hormone levels during a daily cycle. The release and/or amplitude and discharge frequency patterns provide more meaningful information regarding hormone dynamics than simply examining an average concentration at any single time.

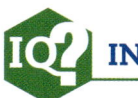

INTEGRATIVE QUESTION

How do hormones act as silent messengers to integrate the body as a unit?

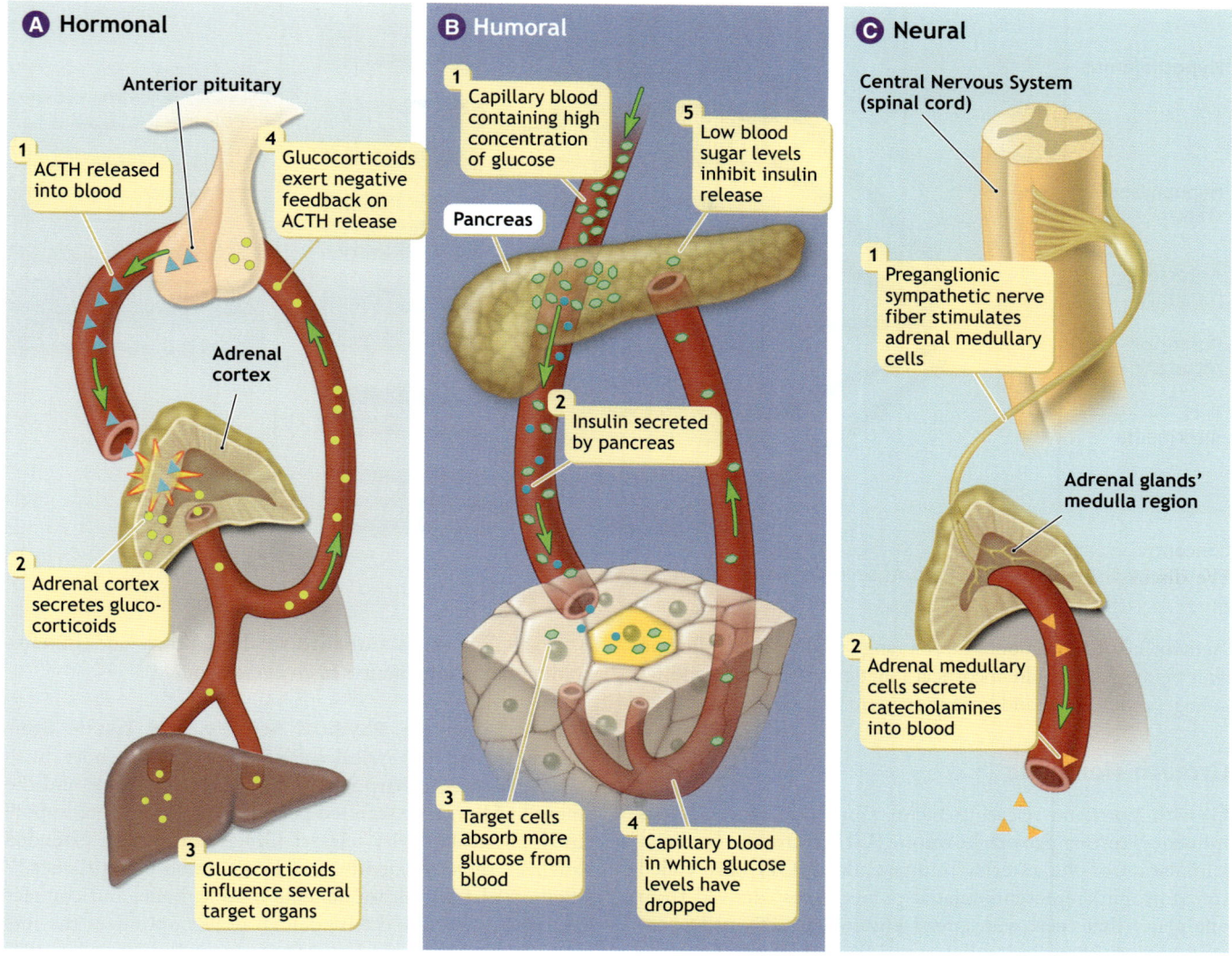

FIGURE 20.4. Endocrine gland stimulation. **(A) Hormonal.** Adrenocorticotropic hormone (ACTH) stimulates glucocorticoid hormone release by the adrenal cortex. **(B) Humoral.** High blood glucose concentrations trigger insulin release, causing rapid cellular glucose uptake. The subsequent decrease in blood glucose removes the stimulus for insulin release. **(C) Neural.** Sympathetic nervous system fibers trigger catecholamine release to blood.
(Reprinted with permission from Marieb E, Hoehn K. *Human Anatomy and Physiology.* 7th ed. Redwood City: Benjamin/Cummings; 2007.)

Resting and Exercise-Induced Endocrine Secretions

TABLE 20.3 lists the different endocrine host organs and nonglandular endocrine tissues, specific hormones secreted, hormone targets, and main effects. The following sections review these hormones, with special emphasis on their immediate response to exertion and adaptations to physical training.

TABLE 20.3 Endocrine organs and their secretions, targets, and main effects

Anterior Pituitary Hormones

FIGURE 20.5 shows the **pituitary gland** (also called the **hypophysis**), its secretions, and various target glands and their specialized hormone secretions. Located beneath the base of the brain, the pituitary secretes at least six specialized polypeptide hormones. With its widespread influence, the **anterior pituitary** gland often was called the body's *master gland*. Researchers now know that the hypothalamus controls anterior pituitary activity, so the hypothalamus should truly claim that distinction. Each primary pituitary hormone has its own hypothalamic-releasing hormone called a **releasing factor**. Neural input to the hypothalamus from anxiety, stress, and physical activity controls the output for these releasing factors.[204,205] In addition to the hormones displayed in Figure 20.5, the pituitary secretes **proopiomelanocortin (POMC**; https://eje.bioscientifica.com/view/journals/eje/149/2/79.xml), a large precursor molecule of other active molecules. POMC provides the source for several neurotransmitters and hormones including ACTH, melanocortin peptides, and several naturally produced opiates such as β-endorphin (see "Opioid Peptides and Physical

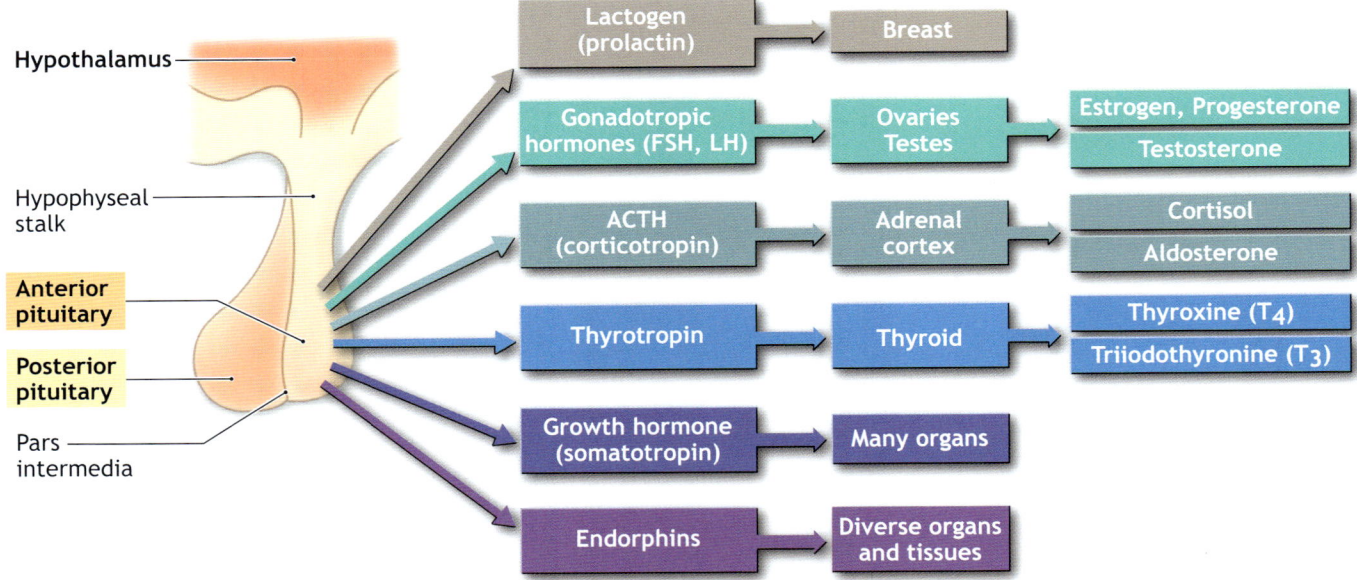

FIGURE 20.5. The pituitary gland, its secretions, and targets.

Activity"). These hormones exert a range of effects including on skin pigmentation, adrenocortical function, food intake and fat storage, and nervous and immune system functions.

Growth Hormone

Growth hormone–releasing factor from the hypothalamus influences resting **growth hormone (GH)** secretions by direct stimulation of the anterior pituitary gland. GH (also called somatotropin) represents related polypeptides (derived from one gene) that exert widespread physiologic activity to promote cell division and cellular proliferation throughout the body. In adults, GH facilitates protein synthesis in three ways:

1. Increasing amino acid transport through the plasma membrane
2. Stimulating RNA formation
3. Activating cellular ribosomes that increase protein synthesis

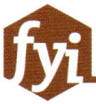 **The True Master Gland**

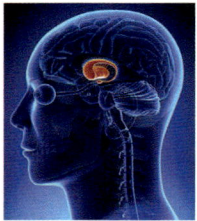

decade3d - anatomy online/Shutterstock

The early Greek physicians, including Galen (131–201 AD), described pituitary gland function in their hundreds of treatises on health and disease. Galen mistakenly proposed that its role was to drain phlegm from the brain to the nasopharynx. Over the next 19 centuries, the pituitary gland had been considered the body's master gland. In reality, the hypothalamus controls anterior pituitary activity, making it the "true" *master gland*.

Source:
Alatzoglou KS, et al. Development of the pituitary gland. *Compr Physiol.* 2020;10:389.

GH also slows carbohydrate breakdown and initiates lipid mobilization and use as an energy source.

Growth Hormone, Physical Activity, and Tissue Synthesis. Increased physical activity for relatively short durations stimulates a sharp rise in GH pulse amplitude and the amount of hormone secreted per pulse.[13,88,193,195] More importantly, physical activity releases GH isoforms with extended half-lives, thereby extending GH's action on target tissues.[137] Augmented GH release benefits muscle, bone, and connective tissue growth and remodeling. It also optimizes the fuel mixture during physical activity, principally decreasing tissue glucose uptake, increasing free fatty acid mobilization, and enhancing liver gluconeogenesis. The net metabolic effect from increased exercise-induced GH production preserves plasma glucose concentration for central nervous system and muscle functions. Many growth-promoting GH effects result from intermediary chemical messengers on different target tissues, rather than a direct GH effect. These peptide messengers produced in the liver are termed somatomedins or **insulinlike growth factors** (IGFs; see next section) from their structural similarity to insulin. These factors exert potent peripheral effects mainly on motor units.

How physical activity stimulates GH release to augment protein synthesis and muscle hypertrophy, cartilage formation, skeletal growth, and cell proliferation remains unclear. The total integrated GH concentration increases with physical activity duration in both males and females.[194] Concurrent measures of circulating lactate, alanine, and pyruvate; blood glucose; and body temperature reveal no association with GH secretory patterns during physical activity.[89] One hypothesis suggests that physical activity directly stimulates GH release (or somatomedins release from the liver or kidneys), which in turn stimulates anabolic processes. Exercise also may indirectly impact GH by stimulating cholinergic pathways to trigger GH

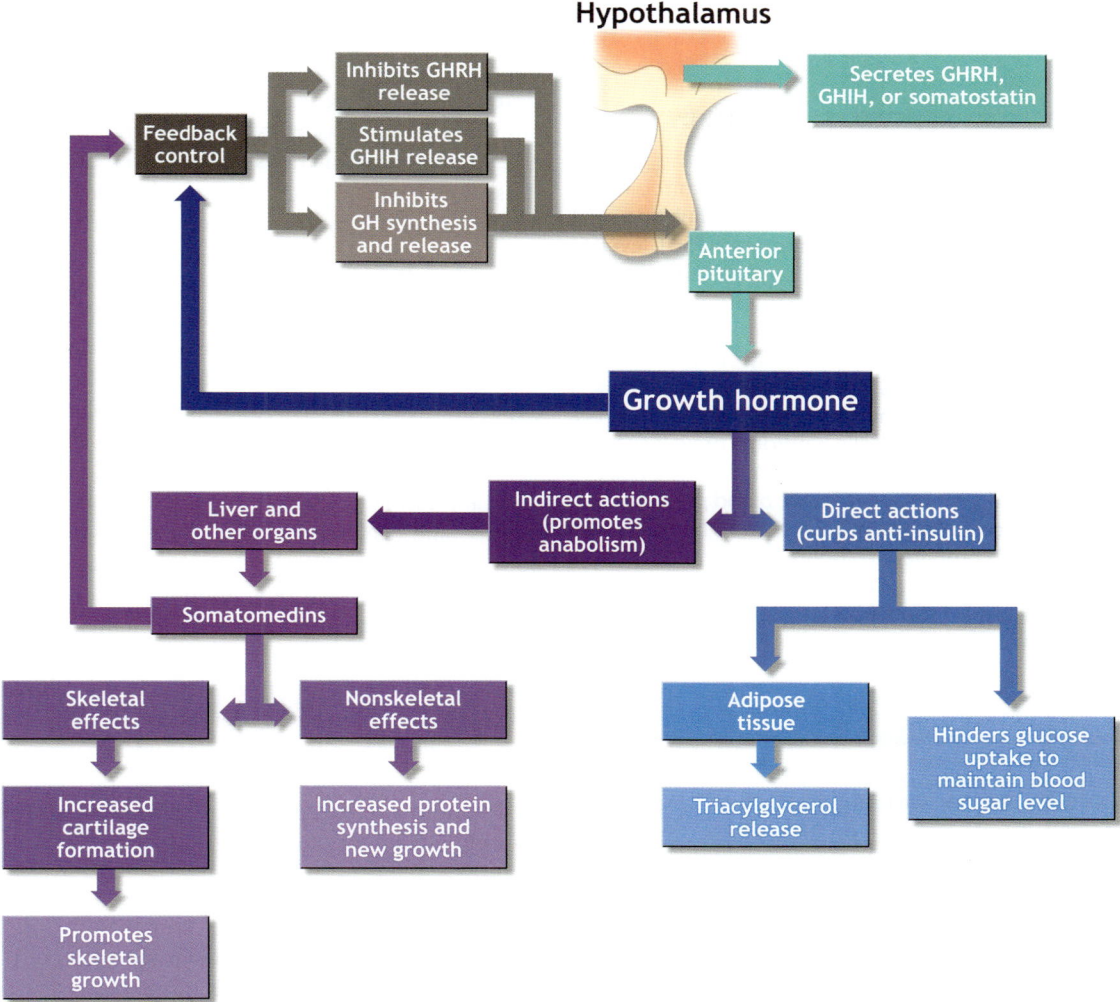

FIGURE 20.6. Overall schema for growth hormone's various direct and indirect metabolic actions.

release. Physical activity stimulates endogenous opiate production that facilitates GH release by inhibiting the liver's production of **somatostatin**, a hormone that blunts GH release.[188]

FIGURE 20.6 outlines the overall schema for GH's various direct and indirect metabolic actions. GH stimulates triacylglycerol breakdown and release from adipose tissue and hinders cellular glucose uptake (anti-insulin effect) to maintain a relatively high blood glucose level. Somatomedins mediate GH's indirect anabolic effects. Elevated GH levels and somatomedins provide feedback to promote GH-inhibiting hormone (GHIH) release while depressing GH-releasing hormone (GHRH), which further inhibits GH release by the anterior pituitary gland (www.vivo.colostate.edu/hbooks/pathphys/endocrine/hypopit/index.html). In essence, GH modulates by feedback control the metabolic mixture during physical activity by stimulating fatty acid release from adipose tissue while simultaneously inhibiting cellular glucose uptake. This glucose-sparing action maintains blood glucose at relatively high levels to augment prolonged exercise performance.

Trained and sedentary individuals show similar increases in GH concentration with exercise to exhaustion. In contrast, the sedentary person maintains higher GH levels for several hours into recovery. Sedentary individuals have a greater GH response during submaximal exertion. The absolute submaximal activity level represents greater stress for the less fit person, allowing GH release to relate more to physical effort's *relative* strenuousness.

Insulinlike Growth Factors. IGFs (somatomedins) mediate many GH effects. In response to GH stimulation, liver cells synthesize IGF-I and IGF-II, a process requiring between 8 and 30 hr. IGFs travel in the blood attached to one of five binding proteins for release as free hormones to interact with specific receptors. The factors that influence IGF transport include binding proteins within muscle, nutritional status, and plasma insulin levels.

Thyrotropin

Thyrotropin, also known as **thyroid-stimulating hormone (TSH)**, controls the thyroid glands hormone secretion. TSH maintains the thyroid gland's growth and development and increases thyroid cell metabolism.

> ### Elevated Thyroid Hormones Predict Metabolic Syndrome in Females
>
> The association between thyrotropin (thyroid-stimulating hormone [TSH]) levels and metabolic syndrome was confirmed in 2760 euthyroid young female volunteers (ages 18 to 39 years) with TSH levels in the normal range (0.3 to 4.5 mU · L^{-1}). The metabolic syndrome prevalence (increased central obesity, hypertriglyceridemia, elevated systolic and diastolic blood pressures) was twofold greater in subjects with higher TSH levels (>2.5 mU · L^{-1}) compared to counterparts with TSH levels less than 2.5 mU · L^{-1}. Healthy young women with TSH levels greater than 2.5 mU · L^{-1} should be assessed for metabolic syndrome, even when TSH levels are within the normal range for their age.
>
> **Sources:**
> Oh JY, et al. Elevated thyroid stimulating hormone levels are associated with metabolic syndrome in euthyroid young women. *Korean J Intern Med*. 2013;28:180.
> Teixeira PFDS, et al. The role of thyroid hormone in metabolism and metabolic syndrome. *Ther Adv Endocrinol Metab*. 2020;11:2042018820917869.

Adrenocorticotropic Hormone

Adrenocorticotropic hormone (ACTH), also known as corticotropin, functions as part of the **hypothalamic-pituitary-adrenal axis** that regulates adrenal cortex hormone output in a manner similar to TSH control of thyroid gland secretion. ACTH acts directly to enhance fatty acid mobilization from adipose tissue, increase gluconeogenesis, and stimulate protein catabolism. Data remain scarce concerning ACTH response during physical activity owing to difficulty in assay methods and the rapid disappearance of this hormone from the blood.[92]

ACTH concentrations may increase proportionately with intensity and duration of effort if intensity exceeds 25% aerobic capacity.[42] Corticotropin-releasing hormone (CRH) and arginine vasopressin (AVP) mediate ACTH release. CRH exhibits a definite diurnal rhythm, with highest levels occurring in early morning just after rising. As the day progresses, CRH levels decline, essentially blocking ACTH release. Factors that alter the normal ACTH rhythm by triggering CRH release include fever, hypoglycemia, and other stressors. CRH is both an ACTH regulator and a central nervous system neurotransmitter, and often is termed the *stress response integrator*. Intense physical activity favors AVP release, while prolonged physical activity favors CRH release, both inhibiting ACTH.[77]

Prolactin

Prolactin principally secretes via the lactotroph cells of the anterior pituitary gland and also from the breast, the decidua (thick layer of modified mucous membrane that lines the uterus during pregnancy), adipose tissue, and parts of the central nervous system as well as some components of the immune system. Prolactin serves as a multifunctional hormone and numerous human tissues express prolactin receptors. Its release and physiological functions connect to emotional and physical stress, water balance regulation, fetal surfactant development, immune system activation, and reproductive function. Prolactin also associates with lactogenesis in mothers and increased levels are associated with gonadal suppression in both women and men. Prolactin displays a diurnal secretion pattern with peak levels during rapid eye movement (REM) sleep.

Prolactin secretion is under a constant inhibition via dopamine from the hypothalamus. Estrogen is another key regulator of prolactin and increases the production and secretion of prolactin from the pituitary gland. In addition to dopamine and estrogen, a whole range of other hormones can both increase and decrease the amount of prolactin released in the body, with some examples being thyrotropin-releasing hormone (TRH), oxytocin, and antidiuretic hormone

Owing to its important role in female sexual function, repeated exercise-induced prolactin release may inhibit ovarian function and contribute to menstrual cycle alterations when females train intensely. Greater increases in prolactin occur in women who run without wearing undergarment support[145]; either fasting or consuming a high-fat diet enhances release of this hormone.[84] Prolactin concentration also increases in males following maximum physical effort.[30]

Gonadotropic Hormones

Gonadotropic hormones stimulate the male and female sex organs to grow and secrete their hormones at a faster rate. The two gonadotropic hormones are **follicle-stimulating hormone (FSH)** and **luteinizing hormone (LH)**. FSH initiates follicle growth in the ovaries and stimulates these organs to secrete the female sex hormone estrogen. LH complements FSH action to cause estrogen secretion and rupture of the follicle, which allows the ovum to pass through the fallopian tube for fertilization. In the male, FSH stimulates germinal epithelium growth in the testes to promote sperm development. LH also stimulates the testes to secrete testosterone.

LH release is normally pulsatile, making it difficult to separate any specific exercise-related change from the normal pulsatile pattern. Generally, LH concentration rises before movement begins and peaks during recovery.

Posterior Pituitary Hormones

The **posterior pituitary** gland forms as a hypothalamic outgrowth resembling true neural tissue (see Fig. 20.5). This tissue, often called the **neurohypophysis**, stores **antidiuretic hormone (ADH)** and **oxytocin**. The posterior pituitary does not synthesize its hormones. Instead, the hypothalamus produces these hormones and secretes them to the neurohypophysis for release as needed via neural stimulation. Posterior pituitary damage or surgical removal does not dramatically affect ADH or oxytocin production.

ADH influences the kidneys' water excretion. Its action limits production of large urine volumes by stimulating water reabsorption in the kidney tubules. Oxytocin initiates muscle contraction in the uterus and stimulates milk ejection during lactation.

Physical activity provides a potent stimulus for ADH secretion. Increased ADH release, stimulated by sweating, helps to conserve body fluids during hot-weather physical activity with accompanying dehydration. The ADH water-conserving effect contributes to efficient cardiovascular response modulation to physical activity.[118] ADH release decreases with fluid overload to increase urine volume and produce more dilute urine (i.e., lighter-color urine).

Thyroid Hormones

Shutterstock: sciencepics; marina_ua; N.Vinoth Narasingam

The 15- to 20-g reddish brown thyroid gland, located nearer the first part of the trachea just below the larynx, comes under the influence of TSH produced by the anterior pituitary gland. In addition to secreting the calcium-regulating hormone **calcitonin**, the thyroid gland secretes two protein-iodine–bound hormones, **thyroxine (T_4)** and **triiodothyronine (T_3)**, the active form of thyroid hormone. These two hormones are often referred to as *major metabolic hormones*. More T_4 is secreted than T_3; although less abundant, T_3 acts several times faster than T_4. The majority of T_3 comes from T_4 deiodination in peripheral tissues, principally liver and kidney. Most receptor cells for T_4 metabolize it to T_3. Both hormones are not readily soluble in water, which means they bind to carrier proteins that circulate in blood. T_4-binding globulin (glycoprotein synthesized in the liver) serves as the main thyroid hormone transporter. This carrier protein (along with two others—transthyretin and albumin) allows for more consistent thyroid hormone availability from which the active, free hormones release for target cell uptake.

Through its stimulating effect on enzyme activity, T_4 secretion raises the metabolism in all cells except in the brain, spleen, testes, uterus, and thyroid gland itself. For example, abnormally high T_4 secretion raises basal metabolic rate (BMR) up to fourfold. This potent thermogenic effect produces large BMR deviations that often indicate thyroid gland abnormality (see Chapter 9). A person may lose weight rapidly with abnormally high thyroid activity. In contrast, depressed thyroid production blunts BMR, which usually leads to gains in body weight and body fat. *Fewer than 3% of obese persons show abnormal thyroid function, so depressed thyroid activity cannot explain excessive body fat gain in most individuals.* For nervous system function, T_3 release facilitates neural reflex activity, whereas low T_4 levels cause sluggishness, where some people often sleep up to 15 hr · d^{-1}. Thyroid hormones provide important regulation for tissue growth and development, skeletal and nervous system formation, and maturation and reproduction. They also play a role in maintaining blood pressure by stimulating an increase in adrenergic receptors in blood vessels.

Whole-body metabolism influences the synthesis of thyroid hormones. Depressing the metabolic rate to some critical value directly stimulates hypothalamic TSH release. This increases thyroid output and increases resting metabolism. Conversely, a chronically elevated metabolism reduces TSH production, causing metabolism to slow. **FIGURE 20.7** illustrates this exquisitely regulated feedback system.

During physical activity, blood free T_4 (T_4 not bound to plasma proteins) levels increase by approximately 35%. This increase could occur from an exercise-induced core temperature elevation, which alters the protein binding of several hormones, including T4. While thyroid disease is common in the general population, particularly in women, it also is prevalent among athletes. Autoimmune malfunctions are the most common cause related to thyroid disorders, but such dysfunction also may be related to insufficient energy intake and micronutrient deficiencies in iodine, selenium, iron, and

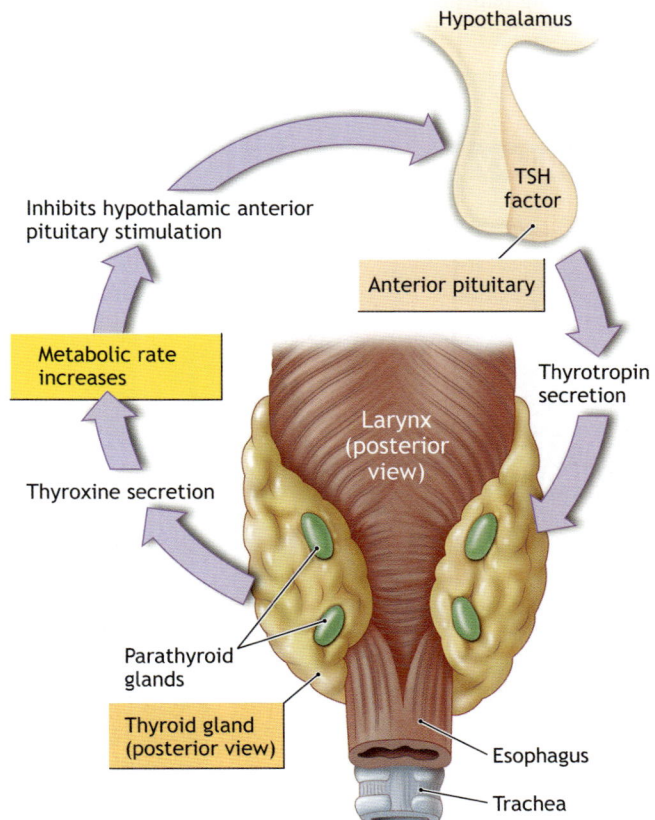

FIGURE 20.7. Feedback system that controls thyroid hormone release.

vitamin D. In addition, strenuous physical activity associates with transient alterations in thyroid hormones to potentially impact health and physical performance.[206]

Thyroid Hormones Can Impact Quality of Life

Thyroid hormones are not essential for life, but they do affect life's quality. In children, full GH expression requires thyroid activity. Thyroid hormones provide essential stimulation for normal growth and development, especially of neural tissues. Thyroid hormone action is most noticeable in people who suffer from either hypersecretion (**hyperthyroidism**) or hyposecretion (**hypothyroidism**).

Thyroid hormone hypersecretion (hyperthyroidism) produces the following four effects:

1. Increased oxygen uptake and metabolic heat production during rest, with heat intolerance being a common complaint
2. Increased protein catabolism and subsequent muscle weakness and weight loss
3. Heightened reflex activity and psychological disturbances that range from irritability and insomnia to psychosis
4. Rapid heart rate (tachycardia)

Hyposecretion of thyroid hormones (hypothyroidism) produces the following four effects:

1. Reduced metabolic rate and cold intolerance from reduced internal heat production
2. Decreased protein synthesis that produces brittle nails, thinning hair, and dry thin skin
3. Depressed reflex activity, slow speech and thought processes, and general fatigue (in infancy causes cretinism marked by depressed mental acuity)
4. Slow resting heart rate (bradycardia)

Parathyroid Hormone

Four parathyroid glands measuring 6-mm long, 4-mm wide, and 2-mm deep are embedded at the thyroid glands' posterior end (see Fig. 20.7). As many as eight glands have been reported in some people, and glands have also been found in neck or thorax regions. **Parathyroid hormone (PTH)**, also known as parathormone, controls blood calcium balance. A decrease in blood calcium levels triggers PTH release; increasing calcium concentrations inhibit its release. PTH's major effect increases ionic calcium levels by stimulating three target organs—bone, kidneys, and small intestine with three main effects:

1. Activation of bone-reabsorbing cells called **osteoclasts**, which digest bone matrix to release ionic calcium and phosphate to the blood
2. Enhanced calcium ion reabsorption and decreased phosphate retention by kidneys
3. Increased calcium absorption by intestinal mucosa

Plasma calcium ion homeostasis also modulates three additional functions:

1. Nerve impulse conduction
2. Muscle contraction
3. Blood clotting

Limited evidence suggests that physical activity increases PTH release in young, middle-aged, and older individuals, an effect contributing to the positive effects of mechanical forces from physical activity on bone mass accretion.[7,16,100,208]

Adrenal Hormones

The adrenal glands appear as flattened; caplike tissues situated just above each kidney (**FIG. 20.8**). The glands have two distinct parts: medulla (inner portion that secretes catecholamines) and cortex (outer portion that secretes mineralocorticoids, glucocorticoids, and androgens). Each functional unit secretes different hormones, so for all practical purposes, these two parts of the adrenal gland are generally considered as two distinct glands.

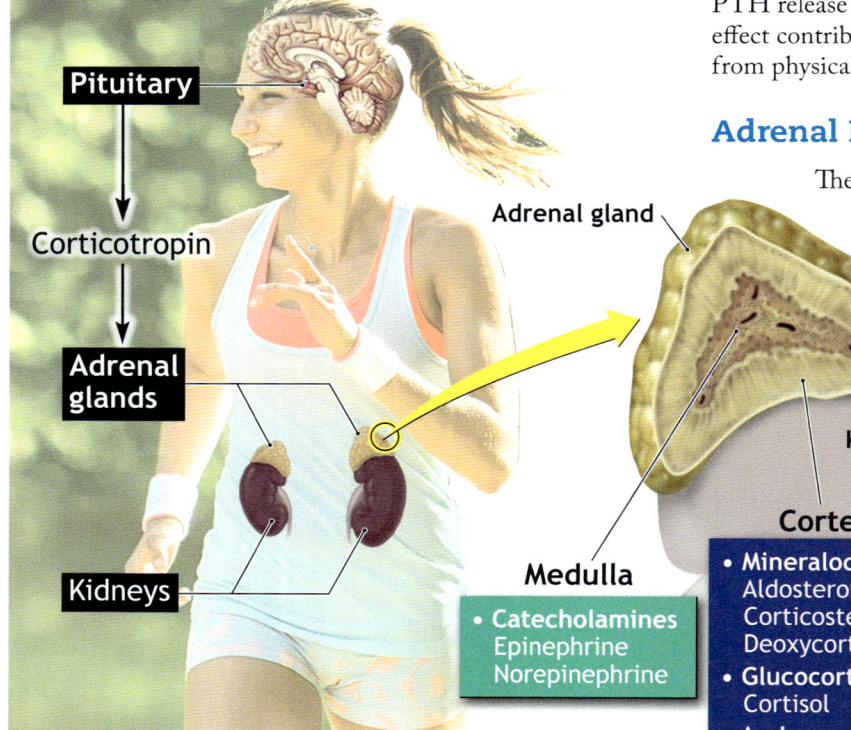

FIGURE 20.8. Adrenal gland secretions.
(BGStock72/Shutterstock)

Adrenal Medulla Hormones

The sympathetic nervous system includes the **adrenal medulla**. This gland acts to prolong and augment sympathetic effects by secreting

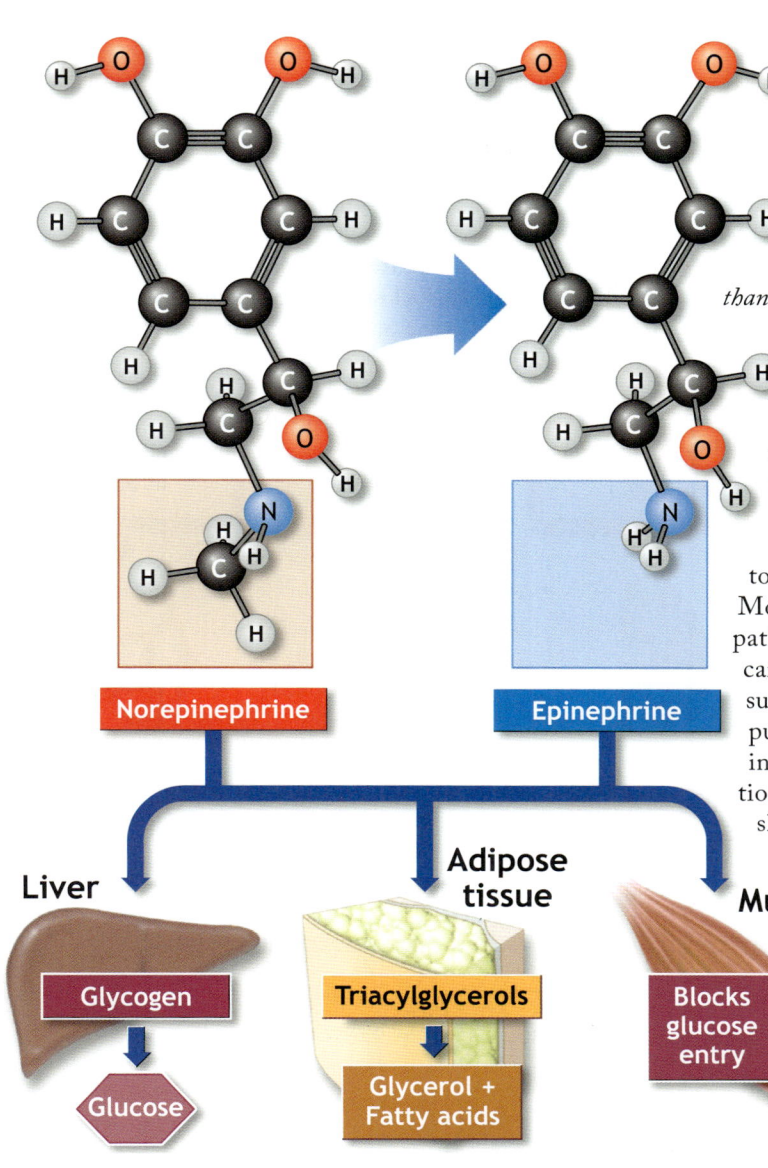

FIGURE 20.9. Chemical structure of epinephrine and norepinephrine and their role in mobilizing glucose from the liver and free fatty acids from adipose tissue (and blunting glucose uptake by skeletal muscle).

provides powerful lipolytic stimulation in adipose tissue.[44,119,169] Sympathetic nerve endings including those to the adrenal gland secrete both epinephrine and norepinephrine, so it is more appropriate to discuss the "sympathoadrenal" response to physical activity and training rather than solely an adrenal gland response. *The **sympathoadrenal response** to physical activity most closely relates to relative rather than absolute activity intensity.*

FIGURE 20.10 illustrates the catecholamine response at various increasing cycling intensities expressed as percent maximum oxygen uptake (% $\dot{V}O_{2max}$) in 10 male subjects. Norepinephrine increases markedly at % $\dot{V}O_{2max}$ intensities that exceed 50%, whereas epinephrine levels remain unchanged until cycling intensity exceeds the 75% level. At maximum effort, an approximate two- to sixfold increase in norepinephrine release occurs. More than likely, increased secretion occurs from sympathetic postganglionic nerve endings and relates to cardiovascular and metabolic adjustments in active tissues. Physical activity also increases epinephrine output from the adrenal medulla, with the magnitude of increase related directly to effort intensity and duration.[26,97,120,170] Athletes involved in sprint-power training show greater sympathoadrenergic activation during maximum exertion than counterparts trained in aerobic activity.[167] This difference relates to the higher anaerobic contribution to maximum energy supply by sprint-power athletes. Age does not affect catecholamine response to physical activity among individuals equal in aerobic fitness.[90,112] The effects of increased adrenal medulla activity on blood flow distribution, cardiac contractility, and substrate mobilization all benefit the physical activity response.

epinephrine and **norepinephrine**, hormones collectively called catecholamines. **FIGURE 20.9** shows epinephrine and norepinephrine's chemical structure and the role each plays in substrate mobilization. Norepinephrine, a hormone in its own right, serves as an epinephrine precursor and neurotransmitter when released by sympathetic nerve endings.

Epinephrine represents 80% of adrenal medulla secretions, whereas norepinephrine provides the principle neurotransmitter released from the sympathetic nervous system. Neural impulse outflow from the hypothalamus stimulates the adrenal medulla to increase catecholamine release, which affects the heart, blood vessels, and glands in the same, albeit slower-acting manner as direct sympathetic nervous system stimulation. Epinephrine's primary function in energy metabolism stimulates glycogenolysis (in the liver and active muscles) and lipolysis (in adipose tissue and active muscles), while norepinephrine

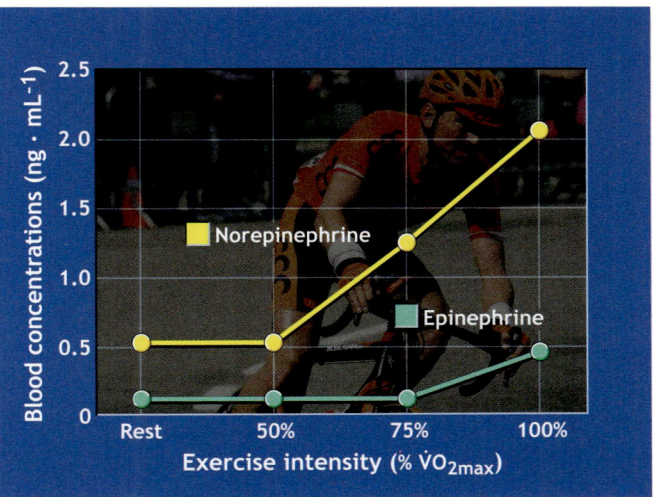

FIGURE 20.10. Catecholamine response to increasing intensity cycling in 10 male collegiate athletes.
(Data with permission from V. Katch. Applied Physiology Laboratory, University of Michigan, Ann Arbor. Maxisport/Shutterstock.)

Catecholamines Implicated in Exercise-Induced and/or Mental Fatigue. Fatigue represents an elusive concept that has important implications for exercise performance. Typically, exercise-induced fatigue can be described in many ways—tiredness, exhaustion, lethargy or weariness, extreme tiredness, and overall lack of energy—each of which promotes impairment during an acute exercise bout. Mental fatigue, coincident with exercise-induced fatigue, is a psychobiological state caused by prolonged exertion with the potential to reduce cognitive awareness to negatively impact overall exercise performance. Perhaps brain catecholamines trigger the onset of fatigue during endurance exercise, which would make the noradrenergic neurotransmitter system hasten central fatigue. This would coincide with a greater increase in perceived exertion ratings often observed during and following endurance activity. Several neurotransmitter systems might also be simultaneously involved, and the summation of such alterations might help to explain the negative impact on performance when one performs strenuous exercise in the mentally fatigued state.[209]

Adrenocortical Hormones

The **adrenal cortex**, stimulated by corticotropin from the anterior pituitary, secretes three **adrenocortical hormone** categories, the hormones of which are produced in a different adrenal cortex zone (layer):

1. **Mineralocorticoids**
2. **Glucocorticoids**
3. **Androgens**

Mineralocorticoids. As the name suggests, mineralocorticoids regulate the mineral salts sodium and potassium in the extracellular fluid, with aldosterone representing almost 95% of all mineralocorticoids.

FIGURE 20.11 shows four major controlling factors for aldosterone release from the adrenal cortex, ending with an increase in blood volume and blood pressure. Aldosterone secretion controls total sodium concentration and extracellular fluid volume. It stimulates sodium ion reabsorption along with fluid in the kidneys' distal tubules and collecting ducts by synthesizing sodium transporter proteins with little sodium or fluid lost in the urine. Increases in cardiac output and arterial blood pressure also accompany increases in plasma volume with aldosterone secretion. In contrast, sodium and water literally flow into the urine when aldosterone secretion ceases. Aldosterone also helps to stabilize serum potassium and pH because the kidneys exchange either a K^+ or H^+ for each Na^+ reabsorbed. Proper mineral balance maintains nerve transmission and muscle function. As with all steroid hormones, cellular response to increased aldosterone production occurs relatively slowly. It

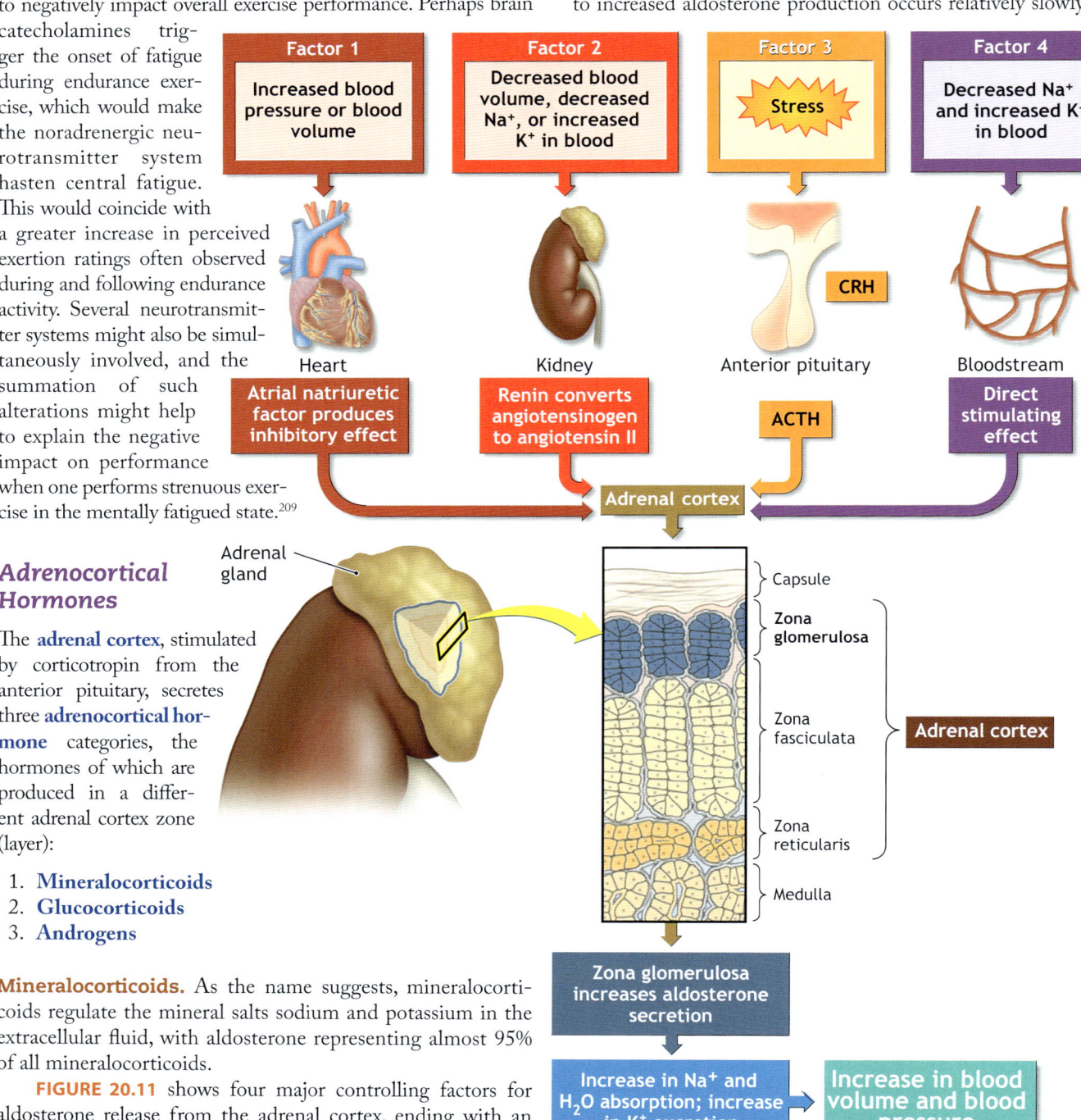

FIGURE 20.11. Major factors controlling aldosterone release from the adrenal cortex: *CRH*, corticotropin-releasing hormone; *ACTH*, adrenocorticotropic hormone.

requires physical activity to exceed 45 min for its major effects to emerge; hence, these effects occur during recovery.

Renin-Angiotensin Mechanism. The renin-angiotensin mechanism stimulates secretion of aldosterone. Increased sympathetic nervous system activity during physical activity constricts blood vessels that serve the kidneys. Reduced renal blood flow stimulates the kidneys to release the enzyme **renin** into the blood. Increased renin concentration stimulates production of two kidney hormones, **angiotensin** II and III. These hormones stimulate arterial constriction and the cortical secretion of aldosterone, which causes the kidneys to retain sodium and excrete potassium. Renal sodium absorption also conserves water, causing plasma volume to expand and blood pressure to increase.

Chronically reduced renal blood flow at rest activates the **renin-angiotensin system**. Hypertension occurs from a prolonged overresponse of this mechanism with resulting excess aldosterone output, as often occurs in teenage obesity[148] and relates to the following three factors:

1. Decreased salt sensitivity and increased water retention
2. Increased sodium intake
3. Decreased sensitivity to the effects of insulin (hyperinsulinemia)

These interrelationships suggest a direct link between obesity as a disease and subsequent adult hypertension development.[35,61]

The Renin-Angiotensin System May Promote Skeletal Muscle Atrophy. Activating the renin-angiotensin system may promote skeletal muscle atrophy in congestive heart failure, chronic kidney disease, and prolonged mechanical ventilation. Recent studies revealed that skeletal muscle fibers do express **angiotensin II type 1 receptors (AT1)**,[210,211] confirming they are more abundant in fast, type II muscle fibers compared with relatively slow, type I fibers.

Glucocorticoids. Physical activity stimulates hypothalamic secretion of **corticotropin-releasing factor**, causing the anterior pituitary to release ACTH. **Cortisol**, also known as hydrocortisone when supplied as a medication, the adrenal cortex major glucocorticoid, affects glucose, protein, and free fatty acid metabolism in six ways:

1. Promotes protein to amino acid breakdown in all cells except the liver; the circulation delivers these "liberated" amino acids to the liver to synthesize glucose by gluconeogenesis
2. Supports action of other hormones, primarily glucagon and GH in the gluconeogenic process
3. Serves as an insulin antagonist by inhibiting cellular glucose uptake and oxidation
4. Promotes triacylglycerol breakdown in adipose tissue to glycerol and fatty acids
5. Suppresses immune system function
6. Produces negative calcium balance

FIGURE 20.12 shows the factors that affect cortisol secretion and its effects on target tissues, which include adipose tissue,

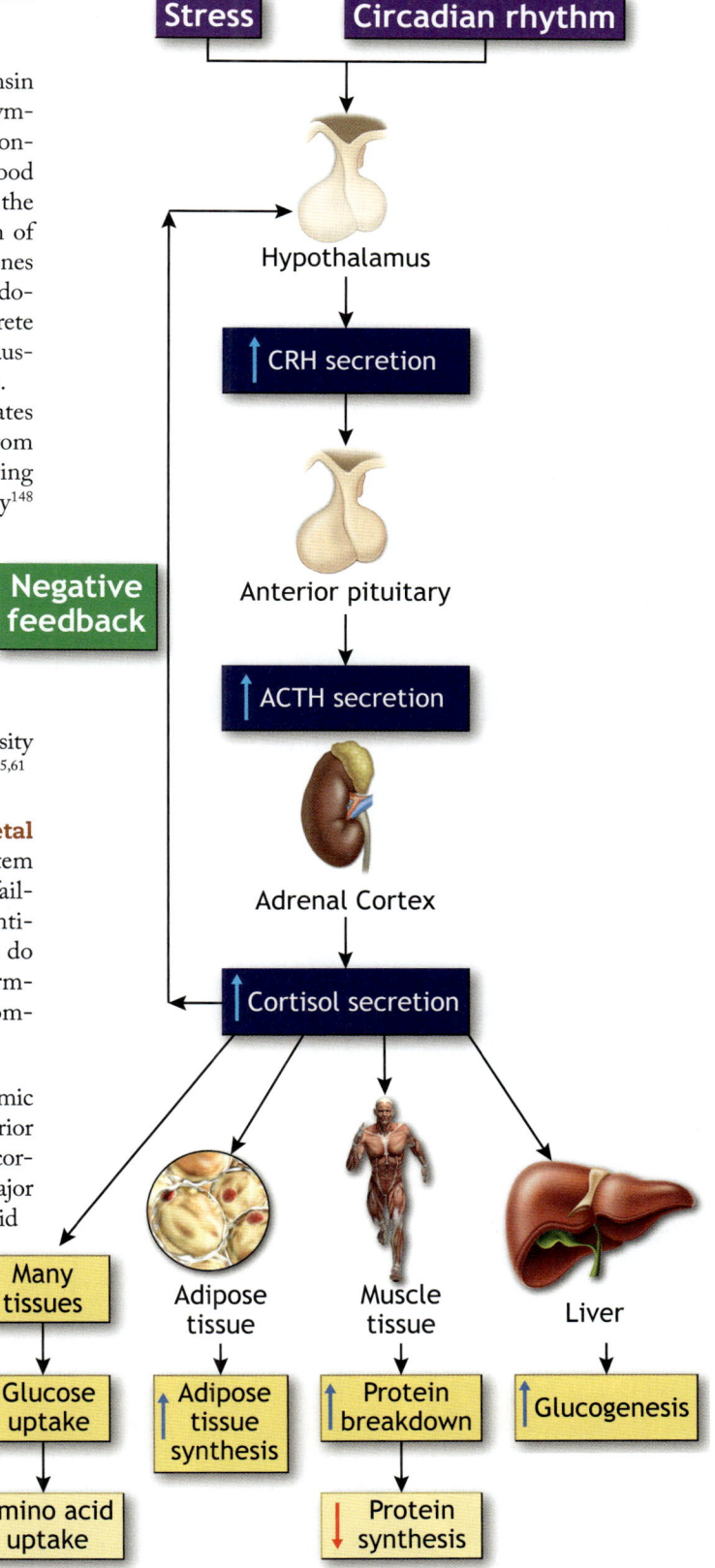

FIGURE 20.12. Factors that affect cortisol secretions and its actions on target tissues. *CRH*, corticotropic releasing hormone; *ACTH*, adrenocorticotropic hormone.
(Shutterstock: Kateryna Kon; Treestons; OrangeVector.)

muscle tissue, and the liver. A strong **diurnal pattern** governs cortisol secretion. Secretions normally peak in the morning and subside at night. Cortisol secretion increases with stress, hence the popular name "stress" hormone. Even though considered a catabolic hormone, cortisol's important effect counters hypoglycemia and is thus essential for life. Animals whose adrenal glands have been removed die if exposed to severe environmental stress. Cortisol exerts a facilitating effect required for full activity of glucagon and the catecholamine hormones.

Chronically high-serum cortisol levels initiate excessive protein breakdown, tissue wasting, and negative nitrogen balance. Cortisol secretion also accelerates lipid mobilization for energy during starvation and prolonged but intense physical activity. With rapid and large increases in cortisol output, the liver splits mobilized lipid into its simple ketoacid components. Excess ketoacid concentrations in the extracellular fluid can lead to the potentially dangerous metabolic state of ketosis (a form of acidosis). Individuals who subsist on very-low-carbohydrate, low-calorie weight-loss diets (*ketogenic diets*; see Chapter 30) can experience ketosis, augmented by elevated cortisol secretion.

Cortisol turnover, the difference between its production and removal, provides a way to study cortisol response to physical activity, which exhibits considerable variability with effort intensity, fitness level, nutritional status, and circadian rhythm.[33,172] Cortisol output increases as exercise intensity increases, which accelerates lipolysis, ketogenesis, and proteolysis. Extremely high cortisol levels occur following marathon running or other, weight-bearing endurance activities[158] and resistance training.[78,143] Plasma cortisol concentration also rises during prolonged-duration moderate physical activity. Highly trained runners maintain a state of hypercortisolism that heightens before competition or intense training.[48,84] Cortisol levels also remain elevated for up to 2 hr following an endurance activity.[189] This suggests that cortisol plays a role in tissue recovery and repair. Unlike the direct, active metabolic effect of epinephrine and glucagon on fuel homeostasis, cortisol exerts a more facilitating effect on substrate use.

Androgens. The reproductive organs (gonads) provide the major source of the so-called sex steroids, but the adrenal cortex produces androgen hormones (gonadocorticoids) with similar actions. For example, the adrenal cortex produces **dehydroepiandrosterone**, which exerts effects similar to the dominant male hormone testosterone. Treatment with dehydroepiandrosterone in women with adrenal insufficiency improves well-being and sexual responsiveness and decreases depression and anxiety compared to placebo treatment. The adrenal cortex also produces some of the "female" hormones estrogen and progesterone.

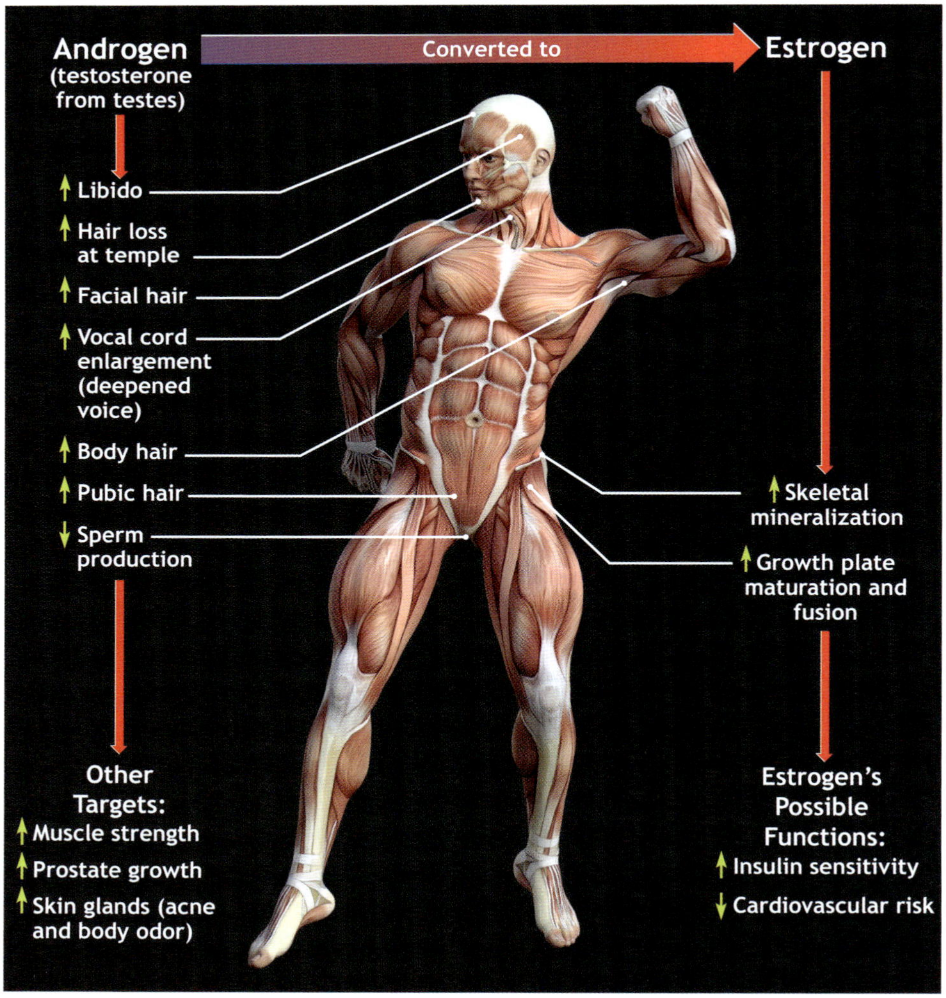

Gonadal Hormones

The male testes and female ovaries are endocrine reproductive glands that release hormones that promote sex-specific physical characteristics and initiate and maintain reproductive function. No distinctly "male" or "female" hormones exist, but rather general differences in hormone concentrations between the sexes. **Testosterone** represents the most important androgen secreted by the testes' interstitial cells. **FIGURE 20.13** shows that among its many functions testosterone initiates sperm production and stimulates development of male secondary sex characteristics by increasing facial, pubic, and body hair, vocal cord enlargement, and altered voice patterns. Testosterone's anabolic, tissue-building role contributes to male-female differences in muscle mass and strength that emerge at puberty onset. Some androgen converts to estrogen in peripheral tissues under aromatase

FIGURE 20.13. Androgen (testosterone) contributes to male secondary sex characteristics and sex differences in muscle mass and strength at puberty onset.
(Valentyna Chukhlyebova/Shutterstock.)

enzyme control (Chapter 2) and gives males a considerable edge over females in maintaining bone mass throughout life.[64]

Estradiol and Progesterone

The ovaries are the primary estrogen source, particularly for **estradiol** and **progesterone**. Estrogens regulate ovulation, menstruation, and physiologic adjustments during pregnancy. Estrogen circulating in the bloodstream and generated locally in peripheral tissues also exerts effects on blood vessels, bone, lungs, liver, intestine, prostate, and testes through action on α- and β-receptor proteins.

Progesterone contributes specific regulatory input to the female reproductive cycle, uterine smooth muscle action, and lactation. Controversy exists concerning estrogen and progesterone's role in substrate metabolism during physical activity.[4,122,123] Estradiol-17β (biologically active estrogen synthesized from cholesterol) increases free fatty acid mobilization from adipose tissue and inhibits glucose uptake by peripheral tissues. In this way, the increases in estradiol-17β and GH during physical activity exert similar metabolic influences.

Testosterone

Plasma testosterone concentration commonly serves as a physiologic marker to characterize anabolic status. In addition to its direct effect on muscle tissue synthesis, testosterone indirectly affects a muscle fiber's protein content by promoting GH release, leading to IGF synthesis and release from the liver. Testosterone also interacts with neural receptors to increase neurotransmitter release and initiate structural protein changes that alter neuromuscular junction size. These neural facilitating effects can enhance a skeletal muscle's force-production capabilities.

Testosterone's effect on the cell nucleus remains controversial. More than likely, a transport protein (sex-hormone–binding globulin) delivers testosterone to target tissues, after which testosterone associates with a membrane-bound or cytosolic receptor. It subsequently migrates to the cell nucleus, where it interacts with nuclear receptors to initiate protein synthesis. Plasma testosterone concentration in females, although only one tenth that in males, increases with physical activity.[111] Physical activity also elevates estradiol and progesterone levels. In untrained males, resistance exercise and moderate aerobic activity after 15 to 20 min increase serum and free testosterone levels.[83] Findings remain equivocal concerning intense endurance exercise effect on testosterone levels.[143,178]

FIGURE 20.14 shows the plasma cortisol and testosterone pattern 4 hr before swimming and immediately following 15 × 200 m freestyle at the swimmer's competitive velocity, with a 20 s rest between swims and 1 hr into recovery. Four 6-wk periods formed the training program, with careful monitoring of training volume. The results show that postexercise cortisol (top left inset) and testosterone (bottom left inset) remain elevated. Values remained higher 1 hr after physical activity, except for testosterone levels in training weeks 6 through 12 and 18 through 24. The generalized decrease in cortisol and testosterone concentrations when the swimmers "peaked" for the championships (weeks 18 to 24) indicates long-term adaptation for these hormones, not the immediate result from excess stress induced by overtraining and poor performance. The depressed performance during weeks 18 through 24 probably indicates overtraining; this period corresponds to a large training volume increase. Chapter 21 provides an in-depth discussion about overtraining and its related syndrome.

INTEGRATIVE QUESTION

Knowing that hormones play crucial roles in normal growth and development and physiologic function regulation, what are some specific examples of why supplementing with an excess of these chemicals is not necessarily better but actually may be harmful?

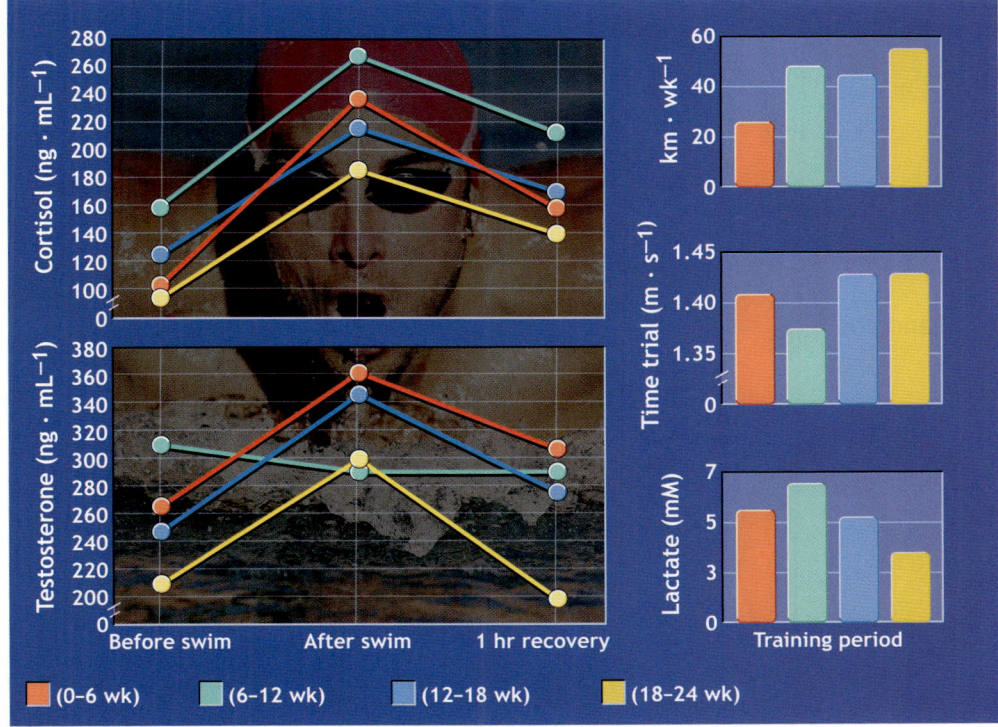

FIGURE 20.14. Plasma cortisol and testosterone concentrations measured at three time intervals (4 hr before swimming, immediately after multiple sprint-swims, and after 1-hr recovery) over a 24-wk swim-training season.
(Adapted with permission from Bonifazi M, et al. Blood levels of exercise during the training season. In: Miyashita M, et al., eds. *Medicine and Science in Aquatic Sports*. Basel, Switzerland: Karger; 1994. Copyright © 1994 Karger Publishers, Basel, Switzerland. Background photo: Maridav/Shutterstock.)

Testosterone Imposter Supplement Use Not Supported by Research

Approximately 50% of American adults consume dietary supplements to try and promote overall health and fill perceived dietary gaps. For men, testosterone (T)-boosting supplements (T-boosters) to improve T levels represents the major supplement purchased without a physician's prescription.

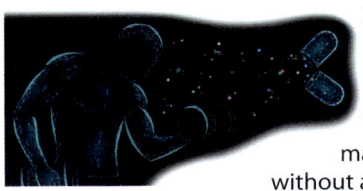
LuckyStep/Shutterstock

There are over 50 different T-booster supplements touted on the Internet each year with different active ingredients and product claims. Recent research evaluated the compositional quality and advertised claims for "T-boosting" supplements with published research evidence. Ninety percent claimed to boost "low T," 50% to "improve libido," and 48% to "feel stronger." In one study, more than 109 unique components were found in the different T-boost supplements evaluated, with 8.3 compounds per product! On PubMed, only 24.8% (27 of 109 individual supplements) had data showing an increase in T, 10.1% had data showing a decrease in T, and 18.3% had no data to show a change in T. The typical supplement contained 1291% of the vitamin B_{12} RDA, 807.6% for vitamin B_6, 272% for zinc, 200% for vitamin B_5, and 187.5% for vitamin B_3. Thirteen products exceeded the U.S. Food and Drug Administration's UL allotment for zinc, vitamin B_3, and magnesium. It seems reasonable that individuals be informed that "T-booster" supplements may not contain ingredients to support their claims and may contain vitamins and minerals above recommended amounts.

Sources:
Balasubramanian A, et al. Testosterone Imposters: An analysis of popular online testosterone boosting supplements. *J Sex Med*. 2019;16:203.
Clemesha CG, et al. Testosterone boosting' supplements composition and claims are not supported by the academic literature. *World J Men's Health*. 2020;38:115.

Pancreatic Hormones

The pancreas gland, approximately 14 cm/5.5 in long and weighing about 60 g/0.132 lb, lies just below the stomach on the posterior abdominal wall. The pancreas has two different tissue types, **acini** and **islets of Langerhans**, the latter named for German pathologist and anatomist Paul Langerhans (1847–1888; www.ncbi.nlm.nih.gov/pmc/articles/PMC1769627/), who first described these cell clusters in 1869 (**FIG. 20.15**). The islets contain about 20% α-cells that secrete glucagon, 75% β-cells that secrete insulin and the peptide **amylin**. The remaining cells are somatostatin-secreting D and PP cells that produce pancreatic polypeptide. The acini serve an exocrine function and secrete digestive enzymes.

Insulin

Insulin regulates glucose entry into all tissues (primarily muscle and adipose) except the brain. Insulin's action aids **facilitated diffusion**, where glucose combines with a carrier protein on the cell's plasma membrane for transport into cells. In this way, insulin regulates glucose metabolism. Any glucose not immediately catabolized for energy either stores as glycogen or synthesizes to triacylglycerol. Without insulin, severely limited glucose enters the cells. **FIGURE 20.16A** illustrates that insulin's anabolic functions promote glycogen, protein, and lipid synthesis. Figure 20.16B outlines insulin's actions on most tissues including specific effects on adipose tissue, liver, and muscle.

See the animation "Insulin Functions" on Lippincott Connect for a demonstration of insulin's activity.

Following a meal, insulin-mediated glucose uptake by cells (and correspondingly reduced hepatic glucose output) decreases blood glucose levels. In essence, insulin exerts a hypoglycemic effect by reducing blood glucose concentration. Conversely, with insufficient insulin secretion or depressed insulin sensitivity, blood glucose concentration can increase from a normal level of about 90 $mg \cdot dL^{-1}$ to a high of 350 $mg \cdot dL^{-1}$

FIGURE 20.15. Pancreatic hormone secretions and actions. (Shutterstock: Liya Graphics; OrangeVector.)

When blood glucose levels remain high, glucose ultimately spills into the urine. Without insulin, fatty acids metabolize as the primary energy substrate.

Insulin also exerts a pronounced effect on lipid synthesis. A rise in blood glucose levels normally occurs following a meal and stimulates insulin release. This causes fat cells to uptake some glucose for triacylglycerol synthesis. Insulin's action also triggers intracellular enzyme activity to facilitate protein synthesis by three possible actions:

1. Increasing amino acid transport through the cell's plasma membrane
2. Increasing cellular RNA levels
3. Increasing protein formation by ribosomes

Transporters to Facilitate Glucose Entry into Cells. Cells possess different glucose transport proteins, termed **glucose transporters (GLUTs)**, depending on the variation in insulin and glucose concentrations.[110,151] Muscle fibers contain GLUT-1 and GLUT-4, with most glucose entering by the GLUT-1 carrier during rest. With high blood glucose or insulin concentrations following eating or during physical activity, muscle cells receive glucose by the insulin-dependent GLUT-4 transporter. GLUT-4 action occurs through a second messenger, which permits migration of the intracellular GLUT-4 protein to the cell surface to promote glucose uptake. The fact that GLUT-4 moves to the cell surface through a separate, insulin-independent mechanism coincides with observations that active muscles can absorb glucose *without* insulin.

Glucose–Insulin Interaction. Blood glucose levels within the pancreas directly control insulin secretion and elevated glucose levels trigger insulin release. This, in turn, causes glucose entry into cells (lowering blood glucose), removing the stimulus for further insulin release. In contrast, a decrease in blood glucose concentration dramatically lowers blood insulin levels to provide a favorable state to increase blood glucose

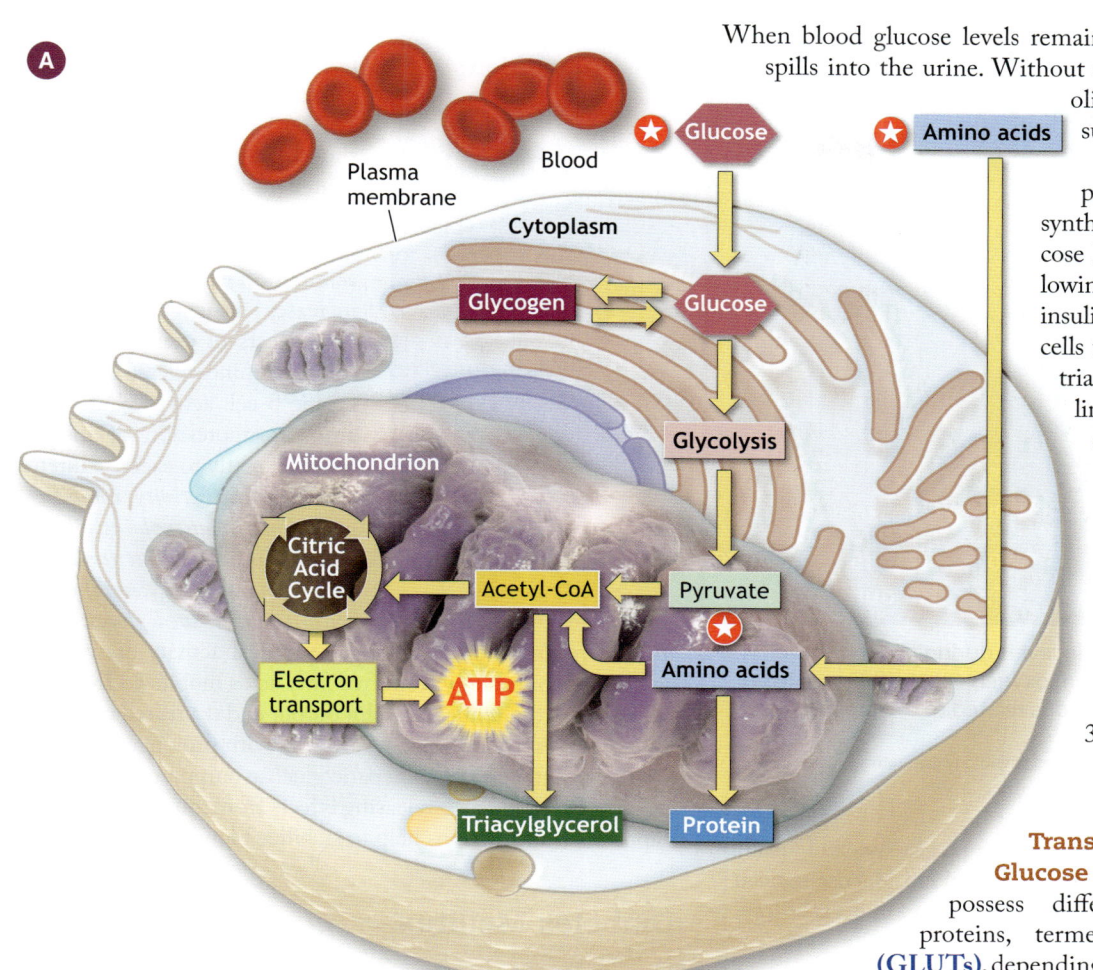

FIGURE 20.16. (A) Insulin's primary functions in the body. The symbol ⭐ shows where insulin exerts its influence in metabolism. **(B)** Target tissues and specific metabolic responses to insulin's action. The anabolic functions of increased insulin promote glycogen, protein, and lipid synthesis.
(Shutterstock: Kateryna Kon; Mitar Vidakovic.)

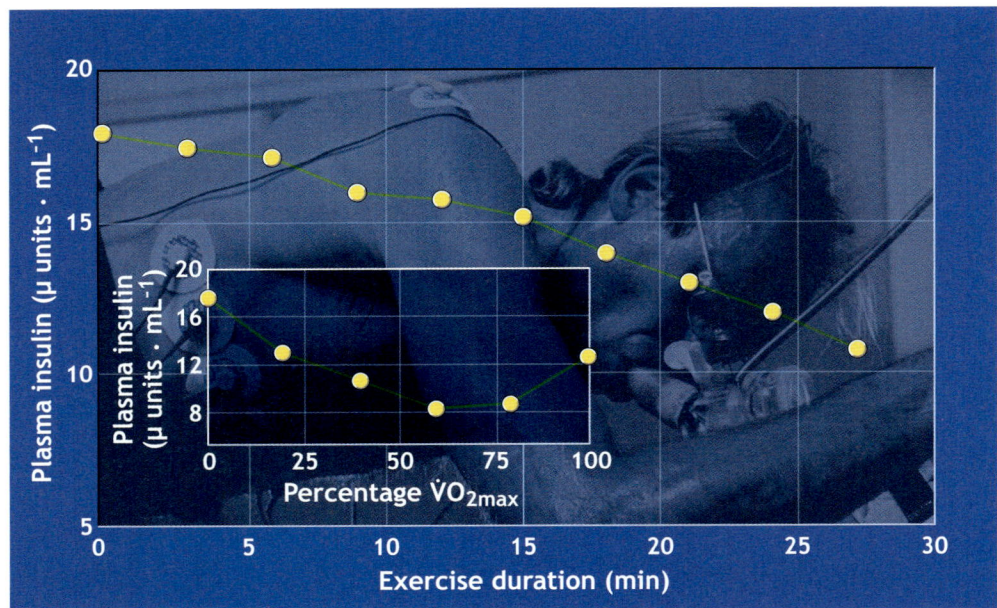

FIGURE 20.17. Plasma insulin levels during cycle ergometry for 30 min at 70% of maximum oxygen uptake ($\dot{V}O_{2max}$). **Inset** data show insulin concentrations related to cycling intensity at percentage $\dot{V}O_{2max}$.
(Data with permission from V. Katch. Applied Physiology Laboratory, University of Michigan, Ann Arbor.)

FIGURE 20.17 relates plasma insulin concentration to physical activity duration for cycling at 70% $\dot{V}O_{2max}$. The inset graph shows plasma insulin response related to exercise intensity (% $\dot{V}O_{2max}$). The decreased insulin concentration below rest values as duration extends or intensity increases results from inhibitory effects of exercise-induced catecholamine release on pancreatic β-cell activity. Catecholamine's suppression of insulin relates directly to exercise intensity. *Physical activity inhibition of insulin output explains why no excessive insulin release (and possible rebound hypoglycemia) occurs with a concentrated glucose feeding during the activity.* Prolonged physical activity draws progressively more energy from free fatty acids mobilized from the adipocytes from reduced insulin output and decreased carbohydrate reserves. Blood glucose lowering with prolonged physical activity directly enhances hepatic glucose output and sensitizes the liver to the glucose-releasing effects from glucagon and epinephrine, whose actions help to stabilize blood glucose levels.

concentration. The interaction between glucose and insulin serves as a feedback loop to maintain blood glucose concentration within narrow limits. Rising plasma amino acid levels also increase insulin secretion.

Diabetes Mellitus

Diabetes mellitus consists of subgroups of disorders with different pathophysiologies. Type 1 and type 2 diabetes are heterogeneous diseases in which clinical presentation and disease progression vary considerably. Classification is crucial in determining therapy strategy, but some individuals cannot be clearly classified as having type 1 or type 2 diabetes as their diagnosis.

Diabetes Classifications

Diabetes mellitus can be classified into four general categories:

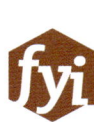 **High Anabolic Steroid Doses Cause Adverse Cardiovascular Side Effects Including Endothelial Cell Dysfunction**

To investigate the effects of supra-physiological testosterone doses on endothelial production of nitric oxide (NO) and oxidative stress, *in vitro* (a process taking place in a test tube, culture dish, or elsewhere outside a living organism) and *in vivo* (process performed or taking place in a living organism) testosterone enanthate was administered as a single 500 mg dose to 27 healthy volunteers. *In vivo* results showed that urinary NO levels and antioxidative capacity were significantly decreased 2 days after testosterone administration. Also, the *in vitro* studies showed that testosterone inhibited endothelial NO synthase (eNOS) gene expression 48 hr later. Supraphysiological testosterone doses may induce endothelial cell dysfunction, which may partly explain the cardiovascular system's adverse side effects observed among anabolic-androgenic steroid abusers.

Aleksandra Gigowska/Shutterstock

Source:
Skogastierna C, et al. A supraphysiological dose of testosterone induces nitric oxide production and oxidative stress. *Eur J Prev Cardiol.* 2014;21:1049.

1. **Type 1 diabetes** (due to autoimmune β-cell destruction, usually leading to absolute insulin deficiency); often develops early in life and represents 5 to 10% of the diabetic population
2. **Type 2 diabetes** (from a progressive decrease in adequate β-cell insulin secretion frequently with insulin resistance); often develops in adult life and associates with obesity, poor dietary practices, and sedentary living
3. **Gestational diabetes mellitus** (diagnosed in the second or third pregnancy trimester; not clearly overt diabetes before gestation)
4. **Specific diabetes types from other causes**, for example, monogenic diabetes syndromes (neonatal diabetes and maturity-onset diabetes in the young), exocrine pancreatic diseases (cystic fibrosis and pancreatitis), and drug-induced or chemical-induced diabetes (from glucocorticoid use, HIV/AIDS treatment, or following organ transplantation)

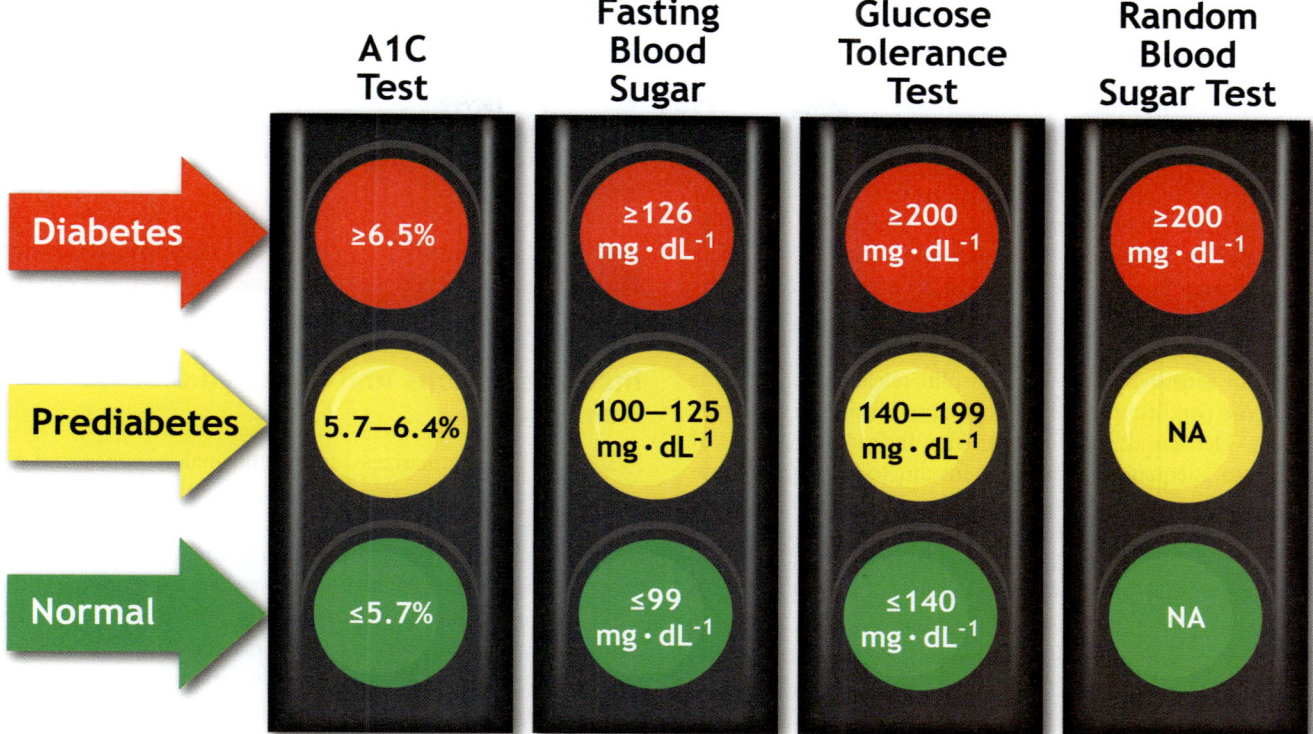

iD_studio/Shutterstock

In both type 1 and type 2 diabetes, various genetic and environmental factors can produce progressive loss of β-cell mass and/or normal function that manifests clinically as hyperglycemia (diagnosed as a fasting blood glucose ≥125 mg · dL^{-1} or blood glucose ≥200 mg · dL^{-1} 2 hr following an oral glucose-tolerance test). Once hyperglycemia is diagnosed, patients are at risk for developing chronic complications, although progression rates vary considerably. The identification of individualized diabetic therapies requires better identification of the paths to β-cell demise or dysfunction.

The most prevalent diabetes symptoms are as follows:

1. Glucose in urine (**glycosuria**)
2. Frequent urination (**polyuria**)
3. Excessive thirst (**polydipsia**)
4. Extreme hunger (**polyphagia**)
5. Unexplained weight loss
6. Increased fatigue
7. Irritability
8. Blurry vision
9. Hands, feet numbness or tingling
10. Slow-healing wounds or sores
11. Abnormally high infection frequency

Diabetes Diagnostic Tests

Different tests diagnose diabetes, including the laboratory-based glucose and insulin clamp methodology, an oral glucose-tolerance test, a simple 8-hr fasting plasma glucose test, and the hemoglobin HbA1c test.

The image below shows cut-off values for different diagnostic tests to determine diabetes mellitus.

Reducing Type 2 Diabetes Risk

Research has confirmed that up to 80 to 90% of type 2 diabetes can be avoided by implementing these lifestyle behavioral changes.

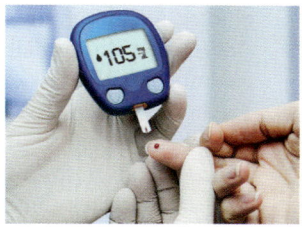

Proxima Studio/Shutterstock

1. Lose excess weight particularly those with excess abdominal fat; at least 80% of diabetics are overweight or obese.
2. Increase daily physical activity.
3. Eliminate *trans* fatty acid and increase polyunsaturated fatty acid and omega-3 fatty acid intake.
4. Lower glycemic load by increasing intake of fiber-rich, unrefined carbohydrates and reducing intake of sugar-laden drinks, and refined breads, cereals, and grains.
5. Increase intake of green leafy vegetables and whole fruit.
6. Decrease intake of foods high in heme iron (e.g., red meats and particularly processed meats) by substituting nonheme iron foods from plants.
7. Maintain moderate coffee and alcohol consumption.
8. Control stress.
9. Lower blood pressure.

Source:
https://www.diabetes.org/diabetes-risk/prevention

1. **Glucose-clamp test** is a method to quantify insulin secretion and the body's resistance to it. The technique measures either how well an individual metabolizes glucose or how sensitive an individual is to insulin's effect. The procedure involves maintaining insulin at a constant, above-normal blood concentration using infusion technology (termed hyperinsulinemic clamp). Once insulin stabilizes at the higher level, the body's glucose use is measured by infusing a known glucose amount into the patient's blood. The clamp maintains blood glucose at a near-normal concentration with insulin production measured. A large glucose uptake for a given insulin concentration reflects increased insulin sensitivity. Increased insulin release to a constant glucose condition relates to augmented insulin responsiveness. Decreased insulin sensitivity indicates inability of cells to adequately respond to insulin to increase glucose uptake. Type 2 diabetes commonly reflects inadequacies in either insulin receptors or cellular response to insulin binding (i.e., a relative insulin resistance). Decreased insulin responsiveness indicates impaired β-cell function evident in some type 2 diabetics and the primary cause in type 1 diabetes. The term *impaired fasting glucose* (IFG) indicates fasting blood glucose values of ≥ 100 mg·dL^{-1} (5.6 mmol·L^{-1}), but less than 126 mg·dL^{-1} (7 mmol·L^{-1}).
2. **Oral glucose-tolerance test** evaluates blood sugar levels 2 hr after drinking 75 g in a concentrated glucose solution. Diabetes is confirmed by delayed ingested glucose removal. The term *impaired glucose tolerance* (IGT) indicates a 2-hr glucose clearance between ≥ 140 mg·dL^{-1} (7.8 mmol·L^{-1}) but less than 200 mg·dL^{-1} (11.1 mmol·mL^{-1}).
3. **Fasting plasma glucose (FPG) test** measures plasma glucose following an 8 hr fast. The American Diabetes Association (www.diabetes.org/a1c/diagnosis) currently recommends the FPG test for suspected type 2 diabetes.
4. The **hemoglobin A1c test (HbA1c)**, also known as the glycated hemoglobin or glycohemoglobin test. With uncontrolled blood glucose, the extra glucose enters red blood cells and glycates (links up) with hemoglobin molecules (www.webmd.com/diabetes/guide/glycated-hemoglobin-test-hba1c). The more excess glucose in blood, the more hemoglobin becomes glycated. In the body, red blood cells constantly form and die, but typically remain for about 3 mo. The A1c test reflects the average of a person's blood glucose levels over the past 3 mo. Test results are reported as a percentage for glucose bound to Hb; the higher the percentage, the higher the blood glucose levels. An A1c level between 5.7 and 6.4% suggests prediabetes. A1c levels below $\leq 5.7\%$ are considered normal.

Diabetes on the Rise

Despite efforts to reduce diabetes incidence, the numbers continue to rise, as diabetes management costs spiral out of control (www.cdc.gov/diabetes/data/index.html). The current diabetes prevalence rates are discouraging—26.9 million people of all ages or 8.2% of the US population had diagnosed diabetes—and suggest that a concerted national public health initiative is required to reduce this disease, particularly in areas with extraordinarily high disease incidence.

 See the animation "Diabetes" on **Lippincott Connect** for an explanation of this disorder and its causes.

Insulin's Actions and Impaired Glucose Homeostasis

FIGURE 20.18 summarizes insulin's normal response and the response under insulin-resistant and type 2 diabetes conditions. The increase in blood glucose concentration following a meal induces insulin release from the islets of Langerhans' β cells. Insulin then migrates in the blood to target cells throughout the body, where it binds to receptor molecules on the cell surface. Insulin-receptor interaction triggers events within the cell that enhance glucose uptake and promote catabolism or storage as glycogen and/or lipid. A defect along the glucose uptake pathway indicates seven possible diabetes causes:

1. β-cell destruction
2. Abnormal insulin synthesis
3. Depressed insulin release
4. Insulin inactivation in blood by antibodies or other blocking agents
5. Altered insulin receptors or decreased receptor number on peripheral cells
6. Defective insulin message processing within the target cells
7. Abnormal glucose metabolism

Type 1 Diabetes

The table below lists the three type 1 diabetes stages.

Type 1 diabetes, formerly called juvenile-onset or child-onset diabetes, typically occurs in younger individuals and represents between 5 and 10% of all diabetes cases (www.nlm.nih.gov/medlineplus/diabetestype1.html). This diabetes form represents an autoimmune response, possibly

Type 1 Diabetes Stages

	Stage 1	Stage 2	Stage 3
Characteristics	• Autoimmunity • Normoglycemia • Presymptomatic	• Autoimmunity • Dysglycemia • Presymptomatic	• New-onset hyperglycemia • Symptomatic
Diagnostic criteria	• Multiple auto-antibodies except IGT or IFG	• Multiple auto-antibodies • Dysglycemia: IFG and/or IGT • FPG 100–125 mg·dL^{-1} • 2-hr PG 140–199 mg·dL^{-1} (7.8–11.0 mmol·L^{-1}) • A1C 5.7–6.4% (39–47 mmol·mol^{-1}) or $\geq 10\%$ A1C increase	• Clinical symptoms • Diabetes by standard criteria

FPG, fasting plasma glucose; IFG, impaired fasting glucose; IGT, impaired glucose tolerance; PG, plasma glucose.
Source: ADA. Classification and Diagnosis of Diabetes: Standards of Medical Care in Diabetes—2020. *Diabetes Care*. 2020;43(suppl 1):S14. Background image: Ezume Images/Shutterstock

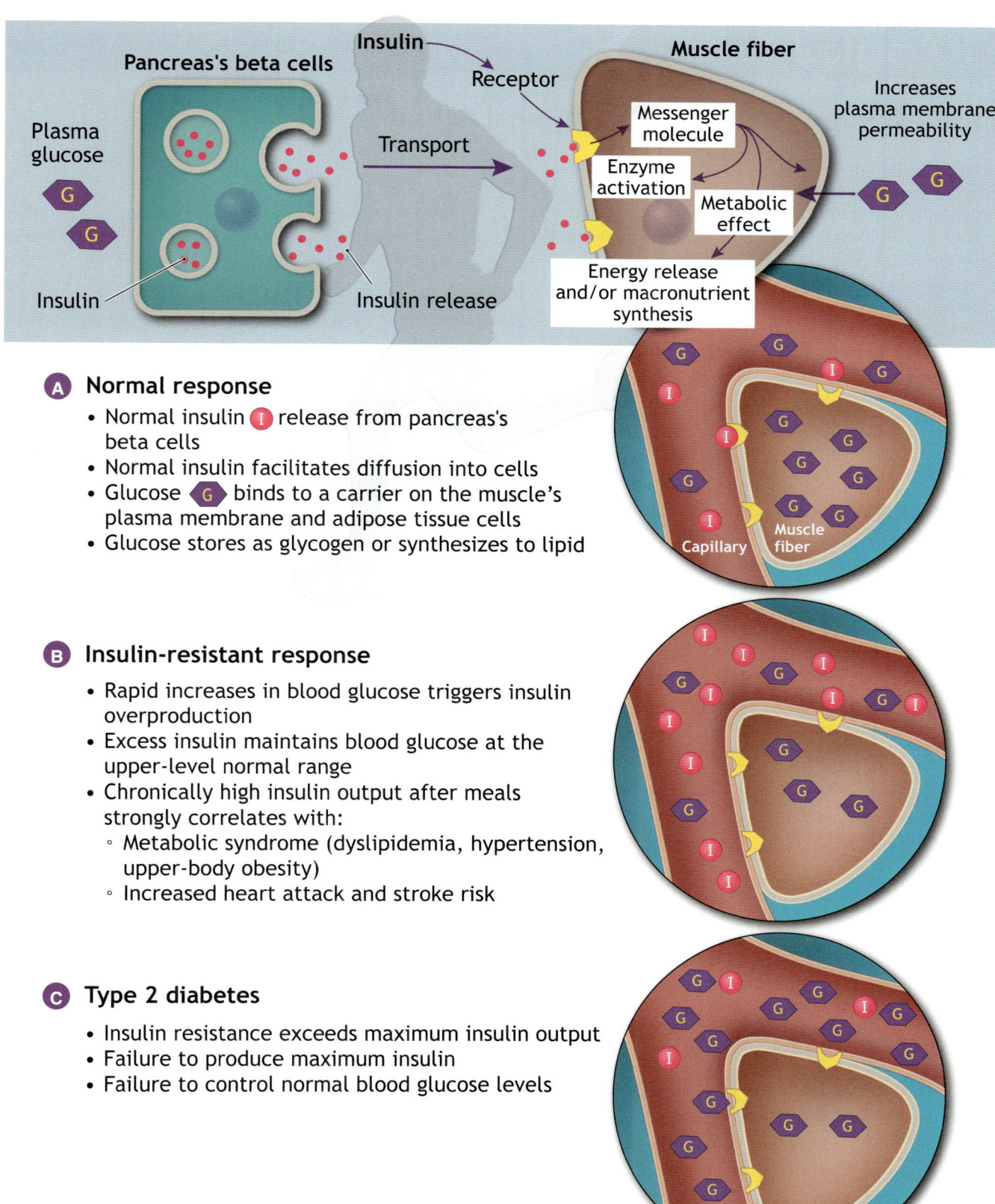

FIGURE 20.18. (A) Normal insulin-glucose interaction, (B) with insulin resistance, and (C) with type 2 diabetes.

In a Practical Sense

Diabetes, Hypoglycemia, and Physical Activity

Persons with type 1 or type 2 diabetes should exercise regularly as part of a comprehensive treatment regimen. Hypoglycemia represents the major risk of physical activity for individuals who take insulin or oral hypoglycemic agents. A physically active diabetic person needs to pay particular attention to the following:

1. Hypoglycemia warning signs
2. Immediate response to a hypoglycemic attack
3. Late-onset hypoglycemia treatment

HYPOGLYCEMIA WARNING SIGNS

Symptoms of moderate and severe hypoglycemia (see Table) result from inadequate glucose supply to the brain. In general, hypoglycemic symptoms appear only after blood glucose concentration drops below 60 mg · dL^{-1}.

Warning Signs of Hypoglycemia

Mild hypoglycemic reactions
- Trembling or shakiness
- Nervousness
- Rapid heart rate
- Palpitation
- Increased sweating
- Excessive hunger

Moderate hypoglycemic reactions
- Headache, irritability, and abrupt mood changes
- Impaired concentration and attentiveness
- Mental confusion
- Drowsiness

Severe hypoglycemic reactions
- Unresponsiveness
- Unconsciousness and coma
- Convulsions

donskarpo/Shutterstock

Low blood glucose symptoms vary considerably. Some diabetic persons with autonomic neuropathy who lose ability to secrete adrenalinelike hormones in response to hypoglycemia experience hypoglycemic unawareness. They require regular blood glucose monitoring during and after physical activity. Individuals who take β-blocker medication also have increased hypoglycemic unawareness risk.

HYPOGLYCEMIA ATTACK: WHAT TO DO

Respond quickly: Hypoglycemic reactions appear suddenly and progress rapidly

1. Stop exercising: Test blood glucose to confirm hypoglycemia
2. Eat or drink carbohydrate immediately (consume 10 to 15 g or 2 to 3 tsp simple sugar). A diabetic person should always carry high-glycemic carbohydrate while exercising (e.g., hard candy, sugar cubes, raisins, juice). Consuming ice cream or chocolates is a poor choice because its high lipid content depresses the glycemic index and impedes glucose absorption.
3. Rest 10 to 15 min to allow for intestinal glucose absorption. Test blood glucose levels before resuming physical activity. If blood glucose registers below 100 mg · dL^{-1}, do not exercise but eat more sugar-rich foods.
4. Remeasure blood glucose following physical activity. After resuming activity, pay close attention to further hypoglycemic signs. If possible, measure blood glucose within 30 to 45 min.
5. Replenish carbohydrate immediately following physical activity with complex carbohydrates. Be prepared to administer glucagon subcutaneously to boost glucose levels.

LATE-ONSET HYPOGLYCEMIA

Late-onset hypoglycemia describes excessively low blood glucose for more than 4 hr (and up to 48 hr) after physical activity. It occurs more frequently in new exercisers or after a strenuous workout. Insulin sensitivity remains high for 24 to 48 hr after physical activity, so late-onset hypoglycemia poses a particular problem for many medicated diabetics. The following four precautions can guard against late-onset hypoglycemia:

- Adjust insulin dosage or other medication before starting physical activity. If needed, increase food intake before and during activity.
- If activity lasts beyond 45 min, monitor blood glucose at 2-hr intervals for 12 hr into recovery or until sleep. Consider reducing insulin or oral hypoglycemic agents until bedtime. Before retiring, eat some low-glycemic food to increase blood glucose levels.
- Use caution when initiating a physical activity program. Start slowly and gradually increase effort intensity and duration over a 3- to 6-wk period.
- If planning activity longer than 45 to 60 min, exercise with a friend who can assist in case of an emergency. Always carry snacks and important phone numbers (doctor, hospital, home) and wear a medical ID bracelet.

ADJUSTING INSULIN LEVELS

For intense physical activity, consider the following:

- Intermediate-acting insulin: Decrease dose by 30 to 35% on the exercise day
- Intermediate- and short-acting insulin: Omit dose if it normally precedes physical activity
- Multiple short-acting insulin doses: Reduce the dose before exercise by 30% and supplement with carbohydrate-rich foods
- Continuous subcutaneous insulin infusion: Eliminate mealtime bolus or insulin increment that precedes or follows physical activity
- Avoid exercising for 1 hr using the muscles that receive the short-acting insulin injection
- Avoid exercising in late evening

Source:
Izquierdo M, et al. International exercise recommendations in older adults (ICFSR): expert consensus guidelines. *J Nutr Health Aging*. 2021;25:824.

from a single protein that renders the β cells incapable of producing insulin and often other pancreatic hormones. Type 1 diabetic patients present a more severe abnormality for glucose homeostasis than individuals in the type 2 subgroup. Physical activity exerts more pronounced effects on the metabolic state in type 1 individuals, and the management of exercise-related problems requires greater attention (see In a Practical Sense: Diabetes, Hypoglycemia, and Physical Activity).

Type 2 Diabetes

Type 2 diabetes tends to occur after age 40, but a sharp increase now occurs in much younger individuals, often less than age 10. This new trend indicates that type 2 diabetes may represent a "pediatric disease" since diabetes has more than tripled over the last 3 to 5 years among children. Physicians consider the spiraling rate of childhood obesity—particularly among African Americans, Native Americans, and Hispanics (most notably children of Mexican descent)—as the predominant factor to explain type 2 diabetes in children. The disease accounts for nearly 95% of all diabetes cases in the United States and is now the leading cause of death from the disease.

Type 2 Diabetes Leading Risk Factors

The seven leading risk factors for type 2 diabetes include the following:

1. Body mass exceeds 20% of ideal
2. First-degree relative with diabetes (genetic influence)
3. Belongs to a high-risk ethnic group (Black, Hispanic American, Pacific Islander, American Indian, Asian)
4. Delivered a baby weighing more than 4.1 kg/9 lb or developed gestational diabetes
5. Blood pressure ≥140/90 mm Hg
6. HDL cholesterol level ≤35 mg · dL^{-1} and/or a triacylglycerol level ≥250 mg · dL^{-1}
7. Impaired fasting plasma glucose or impaired glucose tolerance on previous testing

Obesity, particularly upper-body fat distribution and physical inactivity, are the major risks for type 2 diabetes in both adults and children.[186] An estimated 60 to 80 million Americans show insulin resistance but have not developed overt symptoms of type 2 diabetes. One-third of these "prediabetic" individuals will eventually become full-blown diabetics, and many others are at heightened risk of cardiovascular disease.[58] Insulin's failure to exhibit a normal effect increases glucose conversion to triacylglycerol and storage as body fat. For the insulin-resistant individual, a diet high in simple sugars and refined carbohydrates with a relatively high glycemic index facilitates body fat accumulation.[49] Fat cell enlargement further exacerbates the situation because these cells exhibit insulin resistance from their reduced insulin receptor density. Women with excess body fat and high cardiorespiratory fitness are more insulin sensitive than equally obese but sedentary counterparts.[39]

Three factors can produce high blood glucose levels in type 2 diabetes:

- **Factor 1**. Inadequate insulin produced by the pancreas to control blood sugar (**relative insulin deficiency**)
- **Factor 2**. Decreased insulin effects on peripheral tissue (**insulin resistance**), particularly in skeletal muscle fibers (**FIG. 20.18**)
- **Factor 3**. Combined effect from factors 1 and 2

Dysregulation in glycolytic and oxidative capacities in skeletal muscle also relates to insulin resistance in type 2 diabetes.[73,161,171] The disease most likely results from interactions among genes and lifestyle factors—physical inactivity, weight gain (up to 80% type 2 diabetics are obese), aging, and possibly a high-fat/high animal protein diet. Lifestyle factors have contributed to the 70% increase in the disorder among persons in their 30s during the last decade of the 20th century, and to a 33% overall increase among all adults nationally. Also, the form of insulin resistance in type 2 diabetes has a strong genetic component. Diabetic-prone individuals have a particular gene that directs synthesis of a protein that inhibits insulin's action in cellular glucose transport.

As in type 1 diabetes, the failure of adequate glucose to enter the cells in the type 2 condition triggers abnormally high blood glucose levels, which the kidney tubules filter and void in the urine (glycosuria). Excessive glucose particles in renal filtrate create an osmotic effect that diminishes water reabsorption, which results in large losses in fluid (polyuria). With decreased cellular glucose uptake, a diabetic person relies largely on lipid catabolism for energy. This produces excess

Overweight or Obesity Duration and Cardiometabolic Health

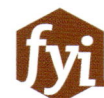
Africa Studio/Shutterstock

A population-based cohort study with 1268 youths aged 3 to 18 years, with follow-up assessment at 3, 6, 9, 12, 21, 27, and 31 years determined the association of obesity and overweight and adult cardiometabolic health. Adulthood outcome measures included type 2 diabetes mellitus, impaired fasting glucose, and plasma insulin levels. Overweight and obesity rates were 7.9% at baseline and 55.9% after 31 years. Longer overweight or obesity duration was associated with increased risk of all adult outcome measures. Detrimental associations with adult body mass index and diabetes outcomes were robust, making overweight or obesity as an adult rather than its acquisition during childhood a more important determinant factor associated with undesirable adult cardiometabolic health outcomes.

Source:
Feitong Wu, et al. Association of body mass index in youth with adult cardiometabolic risk. *J Am Heart Assoc.* 2020;9:e015288.

In a Practical Sense

Are You at Risk for Type 2 Diabetes?

ARE YOU AT RISK FOR TYPE 2 DIABETES?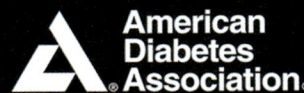

Diabetes Risk Test

1. How old are you?
- Less than 40 years (0 points)
- 40—49 years (1 point)
- 50—59 years (2 points)
- 60 years or older (3 points)

2. Are you a man or a woman?
- Man (1 point)   Woman (0 points)

3. If you are a woman, have you ever been diagnosed with gestational diabetes?
- Yes (1 point)   No (0 points)

4. Do you have a mother, father, sister, or brother with diabetes?
- Yes (1 point)   No (0 points)

5. Have you ever been diagnosed with high blood pressure?
- Yes (1 point)   No (0 points)

6. Are you physically active?
- Yes (0 points)   No (1 point)

7. What is your weight status? (see chart at right)

Write your score in the box.

Add up your score.

Height	Weight (lbs.)		
4' 10"	119-142	143-190	191+
4' 11"	124-147	148-197	198+
5' 0"	128-152	153-203	204+
5' 1"	132-157	158-210	211+
5' 2"	136-163	164-217	218+
5' 3"	141-168	169-224	225+
5' 4"	145-173	174-231	232+
5' 5"	150-179	180-239	240+
5' 6"	155-185	186-246	247+
5' 7"	159-190	191-254	255+
5' 8"	164-196	197-261	262+
5' 9"	169-202	203-269	270+
5' 10"	174-208	209-277	278+
5' 11"	179-214	215-285	286+
6' 0"	184-220	221-293	294+
6' 1"	189-226	227-301	302+
6' 2"	194-232	233-310	311+
6' 3"	200-239	240-318	319+
6' 4"	205-245	246-327	328+
	(1 Point)	(2 Points)	(3 Points)

You weigh less than the amount in the left column (0 points)

If you scored 5 or higher:
You are at increased risk for having type 2 diabetes. However, only your doctor can tell for sure if you do have type 2 diabetes or prediabetes (a condition that precedes type 2 diabetes in which blood glucose levels are higher than normal). Talk to your doctor to see if additional testing is needed.

Image courtesy of the American Diabetes Association, as adapted from Bang H, et al. Development and validation of a patient self-assessment score for diabetes risk. *Ann Intern Med.* 2009;151:775-783. Original algorithm was validated without gestational diabetes as part of the model.

ketoacids and a tendency toward acidosis. In extreme acidotic conditions, diabetic coma occurs as plasma pH falls to as low as 7.0 from a normal 7.6 value. In type 2 diabetes, arteriosclerosis, small blood vessel and nerve disease, and susceptibility to infection occur at increased rates. Obese diabetic women also face an almost threefold greater endometrial cancer risk than normal weight diabetic women, perhaps from persistently high insulin levels (insulin insensitivity).[157]

Type 1 and Type 2 Diabetes Differences. The table below lists different characteristics for type 1 and type 2 diabetes.

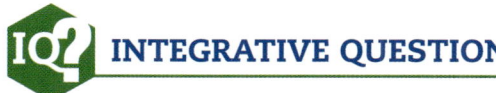

Characteristics	Type 1 Diabetes	Type 2 Diabetes
Age at onset	Usually ≤20 y	Usually ≥40 y
Proportion all diabetics	≤10%	≥90%
Appearance of symptoms	Acute/subacute	Slow
Metabolic ketoacidosis	Frequent	Rare
Obesity at onset	Uncommon	Common
β-cells	Decreased	Variable
Insulin	Decreased	Variable
Inflammatory cells in islets	Initially	Absent
Family history	Uncommon	Common

Background image: UGREEN 3S/Shutterstock

Diabetes and Physical Activity

Hypoglycemia remains the most common disturbance in glucose homeostasis during physical activity in diabetic persons who take exogenous insulin. Hypoglycemia most frequently occurs during prolonged, intense activity when hepatic glucose release does not match an increased active muscle glucose uptake. Individuals with type 2 diabetes often have reduced exercise tolerance independent of glycemic control. Contributing factors include genetics, undesirable lifestyle characteristics, excessive body fat, and poor fitness status.[27,39]

INTEGRATIVE QUESTION

Why do individuals with poorly regulated diabetes mellitus or malnutrition from semi-starvation often have sweet-smelling breath?

Metabolic Syndrome

Metabolic syndrome, a concept first introduced into medical science in the late 1980s, describes a common condition in which obesity, high blood pressure, high blood glucose, and dyslipidemia cluster together in one person. When these syndrome risk factors cluster, the chances of developing coronary heart disease, stroke, and diabetes are greater than when these risk factors develop independently.[10,46,104] Diet-induced insulin resistance/hyperinsulinemia often occurs before metabolic syndrome appears.[5,125,162,201] Diagnosis of the syndrome includes having three or more of the following five indicators:

1. Elevated blood glucose (fasting glucose ≥110 mg·dL^{-1})
2. Overweight with large waist girth in males greater than 102 cm/40 in; females greater than 88 cm/35 in
3. High triacylglycerols (≥150 mg·dL^{-1})
4. Low high-density lipoprotein cholesterol levels in males less than 40 mg·dL^{-1}; females less than 50 mg·dL^{-1}
5. Hypertension (>130 mm Hg systolic; >85 mm Hg diastolic)

Individuals with metabolic syndrome exhibit high risk for cardiovascular disease, type 2 diabetes, Alzheimer disease, and all-cause mortality.[46,103] Some researchers maintain that inappropriate food consumption (e.g., high levels of refined sugar and animal proteins), sedentary lifestyle, and poor muscular strength and cardiorespiratory fitness not only associate with metabolic syndrome but characterize the disease.[81,86,102,147] The most recent 2019 age-adjusted hypertension prevalence in the United States indicates the following: males (24%) and females (23.4%), while Mexican Americans have the highest age-adjusted prevalence (31.9%). The lowest prevalence occurs among whites (23.8%), African Americans (21.6%), and people reporting "other" for race or ethnicity (20.3%). Among African Americans, females exhibit a 57% higher prevalence than males, and Mexican American females have a 26% greater prevalence than male counterparts.

Metabolic syndrome afflicts Western industrialized countries being more prevalent in adult males than in females. Disease occurrence relates to genetic, hormonal, and the lifestyle factors of obesity, physical inactivity, and caloric intake excess, including high saturated and *trans*-fatty acid intakes.[219] Characterized by the clustering of insulin resistance and hyperinsulinemia, dyslipidemia (atherogenic plasma lipid profile), essential hypertension, abdominal (visceral) obesity, and glucose intolerance, the syndrome also relates to blood coagulation abnormalities, hyperuricemia, and microalbuminuria. Psychosocial stress, socioeconomic disadvantage, and abnormal psychiatric traits also link to the syndrome's pathogenesis.[9,10]

Glucagon

The islets of Langerhans' α-cells secrete glucagon known as the "insulin antagonist" hormone. In contrast to insulin's effect in lowering blood sugar levels, glucagon primarily stimulates both glycogenolysis and gluconeogenesis by the liver and increases lipid catabolism (**FIG. 20.19**). The glucose generated by glucagon action then moves into the blood. Glucagon exerts its effect by activating adenylate cyclase. This enzyme stimulates cyclic AMP in liver cells and causes hepatic glycogen breakdown to glucose (glycogenolysis). Glucagon also stimulates gluconeogenesis by promoting the liver's amino acid uptake.

As with insulin, plasma glucose concentration controls pancreatic glucagon output. A decrease in blood glucose concentration from prolonged intense physical activity or food (mainly carbohydrate) restriction stimulates glucagon release.

In a Practical Sense

Metabolic Syndrome: Organs Affected, Common Characteristics, Associated Medical Conditions, and Treatment

MEDICAL CONDITIONS ASSOCIATED WITH METABOLIC SYNDROME

Left untreated, metabolic syndrome increases risk of coronary heart disease, stroke, and type 2 diabetes.

A STROKE

The term *stroke* refers to the sudden death of brain tissue from lack of oxygen. In ischemic stroke, blocked or reduced blood flow occurs in brain tissues. This blockage may result from atherosclerosis and blood clot formation.

B CORONARY HEART DISEASE

Narrowing of the coronary arteries can lead to a heart attack. Atherosclerosis, the buildup of plaque in the lining of the arteries, causes arterial narrowing; all of the metabolic syndrome risk factors can induce atherosclerosis. Heart attacks occur when blood fails to flow through narrowed coronary vessels, which results in ischemic myocardial tissue.

C TYPE 2 DIABETES

In type 2 diabetes, the pancreas produces little or no insulin and/or the body loses the ability to respond normally to insulin (called insulin resistance). Insulin transports glucose into the cells for use as energy; without insulin, body tissues have less access to essential nutrients for energy and storage. Diabetes requires proper management, and if left untreated, it can lead to complications that impact the eyes, mouth, cardiovascular system, kidneys, nerves, and extremities.

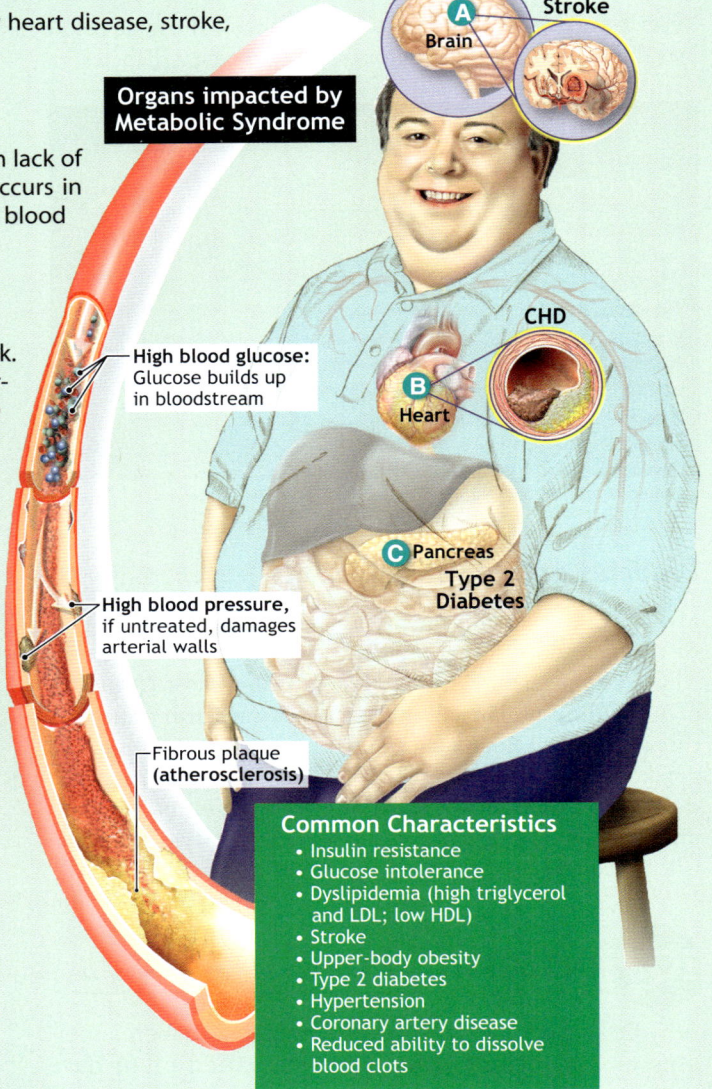

Common Characteristics
- Insulin resistance
- Glucose intolerance
- Dyslipidemia (high triglycerol and LDL; low HDL)
- Stroke
- Upper-body obesity
- Type 2 diabetes
- Hypertension
- Coronary artery disease
- Reduced ability to dissolve blood clots

Treating Metabolic Syndrome

Metabolic syndrome requires long-term management of each risk factor. Poor nutrition and reduced physical activity represent underlying causes of these risk factors. Regular monitoring of blood pressure, cholesterol, and glucose are important for detecting the syndrome, even if an individual fails to experience outward disease symptoms.

- **Weight loss:** A weight loss of 5 to 10% of body weight improves insulin sensitivity.
- **Increased physical activity:** Increased physical activity reverses insulin resistance, reduces blood pressure, lowers "bad" cholesterol, raises "good" cholesterol, and reduces overall type 2 diabetes risk.
- **Eat a heart healthy diet:** Reduce saturated fat, cholesterol, and salt intake. Increase intake of high-fiber fruits, vegetables, and grains.

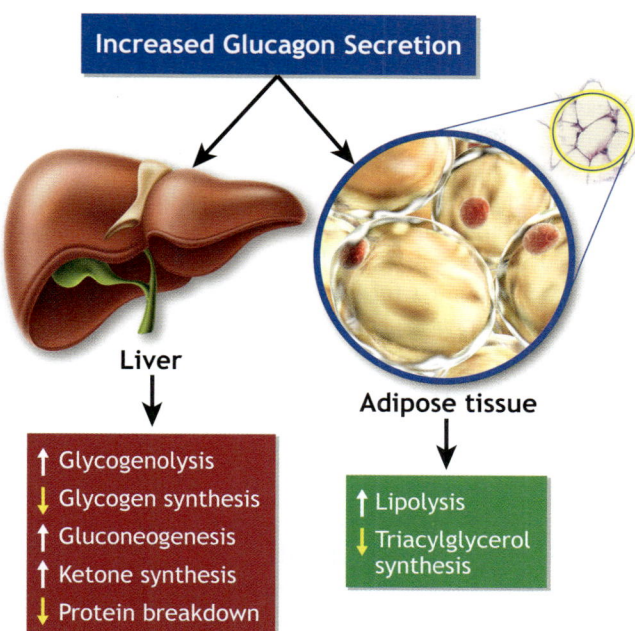

FIGURE 20.19. Glucagon secretion and its actions on target tissues.
(Shutterstock: Kateryna Kon; OrangeVector.)

plays a role in regulating cytokine expression. The myokines IL6, irisin, IGF-1, BDNF, myostatin, and FGF2 exert anabolic/catabolic effects on bone, while osteocalcin and osteokine induce muscle anabolism and the sclerostin osteokine induces catabolism.[212–215]

Both type I and type II muscle fibers express the myokine IL-6, which subsequently exerts its effects both locally within the muscle (e.g., by engaging AMP-activated protein kinase [AMPK]), and when released into the circulation, peripherally in hormonelike fashion. **FIGURE 20.20** illustrates the proposed biological role for interleukin (IL)-6R.

Adipose Tissue as an Endocrine Organ

In addition to energy storage, adipose tissue serves as an important endocrine organ. Research has confirmed that adipose tissue secretes many peptide hormones (see inset figure) including leptin, which influences appetite (see Chapter 30); several cytokines; adipsin and acylation-stimulating protein (ASP); angiotensinogen; plasminogen activator inhibitor-1 (PAI-1); adiponectin (increases insulin sensitivity and fatty acid oxidation in muscle); and resistin (decreases cell sensitivity to insulin's effects). Adipose tissue also produces steroid hormones.

This adipose tissue secretory function has shifted the view about adipose tissue toward being at the nexus of a complex network that influences energy homeostasis, glucose and lipid metabolism, vascular homeostasis, immune response, and reproduction.[216–218] Most known adipose-secreted proteins are dysregulated when the quantity of "normal" body fat becomes markedly altered—either increased in the overfat state or decreased in the underfat (lipoatrophy) state.

Autonomic nervous stimulation does not mediate glucagon release, unlike its effects on insulin secretion. Also, no gender differences exist in the glucagon response to physical activity when individuals exercise at the same aerobic capacity percentage.[2,32,174] Glucagon release occurs later in the activity because this hormone exerts little influence in the early regulation of hepatic glycogenolysis. More than likely, glucagon primarily regulates blood glucose as physical activity progresses and glycogen reserves deplete.

Muscle Tissue as an Endocrine Organ

In 2003, a humoral factor (a cytokine) was first identified as produced and released from contracting muscle cells and appeared to exhibit strong metabolic effects. This discovery opened a new paradigm that views skeletal muscle as an endocrine-secreting organ that influences metabolism in other tissues and organs. The muscle-secreted cytokines (referred to as *myokines*) and other muscle-produced peptides—produced, expressed, and released by muscle fibers—exert autocrine, paracrine, or endocrine effects. Additional research supports muscle as an active endocrine organ with the capacity to produce and express cytokines that belong to distinctly different families. The list currently includes *interleukin* (IL)-6, IL-8, IL-15, LIF, BDNF, follistatinlike 1, and FGF21. A muscle's contractile activity also

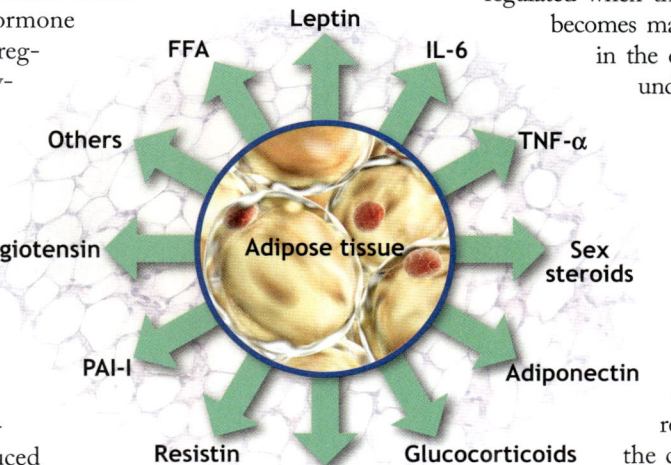

Kateryna Kon/Shutterstock

Leptin and Ghrelin

Leptin is a small peptide considered a pre-inflammatory cytokine belonging to the IL-6 cytokine family that represents an anorexigenic peptide that increases energy expenditure. The leptin receptor expresses not only in the central nervous system but also in some peripheral tissues, suggesting leptin may have functions other than affecting food intake and energy expenditure. Adipose tissue (and plasma) leptin concentrations depend on the energy stored as lipid and energy balance status. As such, leptin levels are higher in obese individuals and increase with overfeeding. Conversely, lean individuals have lower leptin levels, and popular fasting strategies aim to reduce circulating leptin as shown in the inset figure as individuals become satiated. Simultaneously, another hormone from the GI tract **ghrelin** (a 28-amino acid peptide hormone known commonly as the "hunger hormone") is especially active from its release in the stomach. Ghrelin increases in concentration as individuals experience

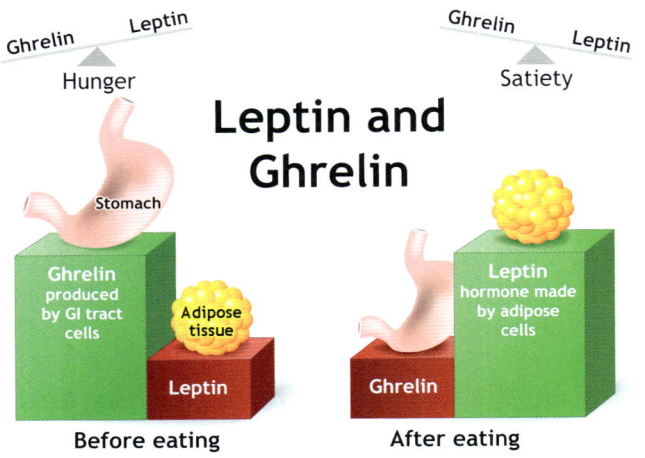

the need to consume food (signaling the brain to eat), which then increases gastric motility to prepare the stomach to assimilate the incoming food intake. In the obese, overactive ghrelin receptor cells (GHS-R [Growth Hormone Secretagogue Receptor]) leads to increased food intake.

Leptin Regulation

Regulation of leptin is mediated in part by insulin; leptin decreases in response to low insulin levels and increases with feeding or in response to insulin stimulation. Leptin synthesis is greater in subcutaneous than in visceral adipose tissue, and the higher circulating leptin concentration in females is likely due to larger subcutaneous fat stores. Leptin has been implicated in other roles, including modulating the brain's neural reward circuitry for feeding, glucose metabolism, lipid oxidation, substrate partitioning, and adipocyte apoptosis (**FIG. 20.21**).

Liver, Gut, and Hypothalamic Hormones

The liver secretes somatomedins, which affect muscle, cartilage, and other tissue growth. The small intestine's mucosal lining secretes **gastrin**, **secretin**, and **cholecystokinin** to promote and coordinate digestive processes. The hypothalamus represents an important endocrine gland that secretes stimulating or releasing hormones to activate or release anterior pituitary hormones. The hypothalamus also releases **somatoliberin** (also known as growth hormone–releasing hormone [GHRH]), which stimulates somatotropin secretion from the anterior pituitary gland.

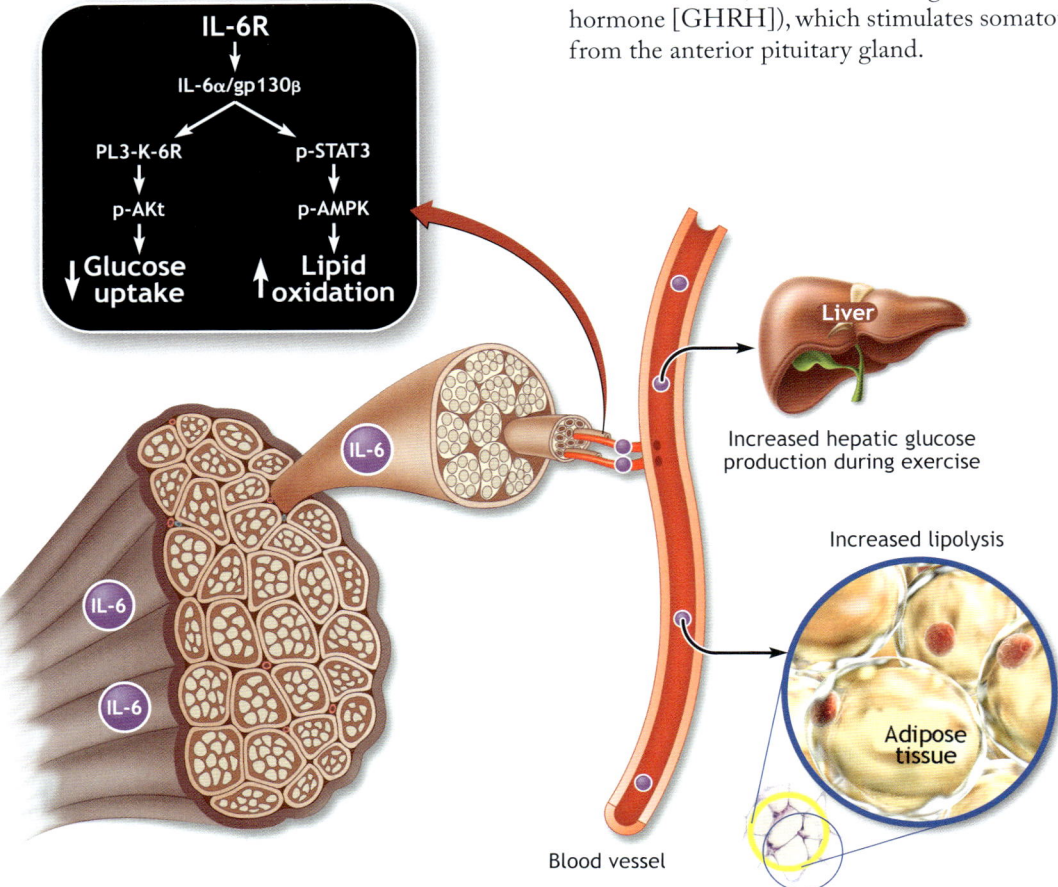

FIGURE 20.20. Proposed biological role for interleukin (IL)-6, expressed in type I and type II muscle fibers, which exerts its effects locally within the specific muscle through activation of AMP protein kinase (AMPK).
(Sources: Pedersen BK, Febbraio MA. Muscle as an endocrine organ: focus on muscle-derived interleukin-6. *Physiol Rev*. 2008;88:1379; Pedersen BK, Edward F. Adolph Distinguished Lecture: muscle as an endocrine organ: IL-6 and other myokines. *J Appl Physiol*. 2009;107:1006; Pedersen BK, Febbraio MA. Muscles, exercise and obesity: skeletal muscle as a secretory organ. *Nat Rev Endocrinol*. 2012;8:457. Shutterstock images: adipose tissue–Kateryna Kon; liver–OrangeVector)

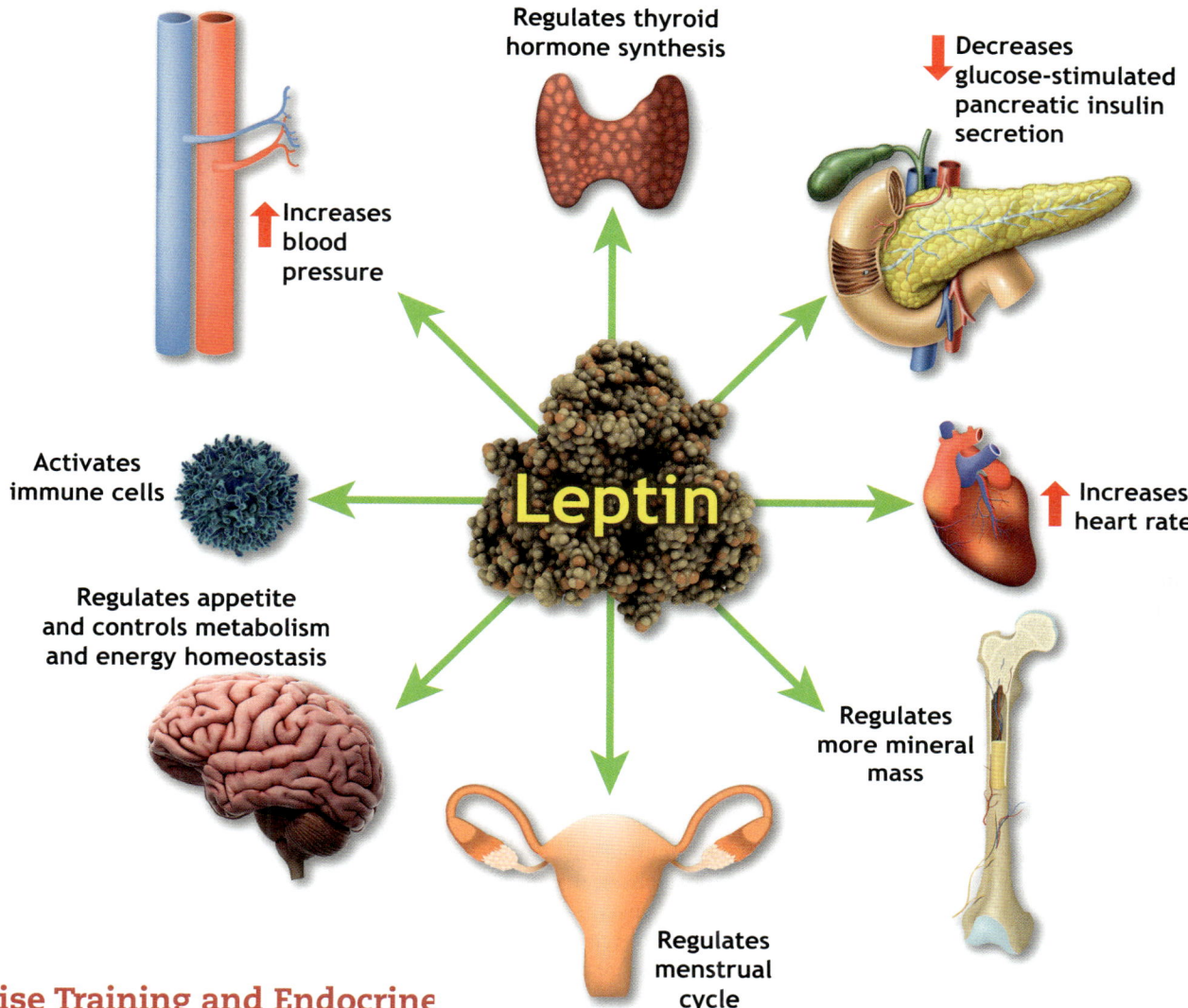

FIGURE 20.21. Leptin's eight primary functions.
(Shutterstock: StudioMolekuul; Designua; Andrea Danti; Aldona Griskeviciene; SciePro; Kateryna Kon.)

Exercise Training and Endocrine Function

Only limited research has evaluated multiple hormone secretions and changes consequent to exercise training because the complex interactions between endocrine secretions and the nervous system can obscure the true relationships. *The hormonal response to a standard exercise load generally declines with endurance training.* For example, when highly trained athletes perform at the same absolute activity level as sedentary individuals, hormonal responses remain lower in the athletes. Improved target tissue sensitivity and/or responsiveness to a given amount of hormone accounts for much of this lowered response.[29,74] A similar level of hormonal response occurs regardless of training state when individuals exercise at the same relative exercise intensity (i.e., same percentage of maximum; lower absolute load in the untrained). With maximum exertion, trained subjects have an identical or greater hormonal response than untrained subjects.[20,37,62]

Anterior Pituitary Hormones

The inset table shows the different anterior pituitary hormone responses to exercise training.

Hypothalamus-Pituitary Hormones	Training Response
Growth hormone	No effect on resting values; less dramatic rise in exercise
Thyrotropin	No known training effect
ACTH	Increased exercise values
Prolactin	Training may lower resting values
FSH, LH, and testosterone	Trained females have depressed values; reduced testosterone in males (may increase with prolonged resistance training)

Background image: Ezume Images/Shutterstock

Growth Hormone

GH stimulates lipolysis and inhibits carbohydrate breakdown, so some maintain that exercise training should enhance GH secretion and conserve glycogen reserves, but this does not occur. Compared with untrained counterparts, endurance-trained individuals show less rise in blood GH levels at a given physical activity intensity—a response attributed to reduced stress as training progresses and fitness improves. Regardless of training status, females typically maintain higher GH levels at rest than males, a difference that disappears during prolonged physical activity.[18]

Adrenocorticotropic Hormone

ACTH secreted by the posterior pituitary gland provides potent stimulation to the adrenal cortex and thus increases free fatty acid mobilization for energy. Training increases ACTH release during physical activity—a response that stimulates adrenal gland activity to promote lipid catabolism and spare glycogen.[14,108] This effect would certainly benefit prolonged, intense exercise performance.

Prolactin

Circulating blood prolactin levels increase during physical activity, with the magnitude of the increase approximately proportional to the intensity of the physical activity. Whether there is a specific intensity threshold required to induce a hormonal response is unclear, but most physical activity above the anaerobic threshold initiates substantial and rapid prolactin elevations.[228] However, if exercise is intense enough, but of a short-term duration, the peak prolactin response may actually occur after exercise ends. Interestingly, excessive emotional stress can cause an anticipatory increase in prolactin even before an exercise session begins.[229,230]

During sustained exercise, the prolactin response is proportional to the exercise intensity. However, extending the duration of the exercise session can result in a gradual increase in the magnitude of the prolactin response.[230]

Intense anaerobic exercise results in greater prolactin responses than typically seen in submaximal aerobic exercise.[230]

The effect of resistance or strength-based exercise on prolactin levels is limited, but some evidence supports the belief that this type of exercise elevates prolactin but the increase may occur during recovery.[231]

Findings are highly contradictory with regard to the effect of chronic exercise training on resting prolactin levels. Some studies report increases in resting levels, whereas others note decreased levels. These ambiguities are likely related to differences in exercise training protocol components (e.g., intensity, frequency, and duration of training sessions). Also, evidence supports that in both men and women who have undergone aerobic exercise training, the prolactin response increases.[231,233]

Gonadotropic Hormones

Regular physical activity depresses reproductive hormone responses in males and females.[36,192] Male endurance athletes generally maintain resting testosterone levels between 60 and 85% of sedentary male values (270 to 1070 ng·dL^{-1}; average of 679 ng·dL^{-1}).

Women. Women with a consistent physical activity participation history have altered FSH and LH levels at different times in their menstrual cycles, often contributing to menstrual dysfunction. For example, FSH levels remain depressed in trained females throughout an abbreviated anovulatory menstrual cycle, whereas LH and progesterone concentrations rise in the cycle's follicular phase. Variations in the menstrual cycle do not affect metabolic and hormonal responses to acute exercise.[48,87]

Men. Endurance training affects a man's pituitary-gonadal function, including testosterone and prolactin levels. One study compared 46 male runners (average weekly running distance: 64 km/40 mi) and 18 nonrunners matched for age, stature, and body mass.[191] The runners showed lower testosterone than nonrunners, with no differences in LH and FSH levels. Reduced testosterone concentration (both increased clearance and lower production) in endurance-trained males parallels the sex-steroid reductions observed in females who undergo endurance training and reduce body fat.[168] No difference exists in LH and FSH levels between trained and untrained men; thus, impaired gonadotropin release from the anterior pituitary does not cause the lower testosterone levels during standard physical activity in the trained state.

Posterior Pituitary Hormones

Posterior Pituitary Hormones	Training Response
Vasopressin (ADH)	Slightly reduced ADH at a given workload
Oxytocin	Helpful dealing with performance stress

Antidiuretic Hormone

Intense physical activity to exhaustion or prolonged submaximal activity maintained at the same relative intensity produces no difference in ADH levels between trained and untrained individuals. **ADH (vasopressin)** concentration decreases with training when exercising at the same absolute submaximal intensity.

While oxytocin's role in exercise and exercise training is limited, most research centers on its role related to elevated production during orgasm, breast-feeding, social recognition, pair bonding, and anxiety. Oxytocin and neuropeptide Y are key indicators of an adaptive approach to motivated performance situations, which enables athletes to respond positively to performance-induced anxiety.[220]

Thyroid Hormones

Thyroid Hormones	Training Response
Thyroxine (T_4)	Reduced total resting T3 and increased free thyroxine concentration thyroxine during rest
Triiodothyronine (T_3)	Increased T_3 and T_4 turnover during exercise

Background image: UGREEN 3S/Shutterstock

Training produces a coordinated pituitary-thyroid response that reflects increased thyroid hormone turnover, which often reflects excessive hormonal action ultimately leading to **hyperthyroidism** (i.e., T_3 and T_4 hormone overproduction). However, no evidence indicates a higher hyperthyroidism incidence in highly trained individuals. For example, inordinately high BMR levels and basal body temperatures rarely occur in the trained state. Consequently, the greater T_4 turnover that accompanies physical training occurs through a mechanism that differs from "normal" thyroid hormone dynamics.

Research on endurance-trained women yields interesting results regarding thyroid turnover. Changing from a baseline of relatively sedentary living to running 48 km/30 mi per week produced a mild thyroid impairment reflected by decreased T_3 and T_4 level.[15] In contrast, nearly doubling the weekly distance increased plasma hormone levels. To explain these apparent conflicting training effects, the researchers suggested that greater body fat loss with more prolonged training produced an exercise-induced increase in thyroid output. Resistance training for 6 months in men slightly reduced T_4 and plasma-free T_4 concentrations without changes in TSH. The magnitude of this change was without clinical or physiologic significance.[139]

Parathyroid Hormone

The significance of a training-induced augmented rise in PTH is inconclusive, and a role for PTH in physical activity-associated health benefits has yet to be established. Acute exercise increases PTH secretion in the late phases of endurance activities and during recovery, regardless of changes in calcium and phosphorous levels.

Endurance training enhances exercise-related increases in PTH in young and elderly adults.[136,175] The exercise-induced PTH rise is driven partially by an exercise-induced increase in calcium levels. A novel research area about exercise-dependent regulation of PTH secretion comes from the apparent "crosstalk" among myokines and skeletal muscle-derived hormones, key mediators in systemic effects of physical activity.[207]

Adrenal Hormones

Adrenal Hormones	Training Response
Aldosterone	No training adaptation
Cortisol/corticosteroid	Elevated during physical activity
Epinephrine/norepinephrine	Decreased secretion at rest and at the same absolute exercise intensity after training

Background image: Ezume Images/Shutterstock

It is well established that adrenal hormone production increases from the stress of both aerobic and resistance exercise, yet the role these hormones play in mediating specific training adaptations in skeletal muscle and other organs is incomplete. Recent evidence suggests that these hormones can induce genomic actions that become relevant to muscle function and subcellular metabolic activity following prolonged exercise training. Training adaptations that appear sensitive to adrenal hormone effects include increased muscle mass, fatigue resistance, increased fatty acid oxidation, increased systemic glucose disposal, and resynchronization (termed core clock entrainment) of skeletal muscles' circadian rhythm.[221]

Epinephrine and Norepinephrine

Sympathoadrenal activity, principally norepinephrine release in response to an absolute submaximal workload, remains lower in trained than untrained individuals.[41] Epinephrine and norepinephrine output in standard exercise falls dramatically during the first several weeks of training. The appearance of bradycardia and a smaller rise in blood pressure during submaximal activity represent the most familiar consequences of the sympathoadrenal training adaptation. Reduced heart rate and blood pressure reflect favorable adaptations because they lower exercise myocardial oxygen demands. For equivalent *relative* exercise intensities, a higher sympathoadrenal response occurs following aerobic training.[57]

FIGURE 20.22 illustrates norepinephrine and epinephrine response during physical activity at intensities ranging between 60 and 85% aerobic capacity in three adult men and six women prior to and following aerobic training for 10 wk where $\dot{V}O_{2max}$ increased by 20%. Plasma norepinephrine levels (top inset) increased progressively with exercise intensity before and after training. Training produced higher plasma norepinephrine levels, particularly at higher exercise intensities. Consistently higher epinephrine values also emerged following training (bottom inset), but the differences did not attain statistical significance. More than likely, greater catecholamine output at the same relative exercise intensity following training reflects three factors requiring greater sympathetic nervous system activation:

1. Greater absolute demand for substrate use from glycogenolysis and lipolysis
2. Increased overall cardiovascular response (e.g., cardiac output)
3. Larger muscle mass activation

Aldosterone

The renin-angiotensin-aldosterone system contributes to homeostatic control of body fluid volumes, electrolytes, and blood pressure, but training does not affect resting levels for these components or their normal response to physical activity.

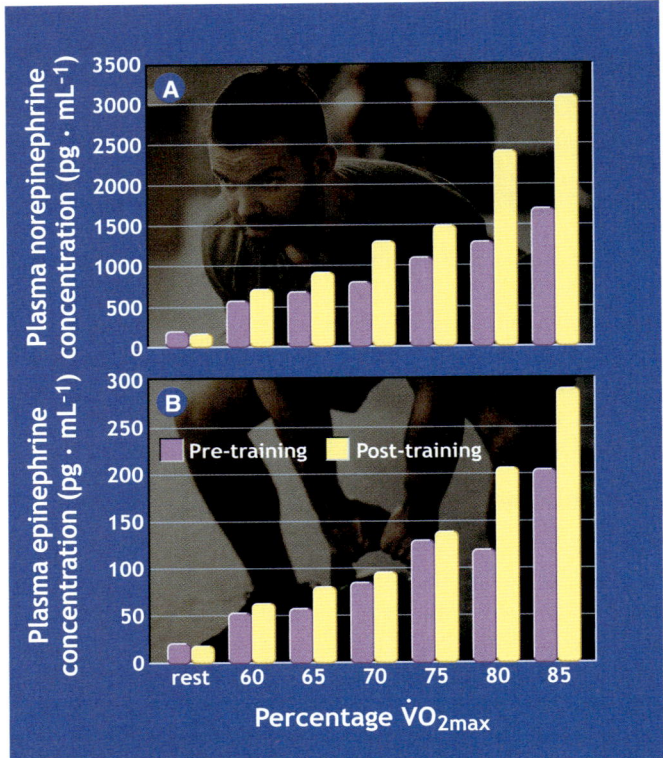

FIGURE 20.22. Plasma norepinephrine (**A**) and epinephrine concentrations (**B**) at rest and after 15 min of exercise at the same relative exercise intensity (%VO) before and after endurance exercise training for 10 wk.
(Adapted with permission from Greiwe JS, et al. Norepinephrine response to exercise at the same relative intensity before and after endurance training. *J Appl Physiol.* 1999;86:531. ©The American Physiological Society (APS). All rights reserved. Background image: Flamingo Images/Shutterstock.)

Cortisol

Plasma cortisol levels increase less in trained subjects than in sedentary subjects who perform the same absolute level of sub-maximal exercise. Adrenal gland enlargement results from both cellular hypertrophy and hyperplasia with repeated intense training bouts with accompanying high cortisol output. Glucocorticoids regulate muscle function following exercise training. These effects reinforce the position that genomic actions related to exercise modulate changes in the genes responsible for increased Na^+ and K^+ pump mRNA expression following exercise training.[221,222]

Pancreatic Hormones

Pancreatic Hormones	Training Response
Insulin	Increased sensitivity to insulin; normal decrease during exercise greatly reduced with training
Glucagon	Smaller increase in glucose levels during exercise at absolute and relative workloads

Background image: UGREEN 3S/Shutterstock

Endurance training maintains blood insulin and glucagon levels during physical activity closer to resting levels. In essence,

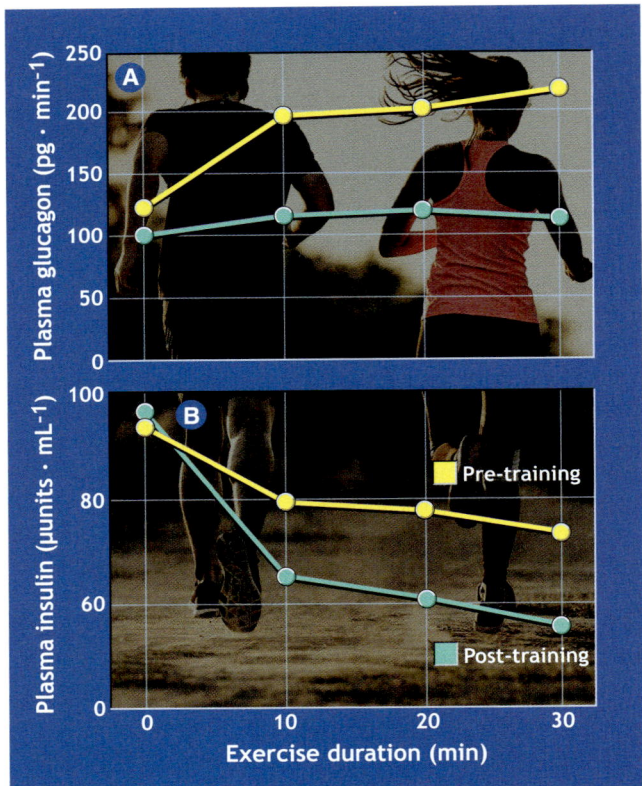

FIGURE 20.23. Pre-post differences in plasma glucagon (**A**) and insulin (**B**) responses to exercise before and after a 20-wk aerobic training program.
(Data from V. Katch. Applied Physiology Laboratory, University of Michigan, Ann Arbor. Background image: GP PIXSTOCK/Shutterstock.)

the trained state requires less insulin at any stage from rest through light to moderately intense activity. **FIGURE 20.23** shows plasma glucagon (A) and plasma insulin (B) responses in 10 young adults before and after training for 20 wk at 60 to 80% $\dot{V}O_{2max}$. Aerobic training depressed the response of both hormones in exercise, with glucagon showing the most pronounced reduction. These findings agree with previous research for adults who trained by running and cycling.[59,60,107,180]

Regular Physical Activity and Type 2 Diabetes Risk

Cross-sectional, retrospective, prospective, and interventional epidemiologic research provide strong evidence that regular physical activity reduces type 2 diabetes prevalence in adolescents and adults with or without concomitant body composition changes.[3,17,68,98,184] (Refer to https://pubmed.ncbi.nlm.nih.gov/10912903 for the ACSM position stands on physical activity and type 2 diabetes.) Those individuals at greatest risk for type 2 diabetes (obese, hypertensive, family history, sedentary lifestyle) gain the greatest benefit from regular physical activity.[1,114,140] For adult men and women, low fitness levels coincide with increased clustering of metabolic abnormalities associated with metabolic syndrome (see section Metabolic Syndrome), the "deadly quartet" of insulin resistance, glucose intolerance, abdominal obesity, and dyslipidemia. For sedentary, middle-age men, aerobic physical activity plus weight loss lowers blood pressure and improves glucose and lipid metabolism.[34,99,166] Resistance exercise also provides benefits—every additional 10% increase in skeletal muscle mass coincides with an 11% reduction in insulin resistance and a 12% lower transitional, prediabetes, or diabetes risk. When researchers compared the one quarter of participants with the most muscle mass with those with the lowest muscle mass, individuals with the greatest muscle mass were 63% less prone to type 2 diabetes.[165]

Regular physical activity may even reduce need for antidiabetic medications to control the disease.[196] A 6-year clinical trial evaluated the effects of a diet and physical activity lifestyle intervention on type 2 diabetes occurrence in individuals with impaired glucose tolerance.[76] Men and women were randomly assigned to either control, diet-only, exercise-only, or diet-plus-exercise groups. Diet modification included 25 to 30 kcal · kg body mass^{-1} (55 to 60% carbohydrate, 25 to 30% lipid, and 10 to 15% protein) for individuals with a BMI below 25. Those with a BMI above 25 maintained the same macronutrient mixture as the leaner group while gradually losing weight at a rate of 0.5 to 1.0 kg per month until their BMI decreased to 23. Physical activity intervention required a progressive increase in mild-to-moderate regular physical activity. The diet-exercise intervention combined both diet and exercise treatments. Clearly, diet, physical activity, and combined diet-exercise decreased diabetes incidence after the 6-year intervention.

A large prospective study evaluated diabetes risk for a cohort of 70,102 female nurses ages 40 to 65 years without diabetes, cardiovascular disease, or cancer at baseline measurements in 1986.[76] In agreement with previous prospective research on men, an 8-year follow-up found increased physical activity associated with a substantially reduced relative risk for type 2 diabetes.

FIGURE 20.24 outlines the possible mechanisms of how exercise training—and its effects on skeletal muscle, pancreatic hormone output, adipose tissue, and liver—improves insulin action and blood glucose control in type 2 diabetes.

Physical Activity Benefits for People with Type 2 Diabetes

Regular physical activity provides considerable benefits for persons with type 2 diabetes.[66,144]

Glycemic Control. Skeletal muscle clears the major amount of glucose transported in blood, generally between 70 and 90% in an oral or intravenous glucose challenge. A single moderate or intense physical activity bout abruptly decreases plasma glucose levels, an effect that persists for up to several days. Extending the weekly physical activity duration from 115 to 170 min produces the greatest increase in insulin sensitivity.[75] The immediate effects of each activity session on increasing the active muscles' insulin sensitivity cause long-term improvement in glycemic control, not any exercise-induced chronic adaptations in tissue function. When resuming a sedentary lifestyle, the muscles' sensitivity to insulin decreases, which requires more insulin to clear a given blood glucose quantity.[132] *Improved insulin sensitivity with regular physical activity provides type 2 diabetics with important "therapy" that ultimately lowers their insulin requirement.* Three factors account for the improved insulin sensitivity for glucose transport in skeletal muscle and adipose tissue following physical activity:

1. Translocation of the glucose transporter protein GLUT-4 from the endoplasmic reticulum to the cell surface
2. Increase in total GLUT-4 quantity
3. Increase in glycogen synthase activity and subsequent glycogen storage independent of any effect on insulin signaling[25,65,72,79,146]

The hyperinsulinemic person who requires the largest insulin release for glucose regulation derives the greatest benefits from regular exercise.[186] This observation supports the theory that regular physical activity acts by reversing insulin resistance (i.e., physical activity increases insulin sensitivity). Combining resistance exercise and endurance training improves markers of insulin resistance and body composition for insulin-resistant individuals more than endurance training alone.[99,179] Benefits of resistance plus endurance training for hyperinsulinemia most likely come

---

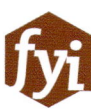

Sport or Recreational Activities Reduce Health Risks

Evidence of prospective associations between participation in sport or recreational activities and health outcomes at the population level was investigated over a 6-year period in 8784 Australian adults age 40 years and older. Mail surveys in 2007, 2009, 2011, and 2013 were used to collect participation data in recreational activities for 12 months, and self-reported height and weight and incidence of hypertension and diabetes. From 2007 to 2013, the cumulative incidence rates were hypertension (14.9%), obesity (11%), and diabetes (3.2%). Running, tennis, team sports, exercise classes, and resistance training associated with reduced hypertension incidence, while running, cycling, resistance training, and yoga/Taiichi associated with reduced diabetes risk. Cycling, tennis, home-based exercises, resistance training, and yoga/Taiichi were related to a lower risk of obesity. Over the 6-year study period, participation in sports and recreational activities revealed a lower hypertension, diabetes, and obesity incidence in middle-age adults.

Rawpixel.com/Shutterstock

Source:
Mielke G, et al. Participation in sports/recreational activities and incidence of hypertension, diabetes and obesity in adults. *Scand J Med Sci Sports*. 2020;30:2390.

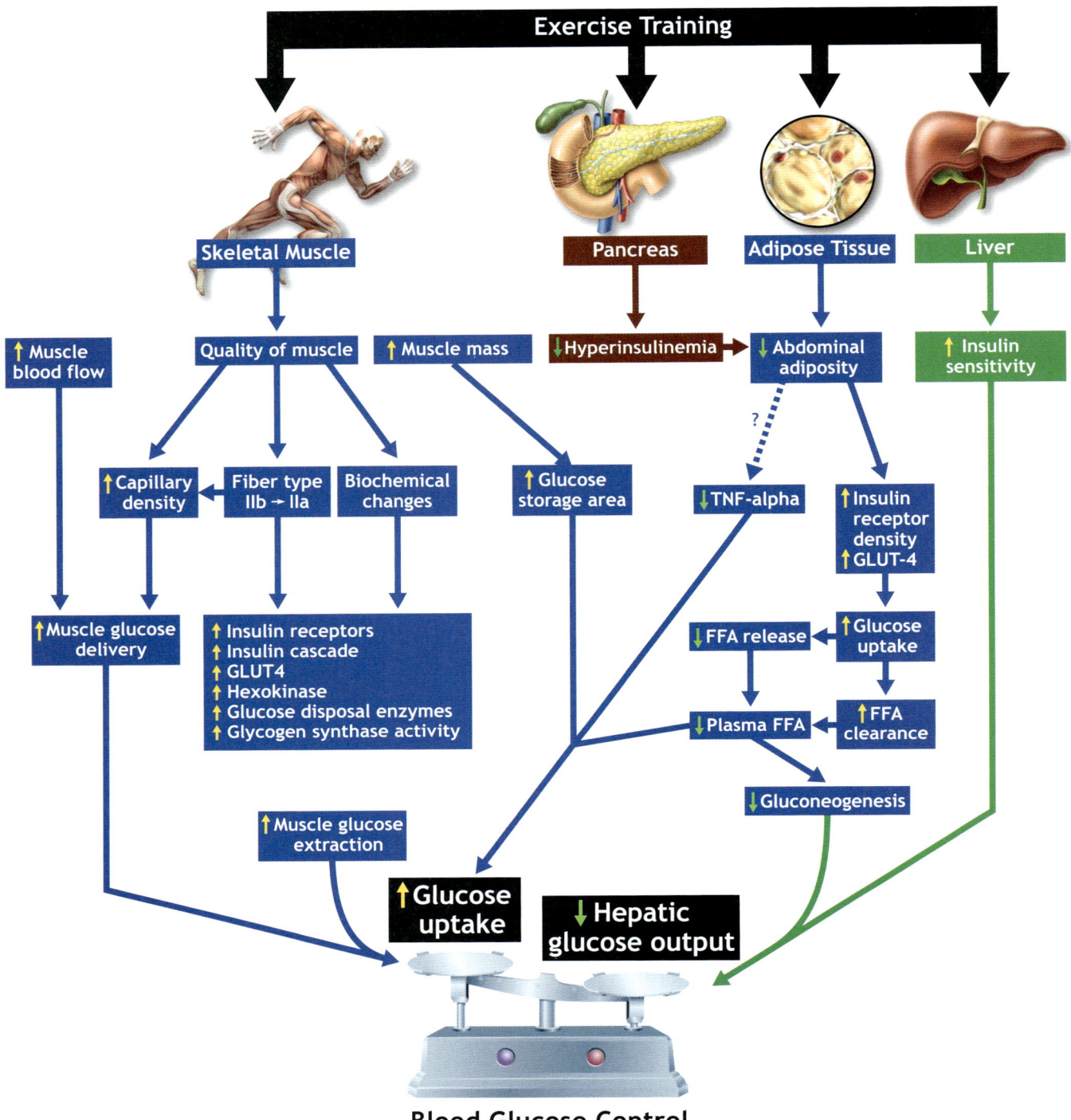

FIGURE 20.24. Possible mechanisms how regular physical activity can improve insulin action and blood glucose homeostasis in type 2 diabetes. TNF-alpha, tumor necrosis factor.
(Adapted with permission from Ivy JL, et al. Prevention and treatment of noninsulin-dependent diabetes mellitus. *Exerc Sport Sci Rev*. 1999;27:1. Shutterstock images: Kateryna Kon; TreesTons; Andrea Danti; OrangeVector.)

from activating a relatively larger muscle mass than with endurance training alone and the additional caloric expenditure. Improvements in blood glucose homeostasis with regular physical activity rapidly decrease once training ceases and completely dissipate within several weeks of inactivity. Reliance on intensive pharmacologic therapy to lower blood glucose levels in high-risk type 2 diabetics decreased mortality but did not reduce cardiovascular events compared with standard therapy.[176]

Reduced Cardiovascular Disease Risk. Excess morbidity and mortality in type 2 diabetes results from coronary heart disease, stroke, and peripheral vascular disease from accelerated atherosclerosis.[38] Disease risk factors that improve with regular physical activity include hyperinsulinemia, hyperglycemia, abnormal plasma lipoproteins, some blood coagulation parameters, and hypertension.[150]

Weight Loss. Weight loss and accompanying reduction in body fat and its distribution enhance glucose tolerance and insulin sensitivity.[6,98] The beneficial physical activity effects on fat loss often are underestimated because changes in body weight with regular exercise do not necessarily reflect the more favorable, exercise-induced body composition changes (fat loss and muscle gain). Combining diet and regular physical activity reduces body fat in diabetic persons more effectively than either treatment alone.

Improved Psychological Profile. Improved physical activity capacity in diabetic persons relates to decreased anxiety, improved mood and self-esteem, increased sense of well-being and psychological control, enhanced socialization, and improved quality of life.[121,177]

Occurrence of Type 2 Diabetes. Regular physical activity contributes to delaying and even preventing the onset of insulin resistance and type 2 diabetes in persons at high risk for developing this disease. Physical activity benefits are particularly pronounced for obese individuals and perhaps all persons with increased abdominal fat deposition.

Physical Activity Risks in Type 2 Diabetics

Type 2 diabetics are subjected to different potential adverse physical activity influences. These include problems associated with the general systemic circulation, cardiovascular dynamics, metabolic functions, and musculoskeletal maladies.

System	Potential Problem
Systemic	• Retinal hemorrhage • Increased proteinuria • Acceleration of microvascular lesions
Cardiovascular	• Cardiac arrhythmias • Ischemic heart disease • Excessive exercise blood pressure • Postexercise orthostatic hypertension
Metabolic	• Increased hyperglycemia • Increased ketosis
Musculoskeletal	• Foot ulcers with neuropathy • Orthopedic injury related to neuropathy • Accelerated degenerative joint disease

Background image: Umpaporn/Shutterstock

Physical Activity Guidelines for People with Type 1 Diabetes

Clinically, the benefits of regular physical activity to improve glucose control in type 1 diabetes remain uncertain. To complicate matters for type 1 diabetics, physical activity can trigger a potentially dangerous dual response:

1. Enhanced glucose uptake by active muscles
2. Greater than anticipated exogenous insulin distributed by more rapid circulation with exercise

These two factors could worsen the imbalance between glucose supply and use, increasing the risk for serious complications from hypoglycemia. "In a Practical Sense: Diabetes, Hypoglycemia, and Physical Activity" offers guidelines for the diabetic patient, including those with well-controlled type 1 diabetes who wish to engage in prolonged and strenuous activity while minimizing the principal risk of hypoglycemia.

Resistance Training and Endocrine Function

Muscle remodeling occurs with resistance training and reflects a complex process involving cell receptor interaction with different hormones and DNA-mediated production of new contractile proteins. The specific response to muscular overload initially links to the configuration of the exercise stimulus—intensity, frequency, volume, sequence, mode, and recovery interval. **FIGURE 20.25** proposes how intense resistance training improves overall muscular size, strength, and power. Hormonal factors responsible for training-induced changes in muscle size and function include these three factors:

1. Changes in hepatic and extrahepatic hormone clearance rates
2. Differential hormone secretion rates with accompanying fluid shifts around receptor sites
3. Altered receptor-site activation via neurohumoral control

In general, early-phase adaptations to resistance training reflect a hormonal response that mediates neuromuscular system adaptations that improve muscle strength. Testosterone and GH are the two primary hormones that impact resistance-training adaptations.[156,190,223] *Testosterone augments GH release and interacts with nervous system function to increase muscle force production.* These roles may be more important than any direct anabolic testosterone effect *per se*. A single resistance training session generally elicits a short-term rise in serum testosterone and decrease in cortisol, with a greater response in males than in females.[32,55,95,173,232] Concurrently, catecholamine release from the adrenal medulla increases with the acute stress of high-force and high-power exercise protocols.[19]

Resistance training in males increases frequency and amplitude of testosterone and GH secretion, thereby creating a favorable hormonal environment for muscular growth (hypertrophy). In contrast, most studies with females fail to demonstrate changes in testosterone and GH concentrations with training. Gender differences in hormone output with resistance

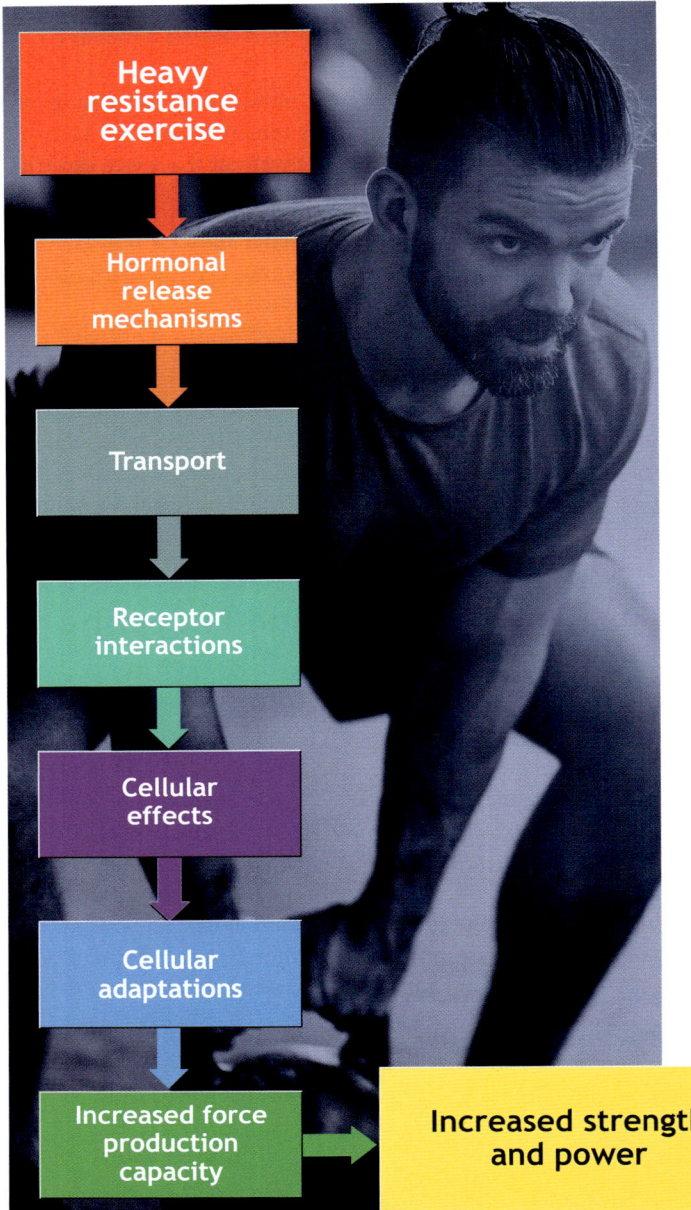

FIGURE 20.25. Model of how heavy resistance training produces favorable adaptations in muscle structure to enhance maximal power and strength.
(Adapted with permission from Kraemer WJ, Ratamess NA. Endocrine responses and adaptations to strength training. In: Komi PV, ed. *Strength and Power in Sport*. 2nd Ed. London: Blackwell Scientific; 2003. Background image: Flamingo Images/Shutterstock.)

Opioid Peptides and Physical Activity

Scientists who studied the pain-relieving effects of opioid peptides such as morphine on brain function in the 1970s reported these substances exhibited neurotransmitter effects and targeted specific opioid brain receptor sites. With this finding came the realization that perhaps the brain itself produced endogenous opioid, mood-altering substances. Evidence for endogenous substances with opiatelike behavior first emerged with the isolation and purification of two opioid pentapeptides, methionine, and leucine enkephalin (Greek, meaning "in the brain"). These opioids form part of a larger propiocortin precursor molecule produced in the anterior pituitary. Other opioid substances include β-lipotropin, β-endorphin, and dynorphin (the most potent of the opioid peptides).

Opioid Effects

The various endogenous opioids exert widespread effects with a range in function from neurohormones to neurotransmitters.[224] Endogenous opiates strongly inhibit hormonal release from the anterior pituitary, principally LH and FSH release. This inhibition may play a key role in menstrual cycle disturbances observed among many physically active women—delay in menarche, dysfunctional uterine bleeding, secondary amenorrhea, and luteal phase inadequacy. In contrast to their inhibitory role, the opioid peptides stimulate GH and prolactin release.

Endorphins also regulate other hormones including ACTH, the catecholamines, and cortisol. Serum β-endorphin and/or β-lipotropin concentrations generally increase with physical activity similarly in men and women, although the response varies among individuals and varies inversely with activity intensity.[40,54,93] Physical activity increases β-endorphin up to five times the resting level and probably even more in the brain itself,[85] particularly region-specific effects in frontolimbic brain areas involved in processing affective states and mood.[12] With resistance exercise, β-endorphin release varies with the exercise protocol; longer duration (lighter resistance) and longer interset rest intervals elicit the greatest response.[94]

Physical activity associates with a reduction in mental depression mediated through the endocannabinoid system's action on neurotrophins such as **brain-derived neurotrophic factor (BDNF)**. BDNF is considered a major candidate molecule for exercise-induced brain plasticity or susceptibility for modification. Eleven healthy trained male cyclists cycled intensely for 60 min at 55% of maximum followed by 30 min at 75% maximum. Plasma levels of the endocannabinoids anandamide (AEA) and 2-arachidonoylglycerol (2-AG) were assessed and their possible link with serum BDNF evaluated. AEA levels increased during cycling and in 15 min of recovery, whereas 2-AG concentrations remained stable. BDNF levels increased significantly during cycling and then decreased during 15 min of recovery. AEA and BDNF concentrations correlated positively at the end of activity and after 15-min recovery, suggesting that increased AEA during exercise might be involved in the exercise-induced increase in peripheral BDNF levels. These findings provide evidence in

training may ultimately explain variations in muscle responsiveness in strength and size to chronic muscular overload.

Testosterone response to resistance exercise reveals several factors that increase its release. The most effective factors include intense activation of large-muscle groups with dead lifts, power cleans, and squats, and other heavy resistance exercises done at 85 to 95% 1-RM or high-volume (total quantity) training with multiple sets and/or exercise with less than 1-min rest intervals.[96] Men who have resistance trained for years show increased resting testosterone levels, which links with their increased strength improvement patterns over time.[63]

humans that acute and strenuous physical activity presents a physiological stressor to increase peripheral AEA levels, and that BDNF might be a mechanism by which AEA influences the neuroplastic and antidepressant physical activity effects.[70]

The Exercise High

The precise physiologic significance of the response patterns observed for the various endogenous opioid peptides to physical activity remains unclear, but several noteworthy effects emerge. These include the postulated opioid effect in triggering the **exercise high**, a state described as euphoria and exhilaration, as moderate-to-intense aerobic activity duration increases. Endorphin secretion also may increase pain tolerance, improve appetite control, and reduce anxiety, tension, anger, and confusion. Interestingly, these effects generally reflect the documented psychological benefits of regular physical activity.

The exercise training effect on endorphin response remains controversial. One study reported no significant change in β-endorphin response to prolonged effort following endurance training for 8 wk. Contrasting research showed that general physical conditioning augmented β-endorphin and β-lipotropin release during physical activity.[22] Greater endorphin release also occurs with sprint-type training, suggesting that anaerobic factors affect endorphin dynamics.[93]

Regular physical activity participation can increase an individual's sensitivity to opioid effects, reducing the amount of hormone required to induce a specific effect. Regular physical activity causes the opioids produced during physical activity to degrade more slowly than in the pretraining condition. A slower hormone disposal rate facilitates and prolongs an opioid response and possibly augments one's tolerance for extended exercise. Taken in total, one could view the endogenous opioid response to regular exercise as a form of "positive addiction."

Endogenous Opioid Peptide Effects on Lower Back Pain

The same mechanisms responsible for the endogenous opioid peptide effects is believed partially responsible for the beneficial exercise training effects on chronic lower back pain. As an example, in one randomized-control study, endogenous opioid mechanisms contributed to the analgesic effects of an aerobic exercise intervention for chronic low back pain. Individuals with chronic lower back pain were randomly assigned to either a 6 wk, 18 session aerobic exercise intervention (n = 38) or a usual-activity control group (n = 44). Before and after the intervention, participants underwent laboratory sessions to assess responses to evoked heat pain after receiving either a saline placebo or intravenous naloxone (opioid antagonist) in double-blinded, crossover fashion. Relative to controls, exercise participants reported significantly greater pre-post intervention decreases in chronic low-pain intensity. Dose-response effects were suggested in the exercise group by a positive association between exercise intensity and an increase in the endogenous opioid response. The researchers concluded that aerobic training in the absence of other interventions appears effective to manage low back pain related in part to the body's endogenous opioid system.[225]

Physical Activity and Immune Function

"Don't exercise when fatigued or you'll get sick" reflects the common perception touted by parents, athletes, and coaches that excessive intense exercise increases susceptibility to certain illnesses. In contrast, some also believe that regular, more moderate physical activity improves health and reduces susceptibility to the common cold.

Studies as early as 1918 reported that most pneumonia cases in boys in boarding schools occurred among athletes, and respiratory infections seemed to progress toward pneumonia after intense sports training. Anecdotal reports also related poliomyelitis (polio) severity to participation in intense exercise at the critical infection time. Current epidemiologic and clinical findings from the **exercise immunology** field—the interactions among the physical, environmental, and psychological factors on immune function—support the belief that short-term, unusually strenuous physical activity affects immune function to increase susceptibility to illness, particularly upper respiratory tract infection (URTI).[52,227] Repeated URTI may signal an overtraining state (see Chapter 21).

The immune system comprises a highly complex and self-regulating grouping of cells, hormones, and interactive modulators that defend the body from invasion from outside microbes (bacterial, viral, and fungal), foreign macromolecules, and abnormal cancerous cell growth. This system has two functional divisions:

1. **Innate immunity system**: Includes anatomic and physiologic components (skin, mucous membranes, body temperature, and specialized defenses—natural killer cells, diverse phagocytes, and inflammatory barriers)
2. **Acquired immunity system**: Consists of specialized B- and T-lymphocyte cells, which regulate a highly effective immune response to a specific infectious agent. When infection occurs, an optimally functioning immune system diminishes illness severity and speeds recovery

 See the animation "Immune Response" on **Lippincott Connect** to view this process.

FIGURE 20.26 proposes a theoretical model for the interactions among the immune system and physical activity, stress, and illness. Within this framework, physical activity, stress, and illness interact, each exerting its separate effect on immunity. For example, physical activity affects susceptibility to illness, while certain illnesses clearly negatively impact exercise capacity. Likewise, psychological factors (via links between the hypothalamus and immune function) include nutritional deficiencies and acute alterations in normal sleep schedule, separately and combined can influence resistance to illness. Also, physical activity can either positively or negatively modulate the stress response. Each factor—stress, illness, and short- and long-duration physical activity—exerts an independent effect on immune status, immune function, and resistance to disease.

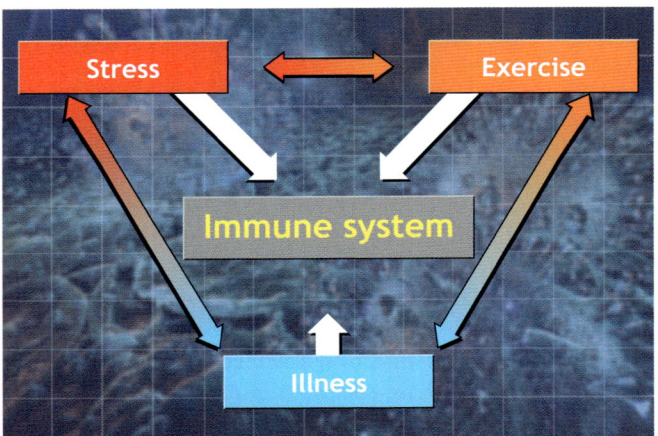

FIGURE 20.26. Theoretical interrelationships among stress, physical activity, illness, and the immune system.
(Adapted with permission from MacKinnon LT. Current challenges and future expectations in exercise immunology: back to the future. *Med Sci Sports Exerc.* 1994;26:191. Background image: 3Dme Creative Studio/Shutterstock.)

Upper Respiratory Tract Infections

FIGURE 20.27 describes the general J-shaped curve relating exercise volume and/or intensity and risk to URTI.[53] Different immune function markers generally follow an *inverted J-shaped curve*.[138,199] Implications drawn from this relationship may be simplistic, but light to moderate physical activity offers more protection against URTI and possibly diverse cancers than a sedentary lifestyle.[109,113,159] Moderate physical activity does not exacerbate illness severity and duration when an infection occurs.[185] In contrast, a marathon run or intense training session provides an "*open window*" (3 to 72 hr) that decreases antiviral and antibacterial resistance and increases URTI risk that manifests within 1 to 2 wk[31,129] particularly for athletes prone to illness.[28] Approximately 13% of the participants in a Los Angeles marathon reported an episode of infectious URTI during the week following the race. For runners of comparable ability who did not compete for reasons other than illness, the infection rate approximated just 2%.[130]

Short-Term Effects of Physical Activity on Immune Function

Moderate Activity. Moderate physical activity boosts natural immune functions and host defenses for up to several hours.[50] Noteworthy effects include increases in natural killer (NK) cell activity. These phagocytic lymphocyte subpopulations enhance the blood's cytotoxic capacity and provide the first line of defense against pathogens. The NK cell does not require prior or specific sensitization to foreign bodies or neoplastic cells. Rather, the cells demonstrate spontaneous cytolytic activity that ultimately ruptures and/or inactivates viruses and also depresses the metastatic potential of tumor cells.

Exhaustive Activity. *Prolonged exhaustive physical activity and other forms of extreme stress or increased training severely depress the body's first line of defense against infection.*[91,105,127,141,187] Repeated cycles of intense activity and sports participation further compound the risk.[197] Impaired immune function from strenuous exertion "carries over" to a second exercise bout on the same day to augment negative changes in neutrophils, lymphocytes, and select CD cells.[152,153,200] Elevated temperature, cytokines, and stress-related hormones (e.g., epinephrine, GH, cortisol, β-endorphins) activated in exhaustive effort may mediate the transient depression of innate mechanisms (NK cell and neutrophil cytotoxicity) and depress adaptive immune defenses (T- and β-cell function).[17,167] Reduced immunity following strenuous exercise remains in the upper respiratory tract's mucosal immune system[5,124,182] and associates with increased URTI risk.[128] This negative effect on immune response clearly supports advising individuals with URTI symptoms to refrain from physical activity (or at least "go easy") to optimize normal immune mechanisms and thus combat infection.

Long-Term Effects of Physical Activity on Immune Function

Aerobic training with accompanying weight loss positively affects natural immune functions in young, and older individuals and obese persons during weight loss.[43,45,164] The training effect includes enhanced functional capacity of natural cytotoxic immune mechanisms (e.g., antitumor NK cell activity) and a diminished age-related decrease in T-cell function and associated cytokine production.[85] The cytotoxic T cells defend directly against viral and fungal infections and help regulate other immune mechanisms.

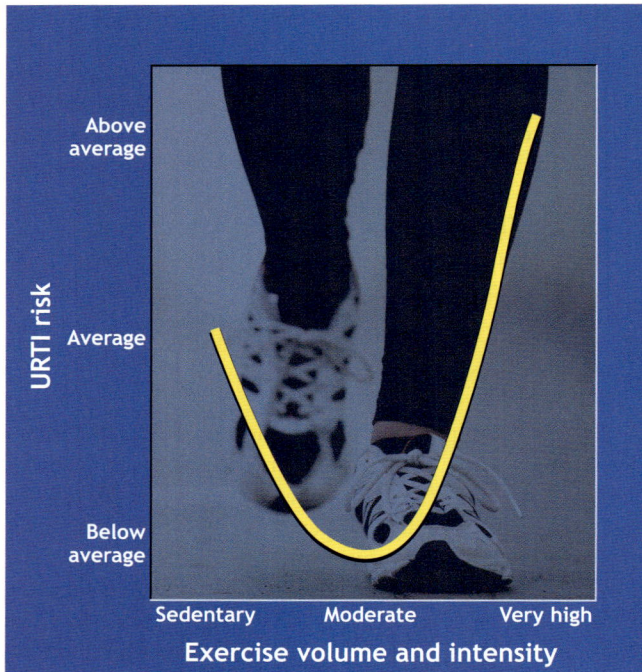

FIGURE 20.27. General relationship between physical activity intensity and susceptibility to upper respiratory tract infection (URTI). Moderate exercise reduces URTI risk, but high training volume and intensity increase the risk.
(Adapted from Nieman DC. Exercise, upper respiratory tract infection, and the immune system. *Med Sci Sports Exerc.* 1994;26:128. Background image: Giovanni G/Shutterstock.)

If exercise training enhances immune function, one might ask why trained individuals show increased URTI susceptibility following intense competition. The **open window hypothesis** maintains that an inordinate increase in training or competition exposes highly conditioned athletes to abnormal stress that transiently but severely depresses NK cell function. The immunodepression period (open window) decreases natural resistance to infection. The inhibitory effect of strenuous physical activity on ACTH and cortisol's maintenance of optimal blood glucose concentrations may negatively affect the immune process. For individuals who are physically active regularly but *only* at moderate levels, the window of opportunity for infection remains "closed," thus maintaining regular physical activity's protective benefits on immune function.

Effects of Resistance Training on Immune Function

Compared to sedentary controls, prior resistance training for 9 years did not affect resting NK cell activity or number,[131] and activated monocytes more than typically observed for aerobic training. Monocyte activation releases prostaglandins that downregulate NK cells following physical activity, blunting the long-term positive effect of physical activity on NK cells. These researchers had previously reported a 225% increase in NK cells following acute resistance exercise,[132] a response similar to the short-term effect from moderate aerobic activity.[47,183]

Effects of Nutrition on Immune Function

Nutrition may optimize immune system function with strenuous physical activity and training.[51,69,115,154]

Macronutrients. Consuming a high-fat diet (62% energy from lipids) negatively affected the immune system compared to a carbohydrate-rich diet (65% energy from carbohydrates). In general, endurance athletes who ingest carbohydrate during a race or prolonged prerace trial experience lower disruption in hormonal and immune measures (indicating diminished physiologic stress levels) than athletes not consuming carbohydrate.[155] Supplementing with a 6% carbohydrate beverage (0.71 L before; 0.25 L every 15 min during, and 500 mL every hour throughout a 4.5-hr recovery) depressed cytokine levels in the inflammatory cascade after 2.5 hr of running at 77% $\dot{V}O_{2max}$.[126] Consuming carbohydrates (4 mL · kg body mass^{-1}) every 15 min during intense running or cycling for 2.5 hr maintained higher plasma glucose levels in 10 triathletes during exercise than a placebo.[134] A blunted cortisol response and diminished proinflammatory and anti-inflammatory cytokine responses accompanied the higher plasma glucose levels with supplementation in both forms of exercise. Similar benefits from carbohydrate ingestion on cortisol and select anti-inflammatory cytokines occur following marathon competition, regardless of age or gender.[135] This suggests a carbohydrate-induced reduction in overall physiologic stress in prolonged intense physical activity. In contrast, carbohydrate ingestion during intense resistance training for 2 hr produced no effect on immune changes compared to similar training with placebo ingestion.[136]

Micronutrients. Combined supplementation with antioxidant vitamins C and E produces more prominent immunopotentiating effects (enhanced cytokine production) in young, healthy adults than supplementation with either vitamin alone.[82] A 200-mg daily vitamin E supplement enhanced several clinically relevant T-cell–mediated indices in healthy elderly subjects.[116] Long-term daily supplementation with physiologic vitamin and mineral doses or with 200 mg of vitamin E did not lower either the URTI incidence or severity of acute respiratory tract infections in noninstitutionalized persons age 60 and older. For individuals with infections, those receiving vitamin E had *longer* total illness duration and activity restrictions.[56]

Daily supplementation with vitamin C benefits individuals engaged in intense physical activity, particularly those predisposed to frequent URTI.[67,142] Runners who received a 600-mg daily vitamin C supplement before and for 3 wk following a 90-km/56 mi ultramarathon competition experienced fewer URTI symptoms—running nose, sneezing, sore throat, coughing, fever—than runners given a placebo. Interestingly, infection risk inversely related to race performance; those with the fastest times suffered more URTI symptoms. Symptoms also appeared most frequently in runners who trained more strenuously. Adding vitamin C and E and perhaps carbohydrate ingestion before, during, and after prolonged stressful exertion may boost immune mechanisms to combat infection.[133] More than likely, other manageable stressors—sleep deficit, mental stress, poor nutrition, weight loss—magnify stress on the immune system from a single or repeated exhaustive exercise bout.

Glutamine. The nonessential amino acid glutamine plays an important role in normal immune function. One protective aspect concerns glutamine's role as an energy fuel for nucleotide synthesis by the disease-fighting lymphocytes and macrophage cells that defend against infection.[21,160,181] In humans, sepsis, injury, burns, surgery, and endurance exercise lower plasma and skeletal muscle glutamine levels. Lowered plasma glutamine levels most likely occur because glutamine demand by the liver, kidneys, gut, and immune system exceeds its supply from the diet and skeletal muscle. The lowered plasma glutamine concentration may contribute to the immunosuppression that accompanies extreme physical stress.[11,71,163] Glutamine supplementation might reduce susceptibility to URTI following prolonged competition or an exhaustive training bout.

Marathoners who ingested a glutamine drink (5 g L-glutamine in 330 mL mineral water) at the end of a race and then 2 hr later reported fewer URTI symptoms than unsupplemented athletes.[23] In subsequent studies by the same researchers to determine a possible protective mechanism, glutamine's effect on postexercise infection risk did not relate to any change in blood lymphocyte distribution.[24] URTI in athletes during intense training does not fluctuate with changes in plasma glutamine concentration. Pre-exercise glutamine supplementation does not affect the immune response following repeated bouts of intense physical activity.[101] Glutamine supplements taken 0, 30, 60, and 90 min after a marathon race prevented the drop in glutamine concentrations following the race but did not influence lymphokine-activated killer cell activity, proliferative responses, or exercise-induced changes in leukocyte subpopulations.[149] Based on current evidence, we cannot recommend glutamine supplements to reliably blunt the immunosuppression associated with exhaustive activity.

Optimizing Immune Function

A lifestyle that emphasizes regular physical activity, maintaining a well-balanced diet, minimizing stress, and obtaining adequate sleep generally can optimize immune function. For weight loss, we recommend a gradual approach because more rapid weight loss with severe caloric restriction suppresses immune function.[114] With prolonged intense activity, consuming about $1\text{-}L \cdot hr^{-1}$ of a typical carbohydrate-rich sports drink lessens negative changes in immune function from the stress of physical activity and accompanying carbohydrate depletion. In general, endurance athletes who consume carbohydrate during a race experience a lower disruption in hormonal and immune measures than athletes who do not consume carbohydrate.

Physical Activity and Cancer

Epidemiologic studies support a protective association between regular physical activity and breast, colon, lung, and prostate cancer risk.[106,117] Enhancement of other natural immune functions with regular physical activity also may contribute to the cancer-protective effect of regular physical activity in addition to its beneficial effects on NK cell activity. Upgraded defenses include augmented phagocytic capacity of the monocyte-macrophage lineage combined with more robust cytotoxic and intracellular killing capacities (T-cell activity) that inhibit tumor growth and destroy cancer cells.[198] Other beneficial effects of regular physical activity on aspects of cancer development include beneficial changes in the body's antioxidant functions, endocrine profiles, prostaglandin metabolism, body composition, and for colon cancer a beneficial increase in intestinal transit time. A meta-analysis using seven prospective cohort studies that included more than 5000 patients concluded that regular physical activity associated with significantly reduced colorectal cancer-specific mortality and all-cause mortality.[80] In Chapter 31, we review the role physical activity plays in preventing and treating different forms of cancer.

Summary

1. The endocrine system consists of a host organ, a transmitted substance (hormone), and a target or receptor organ.
2. Hormones consist of steroids or amino acid (polypeptide) derivatives.
3. Hormones alter cellular reaction rates by acting at specific receptor sites to enhance or inhibit enzyme function.
4. Blood hormone concentration depends on the amount of hormone synthesized and the amount released or taken up by the target organ and its removal rate from the blood.
5. Most hormones respond to peripheral stimulus on an as-needed basis; others release at regular intervals, and some span several weeks while others pattern on a 24-hr cycle.
6. The anterior pituitary secretes prolactin, gonadotropic hormones FSH and LH, corticotropin, TSH, and GH.
7. GH promotes cell division and cellular proliferation, while IGFs (or somatomedins) mediate many of GH effects.
8. TSH controls hormonal secretion by the thyroid gland, ACTH regulates hormone output from the adrenal cortex, prolactin affects reproduction and development of secondary sex characteristics of females; FSH and LH stimulate the ovaries to secrete the estrogens estradiol and progesterone in females and testosterone secretion from the testes in males.
9. The posterior pituitary secretes ADH, which controls water excretion by the kidneys; it also secretes oxytocin for birthing and lactation.
10. PTH controls blood calcium balance. It increases ionic (free) calcium by stimulating three target organs—bone, kidneys, and small intestine.
11. TSH stimulates cellular metabolism in all cells and increases carbohydrate and lipid breakdown in energy metabolism.
12. The adrenal medulla secretes epinephrine and norepinephrine, and the adrenal cortex secretes mineralocorticoids, glucocorticoids, and androgens.
13. Moderate aerobic and resistance exercise increases testosterone in untrained males, and plasma testosterone and estrogen levels during moderate physical activity in females.
14. Insulin, secreted by the pancreas' β cells, increases glucose transport into cells to control blood glucose levels and carbohydrate metabolism.
15. Diabetes mellitus is caused by a diminished supply of insulin, the body's decreased insulin sensitivity, or increased resistance to its action.
16. Pancreatic α-cells secrete glucagon, an insulin antagonist that raises blood sugar levels.
17. Regular physical activity exerts differential effects on resting and exercise-induced hormone production and release.
18. Exercise training elevates the hormone response during physical activity for ACTH and cortisol and depresses the response for GH, prolactin, FSH, LH, testosterone, ADH, T_4, catecholamines, and insulin; no training response occurs for aldosterone, renin, and angiotensin.
19. Exercise-induced β-endorphin elevation contributes to euphoria, increased pain tolerance, "exercise high," and altered menstrual function.
20. Unusually intense physical activity increases URTI susceptibility, while moderate physical activity upgrades immune responses to protect against URTI.
21. Regular physical activity positively affects natural immune functions to protect against URTI and various cancers.

Key Terms

Acini: Exocrine pancreatic cells that produce and transport enzymes into the intestines

Acquired immunity system: Specialized B- and T-lymphocyte cells that regulate immune responses to a specific infectious agent

Adenylate cyclase: Enzyme in cell's plasma membrane; reacts with hormone to form the compound cycle 3'5'-adenosine monophosphate

Adrenal cortex: Adrenal gland outer portion secretes mineralocorticoids, glucocorticoids, and androgens

Adrenal glands: Flattened, caplike glandular tissues situated above each kidney comprises the medulla and cortex

Adrenal medulla: Adrenal gland's inner portion; secretes the catecholamines epinephrine and norepinephrine

Adrenocortical hormone: Provides potent adrenal cortex stimulation to increase free fatty acid mobilization for energy

Adrenocorticotropic hormone (ACTH): Anterior pituitary gland hormone that regulates adrenal cortex output, enhances fatty acid mobilization from adipose tissue, increases gluconeogenesis, and stimulates protein catabolism; also known as corticotropin

Allosteric modulation: Chemical enzyme process that combines with another enzyme to alter its shape and ability to act effectively

Amine: Nitrogen-containing organic compound derived from ammonia (NH_3) that includes the alkaloids present in certain plants and the catecholamine neurotransmitters (i.e., dopamine, epinephrine)

Amylin: Peptide hormone secreted with insulin from the pancreatic β cells; contributes to glycemic regulation by slowing gastric emptying and promoting satiety

Androgens: Hormone group that includes testosterone and androstenedione; play important roles in male traits and reproductive activity

Angiotensin (II and III): Peptide hormone produced by the kidneys that causes vasoconstriction and subsequent increase in blood pressure

Angiotensin II type 1 receptor (AT1): Angiotensin receptor that regulates aldosterone secretion; important in controlling blood pressure and volume

Anterior pituitary: Pituitary gland front portion whose secreted hormones influence growth, sexual development, skin pigmentation, and thyroid and adrenocortical function

Antidiuretic hormone (ADH): Posterior pituitary gland hormone influencing kidneys' water excretion; also known as vasopressin

Brain-derived neurotrophic factor (BDNF): Protein in humans encoded by the BDNF gene, a member of the neurotrophin family of growth factors; relates to canonical nerve-growth factors involved in learning and memory

Calcitonin: Calcium-regulating thyroid gland hormone that promotes calcium deposition in bone and lowers blood calcium levels

Cholecystokinin: A peptide hormone of the gastrointestinal system responsible for stimulating the digestion of lipid and protein

Corticotropin-releasing factor: Releasing hormone found mainly in nucleus of the hypothalamus that regulates the release of ACTH

Cortisol: Adrenal cortex's stress hormone that promotes protein and lipid catabolism, raises blood glucose levels, and supports the body's adaptation to stressors; also known as hydrocortisone when supplied as a medication

Dehydroepiandrosterone: Adrenal cortex hormone that acts similarly to testosterone

Diurnal pattern: Any pattern that recurs every 24 hr (daily)

Downregulation: Cell process that decreases cellular response and/or components when exposed to an external stimulus

Endocrine glands: Possess no ducts (referred to as ductless glands); secrete substances directly into extracellular spaces around the gland

Endocrine system: Consists of a host organ (gland), minute quantities of chemical messengers (hormones), and a target or receptor organ

Estradiol: Ovarian hormone that regulates ovulation, menstruation, and physiologic adjustments during pregnancy

Exercise high: Endorphin secretion related to a state of euphoria and exhilaration as the duration of moderate-to-intense aerobic activity increases

Exercise immunology: An emerging subdiscipline within exercise physiology concerned with the relationship between exercise, immune function, and infection/disease risk

Exocrine glands: Contain secretory ducts that carry substances directly to a specific body compartment or surface

Facilitated diffusion: Process of spontaneous transport of molecules or ions across a biological membrane via specific proteins; does not directly require chemical energy

Fasting plasma glucose (FPG) test: Measure of plasma glucose following an 8-hr fast; recommended as the first test for suspected type 2 diabetes

Follicle-stimulating hormone (FSH): Anterior pituitary gland hormone that initiates follicle growth in the ovaries to stimulate estrogen secretion; in males, stimulates and promotes sperm development

Gastrin: Peptide hormone that stimulates secretion of gastric acid (HCl) by stomach and aids in gastric motility

Ghrelin: Hormone produced by enteroendocrine cells of the gastrointestinal tract, especially the stomach, and is often called a "hunger hormone" because it increases food intake

Glucocorticoids: Adrenal cortex steroid hormones that promote protein and lipid catabolism, raise blood glucose levels, and modulate adaptation to stress

Glucose transporters (GLUTs): Membrane proteins that facilitate glucose transport across the plasma membrane by facilitated diffusion

Glucose-clamp test: Method for quantifying insulin secretion and resistance; measures either how well an individual metabolizes glucose or how sensitive an individual is to insulin; also called euglycemic clamp, and hyperinsulinemic-euglycemic clamp technique

Glycosuria: Glucose in urine

Growth hormone (GH): Peptide hormone that stimulates growth, cell reproduction, and cell regeneration; also known as somatotropin

Hemoglobin A1c test (HbA1c): Hb that chemically links to sugar and represents the 3-month average blood sugar level as a diagnostic diabetes test; also known as the glycated hemoglobin or glycohemoglobin test

Hormones: Chemical messengers produced by endocrine glands affecting all aspects of human function

Hyperthyroidism: Excessive thyroid hormone secretion promotes increased metabolism, protein catabolism, muscle weakness, weight loss, heightened reflex activity, and tachycardia

Hypophysis: Pituitary gland

Hypothalamic-pituitary-adrenal axis: Complex set of feedback interactions among three components: the hypothalamus, the pituitary, and the adrenal glands

Hypothyroidism: Blunted secretion of thyroid hormones; effects include reduced metabolism and cold intolerance, decreased protein synthesis, depressed reflex activity and fatigue, and bradycardia

Innate immunity system: Anatomic and physiologic components (e.g., skin, mucous membranes, body temperature) and the specialized defense mechanisms (e.g., natural killer cells, phagocytes, and inflammatory barriers)

Insulinlike growth factors (IGFs): Mediate growth hormone's potent effects as a chemical messenger

Insulin resistance: Pathological condition where cells fail to respond normally to the hormone insulin

Insulin: Peptide hormone released by pancreatic β cells that lowers blood glucose levels and promotes protein, lipid, and glycogen synthesis

Islets of Langerhans: Pancreatic cells with 20% α cells (secrete glucagon) and 75% β cells (secrete insulin and peptide amylin)

Leptin: Small peptide considered a pre-inflammatory cytokine belonging to the IL-6 cytokine family that represents an anorexigenic peptide that increases energy expenditure

Luteinizing hormone (LH): Anterior pituitary gland hormone; in females, complements FSH action to initiate estrogen secretion and egg follicle rupture; in males, stimulates testes to secrete testosterone

Metabolic syndrome: Cluster of unhealthy conditions (e.g., obesity, high blood pressure, high blood glucose, dyslipidemia), which increases coronary heart disease, stroke, and T2DM risk

Mineralocorticoids: Hormones produced by the adrenal cortex that regulate sodium retention and potassium excretion in the extracellular fluid

Neurohypophysis: Posterior pituitary gland

Norepinephrine: Adrenal medulla sympathetic nervous system hormone that facilitates sympathetic activity, increases cardiac output, regulates blood vessel diameter, and increases glycogen catabolism and fatty acid release

Open window hypothesis: Suggests that an inordinate increase in training or competition exposes highly conditioned athletes to abnormal stress that depresses NK cell function

Oral glucose-tolerance test: Evaluates blood sugar levels 2 hr after drinking a 75 g concentrated glucose solution

Osteoclasts: Bone-reabsorbing cells that digest bone matrix to release ionic calcium and phosphate to the blood

Oxytocin: Posterior pituitary gland hormone that targets breast and uterus tissues, stimulates uterine contractions, and mammary gland milk secretion

Parathyroid hormone (PTH): Regulates blood calcium balance, and promotes calcium release from bone, absorption from small intestine, resorption by the kidneys, and stimulates vitamin D_3 synthesis

Pituitary gland: Endocrine gland the size of a pea and weighing 0.5 g/0.018 oz; comprised of anterior and posterior portions and forms a protrusion from bottom of the hypothalamus at the base of the brain; also known as the hypophysis

Polydipsia: Excessive thirst

Polyphagia: Strong hunger sensations or desire to eat often, triggers overeating

Polyuria: Frequent urination

Posterior pituitary: Glandular tissue formed from hypothalamic neurons; secretes the peptide hormones oxytocin and antidiuretic hormone

Progesterone: Ovarian hormone that promotes endometrial growth to prepare uterus for pregnancy; contributes specific regulatory input to the female reproductive cycle, uterine smooth muscle action, and lactation

Prolactin: Anterior pituitary gland hormone that initiates and supports mammary gland milk secretion

Proopiomelanocortin (POMC): Pituitary gland precursor of circulating melanocyte stimulating hormone (α-MSH), adrenocorticotropin hormone (ACTH), and β-endorphin

Relative insulin deficiency: Inadequate pancreatic insulin production to control blood sugar

Releasing factor: Hormone whose main purpose controls release of other hormones by stimulating or inhibiting their release

Renin-angiotensin mechanism: Diminished renal blood flow stimulates the kidneys to release the enzyme renin into the blood to stimulate angiotensin II and angiotensin III production

Renin: Kidney enzyme that catabolizes protein and produces rise in blood pressure by the renin-angiotensin mechanism

Secreted amount: Describes the plasma concentration of a hormone—represents the sum of hormone synthesis and release by the host gland

Secretin: Hormone that regulates water homeostasis and pH

Somatoliberin: Growth hormone–releasing hormone (GHRH), which stimulates somatotropin secretion from the anterior pituitary gland

Somatostatin: Polypeptide hormone secreted by the delta cells of the islets of Langerhans to inhibit *thyrotropin*, *somatotropin*, and *corticotropin* secretion; regulates gastrointestinal digestion and nutrient absorption

Steroid: Organic compound arranged in a specific molecular configuration; serves as important component of cell membranes

Sympathoadrenal response: Increased activity involving the sympathetic nervous system and adrenal gland, which causes increased adrenal medulla epinephrine secretion and norepinephrine release from postganglionic sympathetic nerve endings

Testosterone: Principal male sex hormone and anabolic steroid secreted primarily by the male testis and female ovary; plays key role in testis and prostate development, and promotes secondary sex characteristics (increased muscle mass, bone mass, and hair growth)

Thyroid-stimulating hormone (TSH): Anterior pituitary gland hormone that controls thyroid gland hormone secretion; maintains thyroid gland growth and development and increases thyroid gland metabolism

Thyroxine (T_4): Thyroid gland hormone; exerts stimulating effect on enzyme activity, increases metabolic rate, and promotes normal physical development

Triiodothyronine (T_3): Most powerful active form of thyroid hormone; significantly impacts growth, body temperature, and heart rate

Upregulation: How cells increase cellular components to an external stimulus

α cells: Pancreatic cells of the islets of Langerhans of the pancreas; serve an exocrine function and secrete digestive enzymes

β cells: Pancreatic cells of the islets of Langerhans; secrete insulin and amylin peptide

References are available online at Lippincott Connect.

Additional References

Aktaş HŞ, et al. The effects of high intensity-interval training on vaspin, adiponectin and leptin levels in women with polycystic ovary syndrome. *Arch Physiol Biochem*. 2022;128:37.

Alkhalaf Z, et al. Markers of vitamin D metabolism and premenstrual symptoms in healthy women with regular cycles. *Hum Reprod*. 2021;36:1808.

Christiansen M, et al. Performance of an automated insulin delivery system: results of early phase feasibility studies. *Diabetes Technol Ther*. 2021;23:187.

Dipla K, et al. Relative energy deficiency in sports (RED-S): elucidation of endocrine changes affecting the health of males and females. *Hormones (Athens)*. 2021;20:35.

Guan YM, et al. A study on the evaluation of the effect of exercise on the treatment of chronic diseases based on a digital human movement model. *J Healthc Eng*. 2022;2022:1984145.

Hopewell S, et al. Progressive exercise compared with best-practice advice, with or without corticosteroid injection, for rotator cuff disorders: the GRASP factorial RCT. *Health Technol Assess*. 2021;25:1.

Iaccarino G, et al. Modulation of insulin sensitivity by exercise training: implications for cardiovascular. *J Cardiovasc Trans Res*. 2021;14:256.

Kraemer WJ, et al. Growth hormone(s), testosterone, insulin-like growth factors, and cortisol: roles and integration for cellular development and growth with exercise. *Front Endocrinol (Lausanne)*. 2020;11:33.

Lendeckel F, et al. Association of cardiopulmonary exercise capacity and adipokines in the general population. *Int J Sports Med*. 2022. doi:10.1055/a-1699-2380.

Lombardi G, et al. Physical activity-dependent regulation of parathyroid hormone and calcium-phosphorous metabolism. *Int J Mol Sci*. 2020;21:E5388.

Martínez-Majolero V, et al. Physical exercise in people with chronic kidney disease-practices and perception of the knowledge of health professionals and physical activity and sport science professionals about their prescription. *Int J Environ Res Public Health*. 2022;19:656.

Meeusen R, et al. Endurance exercise-induced and mental fatigue and the brain. *Exp Physiol*. 2021;106:2294.

Morimoto Y, et al. Web portals for patients with chronic diseases: scoping review of the functional features and theoretical frameworks of telerehabilitation platforms. *J Med Internet Res*. 2022;24:e27759.

Nobari H, et al. The effects of 14-week betaine supplementation on endocrine markers, body composition and anthropometrics in professional youth soccer players: a double blind, randomized, placebo-controlled trial. *J Int Soc Sports Nutr*. 2021;18:20.

Olean-Oliveira T, et al. Menstrual cycle impacts adipokine and lipoprotein responses to acute high-intensity intermittent exercise bout. *Eur J Appl Physiol*. 2022;122:103.

Sandebring-Matton A, et al. 27-Hydroxycholesterol, cognition, and brain imaging markers in the FINGER randomized controlled trial. *Alzheimers Res Ther*. 2021;13:56.

Scheffers LE, et al. Study protocol of the exercise study: Unraveling limitations for physical activity in children with chronic diseases in order to target them with tailored interventions—a randomized cross over trial. *Front Pediatr*. 2022;9:791701.

Terink R, et al. A 2 week cross-over intervention with a low carbohydrate, high fat diet compared to a high carbohydrate diet attenuates exercise-induced cortisol response, but not the reduction of exercise capacity, in recreational athletes. *Nutrients.* 2021;13:157.

Trim WV, et al. The impact of long-term physical inactivity on adipose tissue immunometabolism. J Clin Endocrinol Metab. 2022;107:177.

Yoo JK, Fu Q. Impact of sex and age on metabolism, sympathetic activity, and hypertension. *FASEB J.* 2020;34:11337.

Table 20.1 Storage, Synthesis, Release Mechanism, Transport Medium, Receptor Location and Receptor-Ligand Binding, and Target Organ Response to Peptide, Steroid, and Amine Hormones

	Peptide Hormones	Steroid Hormones	Amine Hormones	
			Catecholamines	Thyroid Hormones
Examples	Insulin, glucagon, leptin, IGF-1	Androgens, DHEA, cortisol	Epinephrine, norepinephrine	Thyroxine (T_4)
Synthesis and storage	Made in advance; stored in secretory vesicles	Synthesized on demand from precursors	Made in advance; stored in secretory vesicles	Made in advance; precursor stored in secretory vesicles
Release from parent cell	Exocytosis	Simple diffusion	Exocytosis	Simple diffusion
Transport medium	Dissolved in plasma	Bound to carrier proteins	Dissolved in plasma	Bound to carrier proteins
Lifespan (half-life)	Short	Long	Short	Long
Receptor location	On cell membrane	Cytoplasm of nucleus; some have membrane receptors	On cell membrane	Nucleus
Response to receptor-ligand binding	Activation of second messenger system; may activate genes	Activate genes for transcription and translation; may have nongenomic actions	Activation of second messenger system	Activate genes for transcription and translation
General target response	Modification of existing proteins and induction of new protein synthesis	Induction of new protein synthesis	Modification of existing proteins	Induction of new protein synthesis

Table 20.2	Hormones Produced by Organs Other Than the Major Endocrine Organs		
Hormone	**Composition**	**Source and Stimulus for Secretion**	**Target and Outcome**
Prostaglandins	20-carbon fatty acid synthesized from arachidonic acid	*Source:* plasma membrane of different body cells *Stimulus:* local irritation, different hormones	*Target:* multiple sites *Outcome:* controls local hormone response; stimulates arterioles to increase blood pressure; increases uterine contractions, HCl and pepsin secretion in stomach, platelet aggregation, blood clotting, constriction of bronchioles, inflammation, pain, and fever
Gastrin	Peptide	*Source:* stomach *Stimulus:* food	*Target:* stomach *Outcome:* release of HCl
Enterogastrin	Peptide	*Source:* duodenum *Stimulus:* food (especially lipids)	*Target:* stomach *Outcome:* inhibits HCl secretion and gastrointestinal motility
Secretin	Peptide	*Source:* duodenum *Stimulus:* food	*Target:* pancreas *Outcome:* release of bicarbonate-rich juice *Target:* liver *Outcome:* release of bile *Target:* stomach *Outcome:* inhibits secretion
Cholecystokinin	Peptide	*Source:* duodenum *Stimulus:* food	*Target:* pancreas *Outcome:* release of bicarbonate-rich juice *Target:* gallbladder *Outcome:* expulsion of bile *Target:* sphincter of Oddi *Outcome:* relaxes sphincter and allows bile to enter duodenum
Erythropoietin	Glycoprotein	*Source:* kidneys *Stimulus:* hypoxia	*Target:* bone marrow *Outcome:* production of red blood cells
Active vitamin D_3	Steroid	*Source:* kidneys activate vitamin D from epidermal skin cells *Stimulus:* parathyroid hormone	*Target:* intestine *Outcome:* active transport of dietary Ca^{2+} across intestinal membranes
Atrial natriuretic hormone	Peptide	*Source:* atrium of heart *Stimulus:* atrial stretching	*Target:* kidneys *Outcome:* inhibits Na^+ reabsorption and renin release *Target:* adrenal cortex *Outcome:* inhibits secretion of aldosterone

Note: The kidneys release an enzyme that modifies a circulating blood protein to produce erythropoietin.

Table 20.3 Endocrine Organs and Their Secretions, Targets, and Main Effects

Location	Gland or Cells	Chemical Type	Hormone	Target	Main Effect
Adipose tissue	Cells	Peptide	Leptin; adiponectin (resistin)	Hypothalamus, other tissues	Food intake, metabolism, reproduction
Adrenal cortex	Gland	Steroid	Mineralocorticoids (aldosterone)	Kidney	Stimulates Na^+ reabsorption and K^+ secretion
			Glucocorticoids (cortisol; corticosterone)	Many tissues	Promotes protein and fat catabolism; raises blood glucose levels; adapts body to stress
			Androgens (androstenedione; dehydroepiandrosterone [DHEA]; estrone)	Many tissues	Promotes sex drive
Adrenal medulla	Gland	Amine	Epinephrine, norepinephrine	Many tissues	Facilitates sympathetic activity; increases cardiac output; regulates blood vessels; increases glycogen catabolism and fatty acid release
Gastrointestinal tract (stomach and small intestine)	Cells	Peptide	Gastrin; cholecystokinin (CCK); secretin; glucose-dependent insulinotropic peptide (GIP)	GI tract and pancreas	Assists digestion and absorption of nutrients; regulates gastrointestinal motility
Heart	Cells	Peptide	Atrial natriuretic peptide (ANP)	Kidney tubules	Inhibits sodium reabsorption
Hypothalamus	Clusters of neurons	Peptide	Trophic hormones (releasing and release-inhibiting hormones: corticotropin-releasing hormone [CRH]; thyrotropin-releasing hormone [TRH]; growth hormone-releasing hormone [GHRH]; gonadotropin-releasing hormone [GnRH])	Anterior pituitary	Releases or inhibits anterior pituitary hormones
Kidney	Cells	Peptide	Erythropoietin (EPO)	Bone marrow	Red blood cell production
		Steroid	1,25 dihydroxy-vitamin D_3 (calciferol)	Intestine	Increases calcium absorption
Liver	Cells	Peptide	Angiotensinogen	Adrenal cortex, blood vessels, brain	Aldosterone secretion; increases blood pressure
			Insulinlike growth factors (IGF-1)	Many tissues	Growth
Muscle	Cells	Peptide	Insulinlike growth factors (IGF-1, IGF-II); myogenic regulatory factors (MRFs)	Many tissues	Growth

Table 20.3 Endocrine Organs and Their Secretions, Targets, and Main Effects (Continued)

Location	Gland or Cells	Chemical Type	Hormone	Target	Main Effect
Pancreas	Gland	Peptide	Insulin	Many tissues	Lowers blood glucose levels; promotes protein, lipid, and glycogen synthesis
			Glucagon	Many tissues	Raises blood glucose levels; promotes glycogenolysis and gluconeogenesis
			Somatostatin (SS)	Many tissues	Inhibits secretion of pancreatic hormones; regulates digestion and absorption of nutrients by GI system
Parathyroid	Gland	Peptide	Parathyroid hormone (PTH)	Bone, kidney	Promotes Ca^{2+} release from bone, Ca^{2+} absorption by intestine, and Ca^{2+} reabsorption by kidney; raises blood Ca^{2+} levels; stimulates vitamin D_3 synthesis
Pineal gland	Gland	Amine	Melatonin	Unknown	Controls circadian rhythms
Pituitary-anterior	Gland	Peptides	Growth hormone (GH) (ACTH)	Many tissues	Growth; stimulates bone and soft tissue growth; regulates protein, lipid, and CHO metabolism
			Thyroid-stimulating hormone (TSH)	Adrenal cortex	Stimulates glucocorticoid secretion
			Prolactin	Thyroid gland	Stimulates secretion of thyroid hormones
			Follicle-stimulating hormone (FSH)	Breast Gonads	Milk secretion *Females:* stimulates growth and development of ovarian follicles and estrogen secretion; *Males:* sperm production by testis
			Luteinizing hormone (LH)	Gonads	*Females:* stimulates ovulation, secretion of estrogen and progesterone; *Males:* testosterone secretion by testis
Pituitary-posterior	Extension of hypothalamic neurons	Peptide	Oxytocin (OT)	Breast and uterus	*Females:* stimulates uterine contractions and milk ejection by mammary glands; *Males:* unknown function
			Antidiuretic hormone (ADH or vasopressin)	Kidney	Decreases urine output by kidneys; promotes blood vessel (arteriole) constriction

(continued)

Table 20.3 Endocrine Organs and Their Secretions, Targets, and Main Effects (Continued)

Location	Gland or Cells	Chemical Type	Hormone	Target	Main Effect
Placenta (pregnant female)	Gland	Steroid Peptide	Estrogens and progesterone Chorionic somatomammotropin (CS) Chorionic gonadotropin (CG)	Many tissues	Fetal and maternal development Metabolism Hormone secretion
Skin	Cells	Steroid	Vitamin D_3	Intermediate hormone form	Precursor of 1,25 dihydroxy-vitamin D_3
Ovaries (female)	Glands	Steroid Peptide	Estrogens (estradiol)	Many tissues	Egg production; secondary sex characteristics
			Progestins (progesterone)	Uterus	Promotes endometrial growth to prepare uterus for pregnancy
			Ovarian inhibin	Anterior pituitary	Inhibits FSH secretion
Testes (male)	Glands	Steroid	Androgen	Many tissues	Sperm production; secondary sex characteristics
		Peptide	Inhibin	Anterior pituitary	Inhibits FSH secretion
Thymus	Gland	Peptide	Thymosin, thymopoietin	Lymphocytes	Stimulates proliferation and function of T lymphocytes
Thyroid	Gland	Iodinated amines	Triiodothyronine (T_3); thyroxine (T_4)	Many tissues	Increases metabolic rate; normal physical development
		Peptide	Calcitonin (CT)	Bone	Promotes calcium deposition in bone; lowers blood calcium levels

PART TWO

Applied Exercise Physiology

SECTION 4 Enhancing Energy Transfer Capacity

SECTION 5 Exercise Performance and Environmental Stress

SECTION 6 Body Composition, Energy Balance, and Weight Control

SECTION 7 Exercise, Successful Aging, and Disease Prevention

SECTION 8 On the Horizon

SECTION 4

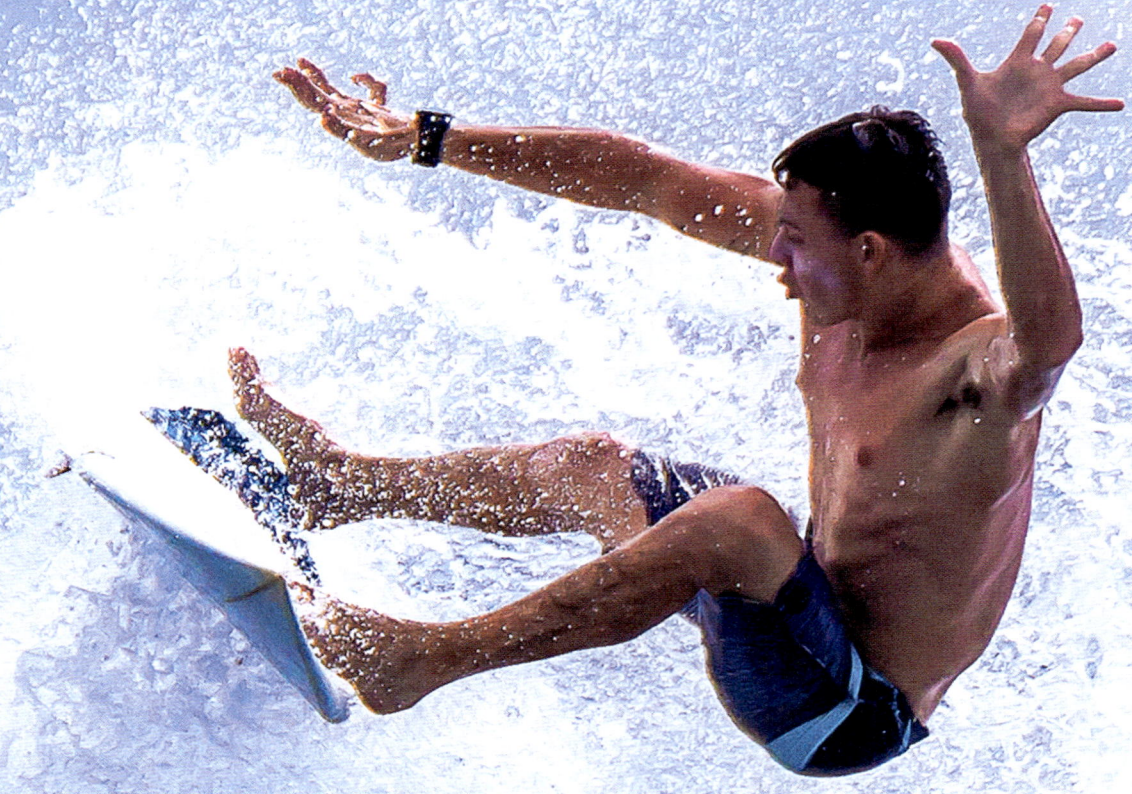

Enhancing Energy Transfer Capacity

Overview

Throughout this book, we underscore that dissimilar physical activities, depending on intensity and duration, activate highly specific energy transfer systems. We recognize difficulty in placing certain activities into only one category.

As an example, as a person increases aerobic fitness, an activity previously classified as anaerobic becomes more aerobic. All three energy-transfer systems—immediate adenosine triphosphate–phosphocreatine (ATP–PCr) system, short-duration lactic acid system, and long-term aerobic system—operate in different time sequences during physical activity, but each remains operational throughout the activity. Their relative contributions to the energy continuum directly relate to the specific activity's duration and intensity.

Intense activities for up to a 6-s duration rely exclusively on "immediate" energy generated from decomposing the stored intramuscular high-energy phosphates ATP and adenosine diphosphate. For that reason, power athletes (e.g., sprinters, American football players, soccer players, shot putters, discus throwers, and pole vaulters) must focus their training toward improving this selective energy-transfer system. This operationalizes the targeted force-generating capacity in the muscles activated in their specific activity. As all-out movement progresses to a 60-s duration and power output decreases, most energy for movement still arises through somewhat slower anaerobic pathways that involve the glycolytic short-term energy system with subsequent blood-lactate accumulation. As intensity diminishes and duration extends to 2 to 4 min, reliance on energy from the intramuscular phosphagens and anaerobic glycolysis decreases, allowing aerobic ATP production to become increasingly more important. As prolonged exercise duration increases, aerobic metabolism contributes 99% to the total energy requirement. Clearly, an efficient training program allocates a proportionate commitment to targeted training using specific energy and physiologic systems set in motion in the activity.

The chapters in this section discuss anaerobic and aerobic conditioning (Chapter 21), including procedures to train muscles to become stronger (Chapter 22), with emphasis on principles, methods, and short-term responses and longer-term training adaptations. In Chapter 23, we explore the safety and efficacy connected with well-defined chemical, nutritional, and physiologic aids to enhance exercise training and physical performance.

CHAPTER 21
Training for Anaerobic and Aerobic Power

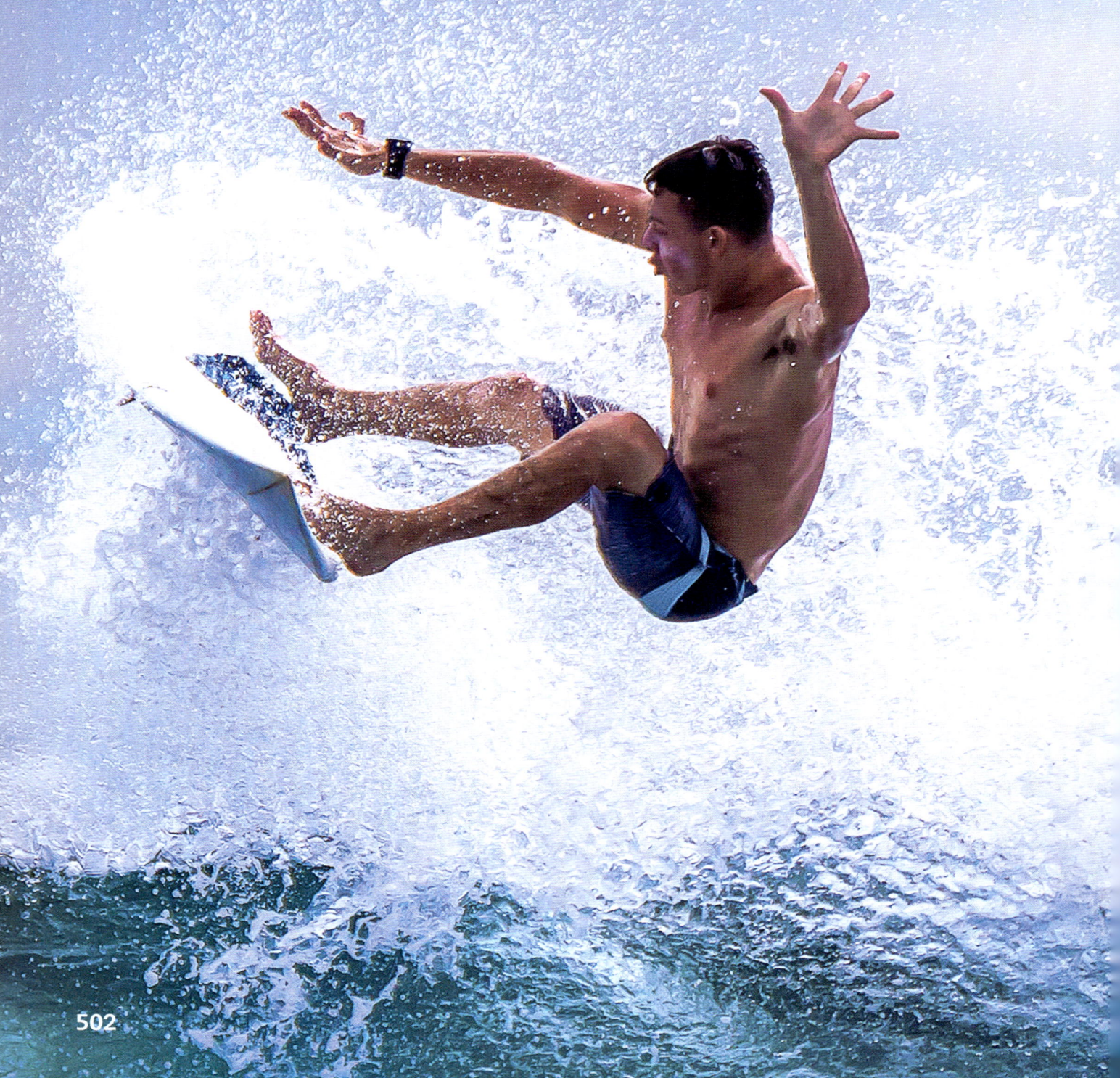

Chapter Objectives

- Discuss and provide examples of the exercise training principles of overload, specificity, individual differences, and reversibility
- Outline metabolic adaptations to anaerobic training and metabolic, cardiovascular, and pulmonary adaptations to aerobic training
- Describe the *athlete's heart* and contrast structural and functional heart characteristics for an endurance athlete versus a resistance-trained athlete
- Describe how initial fitness level, genetics, and training frequency, duration, and intensity influence the aerobic training response
- Discuss the rationale for heart rate to establish aerobic training intensity
- Discuss heart rate variability, how it is measured, and the context in which it is used
- Justify how the "rating of perceived exertion" establishes the aerobic activity intensity
- Give two advantages of training at the lactate threshold
- Contrast continuous and intermittent aerobic training and two advantages and disadvantages for each
- Summarize three important factors to implement interval training exercise prescriptions
- Describe the most common overtraining syndrome, and summarize interacting factors contributing to overtraining in endurance athletes
- Summarize current physical activity guidelines before, during, and after pregnancy

Ancillaries at-a-Glance

Visit Lippincott Connect to access the following resources.

- References: Chapter 21
- Appendix H: Links for Supplemental Animations and Videos
- Focus on Research: Highly Specific Nature of the Training Response

Exercise Training Principles

Stimulating structural and functional adaptations to improve performance in specific physical tasks remains a major exercise training objective. Adaptations require adherence to carefully planned programs with focus on frequency and length of workout; training type, speed, intensity, duration, and activity repetition; rest intervals and appropriate competition. Applying these factors varies depending on performance and fitness goals. *The basic approach to physiologic conditioning applies similarly to men and women within a broad age range—both respond and adapt to training in essentially similar ways.* **FIGURE 21.1** illustrates the four energy-generating pathways and corresponding physical performance examples related to each pathway:

1. Adenosine triphosphate (ATP; strength-power)
2. ATP + phosphocreatine (PCr; sustained power)
3. ATP + PCr + lactate (anaerobic power-endurance)
4. Electron transport-oxidative phosphorylation (aerobic endurance)

The sections that follow discuss physiologic conditioning principles common to improving performance related to these four energy-generating pathways and corresponding physical performance examples.

Overload Principle

Regular specific exercise **overload** enhances physiologic function to induce a training response. Exercising at intensities above normal stimulates highly specific adaptations so that the body functions more efficiently. *Achieving the appropriate overload requires either manipulating training frequency, intensity, and duration, or their combination.*

The individualized and progressive overload concept applies along a broad spectrum from athletes, sedentary persons, disabled persons, and even to cardiac patients. For the latter group, appropriate exercise rehabilitation programs include walking building up to jogging, and eventually running and even competing in marathon and triathlon endurance activities. As we discuss in Chapter 31, achieving regular physical activity's health-related benefits requires lower effort intensity (but greater volume) than required to only improve maximum aerobic fitness.[112,131,213,242,243]

Specificity Principle

Exercise training specificity refers to adaptations in metabolic and physiologic functions that are affected by the intensity, duration, and frequency of the overload. An intense but short-duration overload (e.g., strength-power training) induces specific strength-power adaptations; specific endurance training elicits specific aerobic system adaptations—with only limited interchange between strength-power training benefits and aerobic training benefits.

Nonetheless, the specificity principle extends beyond this broad demarcation. Aerobic training, for example, does not represent a singular entity that requires only cardiovascular overload. Aerobic training that relies on specific muscles in the desired performance improves aerobic fitness for swimming,[58] bicycling,[159] running,[135] or upper-body activities.[25,117] Some evidence suggests a temporal specificity in training response so training improvement indicators will peak when measured at the same time of day when training regularly occurs.[84] Task-specific training that involves practicing the actual motor skill to avoid a fall after losing one's balance may positively affect biomechanical variables among

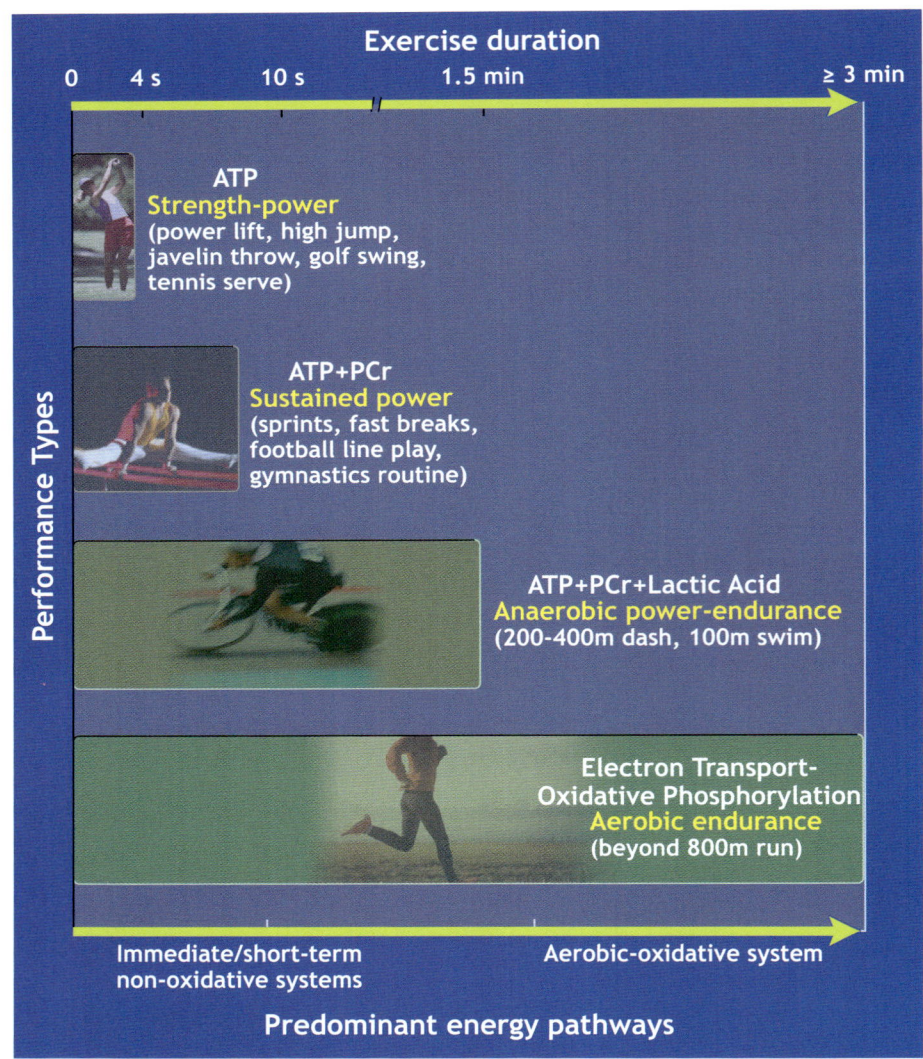

FIGURE 21.1. Classifying physical activity based on all-out effort duration and predominant intracellular energy pathways. ATP, adenosine triphosphate; PCr, phosphocreatine.
(Photo of runner: Izf/Shutterstock.)

older individuals so they avoid falling after purposely being "tripped" under laboratory-controlled conditions.[65] The most effective way to evaluate sport-specific performance is when the laboratory measurement closely simulates the actual sport activity and/or essentially targets the same muscle mass and sport's movement patterns.[13,58,116] *Simply stated, specific exercise elicits specific adaptations to promote specific training effects that produce specific performance improvements.* Put in another easy-to-remember way: specificity refers to the **specific adaptations to imposed demands (SAIDs) principle**.

Maximum Oxygen Uptake Specificity

When training for specific aerobic cycling, swimming, rowing, or running-type activities, the overload must accomplish two objectives:

1. Engage the appropriate muscles required by the activity
2. Provide exercise intensity at a level sufficient to stress the cardiovascular system

Little improvement occurs when measuring aerobic capacity with dissimilar exercise forms; the greatest improvement occurs when the test duplicates the training exercise. These results also apply in movement rehabilitation in coronary artery disease patients.[152] Aerobic training induces a highly specific maximum oxygen uptake ($\dot{V}O_{2max}$) improvement, whereas more general improvements occur in cardiac function. Ventricular contractility, for example, that improves with one mode of training also improves when exercising the untrained limbs.[215] Individuals apparently can train the myocardium equally with diverse "big-muscle" activity modes.[243]

In an experiment in one of our laboratories on aerobic training specificity,[135] 15 men swam 1 hr·d^{-1}, 3 d·wk^{-1}, for 10 wk at heart rates between 85 and 95% of maximum (HR_{max}). $\dot{V}O_{2max}$ was measured during treadmill running and tethered swimming before and after training. Because vigorous swim training overloads the central circulation as reflected by high heart rates, we anticipated at least some transfer in aerobic power improvements from swim training to run training. Yet this did not occur as an almost total specificity accompanied the $\dot{V}O_{2max}$ improvement with swim training.

FIGURE 21.2 illustrates that swim training improved $\dot{V}O_{2max}$ by 11% when measured during swimming, but only 1.5% when measured during running. If only treadmill running had been used to evaluate swim training effects, we would mistakenly have concluded there was *no training effect*. For maximum performance during testing, subjects improved 34% in swim time to exhaustion but only 4.6% for run time on the treadmill test. These findings indicate that training for specific aerobic activities must provide an appropriate general cardiovascular stress *and* overload the *specific muscles* in the specific way required by the activity. Little improvement results when a dissimilar activity measures aerobic capacity or exercise performance. In contrast, considerable improvements emerge when the specific training mode assesses the aerobic adaptations to training.

Local Muscle–Induced Specificity

Overloading specific muscle groups with endurance training enhances performance *and* aerobic power by facilitating oxygen transport and oxygen use in the locally trained muscles.[85,127] For example, well-trained cyclists' vastus lateralis muscle, a muscle highly activated in cycling, has greater oxidative capacity than this muscle in endurance runners. This muscle's oxidative capacity improves considerably following training on a bicycle ergometer. The local metabolic adaptations increase the trained muscle's capacity to generate ATP aerobically before lactate accumulation onset. Aerobic improvement specificity also may result from greater regional blood flow in active tissues from three factors:

1. More effective redistribution of cardiac output
2. Increased microcirculation
3. The combined effect of both factors

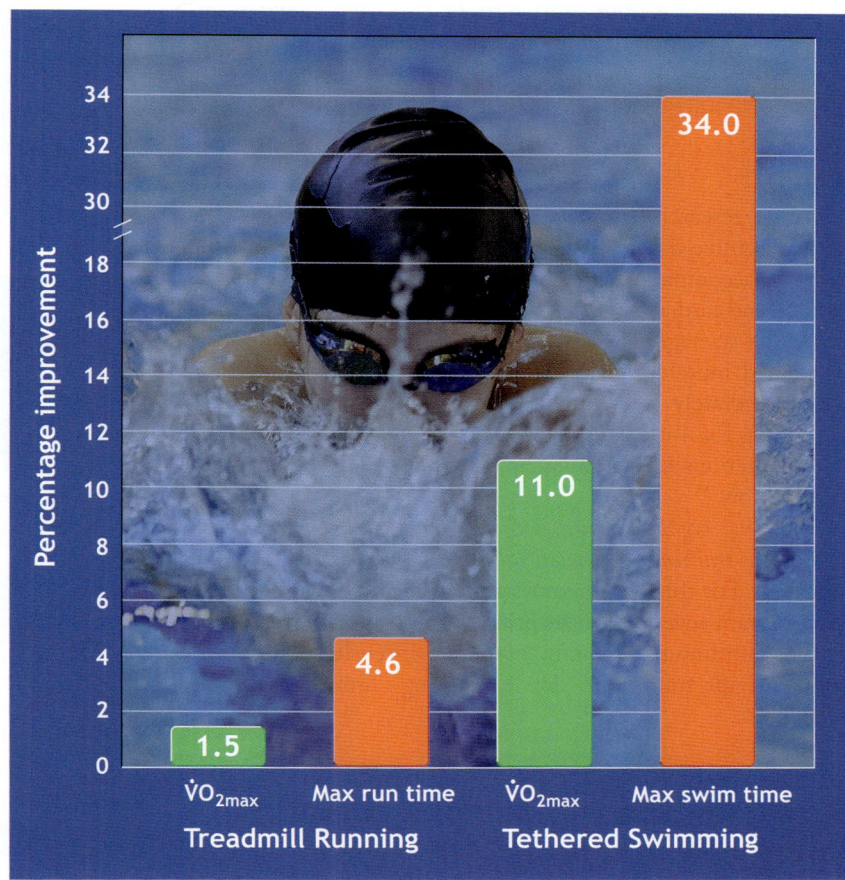

FIGURE 21.2. An example of aerobic training specificity. $\dot{V}O_{2max}$, maximum oxygen uptake.
(Lenar Nigmatullin/Shutterstock)

The mechanism for these three adaptations occurs *only* in specifically trained muscles and *only* becomes apparent in physical activities that activate this musculature.

Individual Difference Principle

The individual difference principle asserts that all individuals do not respond similarly to a given training stimulus. For example, a person's relative fitness level when beginning training exerts an influence. Individuals with lower fitness deliver the greatest training improvement. The individual difference principle encompasses healthy individuals and those with cardiovascular disease or at high risk for the disease.[19,176,235] When a relatively homogenous group begins a training regimen, each person will not achieve the same fitness or exercise performance state after only about 12 wk. *Optimal training benefits occur when exercise programs focus on the participant's individual needs and capacities.*

In Chapter 11, we discuss how genetic factors interact to impact the training response.

Reversibility Principle

Detraining occurs rapidly when a person terminates regular physical activity within only 1 or 2 wk, with many training improvements fully lost within several months.[147,245–247] **TABLE 21.1** shows the biologic consequences of detraining for various short-term (<3 wk) and longer-term (3–12 wk) durations in endurance-trained individuals.

TABLE 21.1 Physiologic and metabolic function changes with various detraining durations

One research group confined five subjects to bed for 20 consecutive days,[189] with $\dot{V}O_{2max}$ decreasing by 25%. This decrease accompanied similar decrements in maximum stroke volume and cardiac output, which decreased maximum aerobic power an average 1% daily. Additionally, capillary number in trained muscle decreased between 14 and 25% within 3 wk immediately following training.[161] For elderly subjects, detraining for 4 mo completely negated the endurance training adaptations on cardiovascular functions and body water distribution.[165]

Among highly trained athletes, even with many years devoted to training, the beneficial results remain transient and reversible. For this reason, most athletes begin a reconditioning program several months prior to the competitive season, or at a minimum, maintain moderate-intensity off-season, sport-specific training to slow detraining's unintended consequences.

How Training Impacts the Anaerobic Energy Systems

The following sections present a detailed discussion about diverse adaptations to anaerobic and aerobic exercise training responses outlined in **TABLE 21.2**.

TABLE 21.2 Typical metabolic and physiologic values for healthy endurance-trained and untrained men

Anaerobic System Changes with Training

FIGURE 21.3 summarizes responses for metabolic adaptations in anaerobic function accompanying anaerobic training. Consistent with the training specificity concept, activities that demand considerable anaerobic metabolism induce specific changes in the immediate and short-term energy systems, generally without concomitant increases in aerobic functions. Three important changes occur with anaerobic power training:

1. Increased anaerobic substrate levels. Muscle biopsy specimens taken before and after resistance training (see inset table below) show increases in the trained muscle's resting ATP, PCr, free creatine, and glycogen levels, accompanied by a 28% improvement in muscular strength.[247,250] All values are averages expressed in mM · g wet muscle^{-1}, and all differences are statistically significant. Other studies have shown higher ATP and total creatine levels in trained muscles of sprint runners and track speed cyclists compared to distance runners and road racers.[151] Speed-power training also increases trained skeletal muscle's PCr content.

2. Increased quantity and activity of key enzymes that control the anaerobic (glycolytic) glucose catabolism phase. These changes do not achieve the magnitude for oxidative enzymes with aerobic training. The most dramatic increases in anaerobic enzyme function and fiber size occur in fast-twitch muscle fibers.

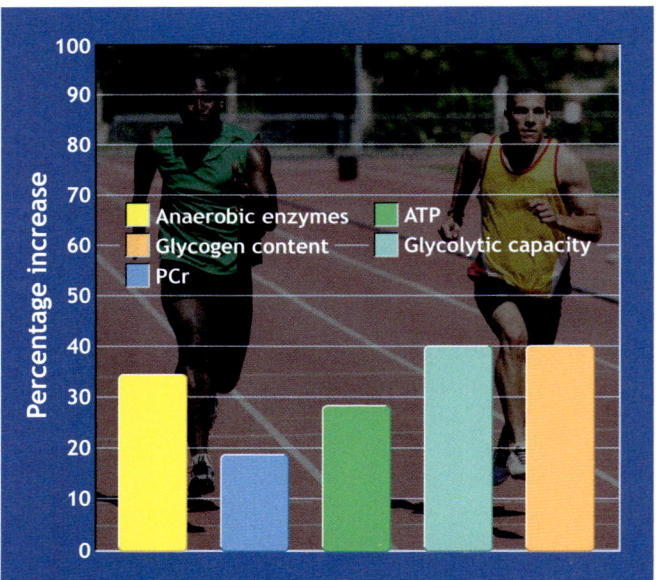

FIGURE 21.3. Generalized potential to increase skeletal muscle anaerobic energy metabolism with sprint-power training. ATP, adenosine triphosphate; PCr, phosphocreatine.
(William Perugini/Shutterstock)

3. Increased capacity to generate and tolerate high blood lactate levels during all-out effort. This adaptation probably results from two factors: increased glycogen and glycolytic enzyme levels, and improved motivation and tolerance to "pain" in fatiguing physical activity. Motivational factors probably account for the improved training-induced tolerance to elevated plasma acidity.

How Training Impacts the Aerobic System

FIGURE 21.4 shows four physiologic and metabolic categories related to oxygen transport and use:

1. Ventilation-aeration
2. Central blood flow
3. Active muscle metabolism
4. Peripheral blood flow

With adequate training, the positive adaptations in these factors remain independent of race, gender, age, and health status.[26,32,196,234]

Muscle Metabolites Before and After Resistance Training

Variable	Pretraining	Posttraining	%Diff
PCr	17.07	17.94	+5.1
Creatine	14.52	10.74	+35.2
ATP	5.07	5.97	+17.8
Glycogen	113.90	86.28	+32.0

ATP, adenosine triphosphate; PCr, phosphocreatine

From MacDougall JD, et al. Biochemical adaptation of human skeletal muscle to heavy resistance training and immobilization. *J Appl Physiol*. 1977;43:700. ©The American Physiological Society (APS). All rights reserved. Andrii Vodolazhskyi/Shutterstock.

Metabolic Adaptations

Aerobic training improves the capacity for respiratory control in skeletal muscle.

Metabolic Machinery

To some extent, mitochondrial potential and not oxygen supply limits untrained muscle's oxidative capacity.[75,238,248] Endurance-

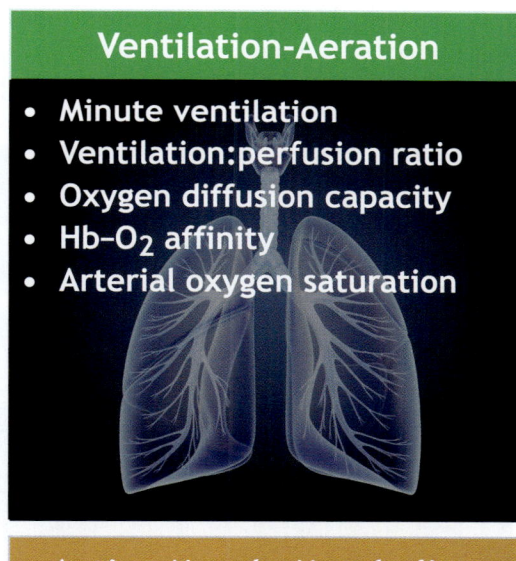

FIGURE 21.4. Physiologic factors limiting $\dot{V}O_{2max}$ and aerobic exercise performance. Hb, hemoglobin. (Shutterstock: decade3d - anatomy online, Andy Gin.)

FYI — Detraining and Muscle Fiber Type Changes

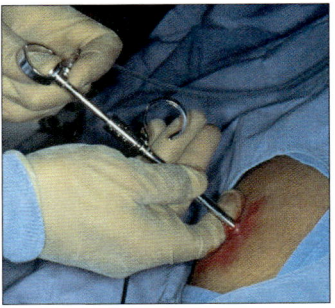

Reprinted with permission from Plowman SA, Smith DL. *Exercise Physiology for Health, Fitness, and Performance*. 5th ed. Baltimore: Wolters Kluwer, 2017.

A systematic literature review examined the effect of reduced muscle activity (detraining, leg unloading, and bed rest) on the relative number (%) of type 1 muscle fibers and any changes in type 2X percentages and muscle fiber cross-sectional area in the human vastus lateralis muscle. A literature review identified 42 studies with 451 participants relevant to this research area. The average type 1 muscle fiber percentage was significantly reduced following both bed rest and restricted muscle use, with no differences between intervention models. No effect emerged for study duration on type 1 fiber percentage. Conversely, the overall type 2X fiber percentage increased after reduced muscle activity. In essence, reduced muscle activity reduces type 1 muscle fiber percentage with only a small effect on fiber size. These results suggest that periods of physical inactivity have their greatest albeit small effect on the type I muscle fiber type distribution.

Sources:
Ekblom B. The muscle biopsy technique. Historical and methodological considerations. *Scand J Med Sci Sports*. 2017;27:458.
Fournier G, et al. Sex differences in semitendinosus muscle fiber-type composition. *Scand J Med Sci Sports*. 2022;32:720. doi:10.1111/sms.14127
Larson ST, Wilbur J. Muscle weakness in adults: evaluation and differential diagnosis. *Am Fam Physician*. 2020;101:95.
Vikne H, et al. Human skeletal muscle fiber type percentage and area after reduced muscle use: a systematic review and meta-analysis. *Scand J Med Sci Sports*. 2020;30:1298.

---

trained skeletal muscle fibers contain *larger* and *more numerous* mitochondria than less active fibers. The enlarged mitochondrial structural machinery and enzyme activity adaptations with aerobic training, sometimes up to 50%, increase within several weeks, greatly *increases* subsarcolemmal and intermyofibrillar muscle mitochondria's capacity to generate ATP aerobically.[67,87,208,238] A nearly twofold increase in **aerobic system enzymes** within 5 to 10 training days coincides with increased mitochondrial capacity to generate ATP aerobically.

Enzyme changes occur from increases in total mitochondrial material, not increased enzymatic activity per unit mitochondrial protein. The increase in mitochondrial protein by a factor of two exceeds the typical 10 to 20% increases in $\dot{V}O_{2max}$ with endurance training. More than likely, enzymatic changes allow a person to sustain a higher aerobic capacity percentage during prolonged effort without blood lactate accumulation.

Lipid Metabolism. Endurance training increases fatty acid oxidation during rest[157] and submaximum exercise, particularly with extended exercise duration as shown in **FIGURE 21.5**.[50,88,224,249,258] Enhanced lipid catabolism becomes apparent at the same absolute submaximum workload without regard to fuel input, either fed or fasted,[10,12,31] and the effect occurs within 2 wk after beginning a training program.[211] Impressive increases also occur in trained muscle's capacity to use intramuscular triacylglycerols as a primary fatty acid oxidation source.[132] This carbohydrate-sparing adaptation results from facilitated release of fatty acids from adipose tissue depots (augmented by a reduced blood lactate level) and an increased amount of triacylglycerol within the endurance-trained muscle fibers. Four factors contribute to a heightened training-induced increased lipolysis:

1. Greater blood flow within trained muscle
2. More lipid-mobilizing and lipid-metabolizing enzymes
3. Enhanced muscle mitochondrial respiratory capacity
4. Decreased catecholamine release at the same absolute power output

Enhanced lipid catabolism in submaximal activity benefits endurance athletes because it conserves the important glycogen reserves during prolonged, intense effort. Improved fatty acid β-oxidation and respiratory ATP production contribute to

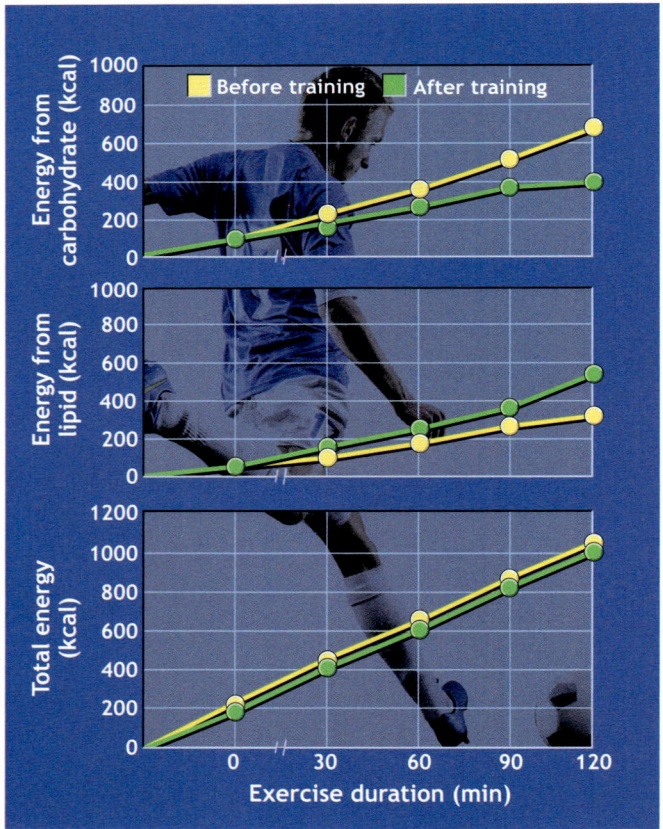

FIGURE 21.5. Aerobic exercise training enhances lipid catabolism in submaximum exercise.
(Reprinted with permission from Hurley BF, et al. Muscle triglyceride utilization during exercise: effect of training. *J Appl Physiol*. 1986;60:562. ©The American Physiological Society (APS). All rights reserved. Eugene Onischenko/Shutterstock.)

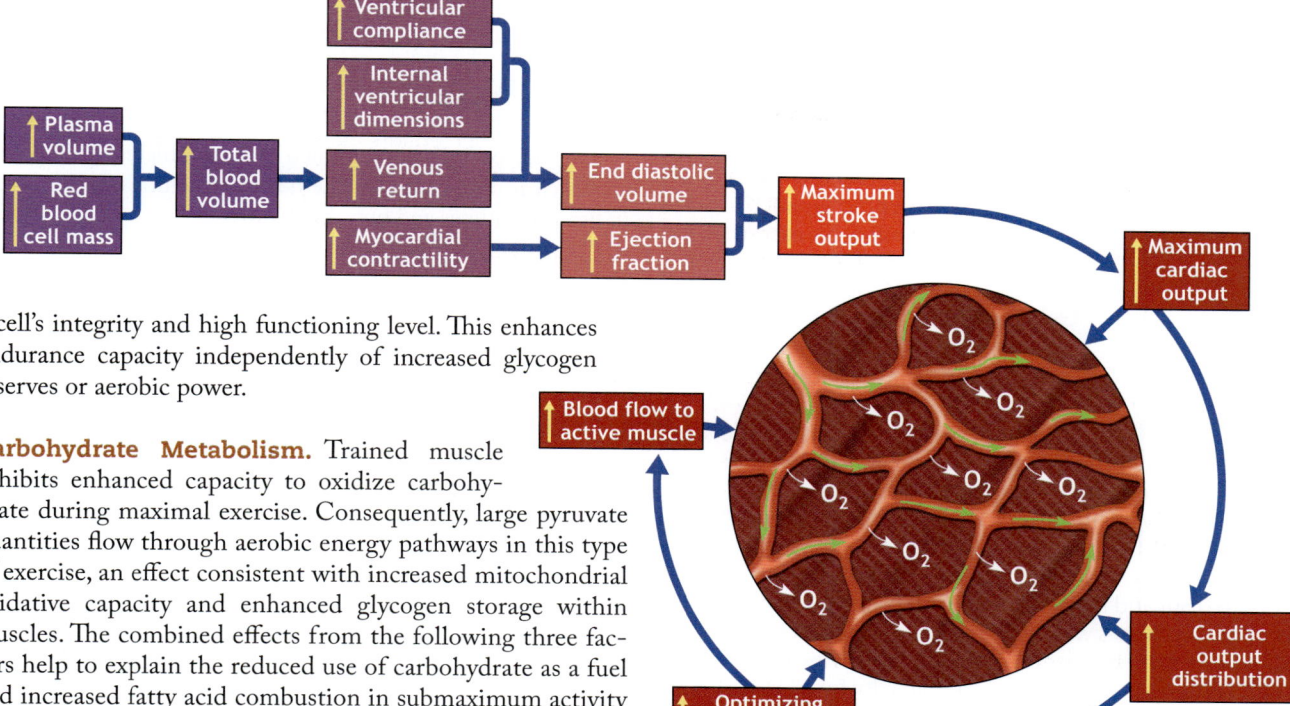

a cell's integrity and high functioning level. This enhances endurance capacity independently of increased glycogen reserves or aerobic power.

Carbohydrate Metabolism. Trained muscle exhibits enhanced capacity to oxidize carbohydrate during maximal exercise. Consequently, large pyruvate quantities flow through aerobic energy pathways in this type of exercise, an effect consistent with increased mitochondrial oxidative capacity and enhanced glycogen storage within muscles. The combined effects from the following three factors help to explain the reduced use of carbohydrate as a fuel and increased fatty acid combustion in submaximum activity with endurance training[31]:

1. Decreased muscle glycogen use
2. Reduced glucose production (decreased hepatic glycogenolysis and gluconeogenesis)
3. Reduced plasma-borne glucose use

Training-enhanced hepatic gluconeogenic capacity provides further resistance to hypoglycemia during prolonged physical activity.[33,42]

Muscle Fiber Type and Size

Aerobic training elicits metabolic adaptations in each muscle fiber type. The basic fiber type probably does not "change" to any great extent; instead, all fibers maximize their already existing aerobic potential.

Selective hypertrophy occurs in the different muscle fiber types with specific overload training.[250] Highly trained endurance athletes have larger slow-twitch (type I) fibers than fast-twitch (type II) fibers in the same muscle. Type II fibers are recruited less during aerobic training than type I counterparts, so their aerobic capacity does not appreciably change with this activity type. With aerobic training, some type II fibers may undergo a transition to exhibit greater aerobic tendencies. This exemplifies muscle fiber "*plasticity*" that likely occurs at the subcellular level.[99]

Slow-twitch muscle fibers with high capacity to generate ATP aerobically contain a relatively large quantity of myoglobin. Among animals, a muscle's myoglobin content relates to their physical activity level.[251] The leg muscles of hunting dogs contain more myoglobin than sedentary house pet's muscles, findings similar for grazing cattle compared with penned animals.[233] In humans, the effect from regular physical activity on myoglobin levels remains undetermined and likely negligible.

FIGURE 21.6. Aerobic training increases oxygen delivery to active muscles.

Cardiovascular Adaptations

FIGURE 21.6 summarizes important aerobic training adaptations in cardiovascular function that increase oxygen delivery to active muscle.

Cardiac Hypertrophy: The "Athlete's Heart"

Long-term aerobic training generally *increases* the heart's mass and volume with greater left-ventricular end-diastolic volumes during rest and physical activity. This exercise-induced remodeling often is referred to as the "**athlete's heart**," first described in 1975.[254] This finding termed the **Morganroth hypothesis** after it's originator posited that regularly increasing cardiac output during exercise caused morphological, functional, and electrical cardiac chamber modifications with modest cardiac hypertrophy secondary to longitudinal myocardial cell enlargement. This response reflected fundamental and normal myocardial training adaptations to an increased workload independent of age.[143,252] The enlargement is characterized by increased left-ventricular cavity size or **eccentric cardiac hypertrophy**, and a modest wall thickening or **concentric cardiac hypertrophy**.[255,256] Despite widespread acceptance of this four-decade old hypothesis, some investigators have questioned whether such a divergent "athlete's heart" phenotype exists or how to effectively diagnose it.[253,257]

Regular training alters cardiac muscle fiber's contractile properties, which include increased sensitivity to activation by Ca^{2+}, changes in force-length relationships, and increased power output.[39] Myocardial overload also stimulates greater

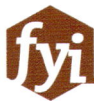

Can Testing Detect the "Athlete's Heart?"

With athletic populations, electrocardiography (ECG), the standard technique to screen for left ventricular hypertrophy (LVH), has proven problematic for a variety of reasons. Retrospective analyses with 196 male Division I college athletes were routinely screened with ECG and echocardiography. Echocardiography determined left-ventricular mass (LVM) and volume, and high-resolution time intervals and QRS voltages were assessed using twelve-lead ECG. Thirty-seven previously published ECG-LVH criteria were applied to diagnose for LVH presence. ECG lead voltages correlated poorly with LVM ($r = 0.18$ to 0.30) and mass/voltage ($r = 0.15$ to 0.25). The proportion of athletes with ECG-LVH varied widely (74 to 90%) across criteria, with between 0 and 91% sensitivity and 27 and 99.5% specificity. The diagnostic capacity for all ECG-LVH criteria was inadequate and clinically deemed nonuseful in screening for LVH or a concentric phenotype in athletes.

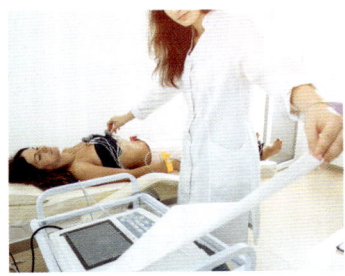
Roman Zaiets/Shutterstock

Sources:
Hedman K, et al. Impact of the distance from the chest wall to the heart on surface ECG voltage in athletes. *BMJ Open Sport Exerc Med.* 2020;6:e000696.
Hedman K, et al. Limitations of electrocardiography for detecting left ventricular hypertrophy or concentric remodeling in athletes. *Am J Med.* 2020;133:123.

---

cellular protein synthesis with associated reductions in protein breakdown. Increasing trained muscle's RNA content accelerates protein synthesis. Individual myofibrils thicken, while contractile filament number increases.

The heart volumes of sedentary men average about 800 mL. In athletes, increases in heart volume relate to the sport's aerobic characteristics—endurance athletes average 25% larger heart volumes than sedentary counterparts. Researchers would still like to more fully understand the degree to which endurance athlete's larger heart volumes reflect genetic endowment, training adaptations, or a combined effect of both factors.

Training duration affects cardiac size and structure, with several studies reporting no cardiac dimensional changes with short-term training despite improved $\dot{V}O_{2max}$ and submaximum exercise heart rate response.[177,215] When endurance training increases left ventricular size, the enlargement does not reflect a permanent adaptation. Instead, heart size decreases to pretraining levels—without deleterious effects as training intensity decreases.[38,83]

Cardiac Enlargement Specificity. The ultrasonic echocardiography technique incorporates sound waves to "map" myocardial dimensions and heart chamber volume (see Chapter 32). This technique evaluates the heart's structural characteristics to determine how various training modes differentially affect cardiac enlargement.[160,209]

Cardiac dimensions in male swimmers, water polo players, distance runners, wrestlers, and shot putters were compared during their competitive seasons with untrained college men. The swimmers and runners represented athletes in "isotonic" or endurance events; the wrestlers and shot putters represented "isometric" or resistance-trained power athletes. **TABLE 21.3** shows clear distinctions in the heart's structural characteristics in healthy athletes and untrained individuals.

> **TABLE 21.3** Comparative average cardiac dimensions in college athletes, world-class athletes, and normal subjects

Differences among athletes relate to how the athletes trained. In swimmers, left-ventricular volume averaged 181 mL and mass equaled 308 g. In wrestlers, left-ventricular volume averaged 110 mL and mass averaged 330 g; nonathletic controls averaged 101 mL for ventricular volume and 211 g for ventricular mass. The resistance-trained athletes had thicker ventricular walls, whereas endurance athletes' heart walls remained within a normal range. Cardiac morphologic and functional adaptations, including resting bradycardia, increased stroke volume, and enlarged ventricular internal dimensions, also occur in prepubertal children who undergo intense endurance training.[153]

One study assessed the distribution for left-ventricular end-diastolic cavity dimensions in 1309 elite male and female Italian athletes ages 13 to 59 years. These dimensions ranged from 38 to 66 mm (average: 48.4 mm) in females and 43 to 70 mm (average: 55.5 mm) in males.[160] In most athletes, ventricular cavity size remained within normal range but 14% showed substantially enlarged dimensions.[161] A large body surface area and participation in endurance cycling, cross-country skiing, and canoeing represented the major determinants of enlarged cavity dimensions. The subjects had no heart problems over the 12-year study period. Other athletic groups also show an enlarged ventricular cavity due to increased end-diastolic volume with normal wall thickness,[139,180] with a less pronounced effect among females.[160]

Training-Induced Plasma Volume. Myocardial structural and dimensional adaptations to regular physical activity generally reflect specific training demands.[114,158,168] As discussed in an upcoming section "Plasma Volume" (see below), a plasma volume increase within several days after endurance training contributes to intraventricular enlargement or eccentric cardiac hypertrophy.[199] Increased plasma volume coupled with a decreased heart rate and increased myocardial compliance dilates or "stretches" the left-ventricular cavity, analogous to pumping water into a balloon.

In contrast to endurance athletes, male and female resistance-trained athletes have the largest intraventricular septum, ventricular wall thickness, and ventricular mass, with little enlargement in the left ventricle's internal cavity.[57,115] These athletes do not experience volume overload with training. Instead, training produces short-term elevated arterial blood pressure episodes from high forces generated by a

IQ INTEGRATIVE QUESTION

How could cardiac hypertrophy with pressure overload training (e.g., resistance training) impact myocardial tissue oxygenation?

limited skeletal muscle mass (see Chapter 15). An increase in ventricular wall thickness that generally falls within the normal range when expressed as ventricular mass per unit body size, particularly fat-free body mass,[160,161] compensates for additional afterload on the left ventricle without affecting ventricular cavity size. More than likely, considerable intra-individual variability exists for the heart's structural response to different training modes, but the implications for myocardial blood supply and long-term cardiovascular health remain unknown. *No compelling scientific evidence indicates that arduous specific physical training damages a healthy heart.*[98] The same conclusion also pertains to cardiac patients.[22]

Functional Versus Pathologic Cardiac Hypertrophy. Disease can induce considerable cardiac enlargement, also called cardiac hypertrophy. In hypertension, for example, the heart chronically works against excessive resistance to blood flow or afterload. This stretches the heart muscle, which in accord with the Frank-Starling mechanism, generates compensatory force to overcome the added resistance to systolic ejection. In addition to ventricular dilation, individual muscle cells hypertrophy to adjust to the increased myocardial work from hypertension. In the untreated hypertensive state, myocardial fibers stretch beyond optimal length so the enlarged, dilated heart weakens and eventually fails. To the pathologist, a "hypertrophied" heart represents an enlarged, distended, and functionally inadequate organ unable to deliver sufficient blood to satisfy minimal resting requirements.

Exercise training, in contrast, imposes only a temporary myocardial stress, so rest periods provide time for "recuperation." Also, dilation and left ventricle weakening, a frequent response to chronic hypertension, does not accompany compensatory myocardial exercise training adaptations. Elite athlete's enlarged heart size generally falls within the upper normal range for either body size or increased end-diastolic volume. *The "athlete's heart" does not represent a dysfunctional organ. Rather, it demonstrates normal systolic and diastolic functions and superior stroke volume and cardiac output capacities.* One possible exception concerns resistance-trained athletes who abuse anabolic steroids. An increase in both systolic and diastolic blood pressure, including exacerbation of normal cardiac hypertrophy, occurs with prolonged steroid abuse.[66,73,96]

Plasma Volume

A 12 to 20% *increase* in plasma volume occurs after three to six aerobic training sessions without any increase in red blood cell mass. In fact, a measurable change occurs within 24 hr after the first exercise bout, with full expansion of extracellular fluid volume requiring several weeks.[191] Intravascular volume expansion directly relates to increased plasma albumin synthesis and retention.[141,149] A plasma volume increase enhances circulatory reserve and increases end-diastolic volume, stroke volume, oxygen transport, $\dot{V}O_{2max}$, and temperature-regulating ability during physical activity.[62,69] An expanded plasma volume returns to pretraining levels within 1 wk following training.[198,229] For endurance athletes in different sports, Hb mass and blood volume averaged 35% higher than in untrained subjects, with little difference in Hb concentration among groups.[78]

Heart Rate

Endurance training creates an imbalance between tonic sympathetic accelerator activity and parasympathetic depressor neurons, which favors greater vagal dominance—a response mediated by increased parasympathetic activity and decreased sympathetic discharge.[61,111] Training also decreases the sinoatrial (SA) nodal tissue's pacemaker intrinsic firing rate.[192] These adaptations contribute to the resting and submaximum exercise bradycardia in highly conditioned endurance athletes or previously sedentary individuals who train aerobically.

Exercise Heart Rate Training Effects. Endurance training depresses submaximum heart rate for a standard physical task by 12 to 15 $b \cdot min^{-1}$, while a smaller decrease occurs for resting heart rate. The heart rate reductions reflect training improvement because they generally coincide with increased maximum stroke volume and cardiac output. **FIGURE 21.7** illustrates the relationship between heart rate and oxygen

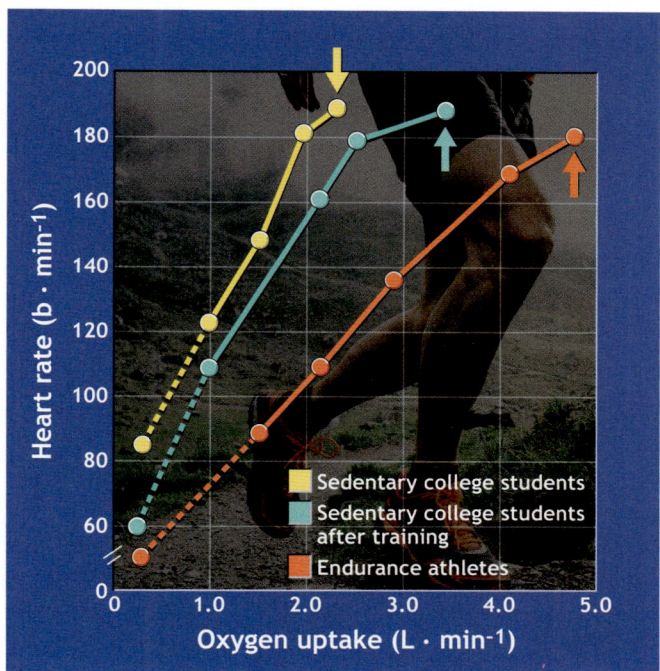

FIGURE 21.7. Heart rate and oxygen uptake during upright exercise in endurance athletes (■) and sedentary college students before (■) and after (■) 55 days of aerobic training (*arrows* = maximum values).
(Giorgio1978/Shutterstock)

uptake during graded exercise for athletes and sedentary students.[188] The six endurance athlete group trained for several year; the other group consisted of three sedentary college students. The researchers evaluated the students' exercise responses before and after a 55-day training program designed to improve aerobic fitness. The lines relating heart rate and oxygen uptake remain essentially linear for both groups throughout the oxygen uptake range. Whereas untrained students' heart rates accelerate rapidly as oxygen uptake increases, the athletes' heart rates rise much less so the rate of change in the HR-$\dot{V}O_2$ lines differs considerably between trained and untrained persons. Consequently, an athlete or trained student performs more intense physical activity and achieves a higher oxygen uptake before achieving a specific submaximum heart rate than a sedentary student. At 2.0 L · min^{-1} oxygen uptake, the athletes' heart rate averaged 70 b · min^{-1} less than the sedentary students. After training 55 days, the difference in submaximum heart rate decreased to about 40 b · min^{-1}. In each example, cardiac output remained essentially unchanged—a stroke volume increase compensated for the lower heart rate.

Heart Rate Variability. Heart rate variability (HRV) represents the beat-to-beat variation in either heart rate or R–R interval duration, also referred to as the *heart period*, has become a popular clinical and investigative tool (www.firstbeat.com/en/blog/what-is-heart-rate-variability-hrv/).

Systematic fluctuations in heart rate exhibit a marked synchrony with respiration—increased during inspiration and decreased during expiration—also called respiratory sinus arrhythmia or RSA. The HRV scores are widely believed to reflect changes in cardiac autonomic regulation.

HRV as a clinical tool to evaluate cardiac autonomic changes in cardiovascular and other disease states can be measured in two ways:

1. Under controlled laboratory conditions with short-term measurements before and after tilt-table maneuvers, drugs, controlled ventilation, or other procedures that challenge the autonomic nervous system
2. From 24 hr electrocardiographic recordings made while subjects perform usual activities of daily living (ADL) and during sleep

HRV is reduced in diabetes, smoking, obesity, stress, hypertension, multiple sclerosis, in patients recovering from myocardial infarction, end-stage renal disease, neonatal distress, and congestive heart failure.[292]

Stroke Volume

Endurance training causes the heart's stroke volume to *increase* during rest and physical activity independent of age or gender. Four factors produce this change[45,102,137]:

1. Increased internal left-ventricular volume (consequent to training-induced plasma volume expansion) and mass
2. Reduced cardiac and arterial stiffness
3. Increased diastolic filling time from training-induced bradycardia
4. Improved intrinsic cardiac contractile function

Exercise Stroke Volume: Trained Versus Untrained.
FIGURE 21.8 shows the stroke volume response during upright exercise for the men depicted in Figure 21.7. Five important training-related observations emerge:

1. The endurance athlete's heart exhibits a considerably larger stroke volume during rest and exercise than an untrained similar-age person.
2. The greatest stroke volume increase during exercise for trained and untrained persons occurs in transition from rest to moderate exercise. Only small increases in stroke volume accompany further increases in exercise intensity.
3. Maximum stroke volume generally occurs between 40 and 50% $\dot{V}O_{2max}$ for untrained persons or at a heart rate of 110 to 120 b · min^{-1} in young adults. Debate has focused on whether the stroke volume decreases, plateaus, or gradually increases during graded exercise to maximum, particularly among endurance athletes where the stroke volume may benefit from an enlarged plasma volume.[63,229] Endurance training minimizes the small decrease in stroke volume often observed during maximum effort. Even at a near-maximum heart rate, sufficient time exists for the trained heart's ventricles to fill during diastole without stroke volume reductions.[60,207] Improved ventricular filling with endurance training results in enhanced ventricular ejection via the Frank-Starling mechanism.
4. For untrained persons, only a small increase in stroke volume occurs during the rest-to-activity transition, while a cardiac output increase occurs from an acceleration of heart rate. For endurance athletes, heart rate and stroke volume *both* increase to increase cardiac output; the athlete's stroke volume generally expands by 60% above resting values. Relatively large stroke volume increases in transition from rest to exercise also occur in endurance-trained children and older men compared with healthy but untrained counterparts.[69,185,187]
5. Aerobic training for 8 wk in previously sedentary individuals substantially increases stroke volume but still remains below that for elite athletes.

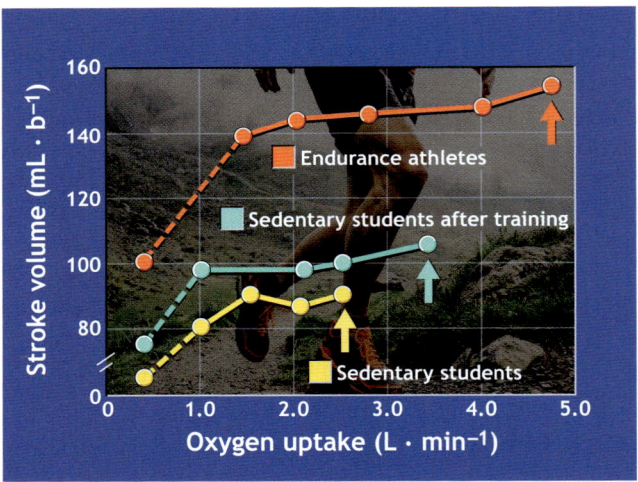

FIGURE 21.8. Stroke volume and oxygen uptake during upright physical activity in endurance athletes (■) and sedentary college students before (■) and after (■) 55 days of aerobic training (*arrows* = maximum values).
(Giorgio1978/Shutterstock)

Stroke Volume and $\dot{V}O_{2max}$. The data in **FIGURE 21.9** amplify the importance stroke volume plays in differentiating among persons with high and low $\dot{V}O_{2max}$ values. The experiment included three groups: athletes, healthy but sedentary men, and patients with a valvular heart disease (mitral stenosis) that causes inadequate left ventricle emptying. The differences in $\dot{V}O_{2max}$ among the groups related closely to maximum stroke volume differences. Patients with mitral stenosis achieved an aerobic capacity and maximum stroke volume half that of sedentary subjects. The importance of stroke volume also emerges in comparisons among healthy groups. Athletes achieved an average 62% larger $\dot{V}O_{2max}$ than sedentary subjects, almost entirely from the athletes' 60% larger stroke volume and cardiac output (see Figs. 21.8 and 21.9).

Cardiac Output

An increase in maximum cardiac output represents the most significant adaptation in cardiovascular function with aerobic training. Maximum heart rate generally decreases slightly with training, while increased cardiac output capacity results directly from improved stroke volume. A large maximum cardiac output, reflected by a larger stroke volume, distinguishes champion endurance athletes from other well-trained athletes and untrained counterparts.

FIGURE 21.10 illustrates cardiac output's important role in achieving a high level aerobic metabolism. In trained athletes and students, cardiac output increases *linearly* with oxygen uptake throughout the major portion of the exercise intensity range with athletes achieving the highest values for both variables. A linear relationship also exists between cardiac output and oxygen uptake in graded exercise in children and adolescents.[35] For these individuals, an increased stroke volume and a proportionate increase in cardiac output closely matches the added oxygen requirement of physical activity during growth.

Early research demonstrated that endurance training, while improving maximum cardiac output, reduced the heart's minute volume during moderate activity. In one study, average

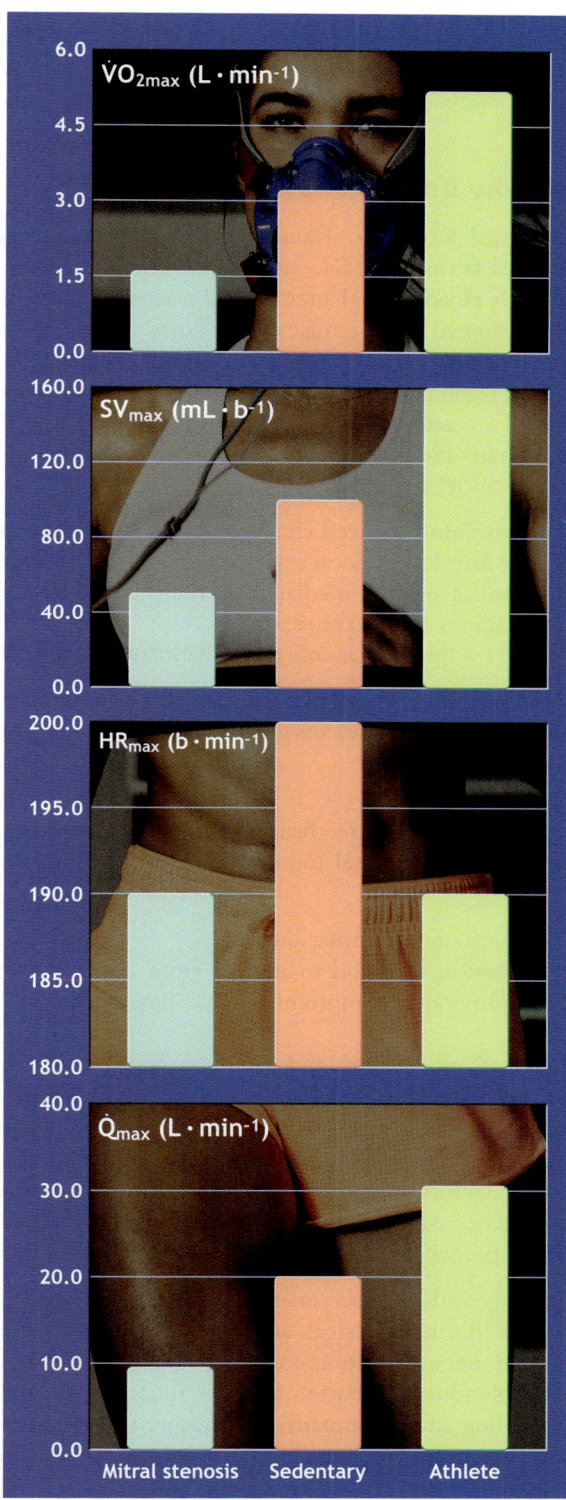

FIGURE 21.9. Maximum values for oxygen uptake ($\dot{V}O_{2max}$, L·min^{-1}), heart rate (HR$_{max}$, b·min^{-1}), stroke volume (SV$_{max}$, mL·min^{-1}), and cardiac output ($\dot{Q}_{max}$, L·min^{-1}).
(Jacob Lund/Shutterstock)

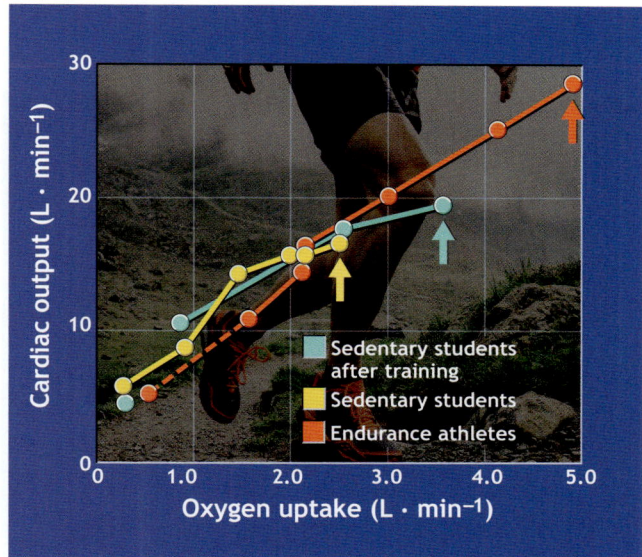

FIGURE 21.10. Cardiac output and oxygen uptake during upright physical activity in endurance athletes (■) and sedentary college students before (■) and after (■) 55 days of aerobic training (*arrows* = maximum values).
(Giorgio1978/Shutterstock)

cardiac output in young men following aerobic training for 16 wk decreased by 1.1 and 1.5 L·min^{-1} at a specific submaximum oxygen uptake.[43] As expected, maximum cardiac output increased 8% from 22.4 to 24.2 L·min^{-1}. With a reduced submaximum cardiac output, a corresponding increase in oxygen extraction in the active muscles achieves the exercise oxygen requirement. A training-induced reduction in submaximum cardiac output reflects two factors:

1. More effective blood flow redistribution
2. Trained muscles' enhanced capacity to generate ATP aerobically at a lower tissue P_{O_2}

Oxygen Extraction: Arterio-Mixed Venous Oxygen Difference

Endurance training *increases* the quantity of oxygen extracted from circulating blood, measured as the arterio-mixed venous oxygen difference or (a-$\bar{v}O_2$ diff).[193] An increase in the maximum a-$\bar{v}O_2$ difference results from more effective cardiac output distribution to active muscles combined with trained muscle fibers' enhanced capacity to extract and process the available oxygen. The a-$\bar{v}O_2$ difference takes on greater importance in contributing to improved aerobic capacity with training in older men and women because the elderly typically show diminished capacity to improve cardiac output with training.[104,195]

FIGURE 21.11 compares the relationship between the a-$\bar{v}O_2$ difference and exercise intensity for trained athletes and untrained students depicted in Figure 21.8. The a-$\bar{v}O_2$ difference for the students increases steadily to a maximum 15 mL·dL^{-1} during graded exercise. Following 55 training days, the students' maximum oxygen extraction increased 13% to 17 mL of oxygen. This indicates that during intense physical activity, arterial blood released approximately 85% of its oxygen content. In fact, active muscles extract even more oxygen because the a-$\bar{v}O_2$ difference reflects an *average* based on mixed venous blood sampling, which contains blood returning from tissues that use much less oxygen during exercise than active muscle. The posttraining maximum a-$\bar{v}O_2$ difference for the students equals that for the endurance athletes. The students' lower cardiac output capacity explains the large difference in $\dot{V}O_{2max}$ that clearly differentiates athletes from students in maximum exercise capacity.

Blood Flow and Distribution

Submaximal Exercise. Trained persons perform submaximum exercise at a lower cardiac output (and unchanged or slightly lower muscle blood flow) than untrained persons. A larger portion of the submaximum cardiac output flows to high oxidative type I skeletal muscle fibers at the expense of blood flow to muscles with a greater type IIb fiber percentage with lower oxidative capacity.[36] Two factors contribute to reduced muscle blood flow in submaximum exercise.[108,214,228,236] Both adaptations support the training specificity principle:

1. Rapid training-induced changes in vasoactive properties of large arteries and local resistance vessels within skeletal and cardiac muscle, mediated by the dilation effects of endothelium-derived nitric oxide
2. Changes within muscle cells that enhance oxidative capacity

As the muscle's ability to deliver, extract, and use oxygen increases, the active tissue's oxygen needs require proportionally less blood flow.

Maximal Exercise. Three factors affect how aerobic training increases total skeletal muscle blood flow during maximum exercise:

1. Larger maximum cardiac output.
2. Distribution of blood to muscle from nonactive areas that temporarily compromise blood flow during all-out effort.
3. Enlargement of large and small arteries (*arteriogenesis*) and veins' cross-sectional areas, and 10 to 20% increase in muscle capillarization (*angiogenesis*).[80,178] This blood flow effect begins rapidly from increased vascular endothelial growth factors produced by skeletal muscle cells to induce angiogenesis following a single exercise bout in trained and untrained persons.[55,101,109]

Training-induced *decreases* in splanchnic and renal blood flow during physical activity occur from reduced sympathetic nervous system outflow to these tissues, which promotes blood redistribution to active muscles.[134] Concurrently, training and accompanying exposure to elevated core temperatures produces heat loss adaptations via enhanced endothelium-dependent increases in skin blood flow at a given internal temperature.[92,103] Augmented cutaneous blood flow facilitates the endurance-trained person's capacity to dissipate the metabolic heat generated in intense physical activity.

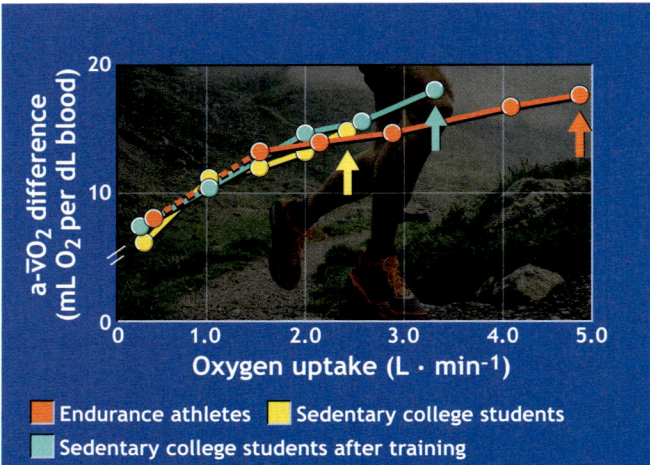

FIGURE 21.11. The a-$\bar{v}O_2$ difference and oxygen uptake during upright exercise in endurance athletes (■) and sedentary college students before (■) and after (■) 55 days of aerobic training (*arrows* = maximum values).
(Giorgio1978/Shutterstock)

Oxygen extraction in skeletal muscle remains near maximum during intense activity and supports the hypothesis that oxygen supply (i.e., blood flow), not oxygen use (extraction), limits muscle tissue's maximum respiratory rate.[11,145,178]

Myocardial Blood Flow. For healthy persons and cardiac patients, structural and functional changes in the heart's vasculature, including modifications in mechanisms that regulate myocardial perfusion, parallel a modest training-induced myocardial hypertrophy.[72,106,107] Structural vascular modifications include increased proximal coronary artery cross-sectional area, possible arteriolar proliferation and longitudinal growth, collateral vessel recruitment, and increased capillary density. These adaptations provide adequate perfusion to support the increased blood flow and energy demands of the functionally improved myocardium.

Two mechanisms help to explain how aerobic training increases coronary blood flow and capillary exchange capacity:

1. Ordered progression of structural remodeling to improve myocardial vascularization when new capillaries form and develop into small arterioles[106]
2. More effective control of vascular resistance and blood distribution within the myocardium[221,228]

The vascular and cellular adaptations' significance to the heart's functional capacity during physical activity remains unclear—mainly because the healthy, untrained heart does not suffer from reduced oxygen supply during maximum exertion. Training adaptations may provide some cardioprotection by enabling myocardial tissue to better tolerate and recover from transient ischemic episodes and thus become more resistant to ischemic injury. Trained myocardial tissue also functions at a lower total oxidative capacity percentage during physical activity. Vascular adaptations do not accompany the myocardial hypertrophy that occurs with chronic resistance training.[143]

Blood Pressure

Regular aerobic training *reduces* systolic and diastolic blood pressure during rest and submaximum physical activity. The largest reduction occurs in systolic pressure, particularly in hypertensive subjects. (Chapters 15 and 32 provide additional discussion about this topic.).

Pulmonary Adaptations

Aerobic training stimulates adaptations in pulmonary ventilation dynamics during submaximum and maximum effort. The adaptations generally reflect a breathing strategy that minimizes respiratory work at a given exercise intensity. This frees oxygen to supply the nonrespiratory active musculature.

Maximal Physical Activity

Maximum exercise ventilation increases from both increased tidal volume and breathing rate as $\dot{V}O_{2max}$ increases. This makes sense physiologically because any increase in $\dot{V}O_{2max}$ raises the body's oxygen requirement and corresponding need to eliminate additional carbon dioxide by alveolar ventilation.

Submaximal Physical Activity

Aerobic training for several weeks *reduces* the ventilatory equivalent for oxygen ($\dot{V}_E/\dot{V}O_2$) during submaximum physical activity and *lowers* the percentage of the total oxygen cost attributable to breathing. Reduced oxygen uptake by the ventilatory musculature enhances endurance for two reasons:

1. Reduces physical activity's fatiguing effects on the ventilatory musculature
2. Any oxygen not used by the respiratory muscles now becomes available to active locomotor muscles

In general, training increases tidal volume and decreases breathing frequency. Consequently, air remains in the lungs for a longer time between breaths, which increases oxygen extraction from inspired air. For example, the exhaled air in trained individuals during submaximum exercise contains only 14 to 15% oxygen, whereas untrained persons expired air averages 18% at the same exercise intensity. This means untrained persons ventilate proportionately more air to achieve the same submaximum oxygen uptake.

Music Positively Impacts Heart Rate Variability

Music therapy (MT), often considered a part of medicine devoted to mind-body interactions, is believed by many to effectively improve holistic health. This includes brain, mind, and body functions through its effects on autonomic and central nervous system neurovisceral integration and its resultant psycho-neuroimmunological impact. More than 1300 subjects in 29 independent studies that included 24 pre-post interventions and 5 randomized, controlled trials were evaluated to determine the immediate and chronic effects of MT on cardiac autonomic regulation measured by heart rate variability and related parameters. The beat-to-beat heart rate variation reflects cardiac autonomic, behavioral, and mental state (stress, fatigue, sleepiness, arousal, and emotional strain or time pressures), on the body's capacity for exercise. While the results were not uniform and of relatively low statistical significance, subjects in 90% of the studies, the majority suffering from some form of health-related condition, reported a positive response to MT, which demonstrated the need for continued research with well-controlled, randomized trials.

Shutterstock: Vasif Maharov, Vectorry

Sources:
Bae IL, et al. The effects of listening to healing beat music on adults' recovery from exposure to stressful stimuli: a randomized controlled trial. *Integr Med Res.* 2022;11:100753.
Mojtabavi H, et al. Can music influence cardiac autonomic system? A systematic review and narrative synthesis to evaluate its impact on heart rate variability. *Complement Ther Clin Pract* 2020;39:101162.

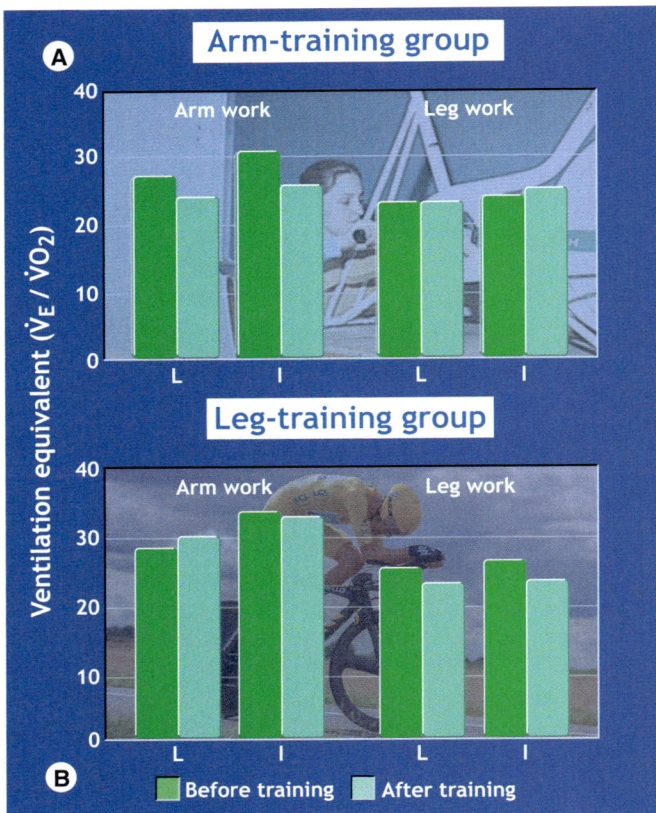

FIGURE 21.12. Ventilation equivalents in light (L) and intense (I) submaximal arm and leg exercise before and after arm **(A)** and leg **(B)** training. $\dot{V}O_2$, oxygen uptake.
(Reprinted with permission from Rasmussen B, et al. Pulmonary ventilation, blood gases, and blood pH after training of the arms and the legs. *J Appl Physiol.* 1975;38:250. ©The American Physiological Society (APS). All rights reserved.)

Substantial specificity exists for ventilatory responses relative to activity mode and training adaptations. When subjects performed arm-only and leg-only exercise, consistently higher ventilatory equivalents occurred for the arms (**FIG. 21.12**), with the ventilatory equivalent decreasing in each mode with training. The reduction occurred only with exercise that engaged the specifically trained muscles. For the group trained by arm-crank ergometry (an exercise that primarily uses the arms), the ventilation equivalent decreased only during arm effort and vice versa for the leg-trained group. The ventilatory training adaptation linked closely to a less pronounced rise in blood lactate and heart rate during the specific training exercise. This suggests that local adaptations in specifically trained muscles affect the ventilatory adjustment to training. In this regard, lower lactate levels with training remove the drive to breathe from any additional carbon dioxide produced from lactate buffering.

Training May Benefit Ventilatory Endurance

Prolonged, intense physical activity induces inspiratory muscle fatigue[9,89,226] and reduces the abdominal muscles' capacity to generate maximum expiratory pressure.[52] *Exercise training allows for sustained, exceptionally high submaximum ventilation levels.*[20,91,203] Endurance training stabilizes the body's internal milieu during submaximum activity. Consequently, exercise causes less disruption in whole-body hormonal and acid-base balance that could negatively impact inspiratory muscle function. The ventilatory muscles also benefit directly from training. For example, run training by healthy males and females for 20 wk improved ventilatory muscle endurance by approximately 16%, characterized by less lactate accumulation during standard breathing exercise. The training-induced increase in aerobic enzyme levels and respiratory musculature's oxidative capacity contribute to an enhanced ventilatory muscle function.[173,206] Training also increases inspiratory muscle capacity to generate force and sustain a given inspiratory pressure level.[27] These adaptations benefit exercise performance in three ways:

1. Less respiratory work by ventilatory muscles reduces overall energy demands
2. Ventilatory muscles produce less lactate during intense, prolonged physical activity
3. Ventilatory muscles more efficiently metabolize circulating lactate as metabolic fuel

Blood Lactate Concentration Adaptations

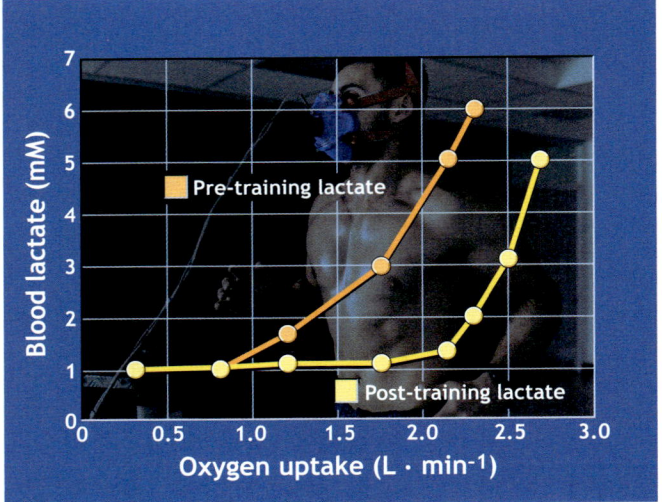

FIGURE 21.13. Generalized response for pretraining and posttraining lactate accumulation and oxygen uptake during incremental treadmill exercise.
(Data from V. Katch, Applied Physiology Laboratory, University of Michigan, Ann Arbor. Jacob Lund/Shutterstock.)

FIGURE 21.13 illustrates the generalized effect of endurance training in lowering blood lactate levels and extending physical effort before the onset of blood lactate accumulation (OBLA) during exercise of increasing intensity. The underlying explanation centers on three possibilities related to central and peripheral adaptations to aerobic training discussed in this chapter:

1. Decreased lactate formation rate during physical activity
2. Increased lactate clearance (removal) rate during physical activity
3. Combined decreased lactate formation and increased lactate clearance effects

Four Additional Aerobic Training Adaptations

1. *Body composition changes*: Regular aerobic activity for the obese or overweight person reduces body mass and body fat and augments a more favorable body fat distribution (see Chapter 30). Exercise only or combined with calorie restriction reduces body fat more than weight loss with dieting by exercise's effect in promoting lean tissue conservation.
2. *Body heat transfer*: Well-hydrated, trained individuals exercise more comfortably in hot environments because larger plasma volumes elicit more responsive thermoregulatory mechanisms to dissipate heat faster and more economically than responses of sedentary individuals.
3. *Performance changes*: Enhanced endurance performance accompanies physiologic adaptations with training. **FIGURE 21.14** depicts cycling performance prior to and following cycling training for 10 wk, 40 to 60 min daily, 4 days weekly at 85% $\dot{V}O_{2max}$. In the performance test, subjects attempted to maintain a constant 265-watt power output for 8 min. Training produced less drop-off from the initial rate in power output during the exercise test.
4. *Psychological benefits*: Regular physical activity from youth through older age creates important potential benefits on psychological state. Adaptations often occur to a degree equal to other therapeutic interventions including pharmacologic therapy.[46,216]

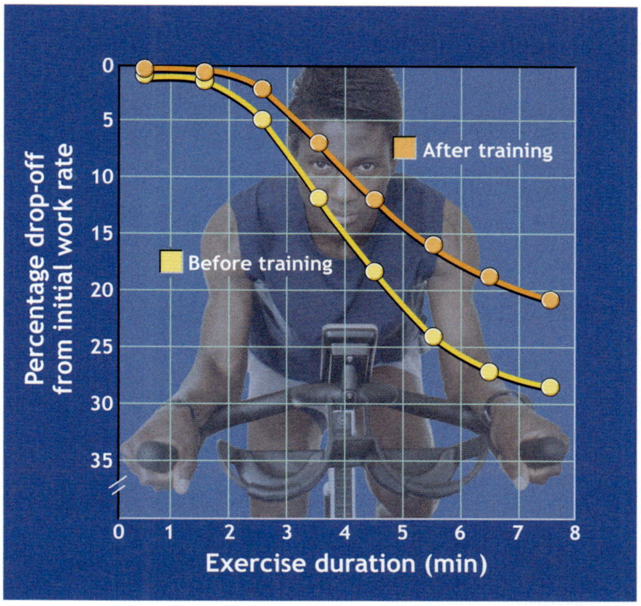

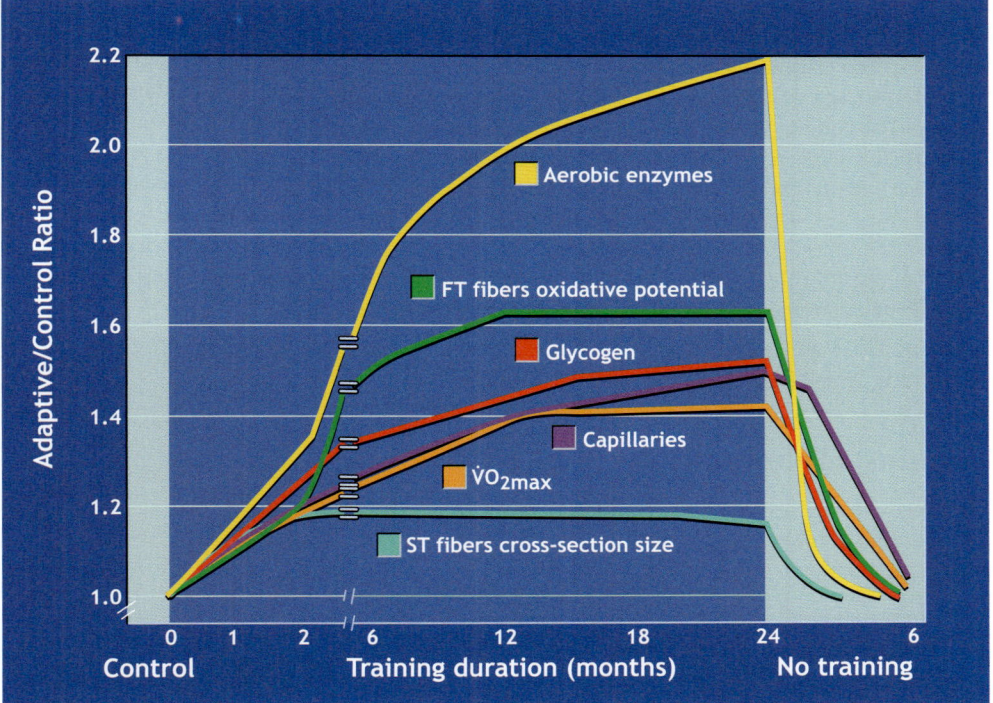

FIGURE 21.14. Percentage drop-off from initial exercise intensity before and after endurance cycling training for 10 wk. (Data from V. Katch, Applied Physiology Laboratory, University of Michigan, Ann Arbor.)

Summary of Training Adaptations

FIGURE 21.15 summarizes adaptive changes in active muscle that accompany $\dot{V}O_{2max}$ improvements with endurance training and detraining. Aerobic capacity generally increases 15 to 25% over the first 3 months of intensive training and may improve by 50% over a 2-year interval depending on initial fitness level. When training ceases, $\dot{V}O_{2max}$ rapidly decreases toward the pretraining level. Even more impressive training effects occur for citric acid cycle and electron transport chain's aerobic enzymes within the trained muscle's mitochondria. These enzymes increase rapidly and substantially throughout training in both fiber types and subdivisions. Conversely, detraining for 2 to 3 wk can substantially reduce a large portion of enzymatic adaptations. Muscle capillary number increases during training, but when training ceases, this adaptation in blood supply probably decreases relatively slowly. The ultimate detraining occurs with aging. Regular physical activity slows but cannot halt the muscle atrophy, weakness, and fatigability that accompany the progression of chronological age.[44]

FIGURE 21.15. Generalized summary for how endurance training duration changes aerobic capacity and adaptations in muscle fiber characteristics. FT, fast-twitch; ST, slow-twitch; $\dot{V}O_{2max}$, maximum oxygen uptake.
(Adapted with permission from Saltin B, et al. Fiber types and metabolic potentials of skeletal muscles in sedentary man and endurance runners. *Ann NY Acad Sci.* 1977;301:3.)

Local metabolic improvement greatly exceeds improvements in capacity to circulate, deliver, and use oxygen, reflected by $\dot{V}O_{2max}$ and cardiac output increases during intense physical activity. With local training adaptations, a muscle's lactate flux remains at lower levels (lower production and/or greater removal rate) than similar submaximum effort before training. These cellular adjustments account for how a trained person performs steady-rate exercise at a greater $\dot{V}O_{2max}$ percentage.

Seven Factors Affecting Aerobic Training Responses

Seven factors influence the aerobic training response, each interrelated and altering how one impacts the other:

1. Initial aerobic fitness level
2. Training intensity
3. Training duration
4. Training volume
5. Training frequency
6. Training mode
7. Training progression

Initial Aerobic Fitness Level

The training response magnitude depends on initial fitness level. Someone who rates low at the start of training has considerable room to improve, but if capacity already rates high, the improvement would remain relatively small. Studies of sedentary, middle-age men with heart disease improved $\dot{V}O_{2max}$ by 50%, while similar training in normally active, healthy adults improved 10 to 15%.[178] However, a relatively small improvement in aerobic capacity represents a crucial change for an elite athlete, where even a 1 to 2% performance change could be the difference between winning gold or coming in last. *As a general guideline, aerobic fitness improvements with endurance training range between 5 and 25%, with some improvement occurring within the first training week.*

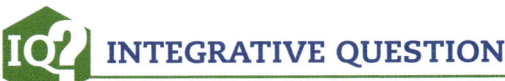 **INTEGRATIVE QUESTION**

How would you respond to someone who asks you, "How long must I exercise to 'get in shape'?"

Training Intensity

Training-induced physiologic adaptations depend primarily on overload intensity, with at least seven different ways to express such effort:

1. Energy expended per unit time (e.g., 9 kcal·min⁻¹ or 37.8 kJ·min⁻¹)
2. Absolute exercise level or power output (e.g., cycle at 900 kg-m·min⁻¹ or 147 W)
3. Relative metabolic level expressed as percentage $\dot{V}O_{2max}$ (e.g., 85% $\dot{V}O_{2max}$)
4. Exercise below, at, or above OBLA (e.g., 4 mM lactate threshold)
5. Exercise heart rate, or percentage HR_{max} (e.g., 180 b·min⁻¹ or 80% HR_{max})
6. Multiples of resting metabolic rate (e.g., 6 METs)
7. Rating of perceived exertion (e.g., RPE = 14)

As an example, absolute training intensity involves all individuals who perform at the same power output or energy expenditure (e.g., 9.0 kcal·min⁻¹) for 30 min. When everyone performs at the same intensity, the task can elicit considerable stress for one person yet fall short of the training threshold for another more fit person. For this reason, *relative intensity* based on a person's physiologic system's response effectively establishes exercise intensity. The assigned relative intensity usually relates to some breakpoint for steady-rate exercise (e.g., lactate threshold, OBLA), some physiologic capacity percentage (e.g., %$\dot{V}O_{2max}$ or %HR_{max}), or maximum exercise capacity. General practice establishes aerobic training intensity by direct measurement or estimation of $\dot{V}O_{2max}$ or HR_{max} and then assigns an exercise level to correspond to some percentage of that maximum.

Establishing training intensity from oxygen uptake provides high accuracy but requires sophisticated monitoring that renders this method impractical for general use. An effective alternative relies on *heart rate* to classify an activity for relative intensity when individualizing training programs. Exercise heart rate is convenient because %$\dot{V}O_{2max}$ and %HR_{max} relate in a predictable way regardless of gender, race, fitness level, activity mode, or age. Training does not affect a particular individual's heart rate at a given %$\dot{V}O_{2max}$. There is little need to frequently adjust the exercise prescription relative to training-induced changes in aerobic capacity if exercise occurs at the %HR_{max}.[202]

The unnumbered figure presents selected values for %$\dot{V}O_{2max}$ and corresponding %HR_{max}.[5,132] The error in estimating %$\dot{V}O_{2max}$ from %HR_{max}, or vice versa, equals approximately ± 8%. One need only monitor heart rate to estimate relative %$\dot{V}O_{2max}$ within the given error range. The relationship between %HR_{max} and %$\dot{V}O_{2max}$ remains the same for arm or leg activities among healthy subjects, normal-weight and obese persons, cardiac patients, and persons with spinal cord injuries.[49,86,100,138] Importantly, upper-body arm exercise produces lower HR_{max} than leg exercise. One must consider this difference when

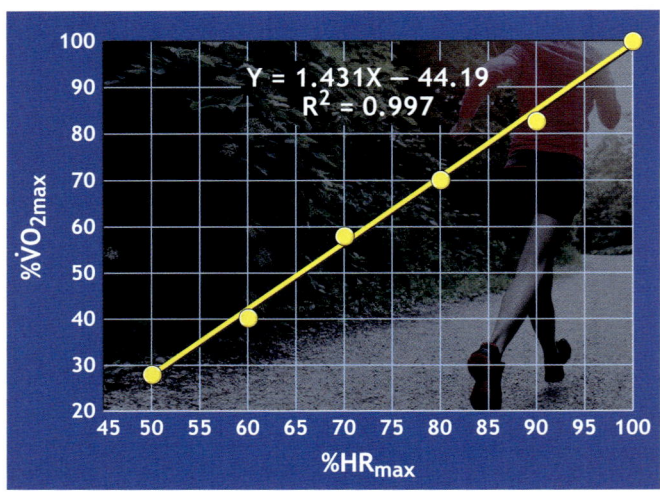

Dasha Petrenko/Shutterstock

formulating an individualized exercise prescription for different exercise modes (see "Running vs. Swimming and Other Forms of Upper-Body Exercise" later in this chapter). For more precise %$\dot{V}O_{2max}$ estimates, use the equation in the unnumbered figure where Y is the predicted %$\dot{V}O_{2max}$ and X is the %HR_{max}.

Train at HR$_{max}$ Percentage

Aerobic capacity improves when heart rate achieves between 55 and 70% of maximum during training regimens. During lower-body cycling, walking, or running, the heart rate increase equals about 40 to 55% of the $\dot{V}O_{2max}$. Consequently, for college-age males and females, training heart rate ranges between 120 and 140 b·min.$^{-1}$

An equally effective method to establish the training threshold, termed the Karvonen method after the researcher who pioneered its use, requires that subjects exercise at a heart rate equal to 60% of the difference between resting and maximum as follows[97]:

$$HR_{threshold} = HR_{rest} + 0.60\,(HR_{max} - HR_{rest})$$

This approach to establishing heart rate training threshold results in a *higher* value than simply computing threshold heart rate as 70% HR_{max}.

Achieving positive training adaptations does *not* require strenuous physical activity. For most healthy persons, a 70% HR_{max} represents "moderate activity" without undue discomfort. This training level (referred to as "**conversational exercise**") establishes a threshold intensity to stimulate a training effect without producing discomfort (e.g., lactate accumulation and associated hyperpnea) that would prevent casual talking during the activity. Previously sedentary individuals need not exercise above this threshold heart rate to improve physiologic capacity.

FIGURE 21.16 illustrates that as aerobic fitness improves, submaximum heart rate decreases 10 to 20 b·min^{-1} at a given oxygen uptake level. Reduced exercise heart rate with training usually reflects an enhanced heart's stroke volume. To keep pace with physiologic improvement, the activity level must increase periodically to achieve the desired "target" heart rate. A person begins training by walking, then walks more briskly; jogging then replaces walking for the workout; and eventually continuous running elicits the desired heart rate level. In each progression, exercise remains at the same "relative intensity." If intensity progression does not increase with training improvements, the exercise essentially becomes an aerobic fitness maintenance program.

Commonly Used HR$_{max}$ Prediction Equations

Population	Equation	Ref #
General	$HR_{max} = 220 - $ Age, y	265
General	$HR_{max} = 216.6 - (0.84 \times $ Age, y$)$	275
General	$HR_{max} = 208 - (0.7 \times $ Age, y$)$	214
General	$HR_{max} = 206.9 - (0.67 \times $ Age, y$)$	56
General	$HR_{max} = 206 - (0.88 \times $ Age, y$)$	276
General	$HR_{max} = 216.6 - (0.84 \times $ Age, y$)$	268
CHD patients	$HR_{max} = 264 - (0.7 \times $ Age, y$)$	261
MR; DS	$HR_{max} = 210 - (0.56 \times $ Age, y$) - 15.5$ DS*	264
Obese	$HR_{max} = 200 - (0.48 \times $ Age, y$)$	267

CHD, coronary heart disease; DS, Down syndrome; MR, mental retardation; HRmax, maximum heart rate
*DS = 1 for patients with DS; 0 for those without DS

Andrii Vodolazhskyi/Shutterstock

Is Strenuous Training More Effective?

Generally, the higher the training intensity above threshold, the greater the training improvement for $\dot{V}O_{2max}$ when controlling for exercise volume.[64] A minimal threshold intensity exists below which no meaningful training effect occurs. A "ceiling" also may exist above which no further gains accrue. More fit males and females generally require higher threshold levels to stimulate a training response than less fit persons. The ceiling for training intensity remains unknown, although about 85% $\dot{V}O_{2max}$, which corresponds to 90% HR_{max}, probably represents a targeted upper limit. Notwithstanding the exertion level selected, more exercise does not necessarily pro-

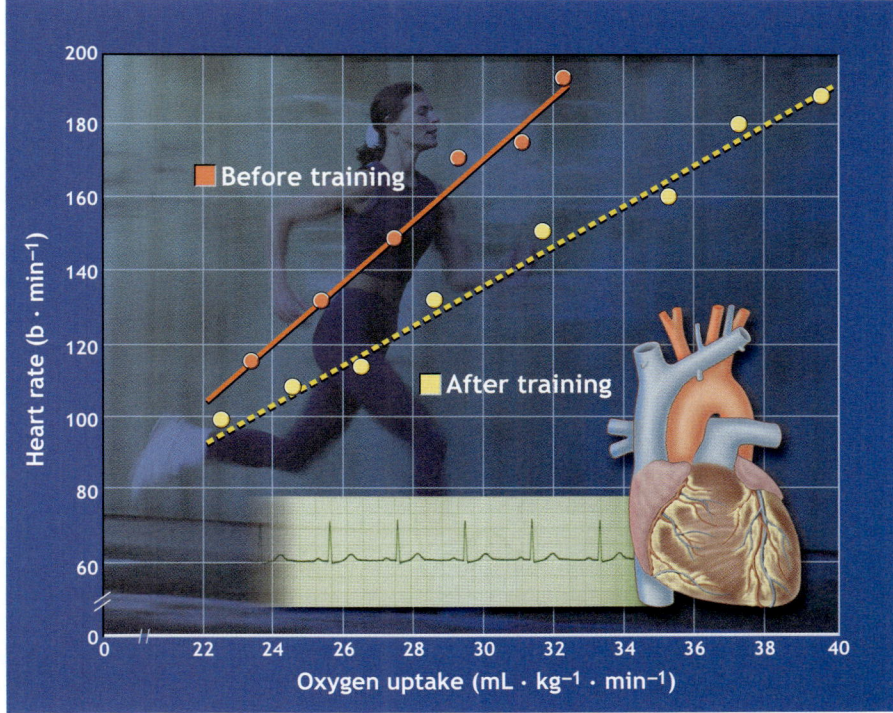

FIGURE 21.16. Aerobic training changes in the heart rate-oxygen uptake relationship.

duce greater results or achieve them more quickly. Excessive training intensity and abrupt increases in training volume increase injury risk to bones, joints, and muscles.[4,93] For adults, miles logged running each week represents the only variable consistently associated with running injuries. In pre-adolescent children, running excessive distances strains the articular cartilage, which could injure the bone's growth plate and adversely affect normal growth and development.

Determining the "Training-Sensitive Zone"

One can determine maximum heart rate immediately following all-out effort for several minutes. This intensity requires considerable motivation and physiologic strain—a requirement inadvisable for adults without medical clearance, particularly those predisposed to heart disease and other documented, underlying conditions. For most individuals, use age-predicted maximum heart rates presented in **FIGURE 21.17** based on averages from population studies grouped by age to establish the proper training threshold.[285]

While different age individuals have varying HR_{max} values, the inaccuracy from individual variation (±10 b·min⁻¹ standard deviation for any age-predicted HR_{max}) has little influence in establishing an effective training regimen for healthy persons. For most individuals, HR_{max} commonly can be estimated as 220 minus age in years, without considering race or gender or in children and adults.[7,90,120,260,272]

$$HR_{max} = 220 - Age\ (y)$$

Modifying the Standard HR_{max} Formula (220 – Age). The standard 220 minus age formula to estimate HR_{max} has been adopted in many studies despite the fact that it often either underestimates or overestimates the actually measured HR_{max}.[56,261,264–266,268,269,270] To improve accuracy, we recommend directly measuring HR_{max}. When this is not feasible, estimate HR_{max} with an equation derived for the specific populations we list in the accompanying table.

A longitudinal study that assessed 132 persons on average seven times over 9 years indicates a bias in the often used 220 – age HR_{max} prediction. The bias overestimates this prediction for males and females under age 40 years and underestimates it in those older than 40 years (**FIG. 21.18**).[56] This prediction equation

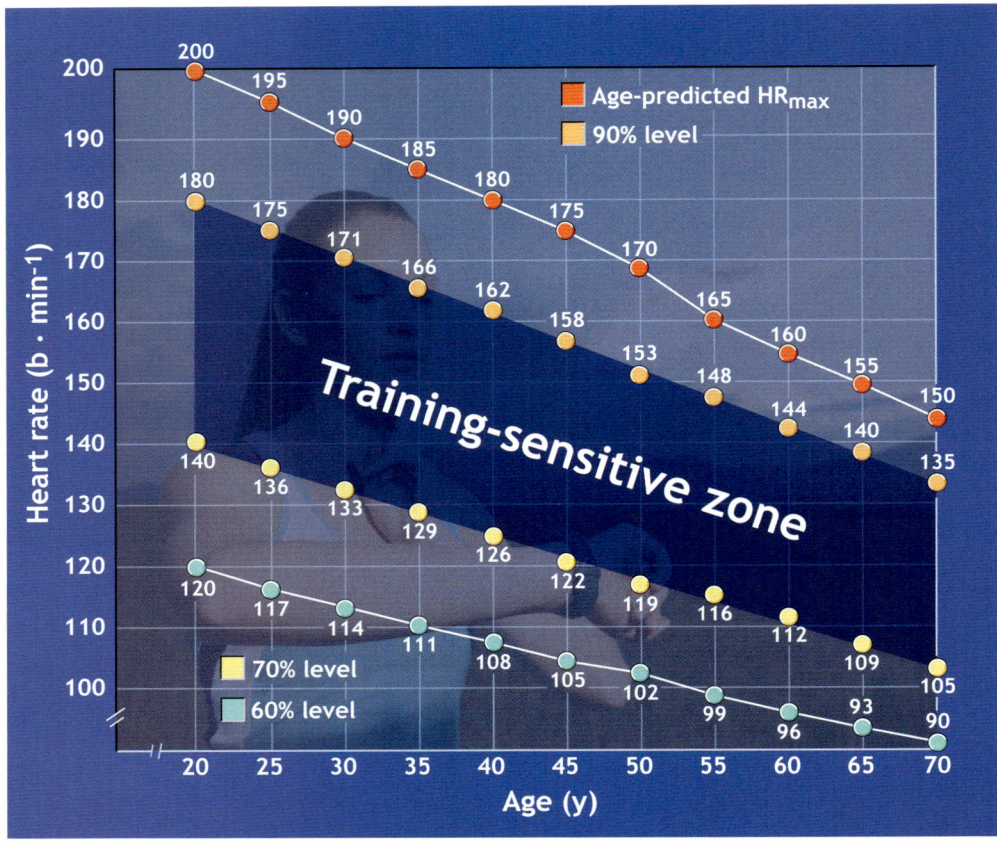

FIGURE 21.17. Age-predicted maximal heart rates and training-sensitive zone for aerobic training of men and women of different ages.

has a ±5 to ±8 beats per minute standard deviation without sex, BMI, and resting heart rate influencing the prediction:

$$HR_{max} = 206.9 - (0.67 \times Age, y)$$

For example, the above equation can estimate maximum heart rate for a 30-year-old male and female:

$$HR_{max} = 206.9 - (0.67 \times 30)$$
$$= 206.9 - 20.1$$
$$= 187$$

This prediction agrees closely with prior research[119,212] to produce acceptable HR_{max} predictions for most individuals.

The prediction formulae associate with a plus or minus prediction error and should be implemented with caution. Each formula represents a convenient rule-of-thumb and does not determine a specific person's maximum heart rate. For example, within normal variation limits and using the 220-minus-age formula, the actual maximum heart rate for 95% (±2 standard deviations) of 40-year-old males and females ranges between 160 and 200 b·min⁻¹. Figure 21.18 also depicts the "training-sensitive zone" related to age.

A 40-year-old person who wants to train at moderate intensity but still achieve the threshold level would select a training heart rate at 70% age-predicted HR_{max}. Using the 220-minus-age formula results in a 126 b·min⁻¹ (0.70 × 180) target activity heart rate. To increase training to 85% maximum, intensity must increase to produce a 153 b·min⁻¹ (0.85 × 180) heart rate.

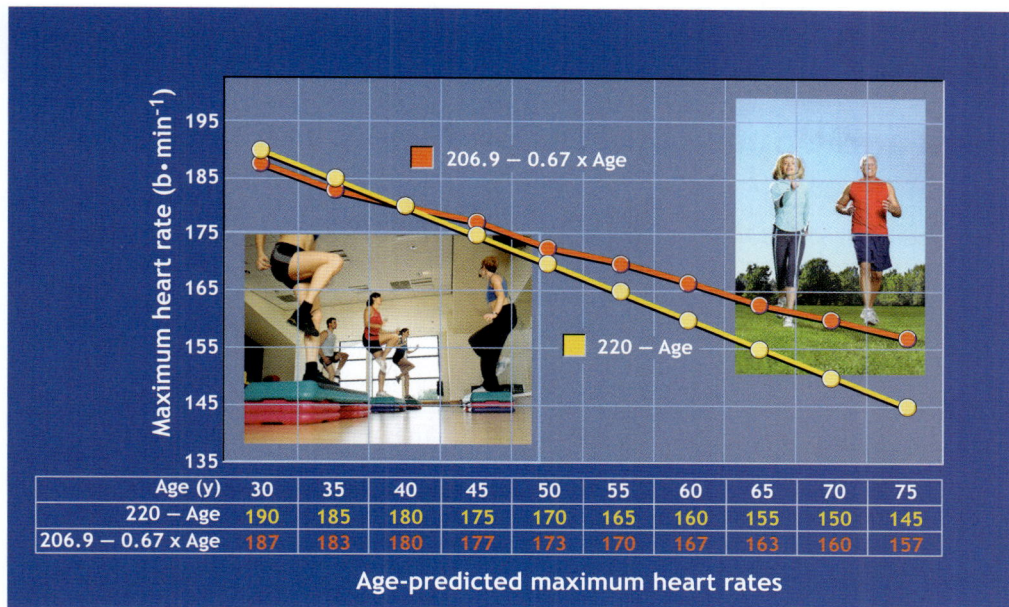

FIGURE 21.18. Modified maximum heart rate versus age prediction compared with the commonly used 220 − age equation.
(Data from Gellish RL, et al. Longitudinal modeling of the relationship between age and maximal heart rate. *Med Sci Sports Exerc.* 2007;39:822.)

Running Versus Swimming and Other Upper-Body Activities. HR_{max} estimation requires an adjustment for swimming or when performing other upper-body activities. HR_{max} during these activity modes averages about 13 b·min^{-1} lower for trained and untrained males and females compared to running.[49,58,135] This difference highlights the less feed-forward stimulation from the motor cortex to the medulla during swimming. There also is less feedback stimulation from the smaller muscle mass in the active upper body. In swimming, the horizontal body position and water's cooling effect also may contribute to a lower HR_{max}.

Establishing the appropriate swimming and other upper-body activity intensities requires subtracting 13 b·min^{-1} from the age-predicted HR_{max} in Figure 21.17. A 30-year-old person who chooses to swim at 70% HR_{max} should select a swimming speed that produces a 124 b·min^{-1} (0.70 × [190 − 13]) heart rate. This would more accurately represent the proper threshold swimming heart rate to induce a positive training effect. Without this adjustment, a prescription utilizing upper-body activity based on %HR_{max} in leg effort *overestimates* the appropriate threshold training heart rate.

Can Less Intense Training be Effective?

The often-cited 70% HR_{max} recommendation as a training threshold for aerobic improvement represents a *general guideline* for effective yet comfortable exertion. The lower limit may depend on the participant's initial exercise capacity and current training state. In addition, older and less fit individuals, including sedentary, overweight males and females have training thresholds closer to 60% HR_{max} (corresponding to about 45% $\dot{V}O_{2max}$). Continuous activity at 70% HR_{max} performed for 20 to 30 min stimulates a training effect—exercise at the lower intensity of 60% HR_{max} for 45 min also proves beneficial. *Generally, longer exercise duration offsets lower exercise intensity benefits.*

Train at Rating of Perceived Exertion

The **rating of perceived exertion (RPE)**, a psychophysiologic scaling approach, allows a person to rate physical activity intensity.[16,156,183] The exerciser rates the perceived feelings of stress relative to the exertion level. In essence, the RPE measures how hard it "feels" based on physical sensations that the person experiences—including increased heart rate, increased respiration or breathing rate, increased sweating, and possibly neuromuscular fatigue. Monitoring and adjusting RPE during activity provides an effective way to prescribe exercise from an individual's perception of effort that coincides with physiologic/metabolic measures, which include %HR_{max}, %$\dot{V}O_{2max}$, and blood lactate concentration.

Methods to Prescribe Exercise Intensity for a Training Effect

Different methods can estimate heart rate to prescribe exercise intensity using an upper and lower effective intensity range.

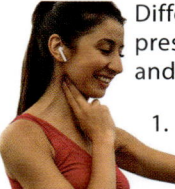

1. **Heart rate (HR) method**

    Target HR = HR_{max} × % intensity desired

    IC Production/Shutterstock

2. **Heart rate reserve method**

    Target HR = [(HR_{max} − HR_{rest}) × % intensity desired] + HR_{rest}

3. **Oxygen uptake ($\dot{V}O_2$) method**

    Target $\dot{V}O_2$ = $\dot{V}O_{2max}$ × % intensity desired

4. **$\dot{V}O_2$ reserve method ($\dot{V}O_{2max}$ − resting $\dot{V}O_2$)**

    Target $\dot{V}O_2$ = [($\dot{V}O_{2max}$ − $\dot{V}O_{2rest}$) × % intensity desired] + $\dot{V}O_{2rest}$

5. **Metabolic equivalent (MET) method**

    Target MET = $\dot{V}O_{2max}$ ÷ 3.5 mL·kg^{-1}·min^{-1}

In a Practical Sense

Computing Lower-Limit and Upper-Limit Target Training Heart Rates

For males and females below age 60, the threshold stimulus or lower-limit target heart rate (LL_{THR}) ranges between 60 and 70% of HR_{max} for cardiovascular improvement, which represents about 50 to 60% of $\dot{V}O_{2max}$. The upper-limit target heart rate (UL_{THR}) represents about 90% HR_{max}, which equals about 85 to 90% of $\dot{V}O_{2max}$. Above age 60, LL_{THR} equals 60% and UL_{THR} equals 75% HR_{max}.

METHOD 1: PERCENTAGE METHOD

This method calculates the lower-limit and upper-limit target heart rates expressed as simple percentages of the age-predicted HR_{max}.

Equations

1. **Calculate LL_{THR}:**

   LL_{THR} = Predicted HR_{max} × Lower-limit percentage for age

   where the lower-limit percentage = 70% for males and females ≤60 years and 60% for males and females greater than 60 years.

2. **Calculate UL_{THR}:**

   UL_{THR} = Predicted HR_{max} × Upper-limit percentage for age

   where the upper-limit percentage = 90% for males and females ≤60 years and 80% for males and females greater than 60 years.

Example

Data: Male, age 55 years

1. **Calculate predicted HR_{max}:**

   $HR_{max} = 208 - (0.7 \times \text{Age, y}) = 170 \text{ b}\cdot\text{min}^{-1}$

2. **Calculate LL_{THR}:**

   LL_{THR} = 170 × Lower-limit percentage for age
   = 170 × 0.70
   = 119 b·min^{-1}

3. **Calculate UL_{THR}:**

   $UL_{THR} = HR_{max}$ × Upper-limit percentage for age
   = 170 × 0.90
   = 153 b·min^{-1}

METHOD 2: KARVONEN METHOD (HEART RATE RESERVE)

Karvonen method, named after the Finnish physiologist who devised the method six decades ago in 1957, provides an equally effective method to calculate the lower-limit and upper-limit training target heart rates. The method uses the percentage difference between resting and maximum HR termed **heart rate reserve (HRR)**. Karvonen method can produce higher values compared with heart rate computed as percentage HR_{max}. The Karvonen method uses about 50% of HRR as LL_{THR} and 85% of HRR as UL_{THR}. The method has been applied in many research experiments, including the conditioning of individuals with diverse conditions such as heart disease and pregnancy.

Rido/Shutterstock

Equations

1. **Calculate predicted HR_{max}:**

   $HR_{max} = 208 - (0.7 \times \text{Age, y})$

2. **Calculate LL_{THR}:**

   $LL_{THR} = [(HR_{max} - HR_{rest}) \times 0.50] + HR_{rest}$

3. **Calculate UL_{THR}:**

   $UL_{THR} = [(HR_{max} - HR_{rest}) \times 0.85] + HR_{rest}$

Example

Data: Male, age 55 years; HR_{rest} = 60 b·min^{-1}

1. **Calculate predicted HR_{max}:**

   $HR_{max} = 208 - (0.7 \times \text{Age, y})$
   = 170 b·min^{-1}

2. **Calculate LL_{THR}:**

   $LL_{THR} = [(HR_{max} - HR_{rest}) \times 0.50] + HR_{rest}$
   = [(170 − 60) × 0.50] + 60
   = 115 b·min^{-1}

3. **Calculate UL_{THR}:**

   $UL_{THR} = [(HR_{max} - HR_{rest}) \times 0.85] + HR_{rest}$
   = [(170 − 60) × 0.85] + 60
   = 154 b·min^{-1}

Sources:
Davis JA, Convertino VA. A comparison of heart rate methods for predicting endurance training intensity. *Med Sci Sports Exerc*. 1975;7:295.
Karandikar-Agashe G, Agrawal RJ. Comparative study of the effect of resistance exercises versus aerobic exercises in postmenopausal women suffering from insomnia. *Midlife Health*. 2020;11:2
Karvonen M, et al. The effects of training on heart rate. A longitudinal study. *Ann Med Exp Biol Fenn*. 1957;35:307.
Khadanga S, et al. Optimizing training response for women in cardiac rehabilitation: a randomized clinical trial. *JAMA Cardiol*. 2022;7:215.

A Borg RPE Scale

RPE	Description	Equivalent % HR$_{max}$	Equivalent % $\dot{V}O_{2max}$
6			
7	Very, very light		
8			
9	Very light		
10			
11	Fairly light	52–66	31–50
12			
13	Somewhat hard	61–85	51–75
14			
15	Hard	86–91	76–85
16			
17	Very hard	92	85
18			
19	Very, very hard		

B Borg CR10 Scale

Score	Level of exertion
0	No exertion as all
0.5	Very, very slight (just noticeable)
1	Very slight
2	Slight
3	Moderate
4	Somewhat severe
5	Severe
6	
7	Very severe
8	
9	Very, very severe (almost maximal)
10	Maximal

FIGURE 21.19. Borg's two rating of perceived exertion (RPE) scales. CR10, category-ratio anchored at number 10; HR$_{max}$, maximum heart rate; $\dot{V}O_{2max}$, maximum oxygen uptake. (Adapted with permission from Borg GA. Psychological basis of physical exertion. *Med Sci Sports Exerc.* 1982;14:377.)

Physical activity pegged to higher energy expenditure and physiologic strain levels produces higher RPE ratings. **FIGURE 21.19A** presents the original visual Likert-type Borg scale and the alternative Borg category-ratio (CR) scale anchored at number 10, which represents an extreme activity intensity. The CR10 scale has proven successful in clinical settings to assess the level of exertion and discomfort.[274,275]

For both scales, the corresponding RPE number indicates activity intensity. Each scale takes seconds to complete and can be researcher- or self-administered and used on single or multiple occasions. For the 20-point scale, an RPE rating (from 6 to 20) multiplied by 10 would correspond to the actual heart rate during physical activity. Consequently, a 12-RPE rating during physical activity in healthy individuals would correspond to a 120 b·min^{-1} heart rate (12 × 10 = 120) (www.cdc.gov/physicalactivity/basics/measuring/exertion.htm).

The RPE also can establish an exercise prescription at intensities that correspond to blood lactate concentrations of 2.5 mM (RPE ~ 15) and 4.0 mM (RPE ~ 18) during a 30-min treadmill run where subjects self-regulated exercise intensity.[210] Similarly, a simple "talk test" that asks whether comfortable speech is possible produces intensities within accepted guidelines to prescribe exercise using treadmill and cycle ergometer methodologies.[162]

Train at the Lactate Threshold

Exercising at or slightly above the lactate threshold provides another effective aerobic training method. The higher intensity levels produce the greatest training benefits, particularly for fit individuals.[118,231,276] **FIGURE 21.20** illustrates how to determine the appropriate activity level by plotting intensity (e.g., running speed) to blood lactate level. In this example, the running speed to produce a blood lactate concentration at the 4-mM OBLA represents the recommended training intensity. Many coaches use the 4-mM blood lactate level as the optimal aerobic training intensity, yet little convincing evidence exists to justify this particular blood lactate level as "ideal." Choosing a target specific blood lactate level for endurance training should be evaluated periodically, with exercise intensity adjusted as fitness improves. If regular blood lactate measurement proves impractical, the heart rate at the initial lactate determination remains a convenient and relatively stable marker to set an appropriate predetermined intensity level. During incremental activity, no systematic training-induced change occurs in the heart rate-blood lactate relationship.[47]

The RPE provides an effective tool to estimate blood lactate threshold when establishing training intensity for continuous physical activity. A change in the blood lactate concentration-RPE relationship does occur with repeated activity bouts. The relationship remains altered from a single bout, even after a 3.5-hr recovery.[232] This limits use of RPE

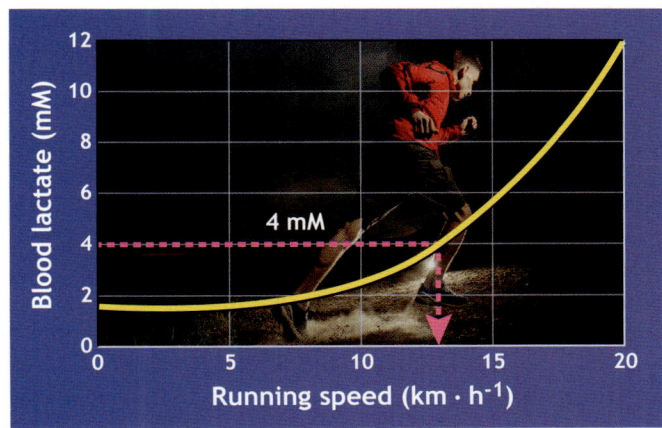

FIGURE 21.20. Blood lactate concentration related to running speed for one subject. At a 4.0 mM lactate level, the corresponding running speed was approximately 13 km·hr^{-1}. This speed establishes the subject's initial training intensity. (Kuznetcov_Konstantin/Shutterstock)

to gauge the intensity for a target blood lactate concentration if repeated exercise bouts occur during the same training session (e.g., during interval training; see "High-Intensity Interval Training" later in this chapter).

One important distinction between %HR_{max} and lactate threshold for setting training intensity lies in the physiologic dynamics each method reflects. The %HR_{max} method establishes a physiologic stress level to overload the central circulation (e.g., stroke volume, cardiac output), whereas the peripheral vasculature and active muscles' capacity to sustain steady-rate aerobic metabolism dictates exercise intensity adjustments based on the lactate threshold.

Training Duration

No threshold for exercise session duration, measured as amount of time per session per workout, exists for optimal aerobic improvement. If a threshold exists, it likely depends on the interaction among total work accomplished (i.e., duration or training volume), exercise intensity, training frequency, and initial fitness level. For previously sedentary adults, a dose-response relationship may exist.[26,286] A 3- to 5-min daily activity period produces some improvements in poorly conditioned people, but 20- to 30-min sessions achieve more optimal results if intensity achieves at least the minimum threshold. For weight management, longer daily training durations (≥60 to 120 min) may be required, particularly for individuals who exhibit sedentary behaviors. Shorter **high-intensity interval training (HIIT)** bouts discussed in a later section have improved many cardiorespiratory health markers including exercise performance.[277–279]

Training Volume

Exercise volume's important role in physical conditioning is to optimize health and fitness outcomes, particularly parameters related to body composition and weight management. Exercise volume generally includes gross energy expenditure expressed in total kcal or METs for a given exercise session. Epidemiological studies and randomized clinical trials have established a dose-response association between training volume and health/fitness outcomes for previously sedentary adults who begin an exercise regimen.[231,281,282] In terms of optimum exercise volume, most studies indicate that a total energy expenditure of between 500 and 1000 METs per wk consistently associates with a lower rate of cardiovascular disease and premature mortality.[282,291] This volume (about 150 min) approximates a weekly expenditure of 1000 kcal in moderate-intensity physical activity. More time and greater total energy expenditure devoted to workouts does not necessarily translate to greater health-fitness benefits, particularly among the physically active. In one experiment with collegiate swimmers, one group trained for 1.5 hr daily while another group performed two 1.5-hr exercise sessions daily. Even when one group trained at twice the daily volume, *no differences* in swimming power, endurance, or performance time improvements emerged between groups.[34]

Training Frequency

Can 2 versus 5 days per week training produce different effects if duration and intensity remain constant for each training session? Some investigators report training frequency influences cardiovascular improvements, while others maintain this factor contributes considerably less than either exercise intensity or exercise duration.[169] Studies with interval training show that training 2 days per week produced $\dot{V}O_{2max}$ changes similar to training 5 days per week.[48] In other studies that maintained a constant total exercise volume, *no differences* emerged in $\dot{V}O_{2max}$ improvement between 2 and 4 or 3 and 5 days per week training frequencies.[201] More frequent training produces beneficial effects when training occurs at a lower intensity.

While the extra time invested to increase training frequency may not improve $\dot{V}O_{2max}$, the extra physical activity (e.g., 3 vs. 6 days a week) often promotes considerable caloric expenditure with improved well-being and health. *To produce meaningful weight loss through physical activity, each activity session should last at least 60 min at sufficient intensity to expend at least 300 kcal*. Training 1 day per week generally does not change anaerobic or aerobic capacity, body composition, or body weight.[6] Typical aerobic training programs occur 3 days per week, usually with a single rest day separating workout days. Does training on consecutive days produce equally effective results? In one experiment about this question, nearly identical $\dot{V}O_{2max}$ improvements occurred despite the sequencing of the 3-day-a-week training schedule.[142] The aerobic training stimulus probably links closely to exercise intensity and total work accomplished, not to the training day sequencing.

Training Mode

Bicycling, walking, running, rowing, swimming, in-line skating, rope skipping, bench stepping, stair climbing, and simulated arm-leg climbing all provide for excellent aerobic system overload.[21,126,227] Training improvement based on the specificity concept varies considerably depending on training type and testing mode. Individuals trained by bicycling show greater improvement when tested on a bicycle than a treadmill.[159] Likewise, swim training and arm cranking show the greatest improvement when measured during an upper-body activity.[58]

Training Progression

Recommendations for training progression rate depend on many factors including the person's health status, initial fitness level, desired training goals, and the individual's training response. Some individuals are classified as fast **responders** and some classify as slower responders. Exercise progressions include increases in training intensity, duration, and frequency. During the initial phase of the exercise program, we recommend increasing the time/duration (i.e., minutes per session). Most individuals tolerate a 5- to 10-min session increase every 1 to 2 wk over the first 4- to 6-wk period.[282] If this increase is well tolerated, the duration per session can be increased considerably after about 6 wk. Gradually increasing and/or varying exercise intensity enhances the training response.

A Well-Rounded Overall Training Program

The primary goal of general physical activity for the adult population seeks to improve and maintain health.[7,76] Centers for Disease Control has issued physical activity guidelines for Americans. The current version was published in 2018 in collaboration with the National Institutes of Health, and the President's Council on Sports, Fitness & Nutrition. This edition builds on the previous *Guidelines*, while incorporating the vast amount of new knowledge regarding physical activity and health. Recommendations are for a "well-rounded training program" for adults age 18 to 65 years (https://jamanetwork.com/journals/jama/article-abstract/2712935?casa_token=l1YEbfCvtqIAAAAA:pGSCKjIZ9-DZzzYUw4c8by15cpinF1nPRzjTwaKQKRRsI7N8P7Vv9T8YjuXQhE6kAhMrEOX8nt8). A combined program of aerobic training (150 min of moderate-intensity activity weekly or 75 min of vigorous activity weekly) and resistance training increases aerobic power and muscular strength, decreases body fat, and increases basal metabolic rate. Additional physical activity produces even greater health benefits. In contrast, singular-focus programs of either resistance *only* or aerobic *only* training produce singularly larger but more limited overall effects.[41,170] For older adults, emphasis should also focus on movements to increase joint flexibility and improve balance to reduce injury risk from slips and falls.[150]

Tracking Aerobic Fitness Improvements

Improvements in aerobic fitness occur within several weeks. **FIGURE 21.21** shows absolute and percentage $\dot{V}O_{2max}$ improvements for subjects who trained 6 days per week for 10 wk. Training included stationary cycling for 30 min, 3 days per week combined with running for up to 40 min on alternate days. The continuous week-to-week improvement in aerobic capacity indicates that training improvement in previously sedentary persons occurs rapidly and progressively. Adaptive responses eventually level off as subjects approach their "genetically predisposed" maximums. The approximate time for the leveling-off remains unknown, particularly for intense training. The data presented in Figure 21.15 indicate that each physiologic and metabolic system responds in a unique and different way.

The data in the unnumbered table reveal the rapidity of maximum cardiovascular adaptations to training.

Five young adult men and five women trained daily for 10 consecutive days. Exercise included cycling for 1 hr—10 min at 65% $\dot{V}O_{2peak}$, 25 min at 75% $\dot{V}O_{2peak}$, and the remaining 25 min of repeat five 3-min intervals at 95% $\dot{V}O_{2peak}$ followed by a 2-min recovery. This relatively brief 10-day training period induced a 9% increase in $\dot{V}O_{2peak}$ and a 10.7% increase

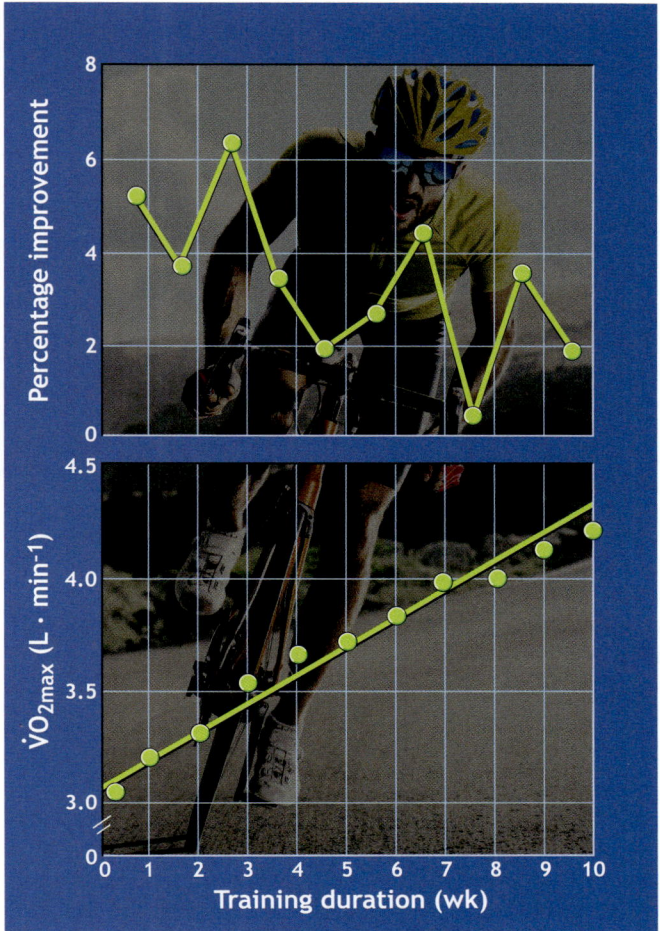

FIGURE 21.21. Continuous percentage improvements in maximum oxygen uptake ($\dot{V}O_{2max}$) during intense aerobic training for 10 wk.
(Reprinted with permission from Hickson RC, et al. Linear increases in aerobic power induced by a program of endurance exercise. *J Appl Physiol*. 1977;42:373. ©The American Physiological Society (APS). All rights reserved. Eugene Onischenko/Shutterstock.)

in cardiac output, 13.3% increase in stroke volume, and 2.7% decrease in peak heart rate. Resting plasma volume increased 8.1% during the 10 training days and correlated with the increased exercise cardiac output and stroke volume. All differences were statistically significant except for the a-$\bar{v}O_{2\,diff}$. This means that cardiovascular adaptations occur rapidly with short-term training in young males and females. The stroke volume increases during physical activity reflected the *combined effects* of increased left-ventricular end-diastolic dimension and increased systolic ejection.

A strenuous training program enhances a person's fitness level without regard to genetic background. The limits for developing fitness capacity appear to link closely to natural endowment. For two individuals in the same training program, one might show 10 times more improvement than the other. A genotype dependency exists for sensitivity in responding to maximum aerobic and anaerobic power training, including most muscle enzyme adaptations.[18,40,70] Stated succinctly, identical twins generally show a similar magnitude in training response.

Maximum Physiologic Responses During Peak Cycle Ergometry Before and After 10 Consecutive Days of Aerobic Training

Variable	Pre	Post	%Diff
$\dot{V}O_{2peak}$, L·min^{-1}	2.54±0.3	2.80±0.3	9.3%
Cardiac output, L·min^{-1}	18.3±1.3	20.5±1.7	10.7%
Heart rate, b·min^{-1}	189±2	184±2	−2.7%
Stroke volume, mL	97±7	112±9	13.3%
a-$\bar{v}O_2$ diff, mL·dL^{-1}	13.6±0.8	13.4±0.6	−1.5%
Plasma volume (rest), mL	2896±175	3152±220	8.1

a-$\bar{v}O_2$ diff, arterio-mixed venous oxygen difference; Diff, difference; $\dot{V}O_{2peak}$, peak oxygen uptake

All differences except a-$\bar{v}O_2$ diff were significant

From Mier CM, et al. Cardiovascular adaptations to 10 days of cycle exercise. *J Appl Physiol*. 1997;83:1900. ©The American Physiological Society (APS). All rights reserved. Photo: Andrii Vodolazhskyi/Shutterstock

days weekly. Both groups maintained their aerobic capacity gains despite a two thirds reduced training frequency.

Another study from the same laboratory evaluated reduced training duration's effect on the maintenance of improved aerobic fitness.[82] Upon completing the same protocol outlined previously for the initial 10 wk of training, subjects continued to maintain training intensity and frequency for an additional 15 wk, but at reduced training *duration* from the original 40-min sessions to either 26 or 13 min a day. Subjects maintained almost all $\dot{V}O_{2max}$ and performance increases despite a two-thirds reduction in training duration. Importantly, if training intensity decreased and frequency and duration remained constant, even a one-third reduction in training intensity reduced the $\dot{V}O_{2max}$.[83]

Aerobic capacity improvement involves different training requirements than its maintenance. *With intensity held constant, the exercise frequency and duration required to maintain a target aerobic fitness level remain lower than required to induce improvement.* In contrast, a small decline in exercise intensity reduces $\dot{V}O_{2max}$, indicating that training intensity plays the principal role to maintain the increased aerobic capacity achieved through training.

Fitness Components Other Than $\dot{V}O_{2max}$

Some fitness components are affected by reduced training volume. Well-trained endurance athletes who normally trained 6 to 10 hr weekly reduced weekly training to one 35-min session over a 4-wk period.[130] $\dot{V}O_{2max}$ remained constant during this time. Nevertheless, endurance capacity at 75% $\dot{V}O_{2max}$ *decreased*, which related to lowered

INTEGRATIVE QUESTION

What factors account for differences in individual responsiveness to the same training program?

FIGURE 21.22 shows a similar $\dot{V}O_{2max}$ training response (both mL·kg^{-1}·min^{-1} and % improvement) among 10 male identical twin pairs who participated in the same 20-wk aerobic training program. If one twin showed high responsiveness to training, a high likelihood existed that the other twin would also be a responder; similarly, a nonresponder to training generally showed little improvement as did his brother. Presence of the muscle-specific creatine kinase gene provides one example for the possible contribution of genetic makeup to individual differences in responsiveness of $\dot{V}O_{2max}$ to endurance training.[181,182]

Maintaining Aerobic Fitness Gains

An important question concerns the optimal exercise frequency, duration, and intensity to *maintain* aerobic improvements with training. In one study, healthy young adults increased $\dot{V}O_{2max}$ 25% by bicycle and run interval training for 40 min, 6 days a week for 10 wk.[81] They then joined one of two groups that continued to exercise an additional 15 wk at the same intensity and duration but at reduced *frequency* to either 4 or 2

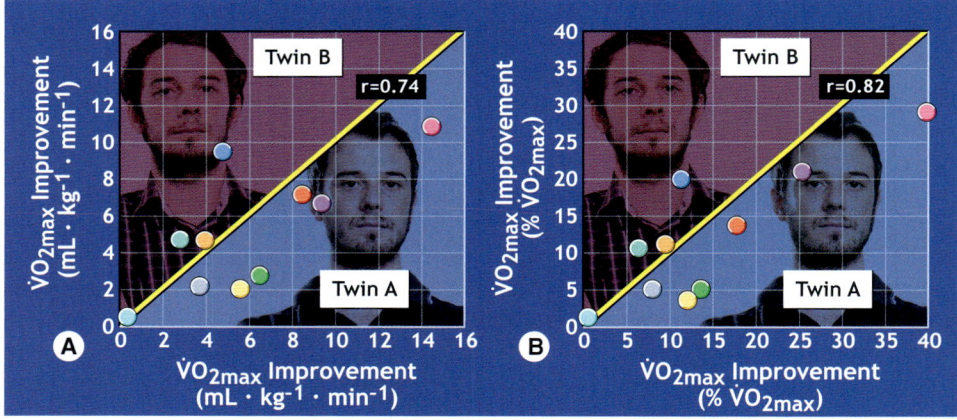

FIGURE 21.22. Maximum oxygen uptake ($\dot{V}O_{2max}$) responsiveness expressed in **(A)** mL·kg^{-1}·min^{-1} or **(B)** as % improvement in 10 identical twin pairs during a 20-wk aerobic exercise training program; *r* = Pearson product–moment correlation coefficient. The 10 colored data points represent a twin pair.
(Reprinted with permission from Bouchard C. Discussion: Heredity, fitness, and health. In: Bouchard C, et al., eds. *Exercise, Fitness, and Health: A Consensus of Current Knowledge* (p. 151). Champaign, IL: Human Kinetics, 1990. Photos: Alessandro de Leo/Shutterstock.)

pre-exercise glycogen stores and diminished lipid oxidation levels during exercise. A single fitness component such as $\dot{V}O_{2max}$ cannot adequately evaluate all of the additional factors that impact exercise training and detraining adaptations.

Tapering for Peak Performance

Little improvement occurs in the aerobic systems *during* the competitive season, as athletes strive to prevent physiologic and performance deterioration as the season progresses. Before major competitions, athletes often **taper** training intensity and/or volume believing that such adjustments minimize the physiologic and psychological stress of daily training and thus optimize competitive performance. The taper period and exact alterations in training vary by sport. A 1- to 3-wk taper that exponentially reduces training volume by 40 to 60%, while maintaining training intensity, provides the most efficient strategy to maximize performance gains.[17,218,219] A 4- to 7-day taper should have the following characteristics:

1. Achieve maximum muscle and liver glycogen replenishment
2. Optimize nutritional support and restoration
3. Alleviate residual muscle soreness
4. Heal minor injuries

In one study involving competitive runners, a 1-wk taper applied either no training (rest), low-intensity running (2 to 10 km daily at 60 $\dot{V}O_{2max}$) or high-intensity running while reducing training volume (five 500-m repeats on day 1, decreasing one repeat each day).[198] Measurements during the taper included blood volume, red blood cell mass, muscle glycogen content, muscle mitochondrial activity, and 1500-m race performance. Compared with rest and low-intensity exercise taper conditions, high-intensity taper produced the most benefit. An optimal taper should include progressively reduced training volume while maintaining training intensity at a moderate-to-high level. With proper tapering, expected performance improvement usually ranges between 0.5 and 6.0%.[148] Tapering does not produce substantial changes in exercise-induced oxidative stress.[225]

Training Methods

Performance improvements occur yearly in almost all athletic competitions, which generally relate to increased opportunities for participation. Individuals with "natural endowment" have opportunities to participate in different sports. Improved nutrition and healthcare, better equipment, and more systematic and scientific approaches to athletic training also bolster performance. The next sections cover general guidelines to effectively enhance the effects of anaerobic and aerobic exercise training.

Anaerobic Training

As previously shown in Figure 21.1, capacity to perform all-out exertion for up to 60 s largely depends on ATP generated by the immediate and short-term anaerobic systems for energy transfer.

Intramuscular High-Energy Phosphates

American football, weightlifting, and other brief sprint-power sport activities rely almost exclusively on energy derived from the intramuscular high-energy phosphates ATP and PCr. Engaging specific muscles in repeated 5- to 10-s maximum bursts of effort overloads the phosphagen pool's energy transfer contribution. Only minimal lactate accumulates, and recovery progresses rapidly. Activity can begin again after a brief 15- to 30-s rest period. Brief all-out exercise interspersed with recovery represents a form of highly specific interval training for anaerobic conditioning.

Physical activities that enhance ATP-PCr energy transfer capacity must engage the sport-specific muscles at the movement speed and power output similar to the sport itself. This strategy enhances the specifically trained muscle fiber's metabolic capacity and also facilitates recruitment and modulation of the neural firing sequence of the appropriate motor units activated in the particular movement.

Lactate-Generating Capacity

Consistent with the specificity principle, training must overload the short-term lactic acid energy system to improve this aspect of energy metabolism. Training the glycolytic energy system demands extreme physiologic and psychological effort. Blood lactate rises to near-peak levels with a 1-min maximum exercise bout. The individual repeats the same exercise bout after a 3- to 5-min recovery period. Repeating this sequence causes "**lactate stacking**," which produces a higher blood lactate level than just one all-out exhaustive effort. As with all training, one must activate the specific muscle groups that require enhanced anaerobic function. A backstroke swimmer trains by swimming the backstroke or using a swim-bench ergometer; a cyclist should bicycle; and basketball, hockey, or soccer players should perform various movement patterns involving movement intensity and directional changes specific to their sport.

Chapter 7 emphasized that the recovery interval requires more time when physical activity involves a large anaerobic component. Considerable recovery time occurs with intense physical activity that elevates core temperature, disrupts internal equilibrium, and elevates blood lactate. For this reason, anaerobic power training of the short-term energy system should occur at the end of the conditioning session so fatigue does not hinder ability to perform subsequent aerobic training.

Aerobic Training: Continuous Versus Intermittent Methods

FIGURE 21.23 illustrates two important factors in formulating aerobic training regimens:

1. Cardiovascular demands must reach an intensity to sufficiently overload stroke volume and cardiac output responses.
2. Cardiovascular overload must activate sport-specific muscle groups to enhance local circulation and the muscle's "metabolic machinery."

Well-planned endurance training overloads components of oxygen transport and use, which incorporates aerobic training's specificity principle. Simply stated, runners must run, cyclists must bicycle, rowers must row, and swimmers must swim. Relatively brief exercise bouts combined with continuous, long-duration exercise sessions will enhance aerobic capacity provided the activity attains sufficient intensity to overload the aerobic system. Interval training, **continuous training**, and **fartlek training** represent three common methods to improve aerobic fitness.

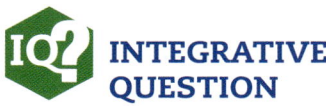

INTEGRATIVE QUESTION

What information would you need to design a program to effectively improve aerobic capacity for the specific physical job performance requirements for (1) firefighters, (2) police officers, and (3) oil field workers?

High-Intensity Interval Training

With optimal exercise-to-rest interval spacing, one can perform considerable intense activity, not normally possible if activity progressed continuously. Repeated intense exercise with brief rest periods or low-intensity relief intervals that typically vary from 2 to 3 s to several min or longer depending on the desired training outcome.[79,108,110,287-290] As few as six sessions of near all-out effort training (e.g., HIIT) over a 2-wk period increases skeletal muscle oxidative capacity and endurance performance.[59,286] The interval training prescription evolves from the following four considerations:

1. Interval intensity
2. Interval duration
3. Recovery duration
4. Exercise-to-relief repetitions

Consider the following example in performing intense physical activity during a workout. Few people can maintain a 4-min mile pace for longer than 1 min, let alone complete a mile in 4 min. Suppose running intervals were limited to only 10 s followed by a 30-s recovery. This scenario makes it reasonably easy to maintain the exercise-to-relief intervals and actually complete running at a 4-min mile pace. This does not parallel a world-class performance but illustrates that a person can accomplish a considerable amount of normally exhausting exercise given proper rest-to-exercise interval spacing. This intense training strategy interspersed with rest intervals would apply to treadmill, stair climbing, and bicycle ergometer workouts performed routinely in health clubs and training centers.

One-Minute Intense Exercise Improves Fitness and Health

Is the question really how much physical activity we need for improved health and fitness or rather how little is required? To answer the question, researchers studied several groups of sedentary but healthy middle-age males and females and middle-age and older patients with cardiovascular disease. Initial stationary bicycle testing quantified maximum heart rate and peak power output, which generally was relatively low. Participants then trained using repetitive HIIT. This routine involved 1-min exercise at about 90% maximum heart rate followed by 1-min easy recovery with 10 total exercise to rest intervals for a total workout duration of 20 min. Participants, particularly the cardiac patients, significantly improved overall health and cardiovascular fitness. The interesting finding was that all participants embraced the routine despite the fact that their perceived exertion ratings during each exercise bout was scored 7 or higher on a 10-point scale.[283] Previous HIIT research has demonstrated increases in cellular proteins involved in energy transfer via aerobic processes (mitochondrial biogenesis and an increased capacity for glucose and fatty acid oxidation), improved insulin sensitivity, and blood sugar regulation, which reduced type 2 diabetes risk.[287,288,289,290,291]

FIGURE 21.23. The two major aerobic training goals: **Goal 1**—develop central circulatory system's functional capacity to deliver oxygen. **Goal 2**—enhance targeted musculature to supply and process oxygen.

Interval Training Rationale. Interval training regimens have a sound basis in physiology and energy metabolism. In the continuous 4-min mile paced run example, anaerobic glycolysis supplies a large part of the energy requirement. Within a minute or two, the lactate level rises precipitously and the runner fatigues. For interval training, repeated 10-s exercise bouts allow the individual to complete the intense exercise without appreciable lactate buildup because the intramuscular high-energy phosphates provide the primary exercise energy source. Minimal fatigue develops during the predominantly short exercise intervals and recovery progresses rapidly (alactacid oxygen debt). The exercise interval can then begin following only a brief rest (**TABLE 21.4**).

In interval training, exercise intensity must activate the particular energy systems that require improvement. **TABLE 21.4** provides practical guidelines to determine the appropriate exercise and recovery intervals for running and swimming different distances.

TABLE 21.4 Guidelines for determining interval training exercise rates for running and swimming different distances

Consider the following four examples:

1. *Exercise interval*: Generally *add* 1.5 to 5.0 s to the exerciser's "best time" for training distances between 55 yd/50.3 m and 220 yd/201.2 m for running and 15 yd/13.7 m and 55 yd/50.3 m for swimming.[48] If a person can run 60 yd/54.9 m from a running start in 8 s, the training time for each repeat equals 8 + 1.5, or 9.5 s. For a 110-yd/100.6-m interval training distance, add 3 s, and for a 220-yd/201.2 m distance, add 5 s to the best running times. This interval training strategy is powered largely by the intramuscular ATP-PCr energy system.

2. *Training for 440-yd/402.3-m running or 110-yd/100.6-m swimming distances*: Determine the exercise intensity by *subtracting* 1 to 4 s from the best 440-yd/402.3-m part in a mile run or 110-yd/100.6-m part in a 440-yd/402.3-m swim. If a person runs a mile in 7 min (averaging 105 s per 440-yd/402.3-m), the interval time for each 440-yd/402.3-m repeat range is 104 s (105 − 1) to 101 s (105 − 4). For training intervals beyond 440 yd/402.3 m, *add* 3 to 4 s for each 440-yd/402.3-m interval distance. In running an 880-yd/804.6-m interval, the 7-min miler runs each interval at about 216 s [(105 + 3) × 2 = 216].

3. *Relief interval*: The relief interval is either passive (rest/relief) or active (work/relief). An exercise-to-recovery duration ratio usually determines relief interval duration. *The 1:3 ratio generally applies to training the immediate energy system.* For a sprinter who runs 10-s intervals, the relief interval equals about 30 s (3 × 10 s). For training the short-term glycolytic energy system, the relief interval averages twice the exercise interval, or a 1:2 ratio. The specific work-to-relief anaerobic training ratios should ensure sufficient restoration of intramuscular phosphates and/or sufficient lactate removal so the next exercise bout can continue with minimal fatigue.

4. *The optimal exercise-to-relief interval of 1:1 or 1:1.5 ratio usually is optimal to train the long-term aerobic energy system.* During a 60- to 90-s high-intensity exercise interval, oxygen uptake increases rapidly to a high level but remains inadequate to meet exercise energy requirements. The recommended relief interval causes the succeeding exercise interval to begin before complete return to baseline resting oxygen uptake. This ensures that cardiovascular and aerobic metabolic stress attains near peak levels with repeated but relatively short exercise intervals. The rest interval's duration takes on less importance with longer intermittent exercise intervals because sufficient time exists for the body to adjust metabolic and circulatory parameters during the activity.

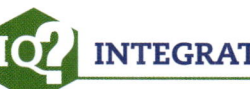

INTEGRATIVE QUESTION

How would you respond to a coach who insists that a single activity mode improves aerobic capacity for all physical activities requiring a high aerobic fitness level?

Sprint-Type Interval Training Impacts Anaerobic and Aerobic Systems. Relatively brief but intense sprint-type interval training increases both anaerobic and aerobic metabolic capacity. For example, a 7-wk training program with 12 young adult men consisted of 30 s of maximum sprint effort (Wingate protocol) interspersed with 2 to 4 min of recovery performed three times a wk.[291] Week 1 began with four exercise intervals and 4 min of recovery per interval and progressed to 10 exercise intervals with a 2.5-min recovery per exercise bout by wk 7. With this relatively brief training stimulus in which exercise duration reached only 5 min per session during wk 7, improvements occurred in $\dot{V}O_{2max}$, short-term power output, and maximum activity of key marker enzymes of aerobic and anaerobic energy pathways. Healthy elderly persons showed positive clinical and cardiovascular adaptations to interval training.[3] HIIT in mice altered cardiac substrate utilization (36% increase in glucose oxidation and associated reduced fatty acid oxidation), improved cardiac efficiency by decreasing work-independent myocardial oxygen uptake, and increased cardiac maximum mitochondrial respiratory capacity. No such changes were observed for animals involved in distance-matched more moderate-intensity training.[68]

Fartlek Training

Fartlek, meaning "speed play" in Swedish, is a training method developed in 1937 by Gösta Holmér (1891–1983 www.newintervaltraining.com/fartlek-training.php), the Swedish

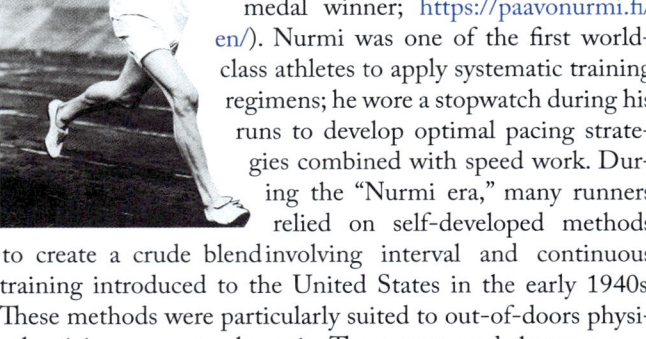

national track coach. Holmér modeled his training system after the training patterns of "The Flying Finn," Paavo Nurmi (1897–1973), perhaps the greatest runner of all time (Finnish world champion and multiple Olympic gold medal winner; https://paavonurmi.fi/en/). Nurmi was one of the first world-class athletes to apply systematic training regimens; he wore a stopwatch during his runs to develop optimal pacing strategies combined with speed work. During the "Nurmi era," many runners relied on self-developed methods to create a crude blend involving interval and continuous training introduced to the United States in the early 1940s. These methods were particularly suited to out-of-doors physical activity over natural terrain. The system used alternate running at fast and slow speeds over both level and hilly landscapes.

Fartlek training workouts do not require systematically manipulating the exercise to relief intervals as prescribed in interval training. In fartlek training, the performer determines the training schema based on "how it feels" at the time, in a way similar to gauging physical activity intensity based on perceived exertion ratings. This training method can overload one or all of the energy-transfer systems. It is ideal, however, for general conditioning and off-season training but lacks the systematic, quantified approaches applied in interval and continuous training.

Continuous Training

Continuous or **long slow distance training** involves steady-paced, prolonged activity at either moderate or high aerobic intensity performed between 60 and 80% $\dot{V}O_{2max}$. The exact pace can vary, but it must minimally meet a threshold intensity to ensure aerobic physiologic adaptations. Previously, we outlined the method to establish the training-sensitive zone that uses HR_{max} (see "Determining the 'Training-Sensitive Zone,'" earlier in this chapter). Continuous training that exceeds 1-hr duration has become popular among fitness enthusiasts, competitive triathletes, and cross-country skiers. Many elite distance runners train twice daily and train by running 100 to 150 mi weekly to prepare for competition.

Continuous submaximum exercise training progresses in relative comfort. This contrasts with the potential intense interval training hazards for coronary-prone individuals and high motivation level required for such vigorous effort. Continuous training ideally suits novices wishing to accumulate a large caloric expenditure, which is an ideal strategy for weight loss. When applied to athletic training, continuous training truly represents "overdistance" training, with most competitors training two to five times the actual distances of their events.

Continuous training allows endurance athletes to participate at nearly the same intensity as actual competition. Specific motor unit recruitment depends on exercise intensity, making this training method desirable for fostering adaptations at the pace-specific cellular level, an important consideration for serious endurance athletes. In contrast, interval training often places disproportionate stress on fast-twitch motor units, not slow-twitch units predominantly recruited in endurance competition.

The Best Training Method?

Little scientific evidence supports proclaiming superiority in any specific training method to improve aerobic capacity and associated physiologic variables, as each training method produces some success with much individual variability and specificity.[144] The various training methods probably can be interchanged, particularly when modifying the training strategy to achieve a diverse and more psychologically acceptable conditioning approach.

fyi Typical Aerobic Training Session

The inset figure illustrates a typical aerobic training session for a 50-year-old female. The sessions begins with a 5- to 10-min warm-up of light to moderate walking or jogging in place. This continues with the conditioning phase (30 to 60 min) with a 70 to 85% of the age-predicted HR_{max}. A 5- to 10-min cool-down of light to moderate-intensity exercise follows as heart rate exponentially declines toward the resting level.

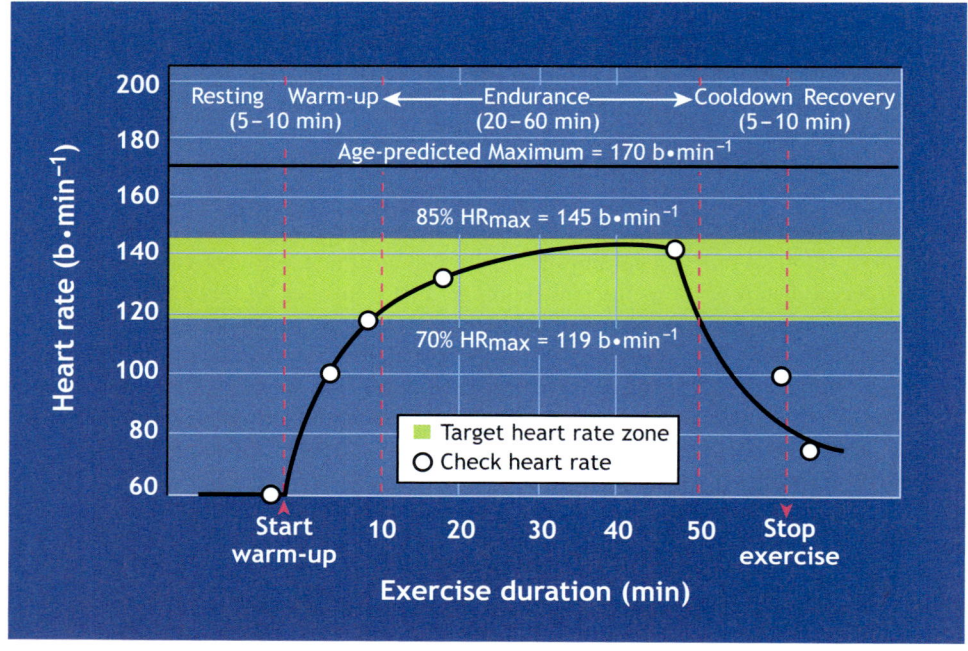

Overtraining Considerations

Ten to twenty percent of athletes experience overtraining or "staleness." The overtrained syndrome represents more than short-term inability to train hard or a slight dip in competition-level performance. Athletes can fail to endure and adapt to training so that normal performance deteriorates, and they encounter increasing difficulty fully recovering following workouts.[23,204,222] Elite athletes cannot afford performance decrements of even 1 to 3%, as this relatively small decrement can prevent a gold medalist from qualifying for competition. Overtraining also relates to increased infection incidence, persistent muscle soreness, general malaise, and lost interest in sustaining high-level training. Injuries also occur more frequently in the overtrained state, so even minor physical setbacks can play havoc in having to deal with the rehabilitation efforts.[223]

There are two clinical overtraining forms:

1. The less common **sympathetic form** (*basedowian* for thyroid hyperfunction patterns), characterized by increased sympathetic activity during rest and generally typified by hyperexcitability, restlessness, and impaired exercise performance. This overtraining form may reflect excessive psychological/emotional stressors that accompany the interaction among training, competition, and normal living responsibilities.[113]
2. The more common **parasympathetic form** (*addisonoid* for adrenal insufficiency patterns), characterized by vagal activity predominance during rest and physical activity. More properly termed **overreaching** in the early stages within as few as 10 days, the syndrome qualitatively is similar in symptoms to the full-blown parasympathetic **overtraining syndrome** but of shorter duration. Excessive and protracted physical overload with inadequate recovery and rest leads to overreaching. Initially, maintaining exercise performance requires greater effort, which eventually leads to performance decrements and deterioration in training quality and competitive performance. Instituting rest intervals for a few days to several weeks usually restores full function. Without appropriate intervention, untreated overreaching eventually leads to the overtraining syndrome.

Parasympathetic overtraining syndrome includes chronic fatigue during workouts and recovery. Associated symptoms include sustained poor exercise performance, disrupted sleep patterns, poor appetite, frequent infections, persistent fatigue, altered immune and reproductive functions, acute and chronic alterations in systemic inflammatory responses, and mood changes that can lead to anger, depression, and anxiety. **FIGURE 21.24** illustrates possible interactive factors that initiate the parasympathetic-type overtraining syndrome. Interactions among chronic neuromuscular, neuroendocrine, psychological, immunologic, and metabolic overload during long-term, high-volume training with insufficient recuperation eventually alter physiologic function and the stress response to produce the overtrained state.[71,128,184] Pre-existing medical conditions; inadequate carbohydrate or dehydration; environmental hot/cold stress, humidity, and altitude; and psychosocial pressures (e.g., monotonous training, frequent competition, personal conflicts) often exacerbate training demands and increase the risk for developing overtraining syndrome.

Significant effects of a chronic imbalance in training load, competition stress, and nontraining stress factors in overtraining include the following:

1. Functional impairments in the hypothalamo-pituitary-gonadal and adrenal axes and sympathetic neuroendocrine system reflected by depressed urinary norepinephrine excretion and β_2-adrenergic system desensitization[51,113,217]
2. Exercise-induced increases in adrenocorticotropic hormone and growth hormone and decreases in cortisol and insulin levels[222]

In some ways, the syndrome reflects the body's attempt to provide the athlete with an appropriate recuperative period from intense training and competition. The eight most common overtraining syndrome indicators include the following:

1. Unexplained and persistently poor performance and high fatigue ratings
2. Prolonged recovery from typical training sessions or competitive events
3. Disturbed mood states characterized by general fatigue, apathy, depression, irritability, and competitive drive deterioration
4. Persistent soreness and stiffness in muscles and joints
5. Elevated resting pulse and increased susceptibility to upper respiratory tract infections (altered immune function) and gastrointestinal disturbances
6. Insomnia
7. Appetite loss, weight loss, and inability to maintain proper body weight for competition
8. Overuse injuries

No simple method diagnoses overtraining in its earliest stages.[53,74] The best indications include physical performance deterioration, mood alterations, a relatively high cortisol/cortisone ratio, and possibly decreased nocturnal HRV.[8,164,197] Conditions that cause some athletes to thrive during intense training initiate an overtraining response in others. Generally, rest relieves the symptoms; if not, symptoms can persist to thwart complete recovery that often requires weeks or months. No reliable strategy can determine the point of complete recovery from the syndrome, but most athletes intuitively seem to know when they can successfully return to competition.

Coaches must allow adequate recuperation during the most intense training cycles or when an athlete attempts to regain peak form following a protracted layoff. Nutrition becomes important during intense training; special emphasis placed on glycogen replenishment, which requires sufficient recovery time, plus high levels of dietary carbohydrate and rehydration reduce symptoms. Nevertheless, nutrition alone cannot prevent the syndrome's progression.[1,175,200]

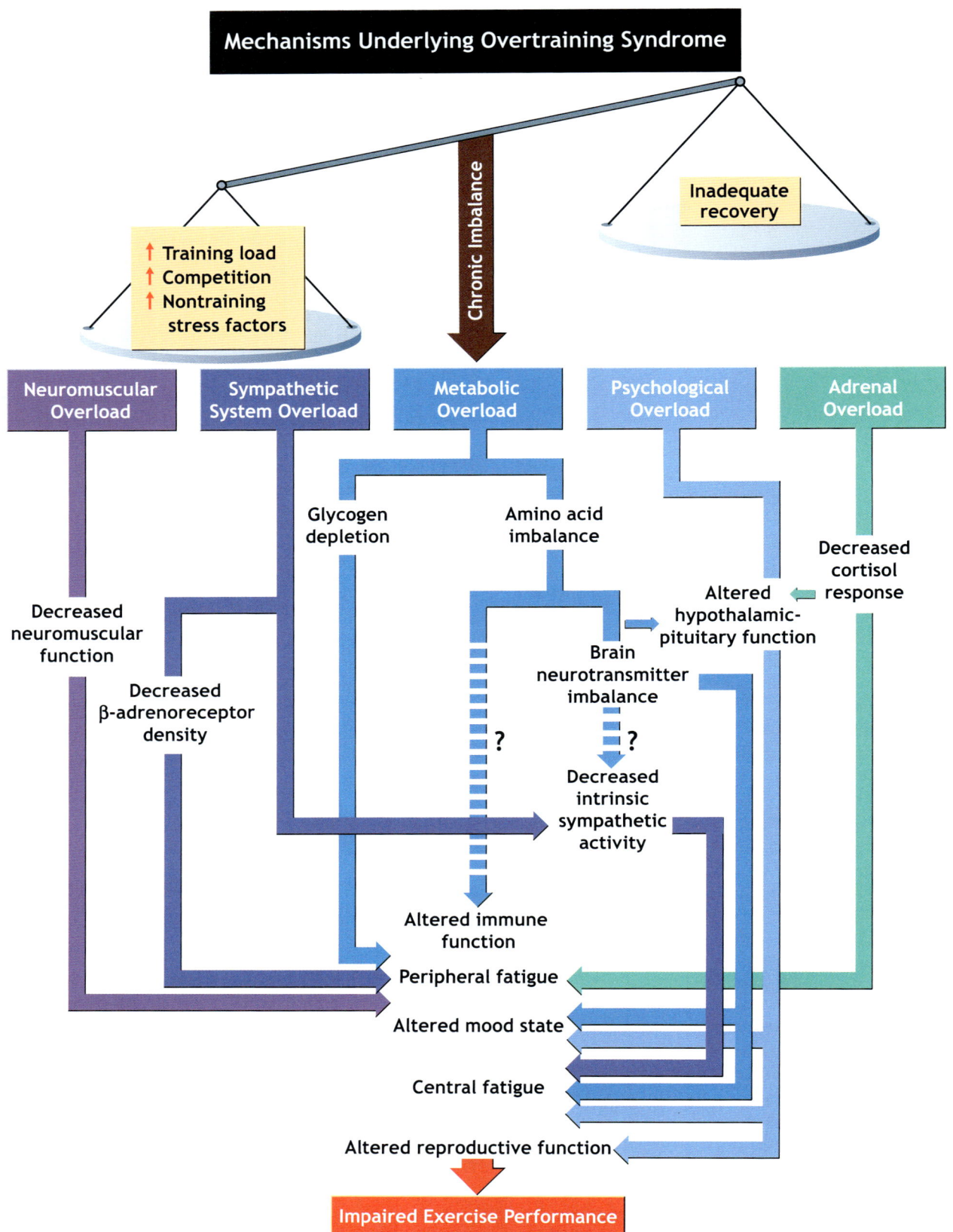

FIGURE 21.24. Schematic overview for developing the overtraining syndrome in endurance sports requiring prolonged high-volume training.
(Adapted with permission from Lehmann M, et al. Autonomic imbalance hypothesis and overtraining syndrome. *Med Sci Sports Exerc.* 1998;30:1140.)

Physical Activity and Exercise Training During Pregnancy

Forty percent or more of women in the United States participate in different physical activities during pregnancy.[77,239] **FIGURE 21.25** illustrates the prevalence and pattern for different activities among pregnant and nonpregnant women. Nonpregnant women are more likely than pregnant women to meet the moderate or vigorous physical activity recommendations. For both groups, walking represented the most common activity (52% for pregnant and 45% for nonpregnant). Pregnant women who engage in either moderate or vigorous physical activity were generally younger, non-Hispanic white, unmarried, more educated, nonsmokers, and had higher incomes than less physically active counterparts.

Maternal Effects

Maternal cardiovascular dynamics follow normal response patterns; moderate physical activity offers no greater physiologic stress to the mother other than the additional weight gain and possible fetal tissue encumbrance. Regular physical activity during pregnancy can reduce maternal weight gain by an average 3.1 kg/6.8 lb compared to relatively sedentary women.[105]

Pregnant women showed similar capacity as postpartum women to cycle for 40 min at 70 to 75% $\dot{V}O_{2max}$. The physiologic responses to this weight-supported activity remained uninfluenced by gestation.[122] Pregnancy does not compromise the absolute aerobic capacity value $(L \cdot min^{-1})$.[123] The increase in maternal body mass and changes in coordination and balance as pregnancy progresses adversely affect movement economy, which adds to the effort in weight-bearing activity. Pregnancy, particularly in the last trimester, also increases pulmonary ventilation at a given submaximum intensity level.[122] The direct stimulating effects of progesterone and increased chemoreceptor sensitivity to carbon dioxide contribute to maternal exercise "hyperventilation."[237] Regular, moderate activity during the second and third trimesters reduces submaximum ventilatory demands and RPE.[154] These training adaptations increase the mother's ventilatory reserve and possibly inhibit exertional dyspnea. The most important maternal metabolic and cardiorespiratory adaptations during pregnancy include the following:

- Blood volume increases 40 to 50%, and hemodilution reduces Hb concentration
- Increase in blood volume dilates the left ventricle
- Slight increase in oxygen uptake during rest and submaximum weight-supported exercise (e.g., stationary cycling)
- Substantial increase in oxygen uptake during weight-bearing exercise (e.g., walking and running)
- Increased heart rate during rest and submaximum exercise
- No change in $\dot{V}O_{2max}$ $(L \cdot min^{-1})$
- Increased ventilatory response—largely progesterone mediated during rest and submaximum exercise
- Possible magnified hypoglycemic response during exercise, especially late in pregnancy
- Possible depressed sympathetic nervous system response to exercise in late gestation

Fetal Effects

Performing physical activity during pregnancy requires adherence to prudent guidelines and recommendations.[5] Epidemiologic evidence indicates that exercise during pregnancy does not increase fetal death risk or induce low birth weights and may reduce preterm birth risk.[94,155,174,194] A moderate program of weight-bearing exercise or recreational activity early in pregnancy through to term enhances fetoplacental growth and reduces pre-eclampsia risk.[30,187] A study of middle-class women evaluated the effects of daily low-to-moderate physical activity (≤ 1000 kcal $\cdot wk^{-1}$), more intense activity (≥ 1000 kcal $\cdot wk^{-1}$), or no physical activity on timely delivery and the safety and potential benefits of regular activity during pregnancy.[77,239] No association emerged between low-to-moderate physical activity and gestation length. A positive finding indicated that higher volume weekly activity lowered rather than raised preterm birth risk. Among births after the projected term, women who performed more intense physical activity had faster deliveries than non exercisers.

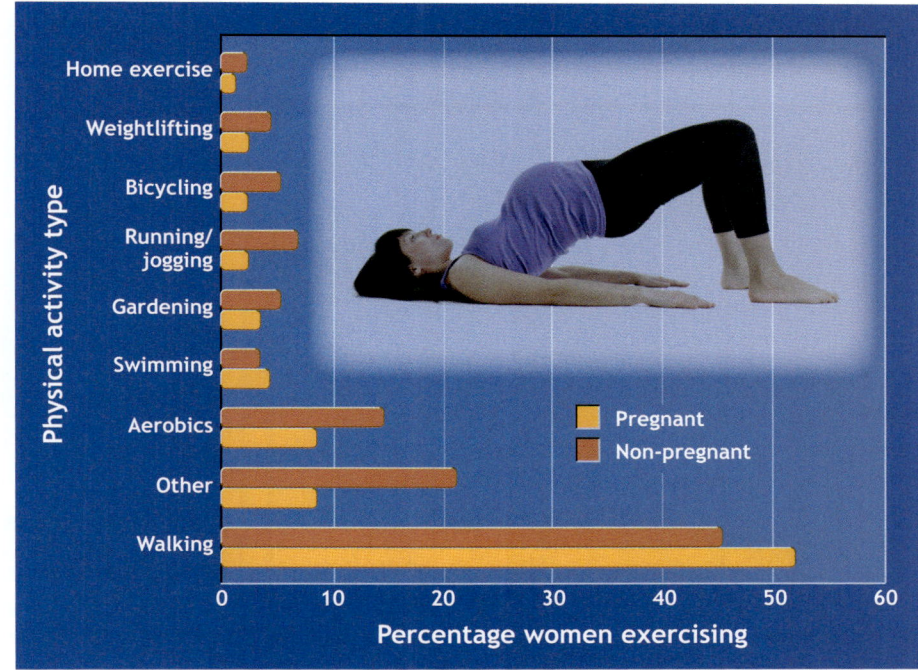

FIGURE 21.25. Common physical activities during pregnancy and nonpregnant controls in combined data from 1994, 1996, 1998, to 2000. (Reprinted with permission from Petersen AM, et al. Correlates of physical activity among pregnant women in the United States. *Med Sci Sports Exerc.* 2005;37:1748.)

The World Health Organization 2020 Physical Activity and Sedentary Behavior Guidelines

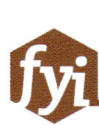
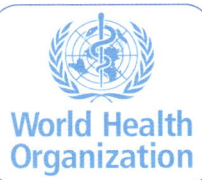

S_E/Shutterstock

The 2020 World Health Organization (WHO) guidelines on physical activity and sedentary behavior updates recommendations about physical activity for various age groups, pregnant and postpartum women, and people living with chronic conditions or disabilities. For the first time, the WHO guidelines modify recommendations for how aerobic physical activity should be accumulated. The previous requirement for a 10-min minimum continuous duration activity has been replaced by "some physical activity is better than none" recommendation. The new guidelines also recommend reducing sitting time to counter the deleterious but adverse sedentary behavior on overall health. The prior WHO physical activity guidelines focused on continuous vigorous aerobic exercise mainly for performance improvement or cardiac rehabilitation, while the new guidelines are more public health focused, shifting from exercise to physical activity as an essential component of daily living. An emphasis on doing any amount of physical activity aims to empower formerly inactive individuals to now reap the benefits of engaging in physical activities, even when the recommended target range is perceived to be out of reach (e.g., 75 to 150 min weekly vigorous-intensity activity or 150 to 300 min a week moderate-intensity physical activity). This new public health focus is particularly relevant to all situations, which impose additional barriers to increasing one's physical activity level.

Source:
Ding D, et al. Physical activity guidelines 2020: comprehensive and inclusive recommendations to activate populations. *Lancet.* 2020;396:1780.

Three potential risks of intense maternal exercise can alter fetal growth and development:

1. Reduced placental blood flow and accompanying fetal hypoxia
2. Fetal hyperthermia
3. Reduced fetal glucose supply

Any factor that might temporarily compromise fetal blood supply raises concern in counseling pregnant women regarding physical activity. Neonates born to physically active mothers exhibit a neurobehavioral profile as early as the 5th day after birth, earlier than neonates from more sedentary counterparts.[29] Active mothers either ran, performed aerobics, swam, or used stair-climbing activities at least three times weekly for at least 20 min at or above 55% aerobic capacity. The women in the control group led active lives that did not include regular, sustained physical activity.

FIGURE 21.26 shows data for five behavioral clusters of the Brazelton Neonatal Assessment Scales (www.brazeltontouchpoints.org/offerings/nbo-and-nbas/) of the offspring of 34 women who exercised regularly and 31 sedentary women who did not exercise. No significant differences emerged between neonates born to physically active women and sedentary controls for clusters of factors to assess motor organization, autonomic stability, and range of state behaviors. Neonates born to physically active women scored higher in orientation behavior and ability to regulate their behaviors (i.e., more alert and interested in their surroundings and less demanding of their mothers). The inset table indicates that axial length and head circumference remained similar between groups, with the offspring of the active women lighter and leaner than the control group offspring. The findings showed that continuing regular physical activity throughout pregnancy modifies neonatal behavior by positively impacting early neurodevelopment.

Current Opinion

Conservative, prudent recommendations apply during a normal pregnancy despite extreme physical activity examples for well-trained women without an apparent negative impact on maternal or fetal health.[10,95,129] Daily moderate aerobic activity for 30 to 40 min for a previously active, healthy, low-risk woman during an uncomplicated pregnancy does not compromise fetal oxygen supply or acid-base status, induce heart rate signs of fetal distress, or produce other adverse

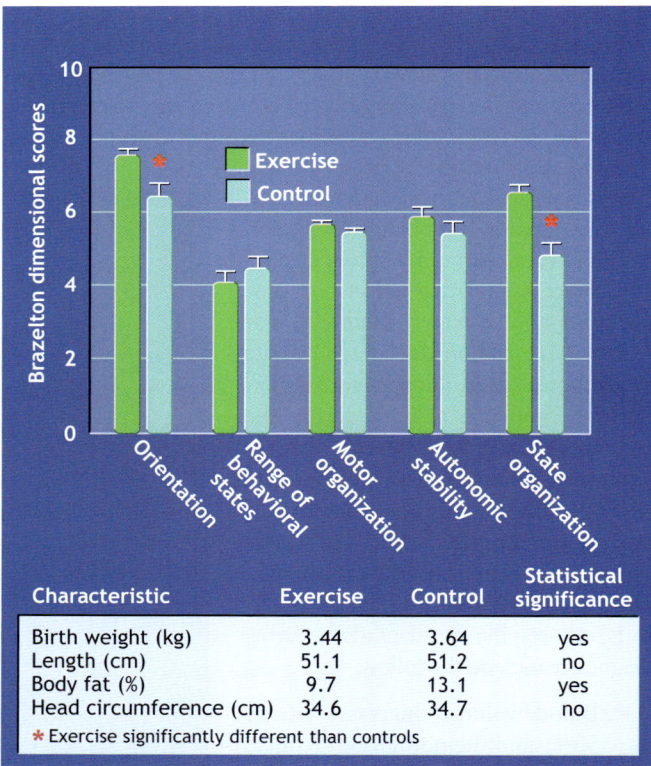

Characteristic	Exercise	Control	Statistical significance
Birth weight (kg)	3.44	3.64	yes
Length (cm)	51.1	51.2	no
Body fat (%)	9.7	13.1	yes
Head circumference (cm)	34.6	34.7	no

* Exercise significantly different than controls

FIGURE 21.26. Behavioral neonate constellation scores in exercise and nonexercise control groups on the Brazelton Neonatal Behavioral Assessment Scales. *Red asterisks* indicate statistical significance ($P = .01$ level). Insert table presents neonatal morphometric values.
(Reprinted with permission from Clapp JF III, et al. Neonatal behavioral profile of the offspring of women who continue to exercise regularly throughout pregnancy. *Am J Obstet Gynecol.* 1999;180:91.)

In a Practical Sense

Exercise Prescription During Pregnancy

Pregnancy alters normal physiology, necessitating some modification in the exercise prescription. During pregnancy, women should consult their physician before initiating a physical activity program or modifying an existing program to rule out possible complications. This pertains particularly to women of low fitness status and little exercise experience prior to pregnancy. Physical activity during pregnancy should heighten awareness about heat dissipation, adequate caloric and nutrient intake, and knowing when to reduce exercise intensity. For a normal, uncomplicated pregnancy, light-to-moderate activity does not affect fetal development negatively, and the exercise benefits generally outweigh the potential risks.

lunamarina/Shutterstock

PHYSICAL ACTIVITY GUIDELINES

Activity mode: Avoid exercise in the supine position, particularly after the first trimester. Supine exercise impairs venous return (mass of the fetus compresses inferior vena cava), which could affect cardiac output and uterine blood flow. Non–weight-bearing activity (e.g., cycling, swimming) minimizes the gravity effect and the added weight effect associated with fetal development. Low-impact, weight-bearing activity in moderation should not pose a risk.

Activity frequency: Exercise 3 days a week, emphasizing continuous, steady-rate effort. Reduce the intensity of more frequent activities.

Activity duration: Exercise 30 to 40 min, depending on how the person feels.

Activity intensity: Pregnancy alters the relationship between heart rate and oxygen uptake, making it difficult to establish guidelines from heart rate. An effective alternative establishes exercise intensity based on the RPE, which should range between 11 ("fairly light") and 13 ("somewhat hard").

Rate of progression: Moderate aerobic activity maintains cardiovascular fitness and often produces a small training effect. Most women should not strive to induce a training effect, but rather maintain cardiorespiratory fitness, muscle mass, and physician-recommended weight gain. The combined effects of pregnancy *per se* and regular physical activity often produce improved fitness following delivery.

WHEN TO STOP EXERCISE AND SEEK MEDICAL ADVICE

Discontinue exercise immediately under the following conditions:

- Any vaginal bleeding
- Any gush of fluid from the vagina (premature rupture of membranes)
- Sudden swelling in the ankles, hands, or face
- Persistent, severe headaches and/or disturbances in vision; unexplained lightheadedness or dizziness
- Elevated pulse rate or blood pressure that does not rapidly return to normal following exercise
- Excessive fatigue, palpitations, or chest pain
- Persistent uterine contractions (more than 6 to 8 an hour)
- Unexplained or unusual abdominal pain
- Insufficient weight gain (<1.0 kg/2.2 lb a month during the last two trimesters)

Contraindications to physical activity:

- Pregnancy-induced hypertension
- History of two or more spontaneous abortions
- Preterm rupture of membranes
- Preterm labor during the prior or current pregnancy
- Incompetent cervix
- Excessive alcohol intake
- Persistent second to third trimester bleeding
- History of premature labor
- Intrauterine growth retardation
- Anemia
- Type 1 diabetes
- Significant obesity
- Multiple pregnancy
- Smoking

Sources:
American Pregnancy Association. Available at: https://americanpregnancy.org/health-fitness/exercise-guidelines/
Davies GAL, et al. Exercise in pregnancy and the postpartum period. *Obstet Gynaecol Can*. 2018;40:e58.
Gregg VH, Ferguson JE II. Exercise in pregnancy. *Clin Sports Med*. 2017;36:741

---

effects to mother or fetus.[2,37,121,146,205] Physical activity performed on a regular basis maintains cardiovascular fitness, promotes a training effect, and inhibits undesirable excessive weight gain for the mother, and is associated with resting fetal heart rate effects similar to a trained response.[54,133,163,166,171,172,186] Four other positive maternal effects include the following:

1. Shorter labor and delivery times
2. Faster recovery following delivery
3. Decreased pregnancy discomforts
4. Fewer pregnancy complications

Hormonal action via the sympathetic nervous system during strenuous effort probably directs some blood from the uterus and visceral organs for preferential distribution to active muscles. This could pose a hazard to a fetus with restricted placental blood flow. In a Practical Sense: Exercise Prescription During Pregnancy presents guidelines to formulate an exercise prescription during pregnancy. This prudent approach dictates that a pregnant woman (in consultation with her healthcare provider) should exercise in moderation, especially for a compromised pregnancy. Physical activity late in pregnancy can magnify the normal maternal hypoglycemic response by increasing glucose uptake by maternal skeletal muscle; in the extreme, this response could adversely affect fetal glucose supply.[15,28]

During pregnancy, women should avoid supine exercise, contact sports, high-altitude exertion, hot tub immersion, and scuba diving. A decrease in uterine blood flow or elevated maternal core temperature with extended-duration activity during environmental heat stress can compromise heat dissipation from the fetus through the placenta.[136] Hyperthermia negatively affects fetal development (e.g., increased neural tube defect risk), particularly in the first trimester, so women should exercise during warm weather in the cool part of the day for shorter intervals while maintaining regular fluid intake.[140] Within this framework, aquatic exercise serves as an ideal venue for maternal physical activity.

Current fitness level and previous physical activity patterns should guide a woman's exercise behavior throughout an uncomplicated pregnancy and postpartum. Regular aerobic activity during pregnancy plays an important role to maintain functional capacity and general well-being. It also optimizes overall weight gain during the later pregnancy stages[28] and may reduce Cesarean delivery risk in women who have never borne children.[24] Controversy remains about whether extremes in physical effort benefit either mother or fetus or whether physical activity during pregnancy benefits labor, delivery, birth weight, and general outcome.[14,167] Beginning a 6- to 8-wk regular exercise program postpartum produces no deleterious effect on lactation volume or composition and improves aerobic fitness without impairing immune function.[37,121,125] Fitness and strength declines in the early postpartum period relative to prepregnancy performance generally return by 27 wk following delivery.[220] Combining moderate physical activity with a 500-kcal reduced daily energy intake allows overweight lactating women to safely lose 0.5 kg/1.1 lb weekly without adversely affecting infant growth.[124]

Summary

1. Specific physical activities are generally classified by their specific energy transfer system requirements.
2. An effective conditioning program trains the appropriate energy system(s) to improve a desired physiologic function or performance goal.
3. Physical conditioning based on sound principles optimizes improvements.
4. The four primary training principles include overload, specificity, individual differences, and reversibility.
5. Exercise training promotes specific cellular adaptations and targeted physiologic changes to enhance functional capacity and physical performance.
6. Anaerobic training increases resting levels of intramuscular anaerobic substrates and key glycolytic enzyme levels with accompanying improvements in short-duration maximum exercise performance.
7. Aerobic training adaptations enhance aerobic ATP production by increasing mitochondrial size and number, aerobic enzymes, muscle capillarization, and lipid and carbohydrate oxidation.
8. A linear relationship exists between heart rate and oxygen uptake from light to moderately intense physical activity in trained and untrained individuals.
9. Improved stroke volume with aerobic training shifts the heart rate-oxygen uptake line to the right to decrease heart rate at any submaximum exercise intensity level.
10. Aerobic training induces functional and dimensional changes in the cardiovascular system by decreasing resting and submaximum exercise heart rate, enhancing stroke volume and cardiac output, and expanding the a-$\bar{v}O_2$ differences.
11. Cardiac hypertrophy represents a fundamental biologic adaptation to increased myocardial workload imposed by training, chiefly by increasing left-ventricular volume and an enhanced stroke volume.
12. Structural and dimensional changes in the left ventricle vary with training modes without harm to normal cardiac function.
13. Exercise intensity is the most crucial factor affecting the magnitude of training improvements; other factors include initial fitness level, training frequency, exercise duration, and training mode.
14. Training intensity can be applied on either an absolute basis for exercise load or relative to a person's physiologic response.
15. Percentage HR_{max} serves as the most practical approach to establish exercise training intensity.
16. Training levels between 60 and 90% HR_{max} induce meaningful changes in aerobic fitness.
17. Training duration and intensity interact to affect the training response; extending duration compensates for reduced intensity.
18. Generally, 30-min exercise sessions are effective for producing an aerobic training response.
19. Two to three days a week represents the minimum aerobic training frequency, but no optimal training frequency has been established.
20. Similar aerobic improvements occur when intensity, duration, and frequency remain constant, regardless of activity mode when training involves large muscle groups, and the evaluation process remains mode specific.
21. The training frequency and duration required to maintain improved aerobic fitness are lower than the frequency and duration required to improve it.
22. Interval, continuous, and fartlek training improve the capacity of different energy transfer systems.
23. Interval training most effectively improves the immediate and short-term anaerobic energy systems.
24. Aerobic training must overload both cardiovascular function and the specific muscles' metabolic capacity.
25. Peripheral adaptations in trained muscle profoundly enhance endurance performance.
26. Prolonged and intense endurance training can precipitate the overtraining syndrome with associated alterations in neuroendocrine and immune system functions.

27. The overtraining syndrome includes chronic fatigue, poor exercise performance, frequent infections, and general loss of interest in training until the athlete stops training for several days to months.
28. Approximately 40% of American women exercise during pregnancy, with walking the most popular (42%), followed by swimming (12%) and aerobics (12%).
29. The most serious potential physical activity risks during pregnancy include reduced placental blood flow and accompanying fetal hypoxia, fetal hyperthermia, and reduced fetal glucose supply.
30. For previously active, healthy women, moderate aerobic activity does not compromise fetal oxygen supply.

Key Terms

Aerobic system enzymes: Enzymes that catalyze the biochemical reactions in aerobic adenosine triphosphate synthesis (e.g., citric acid cycle and electron transport chain)

Athlete's heart: Increased cardiac output during training causes morphological, functional, and cardiac chamber modifications

Concentric cardiac hypertrophy: Modest left ventricular wall thickening from adding new sarcomeres without overall heart enlargement

Continuous training: Physical training involving steady-paced prolonged activity at moderate to high intensity

Conversational exercise: Moderate-intensity physical activity performed without discomfort to achieve sufficient duration and intensity to stimulate a training effect while conducting a conversation

Detraining: Loss of training benefits that occurs rapidly when a person terminates participation in regular physical activity

Eccentric cardiac hypertrophy: Cardiac enlargement characterized by increased left ventricular cavity size; generally related to volume overload

Exercise training specificity: Training principle that incorporates intensity, duration, frequency, and overload to create beneficial adaptations in metabolic and physiologic functions; highly related to specific training mode

Fartlek training: Training type that blends interval and continuous training applicable to outdoor exercise over natural terrain without manipulating exercise or relief intervals

Heart rate reserve (HRR): Exercise training method requiring individuals to exercise at a heart rate at least equal to 60% of the difference between resting and maximum

Heart rate variability (HRV): Variation in time between each heartbeat (R–R interval); used to assess autonomic nervous system heart rate control

High-intensity interval training (HIIT): Enhanced interval training method that alternates short intense anaerobic exercise bouts with less-intense aerobic exercise recovery periods

Individual difference principle: States that all individuals do not respond similarly to a given training stimulus but show variation influenced by age, genetics, and initial fitness level

Lactate stacking: A phenomenon in which blood lactate rises to near-peak levels with a 1-min maximum exercise bout repeated multiple times after 3 to 5 min of recovery

Long slow distance training: Continuous exercise training involving steady-rate activity over extended distances or durations between 60 and 80% of maximum oxygen uptake

Morganroth hypothesis: A theory stating that cardiac output during exercise causes morphological, functional, and electrical cardiac chamber modifications with modest cardiac hypertrophy from myocardial cell enlargement

Overload: Exercising at intensities greater than normal by manipulating training frequency, intensity, and duration, or their combination

Overreaching: Early stages in the overtraining syndrome, occurring within 10 days

Overtraining syndrome: Excessive and protracted physical overload with inadequate recovery produces chronic fatigue, sustained poor exercise performance, altered sleep patterns and appetite, frequent infections, altered immune and reproductive functions, mood disturbances and general malaise, and poor ability for high-level training

Parasympathetic form: Most common overtraining form, characterized predominantly by increased vagal activity during rest and exercise

Rating of perceived exertion (RPE): Scaling method to access an individual's perception of effort

Responders: Individuals with high responsiveness to a training stimulus

Specific adaptations to imposed demands (SAIDs) principle: States that specific exercise elicits specific adaptations to promote specific training effects with highly specific performance improvements

Sympathetic form: Less common overtraining state characterized by increased sympathetic activity during rest, general hyperexcitability, restlessness, and impaired exercise performance

Taper: One to three weeks of reduced training intensity and/or volume prior to competition to minimize the daily physiologic and psychological training stress

References are available online at Lippincott Connect.

Additional References

Adami PE, et al. Physiological profile comparison between high intensity functional training, endurance and power athletes. *Eur J Appl Physiol*. 2022;122:531.

Appel M, et al. Effects of genetic variation on endurance performance, muscle strength, and injury susceptibility in sports: a systematic review. *Front Physiol.* 2021;12:694411.

Boullosa D, et al. Effects of short sprint interval training on aerobic and anaerobic indices: a systematic review and meta-analysis. *Scand J Med Sci Sports.* 2022. doi:10.1111/sms.14133.

Brooks GA, et al. The blood lactate/pyruvate equilibrium affair. *Am J Physiol Endocrinol Metab.* 2022;322:E34.

Brooks GA. Lactate as a fulcrum of metabolism. *Redox Biol.* 2020;35:101454.

Brooks GA. The tortuous path of lactate shuttle discovery: from cinders and boards to the lab and ICU. *J Sport Health Sci.* 2020;9:446.

Burke LM. Ketogenic low CHO, high fat diet: the future of elite endurance sport? *J Physiol.* 2021;599:819.

Cao J, et al. The effect of a ketogenic low-carbohydrate, high-fat diet on aerobic capacity and exercise performance in endurance athletes: a systematic review and meta-analysis. *Nutrients.* 2021;13:2896.

Häfele MS, et al. Quality of life responses after combined and aerobic water-based training programs in older women: a randomized clinical trial (ACTIVE Study). *Aging Clin Exp Res.* 2022. doi:10.1007/s40520-021-02040-.

Hortobágyi T, et al. Effects of exercise dose and detraining duration on mobility at late midlife: a randomized clinical trial. *Gerontology.* 2021;67:403.

Hortobágyi T, et al. Functional relevance of resistance training-induced neuroplasticity in health and disease. *Neurosci Biobehav Rev.* 2021;122:79.

Kaufmann S, et al. Energetics of floor gymnastics: aerobic and anaerobic share in male and female sub-elite gymnasts. *Sports Med Open.* 2022;8:3.

Koay YC, et al. Effect of chronic exercise in healthy young male adults: a metabolomic analysis. *Cardiovasc Res.* 2021;117:613.

Mang ZA, et al. Aerobic adaptations to resistance training: the role of time under tension. *Int J Sports Med.* 2022. doi:10.1055/a-1664-8701.

Martin-Smith R. High intensity interval training (HIIT) improves cardiorespiratory fitness (CRF) in healthy, overweight and obese adolescents: a systematic review and meta-analysis of controlled studies. *Int J Environ Res Public Health.* 2020;17:2955.

Modaberi S, et al. A systematic review on detraining effects after balance and fall prevention interventions. *J Clin Med.* 2021;10:4656.

Petek BJ, et al. Cardiac effects of detraining in athletes: a narrative review. *Ann Phys Rehabil Med.* 2021;65:101581.

Pramkratok W, et al. Repeated sprint training under hypoxia improves aerobic performance and repeated sprint ability by enhancing muscle deoxygenation and markers of angiogenesis in rugby sevens. *Eur J Appl Physiol.* 2022;22:611. doi:10.1007/s00421-021-04861-8.

Ravindrakumar A, et al. Daily variation in performance measures related to anaerobic power and capacity: a systematic review. *Chronobiol Int.* 2022;39:421. doi:10.1080/07420528.2021.

Sapp RM, et al. Changes in circulating microRNA and arterial stiffness following high-intensity interval and moderate intensity continuous exercise. *Physiol Rep.* 2020;8:e14431.

Spiering BA, et al. Maintaining physical performance: the minimal dose of exercise needed to preserve endurance and strength over time. *J Strength Cond Res.* 2021;35:1449.

Verwijs SM, et al. Beneficial Effects of cardiomyopathy-associated genetic variants on physical performance: a hypothesis-generating scoping review. *Cardiology.* 2022;147:90.

Wolf AS, et al. Hourly 4-s sprints prevent impairment of postprandial fat metabolism from inactivity. *Med Sci Sports Exerc.* 2020;52:2262.

Zhang H, et al. Phosphorus recovery in the alternating aerobic/anaerobic biofilm system: performance and mechanism. *Sci Total Environ.* 2022;810:152297.

Table 21.1 Physiologic and Metabolic Function Changes with Various Detraining Durations[a]

Variable	Trained	Detrained	Change, % Short-Term Detraining[b]	Change, % Longer-Term Detraining[c]
$\dot{V}O_{2max}$, mL·kg^{-1}·min^{-1}	62.2 62.1	57.3 50.8	−8	−18
$\dot{V}O_{2max}$, L·min^{-1}	4.45	4.16	−7	
Cardiac output, L·min^{-1}	27.8 27.8	25.5 25.2	−8	−10
Stroke volume, mL	155	139	−10	
Heart rate, b·min^{-1}	148 186 187	129 193 197	4	−13 5
Oxygen pulse, mL·b^{-1}	12.7	10.9		−14
Sum 3-min recovery HR	190	237		25
Plasma volume, L	2.91	2.56	−12	
a-$\bar{v}O_2$ diff, mL·100 mL^{-1}	15.1 15.1	15.4 14.1	−2 (NS)	−7
PCr, mM·(g wet wt)$^{-1}$	17.9	13.0		−27
ATP, mM·(g wet wt)$^{-1}$	5.97	5.08		−15
Glycogen, mM·(g wet wt)$^{-1}$	113.9	57.4		−50
Capillary density, cap·mm^{-2}	511 464	476 476	−7	−2 (NS)
Oxidative enzyme capacity			−29	−32
Myoglobin, mg·(g protein)$^{-1}$	43.3 43.3	41.0 40.7	−5 (NS)	−6
Insulin (rest)			17–120	
Norepinephrine/epinephrine (rest)			No change	
Norepinephrine/epinephrine (exercise)				65–100
Blood lactate			88	
Lactate threshold			−7	−18
Exercise lipolysis			−52	
Muscle glycogen synthesis			−29	−40
Time to fatigue, min			−10	
Swim power, W				−14
Elbow extension strength, ft-lb	39.0	25.5		−35

[a]Represents an average computed from individual studies cited from Wilber RL, Moffatt RJ. Physiological and biochemical consequences of detraining in aerobically trained individuals. *J Strength Cond Res*. 1994;8:110. A change in heart rate represents a functional capacity decline.
[b]Short term, 3 wk or less in primarily aerobically trained individuals.
[c]Long term, 3 to 12 wk in primarily aerobically trained individuals.
ATP, adenosine triphosphate; a-$\bar{v}O_2$ diff, arterio-mixed venous oxygen difference; HR, heart rate; NS, not statistically significant; PCr, phosphocreatine; $\dot{V}O_{2max}$, maximum oxygen uptake.

Table 21.2 — Typical Metabolic and Physiologic Values for Healthy Endurance-Trained and Untrained Men[a]

Variable	Untrained	Trained	Percentage Difference[b]
Glycogen, mM · (g wet muscle)$^{-1}$	85.0	120	41
Number of mitochondria, mmol^3	0.59	1.20	103
Mitochondrial volume, % muscle cell	2.15	8.00	272
Resting ATP, mM · (g wet muscle)$^{-1}$	3.0	6.0	100
Resting PCr, mM · (g wet muscle)$^{-1}$	11.0	18.0	64
Resting creatine, mM · (g wet muscle)$^{-1}$	10.7	14.5	35
Glycolytic enzymes	50.0	50.0	0
Phosphofructokinase, mM · (g wet muscle)$^{-1}$	4–6	6–9	60
Phosphorylase, mM·(g wet muscle)$^{-1}$			
Aerobic enzymes	5–10	15–20	133
Succinate dehydrogenase, mM · (kg wet muscle)$^{-1}$	110	150	36
Max lactate, mM · (kg wet muscle)$^{-1}$			
Muscle fibers			
Fast twitch, %	50	20–30	−50
Slow twitch, %	50	60	20
Max stroke volume, mL	120	180	50
Max cardiac output, L · min^{-1}	20	30–40	75
Resting heart rate, b · min^{-1}	70	40	−43
Max heart rate, b · min^{-1}	190	180	−5
Max a-$\bar{v}$O$_2$ diff, mL · dL^{-1}	14.5	16.0	10
$\dot{V}O_{2max}$, mL · kg^{-1} · min^{-1}	30–40	65–80	107
Heart volume, L	7.5	9.5	27
Blood volume, L	4.7	6.0	28
$\dot{V}_{Emax}$, L · min^{-1}	110	190	73
Percentage body fat	15	11	−27

[a]Trained values represent data from endurance athletes.
[b]Percentage difference: trained versus untrained.
ATP, adenosine triphosphate; a-$\bar{v}$O$_2$ diff, arterio-mixed venous oxygen difference; PCr, phosphocreatine; $\dot{V}_{Emax}$, maximum ventilatory equivalent; $\dot{V}O_{2max}$, maximum oxygen uptake.

Table 21.3 — Comparative Average Cardiac Dimensions in College Athletes, World-Class Athletes, and Normal Subjects

Dimension	College Runners (n = 15)	College Swimmers (n = 15)	World-Class Runners (n = 10)	College Wrestlers (n = 12)	World-Class Shot Putters (n = 4)	Normals (n = 16)
LVID	54	51	48–59	48	43–52	46
LVV, mL	160	181	154	110	122	101
SV, mL	116	NR	113	75	68	NR
LV wall, mm	11.3	10.6	10.8	13.7	13.8	10.3
Septum, mm	10.9	10.7	10.9	13.0	13.5	10.3
LV mass, g	302	308	283	330	348	211

LVID, left-ventricular internal dimension at end diastole; LVV, left-ventricular volume; NR, values not reported; SV, stroke volume; LV wall, left-ventricular wall thickness; Septum, ventricular septal thickness; LV mass, left-ventricular mass.
From *Annals of Internal Medicine*, Morganroth J, et al. Comparative left-ventricular dimensions in trained athletes. *Ann Intern Med*. 1975;82:521. Copyright © 1975 American College of Physicians. All Rights Reserved. Reprinted with the permission of American College of Physicians, Inc.

Table 21.4 — Guidelines for Determining Interval Training Exercise Rates for Running and Swimming Different Distances

Interval Training Distances (yd)		Work Rate for Each Exercise Interval or Repeat
Run	Swim	
55	15	1.5 s *slower* than best
110	25	3.0 times from a running or *swimming* start
220	55	5.0 for each distance
440	110	1–4 s *faster* than the average 440-yd run or 110-yd swim times during a mile run or 440-yd swim
660–1320	165–320	3–4 s *slower* than the average 440-yd run or 100-yd swim times during a mile run or 440-yd swim

Reprinted from Fox EL, Mathews DK. *Interval Training*. Philadelphia: WB Saunders; 1974.

CHAPTER 22

Muscular Strength: Training Muscles to Become Stronger

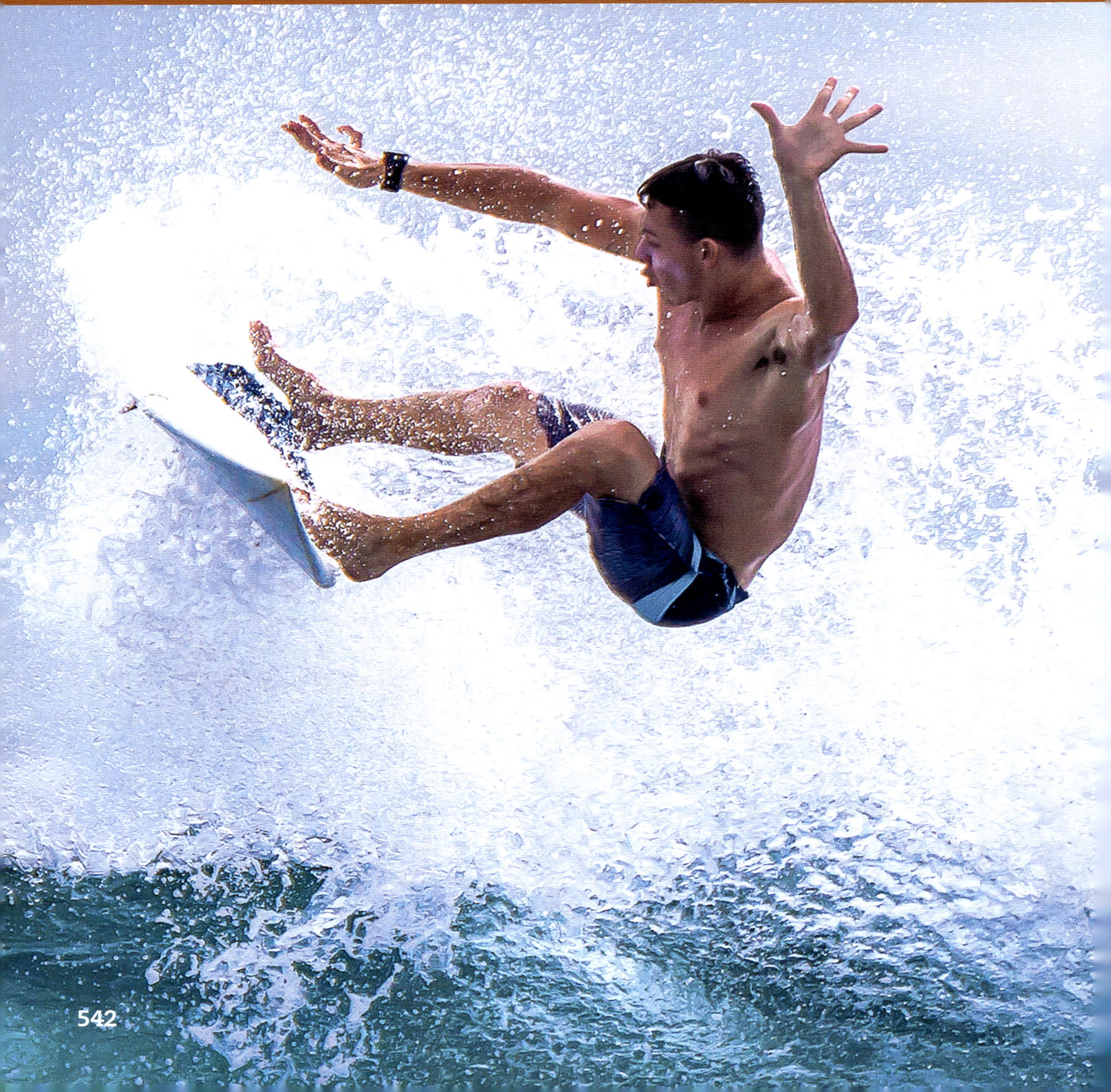

Chapter Objectives

- Describe four standard methods to assess muscular strength
- Outline the one-repetition maximum (1-RM) test procedure for trained and untrained individuals
- Compare absolute and relative upper- and lower-body muscular strength in males and females
- Describe allometric scaling to compare strength and exercise performance characteristics
- Describe two examples for concentric, eccentric, and isometric muscle actions
- Describe optimum sets and repetitions, frequency, and relative intensity for progressive resistance training
- Outline an optimal model for strength-training periodization
- Discuss strength training specificity in sports and occupational tasks
- Differentiate resistance training goals among competitive athletes versus untrained middle-age and the elderly
- Discuss common strength training method that best improves overall muscular strength
- Describe two plyometric training advantages and disadvantages for power athletes
- Describe how "psychologic" and "muscular" factors impact strength capacity
- List six basic adaptations with chronic resistance training
- Explain how resistance training effects muscle fiber type and number
- Take a position and explain—"Should a transwoman compete in sport consistent with her gender identity as a biological male?"
- Design a circuit resistance training program to improve strength and cardiovascular fitness for middle-age males and females
- Explain how specific resistance training can "shape" a muscle's appearance
- Explain the best exercise mode to minimize muscle soreness and enhance intracellular changes
- Explain how to optimize "core strength" to enhance performance

Ancillaries at-a-Glance

Visit Lippincott Connect to access the following resources.

- References: Chapter 22
- Appendix D: The Metric System and Conversion Constants in Exercise Physiology
- Animations: Muscle Contraction Type, RICE Method, Stretch Shortening Cycle
- AFocus on Research: Develop Strength by Increasing Load, Not Repetitions

Part 1: Strength Measurement and Resistance Training

Muscular Strength Development Roots in Antiquity

Strength development programs in athletic training regimens was not new for preparing men for warfare in ancient China, Japan, India, Greece, and Rome. When the Olympic games first began in 776 BC, athletes trained year-round incorporating muscle-strengthening exercises into their training regimens

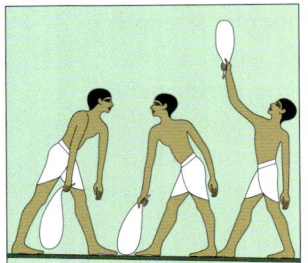

(https://olympics.com/ioc/ancient-olympic-games). The scientific foundations for strength training athletes began with the Chinese in 3600 BC during the Chou dynasty (1122–249 BC), when conscripts had to pass required weightlifting tasks before becoming soldiers. Sculptures and illustrations depict athletes in ancient Egypt and India training with heavy stone weights.

Wall mosaics recovered from Roman villas showed young women exercising with handheld weights, a common practice in early youth education. During the "Age of Strength" in the 6th century, weightlifting competitions routinely took place between soldiers and athletes. Galen, the famous early Greek physician (see book Introduction, section Exercise Physiology: Roots and Historical Perspectives), referred to Greek pentath-

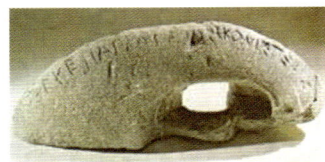

letes exercising with 1.5- to 2.0 kg/3.3 to 4.4 lb handheld weights made from stone or lead (called **halteres** shown at the left) during jumping events.[171]

Other Contributors to Early Strength Science

Early educators set the foundation for including strengthening activities and exercise programs in the schools to improve overall health and well-being. Teachers were trained not only as physical education instructors in the schools and YMCAs (first American YMCA founded in Boston at the Old South Church in 1851; www.ymca.net/history/founding.html) but also for government work as military gymnastics instructors and physiotherapists. In 1887, the YMCA founded a college in Springfield, Massachusetts (first called the International Young Men's Christian Association Training School and now Springfield College), which emphasized gymnastic activities and other individual and dual sport activities. Football was introduced in 1890 by student-instructor Amos Alonzo Stagg (1862–1965), and basketball was developed in 1891 by James Naismith (1861–1938); both men first taught indoor exercise routines and "strengthening" calisthenics at the Springfield YMCA Training School.

Prior to the American popularization about strength-type exercise and calisthenics in schools and colleges, the overseas influence also promoted strengthening activities in Europe and the Nordic countries. Key early pioneers included **Johann Basedow** (1723–1790), German educator, who founded the Philanthropinum (*from Greek:* φιλος = *friend and* ανθροπος = *human*), which literally was founded to embrace philanthropy in society and to promote Mind and Body Education in curriculum emphasizing sports and activity as essential curriculum components in harmony with receiving a sound education (https://en.wikipedia.org/wiki/Johann_Bernhard_Basedow).

Johann Guts Muth (1759–1839), also a German educator and writer, described workout routines for balance on swinging beams, poles, ropes, and vaulting horses shown in this early illustration. Many historians consider him the *grandfather* of gymnastics, the "father" being

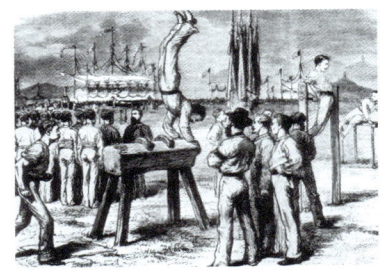

Friedrich Ludwig Jahn discussed in a subsequent section.

In France, Francis Amoros (1770–1848), a Spanish educator, helped to establish gymnastics in that country, emphasizing upper body strength routines on the trapeze, rings, and ropes. In Denmark, Franz Nachtegall (1777–1847) operated a private gymnastic club in Copenhagen, emphasizing mass calisthenics incorporating vaulting and specific routines with dumbbells and small, weighted balls. His facility was the first to focus exclusively on physical training. This successful venture led the government to establish a military institute to train noncommissioned officers. Denmark also introduced physical training into its schools, to prepare future officers in popular gymnastics theory and methods. Another German educator and author, Gerhard Vieth (1759–1839), devised specific exercise routines emphasizing "strength/power movements" on ropes, beams, and horizontal pole vaulting.

The esteemed title "Father of Modern Gymnastics" goes to **Friedrich Ludwig Jahn** (1778–1852) who promoted gymnastic exercise to develop muscular strength and endurance, particularly to prepare France for military readiness through strict physical training.

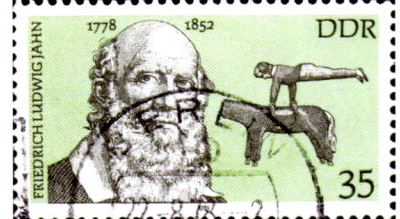

Mirt Alexander/Shutterstock

In 1811, Jahn founded the **Turnverein societies** (German Turnen "to practice gymnastics" and Verein "club or union"), and its members were called "Turners" or gymnasts. The first American **Turnverein** (gymnastics club) was founded in 1848 in Cincinnati, Ohio. Among Jahn's many contributions include inventing the modern vaulting horse (see inset stamp with lineage from Alexander the Great and Roman soldiers in the 4th century who practiced mounting and dismounting wooden horses; www.gymmedia.com/Anaheim03/appa/pommel/history_ph.htm), parallel bars, balance bean, and rings, all "advanced" apparatus to develop muscular strength. The equipment was displayed in Berlin's first open-air gymnasia (Berlin's modern outdoor stadium or "Sportpark" bears his name), as do honors on German stamps and sport medallions.

Above all, Jahn successfully advocated for gymnastics as a competitive sport (https://counter-currents.com/2017/11/friedrich-ludwig-jahn-and-german-nationalism/).

Jahn influenced other leaders in education including Francis Lieber (1800–1872) who immigrated to the United States from Germany in 1824 to manage a gymnasium and swimming pool in Boston. There he met Charles Follen (1796–1840), a life-long educator who started the first college gymnasium (and eventually taught German at Harvard), and another colleague Charles Beck (1798–1866), a German-born United States classical scholar (also taught Latin and Literature at Harvard), a talented gymnast, and strongly believed in preparing for athletic competitions by arduous physical training. Leiber, Follen, and Beck were formidable gymnastic and athletic advocates at this time in American history when understanding the science and physiology of "muscular strength" development began to emerge. In the late 1820s, Beck established

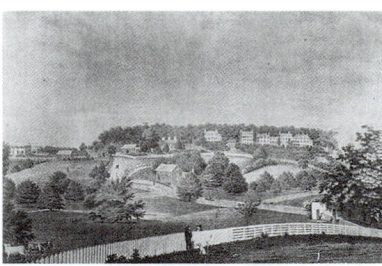

an outdoor gymnasium at the Round Hill School for Boys in Northampton, MA, the first gymnasium in the United States and host to the first secondary school gymnastics program. The school built a half mile track and walking trails to complement its blossoming athletic requirements and strict academic curriculum. Jahn taught physical education classes, creating an athletic curriculum that featured calisthenics modeled after his physical training ideas. Unfortunately, the Round Hill School closed in 1833 due to financial constraints, only 11 years after its creation. A prevailing but short-lived idea in the late 1850s was to incorporate gymnastic apparatus and lifting heavy objects (barbells, weights, stones) into exercise training regimens designed to promote "*Strength is health*" as an ideal educational objective.

America's First Athletic Club

German settlers and educators were instrumental in founding the New York Athletic Club (NYAC) in New York City in 1868, America's first athletic club. This all-male social club, considered by many as the foundation for United States amateur athletics, featured fencing, boxing, and Greco-Roman wrestling. The NYAC was first to compile rules and regulations to govern athletic events, first to offer prizes for open amateur games, and first to hold an amateur championship. Currently, the club fields 22 different teams representing the major sports, along with judo, handball, squash, table tennis, team handball, and platform tennis.

The popularity of sports clubs and athletic events featured mostly "strongmen" (and a few women) and traveling circus performers who showcased their gymnastics talents and unconventional strength feats (www.oldtimestrongman.com/blog/tag/circus-strongman/). Examples include supporting a heavy weight overhead at arm's length, bending steel bars with bare hands, breaking a thick iron chain around the chest by only ribcage expansion, and breaking a steel ring by biting into it using only the jaw muscles.

Weightlifting in Early America

Weightlifting in America in the early 1840s became a spectator sport practiced by strongmen featured in traveling carnivals and sideshows. As pointed out in this text's "Introduction: A View of the Past," military physicians evaluated conscripts' strength during the Civil War, which served as a basic foundation for routine fitness assessments in the prototype college and university physical education programs at the turn of the 19th century, and during the lead up to World War 1.

Pehr Henrik Ling (1776–1839) deserves much credit for introducing strength development "science." Historians consider Ling, a fencing master and teacher of medical-gymnastics (human movement incorporating his studies about anatomy and physiology later evolving into "physiotherapy"), to be the father of "Swedish Gymnastics." In 1813, he founded the current Swedish School of Sport and Health Sciences under the name of the Royal Central Institute of Gymnastics in Stockholm (www.gih.se/In-English/). He and his son Hylmar (1820–1886), both influential writers along with their many disciples, became experts in physical education curriculum design and practice throughout Europe (https://pubmed.ncbi.nlm.nih.gov/19848036/). Their influential strength development techniques migrated to the British Isles and eventually in the early 1800s to the United States. Teachers were trained not only as school physical education instructors, but for government work as military gymnastics instructors and physiotherapists.

FIGURE 22.1 shows late 19th century "strength and exercise machines" popularized by Swedish physician Dr. **Gustav Zander** (1835–1920; www.smithsonianmag.com/smithsonian-institution/gustav-zander-victorian-era-exercise-machines-bowflex-180957758/), whose design was influenced by the Lings' Swedish Gymnastic movement. Zander included standard gymnastic exercise regimens to treat patients and the common person, combined with calisthenics, balance, and core trunk and limb movements. Workouts on his 37 mechanical and steam-powered devices served double duty for general strength development and "mechanical gymnastic treatments" for morbid disorders and diseases of the heart, nerves, respiratory and abdominal organs, obesity, gout, and articular rheumatism, including scoliosis. Dr. Zander's successful treatment clinics in the 1880–1890s featuring his stand-alone machines (some positioned at key locations in Central Park, New York City) provided a new vista and attitude toward self-enhancement through exercise for fitness, therapy, and health. One of the most popular machines was designed to increase "core" strength as part of a vigorous

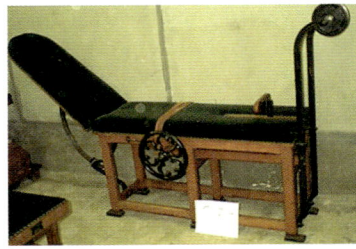

Photo courtesy F. Katch

training regimen. The user would attach a harness to a metal cord to a weight. The metal cord would pass over a pulley so the user could do sit-ups using the weight's added resistance. Four remaining Zander machines from the United States are currently housed in the Hot Springs National Park, AR (www.nps.gov/hosp/learn/historyculture/the-therapy-machines-of-dr-gustav-zander.htm). A full line of Zander equipment is currently available to the public at the Gustav Zander Institute of Mechanotherapy, Yessentuki, Russia (www.localguidesconnect.com/t5/General-Discussion/Exploring-Russia-Zander-Institute-of-Mechanotherapy-in/td-p/1006076).

Perhaps serendipitously (or not), the popular *Nautilus* original exercise equipment line invented by Arthur Jones (1926–2007) was remarkably similar to Zander's machines by employing chain links and a circular cam movement strategy (https://corehandf.com/the-first-name-in-strength/). In the United States at this time, measuring muscular strength became popular to evaluate physical fitness and body development, particularly in schools, colleges, physiotherapy centers, and local gymnasia and training centers. An 1897 meeting with American College Gymnasium Directors (Dr. D. A. Sargent [1849–1924], committee chair from Harvard University) established strength contests to determine overall body strength based on back, leg, arm, and chest strength measurements. The first six college participants included Amherst College, Columbia University, Harvard University, the University of Minnesota, Dickinson College, and Wesleyan College. Harvard was the overall winner followed closely by Columbia.

By the mid-1900s, physical culture specialists, body builders, competitive weightlifters, field-event athletes, and some wrestlers used traditional weightlifting exercises, not the passive massage methods and electrical vibration that also flourished during this time. Research in the late 1950s and early 1960s dispelled the myth that traditional muscle-strengthening exercises reduced movement speed or limited joint **range of motion (ROM)**. Instead, the opposite usually occurred; elite weightlifters, body builders, and "muscle men" exhibited exceptional

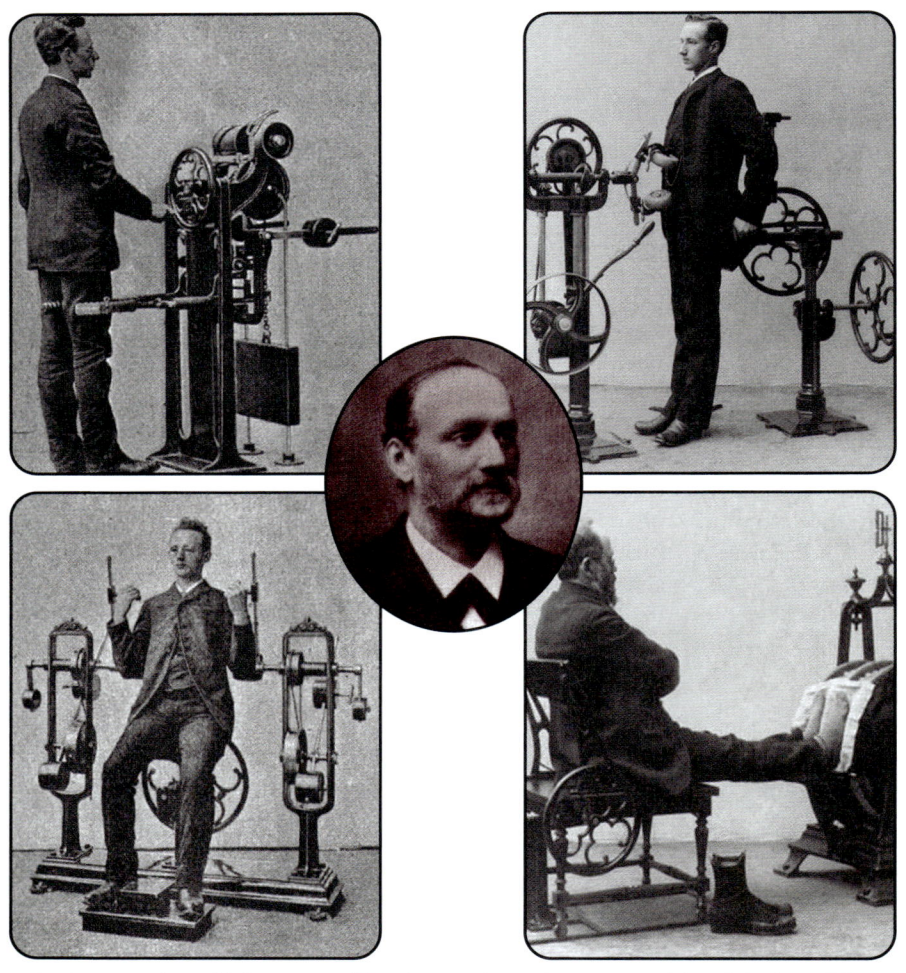

FIGURE 22.1. Late 19th century "Zander mechanotherapy machines" designed for strength, massage, rehabilitation, and strength development in gyms and physical therapy centers in Europe, and for a brief period in the 1880s and 1890s in the Zander Institute in New York City.
(Photos from Levertin A. *Dr. G. Zanders Medico-Mechanical Gymnastics. It's Method, Importance and Application.* Stockholm: P.A. Norstead & Sonner. Printers to the King; 1893.)

Early Strongmen Popularized Body Building and Strength Training

Eugen Sandow (left photo), born Frederick Mueller (1867–1925), emerged as one of the first successful vaudeville

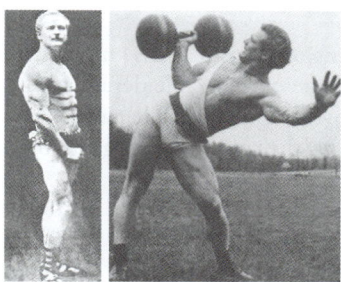

strong-men in the early 1890s, who legendary showman Florenz Ziegfeld (1867–1932) managed and billed as "The Most Perfect Man." Sandow designed a physical fitness training program for the British military, inspiring a future generation of bodybuilders.[40] Sandow published popular magazines, promoted exercise equipment he used (mainly barbells), and promoted "special training foods." John Grimek (right photo) achieved notoriety as a member of the United States 1936 Olympic weightlifting team, two-time Mr. America (1940, 1941), 1948 Mr. Universe, and undefeated in body-building competitions. Most authorities believed Grimek epitomized the first half of the 20th century's "best-built human." In the late 1890s, Daniel L. Dowd (1854–1897) advertised strength equipment targeted for home gym use. Dowd was first to advertise his wall-fixed equipment by showing "before" and "after" selfies of him using the equipment, prepared for self-help books published in 1878 devoted to physical culture, body building, and strength development (Dowd DL. Physical Culture for Home and School; Scientific and Practical. New York: Fowler & Wells, 1889.) *Physical Culture for Home and School; Scientific and Practical*. New York: Fowler & Wells, 1889). Dowd weighed only 138 lb prior to training, but 4 years later gained what he deemed added muscle mass, now weighing 163 lb. To him, the new muscle mass and added weight gain provided ample evidence of the equipment's validity. To sculpt a perfect physique, Dowd advocated many repetitions with light resistance, and his book illustrates numerous exercises to develop neck, trunk, and extremity musculature. By the mid-1800s to late 1800s, rowing machines and strengthening devices became commonplace, eventually leading to studies in the 1890s about the effectiveness of strength building courses in physical education classes at Harvard and Amherst College.

---

joint flexibility without limitations in general limb movement speed. For untrained healthy individuals, heavy-resistance exercises increased muscular effort speed and power without impairing sports performance.

In the sections that follow, we explore the underlying rationale for resistance training and physiologic adaptations that occur when males and females train muscles to become bigger, faster, and stronger. The discussion centers on different muscular strength development methods, gender differences in strength, and different resistance-training programs including "core" strength and power development.

Forerunner to Modern Exercise Machines

Francis Lowndes (1760–1836) invented and patented the **Gymnasticon** in 1798, perhaps the first English patented mechanical device resembling a bicycle designed to activate all body joints and muscles at once or partially. This early exercise machine was designed primarily for individuals unable to exercise on their own or for those in sedentary occupations such as students unable to find the time to move from a sedentary lifestyle to engaging in physically activity on their own. The engraving shows a man holding straps attached to an upper flywheel, while the legs depress foot pedals to turn the lower flywheel. The upper and lower flywheels could work separately. The Gymnasticon, initially targeted for the sick and infirmed, forced involuntary joint movement in diseased, paralyzed limbs, and involuntary body tremors, while more physically active persons could strengthen upper and lower limbs. Unfortunately, Lowndes' invention did not achieve commercial success and his unique engineering attempt to enhance standard rehabilitation practices, and this form of body movement therapy did not materialize.

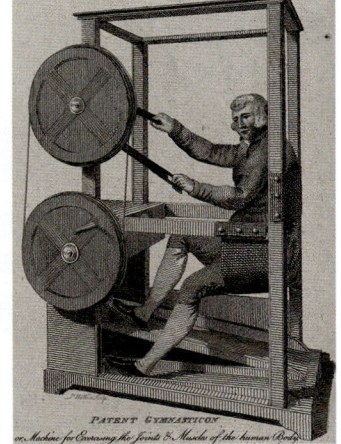

Early 19th century American medicine still included unproven blood-letting procedures to treat unspecified diseases and maladies, including quack devices and "cures" peddled by unscrupulous salesmen. Hence, a new mechanical exercise method to induce movement to improve the human condition was, unfortunately, ahead of its time. It would take at least another 50 to 75 years before fitness/exercise devices invented in Sweden and those sold commercially in the United

States by Dr. Dudley Sargent from Harvard (see Introduction: A View from the Past) gained respectability in physical education and sports training programs both in America and abroad.

Resistance Training Objectives

Six main areas impact strength development through resistance training:

1. Weightlifting and powerlifting competitions
2. Body building to maximize muscular development for aesthetic goals
3. General strength training for fitness and health enhancement
4. Physical therapy for rehabilitation from injury or disease
5. Sport-specific resistance training to maximize sport performance
6. Muscle physiology's practical applications to better understand acute and chronic exercise effects on muscle structure and function

Muscle Strength Measurement

Four muscle strength methods commonly assess maximum force or tension output generated by a single muscle or related muscle groups:

1. Cable tensiometry
2. Dynamometry
3. One-repetition maximum
4. Computer-assisted, electromechanical, and isokinetic methods

Cable Tensiometry

FIGURE 22.2A shows a **cable tensiometer** to assess knee extension muscle force. Increasing force on the cable depresses the riser shown in the inset circle over which the cable passes. This deflects the pointer and indicates the subject's strength score.

Dynamometry

English mathematician and avid inventor **Charles Babbage** (1791–1871; http://mikes.railhistory.railfan.net/r062.html) was first to invent a dynamometer to record the forces over time exerted on a railway car. The ever-inventive Babbage devised a way to track data on a moving paper roll to record the pulling engine's force, plot the railroad car carriage's path, and the carriage's vertical shake. Dynamometry in clinical medicine began in England in 1952 and continued in medical practice to test patients diagnosed with **polio (poliomyelitis),** rheumatic conditions, **myasthenia gravis**, focal cerebral lesions that affect downstream musculature, and various motor dysfunctions.[198]

Figure 22.2B and C illustrate the compression principle using hand-grip and leg and back-lift **dynamometers** to assess

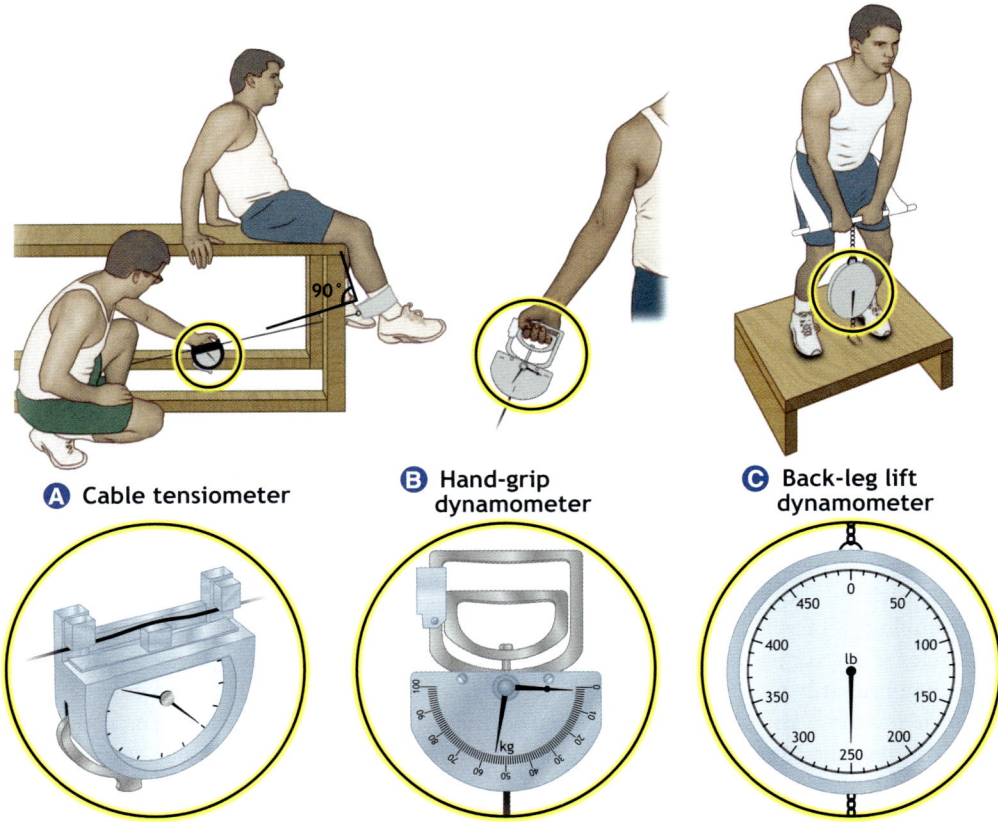

FIGURE 22.2. **(A)** Static strength measurement with a cable tensiometer, **(B)** hand-grip dynamometer, and **(C)** back leg lift dynamometer.

static strength. An external force applied to the dynamometer compresses a steel spring and moves a pointer. The force required to move the pointer a given distance determines the external force applied to the dynamometer.

One-Repetition Maximum

A dynamic procedure to measure muscular strength applies the **one-repetition maximum (1-RM)** method. *1-RM refers to the maximum weight a person can lift one time with proper form during a standard weightlifting movement.* To assess 1-RM for any muscle group, the tester makes a reasonable guess at an initial weight close to, but below, the person's maximum lifting capacity. Weight is progressively added on subsequent attempts until the person reaches maximum lift capacity. The weight increments usually range between 1 and 5 kg/2.2 and 11 lb depending on the muscle group's force-output capacity and equipment type. One-min to 5-min rest intervals usually provide sufficient recuperation before attempting a lift at the next heavier weight.

How to Estimate the 1-RM

Impracticality and/or potential risk in performing 1-RM with preadolescents, the elderly, hypertensives, cardiac patients, and other special populations require a 1-RM *estimate* from submaximal effort. Different **predictive equations** are necessary to estimate 1-RM because resistance training alters the intrinsic relationship between submaximal 7- to 10-RM performance and maximal 1-RM lift capacity. Generally, the weight that one can lift for 7- to 10-RM represents about 68% of the 1-RM score for an untrained person and 79% for the new 1-RM after training.[31] The following equations apply to untrained and resistance-trained young adults:

Untrained

$$1\text{-RM (kg)} = 1.554 \times 7\text{- to }10\text{-RM weight (kg)} - 5.181$$

Trained

$$1\text{-RM (kg)} = 1.172 \times 7\text{- to }10\text{-RM weight (kg)} + 7.704$$

For example, estimate the 1-RM bench press score for a trained person whose 10-RM bench press equals 70 kg/154 lb:

$$1\text{-RM (kg)} = 1.172 \times 70 \text{ (kg)} + 7.704 = 89.7 \text{ kg}$$

Computer-Assisted, Electromechanical, and Isokinetic Methods

Microprocessor technology rapidly quantifies forces, torques, accelerations, and velocities among body segments in numerous movement patterns. Force platforms measure a limb's external muscle force as, for example, in positions vertically, horizontally, and landing following a jump, or horizontal and vertical forces exerted by the feet during the push-off from starting blocks in sprint dashes. Other electromechanical devices assess forces generated during all activity phases (e.g., cycling) or primarily arm (seated press) or leg (leg press) movements.

An electromechanical accommodating resistance instrument or **isokinetic dynamometer** contains a speed-controlling mechanism that accelerates to a preset, constant velocity with force application. Once attaining the preset speed, the isokinetic loading mechanism adjusts automatically to provide a counterforce to variations in force generated by muscle as movement continues throughout the "strength curve." *Thus, maximum force (or any percentage of maximum effort) generates throughout the full ROM at a pre-established limb movement velocity at a continuum from high-velocity (lower-force) to low-velocity (higher-force) conditions.* A microprocessor within the dynamometer continuously monitors the immediate applied force level. An electronic integrator in series with a monitor displays the average or peak force generated during any interval for almost instantaneous feedback about

---

fyi Resistance Exercise Training Effects on Handgrip Strength in the Elderly

A meta-analysis (24 studies from 1995 to 2018) involving 3018 healthy community-dwelling older adults with a mean age of 73.3 years assessed the exercise training effects using maximum handgrip strength as the criterion improvement measure. In general, only small transfer effects occurred from the various exercise programs (aquatic exercise, walking, flexibility, TRX-training, home-trainer exercise, different strength training modes, vibration platform training, dance, Tai Chi, exergames balance training, calisthenics, and multidimensional training regimens). Intervention durations ranged from 4 wk to 36 months (mean 22 wk) with most interventions lasting 8 to 15 wk. Session duration varied between 15 and 72 min/session (average 51 min with most sessions lasting 60 min). Training frequency varied between one session per week and two sessions daily (average 3 sessions a wk) with most 2 to 3 sessions weekly. Handgrip strength changed slightly more with exercise training than control groups, probably related to participants older age, relatively short activity intervention period, lack of weekly training sessions or short-duration single training sessions, or poor grip strength validity as the criterion measure. In essence, older adults who do not train outside of activities of normal daily living (as occurred for control subjects) reduce general body strength and in particular arm strength and by extension handgrip strength, albeit slightly as measured by this criterion.

Ruslan Huzau/Shutterstock

Source:
Labott BK, et al. Effects of exercise training on handgrip strength in older adults: a meta-analytical review. *Gerontology*. 2019;65:686.

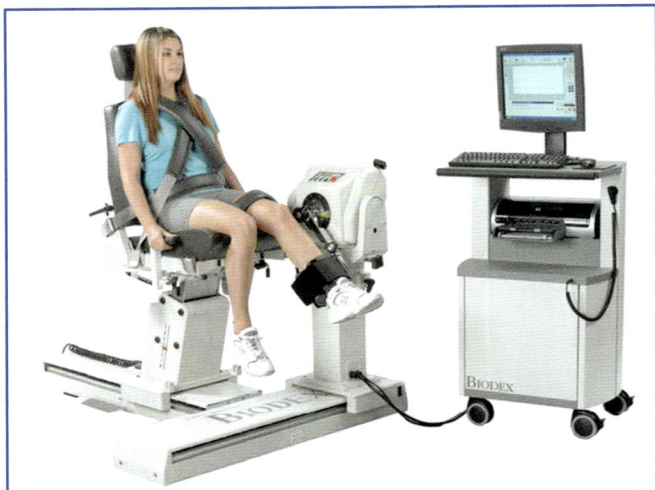

FIGURE 22.3. Biodex advanced isokinetic electromechanical dynamometer.
(Photo courtesy Biodex. Available at: www.biodex.com/physical-medicine/products/dynamometers/system-4-quick-set.)

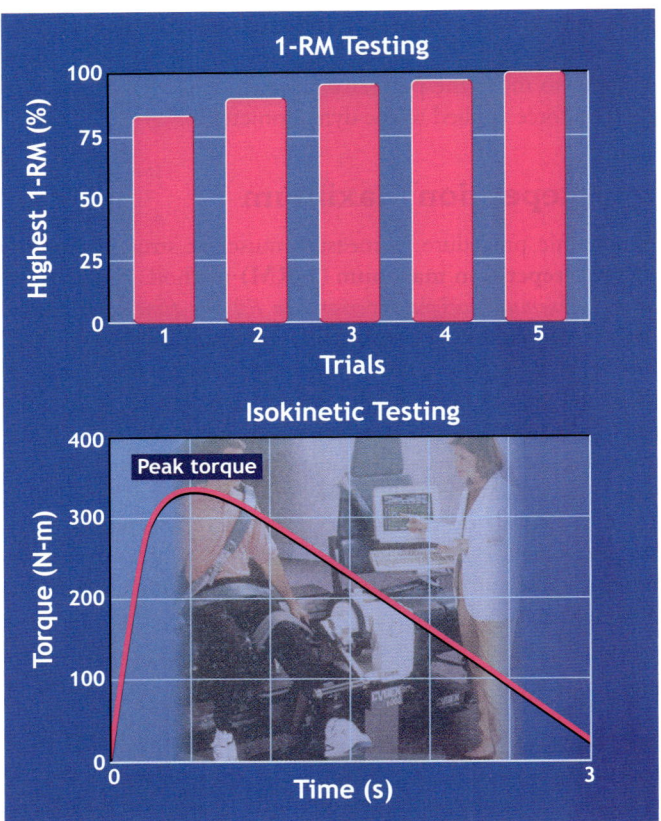

FIGURE 22.4 Top. Conventional 1-RM testing. The heaviest weight lifted constitutes the 1-RM. If 150 kg/331 lb (100%) is the maximum lifted, then 150 kg/331 lb equals the 1-RM. **Bottom.** Force curve obtained during an isokinetic test performed at a 30°·s^{-1} angular velocity over a 3-s interval.

performance (e.g., force, torque, work). **FIGURE 22.3** shows a popular electromechanical accommodating resistance dynamometer.

Interfacing microprocessor technology with mechanical devices provides valuable insights about how to evaluate and rehabilitate injuries. The argument to support isokinetic strength measurement posits that muscle strength dynamics involve considerably more than just the final 1-RM outcome (i.e., the weight lifted). For example, two individuals with identical 1-RM scores could exhibit dissimilar force curves throughout the movement. Individual differences in force dynamics (e.g., time to peak tension) throughout the full ROM may reflect an entirely different underlying neuromuscular physiology that 1-RM fails to assess. **FIGURE 22.4** illustrates the differences between conventional 1-RM knee extension (**top**; pink bars, highest force score during lift 5 represents *only* total weight lifted during that repetition), versus a microprocessor-controlled, isokinetic resistance device that produces a dynamic force curve throughout the ROM (**bottom**; force declines with movement duration). In this example, note that about 350 N-m peak torque occurs in the early movement phase at the most advantageous ROM angle and then declines rapidly to the right; the lowest torque occurs at full knee extension. During an isokinetic test performed at a 30°·s^{-1} angular velocity over a 3-s interval, peak torque would equal 342 N-m. Average torque refers to the force-time integral, or impulse divided by time. Impulse equals 602 N-m·s^{-1}, and average torque equals 200.7 N-m (602 N-m ÷ 3 s). Work equals the product average torque × distance moved (90° or 1.57 radians). Using the data for average torque and distance, work equals 174 N-m × 157 radians = 273 N-m, or 273 joules (J). Power is work per unit time or 273 J ÷ 3 s = 91 W.

TABLE 22.1 lists international system (SI) units to express muscular performance during both linear and angular movements.

TABLE 22.1 International System units to express muscular strength and power during linear and angular motions

New Generation Technology to Assess Muscular Strength Output

Researchers have developed sophisticated force measuring devices to digitally capture and analyze various strength input measures (e.g., 1-RM, 10-RM, fatigue curves over specified durations for single and multiple joint movement patterns). These currently include strain gauge force sensors and piezoelectric force transducers to convert a force or tension associated with the weight lifted based on compression, pressure, or torque output to a "force score" (e.g., see the Biodex dynamometer, next page). New generation sensors can measure and record the output from any selectorized weight stack device that incorporates a belt, band, or cable attached to the weight stack (www.shapelog.com/). The new technology breakthrough is the application to common weight equipment to yield output scores expressed in power (Watts, W), peak force (newtons, N), and total work (milliwatt-hours, mWh).

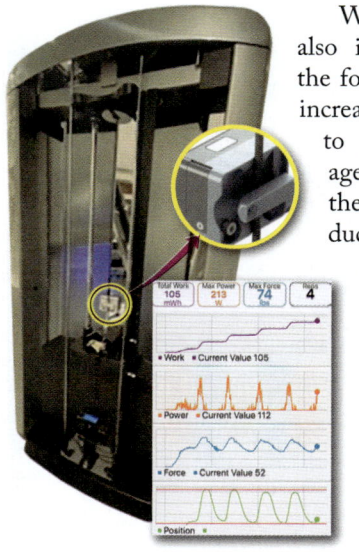

Photo courtesy V. Katch

With the new device, that also includes an accelerometer, the force applied to the load cell increases to allow the transducer to generate an output voltage directly proportional to the force applied to the transducer. These devices can talk directly to a user's smart phone, tablet, or computer, which then can generate a personalized training session to include set and repetition number, and target weight-lifting goals at desired specific movement speeds. Future miniaturized devices applied to home and gym exercise equipment will deliver personalized digital coaching solutions with interactive audio and 3-D, high-definition streaming, and stand-alone workouts for interactive single or group training sessions.

Resistance-Training Equipment Categories

Resistance training typically includes one of four exercise equipment types to manipulate movement speed and/or resistance throughout the ROM.

1. Free weights, **kettlebells**, and barbells, common weight-lifting equipment do not control or measure movement speed or resistance throughout the ROM
2. Isokinetic equipment that provides constant speed and **variable resistance**
3. Isokinetic, air pressure, and hydraulic equipment that provides constant speed and variable resistance, where the individual controls movement speed
4. Cam devices and concentric–eccentric apparatus where movement speed varies with constant resistance

Strength-Testing Considerations

Seven important considerations apply to muscle strength testing methods:

1. Require standardized instructions prior to testing.
2. Ensure warm-up uniformity for duration and intensity.
3. Allow adequate practice prior to testing to minimize "learning" that could compromise initial test results.
4. Require consistency in limb angle and/or body position during testing.
5. Predetermine a minimum trial number (repetitions) to establish a criterion strength score. For example, if administering five test repetitions, what score should represent the individual's strength score? Is the highest or an average from multiple attempts best? In most cases, an average provides a more representative (reliable) strength or power score than a single score.
6. Select test measures with high test score reproducibility. This crucial but often overlooked testing aspect evaluates subject response variability on repeated efforts. Poor test score consistency (unreliability) can mask an individual's most representative performance or change in performance when evaluating strength improvement.
7. Recognize individual differences in body size and composition when evaluating strength scores among individuals and groups.

Consider this legitimate but perplexing question about muscle strength testing: How do you fairly compare the absolute muscular strength for a 130-kg/287-lb football lineman compared to a 62-kg/137-lb distance runner? No clear-cut answer resolves this dilemma; in the section Allometric Scaling, below, we present alternatives to more fairly compare strength scores among individuals.

Learning Factors Affect Strength Measurements

In Chapter 19, we emphasized that initial muscular strength gains with resistance training result largely from neural factors rather than structural changes within muscle *per se*. **FIGURE 22.5** presents data for repetition-by-repetition performance improvements in maximum force (1-RM) at $5° \cdot s^{-1}$ angular velocity during a supine bench press with a 5-s interval between effort repetitions, with strong verbal encouragement provided on each attempt. The improvement averaged 11% between force on attempt 1 and attempt 5, but only 2% between the last two attempts. Strength "improvement" with repeated testing indicates the necessity for at least three attempts before maximum force scores begin to stabilize, or plateau and flatten out. Importantly, using only one or two 1-RM attempts often *underestimates* the "true" 1-RM by as much as 11%. If a single 1-RM trial preceded a 15-wk strength-training program, then

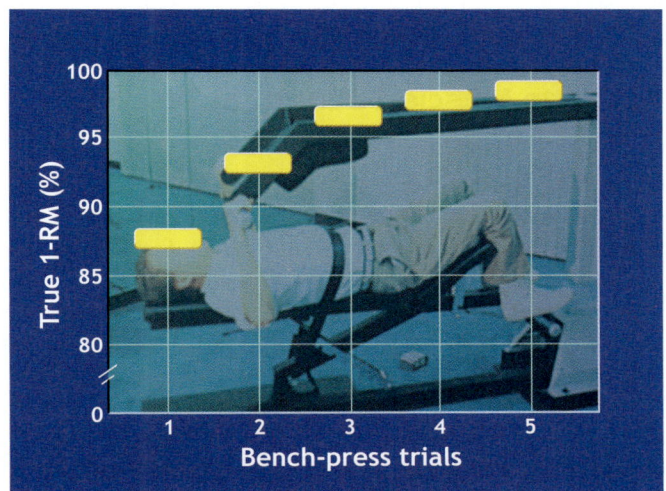

FIGURE 22.5. Five repeated maximal force (1-RM) supine bench press determinations with an electromechanical dynamometer. (Photo from F. Katch, Santa Barbara, CA.)

any strength gains attributable to training would include the 11% "learning" improvement simply from familiarization and not a true training effect!

Gender Differences in Muscle Strength

Four factors help to identify if a true gender difference exists in muscle strength:

1. Muscle cross-sectional area
2. Absolute muscle strength expressed as total force exerted
3. Relative muscle strength indexed to body composition
4. Muscle strength indexed to allometric scaling

Muscle Cross-Sectional Area

Human skeletal muscle generates a maximum 16 and 30 Newtons (N) force per square centimeter of **muscle cross-sectional area (MCSA)** regardless of gender. *In the body, force-output capacity varies depending on the body's bony levers and muscle architecture arrangement* (see Chapter 18). Applying 30 N as a representative force capacity per cm² muscle tissue indicates that a muscle with a 5.0-cm² cross-sectional area develops 150 N maximum force. If all the body's muscles became maximally activated simultaneously with force applied in the same direction, the resulting force would equal 168 kN. This estimation assumes 0.56 m² muscle total cross section.

FIGURE 22.6A compares the absolute arm flexor strength between males and females ages 12 to 20 years related to the flexor muscle's total cross-sectional area. Clearly, individuals with the largest MCSA (10 to 20 cm²) generate the greatest absolute force (30 to 40 kg/66 to 88 lb). In males and females, the near-linear relation between strength and muscle size indicates little difference in arm flexor strength for the same size muscle. Figure 22.6B further demonstrates this point when expressing males' and females' strength per unit MCSA. In addition, women and men matched for absolute muscular strength show similar elbow flexor muscle fatigability during a sustained low-level isometric action.[110]

Absolute Muscle Strength as Total Force Exerted

Comparing muscular strength on an *absolute* score basis, expressed either as total force in lb or kg, shows that males possess considerably greater strength than females for all muscle groups tested. Females score about 50% lower than males for upper-body strength and about 30% lower for leg strength. This gender disparity exists independently from the measuring system and generally coincides with gender-related difference in muscle mass distribution. Exceptions to these general findings usually emerge for strength-trained female track-and-field athletes and bodybuilders who have systematically strength-trained for years, often for a decade or longer.

A unique data set exists on gender differences in weight-lifting competitions in which males and females with identical

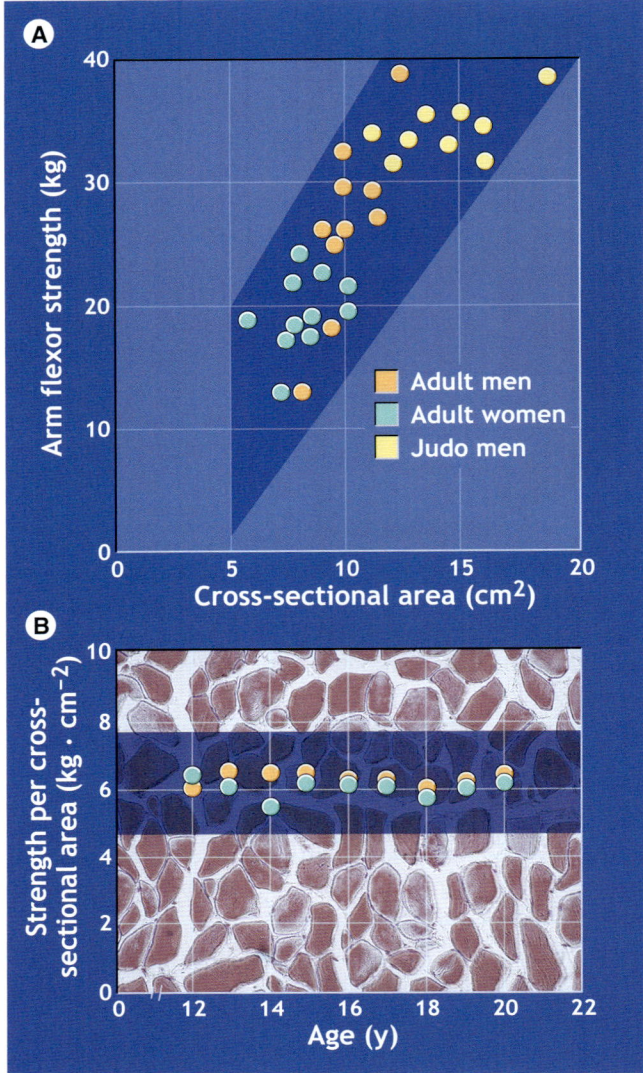

FIGURE 22.6. **(A)** Upper arm flexion strength variability in men and women related to the flexor muscle's total cross-sectional area. **(B)** Strength expressed per unit muscle cross-sectional area against a microscopic view of stained muscle fiber architecture. (Adapted with permission from Ikai M, Fukunaga T. Calculation of muscle strength per unit cross-sectional area of human muscle by means of ultrasonic measurements. Internationale Zeitschrift für angewandte Physiologie einschließlich Arbeitsphysiologie. 1968;26:26. https://link.springer.com/article/10.1007/BF00696087 Background image: Choksawatdikorn/Shutterstock.)

body mass participated in the same weightlifting categories. **FIGURE 22.7** displays percentage differences between males and females in the same body mass categories during national championship competitions for the maximum weight lifted in the combined snatch and clean-and-jerk lifts. These comparisons do not "equate" or "adjust" performance scores based on well-documented gender differences in body composition. The six body weight categories shown in the inset table range from 52 to 82.5 kg/115 to 182 lb. The lighter-weight categories produced the smallest gender difference in strength, with the effect most pronounced in the heavier weight categories. Females with 75 kg and 82.5 kg/155 lb and 182 lb body mass can lift only about 60% of the maximum weight lifted by similar-weight male counterparts. This represents a more

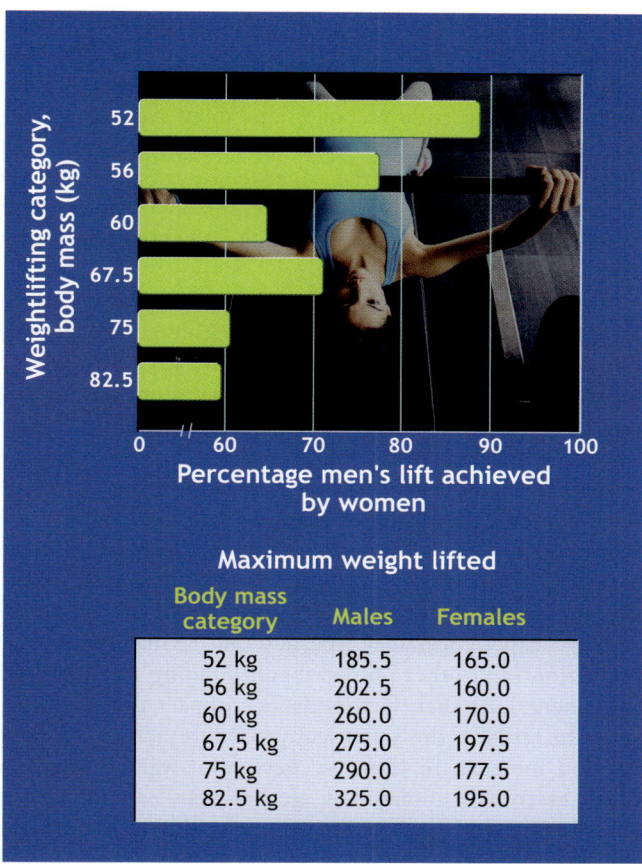

FIGURE 22.7. Difference in maximum weight lifted between males and females in the same body mass categories during a national weightlifting competition. The *inset box* shows the absolute weight lifted for each body mass category.
(Background image: ESB Professional/Shutterstock.)

pronounced gender difference than other comparisons that matched male and female competitors for body composition, chiefly body fat mass and fat-free body mass, not just body mass. In such comparisons, it is impossible to determine what role anabolic steroid use may have impacted gender strength differences.

Relative Muscle Strength Indexed to Body Composition

Relative strength comparisons among individuals involve creating a comparative ratio score by dividing a strength score by a reference measurement (i.e., body mass, FFM, MCSA, or limb volume or girth). In general, such strength ratio scores based on body mass or FFM considerably reduce if not eliminate the large absolute strength differences usually observed between genders.[39]

Consider the following example to determine who is stronger—a male weighing 95 kg/209 lb who bench-presses 114 kg/251 lb or a female weighing 60 kg/132 lb who bench-presses 62% less or 70 kg/154 lb. In absolute terms, the male is stronger. However, the bench-press score divided by body mass yields a much different conclusion. For the male, the strength ratio using the above scores equals 1.20, while the ratio for the female is 1.17—reducing the percentage difference to only 2.5% in bench-press strength! This alternative result would support the argument that little difference exists in muscle "quality" between males and females. Instead, any observed gender difference in absolute muscle strength would reflect differences in muscle quantity expressed by cross-sectional area. Males and females generally do not differ significantly in either upper- or lower-body strength when comparisons are made applying the ratio divisor FFM or MCSA.

We emphasize that this traditional ratio adjustment may not equalize females and males based on their underlying physiology. As with aerobic capacity discussed in Chapter 11, a fair way to evaluate a potential gender difference in a criterion muscular strength or aerobic capacity score includes several strategies:

1. Comparing males and females with similar training histories who do not differ in body size variables such as body mass or FFM
2. Adjusting for body size variables through appropriate statistical control

These two solutions rule out the need to create a ratio score because males and females in essence become equalized for body size and/or body composition. Using this approach, researchers assessed five muscular strength measures using 1-RM concentric muscle actions for bench press and squat and isokinetic dynamometry to assess maximum force during knee flexion and extension and seated shoulder press. **FIGURE 22.8** displays that matching males and females who had the same body mass created larger gender differences in the sedentary group (44% for shoul-

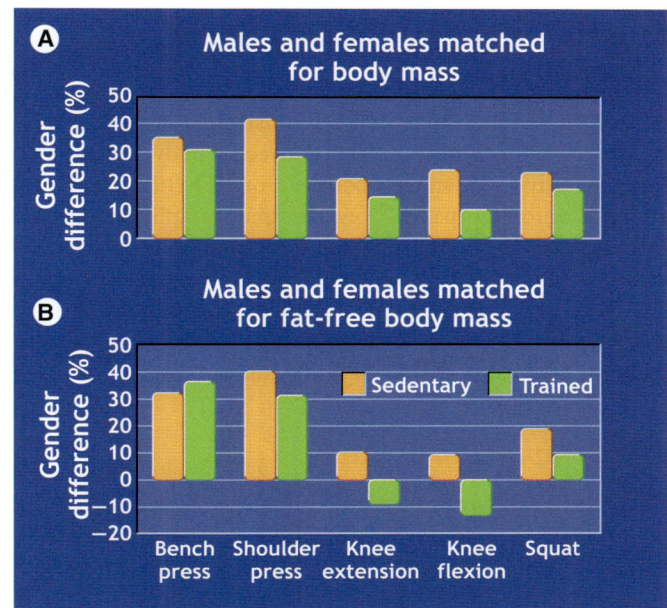

FIGURE 22.8. Five measures of muscular strength for males and females matched for **(A)** body mass and **(B)** fat-free body mass. Above the zero line indicates the percentage by which values for males exceed values for females.
(Data from Dr. Betsy Keller. Unpublished doctoral dissertation, University of Massachusetts, Amherst, 1989.)

ders and 25% for knee flexion) than in the trained group (33% for bench press and 11% for knee flexion). Values above the zero line show the percentage that male values exceed female values. These differences decreased but were not eliminated for both groups by matching subjects for FFM. The shoulder press (39%) and bench press (31%) produced the largest gender differences in the sedentary group, while the corresponding differences for the trained group were 31% (shoulder press) and 35% (bench press). These results differ from prior studies that used the traditional ratio score approach to express male and female strength differences.

Without doubt, ratio scoring supports the argument that few gender differences exist in muscle quality assessed by voluntary force output capacity. In contrast, matching males and females for body size, body composition, and training status before testing yields higher upper- and lower-body strength scores for males.[182] In a study with 2061 male and 1301 female military personnel, mean lift capacity averaged 51% greater in men despite a regression, ratio, or exponential mathematical adjustment in the strength score based on interindividual FFM differences.

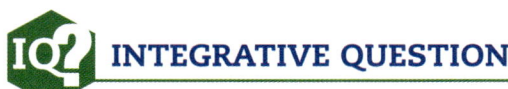

INTEGRATIVE QUESTION

Based on gender-related differences in physical fitness components, what are physical tests that minimize and maximize performance differences between males and females?

Muscle Strength Indexed Using Allometric Scaling

Allometric scaling represents a sophisticated statistical procedure to establish relationships between a body size variable (usually body mass, stature, body fat, or FFM) and muscular strength, aerobic capacity, power output, jumping height, or running speed.[24,55,207,269–271] The adjustment procedure evaluates the relative contribution that diverse independent variables such as gender, maturation, and habitual physical activity contribute to the dependent measure, for example, muscular strength, $\dot{V}O_{2max}$, or pulmonary function variables.

The Comparison Solution

Who is the strongest man and woman in the world, and by how much? If just total weight lifted remains the standard, then obviously the person who lifted the greatest weight would win the title as "strongest." In another approach, if the lifters compete in different flyweight to super heavyweight categories, the strongest person would be the person within the subgroup who lifted the most weight. The above seems reasonable, and indeed, local, national, international weight lifting, and World Master's competitions use some category system to group competitors within a pre-established weight category in the 1980 Rome Olympic competition displayed in **FIGURE 22.9** for the 10 competitive groups. Exercise physiologists have then posed several questions about such open competitions. Is it fair to compare a 23-year old competitor with a 41-year old competitor in the same weight category? Is there an advantage for the 23-year old presumably based on their higher lean body mass and lower body fat content, or greater upper arm MCSA?

It seems intuitive that both age and body composition variables might bias against the older athlete, favoring the younger counterpart. But then one could ask, "Would the older athlete have greater neuromuscular coordination and timing to perform the lifts due to their training and competitive experiences?" Furthermore, would a larger percentage in one fiber type in the shoulder, chest, and thigh musculature confer a performance advantage or disadvantage for either athlete? The allometric scaling method attempts to create a "level playing field" by statistically adjusting whatever conferred advantage or disadvantage there might be from age, experience, fiber type, and muscle maximum force production (and other potential confounding physiological components), so such factors do not impact the final outcome. In essence, the statistical procedure allows the final criterion measure, in this case maximum weight lifted, to remain essentially unbiased by age, body fat, lean body mass, muscle cross-section and force output production, or muscle fiber type.

Neutralizing competing influences creates the level playing field using an adjusted weight lifted value, uninfluenced by those confounding factors. This same logic also applies to 5 km to marathon or ultramarathon runs using an age-adjusted run score[293] (i.e., removing age from the time to run a given distance). The age standard "best" would then be defined as "what is the fastest possible time someone can run a given distance?" This would negate the aging effect, where a 21-year-old should have a clear advantage over a 55-year-old runner because the 21-year-old would surely cover the distance in a faster time. For the marathon and 5 km run, this question was answered affirmatively when allometric scaling was applied to all world records in these races—younger runners' clear advantage was neutralized, and it was possible to determine which runners covered the distance faster without the natural advantage favoring younger runners!

In applying allometric scaling in the athletic world, many organizations (https://more.arrs.run; www.nyrr.org/tcsnyc-marathon), including the world Master's Athletics organization (https://world-masters-athletics.com), use statistically adjusted performance scores for different age athletes within a sporting category www.howardgrubb.co.uk/athletics/wmalookup15.html). In the marathon, where official results are available for each integer age from 5 to 92 years for females and 5 to 93 years for males,[273] some researchers use this statistical technique to determine the fastest age-adjusted marathon world records.[275–277] by including a body weight adjustment to compare performance by age and body weight within the specific sex classification. These methods identify

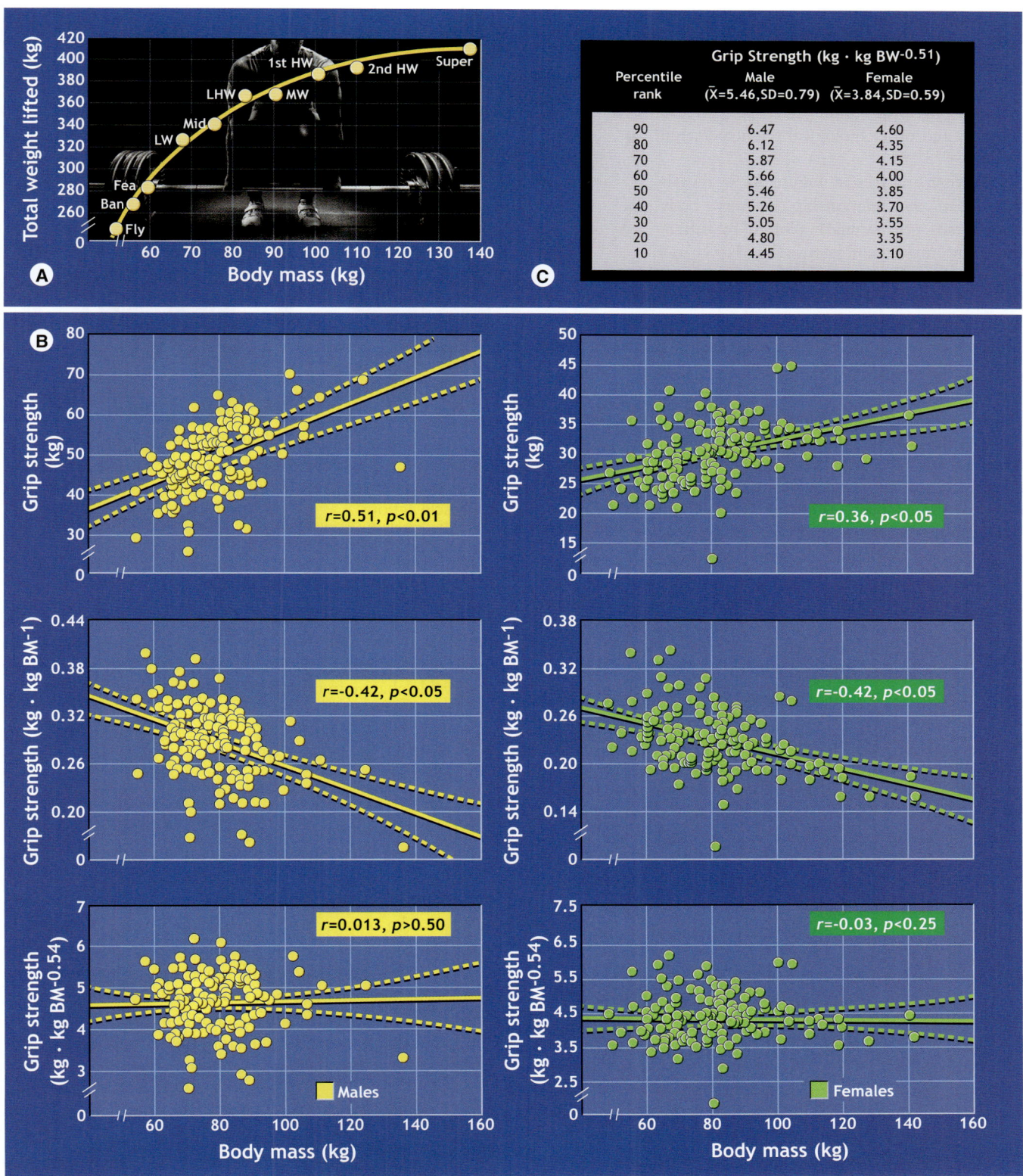

FIGURE 22.9. Relationship between body mass and different expressions for muscular strength. **(A)** Total weight lifted in two Olympic events (1980 Rome Olympic Games) as a function of body mass. Each data point represents the body mass for the top six male finishers in these weight categories: *Fly*, flyweight; *Ban*, bantamweight; *Fea*, featherweight; *LW*, lightweight; *Mid*, middleweight; *LHW*, light-heavyweight; *MW*, middle-heavyweight; *1st HW*, first heavyweight; *2nd HW*, second heavyweight; and *Super*, superheavyweight. **(B)** Maximal absolute grip strength, relative grip strength, and strength scaled allometrically to body mass in 100 college age males (*yellow*) and 105 females (*green*). **(C)** Percentile norms for grip strength scaled to body mass. (Adapted with permission from Lathan and cited by Titel K, Wutscherk H. In: Komi PV, ed. *Strength and Power in Sport*. Oxford, UK: Wiley-Blackwell; 1993. Permission conveyed through Copyright Clearance Center, Inc. Data in **(B)** from Dr. Paul Vanderburgh, University of Dayton. Background photo: Andy Gin/Shutterstock.)

the fastest runners in a particular running event by age, and explore upper limits by age for human endurance race performance.[272,274,278,301] Allometric scaling embodies a well-accepted and valid statistical approach in sports physiology and exercise performance domains and other biological science disciplines.[122,167,238–241,269–278]

Further analyses in Figure 22.9 reveals that when the relationship between body mass versus grip strength plotted by different body mass expressions (kg, kg·kg$_{BM}^{-1}$, and kg·kg$_{BM}^{-0.54}$) for two Olympic weightlifting events during the 1980 Rome Olympic Games. Such "older" data have withstood the test of time as contemporary assessments support these classic analytics. The top left graph in **A** for the Olympic weightlifters plots total weight lifted versus body mass. Each point represents body mass for the top weightlifters by weight category. Importantly, total weight lifted and body mass do not relate linearly but curvilinearly. Weightlifting strength relates proportionally to body mass raised to the exponent 0.7 (the line's slope). The bottom six curves in **B** for college-age males (*yellow*) and females (*green*) depict the relationship between maximum grip strength and body mass. The top graphs illustrate the simple relationship between body mass and grip strength without the body size adjustment. A positive relationship emerges ($r = 0.51$ for males and $r = 0.33$ for females). The middle graphs depict the relationship with grip strength indexed to body mass (i.e., strength divided by body mass in kg). The bottom graphs illustrate the relationship between strength and the allometric scaling with body mass. The resulting strength and body mass correlations with appropriate allometric scaling fall essentially to zero ($r = 0.013$ for males and $r = 0.03$ for females). This satisfies a basic allometric principle—the correlation between the scaled variable (muscular strength) and the scaling factor (body mass) must essentially equal zero. The inset table **C** presents percentile norms for college-age males and females for grip strength adjusted to the allometrically scaled 0.51 body mass exponent (kg·kg$_{BM}^{-0.54}$).

Training Muscles to Become Stronger

A muscle strengthens when trained near its current maximum force-generating capacity. Standard weightlifting equipment, pulleys or springs, immovable bars, resistance bands, or various isokinetic, air pressure, and hydraulic devices and electronic instruments provide effective muscle overload. Importantly, overload intensity (muscle's tension level), not the device type that applies the overload, generally governs strength improvements. Some training approaches lend themselves to precise and systematic overload applications. **Progressive-resistance weight training**, **isometric training**, and **isokinetic training** represent three common and valid muscle training systems to enhance muscular strength. These systems rely on shortening or concentric, lengthening or eccentric (where muscle maintains tension as muscle lengthens), and static or isometric muscle actions, the basic muscle actions illustrated in **FIGURE 22.10A AND B**.

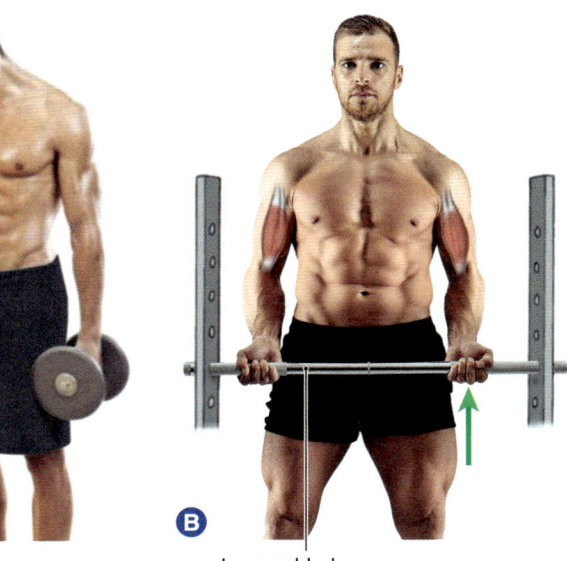

FIGURE 22.10. **(A)** Muscle force generated during concentric muscle actions (shortening; up *green arrows*) and eccentric (lengthening; down *green arrows*). **(B)** Isometric (static) muscle actions.
(Photos: **A**, mihailomilovanovic/iStockphoto; **B**, Slatan/Shutterstock.)

Different Muscle Actions

Neurally stimulating a muscle causes the fiber's contractile elements to shorten along the longitudinal axis. The terms *isometric* and *static* describe muscle activation without any observable change in muscle fiber length.

 See the animation "Muscle Contraction Type" on Lippincott Connect to view these contraction types.

Isometric action (Fig. 22.10B): An isometric action occurs when a muscle generates force and attempts to shorten but cannot overcome the external resistance. From a physics standpoint, this static muscle action does not produce external work. An isometric action does, however, generate considerable force despite the muscle sarcomeres' observable lengthening or shortening and subsequent joint movement. Near-sustained isometric-type muscle actions occur in surfing, kite boarding and wind surfing, alpine ski racing, snowmobiling, bobsleigh, luge, and skeleton, the latter requiring prolonged, static posture during the approximately 1 min race duration while reaching 80 mph/130 kmh lying face down and facing forward without steering or breaking mechanism. This activity requires intense near-maximum isometric muscle actions following the push-off to the finish (www.youtube.com/watch?v=LrOJzowQotw).

Dainis Derics/Shutterstock

A *dynamic* muscle action produces movement usually in the trunk or upper or lower limbs. Concentric and eccentric actions represent two dynamic muscle action types (Fig. 22.10A).

Concentric action: As tension develops, the muscle shortens to produce joint movement. The example shows raising a dumbbell from the extended to the flexed elbow position.

Eccentric action: The muscle lengthens while developing tension. The weight slowly lowers and resists gravity's force. The sarcomeres in the activated muscle's upper arm fibers lengthen eccentrically to prevent the dumbbell from crashing to the surface. In weightlifting, muscles frequently act eccentrically as the weight slowly returns to the starting position to begin the next concentric (shortening) muscle action. Eccentric action during this "recovery" phase adds to exercise repetition effectiveness and thus total work performed. Some "old-time" coaches and trainers still refer to such muscle actions as isotonic, derived from the Greek word *isotonos* (*iso* meaning "the same" or "equal," *tonos* meaning "tension" or "strain"), because concentric and eccentric muscle actions produce movement with a constant resistance. Nevertheless, the term *isotonic* lacks precision when applied to dynamic muscle actions owing to the muscle's ever changing effective force-generating capacity as joint angles change throughout the ROM.

Resistance Training

Raising and lowering an external weight represents the most popular resistance-training mode. Invariably, the weight lifted remains constant (e.g., raising and lowering a 20-kg/44 lb barbell), yet the force generated within the muscle differs as the joint angles change throughout the ROM. This general training application describes **dynamic constant external resistance (DCER) training**. By appropriately and progressively manipulating **training volume**, intensity, and frequency to optimize dose response, DCER selectively strengthens specific muscles to overcome a fixed initial or changing resistance. This resistance typically involves a barbell, kettlebell, dumbbell, or weight plates on a pulley- or cam-type machine.

As with cardiovascular training, muscular strength improvements vary inversely on a continuum with initial training status (less strong individuals experience more improvement than those with greater initial strength). Generally, improvements average 40% for the untrained, 20% in the moderately trained, 15% in the trained, and 10% in the advanced. Only 2% improvements occur in elite, world-class athletes who consistently achieve at the highest competition levels, but comparatively small improvements often produce world record results.[4]

Progressive Resistance Exercise

Progressive resistance exercise (PRE) training provides a practical application about the **overload principle** and forms the basis for most resistance-training programs begun by physical therapists in a rehabilitation hospital in the late 1940s and early 1950s. They devised weight-training regimens to improve the muscular strength in previously injured soldiers returning from World War II. The then "novel" procedure incorporated three exercise sets, each set with 10 repetitions performed continuously. The first set required one half the maximum weight that could be lifted 10 times, or ½ 10-RM; the second set used ¾ 10-RM, and the final 10-RM required maximum weight. As patients trained, the exercised limb muscles became substantially stronger, so the 10-RM resistance was increased periodically to maintain continued strength improvements. Similar improvements occurred even when reversing the intensity progression, so that patients performed the 10-RM as the first set.

PRE Variations

Research has established the optimal number sets and repetitions, including PRE frequency and relative training intensity for optimal strength improvement:

1. Eight- to 12-RM proves effective in novice training, whereas 1- to 12-RM effectively loads for intermediate training, which then increases to more intense loading using 1- to 6-RM.
2. Rest 3 min between exercise sets at moderate movement velocity (1 to 2 s concentric; 1 to 2 s eccentric).
3. For PRE at a specific RM load, increase load 2 to 10% when performing 1 to 2 repetitions above the current workload.
4. Performing one exercise set induces only slightly less strength improvement in recreational weightlifters than performing two or three sets.[38,97]
5. To maximize muscle strength and size gains, higher volume, multiple-set routines emphasizing 6- to 12-RM at moderate velocity with 1- to 2-min rests between sets prove most effective.
6. Single-set programs generally produce the most health and fitness benefits. These "lower-volume" programs also produce greater compliance and reduce financial cost and time commitment.
7. Novices and intermediates should train 2 to 3 d·wk^{-1}, with advanced training boosted to 3 to 4 d·wk^{-1}. The potential downside for greater training frequency extends the transient activation of inflammatory signaling cascades, concomitant with persistently suppressing key anabolic response mediators to blunt a training response.[48]
8. Training twice every other day produces overall superior results compared with daily training,[94] possibly from lowered muscle glycogen content (with training twice every second day) on enhanced gene transcription involved in training adaptations.[216,322]
9. Training with multiple exercises 4 or 5 d·wk^{-1} may produce less improvement than training 2 to 3 d·wk^{-1} because near-daily training impairs muscle recuperation between training sessions.
10. In general, inadequate recovery retards progress in neuromuscular and structural adaptations and subsequent strength development.
11. Fast movement speeds at a given resistance generate more strength improvement than moving at slower speeds.

Neither free weights (barbells, weight plates, dumbbells, kettlebells) nor exercise machines offer inherent superiority for developing muscle strength.

12. Workouts should be sequenced to optimize quality by engaging large before small muscle groups, multiple-joint exercises before single-joint exercises, and higher-intensity exercise before lower-intensity exercise.
13. Combined resistance-training concentric and eccentric muscle actions augment the program's effectiveness, include both single-joint and multiple-joint exercises to enhance a muscle's potential to improve strength and fiber size.[50,118,195,210,229]
14. Overload training that includes eccentric muscle actions preserves strength gains better during a maintenance phase than concentric-only training.[50]
15. Power training should apply a strategy to improve muscular strength (relatively heavy loads) plus include lighter loads (30 to 60% 1-RM) performed at fast contraction velocities.
16. In power training, use 2- to 3 min rest intervals between sets. Emphasize multiple-joint movements that activate larger muscle groups.[319]

Periodization

In 1972, Russian scientist **Leonid Matveyev** (1941-) introduced the *strength-training periodization* concept or sequential training planning[155] incorporated in novice and champion athlete's training regimens.[32,117,133,255] Conceptually, *periodization varies training intensity and volume to ensure that peak performance coincides with major competitions, typically at the competitive season conclusion*. It also proves to be effective in achieving recreational and rehabilitative goals. Periodization subdivides a resistance-training period such as 1 year (*macrocycle*) into smaller periods or phases (*mesocycles*), with each mesocycle again separated into weekly *microcycles*. In essence, the training model progressively decreases training volume and increases intensity as program duration progresses to maximize gains in muscular strength and power. Fractionating the macrocycle into components allows multiple ways to prevent overtraining by manipulating training intensity, volume, frequency, sets, repetitions, and inactive (rest) periods. It also provides a strategy to alter workout variety. Periodization variation can reduce negative overtraining or "staleness" effects so athletes achieve peak performance at competition. **FIGURE 22.11** depicts generalized periodization for a typical macrocycle's four distinct phases, which in turn separate into weekly microcycles. As competition approaches, training volume gradually decreases, while training intensity concurrently increases. Consider the following four phases:

Phase 1. Preparation phase emphasizes modest strength development with *high-volume* (3 to 5 sets, 8 to 12 reps), *low-intensity* workouts (50 to 80% 1-RM plus flexibility and aerobic and anaerobic training).

Phase 2. First transition phase emphasizes strength development with *moderate* workout *volume* (3 to 5 sets, 5 to 6 reps) and *moderate intensity* (80 to 90% 1-RM plus flexibility and interval aerobic training).

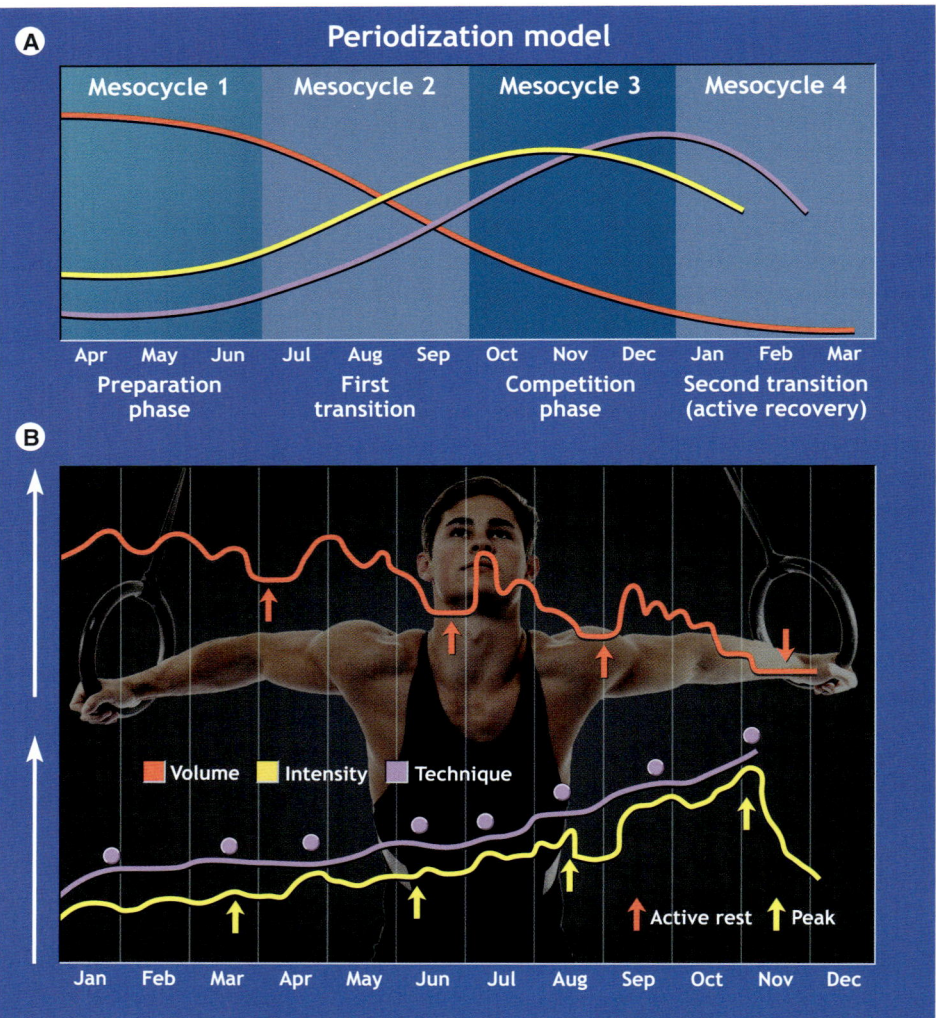

FIGURE 22.11. **(A)** Periodization subdivides a macrocycle into distinct phases or mesocycles. These in turn separate into weekly microcycles. **(B)** Example periodization schedule specifying how volume (*red*), intensity (*yellow*), and technique (*purple*) merge, with the up red arrows denoting "active" rest periods for a college gymnast achieving peak performance at the end of each macrocycle.

(Photo: Nicholas Piccillo/Shutterstock.)

Phase 3. Competition phase strives to achieve a peak for competition, emphasizing selective strength development with *low-volume*, *high-intensity* workouts (3 to 5 sets, 2 to 4 reps at 90 to 95% 1-RM), with short interval, sport-specific movement training.

Phase 4. Second transition phase (active recovery) emphasizes recreational activities and low-intensity workouts that incorporate different activity modes. For the upcoming competition, the athlete repeats the periodization cycle.

Periodization structures an inverse association between training volume and training intensity through the competition phase, which then decreases during the second transition or recuperation period. Note the increase in time devoted to technique training as competition approaches, with training volume at the periodization cycle's lowest point. The bottom in Figure 22.11 illustrates how a Division 1 collegiate gymnast's training volume (*red*), intensity (*yellow*), and technique (*purple*) merge within a mesocycle. Competitions took place throughout the yearly training program to achieve peak performance at each macrocycle's completion. In general, periodization places training into context for strength–power workout intensity, duration, and frequency. The major focus attempts to avoid overtraining (staleness), minimize injury potential, and reduce training monotony, while progressing toward peak competition performance (filled purple circles).

Sport-specific training principles and movement patterns usually apply in periodization to design a training regimen based on a sport's distinct *strength*, *power*, and *endurance* and movement pattern requirements. A detailed metabolic and sport-specific technical requirement analysis also frames the training paradigm. The periodization concept makes intuitive sense, yet limited data exist to verify this training approach's superiority. Several authors questions whether periodized resistance training even is a necessary prerequisite to maximize skeletal muscle hypertrophy beyond nonperiodized programs.[288,]

Researchers have evaluated shorter mesocycles to determine what factors optimize performance improvements. One study that equated training volume and intensity among three approaches to periodization (linear periodization, undulating periodization, and a nonperiodized time interval) found each training method equally effective.[16] The training groups made similar gains in muscular strength (25% squat, 13.1% bench press) and muscular power (7.6% vertical jump). It is not possible to evaluate differences in training effects reported previously without equating training volume and intensity.[225]

Critically reviewing strength training studies concludes that periodization produces greater improvements in muscular strength, body mass, and FFM, and reduced body fat percentage than nonperiodized multiset and single-set training regimens.[77] Additional research must assess how periodization interacts with fitness status,[172] age and gender,[61] and specific motor performance.[184,187] Studies must equate participants on various fitness parameters and then manipulate different linear and nonlinear training protocols to account for factors that impact training response.[286,287] In essence, program evaluation must consider the following four factors either singly or in combination:

1. Biomechanical and motor control sequences in the targeted sport skill
2. Changes in segmental and whole-body composition
3. Biochemical and ultrastructural tissue adaptations
4. How newly acquired strength transfers to subsequent sport performance

Resistance Training Guidelines for Health Enhancement and Disease Prevention

The American College of Sports Medicine (www.acsm.org), American Heart Association (www.americanheart.org), Centers for Disease Control and Prevention (www.cdc.gov), American Association of Cardiovascular and Pulmonary Rehabilitation (www.aacvpr.org), and the US Surgeon General's Office (www.surgeongeneral.gov) currently consider regular resistance exercise an important component in comprehensive, health-related physical fitness programs.[3,78,192] Resistance training goals for competitive athletes focus on optimizing muscular strength, power, and hypertrophy (high-intensity with 1-RM to 6-RM training loads).

Goals for most middle-age and older adults focus on maintenance and a possible increase in muscle and bone mass and muscular strength and **muscular endurance** to enhance the overall health and physical fitness profile. Adequate muscular strength in midlife maintains a safety margin above a threshold to prevent later-life injuries.[28] Among 45- to 68-year-old men, hand grip strength accurately predicted functional limitations and disability 25 years later.[194] Men in the lowest one-third for grip strength showed the greatest risk; those in the middle one-third showed intermediate risk; and men in the top one-third experienced the least disability risk at the 25-year follow-up. The resistance-training program recommended for middle-age and older males and females classifies as "moderate intensity." In contrast to the multiple-set, heavy-resistance approach used by younger athletes, the more moderate program uses single sets of diverse exercises performed between 8- and 15-RM at least twice weekly. The ACSM's Position Stand summarizes current resistance training guidelines for different population groups (https://journals.lww.com/acsm-msse/Fulltext/2011/07000/Quantity_and_Quality_of_Exercise_for_Developing.26.aspx).

Does Resistance Training Plus Aerobic Training Equal Less Strength Improvement?

Research has assessed whether concurrent resistance and aerobic training affects muscular strength and power improvement more than training for strength only.[15,21,132,161,259] This has caused many strength and power athletes and bodybuilders to refrain from including endurance activities in the belief they diminish strength and structural improvements. Advocates for abstaining from aerobic training maintain that the added energy and enhanced protein demands with intense endurance training may limit a muscle's growth and metabolic responsiveness to resistance training. Some data

> ### Concurrent Resistance Exercise Following Endurance Activity Enhances Skeletal Muscle Mitochondrial Biogenesis
>
>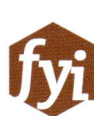
>
> Research tested the hypothesis whether concurrent resistance exercise following endurance exercise augments skeletal muscle mitochondrial biogenesis. Muscle biopsies obtained before and after either endurance exercise only (1 hr cycling at approximately 65% $\dot{V}O_{2max}$) or endurance exercise followed by resistance exercise (6 leg press sets at 70 to 80% 1-RM) with mRNA gene analysis associated with muscle biogenesis and substrate regulation. The mRNA gene prepares a transcripted molecule prior to protein synthesis. Resistance exercise following endurance exercise *amplified* the mitochondrial biogenesis adaptive signaling response compared with single-mode endurance exercise, suggesting that these concurrent training modes benefited muscle oxidative capacity adaptations. Recent endurance training experiments confirm that the mitochondrial fission regulator dynamin and the protein signaling mechanism (Drp1) regulates skeletal muscle function training adaptations, including mitochondrial fragmentation control during apoptosis or programmed cell death.
>
> 3d_man/Shutterstock
>
> **Sources:**
>
> Moore TM, et al. The impact of exercise on mitochondrial dynamics and the role of Drp1 in exercise performance and training adaptations in skeletal muscle. *Mol Metab*. 2019;21:51.
>
> Wang L, et al. Resistance exercise enhances the molecular signaling of mitochondrial biogenesis induced by endurance exercise in human skeletal muscle. *J Appl Physiol*. 2011;111:1335.

support this position. For example, different exercise modes induce antagonistic molecular level, intracellular signaling mechanisms, which may negatively impact a muscle's adaptive responses to resistance training.[177,316] Endurance training also may inhibit signaling to the muscles' protein synthesis machinery, which would definitely be counterproductive to resistance training goals.[27,126,147,260] Brief but intense endurance activity also inhibits performance in subsequent muscular strength activities.[144,185] These findings should not deter the general public from incorporating *both* training modes to achieve a well-rounded conditioning program for overall fitness and health.

Resistance Training for Children

One obvious concern about resistance training in preadolescence regards the injury potential from excessive musculoskeletal loading that includes epiphyseal fractures, ruptured intervertebral disks, lower back bony disruptions, and acute lower back trauma. A child's hormonal profile also lacks full development—particularly the tissue-building hormone testosterone (refer to Chapter 20). One might question whether resistance training in children could even induce meaningful strength improvements.

Supervised resistance training using concentric-only muscle actions with relatively high repetitions and low resistance improves children and adolescents' muscular strength without adversely affecting bone, muscle, or connective tissue.[189] This includes children with disabilities and disease[30,80,125,290] and obesity.[59,66] More than likely, a true learning phase and enhanced neuromuscular activation rather than substantial increases in muscle size account for children's relatively rapid strength improvements. Many national organizations have provided resistance training guidelines for children age 7 and younger and older than 16 (www.heart.org/en/healthy-living/fitness/fitness-basics/aha-recs-for-physical-activity-in-adults; www.cdc.gov/healthyschools/physicalactivity/guidelines.htm; https://health.gov/our-work/physical-activity; www.cdc.gov/physicalactivity/basics/children/index.htm). If children at any age begin a strength training program without prior experience, they should begin at lower levels and advance progressively considering adaptations for exercise tolerance, skill, and training intensity and duration.

Isometric Strength Training

Research in Germany during the mid-1950s showed that isometric strength increased about 5% weekly by performing a daily single, only 1 s duration maximum isometric muscle action, or a 6-s action at two-thirds maximum.[106] Repeating this action 5 to 10 times daily produced the greatest gains in isometric strength.

Isometric Training Limitations

Isometric exercise provides muscle overload and improves strength yet offers limited functional sports training benefits. Without movement, one cannot readily evaluate the overload level and/or training progress. Isometric strength development promotes considerable muscle specificity adaptations. A muscle trained isometrically clearly improves strength when the muscle acts isometrically, particularly at the training joint angle and body position. This means that isometric training to develop "strengths" for a particular movement probably necessitates training at many specific angles through the ROM. This becomes time-consuming and impractical considering conventional dynamic weight training and other functional resistance training methods.

Isometric Training Benefits

Isometric techniques help in muscle testing and rehabilitation. Isometric methods can detect specific muscle weakness at a particular ROM, thus optimizing muscle overload at the appropriate joint angle.

Six Neural Adaptations with Strength Gains

- Enhanced neural recruitment pattern efficiency
- Augmented motor neuron excitability
- Heightened central nervous system activation
- Enriched motor unit synchronization and increased firing rates
- Downgraded neural inhibitory reflexes
- Inhibited autogenic Golgi tendon organ reflexes that regulate muscle contraction force

Which Strength Training Method Is Better: Static or Dynamic?

Static and dynamic resistance training methods each increase muscular "strength." An individual's specific needs determine the optimal resistance training method governed by training response specificity.[173,186,268]

Isometric Training Response Specificity

An isometrically trained muscle shows greatest strength improvement when measured isometrically; similarly, a dynamically trained muscle tests best when evaluated in resistance activities that require movement. Isometric strength developed at or near one joint angle does not readily transfer to other angles or body positions that use the same muscles.[252] In dynamic activities, muscles trained through movement over a limited ROM show the greatest strength improvement when measured in that ROM.[19,88] Even *body position specificity* exists; ankle plantar and dorsiflexor muscular strength developed in the standing position with concentric and eccentric muscle actions showed no transfer with the same muscles evaluated in the supine position.[193] Resistance training specificity makes sense because strength improvement blends two adaptive factors:

1. Inherent muscle fiber and connective tissue harness
2. Motor unit neural organization and excitability to power discrete voluntary movement patterns

A muscle's maximum force output depends on neural factors that recruit and synchronize motor unit firing, not just muscle fiber type and cross-sectional area. A 3-month study involving young adult males and females emphasized the highly specific nature regarding resistance-training adaptations.[68] One group trained the hand adductor pollicis muscle identified in isometrically with 10 daily 5-s duration actions at 1 per min frequency. The other group trained the same muscle dynamically with 10 daily 10-repetition bouts at one-third maximum strength. The untrained muscle served as the control. To eliminate any training influence from psychologic factors and central nervous system adaptations, a supermaximum electrical stimulation applied to the motor nerve evaluated the trained muscle's force capacity. The results were clear—both training groups improved maximum force capacity and peak force development rate. Maximum force improvement for the isometrically trained group nearly doubled the improvements for the dynamically trained group. Conversely, improvement in force development speed averaged about 70% greater in the dynamically trained group. This provided strong evidence that different resistance training modes did not induce all-inclusive *generalized* adaptations in muscle structure and function. Rather, the muscle's maximum force, shortening velocity, and tension development rate with specific training improve in a highly specific manner to the engaged muscle actions. Both static and dynamic training methods produce strength increases, yet no one system rates consistently superior to the other in how best to assess muscle function. The crucial consideration must assess the intended purpose attributed to newly acquired strength.

Practical Implications. The complex interaction between nervous and muscular systems helps to explain why leg muscles strengthened in squats or deep knee bends fail to show equivalent improved force capability in other leg movements requiring jumping or leg extension muscle activation. Low corelationships or statistical correlation coefficients typically occur among dynamic leg extension forces measured at any speed and vertical jumping height. *A muscle group strengthened and enlarged by dynamic resistance training does not demonstrate equal force capacity improvement when measured isometrically or isokinetically.* Strengthening muscles for golf, tennis, rowing, swimming, football, firefighting, or package handling on an assembly line demands more than just identifying and overloading the muscles primarily involved in the activity. *It requires neuromuscular training specifically in the crucial movements necessitating improved strength.* This training mode represents **functional strength training** or functional resistance movement training.[7,9,49] Increasing leg muscle "strength" through general weightlifting does not necessarily improve the same muscles' force-generating capacities activated in a different movement pattern.[160] *Newly acquired strength seldom transfers fully to other strength-type movements, even those that activate the same trained muscles.* A standard weight-training program for leg extension increased leg extension strength by 227%. Evaluating leg extension peak torque in the same leg with an isokinetic dynamometer detected only a 10 to 17% improvement![62,79] *To improve a specific physical performance*

SciePro/Shutterstock

through resistance training, one must train the muscle(s) in movements that mimic the movement requiring force–capacity improvement. This requires laser-focused attention on force, velocity, and power requirements and precise movement patterning rather than simply directing general attention to an isolated muscle action.

Testing Specificity in the Occupational Setting

A comprehensive review outlines physical test validation strategies for pre-employment occupational testing, which requires diverse physical abilities or specific fitness characteristics.[119] Physical performance and physiologic function specificity (e.g., muscular strength and power, joint flexibility, aerobic fitness) combined with specific training response patterns casts serious doubt that broad physical fitness constructs exist to any important extent. This means that no single measure exists to quantify overall muscular strength or aerobic fitness. Instead, an individual expresses many muscular strengths, powers, and aerobic "fitnesses." These muscle function and exercise performance expressions often relate poorly if at all (i.e., poor relationships among different specific fitness components). Likewise, testing someone for aerobic fitness produces different fitness scores depending on the activity mode. For example, it would be undesirable to administer the 12 min run test to assess aerobic capacity in the occupational setting to infer aerobic capacity for firefighting or lumbering (both requiring considerable upper-body aerobic function), or measuring static-grip or leg strength to assess functional dynamic strengths and powers required in these occupations.

Measurements applied in the occupational setting should closely resemble the actual job requirements (i.e., functional tests), not only for specific tasks but that mimics the job's intensity, duration, and pace (i.e., physiologic demands). If such "content testing" remains impractical, one must substantiate alternative testing based on carefully conducted validation studies.

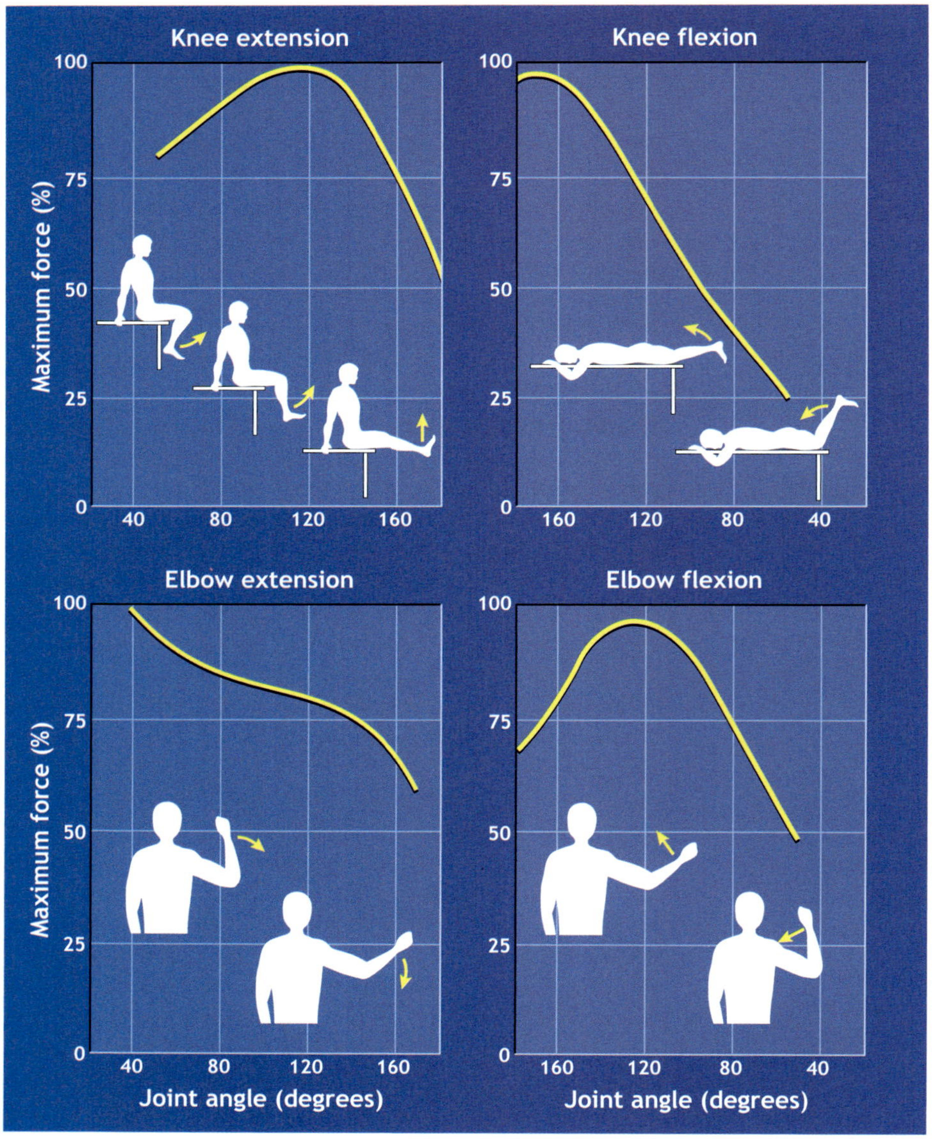

Isokinetic Resistance Training

Isokinetic resistance training combines positive features from isometric exercise and dynamic weightlifting to provide muscle overload at a constant preset speed while the muscle mobilizes force-generating capacity throughout the full ROM. Any effort during the movement encounters an opposing force to that applied to the mechanical device, which represents **accommodating-resistance exercise**. Isokinetic-type training typically targets the motor units to overload muscles consistently—even at relatively "weaker" joint angles throughout the ROM. Maintaining a constant movement speed remains a negative because normal functional-type exercises do not operate at fixed movement speeds.

Isokinetics Versus Standard Weightlifting

An important distinction exists between a muscle overloaded isokinetically and one overloaded using standard weights. **FIGURE 22.12** illustrates that a muscle or muscle groups' force capacity varies with the joint angle as the joint moves through its ROM at approximately 40 to 160° during concentric and 160 to 40° during eccentric movements. During weight training, the external weight lifted usually remains

FIGURE 22.12. Muscle force-generating capacity varies with joint angle throughout the ROM in knee extension and flexion (*top*) and elbow extension and flexion (*bottom*).

fixed at the greatest load to complete the movement. *Resistance cannot exceed the maximum force generated at the weakest point in the ROM.* If it did not, then one could not complete the movement. The term **"sticking point"** describes this ROM area.

Muscles activated during weightlifting do not generate the same absolute maximum force through all movement phases. For professional body builders and top athletes, this limitation requires the athlete to perform many exercise variations but with emphasis on different movement patterns. For the biceps dumbbell curl, for example, one exercise set might be done without supinating or pronating the hand that holds the weight. Another set might be done with alternating hand pronation or supination during the curl, while a third set might engage lateral upper-arm movements during the curling movement. These basic exercise variations target a different force-generating characteristic for the movement. Additional variations can include changes in movement speed—going from a controlled "slow" muscle action to moving rapidly with good form. The most obvious variation alters the weight lifted from light (lifted easily through the ROM) to a heavier lift that necessarily requires a slower movement rate. To reduce such variations, manufacturers have devised training equipment with variable resistance, which adjusts resistance with a particular joint movement's generalized lever characteristics. This equipment still represents a classic weightlifting mode except the *relative resistance* offered to the muscle theoretically remains fairly constant for muscle capacity at a specified shortening velocity in the ROM. With an isokinetically loaded muscle, the desired movement speed occurs almost instantaneously with maximum force application, allowing the muscle to generate peak power output throughout the ROM at a controlled shortening velocity.

Isokinetic Training Experiments

Experiments with isokinetic exercise have explored the force–velocity patterns in different movements related to muscle fiber type composition. **FIGURE 22.13** shows the progressive decline in knee extensor peak torque output with increasing angular velocity in power- and endurance-trained groups who differed in their training regimens and main muscle fiber type. The *dashed line* torque–velocity curves were extrapolated to the approximated maximum knee extension velocity. For movement at $180° \cdot s^{-1}$, maximum torque decrement averaged about 55% of maximum isometric ($0° \cdot s^{-1}$) force. The two curves differ in peak torque depending on the group's muscle fiber composition. Peak force at zero velocity (i.e., isometric force) remained similar for power athletes with relatively high fast-twitch muscle fiber percentages, or endurance athletes with predominantly slow-twitch muscle fibers. This analysis indicated that *both* fast and slow twitch motor units were activated in maximal isometric knee extension. As movement velocity increased, individuals with higher fast-twitch fiber percentages exerted greater torque per unit body mass. This highlights the biologic desirability to inherit predominantly fast-twitch fibers for discus, shot put, hammer, and javelin power activities, where success largely depends on generating considerable torque at the most rapid velocities while maintaining optimal biomechanical movement patterns.

Fast-Speed Versus Slow-Speed Isokinetic Training

Strength and power improvement with isokinetic training at slow and fast limb speeds support the specificity concept related to exercise performance and the training response. For example, strength and power gains from slow-speed isokinetic training relate to the specific angular movement velocity in training. In contrast, exercising at fast speeds facilitates more general improvement—power output increases at fast *and* slow movement speeds, with more improvement in fast angular training velocities.[191] Muscle hypertrophy generally occurs from fast-speed training and mainly in the fast-contracting muscle fibers.[53] Muscle **fiber hypertrophy** may explain the greater generality in strength improvement with fast-speed training. Concentric muscle actions produce greater power increases and concomitant type II fiber hypertrophy from training than eccentric training at equivalent relative power levels.[157]

Isokinetic training benefits include muscular overload through a full ROM at many shortening velocities. Nevertheless, applications to sports movements remain limited because the most rapid isokinetic dynamometer movement velocity approximates $400° \cdot s^{-1}$ where limb speeds in many sports are considerably greater. In professional baseball pitchers, where upper-limb extension velocity exceeds $2000° \cdot s^{-1}$, even the relatively "slow" hip rotators during a pitch move at $600° \cdot s^{-1}$.[35] Also, isokinetic dynamometers cannot simultaneously overload eccentric muscle actions that serve important functions in limb deceleration and "braking" control in normal movements.

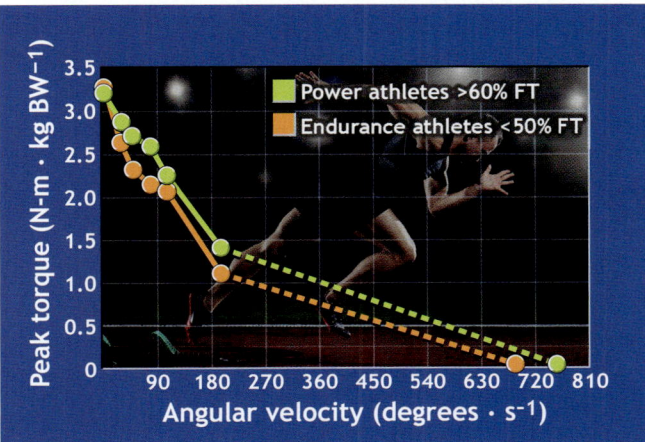

FIGURE 22.13. Peak torque per unit body mass versus joint movement angular velocity in two separate athletic groups with different muscle fiber type predominance.
(Adapted with permission from Thorstensson A. Muscle strength, fiber types, and enzyme activities in man. *Acta Physiol Scand.* 1976;443:1. Permission granted by John Wiley & Sons Books, conveyed through Copyright Clearance Center, Inc. Photo: dotshock/Shutterstock.)

Plyometric Training

For sports that require powerful, propulsive movements as in American football, soccer, volleyball, sprinting, high jump, long jump, and basketball, athletes routinely apply **plyometric training** or explosive jump training to maximize the greatest power outputs.[76,236,257] **Plyometric movements** require various jumps in place or rebound jumping (drop jumping from a preset height, as off a stool) to mobilize the skeletal muscle's inherent stretch–recoil characteristics and its modulation via the stretch or **myotatic reflex**. Plyometric movements involve rapid stretching followed by muscle shortening during a dynamic movement. Consider this analogy for plyometrics when you stretch a rubber band. The stretch within the band creates stored energy, which releases when the band returns to its initial "resting" or unstretched position. *Stretching within a muscle produces a "stretch reflex" and elastic recoil within the muscle.*[54] When combined with a vigorous muscle contraction, plyometric actions overload the muscle's force generating capacity, thereby increasing its absolute strength and power.[258] Plyometric training ranges in difficulty from calf jumps from the ground upward into the air to multiple one-leg jumps to and from boxes ranging in height from 1 foot to 6 ft.

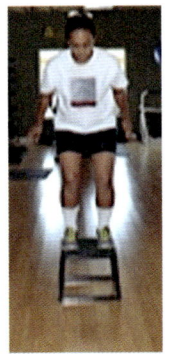

The basic principle for all jumping and plyometric exercises is to absorb the shock with the arms or legs and then immediately contract the muscles just prior to the next jump. When performing consecutive squat jumps, for example, the athlete jumps again into the air immediately after landing, while at the same time thrusting both heels up toward the buttocks. The athlete follows the same technique when jumping from a bench to the floor, followed by an explosive upward jump and thrusting the arms upward. Quicker jumps provide greater muscular overload. *In essence, "fast" dynamic plyometric movements "train" the nervous system and associated, specific musculature to respond quickly to activate and overload muscles to execute desired movement patterns.*

Plyometric maneuvers during a fast movement sustain maximum power production by not having to decelerate a resistance mass in the joint's ROM. **FIGURE 22.14** compares a traditional bench press movement to achieve maximum power output with a ballistic bench throw that maximizes power output by emphasizing that the hands thrust the barbell forcibly upward from the body. The results were unequivocal. During a standard bench press, deceleration begins at about 60% of the bar position relative to total concentric movement distance (*orange line*). In contrast, movement velocity during the bench throw (*yellow line*) continues to increase throughout the ROM and remains higher following the initial movement at all bar positions. This produces greater average force, average power, and peak power outputs. Achieving a faster average and peak velocity throughout the ROM produces greater power output and muscle activation than traditional free-weight lifting movements. The throw condition produced greater muscle activity assessed by EMG for the pectoralis major (+19%), anterior deltoid (+34%), triceps brachii (+44%), and biceps brachii (+27%).

Allowing an athlete to develop greater power at the end of a movement more closely simulates the projection phase when

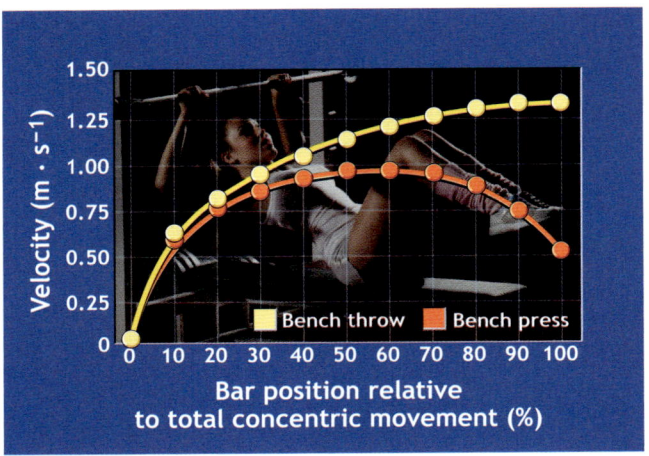

FIGURE 22.14. Mean bar velocity related to total concentric bar movement for bench throw and traditional bench press performed explosively.
(Data from Newton RU, et al. Kinematics, kinetics, and muscle activation during explosive upper-body movements. *J Appl Biomech*. 1996;12:31. Photo: Wallenrock/Shutterstock.)

throwing a baseball, shot put, javelin, or other object, maximum effort jumping movements, impact in striking movements when a golf club contacts the golf ball during forceful, downward arm movements, or in fast, alternate kicking and punching actions when striking a stationary, 32 to 68 kg/70 to 150 lb professional heavy punching bag. Other sports performance examples include overhead soccer throw, push away vigorously from the pole in the pole vault, takeoff jump for a volleyball spike, positioning and jumping for a basketball rebound, and the takeoff in the high jump. In **ballistic resistance training** for these actions, the person moves the object or weight at the fastest possible speed attempting to produce maximum muscular force before releasing it.

Plyometric movement overloads a muscle to provide forcible and rapid stretch (eccentric or stretch phase) immediately before the concentric or shortening recoil phase. The **stretch-shortening cycle (SSC)** represents an important concept that describes how skeletal muscles efficiently function in unrestricted locomotor activities from soccer play,[170,261] to simple sprinting performance,[200] to simpler hopping with a single leg takeoff (or a double leg hop) and same leg landing (or both leg landing).

 View the animation "Stretch Shortening Cycle" on Lippincott Connect to see this process.

When muscle spindles in the gastrocnemius muscle suddenly stretch, their sensory receptors fire with impulses traveling through the dorsal root into the spinal cord to activate the anterior motor neurons and trigger the stretch reflex (see Chapter 19), with timing relying on movement speed.[4,116] The stretching and shortening sequence in muscle fibers, similar to the surface contact phase in running, serves a single purpose—to enhance the final push-off phase. In many sports situations, the rapid lengthening SSC phase produces a more powerful subsequent movement from two main factors[115,143,146,196]:

Factor 1. Attaining a higher active muscle state with enhanced potential energy before the concentric, shortening muscle action

Factor 2. Evoking stretch-induced segmental reflexes to potentiate subsequent muscle activation

These two beneficial effects positively impact the speed–power outcomes from this training mode.[248,262] Improvement likely occurs from *changes* in the muscle–tendon complex's mechanical properties rather than *changes per se* in muscle activation strategies.[135] **FIGURE 22.15** illustrates the sledge ergometer approach for plyometric stretch-shortening cycle exercise and training. The braking phase component and subsequent muscle stretch occurs prior to maximum leg and foot extensor muscle activation accomplished by this ergometer:

1. Quantifies muscle force-generating capacity when impacted by the SSC
2. Offers variety to create different objectives and protocols when training under such conditions
3. Evaluates stretch reflex sensitivity and muscle stiffness under fatiguing physical activity

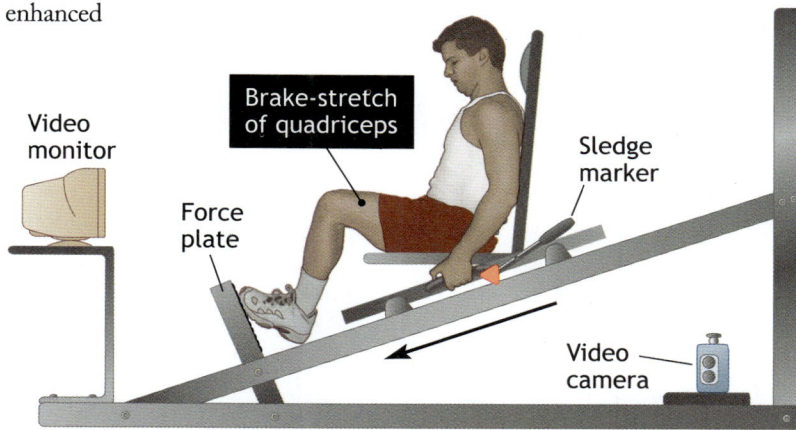

FIGURE 22.15. The sledge ergometer for plyometric (stretch-shortening cycle) exercise, training, and research protocols.
(Adapted with permission from Strojnik V, Komi PV. Fatigue after submaximal intensive stretch-shortening cycle exercise. *Med Sci Sports Exerc.* 2000;32:1314.)

Practical Applications of Plyometrics

A plyometric maneuver uses body mass and gravity for the important rapid SSC pre-stretch or "cocking" phase to activate the muscle's natural elastic recoil elements. Prior stretch augments the subsequent concentric muscle action in the opposite direction. Forcibly dropping the arms to the side before vertical jumping produces an eccentric quadriceps pre-stretch during a natural plyometric movement. Lower-body plyometric maneuvers include a standing jump, multiple jumps, repetitive jumping in place, depth jumps or drop jumping from a 1-m height, single- and double-leg jumps, and various modifications. Repetitive plyometric actions reinforce neuromuscular training to enhance specific muscles and sport-specific power output in jumping.[136,162,266]

Limited controlled experiments from such workouts have considered the benefits versus possible orthopedic risks. Concern for musculoskeletal injury stems partly from estimating that drop jumping generates external skeletal loads up to 10 times body mass. Research with children and older recreational athletes must quantify the appropriate role for plyometric drills in a strength–power training program, particularly during the initial exercise-training phase. A position paper from the National Strength and Conditioning Association (www.nsca-lift.org) suggests that athletes first achieve lifts equal to 1.5 times body weight in the squat exercise before initiating intense plyometric training.[258] An extensive literature review with 153 citations identified key elements for future pediatric youth resistance and plyometric training studies related to different training modes, optimal rest intervals and workout intensities, and maturational status influences.[279]

In **FIGURE 22.16**, plyometric rebound jump training in inset **A** occurs in 3 stages, with the Stage 3 objective to rebound upward following landing from the box. Inset **B** includes four plyometric exercise drills—box jump, cone hop, hurdle hop, and long jump. These routines use two different height boxes, a cone, and miniature hurdles employing polystyrene brick foam blocks or different height hurdles.

Body Weight–Loaded Training

Over the past several centuries, many body weight–loaded exercise systems were created in Europe and United States as a way to facilitate muscular strength acquisition. Over the last few decades, current methods utilize free weights, barbells, and kettlebells, mechanical systems to adjust the load, cams, suspended ropes, and pulleys. Currently, body weight–loaded training using **closed-kinetic chain exercise** to improve sports performance[26,149] has gained popularity and research support to enhance job-related functions[148] and treat pelvic pain following pregnancy.[224,225]

Historical Milestones. The Ling system referred to previously (see Introduction) relied on progressive exercises to strengthen total body musculature. Ling's Swedish system initiated more progressive sling **suspension training** beginning in the 1840s. Between 1914 and 1918, physiotherapists working in English hospitals and rehabilitation facilities during and after World War I developed more advanced suspension and sling

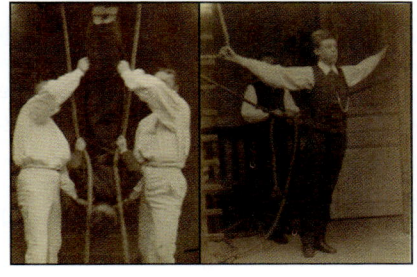

exercise and training methods. This was followed by Norwegian-pioneered sling suspension training methods developed in the early 1990s to complement traditional physical therapy applications, general strength development for athletes, and general and specific fitness training for the recreational participants and fitness-oriented public, and a rapidly expanding fitness industry.

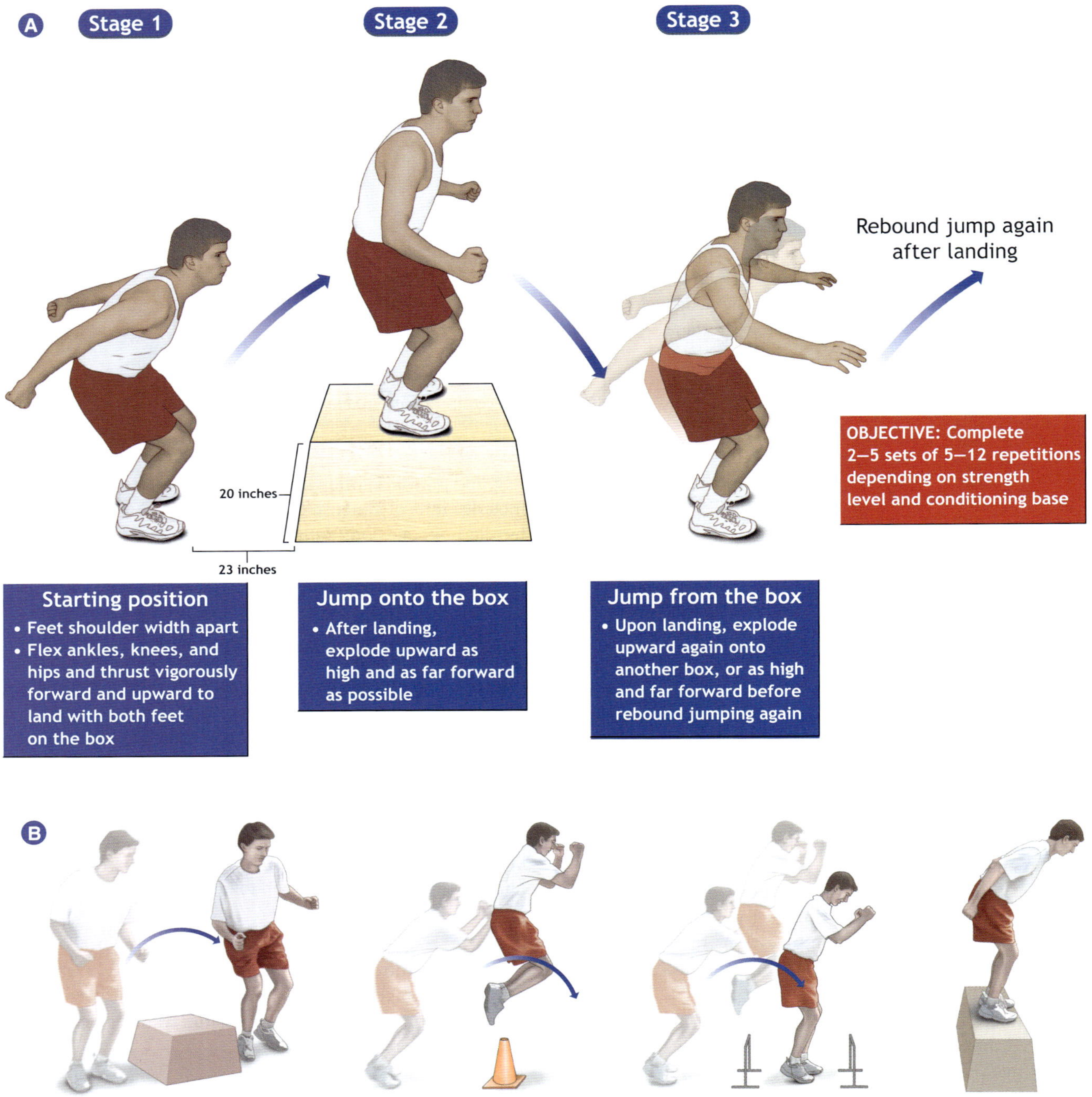

A

Stage 1 — Starting position
- Feet shoulder width apart
- Flex ankles, knees, and hips and thrust vigorously forward and upward to land with both feet on the box

Stage 2 — Jump onto the box
- After landing, explode upward as high and as far forward as possible

20 inches
23 inches

Stage 3 — Jump from the box
- Upon landing, explode upward again onto another box, or as high and far forward before rebound jumping again

Rebound jump again after landing

OBJECTIVE: Complete 2–5 sets of 5–12 repetitions depending on strength level and conditioning base

B

FIGURE 22.16. **(A)** Rebound jumping technique in plyometric training. **(B)** Four plyometric exercise jump examples: (1) box jump, (2) cone hop (3) hurdle hop, (4) box long jump.
(Jump examples courtesy Dr. Thomas D. Fahey, California State University at Chico.)

Sling Suspension Methods and Performance Improvements

Sling suspension methods leverage the person's body weight as resistance increases or decreases by altering the suspension coordinates, sling height, or body position. In weight-supported exercise, the distal segment bears the full or fractional body weight to activate both agonist and antagonist muscles about a joint and other muscle groups along the kinetic chain.[219] Such training is often considered more functional compared to exercises where the distal segment is non–weight bearing as in conventional weightlifting by activating agonists and synergists. In addition, body weight–loaded exercise with the sling-system apparatus introduces an added instability component to further

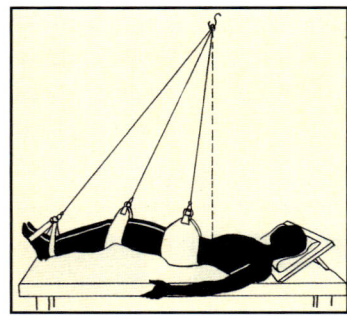

challenge trunk and back neuromuscular control.[220,234,237] Adding manual or mechanical external stimulation during movements with sling training may positively impact the sophisticated signaling patterns involved in neuromuscular control in simple and/or complex movements,[73,154,233,235] and during functional performance training for soccer,[223] golf,[205] team handball,[204] and softball.[206] Improved functional sport movements range from 3 to 5% in limb velocity movement, increased golf club head velocity and hence distance, and static and dynamic balance and shoulder stabilization.

Photo from V. Katch

Enhancing the Core Training Concept

Sports science professionals almost universally concur about the value in promoting "core training"—also referred to as lumbar stabilization, core strengthening, dynamic stabilization, neutral spine control, trunk stabilization, abdominal strength, core "pillar" training, and core-functional strength training.

The core concept does not refer to just the muscles that cross the body's midsection and form the "six-pack" abdominals commonly portrayed in social media advertising. Rather, the core represents a four-sided muscular frame with abdominal muscles in front, paraspinals, and gluteals in back, the diaphragm at the top, and the pelvic floor and hip girdle musculature framing the bottom. The three paraspinal or erector spinae muscle groups include the superficial iliocostalis, longissimus muscles, and the deep but vitally important multifidus muscle adjacent to the spinous process and lamina. A single nerve root innervates this important muscle group, which laterally flex and rotate the spine to the opposite side (www.physio-pedia.com/Lumbar_multifidus). Properly executed core stabilization exercises (as with kettlebells holding the plank position in the inset image) play an essential role in keeping the lower back "strong" to minimize a radiculopathy injury from weaker than desired paraspinal muscles (www.ncbi.nlm.nih.gov/pmc/articles/PMC3806175/; www.ncbi.nlm.nih.gov/pmc/articles/PMC8158512/pdf/ijerph-18-05400.pdf).

wavebreakmedia/Shutterstock

The core region includes 29 muscle pairs that hold the trunk steady, and balance and stabilize the spine, pelvis, thorax, and other bony structures along the kinetic chain that are activated during most movements.[89] The spine frame structures without adequate "strength and balance" can become mechanically unstable. A properly functioning core provides three musculoskeletal benefits[123,164]:

1. Appropriate force distribution along the muscle-joint axis for optimal movement control and efficiency
2. Adequate ground-impact force absorption
3. No excessive compressive, translational, and shearing forces on joints along the kinetic chain

Weakest Link Training and Rehabilitation

Weakest link training began with strength coaches and trainers in American professional football in the early 1970s and previously had been a serious rehabilitative method to assess quadriceps to hamstring "strength deficits" in top professional soccer players worldwide during the same time frame.[300,302,303] The Super Bowl and World Cup events played a major role in how trainers prepared athletes to remain injury free as they prepared for those events. Weakest link training coincided with newer computerized exercise machines applicable to the rehabilitative, therapy, and home market (e.g., see Biodex). Early mechanical devices interfaced with the first affordable Atari and Radio Shack personal computers, which when programmed, assessed the maximum force output and other dynamic muscle indicators through a muscle's ROM at different movement speeds and loads (https://cdn.macrosport.com/videos/01026/adi-vid-01026-revolution-256kbps.mp4).

Assessing Weakest Links. Consider weakest links for hamstrings and quadriceps in the lower leg regions. Each muscle group was assigned a numerical rating on a 10-point scale—from low scores ranging from 1 to 4 (poor strength)—to stronger strength rated 7 to 10. The basic idea was to identify the weakest links through computerized testing and devise training routines to improve the ratios between the weakest and stronger muscle groups.[315] For example, if an athlete scored poor in hamstring strength (rating score 3 based on the computer output score for force) but excellent in quadriceps strength (rating score 8), the hamstring-to-quadriceps ratio would be 3:8. The training objective would be to increase the weakest link rated 3 to a number closer to the higher link score of 8. Following training, the ratio between hamstring-to-quadriceps would typically improve from a 3:8 ratio to a new 8:8 ratio, or 1.0. If the original weakest link indicated a poor hamstring-to-quadriceps strength, then according to the team physician, athletic trainer, and strength coach, the poor hamstring-to-quadriceps ratio would place the athlete in a vulnerable medical and performance situation to tear a hamstring and require months of rehabilitation. Team policy

JoeSAPhotos/Shutterstock

would dictate that an athlete could not attend "contact" team practices until poor (low) H/Q ratios improved substantially. Consequently, targeted weakest link strength/power training (i.e., hamstring strength/power) was believed to demonstrate improved overall athletic performance and reduced injury risk because the new ratio had increased from 3:8 to 1.0—meaning near identical strength between the quadriceps and hamstring muscles. The weakest link would no longer remain a probable predictor for hamstring injury (i.e., high tear probability) or poor performance in movements that demand high level antagonistic muscle action.[305,306] In American football or soccer, simultaneously changing direction and thus the leg muscles' force requirements by planting the foot before the body shifts to the opposite side to avoid the tackle requires an H/Q ratio that avoids compromised weakest links.

Explosive Power Development

The five pillars in the proposed explosive power development model illustrated in **FIGURE 22.17** make important neuromuscular contributions to maximum power training. An efficient adaptation window shrinks for an athlete with well-developed components yet expands for components that require improvement. As an athlete approaches the high-velocity strength potential, that component's contribution to overall maximum power development diminishes. *Maximum explosive power improves the most when training focuses on improving performance in the chain's weakest links to help improve the least-developed performance/skill sets.*

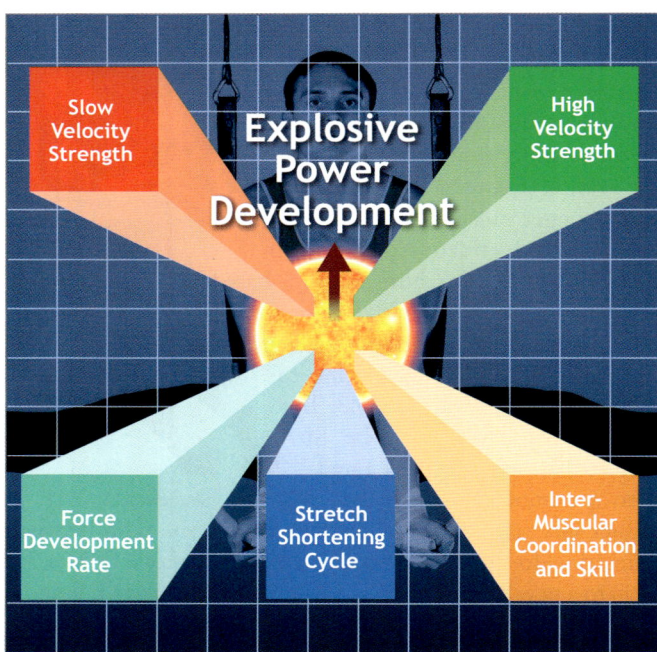

FIGURE 22.17. Five pillars that impact explosive power development.
(Adapted with permission from Kraemer WJ, Newton RU. Training for muscular power. *Phys Med Rehabil Clin.* 2000;11:341. Background photo: Aleksey Mnogosmyslov/Shutterstock; Sun image: silver tiger/Shutterstock.)

Summary

1. The most common methods to measure muscular performance include tensiometry, dynamometry, 1-RM testing with weights, computer-assisted force and work-output determinations, and isokinetic measurements.
2. Human skeletal muscle generates a maximum 30 N force per cm^2 muscle cross section in males and females.
3. On an absolute basis, men almost always exert greater maximum force than women for any given muscular movement pattern.
4. The traditional method to evaluate gender differences in muscle strength creates a ratio score for strength (either strength per unit body mass, FFM, limb volume, or maximum muscle girth).
5. The large strength differences between males and females decrease considerably when adjusting for body size and/or body composition variables with allometric scaling procedures.
6. Optimal overload training to strengthen muscles involves three factors: increased resistance or load to muscle action, increased muscle contraction speed, or combining increased load with increased movement speed.
7. Gains in a muscle's force-generating capacity with training require overload equal to 60 and 80% 1-RM.
8. Three major strength-training systems produce strength gains highly specific to training mode—progressive resistance weight training, isometrics, and isokinetic training.
9. Isokinetic training generates maximum muscular force throughout the full ROM at different limb movement angular velocities.
10. Closely supervised resistance training with concentric muscle actions can improve children's strength without negatively impacting bone, muscle, or connective tissue.
11. Periodization places a training period or macrocycle into smaller training mesocycles, with further subdivisions into weekly microcycles.
12. Compartmentalizing periodization training minimizes staleness and overtraining effects to maximize peak performance coinciding with competition.
13. Resistance training optimizes competitive athletes' muscular strength, power, and hypertrophy.
14. Training goals for middle-age and older adults aim to modestly improve muscular strength and endurance, maintain muscle and bone mass, and enhance overall health and fitness.
15. Concurrent muscular strength and aerobic capacity training inhibit strength improvement compared with only training to increase muscular strength.
16. Neuromuscular system's inherent stretch-recoil characteristics facilitate muscle power development.
17. Specificity related to physiology and performance and their adaptive training response casts doubt about whether *general* fitness components can predict an individual's ability to perform specific tasks or occupations.

18. Functional movement training with body weight–supported sling suspension exercise offers an alternative approach to standard sports training.
19. Core conditioning plays an integral part in sports and physical conditioning to improve muscular balance, strength, and trunk stabilization as a way to reduce injury risk.
20. Weakest link training and rehabilitation assess quadriceps to hamstring (Q/H) "strength deficits" and attempts to increase the Q/H ratios to minimize the high tear probability for injuring hamstring muscles.

Part 2 > Resistance Training: Structural and Functional Adaptations

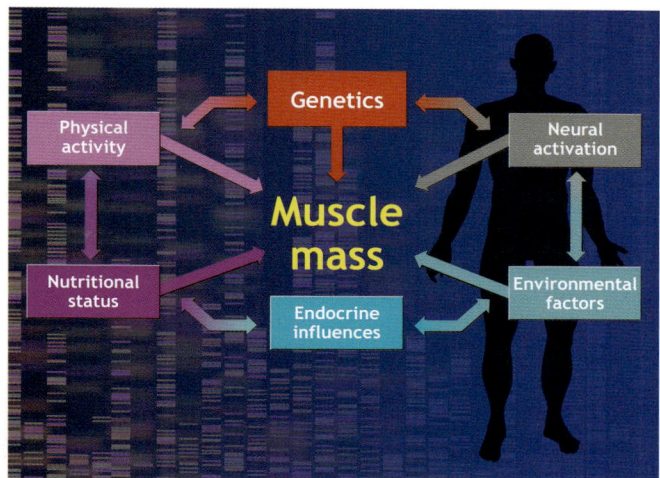

FIGURE 22.18. Six factors interact to develop and maintain muscle mass.
(Background image: Zita/Shutterstock.)

Resistance training produces both **acute responses** and **chronic adaptations**. An acute response refers to immediate changes in muscle or other cells, tissues, or systems during or immediately following a single exercise bout—for example, immediate change in energy stores and cardiovascular dynamics to specific muscle actions. Repeated exposure to a stimulus produces a longer-lasting chronic change to influence the acute response over time (e.g., less disruption in cellular integrity [muscle damage] with a given exercise level). Chronic adaptation refers to how the body adjusts to a repeated, long-term stimulus.

Knowing the acute and chronic responses to resistance training facilitates exercise prescription and program design. Adaptations to repeated muscular overload ultimately determine a training program's effectiveness. Muscle tissues exist in a dynamic state with two general, alternating adaptation characteristics:

1. Amino acid concentration *increases* as proteins continually synthesize.
2. Amino acid concentration *decreases* as proteins continually degrade.

The adaptation time course varies among individuals depending on the nature and magnitude from prior adaptive responses. A resistance-training program must assess individual differences in training adaptation responsiveness.

FIGURE 22.18 shows six influential interacting factors in developing and maintaining muscle mass. Without a doubt, genetic factors provide the underlying reference framework to modulate the other five factors to increase muscle mass and strength.[197] Generalized or specific muscular activity contributes little to tissue growth without appropriate nutrition to provide amino acid availability. Similarly, nervous system activation and systemic and local insulin-like growth factor (IGF) streamline the training response. Successful tension overload dovetails with maintaining a proper balance among testosterone, growth hormone, and cortisol.

Neural and Muscular Adaptations Impact Strength Improvements

FIGURE 22.19 shows that factors broadly characterized as neural (psychologic) and muscular impact human strength improvement. A resistance training program readily modifies many components, while other factors remain training resistant, probably from natural endowment or early life experiences. Note that neural adaptations predominate in the early training phase (this phase encompasses the duration in most research studies).[284,285] Hypertrophy-induced adaptations place the upper limit on longer-term training improvements. This tempts many athletes to use anabolic steroids and/or human growth hormone (upward dashed line of the solid yellow line) to try to induce continual hypertrophy when training alone fails.

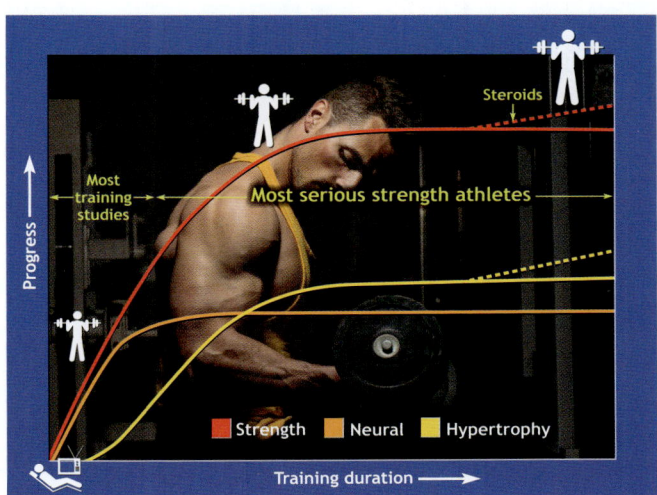

FIGURE 22.19. Neural and muscular adaptations in strength improvement with resistance training.
(Adapted with permission from Sale DG. Neural adaptation to resistance training. *Med Sci Sports Exerc*. 1988;20:135. Photo: Jasminko Ibrakovic/Shutterstock.)

Neural-Psychologic Factors

Adaptive alterations in nervous system function largely account for rapid and large strength increases early in training, often without increased muscle size and cross-sectional area.[1,108,201] In the elderly, resistance training's neural adaptations play an important role to improve muscular strength and power.[92]

FIGURE 22.20 shows the generalized resistance training response curve for gains in muscle strength from neural (*orange*) or hypertrophic (*yellow*) muscular factors. During a typical 8-wk training period, neural factors explain about 90% the strength gained over the first 2 wk. In the subsequent 2 wk, 40 to 50% of any strength improvement still relates to nervous system adaptations. Thereafter, muscle fiber adaptations become progressively more important to strength improvement based on **integrated electromyography (EMG)** recordings in the trained muscle groups. EMG methodology records muscle tissue electrical activity, or its representation as a visual display or audio-amplified signal using skin surface EMG or a needle inserted into the muscle belly (see section below).

Nerve Conduction Velocity

In muscle injuries and related pathologies, where nerve damage often occurred many years before symptoms appear, assessing **nerve conduction velocity (NCV)** measures how quickly a neural signal travels end-to-end through the nerve to evaluate the motor-evoked and sensory-evoked neural responses to the needle stimulation. Nerve conduction velocity is faster in the arms than in the legs, and tapered distal nerve segments conduct more slowly than proximal segments because they are cooler than proximal regions.

The EMG for diagnostic purposes detects neuromuscular abnormalities following a nerve's stimulation to a targeted muscle or muscle groups (www.healthline.com/health/nerve-conduction-velocity). NCV assessment accurately pinpoints nerve damage occurrence using the speed the signal travels along the nerve following a mild but brief electrical impulse through a stimulating electrode shown in red and probe electrode in green. For example, an athlete may have suffered a deep calf (gastrocnemius) muscle bruise, and fortunately, subsequent rehabilitation restored the calf to apparently normal function without loss in leg power to perform a standard toe raise on either one or two legs. Further injury to that calf region decades later can trigger the formerly injured neural and muscular components to relapse, with a power loss in the affected calf. For example, the person could suffer a 75% power loss in the gastrocnemius muscle, unable to jump even a few inches off the floor with both legs, and never able to jump upward with only the injured leg. The nerves responsible for activating the calf muscles cannot mobilize the diminished calf muscle volume (with fewer muscle fibers) to allow the person to execute a floor jump. The EMG and NCV tests help to detect the presence, location, and extent in nerve and/or muscle dysfunction (www.youtube.com/watch?v=s6KIRoNGvFQ). Chronic nerve damage impairs physical performance in many ways, sometimes as routine as walking down stairs, which now necessitates holding onto bannister rails to maintain balance and muscular stability.

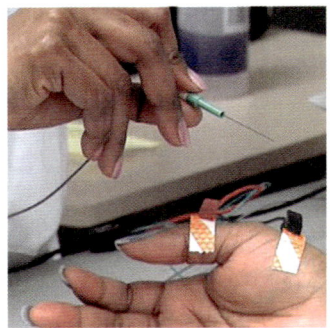
Photo from F. Katch

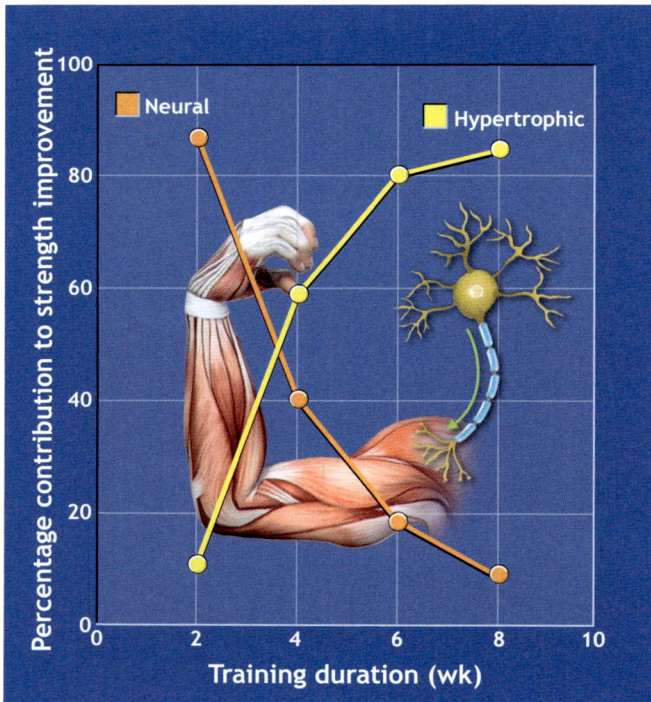

FIGURE 22.20. Resistance training response curve for muscle strength gains from neural (*orange*) or hypertrophic (*yellow*) factors.
(Images: Tefi/Shutterstock (nerve); Valentyna Chukhlyebova/Shutterstock (bicep).)

Training's Impact at the Neuromuscular Junction

Research has considered training's effects on structural changes associated with the synaptic connections between the motor nerve's terminal end with skeletal muscle called the neuromuscular junction (NMJ). In a study with rats, endurance training improved the nerve terminal area-to-muscle fiber size ratio by reducing fiber diameter without altering nerve terminal size.[246] In humans, high- and low-intensity training differentially affected NMJ size.[64] Less-intense, prolonged workouts produced a more expansive NMJ area, whereas intense effort produced greater synaptic dispersion. Aging also interferes with the NMJ's adaptation to training. Clearly, considerable complexity exists in synaptic response coordination patterns among different muscles and their dissimilar fiber types.[65]

Classic experiments have illustrated psychologic factors' importance in muscular strength expression.[113] The researchers

Superhuman Strength Challenges

In their 2006 textbook on strength training, Zatsiorsky and Kraemer describe three broad factors that limit an athlete's lifting potential. The highest potential, called *absolute strength*, represents the theoretical maximum force, which never is reached or exceeded, that muscle fibers, tendons, and bony structures develop under neuromuscular-controlled, precise movement patterns. The lowest maximum force value, termed *maximum strength*, represents the maximum lift under conscious effort, equaling about two thirds of theoretical absolute strength. For someone who can lift 200 lb, for example, the theoretical maximum lift would equal 300 lb—an upper tolerable limit for the body's tissues and bony structures. For experienced weightlifters who routinely train close to maximum during weekly workouts, their upper limit lift capacity exceeds the two-thirds typical limit to about 80% before the muscular system would experience intolerable strain. The third type of lifting potential occurs when weightlifters set a world record at a competitive meet or when heroic efforts are performed under extreme duress. At the highest performance levels during competitions (called *competitive maximum strength*), a top athlete might increase performance by up to 15%, or even more for the most intense competitions. Fred Hatfield (a.k.a. Dr. Squat), one of the world's premier, pure power athletes, set a record in 1984 at age 45 (body weight, 255 lb) by squatting 1014 lb (457.2 kg), a truly superhuman strength feat (www.youtube.com/watch?v=PDOpEtk60C0). A practitioner of self-taught hypnosis learned over a 10-year period, Hatfield put himself into an hypnotic trance, then pre-tensed his muscles (and controlled his breathing) until he believed motor unit recruitment had achieved a maximum. This phenomenon diminishes the brain's fear centers to remove restraints (inhibitions) and subsequently potentiates the rate of force development (disinhibitions).

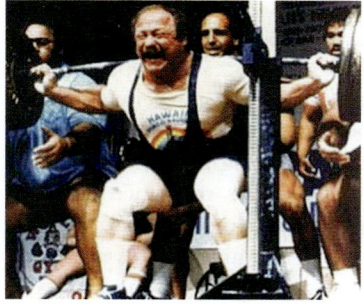
Photo courtesy Fred Hatfield (AKA Dr. Squat)

Sources:
Berger JM, et al. Mediation of the acute stress response by the skeleton. *Cell Metab*. 2019;30:845.
Karsenty G, Mera P. Molecular bases of the crosstalk between bone and muscle. *Bone*. 2018;115:43.
Martinez-Valdes E, et al. Pain-induced changes in motor unit discharge depend on recruitment threshold and contraction speed. *J Appl Physiol (1985)*. 2021;131:1260.

---

measured arm strength in college-age men under five exertion conditions:

1. Normal (no special exertion condition)
2. Immediately following a loud pistol shot near the head with the subject unaware the shot was coming
3. Subject screamed loudly during exertion
4. Under alcohol and amphetamine ("pep pills") influence
5. Under hypnosis (told they possessed considerable strength and should not fear injury)

Each condition generally increased strength above normal levels; hypnosis, the most "mental" treatment, produced the greatest increments. The investigators theorized that temporary modifications in CNS function accounted for strength improvements under the different experimental treatments. They argued that most persons normally operate at neural inhibition levels by protective reflex mechanisms that constrain the true strength expression capacity. Three factors explain strength capacity:

1. Muscle cross-section
2. Fiber type
3. Bone and muscle's mechanical arrangement

Neuromuscular inhibition can arise from unpleasant past physical activity experiences, an overly protective home environment, or fear from injury. Notwithstanding the reason, the person usually cannot achieve maximum strength capacity. The excitement from intense competition or disinhibitory drug influence or hypnotic suggestion can induce a "supermaximum" performance from greatly reduced neural inhibition and optimal motor neuron recruitment.

Highly trained, elite athletes often create a self-induced hypnotic state by intensely concentrating or "psyching" before the competition begins, or immediately before a tense movement when the performance can mean the difference between winning and losing. It sometimes takes years to perfect "blocking out" extraneous stimuli (e.g., crowd noise, peer pressure, or the thought that millions of people worldwide watching the performance) immediately before the performance. The psyching technique has been perfected in elite powerlifting competition where success depends on precise, coordinated movements *with* maximum muscle tension output within a specific, brief time frame. Prior research has confirmed that well-trained athletes have devised mechanisms to divert their attention from stress-filled situations requiring maximum concentration to achieve optimum performance outcomes.[309,310,312] Salient examples could be a Super Bowl game, tied following regulation play with one team attempting a field goal with 1 s remaining on the clock, having to sink a 6-ft putt to win a major professional golf championship, or a final attempt to "stick" a triple summersault in Olympic free-exercise competition.

Enhanced arousal level and accompanying neural disinhibition or facilitation fully activate muscle groups without having to think about their sequence to perform a particular movement, as in the last second game-winning field goal. Hundreds of practice hours mimicking different stressful conditions over many years hopefully makes such "pressure" movements automatic, rather than ending in a performance disaster sometimes referred to as a "choke."

Increased neurologic arousal also may help to explain "unexplainable" strength and power feats during highly charged emergency and rescue situations (e.g., a relatively small person lifting an extremely heavy object off an injured person to save their life).

Muscular and Psychologic Factors in the Early Training Phase

Many factors can impact gains in muscle strength when a strength training program begins, yet anatomic and physiologic factors within the joint–muscle unit ultimately determine a muscle's maximum strength capacity. TABLE 22.2 lists twelve generalized physiologic adaptive responses in muscle with resistance training.

TABLE 22.2 Physiologic adaptations to resistance training

Some modifications occur within weeks, but most adaptations occur over months or years. Resistance training's effects on muscle fibers generally target adaptations in the contractile structures and typically accompany substantial increases in muscular force and power output capacity through a given ROM.

Muscle Hypertrophy

An increase in muscular tension with training provides the primary stimulus to initiate processes related to positive skeletal muscle fiber growth known as hypertrophy. Changes in muscle size become detectable with training after only 3 wk, and remodeling muscle architecture precedes gains in MCSA. Two fundamental adaptations necessary for muscle hypertrophy (increased protein synthesis and satellite cell proliferation) mobilize during the initial resistance training phases.[208,267] Mechanical stress on muscular system components triggers specialized signaling proteins to activate genes that translate messenger RNA to stimulate protein synthesis when it exceeds protein breakdown. Accelerated protein synthesis, particularly when combined with adequate insulin and amino acid availability, increases muscle size during resistance training.[127] Muscle hypertrophy reflects a fundamental biologic adaptation to increased workload independently from gender and age. Improving muscular strength and power capacity does not necessarily require muscle fiber hypertrophy because important neurologic factors initially impact human strength expression. The later, slower-occurring strength improvements generally coincide with noticeable alterations in a muscle's subcellular molecular architecture.

Overload training enlarges individual muscle fibers with subsequent muscle growth. The fast-twitch fibers in weightlifters average about 45% larger than similar fibers in endurance athletes and healthy sedentary individuals. The hypertrophic process couples directly to increased mononuclear number and cellular component synthesis, particularly the protein myosin heavy chain and actin contractile elements.[17,98] Resistance training creates more efficient mRNA translation that mediates myofibrillar protein synthesis stimulation.[253] Muscle growth occurs from repeated muscle fiber injury particularly from eccentric actions followed by protein synthesis overcompensation to produce a net anabolic effect. The cell's myofibrils thicken and increase in number, and additional sarcomeres form from accelerated protein synthesis and corresponding decreased protein breakdown. Considerable increases also occur for intramuscular ATP, PCr, and glycogen. These anaerobic energy stores contribute to the rapid energy transfer required in resistance training. Body build characteristics also help to explain individual differences in responsiveness to resistance training. The greatest increases in muscle mass occur for individuals with the largest relative FFM (corrected for stature and body fat) before training begins.[243] Age also impacts the hypertrophic response to resistance training. Cross-sectional type I and type II muscle fiber areas increased less in older (61 years) compared to younger (26 years) men who resistance trained for 21 wk. The difference in fiber-size enlargement in the older men associated with lower protein and energy intake and greater increases in myostatin gene expression.[168]

FIGURE 22.21 shows the change in muscle fiber size accompanying training-induced hypertrophy in trained and nontrained rat soleus muscle (**A**), while image **B** presents a typical cross section for untrained (control) versus hypertrophied

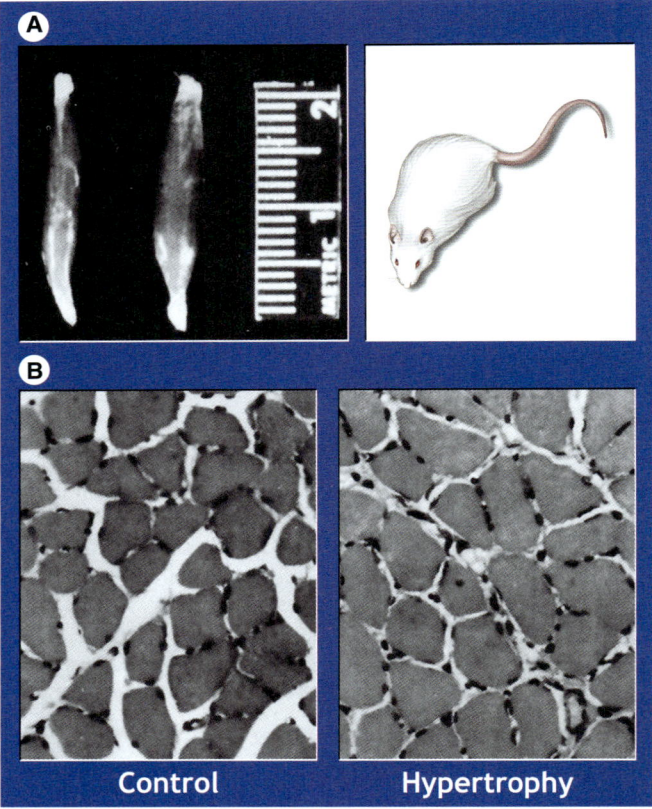

FIGURE 22.21. (**A**) Control (*left*) and hypertrophied (*right*) rat soleus muscle. (**B**) Cross sections for control versus hypertrophied muscles shown in (**A**).
(Reprinted with permission from Goldberg AL, et al. Mechanism of work-induced hypertrophy of skeletal muscle. *Med Sci Sports.* 1975;7(3):185.)

muscle fibers. The average diameter for 50 hypertrophied muscle fibers averaged 30% larger (range 24 to 34%), with the fibers containing 45% more nuclei (range 40 to 52%). These compensatory increases in fiber size relate to marked increases in DNA synthesis and proliferating connective tissue cells and small, mononucleated satellite cells located beneath the basement membrane adjacent to the muscle fibers. The satellite cells, rich among type II muscle fibers, facilitate growth, maintenance, and repairing damaged muscle tissue.[93,100]

Connective tissue cellular proliferation thickens and strengthens muscle's connective tissue components to improve tendon and ligament structural and functional integrity (cartilage lacks sufficient circulation to stimulate growth).[131] Such adaptations help to protect joints and muscles from injury and provide a sound rationale to include different resistance training modes appropriate to preventative, rehabilitative, fitness, and orthopedic strategies.

Resistance-trained muscle fibers have increased total contractile protein and energy-generating compounds while lacking these three components:

1. Parallel increases in vascular capillarization
2. Total mitochondrial volume increases
3. Mitochondrial enzymes

These components' absence decreases the ratio between mitochondrial volume and/or enzyme concentration to myofibrillar (contractile protein) volume. This training response does not hinder performance in strength and power activities because such efforts remain primarily anaerobic. Nevertheless, it impedes endurance in prolonged activity by reducing the fiber's aerobic capacity per unit muscle mass.

Hypertrophic Response Specificity

A single resistance training mode does not create uniform strength improvement or hypertrophic response in the activated muscle(s).[8] For example, biceps curls performed at close to 1-RM do *not* produce equal strength gains from the muscle's origin to its insertion. If they did, then the maximum muscle force–generating capacity would show similar percentage improvements throughout its ROM. This does not occur. Electrical activity measured by surface or needle EMG or MRI to assess a muscle's cross-sectional area does not produce a homogeneous response within the entire muscle when maximally activated.[69,202] A single muscle compartmentalizes into distinct regions, which means the muscle's different regions respond differentially to the imposed adaptive stress. In essence, skeletal muscle remodels its internal architecture, and potentially reconfigures its external orientation and hence its shape. Two primary factors govern the training adaptation to specific resistance exercise modes:

1. Little or no homogeneity in skeletal muscle's overload response
2. Intramuscular differences in fiber type and composition

Significant Metabolic Adaptations Occur

Optimizing muscle fiber distribution governs successful elite performance. The relatively fixed muscle fiber type suggests an apparent genetic predisposition for exceptional physical performance. Considerable *plasticity* exists for metabolic potential because specific training enhances the anaerobic and aerobic energy transfer capacity in both fiber types.

With endurance training, oxidative capacity in fast-twitch fibers brings them to a level nearly equal to the slow-twitch fiber's aerobic capacity present in untrained counterparts. Endurance training does induce some type IIb fiber conversion to more aerobic type IIa fibers.[264] Three well-documented changes occur in fiber subdivisions:

1. Increased mitochondrial size and number
2. Increased citric acid cycle enzymes
3. Increased electron transport enzymes

---

fyi — Ten Functional Test Categories for Personalized Training Assessments

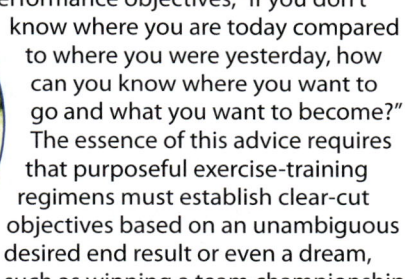
photo_beauty/Shutterstock

A wise track coach once told an "underperforming" yet talented athlete who had not considered clear-cut, long-term performance objectives, "If you don't know where you are today compared to where you were yesterday, how can you know where you want to go and what you want to become?" The essence of this advice requires that purposeful exercise-training regimens must establish clear-cut objectives based on an unambiguous desired end result or even a dream, such as winning a team championship or becoming a gold medal champion. Consider 10 test categories in the exercise physiology, fitness training, physical therapy, and coaching literature about how to assess an athlete's unique, innate capacities throughout training and competitive season—each individual requiring a personalized assessment approach with targeted testing in these areas (agility, anaerobic, power, dynamic balance, sprint/speed, and muscle and aerobic endurance):

1. Self-assessment: past/current goals/objectives; body size status
2. Posture: restrictive musculoskeletal movement patterns
3. Complex movement pattern skills
4. Movement asymmetries: shoulders, arms, legs
5. Leg power: squats, thrusts, directional movement changes
6. Lower body explosive power: vertical/horizontal jumps
7. Upper body power: weighted object maneuvers
8. Agility: coordination/timing/quickness
9. Body weigh supported exercise: timed pullups/pushups
10. Core: strength/endurance

Sources:
https://master-athlete.com
Mazerolle SM, et al. National Athletic Trainers' Association Position Statement: facilitating work-life balance in athletic training practice settings. *J Athl Train*. 2018;53:796.
Onate JA. Normative functional performance values in high school athletes: the functional pre-participation evaluation project. *J Athl Train*. 2018;53:35.

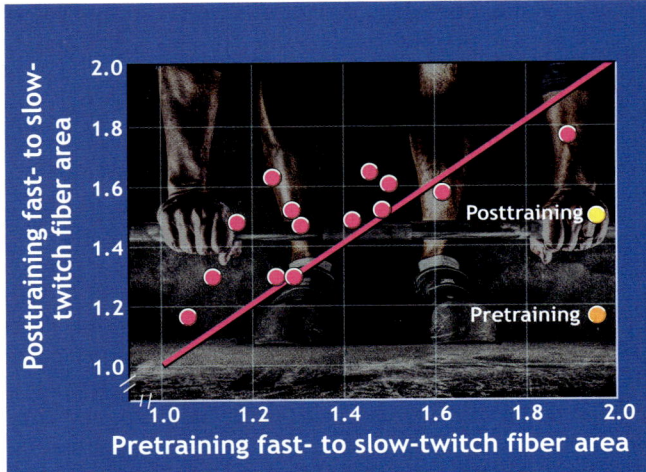

FIGURE 22.22 Fast- and slow-twitch muscle fiber ratios in 14 men before and following resistance training for 8 wk.
(Adapted with permission from Thorstensson A. Muscle strength, fiber types, and enzyme activities in man. *Acta Physiol Scand.* 1976;443:1. Permission granted by John Wiley & Sons - Books, conveyed through Copyright Clearance Center, Inc. Photo: MH STOCK/Shutterstock.)

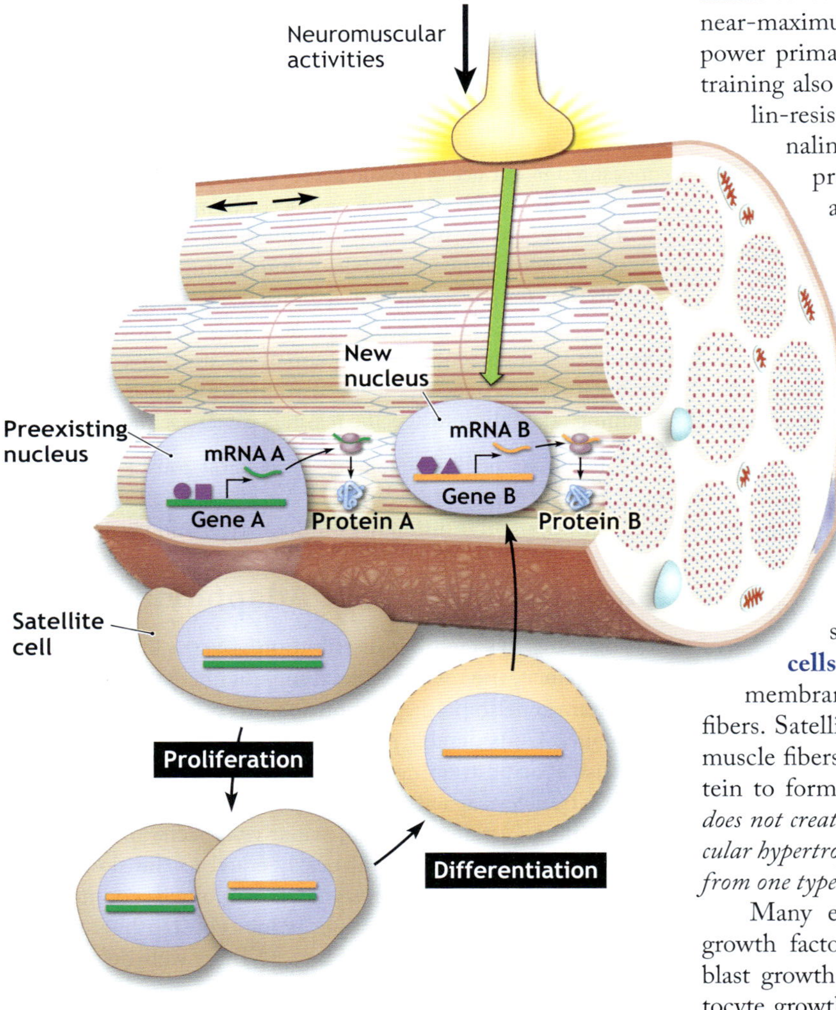

Only the specifically trained muscle fibers adapt to regular training. Within this framework, swimmers or canoeists with well-trained upper-body musculature do not necessarily transfer upper-body strength and performance to a running sport that relies predominantly on highly conditioned, specifically trained lower-body musculature.

Specific fibers and a fiber subdivision's metabolic characteristics undergo modification from targeted resistance training within 4 to 8 wk. This occurs without dramatically changing inherent muscle fiber types. A decrease in the type IIx and corresponding increase in type IIa fiber percentage highlights a more prominent but rapid training adaptations. Furthermore, the volume in trained fast-twitch fibers also increases.[5] **FIGURE 22.22** clearly illustrates this increase for the relative areas for the fast- and slow-twitch muscle fibers before and following resistance training. The *orange circle* position at the lower right indicates the average pretraining FT:ST area ratio, while the *yellow circle* position represents the posttraining average. Considerable fast-twitch fiber hypertrophy occurs in power and Olympic-type lifters who progressive resistance train diligently over many years.[226,228] This observation makes sense considering exercise training specificity because near-maximum resistance exercise requiring high anaerobic power primarily recruits fast-twitch motor units. Resistance training also improves glucose transport in normal and insulin-resistant skeletal muscle by activating the insulin signaling cascade and along with increasing **GLUT-4** protein concentration. These training-induced alterations improve skeletal muscle quality and occur independently from increased skeletal muscle mass.[265]

Muscle Cell Remodeling

Skeletal muscle represents dynamic tissue whose cell populations do not remain fixed throughout life, but rather undergo muscle regeneration and remodeling (changes in structure and function) with resistance or endurance training to alter their phenotypic profile.[101] Activating muscle with specific types and intensities during long-term use stimulates otherwise dormant **myogenic stem cells** positioned under a muscle fiber's basement membrane to proliferate and differentiate to form new fibers. Satellite cell nuclei fuse and incorporate into existing muscle fibers, allowing the fiber to synthesize additional protein to form new myofibril contractile elements. *This process does not create new muscle fibers, but contributes directly to muscular hypertrophy and may stimulate existing fiber transformation from one type to another.*

Many extracellular signal molecules, primarily peptide growth factors (e.g., insulinlike growth factor [IGF], fibroblast growth factors, transforming growth factors, and hepatocyte growth factor) govern satellite cell activity and possibly training-induced muscle fiber proliferation and differentiation. **FIGURE 22.23** proposes a remodeling sequence for muscle cells showing satellite cell incorporation into an existing muscle fiber.

FIGURE 22.23. A model for skeletal muscle adaptations involving satellite cells.
(Adapted with permission from Yan Z. Skeletal muscle adaptation and cell cycle regulation. *Exerc Sport Sci Rev.* 2000;1:24.)

A specific set of genes (gene A in the figure within the preexisting nucleus) is expressed within the fiber. Chronic activation from physical activity stimulates satellite cell proliferation, with some cells differentiating and fusing with preexisting muscle fibers. The new muscle nuclei alter gene expression in the adapting muscle depicted as gene B within the myofibril matrix.

Muscle fiber–type transformations occur with specific-type training. In one study, four athletes trained anaerobically for 11 wk followed by aerobic training for 18 wk. Anaerobic training increased the type IIc fiber percentage (a previous subclassification) and decreased the type I fiber percentage; the opposite occurred during the aerobic training phase.[120] Similarly, sprint training for 4 to 6 wk increased the fast-twitch fiber percentage, with a commensurate decrease in slow-twitch fiber percentage.[60] Increasing daily training duration also increases the fast- to slow-twitch shift in myosin heavy-chain phenotype in rat hind limb muscles.[63] Specific training (and perhaps inactivity) can convert different type I to type II fibers' physiologic characteristics and vice versa,[212,226,227] with genetic code likely exerting a large influence on fiber-type distribution. A muscle's fiber composition (i.e., fast or slow twitch) probably becomes fixed before birth or during the first few years following birth.

Positive Muscle and Tendon Adaptations Occur Independently from Gender or Age

Muscles and tendons, highly adaptable tissues, respond favorably to chronic changes in loading independently from gender or age.[12,134,178]

A study in five active older healthy men with average age 68 years demonstrated human skeletal muscle's remarkable plasticity in **FIGURE 22.24**, with pretraining results shown in red and posttraining results in yellow. Isokinetic and free-weight training for 12 wk increased muscle volume and cross-sectional biceps brachii area (13.9%) and brachialis (26.0%), while hypertrophy increased by 37.2% in type II muscle fibers. Increases in peak **torque** averaged 46.0% and 28.6% in total work output accompanied these cellular adaptations. Older men experienced improvements in these variables similar to younger counterparts in response to a rapid, high-power periodized resistance-training program.[180] Preserving muscle structure and function as one ages provides for a physical reserve capacity above the critical threshold required for independent living.[2,263]

Equally impressive training responses occur for persons 80 years and older. One hundred nursing home residents (average age 87.1 years) trained with resistance exercise for 10 wk.[74] For the 63 female and 37 male participants, muscle strength increased an average 113%. Strength increases paralleled improved function as reflected with an 11.8% increase in normal gait velocity and 28.4% increase in stair-climbing speed, and 2.7% increase in thigh MCSA. Other studies have verified functional strength training benefits to improve **activities of daily living (ADL)** in the older elderly to counter the devastating medical consequences from slips and falls.[14,33] Recent studies confirm prior results for balance training in the elderly to help foil the increased occurrence from slips, trips, stumbles, and balance loss and their associated devastating medical/and rehabilitation costs.[311,313,314]

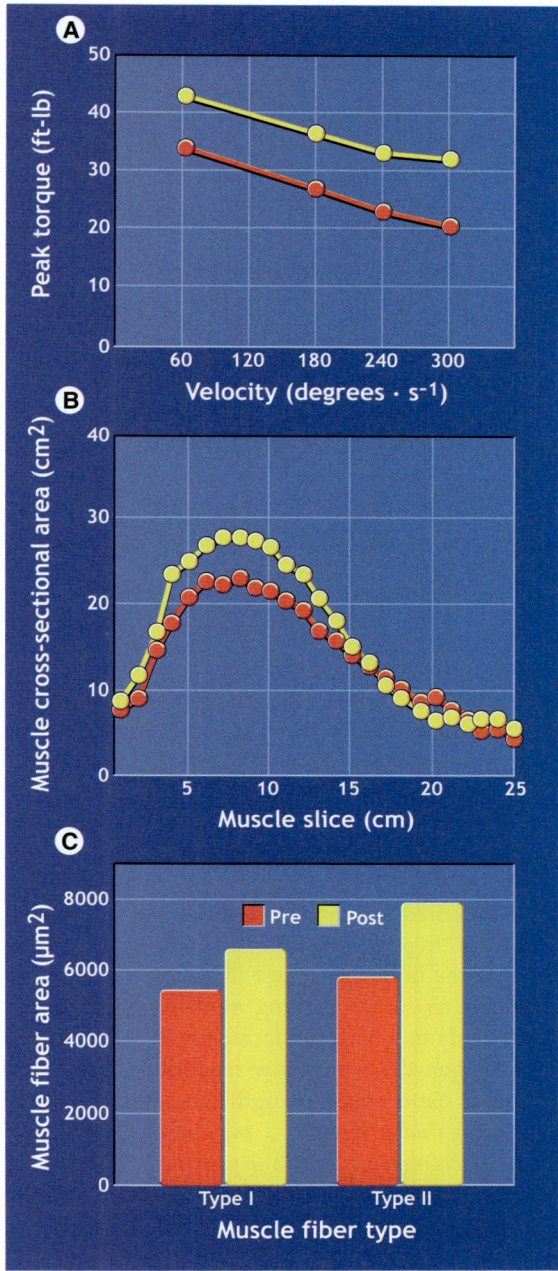

FIGURE 22.24. Aging muscle plasticity in five elderly men pre (*red*) and post (*yellow*) 12 wk of intense resistance training. **(A)** Peak elbow flexor torque versus movement velocity. **(B)** Flexor cross-sectional area from MRI scans from proximal (*right*) to distal (*left*) end of muscle slices. **(C)** Type I and type II average muscle fiber areas.
(Adapted with permission from Roman WJ, et al. Adaptations in the elbow flexors of elderly males after heavy-resistance training. *J Appl Physiol*. 1993;74:750.) ©The American Physiological Society (APS). All rights reserved.

Muscle Hyperplasia: Are New Muscle Fibers Created?

A contemporary question concerns whether training increases muscle fiber number (**hyperplasia**). If this does occur, to what extent does it contribute to human muscle enlargement? Chronic skeletal muscle overload in various animal species stimulates new muscle fiber development from satellite cells or by longitudinally splitting existing cells.[10] The normally dormant satellite cells develop into new muscle fibers under the three conditions featured in Figure 22.23—stress, neuromuscular disease, and muscle injury. With **longitudinal splitting**, a large muscle fiber splits into two or more smaller individual daughter cells through lateral budding. These fibers function more efficiently than the large single fiber from which they originated.[11] In rapidly growing murine models between postnatal day 1 and day 28, large increases occur in myofibrillar packing (2-fold), myofiber cross-sectional area (7-fold), muscle mass (4-fold), and longitudinal myofiber length (5-fold) mainly by adding sarcomeres-in-series during the first 4 to 6 postnatal weeks.[299,304]

Generalizing findings from research on animals to humans poses a problem. The massive cellular hypertrophy created with resistance training in humans does not occur in many animal species. In cats, for example, muscle **fiber hyperplasia** often represents the primary compensatory overload adjustment. Some evidence exists supporting hyperplasia in humans. Autopsy data from young, healthy men who died accidentally show that muscle fiber counts in the larger and stronger leg (leg opposite the dominant hand) contained 10% more muscle fibers than the smaller leg.[213] Cross-sectional studies with bodybuilders with relatively large limb circumferences and muscle masses failed to show they possessed above-normal size individual muscle fibers.[151,152,227] Some bodybuilders may have inherited an initially large number of small muscle fibers (that "hypertrophied" to normal size with resistance training), yet the findings suggest that hyperplasia may occur with different resistance training modes. Muscle fibers may adapt differently to a bodybuilder's high-volume, high-intensity training than the typical low-repetition, heavy-load system favored by experienced strength and power athletes. *Even if other human studies replicate a training-induced hyperplasia (and even if the response reflects a positive adjustment), existing individual muscle fiber enlargement, not new fiber development, represents the greatest contribution from overload training to increased muscle size.*

Muscle Fiber Type Changed by Resistance Training

Research has evaluated resistance training for 8 wk on muscle fiber size and fiber composition for leg extensor muscles in 14 men who completed 6-RM leg squats for 3 sets thrice weekly.[231] Vastus lateralis muscle biopsy specimens before and after training showed *no change* in the percentage distribution in fast- and slow-twitch muscle fibers. This finding agrees with other resistance and endurance training studies and indicates that resistance training for several months in adults *does not alter* skeletal muscle's basic fiber composition. It remains unclear whether specific training early in life or for prolonged durations practiced by elite athletes alters a fiber's inherent shortening speed twitch characteristics. Some progressive fiber-type transformation may occur with longer-duration, specific training discussed in Chapter 18. *Genetic factors largely determine the predominant muscle fiber–type distribution.*

Comparative Male and Female Training Responses

Women now participate successfully in most sports and physical activities, including Japanese sumo wrestlers. Women generally had not incorporated resistance training during workouts to avoid developing overly enlarged muscles similar to men. This hesitation was unfortunate because specific strength acquisition enhances performance in tennis, golf, skiing, dance, swimming, water polo, gymnastics, track and field, and most other sports, including physically demanding firefighting and construction work. The question often arises whether muscular strength acquisition differs between males and females and, if so, what factors might be responsible?

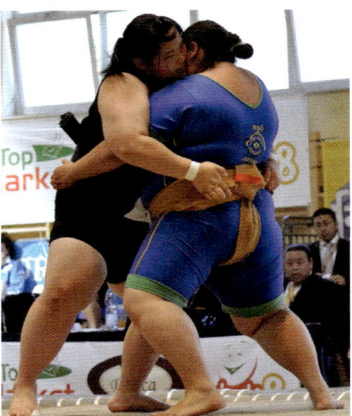
Stanislaw Tokarski/Shutterstock

Muscular Strength, Hypertrophy, and Transgender Athlete Participation

Transgender Competitors. Over the past 10 years, the term gender differences referred solely to males and females at birth in the conventional physical sense (i.e., females have enlarged breasts, unique genitalia, and different hormone profiles [lower testosterone levels] than males), but the term "intersex" describe people as **transgender** when they display some physical traits neither strictly male nor strictly female. In 2004, the International Olympic Committee (IOC) announced that transgender athletes could participate in the Olympics under stringent guidelines—the athletes required sex reassignment surgery, legal gender recognition by appropriate official authorities, and a minimum 2 years verifiable hormone replacement therapy (www.nytimes.com/2016/01/26/sports/olympics/transgender-athletes-olympics-ioc.html). These requirements changed in 2015 when the IOC revised the rules for transgender female competitors—minimum 1 year hormone replacement therapy (rather than 2 year) without a requirement for sex reassignment surgery (athletes transitioning from female to male are allowed to participate without restrictions). In a 2017 summary review featuring eight studies with transgender male and female athletes, the author concluded that there was no direct or consistent research suggesting transgender female individuals (or male individuals) have an athletic advantage at any transitional stage (e.g., cross-sex hormones, gender-confirming surgery). The authors posited that any restrictions on transgender people adopted by governing sports associations require careful consideration and/or potential revision. For the 2021 Tokyo Summer Olympics, the IOC delayed announcing new testosterone limits for athletes in women's events, leaving the issue still unresolved in these emerging social and hotly debated areas. One salient issue involves establishing an acceptable scientific cutoff for female's testosterone levels, which currently range between 0.12 and 1.79 nmol·L^{-1} and for males between 7.7 and 29.4 nmol·L^{-1}. Future research must assess hemoglobin concentration changes, body composition alterations (particularly the impact on lean body mass), endocrine functioning (testosterone and estrogen levels), and psychological, metabolic, strength, and aerobic and anaerobic capacity changes during an athlete's transition period. To create a level playing field among athletes relative to performance, the science must clearly establish that no advantage (or disadvantage) exists in gender considerations.[323,324]

To add more uncertainty to the above controversy, research by Swedish scientists reported that cross-sex hormone treatment markedly affected muscle strength assessed by isokinetic and isometric peak torque determined for knee extensors and flexors using Biodex isokinetic dynamometry, body size, and body composition by MRI imaging in transgender individuals.[169,317] Robust increases occurred in muscle mass and strength in transgender men (female to male), and transgender women (male to female) were still stronger and had more muscle mass following 2-month treatment! The absolute muscle volume levels assessed by MRI and knee extension strength following the intervention still favored the transgender women at the 12-month follow-up. The authors raise a weighty question, "When is it fair to permit a transwoman to compete in sport in line with her gender identity from the lifelong experience being a biological male?" These findings have relevance for sport-governing bodies at all levels, regarding how to evaluate a transwomen's eligibility to compete in the women's athletic competition category.

Males Versus Female Muscle Hypertrophy

A distinct gender difference exists in absolute muscle hypertrophy with resistance training. Computed axial tomography scans (CAT; see Chapter 28) directly evaluates MCSA and verifies that males and females respond similarly in hypertrophic responses to resistance training. Without doubt, males experience a greater absolute change in muscle size due to their larger initial muscle mass, but muscular enlargement on a *percentage* basis remains similar between genders.[56,109,249] Comparisons between elite male and female bodybuilders also indicate substantial muscular hypertrophy in females with considerable resistance training experience.[217,218,222] Gender-related hormonal response differences to resistance exercise (e.g., increased testosterone and decreased cortisol for men) may determine any ultimate gender differences with prolonged training in muscle size and strength adaptations.[140] This intriguing new research area requires longitudinal experiments to assess how "gender" impacts skeletal muscle responses from resistance training.

Muscle Strength's Relationship to Bone Density

A positive relationship exists between muscular strength and bone mineral density (BMD), which indicates that stronger people have greater BMD than less strong counterparts.[46,58,156] Males and females who participate in strength and power activities have as much or more bone mass than endurance athletes.[199,203,262] The lumbar spine and proximal femur bone mass in elite teenage weightlifters[51] and adolescent boys and girls[244,251] exceed representative reference values for fully mature adult bone.

A linear relation exists between increases in BMD and total and exercise-specific weight lifted during a 1-year strength training program.[57] Such findings have raised speculation about the possible positive relationship between muscular strength and bone mass. Laboratory experiments have documented greater maximum flexion and extension dynamic strength in postmenopausal women without osteoporosis than in osteoporotic counterparts.[221] For female gymnasts, BMD correlated moderately with maximum muscle strength and serum progesterone.[105] For adolescent female athletes, absolute knee extension strength moderately associated with total body, lumbar spine, femoral neck, and leg BMD.[69] Women with normal BMD measured by dual-photon absorptiometry in the lumbar spine and femur neck typically exhibit greater strength in 11 of 12 test comparisons for flexion compared to women with low BMD, while only four 12 extension comparisons show higher strength values in women with normal BMD. Subsequent data complement these findings; regional lean tissue mass, often an indication for muscle strength, accurately predicts BMD.[181,291,292] Accordingly, differences in maximum dynamic strength among postmenopausal women should play a routine, clinical role in osteoporosis screening.

Women at risk for osteoporosis or with pre-existing osteoporosis can reduce their fracture risk in two ways[176,291,298]:

1. Strengthen bone by increasing BMD through diet modification, increased physical activity involving strengthening exercises for limbs and trunk, and/or endocrinologist guidance about current pharmacologic therapy options (e.g., bisphosphonate therapy advisability with Alendronate [Fosamax]; Risedronate [Actonel]; Ibandronate [Boniva])
2. Avoid risky activities that increase bone load or spinal compression (e.g., unusually heavy lifting and straining activities involving the lower back/trunk regions)

Detraining Effects on Muscle

Limited data document muscle strength decrements and associated factors when discontinuing resistance training. Training stopped for 2 wk in male power lifters, which reduced their isokinetic eccentric muscle strength by 12% and 6.4% in their type II muscle fiber area without a loss in type I fiber area.[107] Another study evaluated knee extensor muscle strength, muscle volume, and muscle quality in elderly women with a 12-wk strength training program followed by a similar detraining period.[52] No time effect occurred for muscle quality, yet strength increased 33% and muscle volume increased 26% from baseline following post-training. After detraining, knee extensor strength remained 12% higher compared to baseline values, while muscle mass gains returned to baseline values. The authors concluded that muscular strength gains and losses could not solely be determined by changes in muscle mass from resistance training and detraining.

Abstaining for a short time period from resistance training in previously sedentary men caused strength loss within several weeks, most likely from a reversal in training-induced neuromuscular and hormonal adaptations.[50] Some coaches encourage their athletes to "taper" their normal physical routines, including psychological stressors[214] to allow for sufficient recovery before an upcoming competition.[174] In our 2015 eighth edition text, the taper concept remained a fruitful area for future research,[230] as only limited quantitative data existed for different athletic groups' different taper protocols.[87] Recent data now provide more details about the tapering practices in "strongmen" athletes, volleyball players, swimmers, team sport participants, and track and field athletes.[314–318]

Resistance Training and Metabolic Stress

Resistance training produces no improvement in $\dot{V}O_{2max}$ or submaximum exercise heart rate and stroke volume.[111] Limited if any cardiovascular improvement with standard resistance training probably results from the relatively low "whole body" metabolic and circulatory demands and active muscles high anaerobic metabolic requirements by stimulating glucose uptake and lactate release.[70] Maximum isometric and 8- to 10-RM weightlifting exercises in young men elicit only a light-to-moderate heart rate (generally <130 b · min^{-1}) and oxygen uptake (3 to 4 METs) responses.[158]

Resistance training places considerable localized stress on specific muscles. The brief stimulation period and typically small, activated muscle mass create lower heart rates and aerobic metabolic demands than dynamic big-muscle running, hiking, climbing, swimming, or cycling. A person may devote an hour or more to complete a strength-training workout, yet only spend 8 min exercising each hour. For cardiovascular improvement and weight control, traditional resistance-training workouts should still remain an important though lesser part in a program's overall strategy. Resistance training incorporated into a "circuit" routine as described in the next section will produce a substantial caloric expenditure if the participant rotates through 8 to 15 different exercise stations with minimal rest intervals and continues essentially nonstop for 50 to 60 min at a moderate- to high-effort intensity.

Circuit Resistance Training

Modifying the traditional approach to resistance training improves key fitness parameters—body composition, muscular strength and endurance, and cardiovascular fitness.[8,22,83,175,297] The **circuit resistance training (CRT)** approach deemphasizes

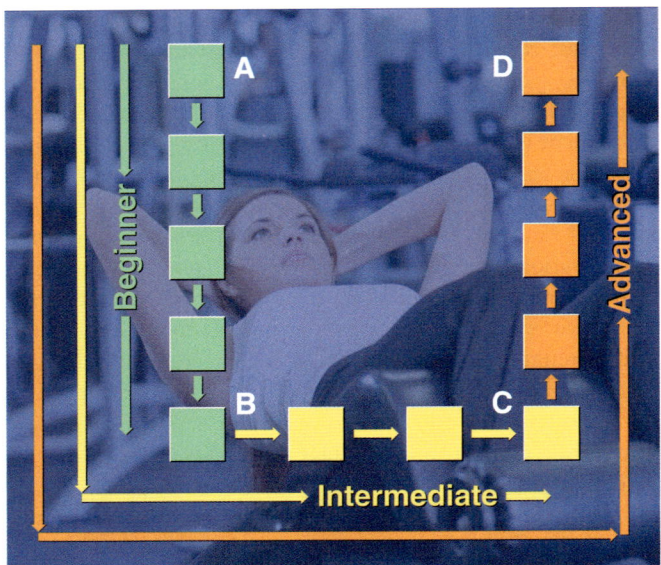

Background photo: AirCam.PRO/Shutterstock

the brief local-muscle overload intervals in standard resistance barbell and free weight training.

Successful CRT programs have incorporated upbeat music tempo during the exercise, with the music lowered to signify the individual should move to the next exercise station. The basic idea is to accomplish as many repetitions during the allotted time with quality movement mechanics during each exercise interval. Beginners can work twice through the circuit from A to B. After several weeks, they progress three times through this circuit, and finally, complete up to six circuits or more. The advanced level, shown in orange, adds several more stations, and participants proceed three to six times through circuit A to D, intermixing exercise load, repetitions, and duration.

With CRT, a person lifts a weight between 40 and 55% 1-RM repeatedly for 30 s with good form. After a 15-s rest, the participant moves to the next station and so on to complete the circuit, usually completing 8 to 15 different exercises. A modification that produces similar CRT energy expenditure uses a 1:1 exercise-to-rest ratios, with either 15- or 30-s exercise bouts.[18] The circuit repeated several times allows for 30 to 50 min continuous exercise, not just the typical 6- to 8-min traditional resistance training workout. As strength increases, a new 1-RM determined for each exercise provides the rationale to increase the resistance while traversing the circuit.

The CRT modification to standard resistance training offers an attractive alternative to those who desire a more general conditioning program. Medically supervised CRT programs effectively train coronary-prone, cardiac, and spinal cord–injured patients for a well-rounded fitness program. CRT supplements off-season conditioning for sports that require maintaining optimal muscular strength, power, and endurance.

Aerobic Improvement Specificity with CRT

Some research indicates that CRT produces nearly 50% less aerobic fitness improvement than typical bicycle or run training.[82] CRT usually involves substantial upper-body exercise, but assessing aerobic benefits for this training mode relied on lower-body musculature involving treadmill or bicycle ergometer testing. To remedy this limitation, one study assessed CRT effects on aerobic capacity with both treadmill running and arm-crank ergometry tests.[96] Aerobic capacity increased 8% with treadmill testing and 21% with arm-crank testing, thus confirming the training specificity principle. These findings take on added significance because they occurred without negative effects in borderline hypertensive subjects. The training program significantly increased muscular strength and decreased blood pressure.

Resistance Exercise Energy Expenditure

TABLE 22.3 displays energy expenditures for exercise performed using free weights, Nautilus (eccentric), Universal Gym (concentric/eccentric), Cybex (isokinetic), and Hydra-Fitness (hydraulic-concentric). Energy expenditure for hydraulic exercises averaged 9.0 kcal·min^{-1}; this averaged 35% higher than exercise with free weights, 29.4% higher than Nautilus exercise, and 11.5% more than CRT using Universal Gym equipment. The energy expenditure values for hydraulic exercise averaged about 6.4% less than slow- and fast-speed isokinetic circuit exercise. For comparison, the last row lists walking energy expenditure at a normal pace on a level surface (5.4 kcal·min^{-1}) for a 68-kg/150-lb person.

TABLE 22.3 Energy expenditure for different resistance exercise modes compared with walking

Muscle Soreness and Stiffness

Following an extended layoff from exercise, or performing unaccustomed exercise or stretching even for a few minutes, most persons usually experience some soreness and stiffness in the exercised joints and muscles. Temporary soreness may persist for several hours immediately following unaccustomed exercise, whereas residual **delayed-onset muscle soreness (DOMS)** usually appears after 12 hr and can last for 3 or 4 days. These six factors singly or in combination contribute to DOMS:

1. Minute tears in muscle tissue or damage to its contractile components with accompanying creatine kinase (CK), myoglobin (Mb) release, and the complex protein troponin I, a muscle-specific indicator for fiber damage
2. Osmotic pressure changes that produce fluid retention in the surrounding tissues
3. Muscle spasms
4. Overstretching and tearing a muscle's connective tissue harness
5. Acute inflammation
6. Alteration in the cell's calcium regulating mechanisms

Eccentric Actions Produce Muscle Soreness

The precise mechanism involved in muscle soreness remains unknown, yet discomfort level, muscle disturbance, and strength loss depends largely on the effort's intensity, duration, and movement performed.[91,103,112,232] The active strain imposed on a muscle fiber (rather than absolute force) precipitates muscle damage and soreness.[145] *Eccentric muscle actions trigger the greatest post-exercise discomfort, particularly in older adults.*[25,242,247] Existing muscle damage or soreness from previous activity does *not* exacerbate subsequent muscle damage or impair the repair process.[183]

In a well-designed study, subjects rated muscle soreness immediately after exercise and 24, 48, and 72 hr later. Greater soreness occurred from repeated and intense straining movements during active lengthening in eccentric actions compared to either concentric or isometric actions. Soreness did not relate to lactate buildup because intense, level running (concentric actions) produced no residual soreness despite significant blood lactate elevations. Downhill running (mostly eccentric actions) precipitated moderate-to-severe DOMS without elevating lactate concentration as occurs in level running. **TABLE 22.4** highlights DOMS and CK activity effects following an exercise circuit with concentric-only or concentric and eccentric muscle actions.

TABLE 22.4 Acute concentric-only and concentric-eccentric exercise effects on delayed-onset muscle soreness 25 hr following exercise

Group 1 performed three sets of eight exercises (concentric–eccentric) at 60% 1-RM on Universal Gym equipment: one set equaled 20 s followed by 40 s rest, with total exercise time 24 min. Group 2 followed the same exercise protocol, but they exercised maximally for each repetition on resistance devices powered by hydraulic cylinders that produced concentric-only actions. Blood samples and perceived muscle soreness ratings were assessed before exercise and 5, 10, and 25 hr following exercise. The major difference in soreness ratings between exercise groups occurred 25 hr post-exercise; the concentric–eccentric workout produced higher perceived soreness ratings for the major muscle groups exercised. The increase in serum CK remained the same between groups from 5 to 25 hr post-exercise. Both exercise modes elevated serum CK, but the concentric-only muscle actions did not cause significant DOMS.

Cell Damage

The first repetitive, unaccustomed physical activity bout disrupts the integrity within the cells' internal environment. This can produce microlesions and temporary ultrastructural damage in stress-susceptible fibers or pool from degenerating muscle fibers. Damage becomes more extensive several days following exercise than in the immediate post-exercise period. A single moderate concentric exercise bout provides a prophylactic effect on muscle soreness from subsequent high-force eccentric exercise, with the beneficial effect lasting up to 6 wk.

Running downhill at a 10° slope for 30 min produced considerable DOMS 42 hr after running.[34] Corresponding increases occurred in serum Mb levels and the muscle-specific CK enzyme, both common muscle injury markers. Acute inflammation also augments greater leukocyte and neutrophil mobilization. Subject testing also took place after 3, 6, and 9 wk. As the data in **FIGURE 22.25** reveal, the highest perceived soreness ratings for the leg muscles related to elapsed post-exercise time for the three study durations measured before exercise and then 8, 16, and 48 hr post-exercise (*yellow*). Bout 2 (*red*) was performed 3, 6, or 9 wk later at the same hours post-exercise. For the 3- and 6-wk comparisons, differences among exercise bouts reached statistical significance, with diminished DOMS in the second bout (*red*). Perceived muscle soreness and CK and Mb levels showed similar patterns. Surprisingly, peak soreness ratings at 48 hr did not relate to absolute or relative CK or Mb changes. Individuals who reported the greatest DOMS did not necessarily score the highest on CK and Mb values. The first repetitive, high-force exercise bout probably disrupts sarcolemma integrity to produce mitochondrial swelling and temporary ultrastructural muscle damage in stress-susceptible or degenerating muscle fibers from increased protein carbonyl markers that reflect oxidative stress.[44–47,139]

Early induced mechanical damage to myocytes from increased CK release 24 hr post-exercise coincides with acute inflammatory cell infiltration within the muscle.[29] The subsequent muscle performance decrease for several days following eccentric injury primarily stems from failure in excitation-contraction coupling and increased myofibrillar **proteolysis**.[114,256] The fast-twitch fibers with low oxidative capacities show particular vulnerability, with more extensive damage several days following exercise than in the immediate post-exercise period. Single preconditioning eccentric exercise bouts performed at least 20% at maximum eccentric contraction and isometric exercise at a long muscle length protect against eccentric contraction–induced muscle damage.[41,42] Resistance to muscle damage in succeeding physical activity may occur from an eccentric exercise–induced increase in muscle fiber sarcomeres connected in series.[150] Such adaptations support a prudent strategy to initiate training with light activity to protect against the muscle soreness that almost always follows an exercise bout that includes an *eccentric* component.[81] Intense *concentric* movements prior to strenuous eccentric exercise does not magnify muscle damage. In fact, it may prepare the muscle to respond more effectively to a following eccentric exercise stress. *Even prior lower-intensity specific exercise does not fully protect from DOMS with more intense movements.*

Altered Sarcoplasmic Reticulum

Four factors produce key alterations in sarcoplasmic reticulum structure and function with unaccustomed physical activity:

1. Changes in pH
2. Changes in intramuscular high-energy phosphates
3. Changes in ionic balance
4. Changes in temperature

These four factors depress Ca^{2+} uptake and release rates and increase free Ca^{2+} concentration as the mineral rapidly moves into the damaged fiber's cytosol. Intracellular Ca^{2+} overload contributes to the **autolytic process** within damaged muscle fibers that degrades the contractile and noncontractile structures. Topographical mapping techniques to investigate sensory and EMG have been investigated 24 and 48 hr following eccentric exercise to produce DOMS in multiple

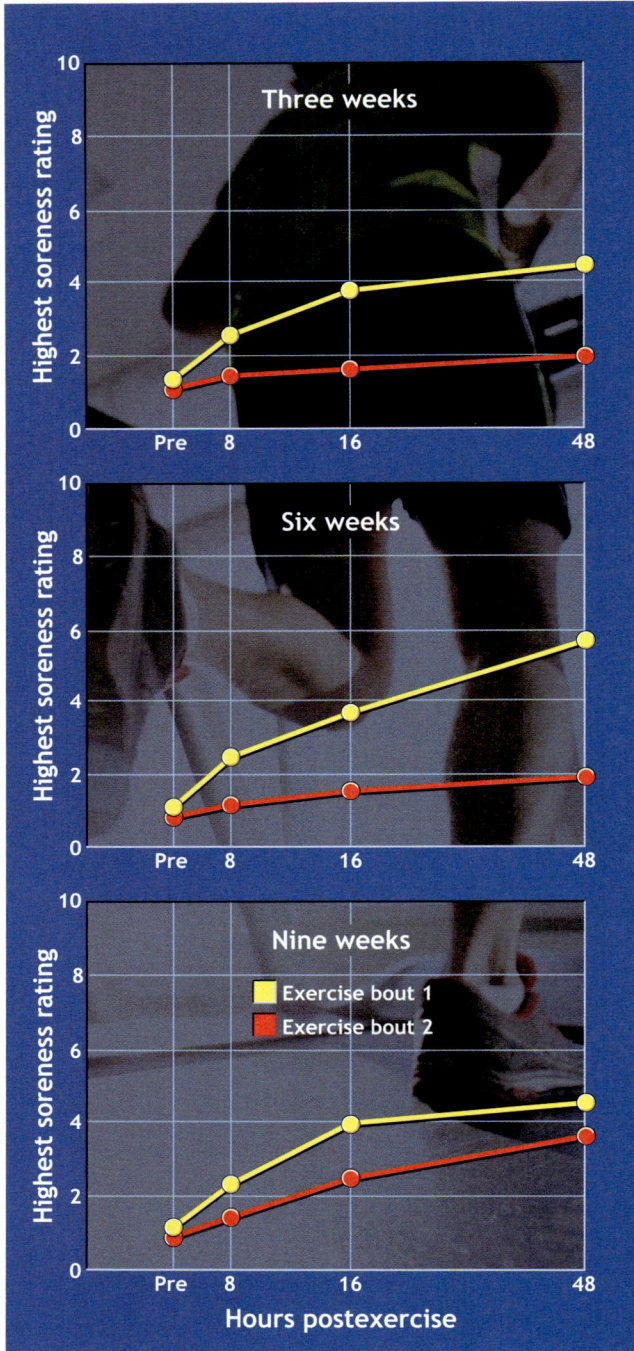

FIGURE 22.25. Highest perceived muscle soreness ratings (scale 1 to 10) before and 8, 16, and 48 hr following downhill running (bout 1, *yellow*) and a subsequent exercise bout (bout 2, *red*) performed either 3, 6, or 9 wk later.
(Adapted with permission from Byrnes WC, et al. Delayed onset muscle soreness following repeated bouts of downhill running. *J Appl Physiol*. 1985;59:710. ©The American Physiological Society (APS). All rights reserved. Photo: Pressmaster/Shutterstock.)

quadriceps muscle locations. Greater DOMS occurred in the quadriceps' distal region, indicating a greater tendency in this region for further injury following eccentric actions along with reduced force capacity.[102]

Vitamin E supplementation, and perhaps vitamin C and selenium, may offer some protection against cellular membrane disruption and enzyme loss from resistance exercise.[86,159] Post-exercise protein supplementation also may protect against muscle soreness in severely exercise-stressed individuals.[75] Compared to a placebo treatment, supplementing daily with either fish oil with high omega-3 and omega-6 fatty acids or isoflavones (soy isolate) 30 days prior to and during the testing wk produced no DOMS benefits (strength, pain ratings, limb girth, and blood measures related to muscle damage, inflammation, and lipid peroxidation) compared to the placebo treatment.[141] Supplementing with 750 mg phosphatidylserine daily for 10 days did not add additional protection against DOMS and muscle damage markers, inflammation, and oxidative stress from prolonged downhill running.[130] Similarly, protease supplements did not impact pain perception with DOMS or blood markers verifying muscle damage.[20]

Current DOMS Model

FIGURE 22.26 presents a six-phase DOMS sequence following unaccustomed exercise. Cellular adaptations to acute exercise provide enhanced resistance to subsequent damage and pain. An undesirable consequence from DOMS interrupts practice sessions, which the athlete, coach, trainer, and physician must confront until soreness diminishes sufficiently to allow continued participation without inducing further muscle damage. Consuming (6 mg · kg^{-1} or 600 mg) caffeine for a 100 kg/220-lb male athlete and 420 mg for a 70 kg/154-lb female counterpart 24 and 48 hr post soreness may confer greater DOMS recovery than without coffee. For reference, one 8-oz cup brewed coffee, in general, contains about 95 mg caffeine (range 70 to 140 mg depending on bean and roast type and brewing method). Ingesting 6 mg caffeine following extreme soreness onset significantly re-established impaired muscle power among elite male and female collegiate athletes, with males exhibiting greater immediate benefits than females.[296]

 See the animation "RICE Method" on **Lippincott Connect** to view this method.

Rationale for Low Back Strengthening

According to the National Center for Health Statistics, including the *Healthcare Cost and Utilization Project, Medical Expenditures Panel Survey* (www.ahrq.gov/data/hcup/index.html), and 2018, Fourth edition "*The Burden of Musculoskeletal Diseases in the United States*" (www.boneandjointburden.org), musculoskeletal disorders impact more than one from every two adults in the United States over age 18, and approximately three of four age 65 and older. Musculoskeletal disorders refer to injuries or

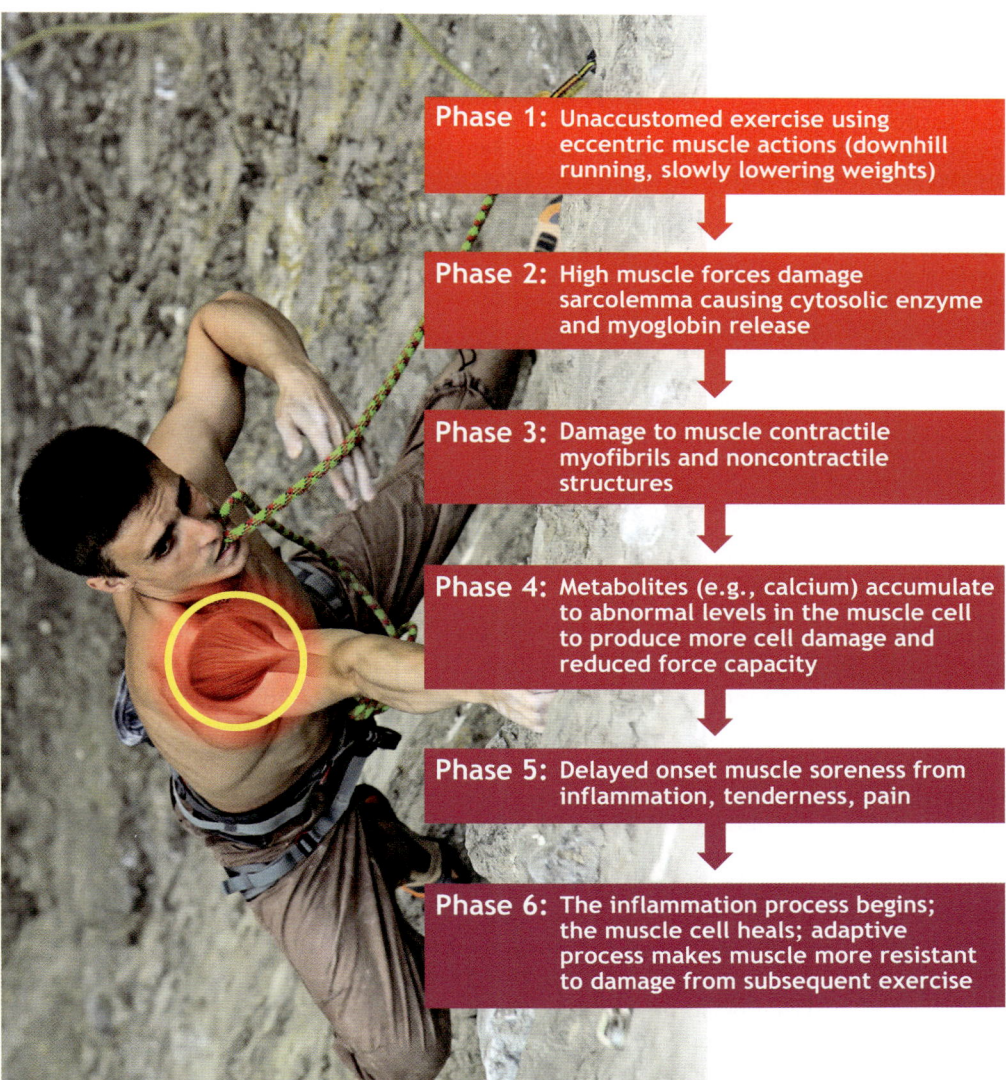

FIGURE 22.26. Six phases in DOMS development and healing provide enhanced resistance to subsequent muscle damage and pain.
(Photo: Photobac/Shutterstock.)

Minimally Invasive Lower Back Surgical Techniques

One microsurgical technique, minimally invasive lumbar discectomy, provides relief from pain and discomfort without extensive rehabilitation, often in an out-patient clinic. Patients are discharged on the same day as surgery and return to a normal lifestyle within a week. The video of neurosurgeons and support staff at a major hospital center presents an up-close tour of the surgery from the first incision to the operation's completion. The problem was caused by a herniated discs pressing on associated nerve root: www.spine-health.com/video/lumbar-micro-endoscopic-discectomy-video. As the video shows, herniated discs typically impinge against a nearby nerve, irritating it with associate radiating pain along the nerve's length. In one report, males and females with decompression lumbar spinal surgery for lumbar low back pain associated with spinal stenosis experienced reduced lower back pain, leg pain, and leg numbness. Females had greater sensitivity to and/or lower tolerance for pain than males.

Lightspring/Shutterstock

Sources:

Brusalis CM, et al. Low back pain versus back-related leg pain: how do patient expectations and outcomes of lumbar spine surgery compare? *HSS J.* 2022 eb;18:83.

Kobayashi Y, et al. Gender differences in pre- and postoperative health-related quality of life measures in patients who have had decompression surgery for lumbar spinal stenosis. *Asian Spine J.* 2020;14:238.

---

illnesses that result from overexertion or repetitive motion, including abdominal trunk muscle weakness and sedentary behaviors.[295] They include soft tissue injuries (sprains, strains, tears, hernias, and carpal tunnel syndrome). Work-related musculoskeletal disorders that result in days away from work most commonly involve the back alone. As reported in an Bureau of Labor Statistics 2020 report, musculoskeletal disorders involving the back accounted for about 38.5% in all work-related musculoskeletal disorders (134,550 back cases out of 349,050 total cases; www.bls.gov/iif/oshwc/case/msds.htm). Further details pointed out that nursing assistants accounted for 10,330 back-related musculoskeletal disorder cases, laborers and hand material movers comprised another 10,660 cases, which accounted for 15.6% of all the back-related cases in 2016. The most common body parts affected by musculoskeletal disorders varied by occupation. Among nursing assistants, more than half their cases affected the back. Compared with other occupations, heavy tractor-trailer truck drivers experienced more injuries that affected the shoulders (19.2%) and legs (16.3%).

Pain and Inflammation

The approximately 150 different musculoskeletal disorders and diseases associate with pain or inflammation. Surprisingly, musculoskeletal injuries account for 50% of chronic medical conditions, more than circulatory (42%), respiratory (24%), and diabetes and cancer (both 9%) (www.who.int/news-room/fact-sheets/detail/musculoskeletal-conditions). The incidence and burden from musculoskeletal conditions are likely to escalate in the next decades from an increasingly aging population with sedentary lifestyles. In particular, back injuries account for one-fourth of all work-related injuries and one-third of all compensation costs, which cost about $90 billion yearly in related health costs. Most cases result from on-the-job injuries, particularly in men in lumber and building retailing (highest risk) and construction (most cases); major risk industries for women include nursing and work in personal care centers (highest risk) and hospitals (most cases). Work in grocery stores and agricultural crop production rank among the top 10 occupations for lower back injury for men and women.

Muscular weakness, particularly in the abdominal and lower lumbar back regions, lumbar spine instability, and poor joint flexibility in the back and legs represent primary external factors related to lower back pain syndrome because movement occurs with a constant resistance. Note that the term *isotonic* inherently lacks precision when applied to functional muscle actions that involve movement because a muscle's effective force-generating capacity varies continually as joint angles change throughout the ROM.

Prevention and Rehabilitation

Preventing and rehabilitating chronic lower back strain commonly uses muscle-strengthening and joint flexibility exercises assessed by **videofluoroscopy**-based tracking algorithms to quantify the time course for intervertebral displacements and other strengthening strategies.[294,308] Continuing normal activities of daily living within limits dictated by pain tolerance yields more rapid recovery from acute back pain than bed rest. Maintaining normal physical activity facilitates greater recovery than specific back-mobilizing exercises performed following pain onset. Prudent resistance-training isolates and strengthens the abdomen and lower lumbar extensor muscles that support and protect the spine through its full ROM. Patients with lower back pain who strengthen these muscle groups experience fewer acute and chronic symptoms, improved muscular strength and endurance, and increased ROM.[307]

Resistance-Training to Prevent and Reduce Lower Back Injury Risk

Resistance-training exercise poses a dilemma for those with lower back syndrome. Improperly performing a typical resistance exercise movement with a relatively heavy load with hips thrust forward and arched back creates excessive lower spine compressive forces. For example, pressing and curling exercises with back hyperextension creates unusually high shearing stress on lumbar vertebrae, often triggering lower back pain accompanied by regional muscle instability. Compressive forces with heavy lifting also can hasten damage to vertebral disks that cushion and protect vertebrae. Performing half squats with barbell loads from 0.8 to 1.6 times body mass produces huge compressive loads on the L3 to L4 spine segment, often the equivalent to 6 to 10 times body mass. For example, a person who weighs 90 kg/198 lb and squats with 144 kg/318 lb can create peak compressive forces exceeding 1367 kg/13,334 N! A sudden amplification in compressive force can precipitate anterior disk prolapse or herniation. A lower-intensity but sustained compressive force that produces muscle fatigue can increase posterior bulging at the lamellas in the posterior annulus. In national-level male and female powerlifters, average compressive loads on L4 to L5 reached 1757 kg/17,192 N. At the practical level during sports training with resistance methods (i.e., functional training with free weights), one must not sacrifice meticulous exercise execution just to lift a heavier load or "squeeze out" additional repetitions. The extra weight lifted through improper technique (**cheating**) does not facilitate muscle strengthening; rather, improper body alignment or unwarranted muscle substitution during the lift can trigger debilitating injury requiring surgery, as often occurs at all golf skill levels.

Practical Example in a High Skill Sport

Golfers with poor initial hip rotation during the downswing often exhibit weak (or deactivated) gluteus medius muscle action. This fan-shaped muscle shown in red (with the unseen gluteus minimus underneath) lies on the ilium's surface, and abducts or stabilizes the thigh and rotates it medially. Reactivating this "athletically important" muscle with closed kinetic chain movements combined with vibration may alleviate the inefficient slide phase during the golf downswing to restore effective hip rotation. Golf swing biomechanical analysis in amateurs and professionals provides insights into golf mechanical injury incidence and provides a rationale for muscular conditioning with resistance training.[71,85,142,245,282] An improper typical resistance exercise movement with relatively heavy load and hips thrust forward with arched back creates excessive lower spine compressive forces. For example, pressing and curling exercises with back hyperextension create unusually high shearing stress on the lumbar vertebrae, often triggering lower back pain accompanied by muscle instability in this body region.

SciePro/Shutterstock

Workplace Disability

At least 32 million adult Americans frequently experience lower back pain sometime in their life, the primary cause for workplace disability.[138,280] Workplace disability from lower back injuries also occurs in common tasks such as refuse collection and other manual handling and lifting tasks.[62,67,128] Muscular weakness, particularly in the abdominal and lower lumbar back regions, lumbar spine instability, and poor joint flexibility in the back and legs represent primary external factors related to lower back pain syndrome.[215,281]

Resistance Training and Joint-Flexibility Exercise

Rehabilitating persistent lower back strain commonly uses muscle strengthening and joint flexibility exercises.[23,72,163] Continuing normal daily living activities (within limits dictated by pain tolerance) yields more rapid recovery from acute back pain than bed rest. Maintaining normal physical activity facilitates greater recovery than specific back-mobilizing exercises performed after pain onset.[153] Prudent resistance-type training isolates and strengthens the abdomen and lower lumbar extensor muscles that support and protect the spine through its full ROM. Patients with lower back pain who strengthen the lumbar extensors with the pelvis stabilized experience less pain, fewer chronic symptoms, and improved muscular strength and endurance and ROM.[37]

An improper typical resistance exercise bouncing movement with or without a load and the hips thrust forward with arched back can create excessive lower spine compressive forces. Also, pressing and curling exercises with back hyperextension create unusually high shearing stress on the lumbar vertebrae, often triggering lower back pain accompanied by muscle instability in this region.[13,99,104] Compressive forces with heavy lifting also can hasten damage to the disks that cushion the vertebrae. A person who weighs 90 kg/198 lb and squats with 144 kg/318 lb can create peak compressive forces in excess of 1367 kg (13,334 N)! A sudden amplification of compressive force can precipitate anterior disk prolapse; a lower-intensity but sustained compressive force that produces fatigue can increase posterior bulging of the lamellas in the posterior annulus.[6] In national-level male and female powerlifters, average compressive loads on L4–L5 reached 1757 kg/17,192 N.[165]

Improper Technique Can Precipitate Injury

During sports training with resistance methods (i.e., functional training with free weights), one should not sacrifice proper execution of an exercise to lift a heavier load or "squeeze out" additional repetitions. The extra weight lifted through improper technique does not facilitate muscle strengthening; instead, improper body alignment or unwarranted muscle substitution during force production can trigger debilitating injury where surgery unfortunately becomes the option of choice. This should encourage proper strengthening of "core" abdominal and lower back muscles (with 12 lower back, abdominal, and hip exercises depicted in the feature In a Practical Sense) to avoid either prolonged reliance on pain-relieving drugs or potentially debilitating surgical alternatives. Wearing a relatively stiff weightlifting belt during heavy lifts (squats, dead

In a Practical Sense

Flexibility and Strengthening Exercises for the Lower Back, Abdomen, and Trunk

The 12 exercises provide abdominal, pelvic region, and lower back general strengthening, and hamstring and lower back flexibility movements for individuals with no apparent lower back and spinal injuries. Symptomatic individuals (including athletes) require specific back exercises[194,206,284,325] to complement the general and specific sport functional movement requirements.

I. LOWER BACK STRETCHES (HOLD EACH EXERCISE FOR 30 TO 60 S)

Knees-to-chest stretch: Lie supine, pull knees into chest while maintaining a flat lower back.

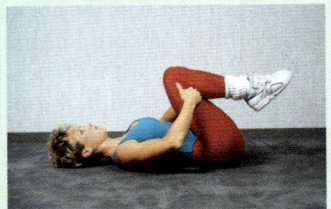

Photo courtesy Dr. Robert S. Swanson, DC

Cross-leg stretch: Cross legs and pull one 90°-flexed knee toward chest. Repeat with the opposite leg.

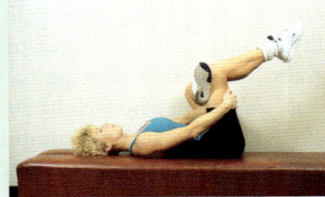

Photo courtesy Dr. Robert S. Swanson, DC

Hamstring stretch: Place strap over foot, keep lower back flat, pull leg upward toward the head.

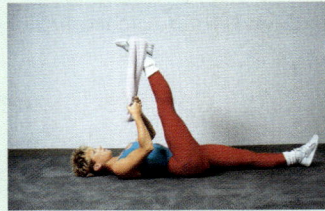

Photo courtesy Dr. Robert S. Swanson, DC

Frog stretch: Sit, buttocks on bilateral heels; move hands forward along floor surface.

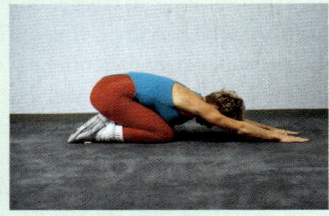

Photo courtesy Dr. Robert S. Swanson, DC

II. ABDOMINAL EXERCISES

Bent-knee sit-up: Hands low on neck (or across chest), head positioned over shoulders, roll up slowly and raise shoulders 4 to 6 in from surface and hold briefly.

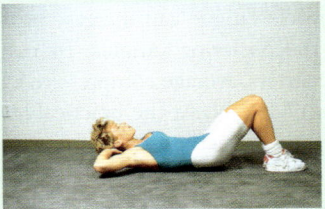

Photo courtesy Dr. Robert S. Swanson, DC

Dying bug: Flatten lower back by flexing pelvis against surface. Bring an extended arm and flexed knee together, extend one arm straight overhead and leg straight backward. Maintain pelvic flexion while alternating opposing arms and legs in this position.

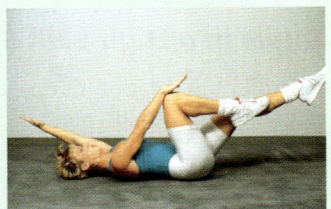

Photo courtesy Dr. Robert S. Swanson, DC

III. PRONE LUMBAR EXTENSION EXERCISES

Dry-land swimming: Lie prone with pelvic flexion, alternately lifting opposite arm and leg.

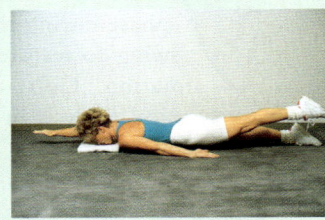

Photo courtesy Dr. Robert S. Swanson, DC

Both legs up: Lie prone with pelvic flexion and lift both legs simultaneously, keeping head on floor.

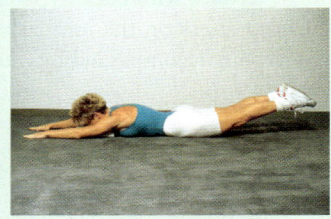

Photo courtesy Dr. Robert S. Swanson, DC

Upper body up: Lie prone with pelvic flexion and arms outstretched or behind back, lift upper torso and keep legs on floor.

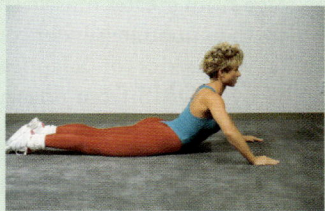

Photo courtesy Dr. Robert S. Swanson, DC

Pointer (bird dog): Hands and knees on floor. Flex pelvis into a counter position. Exchange pointing opposite arm and leg while keeping torso level.

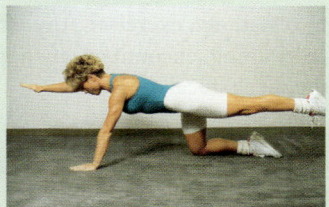

Photo courtesy Dr. Robert S. Swanson, DC

IV. SUPINE PELVIC FLEXION EXERCISES

Leg pointer: Lie supine on floor and flex pelvis with lower abdominals to flatten lower back on surface. Extend one arm upward and one leg outward, keeping quadriceps level.

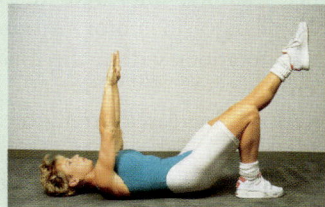

Photo courtesy Dr. Robert S. Swanson, DC

Prone cobra push-up: Keep pelvis on floor, press arms up to produce lower back extension.

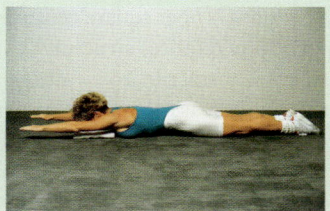

Photo courtesy Dr. Robert S. Swanson, DC

lifts, clean-and-jerk maneuvers) reduces intra-abdominal pressure compared with lifting without a belt.[84,95,137] The belt reduces potentially injurious compressive forces on spinal disks during near-maximal lifting, including most Olympic and powerlifting events and associated training. In one study, nine experienced weightlifters lifted barbells up to 75% body weight under three conditions: (1) while inhaling and wearing a belt, (2) inhaling and not wearing a belt, and (3) exhaling and wearing a belt.[129] Measurements included intra-abdominal pressure, trunk muscle EMG, ground reaction forces, and kinematics. The belt reduced compression forces by about 10%, but only when inhaling before lifting. The authors concluded that wearing a tight and stiff-back belt while inhaling before lifting reduces spinal loading during the lift.

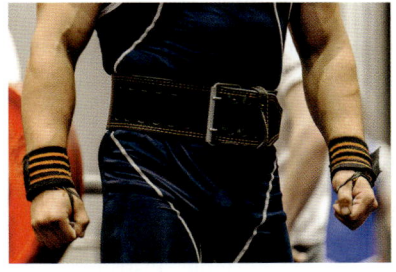

sportpoint/Shutterstock

A person who normally trains wearing a belt should generally refrain from lifting without one. Further recommendations include performing at least some submaximal resistance training without a belt to strengthen the deep abdominal and pelvic stabilizing muscles, which are usually not activated when using a belt. This also develops the proper pattern of muscle recruitment to generate high intra-abdominal pressures when not wearing a belt. Wearing a backbelt to increase intra-abdominal pressure to ameliorate low back injuries in the workplace does not provide a clear-cut biomechanical advantage.[190] A prospective study over 2 years with nearly 14,000 material-handling employees in 30 states evaluated the effectiveness of using back belts to reduce back injury worker's compensation claims and reports of low back pain.[250] Neither frequent back belt use (usually once a day, once or twice a week) nor a store policy that required the continuous use of these belts reduced injury or reports of lower back pain. Researchers continue to probe for answers about the etiology of lower back pain syndrome and how to minimize its severity and reduce its occurrence.[121,209,254] Studies have focused on numerous contributing factors that include intra-disk pressure,[166] facet loads and disk fiber strains,[211] lumbar disk height and cross-sectional area,[179] compressive follower loads,[188] spinal joint force distribution,[43] ligament strain, disk shear, and facet impingement,[81] and prediction models to estimate spinal compression and shear forces.[90,124,283,289]

Summary

1. Muscle fiber size and type and the bone and muscle anatomic lever arrangement govern human muscular strength's upper limit.
2. Central nervous system influences trigger prime movers in a specific action to impact maximum force capacity.

3. Six factors—genetic, exercise, nutritional, hormonal, environmental, and neural—interact with resistance training to regulate skeletal muscle mass and corresponding strength development.
4. Three factors contribute to increased muscle strength with resistance training: improved motor unit recruitment capacity, changes in motor neuron firing pattern efficiency, and alterations within the muscle fibers' contractile elements.
5. Muscular overload increases strength and selectively stimulates muscle fiber hypertrophy.
6. Muscle hypertrophy includes increased protein synthesis with myofibrillar thickening, connective tissue cell proliferation, and increased satellite cell number surrounding each fiber.
7. Human skeletal muscle generates a maximum force between 16 and 30 Newtons (N) per square centimeter MCSA.
8. Muscle hypertrophy requires structural changes within an individual fiber's contractile apparatus, particularly fast-twitch fibers, and increased anaerobic energy stores.
9. The genetic code exerts the greatest influence on muscle fiber-type distribution, with fiber composition largely fixed before birth or during the early growth years.
10. Human muscle fibers adapt to increased functional demands from myogenic satellite stem cells that proliferate and differentiate for muscle remodeling.
11. Relatively brief resistance training periods generate similar percentage strength improvements for women and men.
12. Allometric scaling represents a mathematical procedure to establish a "truer" relationship among a body size variable (usually stature, body mass, FFM) and various muscular strength expressions.
13. Muscle weakness in the core abdominal and lower lumbar back regions, coupled with poor flexibility in the lower back and legs, associate with lower back syndrome.
14. Core muscle strengthening, flexibility, and balance exercises help to protect against and rehabilitate lower back syndrome.
15. For women, increasing bone density and avoiding activities that increase spinal compression and bone stress reduce osteoporosis and fracture risk.
16. Conventional resistance training does not improve aerobic fitness or facilitate weight loss because of its relatively low caloric cost.
17. Circuit resistance training combines muscle training benefits from resistance exercise with the cardiovascular, calorie-burning benefits from continuous dynamic activities in power walking, jogging/running, and vigorous dancing.
18. Eccentric muscle actions provoke greater DOMS than concentric-only or isometric actions.
19. Serum markers for muscle damage (CK and Mb) increase with each form of muscle action (concentric, eccentric, or isometric).
20. A single exercise bout protects against DOMS and muscle damage from subsequent exercise.
21. Beginning a training program that requires considerable muscular force should progress gradually at a lower intensity to minimize eccentric muscle actions and subsequent DOMS.
22. Considerable controversy concerns whether transgender individuals (male to female) obtain an athletic advantage at any transition stage from greater muscle strength, MCSA, or lean body mass than nontransgender counterparts.
23. The body initiates a series of adaptive inflammation responses caused by DOMS from unaccustomed physical activity.
24. Consuming 6 $mg \cdot kg^{-1} \cdot BW^{-1}$ caffeine following extreme soreness onset restores impaired muscle power, with males exhibiting greater immediate benefits than females.

Key Terms

Accommodating resistance exercise: Any effort during isokinetic resistance training encounters an opposing force to that applied to the mechanical device

Activities of daily living (ADL): Self-care daily activities include feeding, bathing, dressing, grooming, work, homemaking, and leisure

Acute responses: Immediate changes in muscle or other cells, tissues, or systems during or immediately following a single exercise bout

Autolytic process: Enzymes from cells and tissues degrade as a "self-digestion" mechanism

Babbage, Charles: English mathematician first to invent a dynamometer to record forces versus time

Ballistic resistance training: Training objective to move a weight or projectile as rapidly as possible through the full range of motion with good form

Basedow, Johann: German educator attempted to reform education, and promoted games and physical exercise as essential school curriculum components

Cable tensiometer: Lightweight, portable instrument to measure tension in a wire or cable from multiple angles about a specific joint's ROM; assesses the muscle's force capacity exerted over the cable during a static muscle action that elicits little or no change in the muscle's external length

Cheating: Breaking from strict form when performing an exercise (e.g., slight upper body swing before lifting allows the person to "help" lift a heavier weight or the same weight more times)

Chronic adaptations: Body's adjustments to repeated, chronic stimulus

Circuit resistance training (CRT): Series of exercises performed sequentially with minimal rest among exercises

Closed kinetic chain exercise: Body weight–loaded exercise or movement where the distal aspect of the extremity remains fixed in constant contact with an immobile surface (e.g., feet anchored to the ground in a squat exercise)

Concentric action: Muscle shortening during force application

Core training: Training of abdominal, gluteal, diaphragm, pelvic floor, hip girdle, and erector spinae musculature (also called paraspinals)

Delayed-onset muscle soreness (DOMS): Soreness and stiffness in exercised joints and muscles that can persist for up to 7 days following unaccustomed exercise

Dynamic constant external resistance training (DCER): External resistance or weight does not change, yet joint flexion and extension occur with each repetition

Dynamometers: Force-measuring instruments to assess a mechanically derived output—force, power, torque, speed, and velocity.

Eccentric action: Muscle lengthening during force application

Fiber hyperplasia: Increase in tissue size from increases in cell number within a tissue

Fiber hypertrophy: Increase in muscle fiber size

Functional strength training: Training requiring neuromuscular adaptations in the important movements that create improved strength.

GLUT-4: Insulin-regulated glucose transporter in adipose and skeletal and cardiac muscle tissues

Gymnasticon: First English patented mechanical device resembling a bicycle designed to exercise all body joints

Halteres: Small 3 to 4 lb handheld stones or lead weights used by the ancients in physical training

Hyperplasia: Increase in muscle fiber number

Hypertrophy: Skeletal muscle fiber growth

Integrated electromyography (EMG): Mathematical integral of the absolute raw signal

Isokinetic dynamometer: Electromechanical accommodating resistance instrument with a speed-controlling mechanism, which accelerates to a preset, constant velocity with applied force regardless of the force exerted on the device movement arm, and where resistance increases or decreases with a muscle's capacity that varies throughout a joint's ROM

Isokinetic training: Provides muscular overload at a preset constant speed while the muscle mobilizes its force-generating capacity throughout the full ROM

Isometric action: Muscle action without change in muscle length

Isometric training: Muscle action performed at a fixed point in the ROM

Guts Muth, Johann: German educator and writer described workout routines for balance on swinging beams, poles, ropes, and other apparatus, and considered the grandfather of early gymnastics

Kettlebells: Cast-iron ball-shaped weight with a single handle used in various strength training movements

Ling, Pehr Henrik: Father of Swedish gymnastics; founded the current Swedish School of Sport and Health Sciences under the name of the Royal Central Institute of Gymnastics, Stockholm

Longitudinal splitting: Muscle fiber splits into two or more smaller individual daughter cells

Matveyev, Leonid: Russian sports scientist introduced in 1962 the concept of strength training periodization or sequential training planning

Muscle cross-sectional area (MCSA): Measured cross-section of the largest diameter in an intact, contracted muscle

Muscular endurance: Sustaining maximum (or submaximum) force, often determined by determining maximum repetition number at a maximum strength percentage

Myasthenia gravis: Autoimmune neuromuscular disorder characterized by disrupted neural signal communication at the neuromuscular junction

Myogenic stem cells: Small multipotent cells within mature muscle that are precursors to skeletal muscle or satellite cells

Myotatic reflex: Monosynaptic reflex in muscle provides automatic regulation of skeletal muscle length

Nerve conduction velocity (NCV): Speed at which an electrochemical impulse propagates down a neural pathway

One-repetition maximum (1-RM): Maximum force generated for one repetition of a movement

Overload principle: Training strategy whereby a muscle makes physiological adaptations to the progressive level of tension placed on it

Periodization: Training planning varies training intensity and volume to ensure optimal conditions so peak performance coincides with major competitions

Plyometric movements: Powerful, propulsive movements to mobilize inherent stretch-recoil skeletal muscle characteristics and modulation via the stretch or myotatic reflex

Plyometric training: Resistance training involving eccentric-to-concentric actions performed quickly so a muscle stretches slightly prior to the concentric action

Polio (poliomyelitis): Crippling and potentially deadly infectious disease caused by the poliovirus

Predictive equations: Mathematical expression provides the best estimate of one variable (e.g., 1-RM) from a predictor variable (e.g., body weight)

Progressive resistance exercise (PRE): Practical application of the overload principle which forms the basis for most resistance training programs

Progressive resistance weight training: Common exercise strategy to train muscles to become stronger using standard

weightlifting equipment, pulleys, slings, springs, immovable bars, resistance bands, and a variety of isokinetic, pneumatic, and hydraulic devices

Proteolysis: Protein breakdown from enzyme action to amino acids

Radiculopathy: Disorder of spinal nerve roots that manifests as pain, weakness, reflex changes, and sensory loss radiating from the spine's affected nerve root

Range of motion (ROM): Maximum movement range through a joint's allowable arc

Sandow, Eugene: One of the first successful muscular vaudeville strongmen in the early 1890s to publish popular magazines, promote barbell exercise equipment, and promote special foods for training

Sticking point: Region in an exercise movement against a set resistance that poses the greatest difficulty to complete the movement

Strength: Maximum force-generating capacity of a muscle or group of muscles

Stretch-shortening cycle (SSC): Sequence of stretching and shortening muscle fibers to reflexly enhance subsequent movement performance

Suspension training: Leveraging a person's body weight during exercise (without reliance on externally fixed weights, pulleys, or cams) by increasing or lessening the suspension coordinates, rope height, pulleys, slings, or bungee cords, relative to the suspension point

Torque: Force that produces a turning, twisting, or rotary movement of bones about a joint in any plane about an axis

Training volume: Total work performed in a single training session

Transgender: Gender identity or gender expression that differs from the sex that they were assigned at birth

Turnverein societies: German-American gymnastic (Turnverein) that promoted German culture, physical culture, and "gymnastics" as an American sport and the field of academic study

Variable resistance: Training with equipment that uses a lever arm, cam, hydraulic system, or pulley to alter the resistance to match increases and decreases in a muscle's capacity throughout a joint's ROM

Videofluoroscopy: Simultaneous movement visualization of internal body structures (e.g., cervical and lumbar spine) with corresponding external body movements using real time and kinematic imaging techniques

Zander, Gustav: Swedish physician (1835–1920) devised methods to treat patients and common persons with standard gymnastic exercise emphasizing mechanical machines, calisthenics, balance, and core trunk and limb strength

References are available online at Lippincott Connect.

Additional References

Aeles J, et al. The effect of small changes in rate of force development on muscle fascicle velocity and motor unit discharge behaviour. *Eur J Appl Physiol.* 2022. doi:10.1007/s00421-022-04905-7.

Almeida AA, et al. Civilians have higher adherence and more improvements in health with a Mediterranean diet and circuit training program compared to firefighters. *J Occup Environ Med.* 2022. doi:10.1097/JOM.0000000000002478.

Andrade MS, et al. Isokinetic muscular strength and aerobic physical fitness in recreational long-distance runners: a cross-sectional study. *J Strength Cond Res.* 2022;36:e73.

Batrakoulis A, et al. Hybrid-type, multicomponent interval training upregulates musculoskeletal fitness of adults with overweight and obesity in a volume-dependent manner: a 1-year dose-response randomised controlled trial. *Eur J Sport Sci.* 2022:1. doi:10.1080/17461391.2021.2025434.

Cannon J, et al. Increased core stability is associated with reduced knee valgus during single-leg landing tasks: investigating lumbar spine and hip joint rotational stiffness. *J Biomech.* 2021;116:110240.

Cao G, et al. The role of oxidative stress in intervertebral disc degeneration. *Oxid Med Cell Longev.* 2022:2166817.

Cognetti DJ, et al. Blood flow restriction therapy and its use for rehabilitation and return to sport: physiology, application, and guidelines for implementation. *Arthrosc Sports Med Rehabil.* 2022;4:e71.

Costa BDV, et al. Does performing different resistance exercises for the same muscle group induce non-homogeneous hypertrophy? *Int J Sports Med.* 2021;42:803.

Eberman LE, et al. Providing transgender patient care: athletic trainers' compassion and lack of preparedness. *J Athl Train.* 2021;56:252.

Fabero-Garrido R, et al. Negative psychological factors' influence on delayed onset muscle soreness intensity, reduced cervical function and daily activities in healthy participants. *J Pain.* 2022:S1526.

Ferreira JP, et al. Effects of combined training on metabolic profile, lung function, stress and quality of life in sedentary adults: a study protocol for a randomized controlled trial. *PLoS One.* 2022;17:e0263455.

Grgic J. Effects of post-exercise cold-water immersion on resistance training-induced gains in muscular strength: a systematic review and meta-analysis. *Eur J Sport Sci.* 2022:1. doi:10.1080/17461391.2022.2033851.

Hackett DA. Acute impairment in respiratory muscle strength following a high-volume versus low-volume resistance exercise session. *J Sports Med Phys Fitness.* 2022;62:395.

Hamarsland H, et al. Equal-volume strength training with different training frequencies induces similar muscle hypertrophy and strength improvement in trained participants. *Front Physiol.* 2022;12:789403.

Hamzeh Shalamzari M, et al. The effects of a self-myofascial release program on isokinetic hamstrings-to-quadriceps strength ratio and range of motion of the knee joint among athletes with hamstring shortness. *J Sport Rehabil.* 2022:1. doi:10.1123/jsr.2020-0487.

Harper J, et al. How does hormone transition in transgender women change body composition, muscle strength and haemoglobin? Systematic review with a focus on the implications for sport participation. *Br J Sports Med.* 2021;55:865.

Heywood SE, et al. The effectiveness of aquatic plyometric training in improving strength, jumping, and sprinting: a systematic review. *J Sport Rehabil.* 2022;31:85.

Hilton EN, Lundberg TR. Transgender women in the female category of sport: perspectives on testosterone suppression and performance advantage. *Sports Med.* 2021;51:199.

Hirono T, et al. Relationship between muscle swelling and hypertrophy induced by resistance training. *J Strength Cond Res.* 2022;36:359.

Holm LW, et al. Vigorous regular leisure-time physical activity is associated with a clinically important improvement in back pain—a secondary analysis of randomized controlled trials. *BMC Musculoskelet Disord.* 2021;22:857.

Homs AF, et al. Relationship between gait complexity and pain attention in chronic low back pain. *Pain.* 2022;163:e31.

Huang YH, et al. The influence of Nordic walking on spinal posture, physical function, and back pain in community-dwelling older adults: a pilot study. *Healthcare (Basel).* 2021;9:1303.

Johansson F, et al. External training load and the association with back pain in competitive adolescent tennis players: results from the smash cohort study. *Sports Health.* 2022;14:111.

Johnston L. Transgender and intersex athletes in single-sex sports. *J Law Med.* 2020;28:197.

Kamandulis S, et al. Increasing the resting time between drop jumps lessens delayed-onset muscle soreness and limits the extent of prolonged low-frequency force depression in human knee extensor muscles. *Eur J Appl Physiol.* 2022;122:255.

Kemmler W, et al. Detraining effects after 18 months of high intensity resistance training on osteosarcopenia in older men-Six-month follow-up of the randomized controlled Franconian Osteopenia and Sarcopenia Trial (FROST). *Bone.* 2021;142:115772.

Konrad A, et al. Relationship between eccentric-exercise-induced loss in muscle function to muscle soreness and tissue hardness. *Healthcare (Basel).* 2022;10:96.

Lucena EG, et al. Isokinetic strength of shoulder rotator muscles in powerlifters: correlation between isometric and concentric muscle actions. *J Sports Med Phys Fitness.* 2022;62:170.

Mang ZA, et al. Aerobic Adaptations to resistance training: The role of time under tension. *Int J Sports Med.* 2022. doi:10.1055/a-1664-8701.

McGill S. Ultimate Back Fitness and Performance. 6th ed., Backfitpro, Inc., 2017. Available at: https://www.backfitpro.com/books/ultimate-back-fitness-and-performance-6th-edition-2017/.

Miller R, et al. The muscle morphology of elite sprint running. *Med Sci Sports Exerc.* 2021;53:804.

Munson EE, Ensign KA. Transgender athletes' experiences with health care in the athletic training setting. *J Athl Train.* 2021;56:101.

Nunes ACCA, et al. Effects of integrative neuromuscular training and detraining on countermovement jump performance in youth volleyball players. *J Strength Cond Res.* 2021;35:2242.

Parra ME, et al. The reliability of the slopes and y-intercepts of the motor unit firing times and action potential waveforms versus recruitment threshold relationships derived from surface electromyography signal decomposition. *Eur J Appl Physiol.* 2021;121:3389.

Pérez-Castilla A, et al. Validity of different velocity-based methods and repetitions-to-failure equations for predicting the 1 repetition maximum during 2 upper-body pulling exercises. *J Strength Cond Res.* 2021;35:1800.

Pigozzi F, et al. Joint position statement of the International Federation of Sports Medicine (FIMS) and European Federation of Sports Medicine Associations (EFSMA) on the IOC framework on fairness, inclusion and non-discrimination based on gender identity and sex variations. *BMJ Open Sport Exerc Med.* 2022;8:e001273.

Posnakidis G, et al. High-intensity functional training improves cardiorespiratory fitness and neuromuscular performance without inflammation or muscle damage. *J Strength Cond Res.* 2022;36:615.

Reece TM, Herda TJ. An examination of a potential organized motor unit firing rate and recruitment scheme of an antagonist muscle during isometric contractions. *J Neurophysiol.* 2021;125:2094.

Reynolds A, Hamidian Jahromi A. Transgender athletes in sports competitions: how policy measures can be more inclusive and fairer to all. *Front Sports Act Living.* 2021;3:704178.

Sato S, et al. Cross-education and detraining effects of eccentric vs. concentric resistance training of the elbow flexors. *BMC Sports Sci Med Rehabil.* 2021;13:105.

Silva JPD, et al. Trajectories of pain and disability in older adults with acute low back pain: longitudinal data of the BACE-Brazil cohort. *Braz J Phys Ther.* 2022;26:100386.

Taber CB, et al. The effects of body tempering on force production, flexibility and muscle soreness in collegiate football athletes. *J Funct Morphol Kinesiol.* 2022;7:9.

Tarabeih N, et al. Deciphering the causal relationships between low back pain complications, metabolic factors, and comorbidities. *J Pain Res.* 2022;15:215.

Thornton JS, et al. Treating low back pain in athletes: a systematic review with meta-analysis. *Br J Sports Med.* 2021;55:656.

Varela-Olalla D, et al. Rating of perceived exertion and velocity loss as variables for controlling the level of effort in the bench press exercise. *Sports Biomech.* 2022;21:41.

Walsh ME, et al. Existing validated clinical prediction rules for predicting response to physiotherapy interventions for musculoskeletal conditions have limited clinical value: a systematic review. *J Clin Epidemiol.* 2021;135:90.

Wang Y, et al. Effect of cold and heat therapies on pain relief in patients with delayed onset muscle soreness: a network meta-analysis. *J Rehabil Med.* 2022;54:jrm00258.

Yoo J, et al. Estimation of 1-repetition maximum using a hydraulic bench press machine based on user's lifting speed and load weight. *Sensors (Basel).* 2022;22:698.

Yu G, et al. Effects of blood flow restriction training on blood perfusion and work ability of muscles in elite para-alpine skiers. *Med Sci Sports Exerc.* 2022;54:489.

Zhao X. Research on athlete behavior recognition technology in sports teaching video based on deep neural network. *Comput Intell Neurosci.* 2022;2022:7260894.

Table 22.1	International System Units to Express Muscular Strength and Power During Linear and Angular Motions
Quantity	**Unit**
Linear Motion	
Force	Newton, N
Velocity	Meters per second, $m \cdot s^{-1}$
Mass	Kilogram, kg
Acceleration	Meters per second squared, $m \cdot s^{-2}$
Displacement	Meter, m
Time	Second, s
Angular Motion	
Torque, T	Newton meter, N-m
Velocity, v	Radians per second, $rad \cdot s^{-1}$
Moment of inertia, I or J	Kilogram meters squared, $kg\text{-}m^2$
Acceleration, a	Radians per second squared, $rad \cdot s^{-2}$
Displacement, θ	Radian, rad
Time, t	Second, s

Appendix D available online at Lippincott Connect includes hundreds of additional interconversion factors.

Table 22.2	Physiologic Adaptations to Resistance Training
System/Variable	**Response**
Muscle fibers	
Number	Equivocal
Size	Increase
Type	Unknown
Strength	Increase
Mitochondria	
Volume	Decrease
Density	Decrease
Twitch contraction time	Decrease
Enzymes	
Creatine phosphokinase	Increase
Myokinase	Increase
Enzymes of glycolysis	
Phosphofructokinase	Increase
Lactate dehydrogenase	No change
Aerobic metabolism enzymes	
Carbohydrate	Increase
Triglyceride	Not known
Basal metabolism	Increase
Intramuscular fuel stores	
Adenosine triphosphate	Increase
Phosphocreatine	Increase
Glycogen	Increase
Triglycerides	Not known
Aerobic capacity	
Circuit resistance training	Increase
Standard resistance training	No change
Connective tissue	
Ligament strength	Increase
Tendon strength	Increase
Collagen content of muscle	No change
Body composition	
Percent body fat	Decrease
Lean body mass	Increase
Bone	
Mineral content and density	Increase
Cross-sectional area	Increase

Adapted with permission from Fleck SJ, Kraemer WJ. Resistance training: physiological responses and adaptations (part 2 of 4). *Phys Sportsmed*. 1988;16:108. Taylor & Francis Ltd., www.tandfonline.com.

Table 22.3 Energy Expenditure for Different Resistance Exercise Modes Compared with Level Walking for a 68-kg/150-lb Person

Mode	Sex	$kJ \cdot min^{-1}$	$kcal \cdot min^{-1}$
Nautilus, circuit	M	29.7	7.1
	F	24.3	5.8
Nautilus, circuit	M	22.6	5.4
Universal, circuit	M	33.1	7.9
	F	28.5	6.8
Isokinetic, slow	M	40.2	9.6
Isokinetic, fast	M	41.4	9.9
Isometric and free-weight	M	25.1	6.0
Hydra-Fitness, circuit	M	37.7	9.0
Level walking	M	22.6	5.4

F, female; M, male.
Data from Katch FI, et al. Evaluation of acute cardiorespiratory responses to hydraulic resistance exercise. *Med Sci Sports Exerc.* 1985;17:168.

Table 22.4 Acute Concentric-Only and Concentric-Eccentric Exercise Effects on Delayed-Onset Muscle Soreness 25 hr After Exercise

	Soreness Ratings	
Site	Concentric $\bar{x}$	Concentric–Eccentric $\bar{x}$
Chest	2.3	5.1
Back (upper)	2.6	2.8
Shoulders (front)	2.2	3.6
Shoulders (back)	1.9	3.6
Biceps (mid)	1.9	4.3
Biceps (lower)	1.8	3.5
Triceps (mid)	1.9	3.4
Triceps (lower)	1.9	3.0
Forearm (front)	1.7	3.4
Forearm (back)	1.7	2.9
Back (lower)	1.7	2.9
Buttocks	1.8	2.5
Quadriceps (mid)	2.0	4.1
Quadriceps (lower)	2.1	3.8
Hamstrings (mid)	2.1	3.5
Hamstrings (lower)	2.1	3.0

	CK Activity ($mU \cdot mL^{-1}$)	
Sample Time	Concentric $\bar{x}$	Concentric–Eccentric $\bar{x}$
Pre	86.7	126.9
5 hr post	344.8	232.0
10 hr post	394.3	368.5
25 hr post	288.0	482.2

Reprinted from Byrnes WC, et al. Muscle soreness following resistance exercise with and without eccentric muscle actions. *Res Q Exerc Sport.* 1985;56:283. Copyright © SHAPE America, reprinted by permission of Taylor & Francis Ltd, www.tandfonline.com on behalf of SHAPE America.

Chapter 23: Special Aids to Exercise Training and Performance

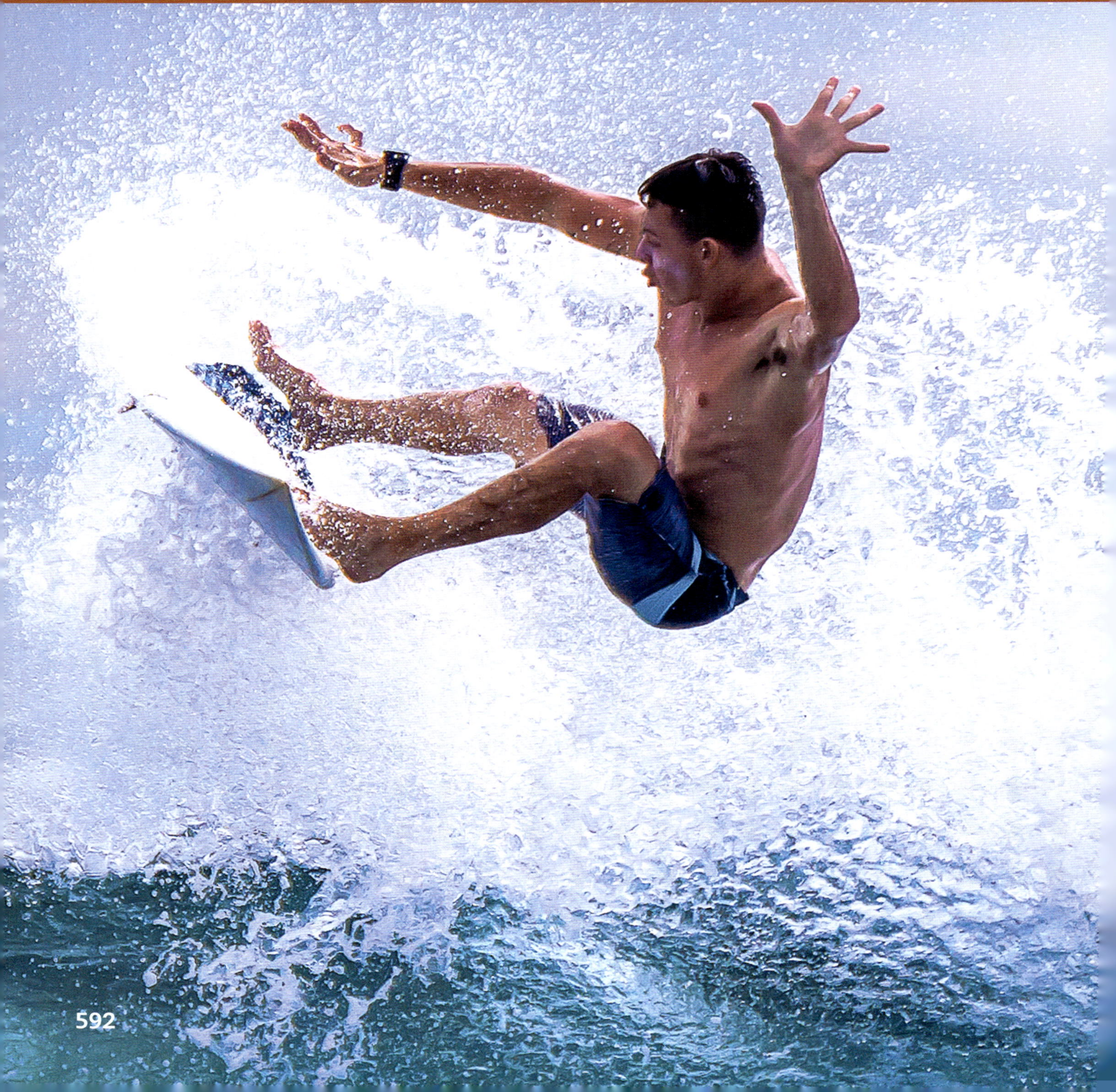

Chapter Objectives

- Define ergogenic aids and outline possible mechanisms and purported effects
- List the categories of substances currently banned by the International Olympic Committee
- List five substances or procedures with alleged ergogenic benefits
- Discuss anabolic steroids' mode of action, their effectiveness to increase muscle size and strength, and health-related risks when used by males and females
- Discuss DHEA as an ergogenic aid and potential health-related risks
- Summarize androstenedione's controversy as a nutritional supplement or harmful drug
- Discuss amino acid, carbohydrate + protein, and carbohydrate-alone effects on hormone secretion and resistance-training responsiveness
- Summarize the ergogenic benefits and risks for amphetamines, caffeine, buffering solutions, chromium picolinate, L-carnitine, glutamine, and HMB
- Describe erythropoietin's medical use by healthy athletes and two potential dangers
- Describe cardiovascular benefits of moderate warm-up prior to physical activity
- Describe how breathing a hyperoxic gas mixture enhances endurance performance and potential to increase tissue oxygenation
- Outline the classic carbohydrate-loading and modified-loading procedures
- Describe the theoretical role for an ergogenic effect for creatine supplements, and two physical activities that benefit from supplementation
- Summarize the main rationale for consuming medium-chain triacylglycerols to enhance endurance performance
- Discuss pyruvate supplementation's effects on endurance performance and body fat loss
- Explain the three phases related to nutrient timing to optimize muscle response to resistance training

Ancillaries at-a-Glance

Visit Lippincott Connect to access the following resources.

- References: Chapter 23
- Appendix I: United States Olympic Committee (USOC) National Anti-Doping Policy Statement of Prohibited Substances and Methods
- Focus on Research: Ergogenic Benefits of Caffeine

Considerable literature exists about **ergogenic aids** and athletic performance—*ergogenic referring to the application of a nutritional, physical, mechanical, psychological, or pharmacologic procedure or aid to improve physical work capacity or athletic performance.* This literature includes studies of potential performance benefits of alcohol, amphetamines, ephedrine, hormones, carbohydrates,[184] amino acids, fatty acids, additional red blood cells, caffeine, carnitine, creatine, phosphates,[37] oxygen-rich breathing mixtures, massage, wheat-germ oil, vitamins, minerals, ionized air, music, hypnosis, and even marijuana and cocaine! Athletes routinely use only a few of these aids, and only a few evoke real controversy. Specific concern focuses on the use of anabolic steroids,[317,318] human growth hormone,[294] dehydroepiandrosterone, and other exogenous hormones and prohormones, some nutritional supplements, amphetamines, and "blood doping."[293] Warm-up and breathing hyperoxic gas are common procedures, so we include these in our discussion of the effectiveness and practicality of ergogenic aids for exercise training and performance. Some sports historians have referred to the 1930s as steroid chemistry's golden age, where that medical era's quest was to discover compounds to alleviate problems related to sexual dysfunction with aging.

In 1934, Polish-born pharmacologist and physician Ernst Laqueur (1880–1947) isolated a tiny amount of crystalline testosterone from bull testes. A few years later, larger quantities (20 mg) were isolated from 18 kg/40 lb of bull testicles obtained from the Chicago stockyards, which quickly promoted testosterone research and development programs. In 1939, the Nobel Prize in Chemistry recognized the joint contributions of German biochemist Adolph Butenandt (1903-1995) and Croatian-Swiss scientist Leopold Ružička (1887-1976) for their work on "sex hormones." In 1929, Butenandt isolated *oestrone* (now called estrogen) in pure, crystalline form, and in 1931 isolated pure androsterone. Both he and Ruzicka working independently obtained testosterone in 1939 (www.nobelprize.org/prizes/chemistry/1939/butenandt/biographical/). This series of experiments and discoveries, culminating in the Chemistry Nobel Prize, began a lively debate in the medical community regarding testosterone replacement therapy that continues to this day—with unintended questions in the sports medicine community about testosterone to "boost" muscle strength in people with low testosterone and other medical maladies. To the sports world, it offered promise as a possible "new" method to gain advantage in athletic events requiring great strength and explosive power. As we discuss in a later section, mostly weightlifters were first to experiment with synthetic testosterone at the 1952 Helsinki Summer Olympics. The notion that such a drug would be tapped by female competitors years later to also gain a performance edge had never been contemplated. To further complicate matters, the side effects from indiscriminately using unknown steroidlike compounds might present adverse, unintended consequences years later.

In today's world, ergogenic substances are used by hundreds of thousands of young and older athletes and nonathletes, which increase the likelihood for experiencing ill effects that range from benign physical discomfort to life-threatening consequences. Many compounds failed to conform to labeling requirements to correctly identify the strength of a product's ingredients and contaminants.[114,140] Supplements available through the Internet and many retail "nutrition shops" often contain steroids and stimulants prohibited in elite sport competition.[138]

An Increasing Challenge to Fair Competition

Ergogenic aids date to antiquity.[308,309] Many early "sports medicine" physicians encouraged Roman and Greek athletes to eat raw meat before competing to enhance their "animal competitiveness." In modern times, the gold medal marathon winner in the 1904 Summer Olympic Games (officially known as the Games of the III Olympiad held in St. Louis, MO), Thomas John Hicks (1876-1952), a Briton running for the United States (www.olympedia.org/athletes/78551), consumed brandy with the stimulant strychnine sulphate (a common rat poison) administered by his physician several times during the race to "supercharge" his marathon performance by juicing his nervous system.[292] Of the 279 medals won by the top 10 nations, the host nation United States won 239 medals (78 gold, 82 silvers, 79 bronze). Over the next 60 years of Olympic competition, a huge reversal occurred in the medal count, primarily from better training methods but also from performance-enhancing substances.

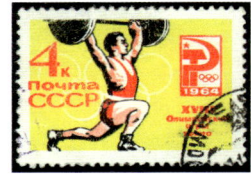
Oldrich/Shutterstock

In the early 1960s, Soviet and American weightlifters used anabolic steroids just prior to competition, and this trend spread rapidly to most strength athletes in weightlifting and track and field.[93]

This was a time before steroids were banned, when world records were changing rapidly,[92] and accomplished world-class athletes admitted to steroid use including Harold Connolly, 1956 Olympic champion in the hammer throw; Dallas Long (1940-), 1964 Mexico City Olympic shotput winner (left in image); Randy Matson (1945-) James E. Sullivan award for best amateur athlete 1967, 1964 silver medal and Mexico City 1968 Olympic shotput champion (right in image); and Russ Hodge (1939-), world decathlon record holder (1966-1967), and silver medalist in the 1967 Cali Columbia Pan American Games. In the 1970s, Olympic athletes were encouraged by their "personal nutritionists" to consume high-carbohydrate foods before competitions held in and near Olympia, WA to decrease

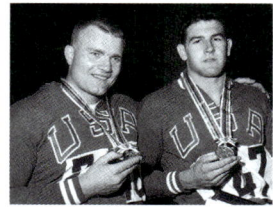
AP/Shutterstock

muscle fatigue (www.perseus.tufts.edu/Olympics/site_1q.html). Even this type of nutritional manipulation was not a unique phenomenon, having been practiced by Greek athletes in the ancient Olympic Games (776 BC–394 AD; www.olympic.org/ancient-olympic-games). Extreme examples included organotherapy (consuming animal and human organs) to improve vigor, vitality, and performance.[10,309]

Recommendations for ergogenic aids combined with illegal drugs to improve competitive achievement in almost all sports have appeared in sports pages and body building magazines for at least the past 60 years. Regrettably, the prohibited use of **performance-enhancing drugs (PEDs)** has not abated.[295] Present-day cycling competitions (including Lance Armstrong's high-profile disqualification for admitted drug use in the 2012 Tour de France discussed later in the chapter), track and field, car racing, boxing, mixed martial arts, cricket, weightlifting and bodybuilding, basketball, baseball, football, and soccer have not been spared from such practices. The practice also has infiltrated into sports where veterinarians and trainers administer powerful steroids (e.g., Winstrol V, Equipoise, Tren, Finaplix) mainly in horse racing,[344,345] but also in racing camels with corticosteroids (e.g., hydrocortisone, flumethasone, methylprednisolone, dexamethasone),[346] and also recombinant human erythropoietin.[347]

Lippincott® Connect Appendix I, available online on **Lippincott Connect**, provides the United States Olympic Committee (USOC) National Anti-Doping Policy Statement of Prohibited Substances and Methods.

Sadly, during the last four Olympiads (IOC; www.olympic.org/ioc), highly celebrated and idolized but now disgraced Olympians were required by the International Olympic Committee to return their medals for illegal doping. High-profile track star Marion Jones, who won five medals (gold in the 100-, 200-, and 1600-m relay and bronze in the long jump and 40-m relay), pleaded guilty to two counts of lying to investigators about her doping abuse and served 6 months in federal prison and probation and community service for 2 years.

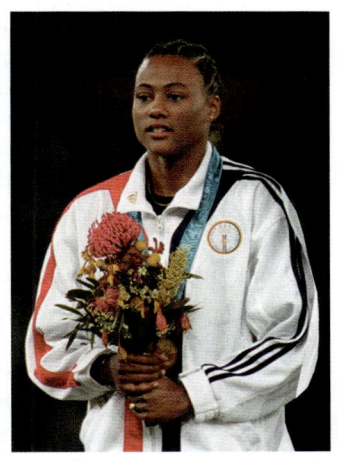

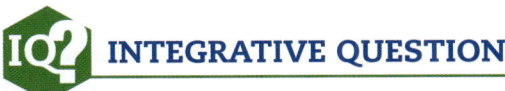 **INTEGRATIVE QUESTION**

What are five points you would make in a talk to a high school football team concerning whether they should consider using performance-enhancing substances?

Levels of Evidence

The National Heart, Lung and Blood Institute (NHLBI; www.nhlbi.nih.gov, part of the National Institutes of Health [NIH; www.nih.gov]) issued guidelines when judging the relevance of evidence about ergogenic aids (**TABLE 23.1**).

TABLE 23.1 Levels of evidence in research

Reproducible results among multiple research studies are an important component in the evaluation process concerning an ergogenic aid's efficacy and safety. The strongest evidence emerges from the cumulative body of scientific literature and not simply the results from anecdotal musings from famous athletes or paid infomercials. Until strong research evidence can support legalized ergogenic substance use, athletes and fitness enthusiasts must strive to understand the relative research credibility about **anabolic adrenergic steroids (AAS)** outlined in **TABLE 23.1**.

On the Horizon

The day may be near when individuals born lacking certain "lucky" genes that augment growth and development and exercise performance will simply add them, doping undetectably with DNA, not drugs. In these instances, "**gene doping**" to change human DNA misappropriates the medical applications afforded by gene alteration therapy to treat atherosclerosis, cystic fibrosis, sickle-cell anemia, and other potentially debilitating and deadly disorders from genetic code "error" mutations. Altering the genetic code of life, which now has been accomplished,[336] is fraught with ethical concerns.[337,338] Who in the society will decide who receives the altered genes, and who will have authority to dictate the promise of increased muscle size,[16] increased contraction speed, or overall muscular strength and power in healthy athletes?[339]

Indeed, inserting altered gene sequences that code for larger and stronger muscles would represent sprinters, weightlifters, and power athletes "holy grail." Endurance athletes would also benefit by altering gene sequences that boost red blood cell production (e.g., targeted genes and novel proteins to produce more erythropoietin) or stimulate blood vessel development from a specific gene that promotes greater vascular endothelial growth factor. The new genetic engineering science pioneered by **CRISPR-Cas9** molecular biology technologies[340,341] may one day allow future generations of athletes to benefit from entirely new categories of genetically engineered substances to enhance physical performance will be hotly debated.

Chapter 33 discusses the science (and scientists) behind the 2020 Nobel Prize in chemistry awarded for developing the CRISPR-Cas9 genetic editing tool (www.nobelprize.org/prizes/chemistry/2020/press-release/) with potential to identify individual genes and the proteins the genes produce. This future role for tailor-made instructional gene programming could establish an individual's body profile and pattern of body fat distribution, as well as how other specific gene patterns impact the sciences as related to muscle physiology, muscle architecture, and nervous system functions.[342,343]

Part 1: Pharmacologic Agents for Ergogenic Effects

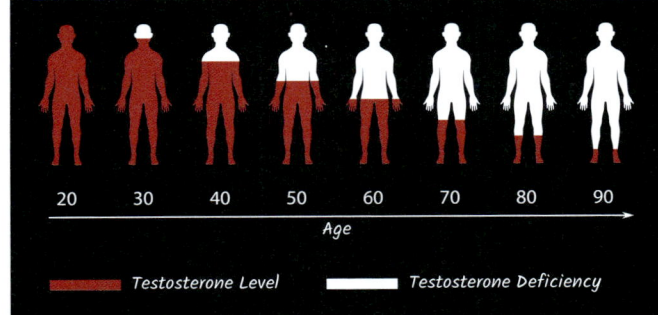
Fancy Tapis/Shutterstock

Athletes go to great lengths to promote all aspects of their health: they train hard; eat well-balanced meals; consume the latest sports drink containing vitamin, mineral, and amino acid megadoses; and seek and receive medical advice for various injuries no matter how minor. Yet ironically, they will ingest synthetic agents, many of which precipitate adverse effects ranging from nausea, hair loss, itching, and nervous irritability to severe consequences such as sterility, liver disease, drug addiction, and even death caused by liver and blood cancers.

The 2021 World Anti-Doping Agency (WADA; www.wada-ama.org/en/content/what-is-prohibited) publishes three categories of well-defined banned substances—those prohibited at all times in-and-out of competition, those prohibited in competition, and those prohibited in particular sports. The prohibited "at-all-times" list includes five broad categories:

1. Anabolic agents[296]
2. Peptide hormones, growth factors and related substances, and mimetics
3. Beta-2 agonists
4. Hormone and metabolic modulators
5. Diuretics and masking agents

Competitive athletes in sanctioned sport competitions are responsible for reading the guidelines and adhering strictly to the list of prohibited compounds and others related to the list. WADA provides educational materials, including the 2021 *Code and Standards* documents, and other technical documents germane to athletes, coaches, and administrative personnel (www.wada-ama.org/en/resources/search?f%5B0%5D=field_resource_collections%3A228).

Anabolic Steroids

AAS gained prominence in the early 1950s for medical purposes to treat patients deficient in natural androgens or with muscle-wasting diseases. Other legitimate steroid uses include treatment of osteoporosis and severe breast cancer in women, and countering the excessive decline in lean body mass and increase in body fat often observed in elderly men, people with HIV, and individuals who undergo kidney dialysis. Male testosterone production shown in the insert image begins early in life, with peak production achieved in late adolescence through age 90 when its production reaches its lowest levels.

Structure and Action

AAS function in a manner similar to the male hormone testosterone by binding with receptor sites on muscle and other tissues and contribute to male secondary sex characteristics. This includes gender differences in muscle mass and strength that develop at puberty onset. Testosterone production takes place mainly in the testes (95%), with the adrenal glands producing the remainder. Synthetically manipulating the steroid's chemical structure to increase muscle growth from anabolic tissue building and nitrogen retention reduces the hormone's androgenic or masculinizing effects. Nevertheless, a masculinizing effect still exists for synthetically derived steroids, particularly in females.

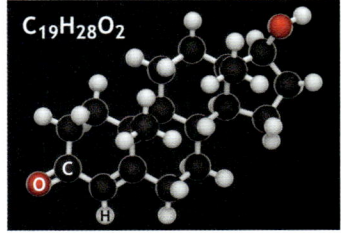
Orange Deer studio/Shutterstock

Steroid Hormone Interactions

Steroid hormones (e.g., testosterone and anabolic steroids) work by entering the cell cytoplasm at step 1 in the image, to bind with specific hormone receptors (step 2). The androgen (steroid) receptor is then activated by binding with testosterone or dihydrotestosterone, which influences DNA to trigger gene activity. This activity promotes muscle hypertrophy, stimulates the sex drive, and facilitates development of primary and secondary sex characteristics.[312] The hormone-receptor complex then enters the nucleus (step 3) and stimulates genes to synthesize proteins (steps 4 and 5). The mRNA single strand shown in red at the bottom of the nucleus refers to messenger RNA, a subtype RNA that carries genetic information between the gene and the ribosomes that translate the genetic information into proteins during the transcription process (see Chapter 33). Also, while the nucleus directs most protein synthesis, a biochemical pathway in the muscle cell's cytoplasm called **mammalian target of rapamycin (mTOR)** regulates protein synthesis as the new amino acids on the ribosomes synthesize new proteins. This pathway is activated by

Shutterstock: Alila Medical Media (muscle cell), Volodymyr Dvornyk (DNA)

Six Ways Ergogenic Substances Might Work

Proposed Mechanisms for Ergogenic Aids

- Stimulate central or peripheral nervous system (e.g., caffeine, choline, amphetamines)
- Increase storage and/or availability of a limiting substrate (e.g., carbohydrate, creatine, carnitine, chromium)
- Serve as supplemental fuel source (e.g., glucose, medium-chain triacylglycerols)
- Minimize performance-inhibiting metabolic byproducts (e.g., sodium bicarbonate or sodium citrate, pangamic acid, phosphate)
- Facilitate recovery from activity (e.g., high-glycemic carbohydrates, water)
- Enhance resistance-training responsiveness (e.g., anabolic steroids, HgH, postexercise carbohydrate/protein supplements)

Background image: jm1366/Shutterstock

---

muscle tension, the androgen dihydrotestosterone (DHT), and other muscle growth factors. This synthesis action occurs faster than that produced by gene stimulation. AAS activate mTOR, which operates inside and outside the nucleus to promote protein synthesis.[181,306] Testosterone binds with androgen receptors throughout the body—not simply within skeletal muscle. A direct linkage exists between testosterone, DHT, and muscle hypertrophy—DHT combined with physical activity triggers greater muscle growth than DHT or physical activity alone.[303] In essence, muscle fibers hypertrophy with resistance training when exposed to DHT, which supports that AAS also contribute to muscle fiber growth thru the mTOR pathway.[304,305]

Testosterone and Growth Hormone

Testosterone and growth hormone trigger muscle growth factor IGF-1 production; together, they play a powerful role to promote muscle hypertrophy. Testosterone and growth hormone work synergistically to stimulate muscle growth.[308,320] Some athletes are naïve enough to believe that judicious adherence to a particular diet plan, excessively consuming nutritional supplements, or taking anabolic drugs by themselves will magically trigger muscle growth.[156] The interaction between arduous training with the body's testosterone and growth hormone production remains essential to elevate protein synthesis and subsequent muscle growth, not a strategy that simply relies on untested methods and/or substances.

Leucine, mTOR, and Muscle Hypertrophy

Leucine and other branch-chain amino acids (BCAAs) stimulate mTOR to promote muscle fiber hypertrophy[301,302] and as a primary protein-building compound. It also is an essential regulator for tissue repair, energy metabolism, blood glucose and energy balance, and food intake. Protein supplements high in leucine content favorably impact protein synthesis in muscle, fat, liver, heart, kidneys, and pancreas tissues.

Satellite Cell Formation Promotes Muscle Cell Hypertrophy

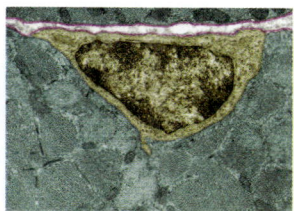
Jose Luis Calvo/Shutterstock

The muscle cell's nucleus directs protein synthesis, which allows the cells to increase in number as they hypertrophy. The image shows a satellite cell depicted in yellow located between the basal lamina (pink) and a striated muscle fiber sarcolemma (blue-green). They initially lie dormant in close proximity to mature muscle fibers.[327] As muscles begin to hypertrophy stimulated by testosterone and/or resistance exercise, the muscle cells acquire and form myoblasts and then myocytes. Integrating these structures into existing muscle fibers help to explain muscle cell hypertrophy,[310,311] in addition to testosterone, growth hormone, insulinlike growth hormone-1, and insulin. Additional contributing factors to hypertrophy include total calorie intake, muscle overload, and rest intervals between high-intensity resistance training workouts. AAS also enhances a muscle cell's neural pathways involved in building and reinforcing the muscle's "memory trace" for a particular movement sequence, a key to perfecting an uncommon, consciously controlled movement pattern into one that becomes automatic or nonconscious. Even following prolonged inactivity or injury, prior learned movement patterns remain relatively intact, making it easier to regain strength or muscle mass. The activated dormant satellite cells migrate to the cells' surface and integrate with existing muscle fibers to increase active cell nuclei.[274,327]

Neural Control Factors, Skilled Practice, and Administering Anabolic Steroids

AAS might exert an ergogenic effect through enhancing neural control involved in all complex human movement activities.[348,349] Over a half century of research has demonstrated that motor control factors regulate movements mediated by neural control mechanisms.[350,351,352]

Perfecting Movement Skills. The concept of timing as the basis to perform and improve motor skills, referred to as the "memory drum" theory of neuromotor reaction,[322,323] demonstrated that complex skilled movements (e.g., golf swing or throwing the discus) were believed to "imprint" in the nervous system and "play back" like a reflex as a function of practice time.[319,321,324] In essence, the brains' memory trace would play back the nonconscious motor pattern as the imprint became stronger with repeated purposeful practice.[192] These ideas at the neural level were impossible to show experimentally[325]—until more recently with advances in neural technologies. Carefully controlled experiments have demonstrated that skill training (i.e., practicing complex, sequenced movements) builds and reinforces nerve tracts that control motor skills by laying down myelin along the nerve fibers.[353–355]

Myelin's Role in Perfecting Motor Skills Without Anabolic Steroids. Myelin, a fatty substance shown in white along the nerve fiber in the 3D rendered image, surrounds neuronal axons throughout the central nervous system. Myelin tremendously increases impulse speed and decreases axon membrane capacitance by increasing the electrical resistance across the cell membrane to prevent the electric current from leaving the axon. Within individual cells, the extracellular and intracellular fluids serve as the conductors, and the lipid myelin membrane acts as the insulator (see Chapter 19). These two inherent factors, independently from AAS, reinforce movement pattern timing and synchronization. Combining AAS with repetitive practice enhances neural activation by increasing myelinated fiber sheath diameter and thickness.[313,315] Continuously practicing specific motor tasks progressively increases the nerve coverings (myelination), which allow faster and smoother performance in demanding skill complexity, particularly in high power sports when combined with therapeutically powerful anabolic steroids (testosterone propionate).[314] Neural feedback from contracting skeletal muscle remains a vital component to enhance endurance exercise capacity (in addition to power-type movements) because muscle perfusion and oxygen delivery determine skeletal muscle fatigability.[316] Stimulating myelin growth with AAS assists nerve grafts[326] in regenerating and degenerating muscles.[327]

Juan Gaertner/Shutterstock

Administrating Anabolic Steroids. The six ways to take steroids include orally, intramuscularly (injected), transdermally (gel or cream), buccally (absorbed under the tongue), intranasally, and as implanted pellets. The method of choice depends on the intended use—legally for therapeutic purposes or illicitly as a PED. In the athletic world, formulated oral AAS resist liver metabolism and cause a high liver toxicity incidence. The most popular oral anabolic steroids include methandienone (Dianabol), oxandrolone (Anavar, Oxandrin), fluoxymesterone (Halotestin), oxymetholone (Anadrol), and stanozolol (Winstrol).

In contrast to "needle" injectables, athletes and middle-age and older adults apply transdermal testosterone (e.g., as gels [Androgel and Testim], solutions [Axiron], and patches [Androderm]) to treat **hypogonadism**, but the gels must be applied frequently due to their short half-life. In contrast, injectables include testosterone in oil solutions (e.g., testosterone cypionate, testosterone enanthate, testosterone undecanoate, nandrolone decanoate [Deca-Durabolin], Sustanon [combination of testosterone propionate, testosterone phenylpropionate, testosterone isocaproate, and testosterone decanoate], and nandrolone phenylpropionate [Durabolin]). Testosterone propionate is no longer prescribed in the United States but is available over the Internet.

triocean/Shutterstock

Athletes typically combine multiple steroid preparations in oral and injectable form, a practice called **stacking**, because they believe that the various androgens differ in physiologic action. They also progressively increase drug dosage, a practice called **pyramiding**, usually in 6- to 12-wk cycles. The drug quantity far exceeds the recommended medical dose, often by 40-fold. The athlete then progressively reduces drug dosage in the months before competition to lower the chance of detection during drug testing.[29]

fyi Warning: Nandrolone Decanoate Toxicity

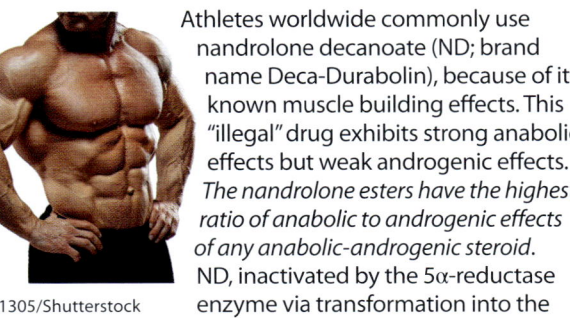

Master1305/Shutterstock

Athletes worldwide commonly use nandrolone decanoate (ND; brand name Deca-Durabolin), because of its known muscle building effects. This "illegal" drug exhibits strong anabolic effects but weak androgenic effects. *The nandrolone esters have the highest ratio of anabolic to androgenic effects of any anabolic-androgenic steroid.* ND, inactivated by the 5α-reductase enzyme via transformation into the low-affinity androgen receptor ligand 5α-dihydronandrolone, helps to explain ND's low androgenicity and possibly lower harmful side effects. Such information has contributed to ND becoming a "drug of choice" to maximize muscle anabolism, while minimizing its androgenic adverse effects. New animal research challenges this assertion by determining the recommended ND and overdose effects on short-term and long-term biochemical markers related to kidney, liver, adrenal, thyroid gland functions, and antioxidant activities. Sixty male rats were randomly assigned to groups treated with ND for either 6 or 12 wk with further assignment to three subgroups: control without ND, and rats injected with either ND 3 mg · kg^{-1} weekly (equivalent to the recommended 240 mg · wk^{-1} dose typically used by an 80 kg/176 lb athlete), or a "high" 15 mg · kg^{-1} weekly dose equivalent for the same size athlete. The results were clear—a high ND short-term or long-term dose significantly elevated kidney dysfunction biomarkers, liver enzymes in serum, cytosol, and mitochondria, decreased adrenal adrenocorticotropic hormone (ACTH), significant up-regulated oxidative stress biomarker balance, and induced higher inflammatory signaling in the male rat's retroperitoneal fat pad. Clearly, ND did not maximize muscle anabolism and minimize adverse side effects.

Sources:

Magalhães SC, et al. High-dose nandrolone decanoate induces oxidative stress and inflammation in retroperitoneal adipose tissue of male rats. *J Steroid Biochem Mol Biol*. 2020;203:105728.

Patanè GD, et al. Nandrolone decanoate: use, abuse and side effects. *Medicina*. 2020;56:606.

Salem NA, Alnahdi HS. The impact of nandrolone decanoate abuse on experimental animal model: Hormonal and biochemical assessment. *Steroids*. 2020;153:108526.

A Drug with a Considerable Following

One often pictures steroid abusers as extremely muscular bodybuilders but abuse also occurs among competitive athletes in road cycling, tennis, track and field, American collegiate and professional football, canoeing, auto racing, swimming, and other highly competitive sport activities. Surveys of United States Powerlifting Team members indicate that up to two thirds used androgenic-anabolic steroids.[70] Many athletes obtain steroids on the black market. Unfortunately, misinformed individuals often take massive and prolonged dosages without medical monitoring and suffer harmful alterations in physiologic function.

Steroid abuse among adolescents and its accompanying risks, including extreme **virilization** and premature cessation of bone growth, remains particularly worrisome. Boys and girls as young as age 11 years have used anabolic-androgenic steroids.[92] Teenagers cite improved athletic performance as the most common reason for taking steroids, yet many acknowledge enhanced appearance as the main reason. In this regard, a body image disturbance may contribute to anabolic steroid abuse among teenagers and adults.[103,201,293] A literature review summarizes the use and abuse of anabolic steroids and growth hormone among athletes.[124]

Anabolic Steroid Sources

While physicians can prescribe testosterone for legitimate medical reasons (e.g., hypogonadism in aging adults, low libido, stunted growth in children), strict regulations prohibit physicians from prescribing drugs to athletes to improve performance and to recreationally active individuals to improve appearance. The Internet is the number one world source of black market anabolic steroids and growth hormone (GH). Numerous websites provide detailed information about the variety of anabolic drugs and their side effects and often tap private lists with fraudulent operators to direct business to their own websites. The United States Food and Drug Administration (FDA; www.usda.gov/topics/opioids) admits that offshore steroid Internet sites are virtually immune from prosecution for illegal or unsafe practices. Several studies by the FDA and European Health Organizations note that about 50% of drugs purchased on the Internet are counterfeit and sometimes contain toxic substances that can cause illness or death. Typical problems with Internet-purchased steroids include products without active ingredients, incorrect quantities of active ingredients, wrong ingredients, fake packaging, copies of original products, products with high levels of contaminants and impurities, and out-of-date drugs purchased from other and/or companies.

Italian researchers surveyed 10 websites selling anabolic drugs.[300] Fifty percent of the websites originated in the United States and 30% in Europe. The most common online anabolic steroids included nandrolone (20%), methandrostenolone (18%), and testosterone (12%). Other typical online performance–enhancing drugs included clenbuterol, growth hormone, IGF-1,[307] thyroid hormones, EPO, and insulin. Recommended dosages were two to fourfold higher than medical recommendations—and the accompanying literature usually did not describe adverse side effects, estrogenicity, or possible toxicity.[145] Dietary supplements for purchase contained mainly DHEA and included several fake compounds. The researchers did not report on the reliability or quality of the products offered on the different sites. They concluded that misleading information and deceiving practices were common on Internet websites selling androgenic anabolic steroids. An Internet search (May 2021) exceeded 1,800,000 sites when including YouTube listings!

Effectiveness Questioned

Much of the confusion regarding AAS's ergogenic effectiveness stems from variations in experimental design, lack of control groups, specific drugs and dosages, treatment duration, accompanying nutritional supplementation, training intensity, evaluation techniques, previous exercise and training experience of subjects, and individual differences in responsiveness to a drug's effectiveness. The relatively small residual androgenic effect of the steroid facilitates central nervous system activation to make the athlete more aggressive (so-called *roid rage*), competitive, and fatigue resistant. Such facilitatory effects allow the person to train harder for a longer time or to believe that augmented training effects have actually occurred. Abnormal mood alterations and psychiatric dysfunction sometimes accompany androgen use.[60,103]

Research with animals suggests that anabolic steroid treatment combined with physical activity and adequate protein intake stimulates protein synthesis and increases muscle protein content for myosin, myofibrillar, and sarcoplasmic factors.[227] In contrast, other research revealed that steroid treatment did not benefit the leg muscle weight of rats subjected to functional overload by surgically removing the synergistic muscle.[175] Treatment with AAS did not complement functional overload to stimulate additional muscular development.

Steroid research with humans is difficult to interpret. Some studies show that steroid use by males who train augments body mass gains and reduces body fat, while other studies show no effect on strength and power or body composition, despite sufficient energy and protein intake to support an anabolic effect.[98] When steroid use produces body weight gains, the compositional nature remains unclear for gains in water, muscle, and/or fat.

Patients receiving dialysis and those infected with HIV commonly experience malnutrition, decreases in muscle mass, and chronic fatigue. Dialysis patients given 6 months of supplementation with the anabolic steroid nandrolone decanoate increased lean body mass and level of daily function.[138] In males with HIV, a moderately supraphysiologic androgen regimen that included the anabolic steroid oxandrolone increased lean tissue accrual and strength gains from resistance training substantially more than physiologic testosterone replacement alone.[255]

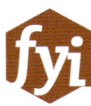

ACSM Position Stand on Androgenic Anabolic Steroids

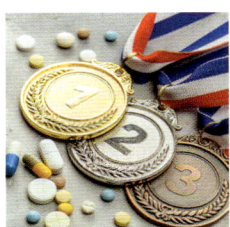

Based on a comprehensive world literature survey and analysis of claims made for and against the efficacy of anabolic-androgenic steroids (AAS) to improve human physical performance, the American College of Sports Medicine (ACSM) has published a position stand regarding athletes and androgenic anabolic steroid use (https://journals.lww.com/acsm-msse/Citation/1987/10000/Position_Stand_on_The_Use_of_Anabolic_Androgenic.23.aspx).[125]

Adragan/Shutterstock

- AAS in the presence of an adequate diet and training can contribute to increased body weight, often the lean muscle mass compartment.
- Muscular strength gains achieved through high-intensity exercise and proper diet can occur by increased anabolic-androgenic steroid use in some individuals.
- AAS do not increase aerobic power or capacity for muscular exercise.
- In therapeutic trials and in limited research on athletes, AASs associate with adverse effects on liver, cardiovascular system, reproductive system, and psychological status. The potential AAS hazards use in athletes must include those found in therapeutic trials.
- AAS use by athletes runs contrary to the basic code and ethical principles ingrained in athletic competition set forth by many of the Sports' governing bodies. The ACSM supports these ethical principles and condemns any athlete who uses them.

Steroid Dosage Important

The difference between dosages used in research studies and those used by athletes contributes to the credibility gap between scientific findings (often, small steroid effect) and what most in the athletic community "know" to be true through trial-and-error self-experimentation. One study focused on 43 healthy males with some resistance-training experience.[15,300] The experimental design accounted for diet (energy and protein intake) and physical activity (standard weightlifting, three times weekly) with steroid dosage (600 mg testosterone enanthate injected weekly or placebo) exceeding values in previous studies with humans. The males who received the hormone for 10 wk while continuing to train gained about 0.5 kg of lean tissue weekly with no increase in body fat. The group receiving the drug without training also increased muscle mass and strength compared with males receiving the placebo. Notably, their increases averaged less than males who trained while taking testosterone. These data indicate a potential for medically supervised anabolic steroid treatment to restore and enhance muscle mass in individuals suffering from tissue-wasting diseases (e.g., over 200 connective tissue disorders related to joints, muscles, skin, eyes, heart, lungs, kidney, GI tract, and blood vessels).

Anabolic Steroid Risks

Whether anabolic steroid use by athletes carries serious long-term health risks remains controversial because risk research generally has involved medical observations with hospitalized patients treated for anemia, renal insufficiency, impotence, or pituitary gland dysfunction. Some athletes take steroids on and off yearly at dosages of 50 to 200 $mg \cdot d^{-1}$ or more versus the usual therapeutic dosage of 5 to 20 $mg \cdot d^{-1}$ Prolonged high dosages can lead to impairment of normal testosterone endocrine function. In male power athletes, for example, 26 wk of steroid administration reduced serum testosterone to less than one half the level when the study began, with the effect lasting throughout a 12 to 16-wk follow-up.[97] Infertility, reduced sperm concentrations (azoospermia), and decreased testicular volume pose additional concerns for the steroid user.[106] Gonadal function usually returns to normal within several months after cessation of steroid use. Other male hormonal alterations during steroid use include a sevenfold increase in estradiol concentration, the major female hormone. The higher estradiol level represented the average value for normal females; this possibly explains the **gynecomastia** (excessive male mammary gland development usually irreversible without plastic surgery) illustrated in this illustration of a male body builder with gynecomastia.

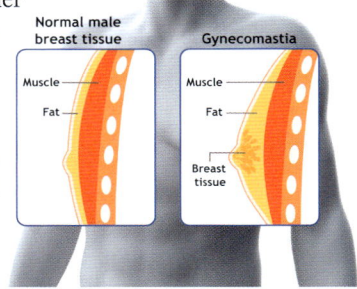

Shutterstock: SciePro (torso), CHEN I CHUN (breast tissue)

Steroid use combined with resistance training may damage connective tissue to decrease tendon tensile strength and elastic compliance.[164] Steroids also are associated with the following five negative side effects:

1. Chronic prostate gland stimulation with possible size increase[5]
2. Injury and alterations in cardiovascular function and myocardial cell cultures[77]
3. Alterations in cardiac structure and function that include diminished cardiac diastolic motion and exacerbation of normal cardiac hypertrophy with resistance training[111]
4. Alterations in normal thyroid gland function and hormone action[98]
5. Increased blood platelet aggregation, which could compromise cardiovascular system health and function and possibly increase stroke and myocardial infarction risk[143,245]

Steroid Abuse and Disease Precursors

Possible links exist between AAS abuse and cardiovascular health, liver function, and plasma lipoproteins. The liver almost exclusively metabolizes androgens so it becomes susceptible to damage from long-term steroid abuse, usually leading to toxic cellular conditions. Developing localized blood-filled lesions shown on the next page as darkened regions in this liver photomicrograph indicating metastasizes in surrounding

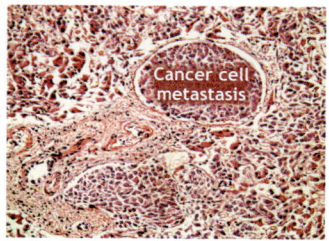
BonD80/Shutterstock

cystlike hepatic capillary vessels, which can produce **peliosis hepatitis** with potentially fatal consequences.

In healthy males and females, taking AAS, particularly the orally active 17-alkylated androgens, negatively impacts blood chemistry and cardiovascular disease ramifications. The most obvious precursor to more serious conditions reduces high-density lipoprotein cholesterol (HDL-C) levels, elevates both low-density lipoprotein cholesterol (LDL-C), and total cholesterol levels and reduces the HDL-C:LDL-C ratio.[62] Weightlifters who take AAS averaged an HDL-C level of 26 mg·dL^{-1} compared with 50 mg·dL^{-1} for weightlifters not taking this drug![143] Reducing HDL-C to this level increases a steroid user's risk of coronary artery disease. The dramatically low HDL-C levels among weightlifters remain low, even after they abstain for at least 8 wk between consecutive steroid cycles.[232] The long-term effects of steroid use on cardiovascular morbidity and mortality remain unknown.

Specific AAS Risks to Females

Testosterone levels normally range 20 to 25 times lower in females than in males, raising additional concerns about AAS abuse among females. As an example, for males at ages 17 to 18 years, testosterone levels average between 300 and 1500 ng·dl^{-1} and approximately 20 and 75 ng·dl^{-1} for females. Medical risks include hirsutism (excessive body and facial hair), virilization (more apparent than in males), disruption of normal growth pattern by premature closure in the plates for bone growth (also for boys), altered menstrual function, dramatic increase in sebaceous gland size, acne, and generally irreversible deepening of the voice, decreased breast size, enlarged clitoris, and hair loss. Serum levels of LH, FSH, progesterone, and estrogens also decline. These may negatively affect follicle formation, ovulation, and menstrual function. The long-term effects require further clarification on reproductive function, including possible sterility.

A4ASHISHMISHRA/Shutterstock

Elite Female Competitors Abuse AAS

A considerable omission from the steroid literature concerns the use and abuse of AAS by female athletes worldwide, particularly in the Olympic Games and other notable competitions. Survey data based on positive doping tests indicate the here-to-fore undocumented common use of AAS use by female athletes compared to well-documented use among males. Historical data from the German Democratic Republic (GDR) and unpublished observations obtained from coaches willing to provide such information attest to these drugs' use and their effectiveness on female athletic accomplishments. GDR reports showed that anabolic steroid use was prevalent among females in power events.

Harvard researchers in 2018 published a seminal paper about the AAS performance enhancing effects on both males and females.[328] They reported that from 1965 to 1989, the German Democratic Republic (GDR) conducted a classified, systematic doping program after the unification of Germany in 1990 involving elite male and female athletes competing in the Olympic Games. Investigative reports by independent researchers verified the existence of scientific reports, secret doctoral theses, and court documents dated to 1966 and sanctioned doping research supervised by physicians and scientists under the guise of "unofficial collaborators" of the Ministry for State Security.

Three key findings from a World Anti-Doping Agency (WADA) report confirmed that the McLaren report (www.theguardian.com/sport/russia-doping-scandal; www.wada-ama.org/sites/default/files/resources/files/mclaren_report_part_ii_2.pdf) validated Russian involvement in sanctioned drug use by over a thousand athletes. Careful analysis of this state-supported conspiracy reveled the following:

1. The Moscow Laboratory operated for the protection of doped Russian athletes, within a State-dictated failsafe drug testing system, described as the "Disappearing Positive Methodology"
2. The Sochi Laboratory operated a unique sample swapping methodology to enable doped Russian athletes to compete
3. The Ministry of Sport directed, controlled, and oversaw the manipulation of athletes' analytical results or provided for sample swapping, with the active participation and assistance of the Russian Federal Security Service, the Center of Sports Preparation of National Teams of Russia, and both Moscow and Sochi laboratories

How Elite Athletes Improved Athletic Performance

The Russian 4-year sanctioned drug program revealed marked improvements in the shotput by 4.5 to 5.0 m, discus throw by 11 to 20 m, 400 m run improvements by 4 to 5 s, and 1500 m run by 7 to 10 s. These performance changes are "off the scale" and simply do not occur without ergogenic involvement. Not surprisingly, the athletes were given 10 to 100 times the therapeutic dosage for the anabolic steroids. Even more revealing was the admission that some female athletes consumed nandrolone and testosterone esters in doses even higher to those administered to male athletic participants in similar events! Even non-Olympic caliber females under medical treatment with androgenic hormones improved when tested for their athletic achievements including performance on bench-press and stair-climbing tasks. Females taking the highest drug dosages showed the greatest increases in muscle mass and physical performance. These females were not dedicated as "world-class" athletes, but their changes were similar to athletes from the GDR. Also, they too exhibited undesirable virilizing side effects (e.g., acne, sexual dysfunction, abnormal hair growth on the face and body [hirsutism], liver damage, alopecia, voice deepening, clitoromegaly, menstrual disturbances, and aggression)

In a Practical Sense

Anabolic Steroid Abuse: Taking a Stand

Anabolic steroid abuse has become common in almost all international, high level sports competitions. We believe the first documented use of synthetic testosterone propionate in sports occurred almost 70 years ago at the 1952 Helsinki Summer Olympics where Soviet Union weightlifters dominated the weightlifting competitions. At that time, most elite athletes were aware of Dianabol's strength-building effects. They also knew how many blue Dianabol pills were needed to lift more "blues," ironically the name given to the blue color 20 kg/45 lb bumper weight plates (shown above) adopted as the official color sanctioned for international weightlifting and powerlifting competitions.

NikSorokin/Shutterstock

To emphasize how widespread anabolic steroid use has become, consider the vast extent of Russian state-sponsored doping that occurred 5 years prior to the Rio 2016 Olympic Games including the 2014 Sochi Winter Olympics. Almost 600 athletes participating in 30 different categories (including 35 athletes in Paralympic Sport and 37 athletes in non-Olympic Sports) were banned from competition because the sanctioned Russian effort falsified drug testing results (or made positive test results "disappear" from investigators)! Track and field and weightlifting had the most offenders (www.nytimes.com/2019/12/09/sports/russia-doping-ban.html), followed by 12 other sport categories. No sport was immune from illicit drug abuse as the inset figure illustrates. The purposeful fraud included nine athletes in less popular sports, which typically field with fewer participants in bobsleigh, judo, volleyball, handball, taekwondo, fencing, triathlon, modern pentathlon, shooting, beach volleyball, curling, sailing, snowboard, table tennis, and ice skating (Beijing Winter Olympics: www.youtube.com/watch?v=CHqE92X1dy8).

BANNING ATHLETES FOR DRUG ABUSE: A LOSING BATTLE

In addition to Olympic Games participation, the internationally recognized athletes banned for documented anabolic use continues to grow, with some suspensions as late as 2022. Four famous transgressors sanctioned for drug infractions are listed by name within the inset figure.

At the 2016 Olympiad in Rio de Janeiro, most observers believed the previously sanctioned athletes would not compete because of their doping ban. Nevertheless, the Rio Olympics set the record for most illegal drug offenses. Of the 974 medals awarded at the Games, older athletes still managed to win 35 medals. The number of athletes with positive drug results was undoubtedly underreported because many countries have lax doping control procedures. Approximately a third of the competing countries entered athletes banned for doping offenses. Russia entered six athletes who failed drug tests

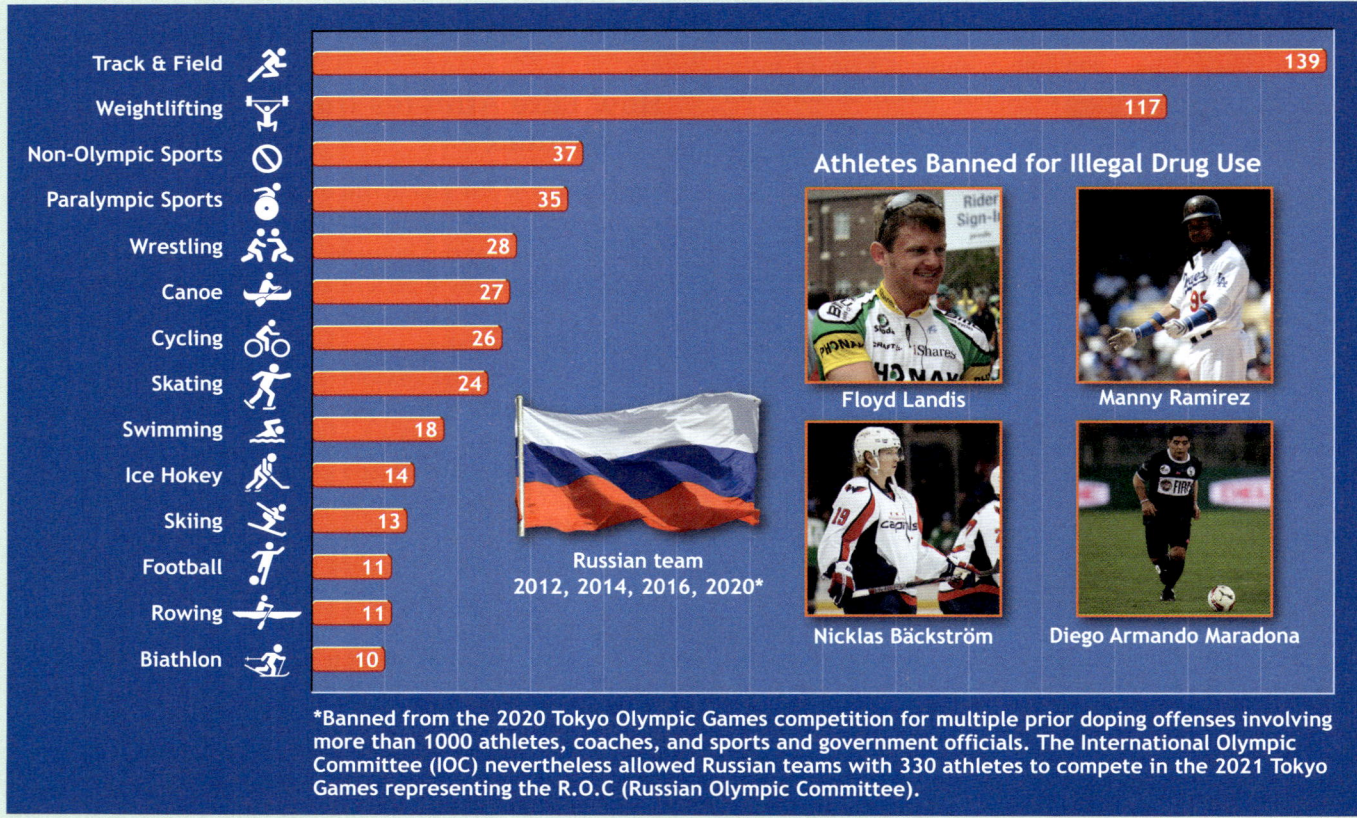

*Banned from the 2020 Tokyo Olympic Games competition for multiple prior doping offenses involving more than 1000 athletes, coaches, and sports and government officials. The International Olympic Committee (IOC) nevertheless allowed Russian teams with 330 athletes to compete in the 2021 Tokyo Games representing the R.O.C (Russian Olympic Committee).

Shutterstock photos: K. Jensen (Landis), Marco Iacobucci Epp (Maradona), Photo Works (Ramirez), Jai Agnish (Backstrom), Slasha (Russian flag)

or were implicated in the Olympic Committee's doping investigation of competing Russian athletes who were previously sanctioned for drug use.

TAKING A STAND

Your textbook authors believe established rules should continue to ban anabolic steroids from sport but not for the reasons cited by most politicians, physicians, sports administrators, and media. The level playing field is a myth. People without key gene variants based on their inherited genetic heritage cannot achieve elite performance levels. Athletic officials propagate the myth that anyone can be a champion if they work hard enough—yet the statistics are overwhelming and convincing that this simply is not true. Consider baseball in 2019–2020. There were approximately 492,000 high school baseball players in the United States and 52,000 college players. This translates to about 9% of high school players competed at the collegiate level, but less than 2% competed at the NCAA Division 1 level. On college baseball's opening day games in 2019, there were roughly 631 players in this exclusive group. Here is a common question, "What are the chances of a college player making it to a major league team roster?" The answer turns out to be only 80 individuals from almost a half a million high school players (roughly 0.02%)! In fact, fewer than 2% of college student-athletes who play college basketball and football ever play professional sports at any level for any amount of time.

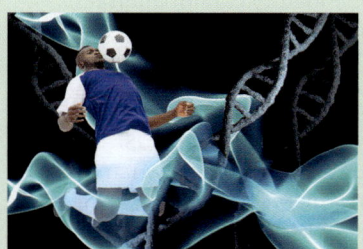
vectorfusionart/Shutterstock

It seems fair to conclude that elite athletic competitors in Olympic sports, professional baseball, football, basketball, golf, and hockey are essentially contests between genetically gifted males and females. Over the past 30 years beginning with the 1992 Heritage Family Study (https://pubmed.ncbi.nlm.nih.gov/7674877/), researchers have thus far identified about 800 genes linked to endurance, strength, power, fat deposition, nutrient fuel use, and many other variables believed to play an important role in elite performance. The evidence seems to point in one direction regarding world-class athletic achievement, "Without a rich genetic endowment, world-class athletic performance is out of reach."[332] This also seems self-evident—parents and coaches should not rely on direct-to-consumer genetic testing to define or alter training to attempt to identify athletic talent aimed at selecting gifted children or adolescents because excessive variability exists in such testing procedures.[333]

While steroids help athletes improve their performance, their use is contrary to the goals of sport in the society, although some have countered that drugs that work should be legalized for both efficacy and safety. The argument posits that this could improve both the athlete's performance and their health, and would be better than athletes trying to subvert drug tests and stay ahead of the scientists who create such tests (https://pubmed.ncbi.nlm.nih.gov/26247087/). Elite athletes serve as role models for millions of athletes worldwide who will never achieve Olympic or professional levels in sport. Rules banning steroid use in sports are justified because they serve society's greater good. The harm caused by allowing widespread drug use by individuals who have almost no chance to excel in sports and win accolades and medals far overpowers the benefits to allow a few elite athletes to misuse powerful drugs with unintended, undesirable consequences while they prepare for competition. Elite athletes world-wide will always try to find a competitive edge because of financial rewards and the sheer competitiveness of sport. Predictably, the cat and mouse game will continue between athletes trying to win at all costs and doping officials and organizations trying to thwart those who break the rules.

---

attributed to their higher-than-normal testosterone levels from both oral and intramuscular AAS injections. At the extreme, reports have verified life-threatening events in elite female athletics, recreational sports, and bodybuilding that include hepatic rupture, multiorgan failure,[329] and thromboembolism, intracardiac thrombosis and stroke, cardiac disturbances including arrhythmias, cardiomyopathies, and sudden death,[330] and hepatotoxicity including adenoma, hepatocellular carcinoma, cholestasis, and peliosis hepatis.[331]

Clenbuterol and Other β_2-Adrenergic Agonists

Extensive, random testing competitive athletes for steroid use have ushered in steroid "substitutes." These have appeared on the health food, mail order, and "black market" drug network as competitors try to circumvent detection. One such drug, the sympathomimetic amine **clenbuterol** (brand names Clenasma, Monores, Novegan, Prontovent, Ventipulmin, and Spiropent), has become popular among athletes because of its purported tissue-building, fat-reducing benefits. When a bodybuilder discontinues steroid use before competition to avoid drug detection and possible disqualification, the athlete substitutes clenbuterol to retard loss of muscle mass and facilitate fat burning to achieve the desirable "cut" look, particularly in the abdominal and back regions. Clenbuterol has particular appeal to female athletes because it does not produce the androgenic side effects of anabolic steroids.

Clenbuterol, one in a group of chemical compounds classified as β_2-adrenergic agonists (albuterol [salbutamol], bitolterol, salmeterol, metaproterenol, pirbuterol, terbutaline, and formoterol), facilitates adrenergic receptor responsiveness to circulating epinephrine, norepinephrine, and other adrenergic amines (www.ncbi.nlm.nih.gov/books/NBK547852/). A review of available animal studies (to our knowledge, no human exercise studies have been conducted) indicates that when fed to sedentary, growing livestock in dosages exceeding those prescribed in Europe for human bronchial asthma, clenbuterol increases skeletal and cardiac muscle protein deposition and slows fat gain by enhanced lipolysis. It also increases FFM and decreases fat mass when administered long term at therapeutic levels to thoroughbred racehorses.[144] Clenbuterol has been used experimentally in animals to counter the effects on muscle of aging, immobilization, malnutrition, and pathologic tissue-wasting conditions. Under these conditions, β₂-agonists show specific growth-promoting actions on skeletal muscle.[82,294] In rats, clenbuterol altered muscle fiber type distribution, inducing enlargement and increased proportion of type II muscle fibers.[69] A decrease in protein breakdown and increase in protein synthesis accounted for the animals' increased muscle size.[2,28]

Clenbuterol's Potential Negative Effects on Muscle, Bone, and Cardiovascular Function (Animal Studies)

Female rats treated with clenbuterol (2 mg·kg⁻¹) injected subcutaneously versus controls sham-injected with the same fluid carrier volume each day for 14 days increased muscle mass, absolute maximal force-generating capacity, and hypertrophy in fast-twitch and slow-twitch muscle fibers.[78] A negative finding indicated hastened fatigue during short-term, intense muscle actions. In contrast, regular physical activity combined with clenbuterol decreased muscular dystrophy progression in mice, reflected by increased muscle force-generating capacity.[81,294] The group receiving clenbuterol experienced increased muscle fatigability and cellular deformities not noted in the exercise-only group. This negative effect may explain why the clenbuterol treatment negated the beneficial training effects on endurance performance, despite increased muscle protein content.[129] Clenbuterol treatment induced muscular hypertrophy in young male rats but also inhibited longitudinal bone growth.[152] Negative clenbuterol and salbutamol effects in animals impacted trabecular bone's mechanical properties and microarchitecture. Increased muscle mass with enhanced bone fragility increases fracture risk when treated with β₂-agonists as part of a doping regimen.[35,36] The negative effect on bone contraindicates its use for prepubescent and adolescent humans.

Echocardiographic evaluations of standard-bred mares showed that chronic clenbuterol administration even at low therapeutic levels alters the heart's structural dimensions, which negatively affects cardiac function.[242] Effects occurred whether the animals exercised or remained inactive. Clenbuterol also caused aortic enlargement after physical activity to a degree that indicated increased risk of aortic rupture and sudden death. Clenbuterol treatment when combined with aerobic training blunts the normal training-induced increase in plasma volume in standard-bred mares; this effect accompanied decreased aerobic performance and ability to recover.[144]

Clenbuterol: Not Approved for Human Use in the United States

Clenbuterol, commonly prescribed in countries other than the United States, functions as an inhaled bronchodilator to treat obstructive pulmonary disorders including asthma, to dilate air passages that become narrowed and filled with mucus. Reported short-term side effects in humans who accidentally "overdosed" from eating clenbuterol-tainted meat include skeletal muscle tremor, agitation, palpitations, dizziness, nausea, muscle cramps, rapid heart rate, and headache. Despite these negative side effects, clenbuterol may benefit humans when used to treat muscle wasting in disease, forced immobilization, and aging. Unfortunately, no data exist for potential toxicity level or its efficacy and long-term safety. Unmistakably, clenbuterol use cannot be justified or recommended for any sport or recreational purpose, especially as an ergogenic aid!

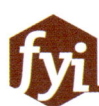 Testing for Performance Enhancing Drugs

The primary "gold-standard" method to detect illicit performance enhance drugs (PEDs) involves a two-stage process. If the initial screening is positive for PEDs, a second step known as the confirmation test is then applied to the positive sample, usually by immunoassay methods. The mandatory confirmation test using mass spectrometry in most laboratories and all testing labs certified by SAMHSA—Substance Abuse and Mental Health Services Administration—a branch of the US Department of Health and Human Services (www.samhsa.gov/newsroom/press-announcements/201709291000). This precise analytical methodology assesses the mass-to-charge ratio of charged particles in a particular chemical substance. The sample, after being vaporized, creates charged particles after electron beam bombardment, and further analyzed into the precise chemical present. The distinct molecular pattern or "signature" is compared with known chemical response patterns. Other banned substances besides AAS include alcohol, amphetamines, methamphetamine, MDMA (Ecstasy), barbiturates, phenobarbital, benzodiazepines, cannabis, cocaine, cotinine (breakdown product of nicotine), morphine, tricyclic antidepressants (TCAs), lysergic acid diethylamide (LSD), methadone, and phencyclidine or PCP (with street names angel dust, supergrass [combined with marijuana], wack, hog, rocket fuel, Tic Tac). Testing time to obtain confirmation can range from 1 day for barbiturates to 3 to 30 days for AAS (https://www.deadiversion.usdoj.gov). More recent antidoping technologies now include retroactive liquid testing, which retroactively analyze previously collected "dormant" samples over a 10-year period. The newer techniques can now identify the popular, most commonly prescribed AAS metabolites. The *Biological Passport* initiated in 2008 has been another World Anti-Doping Agency (www.wada-ama.org) effort to detect and discourage PEDs by establishing typical blood levels for various physiological markers.[29] Changes in the markers "indirectly" reveal prior illegal drug use rather than directly detecting the doping substance or method.

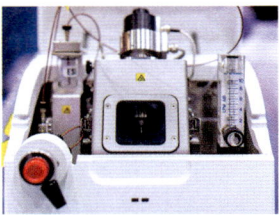
Surasak_Photo/Shutterstock

Other Adrenergic Agonists

Research has focused on possible strength-enhancing effects of **sympathomimetic β$_2$-adrenergic agonists** other than clenbuterol. Males with cervical spinal cord injuries took 80 mg of metaproterenol daily for 4 wk along with physical therapy. Increases occurred in estimated muscle cross-sectional area and elbow flexor and wrist extensor strength compared with a placebo condition.[241] Salbutamol administration (16 mg · d^{-1} for 3 wk) without training improved muscular strength by 10 to 15%.[172] Therapeutic doses of albuterol also facilitated isokinetic strength gains from slow-speed concentric-eccentric isokinetic training.[51,64] The acute administration of either low-dose or high-dose salbutamol produced no beneficial effect on aerobic capacity in normal subjects.[26]

Training State Makes a Difference

Animals

Untrained skeletal muscle of animals responds positively to β$_2$-adrenergic agonists. Increase muscle mass with clenbuterol treatment plus training on a small, continuously rotating exercise wheel is more pronounced in animals without prior training experience than in trained animals that continue training and then receive this drug.[191]

Ingrid Prats/Shutterstock

Humans

Some research with humans shows improved muscle power output with albuterol administration.[240] No ergogenic effect occurred from salbutamol on short-term performance in two 10-min cycling trials.[6] Similarly, no effect occurred in power output during a 30-s Wingate test in nonasthmatic trained cyclists who received 360 mg (twice the normal dose administered by inhaler in four measured doses of 90 mg each) 20 min before testing.[160] For males without asthma, acute therapeutic (200 mg) or supratherapeutic (800 mg) doses of inhaled salbutamol did not affect quadriceps strength, fatigue, and recovery.[72] In other research, twice the recommended dose of salbutamol (albuterol: 400 mg administered in four inhalations 20 min before exercising) failed to enhance anaerobic power output, endurance performance, ventilatory threshold, or dynamic lung function of trained endurance cyclists.[193] The researchers maintained that competitive athletes should not be prohibited from these compounds because they provide no ergogenic benefit, yet "normalize" individuals with obstructive pulmonary disorders.[240] Differences in training status may explain discrepancies among studies concerning albuterol's effect on short-term power output.

Growth Hormone: Genetic Engineering Now Common in Sports

Human growth hormone (GH or hGH), also known as somatotropin, currently competes with anabolic steroids in the illicit market involving alleged tissue-building PEDs. The pituitary gland's adenohypophysis produces GH, a potent anabolic and lipolytic agent in tissue-building processes and growth. Specifically, GH stimulates bone and cartilage growth, enhances fatty acid oxidation, and reduces glucose and amino acid breakdown. Reduced GH secretion accounts for some of the decrease in FFM and increase in fat mass that accompanies aging. This condition reverses somewhat with exogenous recombinant GH supplements produced by genetically engineered bacteria. Healthy elderly males who received GH supplements increased FFM (4.3%) and decreased fat mass (13.1%).[199] *Supplementation did not reverse aging's negative effects on measures of muscular strength and aerobic capacity.* Males receiving the supplement also experienced hand stiffness, malaise, arthralgias, and lower extremity edema. One of the largest studies to date determined the effects of exogenous GH over a 6-month period for changes in body composition and functional capacity of healthy males and females aged mid-60s to late 80s.[33] Males who took GH gained 3.2 kg/7 lb lean body mass and reduced a similar fat mass amount. Females gained about 1.4 kg/3 lb lean body mass and lost 2.3 kg/5 lb of body fat compared with counterparts receiving a placebo. Unfortunately, serious side effects negatively afflicted between 24 and 46% of subjects. Medically related problems included swollen feet and ankles, joint pain, carpal tunnel syndrome (tendon sheath swelling over a wrist nerve), and a diabetic or prediabetic condition. As in prior research, no effects occurred for GH treatment on measures of muscular strength or endurance capacity despite increases in lean body mass.

Excessive GH production during skeletal growth produces **gigantism**, an endocrine and metabolic disorder characterized by abnormal size or overgrowth of the entire body or any of its parts. Excessive hormone production following growth cessation produces the irreversible disorder **acromegaly** that presents as enlarged hands, feet, and facial features. Children who suffer from kidney failure or who produce insufficient GH receive thrice-weekly biosynthetic GH injections until adolescence to help them achieve near-normal size. In young adults with hypopituitarism, GH replacement therapy improves muscle volume, isometric strength, and exercise capacity. Purchasing GH on the black market from foreign regions (e.g., Mexico, Europe, Asia) or from a Google Internet search for "GH sales" (34 million as of February 10, 2021) offers no protection against receiving a counterfeit product, which does not occur when purchased by valid prescription from a US pharmacy. Individuals must remain vigilant when trying to obtain known GH effects from supplements, sprays, pills, and patches that allegedly contain this hormone.

Questionable Benefits

At first glance, GH use seems appealing to strength and power athletes because at physiologic levels, this hormone stimulates amino acid uptake and muscle protein synthesis while enhancing lipid breakdown and conserving glycogen reserves. Unfortunately, few well-controlled studies have examined how GH supplements affect healthy subjects who undertake exercise training. In one study, six well-trained males maintained a high-protein diet while taking either biosynthetic GH or a placebo.[68] During 6-wk standard resistance training with GH, body fat percentage decreased and FFM increased. No changes in body composition occurred for the group training with the placebo. Subsequent investigations failed to replicate these findings. For example, 16 previously sedentary young males who participated in a 12-wk resistance training program received GH supplements (40 mg·kg^{-1}·d^{-1}) or a placebo.[293] FFM, total body water, and whole-body protein synthesis increased more in the GH recipients. However, no significant differences emerged between groups in fractional rate of protein synthesis in skeletal muscle, torso and limb circumferences, or muscle function in dynamic and static strength measures. The authors attributed the greater increase in whole-body protein synthesis in the GH group to a possible increase in nitrogen retention in lean tissue other than skeletal muscle—for example, connective tissue, fluid, and noncontractile protein.

Nonprescription GH only can be obtained on the black market and most likely in an adulterated form. Human cadaver–derived GH (used until May 1985 by US physicians to treat short stature children) greatly increases risk for contracting **Creutzfeldt-Jakob disease**, an infectious, incurable, and fatal brain-deteriorating disorder (www.ninds.nih.gov/disorders/cjd/detail_cjd.htm). Synthetic GH (Protropin and Humatrope) produced by genetic engineering currently treat GH-deficient children. Undoubtedly, child athletes who receive GH believing they gain a competitive edge will suffer increased gigantism incidence, while adults will develop acromegalic syndrome. Additional, less obvious side effects include insulin resistance that leads to type 2 diabetes, water retention, and carpal tunnel compression syndrome created by induced bone growth. Any potential benefits of GH must be weighed against potential adverse effects. Claims that growth hormone enhances physical performance are not supported by the scientific literature. The limited available evidence suggests that growth hormone increases lean body mass, but it may not improve strength; in addition, it may worsen physical capacity and increase adverse events. More research will conclusively determine if and how growth hormone influences athletic performance.[166,179]

INTEGRATIVE QUESTION

A female athlete maintains that a chemical compound added to her diet produced profound improvements in weightlifting performance (or any athletic event). Your review of the research literature indicates no ergogenic benefits for this compound. How would you explain the discrepancy?

Dehydroepiandrosterone

Dehydroepiandrosterone (DHEA) and its sulfated ester DHEA sulfate or DHEAS, the most common hormone in the body, is a weak steroid synthesized primarily by the adrenal cortex from cholesterol in primates. The body produces more DHEA than all other known steroids. Known as the "mother hormone," it has a chemical structure that closely resembles testosterone and estrogen. A small amount of DHEA and related **prohormones**—intermediate substances in the hormone-building process—are naturally derived precursors to testosterone or other anabolic steroids. Athletes consume these products believing they will lead to endogenous testosterone synthesis. **FIGURE 23.1** outlines the major pathways for synthesizing DHEA, androstenedione, and related compounds.[150] The red directional arrows signify one-way and two-way conversions, including intermediate compounds. Those illustrated in dark grey boxes serve as DHEA-precursor products currently available on the market. For example, androstenedione, the popular 19-carbon steroid hormone produced in gonads and adrenal glands, serves as an intermediary step that eventually forms testosterone, estrone, and estradiol.[159] These conversions require specialized enzymes (e.g., 17β-hydroxysteroid dehydrogenase for testosterone, and aromatase for estrone and estradiol). Many of these prohormone compounds only can be purchased with a medical prescription, and in the case of androstenedione, may produce undesirable estrogenic side

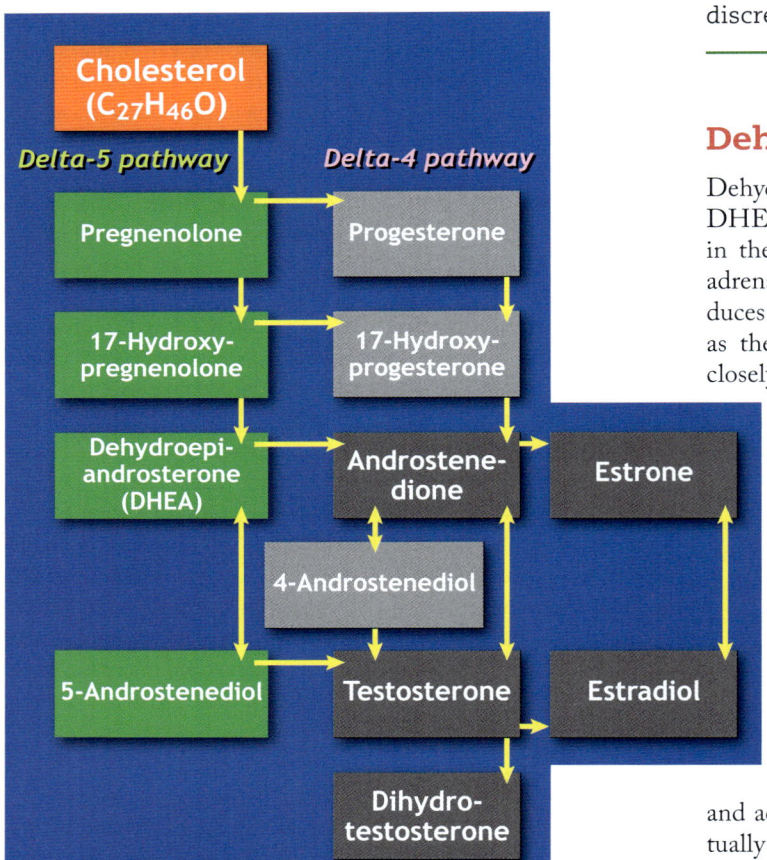

FIGURE 23.1. Metabolic pathways for dehydroepiandrosterone (DHEA), androstenedione, and five DHEA-precursor products currently available as medically prescribed drugs. Directional *arrows* signify one-way and two-way conversions.

effects (breast enlargement or tenderness, ankle and leg swelling, appetite loss, water retention, vomiting, abdominal cramping, and bloatedness). DHEA occurs naturally, curtailing the FDA's control of its distribution or claims for its action and effectiveness. The Drug Enforcement Administration (www.dea.gov) does not consider DHEA an anabolic steroid and does not list it as a controlled substance (www.dea.gov/sites/default/files/2020-06/Steroids-2020.pdf) specified under the Justice Department's Controlled Substances Act (www.dea.gov/drug-information/csa).

The lay press and mail-order, Internet, and health food industry and advertisements tout DHEA as a "superhormone"—a Holy Grail that supposedly increases testosterone production; protects against cancer, heart disease, diabetes, and osteoporosis; bolsters the immune system; preserves youth; invigorates sex life; decreases joint pain and fatigue; facilitates lean tissue gain and body fat loss; enhances mood and memory and generally counters the debilitating effects of aging; and extends life. The hormone's detractors consider it the "snake oil" of the 21st century, and WADA has banned DHEA at zero-tolerance levels.

FIGURE 23.2 illustrates the generalized trend for plasma DHEA levels during a lifetime, with six common claims by manufacturers of supplements. Boys and girls have substantial levels of DHEA at birth, which then decline sharply (not shown). DHEA production increases steadily from age 6 to 10 (may contribute to the beginning of puberty and sexuality) and then rises sharply with peak production (higher in males than in females) between ages 20 and 25. In contrast to the glucocorticoid and mineralocorticoid adrenal steroids whose plasma levels remain relatively high with aging, DHEA levels undergo a steady decline beyond age 30. By age 75, the plasma level averages only about 20% of younger counterparts. This low level means that plasma DHEA levels might serve as a biochemical marker for biologic aging and disease susceptibility.

Popular reasoning concludes that supplementing with DHEA blunts the negative effects of aging by raising its plasma levels to more "youthful" concentrations. Individuals supplement with this "natural" hormone just in case it proves beneficial—typically without considering the potential for biologic harm.

INTEGRATIVE QUESTION

Given that testosterone, growth hormone, and DHEA occur naturally in the body, what harm could come from supplementing with these "natural" compounds?

An Unregulated Compound with Uncertain Safety

Appropriate DHEA dosage for humans remains uncertain. Concern exists about possible harmful effects on blood lipids, glucose tolerance, and prostate gland health, particularly because medical problems associated with hormone supplementation often do not appear until years after drug use initiation.

In humans, cross-sectional observations relating DHEA levels to death risk from heart disease provided early indirect evidence for its beneficial effect. A high DHEA level conferred protection in men; for women, however, elevated DHEA increased heart disease risk. Subsequent research showed only a moderate protective association for males and no association for females. Studies suggest that DHEA supplements may provide cardioprotection during aging (more beneficial in males than in females)[134,135] decrease abdominal fat and improve insulin sensitivity among the elderly to help prevent and treat metabolic syndrome,[275] boost immune function in disease,[271] and provide some antioxidant protection.[7]

In additional research on humans, eight males and eight females aged 50 to 65 years received either 100 mg DHEA or a placebo daily for 3 months and the other treatment for the next 3 months.[189] All subjects showed a small but nonsignificant 1.2% increase in lean body mass during DHEA supplementation with some chemical markers indicating improved immune function. These findings suggest some positive effects of exogenous DHEA on muscle mass and immune function in middle-age males and females. Subsequent research evaluated short-term ingestion of 50 mg of DHEA daily on serum steroid hormones and 8-wk supplementation (150 mg·d^{-1}) on resistance-training adaptations in young adult males.[38] Short-term supplementation rapidly increased serum androstenedione (see next section) concentrations but exerted *no effect* on serum testosterone and estrogen concentrations. Long-term DHEA supplementation elevated serum androstenedione

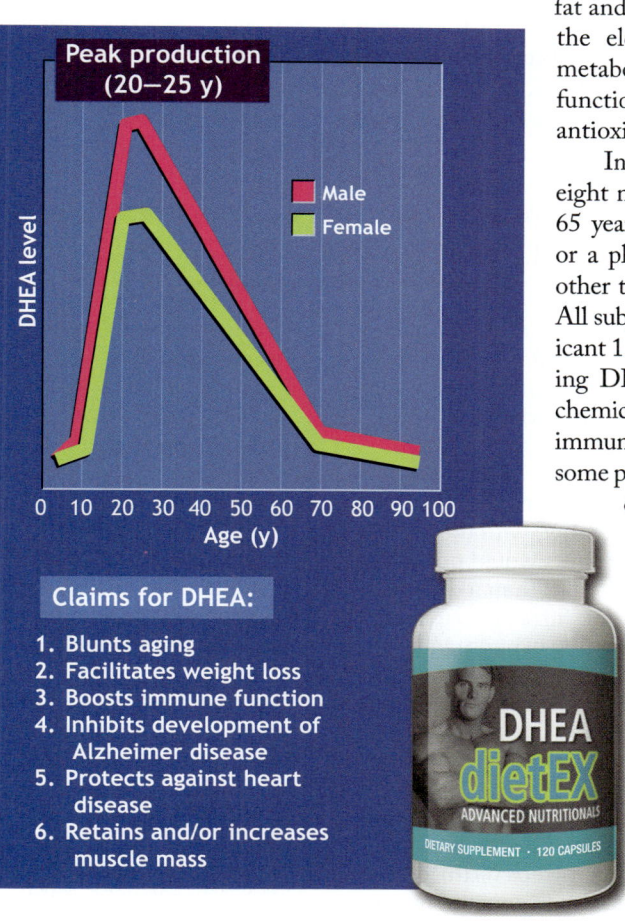

Claims for DHEA:
1. Blunts aging
2. Facilitates weight loss
3. Boosts immune function
4. Inhibits development of Alzheimer disease
5. Protects against heart disease
6. Retains and/or increases muscle mass

FIGURE 23.2. Generalized trend for plasma dehydroepiandrosterone (DHEA) levels for males and females over a lifetime.

levels but did *not* affect anabolic hormones, serum lipids, liver enzymes, muscular strength, and lean body mass, compared with a placebo for males undergoing similar training. These and similar results verify that low-dose DHEA does not increase serum testosterone levels, enhance muscular strength, change muscle and fat cross-sectional areas, or facilitate positive adaptations to resistance training.[203,282]

Concern still exists about the effect of unregulated long-term DHEA supplementation on bodily function and overall health, particularly for levels at or above 50 mg daily. Converting DHEA into the potent androgen testosterone promotes facial hair growth in females and alters normal menstrual function. Like exogenous anabolic steroids, DHEA lowers HDL-C levels to increase heart disease risk. Conflicting data center on its effects on breast cancer risk. Also, clinicians have expressed fear that elevating plasma DHEA by supplementation might stimulate the growth of otherwise dormant prostate gland tumors or cause benign prostate gland hypertrophy—if cancer exists, DHEA accelerates its growth. *Despite its popularity among fitness enthusiasts, no data support an ergogenic effect of exogenous DHEA on young adult males and females.*

Androstenedione: Benign Prohormone Nutritional Supplement or Potentially Harmful Drug?

The over-the-counter prohormone supplement **androstenedione**, popular in the strength training culture (in addition to norandrostenediol and norandrostenedione, which convert to the steroid nandrolone), supposedly confers these four beneficial effects:

1. Stimulates production of endogenous testosterone or forms androgenlike derivatives
2. Enables more intense training
3. Builds muscle mass
4. Rapidly repairs tissue injury

Found naturally in meat and some plant extracts, androstenedione is promoted as a prohormone metabolite only one step away from the biosynthesis of testosterone. The National Football League, National Collegiate Athletic Association, Men's Tennis Association, and WADA ban its use because they believe it provides an unfair competitive advantage and may endanger health. By calling the substance a supplement and avoiding any medical benefit claims, savvy marketers created a lucrative business for androstenedione, mostly by Internet sales and over-the-counter at health food stores. The public can purchase androstenedione-containing chewing gum and steroid lozenges that dissolve under the tongue at grocery and pharmacy stores.

$C_{19}H_{26}O_2$

Bacsica/Shutterstock

Effectiveness

Androstenedione, an intermediate precursor hormone between DHEA and testosterone, aids the liver in synthesizing other biologically active steroid hormones. Androstenedione is normally produced by the adrenal glands and gonads and converted to testosterone enzymatically by 17α-hydroxysteroid

---

Nutritional Supplementation with a Herbal/Botanical Supplement Did Not Enhance Physiological Function or Performance

Researchers assessed the effects of a proprietary supplement containing the botanical *Aphanizomenon flos-aquae* shown in the insert image and several herbal antioxidant and anti-inflammatory substances. The basic idea posited that circulating stem cells (and their number) with these supplements would positively impact muscle damage and muscle strength markers—including decreased inflammation and increased strength adaptations with resistance training. Two experiments were conducted using randomized crossover, double-blind, placebo-controlled trials where subjects in one study received either a placebo or SS (6150 mg · d⁻¹) for 14 days or in the second study received these compounds during a 16-wk strength-training program. Study 1, DOMS was induced on day 7 for both placebo and active conditions in the nondominant elbow flexor group with repeated eccentric repetitions. Muscle swelling (biceps girth), elbow flexor isometric strength (hand-held dynamometer), muscle pain/tenderness (visual analog scale), range of motion (active elbow flexion and extension), and inflammation (high-sensitivity C-reactive protein, interleukin-6, and tumor necrosis factor-α) were measured at baseline and at 24, 48, 72, and 168 hr (1 wk) after eccentric exercise. The crossover washout period was ≥14 days. In experiment 2, 1-RM bench press, 1-RM leg press, vertical jump height, balance (star excursion and center of mass excursion), isokinetic strength (elbow and knee flexion/extension), and perception of recovery were measured at baseline and following the 12-wk strength-training intervention. No statistically significant condition-by-time interactions between placebo and SS supplementation occurred for the main criterion variables. Both studies showed that nutritional supplementation with stem cells did not improve outcome measures related to muscle recovery following acute upper-arm–induced DOMS, nor enhance training-induced adaptations to strength, balance, and muscle function above strength training alone.

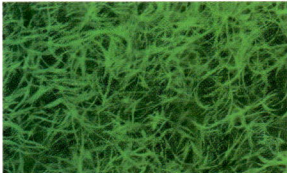

Sources:
Furlong, J, et al. Effect of an herbal/botanical supplement on strength, balance, and muscle function following 12 weeks of resistance training: a placebo-controlled study. *J Int Soc Sports Nutr.* 2014;11:23.
Rynders, C, et al. Effect of an herbal/botanical supplement on recovery from delayed onset muscle soreness: a randomized placebo-controlled trial. *J Int Soc Sports Nutr.* 2014;11:27.

dehydrogenase found in the body's diverse tissues. It also serves as an estrogen precursor. Taking exogenous androstenedione raises testosterone levels. Four-androstene-3,17-dione or 200 mg of 4-androstene-3b,17α-diol in a daily oral treatment increased peripheral plasma total and free testosterone concentrations compared with a placebo.[82] Androstenedione dosages up to 300 mg daily elevated testosterone levels by 34%.[157] Chronic androstenedione administration also elevates serum estradiol and estrone in males and females, perhaps offsetting any potential anabolic effect.[257] *Little scientific evidence supports claims of androstenedione's ergogenic effectiveness or anabolic qualities.* Furthermore, research to date verifies that the prohormone nutritional supplements DHEA, androstenedione, androstenediol, and other prohormone compounds *do not* produce anabolic or ergogenic effects, despite heavily promoted marketing and advertising claims.

Research findings show *no effect* of androstenedione supplementation on basal serum concentrations of testosterone or the training response for muscle size and strength and body composition.[148,282] The potential negative effects of the HDL-C reduction on overall heart disease risk and the elevated serum estrogen levels on risk of gynecomastia and possibly pancreatic and other cancers cause concern when individuals consume 500 to 1200 mg daily for ergogenic purposes.

Modified Versions

Modified androstenedione over-the-counter products include norandrostenedione and norandrostenediol compounds. They are chemically similar to androstenedione and androstenediol with only slight chemical modification without converting to testosterone but do convert to the steroid nandrolone. Researchers assessed the effect of these modifications for a low-dose norsteroid-containing supplement on body composition, girth measures, muscular strength, and mood states of young adult, resistance-trained males.[267] Each subject did resistance training 4 days per week for the study's duration. Norsteroid supplementation provided *no additional effect* on any body composition or exercise performance variables. Recreational and competitive athletes also should be aware that some over-the-counter supplements contain contaminates with trace 19-norandrosterone amounts, the standard marker for nandrolone as a banned substance easily detected by routine urine testing.[54] Additionally, androstenedione preparations often fail to meet quality standards. (See the FYI below.)

Amino Acid Supplementation

An emerging trend involves using nutrition as a "legal" alternative to activate the body's normal anabolic mechanisms. Highly specific dietary changes supposedly create a hormonal milieu that facilitates protein synthesis in skeletal muscle. Weightlifters, bodybuilders, and fitness enthusiasts routinely consume amino acid supplements, believing they boost the body's natural production of testosterone, GH, insulin, or insulinlike growth factor I (IGF-I) to improve muscle size and strength and decrease body fat. The rationale for nutritional ergogenic stimulants comes from clinically infusing amino acids to regulate anabolic hormones in deficient patients.

Research on healthy subjects *does not* provide convincing evidence for an ergogenic effect on hormone secretion, training responsiveness, or physical performance of a *regular dietary intake* of amino acid supplements above the recommended protein intake. In studies with appropriate design and statistical analysis, low-dose oral supplements of arginine, lysine, ornithine, tyrosine, and other amino acids, either singly or in combination, produced no positive effect on GH levels,[63,158] insulin secretion,[40,96] diverse measures of anaerobic power,[95] or all-out running performance at $\dot{V}O_{2max}$.[252] Elite junior weightlifters who regularly supplemented with 20 amino acids did not improve physical performance or change resting or exercise levels of testosterone, cortisol, or GH.[102] Regularly consuming amino acids in the quantities recommended in commercial supplements does not benefit an individual's hormonal profile, body composition and muscle size, or physical performance. Indiscriminately

fyi Competitive Athletes Must Heed This Warning

B Ledger/Shutterstock

Athletes who take androstenedione can fail a urine test for the banned anabolic steroid nandrolone because the supplement often contains contaminates with trace amounts as low as 10 mg containing 19-norandrosterone, the standard marker demonstrating nandrolone presence. Many androstenedione preparations are grossly mislabeled. Analysis of nine different brands of 100-mg doses indicated wide fluctuations in overall androstenedione content ranging from 0 to 103 mg, with one brand contaminated with testosterone, and other supplements with a wide variety of illegal adulterants.

Take-home message—do not even think about taking this supplement!

Sources:

Holubová B, et al. Tailor-Made Immunochromatographic Test for the detection of multiple 17α-methylated anabolics in dietary supplements. *Foods.* 2021;10:741.

Meng Q, et al. A reliable and validated LC-MS/MS method for the simultaneous quantification of 4 cannabinoids in 40 consumer products. *PLoS One.* 2018;13:e0196396.

Micalizzi G, et al. Reliable identification and quantification of anabolic androgenic steroids in dietary supplements by using gas chromatography coupled to triple quadrupole mass spectrometry. *Drug Test Anal.* 2021;13:128.

Wang H, et al. Determination of anabolic androgenic steroids in dietary supplements and external drugs by magnetic solid-phase extraction combined with high-performance liquid chromatography-tandem mass spectrometry. *J Sep Sci.* 2021;44:1939.

consuming amino acid supplements at dosages considered pharmacologic rather than nutritional raises the possibility of direct toxic effects or the creation of an amino acid imbalance.

Specific Timing

Manipulation and intake timing of nutritional variables in the immediate pre-exercise and postexercise periods can affect responsiveness to resistance training (see "In a Practical Sense: Nutrient Timing to Optimize Muscle Response to Resistance Training"). This occurs by mechanisms that alter nutrient availability, enzyme activity, circulating metabolites and hormonal secretions, interactions with receptors on target tissues, and gene translation and transcription.[87,149,262] Resistance training stimulates protein synthesis and protein degradation in exercised muscle fibers. Muscle hypertrophy occurs when a *net increase*

In a Practical Sense

Nutrient Timing to Optimize Muscle Response to Resistance Training

An evidence-based nutritional approach can enhance the quality of resistance training and facilitate muscle growth and strength development. This easy-to-follow new dimension to sports nutrition emphasizes not only the specific type and mixture of nutrients but also the timing of nutrient intake. Its goal—to blunt glucagon, epinephrine, norepinephrine, and cortisol release in the catabolic state to activate natural muscle-building hormones (testosterone, growth hormone, IGF-1, insulin), which facilitates recovery to maximize muscle growth. Three phases optimize nutrient intake:

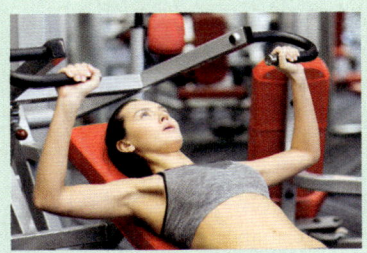

Syda Productions/Shutterstock

PHASE 1

The *energy phase* enhances nutrient intake to spare muscle glycogen and protein, enhance muscular endurance, limit immune system suppression, reduce muscle damage, and facilitate recovery in the postexercise period. Consuming a carbohydrate-protein supplement in the immediate pre-exercise period and during exercise extends muscular endurance; the ingested protein promotes protein metabolism, reducing demand for amino acid release from muscle. The carbohydrates consumed during physical activity suppress cortisol release. This helps to blunt an exercise suppressive effect on immune system function and lessen leucine, isoleucine, and valine branched-chain amino acid use by energy released from protein catabolism.

The recommended energy phase supplement contains these nutrient components: 20 to 26 g high-glycemic carbohydrates (glucose, sucrose, maltodextrin), 5 to 6 g whey protein (rapidly digested, high-quality protein separated from milk in the cheese-making process), 1 g leucine; 30 to 120 mg of vitamin C, 20 to 60 IU vitamin E, 100 to 250 mg sodium, 60 to 100 mg potassium, and 60 to 220 mg magnesium. Consuming more slowly digested whole casein protein after exercise produces similar increases in muscle protein's net balance and net muscle protein synthesis compared with whey protein. Casein and whey protein often are blended as supplements to provide faster-acting and slower-acting protein sources during recovery.[263]

PHASE 2

The *anabolic phase* contains a 45-min postexercise metabolic opening—an interval favoring enhanced insulin sensitivity for muscle glycogen replenishment and tissue repair and synthesis. The shift from a catabolic to anabolic state occurs largely by blunting cortisol's catabolic action and increasing insulin's anabolic, muscle-building effects when consuming a standard high-glycemic carbohydrate-protein supplement in liquid form (e.g., whey protein and high-glycemic carbohydrates). In essence, the high-glycemic carbohydrate consumed postexercise serves as a nutrient activator to stimulate insulin release, and combined with amino acids, increases muscle tissue synthesis and resists protein degradation. The recommended *anabolic phase* supplement profile contains these nutrients: 40 to 50 g high-glycemic carbohydrates (glucose, sucrose, maltodextrin), 13 to 15 g whey protein, 1 to 2 g leucine, 1 to 2 g glutamine, 60 to 120 mg vitamin C, and 80 to 400 IU vitamin E.

PHASE 3

The *growth phase* extends from the end of the anabolic phase to the next workout. It represents the time interlude to maximize insulin sensitivity and maintain an anabolic state to enhance muscle mass and strength gains. The first 2-hr *rapid segment* phase focuses on maintaining increased insulin sensitivity and glucose uptake to maximize glycogen replenishment and eliminate metabolic wastes by increased blood flow. The next 16 to 18 hr *(sustained segment)* maintains a positive nitrogen balance. This occurs with a relatively high daily protein intake between 0.91 and 1.2 g protein per lb body weight, which encourages more sustained but slower muscle tissue synthesis. Adequate carbohydrate intake emphasizes glycogen replenishment. The recommended *growth phase* supplement contains the following nutrients: 14 g whey protein, 2 g casein, 3 g leucine, 1 g glutamine, and 2 to 4 g high-glycemic carbohydrates.

Sources:
Falkenberg E, et al. Nutrient intake, meal timing and sleep in elite male Australian football players. *J Sci Med Sport*. 2021;24:7.
Ivy J, Portman R. *Nutrient Timing: The Future of Sports Nutrition*. Laguna Beach: Basic Health Publications; 2004.
Kume W, et al. Acute effect of the timing of resistance exercise and nutrient intake on muscle protein breakdown. *Nutrients*. 2020;12:1177.

in protein synthesis results from a shift in the body's normal dynamic state of synthesis and degradation. The normal hormonal milieu of insulin and GH levels in the period following resistance exercise stimulates a muscle fiber's anabolic processes while inhibiting muscle protein degradation. Dietary modifications immediately prior to physical activity and/or in the recovery period that increase amino acid transport into muscles, raise energy availability, or increase anabolic hormones, particularly insulin, should theoretically increase the rate of anabolism and/or depress catabolism. Either effect would create a positive body protein balance to improve muscle growth and strength.

Carbohydrate-Protein-Creatine Supplementation in Recovery Augments Hormonal Response to Resistance Exercise

Hormonal dynamics and protein anabolism studies indicate a transient but potential fourfold increase in protein synthesis[212] with carbohydrate and/or protein supplements consumed *prior to*[44,262,292] or *immediately following*[30,130,179] a resistance exercise workout. Supplementation in the immediate postexercise period also can enhance repair and synthesis of muscle proteins following aerobic activity.[19,161,188] Protein sources producing a slow amino acid release when consumed immediately before resistance exercise are as effective as consuming rapidly digested proteins in promoting postexercise muscle protein synthesis.[45]

In one study, drug-free male weightlifters with at least 2 years training experience consumed carbohydrate and protein supplements immediately after a standard workout.[55] Treatment included the following: placebo of pure water or a supplement containing either (1) carbohydrate (1.5 g protein · kg^{-1}); (2) protein (1.38 g protein · kg^{-1}, or carbohydrate-protein (1.1 g carbohydrate with 0.41 g protein · kg^{-1} consumed immediately following and then 2 hr after the training session.

Each nutritive supplement produced a hormonal environment including elevated plasma insulin and GH concentrations during recovery more conducive to protein synthesis and muscle tissue growth than the placebo condition. Subsequent research showed that protein-carbohydrate supplementation before and immediately following resistance training altered the metabolic and hormonal responses to 3 consecutive days of intense resistance training.[154] Changes in the immediate recovery period included increased concentrations of glucose, insulin, GH, and IGF-I and decreased blood lactate concentration. Such data provide indirect evidence for a possible training benefit. This translated to enhanced glycogen and protein synthesis in recovery from increased carbohydrate and/or protein intake immediately following a workout.

Research compared the effects of strategic protein and carbohydrate consumption before and/or after each workout compared with supplementation in the hours not close to the workout on muscle fiber hypertrophy, muscular strength, and body composition. Resistance-trained males matched for strength were placed in one of two groups; one group consumed a supplement (1 g protein · kg^{-1}) containing protein-creatine-glucose immediately before and after resistance training, while the other group received the same supplement dose in the morning and late evening of the workout day. Measurements of body composition by dual energy x-ray absorptiometry (DXA; see Chapter 28), strength (1-RM), muscle fiber type, cross-sectional area, contractile protein, creatine, and glycogen content from vastus lateralis muscle biopsies took place the week prior to and immediately after a 10-wk training program. As **FIGURE 23.3** reveals,

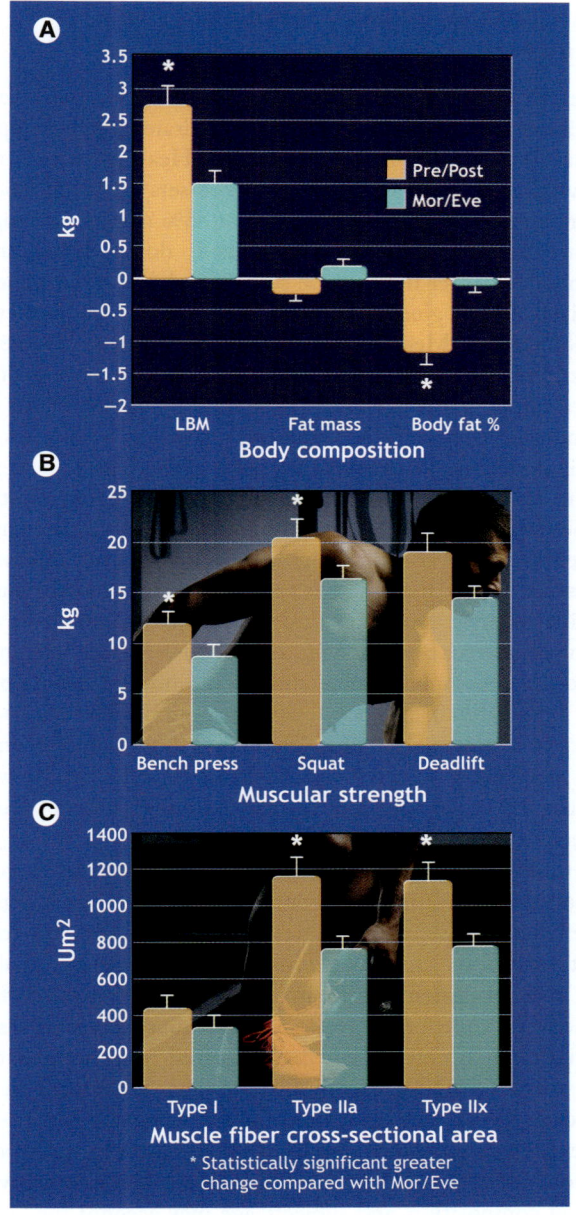

FIGURE 23.3. Effects of receiving 1 g · kg body weight^{-1} of a protein, creatine, and glucose supplement immediately before and after resistance exercise training (**Pre/Post**), or in the early morning (Mor) or late evening (Eve) on the training day for changes in (**A**) body composition, (**B**) 1-repetition maximum strength, and (**C**) muscle cross-sectional area. LBM, lean body mass.
(Adapted with permission from Cribb PJ, Hayes A. Effects of supplement timing and resistance exercise on skeletal muscle hypertrophy. *Med Sci Sports Exerc.* 2006;38:1918. Photo: Paul Biryukov/Shutterstock.)

supplementation in the immediate pre-exercise/postexercise period produced a greater increase in lean body mass and 1-RM strength in two of three measures. Body composition changes were supported by greater increases in muscle cross-sectional area of the type II muscle fibers and their contractile protein content. Supplement timing provides a simple but effective strategy to enhance desirable adaptations from resistance training.

Postexercise Glucose Augments Protein Balance with Resistance Training

Research with postexercise glucose ingestion complements previously described studies of carbohydrate-protein supplementation following resistance training. Healthy males familiar with resistance training performed 8 sets of 10 repetitions of unilateral knee extensor exercise at 85% maximal strength in a placebo-controlled, randomized, double-blind trial. Immediately after the exercise session and 1 hr later, subjects received either a glucose supplement ($1.0 \text{ g} \cdot \text{kg}^{-1}$) or a placebo of Nutrasweet. Measurements consisted of urinary 3-methylhistidine excretion (3-MH) as a marker of muscle protein degradation, vastus lateralis muscle incorporation rate for the amino acid leucine (L-$[1$-$^{13}C]$leucine) to indicate protein synthesis, and urinary nitrogen excretion to reflect protein breakdown. **FIGURE 23.4A AND B** reveals glucose supplementation reduced myofibrillar protein breakdown reflected by decreased excretion of 3-MH and urinary nitrogen. While not achieving statistical significance, glucose supplementation also increased leucine incorporation rate into the vastus lateralis over the 10-hr postexercise period (Fig. 23.4C). These alterations indicated that the supplemented condition produced a more positive body protein balance following exercise. The beneficial effect of a postexercise high-glycemic glucose supplementation most likely occurred from increased insulin release with glucose intake, which should enhance muscle protein balance in recovery.

One should view the effects of immediate postexercise carbohydrate and/or protein supplementation in perspective. One unanswered question concerns the degree that any transient yet positive change in hormonal milieu favoring anabolism and net protein synthesis caused by postexercise dietary maneuvers contributes to long-term muscle growth and strength enhancement. No effect occurred from immediately ingesting an amino acid-carbohydrate mixture postexercise on muscular strength or size gains of older males who did 12-wk knee extensor resistance training.[108] Differences in study population, criterion variables, specific amino acid mixtures, overall diet composition, and subjects' age may account for future discrepancies in research findings.

Dietary Lipid May Affect Hormonal Milieu

The diet's lipid content can modulate resting neuroendocrine homeostasis to modify tissue synthesis and training responsiveness. Research evaluated the effects of an intense resistance exercise bout on postexercise plasma testosterone. In

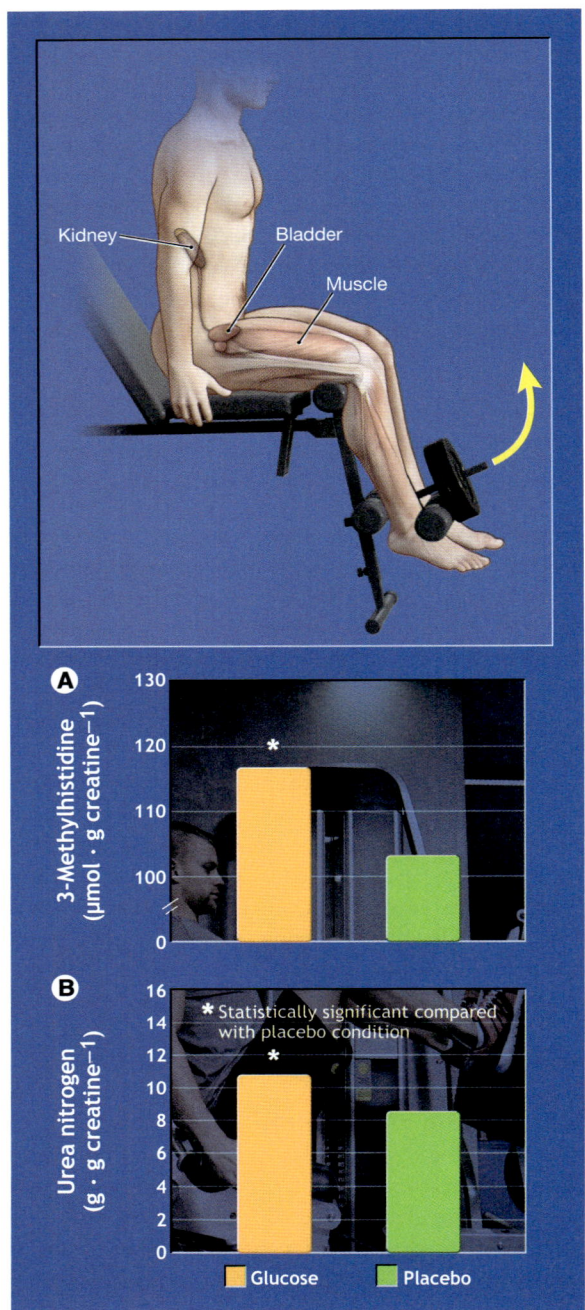

FIGURE 23.4. Effects of 1.0 g · kg body mass^{-1} glucose versus a Nutrasweet placebo ingested immediately after exercise and 1 hr later on protein degradation reflected by 24-hr urinary output of **(A)** 3-methylhistidine, **(B)** urinary urea nitrogen, and **(C)** rate of muscle protein synthesis (MPS) measured by vastus lateralis muscle incorporation of leucine (L-$[l$-$^{13}C]$). *Bars* for MPS indicate difference between exercise and control leg for glucose and placebo conditions.
(Adapted with permission from Roy BD, et al. Effect of glucose supplement timing on protein metabolism after resistance training. *J Appl Physiol*. 1997;82:1882. Figures 5 & 7. ©The American Physiological Society (APS). All rights reserved.)

agreement with prior research, testosterone levels increased 5 min postexercise. A more impressive finding was a close association between the macronutrient composition of the individual's regular diet and resting testosterone levels.

TABLE 23.2 reveals how dietary macronutrients correlate with pre-exercise testosterone concentrations. Dietary lipid and saturated and monounsaturated fatty acid levels best predicted testosterone concentrations at rest—lower levels of each of these dietary components accompanied lower resting levels of testosterone.

TABLE 23.2 Quantity and percentage of dietary macronutrients and the correlations with pre-exercise testosterone concentration

These findings support prior studies that showed that a approximately 20% low-fat diet produced *lower* testosterone levels than a diet with approximately 40% higher lipid content.[212,260] The diet's protein percentage correlated inversely with resting testosterone levels—*higher* dietary protein related to *lower* testosterone levels (see Table 23.2). Many resistance-trained athletes consume considerable dietary protein, so the implications of this association for the training response remain unresolved. If a low dietary lipid intake decreases resting testosterone levels, then individuals who typically consume low-fat diets (e.g., vegetarians, dancers, gymnasts, wrestlers) may experience a diminished training response. Athletes who show low plasma testosterone levels from overtraining may benefit from changing their diet's macronutrient composition to lower protein and higher lipid.

Amphetamines

Amphetamines or "pep pills" comprise a group of pharmacologic compounds that exert powerful stimulating effects on central nervous system function. Amphetamine (Benzedrine) and dextroamphetamine sulfate (Dexedrine) have frequently been used by athletes. Amphetamines exert sympathomimetic β_2-adrenergic effects, mimicking epinephrine and norepinephrine (sympathomimetic)—to increase blood pressure, heart rate, cardiac output, breathing rate, metabolism, and blood glucose.

Five to 20 mg of amphetamine usually exerts its effect for 30 to 90 min following ingestion, although its influence often persists longer. Amphetamines increase alertness, wakefulness, and capacity to perform work by depressing the sensation of muscle fatigue. The deaths of two famed cyclists in the 1960s during competitive road racing were attributed to amphetamine use. In one of these deaths in 1967, British Tour de France rider Tom Simpson overheated and suffered a fatal heart attack during the Mont Ventoux ascent in Provence, France.

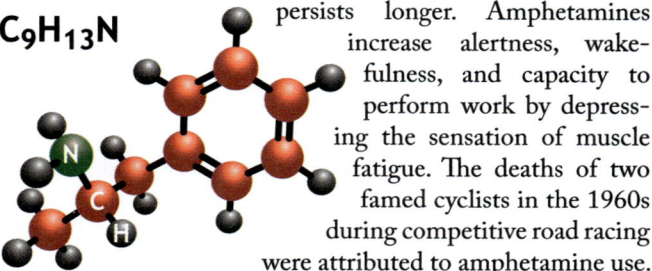

$C_9H_{13}N$

Bacsica/Shutterstock

Amphetamine Dangers and Exercise Performance

Amphetamine use in athletics makes little sense for the following five reasons:

1. Regular use can lead to either physiologic or emotional drug dependency. This causes a cyclical reliance on "uppers" (amphetamines) or "downers" (barbiturates)—the barbiturates reduce or tranquilize the "hyper" state.
2. General side effects include headache, tremulousness, agitation, fever, dizziness, and confusion, all of which negatively affect sports performance that requires rapid reaction and judgment and a high level of steadiness and mental concentration.
3. Larger doses are required to achieve the same effect because drug tolerance increases with prolonged use; this can aggravate and precipitate cardiovascular disorders.
4. Inhibition or suppression of the body's normal mechanisms for perceiving and responding to pain, fatigue, or heat stress jeopardizes health and safety.
5. Effects of prolonged intake at high doses remain unknown.
6. Amphetamines do not affect physical capacity or simple psychomotor tasks performance.

Caffeine

Caffeine represents a possible exception to the general rule against ingesting stimulants to promote ergogenic effects.[270] Caffeine's classification and prior regulatory status depend on its use either as a drug (over-the-counter for migraine headaches), food (in coffee and soft drinks), or dietary supplement (alertness products). The most widely consumed behaviorally active substance in the world, caffeine belongs to a group of lipid soluble purines (proper chemical name: 1,3,7-trimethylxanthine) found naturally in coffee beans, tea leaves, chocolate, cocoa beans, and cola nuts and often added to carbonated beverages, and nonprescription over-the-counter cold remedies, diuretics, pain remedies, stimulants, and weight control aids. Depending on preparation, one cup of brewed coffee contains between 60 and 150 mg caffeine, instant coffee about 100 mg, brewed tea between 20 and 50 mg, caffeinated soft drinks about 50 mg, and diet drinks about 36 mg. For comparison, 2.5 cups of percolated coffee contain 250 to 400 mg of caffeine, or generally between 3 and 6 mg · kg^{-1} of body mass.

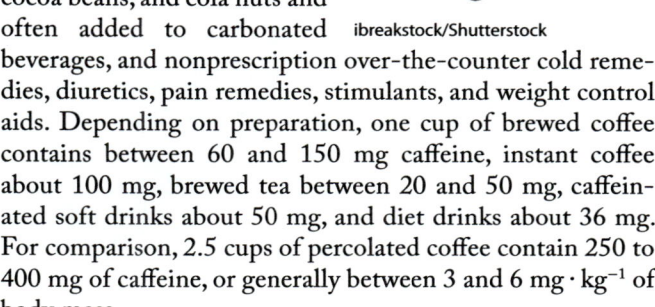

$C_8H_{10}N_4O_2$

ibreakstock/Shutterstock

The intestinal tract absorbs caffeine rapidly; peak plasma concentration is reached within 1 hr. It also clears from the body relatively quickly, taking about 3 to 6 hr for blood caffeine concentrations to decrease by one half, referred to as the substance half-life compared with about 10 hr for the stimulant methamphetamine.

Ergogenic Effects

Drinking 2.5 cups percolated regular coffee up to 1 hr prior to physical activity often extends endurance in strenuous aerobic activities; it also improves higher-intensity, shorter-duration effort and muscular strength and power in longer continuous activity and enhances fatigue resistance, complex cognitive ability, and team sport performance.[73,79,126,183,213,244,298]

Elite distance runners who consumed 10 mg caffeine · kg body mass^{-1} immediately before a treadmill run to exhaustion improved performance time compared with placebo or control conditions.[100] Ergogenic effects during exhaustive exercise at 80% $\dot{V}O_{2max}$ that follows a 5 mg · kg^{-1} caffeine dose are maintained 5 hr later in a subsequent exercise challenge.[21,167] No need exists to ingest an additional dose to maintain high blood caffeine levels and ergogenic effects during subsequent activity within 5 hr. Caffeine ingestion does not impede glycogen resynthesis with carbohydrate supplementation after extreme depletion of muscle glycogen.[18] From a health perspective, drinking either caffeinated or decaffeinated coffee up to 6 cups a day in a dose-response relationship inversely related with total and all-specific mortality (i.e., the greater the coffee intake, the lower the risk of heart disease, respiratory disease, stroke, injuries and accidents, type 2 diabetes, and infections, but not deaths from cancer).[99]

Early research showed that subjects performed on average 90.2 min of physical activity with caffeine (pink triangle) and 75.5 min without it (yellow diamond; **FIG. 23.5**). Consuming caffeine before physical activity increased lipid catabolism and reduced carbohydrate oxidation during exercise. The ergogenic effect of caffeine also applies to physical activity performed at high ambient temperatures.[61]

Caffeine also benefits maximal swimming performance. In a double-blind, crossover research design, seven male and four female competitive distance swimmers (<25 min for 1500 m) consumed caffeine (6 mg · kg^{-1}) 2.5 hr before swimming 1500 m. **FIGURE 23.6** shows that split times improved with caffeine for each 500 m

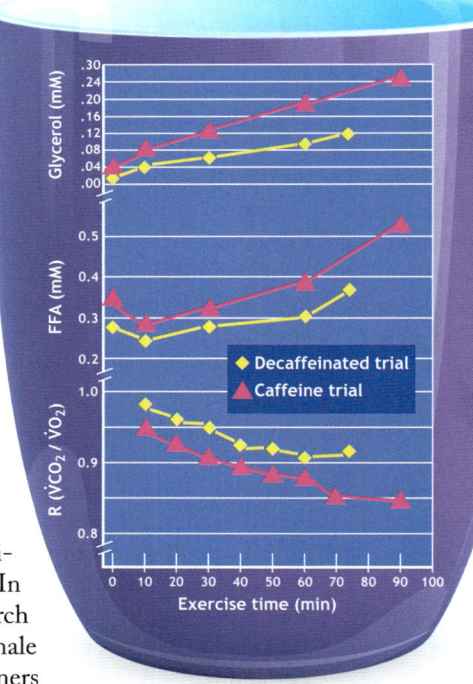

FIGURE 23.5. Plasma glycerol, free fatty acids (FFAs), and respiratory exchange ratio (R) during endurance exercise trials after ingesting caffeine and decaffeinated liquids.
(Adapted with permission from Costill BD, et al. Effects of caffeine ingestion on metabolism and exercise performance. *Med Sci Sports*. 1978;10:155. Photo: vasabii/Shutterstock.)

in the event. Swim time averaged 1.9% faster with caffeine than without it (20:58.6 vs. 21:21.8 min). Enhanced performance with caffeine associated with a lower plasma potassium concentration before the swim and higher blood glucose levels at the end of the trial. These responses suggest a possible caffeine effect on electrolyte balance or glucose availability.[8]

No Dose-Response Relationship

FIGURE 23.7 illustrates the effects of manipulating pre-exercise caffeine dosage on endurance time of nine trained male cyclists. Subjects received a placebo or a capsule containing 5, 9, or 13 mg of caffeine per kg of body mass 1 hr before cycling at 80% of maximum power output on a $\dot{V}O_{2max}$ test. All caffeine trials showed a 24% improvement in performance with no additional benefit from caffeine quantities above 5 mg · kg.$^{-1}$

Proposed Mechanism for Ergogenic Effect

A precise explanation for the ergogenic boost from caffeine remains elusive. The ergogenic effect of caffeine (or related methylxanthine compounds) in intense endurance activity has generally been attributed to facilitated lipid use as an energy fuel, sparing carbohydrate reserves. In the quantities usually administered to humans, caffeine probably affects metabolism in either of two ways:

1. Directly on adipose and peripheral vascular tissues
2. Indirectly by stimulating epinephrine release from the adrenal medulla

Epinephrine then acts as an antagonist of the adenosine receptors on adipocyte cells, which normally repress lipolysis. Caffeine's inhibition of adenosine receptors increases cellular levels of the second-messenger cyclic 3′,5′-adenosine monophosphate or cyclic AMP (refer to Chapter 20). Cyclic AMP then activates hormone-sensitive lipases to promote lipolysis; this effect causes the release of free fatty acids (FFAs) into the plasma. Elevated FFA levels increase lipid oxidation, thus conserving liver and muscle glycogen to benefit intense endurance performance.

Caffeine's ergogenic effects also appear unrelated to hormonal or metabolic changes. This suggests a possible direct action of caffeine on specific tissues, including the nervous system. Caffeine and its metabolites readily cross the blood-brain barrier to produce analgesic

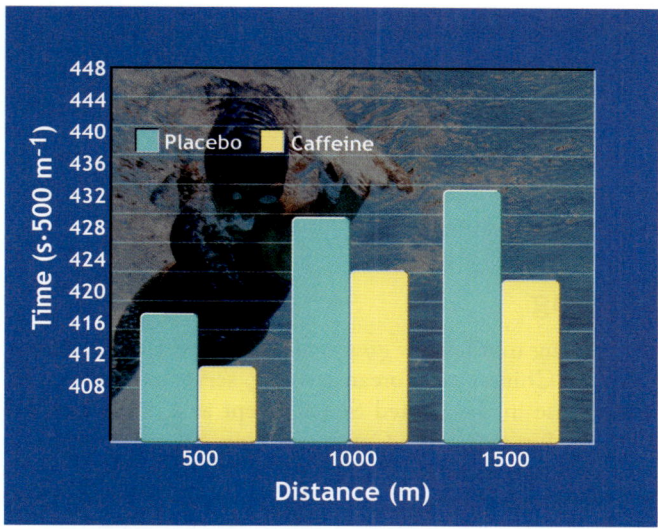

FIGURE 23.6. Split times for each 500 m of a 1500-m time trial with caffeine and placebo. Caffeine produced significantly faster split times.
(Adapted with permission from MacIntosh BR, Wright BM. Caffeine ingestion and performance of a 1500-metre swim. *Can J Appl Physiol.* 1995;20:168. Permission conveyed through Copyright Clearance Center, Inc. Photo: Microgen/Shutterstock.)

effects on the central nervous system, potentially reducing the perception of effort during physical activity. Caffeine enhances motoneuronal excitability to facilitate motor-unit recruitment. The stimulating effects of caffeine do not occur from its direct action on the central nervous system. Instead, caffeine acts indirectly by blocking the receptors for adenosine that also serve a neuromodulator function to calm brain and spinal cord neurons. The following four factors interact to produce caffeine's facilitating neuromuscular activity effects:

1. Lower threshold for motor unit recruitment
2. Alter excitation-contraction coupling
3. Facilitate nerve transmission
4. Increase ion transport within the muscle

Inconsistent Effects Relate to Diet and Habitual Caffeine Use

Prior nutrition partly accounts for why individual differences exist in exercise response after consuming caffeine. Those who normally consume a high-carbohydrate diet show a depressed effect for caffeine on FFA mobilization.[284] Individual differences in caffeine sensitivity, tolerance, and hormonal response from short-term and long-term patterns of caffeine consumption also affect this drug's ergogenic qualities. The ergogenic effects of caffeine occur less for caffeine in coffee than in capsule form.

An athlete should consider "caffeine tolerance" rather than assume that it provides a consistent benefit to everyone. From a practical standpoint, the athlete should omit caffeine-containing foods and beverages 4 to 6 days before competition to optimize caffeine's pre-exercise potential to exert ergogenic effects.

Effects on Muscle

Caffeine acts directly on muscle to enhance physical capacity, particularly repeated submaximum muscle actions.[183,230] A double-blind research design evaluated voluntary and electrically stimulated muscle actions under "caffeine-free" conditions and following orally administered 500 mg caffeine.[177] Electrically stimulating the motor nerve allowed the researchers to remove central nervous system control and quantify caffeine's direct effects on skeletal muscle. Caffeine produced no effect on maximal muscle force during voluntary or electrically stimulated muscle actions. For submaximal effort, caffeine increased force output for low-frequency electrical stimulation before and after muscle fatigue. Pre-exercise caffeine administration also increased by 17% repeated submaximal isometric muscular endurance.[204] Caffeine exerts no ergogenic effect on anaerobic metabolic capacity (glycolysis) assessed during repeated intense Wingate exercise tests.[116]

Warning About Caffeine

Individuals who normally avoid caffeine may experience adverse effects when they first consume it. Caffeine stimulates the central nervous system and in quantities greater than 1.5 g can produce typical **caffeinism** symptoms: restlessness, headaches, insomnia, nervous irritability, muscle twitching, tremulousness, psychomotor agitation, elevated heart rate and blood pressure, and premature left-ventricular contractions. From the standpoint of temperature regulation, caffeine acts as a diuretic, but with moderate caffeine consumption (≤456 mg), it does not produce water-electrolyte imbalances or reduced exercise heat tolerance.[8] Caffeine's effect on fluid loss lessens when consumed

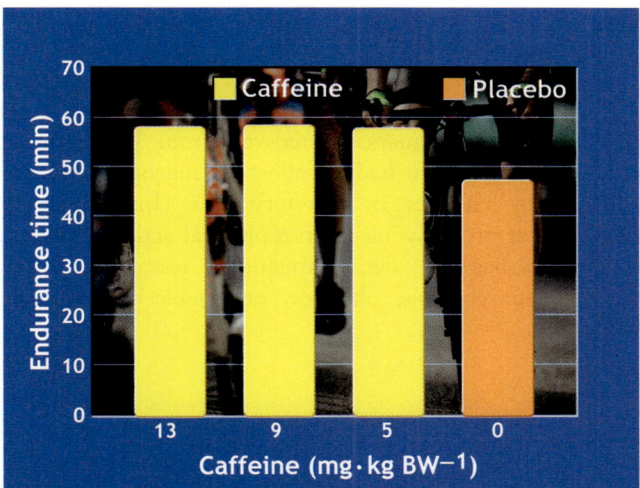

FIGURE 23.7. Time to fatigue endurance performance in nine male cyclists after consuming caffeine in different concentrations before racing. All caffeine trials produced significantly better performance than the placebo condition, with no dose-response association among different caffeine concentrations and performance. BW, body weight.
(Adapted with permission from Pasman WJ, et al. The effect of different dosages of caffeine on endurance performance time. *Int J Sports Med.* 1995;16:225. Photo: Juanan Barros Moreno/Shutterstock.)

during physical activity because catecholamine release in activity greatly reduces renal blood flow and physical activity enhances renal solute reabsorption and consequently water conservation (osmotic effect). Caffeine ingestion at a dose that elicits ergogenic effects during exertion has no detrimental effect on blood platelet function in young healthy individuals.[286]

The effects of excess caffeine generally pose no health risk, yet a caffeine overdose can be lethal. The **LD$_{50}$** or lethal oral caffeine dose required to kill 50% of the population is about 10 g (150 mg·kg^{-1}) for a 70-kg/154-lb person. A 50-kg woman has an acute health risk with a caffeine intake of 7.5 g. Moderate caffeine toxicity exists for small children who consume 35 mg·kg^{-1}. Such observations provide clear indication of the inverted U-shaped relationship between certain exogenous chemicals and health and safety and probably exercise performance. Ingesting even small quantities of caffeine usually produces desirable effects—consuming an excess can wreak havoc.

Consumer Beware: Powdered Caffeine Can Be Fatal

A single teaspoon of powdered (concentrated) caffeine, sold under various names, contains the caffeine equivalent of drinking about 25 consecutive 8-oz/227-g cups brewed coffee, with a total caffeine content of about 6000 mg! Sold as a supplement to mainly boost energy, the recommended 1/16th of a teaspoon dose that invites unintended overdosing because special measuring spoons would be required to exactly measure the correct recommended supplement amount. Although a seemingly benign form of a common substance, two young males in 2014 died almost instantly from a seizure after consuming concentrated powdered caffeine (www.fda.gov/food/dietary-supplement-products-ingredients/pure-and-highly-concentrated-caffeine). Now, consumers can purchase "gummy chews," small candylike chewable "chocolate and other flavored boosts" that each contain 100 mg caffeine and 40 kcal, the equivalent of 1 cup of any coffee brand. The ads tout their fast absorption, "bypassing your stomach and absorbed through the mouth membranes, giving a caffeine kick in as little as 5 min!" The FDA, which does *not* regulate supplement or caffeine-containing drinks or tablets, has previously reported cases documenting dizziness, delirium, nausea, vomiting, and increased heart rate from simply taking a much smaller amount of this compound. Such events have led to initiatives to convince the FDA to ban powdered caffeine. In 2018, the FDA issued a consumer warning regarding powdered caffeine: *"… less than two tablespoons of some formulations of powdered, pure caffeine can be deadly to most adults, while even smaller amounts can be life threatening to children. Regardless of whether the product contains a warning label, such products present a significant and unreasonable risk of illness or injury to the consumer"* (www.fda.gov/news-events/press-announcements/fda-takes-step-protect-consumers-against-dietary-supplements-containing-dangerously-high-levels).

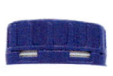
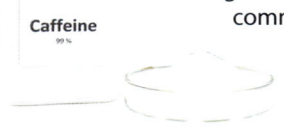
sulit.photos/Shutterstock

Ginseng and Ephedrine

Ginseng and **ephedrine** are commonly marketed as nutritional supplements to "reduce tension," "revitalize," "burn calories," and "optimize mental and physical performance," particularly during periods of fatigue and stress. Ginseng also plays a role as an alternative therapy to treat diabetes and male impotence and stimulate immune function.

Ginseng

The ginseng root (*Panax ginseng*, C. A. Meyer), often sold as Panax or Chinese or Korean ginseng, serves no recognized medical use in the United States except as a component of soothing skin ointments. Commercial ginseng root preparations generally take the form of powder, liquid, chewable tablets or capsules; widely marketed foods and beverages also contain various types and amounts of ginsenosides. Dietary supplements need not meet the same quality control for purity and potency as pharmaceuticals. Thus, considerable variation exists in the concentrations of marker compounds for ginseng, including potentially harmful levels of impurities and toxins such as pesticides and heavy metals.[119]

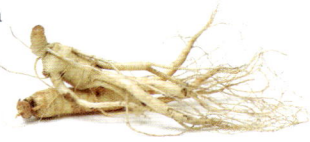
JIANG HONGYAN/Shutterstock

Little objective evidence exists to support ginseng's effectiveness as an ergogenic aid. For example, volunteers consumed either 200 or 400 mg of the standardized ginseng concentrate daily for 8 wk in a double-blind research protocol.[88] Neither treatment affected submaximal or maximal exercise performance, ratings of perceived exertion, or physiologic parameters of heart rate, oxygen uptake, or blood lactate concentrations. No ergogenic effects occurred for physiologic and performance variables following a 1-wk treatment with a ginseng saponin extract administered in doses of either 8 or 16 mg·kg^{-1}.[187] Similarly, 8 wk of ginseng supplementation failed to affect performance or recovery from 30-s Wingate tests. Supplementation had no effect on mucosal immunity indicated by changes in secretory IgA (Immunoglobulin A) at rest or following intense physical activity.[89] When effectiveness has been demonstrated, the research failed to use adequate controls, placebos, or double-blind testing protocols.

Ephedrine

Unlike ginseng, Western medicine recognizes the potent amphetaminelike alkaloid compound ephedrine with sympathomimetic physiologic effects present in several species of the plant ephedra (dried plant stem called ma huang [ma wong; *Ephedra sinica*]). The ephedra plant contains two major active components, first isolated in 1928: ephedrine and **pseudoephedrine**. The medicinal role includes treatment for asthma, common cold symptoms, hypotension, and urinary incontinence, and as a central stimulant to treat depression.

Physicians in the United States discontinued ephedrine use as a decongestant and asthma treatment in the 1930s in favor of safer medications. The milder pseudoephedrine remains common in nonprescription cold and flu medications and clinically treats mucosal congestion that accompanies hay fever, allergic rhinitis, sinusitis, and other respiratory conditions. This drug has been removed from the banned substance list by the IOC and placed on the monitoring program because of lack of convincing evidence for an ergogenic effect.

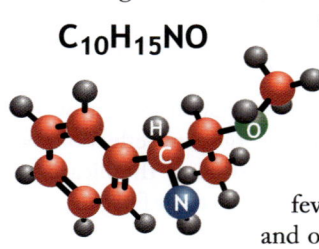
$C_{10}H_{15}NO$
Bacsica/Shutterstock

Ephedrine exerts central and peripheral effects, with the latter reflected in increased heart rate, cardiac output, and blood pressure. Ephedrine produces bronchodilation in the lungs owing to its β-adrenergic effect. High ephedrine dosages produce hypertension, insomnia, hyperthermia, and cardiac arrhythmias. Other side effects include dizziness, restlessness, anxiety, irritability, personality changes, gastrointestinal symptoms, and difficulty concentrating.

Despite the legal and scientific categorizations listing ephedrine as a potent drug, one can legally sell it as a dietary supplement. Its claim for accelerated metabolism and enhanced exercise performance greatly increased ephedrine's popularity as a nutritional supplement. Many commercial weight-loss products have contained high-dosage combinations of ephedrine and caffeine designed to speed up metabolism, yet no credible evidence exists that any initial weight loss lasts beyond 6 months, and the combination may produce adverse side effects.[134,171,238]

The potent physiologic effects of ephedrine have led researchers to investigate its potential as an ergogenic aid. No effect of a 40-mg dose of ephedrine occurred on indirect indicators of physical performance or ratings of perceived exertion (RPE).[75] The less concentrated pseudoephedrine also produced no effect on $\dot{V}O_{2max}$, RPE, aerobic cycling efficiency,[123,256] anaerobic power output (Wingate test), time to exhaustion on a bicycle and a 40-km cycling trial,[107] or physiologic and performance measures during 20 min of running at 70% $\dot{V}O_{2max}$ followed by a 5000-m time trial.[57]

Several double-blind, placebo-controlled studies by the Canadian Defense and Civil Institute of Environmental Medicine using a pre-exercise ephedrine dosage (0.8 to 1.0 mg · kg^{-1}), either alone or combined with caffeine, produced small but statistically significant endurance performance effects[20,22,24] and anaerobic power output during the early phase of the Wingate test.[23] An ergogenic effect of a relatively high dosage of pseudoephedrine (2.5 mg · kg^{-1}) enhanced runners' times by 2.1% in a 1500-m time trial.[124] Ephedrine supplementation also increased muscular endurance during the first set of traditional resistance-training exercise.[134] Whether central mechanisms that increase arousal and tolerance to discomfort, peripheral mechanisms that influence substrate metabolism and muscle function, or the combined effect of both account for any ergogenic effect remains undetermined.

Cardinal Rule for Purchasing Dietary Supplements

In February 2015, the New York State attorney general's office exposed apparent widespread fraud in the dietary supplement industry. Four major retailers (GNC, Target, Walgreens, and Walmart) were accused of selling contaminated herbal products that either failed to contain the major compounds listed on the label or had them only at trivial levels.[297] Many of those products contained significant quantities of fillers of limited nutritional value. Unfortunately, the 1994 federal law that applies to supplements—the Dietary Supplement Health and Education Act or DSHEA (https://ods.od.nih.gov/About/DSHEA_Wording.aspx)—does a better job of protecting the companies that produce the products than protecting the consumers that purchase these products. DSHEA, spearheaded by elected officials with strong financial allegiances to the supplement manufacturing industry, allows companies to attach health claims to their products without providing evidence as to their quality or effectiveness. In essence, the supplement industry is on the "honor system" for self-regulation. Part III—CFR—Code of Federal Regulations Title 21 requires dietary supplement manufacturing facilities to follow strict Good Manufacturing Practices (GMPs). If the FDA identifies violations, the FDA has the authority to issue warning letters, seize products, and shut down facilities. ConsumerLab (www.consumerlab.com) and Labdoor (https://labdoor.com) are independent laboratories that test dietary supplements and, for a fee, provide full reports on a variety of protein powders, fish oil, probiotics, vitamin D, and multivitamins.

© The United States Pharmacopeial Convention

Consumers' Bottom Line: Apply one simple rule before purchasing a supplement—view the label for one of two marks indicating that the product has been verified by a third party as having met strict testing requirements—either the United States Pharmacopeia (USP) Verified Mark, shown here, or the NSF Mark (shown on their website www.nsf.org/about-nsf/nsf-mark/). Do *not* buy the product if neither mark is visible on the product label.

Substantial Adverse Risks

An evaluation of more than 16,000 adverse reactions showed "five deaths, five heart attacks, 11 cerebrovascular accidents, four seizures, and eight psychiatric cases as 'sentinel events' associated with prior ephedra or ephedrine consumption."[238] In general, the cardiovascular toxic effects of ephedra (increased heart rate and blood vessel constriction) are not limited to massive doses but rather to the amount recommended by the manufacturer. Most sports organizations now ban ephedrine, and the National Football League was the first professional sports league to do so. Professional baseball discourages ephedrine use, but it does not ban it. Based on analysis of existing data, the Food and Drug Administration banned ephedra on December 31, 2003, the first time this federal agency banned a dietary supplement.

Buffering Solutions

Maximal exertion for 30 to 120 s dramatically alters the chemical balance between intracellular and extracellular fluids because the active muscle fibers rely predominantly on anaerobic energy transfer. Lactate accumulates with a concurrent fall in intracellular pH. Increased acidity ultimately inhibits energy transfer and contractile dynamics in the active muscle fibers, and physical performance deteriorates.

The bicarbonate aspect of the body's buffering system assessed in Chapter 14 provides a rapid first line of defense against intracellular increases in H^+ concentration. Maintaining extracellular bicarbonate at a high level facilitates H^+ efflux from the cell, which reduces intracellular acidosis. Increasing the bicarbonate reserve before short-term anaerobic exercise might enhance performance by delaying the fall in intracellular pH associated with exhaustive effort. Variations in pre-exercise dosage of sodium bicarbonate and the type of activity to evaluate pre-exercise alkalosis have produced conflicting results about the ergogenic effectiveness of buffering agents.[235,253,269]

To improve experimental design, one study investigated the effects of acute metabolic alkalosis on exhaustive effort that increased anaerobic metabolites.[217] Six trained middle-distance runners ran an 880-m race under control conditions and following alkalosis induced by ingesting a sodium bicarbonate solution (300 mg · kg body mass^{-1}) or a calcium carbonate placebo of similar concentration. The results demonstrated that prior to activity, the alkaline drink elevated pH and standard bicarbonate level. Subjects ran on average 2.9 s faster under alkalosis and exhibited higher postexercise blood lactate, pH, and extracellular H^+ concentration than in the placebo condition.[217] Augmented anaerobic energy transfer and/or delayed onset of intracellular acidification during intense effort most likely explains the ergogenic effect of pre-exercise alkalosis.[32,210,216] Adding **β-alanine** to the bicarbonate supplement, hypothesized to delay muscular fatigue onset, provided no added ergogenic effect.[25] Increased extracellular buffering from pre-exercise sodium bicarbonate ingestion facilitates H^+ efflux from active muscle fibers during physical activity in a dose-dependent manner.[80] This delays the fall in intracellular pH and its subsequent negative effects on muscle function. An improvement of 2.9 s in 800 m race time represents a dramatic performance improvement—a distance of 19 m at race pace brings a last-place finisher to first place in most 800 m races!

The ergogenic effect of pre-exercise alkalosis (use not banned by WADA) also occurs for females (**FIG. 23.8**). Physically active females performed maximal cycling for 60 s on separate days under three conditions in a double-blind research design: (1) control, no treatment; (2) sodium bicarbonate dose of 300 mg · kg body mass^{-1} in 400 mL of low-calorie flavored water 90 min before testing; and (3) placebo sodium chloride equimolar dose (to maintain intravascular fluid status similar to bicarbonate condition) administered like the bicarbonate treatment. Cycling capacity represented total work accomplished in the 60-s ride. The figure's *inset box* shows that total work (kJ) and peak power output (W) reached higher levels with pre-exercise bicarbonate treatment than under either control or placebo conditions. The bicarbonate treatment produced a higher blood lactate level in the immediate and 1-min postexercise period; the effect explains the greater work capacity attained in the short-term, anaerobic exercise trial.

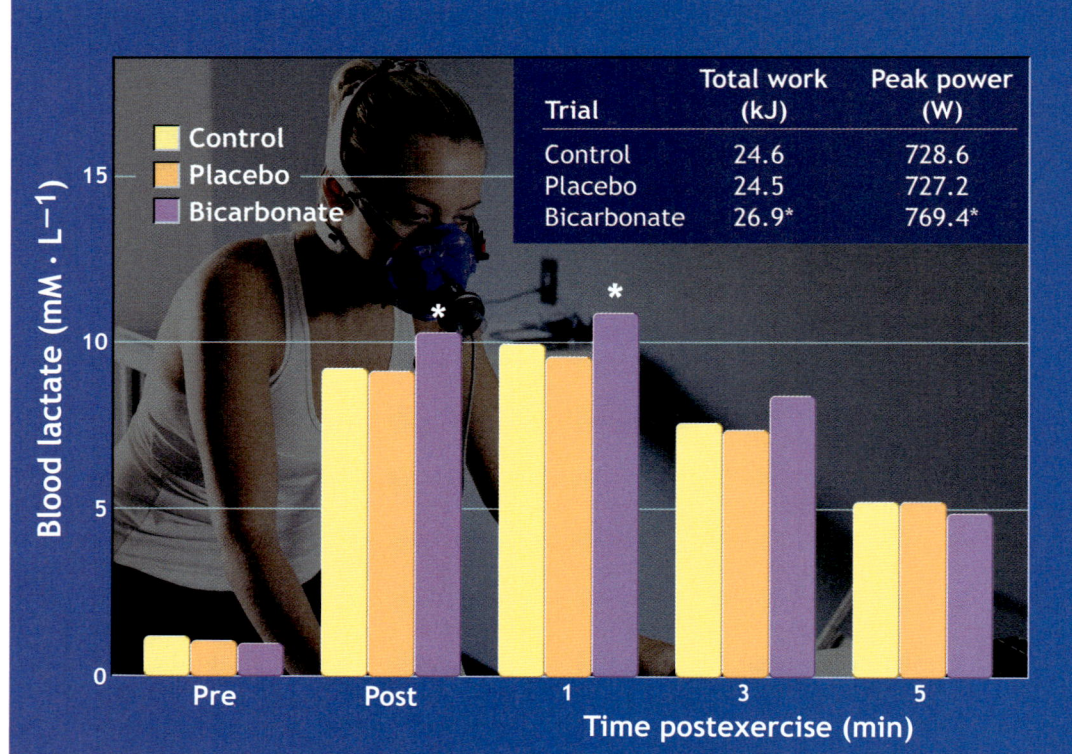

FIGURE 23.8. Bicarbonate loading effects on total work, peak power output, and postexercise blood lactate levels in moderately trained women. *Significantly higher than either control or placebo. (Adapted with permission from McNaughton LR, et al. Effect of sodium bicarbonate ingestion on high intensity exercise in moderately trained women. *J Strength Cond Res*. 1997;11:98. Photo: wavebreakmedia/Shutterstock.)

Effect Related to Dosage and Anaerobiosis

Bicarbonate dosage and the cumulative anaerobic nature of physical activity interact to influence the potential ergogenic effect of pre-exercise bicarbonate loading. Doses of at least 0.3 g·kg^{-1} facilitate H$^+$ efflux from the cell and enhance a single 1- to 2-min maximal effort and longer-term arm or leg exercise that exhausts within 6 to 8 min.[173,177,224] No ergogenic effect emerges for performance typical of intense resistance training from the lower absolute anaerobic metabolic load than in supramaximal whole-body, longer-duration running or cycling.[208] Bicarbonate loading with all-out effort of less than 1 min exerts an ergogenic effect with repetitive, intermittent exercise.[67]

Intense Endurance Performance

Pre-exercise–induced alkalosis does not benefit low-intensity aerobic activity because pH and lactate remain at near-resting levels, but it may enhance aerobic activity of higher intensity. Intense endurance exercise, while predominantly aerobic, increases blood lactate and decreases pH, which negatively affect performance. Eight trained male cyclists consumed sodium citrate (0.5 g·kg^{-1}) before a 30-km time trial.[209] Race times were faster and plasma pH and lactate concentrations higher after sodium citrate ingestion than with the placebo. Despite the relatively small anaerobic component in intense aerobic exercise compared with short-term, maximal activity, ingesting a buffer before such activity facilitates lactate and hydrogen ion efflux and improves muscle function.[178] Individuals who bicarbonate load often endure abdominal cramps and diarrhea about 1 hr after ingestion.[246] This adverse effect would surely minimize any potential ergogenic effect. Substituting sodium citrate (0.4 to 0.5 g·kg^{-1}) for sodium bicarbonate reduces or eliminates adverse gastrointestinal effects while still providing ergogenic benefits.[163,176]

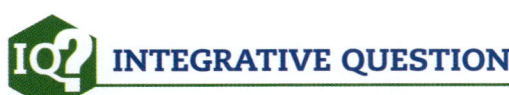

INTEGRATIVE QUESTION

How would you advise an Olympic-caliber weightlifter who plans to bicarbonate load because the competitive event requires an all-out anaerobic effort?

Anticortisol Compounds: Glutamine and Phosphatidylserine

The hypothalamus normally secretes corticotrophin-releasing factor in response to emotional stress, trauma, infection, surgery, and extreme physical exertion. This releasing factor stimulates the anterior pituitary gland to release adrenocorticotropic hormone (ACTH), which induces the adrenal cortex to discharge the glucocorticoid hormone cortisol (hydrocortisone; $C_{21}H_{30}O_5$). Cortisol decreases amino acid transport into the cell, which depresses anabolism and stimulates protein breakdown to its building-block amino acids in all cells except the liver. The circulation transports these "liberated" amino acids to the liver for gluconeogenesis. Cortisol also serves as an insulin antagonist by inhibiting cellular glucose uptake and oxidation. Changes in cortisol concentration are related to exercise intensity. At rest, cortisol averages approximately 250 mmol·L^{-1} and then decreases below 200 mmol·L^{-1} at about 30% $\dot{V}O_{2max}$. It then sharply

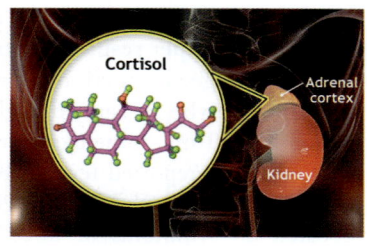

Kateryna Kon/Shutterstock

and progressively increases where it nearly doubles the resting value at close to 400 mmol·L^{-1} at $\dot{V}O_{2max}$.[334,335]

A prolonged, elevated serum cortisol concentration—usually from therapeutic exogenous glucocorticoid intake in drug form—leads to excessive protein breakdown, tissue wasting, and negative nitrogen balance. The potential catabolic cortisol effect has convinced many strength and power athletes to use supplements alleged to inhibit normal cortisol release.[139] They believe that depressing cortisol's normal rise following physical activity augments muscular development by attenuating catabolism. In this way, muscle tissue synthesis progresses unimpeded in recovery. Glutamine and phosphatidylserine are two supplements used to produce an anticortisol effect.

Glutamine

The nonessential amino acid **glutamine**, the most abundant amino acid in plasma and skeletal muscle, accounts for more than half the muscles' free amino acid pool. Glutamine exerts many regulatory functions, one of which provides an anticatabolic effect that augments protein synthesis. From a clinical perspective, glutamine supplementation effectively counteracts the decline in protein synthesis and muscle wasting from repeated glucocorticoid use.[121] Infusing glutamine following physical activity promotes muscle glycogen accumulation, perhaps by serving as a gluconeogenic substrate in the liver.[273]

Bacsica/Shutterstock

The potential anticatabolic and glycogen synthesizing effects of glutamine have promoted speculation that supplementation might augment resistance training effects.[49] Daily glutamine supplementation (0.9 g·kg^{-1} lean tissue mass) during 6 wk of resistance training in healthy young adults did not affect muscle performance, body composition, or muscle protein degradation compared with a placebo.[50]

Immune Response

Glutamine plays an important role in normal immune function. One protective aspect concerns glutamine's use as metabolic fuel by the infection-fighting lymphocytes and macrophages. Glutamine plasma concentration decreases following prolonged intense physical activity, so glutamine deficiency has been linked to immunosuppression from strenuous physical effort (see Chapter 7).[34,52,229]

Glutamine supplementation might lessen increased susceptibility to **upper respiratory tract infection (URTI)** following prolonged competition or a bout of strenuous training. Marathoners who consumed a glutamine drink (5 g L-glutamine in 330-mL mineral water) at the end of a race and then 2 hr later reported fewer URTI symptoms than unsupplemented athletes.[53] More specifically, 65% more athletes reported no symptoms of infection than a placebo group. The mechanism for glutamine's effect on postexercise infection risk remains elusive. For example, subsequent studies by the same researchers showed *no effect* of glutamine supplementation on changes in the blood's disease-fighting white blood cell lymphocyte distribution.[55] Dietary glutamine supplementation did *not* benefit lymphocyte metabolism or immune function with more moderate exercise training in rats.[239] Research with humans indicates that pre-exercise glutamine supplementation does *not* affect the immune response following repeated bouts of intense physical effort.[219,283] Nine equal doses of 100 mg of L-glutamine per kg of body mass taken 30 min before the end of exercise, at the end of exercise, and 30 min into recovery abolished the postexercise decline in glutamine following a race but did *not* impact immune function.[141,218]

Phosphatidylserine

Phosphatidylserine (PS) is a glycerophospholipid typical of a class of natural lipids that compose the structural components of the internal layer of the plasma membrane that surrounds all cells. Through its potential for modulating functional events in the plasma membrane (e.g., number and affinity of membrane receptor sites), PS might modify the neuroendocrine response to stress. In one study, healthy males consumed 800 mg of PS derived from bovine cerebral cortex daily for 10 days.[186] Three 6-min intervals of cycle ergometer exercise of increasing intensity induced physical stress. Compared with the placebo condition, PS treatment diminished ACTH and cortisol release without affecting growth hormone release. These results confirmed that a single intravenous PS injection counteracted hypothalamic-pituitary-adrenal axis activation with exercise.[185] A 750 mg·d^{-1} supplement of PS for 10 days did not protect against delayed-onset muscle soreness or markers of muscle damage, inflammation, and oxidative stress following a bout of prolonged downhill running.[151]

β-Hydroxy-β-Methylbutyrate

β-Hydroxy-β-methylbutyrate (HMB), a bioactive metabolite generated in the degradation of the essential branched-chain amino acid leucine, decreases protein loss during stress by inhibiting protein catabolism. In rats and chicks, less protein breakdown and a slight increase in protein synthesis occurred in muscle tissue (*in vitro*) exposed to HMB.[155] An HMB-induced increase occurred in fatty acid oxidation in mammalian muscle cells exposed to HMB.[56] Depending on the quantity of HMB in food (relatively rich sources include catfish, grapefruit, and breast milk), humans synthesize between 0.3 and 1.0 g HMB daily, with about 5% from dietary leuci catabolism. HMB supplements are taken by fitness enthusiasts because of their potential nitrogen-retaining effects to prevent or slow muscle damage and inhibit muscle breakdown (proteolysis) with intense physical effort.

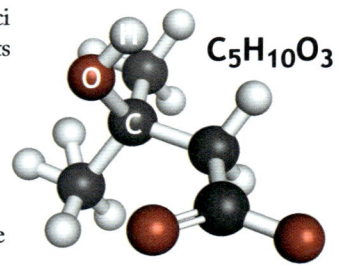

Research has studied the effects of exogenous HMB on skeletal muscles' response to resistance training. In part one of a two-part study (**FIG. 23.9**), young adult males participated in two randomized trials. In

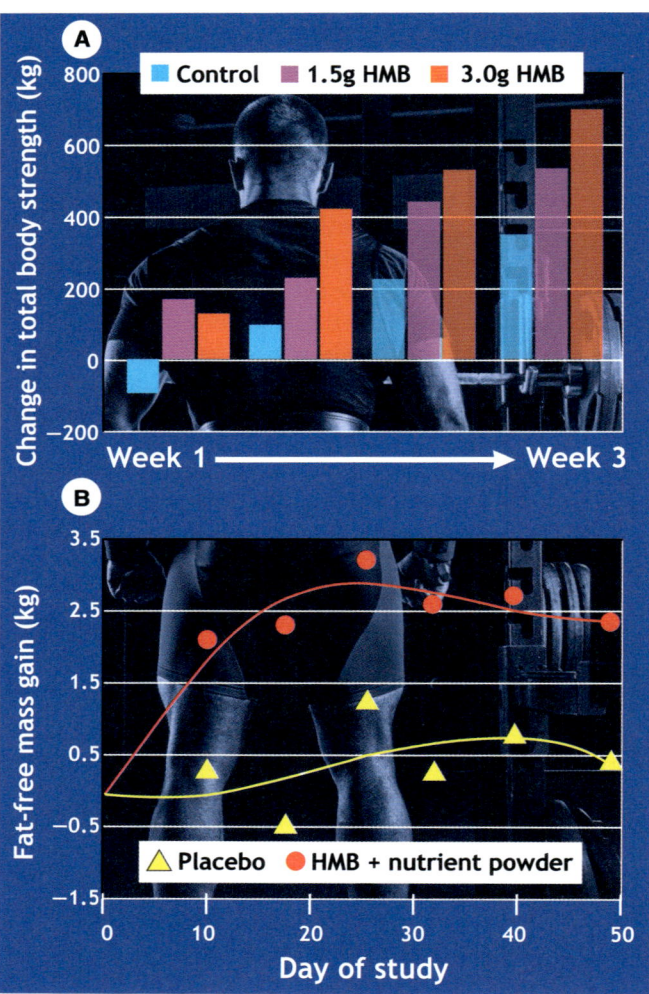

FIGURE 23.9. **(A)** Change in muscle strength as total weight lifted in upper-body and lower-body exercise in *Study 1* (week 1 to 3) in the group supplemented with β-hydroxy-β-methylbutyrate (HMB). Each group of bars represents one complete set of upper-body and lower-body workouts. **(B)** Total body electrical conductivity-assessed change in fat-free mass during *Study 2* for a control group that received a carbohydrate drink (*placebo*) and a group that received 3 g Ca-HMB daily mixed in a nutrient powder (*HMB + nutrient powder*). (Reprinted with permission from Nissen S, et al. Effect of leucine metabolite β-hydroxy-β-methylbutyrate on muscle metabolism during resistance-exercise training. *J Appl Physiol*. 1996;81:2095. Figures 1 & 3. ©The American Physiological Society (APS). All rights reserved. Photo: Andy Gin/Shutterstock.)

the first study, 41 subjects received 0, 1.5, or 3.0 g HMB daily at two protein levels, either 117 or 175 g daily for 3 wk. The males' resistance trained during this time for 1.5 hr, 3 days per week. In the second study, 28 subjects consumed either 0 or 3.0 g of HMB daily and resistance trained for 2 to 3 hr, 6 days per week, for 7 wk. In the first study, HMB supplementation depressed the exercise-induced rise in muscle proteolysis (reflected by urinary 3-methylhistidine and plasma creatine phosphokinase [CPK] levels) during the first 2 wk of training. These biochemical indices of muscle damage were 20 to 60% lower in the HMB-supplemented group. In addition, the supplemented group lifted more total weight during each training week (Fig. 23.9A), with the greatest effect in the group receiving the largest HMB supplement. Muscular strength increased 8% in the unsupplemented group and more in the HMB-supplemented groups (13% for the 1.5-g group and 18.4% for the 3.0-g group). Added protein (not indicated in graph) did not affect any of the measurements; one should view this lack of effect in proper context—the "lower" protein quantity (115 g · d^{-1}) equaled twice the RDA.

Individuals who received HMB supplementation in the second study had higher FFM than the unsupplemented group at 2 and 4 to 6 wk training (FIG. 23.9B). However, at the last measurement during training, the difference between groups decreased and failed to differ from the difference between pretraining baseline values. Subsequent research shows that HMB supplementation augments the response to resistance training to a greater extent when compared to unsupplemented controls. Supplementation increased resting and exercise-induced testosterone and resting GH concentrations and reduced pre-exercise cortisol concentrations.[155] Compared to controls, the supplemented group showed greater training-induced changes in lean body mass and muscle strength and power, including beneficial hormonal responses and markers of muscle damage.

The mechanism for any HMB effect on muscle metabolism, strength improvement, and body composition remains unknown. Perhaps this metabolite inhibits normal proteolytic (breakdown of proteins into smaller polypeptides or amino acids) processes that accompany intense muscular overload. The results demonstrate an ergogenic effect for HMB supplementation, but it remains unclear just what component of the FFM (protein, bone, water) HMB affects. The data in Figure 23.9B indicate potentially transient body composition benefits of supplementation that tend to revert toward the unsupplemented state as training progresses.

Conflicting Results

Not all research shows beneficial effects of HMB supplementation with resistance training. One study evaluated the effects of variations in HMB supplementation (approximately 3 vs. 6 g · d^{-1}) on muscular strength during 8-wk whole-body resistance training in untrained young adult men.[104] The study's primary finding indicated that HMB supplementation, regardless of dosage, produced *no difference* in most of the strength data (including 1-RM strength) compared with the placebo group. In contrast to the findings presented in FIGURE 23.9A, increases in training volume remained similar among groups. In both HMB-supplemented groups, lower creatine phosphokinase levels in recovery indicated some potential effect of HMB to inhibit muscle breakdown.[211] The group that consumed the lower HMB dosage increased more in FFM than the other two groups. Inferences from these findings are limited because skinfolds assessed body composition changes. HMB supplementation with a daily dosage as high as 6 g · d^{-1} during 8 wk of resistance training does not adversely affect hepatic enzyme function, blood lipid profile, renal function, or immune function.[105,142] Age does not affect responsiveness to HMB supplementation.[279] HMB supplementation may prove most effective among untrained individuals with a greater potential for muscle mass and muscular strength accretion than more highly trained counterparts.[195,197,288]

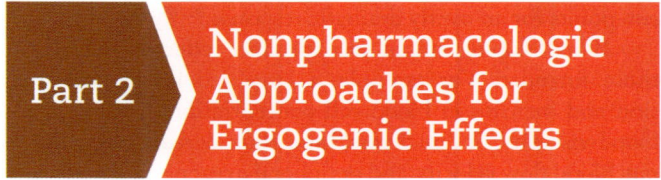

Part 2: Nonpharmacologic Approaches for Ergogenic Effects

Athletes often use physical, mechanical, physiologic, and nutritional means to produce ergogenic effects.

Red Blood Cell Reinfusion—Blood Doping

Red blood cell reinfusion, often called induced erythrocythemia, blood boosting, or blood doping, gained public prominence as a possible ergogenic technique during the 1972 Munich Olympics, when relatively unknown "dark horse" Finnish runner Lasse Artturi Virén (1949-), allegedly used this procedure prior to his two gold medal–winning 5000- and 10,000-m runs, and two more gold medals won at the 1976 Montreal Olympics (https://fasterskier.com/2019/04/limiting-factors-a-genesis-of-blood-doping-part-four/).

How It Works

Red blood cell reinfusion involves withdrawing 1 to 4 units (1 unit = 450 mL whole blood) of a person's blood, immediately reinfusing the plasma, and placing the packed red blood cells in frozen storage for later infusion (autologous transfusion). Homologous transfusion infuses a type-matched donor's blood. To prevent dramatic reductions in blood cell concentration, each unit of blood withdrawal takes place at 3 to 8 wk intervals because it takes this time to reestablish normal red blood cell levels. Stored blood cells are then infused 1 to 7 days before an endurance event; this increases red blood cell count and hemoglobin levels from 8 to 20%.

Hemoconcentration translates to an average hemoglobin increase for males from a normal 15 to 19 g · dL^{-1}, increasing the hematocrit 40 to 60%, which then remains elevated for 14 days or longer. Theoretically, the added blood volume contributes to a larger maximal cardiac output, while red blood cell packing increases the blood's oxygen-carrying capacity. Enhanced oxygen transport and delivery to active tissues provides meaningful performance benefits to endurance athletes.

An ergogenic effect occurs with infusion of 900 to 1800 mL freeze-preserved autologous blood. Each 500-mL whole blood infusion, equivalent to 275 mL of packed red blood cells, adds about 100 mL of oxygen to the blood's total oxygen-carrying capacity—*each 100 mL whole blood carries about 20 mL oxygen*. An elite endurance athlete's total blood volume circulates five to six times each minute in intense activity, so the potential "extra" oxygen available to the tissues from red blood cell reinfusion averages 500 mL (0.5 L). Autologous blood transfusion to boost the blood's hemoglobin/oxygen-carrying capacity to improve athletic performance cannot be detected; nonetheless, it is possible to track an athlete's blood constituents over time to note unreasonable changes based on cut-points for an overly dramatic response.[83,165,168,280]

Blood doping might also produce effects opposite to those intended. For example, a large red blood cell infusion and increase in blood cell concentration could increase blood viscosity, or "thickness," and thus *decrease* cardiac output, blood flow velocity, and peripheral oxygen supply—effects that reduce aerobic capacity and endurance performance. Any increase in blood viscosity could also compromise blood flow through narrowed, atherosclerotic vessels of individuals with artery disease to increase their risk for heart attack or stroke.

Does It Work?

A sound theoretical basis exists for blood doping and experimental evidence justifies its use for physiologic reasons. Early research demonstrated a rapid increase in $\dot{V}O_{2max}$ following whole blood infusion.[85] One study reported a 23% overnight increase in exercise performance and a 9% increase in $\dot{V}O_{2max}$.[86] Subsequent investigations support previous findings showing physiologic and performance improvements.[223,245]

Differences in results among various exercise performance studies following red blood cell reinfusion largely result from variations in blood storage methods. Freezing red blood cells permits storage for more than 6 wk without significant cell loss. With storage at 39.2°F/4°C used in some earlier studies, substantial hemolysis occurs after only 3 wk. This represents an important difference because it usually takes a person 5 to 6 wk to reestablish blood cells lost after withdrawing 2 units whole blood (**FIG. 23.10**).

With appropriate blood storage methods, red blood cell reinfusion elevates hematologic parameters for both males and females. This in turn translates to a 5 to 13% increase in aerobic capacity, decreased heart rate and blood lactate during submaximal effort, and augmented endurance at sea level and altitude. In addition, red blood cell reinfusion benefits thermoregulatory response during physical activity in the heat (reduced body heat storage and improved sweating response). Increased oxygen content in arterial blood in the infused state likely "frees" blood for delivery to the skin for heat dissipation during exertional heat stress while adequately supplying active tissues.

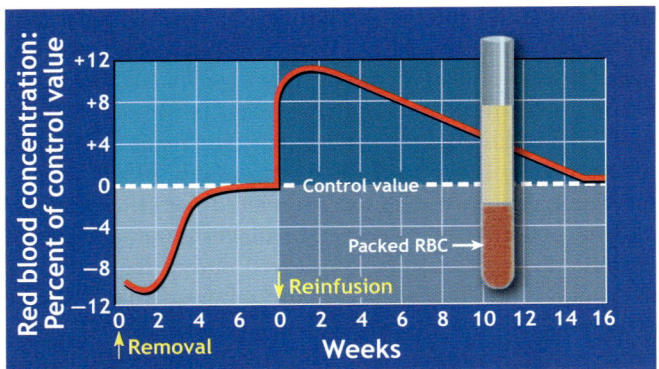

FIGURE 23.10. Time course of hematologic changes after removing and reinfusing 900 mL of freeze-preserved blood. RBC, red blood cells.
(Adapted with permission from Gledhill N. Blood doping and related issues: a brief review. *Med Sci Sports Exerc*. 1982;14:183.)

Hormonal Blood Boosting (EPO)

Endurance athletes now use epoetin, the synthetic erythropoietin (EPO) or recombinant human EPO (rHuEPO), to eliminate the cumbersome and lengthy blood doping process. This complex hormone, produced by the kidneys in response to reduced oxygen pressure in arterial plasma, regulates red blood cell production within the marrow of the long bones but also is essential in the synthesis and proper functioning of several erythrocyte membrane proteins, particularly those facilitating lactate exchange.[9,39,65]

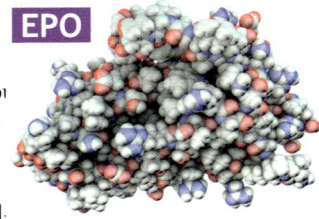

Kateryna Kon/Shutterstock

Medically, exogenous recombinant human EPO commercially available since 1988 has proved useful in combating anemia in patients undergoing chemotherapy or with severe renal disease. Normally, a decrease in red blood cell concentration or decline in the pressure of oxygen in arterial blood—as in severe pulmonary disease or on ascent to high altitude—releases this hormone to stimulate erythrocyte production. The 12% increase in hemoglobin and hematocrit that typically follows 6-wk EPO treatment greatly improves endurance performance.[231,261] Unfortunately, self-administration in an unregulated and unmonitored manner—simply injecting the hormone requires much less sophistication than blood-doping procedures—can increase hematocrit by more than 60%. This dangerously high hemoconcentration (and corresponding increase in blood viscosity) increases the likelihood for stroke, heart attack, heart failure, and pulmonary edema. Other side effects include increased platelet adhesion, arterial hypertension, headache, muscle cramps, URTI, and post-treatment anemia.

EPO use has become particularly prevalent in cycling competition and allegedly contributed to at least 18 deaths among competitive cyclists, mainly from heart attack. While EPO use can be detected in urine, the blood hematocrit serves as a surrogate marker. The International Cycling Union has set a hematocrit threshold of 50% for males and 47% for females;

the International Skiing Federation uses a hemoglobin concentration of 18.5 g · dL^{-1} as the threshold for disqualification. Hematocrit cutoff values of 52% for males and 48% for females (roughly 3 standard deviations above the mean) represent "abnormally high" or extreme values in triathletes.[196] Use of hematocrit level cutoff raises the unanswered question of the number of disqualified "clean" cyclists. Estimates place this number between 3 and 5% due to factors that affect normal variation in hematocrit (e.g., genetics, posture, altitude training, and hydration level).

Enhancing oxygen availability to muscles by EPO analogs and mimetics constitutes a main challenge to successful doping control. Sport governing bodies have now shifted concerns about simple red blood cell reinfusion to concern about transfection (artificially introducing DNA or RNA nucleic acids into cells) and how it might impact an athlete's genes that code for erythropoietin, and thus affect exercise performance.

Additional Ways to Enhance Oxygen Transport

In addition, new classes of substances may emerge to enhance aerobic performance that include emulsions and solutions formulated from bovine (cows, oxen, goats, sheep, bison, buffalo) or human hemoglobin, which improve oxygen transport and delivery to muscle.[146] Despite their potential benefits in clinical use, these substances exhibit potentially lethal side effects that include increased systemic and pulmonary blood pressure, renal toxicity, and impaired immune function.

Warm-Up (Preliminary Exercise)

Coaches, trainers, and athletes at all competition levels generally recommend engaging in some mode of physical activity or "warm-up" prior to vigorous physical effort. Conventional wisdom maintains that preliminary exercise helps the human and animal performer prepare physiologically or psychologically and reduces the likelihood of joint and muscle injury.[233] With animals, injuring a "warmed-up" muscle requires more force and greater muscle length than injuring a muscle in the "cold" condition. The warming-up process stretches the muscle-tendon unit to allow greater length and less tension on exposure to a given external load.

Two Warm-Up Categories

Warm-up generally fits into one of two categories, although overlap exists:

1. **General warm-up** uses body movements or "loosening-up" activities unrelated to the specific neuromuscular actions in the anticipated performance. Examples include multiple calisthenics and stretching movements.
2. **Specific warm-up** applies big-muscle, rhythmic movements that provide skill

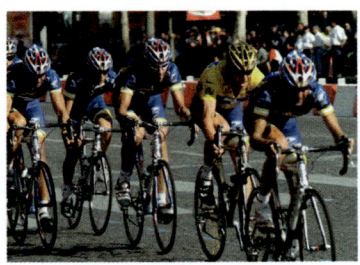

General warm up

F8 studio/Shutterstock

 An International Tour de France Superstar Cyclist's Rise, Fall, and Disgrace

On June 12, 2012, the US Anti-Doping Agency (USADA), a quasi-governmental agency that polices antidoping in sports in the United States, brought formal doping charges against elite cyclist and testicular cancer survivor Lance Armstrong (yellow jersey in image). The accusations alleged that the USADA collected blood samples from him in 2009 and 2010 that were "fully consistent with blood doping including EPO (erythropoietin) use and/or blood transfusions." The charges also alleged that "multiple riders with firsthand knowledge" testified that Armstrong used the blood booster EPO, blood transfusions, testosterone, and masking agents, and that he distributed and administered drugs to other cyclists from 1998 through 2005. In addition to these specific accusations, the charges maintained that his cycling team engaged in a "doping conspiracy" involving "team officials, employees, doctors, and elite United States Postal Service and Discovery Channel riders." In June 2012, the USADA formally charged Armstrong with using performance-enhancing drugs, and in August, 2012 announced his disqualification from all race results since August 1998 (including all seven Tour de France Titles) and a lifetime ban from competition, which applies in all sports that follow the World Anti-Doping Agency code. Also, the Union Cycliste Internationale (www.uci.ch/) governing body endorsed the USADA's verdict and confirmed both the lifetime ban and the stripping of Armstrong's titles. Armstrong paid a $5 million fine, of which one of his coriders and accusers Floyd Landis received $1.1 million—including $1.65 million to cover Landis' lawyer's legal fees. Under the False Claims Act (www.justice.gov/civil/false-claims-act), Armstrong could have paid three times $32 million, the total amount the US Postal Service sponsorship paid to bankroll his first six Tour wins.

Armstrong is but one of many examples where tremendously successful athletes in many sports have fallen from grace for attempting to "game" the system and have been caught and punished—the ultimate price for cheating, corruption, deception, and lying. What really is so sad are the millions of people worldwide who looked up to Armstrong and the US team as ultimate champion athletes and role models who are supposed to embody inspiration, humbleness, unselfishness, respect, and an unrelenting effort to bring out the best in those around them, a colossal disappointment in these important characteristics.

Marc Pagani Photography/Shutterstock

rehearsal in the activity. Examples include swinging a golf club, throwing a baseball or football, tennis practice, basketball shooting and movements, and preliminary lead-up in the high jump or pole vault.

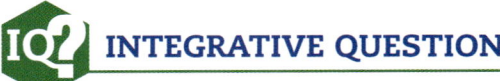

Specific warm up

Ron Alvey/Shutterstock

Psychological Considerations

Competitors at all levels generally believe that performing some prior skill-related activity prepares them mentally to focus on the upcoming performance. A specific warm-up related to the intended activity also may improve the necessary skill and coordination requirements. Consequently, sports requiring accuracy, timing, and precise movements generally benefit from some type of specific or "formal" preliminary practice.

The notion also exists that prior exercise before strenuous effort gradually prepares a person to go "all out" without fear of injury. The ritual warm-up of baseball pitchers exemplifies this belief. Is it conceivable that a pitcher would enter a game, throwing at competitive speeds, without previously warming up? Would any athlete begin competition without first stretching and engaging in a particular form, intensity, or duration of warm-up? Most performers would respond with a definite no, yet objective support for this response remains elusive. One reason is the difficulty of designing a well-controlled experiment with top-flight athletes to determine the necessity of warming up and whether it improves subsequent performance with reduced injury risk. For pre-exercise stretching, research with army recruits indicates that a typical muscle-stretching protocol in the warm-up produces *no* clinically meaningful reductions in risk of exercise-related injury compared with subsequent exercise without warm-up.[207] Strength loss, loss of motion, soreness, or markers of muscle damage from eccentric movements were no different between groups that received pre-exercise passive warm-up with short-wave diathermy, active warm-up with concentric muscle actions, or no warm-up.[91]

Certain sport-related situations require peak performance with little time for warming up. A reserve player entering the last few minutes of a game has no time for stretching, vigorous calisthenics, or taking practice shots; the player must go all out and achieve optimal performance without warm-up except that done before the game or at intermission. Do more injuries occur in such cases? Does physical performance (e.g., shooting, rebounding, or basketball defense) deteriorate during the first few minutes during an "unwarmed" condition from that proceeded by a warm-up? Future research must address such questions.

Psychological factors, including an athlete's ingrained belief in the importance of warming up, establish a definite bias when comparing maximum performance with and without warm-up. It is difficult if not impossible to obtain a maximum effort without warm-up if a subject believes in the importance of preliminary exercise.

IQ? INTEGRATIVE QUESTION

Design an experiment to determine if a psychological or "placebo" ergogenic effect occurs for a particular nutrient, chemical, or procedure.

Physiologic and Performance Effects

One study evaluated the effect of warm-up on 2-min sprint-cycling performance at 120% of the power output at $\dot{V}O_{2max}$. Warm-up produces a higher muscle temperature, increased local muscle oxygen availability and oxygen uptake, lower blood lactate level, and higher oxygen uptake during the early phase of activity than the no-warm-up condition.[74,222]

Warm-up performed at moderate-intensity and high-intensity improved intense cycling performance by 2 to 3%.[46] A pre-exercise warm-up irrespective of intensity enhanced a 3- to 4-min 3-km/1.9 mi cycling time trial. This effect likely resulted from an acceleration of oxygen uptake kinetics from augmented blood flow at exercise onset.[117] An active warm-up 5 min prior to a 30-s maximal sprint on a bicycle ergometer produced less blood and muscle lactate than equivalent effort without a physical warm-up.[113] Differences in muscle temperature with an active warm-up could not account for the ergogenic effect because exercise in the control condition also involved passively heating the muscle to the same temperature. These findings suggest a decreased reliance on anaerobic sources of energy during the activity period preceded by a physical warm-up.

Five mechanisms explain why warm-up "should" improve physical performance and exercise capacity because of subsequent increases in blood flow and muscle and core temperature:

1. Faster muscle contraction and relaxation
2. Greater economy of movement from lowered viscous resistance within active muscles
3. Facilitated oxygen delivery and use by muscles because hemoglobin releases its oxygen more readily at higher temperatures (Bohr effect)
4. Facilitated nerve transmission and muscle metabolism because increased temperature accelerates bodily processes; a specific warm-up may also enhance required motor unit recruitment
5. Increased blood flow through active tissues as the local vascular bed dilates from increased metabolism and higher muscle temperature

Clinical Rationale Prior to Sudden Strenuous Physical Activity

Sudden exertion can trigger the onset of myocardial infarction, particularly in sedentary persons and those with latent coronary artery disease.[41,182] With this in mind, consideration of possible benefits from warming up takes on clinical significance. Several studies have evaluated the effects of preliminary physical activity on the cardiovascular response to sudden, strenuous effort. The findings provide an essentially different physiologic framework to justify warm-up that relates importantly to adult fitness and cardiac rehabilitation programs and occupations and sports that require sudden bursts of physical effort.

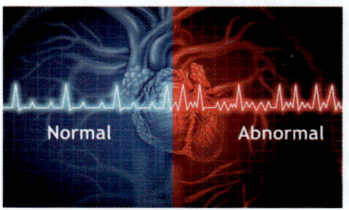

Lightspring/Shutterstock

In one study, 44 males free of overt coronary artery disease symptoms ran on a treadmill at high intensity for 10 to 15 s without prior warm-up.[13] Evaluation of postexercise ECGs revealed that 70% of the subjects displayed abnormal changes attributable to inadequate myocardial oxygen supply unrelated to age or fitness level. To evaluate the effect of a warm-up, 22 of the males with an abnormal ECG from the treadmill run jogged in place for 2 min before treadmill running at moderate intensity (heart rate, 145 bpm). With this warm-up, 10 males showed normal tracings during sudden exertion, while another 10 males displayed improved ECG responses; only two subjects showed significant ECG abnormalities. In a subsequent study, the exercise blood pressure response also improved with prior warm-up.[14] For seven males with no warm-up, systolic blood pressure averaged 168 mm Hg immediately after the 15-s treadmill run. This decreased to 140 mm Hg when the 2-min jog-in-place warm-up preceded exercise.

Coronary blood flow does not adjust instantaneously to a sudden increase in myocardial work; transient myocardial ischemia (poor oxygen supply) can occur in apparently healthy and fit individuals. *Prior warm-up (at least 2 min of easy jogging) benefits the subsequent ECG and blood pressure responses to vigorous physical activity to indicate a more favorable relationship between myocardial oxygen supply and demand.* Warming up before strenuous effort is particularly important for individuals with limited myocardial blood flow from coronary artery disease. A brief warm-up provides more optimal blood pressure and hormonal adjustments at the onset of subsequent strenuous exercise. The warm-up serves two beneficial purposes under these conditions:

1. Reduces myocardial workload and thus the myocardial oxygen requirement
2. Augments blood flow through the coronary arteries

Oxygen Inhalation (Hyperoxia)

Athletes often breathe oxygen-enriched or **hyperoxic gas mixtures** during time-outs, at half-time, or following strenuous activity. They believe this procedure enhances the blood's oxygen-carrying capacity to facilitate oxygen transport to active or recovering muscles when it does not. The fact remains that when healthy persons breathe ambient air at sea level, hemoglobin in blood leaving the lungs normally remains 95 to 98% saturated with oxygen (see Chapter 13). In physiologic terms, consider these two factors:

1. Breathing air with higher than normal oxygen concentration increases oxygen transport by hemoglobin to only a small extent—by about 1 mL of extra oxygen for every deciliter of blood (10 mL $O_2 \cdot L^{-1}$).
2. Oxygen that dissolves in plasma when breathing a hyperoxic mixture also increases by about 0.4 mL · deciliter (dL) of blood^{-1} (4.0 mL $O_2 \cdot L^{-1}$), or from the normal 0.3 mL·dL^{-1} (3.0 mL·L^{-1}) to about 0.7 mL·dL^{-1} (7.0 mL·L^{-1}) of blood.

Based on these two factors, the blood's oxygen-carrying capacity under hyperoxic conditions potentially increases by only about 14 mL of oxygen for every liter of blood—10 mL "extra" attached to hemoglobin and 4 mL "extra" dissolved in plasma.

Pre-Exercise Oxygen Breathing

Blood volume for a 70-kg person averages about 5000 mL (5.0 L). Breathing hyperoxic gas adds about 70 mL of oxygen to the total blood volume (5.0 L of blood × 14 mL "extra" O_2 per liter of blood). Despite any potential psychological benefit for the athlete who believes that pre-exercise oxygen breathing helps subsequent performance, this procedure confers only a trivial physiologic advantage from any additional oxygen *per se*. This small benefit emerges only if subsequent exercise takes place without breathing ambient air in the interval between hyperoxic breathing and exercise. This occurs because ambient air's lower oxygen pressure than its pressure in hyperoxic blood causes any additional oxygen in the blood to exit the body.

The athlete who breathes an oxygen-rich mixture on the sideline before returning to the competition does *not* gain a competitive edge from physiologic benefits. This is particularly ironic in football because metabolic reactions without requiring oxygen generate almost all the energy to power each play.

Breathing hyperoxic gas during submaximal and maximal aerobic activity enhances endurance performance. Oxygen breathing during vigorous exertion accelerates oxygen uptake at the onset of exercise (smaller oxygen deficit in repeated bouts of intense effort); reduces blood lactate, heart rate, and pulmonary ventilation in submaximal effort; and increases $\dot{V}O_{2max}$ and training intensity.[170,202,220] In one study, subjects performed a 6.5-min endurance ride on a bicycle ergometer at an exercise level equal to 115% $\dot{V}O_{2max}$ while breathing either room air or 100% oxygen.[285] Tanks of compressed gas supplied both air and oxygen to mask a subject's knowledge of the breathing mixture. **FIGURE 23.11A** shows superior endurance (less dropoff in pedal revolutions) while breathing 100% oxygen during cycling compared to breathing room air.

Figure 23.11B shows that the hyperoxic condition produced significantly higher oxygen uptakes throughout the 6-min intense activity period.

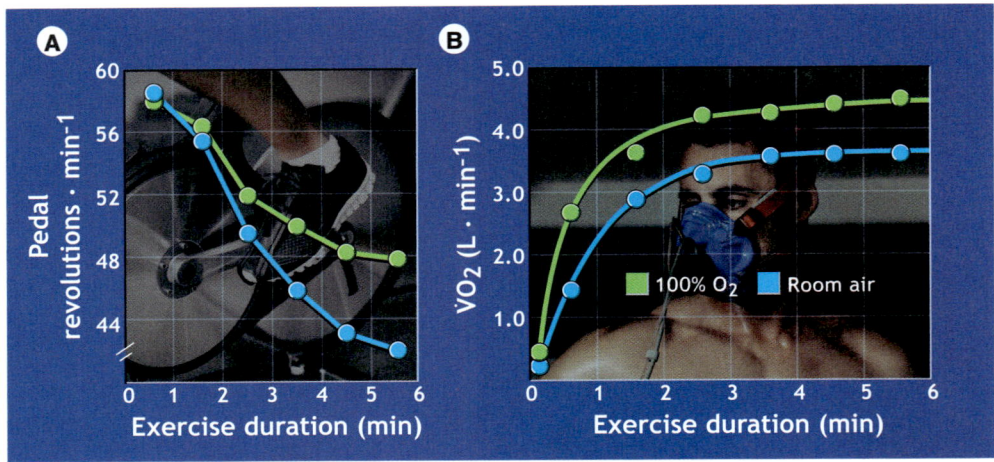

FIGURE 23.11. Endurance in **(A)** assessed by pedal revolutions each minute while breathing 100% oxygen or ambient air. Maximum oxygen uptake ($\dot{V}O_{2max}$) curves in **(B)** during the endurance rides show enhanced oxygen uptake while breathing oxygen. (Data from Weltman A, et al. Effects of increasing oxygen availability on bicycle ergometer endurance performance. *Ergonomics*. 1978;21:427. Photo A: Maridav/Shutterstock; Photo B: Jacob Lund/Shutterstock.)

FIGURE 23.12 shows that the quadriceps muscle's oxygen uptake in seven trained males during maximum knee-extension movement varied with the inspired oxygen level, averaging lower in hypoxia (12% O_2) than in normoxia (21% O_2) and higher in hyperoxia (100% O_2) than normoxia. The figure also includes confirmatory results (*dashed yellow line*) from a previous study of cycle ergometry under comparable conditions.[153] Cycle ergometry produced lower muscle-specific $\dot{V}O_{2peak}$ values than knee-extension exercise. The slopes of the lines relating oxygen delivery to peak muscle oxidative metabolism were remarkably similar for both activity modes. For maximal knee-extension exercise, oxygen content of venous blood leaving the active muscles remained essentially equal among conditions averaging 4 mL · dL^{-1}. Oxygen delivery in arterial blood increased from 17.3 to 19.5 to 21.8 mL · dL^{-1} with increasing concentration levels of oxygen inhalation. The hyperoxic condition during maximal effort produced the largest skeletal muscle a-$\overline{v}O_2$ difference and $\dot{V}O_{2peak}$. Similarly, maximal exercise intensity decreased 25% when breathing 12% inspired oxygen and increased 14% under 100% inspired oxygen compared with normoxic conditions. *Oxygen delivery to active muscles in the circulation, not its use by mitochondrial metabolism, limits aerobic exercise performance.*

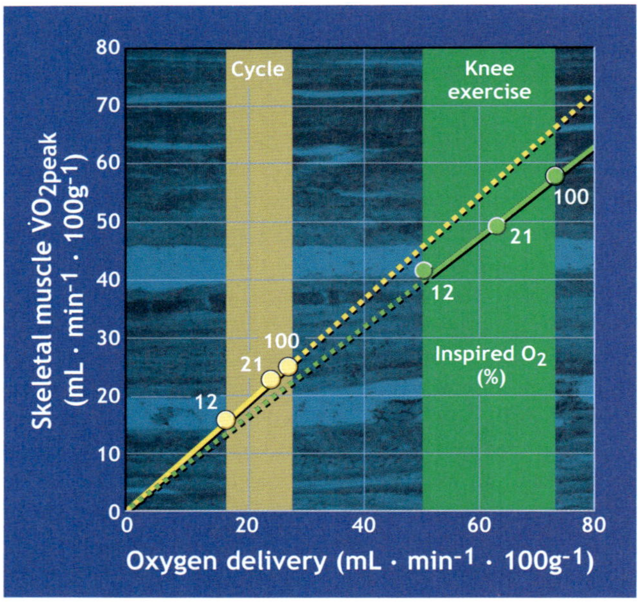

Breathing hyperoxic gas does not increase maximal cardiac output; an expanded a-$\overline{v}O_2$ difference must account for the increased exercise oxygen uptake. The small increases in arterial hemoglobin saturation and dissolved plasma oxygen with hyperoxic breathing increase total oxygen availability as blood volume circulates four to seven times each minute in strenuous effort depending on fitness level. The additional but relatively small 14 mL oxygen in each 1 L of blood from breathing hyperoxic gas represents considerable extra oxygen when exercising at a 20- to 30-L cardiac output. If the muscles metabolized the added oxygen during physical activity, $\dot{V}O_{2max}$ would increase by 5 to 10%. The increased partial pressure of oxygen in solution from breathing hyperoxic gas also facilitates its diffusion across the tissue-capillary membrane into the mitochondria, which may account for the higher oxygen uptake at the onset of activity. Breathing hyperoxic mixtures *during* endurance activity offers positive ergogenic benefits but offers limited practical sports application. The "legality" of using an appropriate breathing system during actual competition seems unlikely.

FIGURE 23.12. Relationship among skeletal muscle and oxygen delivery per 100 g muscle during maximal cycling exercise (*yellow*) and knee-extension exercise (*green*) under hypoxia, normoxia, and hyperoxia.
(Adapted with permission from Richardson RS, et al. Evidence of O_2 supply–dependent in exercise-trained human quadriceps. *J Appl Physiol*. 1999;86:1048. ©The American Physiological Society (APS). All rights reserved. Photo: Aptyp_koK/Shutterstock.)

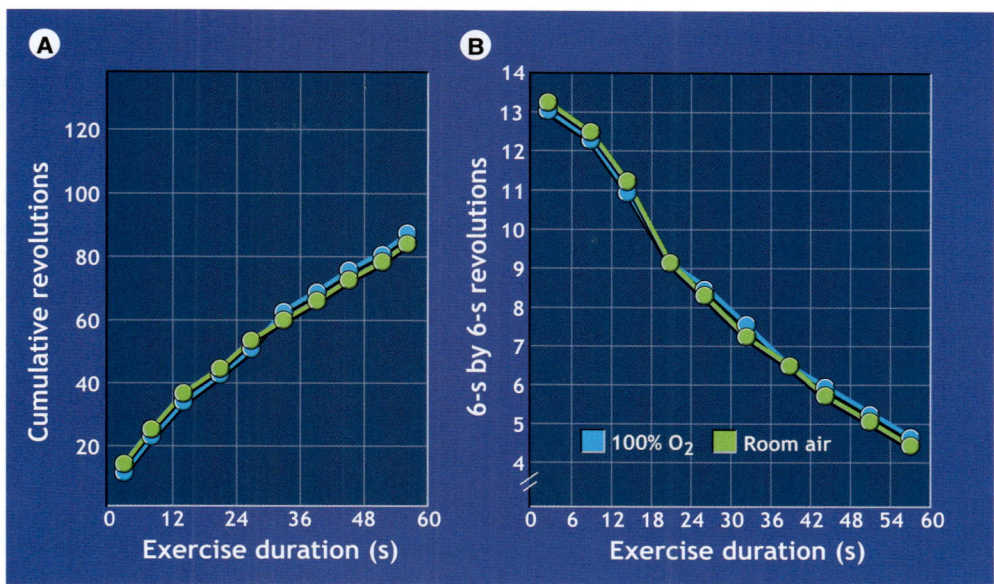

FIGURE 23.13. Cumulative (**A**) and absolute (**B**) 6-s pedal revolutions on a bicycle ergometer during 1-min maximal exercise after breathing either 100% oxygen or ambient air during recovery from a previous maximal exercise bout.
(Adapted with permission from Weltman A, et al. Exercise recovery, lactate removal, and subsequent high-intensity exercise performance. Res Q. 1977;48:786. Copyright © Society of Health and Physical Educators, www.shapeamerica.org; reprinted by permission of Taylor & Francis Ltd, http://www.tandfonline.com on behalf of Society of Health and Physical Educators.)

Postexercise Oxygen Breathing

Breathing hyperoxic mixtures does not facilitate recovery from exercise or improve performance in a subsequent exercise bout (**FIG. 23.13**). Following 1 min of all-out cycling, subjects recovered while breathing either room air or 100% $\dot{V}O_2$ for 10 or 20 min. They then repeated the all-out bicycle ride. No significant differences emerged in cumulative revolutions (*inset A*) and 6-s × 6-s revolutions (*inset B*) for the 1 min ride after breathing room air or 100% oxygen during recovery from previous effort. Breathing either room air or oxygen yielded similar blood lactate levels in the 10- or 20-min recovery periods. This indicated that breathing oxygen in recovery did not facilitate lactate removal. Subsequent research supports these findings; breathing oxygen after short intervals of submaximal and maximal physical effort did not affect recovery kinetics for minute ventilation, heart rate, or serum lactate or the level of ensuing exercise performance.[221,290]

Modifying Carbohydrate Intake

Increased carbohydrate intake before and during intense aerobic physical activity, including periods of strenuous training, is a sound macronutrient manipulation that benefits performance, lowers ratings of perceived exertion, and improves psychological state[1,31,265] (see Chapter 3). Vigilance and mood also improve with a carbohydrate beverage administered during a day of sustained aerobic activity interspersed with rest periods.[162] One of the more popular nutritional exercise modifications used by endurance athletes to augment glycogen reserves involve **carbohydrate loading** or glycogen supercompensation. The procedure produces considerably higher "packing" of muscle glycogen compared to simply maintaining a high-carbohydrate diet. Normally, each 100 g muscle contains about 1.7 g glycogen. Carbohydrate loading packs about three times as much or up to 4 to 5 g glycogen.

Nutrient-Related Fatigue in Prolonged Physical Activity

Glycogen stored in the liver and active muscle supplies most of the energy for intense aerobic activity. Prolonging such activity reduces the body's glycogen reserves. This allows lipid catabolism—from adipose tissue and liver fatty acid mobilization and intramuscular lipid stores—to supply a progressively greater percentage of energy. A substantially lowered muscle glycogen level precipitates fatigue, yet active muscle maintains sufficient oxygen with an almost unlimited potential energy from lipid. Consuming a glucose and water solution near the point of fatigue allows exercise to continue, but for all practical purposes, "the muscles' fuel tank reads empty." Reliance on lipid catabolism decreases power output from the considerably slower mobilization and breakdown of lipid than carbohydrate. The important role of carbohydrate as an energy substrate during 1 to 2 hr of intense exercise has led researchers to search for additional ways to increase pre-exercise glycogen reserves.

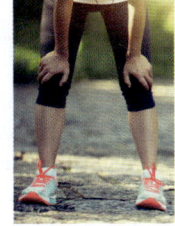
Izf/Shutterstock

Classic Loading Procedure

The classic procedure for achieving the supercompensation effect involves two stages. The first stage requires reducing the muscle's glycogen content with prolonged exercise about 6 days before competition. Glycogen supercompensation occurs only in the specific muscles depleted by exercise, so athletes must engage the muscles activated in their sport. Preparing for marathon running, endurance swimming, or bicycling requires 90 min moderately intense submaximal effort in the specific activity. The athlete then maintains a low-carbohydrate diet (about 60 to 100 g·d^{-1}) for several days to further deplete glycogen

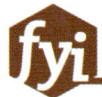

Hitting the Wall

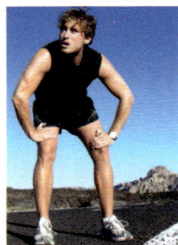
Maridav/Shutterstock

Of the hundreds of thousands of runners who attempted to run a major marathon over the past three decades, more than two fifths experienced severe and performance-limiting depleted physiologic carbohydrate reserves, and thousands dropped out before reaching the finish (approximately 1 to 2% who started). Marathon runners use the term "*hitting the wall*" to describe the fatigue and discomfort sensations associated with severe muscular-glycogen depletion. Factors for marathon success include muscle mass distribution (relatively large leg muscles), high liver and muscle glycogen densities, run speed as a fraction of aerobic capacity, and low oxygen cost (economy of effort) at a particular speed. Successful runners possess large aerobic capacities and store adequate liver and muscle glycogen without depleting carbohydrate below a critical fuel level runs at paces that challenge the current marathon world record 2:03:59 for men and 2:15:25 for women. Runners with lower aerobic capacities or relatively small leg muscle mass must run at slower paces or refuel during the race (or take short rest pauses) to avoid "hitting the wall."

Sources:
Nikolaidis PT, et al. Participation and performance in the oldest ultramarathon-comrades marathon 1921-2019. *Int J Sports Med*. 2021;42(7):638. doi: 10.1055/a-1303-4255.
Scheer V, et al. Age-related participation and performance trends of children and adolescents in ultramarathon running. *Res Sports Med*. 2020;28:507.
Viribay A, et al. Effects of 120 g/h of carbohydrates intake during a mountain marathon on exercise-induced muscle damage in elite runners. *Nutrients*. 2020;12:1367.
Hagerman FC. Energy metabolism and fuel utilization. *Med Sci Sports Exerc*. 1992;24:S309.

Stage	Day(s)	Description
1: Depletion	1	Exhausting exercise to deplete muscle glycogen in specific muscles
	2–4	Low-carbohydrate intake (60–100 g · d^{-1}) High percentage of protein and lipid in daily diet
2: Carbohydrate loading	5–7	High-carbohydrate intake (400–700 g · d^{-1}) Normal percentage of protein in daily diet
Competition day	NA	High-carbohydrate competition meal

Background photo: natali_ploskaya/Shutterstock

depletion, low-carbohydrate diet, and high-carbohydrate diet—but maintain the low-carbohydrate diet for only 1 day. With no adverse effects, the low-carbohydrate diet can gradually extend to a maximum of 4 days.

 INTEGRATIVE QUESTION

What advice would you give to male and female collegiate sprint athletes who plan to carbohydrate load for competition?

Sample Diets to Achieve the Supercompensation Effect

Consider a sample meal plan for carbohydrate depletion (stage 1) and carbohydrate loading (stage 2) preceding an endurance event.

Limited Applicability

Carbohydrate loading's benefits to performance apply only to intense aerobic activities lasting longer than 60 min. Activities

stores. Note that glycogen depletion increases intermediate forms of the glycogen-storing enzyme glycogen synthase within the depleted muscle fibers. Moderate training continues during this time. Then, 3 days before competing, the athlete switches to a high-carbohydrate diet (400 to 700 g · d^{-1}) and maintains this intake up to the precompetition meal (stage 2). The supercompensation diet should also contain adequate daily protein, minerals and vitamins, and abundant water. Supercompensated muscle glycogen levels remain stable for at least 3 days during a maintenance phase in a nonactive individual if the diet contains 60% of calories as carbohydrate.[109,110]

If an athlete decides to supercompensate after weighing the pros and cons, the new food regimen should proceed in stages during training, not for the first time before competition. For example, the track athlete should start with a long run followed by a high-carbohydrate diet. A detailed log should record how the dietary manipulation affects performance. A record of subjective feelings should include exercise depletion and replenishment phases. With positive results, the athlete can try the entire series—

Meal	Stage 1: Depletion	Stage 2: Carbohydrate loading
Breakfast	0.5 cup fruit juice 2 eggs 1 slice whole-wheat toast 1 glass whole milk	1 cup fruit juice 1 bowl hot or cold cereal 1–2 muffins 1 tbsp butter
Lunch	6 oz hamburger 2 sliced bread Salad (normal size) 1 tbsp mayonnaise and salad dressing 1 glass whole milk	2–3 oz hamburger with bun 1 cup juice 1 orange 1 tbsp mayonnaise 1 in slice (pie or cake). 1 cup yogurt, fruit, or cookies
Snack	1 cup yogurt	1–1.5 pieces of chicken, baked
Dinner	2–3 pieces of chicken, fried 1 baked potato with sour cream 0.5 cup vegetables 1 cup iced tea (no sugar) 2 tbsp butter	1 cup vegetables 0.5 cup sweetened pineapple 1 cup iced tea (sugar) 1 tbsp butter 1 glass chocolate milk with cookies
Snack	1 glass whole milk	

During Stage 1, the intake of carbohydrate approaches 60 g or 240 kcal; in Stage 2, the carbohydrate intake increases to 400–700 g or about 1600–2800 kcal.

Background photo: natali_ploskaya/Shutterstock

60 min or less require normal carbohydrate intake and associated glycogen reserves.[169,198] For example, carbohydrate loading did not benefit trained runners in a 20.9-km/13-mi run compared with a run following a low-carbohydrate diet. Similarly, no ergogenic effect emerged for time trial performance, heart rate, and RPE for endurance-trained cyclists in a 100-km trial that simulated continuous changes in cycling intensity typical of competition.[44]

For sports competition and training, a daily diet that contains about 60 to 70% of calories as carbohydrates provides adequate muscle and liver glycogen reserves. This diet ensures about twice as much muscle glycogen as a typical diet of 45 to 50% carbohydrate. For well-nourished athletes, the supercompensation effect remains relatively small. During intense training, athletes who do not upgrade daily calorie and carbohydrate intakes to meet energy demands can experience chronic muscle fatigue and staleness.

Gender Differences in Glycogen Storage and Catabolism During Physical Activity

Gender-related differences in muscle glycogen supercompensation remain controversial. One study reported a relatively small 13% increase in female's muscle glycogen content when they switched from a mixed diet to a high-carbohydrate diet.[280] Other research indicated that females do not increase glycogen storage when dietary carbohydrate increases from 60 to 75% of total caloric intake.[258] Importantly, this increase in carbohydrate intake as a percentage of total calories represents *considerably less total carbohydrate intake* relative to lean body mass (body composition component responsible for considerable glycogen storage) for females than for males.[180] **FIGURE 23.14** illustrates that equalizing daily carbohydrate intake for endurance-trained males and females at 12 g · kg$_{LBM}^{-1}$ for 3 consecutive days produced no gender differences in glycogen loading. *These and other findings show that males and females possess an equal capacity to accumulate muscle glycogen when fed comparable amounts of carbohydrate relative to lean body mass.*[258,259] Females oxidize more lipid and less carbohydrate and protein compared with males during endurance activity.[101,128] The increase in lipid oxidation associates with higher intramyocellular lipid content and use as well as greater adipocyte lipolysis. The greater lipid oxidation for females during submaximal endurance effort seems to occur partly through a sex hormone–mediated enhancement of lipid-oxidation pathways.[258]

Glycogen Supercompensation Enhanced by Prior Creatine Supplementation

A synergy exists between glycogen storage and creatine supplementation.[205,206] For example, preceding glycogen loading with a 5-day creatine loading protocol (20 g · d^{-1}) produced 10% greater glycogen packing in the vastus lateralis muscle than achieved with only glycogen loading.[226] More than likely,

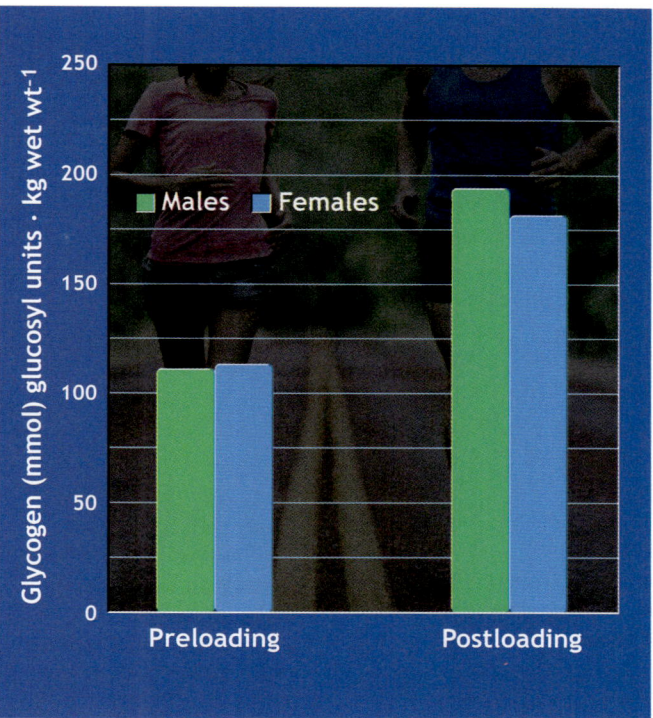

FIGURE 23.14. Muscle glycogen concentrations precarbohydrate and postcarbohydrate loading (12 g carbohydrate · kg^{-1} lean body mass) in exercise-trained males and females.
(Adapted with permission from James AP, et al. Muscle glycogen supercompensation: absence of a gender-related difference. *Eur J Appl Physiol.* 2001;85:533. Copyright © 2001. Photo: Maridav/Shutterstock.)

increases in creatine and cellular volume with creatine supplementation facilitate subsequent muscle glycogen storage.[266]

Modified Loading Procedures

A less stringent **modified loading procedure** displayed in **FIGURE 23.15** eliminates many potential negative aspects of the classic glycogen-loading sequence. The protocol increases glycogen synthase activity without requiring dramatic glycogen depletion with exercise as with the classic loading procedure; it increases glycogen storage to nearly the same level. The 6 days protocol does not require prior exhaustive physical effort. Rather, the athlete trains at about 75% $\dot{V}O_{2max}$ (85%HR_{max}) for 1.5 hr (*red line*) and then, on successive days, gradually reduces (tapers) exercise duration. During the first 3 day, carbohydrates represent about 50% of total calories (*blue line*). Three days before competition, the diet's carbohydrate content increases to 70% of total energy intake.

Rapid Loading Procedure: A One-Day Process

The 2 to 6 days required to achieve supranormal muscle glycogen levels represents a limitation of typical carbohydrate-loading procedures. The desired loading effect can also occur with a shortened duration that combines a brief bout of intense activity with only 1 day of high-carbohydrate intake.

Endurance-trained athletes cycled for 150 s at an intensity of 130% $\dot{V}O_{2max}$ followed by 30 s of all-out cycling. In the recovery period, the males consumed 10.3 g·kg^{-1} of high glycemic carbohydrate foods. Biopsy data presented in **FIGURE 23.16** indicated that vastus lateralis muscle glycogen increased from a 109.1 mmol·kg^{-1} preloading average to 198.3 mmol·kg^{-1} postloading after only 24 hr. This 82% increase in glycogen storage equaled or exceeded values reported by others using a 2- to 6-day regimen. The short-duration loading procedure benefits individuals who do not wish to disrupt normal training with the time required and potential negative aspects of longer loading protocols.[237]

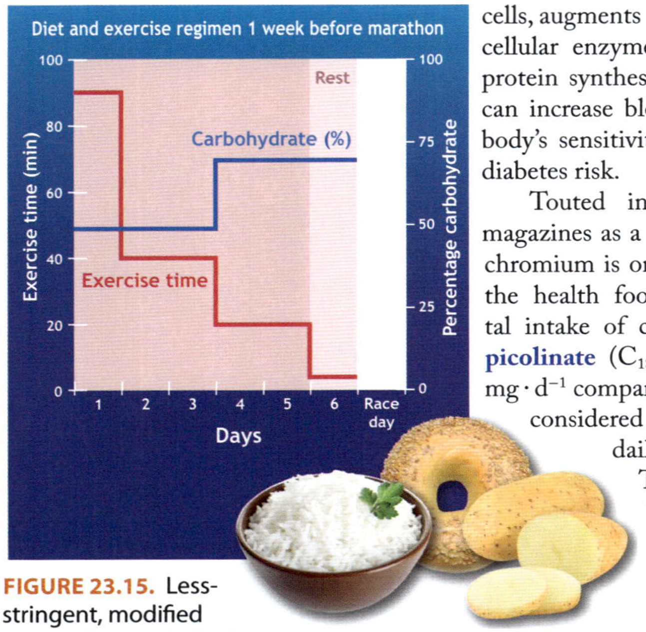

FIGURE 23.15. Less-stringent, modified approach to carbohydrate loading overloads muscle glycogen stores in the week before an endurance contest without requiring dramatic glycogen depletion with exhaustive exercise, while the diet's carbohydrate content increases during the last 3 days. (Reprinted with permission from Sherman WM, et al. Effect of exercise-diet manipulation on muscle glycogen and its subsequent utilization during performance. *Int J Sports Med*. 1981;2:114. © Georg Thieme Verlag KG. Shutterstock photos: New Africa (rice), Binh Thanh Bui (bagel), Anna Kucherova (potato).)

Chromium

The trace mineral chromium serves as a cofactor (as trivalent chromium) for a low–molecular-weight protein that potentiates insulin function, yet its precise mechanism of action remains unclear. Insulin promotes carbohydrate transport into cells, augments fatty acid catabolism, and triggers cellular enzyme activity that facilitates muscle protein synthesis. Chronic chromium deficiency can increase blood cholesterol and decrease the body's sensitivity to insulin, thus raising type 2 diabetes risk.

Touted in popular muscle development magazines as a "fat burner" and "muscle builder," chromium is one of the most hyped minerals in the health food–fitness literature. Supplemental intake of chromium, usually as **chromium picolinate** ($C_{18}H_{12}CrN_3O_6$), often reaches 600 mg·d^{-1} compared to 50 to 200 mg of chromium, considered the estimated safe and adequate daily dietary intake (ESADDI).

This chelated picolinic acid combination supposedly yields better chromium absorption than the inorganic salt chromium chloride. Millions of Americans believe the unsubstantiated claims of health food faddists, television infomercials, and exercise zealots that additional chromium promotes muscle growth, curbs appetite, fosters body fat loss, and even lengthens life. Advertisers target chromium to bodybuilders and other resistance-trained athletes as a safe alternative to anabolic steroids to favorably change body composition. Chromium supplements supposedly potentiate insulin action to increase amino acid anabolism in skeletal muscle. This belief persists despite data that chromium supplements exert no effect on glucose or insulin concentrations in nondiabetic individuals.[4,90]

Some Positive Benefits

Generally, studies suggesting beneficial effects of chromium supplements on body fat and muscle mass infer body composition changes from changes in body weight (or unvalidated anthropometric measurements). One study observed that supplementing daily for 40 days with 200 mg (3.85 mmol) of chromium picolinate produced a small increase in FFM estimated from skinfold thickness and decrease in body fat in young males who resistance trained for 6 wk.[89] The researchers provided no data to show increased muscular strength. Another study reported increases in body mass without changes in strength or body composition in previously untrained female college students (no change in males) who received a daily 200-mg chromium supplement during 12 wk of resistance training compared with unsupplemented controls.[121]

Minimal Benefits

Other research evaluated the effects of a 200 mg·d^{-1} chromium supplement on muscle strength, body composition, and

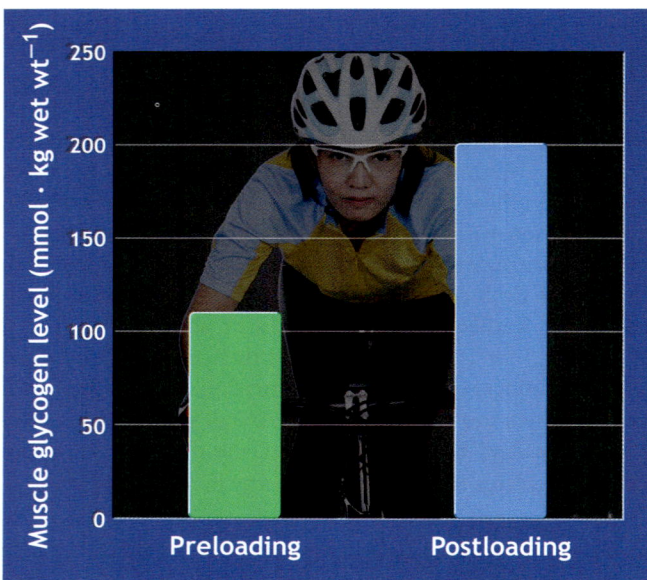

FIGURE 23.16. Vastus lateralis muscle glycogen concentration before (preloading) and after 180 s of near-maximal intensity cycling followed by 1-day high-carbohydrate (postloading) intake. (Reprinted with permission from Fairchild TJ, et al. Rapid carbohydrate loading after short bout of near maximal-intensity exercise. *Med Sci Sports Exerc*. 2002;34:980. Photo: JAKKRIT SAELAO/Shutterstock.)

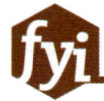

Sports Supplement Manufacturing

The global sports nutrition market size in 2019 was valued at USD 15.6 billion and is expected to grow at a compound annual growth rate of 8.9% between 2020 and 2027 (www.grandviewresearch.com/industry-analysis/sports-nutrition-market). The following four steps provide a general overview for producing a typical sports supplement product.

Step 1. Determine Formula
The supplement creators select premium quality, appropriately selected raw ingredients to create the final product formula to help ensure product efficacy during the creation process.

Step 2. Select Raw Materials
High-quality ingredients must ensure high bioavailability broadly defined as a nutrient's optimal absorption and utilization qualities. All raw ingredients must meet purity and microbiological compliance. Every chemical substance contained in a supplement product (e.g., organic and inorganic compounds, metals, alloys, minerals, elements, proteins and nucleic acids, and polymers) is assigned a unique Chemical Abstracts Service registry number (CAS; www.cas.org). For example, creatine monohydrate has a CAS number 6020-87-7, while the CAS number for caffeine is 58-08-2. This systematic approach allows different agencies world-wide to keep track of the ingredients contained in a product to ensure the product meets required standards during the formulation and manufacturing processes. As a frame of reference, about 177 million organic and inorganic substances reported in the literature have been catalogued since the 1820s!

Step 3. Test Raw Material
Once the raw materials arrive at the manufacturing facility, Current Good Manufacturing Practices (CGMPs) require

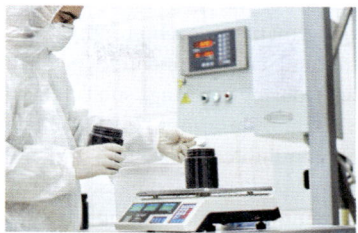

Photo courtesy Anssi Manninen, DOMINUS NUTRITION OY, Finland (www.dominusnutrition.fi).

laboratory testing before they can be released into inventory. This involves determining potency to meet microbiological compliance for safety, including testing for heavy metals (e.g., mercury, lead, cadmium) according to long-established US Pharmacopeia (USP; www.usp.org) standards, established in 1820 and by the 1848 Drug Importation Act.

Step 4. Test and Retest Production Run
The raw materials included in the formula are comixed, and a limited number of tablets, capsules or powder mixtures

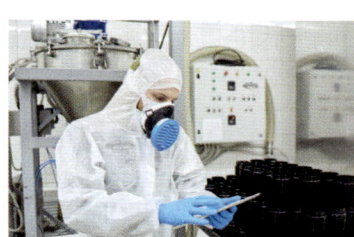

Photo courtesy Anssi Manninen, DOMINUS NUTRITION OY, Finland (www.dominusnutrition.fi).

are produced to certify the formulation for human consumption. This step is followed by production runs in the manufacturing facilities to further establish product quality and safety. This last step may include additional lab testing to validate content uniformity and product stability. Repeat quality control lab tests are performed following steps 2 and 3 before releasing the final product for sale.

---

chromium excretion in 16 untrained males during resistance training for 12 wk.[118] Muscular strength improved 24% for the supplemented group and 33% for the placebo group during training. No changes occurred in any of the body composition variables. The group receiving the supplement did show higher chromium excretion than controls after 6 wk of training. The researchers concluded that chromium supplements provided *no ergogenic effect* on any measured variable. Supplementing with 800 mg of chromium picolinate (plus 6 mg of boron) proved no more effective than a maltodextrin placebo to enhance lean tissue gain or promote fat loss during resistance training.[3] Daily supplementation with 400 mg of chromium picolinate for 9 wk did not promote weight loss in sedentary obese women; it actually caused weight gain during the treatment period.[112]

In support of chromium supplementation, greater body fat loss (no increase in FFM) occurred in subjects "recruited from a variety of fitness and athletic clubs" who consumed 400 mg of chromium daily over 90 days than in subjects who received a placebo.[140] Hydrostatic weighing and DEXA techniques assessed body composition. Body compositional data from hydrostatic weighing do not appear in the report, and the DEXA-derived analysis indicated average body fat values of 42% for both control and experimental subjects, an extraordinary level of obesity for members of fitness clubs. Collegiate football players who received daily 200-mg supplements of chromium picolinate for 9 wk showed no changes in body composition and muscular strength from intense weight training compared with controls receiving a placebo.[59] Similar findings of no benefit on body composition and physical performance emerged from a 14-wk study of NCAA Division I wrestlers that compared combined chromium picolinate supplementation with a typical preseason training program with identical training without supplementation.[281]

Loss of muscle mass commonly affects older individuals so potential ergogenic effect on muscle from chromium supplementation should emerge readily in this age group. This did not occur for older males involved in intense resistance training; a high chromium picolinate dosage ($924 \text{ mg} \cdot \text{d}^{-1}$) did not augment muscle size, strength, or power or FFM accretion above the unsupplemented condition.[48] Obese personnel enrolled in the United States Navy's mandatory remedial physical-conditioning program who consumed an additional 400 mg chromium picolinate daily showed no greater loss in body weight or body fat percentage or increase in FFM than a placebo group.[264]

A comprehensive double-blind study examined the effects of a daily chromium supplement (3.3 to 3.5 mmol as either chromium chloride or chromium picolinate) or a placebo for 8 wk during resistance training in 36 young men. For each group, dietary intakes of protein, magnesium, zinc, copper, and iron equaled or exceeded recommended levels during training; subjects also maintained adequate baseline dietary chromium intakes. Supplementation increased serum chromium concentration and urinary chromium excretion equally regardless of its ingested form. Compared with placebo treatment, chromium supplementation did not affect training-related changes in muscular strength, FFM, or muscle mass. Also, giving middle-age males supplemental chromium (924 mg·d^{-1}) as chromium picolinate for 12 wk did not affect hematologic measures or indices of iron metabolism or iron status.[47] We are unaware of studies that have evaluated the safety of long-term chromium supplementation or the ergogenic efficacy of supplementing in individuals with suboptimal chromium status. Concerning the bioavailability of trace minerals in the diet, excessive dietary chromium inhibits zinc and iron absorption. At the extreme, this could induce iron-deficiency anemia, blunt the ability to train intensely, and negatively affect performance requiring high-level aerobic metabolism.

Creatine

Meat, poultry, and fish provide a rich creatine source containing 4 to 5 g creatine·kg food^{-1}. The body synthesizes only about 1 g nitrogen-containing organic compound daily from the nonessential amino acids arginine, glycine, and methionine in the kidneys, liver, and pancreas. The animal kingdom contains the richest creatine-containing foods, placing vegetarians at a distinct disadvantage for ready sources of exogenous creatine. Skeletal muscle contains approximately 95% of the body's total 120 to 140 g creatine.

Creatine sold in supplemental form as **creatine monohydrate** (CrH_2O) comes as a powder, tablet, capsule, and stabilized liquid. It can be purchased over-the-counter or mail order as a nutritional supplement (but without guarantee of purity).[115] Ingesting creatine monohydrate as a liquid suspension at 20 to 30 g·d^{-1} dosage for 2 wk increases intramuscular concentrations of free creatine and PCr up to 30%. These levels remain high for weeks after only several days supplementation.[128,174] Sports-governing bodies do not consider creatine an illegal substance.

Important Component Present in High-Energy Phosphates

Creatine passes through the digestive tract's intestinal mucosa unaltered for absorption into the bloodstream. Almost all ingested creatine incorporates into skeletal muscle (average concentration, 125 mM·kg^{-1} [range 90 to 160 mM]), with about 40% as free creatine and the remainder

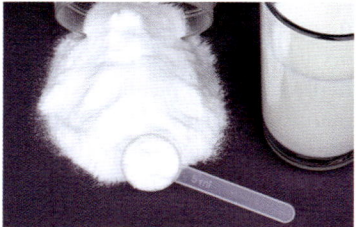
ogichobanov/Shutterstock

readily combining with phosphate to form PCr. Type II, fast-twitch muscle fibers store about four to six times more PCr than ATP. As emphasized in Chapter 5, PCr serves as the cells' "energy reservoir" to make phosphate-bond energy readily available, more rapidly than ATP regenerated in glycogenolysis,[289] to resynthesize ATP in the reversible reaction:

$$PCr + ADP \rightarrow Cr + ATP$$

PCr also shuttles intramuscular high-energy phosphate between the mitochondria and muscle filament cross-bridge sites that initiate muscle action. Maintaining a high sarcoplasmic ATP:ADP ratio by energy transfer from PCr plays an important role in maximum effort lasting up to 10 s. This duration places high demands on ATP resynthesis that exceed energy transfer from intracellular macronutrient breakdown. Improved energy transfer capacity from PCr also lessens reliance on energy from anaerobic glycolysis with associated increase in intramuscular H$^+$ and decrease in pH from lactate accumulation.[12] Increases in PCr provide the following beneficial effects to exercise performance:

1. Accelerate ATP turnover to maintain power output during short-term muscular effort
2. Delay PCr depletion
3. Diminish dependence on anaerobic glycolysis and decrease subsequent lactate formation
4. Facilitate muscle relaxation and recovery from repeated intense, brief efforts from faster ATP and PCr resynthesis
5. Allow rapid recovery to prolong higher-level power output

Documented Human Benefits

Creatine supplementation received notoriety as an ergogenic aid when British sprinters and hurdlers used it in the 1992 Barcelona Olympic Games. Creatine supplementation at recommended levels exerts the following three effects:

1. Improves performance in muscular strength and power activities
2. Augments short bursts of muscular endurance
3. Provides for greater muscular overload to enhance training effectiveness

No serious adverse effects from creatine supplementation for up to 4 years have been reported.[236] Anecdotes indicate a possible association between creatine supplementation and cramping in multiple muscle areas during competition or lengthy practice in American football players. This effect may result from (1) altered intracellular dynamics from increased free creatine and PCr; (2) osmotically induced enlarged cell volume (greater cellular hydration) from the muscle fibers' greater creatine content; and (3) inadequate whole-body hydration. Gastrointestinal tract disturbances (nausea, indigestion, and difficulty absorbing food) have been reported while consuming the product.

Creatine monohydrate supplements substantially increase muscle creatine content and performance during intense physical activity, particularly repeated muscular effort.[215,216,277]

Higher-Dose Arginine Supplementation: An Effective Ergogenic Aid

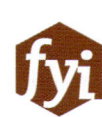

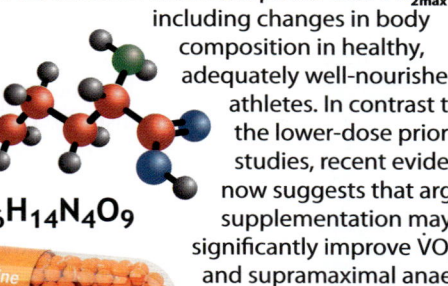

Shutterstock: natatravel (capsule), Bacsica (molecule)

In prior studies, low-dose 3 g · d^{-1} arginine supplementation had little or no effect on anaerobic power and $\dot{V}O_{2max}$, including changes in body composition in healthy, adequately well-nourished athletes. In contrast to the lower-dose prior studies, recent evidence now suggests that arginine supplementation may significantly improve $\dot{V}O_{2max}$ and supramaximal anaerobic performance with proper dosing regimens. A meta-analysis summary of 18 well-controlled studies indicates the following:

- Acute arginine supplementation protocols to improve aerobic and anaerobic performance should now be adjusted to body weight rather than an absolute daily amount). The body weight approach requires 0.15 g · kg$_{BW}^{-1}$ consumed 60 to 90 min before exercise. For a 90-kg/200-lb male 100- to 440-m sprinter (including hurdles), daily arginine intake would be 13.5 g (one-half oz) daily (0.15 g × 90 kg).
- Chronic arginine supplementation with periodization training should include 1.5 to 2 g · d^{-1} for 4 to 7 wk to improve aerobic, endurance-type performance, and 10– to 12 g · d^{-1} for 8 wk to enhance anaerobic, supramaximal performance.

Arginine, a nonessential amino acid, participates in nitric oxide (NO) synthesis and bioavailability. Numerous experiments have verified the NO pathway can serves as an essential physiological mechanism to help to explain improved exercise performance. One might argue that increased NO production also can potentiate arginine supplementation's ergogenic effects in short-term and longer-term athletic performance

Sources:
Hlinský T, et al. Effects of dietary nitrates on time trial performance in athletes with different training status: systematic review. *Nutrients.* 2020;12:2734.
Viribay A, et al. Effects of arginine supplementation on athletic performance based on energy metabolism: a systematic review and meta-analysis. *Nutrients.* 2020;12:1300.

FIGURE 23.17 illustrates creatine supplementation's ergogenic effects on total work accomplished during repetitive sprint cycling performance. Physically active but untrained males performed sets of maximum 6-s bicycle sprints interspersed with various recovery periods (24, 54, or 84 s) to simulate sport conditions. Performance evaluations took place under creatine-loaded (20 g · d^{-1} for 5 days) or placebo conditions. Supplementation increased muscle creatine (48.9%) and PCr (12.5%), which produced a 6% increase in total work accomplished (251.7 kJ presupplement vs. 266.9 kJ creatine loaded) compared to the placebo group (254.0 kJ pretest vs. 252.3 kJ placebo). Creatine supplements have benefited an

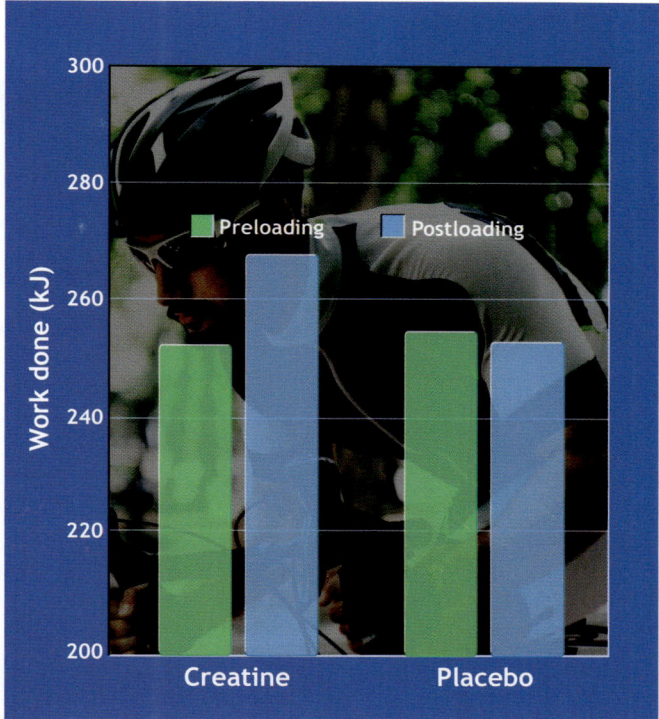

FIGURE 23.17. Creatine loading versus placebo for total work accomplished during an 80-min repetitive sprint-cycling performance.
(Adapted with permission from Preen CD, et al. Effect of creatine loading on long-term sprint exercise performance and metabolism. *Med Sci Sports Exerc.* 2001;33:814. Photo: Forestlife/Shutterstock.)

on-court "ghosting" routine of simulated positional play in competitive squash players.[228]

One research study evaluated a creatine dose of 30 g · d^{-1} for 6 days in trained runners under two conditions: (1) four repeated 300-m runs with a 4-min recovery and (2) four 1000 m runs with a 3-min recovery.[120] Compared with placebo treatment, creatine supplementation improved performance under both conditions, with the most impressive gains in repeated 1000 m runs. Supplementing with 20 g of creatine daily for 4 days also benefited anaerobic capacity in three 30-s Wingate tests with a 5-min rest between trials. For Division I football players, creatine supplementation with resistance training increased body mass, lean body mass, cellular hydration, and muscular strength and performance.[27] Similarly, supplementation augmented muscular strength and size increases during 12 wk of resistance training.[287] The enhanced hypertrophic response with supplementation and resistance training possibly results from accelerated myosin heavy-chain synthesis.[122] For resistance-trained males classified as creatine supplementation "responders" (i.e., a creatine increase ≥32 mmol · kg^{-1}), supplementing for 5 days increased body weight and FFM, and peak force and total force during repeated maximal isometric bench presses.[147] For males classified as creatine supplementation "nonresponders" (i.e., creatine increase ≤21 mmol · kg^{-1}), no ergogenic effect occurred. Research also indicates that creatine supplementation plus resistance training may retard production of the protein myostatin, which inhibits muscle growth, to facilitate muscle mass accretion and reduce the markers of muscle damage after intense endurance effort.[17,214,234]

634 SECTION 4 • Enhancing Energy Transfer Capacity

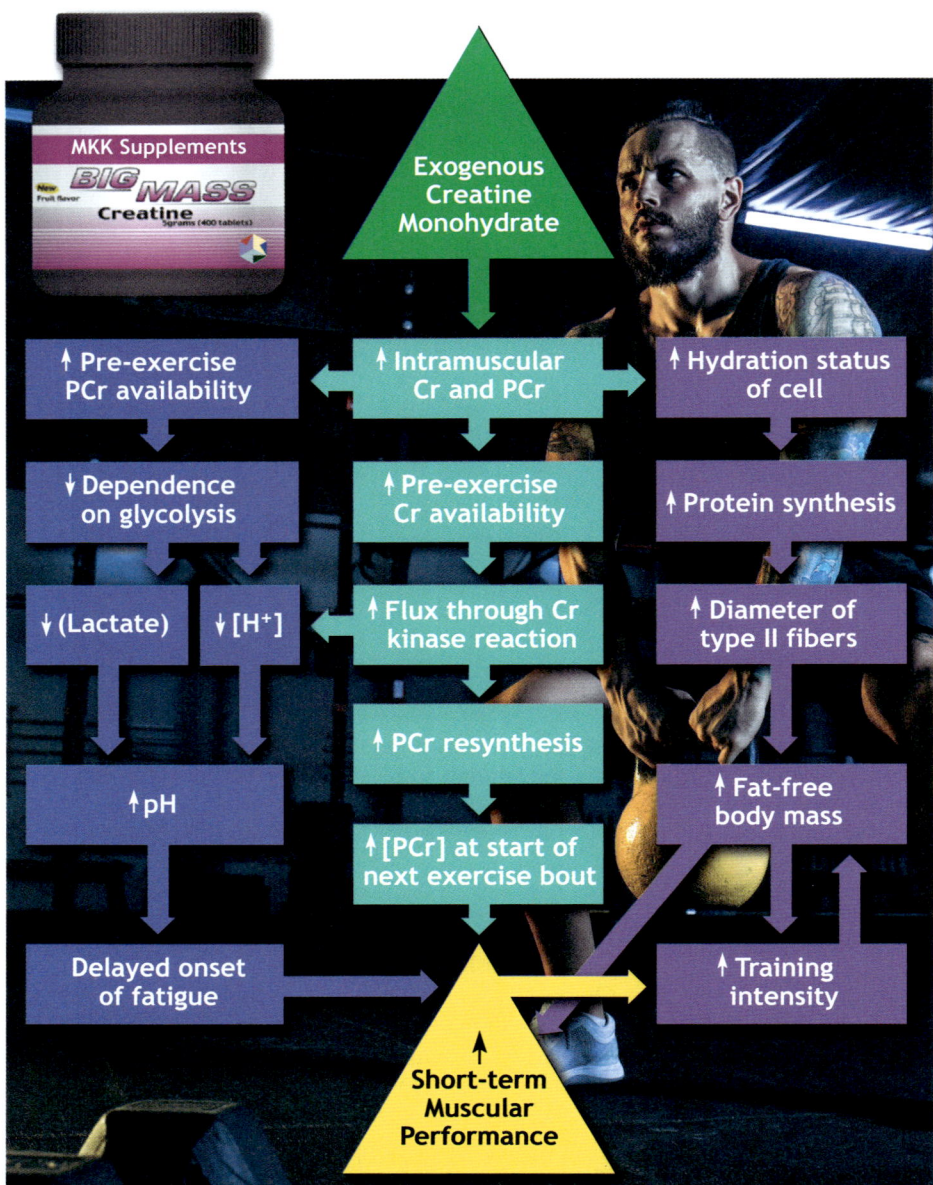

FIGURE 23.18. Mechanisms to explain how increased intracellular creatine (*Cr*) and phosphocreatine (*PCr*) enhance intense, short-duration exercise performance and the training response.
(Adapted with permission from Volek JS, Kraemer WJ. Creatine supplementation: its effect on human muscular performance and body composition. *J Strength Cond Res*. 1996;10:200. Photo: Master1305/Shutterstock.)

FIGURE 23.18 outlines possible mechanisms for enhanced exercise performance and training response by elevating intramuscular free creatine and PCr. Consuming a high dose of creatine increases pre-exercise intramuscular Cr and PCr availability to power short-term effort and helps replenish muscle creatine in recovery. This metabolic "preloading" and "reloading" reduces reliance on glycolytic energy-releasing processes with accompanying lactate formation, helping to replenish muscle creatine following intense physical effort and promotes recovery in muscle contractile capacity, and ability to maintain repeated intense exercise effort and training.[317] A facilitated rate of muscle relaxation may also contribute to the ergogenic action of creatine supplementation.[268]

Besides benefiting weightlifting and bodybuilding, improved immediate anaerobic power output capacity aids sprint running, swimming, kayaking, cycling, jumping, football, and volleyball. Oral creatine supplementation combined with resistance training affects cellular processes in a manner that increases protein deposition within the muscle's contractile mechanism.[287] This response helps to explain increases in muscle size and strength with creatine supplementation.

Creatine supplementation does not improve cardiovascular and metabolic responses with continuous incremental treadmill running or activity requiring high aerobic energy transfer levels.[11,114]

Age Effects Uncertain

Whether creatine supplementation augments the training response in older individuals remains equivocal. For 70-year-old men, a creatine loading phase (0.3 g·kg^{-1} for 5 days) followed by a daily maintenance phase (0.07 g·kg^{-1} for 5 days) increased lean tissue mass, leg strength, muscular endurance, and average power of the legs during resistance training to a greater extent than a placebo.[58] Creatine supplements also benefit muscular performance in normally active older men.[110] In contrast, no enhancement in resistance-training response to creatine ingestion occurred among sedentary and weight-trained older adults, perhaps due to an age-related decline in creatine transport efficiency.[30] Short-term creatine supplementation *per se*, without resistance training, does not increase muscle protein synthesis or FFM.[200]

Effects on Body Mass and Body Composition

Increases in body mass between 0.5 kg/1 lb and 5.2 kg/11.2 lb often accompany creatine supplementation, independent from changing testosterone or cortisol concentrations.[132,278] How much of the weight gain occurs from the anabolic effect of creatine on muscle tissue synthesis, retention of intracellular water from increased creatine stores, or other factors remains unclear.

Resistance-trained males matched for physical characteristics and maximal strength randomly received a placebo or creatine supplement. Supplementation consisted of 25 g daily followed by maintenance at 5 g daily. Both groups engaged in heavy resistance training for 12 wk. **FIGURE 23.19A** shows a greater training-induced increase occurred in body mass and FFM for the creatine-supplemented group compared with controls. The same was true for maximum bench press and squat strength increases in the creatine group than in controls (Fig. 23.19B). Creatine supplementation induced greater muscle fiber hypertrophy with resistance training, indicated by greater enlargement in types I (35 vs. 11%), IIA (36 vs. 15%), and IIAB muscle fiber cross-sectional areas (35 vs. 6%; Fig. 23.19C). The larger volume of weight lifted during weeks 5 to 8 by the creatine supplement group suggests that higher-quality training sessions mediated more favorable adaptations in FFM, muscle morphology, and strength performance. The placebo group trained and consumed Cr supplements identically as the experimental groups.

Creatine Loading

Many creatine users pursue a loading phase by ingesting 20 to 30 $g \cdot d^{-1}$ creatine for 5 to 7 days. Individuals who consume vegetarian-type diets show the greatest increase in muscle creatine levels because of their low dietary creatine content. Particularly large increases characterize individuals with normally low basal levels of intramuscular creatine.[42,50] A maintenance phase follows the loading phase. During this time, the athlete supplements with as little as 2 to 5 g creatine daily.

Practical questions for the athlete desiring to elevate intramuscular creatine levels concern the magnitude and time course of intramuscular creatine increase with supplementation, dosage needed to maintain the creatine increase, and creatine loss or "washout" when supplementation ceases. To provide insight into these questions, researchers studied two groups of men. In one experiment, six males ingested 20 g creatine monohydrate (approximately 0.3 $g \cdot kg^{-1}$) for 6 consecutive days and then stopped supplementing. Biopsies assessed muscle creatine levels before supplement ingestion and at day 7, 21, and 35. Similarly, nine males consumed 20 g creatine monohydrate daily for 6-day consecutively. Instead of discontinuing supplementation, they reduced dosage to 2 g daily (approximately 0.03 $g \cdot kg^{-1}$) for an additional 28 days. **FIGURE 23.20A** shows that total muscle creatine concentration increased approximately 20% (from 122 to 146 mM · kg dry $mass^{-1}$) after 6 days. Without continued supplementation, muscle creatine content gradually declined to near baseline in 35 days. The group that continued to supplement with reduced creatine for an additional 28 days maintained muscle creatine at the higher level (Fig. 23.20B). For both groups, the increase in total muscle creatine content during the initial 6-day supplementation period averaged about 23 mmol · kg^{-1}; this represented about 20 g (17%) total creatine ingested. A similar 20% increase in total muscle creatine concentration occurred with only a 3 g daily supplement (not shown). The increase occurred more gradually and required 28 days rather than 6 days with the 6 g supplement.

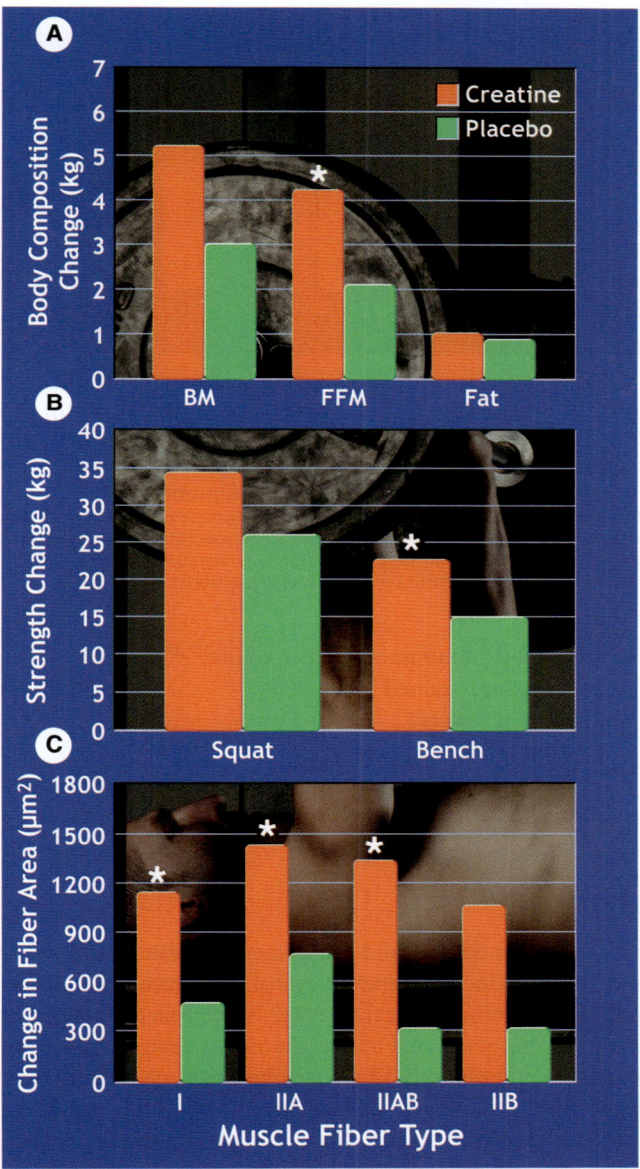

FIGURE 23.19. Creatine supplementation plus heavy-resistance training for 12 wk on changes in **(A)** body mass (BM), fat-free body mass (FFM), and body fat; **(B)** squat and bench press muscular strength; and **(C)** four specific fiber type cross-sectional areas. *Significantly greater change than placebo groups.
(Reprinted with permission from Volek JS, et al. Performance and muscle fiber adaptations to creatine supplementation and heavy-resistance training. *Med Sci Sports Exerc*. 1999;31:1147. Photo: Gorgev/Shutterstock.)

Carbohydrate Ingestion Augments Creatine Loading

Consuming creatine with a sugar-containing drink increases creatine uptake and storage in skeletal muscle (**FIG. 23.21**). For 5 days, subjects received either 5 g creatine four times daily or a 5 g supplement followed 30 min later by 93 g high-glycemic simple sugar four times daily. The creatine-only group increased muscle PCr (7.2%), free creatine (13.5%), and total creatine (20.7%). Much larger increases occurred for the creatine-plus-sugar–supplemented group (14.7% for PCr,

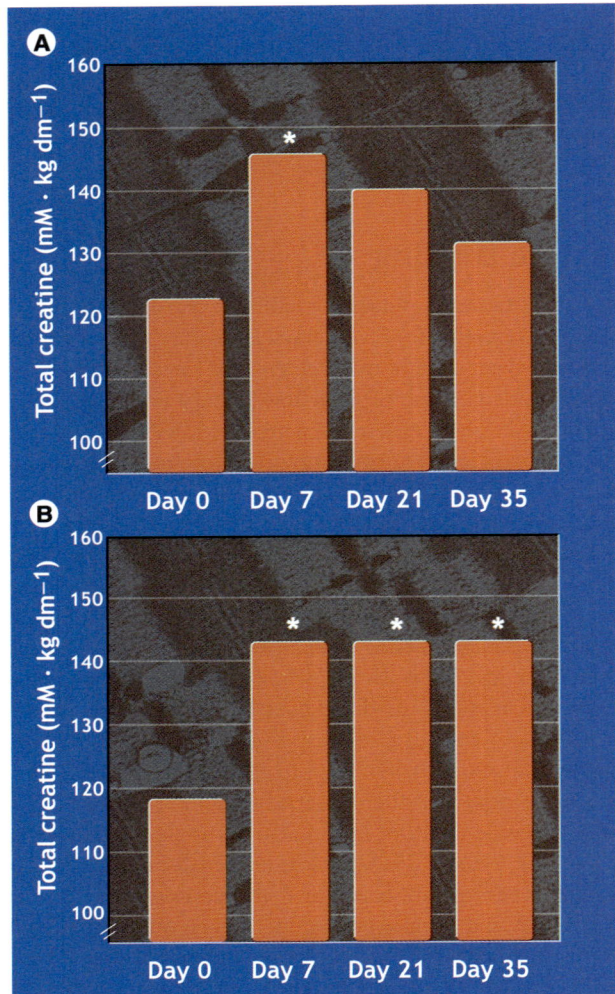

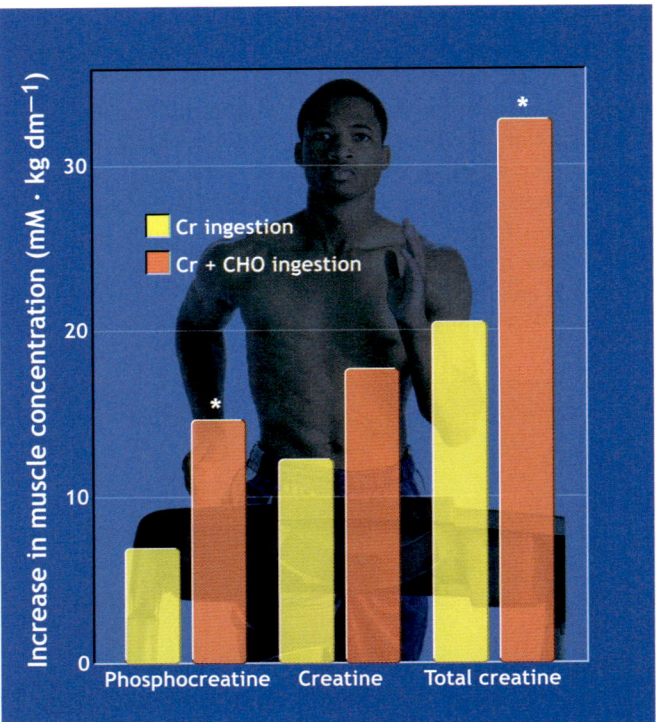

FIGURE 23.20. **(A)** Total muscle creatine concentration in six men consuming 20 g creatine for 6 consecutive days and then stopped the supplement. **(B)** Total muscle creatine concentration ingesting 20 g creatine for 6 days consecutively followed by 2 g daily for 28 days. *Significantly different from day 0.
(Adapted with permission from Hultman E, et al. Muscle creatine loading in men. J Appl Physiol. 1996;81:232.) ©The American Physiological Society (APS). All rights reserved.

FIGURE 23.21. Increases in phosphocreatine, creatine (Cr), and total creatine dry muscle concentrations in one group after 5 days Cr supplementation and after 5 days Cr plus carbohydrate (CHO) supplementation in another group. *Significantly greater than Cr-only supplementation.
(Adapted with permission from Green AL, et al. Carbohydrate ingestion augments skeletal muscle creatine accumulation during creatine supplementation in humans. Am J Physiol Endocrinol Metab. 1996;271:E821. ©The American Physiological Society (APS). All rights reserved. Photo: Flashon Studio/Shutterstock.)

18.1% for free creatine, and 33.0% for total creatine). Creatine supplementation alone did not affect insulin secretion, though adding sugar elevated plasma insulin levels. More than likely, augmented creatine storage with a creatine-plus-sugar supplement resulted from insulin-mediated glucose transport into skeletal muscle, facilitating creatine entry into muscle fibers.[243]

Some Research Shows No Benefits

Not all research confirms positive effects of creatine supplementation. Ergogenic effects may not emerge under the following seven conditions, but the reason for the discrepancies remains unknown:

1. In untrained subjects performing a single 15-s sprint cycling bout[66]
2. In trained subjects performing sport-specific physical activity bouts for swimming, cycling, and running[43,94]
3. In trained and untrained older adults[133,291]
4. In resistance-trained individuals[254]
5. In trained rowers[76]
6. During rapid weight loss[194]
7. When short-term supplementation does not increase muscle PCr[95,190]

Medium-Chain Triacylglycerols

Do high-fat foods or lipid supplements elevate plasma fatty acid levels to increase energy availability from lipid during prolonged aerobic physical activity? Several factors affect the answer to this question. First, consuming triacylglycerols composed of predominantly 12 to 18 carbon long-chain fatty acids delays gastric emptying. This negatively affects the rapidity of lipid availability and slows fluid and carbohydrate replenishment, both crucial factors in intense endurance activity. Second, after digestion and intestinal absorption (normally 3 to 4-hr), long-chain triacylglycerols reassemble with phospholipids, fatty acids, and a cholesterol shell to form a fatty droplet **chylomicron**. These substances travel slowly to the systemic circulation through the lymphatic system. They eventually empty into the systemic venous blood in the neck region via the thoracic duct. Through the action of the enzyme lipoprotein lipase that lines capillary walls, chylomicrons in the bloodstream readily hydrolyze to provide free fatty acids and glycerol for use by peripheral tissues. The relatively slow rate of gastric emptying and subsequent digestion, absorption, and assimilation of long-chain triacylglycerols makes this energy source an undesirable supplement to augment energy metabolism during physical activity.

Medium-chain triacylglycerols (MCTs) provide a more rapid source of fatty acid fuel. MCTs are processed oils, frequently produced for patients with intestinal malabsorption and tissue-wasting diseases. Marketing hypes MCTs as "fat burners," "energy sources," "glycogen sparrers," and "muscle builders." Unlike longer-chain triacylglycerols, MCTs contain saturated fatty acids with 8 to 10 carbon atoms along the fatty acid chain, as for example, lauric acid (coconut oil). During digestion, lipase in the mouth, stomach, and intestinal duodenum hydrolyzes MCTs to glycerol and medium-chain fatty acids (MCFAs). Their water solubility allows MCFAs to move rapidly across the intestinal mucosa directly into the bloodstream (portal vein) without first being transported as chylomicrons by the lymphatic system as long-chain triacylglycerols require. At the tissues, MCFAs move readily through the plasma membrane where they diffuse across the inner mitochondrial membrane for oxidation—they enter the mitochondria largely independent of the carnitine-acyl-CoA transferase system (see Chapter 6). Cellular uptake and mitochondrial oxidation speed contrasts with the relatively slower long-chain fatty acid transfer and oxidation rate. MCTs do not usually store as body fat because of their relative ease of oxidation. Ingesting MCTs rapidly elevates plasma FFAs, making it plausible that these lipids might spare liver and muscle glycogen during aerobic exercise.

Inconclusive MCT Benefits to Physical Activity

Consuming MCTs does not inhibit gastric emptying, as does common lipid, but conflicting research supports their use prior to physical activity.[272,276] In early studies, subjects consumed 380 mg MCT oil per kg body mass 1 hr before exercising at 60 to 70% $\dot{V}O_{2max}$ for 1 hr.[71] Plasma ketone levels generally increased, but the exercise metabolic mixture did not change compared with a placebo trial or a trial after subjects consumed a glucose polymer. Catabolism of 30 g MCTs (estimated maximal amount tolerated in the gastrointestinal tract) consumed before exercising contributed only 3 to 7% to the total energy requirement.[136]

Subsequent research investigated possible metabolic and ergogenic effects of consuming 86 g MCT (surprisingly well tolerated). Six endurance-trained cyclists rode for 2 hr at 60% $\dot{V}O_{2peak}$ while ingesting 2 L of a 4.3% MCT emulsion, 10% glucose plus 4.3% MCT emulsion, or a 10% glucose solution during exercise. They then performed a simulated 40-km cycling time trial. **FIGURE 23.22** shows the effects of the different beverages on average time trial speed. Replacing the carbohydrate

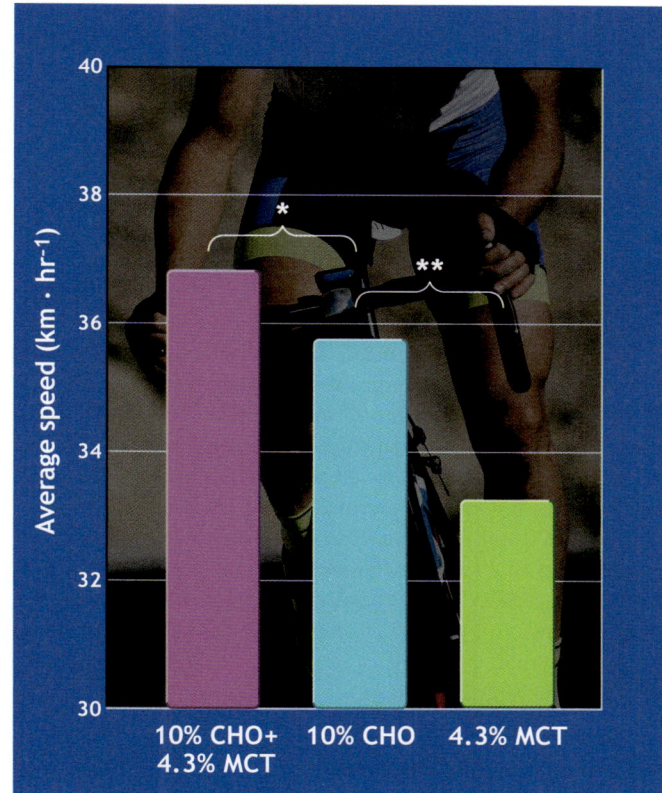

FIGURE 23.22. Effects of ingestion of carbohydrate (CHO; 10% solution), medium-chain triacylglycerol (MCT; 4.3% emulsion), and carbohydrate 1 MCT (10% CHO + 4.3% MCT) during simulated 40-km time-trial cycling speeds after exercising 2 hr at 60% maximum oxygen uptake. *Significantly faster than 10% CHO trials; **Significantly faster than 4.3% MCT trials. (Adapted with permission from Van Zyl CG, et al. Effects of medium-chain triglyceride ingestion on fuel metabolism and cycling performance. *J Appl Physiol*. 1996;80:2217. ©The American Physiological Society (APS). All rights reserved. Photo: Pavel1964/Shutterstock.)

beverage with only MCTs produced an 8% decrement in performance (in agreement with another study), but the combined carbohydrate plus MCT solution consumed throughout the activity produced only a 2.5% cycling speed improvement compared with the two other conditions. This ergogenic effect occurred with reduced total carbohydrate oxidation at a given oxygen uptake level, higher final circulating FFA and ketone levels, and lower final glucose and lactate concentrations.

The small ergogenic enhancement by MCT supplementation probably occurred because this exogenous fatty acid source contributes relatively little to the total energy expenditure (and total lipid oxidation) during sustained effort.[137] MCT ingestion does not stimulate release of bile, the gall bladder's fat-emulsifying agent. Consequently, cramping and diarrhea often accompany excess intake of this lipid. It provides little ergogenic effect.[127]

Pyruvate

Ergogenic effects have been extolled for pyruvate, the three-carbon end product of the cytoplasmic breakdown of glucose during glycolysis. Exogenous pyruvate, as a partial replacement for dietary carbohydrate, supposedly augments endurance performance and promotes fat loss. Pyruvic acid, a relatively unstable chemical, causes intestinal distress, so various forms of the salt of this acid that includes sodium, potassium, calcium, or magnesium pyruvate are manufactured in capsule, tablet, or powder form. Dosage recommendations range between a total of 2 and 5 g pyruvate spread throughout the day and taken with meals. One capsule usually contains 600 mg pyruvate. The calcium form of pyruvate also contains about 80 mg calcium with 600 mg pyruvate. Some advertisements recommend a one capsule dosage per 9.1 kg/20 lb body weight. Manufacturers also combine creatine monohydrate and pyruvate; 1 g creatine pyruvate provides about 80 mg creatine and 400 mg pyruvate. Recommended pyruvate dosages range from 5 to 20 g daily. Pyruvate content in the normal diet ranges from 100 to 2000 mg daily. The largest dietary amounts occur in fruits and vegetables, particularly red apples (500 mg each), with smaller quantities in dark beer (80 mg per 12 oz) and red wine (75 mg per 6 oz).

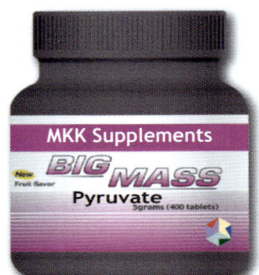

Endurance Performance

Reports indicate beneficial effects of exogenous pyruvate on endurance performance. Two double-blind, crossover studies by the same laboratory showed that 7 days daily supplementation with 100-g mixture pyruvate (25 g) plus 75 g dihydroxyacetone (DHA, another three-carbon compound of glycolysis) increased upper-body and lower-body aerobic endurance by 20% compared with exercise and 100 g supplement of an isocaloric glucose polymer.[247,248] The pyruvate-DHA mixture increased cycle ergometer time to exhaustion in the legs by 13 min (66 vs. 79 min), while upper-body arm-cranking time increased by 27 min (133 vs. 160 min). Exercising with the pyruvate-DHA mixture reduced local muscle and overall body ratings of perceived exertion compared with the placebo condition.[225]

Pyruvate supplementation advocates maintain that elevated extracellular pyruvate augments glucose transport into active muscle. Enhanced "glucose extraction" from the blood provides the important energy source to sustain intense aerobic effort while conserving intramuscular glycogen stores.[131] When the individual's diet contains a normal level of carbohydrate (approximately 55% total energy intake), pyruvate supplementation also increases pre-exercise muscle glycogen levels.[248,249] Both effects—higher pre-exercise glycogen levels and facilitated glucose uptake and oxidation by active muscle—benefit endurance similarly as pre-exercise carbohydrate loading and glucose feedings during exercise exert ergogenic effects.[344]

Body Fat Loss

Consuming pyruvate augments body fat loss when accompanied by a low-calorie diet. Overfat females in a metabolic ward maintained a liquid 1000 kcal daily energy intake (68% carbohydrate, 22% protein, 10% lipid). Adding 20 g sodium pyruvate plus 16 g calcium pyruvate, equal to 13% of energy intake daily for 3 wk, induced greater weight loss (5.9 kg/13.0 lb vs. 4.3 kg/9.5 lb) and fat loss (4.0 kg/8.8 lb vs. 2.7 kg/5.9 lb) than a control group on the same diet but who received an equivalent amount of extra energy as glucose.[250] These findings with obese subjects showed that adding DHA and pyruvate (substituted as equivalent energy for glucose) to a severely restricted low-energy diet facilitated body weight and fat loss without increasing nitrogen loss.[251] Consuming pyruvate may stimulate small increases in futile metabolic activity where metabolism does not couple to ATP production with a subsequent wasting of energy. *Until studies from independent laboratories reproduce existing findings for physical performance and body fat loss, one should view pyruvate supplementation effectiveness with caution.*[84,299]

Summary

1. The term *ergogenic aid* describes substances or procedures to improve physical work capacity, physiologic function, or athletic performance.
2. AAS consist of pharmacologic agents frequently used for ergogenic purposes. These drugs function like the hormone testosterone; they increase muscle size, strength, and power with resistance training in some individuals.
3. Anabolic steroids stimulate protein synthesis by binding with androgen receptor sites on the cells and influence the muscle cell nucleus to create protein.
4. The mTOR pathway creates more muscle protein by a mechanism that does not involve the muscle cell nucleus.
5. Anabolic steroids increase both muscle satellite cells and cell nuclei formation.
6. Anabolic steroid use in female athletes is relatively common (as with males), but objective data are rare on AAS use in female athletes compared to well-documented data in males.
7. AAS abuse has become commonplace in almost all sports in international competitions, particularly the Olympic Games, since their first use at the 1952 Helsinki Summer Olympics.
8. The β_2-adrenergic agonists clenbuterol and albuterol increase skeletal muscle mass and slow fat gain in animals to counter aging, immobilization, malnutrition, and tissue-wasting pathology.
9. Debate exists about whether administration of growth hormone to healthy individuals augments muscular hypertrophy when combined with resistance training. Health risks exist for those who abuse this chemical.
10. DHEA, a relatively weak steroid hormone synthesized from cholesterol by the adrenal cortex, steadily decreases throughout adulthood, prompting individuals to supplement, hoping to counteract the effects of natural aging. DHEA does not produce ergogenic effects.
11. Research indicates no effect of androstenedione supplementation on basal serum testosterone concentration or training response to increase muscle size, strength, and body composition.

12. No ergogenic effects exist for healthy subjects from chronic oral amino acid supplements on hormone secretion, training responsiveness, or physical performance.
13. Hormonal dynamics from carbohydrate and/or protein supplementation immediately following a resistance-exercise workout suggests an ergogenic effect on training responsiveness.
14. Amphetamines, or pep pills, do not aid physical performance or psychomotor skills, other than by a placebo effect. Adverse effects include drug dependency, headache, dizziness, confusion, and gastrointestinal distress.
15. Caffeine ingestion typically exerts an ergogenic effect by extending endurance in aerobic activity from increased lipid use for energy and conservation of glycogen reserves.
16. No compelling evidence supports ginseng supplementation to benefit physiologic function or exercise performance. Significant health risks accompany ephedrine use.
17. Concentrated buffering solutions consumed before physical activity improve anaerobic exercise performance.
18. Further research must determine the benefits and risks of glutamine, PS, and HMB to provide a "natural" anabolic boost with resistance training.
19. The additional blood volume and increased red cell mass and concentration from red blood cell reinfusion contribute to a larger maximum cardiac output and an increase in the blood's oxygen-carrying capacity and $\dot{V}O_{2max}$.
20. A physiologic rationale for why warm-up should enhance exercise performance includes benefits on muscle-shortening velocity and efficiency, enhanced oxygen delivery and use, and facilitated nerve impulse transmission.
21. Moderate warm-up proves beneficial immediately before sudden, strenuous exertion by reducing myocardial work and augmenting coronary blood flow when activity begins.
22. Breathing hyperoxic gas during physical activity extends endurance by increasing oxygen uptake, reducing blood lactate, and lowering pulmonary ventilation but provides no ergogenic effect before or after exercise.
23. Carbohydrate loading augments endurance in prolonged submaximal effort. Athletes should be well informed about this procedure because of potential negative effects.
24. A modification of the classic loading procedure provides the same high level of glycogen storage without dramatic alterations in the diet and exercise routine.
25. No benefits emerge from chromium supplements on training-related changes in muscular strength, physique, or muscle mass for individuals with adequate dietary chromium intake.
26. Creatine supplements increase intramuscular creatine and PCr, enhance brief anaerobic power output capacity, and facilitate recovery from repeated bouts of intense physical effort.
27. MCTs enhance lipid oxidation and conserve glycogen during endurance activity. This procedure enhances performance by an additional 2.5%.
28. Pyruvate supplementation purportedly augments endurance performance and promotes fat loss, but definitive conclusions concerning the supplement's effectiveness requires further verification.

Key Terms

Acromegaly: Excessive hormone production following growth cessation produces an irreversible disorder that presents as enlarged hands, feet, and facial features

Amphetamines: Pharmacologic compounds ("pep pills) exert powerful stimulating effects on central nervous system functions

Anabolic androgenic steroids (AAS): Pharmacologic agents function as testosterone to increase muscle size, strength, and power, usually with resistance training

Androstenedione: Intermediate precursor hormone between DHEA and testosterone produced by the adrenal glands and gonads and converted to testosterone enzymatically by 17α-hydroxysteroid dehydrogenase

Autologous transfusion: Withdrawing and reinfusing the same person's blood

β-Alanine: N-Proteogenic amino produced naturally in the body combines with the amino acid histidine to form dipeptide carnosine

β-Hydroxy-β-methylbutyrate (HMB): Bioactive metabolite generated in degrading the essential branched-chain amino acid leucine

Caffeine: A white, crystalline, bitter alkaloid substance found naturally in coffee beans, tea leaves, chocolate, cocoa beans, and cola nuts and used either as a drug (over-the-counter for migraine headaches), food (in chocolate and soft drinks), or dietary supplement (stimulant products and diuretics)

Caffeinism: Adverse effects when overconsuming caffeine can produce restlessness, headaches, insomnia, nervous irritability, elevated heart rate, and blood pressure

Carbohydrate loading: Procedure produces considerably higher "packing" of muscle glycogen than maintaining a high-carbohydrate diet; also known as glycogen supercompensation

Clenbuterol: $β_2$-Adrenergic agonist purports to have tissue-building, fat-reducing benefits, facilitating adrenergic receptor responsiveness to circulating epinephrine, norepinephrine, and other adrenergic amines

Chylomicron: Lipoprotein rich in triacylglycerol from lipid digestion and assimilation

Chromium picolinate: Salt of the trace metallic element chromium (Cr) essential in glucose metabolism, often touted in supplement form to promote muscle growth, curb appetite, and foster favorable body composition changes

Creatine monohydrate: Supplemental creatine substance sold as a powder, tablet, capsule, and stabilized liquid is a nitrogen-containing organic compound formed in the kidneys, liver, and pancreas from the nonessential amino acids arginine, glycine, and methionine

Creutzfeldt-Jakob disease: Rare, degenerative, fatal brain disorder affects about one person in every one million each year worldwide

CRISPR-Cas9: Unique gene editing technique allows for highly specific and rapid removal, addition, or alteration targeting gene sequences in a genome's DNA, with Cas9 referring to the DNA-cutting enzyme

Ephedrine: Potent amphetaminelike alkaloid compound with sympathomimetic physiologic effects present in several plant ephedra species (dried plant stem called ma huang [ma wong; *Ephedra sinica*])

Ergogenic aids: Substances or procedures that improve physical work capacity, physiologic function, or athletic performance

Gene doping: Manipulating human genes by inserting DNA into cells to produce desirable physical and mental characteristics

General warm-up: Body movements or "loosening-up" activities unrelated to specific neuromuscular actions in the anticipated performance

Gigantism: Endocrine and metabolic disorder characterized by abnormal size or overgrowth of the entire body or any of its parts

Ginseng: Different varieties of a short, slow-growing Asian plant with fleshy roots

Glutamine: Most abundant amino acid in plasma and skeletal muscle accounts for more than half of the muscles' free amino acid pool

Gynecomastia: Excessive male mammary gland development often occurring with chronic anabolic steroid use

Half-life: Time required for the reactant concentration to decrease to half its initial value

Hemoconcentration: Decrease in plasma volume simultaneously increases red blood cell concentration and other commonly tested blood constituents

Homologous transfusion: Infuses a type-matched donor's blood

Human growth hormone (GH or hGH): Potent anabolic and lipolytic agent produced by the pituitary gland's adenohypophysis for tissue-building processes and overall growth

Hyperoxic gas mixtures: Breathing gases with a higher-than-normal oxygen concentration

Hypogonadism: Inadequate testosterone production during masculine growth and development in puberty

Leucine: Dietary amino acid directly stimulates myofibrillar muscle protein synthesis

LD$_{50}$: Lethal oral caffeine dose required to kill 50% of the population (10 g per 150 mg · kg^{-1} at 70-kg/154-lb body weight)

Medium-chain triacylglycerols (MCTs): Contain saturated fatty acids with 8 to 10 carbon atoms along the fatty acid chain

Modified loading procedure: Increases glycogen synthase activity without requiring dramatic glycogen depletion with exercise to increase glycogen storage to nearly the same level as the classic loading procedure

Mammalian target of rapamycin (mTOR): Created by a protein coding gene to regulate translation in the cell nucleus

Peliosis hepatitis: Potentially fatal liver disease characterized by localized blood-filled lesions

Performance-enhancing drugs (PEDs): Substances used illicitly to improve athletic performance

Phosphatidylserine (PS): Glycerophospholipid belonging to a class of natural lipids that help form the plasma membrane's internal layer surrounding all cells

Prohormones: Naturally derived precursors to testosterone or other anabolic steroids serve as intermediate substances in the hormone-building process

Pyramiding: Progressively increasing drug dosage in 6- to 12-wk cycles during a training regimen outside the competition period

Pseudoephedrine: Sympathomimetic drug belonging to the phenethylamine and amphetamine chemical classes

Red blood cell reinfusion: Withdrawing 1 to 4 units whole blood (1 unit = 450 mL) and immediately reinfusing the plasma, then freezing the packed red blood cells for later infusion

Specific warm-up: Big-muscle, rhythmic movements provide a skill rehearsal for the activity

Stacking: Combining multiple androgenic substances simultaneously to create increased anabolic effects

Sympathomimetic β$_2$-adrenergic agonists: β$_2$-Adrenergic receptor agonists that act on the β$_2$-adrenergic receptor to cause smooth muscle relaxation

Upper respiratory tract infection (URTI): Acute infection involving the nose, sinuses, pharynx, or larynx

Virilization: Female develops characteristics associated with male androgenic hormones

References are available online at Lippincott Connect.

Additional References

Adami PE, et al. Cardiovascular effects of doping substances, commonly prescribed medications and ergogenic aids in relation to sports: a position statement of the sport cardiology and exercise nucleus of the European Association of Preventive Cardiology. *Eur J Prev Cardiol*. 2022:zwab198.

Blum TR, et al. Phage-assisted evolution of botulinum neurotoxin proteases with reprogrammed specificity. *Science*. 2021; 371:803.

Burgos J, et al. Long-term combined effects of citrulline and nitrate-rich beetroot extract supplementation on recovery status in trained male triathletes: a randomized, double-blind, placebo-controlled trial. *Biology (Basel)*. 2022;11:75.

Collins FS, et al. Human molecular genetics and genomics—important advances and exciting possibilities. *N Engl J Med*. 2021;384:1.

Corona G, et al. Consequences of anabolic-androgenic steroid abuse in males; sexual and reproductive perspective. *World J Mens Health*. 2021. doi:10.5534/wjmh.210021.

Ding JB, et al. Anabolic-androgenic steroid misuse: mechanisms, patterns of misuse, user typology, and adverse effects. *J Sports Med (Hindawi Publ Corp)*. 2021;2021:7497346.

Dobrowolski H, et al. Nutrition for female soccer players-recommendations. *Medicina (Kaunas)*. 2020;56:28.

Doudna JA. The promise and challenge of therapeutic genome editing. *Nature*. 2020;578:229.

Dvorak AV, et al. An atlas for human brain myelin content throughout the adult life span. *Sci Rep*. 2021;11:269.

Esposito M, et al. Forensic post-mortem investigation in AAS abusers: investigative diagnostic protocol. A systematic review. *Diagnostics (Basel)*. 2021;11:1307.

Fell JM, et al. Carbohydrate improves exercise capacity but does not affect subcellular lipid droplet morphology, AMPK and p53 signaling in human skeletal muscle. *J Physiol*. 2021;599:2823.

Gharahdaghi N, et al. Links between testosterone, oestrogen, and the growth hormone/insulin-like growth factor axis and resistance exercise muscle adaptations. *Front Physiol*. 2021;11:621226.

Hauger LE, et al. Anabolic androgenic steroids, antisocial personality traits, aggression and violence. *Drug Alcohol Depend*. 2021;221:108604.

Havnes IA, et al. Anabolic-androgenic steroid use among women—a qualitative study on experiences of masculinizing, gonadal and sexual effects. *Int J Drug Policy*. 2021;95:102876.

Hlinský T, et al. Effects of dietary nitrates on time trial performance in athletes with different training status: systematic review. *Nutrients*. 2020;12:2734.

Honceriu C, et al. Connections between different sports and ergogenic aids-focusing on salivary cortisol and amylase. *Medicina (Kaunas)*. 2021;57:753.

Huml L, et al. Advances in the determination of anabolic-androgenic steroids: from standard practices to tailor-designed multidisciplinary approaches. *Sensors (Basel)*. 2021;22:4.

Kraemer WJ, et al. Growth hormone(s), testosterone, insulin-like growth factors, and cortisol: roles and integration for cellular development and growth with exercise. *Front Endocrinol (Lausanne)*. 2020;11:33.

Kreider RB, Stout JR. Creatine in health and disease. *Nutrients*. 2021;13:447.

Krzywański J, et al. Elite athletes with COVID-19—predictors of the course of disease. *J Sci Med Sport*. 2022;25:9.

Lamon S, et al. The effect of acute sleep deprivation on skeletal muscle protein synthesis and the hormonal environment. *Physiol Rep*. 2021;9:e14660.

Lima-Silva AE, et al. Caffeine during high-intensity whole-body exercise: an integrative approach beyond the central nervous system. *Nutrients*. 2021;13:2503.

Manoochehri Z, et al. Random forest model to identify factors associated with anabolic-androgenic steroid use. *BMC Sports Sci Med Rehabil*. 2021;13:30.

Martínez-Sanz JM, et al. Nutrition-related adverse outcomes in endurance sports competitions: a review of incidence and practical recommendations. *Int J Environ Res Public Health*. 2020;17:4082.

McCullough D, et al. How the love of muscle can break a heart: impact of anabolic androgenic steroids on skeletal muscle hypertrophy, metabolic and cardiovascular health. *Rev Endocr Metab Disord*. 2021;22:389.

Perry JC, et al. Anabolic steroids and cardiovascular outcomes: the controversy. *Cureus*. 2020;12:e9333.

Płoszczyca K, et al. Effects of short-term phosphate loading on aerobic capacity under acute hypoxia in cyclists: a randomized, placebo-controlled, crossover study. *Nutrients*. 2022;14:236.

Roşca AE, et al. Effects of exogenous androgens on platelet activity and their thrombogenic potential in supraphysiological administration: a literature review. *J Clin Med*. 2021;10:147.

Rothschild JA, et al. Effects of dietary supplements on adaptations to endurance training. *Sports Med*. 2020;50:25.

Sarzynski MA, Bouchard C. World-class athletic performance and genetic endowment. *Nat Metab*. 2020;2:796.

Shawish MI, et al. Effect of atorvastatin on testosterone levels. *Cochrane Database Syst Rev*. 2021;(1):CD013211.

Shivram H, et al. Controlling and enhancing CRISPR systems. *Nat Chem Biol*. 2021;17:10.

Smith SJ, et al. Examining the effects of herbs on testosterone concentrations in men: a systematic review. *Adv Nutr*. 2021;12:744.

Tallis J, et al. The prevalence and practices of caffeine use as an ergogenic aid in English professional soccer. *Biol Sport*. 2021;38:525.

Torrisi M, et al. Sudden cardiac death in anabolic-androgenic steroid users: a literature review. *Medicina (Kaunas)*. 2020;56:587.

Vancini RL, et al. Knowledge and prevalence of supplements used by Brazilian resistance training practitioners before coronavirus outbreak. *Open Access J Sports Med*. 2021;12:139.

Wagener F, et al. Investigations into the elimination profiles and metabolite ratios of micro-dosed selective androgen receptor modulator LGD-4033 for doping control purposes. *Anal Bioanal Chem*. 2022;414:1151.

Wax B, et al. Creatine for exercise and sports performance, with recovery considerations for healthy populations. *Nutrients*. 2021;13:1915.

Yi JY, et al. New application of the CRISPR-Cas9 system for site-specific exogenous gene doping analysis. *Drug Test Anal*. 2021;13:871.

Yinghao L, et al. Effects of a blood flow restriction exercise under different pressures on testosterone, growth hormone, and insulin-like growth factor levels. *J Int Med Res*. 2021;49:3000605211039564.

Table 23.1 Levels of Evidence on Which to Judge Research Findings

Evidence Category	Source of Evidence	Definition and Comment
I	Randomized controlled trials (RCTs) involving a rich body of data	Evidence from end points of well-designed RCTs (or trials that depart only minimally from randomization) that provide a consistent pattern of findings in the population for which the recommendation is made. Requires substantial number of participants. Very high confidence in findings.
II	RCTs involving a limited body of data	Evidence from endpoint of intervention studies that include only a limited number of RCTs, post hoc or subgroup analysis of RCTs, or meta-analysis of RCTs. In general, this line of evidence is less convincing than level I because of some inconsistency in the results between studies.
III	Nonrandomized trials and observational studies	Evidence derived from outcomes of uncontrolled or nonrandomized trials or from observational studies.
IV	Panel consensus judgment	Expert judgment derived from experimental research described in the literature and/or derived from the consensus of panel members based on clinical experience or knowledge that does not meet the above listed criteria on other levels. This category is used only in cases where the provision of some guidance was deemed valuable but an adequately compelling clinical literature addressing the subject of the recommendation was deemed insufficient to justify placement in one of the other categories (I or III).

Table 23.2 Relationships Between Pre-Exercise Testosterone Concentration and Selected Nutritional Variables

Nutrient	Correlation with Testosterone[a]
Energy, kJ	−0.18
Protein, %[b]	−0.71*
CHO, %[b]	−0.30
Lipid, %[b]	0.72*
SFA, g 1000 kcal^{-1} · d^{-1}	0.77[†]
MUFA, g 1000 kcal^{-1} · d^{-1}	0.79[‡]
PUFA, g 1000 kcal^{-1} · d^{-1}	0.25
Cholesterol, g 1000 kcal^{-1} · d^{-1}	0.53
PUFA/SFA	−0.63[‡]
Dietary fiber, g 1000 kcal^{-1} · d^{-1}	−0.19
Protein/CHO	−0.59[‡]
Protein/lipid	0.16
CHO/lipid	0.16

*$p \leq .01$; [†]$p \leq .005$; [‡]$p \leq .05$.
[a]Pearson product-moment correlations.
[b]Nutrient percentage values expressed as percentage of total energy per day.
SFA, saturated fatty acids; MUFA, monounsaturated fatty acids; PUFA, polyunsaturated fatty acids; CHO, carbohydrate.
Reprinted from Volek JS, et al. Testosterone and cortisol in relationship to dietary nutrients and resistance exercise. *J Appl Physiol*. ©The American Physiological Society (APS). All rights reserved.1997;82:49.

SECTION 5

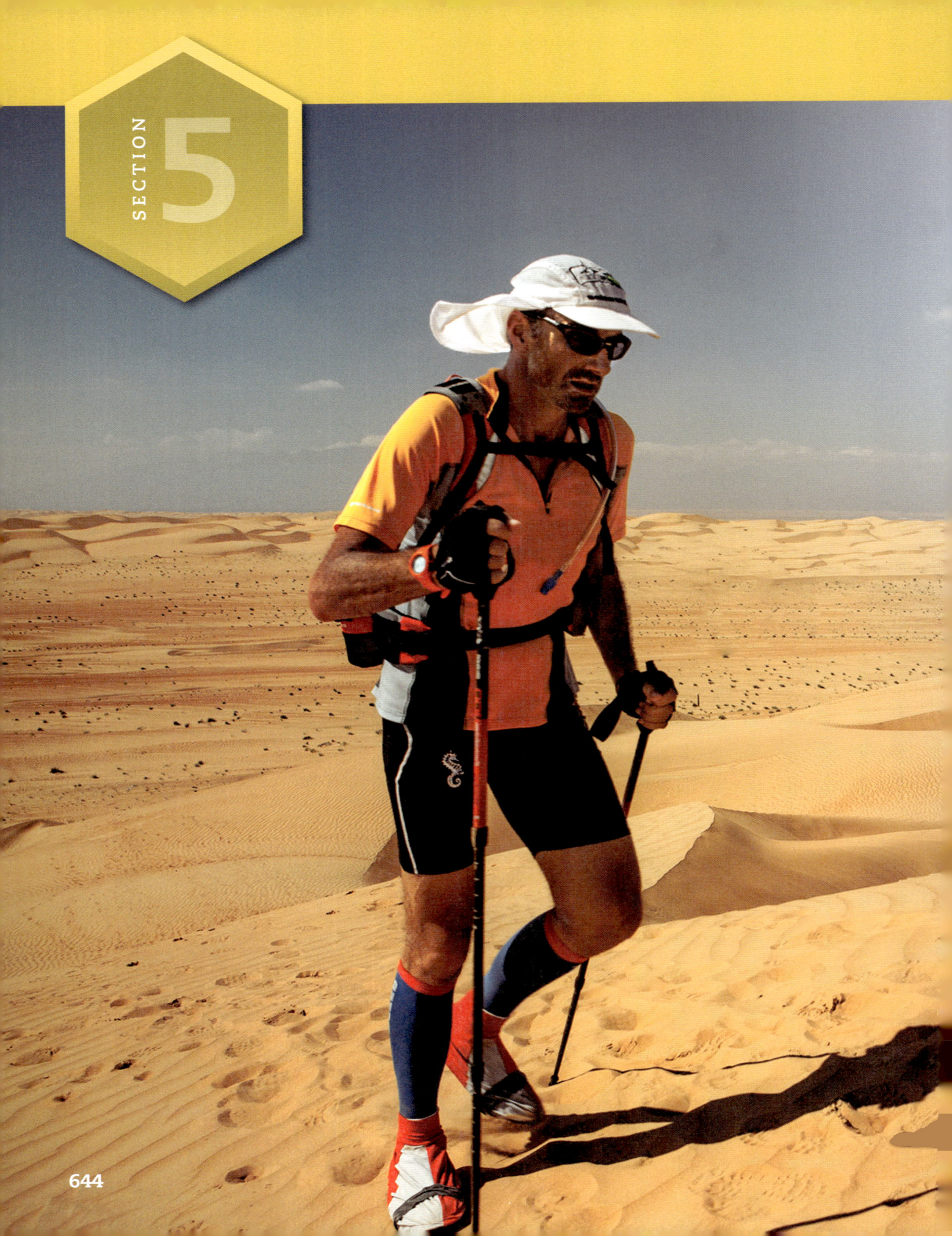

Exercise Performance and Environmental Stress

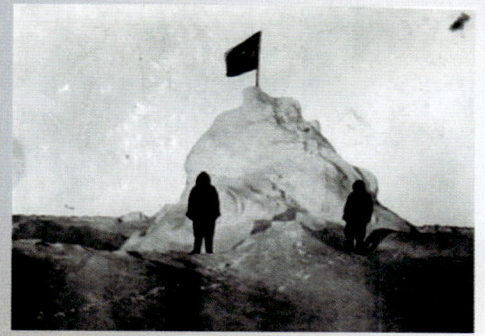

Image from Naval History and Heritage Command
https://www.history.navy.mil/

The true explorer does his work not for any hopes of reward or honor, but because the thing he has set for himself to do is a part of his being, and must be accomplished for the sake of the accomplishment. And he counts lightly hardships, risks, obstacles, if only they do not bar him from his goal.

—Rear Admiral Robert E. Peary (1856–1920), *American polar explorer who discovered the North Pole*

Overview

Sport activities often take place at terrestrial elevations that impair oxygenation of blood flowing through the lungs, which severely limits aerobic exercise energy metabolism. At the opposite extreme, exploration beneath the water's surface poses a different challenge. Divers must transport their sea-level environment in a gas mixture compressed in a scuba tank carried on the back. Some diving enthusiasts use no external assistance, and the underwater excursion time becomes limited by two factors:

1. Inhaled air quantity into the lungs just before the dive
2. Arterial carbon dioxide buildup during the dive

In both breath-hold diving and scuba diving, the environment presents unique challenges and dangers for participants, independently from exercise stress.

Consideration also must focus on the environment's thermal quality. On land, exercising in a hot, humid environment or extreme cold poses severe stress, which can impair exercise capacity and pose an ominous threat to health and safety. Space exploration and accompanying short- and long-term exposures to near-zero gravity produce potent environmental stressors that negatively impact physiologic function, structural mass, and exercise capacity during the mission and the return to terresterial gravity. How each environmental stressor deviates from neutral conditions and the exposure duration determine the total impact on the body. Combined, simultaneous shared stressors (e.g., extreme cold and high altitude exposure) may exceed the additive consequence each stressor imposes separately.

In the four chapters that follow, we explore the specific problems encountered at altitude (Chapter 24), during exercise in hot and cold environments (Chapter 25), and from prolonged microgravity (Chapter 27). We also examine the immediate physiologic adjustments and long-term adaptations as the body struggles to maintain internal consistency despite combined environmental encounters. Chapter 26, on sport diving, assesses the exclusive problems associated with this increasingly popular recreational activity.

Chapter 24: Physical Activity at Medium and High Altitude

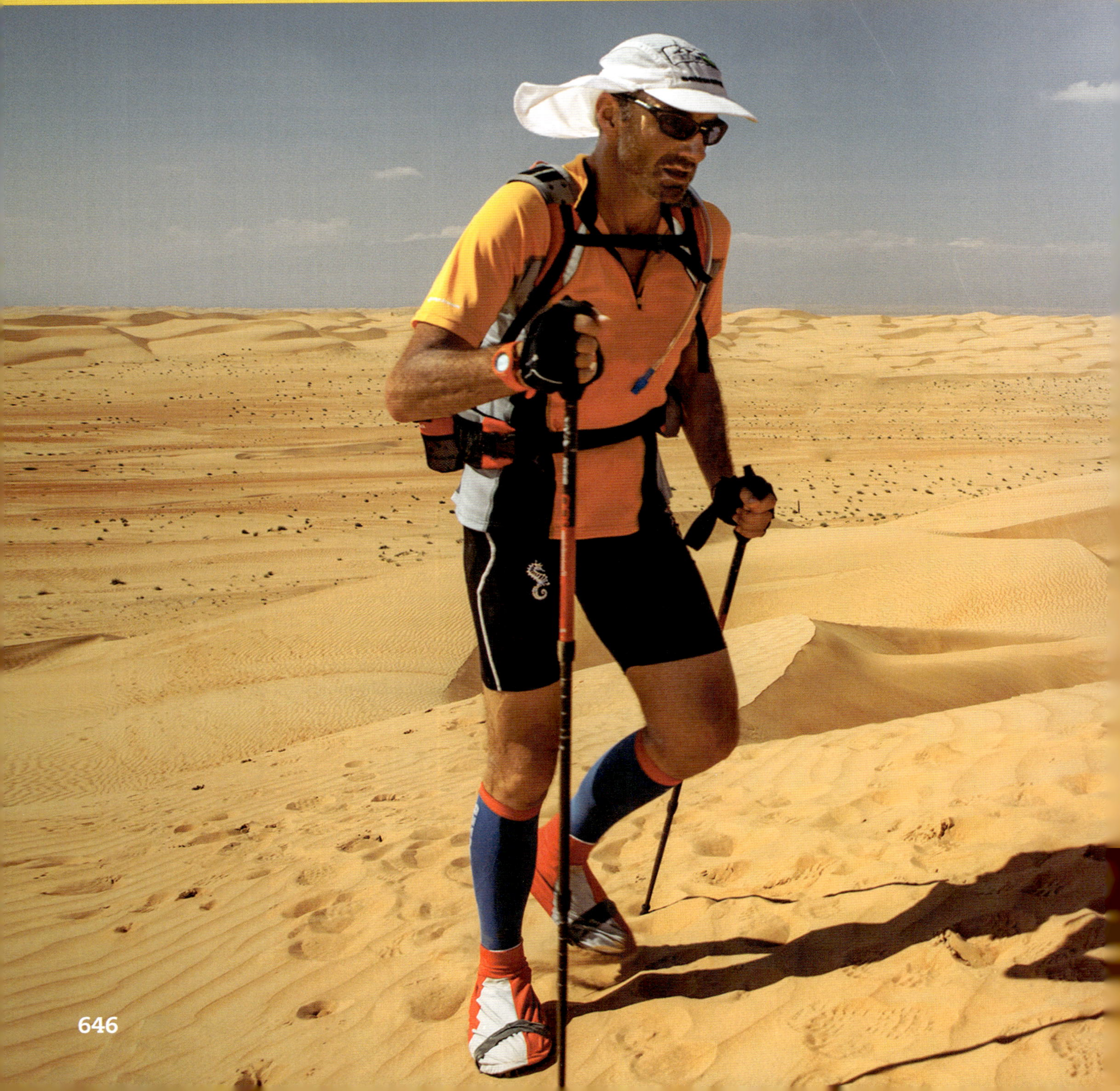

Chapter Objectives

- Outline the effects of increasingly higher altitudes on these three factors: oxygen partial pressure in ambient air, hemoglobin oxygen saturation in pulmonary capillaries, and maximum oxygen uptake ($\dot{V}O_{2max}$)
- Describe and quantify the oxygen transport cascade at sea level and 4300 m/14,108 ft
- Discuss two immediate and two longer-term physiologic adjustments to altitude exposure
- Give symptoms, possible causes, and treatment for acute mountain sickness, high-altitude pulmonary edema, and high-altitude cerebral edema
- Describe the lactate paradox and possible causes for its occurrence
- Summarize factors that affect the time course for altitude acclimatization
- Graph the relationship between increasing altitude exposure and the decrease in $\dot{V}O_{2max}$ (% sea-level value)
- Discuss two main alterations in circulatory function that offset the altitude acclimatization benefits on oxygen transport capacity
- Discuss whether altitude training produces greater improvement than sea-level training on sea-level exercise performance
- Describe the "living high, training low" training concept

Ancillaries at-a-Glance

Visit Lippincott Connect to access the following resources.

- References: Chapter 24
- Focus on Research: High Altitude—A Hostile Environment

More than 40 million people live, work, and recreate at terrestrial elevations between 3048 m/10,000 ft and 5486 m/18,000 ft above sea level. Based on the Earth's topography, these elevations encompass the range generally considered high altitude. High-altitude natives inhabit permanent settlements up to 5486 m in the Andes and Himalayas.[120] Prolonged exposure for an unacclimated person to this altitude causes death from the ambient air's subnormal oxygen pressure (hypoxia), even if the person remains physically inactive. The physiologic challenge from even medium-altitude exposure becomes readily apparent during physical activity.[11]

In the United States, more than 1 million people a year ascend Pikes Peak, Colorado (4300 m/14,108 ft), the most visited mountain peak in North America and second most visited in the world, by train, car, or railroad and by climbing, cycling, and running. Before the tourist boom, female researcher Mabel Purefoy Fitzgerald (1911–1973), who was permitted to attend lectures at Oxford, England, in the late 1890s (women were not allowed to formally enroll), teamed up with physiologist J.S. Haldane (see Introduction: A View From the Past) for his research expedition to Pikes Peak in 1911 (www.ncbi.nlm.nih.gov/pmc/articles/PMC4321126/). Fitzgerald learned how to use his Haldane apparatus to test carbon dioxide pressure in the human lung. Fitzgerald measured hemoglobin and alveolar air from herself and mining staff at altitudes from 1830 to 3810 m/6000 to 12,500 ft and conducted other studies at lower altitudes (1220 m/4000 ft) in nearby mining towns.

The unnumbered image shows Fitzgerald and colleagues (left to right: J.S. Haldane, M.P. Fitzgerald, E.C. Schneider, Y. Henderson, C.G. Douglas) at lower altitudes. The other inset image below shows expedition team member Douglas wearing his "Douglas bag" to collect expired air samples after several minutes upon reaching the Pikes Peak summit. At the time of her research, equipment was transmitted by stagecoach and two horses along a wagon road up to 2895.6 m/9500 ft, continuing on horseback for the final 610 m/2000 ft to the summit. Her results presented pioneering evidence of oxygen's role in the breathing process. One expedition researcher summarized her accomplishments: "She went to great heights to achieve her goals in science." Oxford University awarded her the Master of Arts degree at the age of 100, the oldest physiologist so honored!

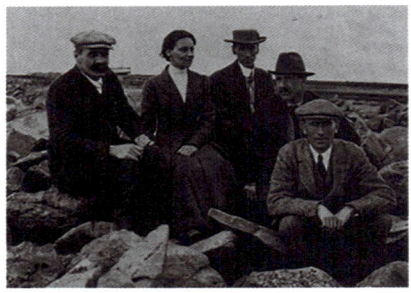
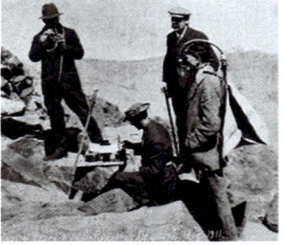

Almost 50 million people worldwide ascend to high altitudes for mountaineering, trekking, tourism, business, and scientific and military excursions. Many altitude newcomers do not take sufficient time to acclimatize to the physiologic challenge of oxygen's reduced partial pressure (P_{O_2}) in ambient air.

Altitude Stressors

Altitude's physiologic challenge comes directly from decreased ambient P_{O_2}, not from reduced total barometric pressure per se or any change in relative gas concentrations (percentages) in inspired (ambient) air. **FIGURE 24.1** illustrates the barometric pressures of respired gases, and percentage hemoglobin saturation at various terrestrial elevations from Denver, CO to Mt. Everest. The dashed line shows the upper limit for permanent residence, the highest being about 4572 m/15,000 ft in the mountainous Aguada Quilcha, region of Chile, a sparsely populated region with only 26 inhabitants per mile. Along the left axis, note the various maladies ranging from mild headache and lightheadedness one might experience around Boulder, CO (1520 m/5000 ft), to possible impending collapse near the Mt. Everest vicinity (7600 m/25,000 ft). Compared to sea level ambient 760 mm Hg barometric pressure, the ambient pressure at Aguada Quilcha is reduced by nearly one-half. **FIGURE 24.2** shows changes that occur in oxygen availability (reflected by P_{O_2}) in ambient air, alveolar air, and arterial and mixed venous blood as one ascends from sea level to Pikes Peak. The oxygen transport cascade refers to the progressive change in the oxygen pressure and in various body areas as oxygen moves from the alveoli to the tissue capillaries.

Air density decreases progressively with ascent above sea level. For example, barometric pressure at sea level averages 760 mm Hg; at 3048 m/10,000 ft, the barometer drops to 510 mm Hg. At 5486 m/17,999 ft elevation, the air pressure at the Earth's surface equals about half its sea-level pressure. Dry ambient air at sea level and altitude contains 20.93% oxygen, while the P_{O_2} (oxygen molecule density) in air decreases directly with the fall in barometric pressure upon ascending to higher elevations ($P_{O_2} = 0.2093 \times$ barometric pressure). Thus, ambient P_{O_2} at sea level averages 150 mm Hg, but only 107 mm Hg at 3048 m/10,000 ft. At the Mt. Everest (8848 m/29,028 ft) summit, ambient air pressure usually ranges between 251 and 253 mm Hg with a concomitant alveolar P_{O_2} of about 25 mm Hg (ambient air P_{O_2} between 42 and 43 mm Hg).[110] This equals only about 30% of the oxygen available in air at sea level. *Arterial hypoxia that accompanies the reduction in P_{O_2} precipitates both the immediate physiologic adjustments to altitude and the longer-term acclimatization process.* Following the International Union of Physiological Sciences (www.iups.org) recommendation, acclimatization refers to adaptations produced by changes in the natural environment, whether through a change in season or residence. In contrast, acclimation concerns adaptations produced in a controlled laboratory environment (in specialized chambers) that simulate high altitude or microgravity, hypoxic environments, and thermal stress extremes.

Altitude m	Altitude ft	Ambient pressure mm Hg	Ambient PO_2 mm Hg
0	0	760	159
1000	3280	674	141
1500	4920	634	133
2000	6560	596	125
3000	9840	526	110
4000	13,120	462	97
5000	16,400	405	85
6000	19,690	354	74
7000	22,970	308	64
8000	26,250	267	56
9000	29,530	230	48

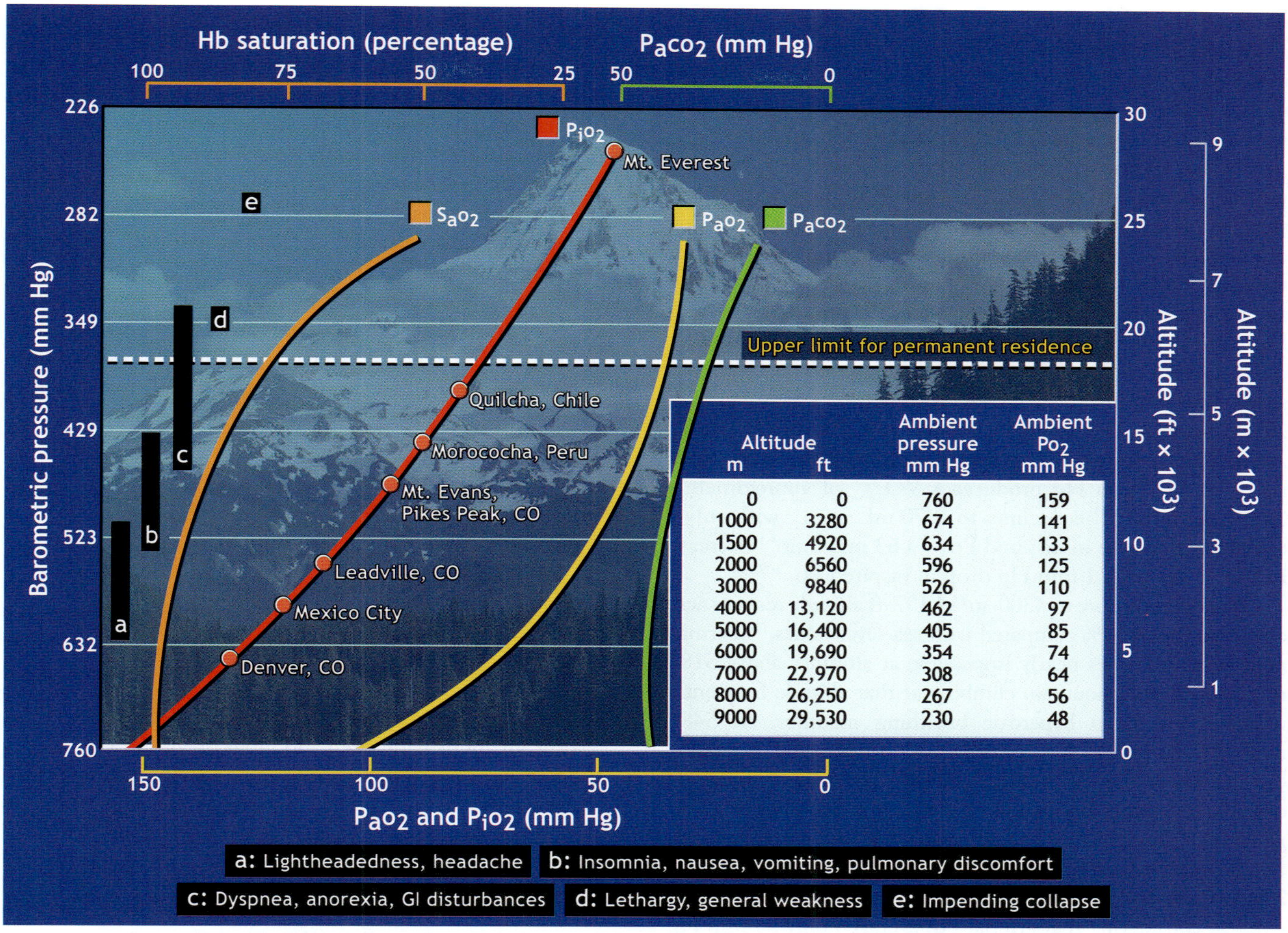

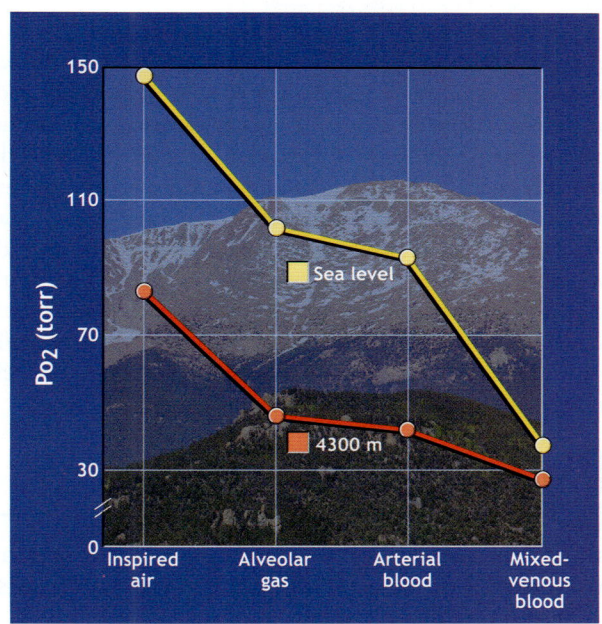

FIGURE 24.1. Changes in environmental and physiologic variables with progressive elevations at various terrestrial elevations from Denver, CO, to Mt. Everest. P_aCO_2, arterial carbon dioxide partial pressure; P_aO_2, arterial oxygen partial pressure; P_iO_2, oxygen partial pressure in inspired air; S_aO_2, hemoglobin oxygen saturation.

Oxygen Loading at Altitude

The S-shaped oxyhemoglobin dissociation curve (see Fig. 13.4) indicates that only a small change occurs in hemoglobin's percentage saturation with oxygen until a 3048-m/10,000-ft altitude. At 1981 m/6500 ft, for example, alveolar PO_2 decreases from 100 mm Hg sea-level value to 78 mm Hg, yet hemoglobin remains 90% saturated with oxygen. This relatively small arterial desaturation exerts little effect on a person during rest or mild physical activity, but severely curtails vigorous activities. Males and females performed relatively poorly in middle-distance and distance running and swimming during the 1968 Olympics in Mexico City (altitude 2300 m/7546 ft), the result of the small reduction in oxygen transport capacity at this altitude. No new world records were established in events lasting longer than 2.5 min. Altitude does *not* impair the short-term anaerobic energy system at moderate altitude (e.g., glycogen storage, glycolysis pathways, and corresponding phosphorylase and phosphofructokinase enzyme activity) or success in sprint-power activities such as sprint-running, speed skating, track cycling, jumping, and discus.[29,33] Performance in single bouts of these activities often improves because lower air density reduces air resistance or drag force more at altitude than at

FIGURE 24.2. Oxygen transport cascade from sea level to Pikes Peak, CO (4300 m/14,108 ft).
(Steve Boice/Shutterstock)

sea level. The lessened air resistance from a 24% reduction in air density at 2300 m/7546 ft should also improve performance in the shot-put, hammer throw, and javelin. Impaired performance has been reported for *repeated short-term power output intervals* (15 s intense training intervals) in elite athletes.[14]

In the transition from moderate altitude to higher elevations, values for alveolar (arterial) Po_2 position on the steep portion of the oxyhemoglobin dissociation curve. This dramatically reduces hemoglobin oxygenation and oxygen transport capacity and negatively affects even mild-intensity aerobic activities. At high elevations in the Andes and Himalayas, oxygen loading of hemoglobin decreases dramatically, and physical activity becomes difficult to sustain. Any small change in inspired Po_2 (i.e., barometric pressure) greatly affects aerobic capacity at the Mt. Everest summit. For well-acclimatized mountain climbers, breathing ambient air with a Po_2 of 48.5 mm Hg produces a $\dot{V}O_{2max}$ of approximately 1450 mL·min^{-1}. This declines to 1070 mL·min^{-1} with only a 6 mm Hg decrease in inspired Po_2—a 63 mL·min^{-1} decrease in $\dot{V}O_{2max}$ for each 1 mm Hg drop in inspired Po_2.[109,110]

Sudden exposure to 4300-m/14,197-ft altitude reduces aerobic capacity by 32% compared with sea-level values.[119] Permanent living becomes nearly impossible at altitudes above 5182 m/17,000 ft and mountain climbing at that altitude frequently requires help from hyperoxic breathing mixtures. At 5486 m/18,000 ft, arterial Po_2 averages 38 mm Hg, and hemoglobin maintains only 73% oxygen saturation. Amazingly, reports describe acclimatized mountaineers who lived for weeks at 6706 m/22,000 ft breathing only ambient air.[45] In fact, members from two Swiss expeditions to Mt. Everest remained at the summit for 2 hr without breathing equipment![74] This represents an impressive feat considering that arterial Po_2 averaged only 25 mm Hg with a corresponding 58% arterial blood oxygen saturation. An unacclimatized person becomes unconscious within 30 s under these conditions. For acclimatized men at simulated extreme altitudes that approach the Mt. Everest summit (8848 m/29,029 ft), $\dot{V}O_{2max}$ decreases by 70%, from 4.13 to 1.17 L·min^{-1}, or from 49.1 to 15.3 mL·kg^{-1}·min^{-1}.[35] These low values reflect the sea-level aerobic capacity for a sedentary 80-year-old man. In addition to impairment in oxygen transport capacity, high-altitude exposure impairs homeostatic regulation of immune balance; this potentially could favor long-term immunological alterations and increase infection risk.[27] In 2006, after 40 climbing days, Mark Inglis (https://en.wikipedia.org/wiki/Mark_Inglis) became the first double amputee to scale Mount Everest. Although remarkable performances at high altitude reflect exceptions and not the rule, they demonstrate the enormous adaptive human capability to survive and achieve extraordinary physical performances without external support at extreme terrestrial elevations.

INTEGRATIVE QUESTION

If altitude has such negative effects on the body, why are certain track and field records broken during competition at higher elevations?

Acclimatization

During the many years that mountaineers attempted to climb the world's highest peaks, they knew it required weeks to adjust to successively higher elevations. *The term altitude acclimatization broadly describes adaptive responses in physiology and metabolism that improve tolerance to altitude hypoxia.* Each adjustment to a higher elevation proceeds progressively, and full acclimatization requires an appropriate time period.[120,121] Successful adjustment to medium altitude affords only partial adjustment to a higher elevation. Moderate altitude residents, however, show less decrement in physiologic capacity and physical performance than lowlanders when both groups travel to a higher altitude.[62]

Immediate Responses to Altitude Exposure

Arrival at 2300-m/2546-ft elevations and higher initiates rapid physiologic adjustments to compensate for thinner air and accompanying reduction in alveolar Po_2. The two more important responses include:

1. Increase in the respiratory drive to produce hyperventilation, an abnormally deep and rapid breathing rate
2. Increase in blood flow during rest and submaximal physical activity

Hyperventilation

Hyperventilation from reduced arterial Po_2 reflects the most important and clear-cut immediate native lowlander response to altitude exposure. Once initiated, the "hypoxic drive" increases during the first few weeks and can remain elevated for a year or longer during prolonged altitude residence.[53] Prior to altitude exposure, specific respiratory muscle training is recommended for strengthening respiratory muscles and minimizing the adverse effects caused by hypoxia-related hyperventilation.[122] The aortic arch and branching carotid arteries in the neck contain peripheral chemoreceptors sensitive to reduced oxygen pressure. Reduced arterial Po_2 at altitudes above 2000 m/6562 ft progressively stimulates these receptors. This modifies inspiratory activity to increase alveolar ventilation, causing alveolar Po_2 to rise toward the level in ambient air. Even small increases in alveolar Po_2 with altitude hyperventilation facilitate oxygen loading in the lungs and provide a rapid defense against reduced ambient Po_2. Mountaineers who respond with a strong, hypoxic ventilatory drive to sudden but extreme altitude exposure perform physical tasks more effectively and reach higher altitude than climbers with a depressed hypoxic ventilatory response.[97] For females, variations in menstrual cycle phase do not affect ventilatory responses and performance decrements during short-term altitude exposure compared with sea level.[8]

IQ4 INTEGRATIVE QUESTION

From a physiologic perspective, what represents a safe altitude for flight in an airplane with a nonpressurized cabin?

Increased Cardiovascular Response

Resting systemic blood pressure increases during early altitude acclimatization. In addition, submaximal heart rate and cardiac output can rise to 50% above sea-level values, while the heart's stroke volume remains unchanged. The increased submaximal blood flow at altitude largely compensates for arterial desaturation. For example, a 10% increase in cardiac output during rest or moderate physical activity offsets a 10% reduction in arterial oxygen saturation in terms of total oxygen transported through the body. **FIGURE 24.3** shows that oxygen cost for cycling at a 100 watt submaximal effort at sea level and high altitude remains unchanged denoted by the dashed line at 2.0 $L \cdot min^{-1}$, but the relative strenuousness of effort to maintain this effort increases dramatically at altitude. In this example, submaximal exercise representing 50% sea-level $\dot{V}O_{2max}$ (orange bar on the left) equals 70% $\dot{V}O_{2max}$ at 4300 m/14,108 ft shown by the right orange bar.

Increased Catecholamine Response

With altitude exposure, sympathoadrenal activity progressively increases over time during rest and physical activity.[63,66,67] Increased blood pressure and heart rate coincide with the

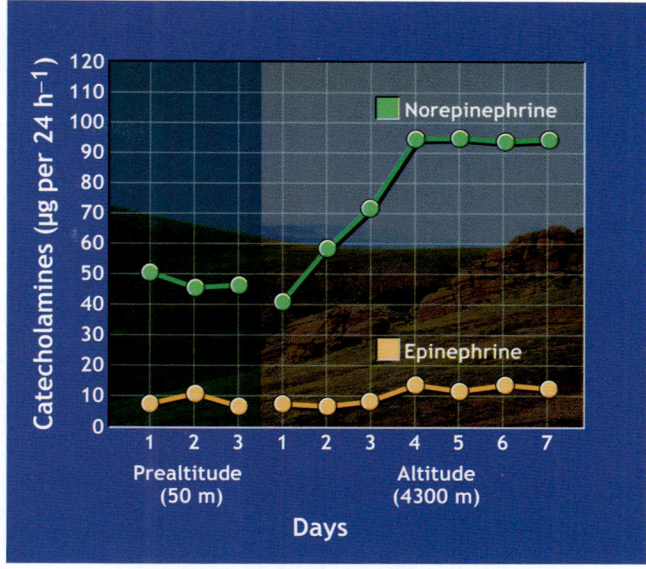

FIGURE 24.4. Generalized response for a short sojourn at 4300-m/14,108-ft altitude on urinary norepinephrine and epinephrine in eight male sea-level residents.
(Adapted from Surks MI, et al. Changes in plasma thyroxine concentration and metabolism, catecholamine excretion and basal oxygen uptake during acute exposure to high altitude. *J Clin Endocrinol Metab.* 1967;27:789. By permission of The Endocrine Society.)

steady rise in plasma levels and excretion rates of epinephrine. Norepinephrine levels peak in females and males after 6 days of high-altitude exposure and remain stable thereafter.[65,117] Increased sympathoadrenal activity also contributes to regulation of blood pressure, vascular resistance, and substrate mixture (enhanced carbohydrate use)[13] during short- and long-term hypobaric exposures. **FIGURE 24.4** shows 24-hr norepinephrine and epinephrine urinary excretion during control (sea-level) measurements and following 4300-m/14,108-ft exposure for 7 days. Epinephrine changed little but norepinephrine excretion increased considerably by the 4th day and remained elevated through day 7. Urinary norepinephrine levels remained elevated for approximately 1 wk following return to sea level.

TABLE 24.1 depicts metabolic and cardiorespiratory responses to moderate and maximal cycling in young men at sea level and during brief exposure to simulated 4000-m altitude. Arterial oxygen saturation decreased from 96% at sea level to 70% during all cycling intensities. In submaximal exercise, increased cardiac output entirely compensated for blood's reduced oxygen content. Greater blood flow occurred from a higher heart rate, while stroke volume remained unchanged. As cardiac output increased, submaximal oxygen uptake remained essentially identical both at sea level and altitude. The greatest altitude effect on aerobic metabolism occurred during maximal exertion when $\dot{V}O_{2max}$ decreased to 72% the sea-level value.

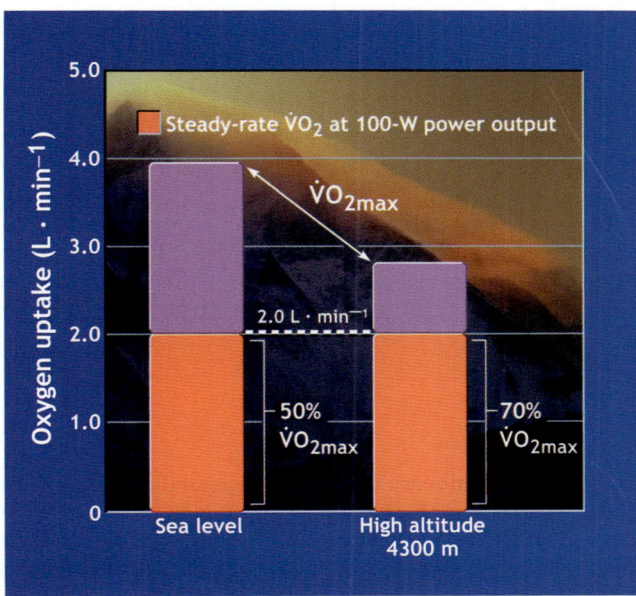

FIGURE 24.3. Oxygen cost and relative submaximal exercise strenuousness at sea level and high altitude (50% sea-level $\dot{V}O_{2max}$ = 70% $\dot{V}O_{2max}$ at 4300 m).

TABLE 24.1 Cardiorespiratory and metabolic response during submaximal and maximal exercise at sea level and 4000-m simulated altitude

In a Practical Sense

Immediate and Longer-Term Adjustments to Altitude Hypoxia

The table reveals that some compensatory responses to altitude occur almost immediately, while other adaptations take weeks or even months to establish. The body's rapid adaptation responses remain largely altitude dependent, exhibiting considerable individual differences for both the rate and success of acclimatization. An individual retains many beneficial submaximal exercise responses with 16 days acclimatization to 4300 m/14,108 ft despite intermittent 8-day sea-level sojourns. This suggests that some acclimatization aspects regress more slowly than their acquisition.

System	Immediate	Longer Term
Pulmonary acid-base	Hyperventilation Bodily fluids become more alkaline from reduced carbon dioxide (H_2CO_3) with hyperventilation	Hyperventilation Base (HCO_3^-) excretion by kidneys, which reduces alkaline reserve
Cardiovascular	Increase in submaximal heart rate Increase in submaximal cardiac output Stroke volume remains the same or decreases slightly Maximum cardiac output remains the same or decreases slightly	Submaximal heart rate remains elevated Submaximal cardiac output falls below sea-level values Stroke volume decreases Maximum cardiac output decreases
Hematologic		Decreased plasma volume Increased hematocrit Increased hemoglobin concentration Increased total red blood cell number
Local		Increased skeletal muscle capillarization Increased red blood cell 2,3-DPG Increased mitochondrial density Increased muscles' aerobic enzymes Loss of body mass and lean body mass

Daniel Prudek/Shutterstock

Source:
Adapted with permission from Beidleman BA, et al. Exercise responses after altitude acclimatization are retained during reintroduction to altitude. *Med Sci Sports Exerc.* 1997;29:1588.

In maximal effort with less than 7 days (short term) altitude exposure, ventilatory and circulatory adjustments fail to compensate the depressed arterial oxygen content. **FIGURE 24.5** illustrates the relationship between pulmonary ventilation and oxygen uptake (and exercise intensity expressed in W, top axis) up to maximum during cycling at sea level and simulated altitudes from 1000 to 4000 m/3280 to 13,123 ft. Each 1000-m/3280-ft increase in altitude proportionately increased exercise ventilation volume. When oxygen uptake exceeded 2.0 L · min^{-1}, pulmonary ventilation increased disproportionately at progressively higher elevations.

Increased Fluid Loss

Ambient air in mountainous regions remains cool and dry, allowing considerable body water to evaporate as inspired air becomes warmed and moistened in the respiratory passages.

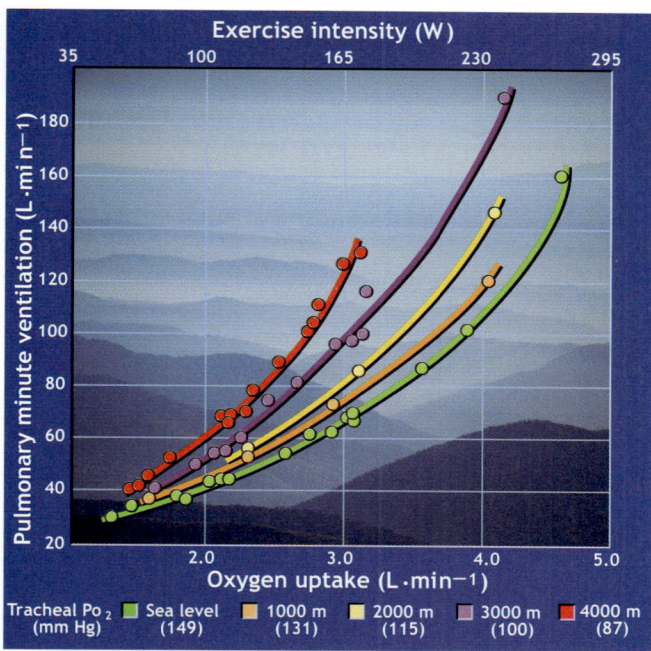

FIGURE 24.5. Increasing simulated altitude's effects when going from sea level (tracheal P_{O_2} = 149 mm Hg) to 4000 m/13,123 ft (tracheal P_{O_2} = 87 mm Hg) on the relationship between pulmonary ventilation and oxygen uptake during cycle ergometry.
(Vitalii Nesterchuk/Shutterstock)

This fluid loss often leads to moderate dehydration and accompanying lip, mouth, and throat dryness. Fluid loss becomes pronounced for physically active people from their large daily total sweat loss and exercise pulmonary ventilation volumes, and hence water loss.[123] For these reasons, individuals should have unlimited access to water.

Decreased Sensory Functions

FIGURE 24.6 displays the percentage deterioration in sensory and mental functions as arterial oxygen saturation decreases with increasing altitude. Neurologic alterations range from a 5% decrease in sensitivity to light at 1524 m/5000 ft to a further 25% decrease in light sensitivity at 6069 m/19,910 ft, a 30% decrease in visual acuity when elevation doubles to 3048 m, and at 6096 m, a 25% deterioration in coding task performance and simple reaction time.

Myocardial Function

Individuals with normal electrocardiograms at sea level including patients with stable chronic heart failure generally show no adverse changes to indicate myocardial ischemia (e.g., arrhythmias, angina, ECG abnormalities) at simulated high altitudes, even during maximal effort.[2,85,100] On Mt. Everest, the heart's contractile function remains stable despite considerable arterial hypoxia.[78] Little information exists about altitude effects on individuals with coronary artery disease; such individuals should not risk high-altitude exposure.

Longer-Term Altitude Adjustments

Hyperventilation and increased submaximal cardiac output provide a relatively effective counter to any short-term altitude exposure challenge. Concurrently, other slower-acting adjustments occur during a prolonged altitude stay. Three important longer-term physiologic adjustments improve tolerance to medium and high altitude hypoxia:

1. Regulation of acid-base balance of body fluids altered by hyperventilation
2. Synthesis of hemoglobin and red blood cells and accompanying changes in local circulation and aerobic cellular functions
3. Elevated sympathetic neurohumoral activity reflected by increased norepinephrine that peaks within 1 wk

Acid-Base Readjustment

Carbon Dioxide Loss Due to Hyperventilation. Hyperventilation's beneficial altitude effect to increase alveolar

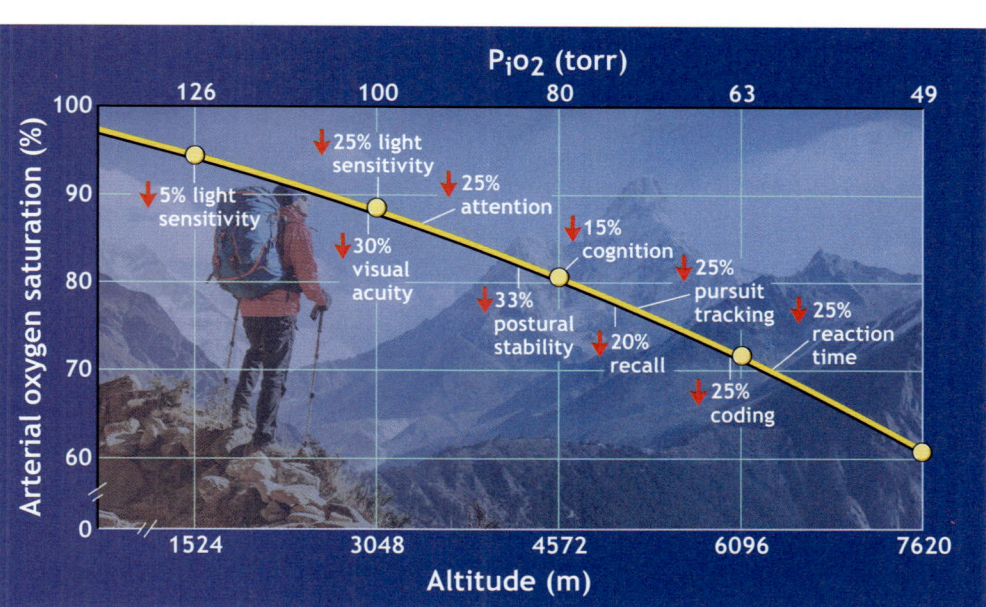

FIGURE 24.6. Arterial desaturation with increasing altitude and corresponding impairment (↓) in sensory and mental functions.
(Adapted from Fulco CS, Cymerman A. Human performance and acute hypoxia. In: Pandolf KB, et al., eds. *Human Performance Physiology and Environmental Medicine at Terrestrial Extremes*. Carmel: Cooper Publishing Group; 1988; Olga Danylenko/Shutterstock.)

In a Practical Sense

Identifying and Treating Altitude-Related Medical Problems

Natives and newcomers who live and work at high altitudes risk many medical problems associated with reduced arterial P_{O_2}. These problems usually remain mild and dissipate within several days depending on ascent speed and exposure time. Other medical complications will compromise overall health and safety, especially three medical conditions that threaten those who ascend to high altitude:

1. *Acute mountain sickness (AMS)*; most common malady
2. *High-altitude pulmonary edema (HAPE)*; reverses if the person returns quickly to a lower altitude
3. *High-altitude cerebral edema (HACE)*; potentially life-threatening condition if not diagnosed immediately

ACUTE MOUNTAIN SICKNESS

Most people experience the discomfort of AMS during the first few days at altitudes of 2500 m/8202 ft and above. Factors that predispose to AMS include individual susceptibility, rapid rate of ascent, and lack of prealtitude exposure.[96] Nonspecific symptoms include headache, nausea, dizziness, fatigue, insomnia, and peripheral edema. This relatively benign condition, which becomes exacerbated by physical activity in the first few hours of exposure,[82] possibly results from acute reduction in cerebral oxygen saturation.[89] Maintenance of hydration and adequate sleep allowance may be critical performance requirements at altitude.[72] It occurs most frequently in those who ascend rapidly to a high altitude without benefiting from gradual and progressive acclimatization to lower altitudes.[124] Symptoms listed in the table by condition usually begin within 4 to 12 hr and dissipate within the first week.[37,42,55] These symptoms are not exacerbated by exertion.[88] Impaired cognitive function and decision-making processes also occur during incremental high altitude ascent.[125]

Headache, the most frequent symptom, probably results from increased cerebral hemodynamics from short-term hyperventilation.[46] Most symptoms become apparent above 3000 m/9800 ft. Rapid ascent to 4200 m/13,800 ft almost guarantees AMS. Poor nutrition also can delay adjustments to altitude exposure.[126]

Decreased thirst sensation and severe appetite suppression occur during early-stage altitude exposure (often with 40% reduction in energy intake and body mass loss). Low salt and high carbohydrate diets are well tolerated during the early stage. Maintaining carbohydrate reserves liberates more energy per unit oxygen with carbohydrate oxidation than with lipid (5.0 kcal vs. 4.7 kcal $\cdot$ L of oxygen^{-1}). High blood lipid levels after a high-fat meal can reduce arterial oxygen saturation. Three benefits from a high-carbohydrate diet:

1. Enhanced altitude tolerance
2. Reduced mountain sickness severity
3. Lessened physical performance decrements during initial altitude exposure

Moderate physical activity becomes intolerable with AMS, but symptoms subside with acclimatizing slowly to moderate altitudes below 3048 m/10,000 ft, followed by a gradual progression to higher elevations (termed *staged ascent*), usually prevents AMS. Climbers should spend several nights at 2500 to 3000 m/8200 to 9800 ft before ascending higher, and an extra night should be added for each additional 600 to 900 m/1968 to 2952 ft climbed. Abrupt increases above 600 m altitude for sleeping should be avoided at 2500 m/8202 ft or above ("climb high-sleep low"). If acclimatization proves ineffective, a 300-m/984-ft descent usually facilitates recovery, as does supplemental oxygen and acetazolamide (*Diamox*).

HIGH-ALTITUDE PULMONARY EDEMA

HAPE can occur at altitudes above 3000 m/9842 ft, with symptoms usually manifesting within 12 to 96 hr following rapid ascent (see Table above). Major predisposing HAPE factors include altitude level, ascent rate, and individual susceptibility.[5,6] Changes in pulmonary function test variables after rapid high altitude ascent cannot predict HAPE susceptibility.[98]

Fluid accumulates in the brain and lungs in this life-threatening condition.[3,81] At first, symptoms do not seem severe, but the syndrome progresses to pulmonary edema with kidney fluid retention. Chest examination reveals wheezy, raspy sounds known as *rales* (excess lung mucus diagnosed as clicking sounds via stethoscope). Even in well-acclimatized persons, HAPE develops with severe exertion above 5486 m/18,000 ft probably from increased pulmonary artery pressure, which damages the blood-gas barrier.[111]

Treatment to prevent severe disability or even death requires immediate descent to lower altitude on a stretcher (or being flown to safety) because physical activity from walking potentiates complications (see table on next page). With proper treatment, symptoms subside within hours, and com-

ALTITUDE-RELATED MEDICAL CONDITIONS AND SYMPTOMS

Condition	Symptoms
Acute mountain sickness	Severe headache, fatigue, irritability, nausea, vomiting, loss of appetite, indigestion, flatulence, generalized weakness, constipation, decreased urine output with normal hydration, sleep disturbance
High-altitude pulmonary edema	Debilitating headache and severe fatigue; excessively rapid breathing and heart rate; rales; cough producing pink frothy sputum; bluish skin color (low blood partial pressure of oxygen); disrupted vision, bladder, bowel functions; poor reflexes; lost trunk muscle coordination; one side body paralysis
High-altitude cerebral edema	Staggered gait, dyspnea upon exertion, severe weakness/fatigue, persistent cough with pulmonary infection, substernal pain/pressure, impaired mental processing, drowsiness, ashen skin color, loss of consciousness

Tappasan Phurisamrit/Shutterstock

plete clinical recovery occurs within days. HAPE poses little or no problem for healthy individuals who recreate without acclimatization at altitudes below 1676 m/5499 ft.

HIGH-ALTITUDE PULMONARY EDEMA PREVENTION AND TREATMENT

Prevention

1. Slow ascent for susceptible individuals (average increase in sleeping altitude of 300 to 350 m · d^{-1}/984 to 1148 ft · d^{-1} above 2500 m/8200 ft)
2. Avoidance of ascent to higher altitude when acute mountain sickness (AMS) symptoms present
3. Descent when AMS symptoms do not improve after 2 hr rest
4. For all persons, avoidance of vigorous activity without acclimatization
5. For susceptible individuals when slow ascent is impossible, taking nifedipine 20 mg slow-release formulation every 6 hr (or 30–60 mg sustained-release formula once daily)

Treatment

1. Descent by at least 1000 m/3280 ft (primary choice in mountaineering)
2. Supplemental oxygen: 2–4 L · min^{-1} (primary choice in areas with medical facilities)
3. When choices 1 and/or 2 are not possible:
   a. Administer 20 mg nifedipine slow-release formula every 6 hr
   b. Use a portable hyperbaric chamber (see Chapter 26)
   c. Immediately descend to low altitude

Roberto Caucino/Shutterstock

HIGH-ALTITUDE CEREBRAL EDEMA

HACE, a potentially fatal neurologic syndrome, develops within hours or days in individuals with AMS. HACE occurs in about 1% of individuals exposed to altitudes above 2700 m/8858 ft and involves increased intracranial pressure, and without immediate treatment, causes coma and death. The early symptoms in the accompanying table are similar to AMS and HAPE, which progressively worsen with altitude stay. Cerebral edema likely results from cerebral vasodilation and elevated capillary hydrostatic pressure, which moves fluid and protein from the vascular compartment across the blood-brain barrier.[38,134] An enlarged cerebral fluid volume eventually distorts brain structures, particularly white matter, which exacerbates symptoms and increases sympathetic nervous system activity. Tissue hypoxia also impacts brain tissue that stimulate angiogenesis (new capillary vessel growth).[118] Immediate, mandatory descent to a lower elevation must occur to adequately diagnose HACE.

OTHER CONDITIONS

Chronic mountain sickness (CMS), prevalent in a small number of altitude natives, develops after months and years at altitude. CMS relates to excessive polycythemia from a genetically linked variation in the EPO response to hypoxic stress.[73] CMS symptoms include lethargy, weakness, sleep disturbance, bluish skin coloring (cyanosis), and changed mental status. **High-altitude retinal hemorrhage (HARH)** affects virtually all climbers at altitudes above 6700 m/21,982 ft. HARH typically progresses unnoticed, with no specific treatment or prevention. Hemorrhage in the eye's macula—the oval "yellow spot" region in the back of the eyeball in close proximity to the optic disc—produces irreversible visual defects. Retinal bleeding occurs from blood pressure surges from increased cerebral blood flow with exercise, causing eye blood vessels to dilate and rupture.

Source:
https://pubmed.ncbi.nlm.nih.gov/28143879/.

P_{O_2} produces opposite effects on carbon dioxide concentrations. Ambient air contains essentially no carbon dioxide ($\leq 0.03\%$), so the increased breathing volumes at altitude dilute normal alveolar carbon dioxide concentrations. This creates a larger than normal gradient for diffusion ("washout") of carbon dioxide from the blood to the lungs, causing a considerable decrease in arterial P_{CO_2}. For example, exposure to 3048 m decreases alveolar P_{CO_2} to about 24 mm Hg, in contrast to its usual 40 mm Hg sea-level value. Alveolar P_{CO_2} decreases to 10 mm Hg during a prolonged high-altitude stay.

Carbon dioxide loss from body fluids in a hypoxic environment creates a physiologic disequilibrium. In Chapter 13, we point out that carbonic acid (H_2CO_3) normally carries the largest carbon dioxide quantity in the body. This relatively weak acid readily dissociates into H^+ and HCO_3^- that move to the lungs in the venous circulation. The H^+ and HCO_3^- recombine in the pulmonary capillaries to form H_2CO_3, which in turn forms carbon dioxide and water; carbon dioxide diffuses from the blood into the alveoli and leaves the body. A decrease in carbon dioxide level with hyperventilation increases the pH from carbonic acid loss, making bodily fluids more alkaline.

Hyperventilation represents a sustained and beneficial response to altitude exposure, with physiologic adjustments proceeding during acclimatization to minimize the accompanying negative disruption in acid-base balance. Ventilatory-induced alkalosis control occurs slowly as the kidneys excrete base (HCO_3^-) through the renal tubules. In turn, restoring normal pH increases respiratory center responsiveness for even greater hyperventilation with altitude hypoxia.

Reduced Buffering Capacity and the Lactate Paradox.

Establishing acid–base equilibrium with acclimatization occurs at the expense of a loss of absolute alkaline reserve. Anaerobic metabolic pathways remain unaffected by altitude, yet the blood's capacity for buffering acid gradually decreases, which lowers the critical level for acid metabolite accumulation.

On immediate high-altitude ascent, a given submaximal exercise load increases blood lactate concentration compared with sea-level values. Greater reliance on anaerobic glycolysis with altitude hypoxia presumably increases lactate accumulation. Surprisingly, after several weeks of hypoxic exposure, the same submaximal and maximal effort with large muscle groups produces *lower* lactate levels (FIG. 24.7).[20,112] This occurs despite no increases in $\dot{V}O_{2\,max}$ or regional blood flow to active tissues. A general depression in maximum lactate concentrations becomes apparent in maximal exertion above 4000 m/13,123 ft. A question arises concerning this apparent physiologic contradiction, termed the lactate paradox: *How is lactate accumulation reduced without a corresponding increase in tissue oxygenation, when the hypoxemia associated with high altitude should promote lactate accumulation?*[107]

Research to resolve the lactate paradox points to reduced output of epinephrine, the glucose-mobilizing hormone, during chronic high-altitude exposure,[10] reduced glucose mobilization from the liver reduces capacity for lactate formation. Diminished intracellular ADP during long-term altitude exposure may also inhibit activation of the glycolytic pathway. In addition, depressed lactate formation during maximal exercise may partly reflect an overall reduced central nervous system drive, which reduces capacity for all-out physical effort.[64] Interestingly, lower blood lactate accumulation at high altitude does not relate to decreased buffering capacity with high-altitude acclimatization.[50]

Hematologic Changes

An increase in the blood's oxygen-carrying capacity provides the most important longer-term adjustment to altitude exposure. Two factors account for this adaptation:

1. Initial decrease in plasma volume, followed by
2. Increase in erythrocytes and hemoglobin synthesis

Initial Decrease in Plasma Volume.

During the first several days at altitude, body fluids shift from intravascular to interstitial and intracellular spaces. The decrease in plasma volume within several hours of altitude exposure increases blood cell concentration.[86] After a week at 2300 m/7545 ft, for example, plasma volume declines by about 8%, whereas red blood cell concentration (hematocrit) increases 4% and hemoglobin 10%. A 1-wk stay at 4300 m/14,107 ft decreases plasma volume 16 to 25% along with increases in hematocrit (6%) and hemoglobin (20%) concentrations. The rapid plasma volume reduction (and accompanying hemoconcentration) increases arterial blood's oxygen content above values observed upon arrival at altitude. Increased urine output, termed *diuresis*, accompanies the plasma fluid shifts to maintain fluid compartment balance despite lower total body water content.

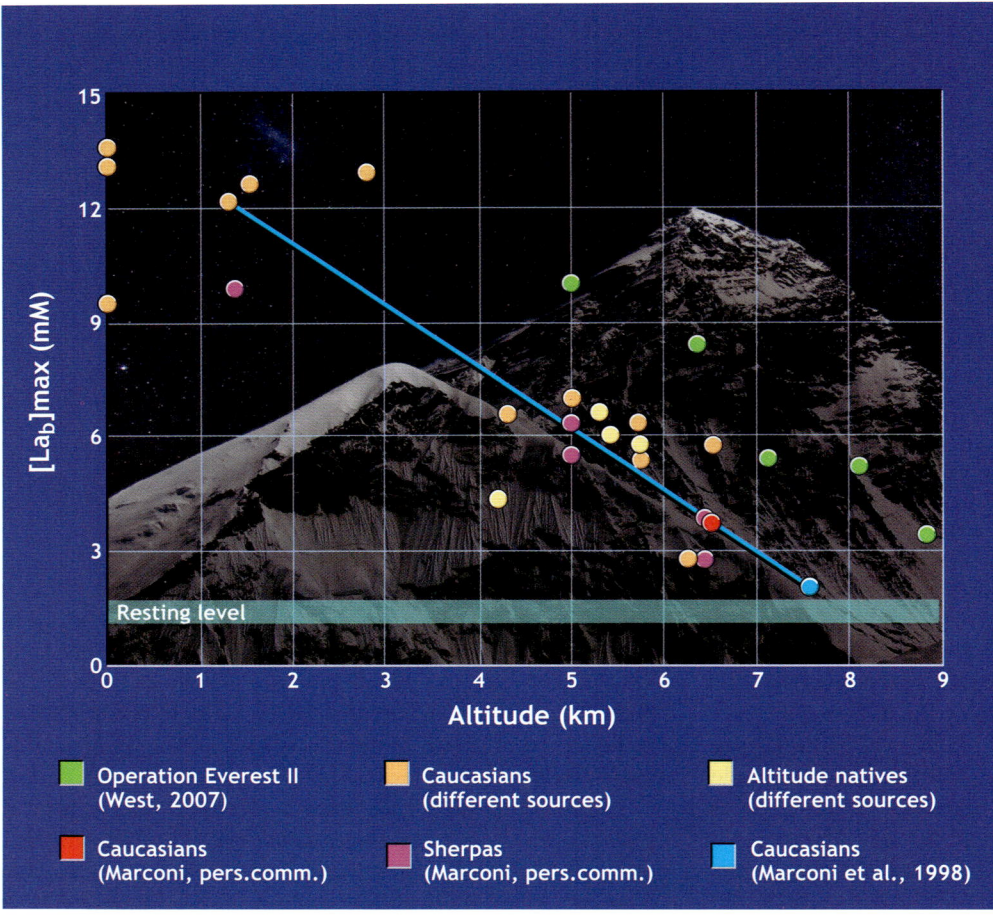

FIGURE 24.7. The lactate paradox: Less oxygen equals less (not more) lactate. Maximal blood lactate concentration ([La$_b$]max) with increasing altitude in acclimatized lowlanders and high-altitude residents. The solid best fit line includes all the points above 1 km altitude, except the four from Operation Everest II.

(Adapted with permission from Ceretelli P, Samaja M. Acid–base balance at exercise in normoxia and in chronic hypoxia. Revisiting the "lactate paradox." *Eur J Appl Physiol.* 2003;90:431; West JB. Point: the lactate paradox does/does not occur during exercise at high altitude. *J Appl Physiol.* 2007;102:2398. Travel Stock/Shutterstock.)

Increase in Red Blood Cell Mass. Reduced arterial P_{O_2} at altitude stimulates an increase in total red blood cell number termed **polycythemia**. The erythrocyte-stimulating hormone **erythropoietin (EPO)** initiates red blood cell formation within 15 hr after altitude ascent. In the weeks that follow, erythrocyte production in the long bone's marrow increases and stays elevated throughout the stay.[36] The blood from a typical copper miner in the Andes contains 38% more erythrocytes than a lowlander. In some apparently healthy high-altitude natives, red blood cell count may reach levels 50% above normal—8 million cells · mm^{-3} compared with 5.3 million for the native lowlander![61] Climbers acclimatized at 6500 m/21,325 ft during a Mt. Everest expedition showed a 40% increase in hemoglobin concentration and a 66% increase in hematocrit.[19] Debate concerns the precise benefits accruing from increased hematopoiesis and whether an optimum exists for hemoglobin concentration at high altitude.[79,106] Clearly, extreme erythrocyte packing increases blood viscosity and restricts tissue blood flow and oxygen diffusion.

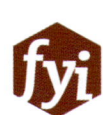

Exogenous Erythropoietin Enhances Blood Parameters and Running Performance for Altitude-Based Kenyan Athletes

The erythropoietin (EPO)-stimulating effects occur whether the hormone is produced naturally in response to altitude exposure or provided exogenously through injection. A recent study compared hematologic responses of highly trained Kenyan endurance athletes (with relatively high basal hemoglobin concentration and hematocrit values) living and training at moderate altitude, to Caucasian athletes living and training at or near sea level for 4 weeks with exogenous EPO injections. Increases of about 10% occurred in hemoglobin and hematocrit for the Kenyan runners, an increase somewhat less than the near-sea level dwelling counterparts. The relative improvement in running performance from EPO treatment for both groups remained similar. The authors concluded that enhanced blood oxygen carrying capacity represented the mechanism to explain the improved exercise performance.

Milan Humaj/Shutterstock

Source:
Haile DW, et al. Effects of EPO on blood parameters and running performance in Kenyan athletes. *Med Sci Sports Exerc.* 2019;51:299.

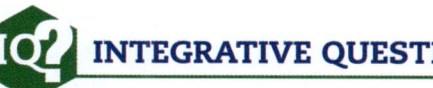

INTEGRATIVE QUESTION

For their assault on Mt. Everest, elite mountaineers spend 3 mo at camps 4877 m/16,600 ft, 5944 m/19,500 ft, 6492 m/21,300 ft, 7315 m/24,000 ft, and 7925 m/26,000 ft before the final ascent. What is the physiologic rationale for this "stage-ascent" approach to mountaineering conquests?

In general, altitude-induced polycythemia translates directly to an increase in oxygen transport capacity. For example, the blood's oxygen-carrying capacity for high-altitude Peruvian residents averages 28% above sea-level values. The blood from well-acclimatized mountaineers carries 10 more mL oxygen per deciliter of blood compared with the total 20 mL average for lowland residents.[75] Despite reduced hemoglobin oxygen saturation, the oxygen *quantity* in arterial blood may approach or even equal sea-level values.[68] **FIGURE 24.8A** illustrates the general trend for increased hemoglobin and hematocrit during acclimatization in eight young women who lived and worked for 10 wk at the Pikes Peak summit (4267 m/14,000 ft). The researchers' previous work showed fewer hematologic changes during acclimatization in women than in men, possibly due to inadequate iron intake. In this experiment, each woman received iron supplementation prior to, during, and on return from altitude. Red blood cell concentration increased rapidly upon reaching Pikes Peak. A reduced plasma volume within the first 24 hr at altitude produced hemoconcentration. Hemoglobin concentration and hematocrit continued to rise in the following month and then stabilized during their remaining stay. Prealtitude values were reestablished within 2 wk after returning to Missouri.

Figure 24.8B shows that iron supplementation progressively increased hematocrit and hemoglobin prealtitude values. One might anticipate this finding because young women frequently suffer from mild dietary iron insufficiency with typically lower iron reserves (see Chapter 2). Comparing the acclimatization curves for the iron-supplemented females and another female group not given additional iron showed greater hematocrit increases for the supplemented group. Iron supplementation enhanced hematocrit increases to a level equivalent to males at the same altitude. Athletes with borderline iron stores may not respond to acclimatization as effectively as those who come to altitude with iron reserves adequate to sustain increased erythrocyte production.[39,60,127]

Cellular Adaptations

Debate concerns whether extreme terrestrial hypoxia stimulates vascular and cellular adaptations that improve local oxygen extraction and maximize oxidative functions.[34,41,43,69] Animals born and raised at high altitude show more concentrated skeletal muscle capillarization (number per mm^2) than sea-level counterparts.[105] Chronic hypoxia can initiate capillary diameter and length remodeling by forming of new capillaries to increase oxygen delivery to neural tissues.[12]

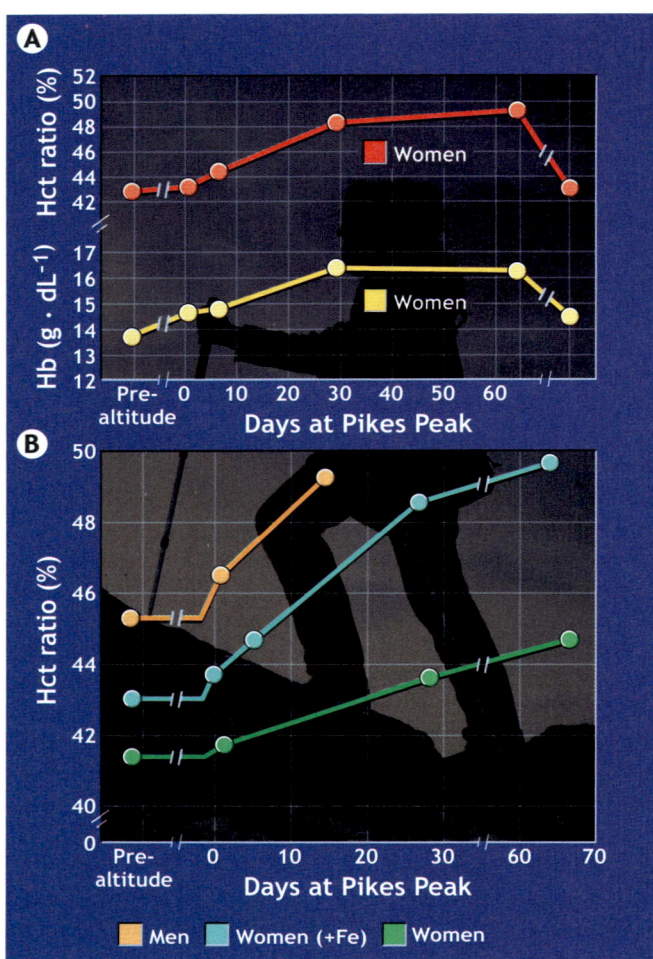

FIGURE 24.8. **(A)** Altitude effects on hemoglobin (Hb; *bottom yellow line*) and hematocrit (Hct; *top red line*) levels for eight young women from the University of Missouri (213 m/699 ft) prior to, during, and 2 wk after exposure to 4267 m/13,999 ft at Pikes Peak, CO. **(B)** Hematocrit response of young women receiving supplemental iron [+Fe] prior to and during altitude exposure compared with male and female subjects receiving no supplemental iron.
(Part A: Adapted with permission from Hannon JP, et al. Effects of altitude acclimatization on blood composition of women. *J Appl Physiol.* 1968;26:540. ©The American Physiological Society (APS). All rights reserved. Part B: Courtesy of Dr. J. P. Hannon.)

Residents living at sea level also increase tissue capillarization at altitude.[70] A more prolific microcirculation reduces the oxygen diffusion distance between blood and tissues to optimize tissue oxygenation with decreased arterial P_{O_2}. Muscle biopsy analysis shows myoglobin increases up to 16% following a period of altitude acclimatization.[80] Additional myoglobin augments oxygen "storage" in specific fibers and facilitates intracellular oxygen release and delivery at a low-tissue P_{O_2}. Researchers are unclear whether the small increase in mitochondrial number and concentration of aerobic energy transfer enzymes that occurs with prolonged altitude exposure and training[59,69,102] reflects the effects of training, the hypoxic environment, or the combination of both factors.[44,91,94]

High-altitude natives benefit from the slight rightward shift for the oxyhemoglobin dissociation curve. This effect decreases hemoglobin's oxygen affinity to favor more oxygen release for a given cellular P_{O_2}. Increased red blood cell 2,3-diphosphoglycerate (2,3-DPG; see Chapter 13) concentration also facilitates hemoglobin's release of oxygen with longer duration altitude exposure. Increased 2,3-DPG coupled with greater circulating hemoglobin and red blood cells favorably impacts the long-term resident's capacity to supply oxygen to active tissues during physical activity. Chronic altitude exposure also may facilitate myocardial adaptations that include interventricular septum thickening, smaller left heart size, and larger right ventricle diameter and thickness.[128]

Body Mass and Body Composition

Prolonged high-altitude exposure reduces lean body mass (muscle fibers atrophy by 20%) and body fat, with the magnitude of weight loss directly related to terrestrial elevation. Six men participated in a 40-day progressive decompression to 249 mm Hg ambient pressure in a hypobaric chamber to simulate a Mt. Everest ascent.[87] Daily caloric intake from depressed appetite decreased by 43% during the exposure period. Reduced energy intake reduced body mass 7.4 kg, predominantly from the muscle component of fat-free body mass. In addition to depressed appetite and food intake during high-altitude exposure, intestinal absorption's efficiency decreases, compounding the difficulty in maintaining body weight.[16,25,113,129,130]

Basal metabolic rate increases upon arrival at altitude to further affect the tendency to lose weight. To some extent, one can override an accelerated metabolic rate and minimize weight loss by consciously increasing energy intake while at altitude.[17] Hypoxic exposure does not induce consistent changes in carbohydrate's or lipid's contribution to the total energy yield compared to similar exercise intensities under normoxic conditions.[131] Carbohydrate feedings during exercise during hypoxia may effectively sustain reaction speed for a cognitive task.[125,126,132]

Required Time for Acclimatization

The time required to acclimatize to altitude depends on terrestrial elevation. Acclimation to one altitude ensures only partial adjustment to a higher elevation. As a broad guideline, it takes about 2 wk to adapt to altitudes up to 2300 m/7545 ft. Thereafter, each 610-m/2000-ft altitude increase requires an additional week up to 4600 m/15,091 ft to fully acclimatize. Athletes who desire to compete at altitude should begin intense training immediately during acclimatization. Rapidly initiating training minimizes detraining effects induced by the normal tendency to reduce physical activity in the first few days at altitude. *Acclimatization adaptations dissipate within 2 or 3 wk after return to sea level.*

Metabolic, Physiologic, and Exercise Capacity at Altitude

High altitude stress considerably restricts exercise capacity and physiologic functions. Even at lower altitudes, exercise performance deteriorates because physiologic and metabolic adjustments do not fully compensate for the reduced ambient oxygen pressures. Stroke volume and maximum heart rate acclimatize in a direction that reduces oxygen transport capacity and $\dot{V}O_{2max}$.[31,90]

Maximum Oxygen Uptake

FIGURE 24.9A describes the relationship between the decrease in $\dot{V}O_{2max}$ (% sea-level value) and increasing altitude or simulated exposures (i.e., hypobaric chambers or normobaric hypoxic gas breathing) reported in many civilian and military studies. The data represent 146 average points from 67 different civilian and military investigations conducted at altitudes from 580 m/1902 ft to 8848 m/29,021 ft. The orange downward regression line represents the best fit curvilinear line. Disparities in experimental design and procedures and physiologic differences among subjects help explain the variation in points about the orange line that captures the relationship. Small declines in $\dot{V}O_{2max}$ become noticeable at 589-m/1932-ft altitude. Thereafter, arterial desaturation decreases $\dot{V}O_{2max}$ by 7 to 9% per 1000-m/3280-ft altitude increase to 6300 m/20,700 ft, where aerobic capacity declines more rapidly and nonlinearly.[23,76] For example, aerobic capacity at 4000 m/13,123 ft averages 75% of the sea-level value. At 7000 m/22,965 ft, $\dot{V}O_{2max}$ averages one half than at sea level. The $\dot{V}O_{2max}$ for relatively fit men atop Mt. Everest averages about 1000 mL · min^{-1};[74] this corresponds to only a 50 watt exercise power output on a bicycle ergometer (equivalent to 0.72 kcal · min^{-1}, 0.14 L O$_2$ · min^{-1}, or less than 0.5 METs for a 72.6-kg person).

Physical conditioning prior to altitude exposure offers little

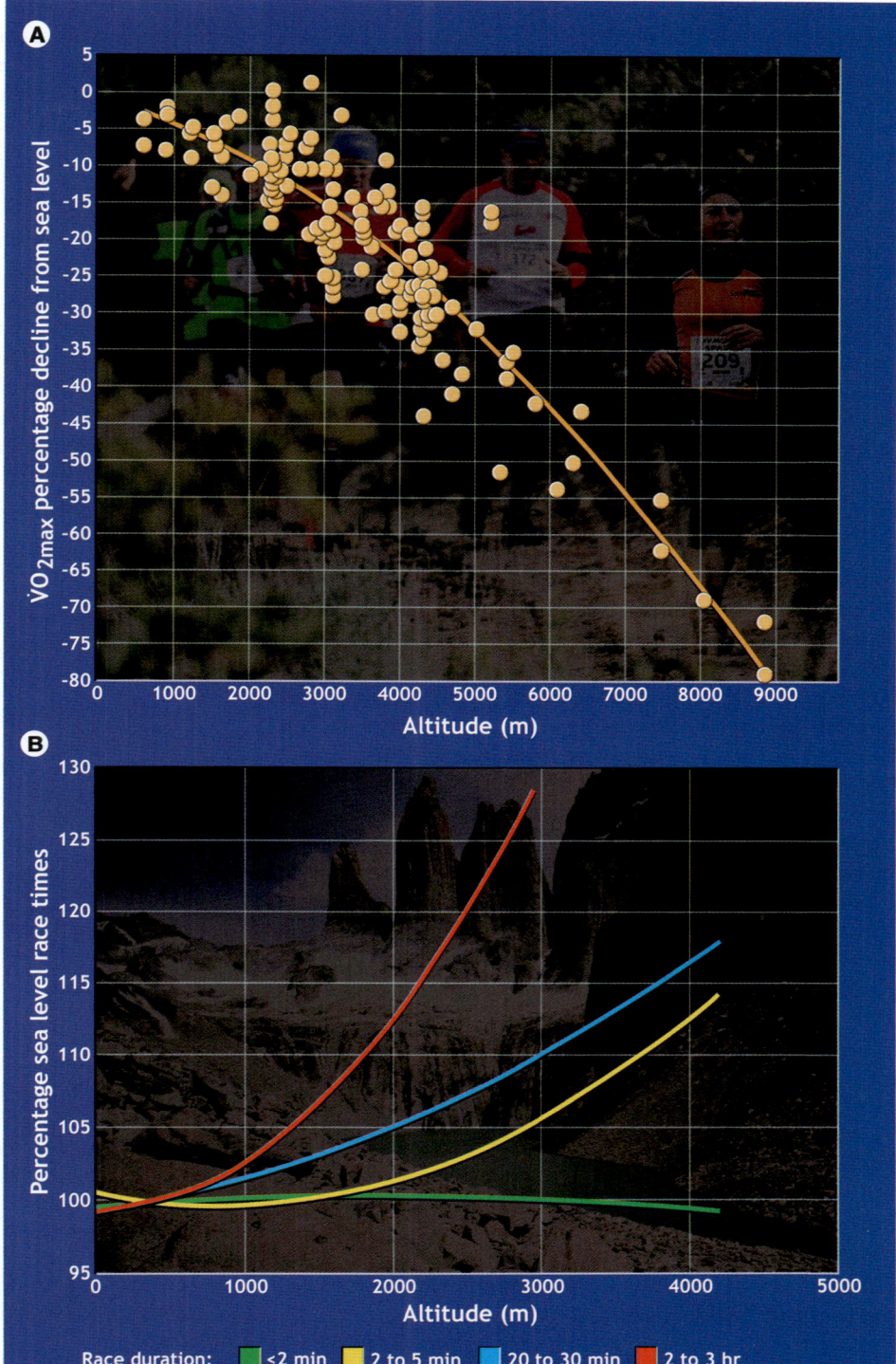

FIGURE 24.9. **(A)** Reduction in $\dot{V}O_{2max}$ as a percentage of the sea-level value related to altitude exposure. **(B)** Generalized trend in performance decrements related to altitude exposure for runners and swimmers primarily during competition.
(Adapted with permission from Fulco CS, et al. Maximal and submaximal exercise performance at altitude. *Aviat Space Environ Med.* 1998;69:793.) Permission conveyed through Copyright Clearance Center, Inc.

protection because the endurance athlete experiences a slightly greater percentage reduction in $\dot{V}O_{2max}$ than an untrained person. In addition, large variability exists among individuals in the decrement in $\dot{V}O_{2max}$ with altitude exposure. Men experience the largest decrease, particularly those with (1) large lean body mass, (2) large sea-level aerobic capacity, and (3) low sea-level lactate threshold.[84] To some extent, arterial desaturation and decrease in $\dot{V}O_{2max}$ become more pronounced in individuals with a depressed hyperventilation response to exertion in a hypoxic environment.[30] Despite any unique altitude exposure effects on aerobically fit individuals, a standard physical task at altitude at a given absolute amount effort still provides relatively less stress for well-conditioned women and men because they perform it at a lower $\dot{V}O_{2max}$ percentage. No change in exercise economy occurs in response to 4 wk of intermittent altitude exposure.[104]

Exercise Performance

Seven days of intermittent (4 hr·day⁻¹) simulated altitude exposure, combined with either rest or training, improves time-trial performance and induces physiologic adaptations during constant-intensity exercise at 4300 m/14,107 ft.[9] Specific nonhematological adaptations to hypoxic exposure that improve sea-level performance include *improved* muscle efficiency at the mitochondrial level from a tighter coupling of intracellular bioenergetic and mitochondrial function, greater muscle buffering, and improved tolerance for lactic acid.[32] Figure 24.9B illustrates the generalized trend in physical performance decrements primarily during competition for athletes at different altitude exposures. Altitude exerts *no* adverse effect on events lasting less than 2 min. For longer-duration events, poorer performance occurs at higher elevations compared sea level. The threshold for decrements appears at about 1600 m/5250 ft for 2- to 5-min events, while only a 600- to 700-m/1970- to 2300-ft altitude induces poorer performance in events longer than 20 min. For the 1- and 3 mile runs, medium altitude (2300 m/7546 ft) decreases performance by 2 to 13% for fit subjects.[28] This coincides with the 7.2% increase in 2-mile run times for highly trained middle-distance runners at the same altitude.[1] After 29 days of acclimatization, high-altitude exposure still increases 3 mile run time, compared with sea-level runs.[77] Three factors help to explain the small improvement in endurance during acclimatization, despite no concomitant $\dot{V}O_{2max}$ increases:

1. Increased minute pulmonary ventilation (ventilatory acclimatization)
2. Increased arterial oxygen saturation and cellular aerobic functions
3. Blunted blood lactate response to physical activity (see the section "Reduced Buffering Capacity and the Lactate Paradox")

Circulatory Factors

After several months of acclimatization to hypoxia, $\dot{V}O_{2max}$ at altitude still remains below sea-level values, even with relatively rapid and pronounced increases in hemoglobin concentration. This occurs because reduced circulatory capacity—combined effect from lowered maximum heart rate and stroke volume—offsets hematologic acclimatization's benefits.

Submaximal Physical Activity

The immediate altitude response to physical activity increases submaximal cardiac output (Table 24.1), but this adjustment diminishes as acclimatization progresses and does not improve with prolonged exposure.[51] A progressive decrease in the heart's stroke volume (associated with diminished plasma volume) during the altitude stay reduces exercise cardiac output. With a lower cardiac output, submaximal oxygen uptake remains stable through an expanded a-$\bar{v}O_2$ difference. To some extent, an increased submaximal heart rate offsets the decrease in stroke volume during submaximal effort.

Inspiratory Muscle Training Benefits Performance at Altitude

Researchers determined whether chronic inspiratory muscle training (IMT) could improve submaximal exercise performance with acute hypoxic exposure. Fourteen endurance-trained male runners completed a 20-km cycling time trial of 30 to 40 min in normobaric hypoxia before and after 6 wk of IMT training. This included inspiratory loads equivalent to 80% sustained maximal inspiratory pressure. The IMT group significantly improved time trial performance compared to endurance athlete controls untrained with inspiratory maneuvers. Significant improvements occurred in maximum minute ventilation and oxygen uptake compared with no changes for the control group. The authors concluded that specific IMT positively affected respiratory efficiency and breathing patterns, lowered dyspneic perceptions, and improved hypoxic exercise performance. Bottom line—preexposure inspiratory muscle training strengthens respiratory muscles to minimize hypoxia-related hyperventilation's adverse effects.

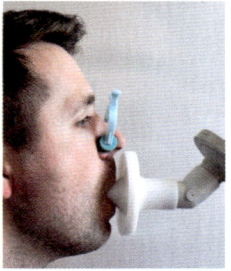

Koldunova Anna/Shutterstock

Sources:
Álvarez-Herms J, et al. Putative role of respiratory muscle training to improve endurance performance in hypoxia: a review. *Front Physiol.* 2019;9:1970.
Hursh DG, et al. Inspiratory muscle training: improvement of exercise performance with acute hypoxic exposure. *Int J Sports Physiol Perform.* 2019;31:1.

Maximum Physical Activity

Maximum cardiac output decreases after about 1 wk above 3048 m/10,000 ft and remains lower throughout one's stay. *Reduced blood flow during maximum effort results from the* combined decreases in maximum heart rate and stroke volume, both of which continue to decrease with the altitude exposure duration and magnitude. The blunted cardiac response does not result from myocardial hypoxia as reflected by normal electrocardiographic and coronary blood flow measurements during vigorous, high altitude activity.[40,90] Decreased plasma volume and increased total peripheral vascular resistance contribute to the reduced maximum stroke volume. Enhanced parasympathetic tone induced by prolonged altitude exposure reduces maximum heart rate.[93]

 INTEGRATIVE QUESTION

If altitude acclimatization improves endurance performance at altitude, why does not it improve similar performance immediately upon return to sea level?

Aerobic Capacity on Return to Sea Level

Sea-level exercise performance does not improve after living at altitude when $\dot{V}O_{2max}$ serves as the improvement criterion.[47,57,70] An 18 day stay at 3100 m/10,500 ft produced no change in the altitude-induced 25% reduction in aerobic capacity in young runners.[36] Also, $\dot{V}O_{2max}$ remained at the same prealtitude value on return to sea level. Even in studies that reported small improvements in $\dot{V}O_{2max}$ or physical performance at altitude and on return to sea level, the change often relates to training effects and/or repeated testing during exposure.[24,52]

Possible Negative Effects

Several physiologic changes during prolonged altitude exposure negate adaptations that could improve physical performance on return to sea level. For example, the residual effects from muscle mass loss and reduced maximum heart rate and stroke volume do not enhance sea-level performance. Any reduction in maximum cardiac output at altitude offsets benefits from an increase in the blood's oxygen-carrying capacity.[95] A depressed circulatory capacity returns to normal after a few weeks at sea level, but so also do potentially positive hematologic adaptations. Within a physiologic context, blood doping (see Chapter 23) mimics the hematologic benefits from altitude exposure without the negative effects on maximum cardiovascular dynamics and body composition.

Altitude Training and Sea-Level Performance

No Evidence of Improved Sea-Level Performance Following Training at Altitude

Endurance training at altitude does not improve subsequent sea-level exercise performance. Altitude acclimatization improves capacity for physical activity at altitude, particularly high altitude. The altitude training effect on aerobic capacity and endurance performance immediately on return to sea level remains unclear. Altitude adaptations in local circulation and cellular metabolism, combined with compensatory increases in the blood's oxygen-carrying capacity, should improve subsequent sea-level performance. Positive pulmonary adaptations and responses during prolonged hypoxic exposure do not regress immediately upon descent from altitude. If tissue hypoxia provides an important training stimulus, altitude plus training should act synergistically, making the total effect exceed similar training only at sea level. Unfortunately, the training-altitude exposure research contains experimental design flaws that limit their conclusions.[58]

Researchers used equivalent groups to compare altitude training's effectiveness (2300 m/7550 ft) and equivalent training at sea level.[1] Six middle-distance runners trained at sea level for 3 wk at 75% sea-level $\dot{V}O_{2max}$ (**FIG. 24.10**). Another six runners trained an equivalent distance at the same percentage $\dot{V}O_{2max}$ at 2300 m/7550 ft. The groups then exchanged training sites (indicated by *red arrows*) and continued to train for 3 wk at the same relative intensity as the preceding group. Initially, 2 mile run times averaged 7.2% slower at altitude than at sea level. Run times improved 2.0% for both groups

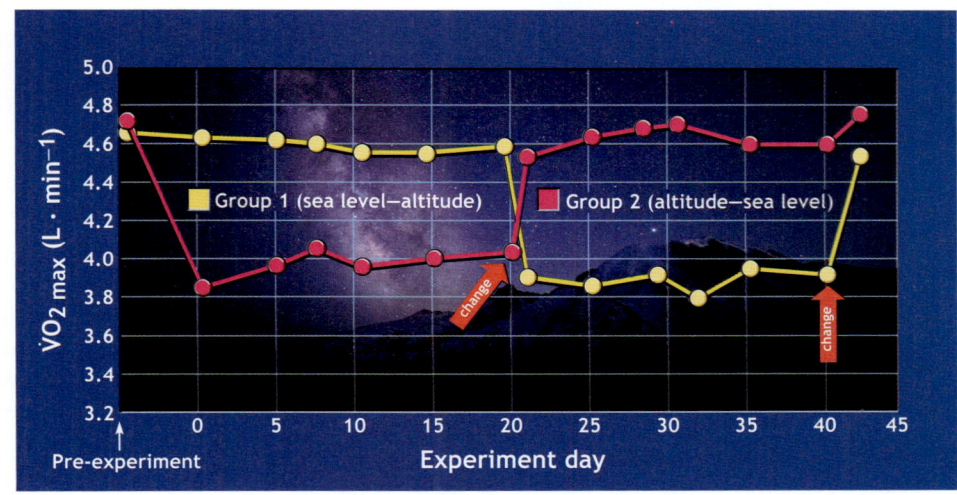

FIGURE 24.10. Maximum oxygen uptake for two equivalent groups during 3 wk altitude training and 3 wk training at sea level.
(Adapted with permission from Adams WC, et al. Effects of equivalent sea-level and altitude training on and running performance. *J Appl Physiol.* 1975;39:262. ©The American Physiological Society (APS). All rights reserved. John T Callery/Shutterstock.)

during altitude training, but postaltitude performance at sea level remained similar to the prealtitude sea-level runs. Short-term altitude exposure decreased $\dot{V}O_{2max}$ 17.4% for both groups and improved only slightly after 20 days of altitude training. When the runners returned to sea level after altitude training, aerobic capacity remained 2.8% *below* prealtitude sea-level values. Clearly, for these well-conditioned middle-distance runners, no synergistic effect developed by combining aerobic training at medium altitude compared with equivalent sea-level training.

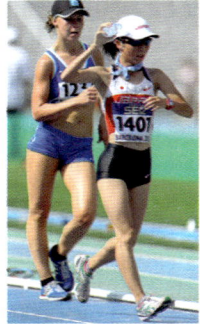

Altitude Natives Exhibit Extraordinary Endurance Performance

Total hemoglobin and blood volume synergistically increase from training and altitude exposure for endurance athletes native to moderate altitude compared to sea-level trained endurance athletes. This unique adaptive response in athletes born and living at altitude (e.g., Kenyan runners, Colombian cyclists, Mexican race walkers) may partially explain the extraordinary endurance performances of these individuals. Longer-term altitude-acclimatized cyclists also have improved aerobic capacity and peak power output during sea-level exercise simulations.

Maxisport/Shutterstock

Sources:
Brothers MD, et al. GXT responses to altitude-acclimatized cyclists during sea-level simulation. *Med Sci Sports Exerc.* 2007;39:1727.
Schmidt W, et al. Blood volume and hemoglobin mass in endurance athletes from moderate altitude. *Med Sci Sports Exerc.* 2002;34:1934.
Sitkowski D, et al. Interrelationships between changes in erythropoietin, plasma volume, haemoglobin concentration, and total haemoglobin mass in endurance athletes. *Res Sports Med.* 2018;26:381.

Other studies have duplicated these observations for $\dot{V}O_{2max}$ and endurance performance at moderate and higher altitudes in athletes from sea level.[26,54] Highly trained male track athletes flew to Nunoa, Peru (altitude 4000 m/13,123 ft), where they trained and acclimatized for 40 to 57 days.[101] $\dot{V}O_{2max}$ decreased 29% below sea-level values after the initial 3 days at altitude; after 48 days, it still remained 26% lower. The 440-yd, 880-yd, and 1- and 2 mile runs during a "track meet" with the altitude natives measured running performance after acclimatization. The race times after acclimatization remained slower than prealtitude sea-level times, particularly for the longer runs. When the athletes returned to sea level, $\dot{V}O_{2max}$ and running performance did not differ from prealtitude measures. On no occasion, did a runner improve his previous prealtitude run time. Run times in the longer events averaged 5% below prealtitude trial run times. In other studies, training in a hypobaric chamber provided no additional benefit to sea-level performance compared with similar training (albeit at a higher absolute exercise level) at sea level. As expected, the "altitude-trained" group achieved better performance at simulated altitude than sea-level residents.

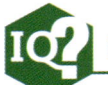 **INTEGRATIVE QUESTION**

What effects would a 2-wk exposure to 3000 m/9842 ft have on maximal 60 s duration exercise performance, and why?

Decrements in Absolute Training Level

One must lower the absolute workload to perform aerobic activity at the same relative intensity at altitude as at sea level. If not, anaerobic metabolism provides a larger portion of the energy required to exercise at altitude (see Fig. 24.3) and fatigue develops. Exposure to 2300 m/7545 ft and above makes it nearly impossible to train at the same absolute intensity as at sea level. The table below shows the reduction in intensity for training relative to sea-level standards for six college athletes. At 4000 m/13,123 ft, the runners could train only at the intensity equivalent to 39% sea-level $\dot{V}O_{2max}$ compared with 78% intensity with sea-level training.

The absolute training level at altitude may become so reduced that an athlete cannot maintain peak condition for sea-level competition.

In this situation, elite athletes benefit from periodically returning from altitude to sea level for intense training to

	Altitude (m)			
	300	2300	3100	4000
Workout intensity (% $\dot{V}O_{2max}$ at 200 m)	78	60	56	39

offset "detraining" during a prolonged altitude stay (see next section). Returning to a lower altitude intermittently does not interfere with acclimatization and might benefit altitude performance.[7,15,24,99] Independent of the training model, athletes who train at altitude should include intense speed work to maintain muscle power.

Combined Altitude Stay with Low-Altitude Training

Benefits

Research has focused on an optimal combination of high-altitude stay plus low-altitude training in competitive runners.[133] Athletes who lived at 2500 m but returned regularly to lower altitudes (1000 to 1250 m/3280 to 4100 ft) to train at near–sea-level intensity (i.e., **live high-train low**) showed greater average $\dot{V}O_{2max}$ and 5000-m run performance increases than athletes who lived and trained only at 2500 m or those who lived and trained only at sea level.[56,108] Strategies that combine altitude acclimatization and maintenance of sea-level training intensity provide *synergistic benefits* to sea-level endurance performance. Regular training exposure to a near–sea-level environment prevents the impaired systolic function (i.e., reduced maximum stroke volume and cardiac output) typically observed during altitude training. Muscular and systemic circulatory capacity for maintaining pH and K^+ balance during intense effort remained unchanged after a 4-wk exposure to this training protocol.[71] Such an approach to training also improves running economy and hypoxic ventilatory drive of elite distance runners, including benefits from hypoxia-induced increases in serum EPO and accelerated erythropoiesis.[49,92,103,116] To remove the inconvenience and cost of the live high-train low strategy, a modification introduces supplemental oxygen during altitude training.[114] Compared with control trials, supplementing with oxygen increases these three factors at moderate altitude:

1. Arterial oxyhemoglobin saturation
2. Exercise oxygen uptake
3. Average power output during high-intensity workouts

This form of training allows athletes to live at altitude yet effectively "train low" with minimal travel expense and inconvenience, and without inducing additional free radical oxidative stress.[115]

Not all individuals benefit to the same degree from the living high, training low strategy.[41,83] Within a group that showed physiologic and performance increases with this protocol, some individuals were "responders," whereas others showed little positive adjustment.[21] The "nonresponders" displayed a smaller increase in plasma concentration for the erythrocyte-producing hormone EPO after 30 hr at altitude than the responders. Such individuals experience a depressed increase in hematocrit during acclimatization to altitude exposure. The benefit from combining altitude living and lower-altitude training depend on three prerequisites:

1. The elevation must be high enough to raise EPO concentrations to increase total red blood cell volume and $\dot{V}O_{2max}$.
2. The athlete must respond positively with increased EPO output.
3. Training must take place at an elevation low enough to maintain training intensity and exercise oxygen uptake at near–sea-level values.

INTEGRATIVE QUESTION

Would periodic breath-holding while exercising at sea level produce physiologic adaptations similar to those produced when training at altitude?

At-Home Acclimatization

Applying the live high-train low training model poses considerable practical and financial hurdles. Unfortunately, some endurance athletes use the banned (and dangerous) procedure of either blood doping or EPO injections to increase hematocrit and hemoglobin concentrations without the potential negative effects of an altitude stay.

A more prudent approach applies the observation that altitude's beneficial effects on erythropoiesis and aerobic capacity may require relatively short-term exposures to hypoxia. For example, daily intermittent exposures for 3 to 5 hr for 9 days to simulated a 4000- to 5500-m/13,123- to 18,044-ft altitude in a hypobaric chamber increased endurance performance, red blood cell count, and hemoglobin concentration in elite mountain climbers.[18,86] This approach also decreases the lactate appearance rate during intense effort.[22] These effects may be time and protocol dependent because a 4-wk intermittent normobaric hypoxia regimen at rest (5:5 min hypoxia-to-normoxia ratio for 70 min, 5 d weekly) did not improve endurance or augment erythropoietic markers in trained runners.[48] Intermittent hypoxic training under normobaric conditions provides an added bonus with clinical and cardioprotective implications—it augments training's effect on selected metabolic and cardiovascular risk factors.[4]

Three alternate approaches without hypobaric chamber use create an artificial "altitude" environment where an athlete, mountaineer, or hot-air balloonist living at sea level stimulates an altitude acclimatization response.

1. **Gamow hypobaric chamber.** A person rests and sleeps for about 10 hr each day. The chamber's total air pressure decreases to simulate the barometric pressure at a preselected altitude. Reduced barometric pressure proportionately reduces the inspired air's P_{O_2} to simulate altitude exposure and induce physiologic adaptations.
2. Simulate altitude at sea level by increasing the air's nitrogen percentage within a man-made enclosure. Increased nitrogen percentage correspondingly reduces the air's oxygen percentage, thus decreasing inspired air P_{O_2}. Nordic skiers have applied this technique by living for 3 to 4 wk in a house that provides "air" with only 15.3% oxygen rather than its normal 20.9% concentration. The system requires mixing nitrogen gas and carefully monitoring the breathing mixture. Interestingly, the Norwegian Olympic Organization has banned these "altitude houses" for its own athletes because they consider this practice "gray-zone" doping.
3. A suitcase-sized unit developed by two-time British Olympic cyclist Shaun Wallace continuously supplies air with an approximate 15% oxygen content to simulate a 2500-m altitude (**FIG. 24.11**). The 70 lb portable **Hypoxico altitude tent** is designed for in-home use as a semipermanent cubicle (a larger unit fits over a double or queen-size bed). A "hypoxic generator" continually feeds altitude-simulating hypoxic air into the tent. The tent material's porosity limits the oxygen diffusion rate

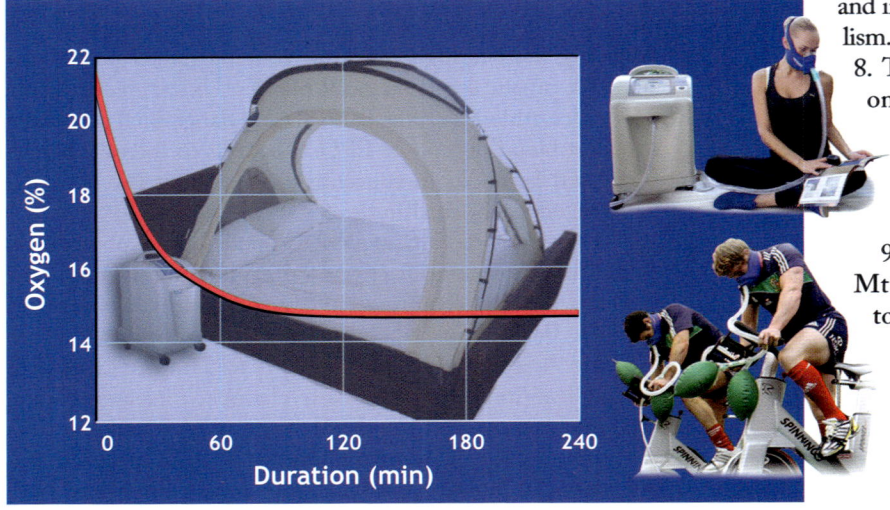

FIGURE 24.11. The Hypoxico Portable Altitude Tent with hypoxic generator (shown left of the tent) continuously supplies "breathable" air with oxygen content that equilibrates within the tent to near 15%. The red curve shows the time course for the air to reach the 15% red level. The top right inset image shows an altitude simulation range from sea level to 6400 m/21,000 ft), ideal for high-altitude training. The bottom inset image shows "altitude training" with cycling, but also can be used for treadmill and other training modes.
(Photos courtesy of Hypoxico Inc., www.hypoxico.com, Cardiff, CA.)

into the tent to maintain the 15% oxygen concentration. Equilibrating the tent's environment at the 15% oxygen level requires about 90 min (orange line). Note that the woman wears an oximeter to continuously monitor oxygen concentration levels.

Summary

1. The progressive reduction in ambient Po_2 with increasing altitude produces inadequate hemoglobin oxygenation of arterial blood. Arterial desaturation impairs aerobic physical activities at 2000-m/6561-ft altitudes and above.
2. Altitude exposure does not adversely affect short-term (anaerobic) sprint and power performances that depend almost entirely on energy from intramuscular high-energy phosphates and glycolytic reactions.
3. Reduced Po_2 and accompanying hypoxia at altitude stimulate physiologic responses and adjustments that improve altitude tolerance during rest and physical activity.
4. Hyperventilation and increased submaximal cardiac output via elevated heart rate provide the primary immediate responses to altitude exposure.
5. Medical problems ranging from mild to life-threatening—AMS, HAPE, and HACE—often emerge during altitude exposure.
6. The potentially lethal HAPE and HACE conditions require immediate removal to a lower altitude.
7. Acclimatization entails physiologic and metabolic adjustments that improve tolerance to altitude hypoxia. The main adjustments involve reestablishing acid-base balance of body fluids, increased hemoglobin and red blood cell synthesis, and improved local circulation and cellular metabolism.
8. The altitude acclimatization rate depends on the terrestrial elevation. Noticeable improvements occur within several days. The major adjustments require about 2 wk, but acclimatization to high altitudes requires 4 to 6 wk.
9. Alveolar Po_2 averages 25 mm Hg at the Mt. Everest summit, reducing $\dot{V}O_{2max}$ by 70% to about 15 mL · kg^{-1} · min^{-1}.
10. Even with acclimatization, $\dot{V}O_{2max}$ decreases about 2% for every 300 m/984 ft above 1500 m/4921 ft. A decrement in endurance-related performance parallels reduced aerobic capacity.
11. Altitude-related declines in maximum heart rate and stroke volume offset any beneficial acclimatization effects; this partly explains the inability to achieve sea-level $\dot{V}O_{2max}$ values, even after acclimatization.
12. Training at altitude provides no greater benefit to sea-level performance than equivalent sea-level training.
13. Athletes benefit from periodically returning from altitude to sea level for intense training to offset "detraining" from lower exercise levels during a prolonged altitude stay.
14. The Gamow hyperbaric chamber and Hypoxico tent system represent two approaches to creating an "altitude" environment under sea-level conditions.

Key Terms

Acclimation: Adaptations produced in a controlled laboratory environment in specialized chambers that simulate high altitude

Acclimatization: Adaptive physiological and metabolic responses that improve altitude hypoxia tolerance

Acute mountain sickness (AMS): Nonspecific symptoms that include headache, nausea, dizziness, fatigue, insomnia, and peripheral edema symptoms experienced during the first few days at altitudes above 2500 m/8202 ft

Arterial hypoxia: Inadequate oxygen at the tissue cells caused by low arterial oxygen pressure

Chronic mountain sickness (CMS): Excessive red blood cell increase (polycythemia) and abnormally low blood oxygen levels (hypoxemia) common prevalent in altitude natives following months and years at altitude

Erythropoietin (EPO): Erythrocyte-stimulating hormone produced by the kidneys in response to reduced oxygen pressure that initiates red blood cell formation

Gamow hypobaric chamber: Person rests for about 10 hr daily in a chamber where total air pressure decreases to simulate a preselected altitude barometric pressure

High altitude: Based on the Earth's topography, terrestrial elevations that range between 3048 m/10,000 ft and 5486 m/18,000 ft above sea level

High-altitude cerebral edema (HACE): Potentially fatal neurologic syndrome that involves disorientation, lethargy, and nausea when the brain swells with fluid in individuals with AMS, which involves disorientation, lethargy, and nausea

High-altitude pulmonary edema (HAPE): Life-threatening condition from fluid accumulation in brain and lungs that occurs within 12 to 96 hr following rapid altitude ascent above 2500 m/8202 ft; from predisposing factors include altitude level, ascent rate, and individual susceptibility

High-altitude retinal hemorrhage (HARH): Affects virtually all altitude climbers above 6700 m/21,982 ft and usually progresses unnoticed without specific treatment or prevention

Hypoxia: Deficiency in oxygen reaching body tissues from ambient air's subnormal oxygen pressure at altitude

Hypoxico altitude tent: An hypoxic generator housed in an airline suitcase continually feeds hypoxic air into the tent to simulate 2500-m/8200-ft altitude

Lactate paradox: Hypoxic exposure for several weeks produces lower lactate levels without increases in either $\dot{V}O_{2max}$ or regional blood flow when high-altitude hypoxemia should promote lactate accumulation

Live high-train low: Training strategy to improve sea level performance in athletes who live at high altitude and train at low altitude to reap altitude acclimatization benefits while maintaining sea-level training intensity

Polycythemia: Reduced arterial oxygen partial pressure at altitude releases erythrocyte-stimulating hormone erythropoietin to stimulate increased total red blood cell number

> References are available online at Lippincott Connect.

Additional References

Allsopp GL, et al. Hormonal and metabolic responses of older adults to resistance training in normobaric hypoxia. *Eur J Appl Physiol.* 2022;122:1007. doi:10.1007/s00421-022-04897-4.

Bao H, et al. Study of brain structure and function in chronic mountain sickness based on fMRI. *Front Neurol.* 2022;12:763835.

Basak N, Thangaraj K. High-altitude adaptation: role of genetic and epigenetic factors. *J Biosci.* 2021;46:107.

Bebic Z, et al. Respiratory physiology at high altitude and considerations for pediatric patients. *Paediatr Anaesth.* 2022;32:118.

Breda FL, et al. Complex networks analysis reinforces centrality hematological role on aerobic-anaerobic performances of the Brazilian paralympic endurance team after altitude training. *Sci Rep.* 2022;12:1148.

Burtscher M, Viscor G. How important is $\dot{V}O_{2max}$ when climbing Mt. Everest (8,849 m)? *Respir Physiol Neurobiol.* 2022;297:103833.

Chen CY, et al. A sports nutrition perspective on the impacts of hypoxic high-intensity interval training (HIIT) on appetite regulatory mechanisms: a narrative review of the current evidence. *Int J Environ Res Public Health.* 2022;19:1736.

Faulhaber M, et al. Effects of acute hypoxia on lactate thresholds and high-intensity endurance performance—a pilot study. *Int J Environ Res Public Health.* 2021;18:7573.

Garrido E, et al. Acute, subacute and chronic mountain sickness. *Rev Clin Esp (Barc).* 2021;221:481.

Graf LC, et al. A prospective cohort study about the effect of repeated living high and working higher on cerebral autoregulation in unacclimatized lowlanders. *Sci Rep.* 2022;12:2472.

Hermand E, et al. Exercising in hypoxia and other stimuli: heart rate variability and ventilatory oscillations. *Life (Basel).* 2021;11:625.

Kong Z, et al. Hypoxic repeated sprint interval training improves cardiorespiratory fitness in sedentary young women. *J Exerc Sci Fit.* 2022;20:100.

Lackermair K, et al. Combined effect of acute altitude exposure and vigorous exercise on platelet activation. *Physiol Res.* 2022;71:171. PMID: 35043652.

Li Y, et al. Methods to match high-intensity interval exercise intensity in hypoxia and normoxia: A pilot study. *J Exerc Sci Fit.* 2022;20:70.

Mateo-March M, et al. Altitude and endurance performance in altitude natives versus lowlanders: insights from professional cycling. *Med Sci Sports Exerc.* 2022. doi:10.1249/MSS.0000000000002890.

Niederseer D, et al. Effects of a 12-week recreational skiing program on cardio-pulmonary fitness in the elderly: results from the Salzburg skiing in the elderly study (SASES). *Int J Environ Res Public Health.* 2021;18:11378.

Park HY, et al. Effects of interval training under hypoxia on the autonomic nervous system and arterial and hemorheological function in healthy women. *Int J Womens Health.* 2022;14:79.

Park HY, et al. Metabolic, cardiac, and hemorheological responses to submaximal exercise under light and moderate hypobaric hypoxia in healthy men. *Biology (Basel).* 2022;11:144.

Parodi JB, et al.; ANDES (Altitude Non-specific Distributed ECG Screening) project investigators. A systematic review of electrocardiographic changes in healthy high-altitude populations. *Trends Cardiovasc Med.* 2022:S1050-1738(22)00015-9.

Pérez-Padilla JR. Adaptation to moderate altitude hypoxemia: the example of the valley of Mexico. *Rev Invest Clin.* 2022;74:4.

Pramkratok W, et al. Repeated sprint training under hypoxia improves aerobic performance and repeated sprint ability by enhancing muscle deoxygenation and markers of angiogenesis in rugby sevens. *Eur J Appl Physiol.* 2022;122:611. doi:10.1007/s00421-021-04861-8.

Prisk GK, West JB. Non-invasive measurement of pulmonary gas exchange efficiency: the oxygen deficit. *Front Physiol.* 2021;12:757857.

Rieger M, et al. Kids with altitude: acute mountain sickness and changes in body mass and total body water in children travelling to 3800 m. *Wilderness Environ Med.* 2022;33:33. S1080-6032(21)00203-9.

Ruggiero L, et al. Neuromuscular fatigability at high altitude: lowlanders with acute and chronic exposure, and native highlanders. *Acta Physiol (Oxf).* 2022;234:e13788.

Schüttler D, et al. Effect of acute altitude exposure on ventilatory thresholds in recreational athletes. *Respir Physiol Neurobiol.* 2021;293:103723.

Shrestha A, et al. Vitreous hemorrhage following high-altitude retinopathy. *Case Rep Ophthalmol Med.* 2021;2021:7076190.

Storz JF, Bautista NM. Altitude acclimatization, hemoglobin-oxygen affinity, and circulatory oxygen transport in hypoxia. *Mol Aspects Med.* 2022;84:101052.

Szymczak RK, et al. Prolonged sojourn at very high altitude decreases sea-level anaerobic performance, anaerobic threshold, and fat mass. *Front Physiol*. 2021;12:743535.

Tymko MM, et al. Acid-base balance at high altitude in lowlanders and indigenous highlanders. *J Appl Physiol (1985)*. 2022; 132:575.

West JB. High altitude limits of living things. *High Alt Med Biol*. 2021;22:342.

West JB. Inspired oxygen: present, past, and future. *Am J Physiol Lung Cell Mol Physiol*. 2021;321:L1131.

Wolff S, et al. Exercise-induced cardiac fatigue in recreational ultramarathon runners at moderate altitude: insights from myocardial deformation analysis. *Front Cardiovasc Med*. 2022;8:744393.

Yang J, et al. Prediction of high-altitude cardiorespiratory fitness impairment using a combination of physiological parameters during exercise at sea level and genetic information in an integrated risk model. *Front Cardiovasc Med*. 2022;8:719776.

Zaman GS, et al. The impact of body resistance training exercise on biomedical profile at high altitude: a randomized controlled trial. *Biomed Res Int*. 2021;2021:6684167.

Table 24.1 Cardiorespiratory and Metabolic Exercise Responses During Submaximum Sea Level and Maximum 4000-m/13,100-ft Simulated Altitude

Exercise Level	$\dot{V}O_2$ (L·min^{-1})		$\dot{V}_E$ (L·min^{-1} BTPS)		Arterial Saturation (%)	
Altitude, m	0	4000	0	4000	0	4000
600 kg-m·min^{-1}	1.50	1.56	39.6	53.7	96	71
900 kg-m·min^{-1}	2.17	2.23	59.0	93.7	95	69
Maximum	3.46	2.50	123.5	118.0	94	70

Exercise Level	$\dot{Q}$ (L·min^{-1})		HR (B·min^{-1})		SV (mL)		a-$\bar{v}O_2$ Diff (mL O_2·dL^{-1})	
Altitude, m	0	4000	0	4000	0	4000	0	4000
600 kg-m·min^{-1}	13.0	16.7	115	148	122	113	10.8	9.4
900 kg-m·min^{-1}	19.2	21.6	154	176	125	123	11.4	10.4
Maximum	23.7	23.2	186	184	127	126	14.6	10.8

a-$\bar{v}O_2$ diff, arteriovenous oxygen difference; B, beats; HR, heart rate; $\dot{Q}$, cardiac output; SV, stroke volume; $\dot{V}_E$, expired volume; $\dot{V}O_2$, oxygen consumption.

Reprinted with permission from Stenberg J, et al. Hemodynamic response to work at simulated altitude 4000 m. *J Appl Physiol*. 1966;21:1589.

CHAPTER 25

Exercise and Thermal Stress

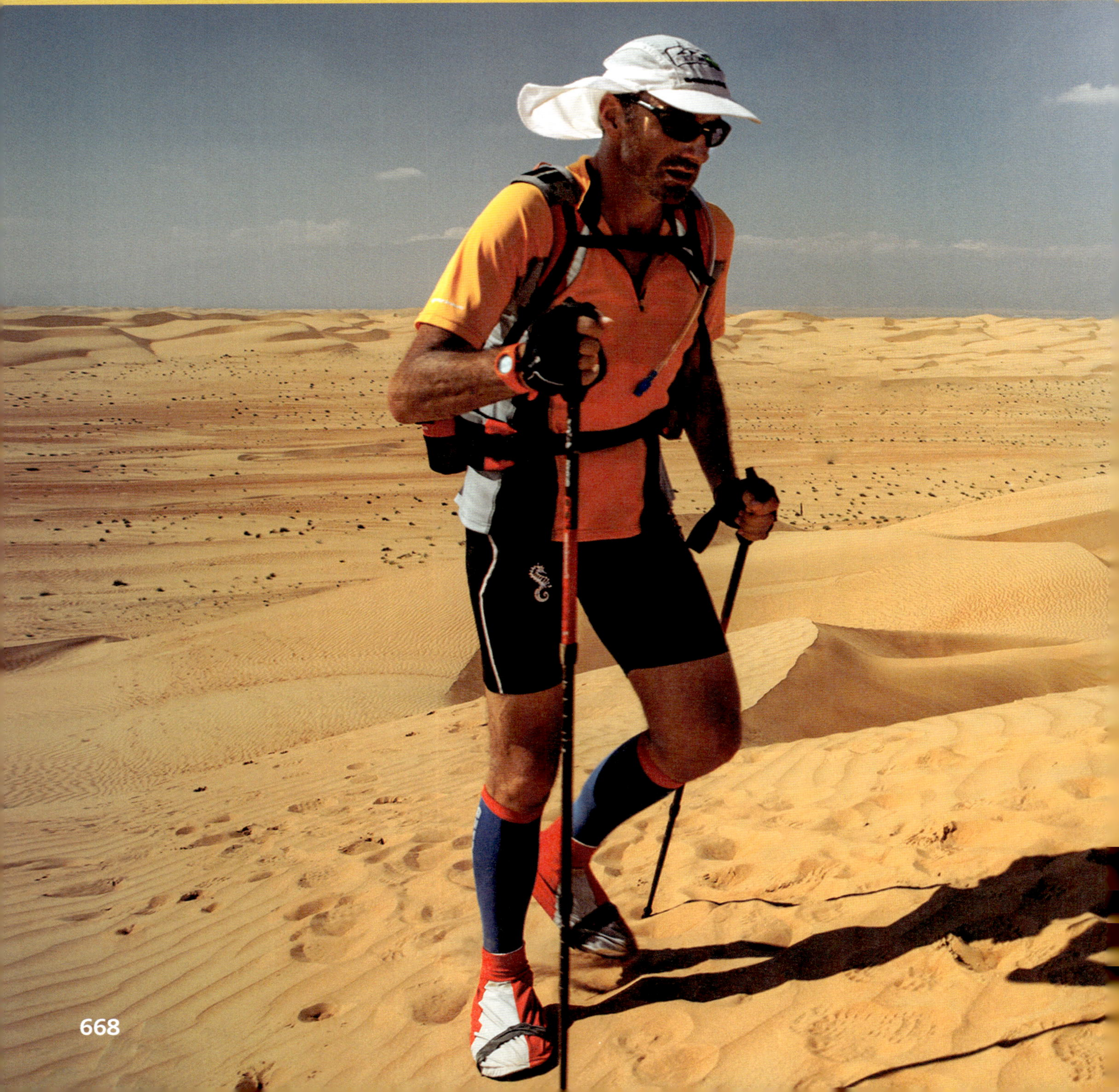

Chapter Objectives

- Explain how the hypothalamus maintains thermal balance
- Explain the four physical factors that contribute to heat gain and heat loss
- Discuss how the circulatory system serves as a thermoregulation "workhorse"
- List six factors that affect clothing's insulation (clo) value and two desirable clothing characteristics when exercising in cold and hot weather
- Discuss two factors that maintain cutaneous and muscle blood flow and blood pressure during hot weather physical activity
- Describe how cardiac output, heart rate, and stroke volume respond during physical activity in hot weather
- Quantify fluid loss during hot weather physical activity, and explain dehydration's effects on physiology and exercise performance
- Describe fluid replacement purposes and the alleged pre-exercise hyperhydration and glycerol supplementation benefits to physical activity in a hot environment
- Explain how acclimatization, training, age, gender, and body fat impact heat tolerance during physical activity
- Describe the main symptoms, possible causes, and treatment for heat cramps, heat exhaustion, and exertional heat stroke
- Describe components of the wet bulb-globe temperature index and the relative importance of each component
- Discuss two immediate and possible longer-term physiologic adjustments to cold stress

Ancillaries at-a-Glance

Visit Lippincott Connect to access the following resources.

- References: Chapter 25
- Focus on Research: Heat Stress and Cardiovascular Dynamics in Exercise

Humans can tolerate a decline in deep body temperature of 10°C/18°F but a body temperature increase of only 5°C/9°F. Temperature technically represents the substance's average kinetic energy of its atoms as they move. The potential for heat exchange between substances (e.g., blood to capillary walls) or objects (e.g., running surface to participant's body) reflects a functional definition for the term temperature. Over the past 30 years, more than 100 American football players at the high school, college, and professional level have died from excessive heat stress during practice or competition, most of them unnecessarily. Corey Stringer (1974–2001), an All-American at Ohio State University and first-round National Football League (NFL) Minnesota Vikings draft choice, died from complications of heat stroke during summer training camp. Stringer's death brought about major changes in how the NFL promoted heat stroke awareness and prevention during early-season practices. The National Center for Catastrophic Sport Injury Research (https://nccsir.unc.edu) prepares three annual reports about death and permanent disability sports injury data that involve the brain and/or spinal cord.

Hyperthermia and dehydration also contributed to how three apparently healthy collegiate wrestlers died just before their competitive season,[141] with numerous accounts worldwide of heat-related deaths during marathon runs and other long-duration events. The people who organize and guide athletic events and physical activity programs bear most of the responsibility for helping to eradicate heat injuries. A proper understanding about thermoregulation and the best ways to support these mechanisms should severely curtail such preventable tragedies.

Weather Versus Climate: Time as a Factor

Time is the factor that differentiates between **weather** and **climate**. Weather defines atmospheric conditions over a short time period, whereas climate describes atmospheric "behavior" over a prolonged period. Numerous factors characterize weather, such as sunshine, rain, cloud cover, wind, hail, snow, sleet, freezing rain, flooding, blizzards, ice storms, thunderstorms, steady rains from a cold front or warm front, excessive heat, and heat waves (https://climate.nasa.gov/ask-nasa-climate/2632/weather-or-climate-change/). Discussions about climate change usually center on long-term average changes in daily weather components for a particular world region or average trend over time.

Part 1 — Thermoregulation Mechanisms

Thermal Balance

FIGURE 25.1. shows that the deeper central tissue or **core** temperature represents a dynamic equilibrium between factors that add and subtract body heat. Integrating mechanisms that alter heat transfer to the periphery (**shell**) regulate evaporative cooling and vary the body's heat production to sustain thermal balance. Core temperature rises when factors that promote heat gain *exceed* the mechanisms for heat loss as during vigorous physical activity in a warm, humid environment. In contrast, core temperature declines in the cold when the body's heat loss *exceeds* heat production.[151] **TABLE 25.1** presents thermal data for heat production and heat loss via sweating during rest and maximal exertion.

TABLE 25.1 Thermodynamics during rest and exercise

The chemical reactions of energy metabolism produce gains in body heat that increase substantially during muscular activity. From shivering alone, whole body metabolism increases threefold to fivefold.[140] Metabolism in elite athletes often rises 20 to 25 times above the resting level to about 20 kcal · min^{-1} during intense aerobic activity; this theoretically can increase core temperature by 1°C/1.8°F every 5 to 7 min. The body also absorbs heat from solar radiation and objects warmer than the body. Heat leaves the body through radiation, conduction, and convection mechanisms, and most importantly from the skin and respiratory passages by water vaporization. Under optimal conditions, evaporative cooling with maximal sweating accounts for an 18 kcal · min^{-1} body heat loss.

Circulatory adjustments provide

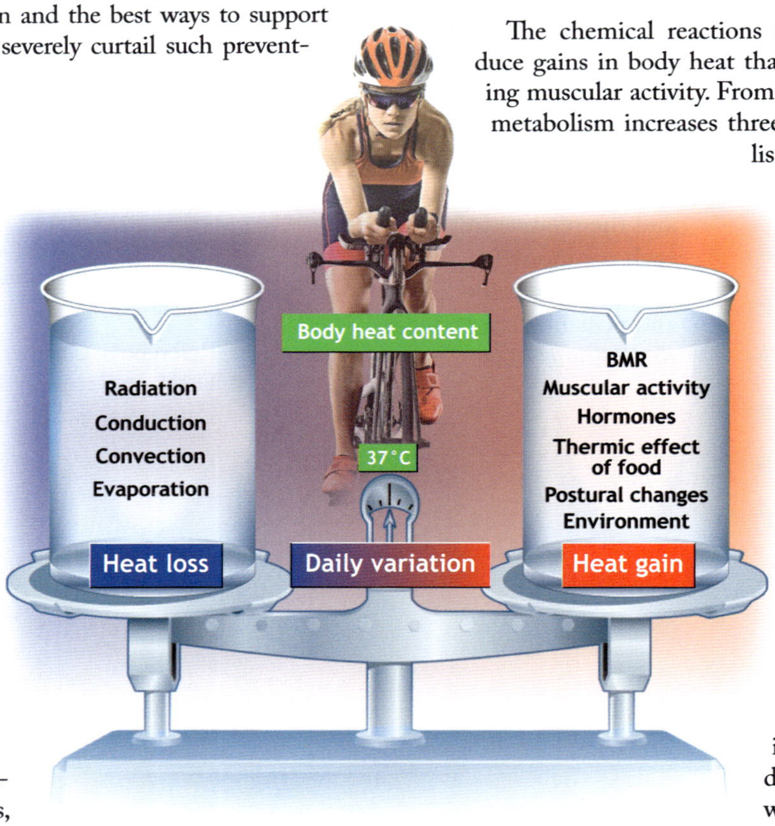

FIGURE 25.1. Contributing factors to heat loss and heat gain to regulate core temperature at 37°C/98.6°F. BMR, basal metabolic rate.
(Photo: OSTILL is Franck Camhi/Shutterstock)

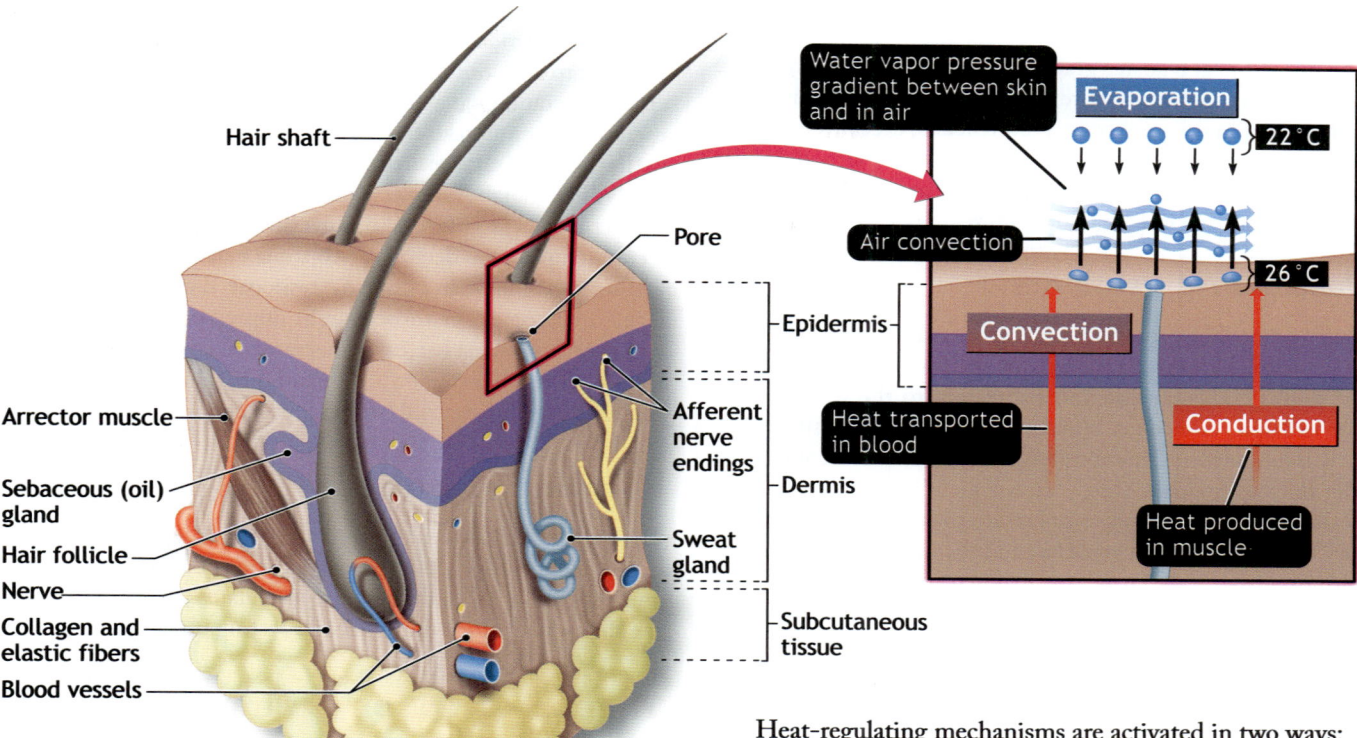

FIGURE 25.2. Left. Skin and underlying dermis, hair shaft, and subcutaneous and sweat gland structures. **Right.** Conduction, convection, and sweat evaporation dynamics for heat dissipation. Each 1 L water evaporated from the skin delivers 580 kcal heat energy to the environment.

"fine-tuning" for effective temperature regulation. Heat conservation occurs when blood shunts rapidly to the deep cranial, thoracic, and abdominal cavities and the body's muscle mass. This optimizes insulation from subcutaneous fat and other shell components. Conversely, increases in internal heat dilate peripheral vessels as warm blood flows to the cooler periphery. The drive to maintain thermal balance remains so strong that it triggers a 2.0 L · hr^{-1} sweating rate during physical activity in the heat or an 1200 mL · min^{-1} oxygen uptake from shivering in response to extreme cold.

Hypothalamic Temperature Regulation

The hypothalamus contains the central coordinating center for temperature regulation. This group of specialized neurons at the brain floor acts as a "thermostat"—usually set and carefully regulated to about 37 ± 1°C/98.6 ± 1.8°F—that continually makes thermoregulatory adjustments to deviations from a temperature norm. Unlike the automatic home thermostat, the hypothalamus cannot "turn off" the heat; it only can initiate responses to protect the body from either a buildup or loss of heat.

Heat-regulating mechanisms are activated in two ways:

1. Thermal skin receptors provide input to the central control center.
2. Temperature changes in the blood perfusing the hypothalamus directly stimulate this area.

FIGURE 25.2 shows the different structures embedded within the skin and subcutaneous tissue. The right *inset* depicts the transfer of heat produced by active muscles for cooling at the body surface by sweat evaporation when the water vapor pressure at the skin surface exceeds that of surrounding air. Peripheral thermal receptors responsive to rapid changes in heat and cold exist predominantly as free afferent nerve endings in the skin. The more numerous cutaneous cold receptors generally exist near the skin surface. Cold receptors play an important role to initiate regulatory responses to a cold environment. The cutaneous thermal receptors act as an "early warning system" to relay sensory information to the brain's hypothalamus and cortex. This direct communication line evokes appropriate heat-conserving or heat-dissipating physiologic adjustments, and the individual consciously seeks relief from any thermal challenge.

The central hypothalamic regulatory center plays the primary role in maintaining thermal balance. Cells in the hypothalamus' anterior portion detect slight blood temperature changes in addition to receiving peripheral input. These cells' heightened activity stimulates the posterior hypothalamus to initiate coordinated responses to conserve heat or the anterior hypothalamus to facilitate heat loss. The blood temperature perfusing the hypothalamus provides the primary monitoring system to assess body warmth, while the peripheral receptors detect cold.

Thermoregulation in Cold Stress

The normal heat transfer gradient flows from the body to the environment. Generally, core temperature regulation involves little or no physiologic strain. Nevertheless, excessive heat loss occurs in extreme cold, particularly at rest. The body's heat production in this case increases, while heat loss slows to minimize any decline in core temperature.

Vascular Adjustments

Cutaneous cold receptor stimulation constricts peripheral blood vessels, which immediately reduces the flow of warm blood to the body's cooler surface and redirects it to the warmer core. For example, cutaneous blood flow averages 250 mL · min^{-1} in a thermoneutral environment; yet with severe cold stress, this flow approaches zero.[61] Consequently, skin temperature declines toward ambient temperature to maximize the insulatory benefits from skin, muscle, and subcutaneous fat. A person with excessive body fat who is exposed to cold stress benefits from this heat-conserving mechanism. For a thinly-clad person with normal body fat content, cutaneous blood flow regulation generally provides effective thermoregulation at ambient temperatures between 25 and 29°C/77 and 84°F.

Muscular Activity

Shivering generates metabolic heat, but physical activity provides the greatest contribution in defending against cold extremes. Energy metabolism during movement sustains a constant core temperature in air as cold as −30°C/−22°F without reliance on a heavy, restrictive clothing barrier. Internal temperature, not the body's heat production *per se*, mediates the thermoregulatory response to cold. Shivering still occurs during vigorous activity if core temperature remains low. Cold stress often induces a larger exercise oxygen uptake from the cost of shivering compared to performing the same exercise in a warmer environment.

When metabolism decreases during more sustained physical activity as fatigue sets in, shivering alone may not prevent a core temperature decline.[138] To some extent, intervariability among individuals in shivering response dictates the many-faceted outcomes for those caught unprepared for accidental wet-cold exposures. Increases in steroid hormones, while having an effect on cardiac structure and functiong,[4] have no beneficial effects during cold (or heat) exposure.

Hormonal Output

Two "calorigenic" adrenal medulla hormones, epinephrine and norepinephrine, increase heat production as cold exposure progresses. Prolonged cold stress also stimulates thyroxine release, the thyroid hormone that increases resting metabolism.

Thermoregulation During Heat Loss

The body's thermoregulatory mechanisms primarily protect against overheating. Dissipating heat efficiently becomes crucial during physical activity in hot weather, when inherent competition exists between mechanisms that maintain a large muscle blood flow versus thermoregulatory mechanisms that redirect flow to the shell. **FIGURE 25.3** illustrates the factors that contribute to

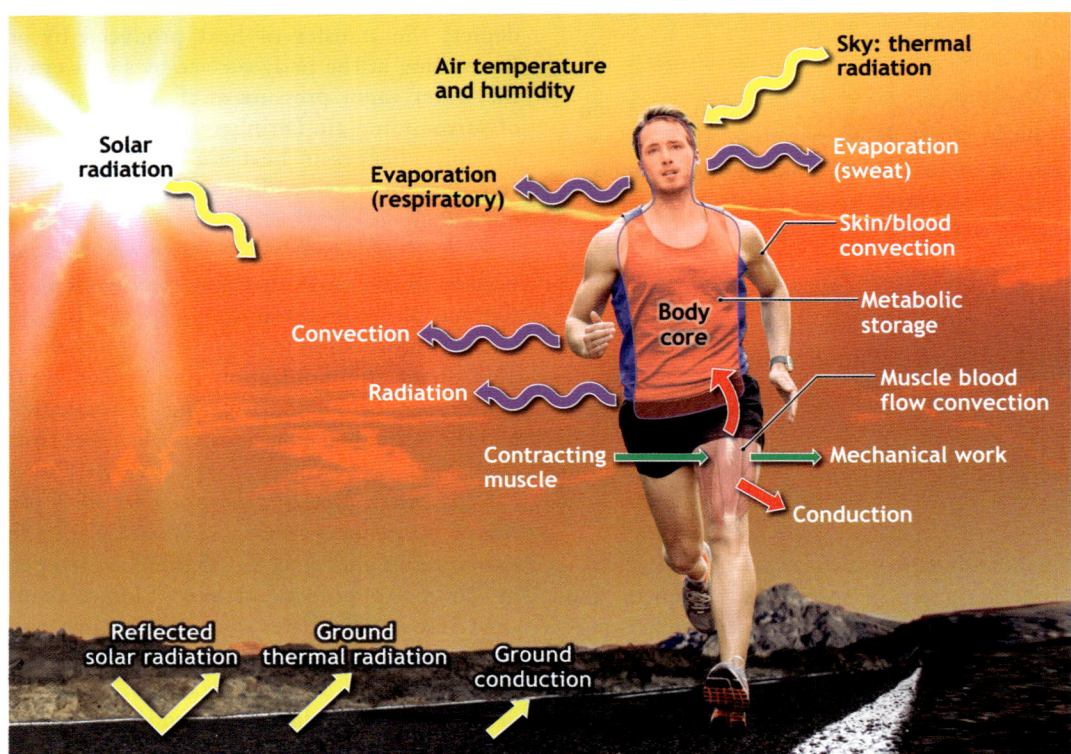

FIGURE 25.3. Heat production within active muscle and its transfer from the core to the skin. Excess body heat dissipates to the environment to regulate core temperature within a narrow range, despite extremes in ambient air temperatures.
(Adapted from Gisolfi CV, Wenger CB. Temperature regulation during exercise: old concepts, new ideas. *Exerc Sport Sci Rev.* 1984;12:339. Photo: Maridav/Shutterstock)

Worldwide Climate Change Concerns

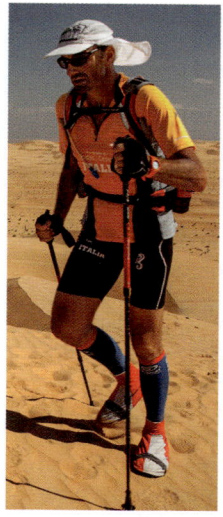
Klemen K. Misic/Shutterstock

Heat waves around the world have been increasing in frequency, intensity, and duration, with all-time records set in numerous countries. Epidemiologic evidence details the heavy toll extreme heat takes on human health and worker productivity. For example:

- Excessive heat has caused more deaths in Australia over the past two decades than the combined effect from all other natural disasters.
- Mortality and morbidity rates during heat waves are highest among the elderly, particularly those with chronic medical conditions, but do not exclude younger, athletic individuals, who often push endurance limits in extremely hot climates during summer months when race temperatures exceed 38°C/100°F.
- A lower sweating capacity in the elderly makes them particularly vulnerable to heat illness, cardiovascular disease, and ischemic events.
- Extreme heat takes a financial toll on businesses by increasing the likelihood workers experience heat strain, which can reduce productivity and adversely impact overall health.
- Increased chronic heat exposure impacts temperature-related excess mortality, disproportionately affecting the most disadvantaged in society, particularly individuals living in warmer and poorer regions.

Sources:
Millyard A, et al. Impairments to thermoregulation in the elderly during heat exposure events. *Gerontol Geriatr Med*. 2020;6:2333721420932432.
Nitschke M, et al. Evaluation of a heat warning system in Adelaide, South Australia, using case-series analysis. *BMJ Open*. 2016;6:e012125.

---

heat gain and heat loss during physical activity. Body heat loss occurs by four physical processes:

1. Radiation
2. Conduction
3. Convection
4. Evaporation

Heat Loss by Radiation

All objects, including humans, continually emit electromagnetic heat waves termed radiant energy. The human body usually remains warmer than the environment, making the net radiant heat energy exchange move through the air to solid, cooler objects in the environment. This heat transfer form, known as **radiation**, does not require molecular contact between objects. In fact, this avenue helps to explain the sun's warming effect on the Earth. A person can remain warm by absorbing radiant heat energy from direct sunlight, or alternatively, by reflection from snow, sand, or water, even in sub-freezing air temperatures. The body absorbs radiant heat energy from the surroundings when an object's temperature exceeds skin temperature.

Heat Loss by Conduction

Conductive heat exchange involves direct heat transfer from one molecule to another through a liquid, solid, or gas. The circulation transports most body heat to the shell, but a small amount continually moves by conduction directly through the deep tissues to the cooler surface. Heat loss by **conduction** involves warming air molecules and cooler surfaces that contact the skin.

Two factors determine the rate of conductive heat loss:

1. Temperature gradient between the skin and surrounding surfaces
2. Thermal properties of the surfaces

As an example, immersing the body in cool water can produce considerable heat loss. Placing one hand in room-temperature water clearly illustrates this phenomenon. Why does the hand in water feel much colder than the hand in air, even though the water and air have identical temperatures? The answer is straightforward—water absorbs several thousand times more heat than air and conducts it away from the warmer body part. Sitting in an indoor swimming pool with water at 28°C/82.4°F provides more discomfort than sitting on the pool deck at the same temperature. Hikers often gain considerable body heat when trekking in a warm environment. Lying on a rock shielded from the sun facilitates some body heat loss by conductance between the rock's cool surface and the hiker's warmer surface.

Heat Loss by Convection

Conductive heat loss effectiveness depends on how rapidly the air (or water) adjacent to the body exchanges once it warms. If air movement or **convection** proceeds slowly, the air next to the skin warms and acts as an "insulation zone" to minimize further conductive heat loss. Conversely, if cooler air continually replaces warmer air about the body on a breezy day, in a room with a fan or when running, heat loss increases because convection continually replaces the insulation zone. For example, air currents at 4 mph are about twice as effective for body cooling as air currents at 1 mph. Airflow's cooling effect forms the basis for the wind-chill temperature index (see "Wind-Chill Temperature Index" later in this chapter). This index indicates the equivalent still-air temperature for a particular ambient temperature at different wind velocities. Convection also exerts an effect on thermal balance in water because the body loses heat more rapidly when swimming than when remaining motionless.

Heat Loss by Evaporation

Water vaporizing from the respiratory passages and skin surface continually transfers heat to the environment (**evaporation**). Convective airflow that moves the moist, humidified air from the skin's surface continues to facilitate heat loss.[99] Each vaporized liter of water extracts 580 kcal from the body and transfers it to the environment.

The body's surface contains approximately 2 to 4 million sweat glands. During heat stress, these eccrine glands—controlled by cholinergic sympathetic nerve fibers—secrete hypotonic saline solution (0.2 to 0.4% NaCl).[158] Sweat evaporated from the skin exerts a cooling effect. The cooled skin in turn cools the blood diverted from interior tissues to the surface. In addition to sweat evaporation, about 350 mL of insensible perspiration seeps through the skin each day and evaporates to the environment. Also, about 300 mL of water vaporizes daily from the respiratory passages' moist mucous membranes, which exhibit as "foggy breath" in cold weather.

Heat Loss at High Ambient Temperatures

Evaporation provides the major defense against overheating. As ambient temperature increases, conduction, convection, and radiation decrease in their effectiveness to facilitate body heat loss. When ambient temperature exceeds body temperature, the body *gains* heat by these three thermal transfer mechanisms. In such environments, or when conduction, convection, and radiation cannot effectively dissipate a large metabolic heat load, sweat evaporation from the skin and respiratory tract provide the only means for heat dissipation. Increases in ambient temperature generally induce proportionate increases in sweating rate.

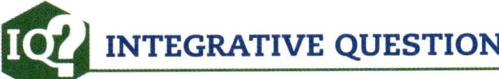

INTEGRATIVE QUESTION

A person walks along a beach on a cloudy day at a constant 4-mph speed. The wind blows from the west at a steady 12 mph. The westerly walk feels cooler than the return walk to the east, which feels warmer. How would you explain this discrepancy based on the physical principles of heat gain-heat loss?

Heat Loss During High Humidity

Three factors influence the total sweat amount vaporized from the skin and/or pulmonary surfaces:

1. Surface exposed to the environment
2. Ambient air's temperature and relative humidity
3. Convective air currents about the body

Relative humidity represents the most important factor in determining evaporative heat loss effectiveness. Relative humidity refers to water's ratio in ambient air at a particular temperature compared to the total moisture that air could contain expressed as a percentage. For example, 40% relative humidity means that ambient air contains only 40% of the air's moisture-carrying capacity at that specific temperature. With high humidity, the ambient vapor pressure approaches that of moist skin of about 40 mm Hg. In this case, evaporation greatly diminishes even though sweat beads on the skin and eventually rolls off. Sweating in this case represents useless water loss that can produce dehydration and overheating. A dangerous rise in core temperature can occur in athletes who compete in moderate- to high-intensity sports that exceed 30-min duration in environments above 35°C/95°F and ≥60% relative humidity. In a Practical Sense: Assessing Environmental Heat Quality: How Hot Is Too Hot?, on the next page, describes how to assess the environment's heat quality, with accompanying recommendations concerning physical activity related to three important factors—ambient temperature, radiant heat, and relative humidity.

Continually drying the skin with a towel while sweating, as some tennis players do between games and sets, thwarts evaporative cooling. *Evaporation, not sweat, cools the skin*. Individuals can tolerate relatively high environmental temperatures provided relative humidity remains low. Most persons find hot, dry desert climates more comfortable than cooler but more humid tropical climates.

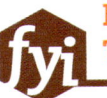 **Body Art Is a Hindrance to Thermoregulation**

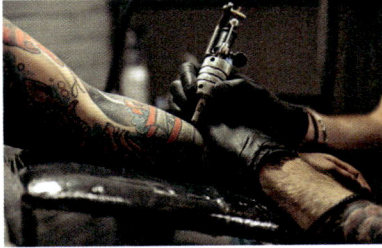

Olena Yakobchuk/Shutterstock

Tattooing skin involves repeatedly inserting a needle to deposit ink into the skin's dermal layer, a process that could potentially damage underlying eccrine sweat glands and accompanying cutaneous vasculature. This study assessed tattooing on reflex sweat rate (SR) increases and cutaneous vasodilation in tattooed skin (TAT) compared with adjacent healthy skin (CON) during passive whole body heat stress (WBH) in five males and five females with relatively large tattooed skin areas. Intestinal temperature (Tint), skin temperature (Tskin), skin blood flow, and SR were continuously measured during normothermic baseline (34C°/93.2°F water perfusing a tube-lined suit) and WBH (up to 48C°/118.4°F water perfusing suit). SR throughout WBH was lower for TAT compared with CON. Accumulated sweating responses during WBH were attenuated in TAT relative to CON. It appears that tattooing skin functionally damages sweat secretion mechanisms to negatively affect the gland's reflex capacity to produce sweat. Decreased sweating could impact heat dissipation, especially when tattooing covers a higher percentage of the body's surface, an occurrence prevalent among basketball, soccer, and American football and baseball athletes.

Source:
Luetkemeier MJ, et al. Skin tattooing impairs sweating during passive whole body heating. *J Appl Physiol.* 2020;129:1033. doi:10.1152/japplphysiol.00427.2019.

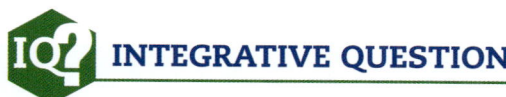

INTEGRATIVE QUESTION

In deciding on the starting time for an upcoming summer marathon, what prior meteorological information would be most valuable and why?

Integration of Heat-Dissipating Mechanisms

The mechanisms for heat loss remain the same whether the heat load originates internally from metabolic heat or externally from environmental heat.

Circulation

The circulatory system represents the "workhorse" to maintain thermal balance. At rest in the heat, heart rate and cardiac output increase, while superficial arterial and venous blood vessels dilate to divert warm blood to the body shell. This manifests as a flushed or reddened face on a hot day or during vigorous activity. With extreme heat stress, about 15 to 25% of the cardiac output passes through the skin. Enhanced cutaneous blood flow greatly increases peripheral tissues' thermal conductance to favor radiative heat loss to the environment, particularly from the hands, forehead, forearms, ears, and tibial areas.

Evaporation

Sweating begins within several seconds of the start of vigorous physical activity. After about 30 min, it achieves equilibrium in direct relation to the exercise load. An effective thermal defense exists when evaporative cooling combines with a large cutaneous blood flow. The cooled peripheral blood then flows to the deeper tissues to absorb additional heat as it returns to the heart.

Hormonal Adjustments

Sweating produces water and electrolytes losses that initiate hormonal adjustments to conserve salts and fluid. Fluid conservation makes urine more concentrated during heat stress. Concurrently, repeated exertion over days in the heat or just a single activity bout stimulates adrenocortical release of the sodium-conserving hormone aldosterone to increase sodium reabsorption. Aldosterone also reduces sweat's osmolality. This decreases sweat sodium concentration during repeated heat exposure to further conserve electrolytes. At the same time, physical activity and/or hypohydration stimulate the hypothalamus' neurohypophysis to release **vasopressin** (antidiuretic hormone). Vasopressin increases the permeability of the kidneys' collecting tubules to facilitate fluid retention. The magnitude of aldosterone and vasopressin release depends on hypohydration severity and physical activity intensity.[94]

How Clothing Impacts Thermoregulation

Clothing insulates the body from its surroundings. It can reduce radiant heat gain in a hot environment or retard conductive and convective heat loss in the cold.

Clothing Insulations (Clo Units)

The U.S. military has made a strong research commitment to develop clothing insulation standards to meet environmental challenges. The **clo unit** represents a thermal resistance index for the insulation provided by clothing. It indicates the insulatory capacity provided by any trapped air layer between the skin and clothing, including the clothing's insulation value. Assuming an environment with negligible air movement and body movement to disturb the air's insulatory layer, a 1 unit clo value maintains a sedentary person at 1 MET indefinitely in a 21°C/68.8°F environment with 50% relative humidity and 0.01 $m \cdot s^{-1}$/20 $ft \cdot min^{-1}$ air movement. Under these environmental conditions, 1 clo unit corresponds to an average-size man wearing a three-piece suit and light undergarments.

An individual's metabolic rate at a given environmental temperature also affects the clo unit requirement. **TABLE 25.2** presents six metabolic intensity categories from sleeping to heavy work expressed in MET units and three environmental temperatures (0°C, −20°C, −50°C/32°F, 4°F, −58°F).

TABLE 25.2 Clo values required to maintain a stable core temperature

Note the inverse relationship, shown in Table 25.2, between metabolic intensity and the insulation requirement (more clothing required for less work). At rest (1 MET) at 0°C/32°F, the clo requirement is 5.4, but when temperature drops to −50°C/−58°F, the clo requirement increases by 130% to 12.4.

Six factors impact clothing's insulation (clo value):

1. *Wind speed*—Increased speed disturbs the insulation zone
2. *Body movements*—Arm and leg pumping action disturb the insulation zone
3. *Chimney effect*—Loosely hanging clothing ventilates the trapped air layers away from the body
4. *Bellows effect*—Vigorous body movements increase ventilation of air layers that conserve body heat
5. *Water vapor transfer*—Clothing resists water vapor passage to decrease heat loss from evaporative cooling
6. *Permeation efficiency factor*—How well clothing absorbs liquid (sweat) by capillary action (wicking); wicking sweat away from the body surface reduces the evaporative cooling effect, thus improving clothing's effectiveness to conserve body heat

TABLE 25.3 presents clo values for common garments related to physical activity level and ambient temperature.

TABLE 25.3 Clo values for common garments

To determine the total insulatory value for what a person wears, add the individual clo values for each garment. Without wind penetration or air movement around the clothing, the clo value for the clothes equals 0.15 times the clothing weight in pounds. For example, wearing clothes weighing 4.5 kg/10 lb produces a clo value 1.5 (0.15 × 10 lb).

In a Practical Sense

Assessing Environmental Heat Quality: How Hot Is Too Hot?

FACTORS AFFECTING ENVIRONMENTAL HEAT STRAIN

Seven important factors determine the physiologic strain imposed by environmental heat:

1. Air temperature and relative humidity
2. Individual differences in body size and fatness
3. Training state
4. Acclimatization degree
5. Environmental influences such as convective air currents and radiant heat gain
6. Physical activity intensity
7. Clothing amount, type, and color

Several football deaths from heat injury occurred with air temperature below 23.9°C/75°F but with relative humidity above 95%. Prevention is the most effective heat-stress injury control. Most importantly, acclimatization minimizes heat injury likelihood. Another consideration requires evaluating the environment for its potential thermal challenge using the **wet bulb-globe temperature (WB-GT) index**. This environmental heat stress index developed by the military provides important information to the National Collegiate Athletic Association to establish thresholds for increased risk of heat injury and physical performance decrements. The WB-GT index depends on ambient temperature, relative humidity, and radiant heat as related in the following equation:

$$WB-GT = 0.1 \times DBT + 0.7 \times WBT + 0.2 \times GT$$

where DBT represents the dry bulb temperature (air temperature) recorded by an ordinary mercury thermometer, and WBT equals the wet bulb temperature recorded by a similar thermometer except that a wet wick surrounds the mercury bulb (see figure below). With high relative humidity, little evaporative cooling occurs from the wetted bulb, so this thermometer's temperature remains similar to the dry bulb. On a dry day, considerable evaporation occurs from the wetted bulb to maximize the difference between the two thermometer readings. A small difference between thermometer readings indicates high relative humidity, whereas a large difference indicates little air moisture and rapid evaporation. GT represents the globe temperature recorded by a thermometer with a black metal sphere enclosing its bulb. The black globe absorbs radiant energy from the surroundings to measure this source of heat gain. Most industrial supply companies sell this relatively inexpensive thermometer. One can also assess ambient heat load from a wet bulb thermometer (WBT) because this reading reflects both air temperature and relative humidity.

WB-GT RECOMMENDATIONS FOR CONTINUOUS ENDURANCE RUNNING AND CYCLING ACTIVITIES

The American College of Sports Medicine proposes the following recommendations concerning heat injury risk with continuous physical activity based on WB-GT (www.rrm.com/Newsarchives/archive11/11heat.htm):

- *Very high risk*: Above 28°C/82°F—Postpone race.
- *High risk*: 23 to 28°C/73 to 82°F—Heat-sensitive individuals (e.g., obese, low physical fitness, unacclimatized, dehydrated, previous history of heat injury) should not compete.
- *Moderate risk*: 18 to 23°C/65 to 73°F
- *Low risk*: Below 18°C/65°F

Without the WBT but knowing relative humidity (local meteorologic stations or media reports), the heat-stress index (see figure) evaluates the relative heat stress. The index should rely on data close to the actual activity/sport location to eliminate potential errors from meteorologic data some distance from the event area.

Relative humidity	Air temperature (°F)									
	70	75	80	85	90	95	100	105	110	115	120
	Heat sensation (°F)									
0%	64	69	73	78	83	87	91	95	99	103	107
10%	65	70	75	80	85	90	95	100	105	111	116
20%	66	72	77	82	87	93	99	105	112	120	130
30%	67	73	78	84	90	96	104	113	123	135	148
40%	68	74	79	86	93	101	110	123	137	151	
50%	69	75	81	88	96	107	120	135	150		
60%	70	76	82	90	100	114	132	149			
70%	70	77	85	93	106	124	144				
80%	71	78	86	97	113	136					
90%	71	79	88	102	122						
100%	72	80	91	108							

- 90°–105°F: Possibility of heat cramps
- 105°–130°F: Heat cramps or heat exhaustion likely, heat stroke possible
- ≥130°F: Heat stroke a definite risk

Cold-Weather Clothing

In providing insulation from cold, cloth fiber mesh traps air that then warms. This establishes a barrier to heat loss because the cloth and air conduct heat poorly. Insulation becomes more effective with a thicker trapped air zone above the skin. For this reason, several light clothing layers or garments lined with animal fur, feathers, or synthetic fabrics with numerous trapped air layers provide better insulation than a single bulky layer. The clothing layer against the skin should also wick moisture from the body's surface to the next insulating clothing layer for subsequent evaporation. Wool or synthetics (e.g., polypropylene) that insulate well and dry quickly serve this purpose. A wool cap contributes considerably to heat conservation; nearly 30 to 40% of body heat dissipates through the highly vascularized head region that represents only about 8% of the body's total surface area. Conversely, cooling the head during physical activity in hot weather reduces thermal discomfort symptoms. When clothing becomes wet, through either external moisture or condensation from sweating, its insulating properties decrease by almost 90%. This facilitates heat loss from the body because water conducts heat 25 times faster than air.

The thermoregulatory challenge when exercising in cold air arises not from inadequate insulation but from inadequate metabolic heat dissipation through a thick air-clothing barrier. Cross-country skiers alleviate this problem by removing clothing layers as the body warms to maintain core temperature without reliance on evaporative cooling. *The ideal winter garment in cold, dry weather blocks air movement but also allows water vapor from sweating to escape through the clothing.*

Warm-Weather Clothing

Dry clothing, no matter how lightweight, retards heat exchange more than the same clothing fully wet. *Switching to a dry tennis, basketball, or football uniform in hot weather makes little sense for temperature regulation.* Evaporative heat loss occurs only when the clothing becomes wet. A dry uniform simply prolongs the time lag between sweating and subsequent evaporative cooling.

Different materials absorb water at different rates. Cottons and linens readily absorb moisture. In contrast, heavy sweatshirts and rubber or plastic clothing produce high relative humidity close to the skin. This retards vaporization from its surface, blunting or even preventing evaporative cooling. Warm-weather clothing should fit loosely to permit free air circulation between the skin and environment to promote convection and evaporation from the skin. Moisture-wicking (breathable) fabrics (e.g., polypropylene, nylon, micromodel, bamboo, Merino wool) optimally transfer heat and moisture from the skin to the environment, particularly during intense activity in hot weather. They also benefit the individual during physical activity in cold environments because dry clothing, in contrast to sweat-drenched clothing, reduces hypothermia risk. Color also exerts an influence—dark colors absorb light rays and add to radiant heat gain, whereas lighter-colored clothing reflects heat rays from the body.

Football Uniforms

Football uniforms and equipment present a considerable barrier to heat dissipation during environmental heat exposure.[87] Even with loose-fitting porous jerseys, the wrappings, padding with its plastic covering, helmet, and other objects of "armor" effectively seal off 50% of the body's surface from evaporative cooling benefits. The 6- or 7-kg equipment barrier, frequently transported over a hot artificial playing surface, adds to the player's total metabolic load. The large size of these athletes further magnifies heat stress, particularly for offensive and defensive linemen with a relatively small surface area to body mass ratio and higher body fat percentage than smaller teammates at the other skill positions.

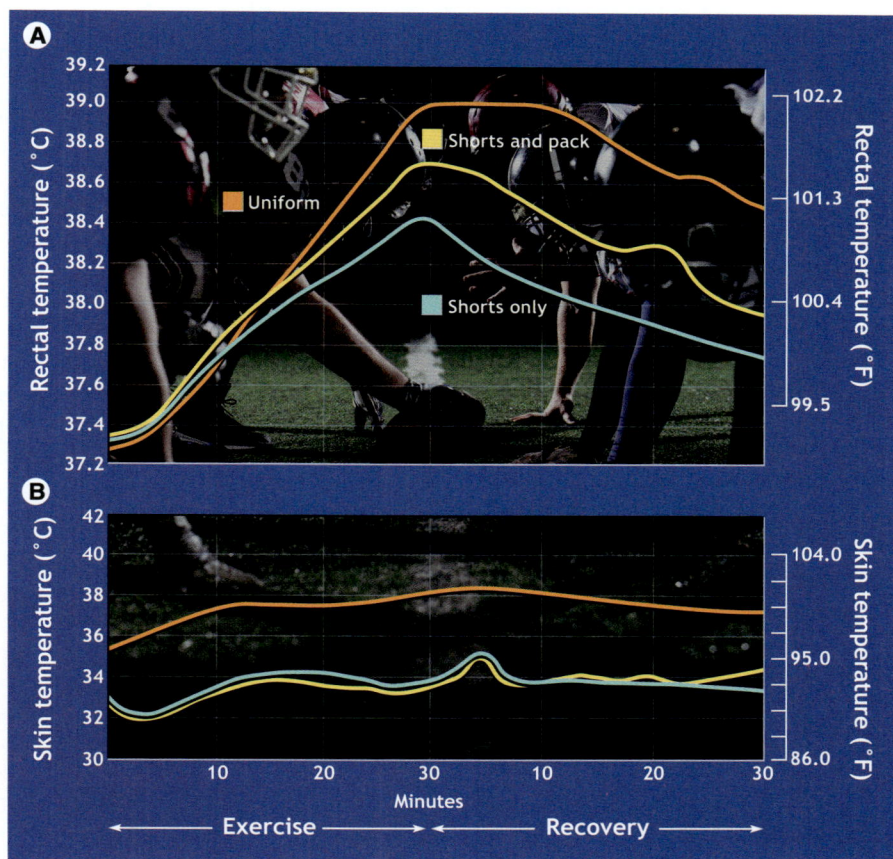

FIGURE 25.4. Full football uniform and its equivalent weight effects on **(A)** rectal temperature and **(B)** skin temperature during a simulated football practice while running on a treadmill at 9.6 km · hr⁻¹ for 30 min at 25.6°C/78°F and 35% relative humidity. The full uniform (*orange line*) caused the largest heat stress in retarding evaporative cooling and significantly elevated rectal and skin temperature.
(Adapted with permission from Mathews DK, et al. Physiological responses during exercise and recovery in a football uniform. *J Appl Physiol.* 1969;26:611. ©The American Physiological Society (APS). All rights reserved. Photo: dotshock/Shutterstock)

FIGURE 25.4 depicts the metabolic and thermal stress provided by a football uniform. In one test, the men wore only shorts; in another, they wore the complete football uniform including helmet and plastic padding. In a third series, they wore shorts and carried a backpack that contained 6.2 kg, the equivalent uniform and equipment weight.

Wearing football gear while exercising produced higher rectal and skin temperatures during physical activity and recovery than the other exercise conditions. Skin temperature directly beneath the padding averaged only 1°C/1.8°F less than rectal temperature. Thus, subcutaneous blood in these areas cooled by only about one fifth compared to blood near the skin surface exposed to the environment. Rectal temperature remained elevated in recovery with uniforms, so a rest period offers limited value to normalize thermal status unless the athlete removes the uniform. The *yellow* line shows that uniform weight accounts for a large portion of the heat load. Not wearing the uniform (*aqua* line in Fig. 25.4A and B) produced cooler skin temperatures and lower sweat rates. Without the uniform, evaporation progressed freely from the skin, whereas the uniform insulated the athlete and reduced the effective evaporative surface.

The Modern Cycling Helmet Does Not Thwart Heat Dissipation

For cyclists, wearing a commercially available helmet provides vital protection against possible head trauma, but does the cycling helmet impede thermoregulatory processes in a hot-dry or hot, humid environment? The head provides an important avenue for heat loss during exercise-induced hyperthermia, so many competitive cyclists believe riding without a helmet reduces thermal strain and physical discomfort. This belief persists even when the commercial protective helmet design retains the aerodynamic and lightweight features with ventilation ports for convective and evaporative cooling. To evaluate the physiologic and perceptual responses to wearing a helmet, 10 male and 4 female competitive cyclists pedaled for 90 min at 60% $\dot{V}O_{2speak}$ in both hot dry (35°C/95°F, 20% relative humidity) and hot humid (35°C/95°F, 70% relative humidity) environments with and without a protective helmet.[128] The results for oxygen uptake, heart rate, core, skin, and head skin temperatures, perceived exertion rating, and perceived thermal sensations about the head and body revealed that cycling in a hot, humid environment produced greater thermal stress than cycling under thermoneutral conditions. Wearing the helmet, nevertheless, did not increase the riders' overall heat strain or perceived heat sensations from the head or body.

Summary

1. Exposure to heat or cold stress initiates thermoregulatory mechanisms that generate and conserve heat at low ambient temperatures and dissipate heat at high temperatures.
2. The "thermostat" for temperature regulation resides in the brain's hypothalamus, which coordinates and initiates adjustments from the skin's thermal receptors and temperature changes of blood perfusing the hypothalamic region.
3. Heat conservation in cold stress results from vascular adjustments that shunt blood from the cooler periphery to the warmer deep body core tissues.
4. If vascular mechanisms prove ineffective during cold stress, shivering provides an input of metabolic heat. Also, prolonged cold stress stimulates hormone release that elevates resting metabolism.
5. Heat stress diverts warm blood from the body's core to the shell.
6. Radiation, conduction, convection, and evaporation are key factors contributing to heat dissipation.
7. Evaporation provides the major physiologic defense against overheating at high ambient temperatures and intense physical activity.
8. Evaporative heat loss effectiveness diminishes dramatically in warm, humid environments, increasing vulnerability to dehydration and spiraling core temperature.
9. Two practical heat-stress indices, the WB-GT index and the heat-stress index, use ambient temperature, radiant heat, and relative humidity to evaluate the environment's potential heat challenge.
10. Three factors influence sweat vaporization from the skin or pulmonary surfaces—surface exposure, ambient air temperature and relative humidity, and convective air currents.
11. Vigorous physical activity generates metabolic heat to maintain core temperature in cold air environments, even if the person wears little clothing.
12. The clo unit reflects thermal resistance from clothing; it quantifies air's insulators capacity trapped between the skin and clothing including the clothing's insulation value.
13. Wearing layers of light clothing traps an air zone against the skin to provide more effective insulation from cold than a single thick clothing layer.
14. Wet clothing loses its insulating properties and thereby facilitates heat flow from the body.
15. Ideal warm-weather clothing is lightweight, loose fitting, and light colored.
16. Football uniforms impose a barrier to heat dissipation because they effectively block about 50% of the body's surface from evaporative cooling's beneficial effects.

Part 2: Thermoregulation and Environmental Heat Stress During Physical Activity

Physical Activity in the Heat

The refrigerating mechanism of evaporative cooling dissipates metabolic heat during physical activity, particularly exposure during hot weather. This places a demand on the body's fluid reserves, often producing a relative hypohydration. Excessive sweating precipitates more serious fluid loss with accompanying reduced plasma volume causing circulatory failure in the extreme when core temperature rises to lethal levels beyond 43°C/104°F.

Circulatory Adjustments

The body encounters two competitive cardiovascular demands when exercising in the heat:

1. Demand muscles require arterial blood (oxygen) delivery to sustain energy metabolism.
2. Demand arterial blood diverts to the periphery to transport metabolic heat for cooling at the skin surface; this blood cannot deliver its oxygen to active muscle.

Submaximal effort produces similar cardiac outputs in hot and cold environments.[118] The heart's stroke volume usually remains lower in the heat in proportion to the fluid deficit and reduced blood volume created in physical activity.[44,97] This effect translates to *higher heart rates* at all submaximal levels of activity in the heat. In contrast, the reflex compensatory increase in heart rate during maximal effort fails to offset the stroke volume decrease, so maximal cardiac output necessarily must decrease.

Vascular Constriction and Dilation

Maintaining adequate cutaneous and muscle blood flow during physical activity under heat stress requires other tissues to temporarily compromise blood supply. For example, during environmental heat stress, compensatory constriction of the splanchnic vascular bed and renal tissue rapidly counteracts active vasodilation of the subcutaneous vessels responsible for 80 to 95% of an elevated skin blood flow.[60,84] A prolonged reduction in renal and visceral tissue blood flow probably contributes to liver and renal complications during exertional heat stress.

Maintaining Blood Pressure

Vasoconstriction in the viscera increases total vascular resistance. A balance between dilation and constriction maintains arterial blood pressure during physical activity in the heat. In intense effort, with accompanying dehydration, relatively less blood diverts to peripheral areas for heat dissipation. Reduced peripheral blood flow reflects the body's attempt to maintain cardiac output because of a diminished plasma volume caused by sweating. *Circulatory regulation and muscle blood flow take precedence over temperature regulation during physical activity in the heat.* When submaximal effort progresses without excessive physiologic strain, a greater dependence still exists on anaerobic metabolism than in cooler conditions.[149] This produces three effects:

1. Earlier lactate accumulation
2. Encroachment on glycogen reserves
3. Premature fatigue during prolonged moderate activity

Two factors increase blood lactate accumulation:

1. Decreased lactate uptake by the liver from reduced hepatic blood flow
2. Reduced muscle catabolism of circulating lactate because heat dissipation diverts a relatively larger portion of the cardiac output to the periphery

Core Temperature During Physical Activity

Heat generated by active muscles can raise core temperature to fever levels that would incapacitate a person if caused by external heat stress alone. Elite endurance athletes, including champions, show no ill effects from rectal temperatures as high as 41°C/105.8°F from a bout of intense physical activity.[13,152] Aerobically fit subjects perform longer in *uncompensably hot environments*, environments where thermoregulatory mechanisms are inadequate, and tolerate higher levels of hyperthermia than less fit subjects.[17] Trained individuals' ability to reach higher core temperatures than untrained counterparts may leave them more prone to experience heat-related problems.[98,100] An abnormally high core temperature for trained and untrained subjects impairs exercise performance. Fatigue generally coincides with core temperatures between 38 and 40°C/100 and 104°F. This temperature range reflects a "critical" high body temperature that impairs muscle activation directly from a high brain temperature that decreases the central drive to exercise. A thermally induced exercise impairment also may result from reduced blood flow to specific gastrointestinal tract regions to produce gastrointestinal barrier dysfunction and increased permeability. This effect allows endotoxins present inside bacterial cells, which upon degradation enter the internal environment and contribute to fatigue.[18,70]

Within limits, the increase in core temperature during physical activity does not reflect a failure of heat-dissipating mechanisms or contributes to early fatigue. To the contrary, it represents a well-regulated response even during physical activity in the cold. **FIGURE 25.5A** illustrates the relationship between core tem-

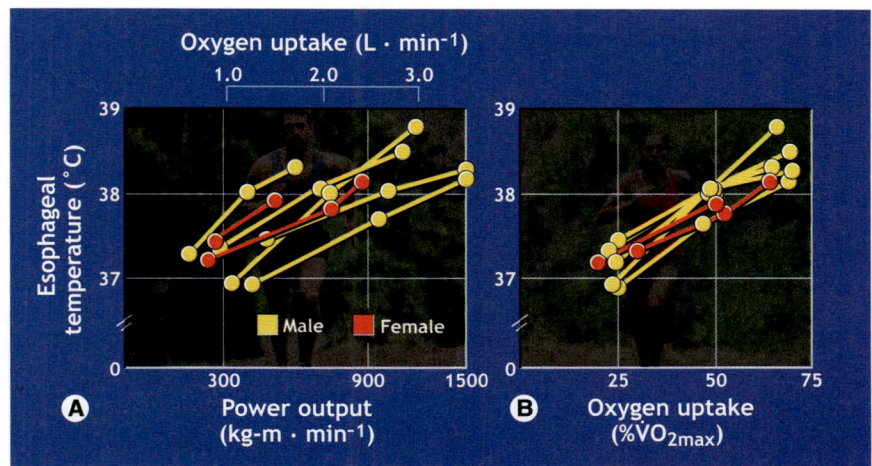

FIGURE 25.5. Relationship among esophageal temperature and **(A)** oxygen uptake (absolute exercise intensity expressed as power output) and **(B)** oxygen uptake as "%$\dot{V}O_2$max."
(Adapted with permission from Saltin B, Hermansen L. Esophageal, rectal, and muscle temperature during exercise. *J Appl Physiol.* 1966;21:1757. ©The American Physiological Society (APS). All rights reserved. Photo: Maridav/Shutterstock)

perature measured in the esophagus and power output expressed as oxygen uptake in five males and two females with different fitness levels during progressively more intense effort. Core temperature increased to a higher level for all subjects with increasing exercise intensity, although considerable intersubject variation occurred in temperature response. Note that the lines move closer together in **FIGURE 25.5B**, which plots core temperature related to oxygen uptake expressed as a percentage of each person's $\dot{V}O_{2max}$. This indicates that relative workload (i.e., percentage capacity) determines the change in core temperature with physical activity. More than likely, a modest rise in core temperature represents a favorable adjustment to optimize physiologic and metabolic functions.

In general, physical effort at 50% $\dot{V}O_{2max}$ in a comfortable environment increases core temperature to a new steady level at about 37.3°C/99°F, whereas work at 75% maximum elevates temperature to 38.5°C/101°F, regardless of the absolute oxygen uptake. This means a fit person generates more total energy (heat) during physical activity than a less-fit person exercising at the same $\dot{V}O_{2max}$ percentage, yet both maintain about the same core temperature. The extra metabolic heat for the trained person dissipates with a larger sweat output. The trained person exercises with a lower core temperature than the untrained person at identical physical activity levels (i.e., same absolute $\dot{V}O_2$).

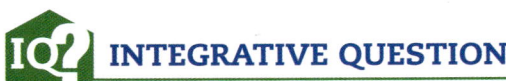

INTEGRATIVE QUESTION

What mechanisms explain how improved aerobic fitness increases exercise tolerance in a warm, humid environment?

Dehydration: Water Loss in the Heat

Dehydration refers to body water loss from a hyperhydrated state to euhydration or from euhydration downward to hypohydration. A moderate workout over 1 hr generally produces a 0.5 to 1.0 L sweat loss. Greater water loss occurs during several hours of intense activity in a hot environment. Sweating still occurs in less challenging thermal environments. For swimmers and divers, water immersion also stimulates fluid loss through increased urine production. Non–exercise-induced water loss occurs when wrestlers, boxers, weightlifters, and rowers aggressively attempt to "make weight" through rapid weight loss induced by common dehydration techniques—external heat exposure from sauna, steam room, hot whirlpool or shower, fluid and food restriction, diuretic and laxative use, and vomiting. Athletes often combine these techniques, hoping to accelerate weight loss. *Heat illness risk greatly increases when a person begins physical activity in a dehydrated state.*

Fluid deficits in the intracellular and extracellular compartments (*hypovolemia*) with hypohydration can reach levels that reduce the body's ability to dissipate heat and increase the rate of heat storage and cardiovascular strain from sweating rate and skin blood flow reductions for a given core temperature. Reduced heat tolerance severely compromises cardiovascular function and physical capacity with intense exertion in hot environments.[96,125,153–155] Sweat remains hypotonic to other body fluids, so hypovolemia from sweating correspondingly increases plasma osmolality.

Rapid weight loss through dehydration does not impair muscular strength or a single bout of anaerobic power performance up to 60-s duration, although the effects on muscular endurance remain equivocal.[19,45,95,144] Reducing body water rapidly before a short-duration activity may even improve muscular power and strength on a relative per kg body mass basis.[58] When intense effort lasts longer than 1 min, dehydration profoundly impairs physiologic function and optimal ability to train and compete.[156] Moderate hypohydration equivalent to 1.5% body mass produces poorer intermittent all-out performance than similar effort when euhydrated.[83] Dehydration associated with a 3% decrease in body weight also slows gastric emptying rate, increasing epigastric cramps and nausea.

Fluid Loss Magnitude

For an acclimatized person, water loss by sweating reaches a 3 L · hr^{-1} peak during intense, hot weather physical activity, and in the extreme, can total nearly 12 L · d^{-1} (about 3.2 gal/406 oz on a daily basis). Intense sweating for several hours produces sweat-gland fatigue that ultimately can interfere with core temperature regulation. Elite marathon runners frequently experience fluid loss in excess of 5 L during competition, a body weight loss equivalent to 6 to 10%. For a slower-paced ultramarathon, the average fluid loss rarely exceeds 500 mL · hr^{-1}. Even in a temperate (10°C/50°F) climate, soccer players lose on average 2 L of fluid during a 90-min game.[80] *Acclimatized humans sustain their exceptional potential for evaporative cooling only with adequate fluid replacement.* **TABLE 25.4** provides the predicted sweating rates for different body weights while running at various speeds in cold/temperate and warm weather conditions.

TABLE 25.4 Predicted sweating rates during running in cool and warm weather

Sports other than distance running induce a large sweat output with accompanying fluid loss. Football, basketball, lacrosse, soccer, and hockey players can lose large fluid quantities during competition. Before a change in certification standards, high school wrestlers often shed 9 to 13% of preseason body weight prior to certification, the greatest portion coming from voluntary water restriction combined with excessive sweating in a sauna prior to the weigh-in. Collegiate wrestlers, excluding heavyweights, regained an average 3.7 kg during the 20 hr between weigh-in and competition.[127] In their desire to "make weight," high school and collegiate wrestlers typically competed while dehydrated (with reduced blood and plasma volume).[1,148] Transient, reversible mood alterations and impaired short-term memory in collegiate wrestlers also are a consequence from rapidly losing weight.[21]

Water Loss Relates to Activity Intensity and Ambient Temperature

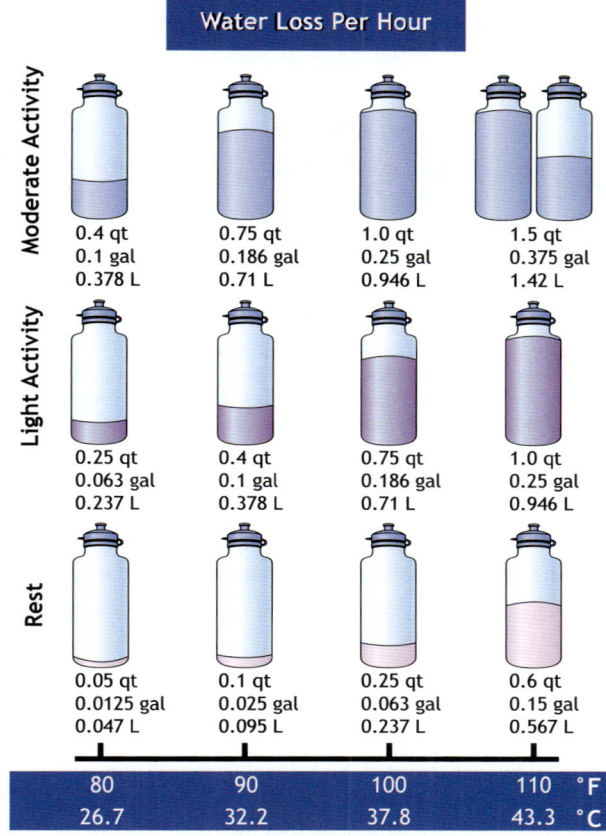

Average water loss per hour for a typical adult caused by sweating at various air temperatures during rest and light and moderate physical activity.

Extreme Ultramarathon Performance in the Heat

Competition across inhospitable environments is not uncommon (www.nps.gov/deva/learn/photosmultimedia/photogallery.htm). For example, the Badwater Ultramarathon-135 (www.badwater.com/event/badwater-135/) is considered the world's most demanding and extreme running race. The competition begins at 282 ft below sea level and covers 217 km/135 mi during mid-July in the hottest and driest North America region in Death Valley National Park, California, when the outside temperature averages 47.8°C/118°F during the day with a low of 32.8°C/91°F.

In this grueling event, the asphalt running surface temperature can reach 93.3°C/200°F (almost the temperature required to boil an egg!) without aid stations along the route. Runners cannot wear "cooling vests" or any other artificial/technological cooling system, including intravenous fluid hookups. Under the carefully controlled and strict adherence for safety requirements by race organizers and State of California, runners have reduced large

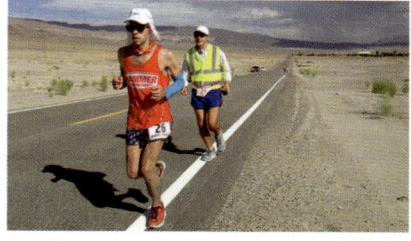

Photo of Pete Kostelnick running in the Badwater 135 in 2015; Photo: Gabe Elizondo

fluctuations in body weight (and thus fluid balance) by judicious water and salt supplementation.

Ultraendurance runners who participate in extreme events worldwide under the most trying, hostile environments can control body weight during continuous activity of 6 or more hours to within about ±2% of their initial prerace weight. They thus maintain "adequate" hydration without a severe hyponatremia calamity and possibly death. During a recent Badwater ultimate endurance challenge, proper fluid ingestion at carefully timed intervals with salt supplements kept runner's body weight loss to only 1.4 kg/3.1 lb. Fluid loss and replenishment represented between 14 and 16 quarts (3.5 to 4 gal) liquid! The record time for the Badwater 135 Basin run with more than 90 invited athletes (only 60 finished) was achieved by Yoshiko Ishikawa from Japan in 2019 (age 31 y) with a time of 21:33:01. The top female competitor in the 2019 race, Patrycja Bereznowska (age 43) from Poland, shattered the prior 2016 record (25:53:07) by almost 1 hr and 20 min to 23:13:24, the overall course record as of July 5, 2022.

Weather's Impact on Running Performance

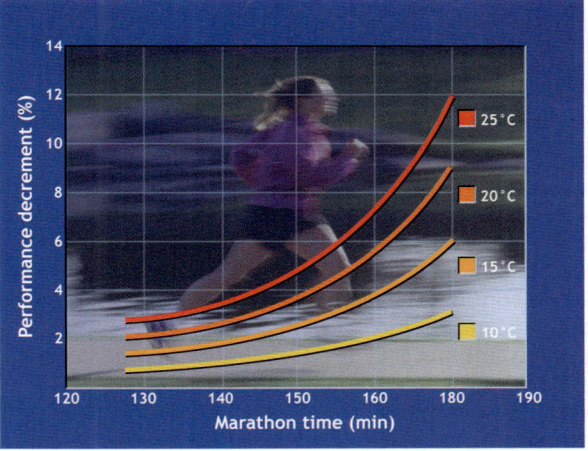

Figure adapted with permission from Ely MR, et al. Impact of weather on marathon-running performance. *Med Sci Sports Exerc.* 2007;39:487.

Marathon running performance's progressive slowing for men and women as wet bulb-globe temperature (WB-GT) increases from 10 to 25°C/50 to 77°F. Slower runners were more negatively impacted.

Significant Dehydration Consequences

Almost any dehydration impairs physiologic function and thermoregulation. Chronic dehydration contributes to hypotension, urinary tract infections, and kidney stones, chronic fatigue, together with diminished mental activity and impaired physical coordination. It may also contribute to damage from inflammation, which increases chronic disease risk. Even a modest 2% body mass fluid loss adversely affects exercise performance.[29,32,93,142] As dehydration progresses and plasma volume decreases, peripheral blood flow and sweating rate diminish, making thermoregulation progressively more difficult. Pre-exercise dehydration equivalent to 5% body mass increases rectal temperature and heart rate and decreases sweating rate, $\dot{V}O_{2max}$, and exercise capacity, while also attenuating multiset-multirepetition resistance exercise performance compared with physical activity under normal hydration.[62,123,130] Reduced central blood volume lowers ventricular filling pressure and helps to explain the elevated heart rate and 25 to 30% stroke volume reduction while dehydrated. An increase in heart rate does not offset the reduced stroke volume, so both cardiac output and arterial blood pressure decline.

Fluid losses increase during physical activity in hot, humid environments because ambient air's high vapor pressure thwarts evaporative cooling. **FIGURE 25.6** shows the linear dependency between sweating rate during rest and activity and the air's moisture content reflected by wet bulb temperature (see In a Practical Sense: Best Rehydration Methods for Physical Activity). Ironically, excessive sweat output in high humidity contributes little to cooling owing to minimal fluid evaporation.

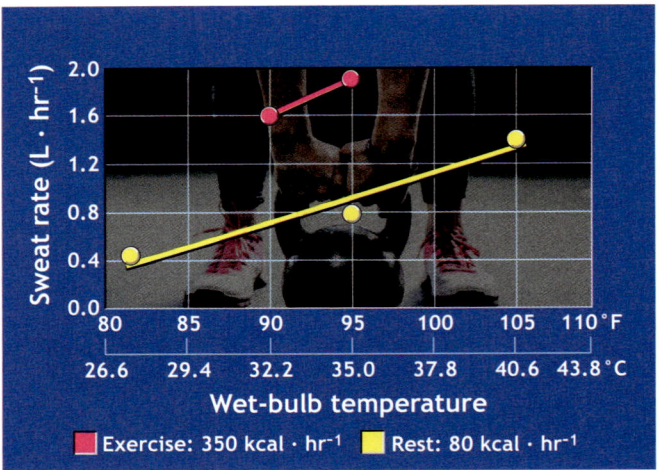

FIGURE 25.6. Humidity's effect (wet bulb temperature) on sweat rate during rest and walking in the heat.
(Adapted from Iampietro PF. Exercise in hot environments. In: Shephard RJ, ed. *Frontiers of Fitness*. Springfield: Charles C. Thomas; 1971. With permission from RJ Shephard. Photo: Goolia Photography/Shutterstock)

 Incredible Fitness Preparation Required!

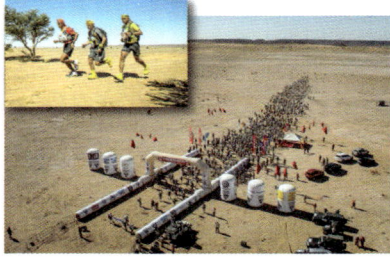

Photo of the 2019 Marathon Des Sables starting gate reprinted with permission from CIMBALY_MDS2019@VCAMPAGNIE.
Photo of three men running in the 2019 Marathon Des Sables reprinted with permission from CIMBALY_MDS2019 @JOSUEFPHOTO.

The Marathon des Sables, a six-stage, 250-kg/155-mi run, is roughly equivalent to running 23.5 mi a day for 6 days in extreme heat over harsh and varied terrain in southern Morocco (www.marathondessables.com/en/marathon-des-sables/race). In the 2021 race, there were 1162 competitors from over 50 countries. The race, held for 35 years, assists children and disadvantaged Moroccan populations with health, education, and sustainable development. Competitors in the 2021 race included highly trained men and women, adventurers only moderately trained, a runner in flip-flops, and even a leg amputee. Each runner, with his or her unique motivation and competitive experience, carried a backpack containing the minimum required for a 6-day desert trek—food, water, sleeping bag, compass, headlamp, and a venom pump to minimize insect bites. A huge volunteer support staff of medical personnel, helicopters, all-terrain vehicles, buses, and 2 camels provided water, painkillers, and miles of salves, compresses, and wraps for foot protection. A special bus provided daily incineration for burning waste.

Being tough, rugged, and highly motivated are traits possessed by just about all high-level ultraendurance competitors. But when the competition demands that the participant, a leg amputee who lost the lower part of her left leg in a motorcycle accident, compete with a leg prosthesis, an additional set of challenges arises. The 46-year-old amputee from Long Island, New York, exemplifies grit, determination, and physical fitness in a quest to conquer this unforgiving challenge. Her greatest hurdle, other than battling the brutal environmental heat, was arriving through trial and error, with a proper carbon fiber leg prosthesis that would not melt in extreme heat and would structurally withstand the uneven undulating terrain without causing unbearable skin irritation from ground heat extremes.

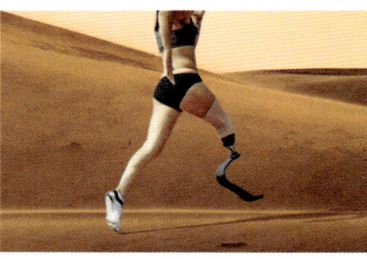

Shutterstock: danm12, sportpoint

A scrap of Goodyear tire, three and a half inches wide, was placed on the running blade for traction. The prosthetic leg included an air chamber to cool its outer and inner layers and was coated in a chalky color with paint to reflect heat. In a note of pre-race encouragement, her 13-year-old daughter wrote, *"Good luck. I love you. Don't die."* The good news is that she did not die and successfully completed the race, and thus became the first female amputee to achieve such a formidable distinction.

Physiologic and Performance Decrements

Physiologic mechanisms contributing to dehydration-mediated performance degradation during physical activity in the heat include the following[124,157]:

1. Augmented hyperthermia
2. Increased cardiovascular strain
3. Altered metabolic and central nervous system functions
4. Impaired cognitive performance
5. Increased perception of effort

Reduced peripheral blood flow and increased core temperature in activity relate closely to dehydration level. A fluid loss equivalent to only 1% body mass increases rectal temperature compared with the same exercise and normal hydration. For each liter of sweat-loss dehydration, exercise heart rate increases 8 b·min^{-1}, with a corresponding 1.0 L·min^{-1} decrease in cardiac output.[22] Water lost through sweating mainly comes from blood plasma, so circulatory capacity progressively decreases as sweat loss progresses. Fluid loss coincides with the following five factors:

1. Decreased plasma volume
2. Reduced skin blood flow for a given core temperature
3. Reduced stroke volume
4. Increased near-compensatory heart rate
5. General deterioration in circulatory and thermoregulatory efficiency during exercise

Dehydration equal to 4.3% body mass reduced walking endurance by 48%; concurrently, $\dot{V}O_{2max}$ decreased by 22%.[23] These same experiments showed decreased endurance performance (−22%) and $\dot{V}O_{2max}$ (−10%) when dehydration weight loss averaged only 1.9% body mass. Clearly, even modest dehydration imposes adverse thermoregulatory effects during physical activity that relate to progressive deterioration in sports performance.[6,7]

Diuretics

Diuretic-induced dehydration draws a greater water percentage from the plasma than body water lost through sweating. In addition, drugs that cause diuresis markedly impair neuromuscular function, which does not occur with comparable fluid loss through physical activity.[145] Chemicals that induce vomiting and diarrhea for sudden weight loss trigger dehydration and promote excessive mineral loss with accompanying muscle weakness and impaired neuromuscular function.

Rehydration and Hyperhydration to Maintain Fluid Balance

Fluid replacement must focus on maintaining plasma volume so circulation and sweating progress at optimal levels. Ingesting fluid during physical activity increases blood flow to the skin for more effective cooling, independent of any change in plasma volume. Such fluid replacement during activity also reverses the sustained postexercise hypotension observed in trained athletes.[40,88,158,159] Dehydration prevention and its consequences, especially hyperthermia, occurs only with an adequate and strictly observed water replacement schedule.[126]

Optimal Goals for Fluid Intake During Physical Activity

- *Prehydrating:* Start the activity euhydrated and with normal plasma electrolyte levels. This should be initiated when needed, at least several hours before the activity to enable fluid absorption and allow urine output to return to normal levels.
- *Drinking during activity:* Prevent excessive dehydration (>2% body weight loss from water deficit) and excessive changes in electrolyte balance to avert compromising performance and health. During activity, consume beverages with electrolytes and carbohydrate to provide benefits over water alone.

Sources:
Cheuvront SN, Kenefick RW. Personalized fluid and fuel intake for performance optimization in the heat. *J Sci Med Sport*. 2021;24:735.
Thomas DT, et al. American College of Sports Medicine Joint Position Statement. Nutrition and athletic performance. *Med Sci Sports Exerc*. 2016;48:543.

Adequate hydration provides the most effective defense against heat stress. The ideal hydration protocol requires balancing water loss with water intake, not dousing the head or body with water. No evidence indicates that constraining fluid intake during training in some way makes an athlete better able to adjust to ensuing work in the heat. *A well-hydrated athlete always functions at a higher level than one who exercises in a dehydrated state.* One should probably refrain from consuming a soft drink (e.g., a high-fructose, caffeinated beverage) during and following physical activity in the heat as this beverage type can signal biomarkers for acute kidney injury.[160] Ingesting "extra" water (**hyperhydration**) before exercising in the heat offers some thermoregulatory protection. Hyperhydration delays hypohydration from inadequate fluid replacement during physical activity, increases sweating, and produces a smaller rise in core temperature in **uncompensable heat stress**, where evaporative cooling is inadequate to maintain thermal balance.[71] Three practical strategies promote acute hyperhydration before exercising in the heat:

1. Consume one-half liter water (500 mL/20 oz) the evening before physical activity.
2. Consume another 500 mL upon awakening.
3. Consume an additional 400 to 600 mL of cold water 20 min before the activity.

An extended, systematic hyperhydration regimen (4.5 L·d⁻¹) 1 wk before soccer competition by elite young soccer players in Puerto Rico increased body water reserves (despite greater urine output) and improved temperature regulation during a soccer match in warm weather.[112] The structured sequence of pre-exercise hyperhydration produced a 1.1-L/37.2-oz greater total body fluid volume compared with the athletes' normal daily 2.5-L/0.7-gal fluid intake.

Pre-exercise hyperhydration does not replace the need for continual fluid replacement during activity, with perhaps fluid temperature playing an augmenting role. Compared with fluid at 37°C/98.6°F body temperature, ingesting a 4°C/39.2°F cold drink before and during physical activity in the heat delayed a rectal temperature increase. This reduced physiologic strain during physical activity, which resulted in a 23% improved endurance capacity.[74] The hyperhydration benefits usually subside if the individual remains euhydrated during the activity. In distance running, matching fluid loss with fluid intake becomes virtually impossible because the stomach only empties a maximum of 800 to 1000 mL each hour. This emptying rate does not match a water loss that can average nearly 2000 mL·hr⁻¹, which makes pre-exercise hyperhydration extremely beneficial.

Does Exogenous Glycerol Provide a Benefit?

The three-carbon glycerol molecule achieved clinical notoriety (along with mannitol, sorbitol, and urea) for its role in producing osmotic diuresis. The capacity to influence water movement within the body makes glycerol effective in reducing edema in the brain and eye.

When consumed with 1 to 2 L of water, glycerol facilitates intestinal water absorption and extracellular fluid retention, mainly in the plasma and interstitial fluid compartments.[39,143] An expanded body fluid volume potentially sets the stage for fluid excretion from increased renal filtrate and urine flow. The proximal and distal kidney tubules reabsorb glycerol, so much of the fluid portion of the increased renal filtrate is also reabsorbed; this averts marked diuresis, while promoting hyperhydration.

Glycerol supplement proponents maintain its hyperhydration effect reduces overall heat stress from increased sweating rate, which leads to a lower exercise heart rate, body temperature, and enhanced endurance performance. Reducing heat stress with augmented hyperhydration before exercise using glycerol plus water supplementation would increase participant safety. The hyperhydration effect persists up to 6 hr by consuming one gram glycerol per kg body mass combined with 1 to 2 L of water.

Not all research demonstrates meaningful thermoregulatory benefits from glycerol hyperhydration over pre-exercise hyperhydration with plain water.[71] For example, exogenous glycerol diluted in 500 mL water consumed 4 hr before exercise failed to promote fluid retention or ergogenic effects.[55] No cardiovascular or thermoregulatory advantages result from consuming glycerol with small water volumes during activity.[102] Exogenous glycerol's side effects include headache, nausea, dizziness, bloating, and light-headedness. We advise caution before recommending ingesting exogenous glycerol for ergogenic and/or thermoregulatory benefits.

Rehydration Adequacy

Changes in body weight indicate water loss and rehydration adequacy during and following physical activity participation. Voiding dark yellow urine with a strong odor qualitatively indicates inadequate hydration. Well-hydrated individuals typically produce large, light-colored urine volumes without an unusual smell.

The ideal condition replaces water losses from sweating at a rate close to or equal to the sweating rate. Athletes can be weighed before and after practice. Each pound of weight

---

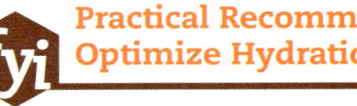 **Practical Recommendations to Optimize Hydration**

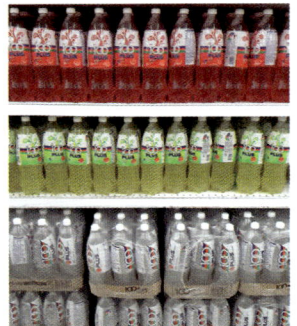

Muhamad Norairin Ngateni/Shutterstock

For most people, water represents an effective beverage for optimal hydration. The National Academy of Medicine recommends that adult women drink at least 2691 mL/91 oz and men at least 3697 mL/125 oz water daily. A steady water intake spread throughout the day rather than guzzling large quantities at predetermined periods (e.g., morning, noon, and night) meets hydration requirements. Urine color is one method to judge hydration effectiveness. A clear color may indicate a poor rehydration beverage retention because water flushes from the body too rapidly—an "overhydration" indicator, typically occurring when ingesting a large fluid volume on an empty stomach. Researchers compared more than a dozen different beverages on hydration effects including a formulated "rehydration solution." They concluded that milk, tea, and orange juice, but not sports drinks, were more hydrating than plain water. This does not mean individuals should forego water to favor other beverages. Water and sports drinks are hydrating. Ingesting water with amino acids, lipids, vitamins, and minerals facilitates water uptake and retention to maintain better hydration levels—important during and following profuse sweating-type activities. Participating in exercise for hours and consuming plain water can excrete excess sodium in urine to create a negative sodium imbalance. In this scenario, beverages with nutrients and sodium are more desirable than plain water to prevent kidney "overload." Slow and steady water intake combined with food helps to maintain optimal fluid balance.

Sources:
Casa DJ, et al. Fluid needs for training, competition, and recovery in track-and-field athletes. *Int J Sport Nutr Exerc Metab.* 2019;29:175.
Maugham RJ, et al. A randomized trial to assess the potential of different beverages to affect hydration status: development of a beverage hydration index. *Am J Clin Nutr.* 2016;103:717.

lost represents 450 mL/15 fl oz of dehydration. Periodic water breaks during activity deter fluid depletion. Coaches and trainers must urge athletes to rehydrate because the thirst mechanism imprecisely monitors dehydration or the body's fluid needs (see "American College of Sports Medicine Clarifies Indicators for Fluid Replacement" [www.acsm-msse.org]). The elderly generally require a longer rehydration time following dehydration.[65] Alcohol-containing beverages generally impede fluid balance restoration, particularly if the rehydration fluid contains 4% or more alcohol.[131,132]

Electrolyte Replacement: Added Sodium May Benefit Rehydration

Restoring water and electrolyte balance in recovery occurs more rapidly by adding between 20 and 60 mmol · L^{-1} sodium to the rehydration drink or combining solid food with appropriate sodium content with plain water.[81,119,120] Adding 2 to 5 mmol · L^{-1} potassium may enhance water retention in the intracellular space and reestablish any extra potassium excretion that accompanies the kidney's sodium retention.[24,122] The ACSM recommends that sports drinks contain 0.5 to 0.7 g sodium · L^{-1} of fluid consumed during activity lasting more than 1 hr. A beverage that tastes good to the individual also contributes to voluntary rehydration during physical activity and recovery.[114,147]

The ingested fluid volume following physical activity must exceed the sweat lost by 25 to 50% to restore fluid balance because the kidneys continually form some urine regardless of hydration status. Pure water absorbed from the gut rapidly dilutes plasma sodium. In turn, decreased plasma osmolality stimulates urine production and blunts the thirst mechanism's normal sodium-dependent stimulus. These responses counter the rehydration objective. Without sufficient sodium in the beverage, excess fluid intake merely increases urine output without fully benefiting rehydration.[133] Maintaining a relatively high plasma sodium concentration by adding sodium to ingested fluid achieves the following:

1. Sustains the thirst drive
2. Promotes ingested fluid retention with lower urine output
3. Rapidly restores lost plasma volume

FIGURE 25.7 illustrates how a rehydration beverage with added sodium affects ingested fluid retention during recovery. Six healthy men exercised in a warm, humid environment until sweating produced about a 2% weight loss. They then ingested one of four test drinks (equivalent to 1.5 times body weight loss or 2045 mL) with either 2, 26, 52, or 100 mmol · L^{-1} containing sodium and matching anion. As a comparison, typical "sports drinks" contain 10 to 25 mmol sodium, while normal plasma sodium concentration ranges between 138 and 142 mmol over a 30-min period beginning 30 min after stopping physical activity. From the 1.5-hr urine sample onward, urine volume inversely related to the rehydration beverage's sodium content. Following the study period, a 787-mL difference in total body water content existed between trials

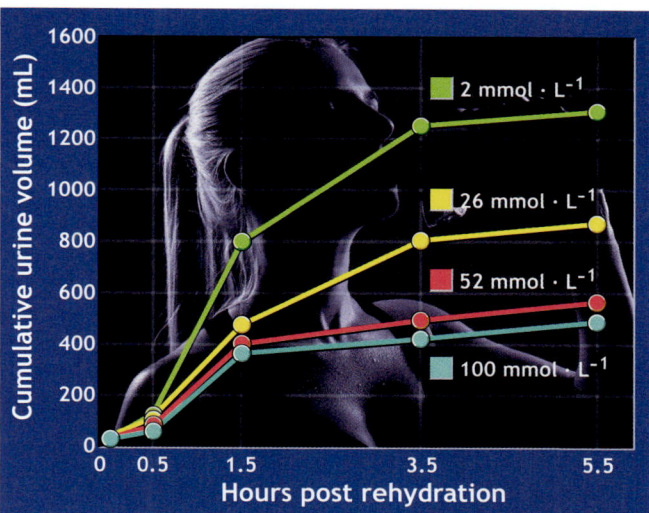

FIGURE 25.7. Cumulative urine output during 5.5-hr recovery from exercise-induced dehydration after drinking one of four test drinks.
(Adapted with permission from Springer: Maughan RJ, Leiper JB. Sodium intake and post-exercise rehydration in man. *Eur J App Physiol*. 1995;71:311. Copyright © 1995 Springer-Verlag. Photo: Dean Drobot/Shutterstock)

using drinks with the lowest and highest sodium content. The drink containing 100 mmol sodium contributed to the greatest fluid retention.

With prolonged effort in the heat, sweat loss can deplete 13 to 17 g of salt daily (2.3 to 3.4 g · L^{-1} of sweat), about 8 g more than typically consumed. In this deficit situation, it seems prudent to replace lost sodium by adding about one-third teaspoon table salt to 1 L water. Moderate activity generally produces a negligible potassium loss in sweat. Even at competitive physical activity levels, potassium losses in sweat range between 5 and 18 mEq, which poses little or no immediate danger.[24] With heavy sweating, increasing potassium-rich citrus fruits and bananas replaces most potassium losses. Minor adjustments in food intake and electrolyte conservation by the kidneys adequately compensate for minerals excreted through sweating.

Whole-Body Precooling

"Cold treatments" that periodically apply cold towels to the forehead and abdomen during physical activity in the heat or a cold shower before exercising improve heat transfer at the body's surface only slightly above the same activity without skin wetting. Whole-body precooling (0.7°C/1.26°F core temperature decrease) with up to 60 min of water immersion at 23.5°C/74°F increases subsequent endurance in a hot, humid environment. Time to exhaustion inversely related to initial body temperature (lowered via precooling) and directly to the heat storage rate.[43] Precooling with cold water immersion facilitated postexercise recovery, enhanced the heat storage rate, and caused less thermoregulatory strain during physical activity.[10,11,34,109,146] In addition, precooling the skin by 5 to 6°C/9 to 10.8°F without reducing core temperature decreased thermal strain and increased distance cycled in 30 min under

In a Practical Sense

Best Physical Activity Rehydration Methods

PRE-EXERCISE HYPERHYDRATION

Start the activity euhydrated and with normal plasma electrolyte levels. Ingesting "extra" water (hyperhydration) before physical activity in the heat offers some protection because it delays hypohydration, increases sweating during physical activity, and creates a smaller increase in core temperature.

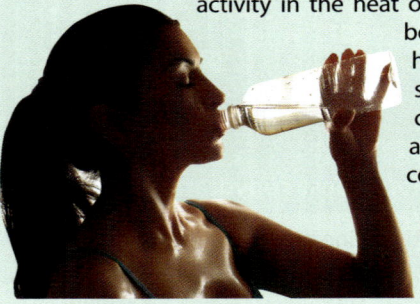

Acute pre-exercise hyperhydration results from consuming (1) at least 500 mL of water before sleeping the night before exercising in the heat, (2) another 500 mL upon awakening, and (3) 400 to 600 mL/13 to 20 oz of cold water about 20 min before exercise. This final pre-exercise fluid intake increases stomach volume for optimal optimize gastric emptying. During intense physical activity in the heat, matching fluid loss with fluid intake becomes virtually impossible because only 800 to 1000 mL/27.1 to 33.8 oz fluid empty from the stomach each hour. This rate of stomach emptying does not match a water loss that may average nearly 2000 mL · hr^{-1}. Consuming beverages containing electrolytes and carbohydrates generally provides benefits over water alone.

REHYDRATION ADEQUACY

Changes in body weight indicate water loss and rehydration adequacy. Voiding dark yellow urine with a strong odor also provides a qualitative inadequate hydration indicator. Well-hydrated individuals typically produce ample urine.

According to the American College of Sports Medicine (ACSM-msse.org/), each pound of weight lost represents 450 mL/15 fl oz dehydration. Periodic water breaks during activity can deter fluid depletion. Alcohol-containing beverages generally impede fluid balance restoration, particularly if the rehydration fluid contains 4% or more alcohol content.

OPTIMIZING HYDRATION

Before Physical Activity

- Drink approximately 502.8 to 591.5 mL/17 to 20 oz 2 to 3 hr before activity
- Consume another 7 to 10 oz after the warm-up (10 to 15 min before exercise)

During Physical Activity

- Drink approximately 800 to 1200 mL/28 to 40 oz every hour of exercise (207 to 561.9 mL/7 to 10 oz every 10 to 15 min)
- Rapidly replace lost fluid (sweat and urine) within 2 hr after activity to enhance recovery by drinking 591.1 to 709.8 mL/20 to 24 oz for every pound of body weight lost through sweating

ELECTROLYTE REPLACEMENT

Ingested fluid loss after exercise must exceed by 25 to 50% the exercise sweat lost to restore fluid balance because the kidneys continually form urine without considering hydration status. Unless the beverage contains sufficiently high sodium content, excess fluid intake merely increases urine output without rehydration benefit. Maintaining a relatively high plasma sodium concentration by adding sodium to ingested fluid sustains the thirst drive, promotes retaining ingested fluid (less urine output), and restores lost plasma volume.

The ACSM recommends that sports drinks contain 0.5 to 0.7 g sodium per liter fluid consumed during exercise lasting more than 1 hr. A beverage that tastes good to the individual also contributes to voluntary rehydration during exercise and recovery. With prolonged physical activity in the heat, sweat loss can deplete the body of 13 to 17 g salt (2.3 to 3.4 g · L^{-1} sweat) daily, about 8 g more than typically consumed. With heavy sweating, increasing potassium-rich citrus fruits and bananas replaces potassium losses. A glass of orange or tomato juice replaces almost all the potassium, calcium, and magnesium excreted in 3 L/101 oz sweat.

Source:
Périard JD, et al. Exercise under heat stress: thermoregulation, hydration, performance implications, and mitigation strategies. *Physiol Rev.* 2021;101:1873.

---

warm, humid conditions.[63] In contrast, whole-body precooling provided no thermoregulatory benefit during a simulated triathlon,[9] or physiologic responses to 90-min soccer activities under normal environmental conditions.[31]

Factors That Modify Heat Tolerance

Five factors interact to improve physiologic adjustments and exercise tolerance during environmental heat stress:

1. Heat acclimatization
2. Training status
3. Age
4. Gender
5. Body fat level

Heat Acclimatization

Relatively easy tasks performed in cool weather become taxing if attempted on the first hot spring day. Early preseason training for warm-weather sports often poses the greatest hazards for heat injury because thermoregulatory mechanisms have not adjusted to the dual challenge of physical activity and environmental heat. Repeated exposure to hot environments when combined with physical activity improves exercise capacity, with less discomfort upon subsequent heat exposure.[106,123,169]

Heat acclimatization describes the collective physiologic adaptive changes to improve heat tolerance. The major portion of acclimatization occurs during the first week of heat exposure, with full acclimatization thereafter. The process requires only 2 to 4 hr of daily heat exposure. The first several sessions in the heat should include 15- to 20-min light-intensity physical activity, with duration and intensity systematically increased thereafter. **TABLE 25.5** summarizes the main physiologic adjustments during heat acclimatization.

INTEGRATIVE QUESTION

Your Maine, U.S.-based soccer team competes in Hawaii in early spring. How would you prepare the team to compete in this hot, humid environment making all pre-competition preparations at your school or elsewhere without considering time, money, and travel?

TABLE 25.5 Physiologic adjustments during heat acclimatization

Optimal acclimatization requires adequate hydration. During physical activity, greater blood flows in the cutaneous vessels to facilitate heat transfer from the core to periphery. A more efficient cardiac output distribution also helps stabilize blood pressure during exertion. A lowered threshold for sweating complements these "circulatory acclimatizations," and cooling begins before core temperature increases appreciably. Sweating capacity, the most significant factor for heat acclimatization, increases early and nearly doubles after 10 days of heat exposure. Sweat also becomes more dilute (less salt lost) and distributes more evenly over the skin surface compared with exercise training without acclimatization.[48] Concurrently, heat acclimatization reduces the kidney's sodium loss. Adjustments in circulation and evaporative cooling enable the heat-acclimatized person to exercise with lower skin and core temperatures and heart rates. A lower exercise core temperature requires less blood flow diversion to skin, freeing a larger cardiac output percentage to supply the active muscles. Acclimatization also reduces carbohydrate use in physical activity, a response consistent with acclimatization-induced plasma epinephrine reduction.[38] The major acclimatization benefits dissipate within 2 to 3 wk following return to a more temperate environment.

Training Status

Exercise-induced "internal" heat stress in a cool environment induces adjustments in peripheral circulation and evaporative cooling qualitatively similar to training in hot ambient temperatures. Such adaptations facilitate metabolic heat elimination generated by physical activity and typically occur following an 8- to 12-wk training period when exercise intensity exceeds 50% $\dot{V}O_{2max}$. Well-conditioned individuals living in a temperate climate respond more effectively to sudden, severe heat stress than sedentary counterparts.[5] Training increases the capacity and sensitivity of the sweating response so sweating begins at a lower core temperature. This produces a greater but more-dilute sweat volume, which conserves a variety of minerals.[20] Concurrently, a training-induced adjustment in cutaneous circulation provides greater skin blood flow at a given internal temperature or percentage of $\dot{V}O_{2max}$, independent of age.[60] Plasma and extravascular fluid volumes also increase during the initial stages of aerobic training, accompanied by better gastrointestinal tract blood flow.[76,82] This maintains a normal barrier to endotoxin movement from the gut lumen into the plasma, blunting the potential for endotoxin-induced fever that could aggravate exercise hyperthermia.[121] Thermoregulatory training benefits occur provided the individual remains fully hydrated during the activity.[123]

Exercise "heat conditioning" in cool weather offers fewer benefits than acclimatization from similar hot weather training. *A physically active person cannot achieve full heat acclimatization without environmental heat stress exposure.* Athletes who train and compete in hot weather have a distinct advantage for thermoregulation over athletes who train in cool climates and rarely compete in hot weather.

Age

What effect does age have on moderate heat stress tolerance and heat acclimatization? An early study exposed men and women ages 60 to 93 years to 70 min of heat stress during physical activity at intensities that ranged from 2 to 5 METs. **FIGURE 25.8** shows the relationship between heart rate and exercise intensity in the heat for age-diverse group adult males and females. The less-fit elderly subjects exercised at higher heart rates than the same gender younger adults. Environmental heat imposed no greater physiologic strain for the older groups because body temperature increased an average of only 0.3°C/0.54°F, compared with 0.2°C/0.36°F for the younger group. Testing elderly subjects in the spring and fall evaluated

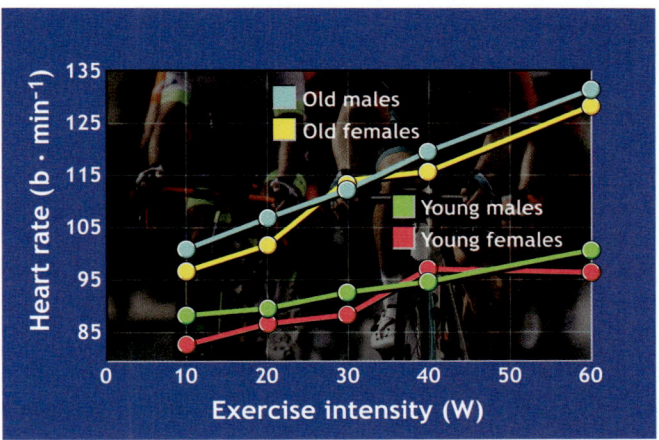

FIGURE 25.8. Heart rate during moderate cycling exercise in hot weather in young and older men and women at dry bulb ambient temperature of 33.5°C/92.3°F and wet bulb temperature of 28.5°C/83.3°F.
(Adapted with permission from Henshel A. The environment and performance. In: Simonsen E, ed. *Physiology of Work Capacity and Fatigue.* Springfield: Charles C. Thomas; 1971. Photo: Juanan Barros Moreno/Shutterstock)

their natural heat acclimatization during the summer months. By fall, all subjects had lower heart rates during the standard thermal-exercise stress.

Comparisons between young and middle-age competitive runners indicated no age-related decrements in thermoregulation during marathon running.[116] Thermoregulatory function was not impaired in trained 50-year-old men compared with younger men.[108] Likewise, sweating capacity for men ages 58 to 84 years adequately regulated body temperature during prolonged desert walks.[27] Research shows little or no age-related decrements in thermoregulatory capacity or heat-stress acclimatization with appropriate controls for body size and composition, aerobic fitness, hydration, degree of acclimatization, and chronological age.

Age-Related Differences Exist

Several age-related factors affect thermoregulatory dynamics despite equivalence between young and older adults in how they regulate core temperature during heat stress. Aging delays sweating onset and blunts the magnitude of the sweating response in one of three ways:[57,64,161]

1. Modified thermoreceptor sensitivity
2. Limited sweat gland output *per se*
3. Dehydration-limited sweat output with insufficient fluid replacement

Aging also alters the intrinsic structure and function of the skin and its vasculature.[51,56,67,79] Aging impairs the mechanisms that mediate cutaneous vasodilation, which results in a diminished vasodilation response. Two factors dampen age-related vascular changes include depressed peripheral sensitivity that impairs cutaneous vasodilation from two factors:

1. Smaller release of vasomotor tone
2. Less active vasodilation when sweating begins

Older athletes show a 25 to 40% lower skin blood flow with increased core temperature than younger athletes.[66] Contributing factors include the combined effects of a lower cardiac output and reduced blood distribution from splanchnic and renal circulations.[91] Older adults do not recover from dehydration as readily as younger counterparts because of a reduced thirst drive. With aging, thirst mechanism sensitivity may decrease from reduced ability to sense hydration level. This places elderly individuals in a chronic hypohydration state with a less-than-optimal plasma volume, which could impair thermoregulatory dynamics. An altered thirst mechanism and shift in the operating point for body fluid volume and composition control also decrease total blood volume in older individuals.[25,78,162]

Children

Children sweat less and maintain higher core temperatures during heat stress than adolescents and adults, even though children possess more heat-activated sweat glands per unit skin area.[8,36] A reduced sweating response likely results from underdeveloped peripheral mechanisms, including the sweat glands and their surrounding tissues, rather than a depressed central drive to sweat.[129] The age difference in thermoregulation lasts through puberty; it generally does not limit physical capacity except during extreme environmental heat stress.[117] Sweat composition differs between children and adults; children's sweat shows higher sodium and chlorine concentrations and lower lactate, H^+, and potassium concentrations.[36,90] *In practice, exercise intensity should decrease for children exposed to a hot environment; they also require more time to acclimatize than older competitors.*

Gender

Early experiments revealed that males exhibited greater tolerance than females to environmental heat stress during a standard physical activity effort. A major flaw in this research, however, required that females exercise at a higher aerobic capacity percentage than males. When researchers controlled for this factor and compared males and females of equal fitness or exercised both groups at the same $\%\dot{V}O_{2max}$, any thermoregulatory differences became less pronounced.[30,54] In essence, women tolerate thermal stress during physical activity at least as well as do men of comparable aerobic fitness and level of acclimatization; both genders acclimatize to the same degree.

Sweating

A distinct gender difference exists in thermoregulation. Women sweat less prolifically than men, despite possessing more heat-activated sweat glands per unit skin area. Women start to sweat at higher skin and core temperatures and produce less sweat than men under comparable heat-exercise loads, even after equivalent acclimatization.

Evaporative Cooling Versus Circulatory Cooling

Women tolerate heat much like men of equal aerobic fitness at the same activity level, despite a lower sweat output. Circulatory mechanisms predominate for heat dissipation in women, whereas evaporative cooling predominates for men. Clearly, producing less sweat to maintain thermal balance protects women from dehydration during exertion at high ambient temperatures.

Body Surface Area-to-Body Mass Ratio

The typically smaller female has a relatively large external surface per unit body mass exposed to the environment, which provides a favorable dimensional characteristic for heat dissipation. Under identical heat exposure conditions, women tend to cool faster than men. Children also possess a similar "geometric" advantage during heat stress from their larger surface area-to-mass ratio than adults.

Menstruation

Different menstrual cycle phases influence cutaneous vascular control that alters skin blood flow and sweating response during rest and physical activity.[16,137,163] For example, a higher core temperature threshold initiates sweating during the luteal phase at 60 and 80% of aerobic capacity.[69] The thermoregulatory setpoint for sweating that resets in an upward direction during the luteal phase and likely reflects a unique feature of hormone dynamics throughout the cycle.[50,137] An upward 0.4°C/0.72°F shift in oral temperature during the luteal phase persists for about 6 d. This change in thermoregulatory sensitivity does *not* impair ability for intense physical activity participation.[77] No changes in exercise performance, lactate threshold, or ventilatory threshold associate with menstrual cycle phases in temperate environments.[134] In hot, humid conditions, exercise performance decreases during the luteal phase, perhaps from physiological and perceptual changes and a greater thermosensitivity at the onset of physical activity.[59]

Body Fat Level

Excess body fat represents a liability when exercising in the heat. Because fat's specific heat exceeds that for muscle tissue, fat increases the insulatory quality of the body shell and retards heat conduction to the periphery. The large, overly fat person also has a smaller body surface area-to-body mass ratio for effective sweat evaporation than a leaner, smaller person with less body fat.

Excess body fat and body weight directly adds to the metabolic cost for weight-bearing activities. A hot, humid environment places the overly fat person at a distinct disadvantage for temperature regulation and physical performance.[107] Additional compounding factors include the added weight of the uniform and protective gear in American football, ice hockey, and lacrosse and the heat generated in intense competition. Fatal heat stroke occurs 3.5 times more frequently in excessively overweight young adults than in individuals of average body size (see next section). Recall the heat-related death during football practice of NFL professional player Corey Stringer mentioned in the introductory section of this chapter. At 1.93 m/6′4″ and 151.9 kg/335 lb, this player was at greater thermal injury risk from his excessively large body size (body mass index of 40.8) that exceeds the most liberal standard for excess body weight.

 **INTEGRATIVE QUESTION**

What are the ideal physical and physiologic characteristics that minimize heat injury risk while exercising in the heat?

Complications from Excessive Heat Stress

According to the Centers for Disease Control and Prevention, more than 600 people die yearly in the United States from excessive heat stress, and about half of these are men and women age 65 and older (www.cdc.gov/pictureofamerica/pdfs/picture_of_america_heat-related_illness.pdf). The most vulnerable groups include older adults over age 65, infants and children, athletes, outdoor workers, and those with chronic medical conditions and low income. If the normal signs of heat stress go unheeded—thirst, tiredness, grogginess, and visual disturbances—cardiovascular compensation mechanisms begin to fail, which initiates disabling complications collectively termed *heat illness*. Heat cramps, heat exhaustion, and heat stroke constitute the major heat illnesses in order of increasing severity. Heat-related disabilities occur more frequently among overweight, unacclimatized, and poorly conditioned individuals, including those who exercise when dehydrated.[2,14,110] No clear-cut demarcation exists between maladies because symptoms often overlap. Exercise-induced heat injury frequently occurs from the cumulative effect of multiple adverse interactions.[136,155,164] **TABLE 25.6** summarizes the cardiovascular response patterns during three distinct stages of exercise hyperthermia.

TABLE 25.6 Cardiovascular responses during three exercise hyperthermia stages

These stages—compensation, crisis, and failure—apply to heat exhaustion and heat stroke. The response patterns broadly classify as central circulatory, peripheral, or central nervous system effects. With serious heat illness, only immediate corrective action reduces heat stress until medical help arrives.[28]

Heat Cramps

Heat cramps—severe involuntary, sustained, and spreading muscle spasms—occur during or after intense physical activity usually in the specifically active muscles, but with core temperature remaining within a normal range. This form of heat illness occurs from an imbalance in the body's fluid level and electrolyte concentrations. Crampers tend to have high sweat rates and/or high sweat sodium concentrations. Prevention should include at a minimum these two factors:

1. Providing sufficient water that contains salt
2. Increasing daily salt intake (e.g., adding salt to foods at mealtime) several days before heat stress

Sweating causes electrolyte loss during prolonged heat exposure. Failure to replenish these minerals often leads to muscle pain and spasm, most commonly in the abdomen and extremities. Drinking more than the usual daily water and increasing salt intake several days before heat stress generally foils this heat-related malady.[33]

Heat Exhaustion

Heat exhaustion can develop in unacclimatized persons during the first summer heat wave or with the first hard training session on a hot day. Exercise-induced heat exhaustion occurs from ineffective circulatory adjustments compounded by depletion of extracellular fluid, principally plasma volume from excessive sweating. Blood usually pools in the dilated peripheral vessels to drastically reduce central blood volume necessary to maintain cardiac output. Heat exhaustion is characterized by a weak and rapid pulse, low blood pressure in the upright position, dizziness, headache, and general weakness. Sweating may decrease somewhat, but core temperature does not increase to 40°C/104°F or higher. A person who experiences heat exhaustion symptoms should stop activity and move to a cooler environment. Replenishment of body fluids should be the immediate goal, often achieved intravenously in a clinic or hospital setting.

Heat Stroke

Heat stroke, the most serious and complex of the heat stress maladies from failure of the body's heat-regulating mechanisms, requires immediate medical attention. An excessively high core temperature can affect seemingly healthy adults in a relatively cool environment.[3,35,111,115,165] The *classic form* of heat stroke—core temperature exceeds 40.5°C/105°F, altered mental status, absence of sweating—typically occurs during heat waves. It particularly affects young children, the elderly, and those with chronic diseases. In classic heat stroke, environmental heat overloads the body's heat-dissipating mechanisms. Severe heat stress produces potentially negative alterations in the immune system and in leukocyte adhesion and activation processes (unrelated to elevated catecholamine levels).[47] One in three individuals who survive a near-fatal classic heat stroke remains permanently disabled with multisystem organ dysfunction.[26]

Exertional heat stroke refers to a state of extreme exercise hyperthermia from two interactive factors:

1. Excessive metabolic heat load in physical activity
2. Inadequate response from heat dissipation mechanisms to a hot, humid environment

When thermoregulation fails, sweating diminishes, the skin becomes dry and hot, and body temperature rises to 41.5°C/106.7°F and above. This places an inordinate strain on cardiovascular function. With intense activity, usually by young, highly motivated individuals, sweating occurs but body heat gain

In a Practical Sense

Recognizing and Treating Heat-Related Disorder Signs and Symptoms

Each year in the United States, extreme heat causes on average 658 deaths—more than tornadoes (www.cdc.gov/disasters/extremeheat/index.html). Men and women age 65 years and older account for about half the fatalities. If the normal heat stress signs are not dealt with—thirst, tiredness, grogginess, and visual disturbances—cardiovascular compensation begins to fail, which then initiates disabling complications collectively termed heat illness.

Heat cramps, heat syncope, heat exhaustion, and heat stroke constitute the major heat illnesses grouped by increasing severity. No clear-cut demarcation exists among these maladies because symptoms often overlap. When serious heat illness symptoms occur, immediate action reduces the heat stress by rehydrating the person until medical help arrives. The table lists the causes, signs, and symptoms and preventive methods for the four heat illness categories.

Heat Illness: Causes, Signs and Symptoms, and Prevention

Condition	Causes	Signs and Symptoms	Prevention
Heat cramps	Intense, prolonged physical activity (PA) in the heat	Tightening, cramps, involuntary active muscle spasms; low serum Na+	Cease PA; rehydrate
Heat syncope	Peripheral vasodilatation and venous blood pooling; hypotension; hypohydration	Lightheadedness; syncope, mostly in upright position during rest or PA; pallor; high rectal temperature	Ensure acclimatization and fluid replenishment; reduce exertion on hot days; avoid standing
Heat exhaustion	Cumulative negative water balance	Exhaustion; hypohydration, flushed skin; reduced sweating in extreme dehydration; syncope, high rectal temperature	Ensure proper hydration before PA and adequate replenishment during PA; ensure acclimatization
Heat stroke	Extreme hyperthermia leads to thermoregulatory failure aggravated by dehydration	Medical emergency requires life-saving countermeasures; includes hyperpyrexia (rectal temperature ≥41°C/105.8°F); severely reduced sweating and neurologic deficit (disorientation, twitching, seizures, coma)	Ensure proper hydration before PA and during PA; ensure acclimatization

overpowers heat loss. Other predisposing factors include poor fitness status, obesity, inadequate acclimatization, sweat gland dysfunction, dehydration, and infectious disease. If left untreated, the disability progresses rapidly, and death ensues from circulatory collapse and central nervous system and other organ system damage. While awaiting medical treatment, aggressive steps must be taken to lower core temperature because mortality relates to hyperthermia magnitude and duration. Immediate treatment includes fluid replacement and body cooling with alcohol rubs, ice pack application to the neck area, and whole-body immersion in cold or even ice water, the latter the "gold standard" treatment for exertional heat stroke.[15,101,103] No attempt should be made to slow the respiratory rate because rapid breathing helps to compensate for metabolic acidosis. Prudent treatment includes specific drug therapy to counter endotoxin effects precipitated by heat stroke pathology.[46]

Oral Temperature Unreliable Following Physical Activity

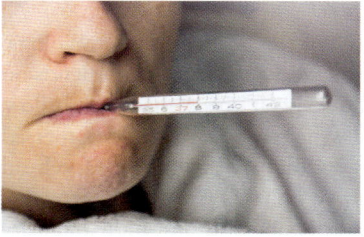

TPROduction/Shutterstock

Following strenuous exercise in trained endurance and ultraendurance competitors, oral temperature does not accurately measure core temperature. Rectal temperature following a 2.5-km/14-mi race or ultramarathon in a tropical climate averaged 39.7°C/103.5°F, while oral temperature surprisingly remained a normal 36.6°C/98°F. The discrepancy was explained by the effects on oral temperature from evaporative cooling in the mouth and airways when ventilating large air volumes.

Sources:
Lavoué C, et al. Analysis of food and fluid intake in elite ultra-endurance runners during a 24-h world championship. *J Int Soc Sports Nutr*. 2020;17:36.
Roy ML, et al. Effect of sodium in a rehydration beverage when consumed as a fluid or meal. *J Appl Physiol*. 1998;85:1329.

Summary

1. Core temperature normally increases during physical activity with relative activity stress determining the temperature magnitude increase.
2. A well-regulated temperature increase creates a favorable environment to support physiologic and metabolic functions.
3. Excessive sweating compromises fluid reserves to create dehydration signs and symptoms.
4. Sweating without fluid replacement decreases plasma volume leading to circulatory dysfunction and a precipitous core temperature rise.
5. Physical activity in a hot, humid environment poses a considerable thermoregulatory challenge because the large sweat loss in high humidity contributes little to evaporative cooling.
6. Fluid loss of more than 4% body weight impedes heat dissipation, compromises cardiovascular function, and diminishes exercise capacity.
7. Adequate fluid replacement maintains plasma volume to optimize the circulatory and sweating response during hot-weather exercise.
8. The ideal replacement schedule during physical activity matches fluid intake to fluid loss, effectively monitored by changes in body weight.
9. The small intestine can absorb about 1000 mL/33.8 oz of water each hour. Adding electrolytes to a rehydration beverage facilitates fluid replacement more than drinking plain water.
10. The diet generally replaces minerals lost through sweating.
11. With prolonged physical activity in the heat, adding 1 tsp $\cdot$ L^{-1} salt to the replacement fluid facilitates sodium and fluid replenishment.
12. Repeated heat stress initiates thermoregulatory adjustments that improve physical capacity and reduce discomfort on heat exposure.
13. Ten days of heat exposure promotes full acclimatization.
14. Aging impacts thermoregulatory function but does not appreciably alter temperature regulation during physical activity or acclimatization to moderate heat stress.
15. Women and men show equivalent thermoregulation during physical activity when controlled for fitness and acclimatization levels. Women produce less sweat than men when exercising at the same core temperature.
16. Heat cramps, heat exhaustion, and heat stroke constitute the major heat illnesses.
17. Heat stroke, a medical emergency, is the most serious and complex heat illness.
18. Oral temperature after physical activity does not accurately measure core temperature because evaporative cooling in the mouth and airways occurs with increased pulmonary ventilation in activity and during recovery.

Part 3: Thermoregulation and Environmental Cold Stress During Physical Activity

Physical Activity in the Cold

Human exposure to extreme cold produces significant physiologic and psychological challenges. Cold ranks high among the differing terrestrial environmental stressors for its potentially lethal consequences. Core temperature becomes further compromised during chronic exertional fatigue and sleep loss, inadequate nourishment, reduced tissue insulation, and depressed shivering heat production.[150] **TABLE 25.7** presents the physiologic changes associated with hypothermia, which range from mild to severe.

TABLE 25.7 Hypothermia stages and physiological changes

Water provides an excellent medium to study physiologic adjustment to cold because it conducts heat about 25 times faster than air at the same temperature. Consequently, immersion in cool water of only 28 to 30°C/82 to 86°F imposes a thermal stress that rapidly initiates thermoregulatory adjustments. Persons frequently shiver if they remain inactive in a pool or ocean environment because of the large conductive heat loss to the water.[166]

Metabolism in exercise often generates insufficient heat to counter the large thermal drain even when exercising at moderate intensity in cold water. This pertains especially during swimming because convective heat transfer increases when water moves over the skin surface.

Light and moderate activity in cold water produces a larger oxygen uptake and lower core temperature than identical activity in warmer water.[85,139] For example, swimming at a submaximal pace in a flume at 18°C/64°F requires 500 mL more oxygen a minute than swimming at the same speed in 26°C/79°F water.[104] The additional oxygen uptake relates directly to the additional energy cost associated with shivering.

Death from Cold Occurs Even if the Body Does Not Freeze

Core body temperature usually averages about 37°C/98.6°F. Hypothermia occurs when this temperature drops to ≤35°C/95°F, which can occur in relatively cool but not freezing ambient temperatures—particularly when a person becomes wet from rain, sweat, or cold water immersion. Exposure to subzero temperatures exacerbates the stress placed on the body's thermoregulatory efforts.

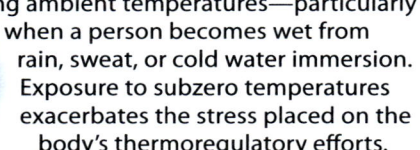
OneSideProFoto/Shutterstock

At −34°C/−30°F, for example, a person improperly dressed for the cold could experience hypothermia within 10 min, triggering physiologic challenges to the brain, heart, liver, and kidneys. Mild hypothermia symptoms—shivering, weakness, and confusion—occur at a core temperature of about 35°C/95°F. Below this temperature, a cascade of negative consequences occurs—amnesia (33°C/91°F), loss of consciousness (28°C/82°F), and death if untreated. Two mechanisms protect the body from cold exposure to counter environment heat loss:

1. Upon exposure to frigid conditions, the body shunts blood via vasoconstriction from the extremities (e.g., face, fingers, toes) toward the inner core tissues.
2. Shivering, a second slower-acting response, generates metabolic heat.

Sources:
Manolis AS, et al. Winter swimming: body hardening and cardiorespiratory protection via sustainable acclimation. *Curr Sports Med Rep.* 2019;18:401.
Tipton MJ, et al. Cold water immersion: kill or cure? *Exp Physiol.* 2017;102:1335

as the body attempts to compensate for the heat loss in colder water. Shivering also serves an important role in recovering from hypothermia; it mitigates the typical postexercise decline in core temperature and facilitates rewarming the core.[42] The body shows remarkable flexibility in oxidative fuel selection during sustained cold exposure, as substrate shifts from lipid to carbohydrate during intense cold stress.[49]

Body Fat and Cold Stress

Differences in body fat content among individuals influence physiologic function in the cold during rest and physical activity.[86,140] Successful ocean swimmers possess a larger subcutaneous fat content than highly trained nonocean swimmers. The additional fat increases the effective insulation in cold water when peripheral blood reroutes from the shell to the core. With this advantage, athletes with greater thermal insulation from fat swim in cool ocean water with almost no decline in core temperature. For leaner swimmers, exercise does not generate sufficient heat to offset heat drain to the water, and the body's core cools.

Consider the stress from "cold" as relative. The physiologic strain from cold water and cold land environments depends on one's metabolism level and the body fat's resistance to heat flow. A person with excess body fat who rests comfortably immersed to the neck in 26°C/78.8°F water may sweat about the forehead during vigorous physical activity. For this person, 18°C/64.4°F provides a more favorable water temperature for high-intensity effort. For a lean person, water at 18°C/64.4°F proves debilitating during both rest and activity. An optimum water temperature exists for each person and for each activity. Water temperatures between 26°C/78.8°F and 30°C/86°F usually allow for effective heat dissipation in sustained exertion without compromising capacity from large deviations in core temperature. Water temperatures ranging between 16 and 18°C/60.8 and 64.4°F have been deemed too cold for marathon swim racing. Rules were changed in 2017 that made wet suits compulsory in water temperatures below 18°C/64.4°F and optional in temperatures between 18 and 20°C/64.4 and 68°F.[167] Even colder water may optimize performance in shorter-term, near-maximal effort, particularly in individuals with greater body fat. Older adults do not withstand the cold challenge during rest and low-intensity activity as effectively as younger counterparts with similar aerobic capacities.[37] Age-related variations in body composition or hormonal functions may help to explain the differences.

Children and Cold Stress

Cold water for children provides an exceptionally stressful thermoregulatory environment. A child's distinctly large ratio of body surface area-to-body mass facilitates heat loss in a warm environment, yet becomes a liability during cold stress because body heat dissipates rapidly. During the less stressful cold air environment, exercising children rely on two mechanisms to compensate for their relatively large body surface area[135]:

1. Increased energy metabolism
2. More effective peripheral limb vasoconstriction

Cold Acclimatization

Humans possess much less capacity to adapt to long-term cold exposure than to prolonged heat exposure. The indigenous Arctic inhabitants from North America, Greenland, and Asia have learned over the centuries to avoid the cold and to minimize its effects. Their clothing provides a near-tropical microclimate; the temperature inside an igloo catenary shelter (snow house or snow hut carved in an arch shape) typically averages 15.6°C/60°F despite freezing outside temperatures with gale-force winds or freezing rain (www.youtube.com/watch?v=1L7EI0vKVuU).

The Ama

Studies of the Ama, the women divers of Korea and southern Japan (www.youtube.com/watch?v=sTIf2vA-_JQl; see Chapter 26), indicate some human cold adaptation.[53] These women tolerate daily prolonged exposure to diving for food in cold water that in winter averages 10°C/50°F. During the summer, when water temperature rises to 25°C/77°F, the Ama perform three diving bouts each 45 min long. In winter, they perform only one 15-min dive daily. The women generally remain in the water until oral temperature declines to about 34°C/93.2°F. **FIGURE 25.9** shows the Ama skin and core (rectal) temperature responses to total time in the water. Mean skin and mean body temperatures always remained lower during the winter dives. Earlier research described the relationship between water temperature and coldest water temperatures when at least 50% of the Ama and nondiving Korean women and men started shivering.[52] The response curve (not shown) for the Ama shifted

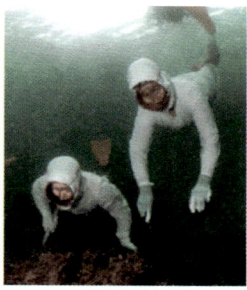

FIGURE 25.9. Differences in rectal temperature, mean skin temperature, and mean body temperature related to water temperature during summer and winter in Ama divers upon resurfacing from a dive.
(Adapted with permission from Kang DH, et al. Energy metabolism and body temperature of the *Am J Appl Physiol*. 1965;18:483. ©The American Physiological Society (APS). All rights reserved.)

to the right, clearly indicating a blunted thermogenic response (higher shivering threshold) until water temperature reached 28°C/82.4°F. An elevated resting metabolism may contribute to how the Ama tolerate extreme cold. In winter, resting metabolic rate increased by about 25% compared with nondiving women from the same country. Interestingly, the Ama and nondiving female counterparts had equivalent body fat percentages. This suggests that circulatory adaptations aid the Ama by retarding heat transfer from the core to the skin during cold water immersion.

Other Cold Adaptation Examples

One hour of daily cold water immersion (14°C /57.2°F) for 7 consecutive days in adult humans substantially reduced shivering intensity and increased nonshivering thermogenesis.[168] This cold adjustment reduced total shivering intensity by 36% without affecting whole-body heat production, double that previously shown from a 4-wk mild cold adjustment. This implies that nonshivering thermogenesis increased to supplement the reduction from shivering's thermogenic contribution.

A type of general cold adaptation also occurs with regular and prolonged cold air exposure. Here, heat production does not balance heat loss, and the person regulates at a lower

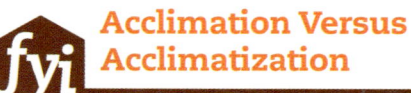 **Acclimation Versus Acclimatization**

Acclimation occurs when a human or animal is subjected to a changed condition in the laboratory and shows compensatory adjustments to the new condition. Acclimation can be studied for long-term and short-term exposures to hot or cold conditions or simulated exposures to hypoxic conditions via chamber-mediated alterations in barometric pressure, or through alterations in respired gas concentrations. In acclimatization, normal compensatory adjustments occur to environmental changes in nature or under natural conditions (e.g., adjustments to seasonal changes in temperature or as result of exposure to higher terrestrial elevations).

Ingus Kruklitis/Shutterstock

core temperature during cold stress. Some peripheral circulatory adaptations also reflect a form of acclimation with severe local cold exposure.[72,73,75] Repeated cold exposure of hands or feet increases blood flow through these tissues. Fisherman routinely experience this common occurrence when handling fishing nets.[105] Local tissue adaptations facilitate heat loss from the periphery but do provide a self-defense mechanism because warmed blood in exposed tissue thwarts tissue damage from localized hypothermia. Longer-term cold exposure may also blunt the depression of the immune response typically observed with acute cold stress.[68] Improved physical fitness expressed by a relatively large aerobic capacity and muscle mass enhances thermoregulatory defenses against cold stress to produce a substantial shivering response and earlier more sensitive shivering onset with cold exposure.[9]

Three responses provide some indication for mild acclimatization to chronic cold exposure:

1. Shivering occurs at a lower body temperature because more heat is generated without shivering (i.e., nonshivering thermogenesis)
2. Improved ability to sleep in the cold
3. Change in peripheral blood flow distribution that either conserves heat in the core or warms the extremities to prevent cold injury

How Cold Is Too Cold?

Cold injuries from overexposure continue to rise from worldwide participation in ice skating and outdoor ice hockey, ice fishing, Alpine and Nordic skiing, snowboarding, snowmobiling, and all-season walking, hiking, jogging, and cycling. Pronounced peripheral vasoconstriction with severe cold exposure causes dangerously low skin and extremity temperatures, particularly when compounded by marked increases in convective and conductive heat loss. Predisposing factors to frostbite include alcohol use, low physical fitness, fatigue, dehydration, and poor peripheral circulation.[113] Early cold injury warning signs include tingling and numbness in the fingers and toes or a burning sensation in the nose and ears. Overexposure from failure to heed these warning signs leads to frostbite; in the extreme, irreversible damage occurs requiring surgical removal of damaged tissue, sometimes involving an entire hand or foot, and even ears, nose, and lips. From military operations and occupational jobs during extensive and prolonged cold exposure, applying external heat to the torso can maintain fingers and toes at a relatively comfortable temperature for up to 3 hr with exposure to −15°C/5°F.[12]

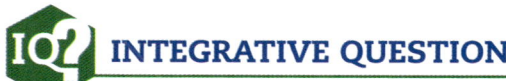 INTEGRATIVE QUESTION

What specific information predicts an individual's survival time during extreme cold exposure?

In severe cold stress (e.g., near drowning with cold water submersion), brain temperature significantly decreases, which reduces its oxygen needs. The central nervous system also

Three Frostbite Stages

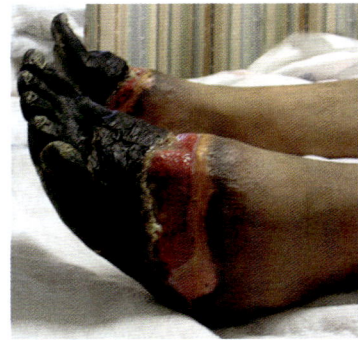

Image reprinted with permission from Southerland J, et al. *McGlamry's Comprehensive Textbook of Foot and Ankle Surgery*. 4th Ed. Philadelphia: Wolters Kluwer Health; 2012.

Stage 1: Skin appears yellow or white, often with slight burning sensations. This relatively mild stage can be reversed by gradual warming the affected area.

Stage 2: Pain disappears with skin reddening and swelling. Treatment may produce blisters and skin peeling.

Stage 3: Skin becomes waxy and hard, skin dies, and edema occurs when blood flow to the area stops.

Without immediate treatment, damage usually becomes permanent, with nerve loss from oxygen deprivation. Frostbitten areas turn discolored—purplish at first and then black. Nerve damage produces a loss of feeling in the frostbitten areas. Without feeling in the damaged area, checking it for cuts and breaks in the skin is vital. Infected open skin can lead to gangrene (tissue necrosis) and amputation. The image shows deep bilateral frostbite injury to both feet. Rewarming and preventing infection over a 6-wk or longer duration determine if the tissue survives following frostbite. When irreversible damage occurs, the tissue must be removed surgically.

benefits from a blood redistribution from tissues that can compromise their supply for relatively long periods. Other responses include potential benefits from the mammalian dive reflex (see Chapter 26, "Diving Reflex in Humans") and possibly cold-induced changes in neurotransmitter release.[41]

 **INTEGRATIVE QUESTION**

Why does a person have a greater likelihood for resuscitation and survival drowning in cold water than in warmer water?

Wind-Chill Temperature Index

One dilemma in evaluating an environment's thermal quality relates to the inadequacy of ambient temperature alone to assess coldness. Many of us have experienced the chilling winds of a spring day even though air temperature remained well above freezing. In contrast, a calm subfreezing day may feel comfortable. Wind makes the difference—air currents on a windy day magnify heat loss because the warmer insulating air layer surrounding the body continually exchanges with cooler ambient air.

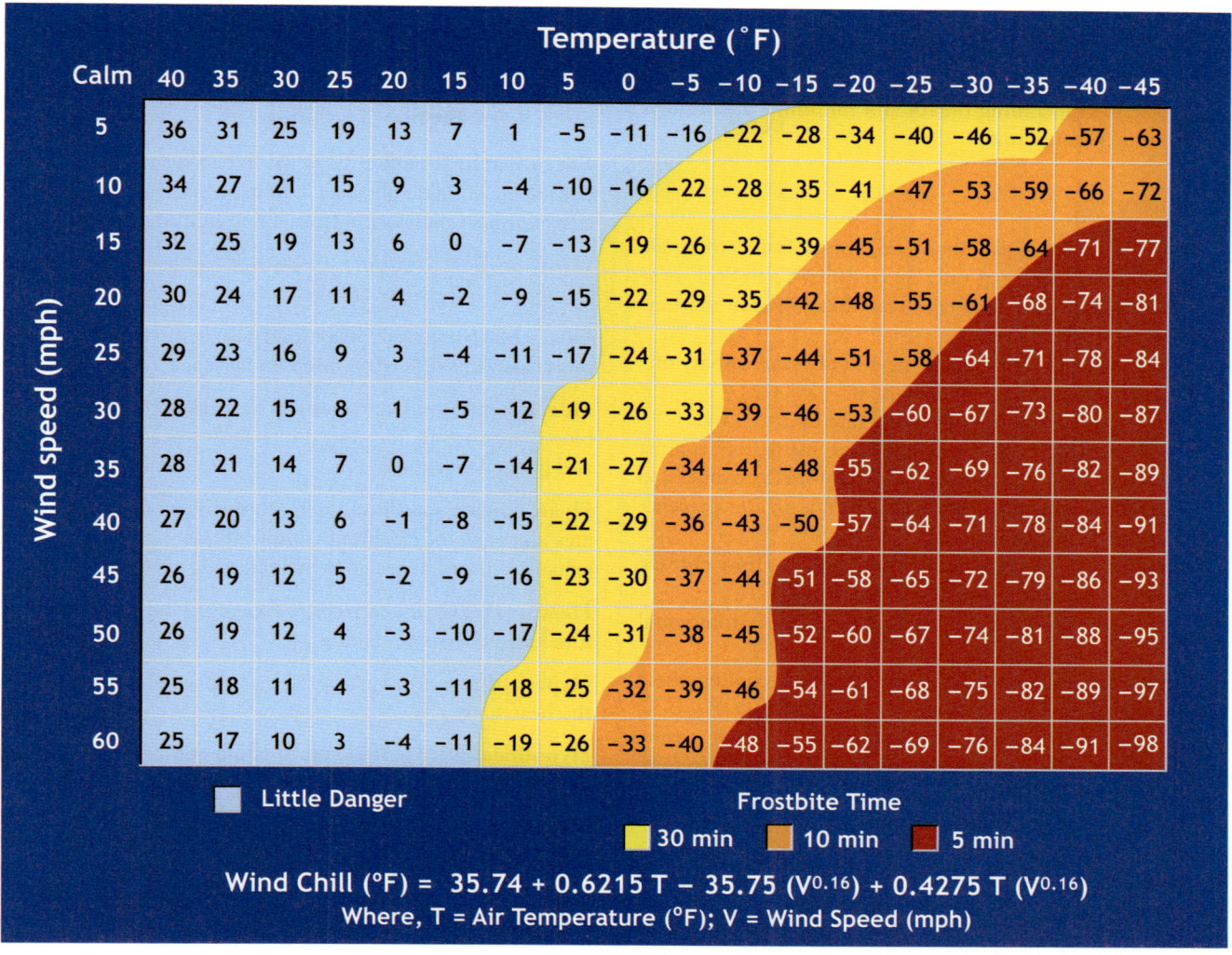

FIGURE 25.10. The wind-chill temperature index provides wind-chill temperatures for relative frostbite risk and predicted times to freezing for exposed facial skin.
(Reprinted with permission from American College of Sports Medicine Position Stand. Prevention of cold injuries during exercise. *Med Sci Sports Exerc.* 2006;38:2012.)

The National Weather Service has used the wind-chill temperature index displayed in **FIGURE 25.10** since 1973 and modified in 2001 (www.weather.gov/safety/cold-wind-chill-chart). Based on advances in science, technology, and computer modeling, the 2001 revised formula provides a more accurate, understandable, and useful way to recognize the dangers from winter winds and freezing temperatures to provide frostbite threshold values.[92] For example, a −1°C/30°F ambient air reading is equivalent to −12.7°C/9°F with a wind speed of 25 mph, while a 12.2°C/10°F reading equals −23.8°C/−11°F at the same wind velocity. If a person runs, skis, or skates into the wind, the effective cooling increases directly with forward velocity. Running at 8 mph into a 12-mph headwind creates the equivalent 20-mph wind speed. Conversely, running at 8 mph with a 12-mph wind at one's back creates only a relative 4-mph wind speed. The *blue zone* denotes relatively little danger from cold injury for a properly clothed person. In contrast, the *yellow-* and *orange-shaded zones* indicate frostbite threshold values. The danger to exposed flesh increases, especially for the ears, nose, and fingers, when moving to the right of the chart.

Wet skin exposed to wind cools even faster, and if the skin is wet and exposed to wind, the ambient temperature should be 10°C/50°F lower than the actual ambient temperature. In the *red-shaded zone*, the equivalent wind-chill temperatures pose serious risk to exposed flesh freezing within minutes.

Respiratory Tract During Cold-Weather Physical Activity

Cold ambient air generally poses no special danger of damaging the respiratory passages. Even in extreme cold, incoming air warms to between 26°C/78.8°F and 32°C/89.6°F as it reaches the bronchi, with values as low as 20°C/68°F observed with breathing large volumes of cold, dry air.[89] Warming an incoming breath of cold air greatly increases its capacity to hold moisture. Humidification of inspired cold air produces considerable water and heat loss from the respiratory tract with large ventilatory volumes during physical activity. Airway moisture loss during cold-weather activity contributes to mouth dryness, a burning sensation in the throat, irritation of the respiratory passages, and general dehydration. Wearing a scarf or cellulose mask-type baklava that covers the nose and mouth and traps the water in exhaled air helps to warm and moisten the next incoming breath and minimize uncomfortable respiratory symptoms.

Summary

1. Water conducts heat about 25 times faster than air. Immersion in water at only 28 to 30°C/82 to 86°F provides considerable thermal stress that initiates thermoregulatory adjustments.
2. Heat production from shivering and physical activity offsets heat flux to a cold environment.
3. Shivering increases the metabolic rate by 3 to 6 METs.
4. Subcutaneous fat provides excellent insulation against cold stress. It greatly enhances vasomotor effectiveness, so individuals with excess body fat retain a greater percentage of metabolic heat.
5. Much less physiologic adaptation occurs from chronic cold stress than prolonged heat exposure.
6. Ambient temperature and wind influence environmental coldness.
7. The wind-chill index determines the wind's cooling effect on exposed tissue.
8. Pronounced peripheral vasoconstriction during severe cold exposure causes dangerously low skin and extremity temperatures when compounded by marked increases in convective and conductive heat loss.
9. Considerable water loss occurs from the respiratory passages during physical activity on a cold day, but inspired air temperature generally does not pose a danger to respiratory tract tissues.
10. The Ama, the women divers of Korea and southern Japan, display cold adaptation from a blunted thermogenic response to prolonged diving that allows them to effectively tolerate extreme cold.

Key Terms

Adequate hydration: Most effective heat stress defense

Climate: Describes atmospheric "behavior" over a prolonged time period

Clo unit: Thermal resistance value to describe the insulation provided by any trapped air layer between the skin and the clothing's insulation value

Conduction: Heat exchange involving direct heat transfer from one molecule to another through a liquid, solid, or gas

Convection: Heat transfer from the body to cooler molecules in the environment with effectiveness depending on how rapidly air or water adjacent to the body exchanges as it warms

Core: Deeper central tissues' temperature that represents a dynamic equilibrium between factors that add and subtract body heat

Dehydration: Body water loss from a hyperhydrated state to euhydration or from euhydration downward to hypohydration

Diuretic-induced dehydration: Greater percentage water drawn from plasma than water lost through sweating

Evaporation: Change from liquid to vapor; provides the major defense against overheating

Exertional heat stroke: Extreme hyperthermia from interactive effects of metabolic heat load in physical activity and challenge for heat dissipation from a hot, humid environment

Heat acclimatization: Collective physiologic adaptive changes to improve heat tolerance

Heat cramps: Severe involuntary, sustained, and spreading muscle spasms following intense physical activity

Heat exhaustion: Characterized by weak and rapid pulse, low blood pressure in the upright position, headache, dizziness, and general weakness

Heat illness: Cardiovascular compensation's failure initiates a cascade of disabling complications—heat cramps, heat exhaustion, and heat stroke by increasing severity

Heat stroke: Characterized by excessively high core temperature leading to organ failure

Hyperhydration: Ingesting "extra" water before exercising in the heat

Hypothalamus: Central coordinating center for temperature regulation

Hypovolemia: Fluid deficits in the intracellular and extracellular compartments

Radiation: Heat transfer by electromagnetic heat waves or radiant energy

Shell: Body's peripheral tissue mass

Uncompensable heat stress: Inadequate evaporative cooling that fails to maintain thermal balance

Vasopressin: Hormone released from the hypothalamic neurohypophysis to increase permeability of kidney's collecting tubules to facilitate fluid retention

Weather: Defines atmospheric conditions over a short time period

Wet bulb-globe temperature (WB–GT) index: Heat stress in direct sunlight based on temperature, humidity, wind speed, and solar radiation

References are available online at Lippincott Connect.

Additional References

Alexander J, et al. Utilisation of performance markers to establish the effectiveness of cold-water immersion as a recovery modality in elite football. *Biol Sport*. 2022;39:19.

Amano T, et al. Influence of exercise intensity and regional differences in the sudomotor recruitment pattern in exercising prepubertal boys and young men. *Physiol Behav*. 2022;243:113642.

Belzile D, et al. Heart rate variability after bariatric surgery: the add-on value of exercise. *Eur J Sport Sci*. 2022;6:1.

Benjamin CL, et al. The efficacy of weekly and bi-weekly heat training to maintain the physiological benefits of heat acclimation. *J Sci Med Sport*. 2022;25:255.

Cao Y, et al. Head, face and neck cooling as per-cooling (cooling during exercise) modalities to improve exercise performance in the heat: a narrative review and practical applications. *Sports Med Open*. 2022;8:16.

Eser P, et al. Acute and chronic effects of high-intensity interval and moderate-intensity continuous exercise on heart rate and its variability after recent myocardial infarction: a randomized controlled trial. *Ann Phys Rehabil Med*. 2022;65:101444.

Foster J, et al. Quantifying the impact of heat on human physical work capacity; part II: the observed interaction of air velocity with temperature, humidity, sweat rate, and clothing is not captured by most heat stress indices. *Int J Biometeorol*. 2022;66:507.

Kasza I, et al. Contrasting recruitment of skin-associated adipose depots during cold challenge of mouse and human. *J Physiol*. 2022;600:847.

Kounalakis SN, et al. Exercise temperature regulation following a 35-day horizontal bedrest. *Exp Physiol*. 2021;106:1498.

Lankford HV, Fox LR. The wind-chill index. *Wilderness Environ Med*. 2021;32:392.

Mantzios K, et al. Effects of weather parameters on endurance running performance: discipline-specific analysis of 1258 races. *Med Sci Sports Exerc*. 2022;54:153.

McCubbin AJ. Exertional heat stress and sodium balance: leaders, followers, and adaptations. *Auton Neurosci*. 2021;235:102863.

McGarr GW, et al. Influence of uncomplicated, controlled hypertension on local heat-induced vasodilation in non-glabrous skin across the body. *Am J Physiol Regul Integr Comp Physiol*. 2022. doi:10.1152/ajpregu.00282.2021.

Okamoto Y, Amano T. Effects of sex and menstrual cycle on sweating during isometric handgrip exercise and postexercise forearm occlusion. *Exp Physiol*. 2021;106:1508.

Périard JD, et al. Exercise under heat stress: thermoregulation, hydration, performance implications, and mitigation strategies. *Physiol Rev*. 2021;101:1873.

Racinais S, et al. Association between thermal responses, medical events, performance, heat acclimation and health status in male and female elite athletes during the 2019 Doha World Athletics Championships. *Br J Sports Med*. 2022:bjsports-2021-104569.

Ravanelli N, Jay O. The change in core temperature and sweating response during exercise are unaffected by time of day within the wake period. *Med Sci Sports Exerc*. 2021;53:1285.

Rodriguez-Giustiniani P, et al. Fluid and electrolyte balance considerations for female athletes. *Eur J Sport Sci*. 2021:1. doi:10.1080/17461391.2021.1939428.

Siegler JC, et al. The hyperhydration potential of sodium bicarbonate and sodium citrate. *Int J Sport Nutr Exerc Metab*. 2021;7:1.

Spadaro O, et al. Caloric restriction in humans reveals immunometabolic regulators of health span. *Science*. 2022;375:671.

Stark C, et al. Systematic investigation of the link between enzyme catalysis and cold adaptation. *Elife*. 2022;11:e72884.

Stone T, et al. Menstrual cycle effects on cardiovascular drift and maximal oxygen uptake during exercise heat stress. *Eur J Appl Physiol*. 2021;121:561.

Szymczak RK, et al. Comparison of environmental conditions on summits of Mount Everest and K2 in climbing and midwinter seasons. *Int J Environ Res Public Health*. 2021;18:3040.

Tsadok I, et al. Assessing rectal temperature with a novel non-invasive sensor. *J Therm Biol*. 2021;95:102788.

Wagner DR, Cotter JD. Ultrasound measurements of subcutaneous fat thickness are robust against hydration changes. *Int J Sport Nutr Exerc Metab*. 2021;31:244.

Watkins ER, et al. Extreme occupational heat exposure is associated with elevated hematological and inflammatory markers in fire service instructors. *Exp Physiol*. 2021;106:233.

Wickham KA, et al. Sex differences in the physiological adaptations to heat acclimation: a state-of-the-art review. *Eur J Appl Physiol*. 2021;121:353.

Yu TY, et al. Delayed heart rate recovery after exercise predicts development of metabolic syndrome: a retrospective cohort study. *J Diabetes Investig*. 2022;13:167.

Zheng H, et al. Menstrual phase and ambient temperature do not influence iron regulation in the acute exercise period. *Am J Physiol Regul Integr Comp Physiol*. 2021;320:R780.

Table 25.1 Thermodynamics During Rest and Exercise

Condition	Rest	Maximal Exercise
Body's heat production (1 L O_2 uptake = 4.82 kcal)	~0.25 L $O_2 \cdot min^{-1}$ ~1.2 kcal $\cdot min^{-1}$	~4.0 L $O_2 \cdot min^{-1}$ ~20.0 kcal $\cdot min^{-1}$
Body's capacity for evaporative cooling (each 1 mL sweat evaporation = ~0.6 kcal body heat loss)	Maximal sweating ~30 mL $\cdot min^{-1}$ = 18 kcal $\cdot min^{-1}$	
Core temperature increase	None; remains stable	~1°C every 5–7 min

Table 25.2 Maintaining Core Temperature at Different Clo Values for Different Physical Activity Levels and Ambient Temperatures

Activity	Temperature, °C		
	0	−20	−50
Heavy work, 6.0 METs	1.0	1.6	2.2
Moderate work, 3.0 METs	1.6	2.8	4.2
Light work, 2.0 METs	2.6	4.0	6.2
Very light work, 1.5 METs	3.4	5.6	8.2
Rest, 1.0 MET	5.4	8.3	12.4
Sleep, 0.8 METs	6.7	10.6	15.5

Table 25.3 Common Garment Clo Values

Garment Description	Clo Value	Garment Description	Clo Value
Underwear, pants		**Coats, jacket, overtrousers**	
Pantyhose	0.020	Coat	0.6
Panties	0.30	Down jacket	0.55
Briefs	0.40	Parka	0.7
Pants, long legs	0.1		
Underwear, shirts		**Accessories**	
Bra	0.01	Socks	0.02
Shirt, sleeveless	0.06	Ankle socks (thick)	0.05
T-shirt	0.09	Long socks (thick)	0.1
Shirt with long sleeves	0.12	Slippers, quilted fleece	0.03
Half-slip, nylon	0.14	Shoes (thin soled)	0.02
		Shoes (thick soled)	0.04
		Boots, gloves	0.05
Shirts		**Skirts, dresses**	
Tube top	0.06	Light skirt, 15 cm above knee	0.10
Short sleeve	0.09	Light skirt, 15 cm below knee	0.18
Lightweight blouse, short sleeves	0.15	Heavy skirt, knee-length	0.25
Lightweight blouse, long sleeves	0.20	Light dress, sleeveless	0.25
Normal, long sleeves	0.25	Winter dress, long sleeves	0.4
Flannel shirt, long sleeves	0.3		
Trousers		**Sleepwear**	
Shorts	0.06	Long gown, long sleeves	0.3
Walking shorts	0.11	Short gown, thin-strap	0.15
Lightweight trousers	0.20	Hospital gown	0.31
Normal trousers	0.25	Long pajamas, long sleeves	0.50
Flannel trousers	0.28		
Overalls	0.28		
Sweaters		**Robes**	
Sleeveless vest	0.12	Long sleeve, wrap, long	0.53
Thin sweater	0.2	Long sleeve, wrap, short	0.41
Turtleneck, long sleeves (thin)	0.26		
Sweater	0.28		
Thick sweater	0.35		
Turtleneck, long sleeves (thick)	0.37		
Jacket		**Coveralls**	
Vest	0.13	Daily work wear, belted	0.49
Light summer jacket	0.25	Highly insulating, multicomponent, filling coveralls	1.03
Jacket	0.35	Fiber-pelt	1.13

Note: higher numbers indicate greater insulatory capacity.

Table 25.4	Predicted Sweating Rates (L·hr⁻¹) for Running at 8.5 to 15.0 km·hr⁻¹ in Cool/Temperate (TDB = 18°C) and Warm (TDB = 28°C) Weather				
Body Weight, kg	Climate	8.5 km·hr⁻¹/5.3 mph	10 km·hr⁻¹/6.3 mph	12.5 km·hr⁻¹/7.9 mph	15 km·hr⁻¹/9.5 mph
50	Cool/temperate	0.43	0.53	0.69	0.86
	Warm	0.52	0.62	0.79	0.96
70	Cool/temperate	0.65	0.79	1.02	1.25
	Warm	0.75	0.89	1.12	1.36
90	Cool/temperate	0.86	1.04	1.34	1.64
	Warm	0.97	1.15	1.46	1.76

Note: TDB, temperature of dry bulb thermometer.

Reproduced from Montain SJ, et al. Exercise-associated hyponatremia: quantitative analysis for understanding the aetiology. *Br J Sports Med*. 2006;40:98. With permission from BMJ Publishing Group Ltd.

Table 25.5 Physiologic Adjustments During Heat Acclimatization

Acclimatization Response	Effect
• Improved cutaneous blood flow	• Transports metabolic heat from deep core tissues to shell
• Effective cardiac output distribution	• Appropriate circulation to skin and muscles to meet metabolic and thermoregulation demands; greater blood pressure stability during exercise
• Lower threshold to begin sweating	• Evaporative cooling begins early in exercise
• More effective sweat distribution over skin surface	• Optimum body surface for effective evaporative cooling
• Increased sweat output	• Maximizes evaporative cooling
• Lower salt concentration in sweat	• Dilute sweat preserves extracellular fluid electrolytes
• Lower skin and core temperatures and heart rate during standard exercise	• Allows greater cardiac output to active muscles
• Less carbohydrate catabolism during exercise	• Carbohydrate sparing

Table 25.6 Cardiovascular Responses During Three Exercise Hyperthermia Stages

	Central Circulation	Peripheral Circulation		Rectal Temperature	Central Nervous System Status
Compensation	↑CO ↑SV, ↑HR ↓PV Respiratory alkalosis	↓Low SPBF ↓PV	↓Low TPVR ↑Skin BF ↑Muscle BF	37.0°C–39.5°C	Premonitory signs Dizziness Headache Euphoria Psychoses
Crises	↑↓CO ↑MABP ↓SV ↑↑HR Tachycardia (180 b·min^{-1}) Metabolic acidosis	↑↓SPBF ↓PV Moderate CVP	↓TPVR ↑↓Skin BF	39.5°C–41.5°C	↘Cerebral congestion ↘Cerebral edema Intracranial hypertension
Failure	↓↓CO ↓↓MABP ↑HR Tachycardia Metabolic acidosis	↑↑SPBF (autoregulatory escape); high CVP but low if hypovolemic	↓TPVR ↓Low skin BF	41.5°C	↘Coma, decreased cerebral perfusion ↘Cerebral ischemia Neurologic damage, seizures

Note: CO, cardiac output; SV, stroke volume; HR, heart rate; SPBF, splanchnic blood flow; PV, plasma volume; TPVR, total peripheral vascular resistance; BF, blood flow; MABP, mean arterial blood pressure; CVP, central venous pressure. ↑ = moderate increase; ↑↑ = strong increase; ↓ = moderate decrease; ↓↓ = strong decrease; ↑↓ = increase then decrease; ↘ = progressing to.

Data from Hubbard RW, Armstrong LE. The heat illnesses: biochemical, ultrastructural, and fluid-electrolyte considerations. In: Pandolf K, et al., eds. *Human Performance Physiology and Environmental Medicine at Terrestrial Extremes*. Carmel: Cooper Publishing Group; 1994; original data from Kielblock AJ, et al. Cardiovascular origins of heatstroke pathophysiology: an anesthetized rat model. *Aviat Space Environ Med*. 1982;53:171.

Table 25.7 Core Temperature and Physiological Changes When Core Temperature Declines

Stage	Core Temperature °F	Core Temperature °C	Physiological Changes
Normothermia	98.6	37.0	No noticeable effect
Mild hypothermia	95.0	35.0	Maximal shivering, increased blood pressure
	93.2	34.0	Amnesia; dysarthria; poor judgment; behavior change
	91.4	33.0	Ataxia; apathy
Moderate hypothermia	89.6	32.0	Stupor
	87.8	31.0	Shivering ceases; pupils dilate
	85.2	30.0	Cardiac arrhythmias; decreased cardiac output
	85.2	29.0	Unconsciousness
Severe hypothermia	82.4	28.0	Ventricular fibrillation likely; hypoventilation
	80.6	27.0	Loss of reflexes and voluntary motion
	78.8	26.0	Acid-base disturbances; no response to pain
	77.0	25.0	Reduced cerebral blood flow
	75.2	24.0	Hypotension; bradycardia; pulmonary edema
	73.4	23.0	No corneal reflexes; areflexia
	66.2	19.0	Electroencephalographic silence
	64.4	18.0	Asystole
	59.2	15.0	Lowest infant survival from accidental hypothermia
	56.7	13.7	Lowest adult survival from accidental hypothermia

Note: Individuals respond differently at each core temperature level.

Reprinted from American College of Sports Medicine Position Stand. Prevention of cold injuries during exercise. *Med Sci Sports Exerc*. 2007;38:2012

Chapter 26: Sport Diving

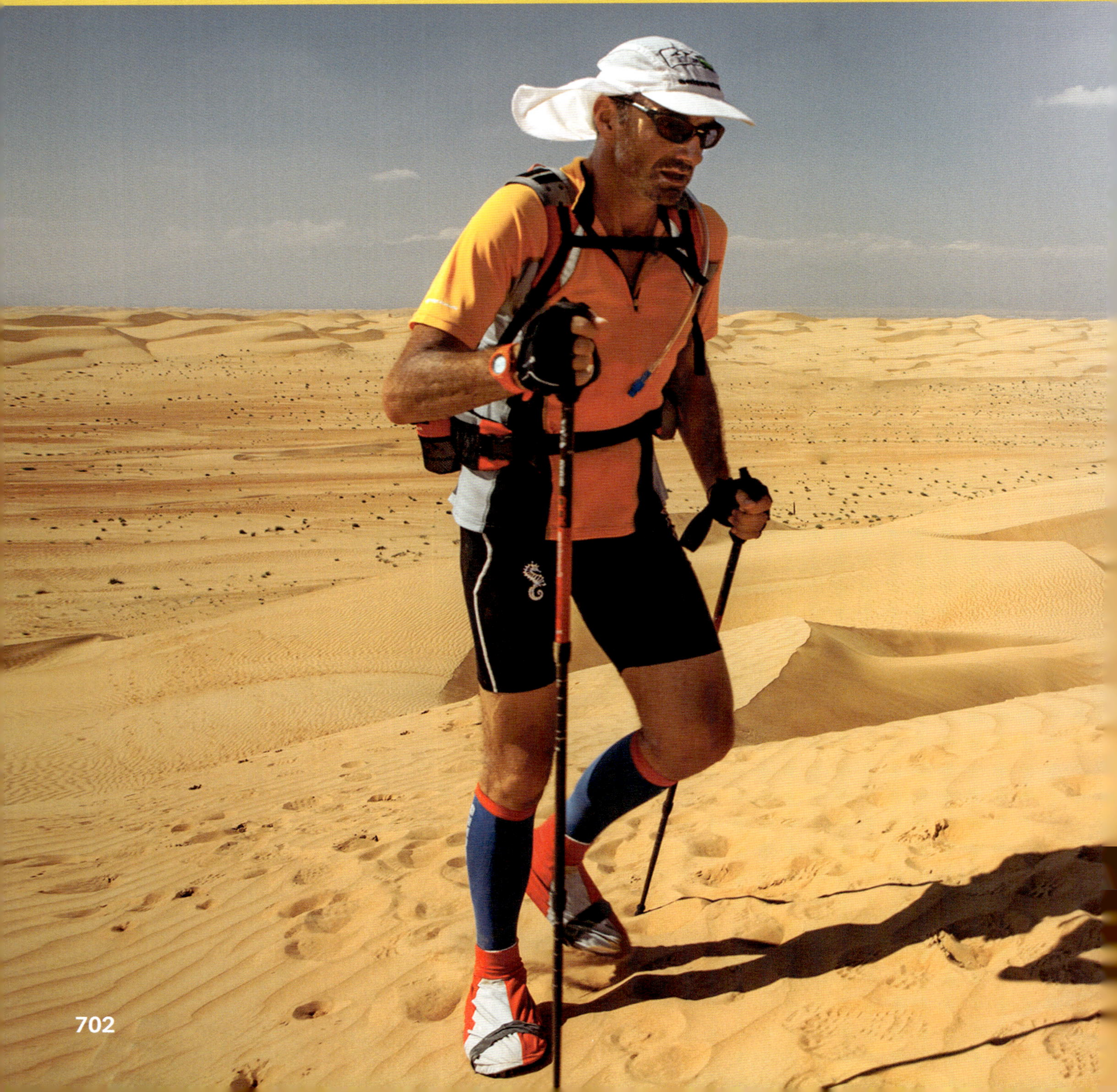

Chapter Objectives

- Give two examples describing the relationship among depth underwater and gas pressure and gas volume
- Discuss the rationale for snorkel size and underwater breathing depth
- Describe two factors that limit the depth of a breath-hold dive
- Describe hyperventilation's effect before diving on breath-hold duration and potential risks
- Outline evidence that supports a "diving reflex" in humans
- Contrast the main differences between open-circuit and closed-circuit scuba systems
- List causes, symptoms, and treatment for air embolism, lung burst, pneumothorax, mask squeeze, aerotitis, nitrogen narcosis, decompression sickness, and oxygen poisoning
- Explain the rationale influencing the decompression schedule for diving with compressed air
- Present two reasons for saturation diving and the environment where the diver lives for prolonged dives to extreme depths
- Give reasons for and describe limitations of breathing helium-oxygen mixtures during dives to deep depths
- Describe the closed-circuit, mixed-gas system used by the U.S. Navy in technical diving
- Describe the four free dive categories, and outline a general training strategy for diving success

Ancillaries at-a-Glance

Visit Lippincott Connect to access the following resources.

- References: Chapter 26
- Appendix H: Links for Supplemental Animations and Videos
- Focus on Research: The Oxygen Cost of Swimming Underwater

An estimated 6.2 million individuals in the United States scuba dive for work or recreation, and over 510,000 divers are trained yearly in formal certification courses. In the United States, there are approximately 11 million snorkelers (60% male, 40% female) and 20 million worldwide (https://medium.com/scubanomics/scuba-diving-participation-rate-statistics-36b9eecd8540). In economic terms, recreational scuba diving and snorkeling contribute $11 billion to the U.S. gross domestic product. With diving's unquestioned popularity, its safe practice requires thorough knowledge about diving physics and physiology basics. In this chapter, we emphasize relationships among diving depth, pressure, and gas volume and the potentially toxic effects from various gases breathed at high pressures in diving.[8,32,34,43]

Diving History: Antiquity to the Present

Men and women have practiced breath-hold diving for centuries as they hunted for sponges and food, salvaged artifacts and treasures, repaired ships, observed marine life, and participated in military maneuvers. The 5th century Greek historian Herodotus tells about the underwater exploits in 480 BC of the Greek patriot Scyllias and his daughter Hydna during the war against the Persians. When Scyllias, taken as prisoner aboard a ship, learned that Xerxes planned to attack a Greek flotilla, they escaped by jumping overboard. The Persians presumed they had drowned. To the contrary, Scyllias used a hollow reed as a snorkel and remained undiscovered, surfacing at night to cut each enemy ship loose from its moorings—saving the Greek Navy from sure disaster.

Understandably, each dive could last only a few minutes until the discovery that permitted dives for longer durations. Using longer "snorkels" did not work because the diver could not inhale against water pressure at depths greater than several feet (see "Snorkeling and Breath-Hold Diving," later in this chapter). Rebreathing from an air-filled bag submerged underwater also failed because the exhaled carbon dioxide buildup caused the diver to react erratically and lose consciousness.

The first solutions to these problems occurred in the 1530s with the invention allowing diving bells to supply surface air. The bell, positioned a few feet from the surface, had its bottom open to water and its top portion containing air compressed by water pressure. A diver in the bell with his head surrounded by air could then hold his breath, swim from the bell for a few minutes, and return, repeating the breath-hold process until the bell's remaining air became toxic.

In England and France in the 16th century, leather diving suits allowed descent to 18.3-m/60-ft depths. Manual pumps delivered fresh air from the surface to the diver. Soon metal helmets could withstand greater water pressures, and divers could descend further. By the 1830s, perfecting the surface-supplied air helmet allowed extensive underwater salvage work.

Starting in the 19th century, two main investigative avenues—one scientific and the other technologic—accelerated underwater exploration. French physiologist Paul Bert (1833–1886) and Scottish physiologist John Scott Haldane (1860–1936) explained water pressure's physiologic effects on body tissues and also defined safe limits for compressed air diving using a decompression chamber and accompanying decompression tables based on numerous animal experiments. Technologic improvements with compressed air pumps, carbon dioxide scrubbers (machines that capture the carbon for elimination), and demand valve regulators allowed prolonged underwater explorations. The next section presents a chronology in diving history, highlighting the inventors and technological innovations that improved human and robotic underwater exploration.

Diving History Chronology

Diving history is rich in legend and scientific discovery, with ready access to worldwide diving records (www.timetoast.com/timelines/history-of-scuba-diving).

4500 BC: Archeologists unearth shells in Mesopotamia dated to this period that must have originated from the sea floor.

3200 BC: Archeologists discover mother-of-pearl (abalone) shell ornaments dated to this period from the Egyptian Theban VI dynasty.

2500 BC: Greek divers make sponges widely available in commerce; *The Iliad* and *The Odyssey* mention diving and sponges.

550 BC: Pearl diving is documented in India and Ceylon.

480 BC: Scyllias and his daughter Hydna swim underwater using snorkels and knives to cut enemy moorings to help a Greek fleet defeat invading Persian naval forces before the Battle of Salamis.

100 BC: The Ama, Japan's women breath-hold divers of antiquity and modern times, gather pearl oysters, shellfish, sea cucumbers, and edible seaweed. The divers held their breath, then surfaced and opened their mouths slightly, and exhaled slowly before inhaling for another dive.

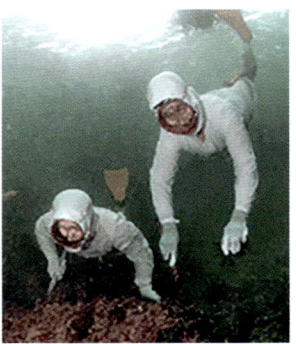

1500: Da Vinci designs the first "snorkel" device and dive fins for the hands and feet.

1530: First diving bell invention by Italian Guglielmo de Lorena. From 1531 until 1535, de Lorena built a large "bell" that rested on the diver's shoulders with a tube running from the surface into the bell to supply fresh air during commercial sponge fishing and salvaging operations and sunken treasure explorations.

1650: First effective air pump developed by German scientist and inventor Otto Von Guericke (1602–1686), which physicist Robert Boyle (1627–1691) uses in animal compression and decompression experiments.

1667: Robert Boyle makes first records of decompression sickness or "bends" by documenting a gas bubble in a viper's eye before he compressed and then decompressed it.

1690: Sir Edmund Halley (1656–1742; discovered Halley's comet) patents a practical diving bell with lead-coated wood and a glass top to allow light to enter (1.7 m³/60 cubic ft in volume) and connected by a pipe to weighted barrels that replenished with surface air, allowing dives to 18.3 m/60 ft for 90 min.

1715: John Lethbridge (1675–1759) constructs a "diving engine" or underwater "diving machine" built from an oak cylinder 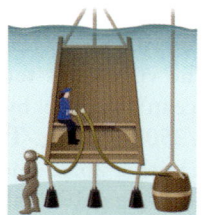 and supplied with compressed surface air. The diver remained submerged for 30 min at 18.3 m/60 ft; holes in the cylinder sealed by greased leather cuffs allowed his arms to protrude into the water while performing salvage work.

1788: John Smeaton's (1724–1792) popular diving bell uses a hand pump to supply fresh surface air and a one-way valve to prevent air from returning to the pump when it stops.

1808: Friedrich von Drieberg (1780–1856) invents a bellows-in-a-box device named Triton. Worn on the diver's back, it delivered compressed air from the surface. The device never worked successfully yet suggested that compressed air could be used in diving, an idea conceived by Halley in the late 1690s.

1823: Charles Anthony Deane (1796–1848) patents the "smoke helmet" for fighting structural fires. Later modified for diving, the helmet fastened over the head with weights and received surface air through a hose. In 1828, Deane and his brother John market the helmet with a loosely attached "diving suit" so the 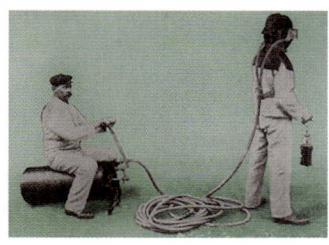 diver could perform salvage work, but only in the full vertical position to prevent water from entering the suit.

1825: First prototype for "scuba" invented by Englishman William H. James incorporates a cylindrical belt (air reservoir) around the diver's trunk that supplies air to a helmet at 450 psi (lb per in²) by a hand-operated valve and rubber tube. This 1873 newspaper illustration from a London paper shows the diver in full suit ensemble while a crew member straightens the air hose. 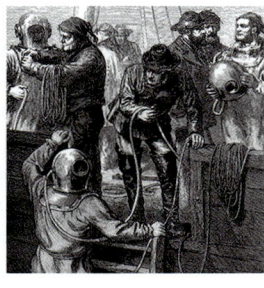 The diver inhales through the nose and exhales through a mouthpiece connected by a short tube to an escape valve in the helmet's crown. With the reservoir charged to 30 atm, James believed a diver would have enough air to last 60 min.

1837: Augustus Siebe (1788–1872), the father of diving, seals Deane brothers' diving helmet to a waist-length jacket to create a full, watertight rubber suit that received surface air. This suit served as the forerunner for modern hardhat diving gear.

1839: Siebe's diving suit is used in salvaging the British warship HMS *Royal George*, sunk in 1782 to a depth of 19.8 m/65 ft; divers report the first decompression sickness symptoms.

1843: From experience salvaging the HMS *Royal George*, the British Royal Navy establishes the first diving school.

1865: Benoît Rouquayrol (1826–1875) and Auguste Denayrouze (1837–1883) patent an underwater breathing apparatus called the 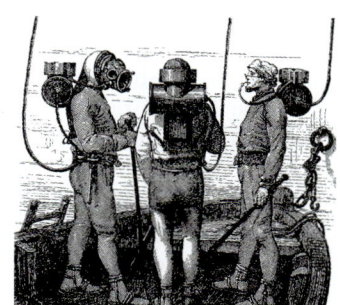 "aerophore," a steel tank containing compressed air at 250 to 350 psi worn on the back and connected through an automatic demand valve to a mouthpiece (www.divinghelmet.nl/divinghelmet/1860_Rouquayrol_Denayrouze_2.html). This forerunner of modern scuba enabled the diver to disconnect from a tether that supplied surface air and swim freely with the tank for several minutes.

1873: Dr. Andrew H. Smith, surgeon to the New York Bridge Company (the builders of the Brooklyn Bridge), reports regarding compressed air sickness in workers who leave their pressurized caisson. Smith recommends chamber recompression for future projects but does not mention nitrogen bubbles for causing decompression sickness.

1878: Henry A. Fleuss, an engineer, develops the first self-contained diving apparatus with compressed oxygen, not compressed air, based on the closed-circuit principle. Rope soaked in caustic potash absorbed carbon dioxide so the diver rebreathed exhaled air without bubbles entering the water. The apparatus provided divers up to 3 hr "bottom time."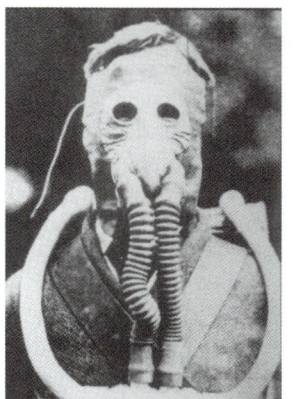

1878: Paul Bert (1833–1886), a French zoologist, physiologist, and politician, publishes *La Pression Barométrique*, describing physiologic studies with pressure changes. Bert proves that nitrogen gas bubbles cause decompression sickness (the "bends" or caisson disease), while gradual ascent prevents the problem and recompression relieves pain. Deep sea pearl divers during that era experienced the bends.

1908: John Scott Haldane (1860–1936), Arthur Boycott, and Guybon Damant publish "The Prevention of Compressed-Air Illness," a landmark paper describing staged decompression to combat decompression sickness. The British Royal Navy and United States Navy subsequently develop diving tables for compressed air diving up to a 61-m/200-ft depth.

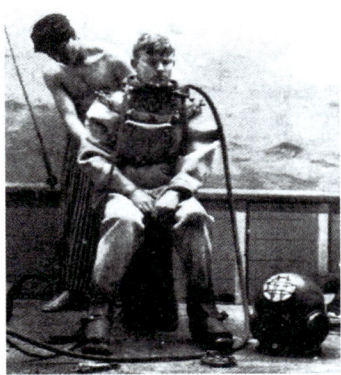

1910: English inventor Sir Robert Davis (1870–1965) patents the Davis Submerged Escape Apparatus (DSEA), a device that allowed British submarine crews about 30 min to escape from a sinking ship.

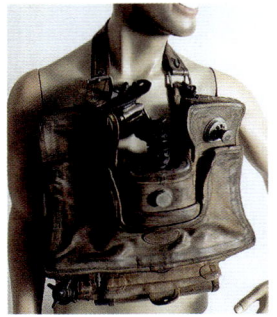

The DSEA rig shown in the left inset figure contained a rubber breathing/buoyancy bag with a barium hydroxide canister to scrub exhaled CO_2. The DSEA included a steel pressure cylinder with a control valve connected to the breathing bag with approximately 56 L oxygen at 120 ata pressure. Opening the cylinder's valve admitted oxygen to the bag and charged it to the surrounding water pressure. The CO_2 absorbent canister inside the breathing bag connected to a mouthpiece and goggles by a flexible corrugated tube, with breathing done by mouth only with the nose closed by a clip.

1917: The U.S. Bureau of Construction and Repair first introduces the Mark V diving helmet, revolutionizing World War II salvage operations

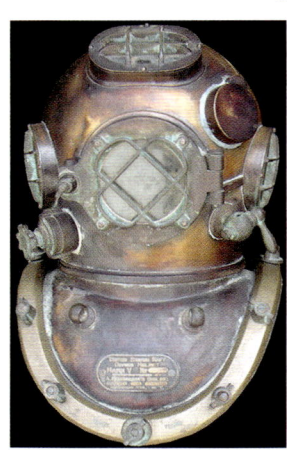

This "gold standard" in helmet design served five purposes: it sealed the whole of the diver's head from the water, it allowed the diver to see clearly underwater, it provided breathing gas, it protected the diver's head when doing heavy or dangerous work, allowing for voice communications with the surface during the dive. If a diver became incapacitated during a dive but was still breathing, the helmet remained in place and continued to deliver breathing gas until a rescue took place.

1920s: U.S. researchers experiment with helium-oxygen mixtures for deep dives.

1924: The U.S. Navy and Bureau of Mines conduct the first experiments with helium-oxygen mixtures.

1930: Dr. Charles William Beebe (1877–1962) and Lieutenant and submariner Otis Barton (1899–1992) descend 435 m/1426 ft in a 1.4-m/4-ft bathysphere attached to a barge by a steel cable. In the photo, Beebe is on the left, and Barton on the right (https://sites.google.com/site/cwilliambeebe/Home/bathysphere).

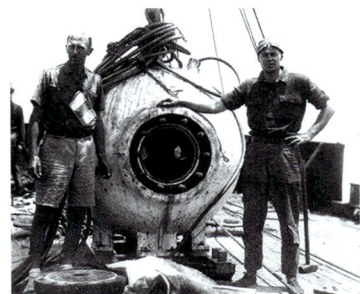

The bathysphere walls measured 0.457-m/1.5-ft thick made from a single casting. The vessel was tethered from a mother ship at the ocean's surface by a single, nontwisting cable 1066.8 m/3500 ft long. The steel cable was 2.22-cm/7/8-in thick with a 26.31-metric ton/29-ton breaking strain. An additional 100 cable strands were interwoven around the steel central core to ensure the cable would not rotate the sphere upon descent or on return to the ocean's surface. Electric lines for light and a telephone line were wrapped inside a rubber hose, which entered through a small hole at the bathysphere's top. Oxygen tanks with automatic valves were installed. Trays of calcium chloride to absorb moisture were placed on racks alongside soda lime trays to remove excess CO_2. The two explorers were sealed inside using a 38.1-cm/15-in, 181.4-kg/400-lb circular door put in place by a winch and then hand-tightened with 10 bolts. The Beebe and Barton dive, one of the great exploration triumphs of the 1930s, received worldwide notoriety. Beebe wrote a riveting account about the historic dive in 1951, which can be read online at http://archive.org/stream/halfmiledown00beeb#page/n0/mode/2up.

1930s: American pilot and writer Guy Gilpatric (1896–1950) pioneers using rubber goggles with glass lenses for skin diving. He added putty to aviator goggles for eye protection from salt water. By the mid-1930s, face masks, fins (also called "swimming propellers"), and snorkels were in common use.

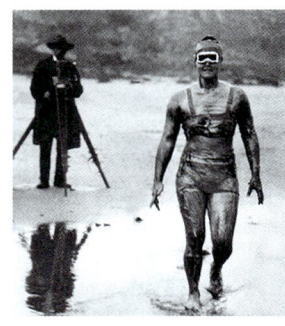

The famous female 1924 Olympic champion and competition swimmer Gertrude Ederle (1905–2003) broke the prior men's Channel record on August 6, 1926, by 2 hr, becoming the first woman to swim the Channel and the first person (male or female) to swim the front crawl the entire distance. What made her swim possible were the motorcycle goggles she waterproofed with a paraffin seal.

1933: French Navy captain Yves Le Prieur (1885–1963) modifies the Rouquayrol-Denayrouze "aerophore" by combining a new demand valve with a 1500-psi high-pressure air tank without a regulator to eliminate restricting effects from hoses and lines. The diver breathes fresh air by opening a tap, while exhaled air escapes under the diver's mask edge.

1934: William Beebe and Otis Barton descend 922.9 m/3028 ft in their bathysphere near Bermuda, setting a depth record that remained until 1948.

1935: French Navy adopts Yves Le Prieur's "scuba" equipment.

1936: Le Prieur establishes the world's first scuba diving club called the "Club of Divers and Underwater Life."

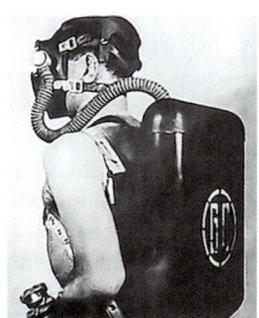

1937: Georges Commeinhes (1911–1944) patents the first two-cylinder open-circuit breathing apparatus (model CG-42) with a novel demand regulator between two cylinders tied to a full face mask demonstrated for the French Navy with a 53-m/174-ft dive in the Mediterranean Sea near Marseilles, France.

1937: Edgar End, MD, and Max E. Nohl establish a new world record in diving history achieving a 128-m/420-ft descent using a helium-oxygen breathing mixture in an open water environment. Dr. End calculated the helium-oxygen breathing mixture concentrations and decompression schedules (www.mejeme.com/dive/articles/mixhistory.htm).

1938: Dr. Edgar End and Max E. Nohl make the first intentional saturation "dive" in a Milwaukee hospital hyperbaric chamber (27 hr at a 31-m/101-ft depth). Decompression took 5 hr, and Nohl suffers the bends. Dr. End believes helium can replace nitrogen to reduce nitrogen narcosis.

1939: A new diving bell, the McCann–Erickson Rescue Chamber, makes the first successful rescue aboard the submarine USS *Squalus*, a new 94.5-m/310-ft submarine sunk in 74 m/243 ft of water in the North Atlantic. The chamber fit over the submarine's escape hatch, which four men at a time entered under one atm pressure. The rescue involved attaching salvage pontoons along the submarine sides with chains slung under the hull. The pontoons inflated to lift the boat off the bottom and moved to shallower water where the pontoons were reset. The process was repeated until *Squalus* was shallow enough to enter the river at Portsmouth. The subsequent rescue and salvage operations ushered in several new technologies, including the McCann Rescue Chamber designed specifically to rescue sailors trapped in submarines but never tested outside a controlled training environment. In the first operational use of helium diving by the U.S. Navy,

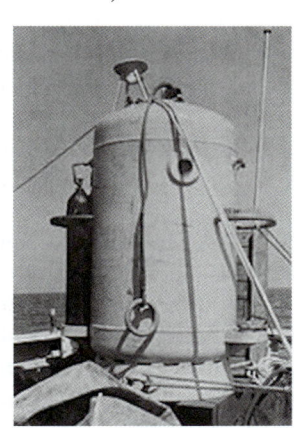

Dr. Albert Behnke (see Chapter 28, "Reference Man and Reference Woman") helped to supervise the successful rescue efforts (https://coffeeordie.com/squalus-rescue/) and provided operational support as one of the medical officers. The 39-hr operation saved 33 sailors, but 25 died and 1 was never found. Salvaging the *Squalus* took 113 days, and it was raised on September 13, 1939, using compressed air tanks for flotation.[53]

1941–1944: Italian divers, working out of midget submarines during World War II, use closed-circuit scuba to place explosives under British naval and merchant marine vessels. The British adopt this technology after almost five years trying to sink German submarines, finally sinking the killer 52,000-ton/23.2-imperial ton armored German battleship *Tirpitz* on November 12, 1944 (www.thehistorypress.co.uk/articles/the-sinking-of-hitler-s-battleship-tirpitz/). The effort required about 400 bombers, torpedo bombers, fighter planes, and reconnaissance aircraft.

1942–1943: Jacques-Yves Cousteau (1910–1997; French naval lieutenant) and Emile Gagnan (1900–1979; engineer for a Parisian natural gas company) redesign a car regulator to supply compressed air to a diver when they initiate the breathing cycle. They attach their new demand valve regulator to hoses, a mouthpiece, and a pair of compressed air tanks, which they patent as the

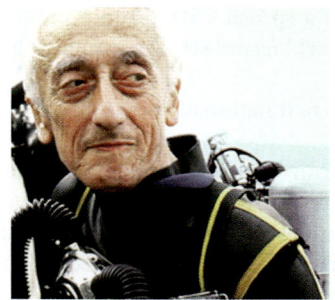

AquaLung. Frederic Dumas (1913–1991) descends to 64 m/210 ft in the Mediterranean Sea and experiences *l'ivresse des grandes profondeurs* ("the rapture of the great depths"). Cousteau achieves worldwide acclaim for his underwater explorations, movies, books, and dedication to environmental causes (www.cousteau.org).

1947: Frederic Dumas uses the AquaLung and dives to 94 m/307 ft in the Mediterranean Sea.

1948: Otis Barton (1899–1992) descends in a modified bathysphere to 1370 m/4500 ft off the California coast.

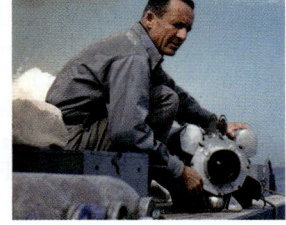

1950s: August Picard and Jacques Picard develop the Swiss-designed, Italian-built research bathyscaphe (www.nationalgeographic.org/encyclopedia/bathyscaphe/), a completely self-contained vessel. In 1954, the bathyscaphe sets a diving record to 4050 m/13,287 ft.

For submarine survival equipment, a British company in 1952 pioneered submarine escape technology (https://survitecgroup.com/about-us/

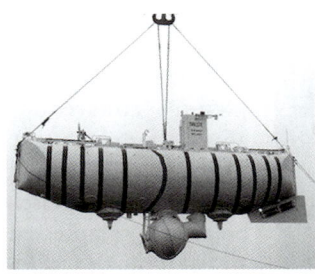

our-history/). Designed to provide protection for submariners in a damaged submarine, the products include single-skinned suits with integrated life rafts, escape jerkins, inflatable abandonment suits, external submarine life raft systems, and freeboard extenders. There are in excess of 30,000 units of submarine escape equipment in use currently, and 30 of the world's navies (including the U.S. Navy) use the latest Submarine Escape Immersion Equipment (SEIE) MK-11. The suit allows survivors to escape a disabled submarine at depths down to 183 m/600 ft, at a rate of eight or more men per hour.

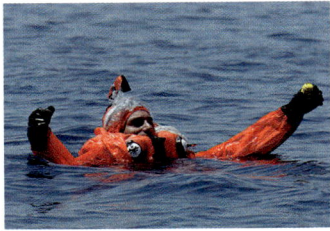

1958-2021: World records for breath-hold diving chronicled by the World Underwater Federation (www.cmas.org/cmas/about), U.S.A. Freediving (www.usafreediving.com/about/), Livingdreams.TV (www.livingdreams.tv/oceans/freediving-and-amazing-records), and a special CBS 60-min program featuring the free-diving world record sets the current record at a 101-m/331-ft depth.

1959: The YMCA begins the first nationally organized course for scuba certification.

1960: Jacques Picard and Don Walsh descend to approximately 10,916 m/35,820 ft, 10.9 km/6.78 mi; water pressure 16,883 psi, temperature 3°C/37.4°F in the August Picard–designed, Swiss-built, U.S. Navy–owned bathyscaphe *Trieste*, to the Mariana Trench in the Pacific Ocean (deepest known seafloor depression on Earth). Listen to a first-person account by Don Walsh about this Picard and Walsh 1960 dive, including a historical perspective of the dive and its accomplishments for science (www.youtube.com/watch?v=5uRozfExtYo).

1960s: As accident rates for scuba divers climb, the first national agencies form to train and certify divers: the National Association of Underwater Instructors (NAUI) forms in 1960 and the Professional Association of Diving Instructors (PADI) forms in 1966.

1962: Albert Falco and Claude Wesley, in the first of three planned experiments called Conshelf (continental shelf), sought to establish that humans can live underwater for an extended period. Falco (Cousteau's lead diver) and Wesley spent 7 days under 10 m/33 ft in the open sea near Marseilles, France, in an underwater living habitat named *Diogenes* (https://scubadiverlife.com/diving-history-jacques-cousteaus-conshelf-missions/). They ate, worked, and slept in the vessel, breathing compressed air fed through surface pipes. TV monitors recorded their activities, and other divers including Jacques Cousteau, at left in the image, paid regular visits to the "oceanauts." No ill physiological effects occurred from that first sojourn.

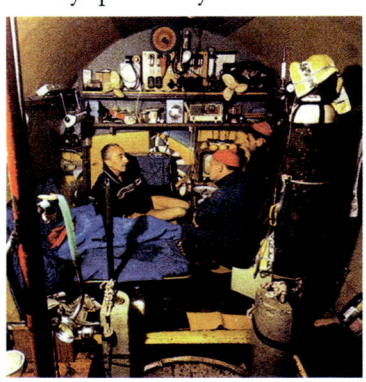

1963–1965: Divers live and work in underwater habitats for a month at a time at 60 m/197 ft.

1963: Whitey Stefens (*left*) and Bob Ratcliffe (*right*), commercial abalone divers from Santa Barbara, California, pose in the photo below with the first prototype diving helmet converted for deep diving use by commercial construction and oilfield divers

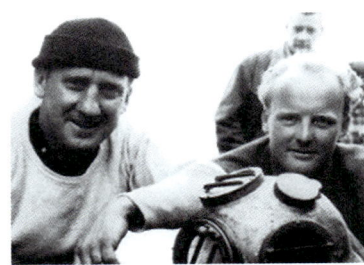

The DESCO commercial abalone helmet (www.divedesco.com/P/151/Lightweight-AbaloneDiversHelmet) had been fitted with a newly developed second-stage scuba breathing regulator, which conserved the expensive oxygen and helium breathing mixture required for ultra-deep (61+ m/200+ ft) commercial construction and offshore oilfield diving

1964: Abalone diver and young entrepreneur Danny Wilson (see Deep-Water Diving's Historical Roots, below) dove 76.2 m/250 ft to 152.4 m/500 ft off the Santa Barbara channel without conventional heavy gear limitations and built the Purisima diving bell shown in the photo at left with diver Bob Ratcliffe. This represented the world's first oxy-helium–equipped, deep capability commercial diver lockout bell.

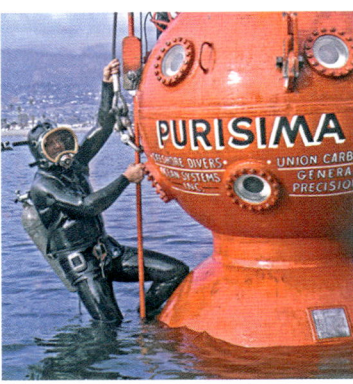

Purisima's goal was to provide relatively short-duration "bounce" dives to the extreme depths that required an oxy-helium mixture.

With the divers safely back in the diving bell after completing their tasks, a similar bell was quickly raised to the surface by an overhead hoist and carefully mated to the cylindrical, deck decompression chamber (photo *left*) for lengthy decompression to avoid the bends.

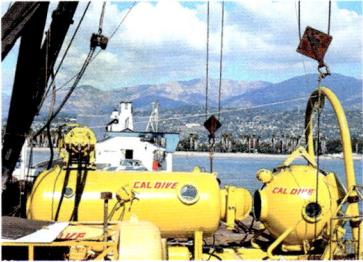

1968: John J. Gruener and R. Neal Watson dive to 133 m/436 ft breathing compressed air.

1969: Following the Purisima diving bell's commercial success, divers Bob Ratcliffe, Lad and Gene Handelman, and Ken Lengyel formed California Divers Inc. (known as *Cal Dive*), which later evolved into *Oceaneering International Inc.* (www.oceaneering.com), an acknowledged world leader in subsea engineering and applied technology.

1970s: Diving safety standards include certification cards to indicate a minimum training level and as a requirement for tank refills, change from J-valve reserve systems to nonreserve K-valves, adopting submersible pressure gauges, buoyancy compensators, and single-hose regulators.

1980: *Divers Alert Network* is founded at Duke University as a nonprofit organization to promote safe diving (https://dan.org).

1981: Record 686-m/2250-ft "dive" made in a Duke Medical Center chamber. Stephen Porter, Len Whitlock, and Erik Kramer live in the 2.74-m/8-ft chamber for 43 days, breathing a nitrogen, oxygen, and helium mixture.

1983: First commercially available dive computer (Orca Edge; http://divemagazine.co.uk/kit/6597-history-of-the-dive-computer).

1985: Oceanographer, Naval Intelligence Officer, and explorer Robert Ballard (Institute for Exploration at Mystic Aquarium, Mystic, Connecticut; www.mysticaquarium.org) and Ralph White use a remote-controlled camera to explore the wreck of the *Titanic* shown in the inset (3810-m/12,500-ft depth) located about 1609.34 km/1000 mi due east of Boston.

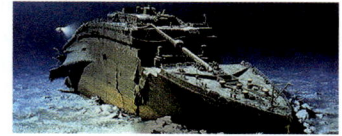

In this brief video (https://achievement.org/achiever/robert-d-ballard-ph-d/), Ballard discusses exploring underwater wrecks, including deep-sea hydrothermal vents (massive formations that spew superheated fluids from the ocean floor). Ballard also discovered the *Bismarck* and the USS *Yorktown* wrecks during his 135 expeditions.

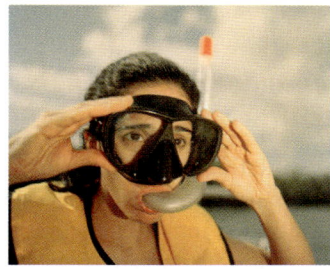

1990s: An estimated 500,000 new scuba divers are certified yearly in the United States as this activity's popularity for recreational and commercial purposes increases.

Numerous scientific experiments using submersibles explored worldwide deep-diving sites in the Atlantic and Pacific oceans. The journeys included probing deep-sea volcanism, deep geology, and searching for artifacts from sunken vessels, including 2000-year-old shipwrecks in the Mediterranean Sea.

2003: Tanya Streeter, a world champion freediver, shatters the men's and women's variable ballast free-diving world records by descending 122 m/400 ft in 3 min 38 s to capture the variable ballast record. Streeter becomes the first person to break all four deep free-diving world records.

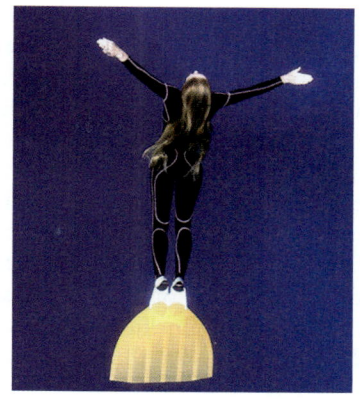

2004–2006: Technical diving by nonprofessionals expands for mixed gas use, new propulsion systems, full-face masks, underwater voice communication, and digital cameras.

2012: Deepest no-limit free dive world record by Austrian Herbert Nitsch (253.2 m/831 ft; www.guinnessworldrecords.com/world-records/673884-deepest-no-limit-freedive-male).

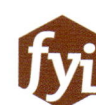 **First Submarine "Turtle" Invented in 1776**

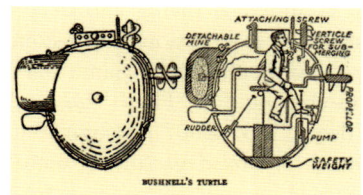

The first confirmed submarine "Turtle" invented by David Bushnell (1740–1824) was planned between 1771 and 1775 for use in the war against the British in New York harbor in 1776 (www.history.navy.mil/research/library/online-reading-room/title-list-alphabetically/s/submarine-turtle-naval-documents.html#item10). Bushnell's submarine never saw battle, but his expectations and forward thinking were clear—"one man could carry out the combined duties of diving officer, navigator, torpedoman, and engineer, while at the same time fighting tides and currents and propelling the boat with his own muscles." The Turtle embodied basic requirements for a successful military submarine: ability to submerge, maneuver underwater, maintain an adequate air supply to support the craft's operator, and carry out effective offensive operations against an enemy surface vessel. The self-pedaled device could be packed with 150 lb of gunpowder called a *keg mine* (about 0.76 m/2.5 ft long and 0.30 m/1.5 ft in diameter), which when detonated underwater would destroy a British warship's wooden hull. In practice, the submariner was to pedal toward an intended vessel during the middle of the night in darkness and relative silence with less chance for detection. The submariner would attach a sharp screw cranked into the wooden hull just above the water line, and activate the keg mine with a timed fuse. For his insights about naval warfare's future, Bushnell is rightfully remembered by historians as the "Father of Submarine Warfare."

Sources:
Barber FM. *Lecture on Submarine Boats and their Application to Torpedo Operations.* Newport: U.S. Torpedo Station; 1875.
Papers of Thomas Jefferson, vol. 13, Library of Congress, Washington, DC. Printed in Thomas Jefferson, *The Papers of Thomas Jefferson*, ed. by Julian Boyd, et al., 34 vols. to date. Princeton: Princeton University Press; 1950-, 12: 303-4.

2012: Oceanographer and filmmaker James Cameron completes record-breaking nearly 11,270-m/7-mi Mariana Trench solo submersible dive. Cameron achieved this milestone on March 25, 2012, descending to the deepest part of the world's oceans located in the western Pacific Ocean to the east of the Mariana Islands in a 12-ton/0.0893-imperial ton submarine vessel called the *Deepsea Challenger* (www.theguardian.com/film/australia-culture-blog/2014/aug/21/james-cameron-on). The trench is about 2550 km/1580 mi long with an average 69 km/43 mi width. The maximum-known depth is 10.911 km (±40 m)/6.831 mi (±131 ft) at the Challenger Deep, a small slot-shaped valley in its floor. The dive was part of Deepsea Challenge, a scientific expedition by Cameron, the National Geographic Society, and Rolex to conduct deep-ocean research.

Deep-Water Diving's Historical Roots

Santa Barbara, California

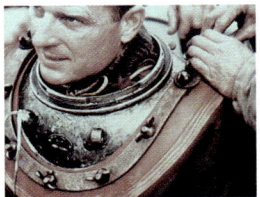

Santa Barbara, California, can rightfully lay claim to a historic dive that revolutionized commercial diving and deep-water oil exploration expansion. On November 3, 1962, Santa Barbara abalone diver Hugh "Danny" Wilson (1931–2007), recognizing a need for mixed-gas diving techniques to support offshore petroleum exploration, modified his abalone diving helmet with an oxygen and helium mixture and dove to about 122 m/400 ft off Santa Cruz Island in the Santa Barbara Channel.

Prior to the 1960s and Wilson's historic dive, diving depths were severely limited by the narcotic effects from high nitrogen pressures and deleterious central nervous system toxicity from high oxygen pressures in typical compressed air diving. The large support vessel and numerous support crew required for the U. S. Navy's equipment and approach to deep-water diving were neither cost-effective nor practical for commercial construction or offshore oilfield diving. The Navy's helmet and procedures had been used successfully in 1939 in the *USS Squalus* submarine rescue off the New Hampshire coast that saved 33 lives (see Salvaging the Squalus: A Historic Undersea Rescue, below). The Navy system was largely viewed as impractical for the needs of deep-water commercial operations. Wilson hoped the dive would convince oil company executives that drilling in the Santa Barbara Channel would offer a better opportunity for dive operations and business viability.

The oil companies and petroleum geologists were convinced that vast oil and gas reserves were available at ocean depths beyond 91.4 m/300 ft, yet they could not drill at those depths without better diving support from workable, lightweight diving gear and appropriate gas mixtures. Wilson, hoping to enter the then "closed" cadre of divers who worked for the Associated Divers Company in the 1950s and

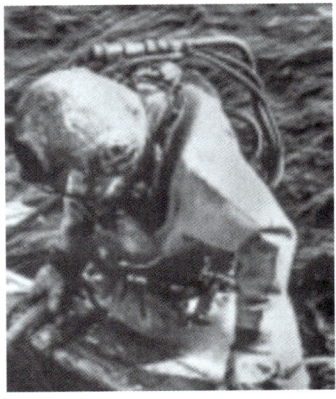

1960s, was told his proposed methods would not work. Now motivated to succeed and break market domination, he modified his open-circuit air free-flow abalone helmet into an open-circuit demand/free-flow system fed with a heliox mixture. Wilson did not publicize his final "test" dive to avoid alerting competing local divers. When the diving community later learned about the dive, they considered it foolish and dangerous because Wilson dove using untried and unproven equipment and gas mixtures and made the dive from a relatively small fishing boat that lacked space for a decompression chamber in the event of decompression problems.

Wilson, who had risked his life on the dive, successfully demonstrated the prototype helmet design permitted working in deep water for 60 min without deleterious nitrogen narcosis effects (mental torpidity or euphoria similar to altitude anoxia or alcoholic intoxication) that typically hinder such tasks. In the diving operations offered by competitor Associated Divers, their divers only remained working at depth for about 25 min breathing ordinary compressed air. And so the gamble had paid off—the diving David had slain Goliath, and the stranglehold on offshore diving in the Santa Barbara channel had been defeated. Wilson's breakthrough demonstration dive using his newly designed helmet—relying on a 80% helium, 20% oxygen breathing mixture for descent, and a bottom 90% helium and 10% oxygen mixture—collapsed an important barrier in diving technology with a lasting economic impact. Wilson's contribution served as the forerunner to the modern-day open-circuit demand/free-flow helmets (https://b2b.partcommunity.com/community/knowledge/en/detail/7837/Diving+helmet).[6]

The Man and the Dive: Reflections from Pioneer Diver Bob Ratcliffe

Bob Ratcliffe, inventor of the "Rat-Hat" diving helmet in use worldwide (www.divescrap.com/DiveScrap_INDEX/Oceaneering.html) and 2010 inductee into the Commercial Diving Hall of Fame (https://aquadocs.org/bitstream/handle/1834/31134/The_Journal_of_Diving_History_65_2010.pdf?sequence=1&isAllowed=y), spent about a decade diving with Danny Wilson for abalone and participated with him in commercial oxy-helium diving along the California coast. He provides the following reflections on his experience:

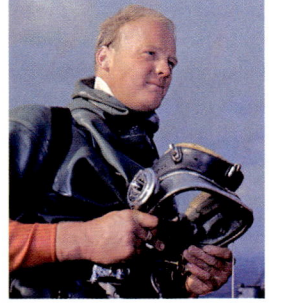

Oil companies that want to drill in deep water are not interested in paying commercial divers to descend to their sea floor equipment in 250 FSW (feet of salt water) to blow bubbles! They want the highly paid divers to perform the work on the sea floor assigned to them. Nitrogen narcosis severely reduces the amount of time of useful work that a diver can accomplish. Use of oxygen and helium mixtures for the diver's breathing gas allows the diver to perform the amount of work in very deep water comparable to what he could accomplish in very shallow water. He is as clear headed at depth as he is working in his own back yard. Dan Wilson's purpose was to allow him to break into oilfield diving (for lucrative pay) by being able to perform more useful work in deep water as an inexperienced oilfield diver using oxy–helium than the experienced, excellent divers could accomplish breathing compressed air.

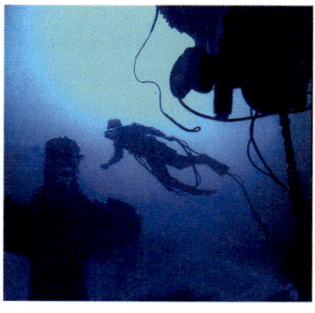

This was in fact what happened. The new oxy–helium divers accomplished much more for each dive, when calculated per dollar paid, than the compressed air divers. The inset photo (see the prior page) shows me leaving through the lower hatch of our diving bell *Purisima*, and swimming to a sub-sea wellhead (consisting of valves and pipes) on the sea floor in the Santa Barbara channel in the early 1960s. Wilson did these many times during contract work for oil companies, due in part to the effective use of oxy–helium mixtures during deep-water dives.

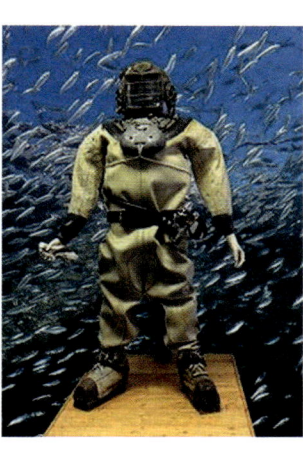

The photo shows a model of the diving suit and gear Wilson wore during his historic dive on November 3, 1962, that paved the way for future endeavors in commercial deep-sea diving.

Salvaging the Squalus: A Historic Undersea Rescue

When the submarine USS Squalus (SS 192) and her 59 crewmen sank off New Hampshire on May 23, 1939, the crew's struggle for survival and the courage of rescuers kept Americans close to their radio dials. Before television, the public was gripped by compelling events far beneath the sea in what became the greatest submarine rescue in U.S. history.

—Robert F. Dorr, February 18, 2010
(www.defensemedianetwork.com/stories/squalus-disaster-rescue-gripped-a-nation-on-the-eve-of-war/)

Rescuing the submarine *Squalus* in 1939, the last Naval salvage operation prior to World War II, provided a unique opportunity for then Lieutenant Commander Albert R. Behnke, Jr. MC (U.S. Navy), to assist in the medical operations that saved 33 men when the submarine sank in 74 m/243 ft of water off the Isles of Shoals along the New Hampshire coast during a "crash" test requiring the rapid vessel submersion to avoid enemy detection.

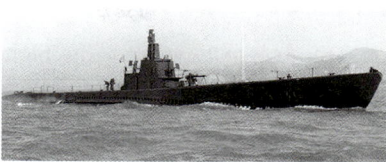

During the initial dive, a valve that supplied air to the diesel engine apparently remained open. This caused immediate flooding in the aft torpedo room, both engine rooms, and the crew's quarters—forcing the submarine to sink to the ocean floor. It took the Navy rescue workers using the relatively untested Monson-McCann rescue chamber and four dives over 13 hr, including a full day, to reach the submarine and to rescue the 33 submariners (www.history.navy.mil/content/history/nhhc/our-collections/art/exhibits/conflicts-and-operations/the-rescue-of-the-uss-squalus-ss-192.html).

As part of an invited Harvard Lecture about research related to deep-sea diving physiology and its risks, subsequently published in 1942 in the *Bulletin of the New York Academy of Sciences*, Behnke provided details about two rescue operations, each relating to how divers used breathing heliox gas mixtures that permitted them to work effectively at depths below 60.9 m/200 ft without experiencing the narcoticlike, intoxicating submersion effects while breathing compressed air for extended periods. Behnke first discussed an ergometer test to assess the effects of working while breathing different gas concentrations had on performance and then provided details about practical applications during rescue missions.[9]

The observations made in the laboratory soon governed field practice during diving operations in submarine disasters. In 1939, divers breathing air at 73.2 m/240 ft depth in salvage work on the USS Squalus suffered memory lapses, mental confusion, and occasionally became unconscious.

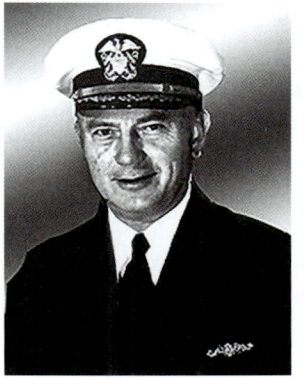

It proved to be not only dangerous but futile to work within jumbled hoses and cables at a depth of 240 ft in an air atmosphere. As in the laboratory, so also in the field—substituting helium for nitrogen rendered the impairment in neuromuscular coordination negligible and enabled divers to work efficiently when under 7 ATM. The successful termination of the salvage operations was made possible only by the employment of helium. In 1940 a second submarine disaster occurred in water 440 ft deep. Although the pressure at this depth was sufficient to crush the disabled craft's hull, divers breathing heliox reached the bottom and surveyed the sunken vessel. These divers, despite 14 ATM pressure, felt well and had little difficulty in performing the work required in descent and ascent to a depth corresponding closely to the 159.2 m/555 ft tall Washington monument.[7]

Pressure-Volume Relationships and Diving Depth

Diving Depth and Pressure

Water remains essentially noncompressible owing to its high density relative to air. Consequently, its pressure against a diver's body increases directly with dive depth. Two forces produce increased external pressure (**hyperbaria**) in diving:

1. Weight of a water column directly above the diver called *hydrostatic pressure*
2. Weight of the atmosphere (*ata* or *bar*) at the water's surface

TABLE 26.1 shows that a seawater column exerts a force equal to 1 sea-level ata (760 mm Hg/14.7 psi) for each 33-ft/10-m descent below the water's surface.

TABLE 26.1 Relationships among water depth, external pressure, lung volume, and inspired gas pressure

Freshwater is less dense than seawater, so a depth at about 10.4 m/34 ft corresponds to 1 ata in freshwater diving. Hence, a dive to 10.4 m/33 ft in seawater exposes the diver to 2 ata pressure: 1 ata from the ambient air weight at the surface and the other from the water column weight itself. Diving from sea level to 20 m/66 ft exposes a diver to an absolute 3 ata external pressure; the 30-m/99-ft pressure is 4 ata, and so on. Clearly, considerable external pressure builds up when diving relatively short distances below the surface.

The body's tissues contain a large water component, so they too remain noncompressible and not particularly susceptible to increased external pressure during diving. The body also contains air-filled cavities in the lungs, respiratory passages, and sinus and middle ear spaces. Volume and pressure in these cavities change considerably with any increase or decrease in diving depth. The consequences, without adjustments to *equalize* the rapid and large changes in pressure that occur in a hyperbaric environment, can lead to pain, injury, and ultimately death.

Diving Depth and Gas Volume

Boyle's law *(formulated in 1662 by chemist/physicist Robert Boyle; see Introduction: A View From the Past) states that at constant temperature, the volume for a given mass of gas varies inversely with pressure.* When pressure doubles, volume halves; conversely, reducing pressure by half expands any gas volume to twice its previous size. **FIGURE 26.1** (as well as **TABLE 26.2**) shows that if divers fill their lungs with 6 L of air at the surface and then descend to 10 m/33 ft, the lung volume compresses to 3 L.

TABLE 26.2 Recommended depth-time limits breathing pure oxygen during working dives

Diving an additional 10 m/33 ft to 20 m/65.6 ft, the external pressure now at 3 ata reduces the original 6-L lung volume by two thirds to 2 L. At 91 m/300 ft and 10 ata, the lung volume compresses to 0.6 L, simply from the compressive water force against the air-filled thoracic cavity. The basic principle states that gas volume varies inversely with the pressure acting upon it, whether in an open bell or in the flexible thoracic cavity. The inset figure graphically illustrates the curvilinear relation in seawater between lung volume at the surface and water depth. For most individuals, further increases in diving depth reduce the pulmonary air volume and seriously damage the chest wall and lung tissue. As the diver ascends to the surface, the air volume re-expands to its *original* 6-L volume. For the scuba diver who breathes pressurized air beneath the water, a 6-L lung volume at a 10-m/33-ft depth expands to 12 L at the water's surface; this same 6-L volume at 50-m/16.4-ft depth occupies 36 L at sea-level pressure. Lung tissues will rupture during ascent from the powerful expanding gas forces if the "extra" air volume cannot escape through the nose or mouth.

Snorkeling and Breath-Hold Diving

Swimming at the water's surface with fins, mask, and snorkel provides recreation and sport for spear fishing and exploring shallow clear water areas. A J-shaped tube or snorkel allows the swimmer to breathe continually with the face immersed in water. The swimmer periodically inhales fully and dives to explore beneath the water's surface. After about 30 s, the carbon dioxide level in arterial blood builds up, causing the diver to sense a need to breathe and return quickly to the surface. In snorkeling, the swimmer's breath-holding ability determines success in prolonging the underwater stay.

Limits to Snorkel Size

Novice skin divers often speculate that if they had a longer snorkel, they could swim deeper under the water and still breathe ambient air through the snorkel. Some neophytes believe they can sit at a pool bottom and breathe through a garden hose extending to the pool deck! The idea of a longer snorkel seems intriguing, but two factors limit snorkel length and volume:

1. Increased hydrostatic pressure on the chest cavity as one descends beneath the water
2. Increased pulmonary dead space by enlarging the snorkel's volume

Inspiratory Capacity and Diving Depth

When breathing through a snorkel, the diver inspires air at atmospheric pressure. At about a 1-m/3-ft depth, water's compressive force against the chest cavity becomes so large that the inspiratory muscles cannot overcome external pressure to expand thoracic dimensions. This makes inspiration impossible without external air at sufficient pressure to counter water's compressive force at the particular depth. This reality forms the basis for using the scuba apparatus discussed in the section "Scuba Diving."

Snorkel Size and Pulmonary Dead Space

In Chapter 12, we explain that not all inspired air enters the alveoli. About 150 mL air fills the nose, mouth, and other

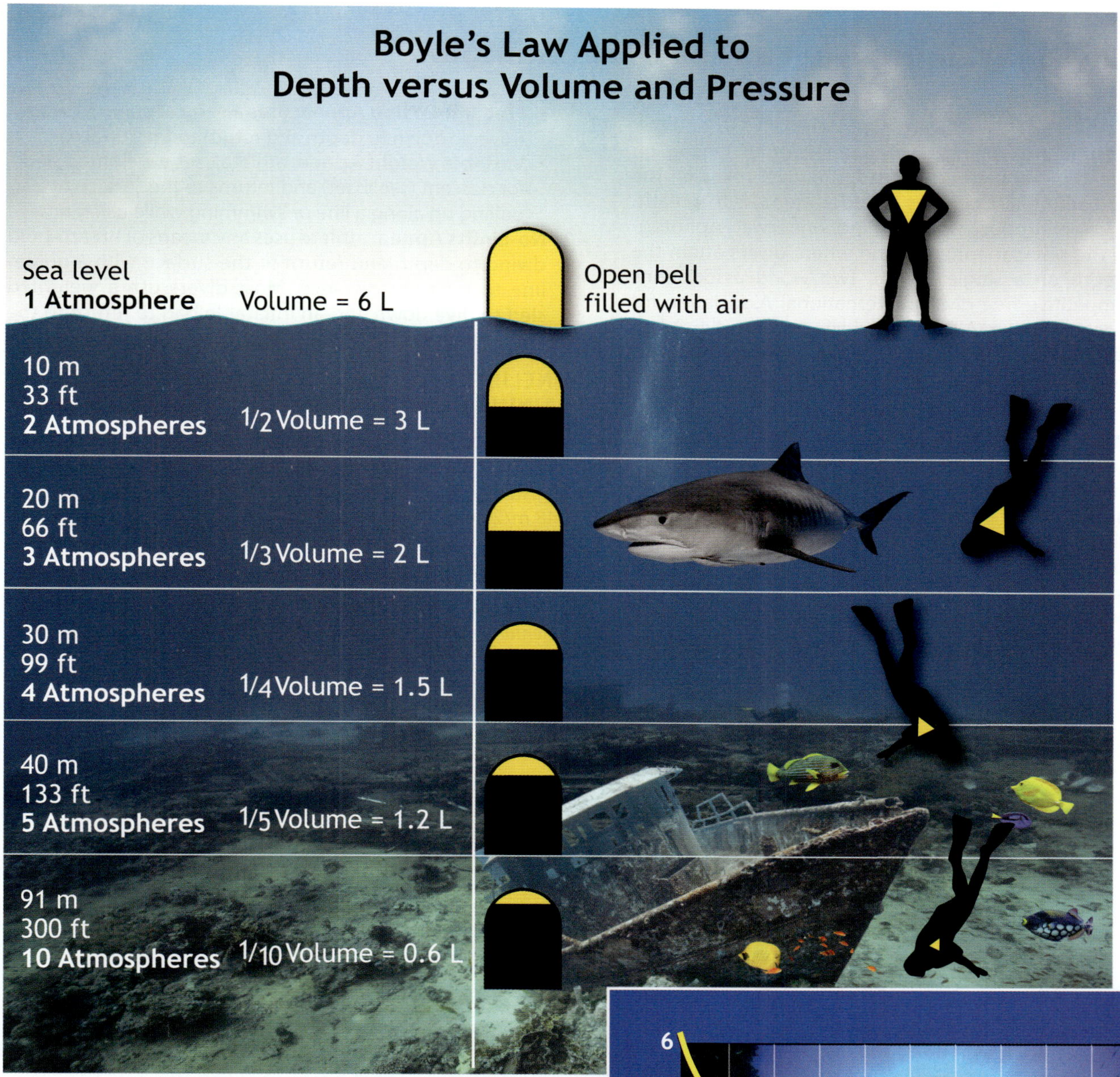

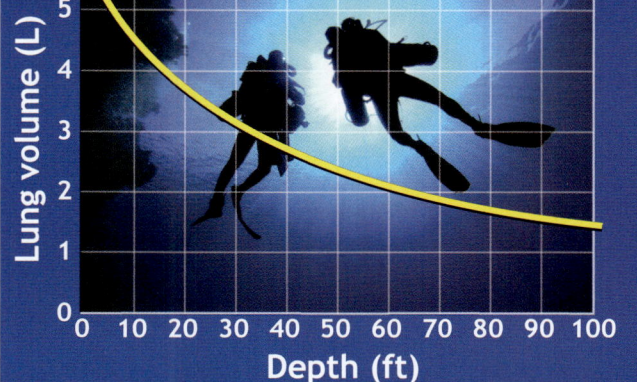

FIGURE 26.1. Gas volume varies inversely with the pressure acting upon it. The inset figure shows that the lung volume change (L) per unit depth change (ft) is greatest near the water's surface, designated zero on the bottom axis, and lowest at a 30-m/100-ft depth.
(Shutterstock photos: kaschibo, RoBayer, Martin 175, Stubblefield Photography, Rich Carey.)

or volume increases anatomic dead space volume, thereby encroaching on alveolar ventilation.

Breath-Hold Diving

Two factors determine breath-hold dive duration and depth:

1. Breath-hold duration until arterial carbon dioxide pressure reaches the breath-hold breakpoint
2. Relationship between a diver's total lung capacity (TLC) and residual lung volume (RLV)

In a Practical Sense

Free-Diving Training from a Free Dive Champion

BACKGROUND

Free diving refers to diving underwater without relying on external breathing apparatus; instead, the diver relies on the ability to breath-hold. Examples include attempts to breath-hold in a swimming pool, spear fishing, underwater photography, and the popular apneic diving where divers attain the deepest depth on a single breath. Two world associations govern competitive free diving: International Association for Development of Apnea (AIDA; www.aidainternational.org) and World Underwater Federation (CMAS; www.cmas.org). AIDA has established the depth disciplines for the following free-diving competitions:

1. **Constant Weight Apnea**: athlete dives to the depth following a guideline he or she cannot actively use during the dive. "Constant Weight" (French: "*poids constant*") means the athlete cannot drop any diving weights during the dive. The diver can use either bifins or a monofin for propulsion.
   - **Constant Weight Apnea Without Fins:** follows the identical rules as Constant Weight but without use of swimming aids (fins).
   - **Free Immersion Apnea:** uses a vertical guide rope to traverse down to depth and return to the surface.
   - **Variable Weight Apnea:** athlete uses a weighted sled for descent (see inset) and returns to the surface by pulling up along a line or swimming while using fins.
2. **No-Limits Apnea:** athlete uses any means of breath-hold diving to depth and return to the surface with a guideline to measure distance. Most divers use a weighted sled to dive down and an inflatable bag to return to the surface.

ANNELIE POMPE, SWEDISH CHAMPION FREE DIVER TRAINING REGIMEN

In addition to free diving, Annelie Pompe (1981–) is an accomplished mountain climber; in 2011, she became the first Swedish woman to climb the north side of Mt. Everest, Tibet (8848 m/29,029 ft).

The best way to become a good climber and freediver is of course to climb and freedive. But sooner or later you will reach your limit within equalization, oxygen consumption, squeeze, physical or mental ability. Now it's only for you to determine: which one of these stops you from going higher and deeper?

—Annelie Pompe

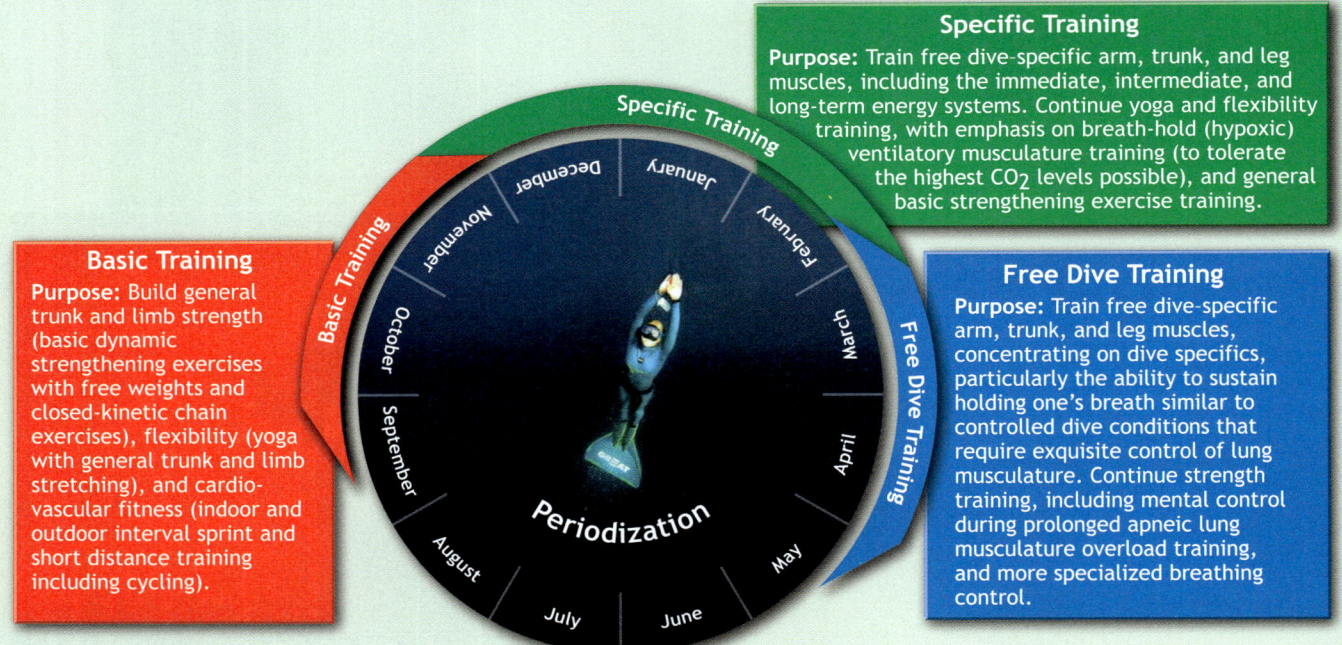

Specific Training
Purpose: Train free dive-specific arm, trunk, and leg muscles, including the immediate, intermediate, and long-term energy systems. Continue yoga and flexibility training, with emphasis on breath-hold (hypoxic) ventilatory musculature training (to tolerate the highest CO_2 levels possible), and general basic strengthening exercise training.

Basic Training
Purpose: Build general trunk and limb strength (basic dynamic strengthening exercises with free weights and closed-kinetic chain exercises), flexibility (yoga with general trunk and limb stretching), and cardiovascular fitness (indoor and outdoor interval sprint and short distance training including cycling).

Free Dive Training
Purpose: Train free dive-specific arm, trunk, and leg muscles, concentrating on dive specifics, particularly the ability to sustain holding one's breath similar to controlled dive conditions that require exquisite control of lung musculature. Continue strength training, including mental control during prolonged apneic lung musculature overload training, and more specialized breathing control.

Photo of diver courtesy of and used with permission from Sebastian Naslund, www.freediving.biz/education/1trainer.html

A full inspiration of ambient air causes 1-L oxygen to move into the respiratory passages and lungs. Upon breath-hold, 650-mL oxygen sustains metabolism before arterial carbon dioxide (PCO_2) partial pressure signals the need to renew breathing.[10,45] With some practice, most persons can breath-hold for up to 1 min, and 2 min represents a typical upper limit.

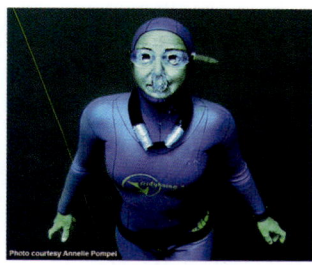

During this time, arterial PO_2 drops to 60 mm Hg, whereas PCO_2, the most important factor controlling breath-holding, rises to 50 mm Hg and signals the urgency to breathe. Physical activity greatly reduces breath-holding time because oxygen uptake and carbon dioxide output increase with exercise intensity.

Hyperventilation and Breath-Hold Diving: Blackout

Hyperventilation before breath-hold diving extends the breath-hold period, greatly increasing the diver's **blackout** *risk.* This risk, including **shallow water blackout (SWB**; http://shallowwaterblackoutprevention.org), refers to a sudden loss of consciousness that usually afflicts those who try to extend the underwater duration beyond reasonable limits. Unfortunately, SWB also can occur regardless of water depth in any pool, lake, or even when body surfing. A critical reduction in arterial PO_2 (and lowered PCO_2 to the brain with prolonged hyperventilation) can cause blackout, a condition that contributes to total respiratory muscle relaxation.

The breakpoint for breath-holding corresponds to an increased arterial PCO_2 to 50 mm Hg. Some persons can ignore this stimulus and continue breath-holding until arterial carbon dioxide reaches levels that cause severe disorientation and even blackout. When hyperventilation precedes breath-hold, arterial PCO_2 decreases from its normal 40 to 15 mm Hg. Lowering the body's carbon dioxide content before the dive extends the breath-hold duration until arterial PCO_2 reaches a trigger level to stimulate ventilation. The current world record breadth-hold dive, established March 27, 2001, is 24 min:37.36 s, which surpassed the previous record by 34 s (https://www.guinnessworldrecords.com/news/2021/5/freediver-holds-breath-for-almost-25-minutes-breaking-record-660285). Breath-holds of 15 to 20 min routinely occur in free divers with hyperventilation followed by breathing pure oxygen for several deep breaths.[24,46]

Combining hyperventilation, breath-holding, and exercise in the underwater environment poses serious risks. Consider the following scenario: A skin diver hyperventilates at the surface before a dive to reduce arterial PCO_2 to augment breath-hold duration. The diver now takes a full inhalation and descends under the water. Alveolar oxygen continually moves into the blood for delivery to active muscles. Owing to previous hyperventilation, arterial carbon dioxide levels remain low, freeing the diver from the urge to breathe. Concurrently, as the diver swims deeper, external water pressure compresses the thorax and increases gas pressure within this cavity. Increased intrathoracic pressure maintains a relatively high alveolar PO_2. Even though absolute alveolar oxygen quantity decreases as oxygen moves into the blood during the dive, PO_2 continually loads hemoglobin as diving progresses. When the diver senses the need to breathe from carbon dioxide buildup and begins to ascend, reversals occur in intrathoracic pressure. As water pressure on the thorax decreases with ascent, lung volume expands and alveolar PO_2 decreases to a level where no gradient exists for oxygen diffusion *into* arterial blood, placing the diver in a hypoxic state. Near the surface, alveolar PO_2 reaches levels so low that dissolved oxygen diffuses *from* venous blood returning to the lungs and flows *into* the alveoli, causing the diver to suddenly lose consciousness before surfacing.

Two additional risks occur from hyperventilation before a breath-hold dive:

1. A normal arterial carbon dioxide concentration maintains the blood's acid-base balance, mediated by H^+ release as carbonic acid forms from carbon dioxide joining with water. By reducing the blood's carbon dioxide content through hyperventilation, H^+ concentration decreases while pH and alkalinity increase.
2. Normal arterial PCO_2 stimulates arteriole dilation in the brain.[29,32,47] A decrease in arterial carbon dioxide with hyperventilation reduces cerebral blood flow, producing dizziness or possible loss of consciousness.

Depth Limits with Breath-Hold Diving: Thoracic Squeeze

Progressing deeper beneath the water subjects the body's air cavities to tremendous compressive forces. Generally, when lung volume compresses below 1.5 to 1.0 L (i.e., to RLV), internal and external pressures fail to equalize causing **lung squeeze**. Excessive hydrostatic pressure on pulmonary air volume causes extensive damage to the pulmonary tissues.

Commercial breath-hold diving generally does not exceed 30.5-m/100-ft depths in salt water, and lung squeeze generally occurs at depths between 45.7 m/150 ft and 61 m/200 ft of salt water. Nevertheless, individuals show considerable variability in the safe depth for breath-hold diving without lung squeeze danger. New Zealander William Trubridge (1980–) in 2016 re-established his world record by swimming to a 122-m/400-ft depth on a single breath and with only hands and feet for propulsion (www.theguardian.com/sport/video/2016/may/02/freediver-plunges-122m-into-blue-hole-to-set-new-world-record-video). The world record for "no-limits" breath-hold diving depth following a single breath of air for men is an amazing 253 m/830 ft, a level below the typical cruising depth of nuclear submarines. The external water pressure against the diver's thoracic cavity at this depth compresses chest girth to less than 20 in/50.8 cm. Austrian Herbert Nitsch (1970–) achieved this remarkable physiologic feat on June 6, 2012, off the coast of the historic Greek island of Santorini, but not without serious injury after his ascent. Unconscious, he was brought to the surface by rescue divers after reaching his record-breaking depth. For almost a year afterward, no information emerged about the accident or Nitsch's condition. He fully recovered and continues his attempts at achieving an unthinkable "304.8-m/1000-ft dive."

Tanya Streeter (1973–) of the Cayman Islands in 2003 redefined the limits of achievement for a woman by setting the world record for no-limits breath-hold diving when she reached 160 m/524 fsw. At this depth, the lungs compress to about 1/17th their normal volume—a threat for lung collapse. Of the six men and women who have dived to depths deeper than 160 m/520 ft, two have died during sled diving (use of a weighed sled for descent and an inflatable bag to return to the surface), with four serious cases of decompression sickness (http://freediving.biz/nolimit/).

The ratio of the diver's TLC to RLV at the surface generally determines the critical diving depth before lung squeeze; this ratio typically averages 4:1 at the surface. For example, for a diver with a 6.0-L TLC and 1.5-L RLV, Boyle's law predicts that TLC would compress to RLV at 30 m/98 ft or 4 ata external pressure. No danger from lung squeeze exists if lung volume remains greater than RLV because sufficient air remains in the lungs and more rigid respiratory passages to equalize pressure and prevent damage from compression. If TLC during a dive decreases below RLV (i.e., if the TLV to RLV ratio falls below 1.00), pulmonary air pressure becomes less than the external water pressure, and this unequalized pressure creates a relative vacuum within the lungs. In severe lung squeeze cases, blood literally spurts from the pulmonary capillaries through the alveoli flooding the lungs. In this situation, divers drown in their own blood. Further increases in depth cause compression fractures of the ribs as the chest cavity collapses from excessive external pressure.

In many cases, the TLV to RLV ratio at the surface considerably *underestimates* the actual impressive depths achieved by trained breath-hold divers. The explanation may partially relate to reduced RLV as immersion progresses from increased intrathoracic blood volume. A smaller RLV underwater increases the TLV to RLV ratio, allowing the individual to increase maximal depth before reaching this critical ratio.

Other Problems

If pressures within internal air spaces do not continually equalize with external hydrostatic pressures, problems other than lung squeeze limit the depth for a breath-hold dive. For example, if air at ambient pressure remains trapped within the middle ear from inflamed tissue or a mucous plug and cannot equilibrate with air in the lungs, external hydrostatic pressure forces the eardrum inward and it ruptures. A ruptured eardrum frequently occurs at relatively shallow depths.

The sinus cavities also present difficulty for skin divers. Air compressed in the lungs by water's external force attempts to move into the paranasal sinuses. Sinuses inflamed and irritated from infection provide extremely narrow openings that hinder sinus space equilibration with pressure changes in the respiratory tract. Failure to equilibrate creates a relative vacuum in the sinus cavities that distorts their tissues' shape and causes intense sinus pain. With severe disequilibrium, fluid and blood move into the sinuses to fill the vacuum.

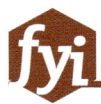

Mammals' Adaptations to Deep Dives

Seals and whales that descend to great depths with a single breath of air have evolved with special survival adaptations. Based on sonar readings, the endangered sperm whale, with a 19.8-m/65-ft length and 36,287- to 45,359-kg/40- to 50-ton weight—larger than a school bus—can dive to 1000-m/3300-ft depths in about 27 min. At this depth, the pressure on the animal exceeds 3500 psi. Older estimates indicated that a typical dive lasted 90 min while the whale consumed about 900-kg/1980-lb fish and squid daily, with extended breath-hold times to 120 min. Recent research has now revised the record for dive limits in Cuvier's beaked whales (https://jeb.biologists.org/content/223/18/jeb222109). Marine biologists from the Nicholas School of the environment at Duke University analyzed 3680 dives from 23 satellite-linked tags to assess long-duration dives to estimate aerobic dive limit. The new record for the deepest dive ever recorded has been extended to 3048 m/10,000 ft with 3 hr 42 min submersion time, extending the prior record by more than an hour! Whales cruise the oceans at about 37 km/23 mi per hour. These elegant aquatic mammals have more elastic chest cavities than humans; their lungs, even when reduced from external pressure, do not separate from the chest wall and have adapted to use the oxygen in their bloodstream with high efficiency owing to redirected blood to vital organs (www.ftexploring.com/askdrg/askdrgalapagos2.html; www.amnh.org/explore/news-blogs/on-exhibit-posts/sperm-whales-amazing-adaptations). The deep-diving whales have low metabolic rates, high oxygen storage capacities, and enhanced acid buffering to counteract the byproducts from aerobic and anaerobic metabolism—the necessary adaptations to extend their continual food foraging habits at extreme depths.

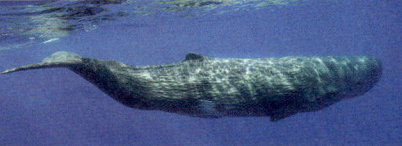

wildestanimal/Shutterstock

Sources:

Apprill A, et al. Marine mammal skin microbiotas are influenced by host phylogeny. *R Soc Open Sci.* 2020;7:192046.

Quick NJ, et al. Extreme diving in mammals: first estimates of behavioural aerobic dive limits in Cuvier's beaked whales. *J Exp Biol.* 2020;223:jeb222109. doi:10.1242/jeb.222109

Tønnesen P, et al. The long-range echo scene of the sperm whale biosonar. *Biol Lett.* 2020;16:20200134.

Diving Reflex in Humans

Physiological responses to water immersion, collectively termed the *diving reflex,* enable diving mammals to spend considerable time underwater. These four responses include the following:

1. Bradycardia
2. Decreased cardiac output
3. Increased peripheral vasoconstriction
4. Lactate accumulation in underperfused muscle

A modified diving response also has been noted for humans during face immersion, breath-hold face immersion, and dives to modest depths.[1,15,19,25] Human research has primarily documented increased vagal activity that induces bradycardia during face immersion and diving, particularly in cool and cold water. Elevated blood lactate concentration during breath-hold dives to 65 m/213 ft at energy expenditures only slightly above rest suggests that a diving-mediated peripheral vasoconstriction decreases blood flow (oxygen supply) to skeletal muscles and compromises performance.[14]

Some research has expanded findings on blood lactate concentration to include breath-hold diving hemodynamics in thermoneutral and cool water by elite divers to depths of 40 m/131 ft to 55 m/180 ft. **FIGURE 26.2A** illustrates the responses for one diver during descent to 40 m/131 ft, bottom stay, and ascent (depth indicated by *green line*) in water at 25°C/77°F and 35°C/95°F. The electrocardiographic tracing (**FIG. 26.2B**) shows the longest R–R interval recorded during the cool-water dive. After an initial tachycardia, bradycardia became most pronounced in cool water, where heart rate decreased to 16 bpm near the dive's bottom. Because stroke volume did not change appreciably during the dive, lower heart rates reduced cardiac output (yellow line). Output decreased to a low of 3 L·min^{-1} (25°C/77°F) compared with 6.4 L·min^{-1} at the surface. A large number of diverse arrhythmic beats, often more frequent than true sinus beats, accompanied bradycardia mainly during cool-water dives. Arterial blood pressure increased suddenly and dramatically, reaching 280/200 and 290/150 mm Hg in two divers. The hypertensive response reflected overall peripheral vasoconstriction, while the large increase in blood lactate concentrations reflected increased anaerobic metabolism.

The intense cardiovascular responses to breath-hold diving in elite divers resemble response patterns of diving mammals.[23,28,48] The undesirable occurrence in arrhythmias and large blood pressure increases probably reflect species differences and less than perfect human adaptation.

Scuba Diving

Snorkeling cannot take place at depths below 1 m/3 ft because inspiratory muscle power cannot overcome water's compressive force against the thoracic cavity. Air under pressure from an

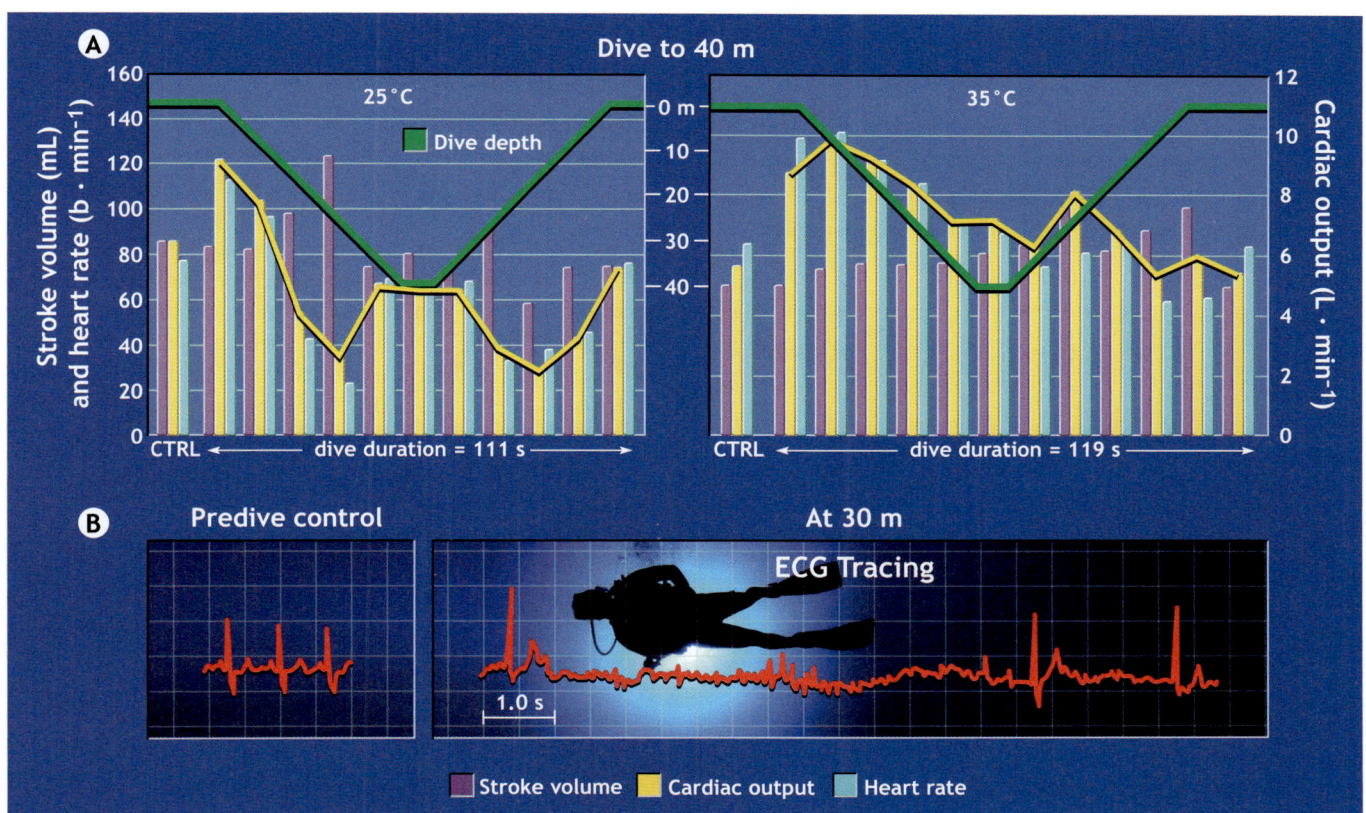

FIGURE 26.2. **(A)** Heart rate, stroke volume, and cardiac output for an elite breath-hold diver throughout a dive to 40 m/131 ft in warm (35°C/95°F) and cool (25°C/77°F) water. CTRL, control measures prior to dive. **(B)** Electrocardiographic (ECG) tracing. (Adapted with permission from Ferrigno M, et al. Cardiovascular changes during deep breath-hold dives in a pressure chamber. *J Appl Physiol* 1997;83:1282. ©The American Physiological Society (APS). All rights reserved. Photo: Rich Carey/Shutterstock.)

external source to promote inspiratory action counteracts the external hydrostatic force. The modern **scuba (self-contained underwater breathing apparatus)** was principally developed in 1943 by French oceanographer/ecologist/researcher Jacques-Yves Cousteau (1910–1997; www.cousteau.org) and National Inventors Hall of Fame inductee Emile Gagnan (1915–2003; www.invent.org/inductees/emile-gagnan). Their invention represents the most common apparatus to supply air under pressure to achieve complete independence from atmospheric air at the surface. *Sport divers should use only this form of scuba*. The scuba system, strapped to the diver's chest or back, includes a compressed air tank and demand regulator valve with hose and mouthpiece or full face mask to deliver air the diver requires at a particular depth. There are two basic scuba designs:

1. Common open-circuit system
2. **Closed-circuit system** used primarily for clandestine military operations and special applications that require mixed gases

Underwater commercial operations frequently apply surface-demand diving techniques in operations below a 50-m/164-ft depth. This approach supplies air directly from a compressor at the surface to the diver via a direct reinforced hose. German-born British engineer/inventor Augustus Siebe (1788–1872; www.divinghelmet.nl/divinghelmet/1839_Augustus_Siebe.html) provided the original design for this system in 1819. His design consisted of a copper helmet (called a *hard hat*) riveted to a leather jacket, with air delivered continuously from the surface. The excess supplied air and the diver's expired air bubbled out from the jacket's bottom. If the diver moved substantially from the vertical position, water would rush in through the jacket and fill the headpiece. Siebe modified this design in 1837 (see Siebe's early diving suit in "Diving History Chronology"); he constructed a full waterproof diving suit bolted to a breastplate and helmet that allowed a diver to work in any position because the suit encapsulated the entire body. Valves admitted air through the diver's helmet as needed, and expired air exited the helmet through valves.[22] Siebe's "closed" diving helmet allowed divers to dive safely to depths previously deemed impossible.

Open-Circuit Scuba

FIGURE 26.3 illustrates the typical open-circuit scuba system for submerged swimming with neutral buoyancy in relatively shallow water. Compressed air flows through a two-stage regulator valve that reduces tank pressure to a near breathable pressure at a given depth and releases air to the diver on demand at a pressure equal to "ambient" so the diver breathes without difficulty. For most diving purposes, steel or aluminum tanks (and lightweight titanium that withstands high pressures) contain 2000 L/70–80 ft^3 air compressed to about 3000 psi; deeper and longer exposures require 3500 L/120 ft^3 compressed air. One tank supplies enough air for a 0.5- to 1-h dive to moderate depths. Inspiration creates a slight negative pressure. This opens the demand valve shown in the diagram with orange tank, which releases air to the diver at a pressure nearly equal to the water's external pressure. The positive pressure created with exhalation closes the inspiratory valves and discharges the exhaled air into the water. The scuba gear contains gauges to continually monitor tank pressure and diving depth.

Open-circuit scuba presents several drawbacks. The air exhaled into the water generally contains approximately 17% oxygen, so the open-circuit system "wastes" about 75% of the tank's total oxygen. The diver requires a considerable air mass at increased depths to provide adequate tidal volume for pulmonary ventilation. As an extreme example, inhaling a 5-L volume at 90 m/300 fsw requires the equivalent of 50-L sea level air!

This dramatic pressure effect on air volume greatly limits "bottom time" at great depth before depletion of the scuba tank's air. Factors that influence underwater swimming's energy cost and thus pulmonary ventilation include gender (lower in women than in men), number of tanks (25% higher with two tanks), fin type (flexible fin lower than rigid fin), and diver's experience (lower in advanced divers).[31] Diving tanks contain moisture-free compressed air, making each breath produce heat and moisture loss as the inspired air warms and humidifies on its passage down the respiratory tract, causing substantial body heat loss during prolonged diving. To counter heat loss, the diver breathes a *heated* compressed helium-oxygen gas mixture to avoid hypothermia during deep diving (see "Helium-Oxygen Mixtures," later in this chapter).

FIGURE 26.4 shows the theoretical air time limits for a diver who performs similar work at various underwater depths. These time limits for bottom time (red dashed line) and time for descent plus time on the

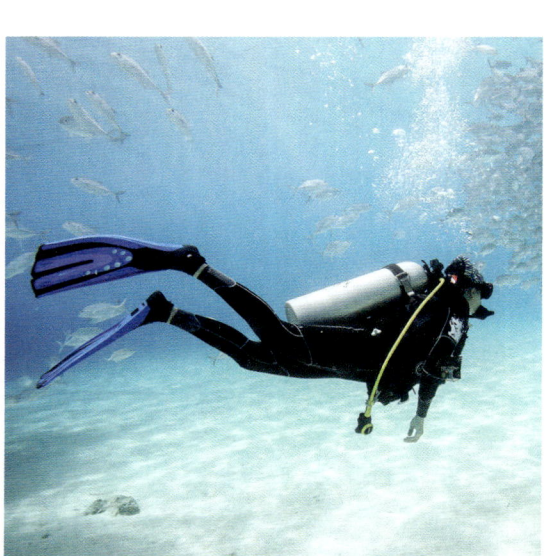

FIGURE 26.3. General design of an open-circuit scuba unit. (littlesam/Shutterstock)

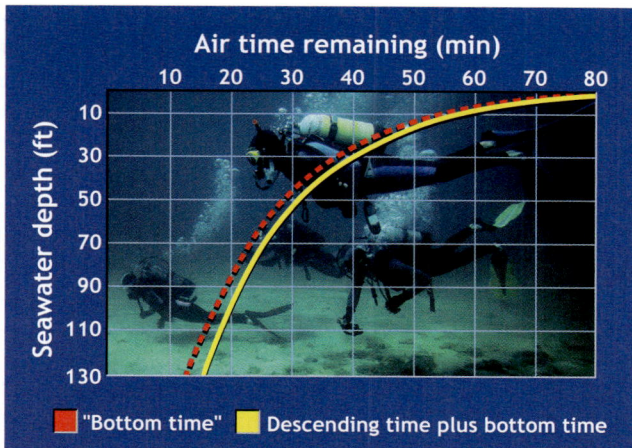

FIGURE 26.4. Theoretical air time for a single tank containing 80 cubic ft of air. The *yellow line* includes the time spent descending at a rate of 60 ft · min^{-1} plus time on the bottom; *dashed line*, only "bottom time."
(Popartic/Shutterstock)

bottom (yellow solid line) assume a completely filled standard compressed air tank and ascent and descent at 18 m/60 ft per min. For example, a single aluminum tank that contains 80 ft^3 of air compressed to 3000 psi normally sustains an 80-min dive near the surface. At a 10-m/33-ft depth, this tank supplies enough air for about 40 min, whereas at 3 ata (20 m/66 ft), dive duration decreases by one third, to 27 min. These time limits vary with the diver's body size, physical activity type and intensity, fitness level, and diving experience, all affecting exercise energy cost and ventilatory volumes.

The **wet suit**, the most common protective garment worn by recreational scuba divers and surfers, counters cold stress during diving. This garment, containing air-impregnated neoprene foam, traps water against the diver's skin, warming it to body temperature to provide the insulating boundary. Wet suits generally furnish sufficient thermal protection for relatively short dives, even in ice water. For longer dives in moderately cold water (17 to 18.5°C/63 to 65°F), a full wet suit offers insufficient thermal protection.[4] As the diver descends, wet suit compression progressively diminishes the suit's insulating properties.

The modern **dry suit**—made from foam neoprene, crushed neoprene, vulcanized rubber, or heavy-duty nylon with laminated waterproof materials and often worn over insulating garments—maximizes protection against cold stress. The protective clothing ensemble keeps the diver dry by sealing at the neck, wrists, and ankles, with a waterproof zipper that prevents water from entering the suit. For additional insulation, dry-suit underwear traps an air layer between the diver and water. Layering with underwear adjusts insulation to water temperature.

Closed-Circuit Scuba

The need for undetectable shallow diving maneuvers during World War II produced new diving strategies that relied on pure oxygen rebreathing with carbon dioxide absorption within a closed system. The closed-circuit underwater breathing apparatus operates similarly to the closed-circuit spirometer described in Chapter 8. The diver breathes from a small cylinder that feeds pure oxygen into a small bellows or bag, which acts as a pressure regulator. Valves in the breathing mask direct the exhaled gas through a carbon dioxide–absorbing canister containing soda lime; the carbon dioxide–free gas then passes back to the diver. The oxygen cylinder replenishes the oxygen uptake in energy metabolism, allowing the diver to continually rebreathe oxygen, the only gas removed from the breathing bag. A small oxygen cylinder sustains the submerged diver for 3 hr or longer. No expired air releases into the water, so the system provides a near-silent and bubble-free operation for clandestine activities. **FIGURE 26.5** illustrates a closed-circuit scuba design used by the U.S. Navy that requires only a single compressed oxygen cylinder shown in green. Another closed-circuit system design uses mixed gas—one pure oxygen bottle and a second mixed gas bottle containing helium and oxygen (**heliox**) or nitrogen and oxygen (**nitrox**; see "Dives to Exceptional Depths: Mixed-Gas Diving," later in this chapter).

The closed-circuit system requires high-level proficiency. Two main problems exist with using it. First, a serious medical emergency occurs if carbon dioxide output exceeds its absorption rate or if absorption fails altogether. With a faulty rebreathing system, the diver may not receive warning symptoms, becoming sedated by arterial carbon dioxide buildup, with drowning the end result. Second, a high inspired oxygen concentration, particularly when breathed under high pressures beneath the water, produces adverse effects on physiologic functions, particularly those related to central nervous system functions. These problems remain minimal if

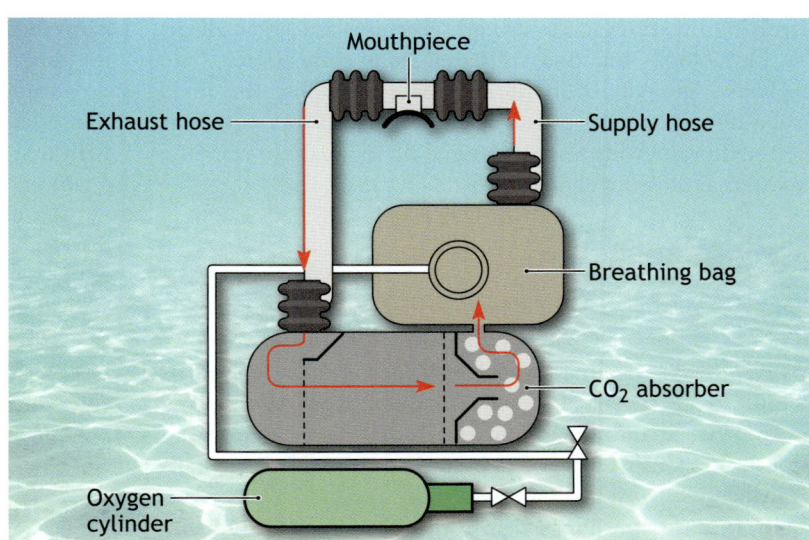

FIGURE 26.5. General closed-circuit scuba system design used by the U.S. Navy. The breathing bag acts as a pressure regulator and an absorber removes the expired CO_2 from the circulating air.
(Arctic ice/Shutterstock)

the depth–time limits do not exceed the recommendations in Table 26.2 developed by the U.S. Navy. Closed-circuit oxygen breathing generally should not exceed a maximum 25 fsw and definitely not beyond 50 fsw. At this point, oxygen poisoning produces a high risk to trigger central nervous system seizures.

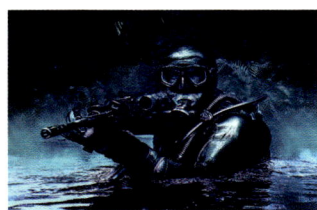
Getmilitaryphotos/Shutterstock

Minimal risk usually exists in military diving because most clandestine operations require specially trained individuals swimming underwater with munitions in relatively shallow depths at night to avoid detection. Decompression sickness does not pose a problem because no inert gas absorption occurs when rebreathing pure oxygen. The increased resistance to breathing and generally large dead space typically characterized by closed-circuit systems limit intense physical effort.

Special Problems Breathing Gases at High Pressures

Henry's law (first proposed in 1803 by English physician and chemist William Henry [1734–1816]) states that a gas dissolved in a liquid at a given temperature varies directly with two factors:

1. Pressure differential between the gas and liquid
2. Gas solubility in the liquid

Underwater breathing systems must supply air, oxygen, or other gas mixtures at sufficient pressure to overcome water's force against the diver's thorax. For example, at 3 ata (20-m/66-ft depth), the respired gas requires delivery at approximately 2280 mm Hg (3 × 760 mm Hg), whereas gas delivery at 60 m/197 ft requires 5320 mm Hg pressure. The material that follows considers the specific dynamics involving breathing gases at high pressures and their effects on physiologic functions. **FIGURE 26.6** summarizes (and explained more fully in the following sections) the main scuba diving hazards posed by improper pressure equalization within the body's air spaces and diving mask in response to external pressure changes.

Air Embolism

An air volume breathed underwater expands directly proportional to the reduced external pressure as the diver ascends to the surface. Air breathed at a 10-m/33-ft depth doubles its volume at the surface. If normal breathing continues during ascent, the expanding air vents freely through the nose and mouth. If a diver takes a full breath at 10 m/33 ft but fails to exhale while ascending, the rapidly expanding gas eventually ruptures the lungs before the diver reaches the surface. Lung burst becomes a potential reality in scuba diving. Many inexperienced divers react to a perceived underwater danger by filling their lungs and then holding their breath while swimming rapidly to the surface. This particular diving hazard does not necessarily require a deep dive. Accidents caused by breath-hold ascent with scuba frequently occur in relatively shallow dives. Changes in pressure exert the greatest effect on the expanding lung volume near the water surface (see inset box Fig. 26.1). *Inhaling a full breath of compressed air in 1.8 m/6 ft of water causes serious lung tissue overdistension if the diver fails to exhale while ascending.* Fatal air embolism can occur in swimming pools as shallow as 2.4 m/8 ft for a novice scuba diver. Air embolism from pulmonary barotrauma ranks second only to drowning among recreational scuba divers.

If air expansion in the respiratory tract causes lung tissue to rupture during ascent—from either breath-holding or pulmonary obstruction (bronchospasm, excessive pulmonary secretions, or bronchial inflammation)—air bubbles or **emboli** enter the pulmonary venous system (www.healthline.com/health/air-embolism). Emboli then flow to the heart and enter the systemic circulation. The diver usually maintains a head-up, vertical position on ascent, causing the air bubbles to move upward in the body. Eventually, they lodge in the small arterioles or capillaries and restrict vital tissue's blood supply. General air embolism symptoms include confusion, weakness, dizziness, and blurred vision. Severe blockage in the pulmonary, coronary, and cerebral circulation causes collapse, unconsciousness, and frequently death. Effective air embolism treatment requires rapid decompression to reduce bubble size and force them into solution to open the plugged vessels. Even with rapid, expert treatment, 16% of air embolism victims die (www.encyclopedia.com/topic/Embolism.aspx).

Pneumothorax: Lung Collapse

Air forced through the alveoli when lung tissue ruptures sometimes migrates laterally to burst through the lung's pleural sac. In approximately 10% of patients with pulmonary barotrauma, an air pocket forms in the chest cavity outside the lungs between the chest wall and lung itself. Continued expansion during ascent collapses the ruptured lung, a condition called *pneumothorax*, which requires surgical intervention with a syringe to extract the air pocket (www.ncbi.nlm.nih.gov/pmc/articles/PMC2600088/).

To eliminate air embolism danger and pneumothorax, instructors teach divers to ascend slowly and breathe normally when using scuba gear (www.ncbi.nlm.nih.gov/pmc/articles/PMC5126790/). The diver's lungs also must remain free from any disease (e.g., chronic obstructive pulmonary disease) that could lead to air trapping, which creates difficulty during ascent equalizing alveolar pressure and external pressure.

Facemask "Squeeze"

Air in a facemask or goggles before a dive equals ambient air pressure at the surface.[49] As the diver progresses deeper, a greater pressure differential develops between the mask's inside

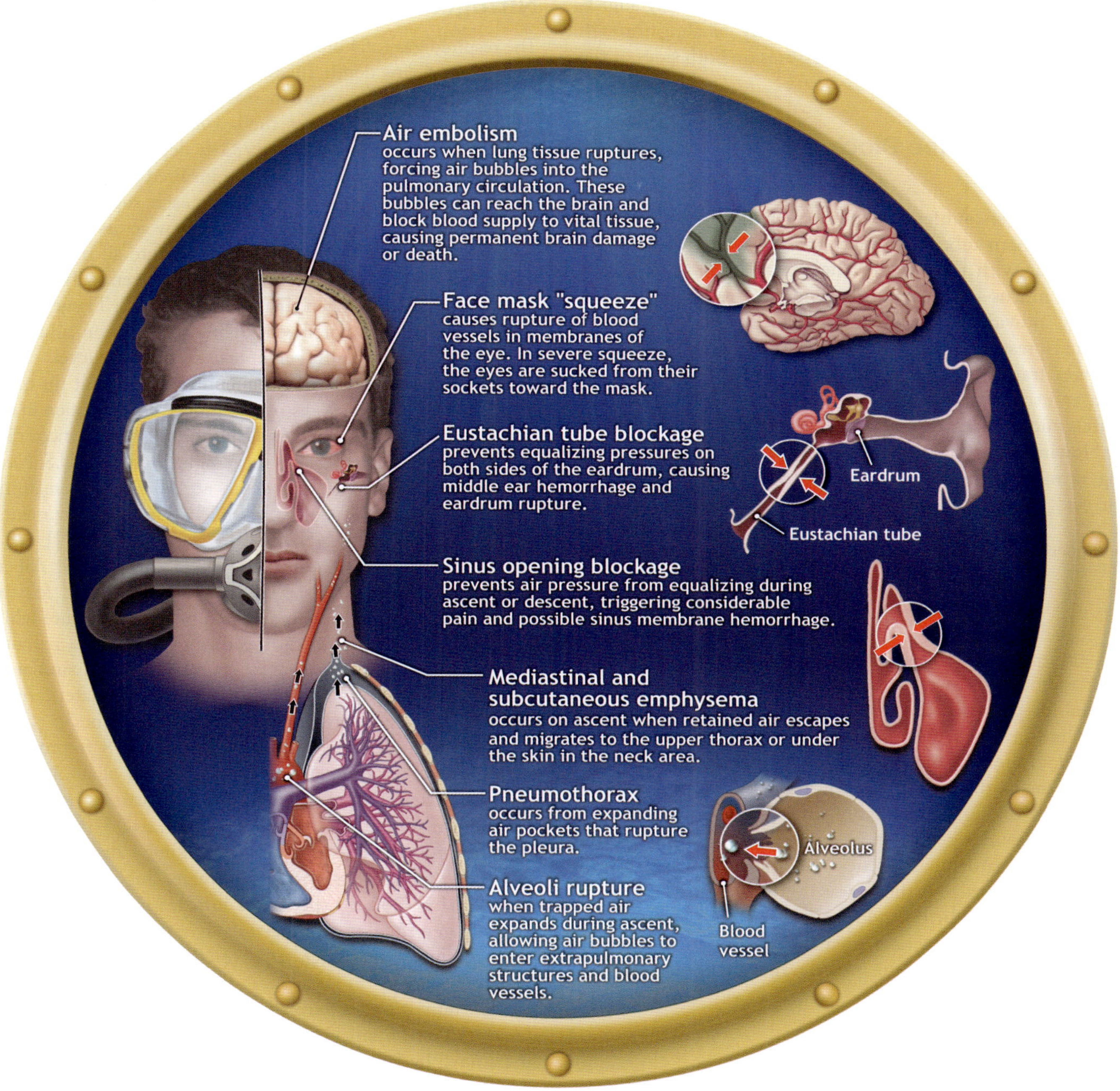

FIGURE 26.6. Scuba diving hazards from failure to equalize internal and external gas pressures.

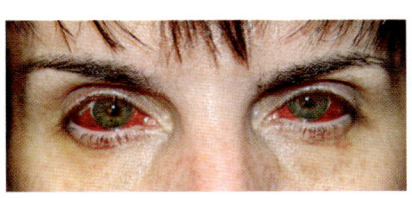

and outside to create a relative vacuum within the mask. For example, wearing swim goggles to improve vision and protect the eyes from irritants during even a shallow dive can cause the eyes to bulge or squeeze from their sockets.

This leads to capillary rupture and hemorrhage in the eyes and surrounding soft tissue. The facemask squeeze effect occurs because most goggles are constructed from rigid materials. Soft tissue displacement into the air space between the eye and the goggle interior provides the only way to equalize the difference in air pressure between the goggle space and external water pressure during breath-hold diving (https://pubmed.ncbi.nlm.nih.gov/27462262/). As newer pools with separate diving areas reach 4.3-m/14-ft depths, wearing goggles poses a serious risk diving to this depth.

Breath-hold diving with a facemask that covers the eyes and nose represents a somewhat different situation than diving with only swim goggles. Air pressure within the mask that covers the eyes and nose readily equalizes to external water pressure as air flows freely between the nasal passages and the lungs' relatively large air volume. In breath-hold diving, air in the lungs compresses and passes through the nose to equalize mask pressure. With scuba, inspired air automatically adjusts to the external water pressure. Periodically exhaling through the nose into the mask balances pressures on both sides of the facemask.

Eustachian Tube Blockage: Middle-Ear Squeeze

Divers often encounter problems equalizing pressure within the Eustachian tube's air spaces (passages that connect the middle ear with the back of the throat).[40] These relatively narrow, mucus-lined channels generally resist air flow. In healthy individuals, the tubes remain clear and changes in external pressure against the eardrum equalize by pressure changes transmitted from the lungs through the tubes. In skin and scuba diving (and air travel in nonpressurized aircraft), middle-ear pressure equalizes with external pressure by blowing gently against closed nostrils. Swallowing, yawning, or moving the jaws from side to side also helps to "pop" the ears.

Lippincott® Connect   Appendix H, available online at Lippincott Connect, provides supplemental animations and videos on this topic.

In upper-respiratory tract infection, the Eustachian tube membranes swell and produce mucus that can plug cranial air passages. The greatest difficulty involves equalizing middle-ear pressure during descent because an equal force from the ear canal does not match the pressure change against the eardrum's outer surface. Pressure changes experienced in diving considerably exceed those in air travel. Divers can suffer severe pain only a few feet underwater because the eardrum stretches and moves inward toward the plugged canal. Further pressure disequilibrium creates a relative vacuum in the middle ear that hemorrhages tissues. Completely blocked Eustachian tubes can rupture the eardrum, forcing water into the middle ear as pressure equalizes.

Never Use Earplugs

WARNING—NEVER WEAR EARPLUGS WHILE DIVING! During a dive, the external water pressure pushes the earplug deep into the external ear canal. An ambient air pocket trapped between the plug and eardrum can rupture the eardrum outward during descent.

Aerosinusitis

Inflamed, congested sinuses prevent air pressure in these cavities from equalizing during diving. Sinus air pressure that does not equalize during descent remains at atmospheric pressure while external pressure increases.[50] This relative vacuum creates "sinus squeeze," causing sinus membranes to bleed as blood occupies the space to equalize the pressure differential.[30]

Nitrogen Narcosis: "Rapture of the Deep"

The respired gas total pressure during diving increases proportionately to diving depth. Likewise, the partial pressure for each gas in the breathing mixture increases: at 10 m/33 ft, the nitrogen partial pressure doubles the sea-level value to 1200 mm Hg. With each additional 10-m/33-ft depth, nitrogen partial pressure increases by 600 mm Hg—inspired P_{N_2} equals 4200 mm Hg at a 60-m/197-ft depth. At each successive depth, the gradient increases for net nitrogen flow across the alveolar membrane into the blood and eventually into all tissue fluids for equilibration. At 20 m/66 ft, all tissues eventually contain three times more nitrogen than before the dive. Tissue perfusion, tissue solubility coefficients, body composition, and temperature all influence nitrogen uptake at the tissue level.

Three-hundred fsw generally represents the limit for compressed air diving because dissolved nitrogen accumulation in the body's fluids and tissues renders all but the most experienced divers incapable of accomplishing meaningful work. The U.S. Navy sets the maximum operating depth at 190 fsw for breathing compressed air (www.navsea.navy.mil/Portals/103/Documents/SUPSALV/Diving/US%20DIVING%20MANUAL_REV7.pdf?ver=2017-01-11-102354-393). In 1935, Dr. Albert Behnke and coworkers (see Chapter 28) discovered for the first time that the increase in inspired nitrogen pressure while breathing compressed air during diving produced a narcotic effect characterized by a general state of euphoria similar to alcohol intoxication, which Cousteau and Dumas later termed *rapture of the deep* ("I'vresse des grandes profondeurs").

Dissolved nitrogen at a depth of 30 m/98 ft produces effects similar to those felt after consuming alcohol on an empty stomach. Divers often speak of "Martini's Law." This well-known dictum states that every 15.2-m/5-ft depth in seawater produces effects equal to drinking 1 dry martini on an empty stomach. As a rough estimate, this would mean a diver at 61 m/200 ft experiences intoxication from pressurized nitrogen equal to four martinis! Eventually, high nitrogen levels produce a numbing, sedative effect on central nervous system functions.

The term *nitrogen narcosis* or "*inert gas narcosis*" collectively describes these mimicking intoxication effects. The term was first coined by Jacques Cousteau (1910–1997; www.cousteau.org) in his 1953 book, *The Silent World*. Cousteau's colleague Frederic Dumas (1919–1991; www.visitcaymanislands.com/en-us/isdhf/isdhf-bios/frederic-dumas) was diving to about 73 m/240 ft in the Mediterranean Sea. The following quote from Dumas was the first widely read description about breathing nitrogen under pressure and its intoxicating consequences.

I'm anxious about that line, but I really feel wonderful. I have a queer feeling of the beatitude. I am drunk and carefree. My ears buzz and my mouth tastes bitter. The current staggers me as though I had too many drinks. I [have] forgotten Jacques and the people in the boats. My eyes are tired. I lower on down, trying to think about the bottom, but I can't. I'm going to sleep, but I can't fall asleep in such dizziness. At the extreme, mental processes deteriorate so that a diver may feel that the scuba serves little purpose and remove it or swim deeper instead of toward the surface (The Silent World).

Nitrogen diffuses slowly into body tissues so the narcotic effect depends on dive depth and duration. Considerable individual variation exists for nitrogen sensitivity, but a mild narcosis usually appears after an hour or more at 30 to 40 m/98 to 131 ft—the maximum recommended depth for recreational scuba divers. Treatment requires the diver ascend to a shallower depth, where complete recovery usually occurs rapidly. There is little doubt that overweight and obesity link to nitrogen narcosis susceptibility because inert gases like nitrogen store readily in fatty tissues (https://pubmed.ncbi.nlm.nih.gov/1226586/).

Decompression Sickness

With rapid ascent, the external pressure against the diver's body decreases dramatically. Excess dissolved nitrogen in the body tissues begins to separate from the dissolved state; it eventually forms bubbles in the tissues, an effect not unlike carbon dioxide bubbles in carbonated beverages. With the bottle cap in place, the gas remains dissolved under pressure. Removing the cap suddenly reduces pressure above the fluid causing bubble formation. *Decompression sickness occurs when dissolved nitrogen moves out of solution to form gas bubbles in body tissues and fluids.* It results from ascending to the surface too rapidly following a deep, prolonged dive, often made possible with double and triple air tanks.

Lippincott® Connect Appendix H, available online at Lippincott Connect, provides a list of supplemental animations and videos on the topic.

Nitrogen reaches equilibrium slowly in many tissues, particularly fatty tissues, so it leaves the body slowly.[20,42] This means that females with greater average percentage body fat than males (and overfat males) face greater risk for decompression sickness. **FIGURE 26.7** compares nitrogen elimination following a simulated "dive" by two dogs differing in fat content. The dog with relatively high body fat content (*yellow line*) eliminated considerably more nitrogen over the 4-hr decompression than the leaner dog.

The term *bends*, a synonym for decompression sickness, was coined during pier construction for the Brooklyn Bridge (1869–1883) to reflect a limping worker's bent-over position upon emerging following work from the pressurized, watertight chambers. The following poignantly describes the time course and fatal decompression sickness consequences in an early history of this malady[41]:

> In 1900 … a Royal Navy diver descended to 150 fsw in 40 minutes, spent 40 minutes at depth searching for a torpedo, and ascended to the surface in 20 minutes without apparent difficulty. Ten minutes later, he complained of abdominal pain and fainted. His breathing was labored, he was cyanotic, and he died after 7 minutes. An autopsy the next day revealed the organs to be healthy, but gas was present in the liver, spleen, heart, cardiac veins, venous, subcutaneous, and cerebral veins and ventricles.

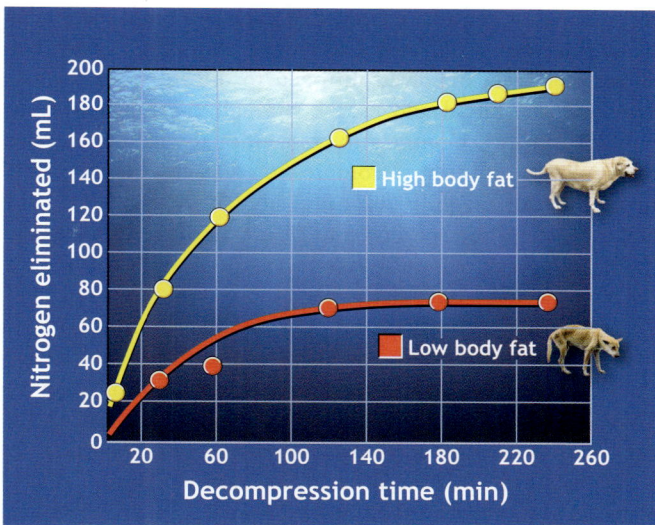

FIGURE 26.7. Nitrogen elimination from body tissues in a relatively lean dog and one higher in body fat during decompression in a chamber.
(Data courtesy Dr. A. R. Behnke. Shutterstock photos: Rich Carey, Phatthanit, Clock Is Ticking.)

Nitrogen Elimination: Zero Decompression Limits

Diving at a depth of 30 m/98 ft for up to 30 min represents the time limit before sufficient nitrogen dissolves to pose danger from decompression sickness. About 18 min is the limit at 40 m/131 ft, and one can spend almost an hour at 20 m/66 ft without danger from decompression sickness. If a diver exceeds the depth-duration recommendations for compressed air diving shown in **FIGURE 26.8** in the area to the right of the yellow line, the ascent to the surface must progress in a pre-established manner specified in the U.S. Navy diving table for diving medicine and recompression chamber operations. (www.uhms.org/images/DCS-and-AGE-Journal-Watch/recompression_therapy_usn_di.pdf). With this approach, a

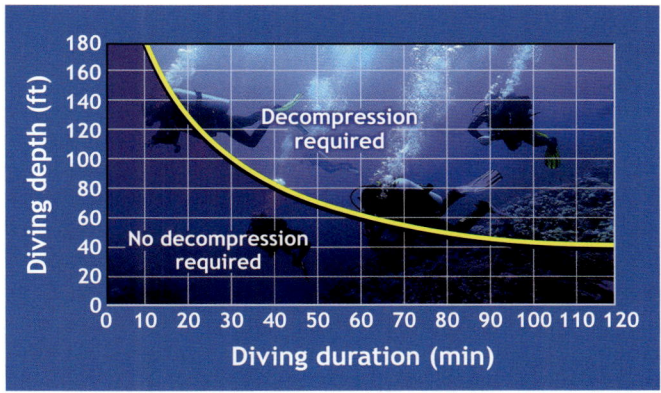

FIGURE 26.8. Zero decompression limits for any single dive that falls below the curve, provided the ascent rate does not exceed 60 ft · min^{-1} (m = ft × 0.34048). Dives above the line for dive duration require the decompression period specified in standard decompression tables.
(Kichigin/Shutterstock)

recreational or commercial diver ascends at a prescribed, relatively slow rate designed not to require stops. This ascent rate allows all excess dissolved nitrogen to diffuse from the tissues into the blood and escape through the lungs without bubbles forming. Contrary to conventional wisdom, exercise before diving or during decompression does not increase bubble number or magnify decompression sickness risk.[12,41,42] In fact, mild continuous exercise (30% maximum oxygen uptake [$\dot{V}O_{2max}$]) during a 3-min decompression period may reduce postdive gas bubble formation.[11]

Stage decompression requires the diver to make one or more stops on ascent to the surface. The time required for the slowest tissue compartment to lose sufficient nitrogen to allow ascent to the next depth determines the duration for such pauses (termed *stage-decompression stops*). For example, a dive to 30 m/98 ft for 50 min requires one 2-min decompression stop at 6 m/20 ft and a 24-min stop at 3 m/10 ft. Surface stage decompression transfers the diver from the water (after several in-water stops) to a decompression chamber at the surface. A hyperoxic breathing mixture facilitates recompression.

A conservative approach recommends that the sport diver not exceed a 20- to 25-m/66- to 82-ft depth (30-m/98-ft maximum). During single or repetitive dives, the diver should never approach the time limits indicated by the decompression tables. The recommendations in Figure 26.8 assume a single dive, with a 12-hr minimum between dives. For repeated dives within 12 hr, the diver must consult the appropriate repetitive dive decompression schedules.[38,39] These recommendations account for residual nitrogen remaining in the body when the next dive begins if it occurs within the 12-hr period. Interestingly, air travel within 24 hr of scuba diving increases decompression sickness risk because commercial airlines usually pressurize cabins to an equivalent of 2130-m/7000-ft altitude. This reduced ambient atmospheric pressure may initiate bubble formation from excess nitrogen dissolved in body tissues during the prior preflight dive(s).[21]

Inadequate Decompression Consequences

Bubbles within the vascular circuit initiate complications from decompression injury.[5,13,27] Except for bubbles formed in central nervous tissue that cause brain and spinal cord lesions and damage intervertebral disks,[16] the primary bubbles form in the venous and arterial vascular bed. Decompression sickness symptoms usually appear within 4 to 6 hr following a dive. Significant decompression procedure violations (e.g., diver runs out of air and ascends too rapidly) trigger immediate, observable symptoms that can quickly progress to paralysis within minutes. Indicators for inadequate decompression include dizziness, itchy skin, and aching pain in the legs and arms, particularly in ligaments and tendons, the classic and most commonly afflicted areas. Injury magnitude depends on bubble size and where they form. Bubbles in the lungs cause choking and asphyxia; bubbles in the brain and coronary arteries block blood flow and deprive oxygen and nutrient delivery to these vital tissues, ultimately producing cellular damage and death. Central nervous system bends occur with some frequency—failure to initiate immediate treatment produces permanent neural damage.

Treatment

Treatment for the bends involves lengthy recompression in a **hyperbaric chamber**. This specialized device elevates external pressure to force nitrogen gas back into solution. Gradual decompression then follows to provide time for the expanding gas to leave the body as the diver returns to the "surface." Immediate recompression offers the best chance for success; any delay decreases prognosis for complete recovery. **FIGURE 26.9** shows a collapsible, lightweight, transportable, rapid-deployment chamber for transporting a single diver to an appropriate facility to treat decompression accidents. A larger chamber can accommodate 3 to 4 occupants at 6 ata (5 bar) pressure for full treatment. For a single person, a compressed air cylinder provides a working 2.1 ata/2.3 bar pressure differential or 70 fsw, between the chamber environment and ambient conditions. The diver receives oxygen via a breathing mask. The emergency tube is constructed from para-aramid Kevlar-like fiber in a matrix of silicone rubber. This provides flexibility, can fold when not in use, and provides considerable strength under pressure. Chances are slim for a sport and recreational diver to have ready access to such a recompression chamber, which makes it imperative that all divers, novice and experienced, adhere *meticulously* to diving depth and duration recommendations.

Higher Prevalence with a Patent Foramen Ovale

Decompression sickness sometimes occurs after uneventful dives, without any reported errors in recommended decompression procedures. Divers with lesions localized in the high cervical spinal cord and brain areas show a higher patent foramen ovale (PFO; www.heart.org/en/health-topics/congenital-heart-defects/about-congenital-heart-defects/patent-foramen-ovale-pfo) prevalence in the myocardium than divers who experience decompression sickness that ultimately localizes in the lower spinal cord.[17] PFO

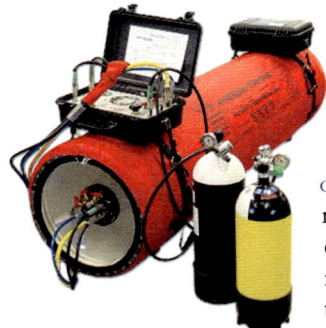

FIGURE 26.9. Portable, collapsible recompression chamber for transferring a stricken diver under pressure for treatment in an emergency. Manufactured by SOS Limited, London, England.

(Photo courtesy John Selby, SOS Hyperlite of Douglas, Isle of Man.)

consists of an interatrial septum channel that creates a functional valve between the right and left atria. This channel could cause localized decompression sickness because nitrogen bubbles that the pulmonary vasculature normally filters pass through the PFO into the arterial circulation. The bubbles then migrate preferentially into the carotid and/or vertebral arteries. Divers should be evaluated for PFO with unexplained decompression sickness, but exhibit cerebral or high spinal localized symptoms.[18]

Oxygen Poisoning

Inspiring a gas with a P_{O_2} above 2 ata (1520 mm Hg) greatly increases a diver's susceptibility to **oxygen poisoning**, particularly with elevated metabolic rates during physical activity.[2] For this reason, closed-circuit scuba that uses pure oxygen severely restricts both diving depth and duration (**TABLE 26.3**). At depths greater than 25 fsw (7.6 m/25 ft), the diver should *not* rebreathe pure oxygen except in extraordinary circumstances. A decreased vital capacity strongly indicates impaired pulmonary function under hyperoxic conditions.[9]

TABLE 26.3 Depth–time limits for closed-circuit diving

Breathing oxygen at high pressures negatively affects bodily functions in three ways:

1. Irritates respiratory passages and eventually induces bronchopneumonia with continued exposure
2. Constricts cerebral blood vessels at pressures above 2 ata and alters central nervous system function
3. Depresses carbon dioxide elimination

For carbon dioxide elimination, an elevated inspired P_{O_2} may force sufficient oxygen into solution in the plasma to supply the diver's metabolic needs. In this case, oxygen remains combined with hemoglobin (called oxyhemoglobin) as blood returns to the pulmonary capillaries. This causes carbon dioxide buildup because deoxygenated hemoglobin normally transports considerable carbon dioxide as carbaminohemoglobin from the tissues. The common treatment for oxygen poisoning reduces exposure to increased oxygen levels by breathing air at sea-level pressure (www.ncbi.nlm.nih.gov/books/NBK430743/). Damage from oxygen-induced pulmonary toxicity is reversible in most adults.[51,52]

Carbon Monoxide Poisoning

Potentially lethal carbon monoxide gas with only one carbon and oxygen atom (CO) combines about 200 times more readily with hemoglobin than does oxygen with two oxygen and one carbon atom. Accordingly, a minute CO quantity in the inspired mixture can induce tissue hypoxia. This odorless, colorless molecule is invisible. Carbon monoxide poisoning heightens concern during deep dives because the partial pressures of all gases in the breathing mixture, including impurities, increase greatly.

The air in urban areas likely contains high contaminant levels including CO and sulfur oxides from automotive and industrial exhausts.

ALERT: NEVER FILL A SCUBA TANK DURING AIR POLLUTION OR "UNHEALTHY AIR" ALERTS!

Aside from contaminants present in ambient air, operating gasoline or diesel engine compressors contributes additional CO and oil impurities. Placing the compressor's engine exhaust downstream from the air intake eliminates this potential contamination source. The antidote for CO poisoning requires immediate hyperbaric oxygen breathing. High inspired oxygen pressures hasten CO dissociation from hemoglobin molecules.

Females at No Greater Diving Risk than Males

Approximately 35% of recreational scuba divers in the United States are female. They do *not* experience a greater risk than males of about equivalent fitness levels for decompression sickness, nitrogen narcosis, oxygen toxicity, air embolism, or diving accidents.[36]

Limited research has assessed the risks of open-circuit scuba diving to the fetus during pregnancy. According to the Divers Alert Network (https://dan.org/safety-prevention/diver-safety/divers-blog/scuba-diving-and-pregnancy/), women should *refrain* from scuba diving when trying to become pregnant and during pregnancy to eliminate fetal injury risk from breathing compressed air at elevated pressures. The consequences can lead to low birth weight, fetal abortion, bubbles in the amniotic fluid, premature delivery, abnormal skull development, malformed limbs, abnormal cardiac development, changes in fetal circulation, limb weakness associated with decompression sickness, and blindness. The science is fairly conclusive to support the general recommendation about abstaining from recreational scuba during pregnancy, yet more studies are needed in this area.[35,37]

Dives to Exceptional Depths: Mixed-Gas Diving

Commercial, military, scientific, rescue, and technical divers often descend to depths in excess of 160 fsw. At depths greater than 60 fsw, recall that diving with compressed air and saturation diving increase oxygen toxicity risk. Diving beyond this depth requires breathing compressed mixed gases (nonair) with a lower P_{O_2}. **FIGURE 26.10** lists the main advantages using nonair mixtures for dives to great depths—specifically the reduced nitrogen narcotic effects and reduced oxygen toxicity risk. Oxygen always exists in the breathing mixture in mixed-gas diving but represents only a small fraction of the total gas mix in dives to extreme depths. Precise oxygen concentration management remains the primary consideration in **mixed-gas diving**. Three mixtures of oxygen, nitrogen, and helium are used for deep and saturation diving:

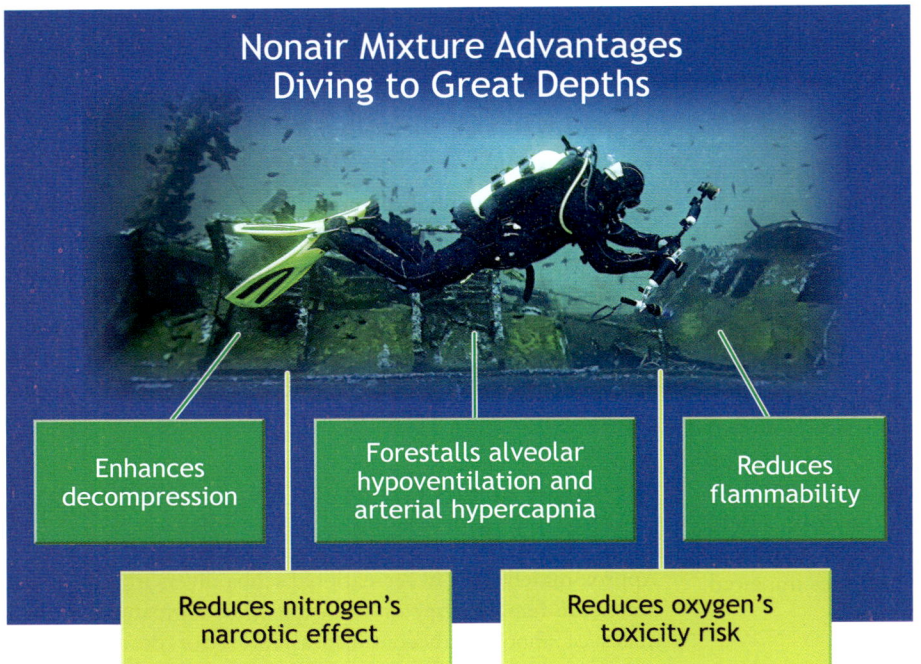

FIGURE 26.10. Rationale for breathing gas mixtures other than compressed air when diving to great depths. Avoiding nitrogen narcosis and oxygen poisoning is the overwhelming reason to breathe nonair mixtures.
(Kichigin/Shutterstock)

1. *Nitrox* (nitrogen + oxygen)
2. *Heliox* (helium + oxygen)
3. *Trimix* (helium + nitrogen + oxygen)

Relatively shallow recreational dives employ nitrox, while heliox is used for deep diving, and trimix for dives to depths that may produce high-pressure nervous syndrome (see next section).[3]

Helium-Oxygen Mixtures

Helium, the second lightest known element, is the most common inert gas substituted for nitrogen in deep diving. The gas remains colorless, odorless, tasteless, nonexplosive, and relatively nontoxic and does not induce narcosis at any inspired pressure.[33]

Helium in the breathing mixture in diving proved its usefulness in 1939 during the submarine *Squalus* rescue and salvage operations (see "Diving History Chronology," earlier in this chapter). For this purpose, a compressor at the water's surface continually supplied the divers with a helium-oxygen (heliox) mixture. Because of helium's low density, breathing heliox reduced the typical increased breathing resistance imposed by nitrogen.

During rapid descent to depths in excess of 300 fsw up to 2280 fsw, divers breathing heliox can experience potentially incapacitating nausea, muscle tremors, and other central nervous system consequences. This phenomenon, first noted in the 1960s and called **high-pressure nervous syndrome (HPNS;** www.ncbi.nlm.nih.gov/books/NBK513359/), was previously known as helium tremors from the direct hydrostatic pressure extremes on excitable nerve cells. Slowing the descent compression rate and adding 5% nitrogen to the heliox breathing mixture relieve the tremor associated with HPNS.

Two additional negative effects occur when breathing helium:

1. Changes in voice characteristics (high-pitched, cartoonlike quality), which interfere with voice communication among divers and remedied by technologically advanced electronic voice unscramblers (www.jfdglobal.com/products/electrical-diving-equipment/diver-communications/helicom-helium-unscramblers/).
2. Considerable heat loss for divers living in a heliox environment occurs from helium's high thermal conductivity (six times that of air).[26] The thermal challenge also contributes to weight loss, common among saturation divers.

Increased central nervous system oxygen toxicity risk when breathing surface-supplied heliox gas makes it crucial that the diver not exceed the oxygen exposure limits established in **TABLE 26.4**.

TABLE 26.4 Oxygen partial pressure limits for surface-supplied heliox diving

Saturation Diving

Breathing a heliox mixture supports a safe dive to depths greater than 300 fsw, but the time the diver must remain "in-water" for decompression becomes prohibitive. Thus, dives below 300 fsw generally take place with **saturation diving** in a deep-diving system using a helium-oxygen-nitrogen (trimix) breathing mixture that maintains oxygen pressure between 0.4 and 0.6 ata (P_{O_2}, 300 to 450 mm Hg). In saturation diving, each inert gas in a mixture begins to concentrate in body tissues as depth and duration progress. Within 24 to 30 hr, the gases equilibrate and *saturate* body tissues to equal the inspired gas pressures. Once the tissues saturate, the decompression procedure remains identical regardless of the dive's duration.

The deep-diving system includes a chamber so divers can live under pressure for up to 4 wk. The system also contains a deck decompression chamber and transfer capsule (diving bell) to transport personnel under pressure to and from the

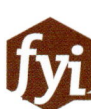

Three Recommendations to Avoid High-Pressure Nervous System Injury During Diving

The National Association of Underwater Instructors (NAUI; www.naui.org/) has been a premier diving organization for

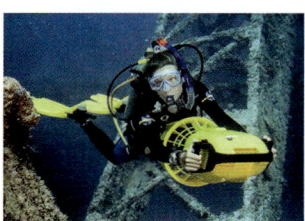

underwater diver certification since the early 1950s. NAUI's first elected Board of Directors included two diving pioneers we feature in this chapter, Captain Albert Behnke, Jr and Captain Jacques-Yves Cousteau. The NAUI features formal courses in technical diving skills, mixed gases and decompression diving, rebreather diving, diver propulsion vehicles, and gas blender services (www.naui.org/certifications/technical/). The NAUI advocates following strict guidelines to avoid high-pressure nervous system (HPNS) injury.

1. Do not dive with heliox (He + O_2) mixtures deeper than 400 fsw.
2. Do not dive with trimix (He + N_2 + O_2) deeper than 600 fsw. Adding 10% nitrogen to a He + O_2 mixture buffers mix for use to 600 fsw to avoid experiencing HPNS injury.
3. Use slow descent rates. Descending slower than 1 fsw per min beyond 400 fsw on heliox and 600 fsw on trimix keeps HPNS injury at bay. Unfortunately, this slow decent rate is only practical in commercial diving and is of no use in technical diving.

Source:
January 13, 2020 update; www.ncbi.nlm.nih.gov/books/NBK513359/.

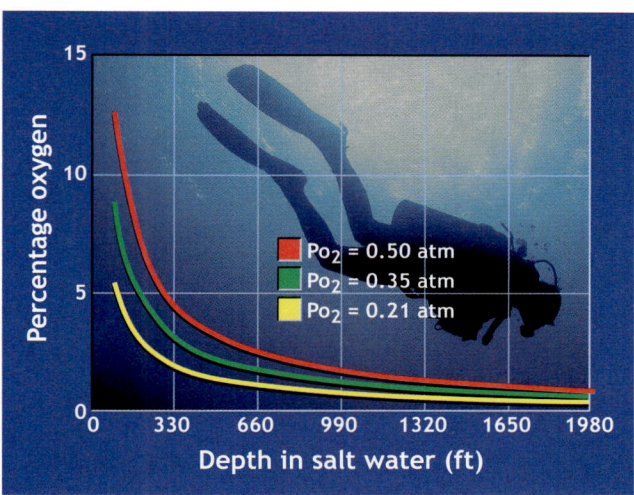

FIGURE 26.11. Range of percentage oxygen concentrations for P_{O_2} at 0.50, 0.35, and 0.21 ata in saturation diving to 1980 FSW. (Adapted with permission from Hamilton RW. Mixed-gas diving. In: Bove AA, Jefferson CD, eds. *Diving Medicine*. 4th Ed. Philadelphia: WB Saunders, 2004. Photo: Marjan Schmit Visser/Shutterstock.)

worksite. Once at the worksite, the divers exit while tethered to an umbilicus-supplied breathing apparatus. Saturation diving provides benefits in offshore oil-field work with dives up to 30 days at 1500-fsw depths. Successful dives to 2300-fsw depths in a dry chamber apply saturation diving principles with a hydrogen, helium, and oxygen breathing mixture. Decompression from a saturation dive takes 8 to 24 hr per 10 m/33 ft ascent.

The main objective in saturation diving with heliox mixtures must maintain normoxic P_{O_2} with great precision. Breathing the wrong mixture or the correct mixture at the wrong pressure creates the potential for a tragic fatality. Oxygen percentages must remain within ±0.10% the desired value to avoid either hypoxia or oxygen toxicity. **FIGURE 26.11** shows the typical recommended percentage for oxygen in heliox up to 1980 fsw for saturation diving depths. For example, the oxygen concentration to obtain a desired 0.35 ata for P_{O_2} at a 1200 fsw (P_{O_2}, 270 mm Hg; green curve) requires a breathing mixture with approximately 0.7% oxygen. The *yellow line* represents the oxygen needed to provide a normoxic level at 0.21 ata. The *red line* represents 0.5 ata (P_{O_2} = 380 mm Hg), the upper limit for continuous exposure to avoid whole-body oxygen toxicity. The low oxygen concentrations needed at great depths become difficult to mix and analyze within acceptable tolerance limits; accordingly, they are usually mixed while the diving chamber becomes pressurized.

Technical Diving

Technical diving defines untethered dives (scuba or closed-circuit rebreathing) beyond the traditional compressed air range for military operations, science, salvage, and recreational pursuits. Many recreational scuba divers now consider too restrictive the typical 130-fsw depth limit imposed by compressed air diving. They wish to expand diving depths for personal achievement, recreation, and exploration (e.g., cave diving). Technical diving requires special equipment, expertise, and vigilant gas mixture management. Technical divers routinely use various trimix compressed gas mixtures to dive below 300 fsw. Blending a depth-specific gas mixture allows the diver to control hyperoxia risk and nitrogen's narcotic potential.

Closed-circuit nitrogen-oxygen and helium-oxygen scuba originally developed for military operations now appear in the recreational technical-diving community. These highly sophisticated systems maintain a constant oxygen partial pressure in the inhaled mixture independent of depth. **FIGURE 26.12** illustrates a closed-circuit mixed-gas system used by U.S. Navy divers and Navy SEALS (www.americanspecialops.com/equipment/SEAL-diving-gear/). An oxygen sensor (*#19*) and microprocessor (*#21*) in the breathing loop continually detect and regulate falling P_{O_2}. The sensors activate valves that add 100% oxygen at the precise quantity to regulate inspired P_{O_2} at 0.75 ata (427 mm Hg). One of two high-pressure gas bottles (*#9* and

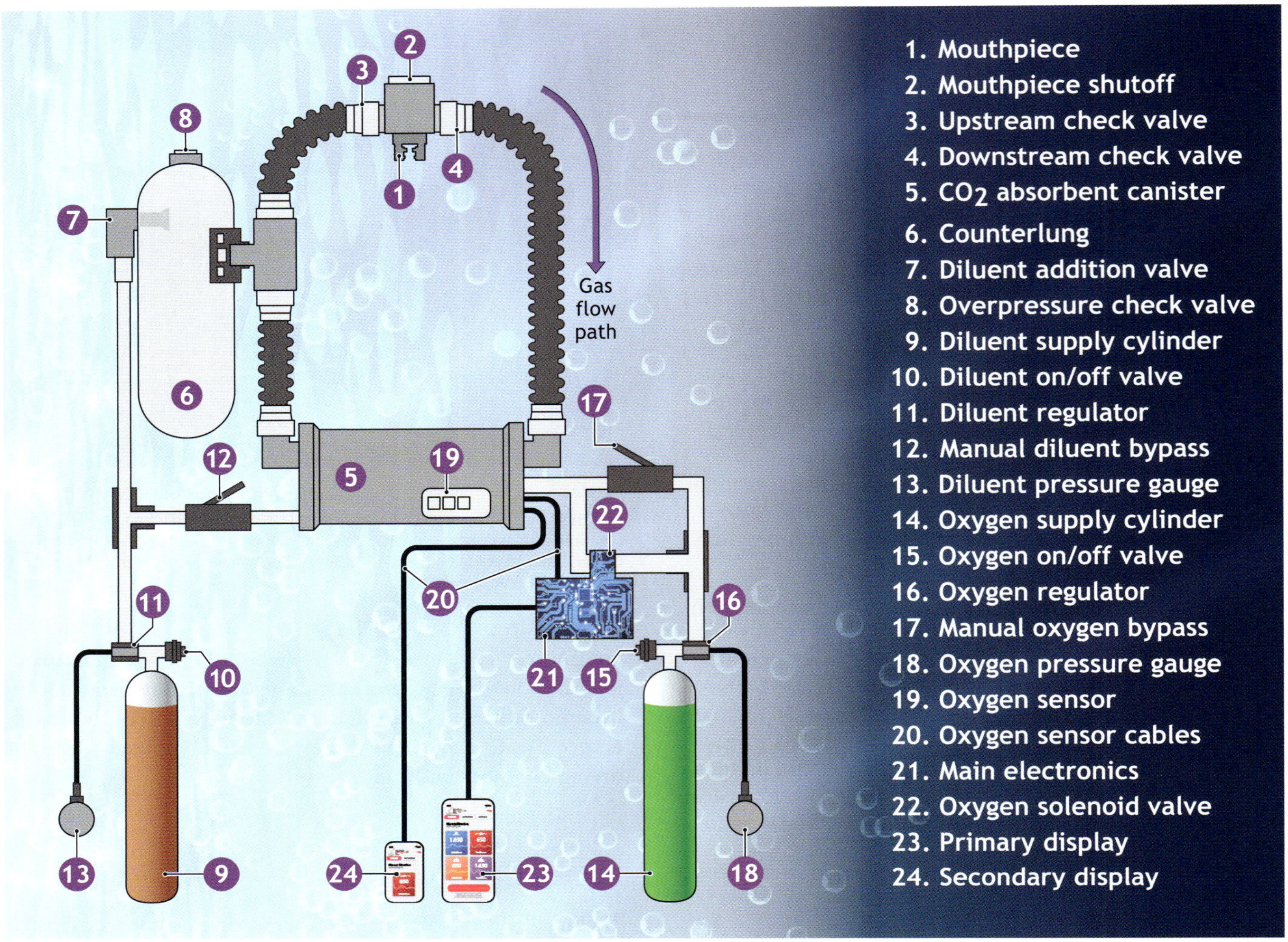

FIGURE 26.12. Closed-circuit mixed-gas system for technical diving to great depths.
(Shutterstock: K3Star, ZinetroN, bestfoto77)

#14) supplies pure oxygen, and the other provides either air or a heliox mixture as the diluent gas. As with the typical closed-circuit system, a chemical bed absorbs carbon dioxide continually produced by metabolism. Monitors within the facemask provide feedback about P_{O_2} and diving depth. A fiberglass casing worn on the diver's back contains the microprocessor, gas bottles, breathing bag, and insulated carbon dioxide absorbent canister (cold decreases CO_2 absorbent life).

Underwater Swimming Energy Cost

As with surface swimming, drag forces impede the diver's forward movement and greatly increase underwater swimming's energy cost. **FIGURE 26.13** shows the curvilinear relationship between oxygen uptake and underwater swimming speed. For example, a swimmer with a 35 mL · kg^{-1} · min^{-1} $\dot{V}O_{2max}$ could swim underwater at 1.2 knots/1.4 mph for only a few minutes. This speed creates minimal stress for a diver with a 65 mL · kg^{-1} · min^{-1} $\dot{V}O_{2max}$. The gear's location and density can alter the diver's positioning in the water and increase the swimming energy cost by up to 30% at slower speeds. The fin type worn by the diver affects the kick's depth and frequency, thus influencing drag and swimming economy.[31]

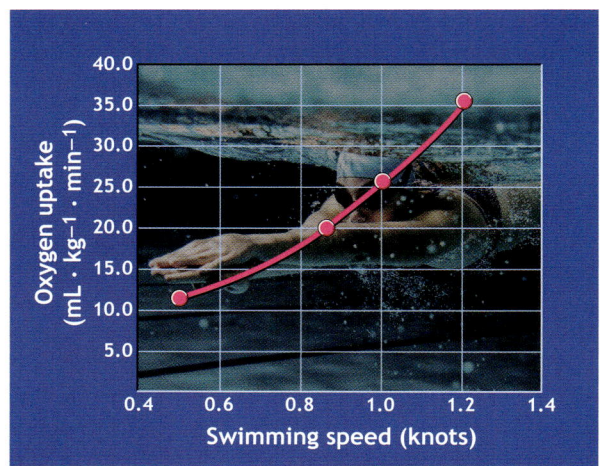

FIGURE 26.13. Generalized curvilinear relationship between oxygen uptake (mL · kg^{-1} · min^{-1}) and underwater swimming speed (1.0 knot = 1.15 mph).
(BalanceFormCreative/Shutterstock)

Summary

1. Breath-hold diving has been practiced for centuries, while deep-sea diving had its origins in the 14th century with the invention of diving bells supplied with surface air.
2. The underwater environment exposes divers to high pressures (hyperbaria) and the possibility of rapidly changing pressures and can produce severe injury or death unless the diver equalizes pressures in the body's air-filled cavities.
3. Two factors limit snorkel size—increased hydrostatic pressure on the chest cavity during descent and increased pulmonary dead space from enlarging the snorkel's internal volume.
4. Breath-hold dive duration depends on time until arterial P_{CO_2} reaches the breath-holding breakpoint.
5. Hyperventilation considerably lowers arterial P_{CO_2} and increases breath-holding time—it also increases likelihood for underwater blackout.
6. Compressing the lung volume to RLV determines maximum breath-hold diving depth; lung squeeze occurs below this critical depth because internal and external pressures cannot equalize.
7. Breath-hold diving by elite divers produces intense cardiovascular changes that resemble diving mammals' response patterns.
8. Free diving has different dive categories where the diver attempts to achieve maximum depth with a single breath before descending and returning to the surface.
9. Free dive periodization training focuses on general strength training principles, cardiovascular, flexibility, and yoga, and specific dive training to optimize breath-hold ability by focusing on ventilatory musculature and tolerating high CO_2 levels.
10. Four major scuba hazards from improper pressure equalization in lungs, sinus, and middle-ear spaces with the external water pressure include air embolism, pneumothorax, mask and middle-ear squeeze, and aerosinusitis.
11. Gases breathed at high pressures move across the alveolar membrane to dissolve and equilibrate in fluids within all tissues.
12. The maximum recommended diving depth for breathing compressed air is about 30 m/98 ft, beyond which high tissue oxygen and nitrogen pressures exert profound negative physiologic effects.
13. Prolonged breathing of a gas with a P_{O_2} above 2 ata increases a diver's susceptibility to oxygen poisoning.
14. Closed-circuit scuba systems that use pure oxygen severely restrict dive depth and duration.
15. Nitrogen bubbles form in tissues when excess nitrogen fails to exit through the lungs if ascent progresses too rapidly causing painful decompression sickness or bends.
16. Diving to depths below 60 fsw requires inhaling compressed mixed gases with technical precision to safely manage optimal oxygen concentrations.
17. Breathing helium and oxygen mixtures (heliox) allows dives to 2000 fsw, eliminating nitrogen narcosis risk and minimizing oxygen-poisoning risk.
18. Rapid descent to depths from 300 to 2800 fsw from breathing heliox mixtures produces nausea, muscle tremors, and other potentially dangerous central nervous system effects termed *HPNS*.
19. Drag forces that impede a diver's forward movement considerably increase underwater swimming's energy cost.

Key Terms

Bends: Dissolved gases (mainly nitrogen) escape solution as bubbles in the vascular system during ascent to sea level directly relate to dive depth, time under pressure while submerged, and ascent rate to the surface causing decompression illness mainly pain in shoulder and elbow joints

Blackout: Loss of consciousness due to cerebral hypoxia when a swimmer does not experience an urgent breathing need toward the end of a breath-hold free dive

Boyle's law: Gas volume varies inversely with its pressure at a constant temperature

Closed-circuit system: Apparatus that absorbs carbon dioxide from exhaled air to allow continuous rebreathing of unused oxygen content while an oxygen cylinder replenishes the diver's metabolized oxygen

Decompression sickness: Illness in which rapid pressure decrease causes dissolved nitrogen to move from solution to form gas bubbles in body tissues and fluids

Diving reflex: Physiologic responses to cold water submersion that enable diving mammals to spend considerable time underwater

Dry suit: A close-fitting, double-layered synthetic garment worn during cold water immersion to protect the skin from water contact

Emboli: Blood clots, air bubbles, or fatty deposits carried in the bloodstream that lodge in a blood vessel

Heliox: Helium (H_e) and oxygen (O_2) gas mixture used in deep-water diving

High-pressure nervous syndrome (HPNS): Neurological and physiological diving disorder that can occur when a diver descends below about 150 m/500 ft using a breathing gas containing helium-oxygen mixtures

Hyperbaria: Pertaining to gas pressures greater than 1 atmosphere pressure

Hyperbaric chamber: Specialized chamber that elevates external pressure to force nitrogen gas back into solution to provide sufficient time for dissolved gas to leave the body without forming bubbles as the diver ascends to the surface

Lung squeeze: Lung and thoracic cavity compression during a breath-hold dive when increased external pressure causes air spaces and gas pockets to compress

Mixed-gas diving: Saturation diving in which different oxygen, nitrogen, and helium mixtures are used—nitrogen + oxygen (nitrox); helium + oxygen (heliox); helium + nitrogen + oxygen (trimix)

Nitrogen narcosis: Reversible alteration in consciousness (intoxication effect) while diving at depth caused by nitrogen's anesthetic effect from breathing gas mixtures at pressures exceeding 300 fsw; also known as rapture of the deep ("I'vresse des grandes profondeurs")

Nitrox: Nitrogen and oxygen gas mixtures where oxygen concentration exceeds the percent normally found in ambient air

Oxygen poisoning: Sickness due to prolonged oxygen breathing at increased partial pressures

Pneumothorax: Abnormal air collection in the pleural space between the lung and chest wall causing lung(s) to collapse

Raptures of the deep: Condition caused when a diver goes deeper into the water, where the nitrogen partial pressure increases and releases more nitrogen into the bloodstream, causing an intoxicating effect seriously impairing judgment underwater

Saturation diving: Prolonged deep diving while breathing a helium-oxygen-nitrogen trimix that maintains oxygen pressure between 0.4 and 0.6 ata (Po_2, 300 to 450 mm Hg)

Scuba (self-contained underwater breathing apparatus): Portable compressed gas supply delivered at a regulated pressure during underwater breathing

Shallow water blackout (SWB): Sudden loss of consciousness afflicts those who extend their underwater depth duration too long

Technical diving: Extending diving beyond recreational "no stop" limits to plan longer dives at shallower depths, or plan dives to advanced depths and diving environments, using specialized gas mixtures and decompression procedures

Wet suit: Close-fitting diving garment made with closed-cell neoprene foam filled with gas bubbles reduces heat conduction and offers thermal protection during cold water immersion

References are available online at Lippincott Connect.

Additional References

Aragaki-Nakahodo A. Management of pneumothorax: an update. *Curr Opin Pulm Med*. 2022;28:62.

Balestra C, et al. Physiology of repeated mixed gas 100-m wreck dives using a closed-circuit rebreather: a field bubble study. *Eur J Appl Physiol*. 2022;122:515.

Bao XC, et al. Human physiological responses to a single deep helium-oxygen diving. *Front Physiol*. 2021;12:735986.

Buzzacott P, et al. Incidence of cardiac arrhythmias and left ventricular hypertrophy in recreational scuba divers. *Diving Hyperb Med*. 2021;51:190.

Buzzacott P, et al. Mortality rate during professionally guided scuba diving experiences for uncertified divers, 1992–2019. *Diving Hyperb Med*. 2021;51:147.

Chishti EA, et al. Severe acute kidney injury caused by decompression sickness syndrome. *Clin Nephrol*. 2022. doi:10.5414/CN110662.

Di Giacomo A, et al. Cardiovascular responses to simultaneous diving and muscle metaboreflex activation. *Front Physiol*. 2021;12:730983.

Edgar M, et al. Case series of arterial gas embolism incidents in U.S. Navy pressurized submarine escape training from 2018 to 2019. *Mil Med*. 2021;186:e613.

Fichtner A, et al. A doppler ultrasound self-monitoring approach for detection of relevant individual decompression stress in scuba diving. *Intern Emerg Med*. 2022;17:173.

Fico BG, et al. Vascular responses to simulated breath-hold diving involving multiple reflexes. *Am J Physiol Regul Integr Comp Physiol*. 2022;322:R153.

Giaconi C, et al. Post-mortem computer tomography in ten cases of death while diving: a retrospective evaluation. *Radiol Med*. 2022. doi:10.1007/s11547-022-01448-x.

Gibert L, et al. Comparing meditative scuba diving versus multisport activities to improve post-traumatic stress disorder symptoms: a pilot, randomized controlled clinical trial. *Eur J Psychotraumatol*. 2022;13:2031590.

Goldbogen JA, Madsen PT. The largest of August Krogh animals: physiology and biomechanics of the blue whale revisited. *Comp Biochem Physiol A Mol Integr Physiol*. 2021;254:110894.

Hallifax R. Aetiology of primary spontaneous pneumothorax. *J Clin Med*. 2022;11:490.

Karakaya H, et al. Effects of hyperbaric nitrogen narcosis on cognitive performance in recreational air SCUBA divers: an auditory event-related brain potentials study. *Ann Work Expo Health*. 2021;65:505.

Levenez M, et al. Full-face mask use during scuba diving counters related oxidative stress and endothelial dysfunction. *Int J Environ Res Public Health*. 2022;19:965.

Lovering AT, et al. Implications of a patent foramen ovale for environmental physiology and pathophysiology: do we know the "hole" story? *J Physiol*. 2022. doi:10.1113/JP281108.

Lundell RV, et al. Diving responses in experienced rebreather divers: short-term heart rate variability in cold water diving. *Front Physiol*. 2021;12:649319.

Marlinge M, et al. Blood adenosine increase during apnea in spearfishermen reinforces the efficiency of the cardiovascular component of the diving reflex. *Front Physiol*. 2021;12:743154.

Monnoyer R, et al. Functional profiling reveals altered metabolic activity in divers' oral microbiota during commercial heliox saturation diving. *Front Physiol*. 2021;12:702634.

Patrician A, et al. Breath-hold diving. The physiology of diving deep and returning. *Front Physiol*. 2021;12:639377.

Patrician A, et al. Case studies in physiology: breath-hold diving beyond 100 meters. Cardiopulmonary responses in world-champion divers. *J Appl Physiol* (1985). 2021;130:1345.

Patrician A, et al. Temporal changes in pulmonary gas exchange efficiency when breath-hold diving below residual volume. *Exp Physiol*. 2021;106:1120.

Piispanen WW, et al. Assessment of alertness and cognitive performance of closed-circuit rebreather divers with the critical flicker fusion frequency test in arctic diving conditions. *Front Physiol*. 2021;12:722915.

Ponganis PJ. A Physio-logging journey: heart rates of the emperor penguin and blue whale. *Front Physiol*. 2021;12:721381.

Rosén A, et al. Protein tau concentration in blood increases after SCUBA diving: an observational study. *Eur J Appl Physiol*. 2022. doi:10.1007/s00421-022-04892-9.

Shapiro SD, et al. Stereotactic intracerebral underwater blood aspiration (SCUBA) improves survival following intracerebral hemorrhage as compared to predicted mortality. *World Neurosurg.* 2022. doi:10.1016/j.wneu.2022.01.123.

Sundal E, et al. Long-term neurological sequelae after decompression sickness in retired professional divers. *J Neurol Sci.* 2022;434:120181.

Taylor SE, et al. Regular medication use by active scuba divers with a declared comorbid medical condition and victims of scuba and snorkeling-related fatalities. *Diving Hyperb Med.* 2021;51:264.

Tetzlaff K, et al. Going to extremes of lung physiology-deep breath-hold diving. *Front Physiol.* 2021;12:710429.

Table 26.1 Relationships Among Water Depth, External Pressure, Lung Volume, and Inspired Gas Pressure

Depth		Pressure		Hypothetical Lung Volume	Inspired Air (mm Hg)	
ft	m	atm	mm Hg	mL	P_{O_2}	P_{N_2}
Sea level		1	760	6000	159	600
33	10	2	1520	3000	318	1201
66	20	3	2280	2000	477	1802
99	30	4	3040	1500	636	2402
133	40	5	3800	1200	795	3003
166	50	6	4560	1000	954	3604
200	60	7	5320	857	1113	4204
300	90	10	7600	600	1590	6006
400	120	13	9880	461	2068	7808
500	150	16	12,160	375	2545	9610
600	180	19	14,440	316	3022	11,412

Table 26.2 U.S. Navy–Recommended Depth–Time Limits Breathing Pure Oxygen During Working Dives

Depth		Time (min)
ft	m	
Normal Operations		
10	3.0	240
15	4.6	150
20	6.1	150
25	7.6	75
Exceptional Operations		
30	9.2	45
35	10.7	20
40	12.2	10

No symptoms of oxygen poisoning were noted at these depths and durations.

Table 26.3 Representative Depth–Time Limits for Closed-Circuit Diving with 100% Oxygen

Depth (fsw)	Maximum Time (min)
25	240
30	80
35	25
40	15
50	10

fsw, feet of sea water.

Adapted from *U.S. Navy Diving Manual*, Vol. 5. Washington, DC: Superintendent of Documents, U.S. Government Printing Office, 2008.

Table 26.4 Representative Oxygen Partial Pressure Limits for Surface-Supplied Heliox Diving

Exposure Time (min)	Maximum Oxygen Partial Pressure (ata)
13	1.8
20	1.7
30	1.6
40	1.5
80	1.4
Unlimited	**1.3**

ata, atmosphere absolute.

Adapted from *U.S. Navy Diving Manual*, Vol. 5. Washington, DC: Superintendent of Documents, U.S. Government Printing Office, 2008.

Chapter 27
Microgravity: The Last Frontier

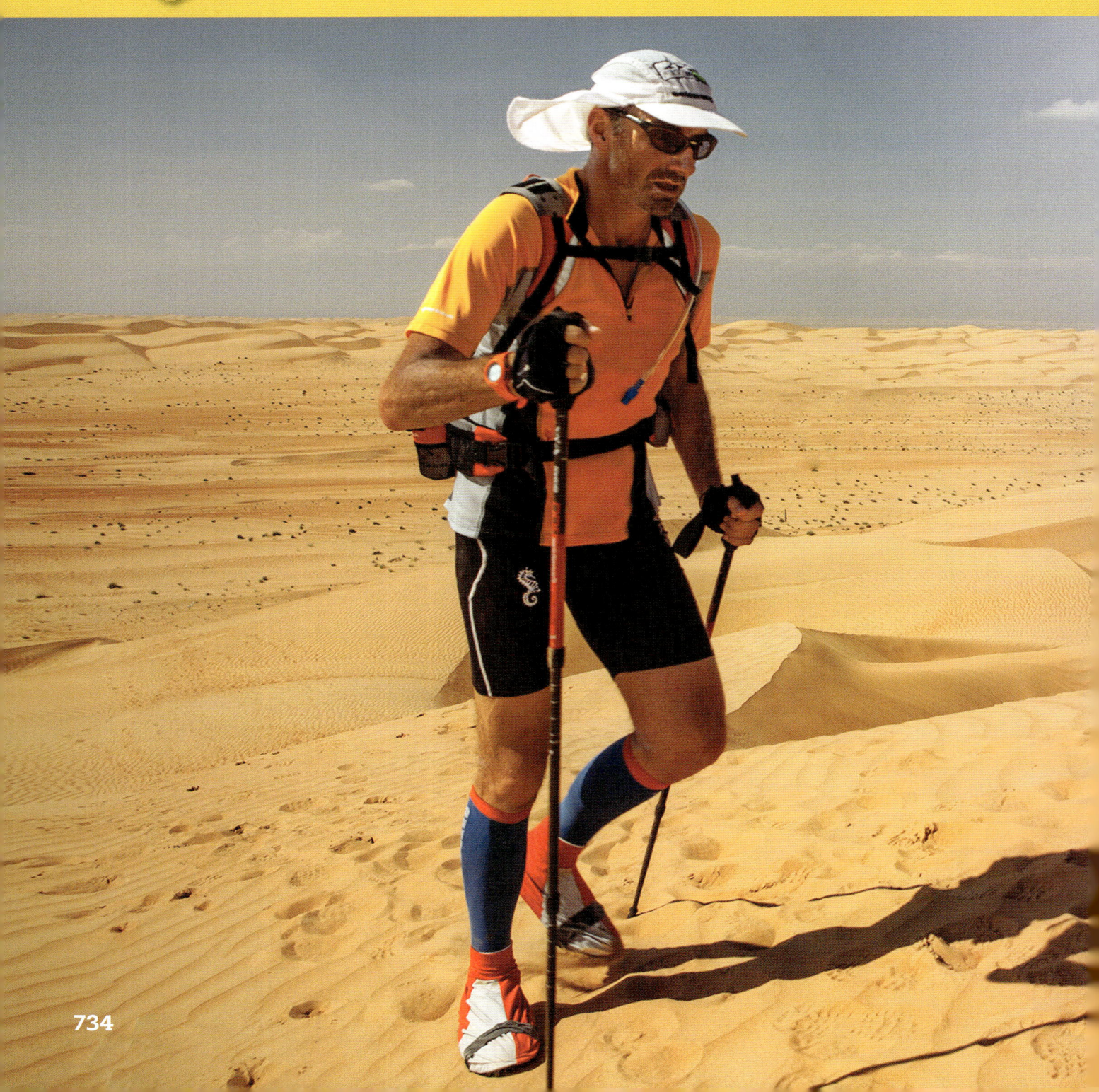

Chapter Objectives

- Define gravity and list three key factors impacting gravitational forces
- Differentiate between zero-g and weightlessness
- Explain the "Vomit Comet's" function for training astronauts for space missions
- List five physiologic/anatomic responses to microgravity exposure, and differentiate between short-term (≤30 days) and long-term (≥3 mo) responses
- Give three reasons for denitrogenation prior to extravehicular activity in space and the procedures to achieve this effect
- Outline four exercise countermeasure goals to ensure astronaut health and safety during different duration space missions
- Describe the rationale for applying lower-body negative pressure and its role as a countermeasure during spaceflight
- Outline three interactions among energy balance, nutrition, and protein dynamics during space missions
- Describe the time course for postflight recovery for different physiologic systems from 2-wk and 1-year space missions
- List 10 beneficial spin-off technologies from space biology research
- Describe the Artemis Moon Mission's three exploration phases
- List three important physiological concerns astronauts would confront during a 7-mo space mission from the moon to Mars

Ancillaries at-a-Glance

Visit Lippincott Connect to access the following resources.

- References: Chapter 27
- Appendix J: Accomplishments of the United States and Soviet Human Space Programs: From Project Mercury to the International Space Station
- Focus on Research: Microgravity's Effects on Muscle Fibers; James Webb Space Telescope Launches and Deploys

The Weightless Environment

The pioneering efforts of mainly American, German, and Russian scientists and engineers advanced **aerospace medicine** from the early rocket-propelled "X" jet aircraft test flights in the 1940s to the game-changing **International Space Station (ISS)** constructed with international partners and the U.S. space shuttle fleet (Columbia, Challenger, Discovery, Atlantis, and Endeavour; www.nasa.gov/mission_pages/station/main/index.html; https://www.issnationallab.org), to the currently active Mars Perseverance and Curiosity rover missions and the first powered helicopter flight from Mars' surface (https://mars.nasa.gov/technology/helicopter/).

The remarkable successes of human's escape from Earth's atmosphere at approximately 25,000 mph/40,233.6 km · hr^{-1}/7 mi · s^{-1}/11,265.4 km · s^{-1}, or 34 times the speed of sound and subsequent return, had its origins in antiquity when prophets and philosophers could only dream of contacting celestial bodies. From da Vinci's flying machine drawings five centuries ago to when modern science began successful hot-air balloon ascents during the mid-1700s, the obsession has not waned to explore the universe. By 2011, powerful rocketry and new aircraft design and composite materials kindled the possibilities for suborbital commercial "space tourism" adventures (www.cnbc.com/2020/09/26/space-tourism-how-spacex-virgin-galactic-blue-origin-axiom-compete.html).

The early jet flights were unable to test human responses to changing gravitational forces because that era's test aircraft could not accommodate specialized laboratory equipment. Nevertheless, knowing how to cope with the unique environmental stressors[24] (and health challenges) during high-altitude exposure still required new understanding unavailable from traditional medicine. The aerospace medicine field (www.asma.org) emerged from a need to deal with unconventional situations not encountered in normal **gravity (g or G)** but in **microgravity (µG)**. Aerospace medical research progressed using responses from mice, cats, dogs, monkeys, and eventually humans to spaceflight in µG. Throughout this chapter, we use the terms microgravity and µG interchangeably.

Research in µG progressed by creating space cabin simulators on Earth. Scientists focused on human psychophysiologic responses to changing gravitational forces and prolonged isolation while performing complex motor and mental tasks. The experience from simulations and manned suborbital flights provided new understanding about spaceflights' impact on human structure, function, and adaptation.

The United States is not the only country committed to future space exploration.

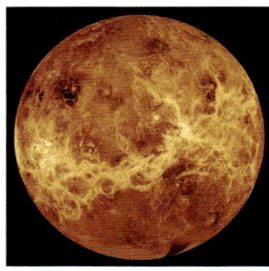
Credit: NASA/JPL-Caltech

Currently, 72 different government-sponsored space agencies have committed to long-duration mission (LDM) explorations into deep space, and a recent NASA goal is to land a rover on the planet Venus by 2030 (www.nasa.gov/press-release/nasa-selects-2-missions-to-study-lost-habitable-world-of-venus).

The Chinese National Space Administration (CNSA), European Space Agency (ESA), Indian Space Research Organization (ISRO), Japan Aerospace Exploration Agency (JAXA), the National Aeronautics and Space Administration (NASA), and Russian Federal Space Agency (RFSA or Roscosmos) can launch and recover multiple satellites, deploy cryogenic rocket engines, operate space probes, and conduct technical and animal and human research experiments in µG.[172,173]

Gravity

On Earth's surface, gravity provides an invisible attraction force that makes any mass exert downward force or have weight. Gravity behaves in the same fundamental way between Earth and any object on it, between any of the planets that revolve about the sun in our solar system, or between a planet and its moons. The gravitational law's universality, first proposed in 1687 by English physicist and mathematician **Sir Isaac Newton** (1642–1727), can be stated as follows and depicted in the **FIGURE 27.1** upper yellow insert.

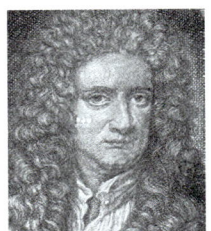
Morphart Creation/Shutterstock

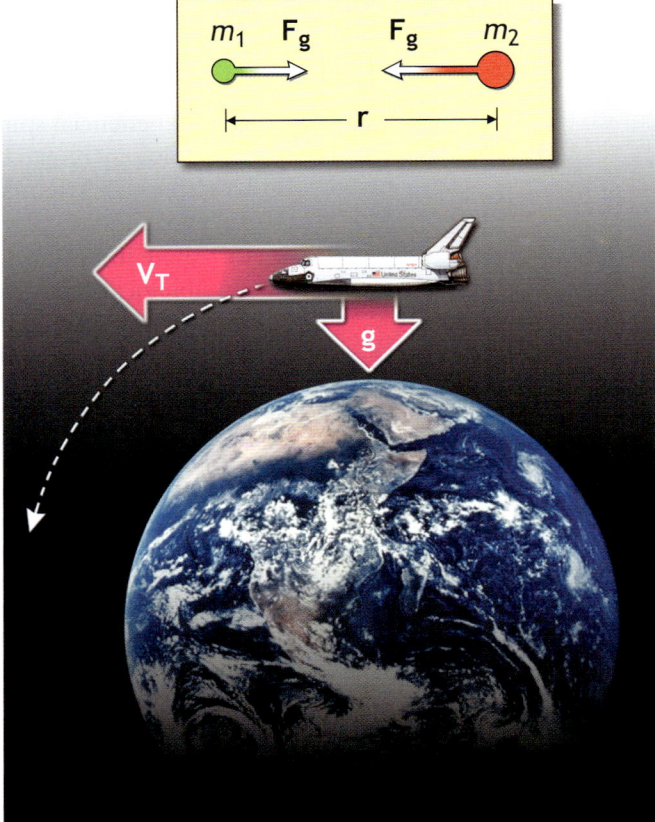

FIGURE 27.1. (Top yellow inset). Two different size masses (m_1 green and m_2 red), separated by a distance r, exert attractive gravitational forces (F_g) on each other. The forces on each particle have equal magnitude even when their masses differ markedly. No perceived force (i.e., weight) exists because nothing counteracts gravity's force.

Every particle within matter in the universe attracts every other particle with a force directly proportional to the product of the masses of the particles and inversely proportional to the square of the distance separating them.

—Sir Issac Newton

When a person sits in a chair on Earth, gravity's force pulls the person into the seat because the fixed chair provides an equal and opposite force (**Newton third law**). Every mass (m) on Earth requires support from a force (F) equal to its weight (w, in Newtons), such that $F_w = mg$, where m is mass in kg and g is acceleration of gravity (9.8 m·s^{-2}). Stated differently, the constant acceleration force per second of descent on a freely falling body at or near Earth's surface has a 1 g value or the acceleration due to gravity, with an equivalent magnitude = 9.80665 or 9.80 m·s^{-2}, 980 cm·s^{-2}, or 32 ft·s^{-2}. On the moon's surface, in contrast, the moon's attractive force but not Earth's causes gravity's acceleration, where g = 1.6 m·s^{-2}. Thus, someone on Earth who weighs 68 kg/150 lb would weigh 160.5 kg/354 lb on planet Jupiter (about 5.2 times farther away from the sun than Earth). Near the sun's surface, with a much larger mass than Earth, the moon, or Jupiter, the g value increases tremendously by a factor nearly 169 to equal 270 m·s^{-2}. In the near future when humans land on another planet or asteroid, as NASA's OSIRIS-REx mission did in 2018 to retrieve dust and pebble samples from the asteroid Bennu for return to Earth planned in 2023 (www.nasa.gov/press-release/nasa-s-osiris-rex-spacecraft-successfully-touches-asteroid), and to launch an unmanned spacecraft to asteroid 16 Psyche in August 2022 (www.smithsonianmag.com/smart-news/asteroid-16-psyche-may-be-worth-more-than-planet-earth-at-10-quintillion-in-fine-metals-180979303/). In the next decade when humans land on Mars, an astronaut's mass will remain the same as on Earth, yet the change in mass will be 38% the surface gravity on Earth—so the person's mass will be 38% the mass on earth.

When the first **astronaut**, Commander Neil Armstrong (1930–2012), stepped onto the moon' surface on July 20, 1969, he weighed one-sixth his 74 kg/165 lb Earth weight, or 12.5 kg/27.5 lb, because the moon's gravity is one sixth that of Earth. In essence, knowledge about an object's mass allows computing its weight; conversely, knowing weight allows for computing mass. The general equation $F_w = mg$ allows the conversion between mass and weight or weight and mass while accounting for the pull of g.

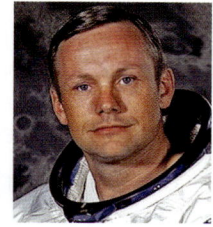
Credit: NASA

Microgravity and Weightlessness

To achieve an orbit around Earth or move away from it, the rocket velocity must exceed the downward pull attributable to Earth's gravity. The gravitational pull on a rocket decreases as it moves farther from Earth. When the rocket reaches a specified distance from Earth sufficient for orbit, a traveler experiences a weightless feeling because *nearly* all forces acting on the

fyi Gravity on the Moon and Mars

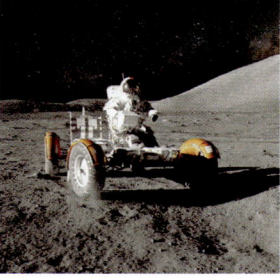
Castleski/Shutterstock

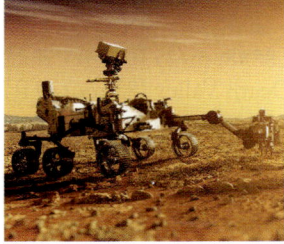
Evgeniyqw/Shutterstock

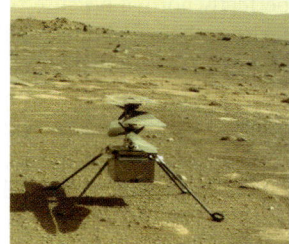
Credit: NASA

Gravity's effect on celestial bodies always remains a positive number because it represents the magnitude of a vector quantity. The attractive force on the moon's surface experienced by the 12 astronauts who walked there from the Apollo 11 to 17 missions produces a 1.6 m·s^{-2} g force, or approximately one sixth that on Earth. At the surface of Mars, the atmosphere is just 1/100th as dense as Earth's. This obstacle must be overcome because future Mars missions will require a spaceship to take off from the Martian surface, a feat comparable to flying at an altitude of 100,000 ft on Earth. Such a mission is conservatively scheduled for mid-2030 (the image shows Mars rover Perseverance, which landed successfully on Mars February 18, 2021). During this mission, astronauts will experience a g force of 3.7 m·s^{-2}, approximately 40% that on Earth's surface at sea level. On Mars, the lesser gravity—one third that on Earth—helps with getting airborne. But taking off from the Martian surface requires new technological advances and will be a monumental breakthrough comparable to flying at 100,000 ft above the Earth, more than two times the typical jetliner's average cross-country flying altitude. As a first step to achieve this goal, 117 years on April 19, 2021, after the Wright brothers succeeded in making the first flight on Earth, NASA's Ingenuity 49-cm/19.3-in-tall, 1.8 kg/4 lb solar-powered rotorcraft helicopter separated by 173 million miles from Earth, succeeded in lifting off the Martian surface to achieve another first "Kitty Hawk" moment in aviation history by achieving powered flight on a distant planet. (www.youtube.com/watch?v=GUqsH5y1j1M; www.youtube.com/watch?v=xVuk7vdurAw) Ingenuity achieved its planned maximum 3-m/10-ft altitude, maintaining a stable hover for 30 s before descending back to the Martian surface—overcoming substantially reduced gravity to achieve its primary and required objective.

Sources:
www.youtube.com/watch?v=qwdfdE6ruMw; www.nasa.gov/feature/jpl/nasa-s-ingenuity-mars-helicopter-reaches-a-total-of-30-minutes-aloft

body remain in balance. To reach a point in space where the gravitational pull from Earth equals one-millionth the force at Earth's surface requires traveling 6.37 million km/3.958 million mi, 16.6 times the distance from Earth to the moon, or 1400 times the highway round-trip distance between Olive Bridge, New York, and Orlando, Florida. In a practical sense, a rock dropped from a window 5 m/16 ft 3 in above the ground requires 1 s to touch the ground. In an environment with only 1% Earth's gravitational pull, the same drop would take 10 s. In a microgravity environment equal to one-millionth Earth's gravity, the same 5-m drop would take 1000 s or nearly 17 min.

Apparent Sense of Weightlessness

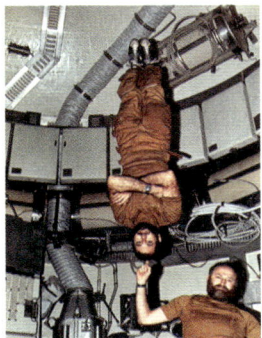

Credit: NASA

Spacecraft orbit Earth at a relatively close distance (typically 200 to 450 km/155/248 mi), so astronauts experience only an *apparent* sense of weightlessness. In essence, the force of gravity never truly reaches an absolute zero value (called **zero-g**) because some gravitational force still exists. Consequently, the term microgravity (µG), not weightlessness (or zero-g), correctly describes what astronauts feel during spaceflight in Earth's orbit when the rocket's altitude exceeds approximately 160 km/100 mi at a 28,200 kmh/17,500 mph velocity. In µG, as in this vintage Spacelab image, there is no "up" or "down." On Earth, we would view an astronaut static image (or video) who seems to us to be turned "upside down," yet the astronaut does not perceive this condition. To them, upside down seems perfectly normal because from their perspective it does not differ from being right side up! The same holds true if the image were turned horizontally or rotated 90° and viewed from a sideways perspective to literally defy our vision regarding what is "normal." The rotated image reveals that there would be no "correct" up or down. In effect, astronauts do not feel the gravity's effects as they are not pulled in any one direction, so they "float."

The ISS orbiting laboratory can carry a 29,479-kg/64,990-lb payload into orbit, with each main engine producing 170,068-kg/374,900-lb thrust at sea level burning a liquid oxygen and hydrogen mixture. After achieving orbital velocity, the astronaut and spacecraft continually accelerate toward a single point at Earth's center. They do not fall to Earth due to the planet's curved surface and because both craft and crew move at a fast enough tangential velocity (V_T) to the Earth (V_T and g shown in pink in Fig. 27.1). The spacecraft's speed creates an outward **centrifugal force** that "balances" the downward gravitational force on the spacecraft.

Microgravity refers to the perceived "weightlessness" associated with free fall. The forces acting on an astronaut orbiting Earth in a spacecraft are not balanced—both astronaut and spacecraft accelerate toward Earth's center. They do not "fall" to Earth because Earth's surface is curved and they move at a tangential velocity (V_T) high enough to "balance" gravity's downward force on the spacecraft. When spacecraft velocity decreases (reduced V_T)—a planned maneuver during reentry—the craft "plunges" toward Earth under gravity's pull.

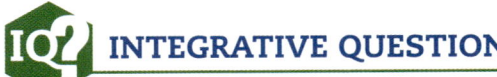

INTEGRATIVE QUESTION

How would a person's hemodynamic responses when moving from the upright to the upside-down position on Earth differ from those in a microgravity environment?

The International Space Station's 20th Anniversary

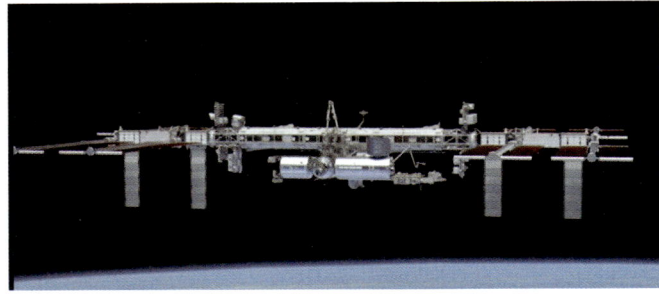

Credit: NASA

The International Space Station (ISS), one of the most ambitious engineering feats ever attempted, was a coordinated project involving the United States, Russia, Canada, Japan, and the European Space Agency's participating countries (www.nasa.gov/station20; www.nasa.gov/astronauts). On November 2, 2020, the ISS celebrated 20 continuous years in low Earth orbit, with NASA and university researchers contributing 2000 peer-reviewed journal articles (from more than 4000 scientists in multiple disciplines) detailing ISS research efforts to understand fundamental phenomena about the impact of spaceflight on humans and machines and to pave the way for future space exploration efforts. In 2005, the U.S. Congress designated the ISS a U.S. National Laboratory, to manage all non-NASA research and investigations involving microgravity and ISS-specific experiments to benefit the Earth and all its inhabitants.

Practical Example on Earth. Why does an apple hanging from a tree branch have a different gravity status than an apple lying below it on the ground? The gravitational force depends on the apple's mass and its distance from the Earth's center of mass. The apple hanging from the tree has *less* gravitational force acting on it than the fallen apple on the ground because it is farther from the center of the Earth's mass. Thus, a person would weigh less standing at the top of Earth's tallest mountain (e.g., Mt. Everest; 8848 m/29,030 ft) than when standing at the low point in Death Valley (85 m/279 ft) below sea level.

Parabolic Flights Simulate Microgravity. FIGURE 27.2A illustrates NASA's Reduced Gravity Program strategy to evaluate physiologic responses to microgravity produced when NASA's original Boeing KC-135 aircraft climbed rapidly at a 45° angle and then followed a parabolic path downward (www.nasa.gov/missions/research/kc135.html). The turbojet aircraft, originally designed for inflight refueling, produced a near–zero-g effect (1×10^{-3} g) for about 30 s (*center orange area* in the figure) when the aircraft achieved 9500 m/31,200 ft during the 10,000-m/32,800-ft ascent (termed *pull-up*) before it slowed. Air speed is referenced as KIAS (knots indicating air speed). The plane then traces a parabola (termed *pushover*), descending rapidly at a 45° angle (termed *pull-out*) to 7300 m. The acceleration and deceleration forces produce 2 to 2.5 times normal gravity (g) during pull-up and pull-out; the brief pushover at the apogee generated an environment with less than 1% Earth's gravity. In space, centrifugal force cancels the gravitational force and the orbiting spacecraft remains in continuous freefall (or microgravity). Figure 27.2B and C show tethered treadmill walking (B) and dynamic resistance training (C) during parabola practice.

Parabolic Flights and Astronaut Training

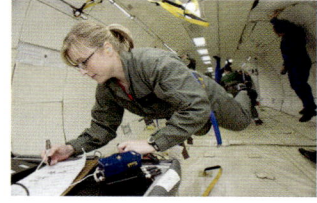
Credit: NASA

The nickname "**Vomit Comet**" aptly describes the gut-wrenching sensations produced during repeated brief parabolic roller coaster–like training maneuvers in a special aircraft to prepare astronauts for their microgravity space experience. These maneuvers met the need to evaluate how humans and on-board equipment functioned during intermittent forces ranging from 1.8 g to near–zero-g. The specialized flight training produced high g-forces equivalent to lift-off at 11,000 m·s^{-1} escape velocity (40,000 kmh/24,850 mph) when pulling away from Earth's downward gravitational pull.

Depending on the mission, astronaut training included up to 60 **parabolic flights** daily for a week, providing about 3-hr cumulative weightlessness while they performed simple to complex tasks.[126] From September 1995 to its final flight on October 29, 2004, the KC-135 had flown 34,757 training flights, an equivalent 300 flight hours yearly. Its DC-9 replacement remains useful as valuable training to understand microgravity's effect on humans and hardware in space. The European Space Agency, a valued NASA partner, relies on a "Zero-G" Airbus A300 so its passengers and cargo experience longer freefalling weightlessness in the parabolic arc maneuvers. The Airbus flies 31 parabolas daily, which equates to an annual microgravity effect achieved by a spacecraft during a 90-min Earth orbit (www.esa.int/Science_Exploration/Human_and_Robotic_Exploration/Research/Experience_weightlessness_on_board_the_Zero-G_Airbus). The Zero-G experience now is available to individuals living in the United States with flights from select airport destinations (www.gozeroG.com).

Bioastronautics and Space Research

Bioastronautics focuses on how spaceflight impacts biological and medical processes. The National Space Biomedical Research Institute (NSBRI) developed long-range research plans to mitigate the known and potentially unknown risks to astronaut health, safety, and mission performance.[36,41,128] In 2008, the NSBRI and NASA selected 33 research proposals to investigate questions about astronaut health and performance on future space exploration missions. The NSBRI supports research

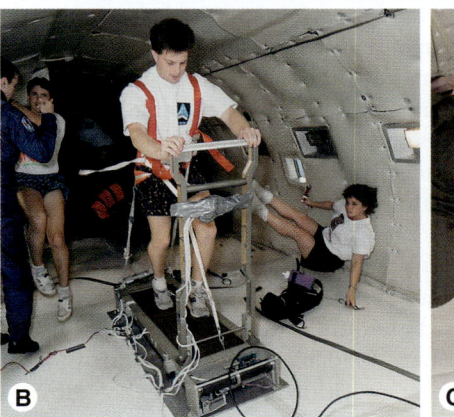
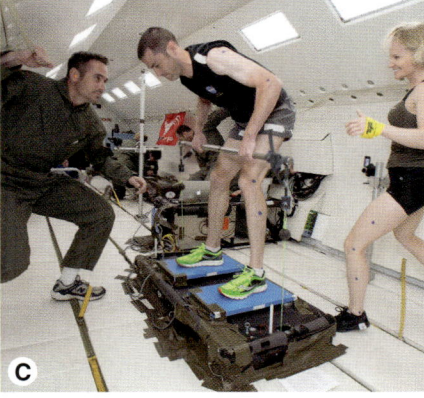

FIGURE 27.2. **(A)** Parabolic (Keplerian trajectory) flight profile of NASA's KC-135 aircraft to achieve brief periods of weightlessness. **(B)** Evaluating vibrations while treadmill running. **(C)** Evaluating static and dynamic balance during microgravity. (Graph: Reprinted from Nicogossian AE, et al. *Space Physiology and Medicine*. 3rd ed. Philadelphia: Lea & Febiger; 1994. Photos: NASA.)

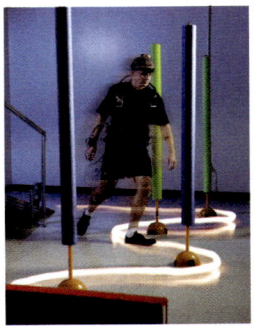
Credit: NASA

relevant to many exercise physiology topics. For example, the Human Factors and Performance Team studies ways to improve daily living and keep crewmembers and other personnel healthy, productive, and safe during exploration missions. The overall aims are to reduce performance errors and mitigate habitability, environmental, and behavioral factors that pose risks to mission success. NSBRI developed the initial guidelines for human systems design and information tools to support crew performance. They examined methods to improve sleep and work shift schedules,[102] including how lighting inside the spacecraft and the outside habitat effect an astronaut's alertness and performance. Other projects addressed improving interactions among spacecraft operation in automated and manual control modes, and how environmental factors such as dust and pollutants affect crew health. When the NSBRI was congressionally mandated by congress to end in 2017, a continuation program renamed TRISH (Translational Research Institute for Space Health; www.nasa.gov/hrp/tri) was created to promote relevant microgravity-related topic areas involving balance and coordination (www.bcm.edu/academic-centers/space-medicine/translational-research-institute; www.nasa.gov/sites/default/files/atoms/files/space_portal_trish.pdf).

Aerospace Physiology and Medicine Historical Overview

Astronauts must overcome numerous challenges as they prepare to live in space for extended durations. Perhaps during the middle of this century, thousands of individuals will routinely travel into space, some establishing permanent space colonies relatively near Earth orbit as in the current moon to Mars exploration approach with **Artemis missions** to the moon to prepare for future human Mars explorations (www.nasa.gov/artemisprogram).

Early Years

The first national civil aeronautics laboratory, now known as the National Aeronautics and Space Administration Langley Research Center, was established in 1917 in Hampton, Virginia. This facility currently focuses on aeronautics, earth science, space technology and structures, and materials research (www.larc.nasa.gov). In 1951, the Aeromedical Association created a Space Medicine Branch for systematic human function evaluation in a weightless environment (www.wpafb.af.mil). Two research laboratories, the U.S. Air Force School of Space Medicine and the Naval Aerospace Medical Institute (www.hq.nasa.gov/office/pao/History/SP-60/cover.html), also devoted time and resources to study space medicine. These military research facilities partnered with universities and private-sector laboratories to create a formidable team to study high-performance aircraft and unmanned guided missiles at high altitudes. Research eventually covered human adaptation to high-altitude exposure. This included development in the 1930s with pressurized suits to allow pilots to achieve higher altitudes than previously (15,240 km/9470 mi), paving the way for the 1961–1963 Mercury suborbital flights and eventual lunar missions.[93] From 1951 to 1957, the two laboratories produced information mostly about spaceflight "hardware" and also biomedical evaluations during suborbital flights with lower animal forms (bacteria, mice) and primates.[60]

Suborbital Flights

In December 1946, experiments sponsored by the National Institutes of Health at Holloman's Aeromedical Field Laboratory (and later at Wright-Patterson Air Force Base, Ohio, and White Sands Air Force Base, New Mexico) studied cosmic radiation's effects on fungus spores (unsuccessful, as the cylinders carrying the microbes vanished on re-entry) and how fruit flies survived without deleterious effects at 171-km/106-mi altitude. The **Albert Project** named for the monkey sealed in the V-2 rocket nose cone attempted to record respiration during spaceflight, but the mechanical apparatus failed just before launch and Albert perished. The mission was doomed anyway because the parachute recovery apparatus also failed on re-entry.

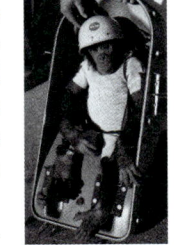
Credit: NASA

A second launch (Albert II) occurred 1 year later on June 14, 1949, but the primate died on impact when the recovery chute again failed to open. The first chimpanzee and hominid launched into space named HAM was trained at Holloman's Air Force Base, NM—hence, the name HAM for Holloman Aero Medical. Fortunately, respiratory and electrocardiographic instruments verified that the primate functioned well during the 83-mi ascent and return. Two additional V-2 rocket flights provided supportive evidence that a primate could successfully withstand 5.5-g re-entry forces and exposure to cosmic radiation.[108] A fifth V-2 launch substituted a mouse for the monkey, and an onboard camera photographed the mouse at fixed intervals.

The mouse died on impact (once again the recovery system failed), but the mouse displayed normal muscular function and coordination during the subgravity flight. Additional flights in 1951 that monitored cardiovascular and respiratory dynamics in primates showed no negative responses during these relatively brief missions.

With subsequent travel, rocketry systems improved and the onboard "animalnauts" survived intact during suborbital flights to 58-km/36-mi altitude (www.abc.net.au/radionational/programs/archived/animalpeople/animalnauts3a-animals-in-space/5617630). High-altitude balloon flights also proved successful. In September 1950, eight white mice withstood a 29,600-m/97,000-ft ascent without negative physiologic consequences. The balloon experiments continued with fruit flies, mice, hamsters, cats, and dogs for up to 24 hr. Most experiments ended in failure, mainly from equipment malfunction. Nonetheless, the invaluable experience gained from rocket and balloon launchings, instrumentation and recovery techniques, and considerable scientific about cosmic radiation and subgravity physiologic responses would greatly benefit subsequent human endeavors. The years 1946 through 1952 marked when Air Force research devoted time and resources to space biology (mostly with animals), setting the stage for future experimentation with more powerful rocketry (https://oarklibrary.com/search/result/fb328088-3653-4b4b-951e-612785e41d07?title=BIOSPEX3A20Biological20Space20Experiments).

High-Altitude Explorations

Between 1952 and 1957,[43] high-altitude research included human reaction to near–zero-g conditions, human re-entry into Earth's atmosphere, abrupt and sustained acceleration and deceleration on human response to rocket flight, and equipment design to better accommodate primate and human explorers as they pushed the envelope by ascending higher (36,576-m/120,000-ft balloon ascent) and for longer durations, up to 74 hr. In 1952, the National Advisory Committee for Aeronautics (NACA; established in 1915 to foster aviation) proposed new research to extend airplane velocity to Mach 10, from 19.3-km/12-mi to 80-km/50-mi altitude, and identify problems with spaceflights at speeds requiring escape velocity conditions from Earth's gravity.

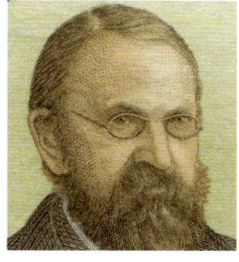

rook76/Shutterstock

Mach numbers were named to honor Austrian physicist Ernst Mach (1838–1916) who established basic principles in supersonics and ballistics. The Mach number represents the ratio of an object's velocity to the velocity of sound, which travels at 1089 ft·s^{-1}/331.9 m·s^{-1} at 0°C. For example, Mach 10 refers to 10 times the speed of sound. Interestingly, Professor Mach rejected Newton's concepts about absolute time and space before Einstein, who cited Mach's inertial theories in the early 1900s to develop his revolutionary theory about relativity.

By 1954, the flight characteristics for a new hypersonic research aircraft had been defined, and the North American Aviation manufacturing company won the competition to build the X-15 airplane (https://history.nasa.gov/x15/cover.html). Construction began in September 1957, ushering in a new era that featured high-performance aircraft capable of hypersonic speeds (6840 kmh/4250 mph) at altitudes close to 1079 km/671 mi/353 at the atmosphere's outer edges. Concurrently, the United States had committed to launch an Earth-orbiting satellite in the International Geophysical Year (July 1, 1957, to December 31, 1958) to gather scientific information about Earth. At the same time, developing a potential space vehicle and sophisticated satellite program were about to change in sudden and spectacular fashion.

Sputnik: The Rocket Launch That Shocked the World

On October 4, 1957, the Russians surprised the world when their 83.6-kg/184-lb, 58-cm/22.8-in-diameter aluminum alloy **Sputnik 1** became the first Earth-orbiting satellite. This beach ball–sized sphere took just 98 min to orbit the Earth on its elliptical path—and its journey sent shockwaves around the globe. As a technical achievement

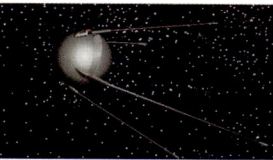

Okaypixel/Shutterstock

(www.nasa.gov/externalflash/SpaceAge/), Sputnik caught the world's attention and the American public and most public officials off-guard. Of major concern was the Soviets' ability to launch satellites translated into the capability to launch ballistic missiles that could carry nuclear weapons from Europe to the United States. After 57 days in orbit, Sputnik 1 was destroyed during its re-entry to Earth's atmosphere. One month later on November 3, a larger 508-kg Sputnik 2 remained in orbit for almost 200 days with a dog on board. These space milestones—achieved 4 mo before the Naval Research Laboratory launched its inaugural, tiny 1.6-kg/3.5-lb Vanguard 1 orbiting, unmanned satellite—jolted the United States' scientific and government establishments into a sense of urgency to surpass Russia's apparent space technology supremacy. Two factors contributed to a "space race" to achieve dominance in this new frontier:

1. Fear in relinquishing potential military superiority in space
2. Fear in trailing the "education race" to an enlightened Russian youth who excelled in mathematics and science

Modern Era

National Aeronautics and Space Administration

Reacting swiftly to the perceived Soviet technological superiority, the U.S. Congress passed the National Aeronautics and Space Act signed into law on July 29, 1958, by President Dwight D. Eisenhower. As a new federal agency, NASA began operation on October 1, 1958, less than a year after the successful Sputnik-1 launch. For the first time in U.S. history, a single government agency had responsibility for conquering a new frontier only dreamt about by the early aeronaut explorers.

Rapid Expansion

At its inception, NASA inherited 8000 employees and a $100 million budget; it supervised three major research laboratories (Langley Aeronautical Laboratory, Virginia, established in 1918; Ames Aeronautical Laboratory, California, founded in 1940; and Lewis Flight Propulsion Laboratory–officially renamed the NASA John H. Glenn Research Center at Lewis Field, Ohio, in 1999 created in 1941). NASA also supervised two smaller facilities at Monroc Dry Lake in the California desert for high-speed flight research and Wallops Island, Virginia, for testing rockets. NASA absorbed the Jet Propulsion Laboratory, managed by the California Institute of Technology, and the Army Ballistic Missile Agency, whose engineers were developing the massive rocket engines required for spaceflight. NASA assimilated the technical resources obtained from 13 prior years of jet aircraft research with the X-1 (achieved Mach 1) and X-2 rocket airplanes (achieved Mach 3), including engineering information gleaned from hundreds of other rocket and jet airplane flights.

Race to Become First in Space. NASA had two main goals in the race to become first in space:

1. Launching a man into space and returning him safely to Earth
2. Developing human capability to endure space missions[88]

Achieving the second goal had been a Herculean task because the current knowledge about how microgravity impacted human responses to actual spaceflight remained restricted to laboratory simulations. Scientists knew little about how humans would act in response to the rigors plaguing μG and what might happen during extended sojourns beyond Earth's gravitational field. Experts publicly expressed concern about possible deleterious spaceflight effects on human functions and overall health. In 1958, the National Academy of Sciences–National Research Council Committee on Bioastronautics listed 30 potential adverse outcomes shown in **TABLE 27.1** from human exposure to the space environment during launch and re-entry. Many of these concerns proved justified and are discussed in subsequent sections.

TABLE 27.1 Potential deleterious weightlessness effects launch through re-entry

In the competition to achieve status as the first major country to launch humans into space, scientists could not afford the luxury to conduct systematic research. Instead, a test pilot's prior flight experience provided "seat-of-the pants" solutions to important aeronautical questions. The fully pressurized flight suits Navy test pilots used during high-altitude reconnaissance became the first "space suits" during the early rocket missions. This allowed NASA to proceed on a fast track toward eventually rocketing the first human into space.

Experimental Aircraft Push the Flight Frontiers

The experimental X-1, X-2, and X-15 rocket aircraft were the predecessors of NASA's successful shuttle aircraft. The X-1 (top image) piloted by Air Force test pilot Chuck Yeager (1923–2020; https://history.nasa.gov/x1/chuck.html) made the world's first supersonic flight (Mach 1.45) by breaking the sound barrier on October 14, 1947. The X-2 (middle image) achieved Mach 3 on September 27, 1956. The X-15 achieved a world record 354,200-ft/67.1-mi altitude on August 22, 1963.

U.S. Races into Space

NASA's top priority besides initiating human spaceflight centered on a plan to allow humans to work for extended periods during prolonged space missions. NASA's two goals required advanced technologies in rocket design and effective approaches to prepare test pilots for missions never attempted previously. To put a human into Earths' orbit required new ways of looking at the man–machine interface. On the human side, engineers had to design a fail-safe life-support system, provide for food and water, integrate an efficient

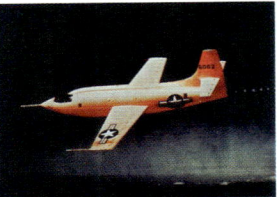
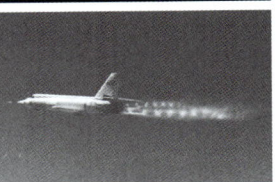
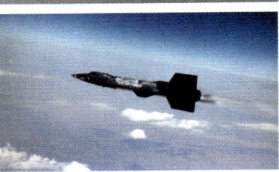

Credit: NASA

method to remove metabolic byproducts, and implement temperature control to ensure crew safety during liftoff, flight, and re-entry. Research had to determine physiologic responses to extremes of acceleration and reduced gravity, including short-term and long-term adjustments to prolonged weightlessness. Could a human function competently during liftoff, propelled upward at thousands of miles per hour, and then perform flawlessly in maneuvering the space vehicle and returning it to Earth safely? Engineers needed to develop rocket engines with sufficient thrust to achieve escape velocity. The pilot's capsule required intricate communication and navigation controls. The capsule's weight and size had to dovetail with rocket design and launch requirements. In addition, a capsule recovery system required development for safe re-entry. The human and engineering requirements facing NASA provided considerable challenges to say the least, and the race into space was on with no turning back.

U.S. Human Space Program

The key achievements of the U.S. and Russian space programs relate to advances in space medicine and physiology. These superpowers played the dominant role in the space effort but not without significant contributions from European, Japanese, and Canadian human space programs. Their remarkable successes culminated in the two 1998 launches of Russian and U.S. rockets to initiate assembling the ISS.

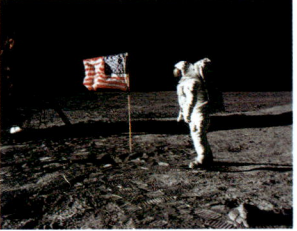

Perhaps the most significant technologic achievement of the 20th century took place on July 20, 1969, when **Apollo 11** astronauts Edwin "Buzz" Aldrin (1930–; www.buzzaldrin.com) and Neil Armstrong (1930–2012; www.nasa.gov/centers/glenn/about/bios/neilabio.html) landed on the moon's surface in the lunar module **Eagle**

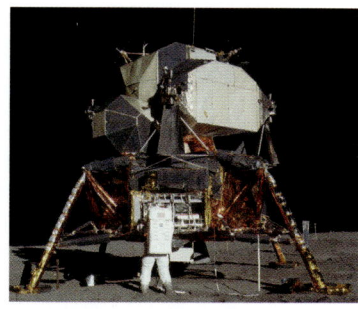
Credit: NASA

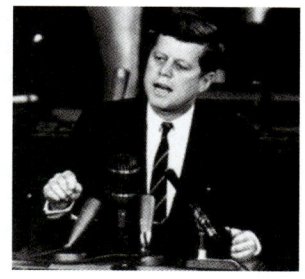

after it separated from the main spacecraft at 50,000 ft. The photo shows Aldrin, the lunar module pilot on the first moon landing mission, posing beside the deployed U.S. flag stiffened by inserts during the Apollo 11 moon mission on July 20, 1969. The module is darkly outlined on the left, and the astronaut's footprints are visible in the soil (foreground). With these words, "Houston, Tranquility Base here. The Eagle has landed," the world knew a momentous accomplishment had taken place.

Seven hours later, Armstrong's hopeful words as he set foot on the lunar surface—"*One small step for man, one giant leap for mankind*"—resonated worldwide to demonstrate that humans could travel to the moon, explore its surface, and return safely to Earth. Aldrin joined him on the surface several minutes later, and for 2 hr they collected rocks and took photographs. The image shows Aldrin removing the passive seismometer from a compartment from the Lunar Lander.

For this remarkable achievement, it had taken almost a decade and $25.4 billion to achieve the goal of putting a man on the moon.

During prior time periods, 12 early space milestones between October 1, 1958 and May 5, 1961 preceded President Kennedy's congressional moon speech to Congress committing to putting a man on the moon and return the crew safely to Earth.

On May 25, 1961, President Kennedy first stated the following to both houses of Congress:

*I believe that this nation should commit itself to achieving the goal, before this decade is out, of landing a man on the Moon and returning him safely to the Earth. No single space project in this period will be more impressive to mankind, or more important for the long-range exploration of space, and none will be so difficult or expensive to accomplish. (*www.youtube.com/watch?v=8ygoE2YiHCs*).*

Indeed, the Apollo program achieved its three main objectives with the highest marks of excellence: (1) ensuring crew member's safety and health, (2) preventing Earth's contamination by extraterrestrial organisms, and (3) studying how space exposure impacts the human body. During the pioneering and successful Apollo program, 12 astronauts walked on the moon during six lunar landings.

First Astronauts

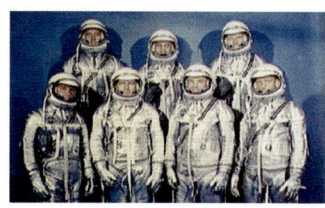
Credit: NASA

The test battery identified a final group of astronaut candidates believed best qualified to achieve the following five goals:

1. *Survive*: Demonstrate ability to fly in space and return safely
2. *Perform*: Demonstrate effective performance under spaceflight conditions
3. *Serve as backup for automatic controls and instrumentation*: Increase flight system reliability
4. *Serve as a scientific observer*: Go beyond what the instruments and satellites can observe and report
5. *Serve as an engineering observer and true test pilot*: Improve the flight system and its components

In April 1959, NASA pronounced that the final seven **Mercury astronauts** would only be males with commissions in the armed services and with considerable prior fighter pilot training and experience (www.nasa.gov/mission_pages/mercury/missions/astronaut.html). This elite group, selected from among hundreds of well-qualified candidates during an extraordinarily elaborate search and selection process, began training to enter an unknown environment with a life-support system previously tested only during high-altitude balloon flights. Those early balloon pioneers had been known as *Argonauts*.

Oct 1, 1958: Under the 1958 National Aeronautics and Space Act, NASA announces a manned spaceflight program six-days after its official formation
Jan 2, 1959: The U.S.S.R. launches Luna 1, which misses the moon but becomes the first artificial object to leave Earth orbit
Jan 12, 1959: NASA awards McDonnell Corporation the contract to manufacture the Mercury space capsules
Feb 28, 1959: NASA launches Discover 1, the first U.S. spy satellite
May 28, 1959: The U.S. launches the first primates, Able and Baker, who survive a 480 km/300 mi suborbital flight traveling 2700 km/1700 mi in 15 min
Aug 7, 1959: NASA launches Explorer 6, providing the first Earth photographs from space
Sept 12, 1959: The Soviet Union launches Luna 2 and then intentionally crashes it into the Moon
Sept 17, 1959: NASA's X-15 first powered hypersonic research plane flight
Oct 24, 1960: A Russian ICBM rocket explodes during launch preparations to send a vehicle into space killing 126 people
Feb 12, 1961: The Soviet Union launches a spaceship Venera to Venus, but the probe stops responding after a week
April 12, 1961: Yuri Gagarin (1934–1968) becomes the first man in space with a one orbit, 108-min flight on vehicle Vostok 1
May 5, 1961: Mercury Freedom 7 launches on a Redstone rocket for a 15-min suborbital flight with Astronaut Alan Shepard

Dotted Yeti/Shutterstock

In addition to medical screening and testing, NASA conducted retrospective and longitudinal studies of most male and female astronauts matched against a large control group of Johnson Space Center employees. A behind-the-scenes view of astronaut training, written by the astronaut candidates in the form of journals, provides insights from the time they entered the program through spaceflight (www.nasa.gov/centers/johnson/astronauts/journals_astronauts.html).

Decision to Exclude Females. While not made public at the time, a special flight-training program included a program for a final group of 13 highly qualified female aviators with extensive flight experience for future space missions. Shortly before the 13 finalists, referred to as **first lady astronaut trainees (FLATS)** were scheduled to report for testing, the Navy unceremoniously scuttled this effort, in part because of bureaucratic cronyism at the highest levels of the space agency.[2,61] Without official NASA support to conduct the tests, the Navy prohibited the use of their test facilities for this purpose. NASA's official position required that all astronauts be jet-test pilots and have engineering degrees. Because no women could meet those requirements (although by every account they were as qualified for flight status as their male counterparts), no women could qualify to become an astronaut! Interestingly, test pilot Geraldine (Jerrie) Cobb was the first and only woman to undergo and successfully pass all three phases of Mercury astronaut testing.[25]

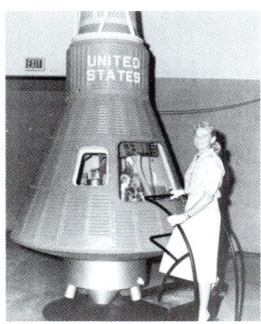

Cobb passed all of the training exercises and demanding medical tests, ranking in the top 2% compared with all astronaut candidates considered for the Mercury 7 crew (www.mercury13.com)! The lower image shows Cobb in the wind tunnel piloting the Gimbal Rig that trained astronauts to control a tumbling spacecraft's spin. Cobb's autobiography and other books provide insights into the male-dominated test pilot world and these women's zeal to become the first female NASA astronauts.[10,64,98]

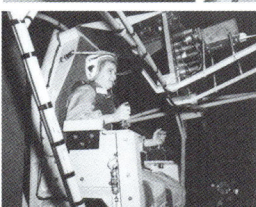

Credit: NASA

In October 1962, in its annual report to Congress, the House Committee on Science and Astronautics issued these recommendations from the subcommittee on astronaut qualifications:

After hearing witnesses, both Government and non-Government, including Astronauts Glenn and Carpenter, the subcommittee concluded that NASA's program of selection was basically sound and properly directed, that the highest possible standards should continue to be maintained, and that in the future, consideration should be given to inaugurating a program of research to determine the advantages to be gained by utilizing women as astronauts. (Report of the Special Subcommittee on the Selection of Astronauts: Qualifications for Astronauts. Committee on Science and Astronautics. U.S. House of Representatives. 87th Congress. Second Session. Serial S. Washington, DC: U.S. Government Printing Office, 1962.)

Ironically, it was Colonel John Glenn Jr (1921–2016) who did not have an engineering degree before he became one of the Mercury astronauts (and would have been eliminated from the program had NASA strictly enforced its regulations) testified to the committee as follows: "It is just a fact. The men go off and fight the wars and fly the airplanes and come back and help design and build and test them. The fact that women are not in this field is a fact of our social order. It may be undesirable."[114]

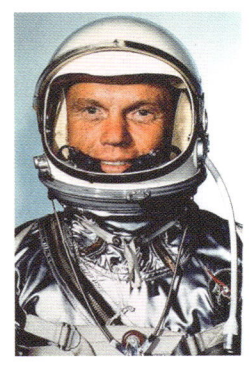

Glenn became the first American astronaut to circumnavigate Earth, piloting the 1962 Friendship 7 Earth orbit space mission (https://commons.wikimedia.org/wiki/File:KSC-JohnGlenn-0016_(31144904130).jpg). This historic flight was the longest duration studying physiologic responses following μG exposure. Thirty-six years later on October 29, 1998, at age 77, Glenn served as a Payload Specialist 2 on Shuttle Discovery STS-95 for an 8-day mission, becoming the oldest person at that time to be part of a scheduled space mission, which included studies involving bone and muscle loss, balance, and sleep disorders (www.nasa.gov/mission_pages/shuttle/shuttlemissions/archives/sts-95.html). Sixty years later, that age barrier was broken on July 20, 2021 (the same day of the Apollo 11 moon landing), when one of the original 13 FLATS pilots, Mary Wallace Funk, an 82-year-old female aerospace pioneer who had trained for the Mercury Program but was denied astronaut status because of her sex.[161] She broke Colonial John Glenn's age barrier a passenger aboard the first suborbital flight voyage on the private Blue Origin Space project (www.blueorigin.com/news/wally-funk-will-fly-to-space-on-new-shepard).

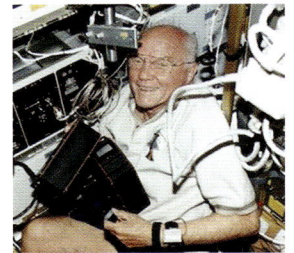

Credit: NASA

1978: Females Finally Become Astronauts It was not until 1978 that NASA first selected 6 women (then increased to 13) as astronaut candidates (www.thoughtco.com/mercury-13-first-lady-astronaut-trainees-3073474), 15 years *after* cosmonaut and engineer **Valentina Tereshkova** (1937-2019) from the USSR became the first woman at age 26 to rocket into space. During her 70.8-hr spaceflight on Vostok 6 over 3 days, she orbited Earth 48 times from June 17 to 19, 1963 (https://airandspace.si.edu/people/historical-figure/valentina-tereshkova).

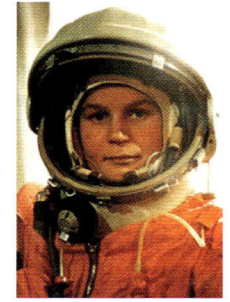

Her flight served as the first space mission where physiological measurements were collected about a female's acute μG responses.

Extravehicular Mobility Unit

The **extravehicular mobility unit (EMU)** astronaut space suits designed in the 1980s combined soft and hard components to provide support, mobility, and comfort compared to early spacesuits constructed entirely from soft fabrics. The 127-kg/280-lb suit (weight on Earth) has 13 different layers, including an inner cooling garment (two layers), pressure garment (two layers), thermal micro-meteoroid garment (eight layers), and outer cover (one layer). The materials include Kevlar used in bulletproof vests. The suits were designed to be fail-proof when the astronaut ventures outside the airlock into space to perform **extravehicular activity (EVA)**. The EMU has component pieces to fit astronauts of any size. In essence, the EMU serves as a "spacecraft" in and of itself, independent of the type of shuttle vehicle or space station.

Credit: NASA

Next-Generation Space Suits The latest generation spacesuit, the **exploration extravehicular mobility unit (xEMU)**, is designed for continuous EVA future deep space exploration missions, on the lunar surface, and eventually on Mars. (www.nasa.gov/image-feature/exploration-extravehicular-mobility-unit-xemu) The history surrounding the new spacesuit reveals a tale of engineering evolution traced from the Mercury spacesuits and upgraded Navy high-altitude flight suits.

Current suit testing takes place in the desert, underwater, and in specialized laboratories to simulate various gravity conditions. The red text bars describe the xEMU's various components and capabilities.

In the Anthropometry and Biomechanics Facility at NASA's Johnson Space Center (www.nasa.gov/hhp/index.html), astronauts undergo full-body, 3-D scans while performing basic motions and postures to be encountered during spacewalks. With a complete 3-D animated model, NASA can match the astronaut to the modular space suit components to provide the most comfort and broadest range of motion. The laboratory performs multi-joint motion tracking in complex environments (cockpits and cramped quarters, various depth craters) and maintains an anthropometry resource database based on suited and unsuited crewmember movement patterns.

Before the first astronauts reach the moon's lunar South Pole in 2024 (planned for one male and female), a $3.2 billion project in NASA's long-range Artemis moon shot program (www.space.com/artemis-program.html), the new suits and several of its components will undergo evaluation on the ISS to confirm their overall performance in a spaceflight environment.

NASA's Exercise Physiology Laboratory Countermeasures Program A guiding objective of NASA's Exercise Physiology Laboratory Countermeasures team (ExPC) is to assess astronaut's physiological responses to critical mission tasks (www.nasa.gov/content/exercise-physiology). Increasing time in the space environment has the potential to reduce overall fitness, which facilitates muscle and bone loss[197] and diminishes overall cardiovascular, pulmonary, endocrine, and basic metabolic functions. Consequently, understanding how exercise countermeasures per se,[119,185,202] or combined with other therapies, becomes crucial in mitigating such changes in future longer-duration missions to Mars whether directly from Earth or a spaceflight originating from the moon.

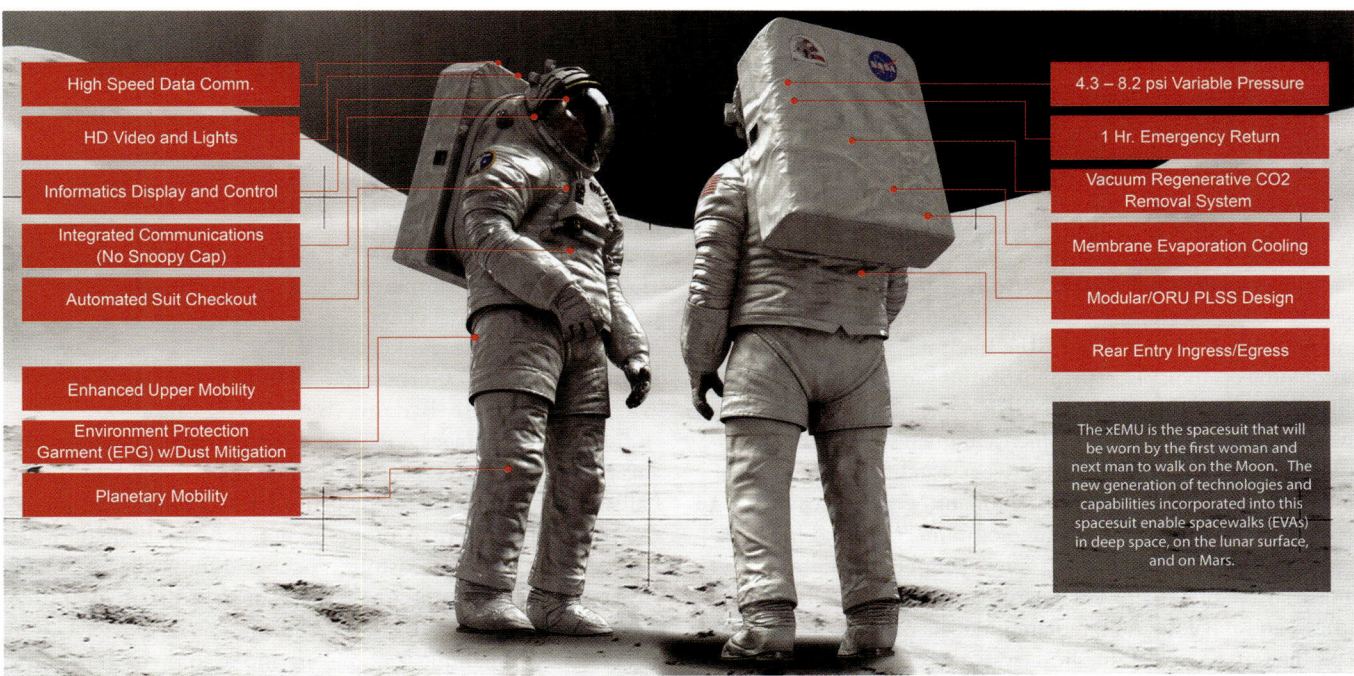

Credit: NASA

The ExPC has three main objectives:

1. Complete astronaut health and medical assessment testing requirements about musculoskeletal and aerobic fitness
2. Evaluate and validate new exercise countermeasures hardware and monitoring tools, exercise protocols, and conditioning programs to maintain crew health and performance during ISS missions and future longer-duration exploration missions
3. Quantify microgravity's effects on human physiology and performance during and following spaceflight

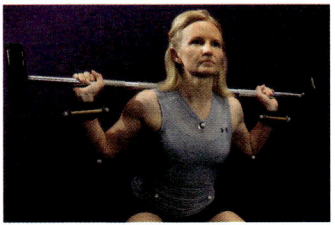

Credit: NASA

The ExPC has created multiple videos with detailed information about these three objectives. One example video explains the "Sprint" experiment with higher-intensity, lower-duration exercise techniques on the space station using a resistance device to simulate weight lifting workouts, an exercise bicycle, and workouts at different speeds and durations on the COLBERT (Combined Operational Load Bearing External Resistance Treadmill) treadmill (www.nasa.gov/hhp/exercise-physiology-videos). Astronauts on the Sprint protocol exercise half the number of times weekly (3-day instead of the 6-day adhered to by the "control" group), but the 3-day workouts were more intense and followed four different durations from 30 s to 30 min. The protocols were developed and funded by NASA based on 20-year ground research and 50-year prior spaceflight experience. Astronauts currently in training for future space missions gain considerable ground experience to optimize their individualized intense interval training countermeasure protocols to prepare them for "normal" 2.5 hr · d⁻¹ exercise currently undertaken on the space station.

National Space Biomedical Research Institute The NSBRI Research Program created in 1946 was eventually disbanded due to mandated NASA budget cuts. It represented an initial consortium involving 12 institutions that worked diligently on physiological and medical solutions to health problems related to longer-duration space travel and prolonged μG exposure.[192] The Institute's research and education projects took place at 75 institutions in 22 states involving almost 300 investigators. The NSBRI's primary mission objective was to ensure safe and productive human spaceflight. Established in 1997, the NSBRI had active research programs in bone loss, cardiovascular alterations, human performance factors, sleep, and chronobiology, immunology, infection, and hematology, muscle alterations and atrophy, neurobehavioral and psychosocial factors, neurovestibular adaption, nutrition, physical fitness, and rehabilitation, radiation effects on male and female reproduction,[187] smart medical systems, technology development, space medicine, and prolonged bed rest to determine its value as a nutritional countermeasure to muscle loss.[55,177,193]

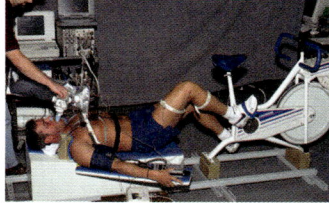

Credit: NASA

U.S. Air Force School of Space Medicine

The first national civil aeronautics laboratory, now known as National Aeronautics and Space Administration Langley Research Center, was established in 1917 in Hampton, Virginia. This facility currently focuses on aeronautics, earth science, space technology and structures, and materials research (www.nasa.gov/langley). In 1951, the Aeromedical Association created a Space Medicine Branch to evaluate human function in a weightless environment. Two new research laboratories (U.S. Air Force School of Aerospace Medicine [www.afrl.af.mil] and Naval Aerospace Medical Institute [www.med.navy.mil/Navy-Medicine-Operational-Training-Command/Naval-Aerospace-Medical-Institute/]) devoted resources to study space medicine. These facilities partnered with universities and private sector laboratories to create a formidable team to study high-performance aircraft and unmanned guided missiles at high altitudes, which eventually included human adaptation to this unconquered environment made possible by new pressurized suits, which allowed pilots to achieve altitudes up to 15.3 km/9.5 mi/50,000 ft higher than ever before. This breakthrough technology paved the way for the 1961–1963 Mercury suborbital flights and eventual lunar missions.[82]

From 1951 to 1957, the two new laboratories and auxiliary support facilities produced information mostly about "hardware" penetration into space and also biomedical evaluations during suborbital flights between 1948 and 1969 with lower animal forms (bacteria, microscopic invertebrates, fruit flies, tortoises, frogs, spiders, mice, dogs) and 33 monkeys and apes (https://history.nasa.gov/animals.html). A biological payload record was set on April 17, 1998, when Shuttle Columbia (STS-90) included two thousand creatures onboard for a 16-day mission involving intensive neurological animal testing on project Neurolab[178] in cooperation with the U.S. National Institutes of Health (NIH) and international partners (https://humans-in-space.jaxa.jp/en/).

German Rocket Scientists Strengthen NASA's Efforts

Progress in the embryonic aerospace physiology[97] and medicine fields accelerated following World War II, primarily from impetus provided by the successful bomb-carrying rockets launched by the German Air Force against Britain

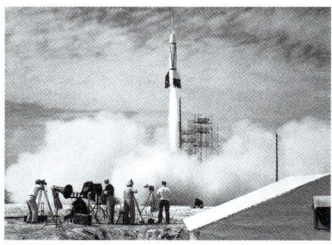

Everett Collection/Shutterstock

in the war's late stages. German scientists who pioneered the successful V-2 rocket, the world's first operational long-range ballistic missile, immigrated to the United States and joined the rocket development program at the Army Ballistic Missile Agency of the Redstone Arsenal, Huntsville, Alabama (https://nasa.fandom.com/wiki/Army_Ballistic_Missile_Agency). After the war, the United States and Soviet Union seized many remaining V-2 rockets and used them in research that culminated in future space exploration programs. On October 24, 1946, a V-2 rocket took the first-ever photo of

Earth from space. Launched from the White Sands Missile Range in New Mexico (featuring a museum "Missile Park" with early rockets on display; www.nps.gov/whsa/learn/historyculture/white-sands-missile-range.htm), the rocket carried a 35-mm motion picture camera to an 105-km/65-mi altitude, where a brief video shows that launch (www.youtube.com/watch?v=REDFzXoagqY). By 1950, the U.S. military had capitalized on German rocket technology and launched new V-2 style rockets and advanced high-altitude balloons that carried primates and other animals into suborbital space. With war no longer a major threat, research concentrated on developing more-sophisticated and powerful rocket engines capable of catapulting humans into Earth orbit.

Early Soviet Human Space Program

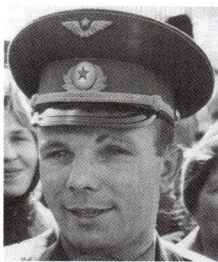

The Soviet human space program began in 1957 when Sputnik 1 crystallized the United States' efforts to join the race into space. The first Soviet cosmonaut in space, Lt. Colonel **Yuri Gagarin** (1934–1968), prepared for manned spaceflight as a test pilot in the Vostok program. On April 12, 1961, Gagarin completed a single Earth orbit in 108 min and ejected from the Vostok spacecraft at 7000 m/23,000 ft in a parachute landing. The Soviets withheld the news that Gagarin might have perished when the Vostok spacecraft malfunctioned on re-entry. His safe return scored another key space victory for the Soviet Union in their quest for space supremacy. Longer-duration missions for up to 5 days followed this historic flight. Following the Vostok missions, the two succeeding Soviet missions, named Voskhod, advanced space science by completing the first EVA that lasted 8 min by cosmonaut Alexei Leonov (1934–2019), who exited the spacecraft through a canvas tube attached to Voskhod 2, and medical lung function and middle-ear (vestibular) function studies, blood pressure, muscular strength (hand grip), and blood composition from the first blood sample taken during weightlessness by Dr. Boris Yegorov (1937–1994), the first space physician.

Soviet Manned Flight Space Missions

The next period of Soviet exploration included manned flight aboard the advanced Soyuz 1 spacecraft, but a tragic accident stalled several planned rendezvous and docking missions. In January 1969, Soyuz flights 4 and 5 completed mission-critical maneuvers (rendezvous, docking, EVA transfer) for a future moon landing. Unfortunately, four unmanned spacecraft designed to test a powerful booster rocket needed to achieve moon orbit exploded on launch, canceling that phase of the program. One year later, the 18-day Soyuz mission included extensive experiments to evaluate microgravity's

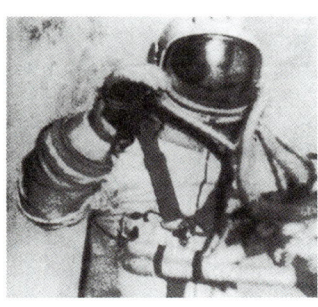

effects on heart function, vision, muscular strength, and hematologic variables[151]. Unfortunately, an inflight exercise countermeasures effort did *not* reduce problems experienced with balance (one aspect of **orthostatic intolerance**) and muscle weakness.

April 19, 1971, marked the launch of the world's first space station Salyut-1. Forty-nine days later, three cosmonauts from Soyuz-11 boarded Salyut-1 to become the space station's first crew. Over the next 6 years, the Soviets launched four additional Salyut space stations, the cosmonauts performing biomedical experiments on 24 missions, 10 involving humans, yet only 5 experiments categorized as successful. The longest

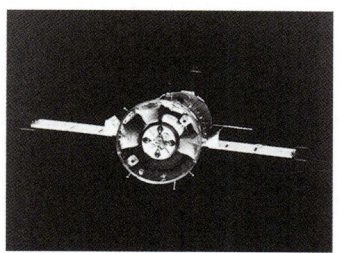

mission (Soyuz-18) lasted 63 days. Subsequent missions on advanced Salyut-6 and Salyut-7 space stations lengthened flight duration and increased the number of crew members. Between 1977 and 1981, five, two-man crews completed flights ranging from 96, 140, 175, 185, and 74 days. Thirteen other crews completed shorter flights. During the Salyut-6 program, the Soviets accumulated about 3-year flight experience and 5-hr devoted to EVA. In 1982, two cosmonauts accumulated 211 days in orbit. American and Soviet cooperation in space commenced during July 15–24, 1975, with the first docking of an Apollo spacecraft with a Soyuz spacecraft (Apollo–Soyuz Test Project or ASTP). This mission established the basis for future American-Russian cooperation between the American Space Shuttle and Mir Space Station. The 143-ton Mir, almost twice as heavy as Skylab (76 tons/152,000 lb) and the largest manufactured object in space ($4.2 billion to build and maintain), was purposely deorbited after 15-year achieving unprecedented scientific advances (46 expeditions and 23,000 experiments, including the longest continuous space mission [438 days] and 16 spacewalks totaling 77 hr). Mir plunged in fiery descent from the Earth's atmosphere into the Pacific Ocean on March 22, 2001. Twenty-two years earlier, the United States first space station Skylab, despite three repair attempts to save this science space station from failure after only 6 years in orbit, also met a fiery re-entry from Earth's atmosphere (www.nasa.gov/mission_pages/skylab). A recent Soyuz MS-18 successful flight occurred on April 9, 2021, nearly 60 years following the first Soyuz-1 orbital flight on April 23, 1967, which ended in a crash landing, killing the pilot Vladimir Komarov (1927–1967: www.nasaspaceflight.com/2021/04/soyuz-ms18-launch-docking/).

Early Chinese Human Space Program

China has established an extensive Human Space Program (www.space.com/topics/china-space-program). On October 15, 2003, China became the third nation to independently launch an astronaut into Earth orbit from the Jiuquan Satellite Launch Center (JSLC) in northwest China's Gansu Province. Ten minutes after lift-off, the modified Russian Soyuz capsule module entered an initial 200- to 343-km/120- to 250-mi orbit piloted by 38-year-old Lt. Col. Yang Liwei (1965–),

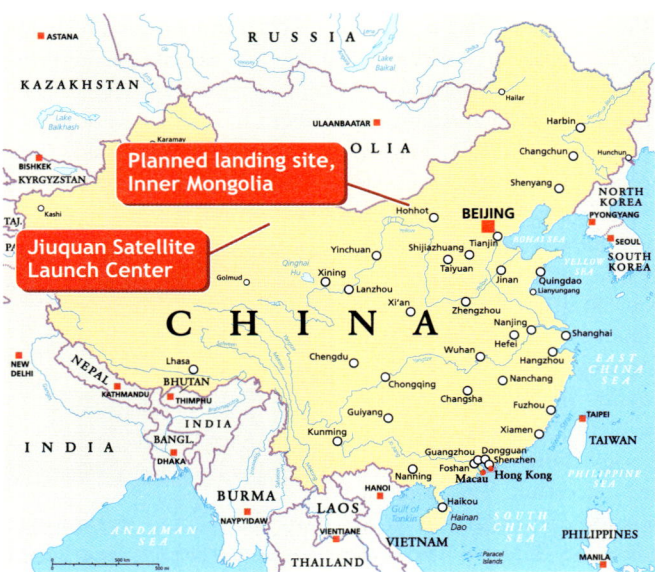

Peter Hermes Furian/Shutterstock

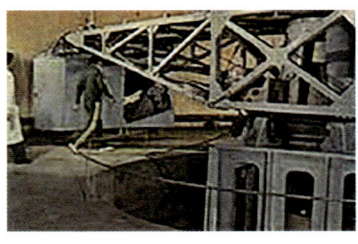

China's first man in space. The map shows the JSLC location and the anticipated grasslands landing site in Inner Mongolia for the re-entry, kettle-shaped capsule, which ended up touching down only 4.8 km away. The single-pilot flight circled the globe 14 times in the 21-hr, 31-min–long mission, which catapulted China into an initial elite three-nation group capable of independent human spaceflight.

The unmanned ShenZhou-3 flight, a precursor flight to a manned mission, launched in March 2002, lasted 6 days, 18 hr, 51 min during 107 orbits with life-support and emergency escape systems and a dummy astronaut to test life-support system reliability. Nine months later (December 30, 2002), ShenZhou-4 launched carrying a fully functioning crew module with two dummy astronauts to assess viability for the planned ShenZhou-5 manned launch. The spaceship carried 52 science payloads for Earth observation, space environment monitoring, microgravity fluid physics, and biotechnology research. The spacecraft remained in Earth orbit for 7 days and completed 107 orbits.

Chinese Astronauts

Training Chinese astronauts began in 1968 at China's Spaceflight Medical Research Institute to investigate physiological responses to the space environment (https://chinaspacereport.wordpress.com/programmes/astronaut-selection-training/). The once secret program, named *Project 714*, began with 80 candidates from a pool of 1800 fighter pilots. A final group of 20 astronaut trainees continued to train until the program was cancelled in 1975 from poor funding and minimal political support. In 1995, China and Russia signed a cooperative agreement to share aerospace technologies that included spacecraft capsule design and life-support systems. Twenty astronauts currently comprise the Chinese Astronaut Corp.

In the 1980s, the first Chinese astronauts trained on a spaceflight dynamic simulator (centrifuge; shown in the image) and vacuum chamber testing to monitor physiological responses to increasing G forces and confined space activities. Current astronaut training and space medical research take place at its primary training facility inside the Beijing Aerospace City facility (https://chinaspacereport.wordpress.com/facilities/beijing/), a square-mile campus located in Tang Jialing in the northwest Beijing suburbs. In April 2021, the China Space Agency (CAST) announced plans to take their astronauts to the moon (www.space.com/china-new-spacecraft-crewed-moon-missions.html) with a new next-generation spacecraft (www.space.com/34077-china-launches-tiangong-2-space-lab.html) and a future competing **Hubble Space Telescope** (www.space.com/china-space-station-module-tianhe-ready) as part of their own orbiting Tiangong space station (www.space.com/china-space-station-core-module-launch-spring-2021), in which three Chinese astronauts successfully boarded the space station's core module for a 3-mo mission that began June 17, 2021 (https://spaceflightnow.com/2021/06/17/chinese-astronauts-enter-tiangong-space-station-for-first-time/).

Spaceflight Physiology

On Earth, the human body remains remarkably adaptable to almost all environmental challenges from deep sea free diving to hostile desert climate survival to frozen ice sheets in high-altitude mountain climbing. Space physiology and medicine is now a mature discipline, having made great strides during a half century of human spaceflight. Researchers have a good appreciation about the medical problems associated with short-duration spaceflights and for the most part have successfully developed effective **countermeasure strategies**. The new challenge for nations preparing for longer-duration space missions is first to re-explore the moon in 2024 and then to develop a viable plan to travel from the moon's surface to Mars, hopefully within the next two decades (www.nasa.gov/topics/moon-to-mars/overview).

The major challenges currently facing space medicine researchers is to focus efforts on the physiologic consequences of establishing suitable working environments in µG where normal gravitational loading essentially does not exist as it does on Earth.[179] This single challenge focuses on how best to mitigate health risks astronauts must overcome through a well-designed, validated countermeasures program. In the sections that follow, we give an overview of how the body's major physiological systems respond to short-duration and longer-duration space missions conducted over the past 50 years.

Bone

Spaceflight has produced considerable biomedical information regarding human physiology during µG, beginning on May 5, 1961, with astronaut Alan Shepard's (1923–1998) solo flight aboard Freedom 7 (http://history.nasa.gov/40thmerc7/shepard.htm). This capstone event launched suborbitally to 187 km/116 mi above and 488 km/303 statute

Three Tissues on a Chip Microgravity Research Projects

Study 1. Disease and Drug Research. Tissue chips contain small cell clusters or tiny organoids that grow on chip scaffolding, a new method in regenerative medicine, to form 3-D structures to allow astronaut-researchers to manipulate the chips to mimic different disease types (www.issnationallab.org/iss360/revolutionizing-medicine-with-organs-on-chips/). The primary aim is to discover new pharmaceutical treatments as countermeasure strategies. This experimental paradigm should lead to a better understanding about how the body's major organ systems—heart, liver, kidney, gut, muscle, and lung—might respond on two space exploration missions: travel to and from Mars, and living for extended durations in newly established moon habitats and eventually permanent base camps on Mars.

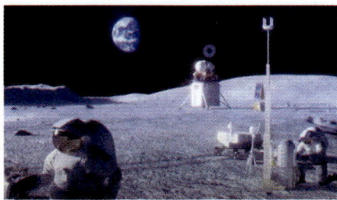
Credit: NASA

Study 2. Kidney Stones. Chip research is investigating kidney stone formation, a hard mass formed in one or both kidneys from minerals in urine. Various size stones form when urine cannot dilute the waste chemicals calcium, oxalate, and phosphorous, which then become concentrated to create mainly calcium oxalate crystal stones. Prior research on 8- to 16-day missions had planned for an unexpected kidney stone attack, prompting astronaut training before the mission to include a surgical procedure with sound waves to destroy the stones until they would become small enough to pass. Now, researchers want to understand *why* microgravity might rapidly produce kidney stones, and if they occur on a long-duration exploration mission, what technical strategy can mitigate the medical emergency.

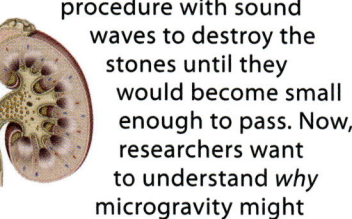
ilusmedical/Shutterstock

Study 3. Muscle Atrophy in Space. Analysis will include 16 skeletal muscle tissue samples from younger physically active individuals and 16 older more sedentary volunteers. Half the tissue samples in each group will receive electrical stimulation to determine how microgravity alters muscle tissue contractility, and in additional separate experiments, alters muscle tone, viscoelasticity, and biomechanical properties of the myofascial system reflected by changes in bloodborne biomarkers (e.g., matrix metalloproteinases) related to connective tissue and extracellular matrix component remodeling. On-going research serves as a starting point to assess how different pharmacologic and exercise therapies could mitigate muscle's ultrastructural component degradation in space and rehabilitation on Earth.

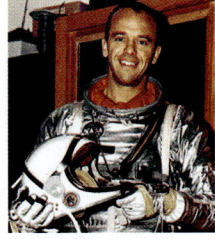
Credit: NASA

mi downrange from the Cape Canaveral launch complex. His 15-min, 28-s flight attained a final 8262-kmh/5134-mph velocity and pulled a maximum 11 g. From this point on, the race had begun for NASA to explore uncharted paths outside of Earth's gravitational pull. In the ensuing 50 years, researchers quantified physiologic adaptations to relatively brief space missions (1 to 14 days) and flights lasting longer than 2 wk, including postflight adaptations.

FIGURE 27.3 displays a generalized schema involving two physiologic function dynamics during μG exposure:

1. Reduced hydrostatic gradients (purple box left with white text)
2. Reduced loading and disuse of weight-bearing tissues (purple box right with white text)

The figure reveals how these two factors impact the following six systems:

1. Cardiovascular and cardiopulmonary (orange)
2. Hematologic (dark blue)
3. Fluid, electrolyte, and hormonal (red)
4. Muscle (green)
5. Bone (light blue)
6. Neurosensory and vestibular (aqua)

Each color-coded system has arrows indicating how one system might influence another. For example, trace the pathways between a decrease in hydrostatic gradients and reduced total blood volume. How many different pathways interact to reduce total blood volume? Similarly, trace how altered sensory and balance information also affects blood volume and maximal exercise capacity. All of the different systems impact singularly yet often interact with each other, with all being impacted by the two main factors: reduced hydrostatic gradients and unloading and disuse in weight-bearing tissues, attempting to unravel the separate yet compounding influences the six main systems impact. Two of NASA's main research efforts focus on the impact related to reduced bone density on bone fracture risk and functional impact risk of skeletal muscle atrophy (reduced strength) on performing mission-related tasks.[87,118]

These physiologic responses to microgravity, in addition to the heart's reduced stroke volume related to orthostatic hypotension and possible syncope,[39] have implications for developing and testing effective countermeasure strategies. Excellent summary resource materials exist about the body's cardiovascular, pulmonary, body fluid, sensory, bone loss, and musculoskeletal responses to microgravity.[18,29,44,45,47,52,56,77,131,148,162]

Lippincott® Connect Appendix K, available online at Lippincott Connect, provides a list of popular Web sites related to microgravity.

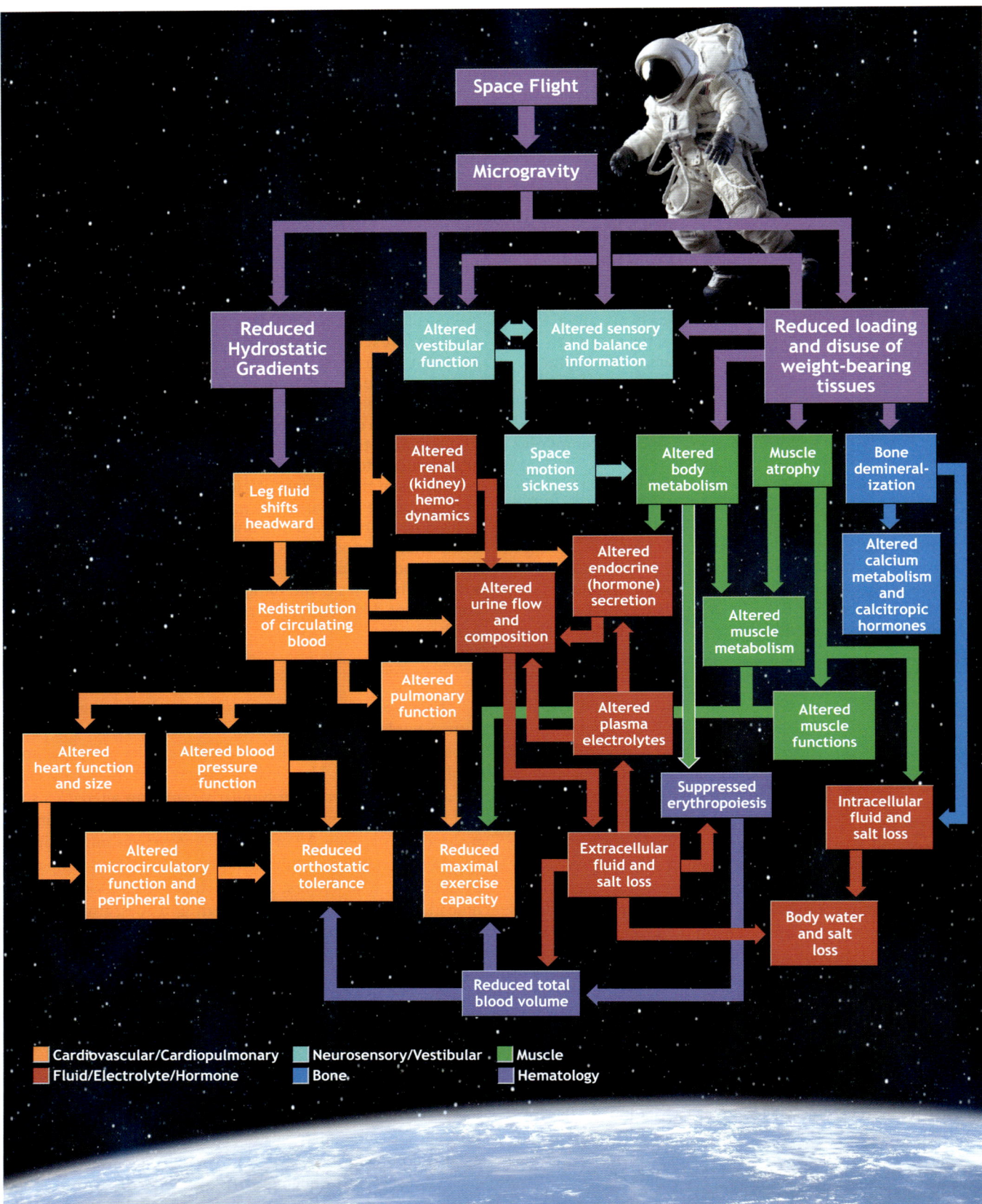

FIGURE 27.3. NASA's general schema of microgravity's effects on physiologic alterations from reduced hydrostatic gradients and reduced loading and disuse of weight-bearing tissues.
(Adapted from NASA. Earth photo: Tony_Traveler85/Shutterstock.)

Cardiovascular Adaptations

The decrease in total fluid volume during the first few days in µG reduces the heart's total work effort. With continued µG exposure, overall heart size decreases mainly from reduced left ventricular end-diastolic volume. Such adaptations represent an appropriate response to microgravity without compromising a mission's "normal" cardiovascular functions.[54]

TABLE 27.2 summarizes adaptations in 15 cardiovascular variables during pioneer space missions, while **FIGURE 27.4A** displays preflight-to-postflight changes in stroke volume in upright exercise expressed as a percentage of preflight baseline. Figure 27.4B also displays changes in $\dot{V}O_{2max}$ related to exercise intensity and frequency during 20-min inflight cycle ergometer exercise bouts on four different missions.[191] The $\dot{V}O_{2max}$ declined in the training regimen, except for group 1, which maintained HR above 130 b·min^{-1} and exercised longer than 20 min more than three times weekly.

> **TABLE 27.2** Cardiovascular adaptations during pioneer space missions

Experiments have measured changes in cardiac function (left and right ventricular mass and left ventricular end-diastolic volume) assessed by magnetic resonance imaging to isolate whether microgravity *per se* or frank atrophy from physical inactivity produced changes in cardiac loading functions. In four astronauts on a 10-day mission and in controls on Earth measured at 2-, 6-, and 12-wk bed rest and 6-wk routine daily activities, left ventricular mass declined by 12% (67.9%). Cardiac atrophy occurs both during relatively long 6-wk horizontal bed rest periods (inactivity) and after short-term spaceflight (microgravity). These findings suggest that physiologic adaptation to reduced myocardial load and work in real or simulated microgravity produces the cardiac atrophy, demonstrating the plasticity of cardiac muscle under different loading conditions.[105]

Pulmonary Adaptations

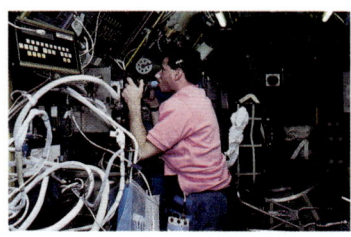

A tight linkage exists between the cardiovascular, pulmonary, and metabolic systems. The cells' demand for oxygen during rest and physical activity remains invariant in all environments. Any increase in external work above a resting baseline immediately triggers an increase in breathing rate and tidal volume. Consequently, augmented alveolar ventilation maintains an adequate pressure differential for oxygen diffusion across lung tissues delivered in response to increased energy metabolism. The image shows an astronaut performing automated lung function testing. This included rib cage and abdominal movements during deep breathing to assess lung gas distribution patterns when inhaling different gas mixtures and different inhaled and exhaled gas volumes and concentrations before and following different exercise durations and exercise modes. **TABLE 27.3** summarizes changes in pulmonary variables during two Spacelab missions.

> **TABLE 27.3** Changes in pulmonary variables during two Spacelab missions

FIGURE 27.5 depicts changes in pulmonary carbon monoxide (CO) diffusing capacity measured preflight on days 2, 4, and 9 during the mission and within 6 hr before or after landing, and then at days 1, 2, 4, and 6 postflight. Values are presented as a percentage of preflight standing CO diffusing

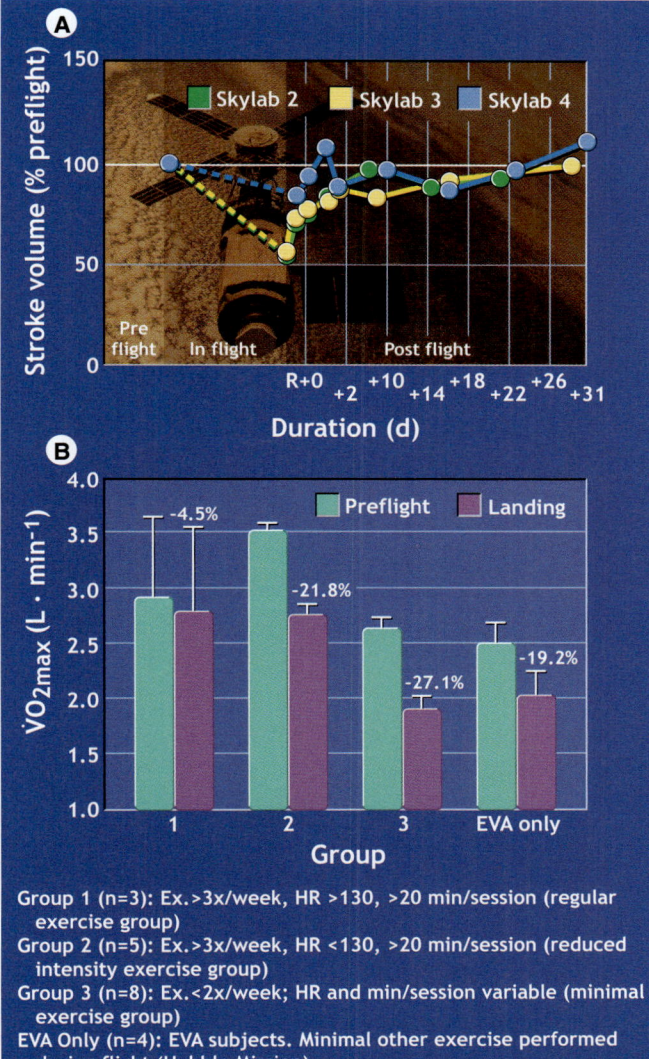

FIGURE 27.4. Postflight to preflight changes in **(A)** stroke volume during upright exercise (Skylab 2 to 4; R, return to Earth) and **(B)** aerobic capacity related to 20-min inflight cycle ergometry intensity and frequency.
(Data for **A** from Michel EL, et al. *NASA SP-377*. Washington, DC: U.S. Government Printing Office; 1977, and data for **B** from Sawin CF. Biomedical investigations conducted in support of the extended duration orbiter medical project. *Aviat Space Environ Med.* 1999;70:169. Background photo: Everett Collection/Shutterstock.)

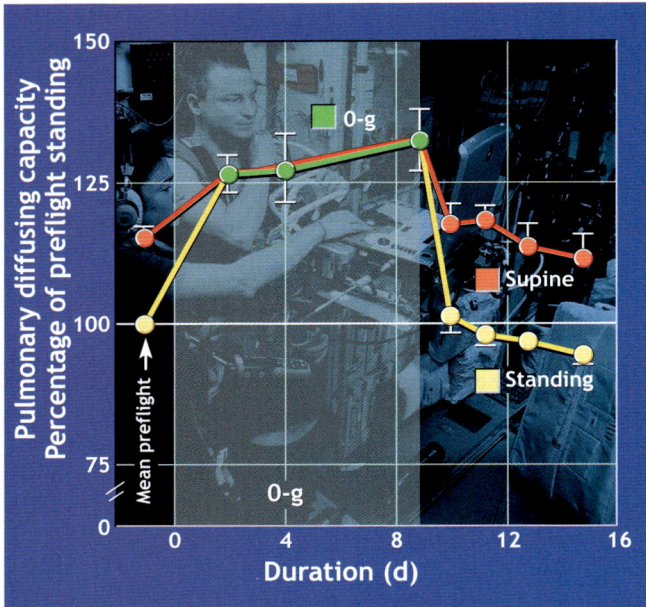

FIGURE 27.5. Pulmonary diffusing capacity for carbon monoxide preflight on flight days 2, 4, and 9 and 6 hr following landing and on days 1, 2, 4, and 6 postflight. (Data referenced to the preflight standing value.)
(Graph: adapted with permission from Prisk GK, et al. Pulmonary diffusing capacity, capillary blood volume, and cardiac output during sustained microgravity. *J Appl Physiol*. 1993;75:15. ©The American Physiological Society (APS). All rights reserved. Photo: NASA.)

capacity. Note that diffusing capacity increases in the sitting and standing positions during 3 days in microgravity and then returns to preflight baseline values.

Denitrogenation and EVA

Before astronauts perform EVA maneuvers, they must "wash out" the nitrogen from their fluids and tissues to prevent decompression sickness (DCS or bends) from differentials in gas pressures within the cabin and EVA garment.[19,40,112] They do this by using a 10.2 lb per square inch atmosphere (psia) staged decompression of the shuttle for at least 12 hr. This also includes 100 min of **preoxygenation**, breathing 100% O_2 at 14.7 psia prior to decompression and before decompression to the suit pressure of 4.3 psia (equivalent to 9144-m/5.7-mi altitude). Scientists have proposed several ways to induce **denitrogenation**. First, reduce the total pressure inside the spacecraft from 760 to 630 torr, the approximate barometric pressure of Denver, Colorado, to shorten overall time for denitrogenation prior to EVA. Second, have astronauts sleep in a special low-pressure compartment prior to EVA. One-hr preoxygenation during exercise improves resistance to DCS, illustrating the potentially positive exercise effect on ameliorating DCS during critical mission EVA maneuvers.

Body Fluid Adaptations

FIGURE 27.6 shows data for percentage changes in plasma volume and red cell mass (A), total hemoglobin (B), and orthostatically stressed heart rate percentage change versus blood volume percentage change (C) on different duration

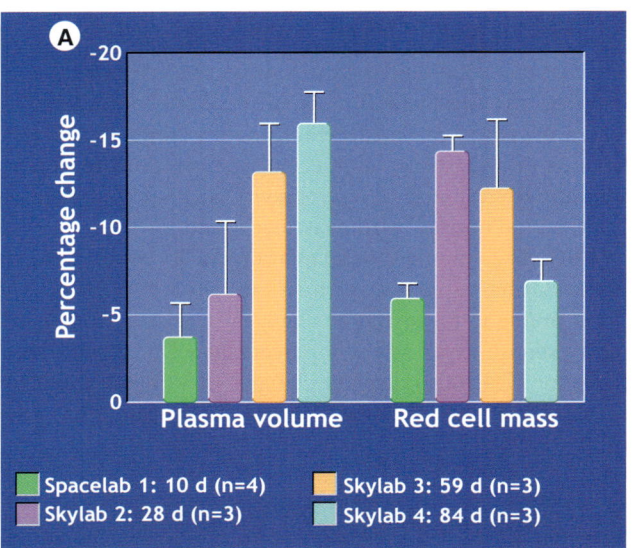

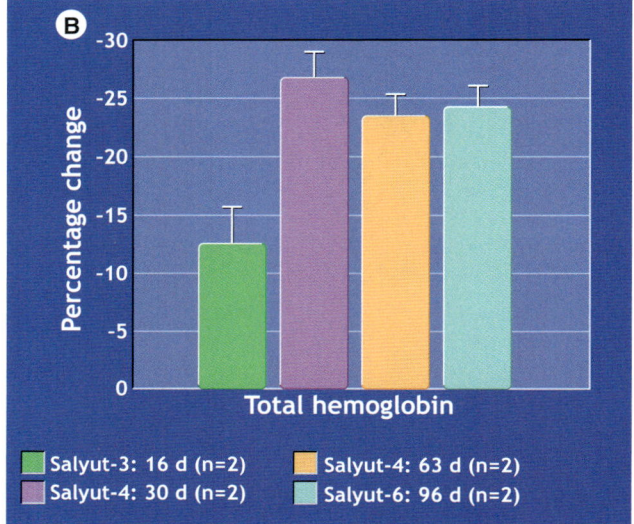

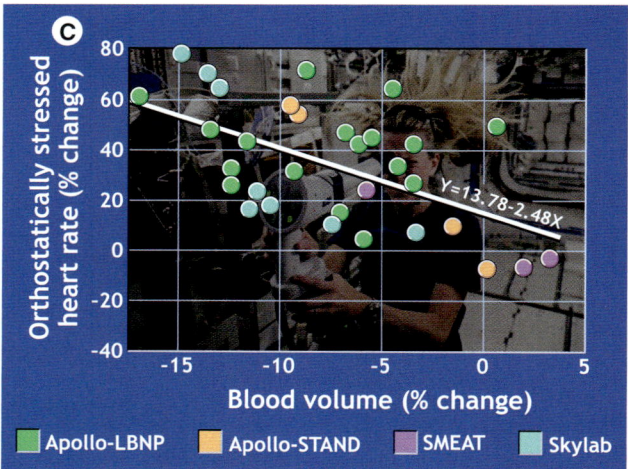

FIGURE 27.6. Postflight to preflight changes in **(A)** plasma volume and red blood cell mass (Spacelab 1; Skylab 2 to 4), **(B)** total hemoglobin (Salyut 3 to 4, 6), and **(C)** blood volume related to orthostatically stressed heart rate. Error bars in **A** and **B** represent standard errors of measurement.
(Data in **A** and **B** from Convertino VA. Physiological adaptations to weightlessness: Effects on exercise and work performance. *Exerc Sports Sci Rev*. 1990;18:119. Photo: NASA.)

(10 to 16 days) and longer-duration (>2 wk) spaceflights on Apollo, Skylab, and Russian science missions. The longest space mission (96 days) at that time to assess fluid adaptation changes took place on the Salyut 6 mission.

TABLE 27.4 summarizes preflight to postflight adaptations in microgravity for 23 body fluid–associated variables[84] based on various American (Mercury, Gemini, Apollo, Shuttle, Spacelab SMEAT [Skylab Medical Experiments Altitude Tests]), Russian (Vostok, Voskhod, Soyuz, Mir), and ASTP-Apollo joint American and Soviet Union space missions (https://history.nasa.gov/apollo/apsoyhist.html).

> **TABLE 27.4** Body fluid changes during American and Russian space missions

Sensory System Adaptations

FIGURE 27.7A shows an overview detailing multisensory interactions that readjust the sensory responses disturbed by microgravity. **Sensorimotor integration** plays a pivotal role in posture and movement control, ambulation, and manipulating objects at 1 g, which necessitate proper adjustment in body orientation. In essence, the sensorimotor control system consists of highly complex, tightly integrated neural complexes that modulate vestibular, visual, somatosensory, tactile, and proprioceptive input within a central command-processing center. Disturbance in one part of the system usually initiates an override, readjustment, or temporary substitution by other system components to maintain the system's functional integrity.[50,81,106,156,194]

Considerable research has assessed how microgravity affects spatial orientation, postural control,[80] vestibulocochlear reflexes, and vestibular processing.[57] Studies have also focused on mechanisms related to **space motion sickness (SMS)** and perceptual motor performance.[100,101,209,210]

Figure 27.7B displays the immediate spaceflight effects on postural reflexes in crew members from eight missions that lasted 4 to 10 days. Immediate postflight measurements were made within 1 to 5 hr in 10 of the 13 crewmembers. The greatest postural instability occurred in tests that required vestibular information pertaining to posture, balance, and eye movements. Note that few responses occurred below the established lower critical normalized composite equilibrium score. In total, the experiments demonstrated a two-stage readaptation process that followed microgravity exposure. The first stage occurred quickly, within a few hours after landing; in a second, slower stage, stability returned to near normal in approximately 4 days. On longer Russian Mir missions (140 and 175 days), recovery of postural parameters to preflight levels required approximately 6 wk. Apparently, readaptation of postural control upon return from space coincides with mission duration, with a prominent role played by visual cues.[195]

TABLE 27.5 summarizes spaceflight adaptations in audition, taste (gustation) and olfaction, somatosensory, and vision sensory system categories in relatively short (≤14 days) and longer (≥14 days) during early American space missions. The bottom of the table lists general vestibular system changes.

> **TABLE 27.5** Adaptations in audition, gustation, and olfaction for short (≤14 days) and longer (≥14 days) space missions

Musculoskeletal Adaptations

FIGURE 27.8A illustrates how the digestive (intestine), cardiovascular (kidney), and skeletal (bone) systems adjust calcium distribution in response to reduced (microgravity), normal (1 g), and increased (2 g) gravitational skeletal loading. The degree of shading within the circles in the right panel represents the adaptation in whole-body bone mineral (darker shading, greater calcium accretion) to the different loading conditions. Under normal gravity conditions, the small intestine absorbs approximately 250- to 500-mg calcium for every 1000-mg consumed, with the remainder excreted in feces. In a microgravity environment, reduced calcium intestinal absorption exacerbates calcium fecal loss. Abnormal calcium excretion from bone resorption disrupts calcium homeostasis, which in turn decreases total body calcium and bone mass. With increased gravitational loading, calcium absorption by bone increases to spare overall calcium loss. In Figure 27.8, the flow diagram shows proposed parallel dynamics among calcium-endocrine response and skeletal adaptation and altered bone composition and architecture to altered gravitational loading with adequate diet and endocrine balance.[65]

Without suitable countermeasures, progressive calcium losses during future missions lasting several years' duration will compromise astronaut well-being, increasing bone fracture risk upon return to Earth. Onboard, multimode exercise training and lower limb exercise have not prevented BMD loss, despite United States and Soviet crewmembers' commitment to intense resistance-type daily workout regimens. Prior research using valid animal and bed rest models has documented the basic bone remodeling mechanism during prolonged microgravity exposure.[26,129,149,169,171] Biochemical markers of bone turnover during 120-day bed rest (skeletal unloading) showed the combined effects of accelerated bone resorption and retarded bone formation accounted for bone loss.[66] BMD measurements at the distal radius and tibia in 15 cosmonauts on Mir space station missions for 1, 2, and 6 mo revealed the following[154]:

1. Cancellous and cortical radius bone decreased progressively at each of the time points during shorter-duration missions, while astronauts on the longest duration missions seemed to resist the greater initial bone loss compared to shorter-duration flights.
2. For the weight-bearing tibial site, cancellous BMD appeared normal after 1 mo and deteriorated thereafter. After 2 mo, bone loss became noticeable in the tibial cortices.
3. At 6 mo, cortical bone loss was less evident than cancellous bone loss; cumulative time in μG did not relate to BMD changes.
4. Tibial bone loss still persisted after return to Earth for durations similar to 1- to 6-mo time in space.

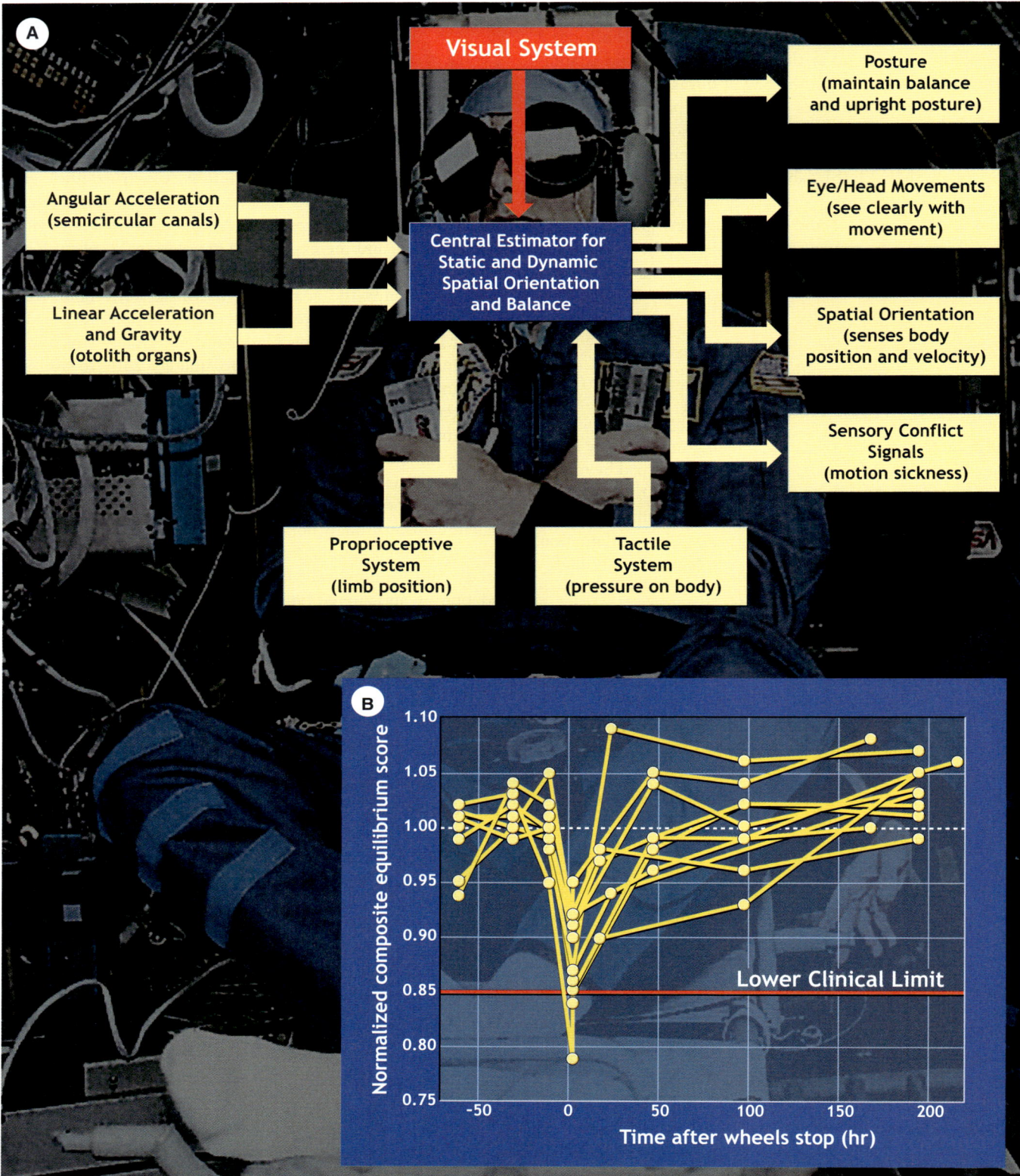

FIGURE 27.7. (A) Schematic representation of sensory motor system that controls eye movements for orientation and posture motion perception. **(B)** Changes in anterior-posterior sway composite equilibrium score in 10 astronauts at target times after the space shuttle returned to Earth. The tests involved posture platform perturbation for differing visual, vestibular, and proprioceptive input. *Dashed horizontal line* at 1.00 represents normal response.
(Data from Fregly MJ, Blatteis CM, eds. *Handbook of Physiology. Section 4, Environmental Physiology*, Vol. 1. American Physiological Society. New York: Oxford University Press; 1996. Photo courtesy F. Katch.)

Alterations in circulation to bone during microgravity exposure can alter the balance between bone resorption and bone formation. Bone blood flow may play an important role in bone remodeling in microgravity.[22] Part of the solution to the problem of bone loss in prolonged microgravity lies in selecting crew members with the greatest resistance to bone loss, including applying targeted prevention and/or treatment strategies.[150] Carefully controlled, longitudinal studies in a microgravity environment (i.e., long-term studies on the ISS and eventual missions to Mars) become crucial to better understand the deleterious consequences on skeletal biology and apply appropriate countermeasure strategies, which daily include aerobic and resistance exercise sessions (www.nasa.gov/mission_pages/station/research/station-science-101/bone-muscle-loss-in-microgravity/). Altering the ratio of animal protein intake to potassium intake can affect bone metabolism in ambulatory and bed rest subjects, so changing this ratio may help attenuate bone loss on Earth and spaceflight.[170]

Future studies must quantify how to best disrupt bone loss associated with increased calcium excretion in urine and feces, in addition to increased calcium absorption from bone. This also reveals the important role bone/calcium homeostasis must play during missions, including how parathyroid hormone (PTH), calcitonin, the various vitamin D metabolites, osteocalcin, a calcium sensor mechanism, and bone-specific alkaline phosphatase interact on space missions.

TABLE 27.6 examines musculoskeletal adaptations during exposure to microgravity for short-duration spaceflights (1 to 14 days) and longer flights (≥2 weeks). The degree of shading within the circles in the right panel represents the adaptation in whole-body bone mineral (darker shading, greater calcium accretion) to the different loading conditions. One of NASA's greatest biomedical concerns still involves the 1 to 9% loss in weight-bearing bone mass shown in the image during space missions.[109,174–176] A recent study measured the overall change in seated height and overall stature for crewmembers

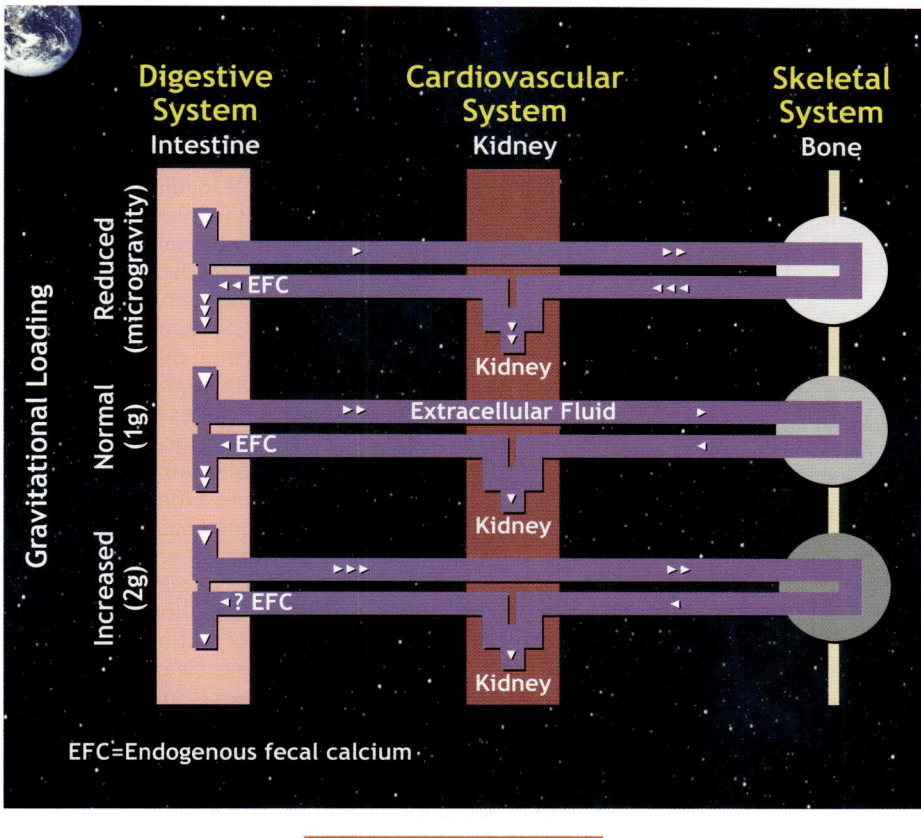

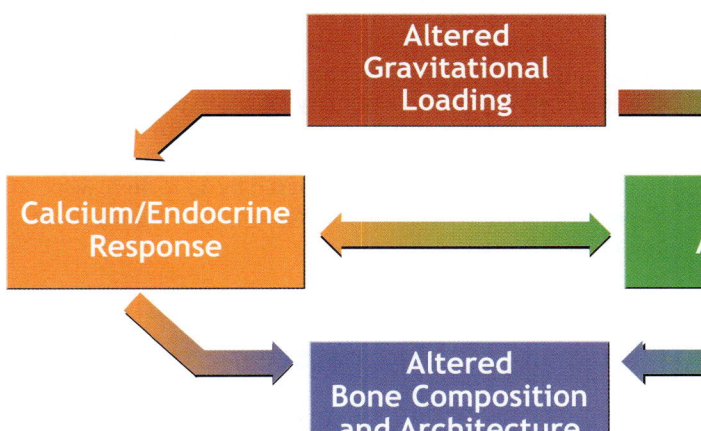

FIGURE 27.8. Influence of gravitational loading (mechanical stress) on calcium balance to reduced microgravity and normal (1 g) and increased (2 g) gravitational skeletal loading, and how it would impact digestive, cardiovascular, and muscular factors with adequate diet and stable endocrine balance.
(Adapted from Morey-Holton ER, et al. The skeleton and its adaptation to gravity. In: Fregly MJ, Blatteis CM, eds. *Handbook of Physiology. Section 4, Environmental Physiology*, Vol. 2. American Physiological Society. New York: Oxford University Press; 1996. Photo: NASA.)

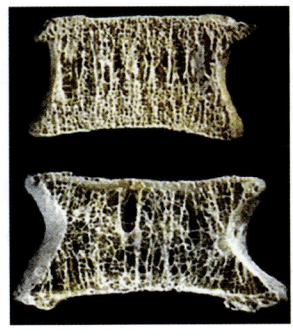

Credit: NASA

A systematic review of microgravity-induced bone loss in space travelers revealed that the amount of bone loss via bone density measurements depends on the skeletal region evaluated (i.e., skull and cervical spine, upper limbs and thorax, pelvis and lumbar spine, and limbs). Postflight recovery of bone loss can take up to 2 to 5 years[200,201] and in shorter-duration flights (≤30 days) when bone loss exceeds its resorption.[199]

exposed to microgravity. Seated height from 29 crewmembers included 8 ISS increment crew (2 females and 6 males) and 21 Shuttle crew (1 female and 20 males). All participants experienced a statistically significant 6% decrease from preflight seated height.[189]

TABLE 27.6 Musculoskeletal adaptations in short and longer missions

Increased Calcium Loss

TABLE 27.7 summarizes data from 18 male crew members aboard Russian Mir station missions lasting between 4 and 14.4 mo. **Bone mineral density (BMD)** declined at all seven sites measured, with spine, neck of the femur, trochanter, and pelvis decreasing more than 1% per mo. On the shorter 4- to 14-day Gemini flights, BMD decreased 3 to 9% in the os calcis (heel bone).[158] BMD loss at the os calcis and radius occurred during Apollo Skylab missions and showed no recovery, even 97 days postflight.[147,157] During the Skylab 2, 28-day orbital mission, crew members experienced a daily negative 50-mg calcium imbalance.[163] Increased bone calcium loss, if coupled with a high fluid and salt intake, could alter plasma filtrate composition and pH to favor supersaturation in kidney stone–forming salts.[164]

TABLE 27.7 Monthly bone loss on Mir Space Station missions

Skeletal Muscle Adaptations

Bone loss during prolonged microgravity exposure coincides with considerable decrements in muscle mass and strength.[167] Deterioration in muscle structure and function could compromise crew health and safety, including critical EVA task performance, landing maneuvers, and procedures for leaving orbit on return to Earth. Gravity's absence virtually eliminates any load-bearing effects on antigravity muscles, rendering them susceptible to impaired performance in emergencies. Preserving crew member health and fitness remains a major objective because astronauts can now spend 6 mo on the ISS and from one or more years on future missions.[95] As such, **exercise countermeasures** remain a primary way to protect cardiovascular, bone, and skeletal muscle health and function. NASA[203] and European Space Agency partners[202] have developed advanced resistance training countermeasures to preserve muscular strength and retard bone loss during flight and on return to Earth.

Concentric and Eccentric Strength

Research on the important role of concentric and eccentric muscle actions during space missions has focused on preflight and postflight submaximal and maximal muscle functions.[4,15,20,23,27,30,37,38,58] The preponderance of research

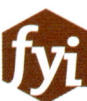

Advanced Resistive Exercise Device

An **advanced resistive exercise device (ARED)** uses adjustable resistance piston-driven vacuum cylinders with a flywheel system to provide muscle loading to build and maintain muscle strength and mass (www.nasa.gov/mission_pages/station/research/experiments/explorer/Facility.html?#id=973). ARED became operational in January, 2009, on the International Space Station (ISS) during up to 6-mo long-duration missions (LDM). Its major instrumentation feature includes triaxial force sensors located in the exercise platform to record the x, y, and z forces in three dimensions. Load sensors in the main lift arm and the arm base assembly measure unidirectional forces, and the arm base assembly has rotational sensors to record arm range of motion. The ARED has the capability to exercise all major muscle groups while focusing on the primary resistive exercises—squats, bench press, deadlifts, and heel raises. The ARED can accommodate crew members from the 5th percentile Japanese female to the 95th percentile American male. The ARED provides a load of up to 600 lb for bar and 250 lb for cable shoulder presses, bench presses, seated or lying exercises, sit-ups, and other abdominal/lower-back core strengthening exercises. NASA and the ESA (European Space Agency) developed the exercise protocols as a primary means to protect cardiovascular, bone, and skeletal muscle health while in space on LDM. The relative contribution from ARED exercise to daily total inflight exercise increased by 33 to 46%, with squat, deadlift, and heel raises increasing significantly more than bench press.

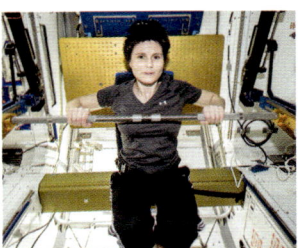

Credit: NASA

Sources:
https://blogs.nasa.gov/ISS_Science_Blog/tag/bone-strength/. Credit: NASA.

in exercise countermeasures supports the use of resistance exercise training on various modes of exercise equipment to increase "space-bound" muscle mass to improve its force-generating capacity and produce positive ultrastructural changes and complimentary neural components.[1,3,8,9,42,63,144] Standard concentric and eccentric methods, including isokinetic loading devices and newer onboard equipment,[5–7,124,127,143] produce such improvements. For example, concentric strength of Skylab crews tested isokinetically before and 5 days after the 28-day flight showed decrements of approximately 25% in leg extensor strength.[146] Greater losses would probably have occurred had testing been conducted immediately upon landing. Subsequently, longer Skylab missions (59, 84, and 59 days) provided preflight fitness and conditioning that emphasized strengthening exercises for the lower extremities. This emphasis on preflight fitness produced smaller strength decrements during flight than during Skylab 2. On

extensor musculature. On longer 110- to 237-day missions, cosmonauts' average triceps strength loss ranged between 20 and 50%.

FIGURE 27.9 reveals considerable losses in peak torque occurred for isokinetic ankle flexion and extension at all measured angular movement velocities. From studies in cosmonauts, **functional electrostimulation (FES)** minimized atrophy, morphologic changes, and decreased neuromuscular coordination patterns during prolonged space missions.[92] FES trains lower extremity muscle groups using 1-s tetanic muscle actions followed by 2 s of relaxation continuously at 20 to 30% of maximum tetanic muscle force up to 6 hr daily.

Muscle Ultrastructural Changes

Permanent neuromuscular dysfunction has not yet been demonstrated during prolonged space missions.[21] Nevertheless, inflight and postflight changes during missions of nearly 1 year reveal altered muscular coordination patterns, some delayed-onset muscle soreness (DOMS), and generalized muscular fatigue and weakness. Many unanswered questions remain about muscle physiology and biochemical adaptations related to microgravity exposure in humans. Animal models using head-down, tail-suspended, non–weight-bearing rodents rely on reduced gravity's effects on skeletal muscle contractile morphology and physiology.

Placing a rodent in a harness in an uploading technique shown in **FIGURE 27.10A** elevates the hindquarters or tail, which limits the animal's movements to simulate microgravity's non–weight-bearing effects. The model mimics microgravity's fluid shifts by reducing sensory input to the motor centers and less mechanical stimulation in connective, muscular, and osseous tissues.[196] Figure 27.10B depicts a partial weight-bearing rodent model (hypodynamic or graded gravitational loading), which can "unweight" the animal to a desired percentage of full body weight measured on the platform by adjusting movable rods at the top of the balance. Both spaceflight and non–weight-bearing confinement atrophies rat skeletal muscles, mainly the slow-twitch (type 1) leg-extensor fibers.[69,70,117,120,168] Also, non–weight bearing in microgravity reduces contractile activity assessed by EMG of male rat hindlimb soleus muscle by 75%.

Maximum Explosive Leg Power Before and After Space Missions

FIGURE 27.11 shows different duration spaceflight effects on maximal explosive power (MEP) and maximal cycling power (MCP) assessed preflight and 26 days postflight for astronauts exposed to microgravity for up to 180 days.[198] Part A shows the percentage of premission scores for MEP and MCP for four astronauts at four periods after mission completion. Astronaut 1, who spent 31 days in orbit, recovered nearly all MEP by 11 days postflight. For the other three astronauts, whose missions lasted 169 to 180 days, MEP recovery approached preflight values by only 77%. For the two astronauts tested 26 days

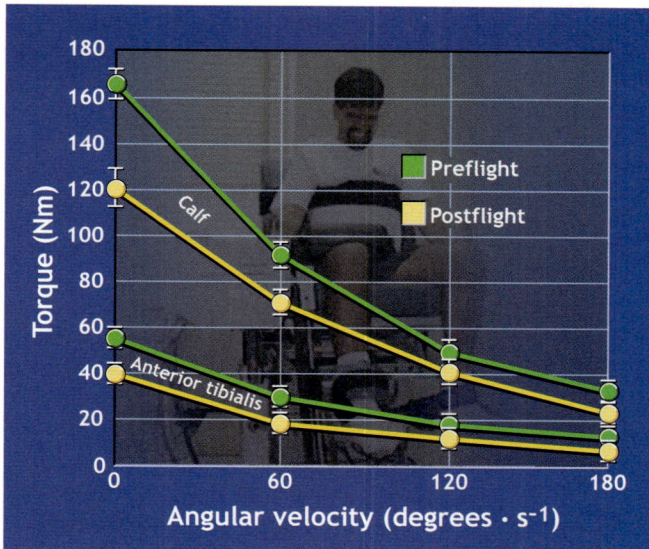

FIGURE 27.9. Force-velocity relationship of ankle flexors (anterior tibialis) and extensor calf muscles measured by isokinetic dynamometry at four angular velocities in six cosmonauts before and after 110 to 237 days in microgravity on Salyut 7.
(Data from Convertino VA. Effects of microgravity on exercise performance. In: Garrett WE, Kirkendall DT, eds. *Exercise and Sport Science.* Philadelphia: Lippincott Williams & Wilkins; 2000.)

longer (110 to 237 days) and short (7 days) Russian missions, isokinetic concentric strength declined up to 28%.[59] The 7-day Salyut 6 mission decreased torque-velocity relationships in the gastrocnemius/soleus, anterior tibialis, and ankle

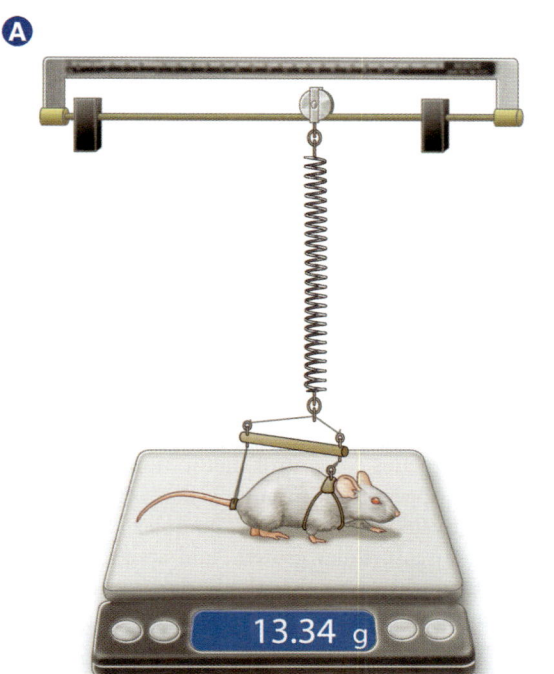

FIGURE 27.10. (A) Partial weight-bearing **(B)** hindlimb suspension mouse model suspension methods limit the animal's activity or movement by immobilizing or restraining its hind limbs or tail to simulate the non–weight-bearing effects of microgravity.
(Based on photos provided courtesy Dr. Susan Bloomfield, Bone Biology Lab, Texas A&M University.)

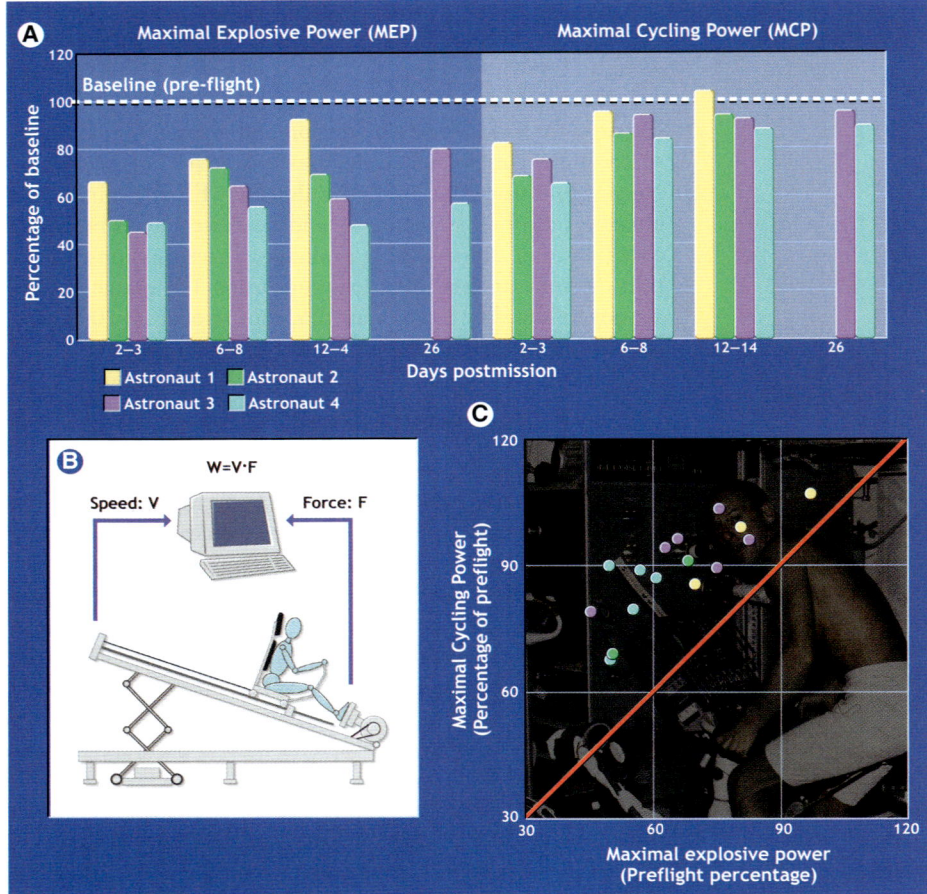

FIGURE 27.11. (A) Effects of up to 180 days in microgravity on changes in maximum explosive power (MEP) and maximal cycling power (MCP). **(B)** The ergometer-dynamometer assessed MEP of the lower limbs by varying either force or velocity. **(C)** Plot of MCP versus MEP scores expressed as a percentage of premission values.

(B and C adapted with permission from Figures 1 and 5 in Antonutto G, et al. Effects of microgravity on maximal power of lower limbs during very short efforts in humans. *J Appl Physiol.* 1999;86:85. ©The American Physiological Society (APS). All rights reserved.)

postflight, MEP for astronaut 3 was 80% of his premission score, while astronaut 4 achieved only 57%. In contrast, each astronaut's MCP, a measure of sustained power output, recovered more rapidly throughout the postflight measurement period, with final scores within premission values by 10%. Figure 27.11B shows the ergometer-dynamometer to assess MEP. Part C shows the relation between MCP and MEP in five to seven "all-out" pedal revolutions for 5 to 6 on a bicycle ergometer following either 5- to 7-min mild aerobic exercise or free-wheel pedaling expressed as a percentage of premission values. Subjects made six maximal pushes with both feet against the force platform for approximately 250 ms at a knee angle of 110° with a 2-min rest between pushes.

On average, MCP deterioration exceeded MEP loss. The researchers attributed the differential deterioration in the two forms of maximal exercise to muscular and neurologic factors involved in each form of effort. In essence, the absence of gravity appears to rearrange postural muscle tone and locomotor coordination substantially. This adversely affects the motor control system; in one astronaut, it negatively affected the normal pattern of motor unit recruitment. Changes in neural drive during long-term missions of 90 to 180 days could negatively impact lower limb musculature's contractile and elastic characteristics.[71]

Immune System Changes

Over the past three decades, approximately 250 experiments conducted during short-term and long-term space missions have verified dramatic changes in immune-functioning cells (e.g., lymphocytes, macrophages, T cells, IL-2, and IL-2 receptor alpha [IL2Rα]).

Microgravity exposure negatively impacts human immune response during extended-duration missions,[1,2] particularly the loss of T-cell activation and diminished gene expression. A 5-mo experiment provided insights into immune cellular response by studying two cultures of human cells under two conditions: one with the culture free-floating in weightlessness without constraints, and the other in simulated microgravity using an onboard centrifuge that generated a 1-g simultaneous control to isolate microgravity's effects from other potentially confounding spaceflight variables. On return to Earth, the cells preserved in microgravity fared more favorably than the ones maintained in simulated microgravity.[103] The researchers hypothesized that the protein complex Rel/NF-κB, an important cellular signaling pathway active in human cells to control DNA transcription in regulating infection's immune response, failed to function properly. This protein complex normally participates in lymphatic β cell and T-cell functions, the latter shown in the unnumbered figure as red spheres attacking an unknown carcinogen. When these cells receive the "correct" external stimulation, they activate a cascade of events that end with NF-κB entering the nucleus to "turn on" genes to control maturation, activation, and proliferation of specialized immune cells. Unfortunately, microgravity deactivated the protein complex regulating inflammatory responses, cellular growth, and apoptosis (Rel/NF-κB pathway), which meant that the body's immune cells would remain compromised in the event of infection during a space mission. This poses serious concern, particularly for future 7-mo, one-way Mars missions. Immune function dysregulation can lead to ineffective proinflammatory host defenses against infectious

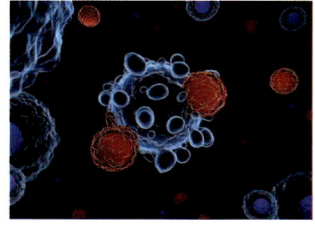

Meletios Verras/Shutterstock

pathogens. Research continues to study means to productively combat this negative down-regulation effect, particularly because of its deleterious effects on bone mass during prolonged microgravity exposures.[138,206]

In another key experiment,[204] various adaptive immune parameters were assessed in astronauts at three intervals during a 6-mo spaceflight on the ISS. Leukocyte subset redistribution occurred during flight, including an elevated white blood cell count and alterations in CD8+ T-cell maturation. Generally, reduced T-cell function in CD4+ and CD8+ persisted throughout the mission, with differential responses between mitogens suggesting an activation threshold shift. The authors concluded that immune alterations persist during long-duration spaceflight. This phenomenon, without appropriate countermeasures, can increase clinical risks to crewmembers from radiation, microbes, stress, altered sleep cycles, and isolation during long-duration space missions.[165,166,205,207,208]

Countermeasure Strategies

Countermeasures systematically attempt to neutralize or minimize spaceflight's potentially harmful deconditioning effects on crew physiologic function, performance, and overall health during mission-critical maneuvers, particularly re-entry and landing.[82] In the absence of gravity, no linear, downward head-to-foot acceleration forces (referred to as 1 Gz) act on the body. This makes normal biologic functions more susceptible to short-term and long-term maladaptations such as SMS. This syndrome usually manifests within the first 72 hr of a mission and is often characterized by clumsiness, difficulty concentrating, disorientation, persisting sensation aftereffects, nausea, pallor, drowsiness, vomiting, vertigo while walking and standing, difficulty walking a straight line, blurred vision, and dry heaves. Some symptoms resemble those of terrestrial motion sickness. SMS symptoms often dissipate on their own or with medication during the first few days of spaceflight. On re-entry after short-duration missions, SMS can manifest as a **general re-entry syndrome (GRS)** that imposes potentially deleterious effects on astronaut performance. GRS symptoms include vertigo, nausea, instability, and fatigue induced by reimposition of increased +Gz during re-entry and landing. In contrast to the relatively acute emergence of SMS, weeks and months of prolonged absence of normal gravitational loading adversely affect bone and muscular structure and function. Concurrently, fluid shifts within the vascular system produce considerable loss of electrolytes and bone minerals. Cumulative negative effects during sustained missions could trigger more severe medical complications that include increased risk for developing renal stones, orthostatic intolerance, neurosensory and motor dysfunctions, and musculoskeletal injuries (including bone fracture) in the weeks and months following return to Earth.[110,111]

Without appropriate countermeasures, microgravity's deleterious effects mimic the adverse changes with prolonged bed rest. For example, bed rest for 30 days dramatically impairs skeletal muscle function; knee extensor strength declines nearly 23%, while knee flexor strength and leg volume decrease 10 to 12%. Reductions in limb volume result from decreased muscular cross-sectional area from muscle fiber protein loss. The 28-day Skylab 2 mission decreased muscular function and leg volume to an extent comparable with bed rest. The protein loss has been attributed in part to a normal adaptive response to decreased workload on weight-bearing muscles.[140] Decrements in cardiovascular function generally parallel losses in muscle strength and size,[142,145] including problems related to low back pain.[122] Projected travel time for an exploration-class mission to Mars requires approximately 6-mo isolation in microgravity, more than a year of planetary habitation at 0.38 g, followed by a 6-mo return trip to Earth during microgravity. Onboard countermeasures play a critical role in minimizing pathology or impaired motor task performance to preserve crew health and safety.[123,125,133] More than likely, gender-related factors affect these health and performance goals.[51] *Inflight resistance and endurance exercises show the greatest overall potential as exercise countermeasures to combat microgravity's sustained deleterious effects.* TABLE 27.8 lists examples of adverse effects in four functional body areas with different countermeasure strategies during prolonged microgravity. Countermeasure strategies, which include fluid loading, G-suit inflation, pharmacologic agents, **artificial gravity**, and short-term physical exertion to elicit maximal effort, help to minimize microgravity-induced orthostatic intolerance.[33] A compelling argument posits that combining multiple countermeasures could afford astronauts optimal protection against potential adverse effects of long-duration space missions.

> **TABLE 27.8** Adverse effects in four functional body areas with countermeasure strategies in prolonged microgravity

On an ISS mission in September 2012, NASA astronaut Sunita "Suni" Williams completed the first simulated triathlon in space. Only the second female commander of the ISS, she also ran a simulated Boston Marathon during her last extended ISS stay in 2007. Williams holds the female record for the longest continuous spaceflight (195 consecutive days on ISS). She competed in the 2012 Malibu triathlon using ISS equipment—exercise bike, treadmill, and **interim resistive exercise device (iRED)**—to simulate

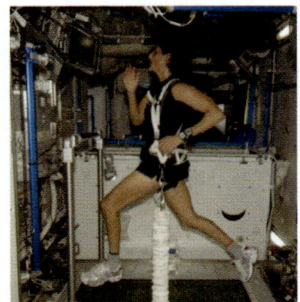

Credit: NASA

the workout type in a half-mile ocean swim. Williams, a committed fitness enthusiast, also holds the women's world records for six spacewalks and a record 44 hr 2 min for EVA (www.youtube.com/watch?v=k-uS29WjmQU). Her workouts in NASA's Houston exercise physiology laboratory (ExPC) illustrate the high value NASA places on fitness status as a primary countermeasures strategy to combat cardiovascular deconditioning, maintain muscle mass, and minimize bone mass loss.

Inflight Space Station Daily Exercise

Four predominant exercise modes shown in **FIGURE 27.12A**[173–175] have played crucial roles during inflight microgravity workouts.[9,34,40,180,181]

1. Treadmill walking and running
2. Cycle ergometry, including maximal effort performed 24 hr before landing[94]
3. Leg rowing
4. Upper and lower body multi-joint dynamic resistance exercise

For treadmill exercise (Fig. 27.12A), note the strap arrangement around the upper body and straps anchored to the hips to keep the astronaut tethered to the treadmill. The iRED (Part B), the resistance exercise training equipment aboard the ISS, allows astronauts to exercise dynamically with increasing resistance throughout a full range of motion (ROM) for three basic movements that stress the hip, back, and spine. For each repetition, measurements includes peak force, average force, and limb ROM.[124]

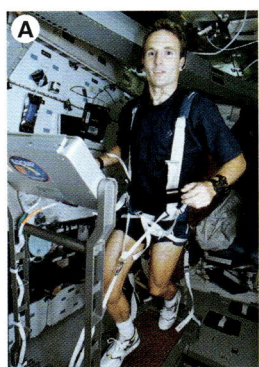
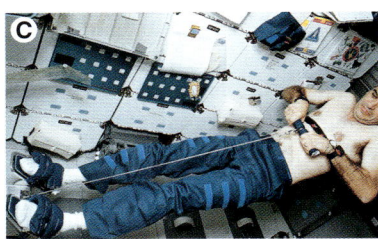
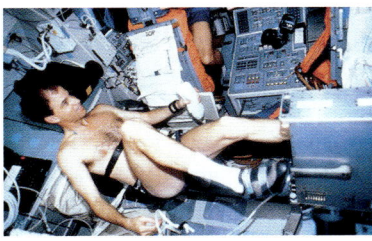
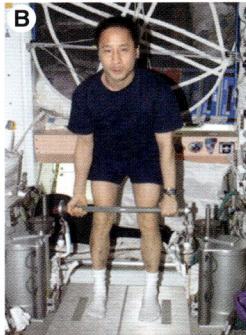
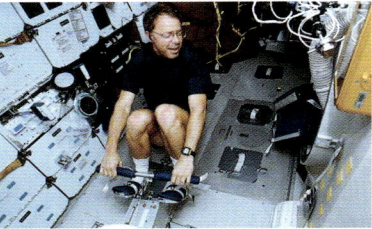

FIGURE 27.12. Five examples of exercise training for different exercise modes during microgravity conditions. Note the strap arrangement in **(A)** around the upper body and straps anchored to the hips to keep the astronaut tethered to the treadmill. The astronaut in **(B)** uses the short bar for the interim resistive exercise device (IRED) to perform upper body strengthening exercise. The images in **(C)** show examples of exercise training during different space shuttle missions, including back and arm, cycling, and rowing activity modes. A NASA video (www.youtube.com/watch?v=doN4t5NKW-k) tours the International Space Station, with an explanation of exercise workouts beginning at 3 min 20 s.
(Photos: NASA.)

Countermeasures on Longer-Duration Missions

The prolonged Russian Mir missions extensively relied on exercise countermeasures based on considerable prior experience with extended space missions. Like their American counterparts, cosmonauts did not exercise during the flight's first 48 to 72 hr to provide sufficient recovery from SMS that 70% of astronauts and cosmonauts experience on their first space mission. On current shuttle missions, an intramuscular Phenergan injection relieved SMS, replacing Dexedrine and other drug combinations that evoke strong negative central nervous system responses.

Toward the end of the flight's first week and over the next 24 days, cosmonauts exercised twice daily, progressing to continuous ergometer cycling for 1 hr at an initial 900 kg-m · min^{-1} workload. Exercise intensity progressively increased to maintain heart rate between 80 and 90% of age-predicted maximum. They added 5- to 15-min daily strengthening exercise (hamstrings, trunk extensors) with bungee cord devices. On missions exceeding 1 mo, cosmonauts exercise twice daily for 1 hr on a passive (subject-driven) treadmill with a restraint system similar to that used by space shuttle astronauts depicted in the schematic for a U.S. Space Shuttle passive treadmill in which a rapid-onset centrifugal brake provided seven braking levels to control drag forces on the running track. On each daily orbit on the ISS, each station crew member exercised aerobically for 1 hr on a treadmill or cycle ergometer (www.youtube.com/watch?v=irCmnn5vIRQ&list=PLiuUQ9asub3S34pyIicCQgHyFUErfpxSz) and 1 hr with dynamic resistance exercise similar to lifting weights with the iRED device (www.youtube.com/watch?v=gzynkaHuHwY&list=PLiuUQ9asub3S34pyIicCQgHyFUErfpxSz&index=2). To simulate gravitational forces, straps from their side—called subject load devices—secured the astronaut to the treadmill. Treadmill exercise using a harness and bungee tether system generated 0.5 to 0.7 g gravitational pull, while exercise on Salyut and Mir treadmills generated 0.62 g "gravitational" pull. The nonmotorized treadmill required astronauts to run at a positive percentage grade to overcome frictional resistance. Several of the exercise modes that served as a cornerstone for countermeasures on shuttle missions now will extend their important role on ISS missions and remain a part of future travel to asteroids and Mars in the decades to come.

FIGURE 27.13 compares heart rate during continuous treadmill exercise at 60, 70, and 80% $\dot{V}O_{2max}$ on an 11-day shuttle mission. The light-blue shaded area under the green line shows the exercise HR during workout on days 3 to 11. The orange circles represent heart rate for the 30-min familiarization run on flight day 2, including the expected immediate, exponential decline in recovery heart rate for a 5-min period after exercise stopped. The astronauts did not attain their assigned target heart rates when exercising continuously for 30-min daily during the mission. More than likely, altered running mechanics while wearing a bungee apparatus for stability during the run reduced ability to attain the target heart rates. The intense workouts were intended to minimize orthostatic dysfunction more often than not experienced upon Earth landing.

Space Pharmacology

SMS remained the most persistent short-term problem during spaceflight missions, and future research with countermeasures will attempt to mitigate this problem on ISS and future NASA missions. Approximately 50% of cosmonauts, 60% of Apollo astronauts, and 71% of first-time shuttle astronauts encountered mild-to-severe SMS. **TABLE 27.9** lists SMS incidence and severity during 36 space shuttle flights. Note the decline in mild, moderate, and severe prevalence from 77 episodes to 34 episodes on crewmember's second shuttle flight. On Space Shuttle Life Sciences mission (SLS-2), only one astronaut experienced nausea without sickness during the mission's first few days.[135]

TABLE 27.9 Space motion sickness incidence and severity during 36 space shuttle flights

SMS is not confined to orbital flight; nearly 10% of astronauts experience it during re-entry or immediately upon landing, including training during parabolic flights. Ninety-two percent of cosmonauts report SMS upon return from missions that last several months or longer.[68] To date, no single pharmacologic treatment prevents or cures SMS. On shuttle missions, the disorder shows no preference for commanders, pilots, or mission specialists, gender or age, career versus noncareer astronauts, or first-time versus repeat flyers. Incomplete understanding about SMS hampers its treatment as pharmacologic remedies usually relieve most symptoms within the first 3 days in the space environment. Additional countermeasure strategies to minimize SMS effects include mechanical and electrical stimulation and biofeedback techniques. Despite these efforts, medication still provides the most effective pharmacologic therapy against SMS. These drugs most effectively provide the best outcomes—meclizine, scopolamine, promethazine, and lorazepam.[190]

Lower Body Negative Pressure

The inflight **lower body negative pressure (LBNP)** apparatus used aboard Skylab and Shuttle missions serves two functions. First, to assess orthostatic deconditioning during spaceflight and postlanding, and second as a countermeasure against adverse orthostatic changes with short and longer missions. The LBNP device applies negative pressure to the lower limbs,[46,160] achieved by a leg volume measuring system (LVMS) leg band (upper left of the image). The waist seal shroud maintains controlled and regulated negative pressure from 0 to 50 mm Hg below ambient pressure. During ground tests, a vacuum provides negative pressure; during flight, negative pressure occurs from the space vacuum. The 50.8-cm/20-in-diameter, 122-cm/48-in-long cylindrical chamber separates longitudinally to provide access to the legs, beginning at the subject's waist at the iliac crests, and ease for securing leg bands to measure change in lower calf volume. Lower leg volume changes with negative pressure occur from the caudal displacement of blood and other fluids.[85] Fluid in the vascular system migrates downward from the upper torso to the lower body—an effect that counters any inflight response to microgravity.

During three 6-mo Mir missions, cosmonauts wore thigh cuffs (rather than rely on an LBNP device) at 1, 3 to 4, and 5 to 5.5 mo and assessed cardiovascular parameters with echocardiography. Data were contrasted with control sessions 30 days preflight and 3 and 7 days postflight.[62] All cosmonauts had reduced vasoconstrictive responses and a less efficient blood flow redistribution toward the brain, which coincided with orthostatic intolerance during postflight stand tests.[35,128] The vascular response to LBNP tests remained depressed during the flights. Thigh cuffs compensated partially for the cardiovascular changes induced by microgravity but not for microgravity deconditioning. Up-regulation of nitric oxide (NO; a potent vasodilator and natriuretic) may explain orthostatic intolerance in microgravity.[152] The vintage image shows the LBNP device during one of the Skylab flights. If this mechanism proves correct, administering an inducible nitric oxide

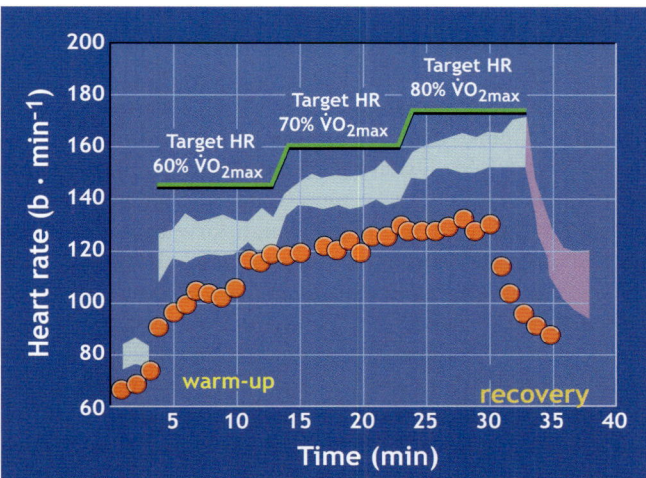

FIGURE 27.13. Heart rate during continuous treadmill exercise at 60, 70, and 80% on an 11-day shuttle mission. (Data courtesy SL Lee, NASA.)

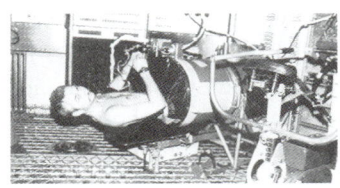

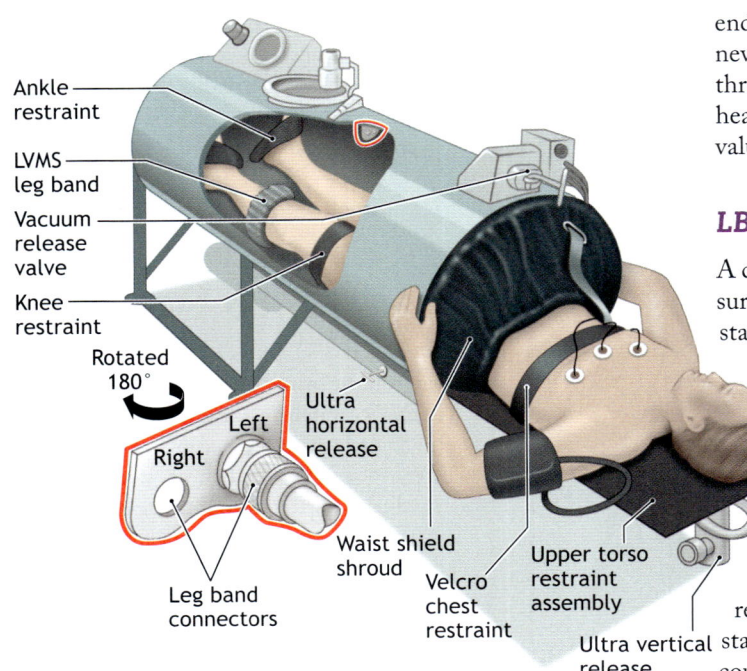

Reprinted with permission from Nicogossian AE, et al., eds. *Space Physiology and Medicine*. 3rd ed. Philadelphia: Lea & Febiger; 1994.

synthase (iNOS) inhibitor may attenuate orthostatic intolerance when astronauts return to Earth; it also benefits patients following extended bed rest.

Assessing Orthostatic Deconditioning Effects

Disruptions in cardiovascular dynamics—heart rate, blood pressure, and leg volume changes—during space missions could compromise crew performance and mission success.[17,33] For example, FIGURE 27.14 displays results for orthostatic testing conducted after Gemini (14 days) and during Skylab (80 days) missions documented orthostatic deconditioning's effects. The Gemini vehicles (including Mercury and Apollo) barely had enough room for the astronauts, so the mission could not accommodate an onboard LBNP chamber. Testing on Gemini took place only before and after flights (Fig. 27.14A). Also, Gemini flights used a tilt table rather than the LBNP device. A 15-min, 70° vertical LBNP tilt test produced dramatic changes in heart rate, systolic and diastolic blood pressure,[32] and leg volume during the prolonged Skylab mission compared with the same variables assessed 3 wk prior to liftoff. Heart rate increased 100% from 70 b·min^{-1} at rest at the start of the LBNP tilt test to 140 b·min^{-1} at the end of the procedure. Systolic blood pressure declined more (30%) than diastolic blood pressure (<10%) during the tilt, whereas leg volume increased 10-fold.

Figure 27.14B shows the resting heart rate pattern in a 250-mm Hg LBNP test in one crew member during the 80-day Skylab 4 mission and 2 mo postflight. While not as dramatic as the shorter-duration Gemini experiments, the resting heart rate increase in response to the LBNP Skylab challenge confirmed the relative heart rate instability (and variability), particularly in the first month compared with the end of the mission. Heart rate with LBNP during preflight never exceeded 75 b·min^{-1} and always surpassed this value throughout the mission. On Skylab missions 2 and 3, resting heart rate averaged 109 b·min^{-1}, a 55% increase over preflight values.

LBNP Combined Countermeasures

A combined LBNP and increased fluid ingestion countermeasure during spaceflight improved performance on an upright standing posture test postflight.[153] For example, two groups of 26 male astronauts consumed either no fluid or a 32-oz water or juice loading volume plus eight salt tablets (to facilitate fluid retention) 1 hr before leaving Earth orbit during shuttle missions 1 through 8.[22] Crew members who used the liquid countermeasures did not experience syncope after landing mainly because about 40% of the ingested fluid increased plasma volume for nearly 4 hr. Astronauts who loaded fluid before re-entry also had lower heart rates and maintained a more stable mean blood pressure. Overall, the hyperhydration countermeasures were more effective during short 3- to 7-day missions than during longer 10-day ones.

The protective benefits of *combined countermeasures* reduce the incidence of orthostatic intolerance assessed by postural tests postflight to only 5%.[121] In contrast, fluid loading alone prior to re-entry loses its effectiveness after 7 days in microgravity[31] or during a 7-day, 6° **head-down bed rest**[28] because the vascular space cannot maintain enough fluid to restore plasma volume to a level that provides benefits.[91] Another countermeasure tactic reduces air temperature inside the space cabin the night before landing. Keeping the cabin "as cold as tolerable" helps to dissipate cabin heat and ultimately in the space garments during re-entry and postlanding when cabin air temperature can reach 26.7 to 32°C/80 to 90°F. The astronaut's liquid cooling garment uses a thermoelectric cooler to keep the precirculated water cool before it circulates through the full-torso garment. Reducing sweating response during re-entry and landing minimizes fluid loss.

Spaceflight Nutrition

An optimal diet for spaceflight should theoretically provide energy intake equal to the energy required for the mission.[11,12,14,72–74,105,116] Dietary management also may counter the many adverse effects of physiologic adaptation to microgravity.[48,148] This goal, seemingly straightforward, has not been reached successfully on most missions. *Almost every space journey produced weight loss compared with similar–duration ground-based activities on Earth.*[71,115,135,155] Disruption in energy balance results from two combined factors: (1) demands of spaceflight's physical requirements and (2) decreased food intake during microgravity exposure. Both factors negatively affect an astronaut's energy balance.[136] A negative energy balance became apparent not only in weight loss but in impaired fluid, electrolyte, and mineral balance.[76,79] Each of these factors influences cardiovascular, musculoskeletal, immunologic, and endocrinologic functions. Cosmonauts in the Russian space program also have experienced weight loss during extended missions.

Effects on Body Weight

Large individual variations in body weight occurred for crewmembers during three Skylab missions lasting 24, 56, and 84 days. On each mission, all crewmembers lost weight and did not regain it except for the commander whose weight returned to prelaunch values by mission's end. The most dramatic 3 to 4% weight loss generally occurred over the first 10 days on each mission mainly from fluid loss. Weight loss reversed within 5 days after returning to Earth.[53] The same weight loss pattern in spaceflight and weight regain postflight occurred on almost every space mission except one (Euro-Mir, 1994). This response is shown independently from flight duration depicted in the figure showing flight duration (top) and body mass change (bottom) for 12 Shuttle missions through ISS using data from various research publications.[182–184]

INTEGRATIVE QUESTION

How would you measure an astronaut's body weight in microgravity? (Hint: Refer to Lippincott Connect references[53,121]).

Altered Protein Dynamics *Atrophy of skeletal muscles that support posture and locomotion represents a characteristic maladaptation to microgravity during short-duration and long-duration exposures.*[49] Decreases in lean body mass, muscle volume, and muscle strength and changes in muscle fiber microarchitecture[168] accompany space-induced muscle atrophy. Such changes suggest poor adaptation in whole-body protein (nitrogen) balance.[88,135,137] Isotopic methods that assess tissue protein turnover show that astronauts increase protein breakdown rate by approximately 30% on mission days 2 to 8, thereby producing negative nitrogen balance. In addition, increases occur in urinary cortisol, fibrinogen, and interleukin-2 (IL-2). These changes suggest that spaceflight triggers a stress response similar to response patterns from physical injury. In both stressful situations, tissue protein serves as a substrate for energy metabolism that fosters a negative nitrogen balance from protein catabolism. This supports the recommended daily 1.5 g · kg^{-1}/2.2 lb body mass protein intake during space travel.[78,89] In addition, long space missions (4 to 9 mo on the Russian Mir Space Station) and shorter-duration space shuttle flights (up to 15 days) were associated with decreased oxidative damage from reduced oxygen radical

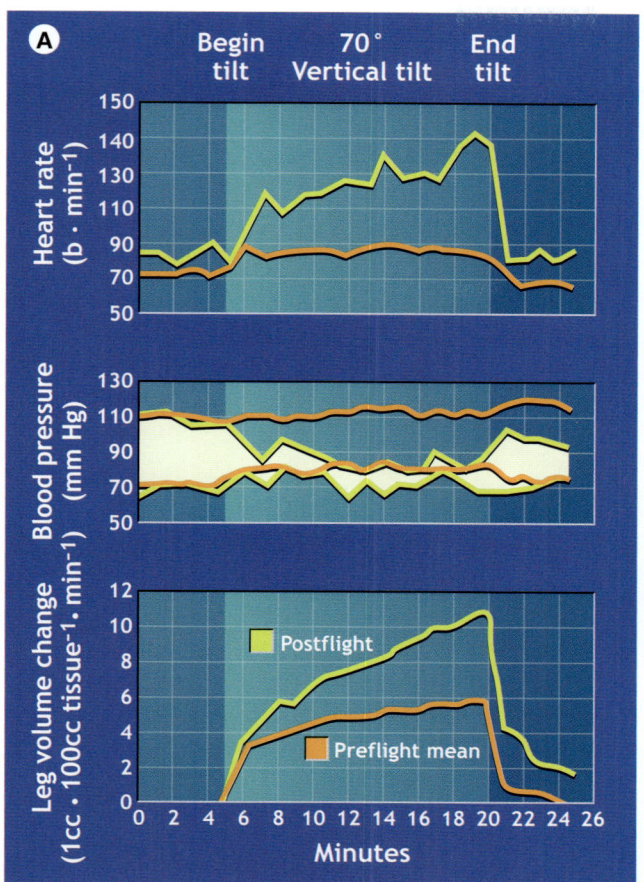
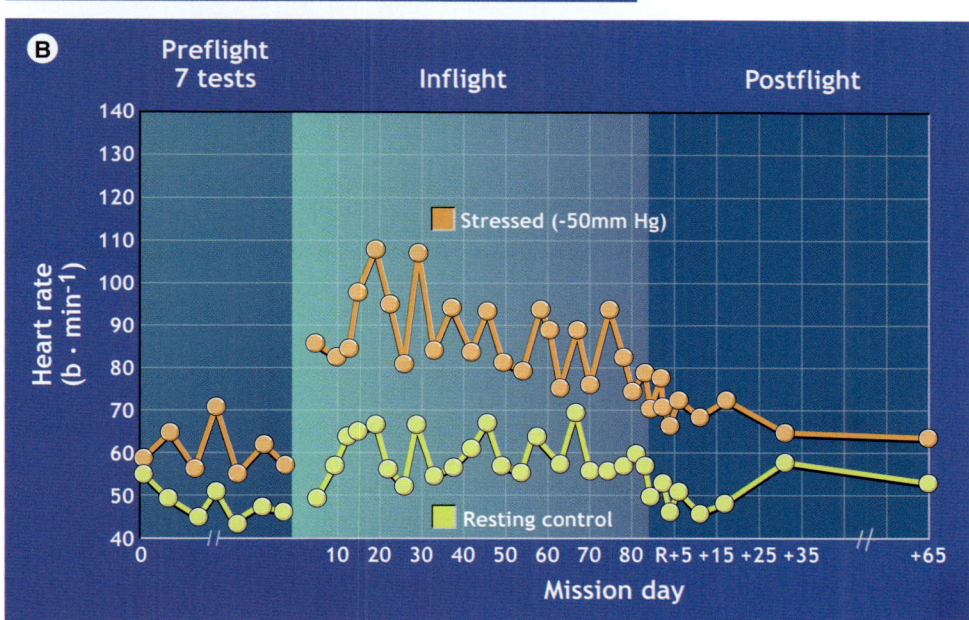

FIGURE 27.14. Lower body negative pressure (LBNP) evaluation of cardiovascular dynamics during space missions. **(A)** Gemini 14-day postflight to preflight changes in heart rate, blood pressure, and leg volume. **(B)** Resting heart rate in a −50 mm Hg LBNP test in one crew member during an 80-day Skylab mission.
(From Schnieder VS, et al. Cardiopulmonary system: Aeromedical considerations. In: Nicogossian A, et al. *Space Physiology and Medicine.* 4th Ed. New York, NY: Springer, 2016.)

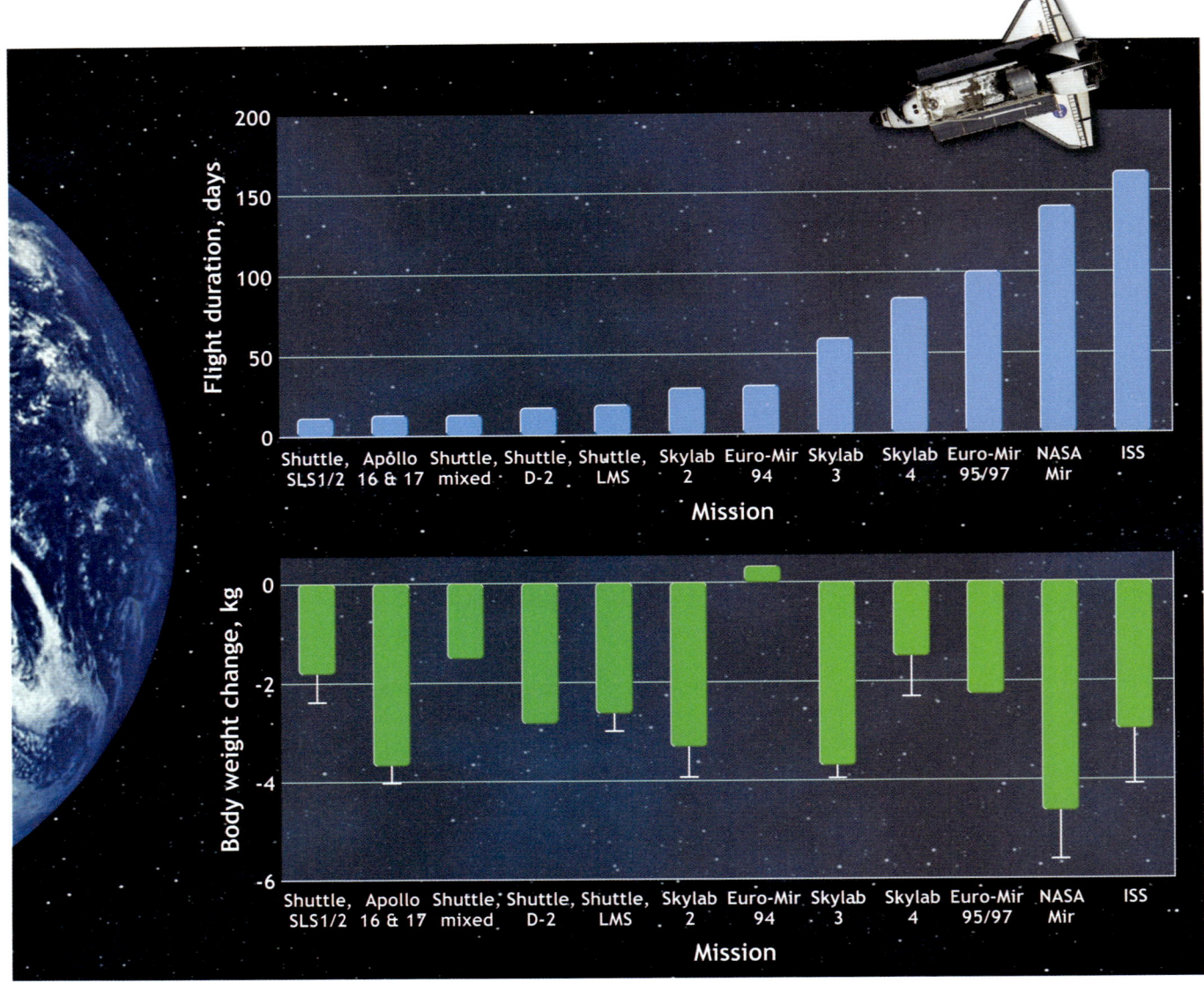

Data from Laurens C, et al. Revisiting the role of exercise countermeasure on the regulation of energy balance during space flight. *Front Physiol*. 2019;10:321. doi: 10.3389/fphys.2019.00321. Photos: NASA.

production in the electron transport chain from reduced energy intake. Increased oxidative damage occurs postflight from combined increases in metabolic rate and possibly losing inflight host antioxidant defenses.[139] The potential postflight antioxidant supplementation beneficial effects remain unknown. On the two shuttle missions, daily calorie intake and nitrogen balance were affected negatively compared with preflight values. Based on Russian data aboard the Salyut 7 space mission, the estimated energy cost from twice-daily inflight exercise sessions was approximately 20 kcal · kg^{-1}/2.2 lb body mass. Adding this energy requirement to an already inadequate daily energy intake would provoke further protein loss to absorb the energy deficit.[67] Research must determine effective combinations with exercise and nutritional supplementation to stabilize energy and protein balance during space missions, including developing renal stones that can negatively impact crew member health and ultimately the mission.[107]

Space Shuttle Energy Expenditure and Energy Balance Dynamics The 1996 LMS shuttle mission quantified energy expenditure and energy balance in four crew members for 12 days before liftoff, during the 17-day flight, and 15-day postflight.[136] A complementary bed rest study assessed a 6° head-down tilt to simulate microgravity to evaluate energy expenditure and energy balance in eight subjects. The bed rest study had three phases: (1) 15-day pre–bed rest ambulatory period, (2) 17-day bed rest (except when subjects exercised to match the inflight exercise routines), and (3) 15-day recovery period. Subjects in both experiments performed submaximal and maximal bicycle cycling tests on days 13 and 8 before launch and days 4 and 8 postflight. During spaceflight days 2, 8, and 13, crewmembers performed an additional ergometer test to assess cardiorespiratory responses to exercise at 85% VO_{2max}.

FIGURE 27.15A shows the results for doubly labeled water (DLW; $^2H_2^{18}O$) and body composition by dual-energy x-ray absorptiometry (DXA) before and after spaceflight/bed rest to quantify positive energy balance (lipid stored) or negative energy balance (lipid catabolized). There were three energy intake periods expressed as $kcal \cdot kg^{-1} \cdot d^{-1}$ during preflight, flight, and postflight. Within each period, a relative stabilization took place for energy intake. This probably occurred from resetting set point mechanisms to regulate energy balance. The lower right histogram inset expresses average daily energy intake ($kcal \cdot d^{-1}$) to highlight the dramatic 45% lower inflight energy intake (1708 $kcal \cdot d^{-1}$) compared with remarkably similar preflight values (3025 $kcal \cdot d^{-1}$) and postflight (3151 $kcal \cdot d^{-1}$). Subjects quantified each food item consumed and not consumed with a bar code reader and verbal description using a cassette recorder to estimate the contents remaining in the individual food package. During preflight and postflight periods, subjects consumed prepared meals with known nutrient content.[104] Spacelab collected, measured, and saved a 20-mL daily urine sample to estimate nitrogen balance from nitrogen and creatinine excretion.

The results in Figure 27.15B contrast the energy intake during the first 2 wk in spaceflight for Skylab missions 2 (28 days), 3 (56 days), and 4 (84 days); two shuttle missions (SLS-1 and SLS-2 combined); and shuttle LMS. The histogram inset in A expresses the data as average $kcal \cdot d^{-1}$ during each mission phase. Astronauts on the shuttle LMS (*bottom red curve*) remained in substantial negative energy balance throughout the flight. Astronauts on the previous three Skylab missions participated in a metabolic balance study, so daily energy intakes remained fairly stable during the different-duration missions. In contrast, astronauts on shuttle LMS consumed food *ad libitum*. At the same time, they performed vigorous daily exercise that contributed to their relatively high average total 40.8 $kcal \cdot kg^{-1} \cdot d^{-1}$ (3238 kcal) daily energy expenditure. No differences occurred among the three methods to estimate energy balance. The results supported the methodology validity, and a more recent study added a third suggestion about how best to maintain energy balance to ameliorate body weight loss[182]:

1. Severe negative energy balance and corresponding body mass, body fat, and protein loss could compromise a mission and adversely affect an astronaut's health in a manner resembling prolonged malnutrition.
2. High physical activity levels during spaceflight may disrupt mechanisms that maintain energy balance.
3. The countermeasure program should exert minimal impact on total energy expenditure, not induce appetite loss and reduced energy intake, yet benefit muscle mass by reducing muscle fiber-type reversal, and preserve bone mass, intermediary metabolism, cardiovascular function, and aerobic fitness. Resistance exercise could help prevent muscle mass and function loss without inducing a large increment in energy expenditure, coupled with high-intensity interval training (HIIT), which relies more on carbohydrate as a preferred fuel rather than lipid to limit body mass loss.[186]

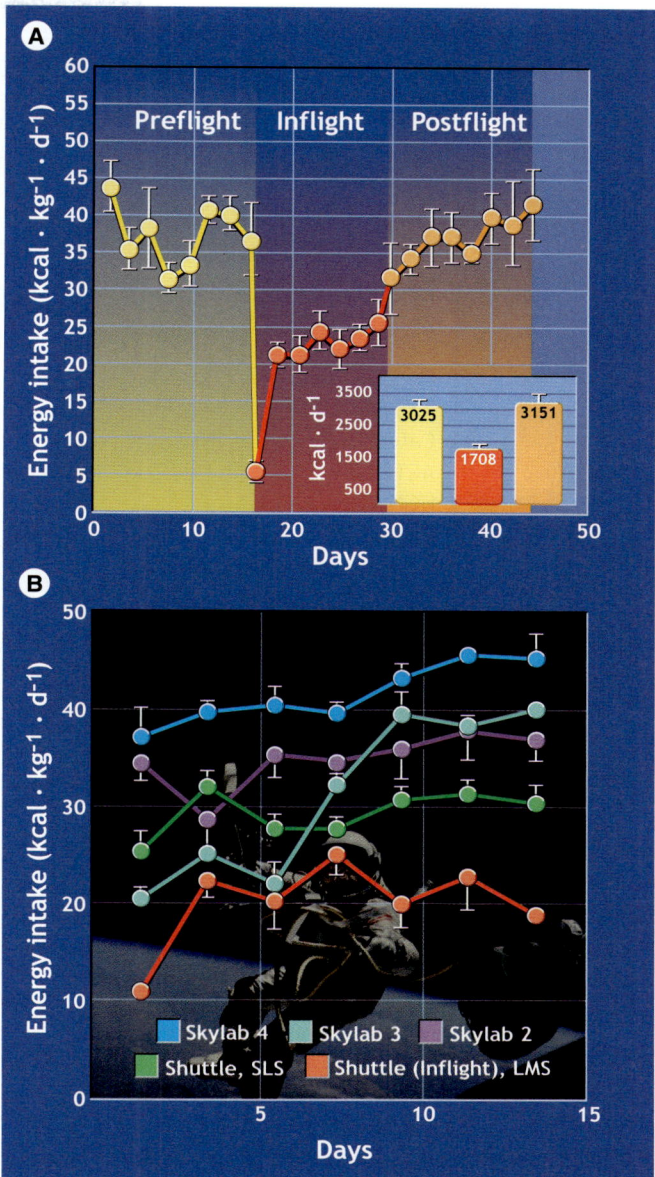

FIGURE 27.15. **(A)** Daily energy intake before, during, and after spaceflight on the Life and Microgravity Spacelab (LMS) shuttle. The histogram inset expresses the data as average $kcal \cdot d^{-1}$ during each mission phase. **(B)** Daily energy intake during different spaceflight missions.
(Data from Stein TP, et al. Energy expenditure and balance during spaceflight on the space shuttle. *Am J Physiol*. 1999;45:R1739.)

ISS Nutrition and Body Composition Experiments One difficulty facing space medicine scientists is how to plan for optimal nutrient requirements during long-duration space missions.[75] The ISS provides a unique vehicle to assess nutritional changes during prolonged 128- to 195-day spaceflights. Experiments aboard the ISS have examined body composition, bone metabolism, hematology, general blood chemistry, and selected vitamin and mineral blood levels in 11 astronauts before and after such longer-duration flights. Crewmembers consumed an average 80% their recommended energy intake, and on landing day, their body weight registered significantly lower than before flight. Hematocrit, serum iron, ferritin saturation,

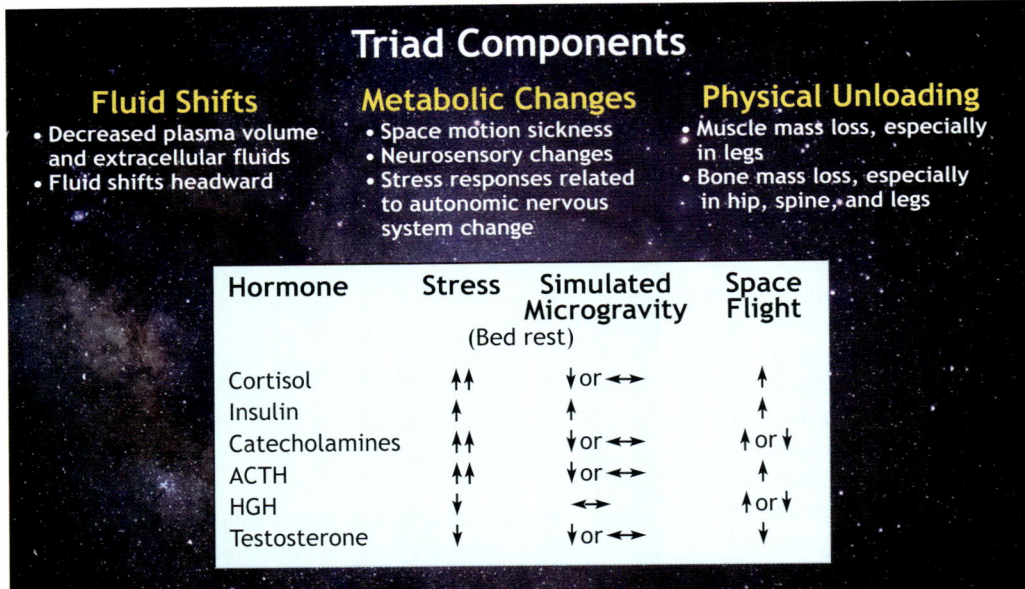

FIGURE 27.16. Triad of nutritionally related effects of spaceflight on physiologic systems. The **inset** shows endocrine changes during stress, simulated microgravity (bed rest studies), and spaceflight. ↑, increase; ↑↑, large increase; ↓, decrease; ↔, no change.
(Adapted with permission from Lane HW, Gretebeck RJ. Nutrition, endocrinology, and body composition during space flight. *Nutr Res.* 1998;18:1923. Background image: sripfoto/Shutterstock.)

that spaceflight's endocrine effects relate more to nutritional changes characterized by stress-related models, not a model that includes bed rest. The similarity between the increased catabolic demands on energy metabolism (and negative energy balance) and spaceflight's catabolic "stress" effects help to explain space-induced decreases in body mass, lean body mass, and bone density. This includes shifts in extracellular and intracellular water compartments.

Body Composition Changes

FIGURE 27.17 shows percentage changes in body composition variables in 10 astronauts assessed by densitometry and bioelectrical impedance before and 2 days following 7- to 16-day missions. No changes occurred in body fat or extracellular water, with the 2.3% decline in body mass attributable to a loss in fat-free body mass (FFM). Note that all three FFM (water, protein, and mineral) components declined from 3 to 4% when measured postflight. The 3% loss in intracellular water—attributable to decreased protein and mineral levels within other tissues including muscle—explains the total body water decrease. An integrative approach assesses regional body composition (calf muscle volume)[159] and MRI-derived muscle (transverse calf muscle relaxation) characteristics following multiple shuttle/Mir missions lasting 16 to 28 wk.[86]

and transferrin were decreased and serum ferritin increased after flight. The finding that other acute phase proteins were unchanged postflight suggests that iron metabolism changes could not solely account for an inflammatory response. Urinary 8-hydroxy-29-deoxyguanosine concentration was greater and red blood cell superoxide dismutase lower postflight, signaling increased oxidative damage. The astronauts consumed vitamin D during flight, nonetheless serum 25-hydroxycholecalciferol decreased after flight. Bone resorption was increased after flight, yet bone formation did not consistently rise 1 day after landing. Bone loss, compromised vitamin D status, and oxidative damage are among critical nutritional concerns that require resolution for long-duration space travelers.[132]

Nutrition Related to Spaceflight Physiological Functions From the first space missions, researchers have tracked adaptations in physiologic function in the microgravity environment. A prevailing theory to explain such changes involves interactions among nutritional variables and endocrine functions and their combined effects on cardiopulmonary, hormonal, skeletal, and body fluid functions, and body mass and composition.[34,99,130,141] **FIGURE 27.16** shows the nutritionally related triad effects from spaceflight on different physiologic systems. The interrelated triad components—fluid shifts, physical unloading in weight-bearing structures, and metabolic changes—in many ways link to shifts in endocrine function. The inset table shows endocrine changes during stress, simulated microgravity (bed rest), and spaceflight. Note the responses to bed rest do not generally mirror endocrine changes in spaceflight and instead mimic stress-mediated responses. An attractive hypothesis posits

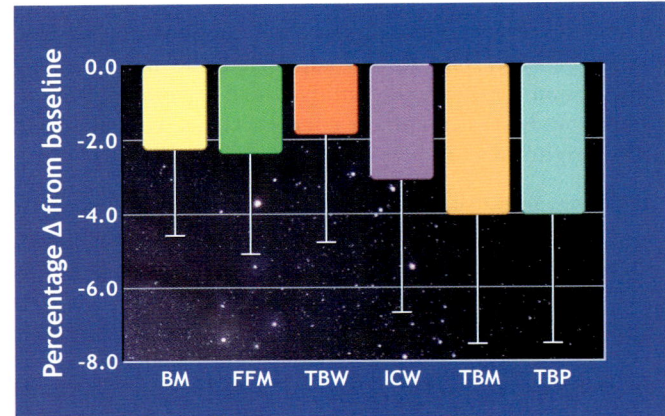

FIGURE 27.17. Percentage changes (Δ) in body composition variables in 10 astronauts assessed by densitometry and multifrequency bioelectrical impedance analysis before and 2 days after 7- to 16-day missions. BM, body mass; FFM, fat-free body mass; TBW, total body water; ICW, intracellular water; TBM, total body mineral; TBP, total body protein.
(Data from Greenisen MC., et al. Functional performance evaluation. In: *Extended Duration Orbiter Medical Project. NASA Johnson Space Center final report. 1989–1995. [NASA/SP-1999-534]* NASA. Houston: Lyndon B. Johnson Space Center; 1999. Background image: sripfoto/Shutterstock.)

INTEGRATIVE QUESTION

Would consuming additional protein during a 2-mo space mission restore fat-free body mass? Why or why not?

Overview of Physiologic Responses to Spaceflight

Numerous research reports discuss short-term and long-term spaceflight consequences on human physiology.[16,83,113] From the first single-pilot Project Mercury flights in the early 1960s to the extended Soviet Soyuz missions in the 1990s and latest manned Chinese space missions, scientists have pondered how best to minimize deleterious microgravity effects during flight and upon return to Earth. **FIGURE 27.18** diagrams two main physical stressors from space travel. Both factors ultimately *increase* physiologic strain indicated in the bottom blue box and negatively impact or *decrease* an astronaut's physical performance noted in the bottom red box:

1. Decreased hydrostatic pressure gradients within the cardiovascular system (displayed on left)
2. Decreased weight loading on muscles (displayed on right)

Note that $\dot{V}O_{2max}$, muscular strength, and increased fatigability, combined with an increased thermal load, add substantially to the body's total physiologic strain. Exercise countermeasures, principally site-specific lower body eccentric and concentric resistance exercise coupled with intense cardiovascular workouts mitigate deleterious effects from prolonged microgravity sojourns when astronauts return to a 1-g Earth environment.

Short-term and Long-term Responses

Short-term and long-term categories describe the physiologic responses and adaptations during transition from Earth's 1-g environment to microgravity in low-Earth orbit and then return to 1 g following a mission. Short-term responses occur within 24 hr or the first few mission days. The second category describes long-term changes following a mission. **FIGURE 27.19** presents a generalized model expressed as a flow diagram for both immediate or short-term (<24 hr) and delayed or long-term (>24 hr) responses. Both response effects eventually contribute to **orthostatic hypotension** (*bottom red box*), the most common problem following spaceflight.

In space, body fluids no longer move "downward" from gravity's pull, so fluids redistribute toward the chest and upper body (note facial puffiness from cranial edema in the two inset photos on the left). Lower body fluid loss gives the legs a birdlike appearance. Excess fluid buildup in the torso triggers fluid elimination by the kidneys. Mean arterial pressure increases in the cranial region from a normal preflight 70 to 100 mm Hg in space (Top), while mean pressure at the feet declines 50% from its normal 200 mm Hg; heart volume also decreases slightly in microgravity. The immediate change in body fluid distribution activates many additional responses while lowering sympathetic nervous system activity. Restricted stimulation environments such as spaceflight and other stress-inducing situations from prolonged confinement and isolation share many similar responses and adaptations.[90,187,188]

Inflight Adaptations

FIGURE 27.20 depicts the proposed immediate (≤24 hr) and delayed (≥24 hr) time course for shifts in physiologic responses to microgravity compared with those under 1 g preflight (1 g) and postflight conditions for up to 1 year. The *green horizontal line* represents baseline function on Earth (denoted as 0% change). Within the first 3 wk, up to a 10% change in cardiovascular function reflects a deconditioning response; within 14 days, a 10% change occurs in body fluid redistribution; and within 3 mo, bone mass declines by 5%. Bone mass declines further to 15% between months 5 and 6 when it stabilizes for several months before decreasing farther to 17% after 1 year. Like bone mass, muscle structure and function deteriorate at a slower rate than do cardiac deconditioning and fluid redistribution; the decrement reaches higher values that approach 20% from baseline values. Note the similar, parallel decline in bone and muscle mass with deconditioning throughout a year.

Postflight Readaptations

FIGURE 27.21 shows how 3-mo recovery (readaptation) impacts neurovestibular and cardiovascular functions, fluid and electrolyte balance, red blood cell mass, and lean body mass. For reference, the *lower horizontal line* indicated by the *arrow at bottom left* (*1 g set point*) represents baseline measures expected under normal 1 g conditions. The *colored lines* for each variable indicate average trends with considerable interindividual and intraindividual differences existing in the basic response variables.

Analyzing the recovery curves in microgravity illuminates two prominent findings:

1. The nonlinear response rate appears bimodal for some processes with relatively large rate constants
2. Recovery time varies depending on the variable

For example, the rapid change in fluid distribution during the first few weeks recovers to baseline within the first week following return to 1 g (*yellow curve*). In contrast, the *aqua curve* for lean body mass and top *magenta curve* representing cardiovascular system deconditioning require approximately 6 wk to move toward baseline.

NASA's Ambitious Vision for Future Space Exploration

NASA has begun to implement new exploration programs begun in the late 2018–2021 time frame (www.nasa.gov/feature/nasa-perseveres-through-pandemic-looks-ahead-in-2021;

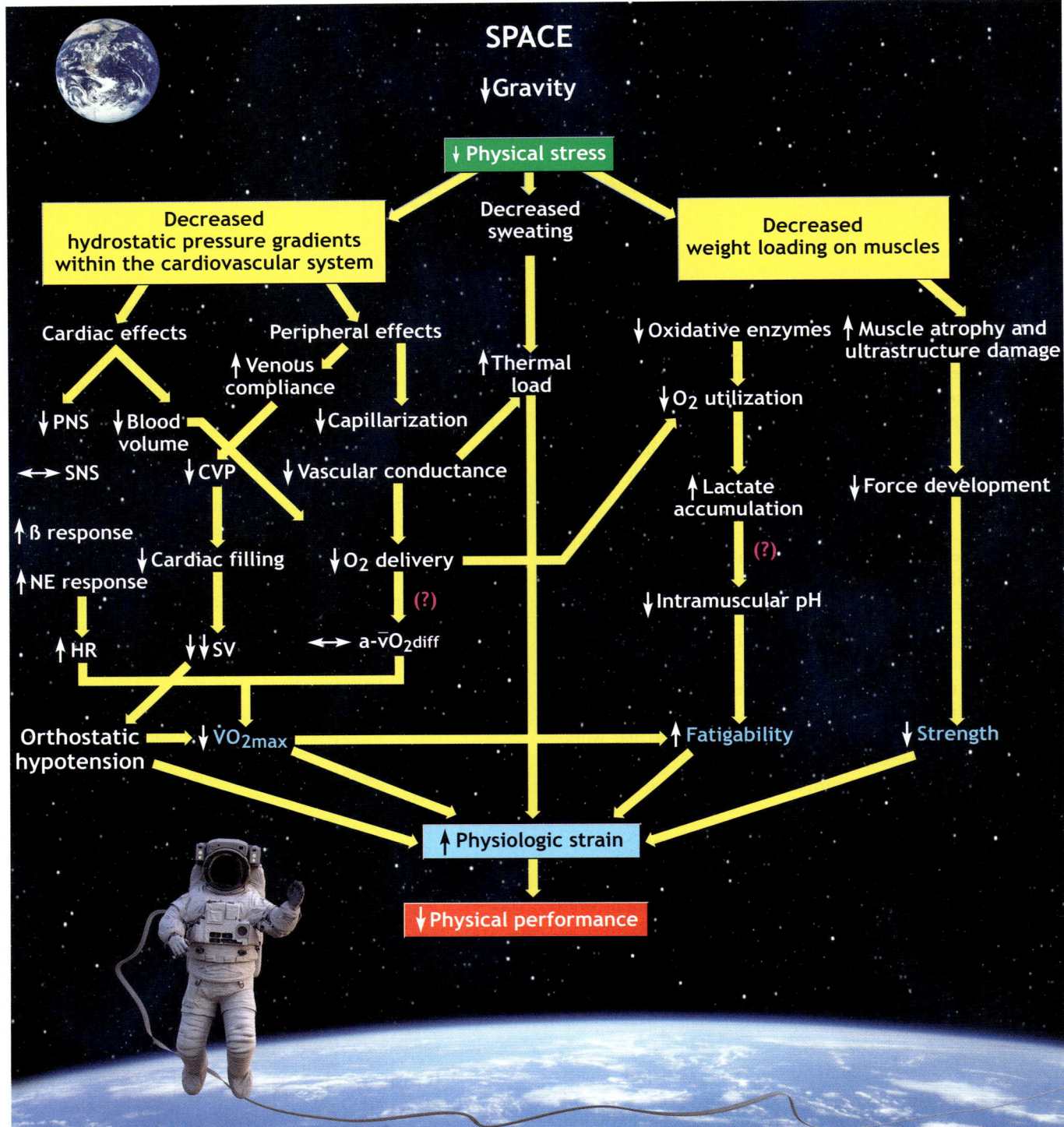

FIGURE 27.18. Model of the relationship between physical stress of the space environment and adaptation of cardiovascular and muscular systems, with resulting increased physiologic strain and decreased physical performance. SNS, sympathetic nervous system; CVP, central venous pressure; β, beta-adrenergic; NE, norepinephrine; HR, heart rate; SV, stroke volume; aV-O_2 diff, arteriovenous oxygen difference; ↑, increase; ↓, decrease; ↓↓, large decrease; ↔, no change.
(Reprinted with permission from Convertino VA. Effects of microgravity on exercise performance. In: Garrett WE, Kirkendall DT, eds. *Exercise and Sport Science*. Philadelphia: Lippincott Williams & Wilkins, 2000. Background image: Dotted Yeti/Shutterstock.)

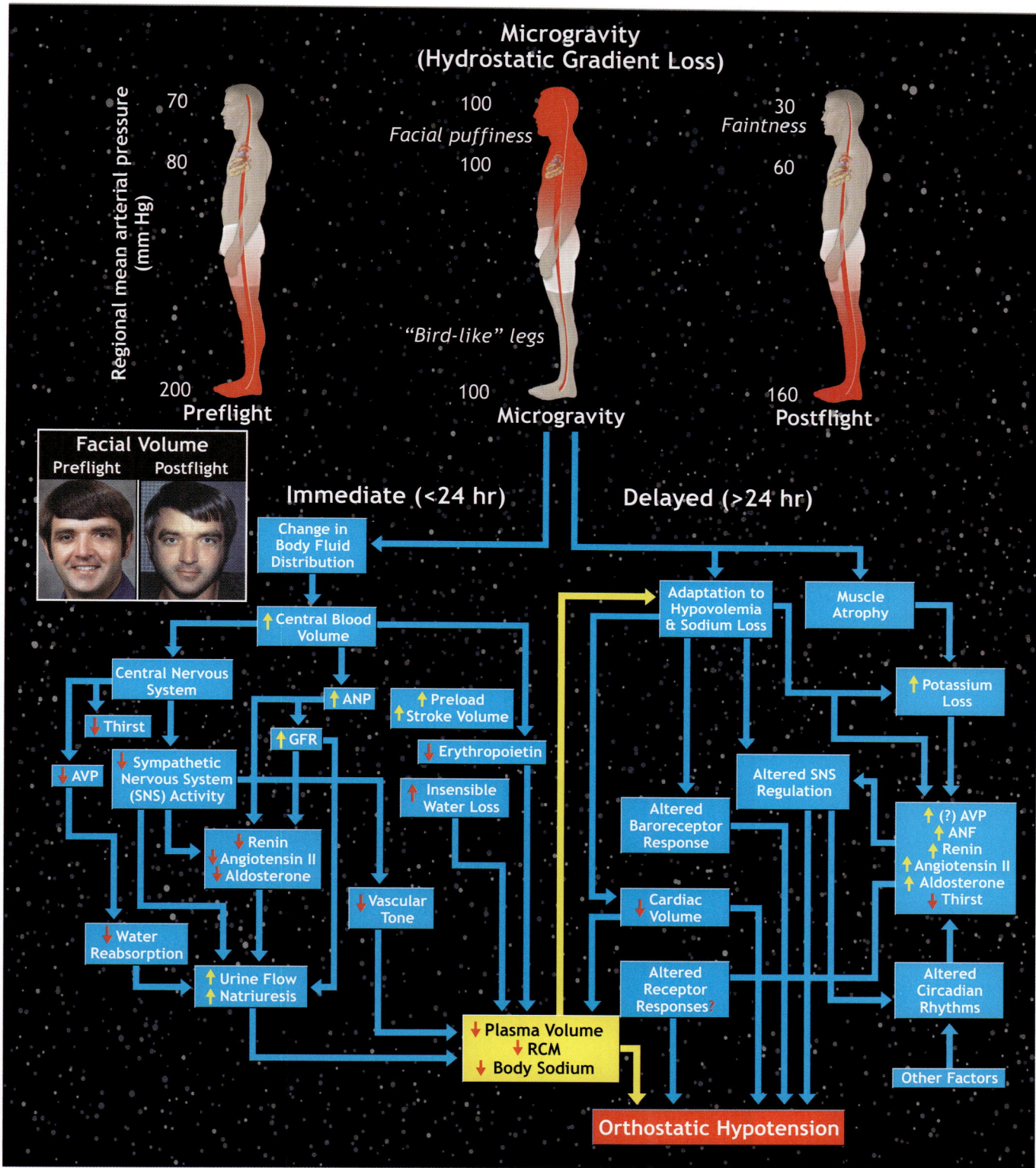

FIGURE 27.19. Proposed immediate (<24 hr) and delayed (>24 hr) responses to microgravity compared with preflight (1 g) and postflight (1 g) conditions. AVP, arginine vasopressin; ANP, atrial natriuretic peptide; GFR, glomerular filtration rate; RCM, red cell mass; ↑, increase; ↓, decrease, ?, possible.
(**Top figures** adapted with permission from Hargens AR, et al. Control of circulatory function in altered gravitational fields. *Physiologist*. 1992;35:S80. ©The American Physiological Society (APS). All rights reserved. **Bottom figure** adapted from Maillet A, et al. Cardiovascular and hormonal changes induced by isolation and confinement. *Med Sci Sports Exerc*. 1996;28:S53. Photos: NASA.)

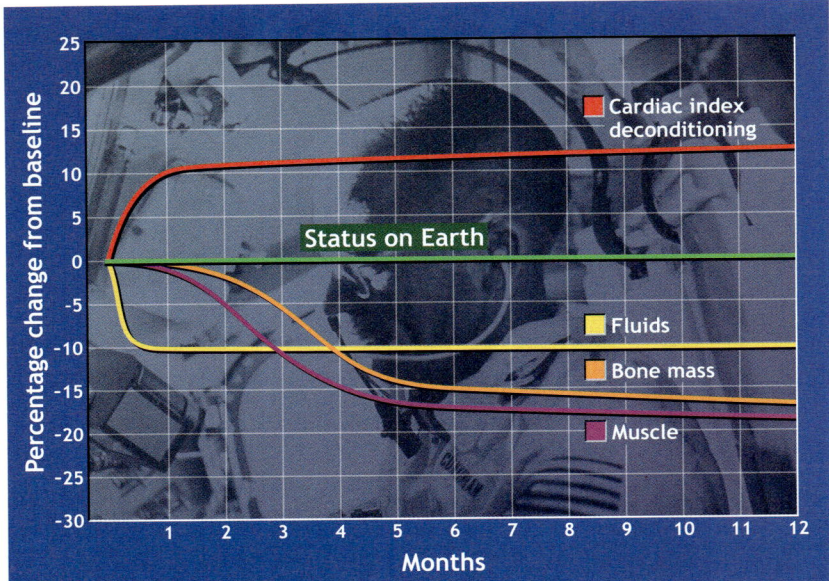

FIGURE 27.20. Proposed immediate (<24 hr) and delayed (>24 hr) time course for shifts in physiologic function during 1 yr in microgravity. The cardiac deconditioning index (*top red line above the green Status on Earth line*) reflects orthostatic intolerance severity to gravitational stress.
(Adapted with permission from Nicogossian A, et al. Overall physiologic response to space flight. In: Nicogossian AE, et al., eds. *Space Physiology and Medicine*. 3rd ed. Philadelphia: Lea & Febiger; 1994.)

www.nasa.gov/feature/nasa-confirms-new-simplex-mission-small-satellite-to-blaze-trails-studying-lunar-surface). Ongoing programs not discussed previously include the following:

- Mars Perseverance rover exploration (https://mars.nasa.gov/mars2020/)
- First commercial moon missions (www.nasa.gov/content/commercial-lunar-payload-services; https://www.jpl.nasa.gov/news/press_kits/mars_2020/landing/)
- Double Asteroid Redirection Test (DART; https://dart.jhuapl.edu/Mission/index.php)
- Mission to Metal Asteroid Psyche (www.jpl.nasa.gov/missions/psyche)
- First mission LUCY to the Trojan asteroid (www.nasa.gov/mission_pages/lucy/main/index)
- James Webb Space Telescope Launch (www.jwst.nasa.gov)

NASA's most ambitious program scheduled for 2024 is for the first woman and next man to land on the moon, with follow-up missions to establish sustainable lunar exploration by decades end (Artemis program; www.nasa.gov/specials/artemis/). Simultaneously, NASA has been planning an ambitious human Mars exploration mission with a 2030 time frame (www.nasa.gov/content/nasas-journey-to-mars).

Exploring Beyond Earth

NASA with several European partners plan to send humans to destinations beyond low Earth orbit (LEO), near-Earth asteroids (NEAs), the moon, and beyond to Mars and its two moons Phobos and Deimos (www.space.com/20413-phobos-deimos-mars-moons.html). Initially, exploring the vast expanse in space surrounding the Earth and moon, including the Lagrange points—locations in space where gravitational forces and body orbital motions balance each other—would establish a human presence outside LEO in preparing to undertake more complex missions beyond Earth's gravitational influence. Exploring an NEA could reveal information about how the solar system formed, how life started on Earth, and how to predict and mitigate the threat from asteroid impacts. NASA also established a longer-range plan to land humans on the Martian surface. A future Mars exploration would represent the first step to long-term human space exploration beyond the inner solar system by driving technology innovation necessary to sustain humans on another planet (https://solarsystem.nasa.gov/news/1652/10-things-to-expect-in-planetary-science-for-2021/).

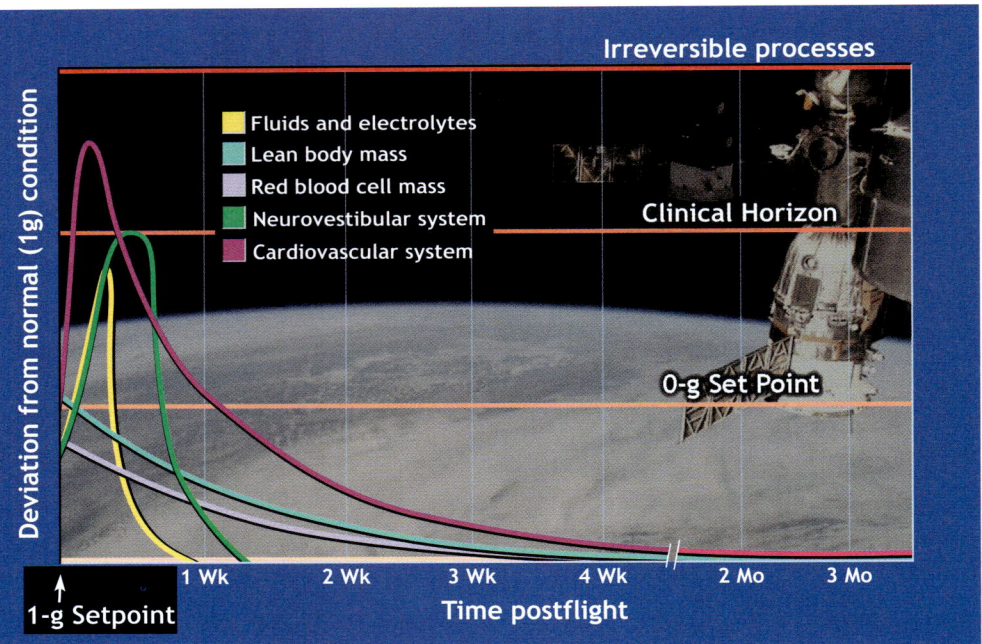

FIGURE 27.21. Physiologic shifts in the time course during 3-mo readaptation to 1 g, where flight duration only minimally affected readaptations.
(Adapted with permission from Nicogossian AE, et al., eds. *Space Physiology and Medicine*. 3rd ed. Philadelphia: Lea & Febiger, 1994. Photo: NASA.)

In a Practical Sense

Initially Against All Odds, African American Astronauts Now Fly into Space

To our readers: This "In a Practical Sense" differs from those in other chapters because we pay homage to all United States and foreign-trained astronauts for their extraordinary contributions to the diverse exploratory space programs since their inception. The astronauts express the very best in following their dreams and public service, while still serving as an inspiration to all who strive to pursue excellence in their chosen field, coupled with love and dedication to explore science at the highest levels.

On July 29, 1958, Congress passed the legislation and President Eisenhower signed the National Aeronautics and Space Act into law (https://history.nasa.gov/spaceact.html). Since then, there have been 336 astronaut candidates selected for training, a new group of carefully selected aspirants chosen every 5 years (www.space.com/37110-becoming-a-nasa-astronaut-surprising-facts.html), but it would take another decade before NASA accepted minorities for future space assignments. Currently, 17 African American astronauts from different backgrounds as military pilots, engineers, scientists, and physicians have flown in space on both short-duration and longer-duration missions. In the current Artemis Moon Exploration Program, two African American astronauts with considerable prior mission experience (Astronauts Wilson and Glover) will join current astronaut Jennifer Watkins (without onboard flight experience) among the candidates selected for the future Artemis missions (Watkins video profile; https://spacecenter.org/artemis-astronaut-feature-jessica-watkins/). These three were selected from a group of more than 18,000 applications just for a chance to become part to the Artemis program!

NASA MILESTONES

Former astronaut Robert H. Lawrence holds the honor as the first African American selected for NASA's space program. In June 1967, the U.S. Air force selected him as an aerospace research pilot for the Manned Orbiting Laboratory (MOL) Program (https://spacecenter.org/artemis-astronaut-feature-jessica-watkins/). Tragically, Lawrence was killed in an aircraft accident 6 mo after his selection and the Air Force cancelled the MOL Program. NASA administrators were planning to select Lawrence for a future space mission, and he would have been the first African American astronaut to fly in space. In January 1978, NASA for the first time included women and minorities for the Space Shuttle program—three African Americans, one pilot and two mission specialists. Astronaut Guion S. Bluford Jr, who we also profile, was the first African American in space as a mission specialist aboard space shuttle Challenger's STS-8 1983 mission (www.nmspacemuseum.org/inductee/guion-s-bluford-jr/).

ASTRONAUTS' EXTRAORDINARY ACHIEVEMENTS

Michael Anderson. In Memoriam. *Education*: BS physics/astronomy, University of Washington (1981); MS physics, Creighton University (1990). *NASA Service*: Selected as an astronaut (1994); first African American in space aboard space shuttle Endeavor STS-89 (1998) and payload commander on STS-107, logging 593 hr in space; killed February 1, 2003 when Space Shuttle Columbia disintegrated during re-entry.

All images courtesy of NASA.

Guion S. Bluford Jr. *Education*: BS aerospace engineering, Pennsylvania State University (1964); MS with distinction in aerospace engineering, Air Force Institute of Technology (1974); PhD in aerospace engineering and minor in laser physics, Air Force Institute of Technology (1978); MBA, University of Houston-Clear Lake (1987). *NASA Service*: Selected as astronaut (1979); Mission Specialist STS-8, STS-61-A, STS-39, STS-53.

Charles F. Bolden Jr. *Education*: BS electrical science, U.S. Naval Academy (1968); MS systems management, University of Southern California (1977). *NASA Service:* Selected as astronaut (1980). Veteran of four spaceflights with over 680 hr in space. Served as Pilot on STS-61C and STS-31 and Commander on STS-45 and STS-60. Selected as 12th NASA administrator and first African American administrator (2009); Retired (2017).

Yvonne Darlene Cagle, MD. BA biochemistry San Francisco State University (1981); MD University of Washington (1985); Received aerospace medicine certification School of Aerospace Medicine, Brooks Air Force Base, TX (1988); Completed residency in family practice Ghent FP Eastern Virginia Medical School (1992). Received certification as senior FAA aviation medical examiner (1995). *NASA Service*: Selected as astronaut (1996); currently at Ames Research Center as Astronaut Science, Liaison, and Strategic Relationships coordinator; Strategic Relationships Manager for Google and other Silicon Valley programmatic partnerships.

Robert L. Curbeam Jr. *Education*. BS aerospace engineering U.S. Naval Academy (1984); MS aeronautical engineering Naval Postgraduate School (1990) and astronautical engineering Naval Postgraduate School (1991). *NASA Service*: Selected as astronaut (1994). Flew on STS-85, STS-98, STS-116, logging over 593 hr in space, including 19 spacewalk hr during three spacewalks.

Benjamin Alvin Drew. BS astronautical engineering and BS physics U.S. Air Force Academy (1984); MS aerospace science Embry Riddle University (1995). *NASA Service*: Selected as Mission Specialist (2000); flew on STS-118 (2007) and STS-133 (2011).

Jeanette J. Epps. *Education*: BS physics Le Moyne College (1992); MS and PhD aerospace engineering, University of Maryland (1994 and 2000). *NASA Service*: Selected as astronaut (2009). Graduated from Astronaut Candidate Training (instruction in ISS systems, spacewalk training, robotics, T-38 flight training, and water and wilderness survival training).

(Continued)

In a Practical Sense

Initially Against All Odds, African American Astronauts Now Fly into Space (Continued)

Victor J. Glover Jr. *Education*: BS general engineering California Polytechnic State University San Luis Obispo (1999), MS flight test engineering Air University, Edwards Air Force Base, CA (2007); MS systems engineering Naval Postgraduate School (2009); Master of Military Operational Art and Science Air University (2010). *NASA Service:* Selected 2013 and training for first post-certification mission on SpaceX's Crew Dragon spacecraft and a long-duration mission aboard ISS.

Frederick D. Gregory. *Education*: BS U.S. Air Force Academy (1964); MS information systems George Washington University (1977). *NASA Service*: Selected as astronaut candidate (1978). Logged over 455 hr in space on three shuttle missions. Served as Pilot on STS-51B and Commander on STS-33 and STS-44. Led NASA's Safety and Mission Assurance Effort and Office of Space Flight. Retired 2005 as NASA's Deputy Administrator.

Bernard A. Harris Jr. *Education*: BS biology University of Houston (1978); MD Texas Tech University School of Medicine (1982). Completed Mayo Clinic internal medicine residency (1985). Flight Surgeon Aerospace School of Medicine, Brooks Air Force Base (1988); MS in biomedical science University of Texas Medical Branch at Galveston (1996). *NASA Service*: Selected as astronaut (1990); logged more than 438 hr in space on STS-55 and STS-63.

Joan E. Higginbotham. *Education*: BS electrical engineering Southern Illinois University, Carbondale (1987); MS management Florida Institute of Technology (1992); MS space systems from Florida Institute of Technology (1996). *NASA Service*: Selected as astronaut (1996); flew on STS-116 (2006).

Mae C. Jemison, M.D. *Education*: *NASA Service*: BS chemical engineering (and fulfilled the requirements for BA African and Afro-American studies) Stanford University (1977); doctorate in medicine Cornell University (1981). *NASA Service*: Selected as astronaut (1987); science Mission Specialist STS-47 Spacelab-J, logging 190 hr in space.

Ronald E. McNair, PhD. In Memoriam. *Education*: BS physics North Carolina A&T State University (1971); PhD physics MIT (1976); honorary doctorate of laws North Carolina A&T State University (1978); honorary doctorate of Science Morris College (1980); honorary doctorate of science University of South Carolina (1984); Presidential Scholar (1971–1974); Ford Foundation Fellow (1971–1974); National Fellowship Fund Fellow (1974–1975); NATO Fellow (1975); sixth-degree karate black belt; accomplished saxophonist. *NASA Service*: Selected as astronaut (1978); STS 41-B, logging 191 hr in space before he perished aboard Space Shuttle Challenger.

Leland D. Melvin. *Education*: BS chemistry University of Richmond (1986); MS materials science engineering University of Virginia (1991). *NASA Service*: Selected as astronaut (1998); flew on STS-122, delivering the Columbus Laboratory to the ISS; flew on STS-129 (2009); served as NASA's Associate Administrator for the Office of Education (2010–2014).

Bobby Satcher. *Education*: BA and PhD chemical engineering MIT; MD Harvard University; Orthopedic surgeon Northwestern University Illinois. *NASA Service*: Selected as astronaut (2004); Mission Specialist STS-129 (2009).

Winston E. Scott. *Education*: BA music Florida State University (1972); MS aeronautical engineering U.S. Naval Postgraduate School (1980). *NASA Service*: Selected as astronaut (1992); flew on STS-72 (1996) and STS-87 (1997); logged 24 days, 14 hr, 34 min in space; three spacewalks totaling 19 hr 26 min.

Stephanie D. Wilson. *Education*: BS engineering science Harvard University (1988); MS aerospace engineering University of Texas (1992). *NASA Service*: Selected as astronaut (1996); first spaceflight STS-121 (2006), STS-120 (2007), and STS-131 (2010).

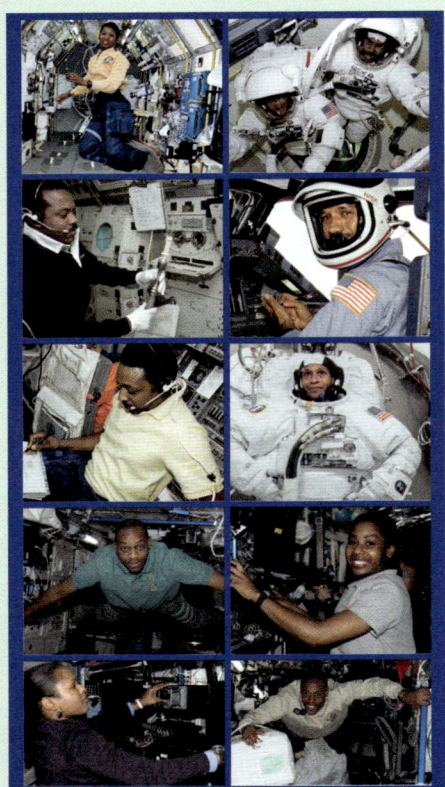

All images courtesy of NASA.

Future Mars Missions

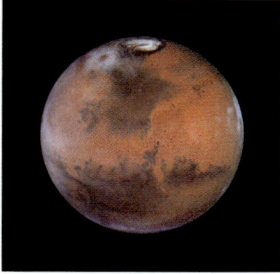
Credit: NASA

The first successful human Mars mission will require a voyage built on new technological and operational complexities. The distance from Earth to the moon is a relatively manageable 240,000 miles and can be travelled in about 3 Earth days. In contrast, Mars is nearly 140 million mi from Earth depending on their orientation from the sun. The challenging Mars mission originating from the moon is compounded by these huge travel distances, the near 7-mo travel time from the moon to Mars, and dangerous radiation types encountered in deep space.[134]

Dangerous Radiation Effects on Mars and the Moon

Mars' atmosphere presents distinct challenges for getting humans to and from its surface. The main challenge is that Mars has no global magnetic field, which allows the sun over billions of years to eradicate the Martian atmosphere and leave its surface vulnerable to deadly radiation. This was confirmed when the Mars Curiosity rover on its deep space mission in 2011–2012 revealed that the radiation dose was about 0.66 **sievert units (Sv)**, the equivalent of an astronaut receiving a whole body CT scan every week spent on the Martian surface (https://mars.nasa.gov/msl/home/). As a comparison, a 1-sievert radiation dose associates with a 6% increase in fatal cancers,[13] cataracts and vision impairment, and degenerative cardiac disease, whereas the normal daily dose on Earth is about 10 microsieverts (mSV) or 0.00001 sievert (Sv). NASA has mapped the radiation effect on Mars from above and below 8 km/5 mi (www.nasa.gov/hrp/elements/radiation/risks) as a first step in developing eventual radiation protective measures. At lower altitudes (farther from the sun), the radiation effect is less (0.20 to 0.26 Sv) or about 0.30 Sv yearly. Nevertheless, radiation carcinogenesis is still unavoidable and deadly and will require perfecting an effective countermea-

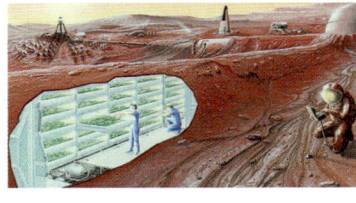
Credit: NASA/JPL-Caltech

sures strategy.[96] Currently, lifetime exposure limits established by NASA range from 180 Sv for a 30-year-old female to 700 Sv for a 60-year-old male. Those limits are based on models intended to set a limit no more than a 3% **radiation exposure–induced death (REID)** risk at the 95% confidence level. NASA has now proposed changing to a 600 millisievert limit regardless of age or gender (https://spacenews.com/report-backs-nasa-proposal-to-change-astronaut-radiation-exposure-limits/).

The first phases in the planned three Artemis Moon Missions in the middle to late 2020s will pave the way for an eventual epic Mars journey and future planet colonization. The Artemis III mission and four-member Orion spacecraft will be the mission that lands on the moon to establish a working basecamp following the successful Apollo missions almost 50 years ago. Because the moon has no atmosphere and a weak magnetic field, astronauts must wear space suits to protect them from outside radiation and will have to bury their living habitats underground.

Lippincott® Connect — Appendix J, available online at **Lippincot Connect**, lists science-based podcasts produced by NASA, in conjunction with public and private agencies and sponsoring partners, available on the Apple, Soundcloud, and Google platforms that cover the spectrum from early NASA historical milestones to the latest updates from the scientists, engineers, and astronauts who create cutting-edge technologies and fly on the NASA space missions.

NASA Space Biology Research Pays Big Dividends

Conducting space biology research remains a costly endeavor. NASA's budget is established annually that begins with the White House and concludes with legislation passed by Congress and signed by the President. The budget specifies funding amounts for programs and projects in human spaceflight, space science, aeronautics, technology development, and education.

NASA's budget peaked during the Apollo program in the 1960s. After the United States won the race to the moon, space exploration lost political support and NASA's budget was cut significantly. From about 1970 to 2018, the NASA budget has hovered between 1 and 0.5% of all U.S. government spending, which translates to less than 1% spent on the entire U.S. space program! That amounts to less than one penny for every dollar the government spends on different programs. The average American spends more on a monthly cable bill or eating out at fast-food restaurants. As pointed out in the section on spin-off technologies, the investment in space biology has been a huge benefit to the United States and other countries worldwide. For every dollar the United States spends on research and development in the space program, seven dollars come back as corporate and personal income taxes from increased jobs and economic growth (http://spinoff.nasa.gov/).

NASA Budget Process for Space Biology Research

Conducting space biology research remains a costly endeavor. NASA's budget is established annually that begins with the White House and concludes with legislation passed by Congress and signed by the President. The budget specifies funding amounts for programs and projects in human spaceflight, space science, aeronautics, technology development, and education.

NASA 2022 Budget NASA is internally separated into major program areas, each receiving funding to administer their own projects. Funding varies yearly, with generally about 50% in the annual budget concerns human spaceflight activities, 30% for robotic missions and scientific research, and the remainder allocated among aeronautics, technology development programs, staff salaries, facilities management, and facilities and overhead.

NASA's budget is not used for national defense nor intelligence gathering programs, and as a civilian agency, is responsible for peaceful space exploration. National security space programs are the responsibility of the Armed Forces under the newly created Space Force (www.spaceforce.mil) and existing National Reconnaissance Office (www.nro.gov). NASA's space technology program, which received $1.1 billion in 2021, was to receive a 27% increase to $1.4 billion in 2022 (www.nasa.gov/news/budget/index.html). The added funding enhances NASA's space exploration programs and provides new technologies to help the expanding commercial space industry grow, including novel early-stage space technology research to support developing clean energy Earth resources (https://spacenews.com/biden-administration-proposes-24-5-billion-budget-for-nasa-in-2022/). Three private companies have been developing their own programs using newly designed spacecraft and launch facilities to fly humans into space beginning in July, 2021 (www.blueorigin.com; www.spacex.com; www.virgingalactic.com). These three companies are not the only privately funded companies with an interest in either exploring space or developing new technologies to assist in eventual space settlement. As of July, 2021, 30 companies have announced plans related to space exploration efforts (www.space-settlement-institute.org/space-companies.html).

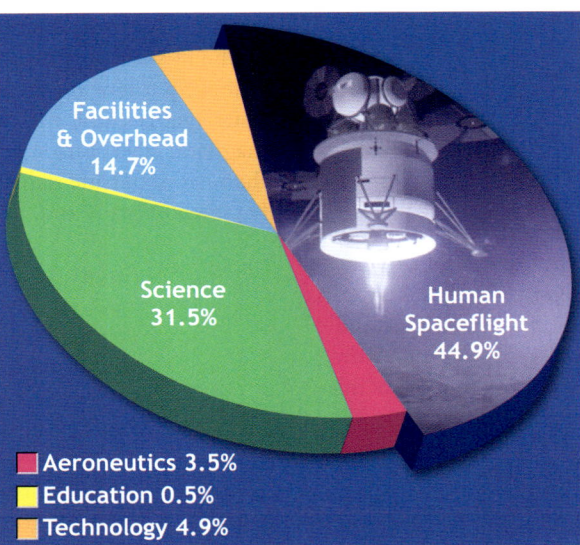
Photo: NASA

Practical Benefits from Space Biology Research

Companies that apply NASA technology in non–space-related areas create thousands of jobs that ultimately impact citizens worldwide (https://spinoff.nasa.gov/sites/default/files/2020-12/NASA_Spinoff-2021.pdf). Technologies developed over the half century to meet space exploration challenges have produced more than 30,000 secondary commercial applications in seven categories dating from 1976 to the present (https://spinoff.nasa.gov):

1. Computer Technology
2. Consumer/Home/Recreation
3. Environmental and Resource Management
4. Health and Medicine
5. Industrial Productivity/Manufacturing
6. Public Safety
7. Transportation

NASA maintains an active database and detailed archives from all its programs and over 2000 spin-off technologies, providing commercial potential and benefits to improve life on Earth (https://spinoff.nasa.gov/spinoff/archives). The two most celebrated prior space undertakings, the Apollo and Space Shuttle programs, provided a treasure trove in new technologies that now have become ubiquitous in most people's daily lives. **TABLE 27.10** lists 20 examples from the Apollo and Space Shuttle Programs that the reader will recognize from their own life experiences, from wearing heart rate monitors embedded in smartphones and exercise equipment, to athletic shoes to lightweight prosthetic devices and MRI technology to kidney dialysis machines. The cost-to-benefit ratio surely favors the benefit side of the equation—justification enough to prove the worth from the international community for continued economic and political support for space exploration in the coming decades and beyond.

TABLE 27.10 Significant spin-off contributions from the Apollo and Space Shuttle Programs

Final Words

As we close this chapter, the Mars 2020 Perseverance rover expedition has begun to search for ancient microbial life, which will advance NASA's quest to explore Mars' past habitability. The rover applies a drill to collect core rock and soil samples, then store them in sealed tubes for pickup by a future mission to ferry them back to Earth for detailed analyses. Perseverance also will test technologies to pave the way for future human Mars exploration. Strapped to the rover's belly for the journey and a technology demonstration—the Mars Helicopter Ingenuity achieved a "Wright Brothers' moment" on the Red Planet akin to their historic first controlled flight in 1903. That single event and others, captured in a real-time video on the Martian surface (https://mars.nasa.gov/resources/25838/mastcam-z-video-of-ingenuity-taking-off-and-landing/; credit to NASA/JPL-Caltech/ASU/MSSS) represents a major milestone—the first rotor-powered craft in Mars' extremely thin atmosphere. This seminal event achieved its prescribed maximum

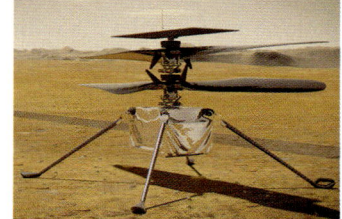
Credit: NASA/JPL-Caltech

NASA's Considerable Data Resources

Five publicly available, free open-source data resources are available at NASA's Open Data Portal (https://data.nasa.gov) covering numerous research endeavors sponsored by multiple NASA agencies.

1. **EarthData** (earthdata.nasa.gov): The NASA Earth Observing System Data and Information System (EOSDIS) provides Earth science data to users from satellite, airborne, and ISS missions for long-term global observations of the land surface, biosphere, solid Earth, atmosphere, and oceans.
2. **HICO—NASA Ocean Color Database** (https://oceancolor.gsfc.nasa.gov/data/hico/): The Hyperspectral Imager for the Coastal Ocean (HICO) was an imaging spectrometer, collecting more than 10,000 images of Earth from 2009 to 2014 at selected coastal regions at 90 m with full spectral coverage (380 to 960 nm sampled at 5.7 nm) with a high signal-to-noise ratio to resolve the coastal ocean's optical complexity.
3. **GeneLab** (https://genelab.nasa.gov/): Comprehensive space-related biology database allowing users to upload, download, share, store, and analyze spaceflight relevant data from experiments using model organisms.
4. **Life Sciences Data Archive** (https://lsda.jsc.nasa.gov/): Public archive of spaceflight, flight-analog, and ground-based life sciences research investigations.
5. **Physical Science Informatics** (https://www.nasa.gov/PSI): A data repository for physical science experiments performed on the ISS and space shuttle flights coordinated through NASA's Physical Sciences Research Program at the Glenn Research Center (GRC), Jet Propulsion Laboratory (JPL), and Marshall Space Flight Center (MSFC).

3-m/10-ft altitude, maintaining a stable hover for 30 s before descending again, becoming the first ever rotorcraft to fly on another planet. Five additional flights accomplished incrementally farther distance and altitude targets (www.space.com/mars-helicopter-ingenuity-19th-flight-preview). The Perseverance rover will continue its scientific mission for at least 1 Mars year or about 687 Earth days.

Future Missions

A key objective for Perseverance's future Mars missions is **astrobiology** (www.nasa.gov/feature/what-is-astrobiology), which included the search for ancient microbial life. The rover will characterize the planet's geology and past climate, chart a way for future Mars human exploration, and become the first mission to collect and cache Martian rock and regolith (broken rock and dust). In addition, Perseverance will test a technology to extract oxygen from the Martian atmosphere, which is 96% carbon dioxide. The aim is to test ways to use Mars' natural resources to support human explorers and improve designs for life-support, transportation, and other systems to allow humans to eventually live safely by controlling radiation's deadly consequences and to continue scientific explorations for humankind's future benefits (https://mars.nasa.gov/mer/mission/timeline/).

Subsequent NASA missions, in cooperation with ESA (European Space Agency), would send spacecraft to Mars to collect these sealed samples from the surface and return them to Earth for in-depth analysis. The Mars 2020 Perseverance mission supports NASA's moon-to-Mars exploration approach, which includes Artemis missions to the moon that will help prepare for human exploration on the Red Planet (http://www.nasa.gov/specials/artemis/; www.youtube.com/watch?v=_T8cn2J13-4; www.nasa.gov/sites/default/files/atoms/files/artemis_plan-20200921.pdf). A trip to our nearest neighboring Earthlike planet Venus (only 38.2 million km/27 million mi compared to 55.7 million km/34.6 million mi for Mars) remains a goal far into the future. Scientists will have to overcome the physiological challenges that life on Venus for 1 day is equal to 243 Earth days!

 ## NASA Explores Winter Sports Technology

NASA has developed new materials and technologies to overcome the extreme thermal challenges in the space environment required for high-thrust propulsion for crew and cargo capsules. NASA developed unique **aerogel material** to limit cryogenic propellant from boiling away in spacecraft elements during the liftoff cryogenic propulsion stage in a space mission (www.nasa.gov/pdf/657307main_Exploration%20Report_508_6-4-12.pdf).

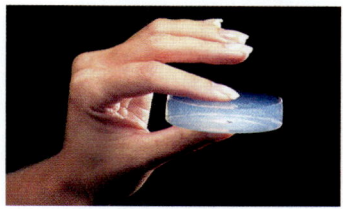

Credit: NASA

The aerogel insulating material serves a dual purpose—it was applied to terrestrial applications in extreme winter sports equipment that warms snowboarders and skiers hands and feet. The material is currently available commercially in many products available to the public via Internet searches. The next-generation cryogenic propulsion systems will require more advanced materials than current aerogels. Newer materials will enable zero-boil-off propellant storage, saving more than 10 metric tons in launch mass, roughly the equivalent weight of a crew capsule. Increased efficiency during space launches will be necessary for humans to travel to Mars and most Near-Earth Orbit (NEA) asteroids.

Source:
An L, et al. An all-ceramic, anisotropic, and flexible aerogel insulation material. *Nano Lett.* 2020;20:3828.

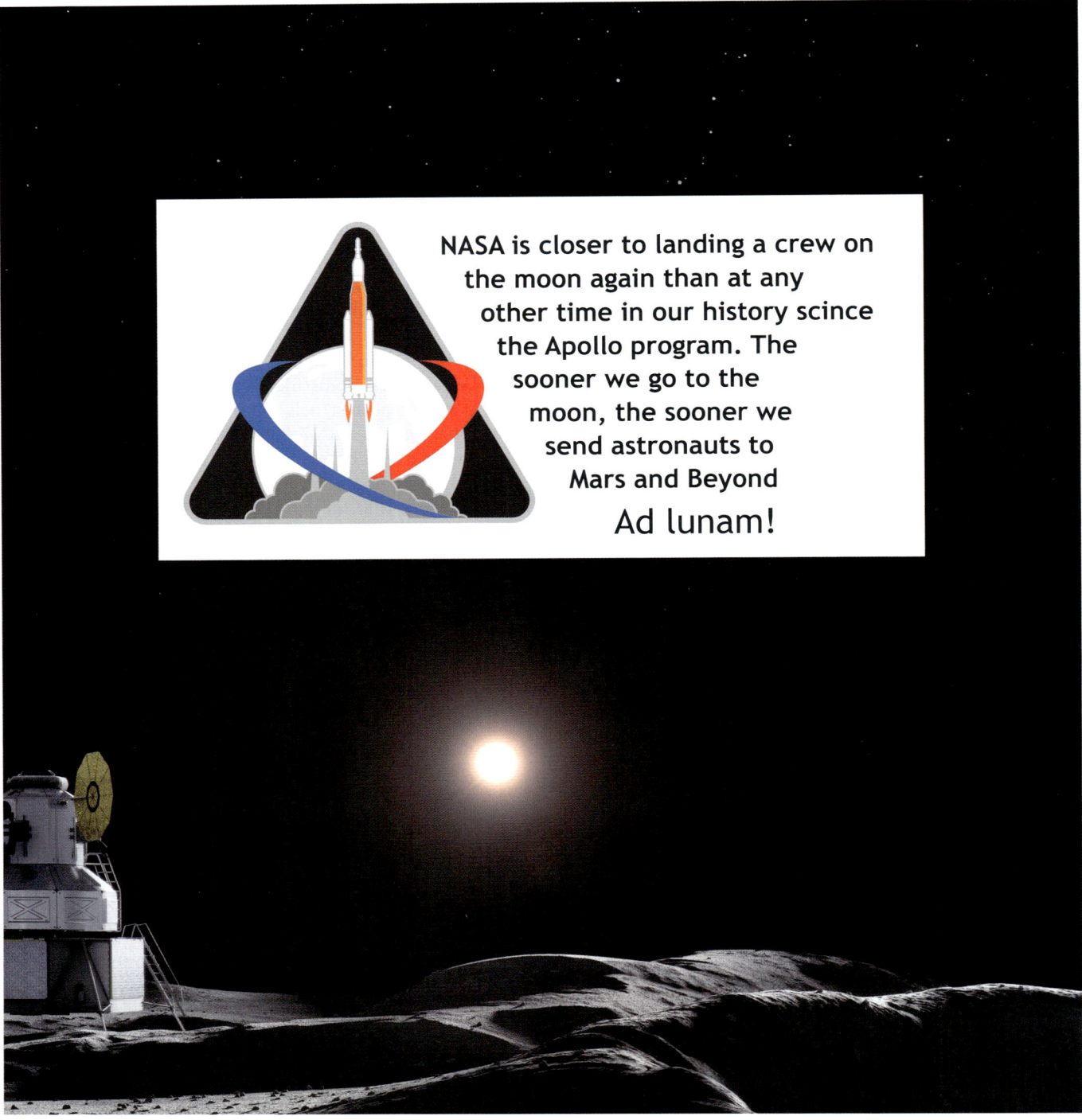

Credit: NASA

Summary

1. On Earth's surface, gravity provides an invisible attraction force that makes any mass exert downward force or have weight. Sir Isaac Newton (1642–1727) discovered the universality of the gravitational law.
2. An object or celestial body's escape velocity depends on the mass and radius of that body. Escape velocity from Earth equals 40,296 kmh/25,039 mph.
3. The force of gravity never reaches an absolute zero value (called zero-g) because a gravitational force still exists. The term *microgravity*, not weightlessness or zero-g, best describes what an astronaut perceives during spaceflight.
4. On October 4, 1957, the Russians' Sputnik 1 became the first Earth-orbiting satellite. One month later, Sputnik 2 remained in orbit for almost 200 days with an on-board dog.
5. NASA established two main early goals: first, launch a man into space and return him safely to Earth and, second, develop human capability to endure space missions.
6. The most significant technological achievement in the 20th century took place when Apollo 11 astronauts first landed on the moon's surface on July 20, 1969.

7. During the first few days in microgravity, fluid shifts from the lower body to the upper body. Total fluid volume also decreases to reduce the heart's work effort.
8. The greatest postural instability in microgravity occurs in tests that require vestibular information.
9. Among NASA's greatest biomedical concerns during space missions involves the 1 to 6% monthly loss in weight-bearing bone mass among male and female astronauts on flights differing in duration.
10. Permanent neuromuscular dysfunction has not occurred as a result from prolonged space missions.
11. Inflight and postflight changes during nearly 1-year missions reveal altered muscular coordination patterns, delayed-onset muscle soreness, and generalized muscular fatigue and weakness.
12. Countermeasure strategies attempt to minimize spaceflight's potentially harmful deconditioning effects on crew physiologic function, performance, and overall health during mission-critical maneuvers with re-entry and landing.
13. Without gravity, normal biologic functions become more susceptible to short-term and long-term maladaptations such as space motion sickness (SMS).
14. The energy balance equation has not been satisfied successfully on most missions related to spaceflight's increased energy demands and decreased food intake.
15. Maladaptations to microgravity include decreases in lean body mass, muscle volume, and muscle strength; altered muscle fiber microarchitecture; and skeletal muscle atrophy to support posture and locomotion.
16. New technologies developed for the space program over the past 50 years have produced more than 30,000 secondary commercial spin-off applications.
17. For every dollar the United States spends on research and development in the space program, seven dollars come back as corporate and personal income taxes from increased jobs and economic growth.
18. Most advances in space biology research provide life-altering breakthroughs in computer technology, consumer/home/recreation, transportation, environmental and resource management, industrial productivity/manufacturing, health and medicine, and public safety.
19. The next-generation spacesuit, the exploration extravehicular mobility unit or xEMU, plays a crucial role in NASA's many future planned space exploration programs.
20. The Mars 2020 Perseverance mission, integral to NASA's new moon to Mars exploration Artemis strategy, includes the first three missions to the moon beginning 2024–2026 depending on Congressional budget allocations; it will help prepare for future human Mars explorations in the 2030 time frame.

Key Terms

Advanced resistive exercise device (ARED): Adjustable resistance piston-driven vacuum cylinders and flywheel provide muscle loading for crew members to maintain muscle strength during space missions akin to conventional "weight-lifting" exercise on Earth

Aerogel material: Synthetic porous ultralight material derived from a gel, resulting in a solid with extremely low density and extremely low thermal conductivity

Aerospace medicine: Focuses on the clinical care, research, and operational support of the health, safety, and performance of crewmembers and passengers of air and space vehicles, together with the support personnel who assist operation of such vehicles

Albert Projects: Named for the monkey sealed in the nose cone of the V-2 rocket during an exploratory space mission before human flight

Apollo 11: First American spacecraft lands on the moon, July 20, 1969

Artemis missions: Three-phase new program for future moon exploration

Artificial gravity: Creation of an inertial force that mimics the effects of a gravitational force, usually by rotation; sometimes referred to as pseudogravity or rotational gravity

Astrobiology: Study of life in the universe, including the search for beyond earth

Astronaut: Derives from the Greek words meaning "space sailor" and refers to all who have been launched as crew members aboard NASA spacecraft bound for orbit and beyond

Bioastronautics: Field of study that focuses on biologic and medical effects of spaceflight on human systems and encompasses numerous aspects of biological, behavioral, and medical concerns governing humans and other living organisms in a spaceflight environment

Bone mineral density (BMD): Amount of bone mineral in bone tissue reflects the mass of mineral per volume of bone

Centrifugal force: Outward force on a rotating mass

Countermeasure strategies: Systematic attempts to neutralize or minimize spaceflight's potentially harmful deconditioning effects on physiologic function, performance, and overall health during mission-critical maneuvers, particularly re-entry and landing

Denitrogenation: Removal of nitrogen from the body by breathing nitrogen-free gases

Eagle: Spacecraft that served as the crewed Apollo 11 lunar lander, the first mission to land humans on the moon on July 20, 1969

Exercise countermeasures: Site-specific lower body eccentric and concentric resistance exercise coupled with relatively intense cardiovascular workouts on a cycle ergometer and treadmill

Exploration extravehicular mobility unit (xEMU): Latest generation astronaut space suit designed for continuous EVA use in future deep space exploration missions, on the lunar surface, and eventually for use on Mars

Extravehicular activity (EVA): Activity done by an astronaut outside a spacecraft beyond the Earth's appreciable atmosphere

Extravehicular mobility unit (EMU): Second-generation astronaut spacesuit that combines soft and hard components to provide support, mobility, and comfort

First lady astronaut trainees (FLATS): Special flight-training program for a group of 13 highly qualified female aviators with extensive flight experience for future space missions.

Functional electrostimulation (FES): Treatment applies small electrical charges to a muscle paralyzed or weakened from brain or spinal cord damage

Gagarin, Yuri: First Soviet cosmonaut in space

General re-entry syndrome (GRS): Symptoms include vertigo, nausea, instability, and fatigue induced by reimposing increased +Gz during re-entry and landing

Gravity (G or g): Net acceleration imparted to objects due to the combined effect of gravitation (from mass distribution within Earth) and centrifugal force (from the Earth's rotation); measured in meters per second squared (m/s2 or m·s^{-2}) or equivalently in newtons per kilogram (N/kg or N·kg^{-1})

Head-down bed rest: Subjects remain confined to bed for extended time (weeks, months, or a year) in a horizontal or head-down tilt position ($-3°$ to $-12°$)

Hubble Space Telescope: Space telescope named after renowned astronomer Edwin Hubble launched in 1990 by NASA

International Space Station (ISS): Modular space station in low Earth orbit (220 nautical miles; 1 nautical mile = 1.852 km) above Earth

Interim resistive exercise device (iRED): Exercise device designed by NASA to allow for more intense workouts in zero gravity using a system of vacuum tubes and flywheel cables to simulate free weight exercises

Lower body negative pressure (LBNP): Special device applies negative pressure to lower limbs to force fluid in the vascular system to migrate downward from the upper torso to the lower body

Mach numbers: Named to honor Austrian physicist Ernst Mach who established basic principles associated with supersonics and ballistics, determined the ratio of an object's velocity to the velocity of sound (which travels at 1089 ft·s^{-1} or 331.9 m·s^{-1} at 0°C/32°F)

Mercury astronauts: First seven astronauts selected for the human space program; Scott Carpenter, Gordon Cooper, John Glenn, Gus Grissom, Wally Schirra, Alan Shepard, and Deke Slayton

Microgravity (µG): Synonymous with *weightlessness* and *zero-g*, but with an emphasis that g-forces are never exactly zero—just very small

Newton, Sir Isaac: English mathematician, physicist, astronomer, theologian, and author widely recognized as one of the most influential scientists of all time and key figure in the scientific revolution; formulated the laws of motion and universal gravitation that formed the dominant scientific viewpoint until introduction of relativity theory

Newton third law: When one object exerts a force on a second object, the second object exerts a force equal in magnitude and opposite in direction on the first object

NSBRI Research Program: Consortium of 12 institutions that worked on physiological and medical solutions to health problems related to longer-duration space travel and prolonged microgravity exposure

Orthostatic hypotension: Minimum 20 mm Hg systolic blood pressure decrease and at least 10 mm Hg diastolic blood pressure decrease within 3 min of standing

Orthostatic intolerance: Compromised venous return to the heart during upright posture in a gravity environment

Parabolic flights: Aircraft trajectory provides freefall for up to 30 s where when aircraft acceleration cancels acceleration due to gravity

Preoxygenation: Oxygen administered prior to decompression

Radiation exposure-induced death (REID): Quantifies lifetime death risk from radiation-induced cancer in an exposed astronaut

Sensorimotor integration: Capability of the central nervous system to integrate different sources of stimuli, and parallelly, to transform such inputs in motor actions

Sievert units (Sv): Derived ionizing radiation dose unit in the International System of Units to measure the health effect of low ionizing radiation levels on the human body

Space motion sickness (SMS): Usually occurs within the first 72 hr in spaceflight; characterized by clumsiness, difficulty concentrating, disorientation, persisting sensation aftereffects, nausea, pallor, drowsiness, vomiting, vertigo while walking and standing, difficulty walking a straight line, blurred vision, and dry heaves

Sputnik 1: First Russian spacecraft to orbit Earth

Tereshkova, Valentina: Russian cosmonaut was the first woman into space

Vomit Comet: Repeated roller coaster–like training maneuvers, with up to 60 parabolic flights daily for a week, providing about 3-h cumulative weightlessness while performing simple to complex movement tasks on NASA's KC-135 aircraft

Zero-g: Complete or near-complete absence in sensing weight

> **References are available online at Lippincott Connect.**

Additional References

Acres JM, et al. The influence of spaceflight and simulated microgravity on bacterial motility and chemotaxis. *NPJ Microgravity*. 2021;7:7.

Bailey JF, et al. Biomechanical changes in the lumbar spine following spaceflight and factors associated with post spaceflight disc herniation. *Spine J*. 2022;22:197.

Berrios DC, et al. GeneLab: interfaces for the exploration of space omics data. *Nucleic Acids Res*. 2021;49:D1515.

Buoite Stella A, et al. Neurophysiological adaptations to spaceflight and simulated microgravity. *Clin Neurophysiol*. 2021;132:498.

Buravkova L, et al. Microgravity effects on the matrisome. *Cells*. 2021;10:2226.

Cao Z, et al. Comprehensive circRNA expression profile and function network in osteoblast-like cells under simulated microgravity. *Gene*. 2021;764:145106.

Carriot J, et al. Challenges to the vestibular system in space: how the brain responds and adapts to microgravity. *Front Neural Circuits*. 2021;15:760313.

Desai RI, et al. Nonhuman primate models in the study of spaceflight stressors: past contributions and future directions. *Life Sci Space Res (Amst)*. 2021;30:9.

Dhar S, et al. Mechano-immunomodulation in space: mechanisms involving microgravity-induced changes in t cells. *Life (Basel)*. 2021;11:1043.

Domnin PA, et al. Combined impact of magnetic force and spaceflight conditions on Escherichia coli physiology. *Int J Mol Sci*. 2022;23:1837.

Doroshin, A, et al. Brain connectometry changes in space travelers after long-duration spaceflight. *Neural Circuits*. 2022; doi.org/10.3389/fncir.2022.815838.

ElGindi M, et al. May the force be with you (or not): the immune system under microgravity. *Cells*. 2021;10:1941.

Genah S, et al. The effect of space travel on bone metabolism: considerations on today's major challenges and advances in pharmacology. *Int J Mol Sci*. 2021;22:4585.

Goodenow-Messman DA, et al. Numerical characterization of astronaut CaOx renal stone incidence rates to quantify in-flight and post-flight relative risk. *NPJ Microgravity*. 2022;8:2.

Green MJ, et al. Immunity in space: prokaryote adaptations and immune response in microgravity. *Life (Basel)*. 2021;11:112.

Greene KA, et al. Trunk skeletal muscle changes on CT with long duration spaceflight. *Ann Biomed Eng*. 2021;49:1257.

Grimm D. Microgravity and space medicine. *Int J Mol Sci*. 2021 22:6697.

Hearon CM Jr, et al. Effect of nightly lower body negative pressure on choroid engorgement in a model of spaceflight-associated neuro-ocular syndrome: a randomized crossover trial. *JAMA Ophthalmol*. 2022;140:59.

Hides JA, et al. The effects of exposure to microgravity and reconditioning of the lumbar multifidus and anterolateral abdominal muscles: implications for people with LBP. *Spine J*. 2021;21:477.

Hughes L, et al. Optimization of exercise countermeasures to spaceflight using blood flow restriction. *Aerosp Med Hum Perform*. 2022;93:32.

Hupfeld KE, et al. Brain and behavioral evidence for reweighting of vestibular inputs with long-duration spaceflight. *Cereb Cortex*. 2022;32:755.

Hupfeld KE, et al. Microgravity effects on the human brain and behavior: dysfunction and adaptive plasticity. *Neurosci Biobehav Rev*. 2021;122:176.

Jamšek M, et al. Effects of simulated microgravity and hypergravity conditions on arm movements in normogravity. *Front Neural Circuits*. 2021;15:750176.

Jirak P, et al. How spaceflight challenges human cardiovascular health. *Eur J Prev Cardiol*. 2022:zwac029. doi:10.1093/eurjpc/zwac029.

Jordan J, et al. Cardiovascular autonomic nervous system responses and orthostatic intolerance in astronauts and their relevance in daily medicine. *Neurol Sci*. 2022. doi:10.1007/s10072-022-05963-7.

Juhl OJ IV, et al. Update on the effects of microgravity on the musculoskeletal system. *NPJ Microgravity*. 2021;7:28.

Kim DS, et al. The effect of microgravity on the human venous system and blood coagulation: a systematic review. *Exp Physiol*. 2021;106:1149.

Krachtis A, et al. Arterial stiffness alterations in simulated microgravity and reactive sledge as a countermeasure. *High Blood Press Cardiovasc Prev*. 2022;29:65.

Kramer LA, et al. Cerebrovascular effects of lower body negative pressure at 3t MRI implications for long-duration space travel. *J Magn Reson Imaging*. 2022. doi:10.1002/jmri.28102.

Kuehnast T, et al. The crewed journey to Mars and its implications for the human microbiome. *Microbiome*. 2022;10:26.

Kuga T, et al. Enzymatic synthesis of cellulose in space: gravity is a crucial factor for building cellulose II gel structure. *Cellulose (Lond)*. 2022:1. doi:10.1007/s10570-021-04399-0.

Kunavar T, et al. Effects of local gravity compensation on motor control during altered environmental gravity. *Front Neural Circuits*. 2021;15:750267.

Lan M, et al. Proposed mechanism for reduced jugular vein flow in microgravity. *Physiol Rep*. 2021;9:e14782.

Lebedeva, S, et al. Assessment of the psychophysiological state of female operators under simulated microgravity. *Front Physiol*. 2022; doi.org/10.3389/fphys.2021.751016.

Lee PHU, et al. Factors mediating spaceflight-induced skeletal muscle atrophy. *Am J Physiol Cell Physiol*. 2022 6. doi:10.1152/ajpcell.00203.2021

Limper U, et al. A 20-year evolution of cardiac performance in microgravity in a male astronaut. *Clin Auton Res*. 2021;31:139.

Liu HY, et al. Simulation study on the effect of resistance exercise on the hydrodynamic microenvironment of osteocytes in microgravity. *Comput Methods Biomech Biomed Engin*. 2022:1. doi:10.1080/10255842.2022.2037130.

Ludtka C, et al. Macrophages in microgravity: The impact of space on immune cells. *NPJ Microgravity*. 2021;7:13.

Mahadevan, AD, et al. Head-down-tilt bed rest with elevated CO_2: effects of a pilot spaceflight analog on neural function and performance during a cognitive-motor dual task. *Front Physiol*. 2021. doi.org/10.3389/fphys.2021.654906.

Marshall-Goebel K, et al. Mechanical countermeasures to headward fluid shifts. *J Appl Physiol (1985)*. 2021;130:1766.

McFarland AJ, et al. RNA sequencing on muscle biopsy from a 5-week bed rest study reveals the effect of exercise and potential interactions with dorsal root ganglion neurons. *Physiol Rep*. 2022;10:e15176.

Mhatre SD, et al. Neuro-consequences of the spaceflight environment. *Neurosci Biobehav Rev*. 2022;132:908.

Möller F, et al. Physical exercise intensity during submersion selectively affects executive functions. *Hum Factors*. 2021;63:227.

Montandon D, Malvido F. Microgravity, levitation and plastic surgery. *J Craniofac Surg*. 2021. doi: 10.1097/SCS.0000000000008387.

Moosavi D, et al. The effects of spaceflight microgravity on the musculoskeletal system of humans and animals, with an emphasis on exercise as a countermeasure: a systematic scoping review. *Physiol Res*. 2021;70:119.

Mortreux M, et al. Hindlimb suspension in Wistar rats: sex-based differences in muscle response. *Physiol Rep*. 2021;9:e15042.

Nguyen HP, et al. The effects of real and simulated microgravity on cellular mitochondrial function. *NPJ Microgravity*. 2021; N7:44.

Okada R, et al. Transcriptome analysis of gravitational effects on mouse skeletal muscles under microgravity and artificial 1 g onboard environment. *Sci Rep*. 2021;11:9168.

Pavletić B, et al. Spaceflight virology: what do we know about viral threats in the spaceflight environment? *Astrobiology*. 2022;22:210.

Riwaldt S, et al. Role of apoptosis in wound healing and apoptosis alterations in microgravity. *Front Bioeng Biotechnol*. 2021;9:679650.

Sathasivam M, et al. Plant responses to real and simulated microgravity. *Life Sci Space Res (Amst)*. 2021;28:74.

Saveko A, et al. Adaptation in gait to lunar and Martian gravity unloading during long-term isolation in the ground-based space station model. *Front Hum Neurosci*. 2022;15:742664.

Shankhwar V, et al. Effect of countermeasure bodygear on cardiac-vascular-respiratory coupling during 6-degree head-down tilt: an earth-based microgravity study. *Life Sci Space Res (Amst)*. 2022;32:45.

Shymanovich T, Kiss JZ. Conducting plant experiments in space and on the moon. *Methods Mol Biol*. 2022;2368:165.doi: 10.1007/978-1-0716-1677-2_12.

Siddiqui R, et al. Effect of microgravity environment on gut microbiome and angiogenesis. *Life (Basel)*. 2021;11:1008.

Siddiqui R, et al. Gut microbiome and human health under the space environment. *J Appl Microbiol*. 2021;130:14.

Smith K, Mercuri J. Microgravity and radiation effects on astronaut intervertebral disc health. *Aerosp Med Hum Perform*. 2021;92:342.

Smith SM, Zwart SR. Nutrition as fuel for human spaceflight. *Physiology (Bethesda)*. 2021;36:324.

Strollo F, Vernikos J. Aging-like metabolic and adrenal changes in microgravity: state of the art in preparation for Mars. *Neurosci Biobehav Rev*. 2021;126:236.

Tays GD, et al. The Effects of long duration spaceflight on sensorimotor control and cognition. *Front Neural Circuits*. 2021; doi.org/10.3389/fncir.2021.723504.

Topal U, Zamur C. Microgravity, stem cells, and cancer: a new hope for cancer treatment. *Stem Cells Int*. 2021;2021:5566872.

Tran KN, Choi JI. Mimic microgravity effect on muscle transcriptome under ionizing radiation. *Life Sci Space Res (Amst)*. 2022;32:96.

Trudel G, et al. Hemolysis contributes to anemia during long-duration space flight. *Nat Med*. 2022;28:59.

Weber B, et al. Sensorimotor impairment and haptic support in microgravity. *Exp Brain Res*. 2021;239:967.

Weber B, Proske U. Limb position sense and sensorimotor performance under conditions of weightlessness. *Life Sci Space Res (Amst)*. 2022;32:63.

Wostyn P, et al. The odyssey of the ocular and cerebrospinal fluids during a mission to Mars: the "ocular glymphatic system" under pressure. *Eye (Lond)*. 2021; doi: 10.1038/s41433-021-01721-9.

Wu XT, et al. Cells respond to space microgravity through cytoskeleton reorganization. *FASEB J*. 2022;36:e22114.

Yuzawa R, et al. VDR regulates simulated microgravity-induced atrophy in C2C12 myotubes. *Sci Rep*. 2022;12:1377.

Table 27.1 Potential Deleterious Weightlessness Effects Launch through Re-entry

• Anorexia	• Motion sickness
• Bone demineralization	• Muscular incoordination
• Cardiac arrhythmia	• Muscle atrophy
• Decreased g tolerance	• Nausea
• Decreased work capacity	• Postflight syncope
• Dehydration	• Pulmonary atelectasis
• Disorientation	• Reduced blood volume
• Diuresis	• Reduced plasma volume
• Euphoria	• Renal calculi
• Fatigue	• Restlessness
• Gastrointestinal disturbance	• Sleepiness
• Hallucinations	• Sleeplessness
• Hypertension	• Tachycardia
• Hypotension	• Urine retention
• Infectious illnesses	• Weight loss

Adapted from Dietlein LF. Skylab: a beginning. In: Johnston RS, Dietlein LF, eds. *Biomedical Results from Skylab (NASA SP-377)*. Washington, DC: U.S. Government Printing Office; 1977.

Table 27.2 Changes in Cardiovascular Variables Associated with Microgravity

Physiologic Measure	Short Spaceflights (1–14 d)	Long Spaceflights (≥2 wk) Preflight vs. Inflight	Long Spaceflights (≥2 wk) Preflight vs. Postflight
Heart rate (resting)	Variable inflight; increased after flight; peaks during launch and re-entry; RPB up to 1 wk	Normal or slightly increased	Increased; RPB 3 wk
Blood pressure (resting)	Normal; decreased after flight	Diastolic blood pressure reduced or unchanged	Decreased mean arterial pressure
Orthostatic tolerance	Decreased after flights longer than 5 hr; exaggerated cardiovascular responses to tilt test, stand test, and LBNP after flight; RPB 3–14 d	Exaggerated cardiovascular responses to inflight LBNP (especially during first 2 wk); last inflight test comparable to recovery day test	Exaggerated cardiovascular responses to LBNP; RPB up to 3 wk
Total peripheral resistance	Decreased inflight; no increase at landing despite drop in stroke volume and increase in HR	Tendency toward decrease	Increased after landing
Cardiac size	Normal or slightly decreased C/T ratio after flight	C/T ratio decreased after flight	
Stroke volume	Increased inflight by as much as 60% (SLS-1); compensated by decreased HR	Increased early inflight then decreased	12% decrease on average
Left end-diastolic volume	Same as stroke volume	Same as in short-duration missions	16% decrease on average
Cardiac output	Elevated 30–40% inflight (SLS-1); reduced immediately postflight	Unchanged	Variable; RPB 3–4 wk
Central venous pressure	Elevated above resting supine level before launch; transient increase followed by levels below preflight upon attaining orbit	Not measured	Not measured
Left cardiac muscle mass thickness	Unchanged	Unchanged	11% decrease; return to normal after 3 wk
Cardiac electrical activity (ECG/VCG)	Moderate rightward shift in QRS and T waves after flight	Increased P-R interval, QT interval, and QRS vector magnitude	Slight increase in QRS duration and magnitude; increase in P-R interval duration
Arrhythmia	Usually PABs and PVBs; isolated nodal tachycardia cases, ectopic beats, and inflight supraventricular bigeminy	PVBs and occasional PABs; sinus or nodal arrhythmia at release of LBNP inflight	Occasional unifocal PABs and PVBs
Systolic time intervals	Not measured	Not measured; PEP/ET ratio RPB 2 wk	Increase in resting and LBNP stressed
Exercise capacity	No change or decreased <12% after flight; increased HR for same VO_2; no change in efficiency; RPB 3–8 d	Submaximal exercise capacity unchanged	Decreased postflight; recovery time inversely related to amount of inflight exercise rather than mission duration
Venous compliance in legs	Not measured	Increased: continues to increase for ≥10 d; slow decrease later inflight	Normal or slightly increased

RPB, return to preflight baseline; LBNP, lower body negative pressure; C/T, cardiothoracic; ECG, electrocardiogram; VCG, vectorcardiogram; PAB, premature atrial beat; PVB, premature ventricular beat; HR, heart rate; SLS-1, Spacelab Life Sciences 1.
Data from Nicogossian AE, et al. *Space Physiology and Medicine*. 3rd ed. Philadelphia: Lea & Febiger; 1994:216.

Table 27.3 Changes in Pulmonary Variables Associated with Microgravity During Two Spacelab Missions

Physiologic Response to Microgravity (1–14 d)	Reference Letter	Number of Subjects	Changes in Microgravity (Inflight vs. Preflight Standing Measurements)
Pulmonary Blood Flow			
Total pulmonary blood flow (cardiac output)	A	4	18% increase
Cardiac stroke volume	A	4	4% increase
Diffusing capacity (carbon monoxide)	A	4	28% increase
Pulmonary capillary blood volume	A	4	28% increase
Diffusing capacity of alveolar membrane	A	4	27% increase
Pulmonary blood flow distribution	C	7	More uniform but some inequality remained
Pulmonary Ventilation			
Respiration frequency	E	8	9% increase
Tidal volume	E	8	15% decrease
Alveolar ventilation	E	8	Unchanged
Total ventilation	E	8	Small decrease
Ventilatory distribution	B	7	More uniform but some inequality remained
Maximal peak expiratory flow rate	E	7	Decreased by ≤12.5% early in flight, then returned to normal
Pulmonary Gas Exchange			
O_2 uptake	E	8	Unchanged
CO_2 output	E	8	Unchanged
End-tidal P_{O_2}	E	8	Unchanged
End-tidal P_{CO_2}	E	8	Small increase when CO_2 concentration in spacecraft increased
Lung Volumes			
Functional residual capacity	D	4	15% decrease
Residual lung volume	D	4	18% decrease
Closing volume	B	7	Unchanged as measured by argon bolus

Note: Pulmonary blood flow in normal subjects equals cardiac output. How well carbon monoxide diffuses into the blood is a standard clinical test of the integrity of the alveolar membrane and its surrounding capillary blood supply. The data indicate that more alveoli are expanded and ventilated in space than on Earth. Closing volume refers to the volume in the lung where the alveoli close in significant numbers.

A. Prisk OK, et al. Pulmonary diffusing capacity, capillary blood volume and cardiac output during sustained microgravity. *J Appl Physiol*. 1993;75:15.
B. Guy HJB, et al. Inhomogeneity of pulmonary ventilation during sustained microgravity as determined by single-breath washouts. *J Appl Physiol*. 1994;76:1719.
C. Prisk OK, et al. Inhomogeneity of pulmonary ventilation during sustained microgravity on Spacelab SLS-1. *J Appl Physiol*. 1994;76:1730.
D. Elliott AR, et al. Lung volumes during sustained microgravity on Spacelab SLS-1. *J Appl Physiol*. 1994;77:2005.
E. Prisk OK, et al. Pulmonary gas exchange and its determinants during sustained microgravity on Spacelab SLS-1. *J Appl Physiol*. 1995;76:1290.
Adapted from West JB, et al. Pulmonary function in space. *JAMA*. 1997;277:1957.

Table 27.4	Body Fluid Changes Associated with Space Missions in Microgravity		
		Long Spaceflights (≥2 wk)[b]	
Physiologic Measure	Short Space flights (1–14 d)[a]	Preflight vs. Inflight	Preflight vs. Postflight
Total body water	3% decrease by flight day 4 or 5		Decreased postflight
Plasma volume	Decreased postflight (except Gemini 7 and 8); decreased inflight (SLS-1)		Markedly decreased after flight; RPB 2 wk increased at R + 0; decreased R + 2 (hydration effect)
Hematocrit	Slightly increased after flight		Decreased postflight; RPB 2–4 wk after landing
Hemoglobin	Normal or slightly increased postflight	Increased in first inflight sample; slowly declines later inflight	Decreased from near-preflight values on landing day; RPB 1–2 mo
Red blood cell (RBC) mass	Decreased postflight (~9% on SLS-1); RPB at least 2 wk	Decreased ~15% during first 2- to 3-wk inflight; begins to recover after about 60 d; recovery RBC mass independent of time in space	Decreased after flight; RPB 2 wk to 3 mo post landing
Red blood cell morphology	No significant changes postflight	Increased percentage of echinocytes; decrease in discocytes	Rapid reversal of inflight changes in distribution of red blood cell shapes; increased potassium influx; RPB 3 d
Red blood cell half-life (^{51}Cr)	No change; verified on SLS-1		No change
Reticulocytes	Decreased postflight; RPB 1 wk		Decreases at landing, then shifts to increases over preflight values by 7 d after landing; greatest changes seen after longer flights
Iron turnover	No change		No change
Mean corpuscular volume	Increased after flight; RPB at least 2 wk		Variable, but within normal limits
White blood cells	Increased after flight, especially neutrophils; lymphocytes decreased; RPB 1–2 d; no significant change in T/B lymphocyte ratio		Increased, especially neutrophils; postflight reduction in number of T cells and T-cell function measured by PHA responsiveness, RPB 3–7 d; transient postflight elevated B cells, RPB 3 d
Plasma lipids	Decreased cholesterol and triacylglycerols inflight		
Plasma glucose	Decreased during and immediately postflight	Decreased for first 2 mo, then leveled off	Postflight hyperglycemia with increased lactate and pyruvate
Plasma proteins	Occasional postflight elevations α_2-globulin from increased haptoglobin, ceruloplasmin, and α_2-macroglobulin; elevated IgA and C_3		No significant changes

Table 27.4	Body Fluid Changes Associated with Space Missions in Microgravity (Continued)		
Physiologic Measure	**Short Space flights (1–14 d)**[a]	**Long Spaceflights (≥2 wk)**[b]	
		Preflight vs. Inflight	**Preflight vs. Postflight**
Red blood cell enzymes	No consistent postflight changes	Decreased phosphofructokinase; no lipid peroxidation evidence or RBC damage	No consistent postflight changes
Serum/plasma electrolytes	Increased K and Ca inflight (SLS-1); decreased Na inflight; decreased K and Mg postflight	Decreased Na, Cl, and osmolality; slight increase in K and PO_4	Postflight decreases in Na, K, Cl, Mg; increase in PO_4 and osmolality
Serum/plasma hormones	Decreased ANF, aldosterone, and ADH inflight (SLS-1); increased cortisol and angiotensin 1 inflight (SLS-1)	Increased cortisol; decreased ACTH, insulin	Postflight increases in angiotensin, aldosterone, thyroxine, TSH, and GH; decrease in ACTH
Insulin		Decreased during long missions	Decreased postflight
Serum/plasma metabolites and enzymes	Postflight increases in blood urea nitrogen, creatinine, and glucose; decreases in lactic acid dehydrogenase, creatinine phosphokinase, albumin, triacylglycerols, cholesterol, and uric acid		Postflight decrease in cholesterol, uric acid
Urine volume	Decreased after flight	Decreased early inflight	Decreased after flight
Urine electrolytes	Postflight increases in Ca, creatinine, PO_4, and osmolality; decreases in Na, K, Cl, Mg	Increased osmolality, Na, K, Cl, Mg, Ca, PO_4; decrease in uric acid excretion	Increased Ca excretion; initial postflight decreases in Na, K, Cl, Mg, PO_4, uric acid; Na and Cl excretion increased in second and third wk postflight
Urinary hormones	Inflight decreases in 17-OH-corticosteroids, increase in aldosterone; postflight increases in cortisol, aldosterone, ADH, and pregnanediol; decreases in epinephrine, 17-OH-corticosteroids, androsterone, and etiocholanolone	Inflight increases in cortisol, aldosterone, and total 17-ketosteroids; decrease in ADH	Increased cortisol, aldosterone, norepinephrine; decreases in total 17-OH-corticosteroids, ADH
Urinary amino acids	Postflight increases in taurine and β-alanine; decreases in glycine, alanine, and tyrosine	Increased inflight	Increased postflight

SLS, Spacelab Life Sciences; RPB, return to preflight baseline; R, return to Earth.
[a]Biomedical data from Mercury, Gemini, Apollo, ASTP, Vostok, Voskhod, Soyuz, Shuttle, Spacelab.
[b]Biomedical data from Skylab, Salyut, Mir missions.
Data from Nicogossian AE, et al. *Space Physiology and Medicine*. 3rd ed. Philadelphia: Lea & Febiger; 1994:217.

Table 27.5 Sensory System Adaptations with Microgravity

Physiologic Measure	Short Spaceflights (1–14 d)	Long Spaceflights (≥2 wk) Preflight vs. Inflight	Long Spaceflights (≥2 wk) Preflight vs. Postflight
Audition	No change in thresholds after flight	One report of lowered thresholds during a 1-year flight	No change in thresholds after flight
Gustation and olfaction	Subjective and varied human experience; no impairments noted	Same as shorter missions	Same as shorter missions
Somatosensory	Subjective and varied human experience; no impairments noted	Subjective experiences (e.g., tingling in feet)	
Vision	Intraocular tension tends to increase during flight and decrease at landing; postflight decreases in visual field; retinal blood vessels constricted after flight; dark-adapted crews reported light flashes with eyes open or closed; decrease in visual motor task performance and contrast discrimination; no change in inflight contrast discrimination or distant and near visual acuity	Light flashes reported by dark-adapted subjects; frequency related to latitude (highest in South Atlantic, lowest over poles)	No significant changes except transient decreases in intraocular pressure
Vestibular system	Forty to seventy percent of astronauts/cosmonauts exhibit inflight neurovestibular effects including immediate reflex motor responses (postural illusions, sensations of tumbling or rotation, nystagmus, dizziness, vertigo) and space motion sickness (pallor, cold sweating, nausea, vomiting); motion sickness symptoms appear early inflight and subside or disappear in 2–7 d; postflight difficulties in postural equilibrium with eyes closed or other vestibular disturbances	Inflight vestibular disturbances are the same as for shorter missions; markedly decreased susceptibility to provocative motion stimuli (cross-coupled angular acceleration) after adaptation period of 2–7 d; cosmonauts reported occasional reappearance of illusions during long missions	Immunity to provocative motion continues for several days after flight; marked postflight disturbances in postural equilibrium with eyes closed; some cosmonauts exhibit additional vestibular disturbances after flight, including dizziness, nausea, and vomiting

Data from Nicogossian AE, et al. *Space Physiology and Medicine*. 3rd ed. Philadelphia: Lea & Febiger; 1994:219.

Table 27.6 — Musculoskeletal Adaptations in Short (1–14 d) and Longer (>2 wk) Space Mission Durations

Physiologic Measure	Short Spaceflights (1–14 d)	Longer Spaceflights (>2 wk) Preflight vs. Inflight	Longer Spaceflights (>2 wk) Preflight vs. Postflight
Stature	Slight increase during first wk inflight (~1.3 cm); RPB 1 d	Increased during first 2 wk in light (max 3–6 cm); stabilizes thereafter	Height returns to normal on R + 0
Body mass	Postflight weight losses average about 3.4%; about 2/3 loss occurs from water; remainder from lean body mass and fat loss	Inflight weight loss average 3–4% during first 5 d; thereafter, weight either declines or increases for mission remainder; early inflight losses probably occur from fluid loss, with later losses metabolic	Rapid weight gain during first 5 d postflight, mainly fluid replenishment; slower weight gain from R + 5 d to R + 2 or 3 wk; postflight weight loss inversely relates to inflight caloric intake
Protein synthesis	Elevated 40% on flight day 8 (SLS-1) suggests a "stress response"		
Body composition		Lipid probably replaces muscle tissue, and muscle mass partially preserved based on exercise regimen	
Total body volume	Decreased postflight	Center of mass shifts headward	Decreased postflight
Limb volume	Inflight leg volume decreases exponentially during first flight day; thereafter, rate of decrease declines and plateaus within 3–5 d; postflight leg volume decrements rapidly increase up to 3%; slower RPB occurs immediately postflight	Same as short missions early inflight; leg volume continues to decrease slightly throughout mission; arm volume decreases slightly	Rapid increase in leg volume immediately after flight followed by slow RPB
Muscle strength	Decreased during and after flight; RPB 1–2 wk		Postflight decrease in leg muscle strength, particularly extensors; increased inflight exercise reduces postflight losses in strength regardless of mission duration; arm strength normal or slightly decreased postflight
EMG analysis	Postflight gastrocnemius EMG suggests increased fatigue susceptibility and reduced muscular efficiency; arm muscle EMG shows no change		Postflight gastrocnemius EMG shifts to higher frequencies, suggesting muscle tissue deterioration from increased fatigue susceptibility to RPB in about 4 d
Reflexes (Achilles tendon)	Reflex duration decreased postflight		Reflex duration decreased postflight by ≥30%; reflex magnitude increased; compensatory reflex duration increases in about 2 wk postflight; RPB about 1 mo

Table 27.6 Musculoskeletal Adaptations in Short (1–14 d) and Longer (>2 wk) Space Mission Durations (Continued)

Physiologic Measure	Short Spaceflights (1–14 d)	Longer Spaceflights (>2 wk)	
		Preflight vs. Inflight	Preflight vs. Postflight
Nitrogen and phosphorus balance		Negative balances early inflight shift to less negative or slightly later positive balances	Rapid return to positive balances postflight
Bone density	Os calcis density decreased postflight; radius and ulna show variable changes depending on measurement method		Os calcis density decreased postflight; loss correlates with mission duration; little or no loss from non–weight-bearing bones; RPB is gradual; time course undetermined
Calcium balance	Progressive negative inflight calcium balance	Urine Ca^{++} excretion increases during first month inflight, then plateaus; fecal Ca^{++} excretion declines until day 10, then increases continually throughout flight; Ca^{++} balance becomes increasingly negative throughout flight	Urine Ca^{++} content drops below preflight baseline by day 10; fecal Ca^{++} content declines but does not reach preflight baseline by day 20; markedly negative Ca^{++} balance postflight becomes less negative by day 10; Ca^{++} balance remains slightly negative on day 20; RPB at least several weeks

RPB, return to preflight baseline; SLS, Spacelab Life Sciences; R, return to Earth; EMG, electromyography.
Data from Nicogossian AE, et al. *Space Physiology and Medicine*. 3rd ed. Philadelphia: Lea & Febiger; 1994:220.

Table 27.7 Bone Loss on Mir Space Station Related to Percentage of Bone Mineral Density Lost Monthly

Variable	Crew Members (n)	Mean Loss (%)	SD[a]
Spine	18	1.07[b]	0.63
Neck of femur	18	1.16[b]	0.85
Trochanter	18	1.58[b]	0.98
Total body	17	0.35[b]	0.25
Pelvis	17	1.35[b]	0.54
Arm	17	0.04[b]	0.88
Leg	16	0.34[b]	0.33

[a]Standard deviation.
[b]$p < 0.01$.
Reprinted from LeBlanc A, et al. Bone mineral and lean tissue loss after long duration space flight. *J Musculoskelet Neuronal Interact*. 2000;1:157.

Table 27.8	Adverse Spaceflight Effects in Four Functional Body Areas and Proposed Countermeasure Strategies			
Area	Major Findings	Clinical/Operational Consequences	Countermeasures under Evaluation	
Cardiovascular	Fluid loss Electrolyte changes Electrical activity disturbances Neuroreflex readjustments	Orthostatic intolerance	Fluid/electrolyte replenishment Exercise	
Neurovestibular	Motion sickness Gait disturbances Motor performance degradation	Decreased productivity	Palliative treatments (intramuscular promethazine) Adaptation trainers	
Musculoskeletal	Bone mass loss Muscle mass loss	Renal stone formation Muscle/joint injuries Bone fractures	Diet Exercise; lower body negative pressure Drugs (bisphosphonates, etc.)	
Immunologic endocrinologic	Changes in immune response *in vitro* Inappropriate hormonal secretion or metabolism	Susceptibility to infection (?) Synergistic radiation effects Allergic reactions and disorders	Growth factors (?)	

Note: Third column lists factors (renal stone formation, muscle/joint injuries, bone fractures) undocumented in NASA reports.
Reprinted from Nicogossian AE, et al. Countermeasures to space deconditioning. In: Nicogossian AE, et al., eds. *Space Physiology and Medicine.* 3rd ed. Philadelphia: Lea & Febiger; 1994:447.

Table 27.9	Space Motion Sickness Incidence and Severity During 36 Space Shuttle Flights		
	Number of Crew Members		
Motion Sickness Rating	First Shuttle Flight	Later Shuttle Flight	Totals
None	32 (29%)	28 (45%)	60 (35%)
Mild	36 (33%)	24 (39%)	60 (35%)
Moderate	29 (27%)	10 (16%)	39 (23%)
Severe	12 (11%)	0 (0%)	12 (7%)
Total	**109 (64%)**	**62 (36%)**	**171 (100%)**

Reprinted from Nicogossian AE, et al. Countermeasures to space deconditioning. In: Nicogossian AE, et al., eds. *Space Physiology and Medicine.* 3rd ed. Philadelphia: Lea & Febiger; 1994:230.

Table 27.10	Significant Spin-off Technologies from the Apollo and Space Shuttle Programs
Spin-off Device	**Description**
Apollo Program	
CT and MRI scans	Digital signal-processing techniques, originally developed to computer-enhance pictures of the moon for the Apollo program, are an indispensable part of CT and MRI scans in hospitals worldwide. As a medical CT scan searches the human body for tumors or other abnormalities, the industrial or advanced CT inspection system finds imperfections in aerospace castings, rocket motors, and nozzles.
Protective suits	Cool suits, which kept Apollo astronauts comfortable during moon walks, are worn by race car drivers, nuclear reactor technicians, shipyard workers, persons with multiple sclerosis, and children with a congenital disorder known as hypohidrotic ectodermal dysplasia.
Kidney dialysis machines	Kidney dialysis machines were developed from an NASA-developed chemical process that removed toxic waste from used dialysis fluid.
Cardiovascular conditioner	A cardiovascular conditioner developed for astronauts in space led to the development of a physical therapy and athletic development machine used by football teams, sports clinics, and medical rehabilitation centers.
Cordless power tools and appliances	N/A
Athletic shoes	Athletic shoe design and manufacture incorporated technology from NASA spacesuits into a shoe's external shell. A stress-free "blow molding" process is used in the shoe's manufacture.
Insulation barriers in cars and trucks	Insulation barriers made of aluminum foil laid over a core of propylene or Mylar, which protected astronauts and their spacecraft's delicate instruments from radiation, protect cars and trucks and dampen engine and exhaust noise.
Space Shuttle Program	
Artificial heart	Technology used in space shuttle fuel pumps led to the development of a miniaturized ventricular assist pump.
Automotive insulation	NASCAR racing cars use materials from the space shuttle thermal protection system to protect drivers from extreme engine heat.
Balance evaluation systems	Medical centers use balance systems to measure the equilibrium of space shuttle astronauts upon return from space; the balance systems diagnose and treat patients who suffer from head injury, stroke, chronic dizziness, and central nervous system disorders.
Bioreactor	A rotating cell culture apparatus simulates some aspects of the space environment or microgravity on the ground. Tissue samples grown in the bioreactor help to design therapeutic drugs and antibodies.
Diagnostic instrument	NASA technology created a compact laboratory instrument for hospitals and doctors' offices that analyzes blood in 30 s, which once required 20 min.
Gas detector	Ford Motor Company uses a gas-leak detection system, originally developed to monitor the shuttle's hydrogen propulsion system, to produce a natural gas-powered car.
Infrared camera	A sensitive infrared handheld camera that observes the blazing plumes from the shuttle can scan for fires. The camera localizes hot spots for firefighters.
Infrared thermometer	Infrared sensors developed to remotely measure distant star and planet temperatures led to developing the handheld optical sensor thermometer. Placed inside the ear canal, the thermometer provides an accurate reading in 2 s or less.
Land mine removal device	The same rocket fuel that helps launch the space shuttle destroys land mines. A flare device, using leftover fuel donated by NASA, is placed next to the uncovered land mine and ignited from a safe distance with a battery-triggered electric match. The explosive burns away, neutering the mine and rendering it harmless.

Table 27.10	Significant Spin-off Technologies from the Apollo and Space Shuttle Programs (Continued)
Spin-off Device	**Description**
Lifesaving light	Special lighting technology developed for plant growth experiments on space shuttle missions treats brain tumors in children. Physicians use light-emitting diodes to eradicate cancerous tumors.
Prosthesis material	The foam insulation to protect the shuttle's external tank replaced the heavy, fragile plaster to produce light, virtually indestructible master molds for prosthetics.
Video stabilization software	Image-processing technology that analyzes space shuttle launch video and studies meteorologic images helps law enforcement agencies improve crime-solving video. The technology removes defects from image jitter, image rotation, and image zoom-in video sequences.

CT, computed tomography; MRI, magnetic resonance imaging.

SECTION 6

Body Composition, Energy Balance, and Weight Control

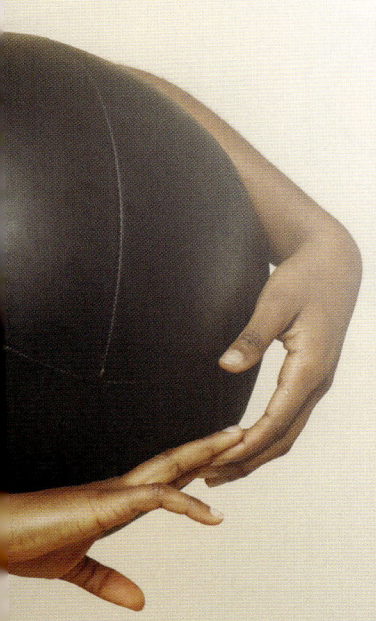

Overview

Obesity rates since 1980 have skyrocketed threefold in some North American areas and in the United Kingdom, Eastern Europe, the Middle East, the Pacific Islands, Australia, and China. Worldwide, more than 1 billion people now are defined as overweight, with 300 million classified as clinically obese. And the number continues to increase annually.

Six major reasons justify an accurate body composition appraisal in a comprehensive total physical fitness program:

1. Provides a starting point to base current and future decisions about weight loss and weight gain
2. Provides realistic goals about how to best achieve an "ideal" balance between the body's fat and nonfat compartments
3. Relates to general health status and plays an important role in all individuals' health and fitness goals
4. Monitors changes in the body's fat and lean components during different duration and intensitiy physical activity regimens
5. Allows allied health practitioners (sports nutritionist, dietician, personal trainer, chiropractor, coach, athletic trainer, physical therapist, physician, health coach, exercise leader) to interact with the individuals they deal with to provide quality information about exercise training, nutrition, weight control, exercise, and rehabilitation
6. Provides objective information that connects body composition assessment to sports performance and the changes in body composition from different exercise training regimens

This section discusses body composition, its assessment, and differences in body size and composition between sedentary and physically active males and females. We also consider topics germane to obesity and discuss how diet and physical activity impact weight management.

CHAPTER 28
Body Composition Assessment

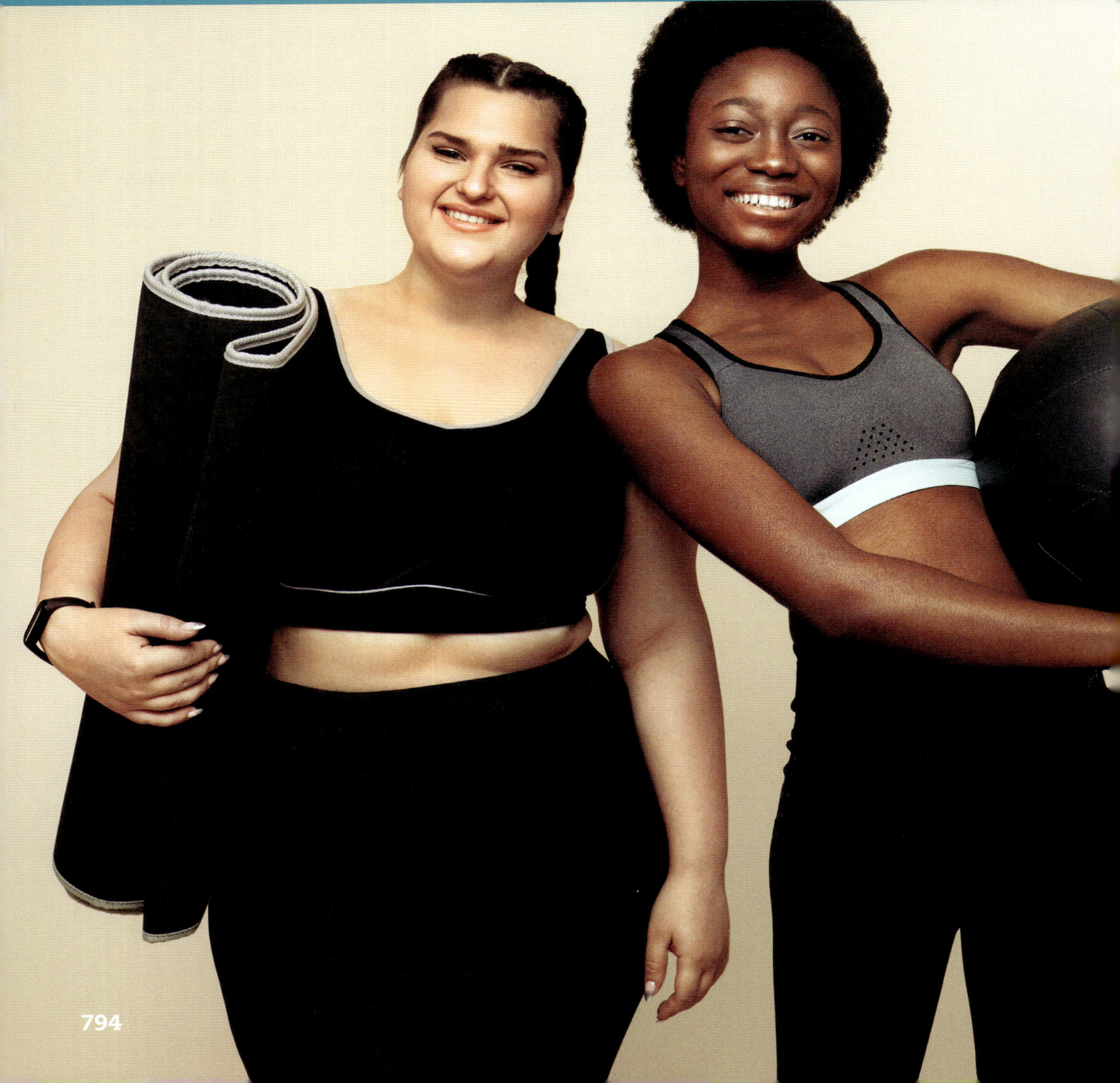

Chapter Objectives

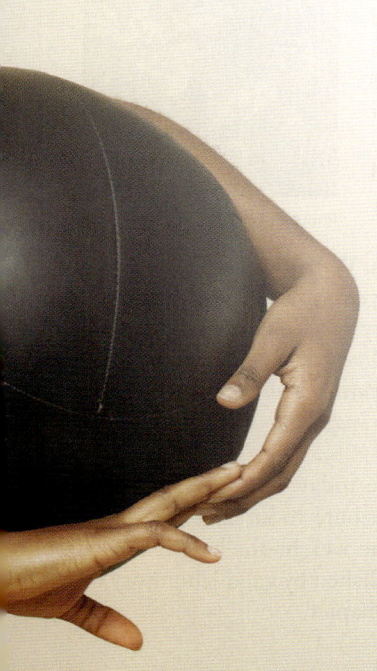

- Summarize the early research concerning inadequacies in the weight-for-height tables
- Compare and contrast the terms *overweight*, *overfat*, and *obesity*
- Outline two current systems to classify the overweight and obese conditions
- List values for storage fat, essential fat, and sex-specific essential fat for the "reference male" and "reference female"
- Discuss menstrual irregularity prevalence within the general population and specific athletic groups, and factors associated with their occurrence
- Explain Archimedes' principle applied to measuring human body volume by densitometry
- Discuss two limitations and two assumptions in computing percentage body fat from body density measurements
- Summarize the rationale and three strengths and weaknesses for air-displacement plethysmography (BOD POD) to assess body composition
- Describe the anatomic locations for six frequently measured skinfolds with a caliper and girths with a tape measure
- Describe two ways skinfolds and girths provide meaningful information about body fat and its distribution
- Summarize the rationale for bioelectrical impedance analysis and three factors that may negatively impact body composition estimates with this technique
- Summarize the rationale and two strengths and two weaknesses to assess body composition using near-infrared interactance spectroscopy, computed tomography, magnetic resonance imaging, dual-energy x-ray absorptiometry, and ultrasonography
- Describe the "average" percentage body fat and variation limits for young and older adult males and females
- Discuss two conditions from the environment, epigenetics, and genetics tied to obesity and disease dysregulation

Ancillaries at-a-Glance

Visit **Lippincott Connect** to access the following resources.

- References: Chapter 28
- Appendix D: The Metric System and Conversion Constants in Exercise Physiology
- Appendix H: Links for Supplemental Animations and Videos
- Appendix L: Body Composition Evaluation
- Focus on Research: Overweight but Not Overfat

Introduction

The life insurance actuary-based-weight-for-height tables (weight measured with normal indoor clothing and height measured with 2.54-cm/1-in. heels) provide a popular practice to assess "overweightness" based on gender and body frame size. These tables do not provide reliable information about an individual's relative body composition (muscle, bone, and fat). Rather, they offer statistical landmarks based on an average body mass range related to **stature** associated with the lowest mortality rate for persons' ages 25 to 59. They do not consider cause related to death or health quality before death.

A person may weigh considerably more than the average weight-for-height standard yet still rate "underfat" for body composition, the "extra" weight chiefly existing as muscle mass. According to the tables, the desirable body weight for a large frame size professional American football player 188 cm/74 in. tall and weighing 116 kg/255 lb ranges between 78 kg/172 lb and 88 kg/194 lb. Similarly, body weight without regard for frame size for young adult men 188 cm/74 in. tall averages 85 kg/187 lb. Using either criterion, conventional standards would classify this player as overweight, implying that he needed to reduce at least 28 kg/62 lb just to achieve the upper desirable body weight range. He must lose an additional 3 kg/6.6 lb to match his "average" American male counterpart. Body fat percentage for the football player (even though he weighed 31 kg/68 lb more than the average) was only 12.7%, compared with about 15.0% body fat for an untrained "normal-weight" young male.

Four Limitations in Using the Weight-for-Height Tables

1. Uses unvalidated estimates for body frame size
2. Developed from data derived primarily from White populations
3. Specific focus on mortality data may not reflect obesity-related comorbidities
4. Provides no body composition assessment information

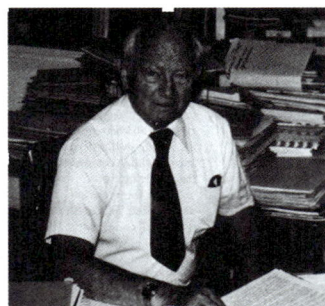
Photo: F. Katch

Navy physician and research scientist **Albert Behnke** (1898–1993; see a brief profile in the Preface) with other Navy physicians in 1942 first observed body composition variations between untrained individuals and 25 elite National Football League (NFL) Washington Redskins players.[211,230] Their classic publication from 80 year ago remains a "classic," one of the most cited studies in the body composition and exercise physiology literature.

These naval physician-researchers tested the hypothesis that differences in body fat content related chiefly to specific gravity differences (essentially to body density) and not body mass *per se*. The hypothesis predicted that heavy but lean men would have higher body specific gravity values than counterparts with similar body mass but with substantially more body fat. If their reasoning was correct, a large body mass would not always provide an appropriate assessment related to excessive fatness. According to the standard weight-for-height tables in use for decades before the Behnke experiments, 17 players failed to qualify for military service because their "overweight" status incorrectly assumed they were "excessively fat" and therefore not qualified under the existing military service regulations. Applying Archimedes' water submersion principle to assess the player's specific gravity (assessed by densitometry discussed in a later section) revealed their excess weight (which disqualified them for life insurance and also from entering the military) consisted primarily of muscle mass not fat mass! For the six heaviest players, body mass averaged 104.5 kg/230 lb with body density averaging 1.059 $g \cdot cm^{-3}$.

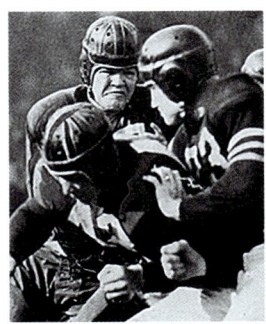
Photo: F. Katch

Behnke's insightful research showed that variability in body specific gravity related mainly to individual differences in the body's fat content and illustrated the weight-for-height table inadequacies to deduce body fatness or determine a desirable body weight among highly trained, large individuals. The researchers suggested that a 1.060 $g \cdot cm^{-3}$ body density should serve as the lower demarcation for excessive fatness in males. With this criterion, 23 of the 25 heavy but lean football players would have qualified as fit (and not overly fat) for military service. *This intuitive discovery clearly meant that the term "overweight" should refer only to body mass greater than some standard, usually the average body mass for a given stature—and not to body fat levels or risks related to serious medical illness.*

The bottom line remains true today—extreme muscular development very often can contribute to an excess in body mass.[282,283] As an alternative to the weight-for-height tables, body composition should be established by valid laboratory or field techniques reviewed in this chapter.

Overweight, Overfat, and Obesity Prevalence

Confusion surrounds the precise meaning for the terms *overweight*, *overfat*, and *obesity* applied to the body's structural components. Each term often takes on a different meaning depending on the situation and context, particularly when considering their prevalence even to the physicians in antiquity.[145] Research and contemporary discussion among diverse disciplines reinforces the need to more clearly articulate what these three terms mean.

The overweight condition refers to a body weight that exceeds some average weight for height aligned with age, usually by standard deviation limits. The overweight condition frequently accompanies an increase in body fat, but not always (e.g., male power athletes), and may or may not coincide with glucose intolerance, insulin resistance, dyslipidemia, and hypertension comorbidities. The medical literature often assigns the term *overweight* to an overfat condition despite accompanying body fat measurements. In contrast, obesity refers to individuals at the extreme along an overweight (overfat) continuum. The obesity prevalence rate in adults above age 20 is defined as BMI ≥ 30, which translated to 31% prevalence rate in 2000, and 15-year later spiked to nearly 40% in the U.S. population.[248] As of July 2021, approximately 93 million American adults were classified as obese using the BMI obesity threshold cutoffs shown in the inset figure using average weight and height

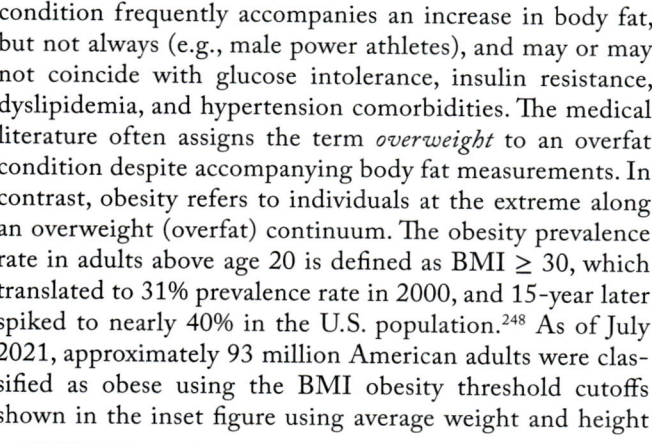

in increments of 3 in./0.08 m to establish the threshold body weight range from 69.3 kg/253 lb to 1091 kg/240 lb. Unfortunately, in children and adolescents obesity prevalence increased from about 14% in 2000 to almost 19% over a 16-year period.

Severe obesity (BMI ≥ 40) prevalence increased from 4% in 2000 to about 7% in 2010, and for the first time exceeded 40% (42.3%) in 2021. This translates to 15.5 million more obese adult Americans within the last decade. This shocking number shows that the increased BMI prevalence is occurring at a faster rate than predicted.[249] To make matters more ominous, if recent projections prove accurate, 50% in the adult U.S. population will achieve obesity status during the next decade with BMI ≥ 35 becoming the most common category for female, non-Hispanic, Black, and low-income adults. The inset image displays the new standards to identify an obesity threshold defined by BMI ≥ 30 for six heights ranging from 1.52 m/66 in. to 1.9 m/63 in. For example, a male 1.83 m/6.0 ft weighing 100.2 kg/221 lb and a female weighing 84.4 kg/186 lb at 1.68 m/66 in. would both have a calculated BMI 30, and both would be approximately 14 kg/30 lb *overweight*.

We acknowledge that individuals may indeed be overweight or overfat yet not exhibit obese syndrome components. For this reason, we urge caution in applying the term *obesity* to pigeon hole an individual into that category—rather, the correct term would be *overweightness*.

Obesity and Comorbidities

Obesity refers to the overfat condition with many comorbidities, which include one or all nine "**obese syndrome**" components:

- Glucose intolerance
- Insulin resistance
- Dyslipidemia
- Type 2 diabetes
- Hypertension
- Elevated plasma leptin concentrations
- Visceral adipose tissue accumulation
- Increased coronary heart disease risk
- Increased cancer risk

In all likelihood, excess body fat, not excess body weight by itself, explains the relationship between above average body weight and disease risk. This distinction underscores the importance to distinguish the excess body weight and excess body fat level linked to comorbidities and disease risk.[210,225]

The Body Mass Index: A Popular but Imprecise Clinical Standard

Clinicians and researchers use **body mass index (BMI)**, derived from body mass and stature, to assess "normalcy" applied to body weight. The BMI, originally derived in 1832 by Belgian mathematician, musician, astronomer, and statistician Adolphe Quetelet (1796–1874; https://mathshistory.st-andrews.ac.uk/Biographies/Quetelet/), applied his interest in probability calculus about the "normal curve" to study physical characteristics and social aptitudes including crime rates and mortality. Quetelet used the BMI to explain his observations in the Belgian population that body mass increased relative to stature squared. For the next 142 years, BMI was termed the "**Quetelet Index**" (https://pubmed.ncbi.nlm.nih.gov/17890752/; https://pubmed.ncbi.nlm.nih.gov/17890752/0). Then in 1972, American physiologist Ancel B. Keys (1904–2004) studied diet's impact on health and first applied the term "body mass index" in referencing the Quetelet Index in his studies about health and disease.[212] Keys believed this term was the best proxy for body fat percentage among various body mass and stature ratios then in use. This measure exhibits a somewhat higher yet still moderate association with body fat and disease risk than other estimates based simply on stature and body mass.

A new body shape index incorporating waist girth adjusted for body mass and stature provides an alternative to identify risk factors for premature mortality across the range for age, sex, BMI, and for White and Black (but not Mexican) ethnicities.[96] Adding abdominal girth to the BMI assessment also has been successfully tested among Canadians.[169] A PubMed search in July 2021 covering the past two decades has identified approximately 10,100 research publications dealing with the search, "BMI related to health status." The more recent 2021 studies acknowledge BMI's contribution to overall metabolic health.[213,214]

Computing BMI

Compute BMI as follows:

$$\text{BMI} = \text{body mass (kg)} \div \text{stature (m}^2)$$

Example

Male: stature: 175.3 cm or 1.753 m/69 in.; body mass: 97.1 kg/214.1 lb

$$BMI = 97.1 \div (1.753)^2$$
$$= 31.6 \text{ kg} \cdot \text{m}^{-2}, \text{ or simply } 31.6$$

The importance of this easily obtained index relates to its curvilinear relationship with all-cause mortality. As the figure at right illustrates, the BMI increases throughout the range in moderate, high, and very high categories for overweight, so also does increased risk expressed as the mortality ratio for cardiovascular complications (including gallstones, diabetes, hypertension, and stroke), certain cancers, Alzheimer disease, sleep apnea, osteoarthritis, rheumatoid arthritis, and renal disease.[90,127,135,157]

A large prospective study involving more than 1 million United States adults with 14-year follow-up revealed the relationships between BMI and mortality risk.[26] Smoking status and disease presence or absence substantially modified the association between BMI and premature death risk from all causes. Males and females who never smoked and remained disease free at the study's start experienced the greatest health risk from excess weight. Excessive leanness related to increased death risk among current and former smokers with disease history. In healthy people, the lowest relationship between BMI and mortality occurred at a BMI between 23.5 and 24.9 for males (e.g., 177.8 cm/70 in. at 78.9 kg/174 lb) and 22.0 and 23.4 for females (e.g., 165.1 cm/65 in. at 68 kg/150 lb). A gradient exists between increasing risk, then beginning to accelerate with low-moderate to moderate overweight through very high risk. Among white males and females with the highest BMI, relative death risk was 2.58 for males and 2.00 for females compared with counterparts with BMI 23.5 to 24.9 and relative risk 1.00.

New Standards for Overweight and Obesity

In 1998, the expert panel from the National Heart, Lung and Blood Institute lowered the BMI demarcation point for "overweight" from 27 to 25. Based on the close association between excess body weight and disease, individuals with a BMI ≥ 30 or more were categorized as obese. Persons with a 30 BMI averaged 14-kg/30-lb overweight.

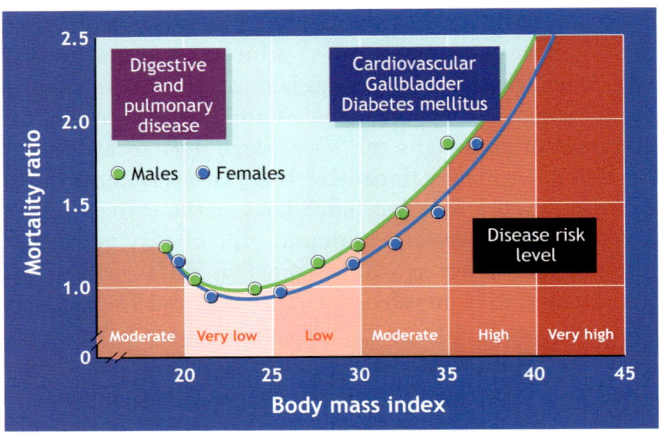

These revised standards place nearly 130 million Americans in the overweight and obese categories—a whopping 62%—up from 72 million under the previous standard. Of this total, 30.5% (59 million) classify as obese. *For the first time, overweight persons with a BMI ≥ 25 outnumber persons with desirable body weight!* More Black, Mexican, Cuban, and Puerto Rican males and females classify as overweight than White contemporaries. **FIGURE 28.1** shows the BMI and accompanying

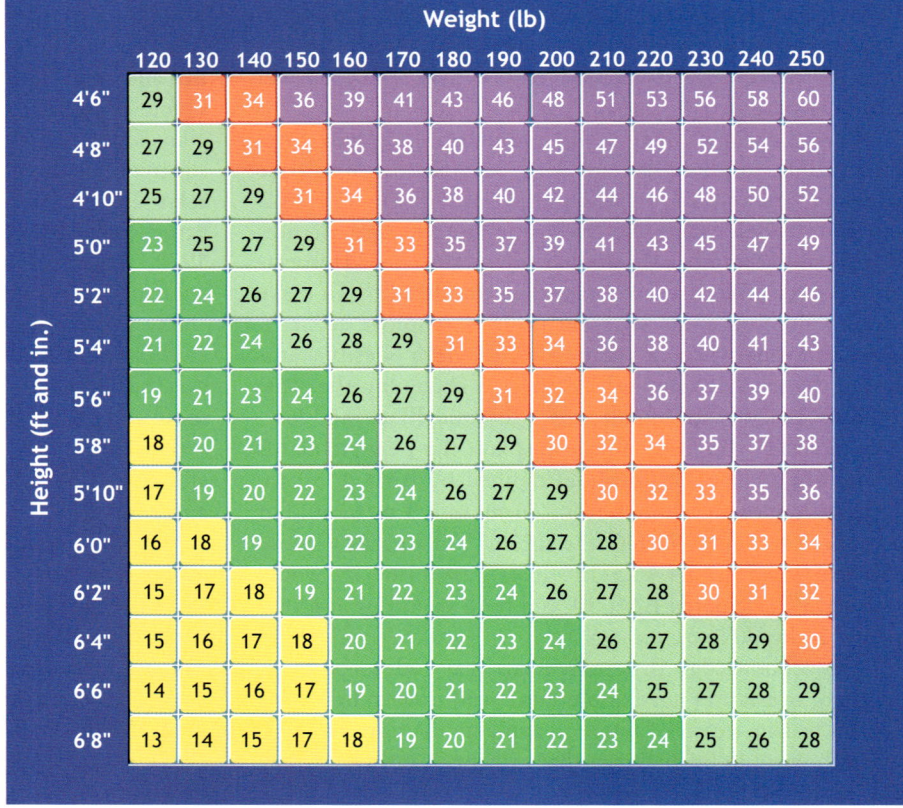

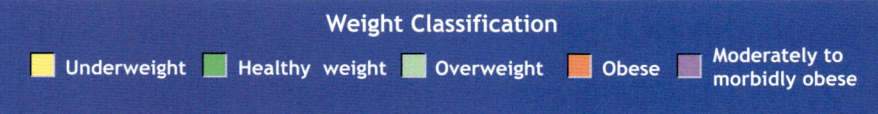

FIGURE 28.1. Body mass index (BMI), weight classifications, and associated health risks depicted by color from yellow (lower risk) to purple (highest risk).

weight classifications with associated health risks arranged by color. An accelerated diabetes and gallstone risk also occurs in persons moderately to morbidly obese.

FIGURE 28.2 presents the revised growth charts for boys and girls in the United States ages 2 to 20. No absolute BMI standard exists to classify children and adolescents as overweight and obese. Expert panels recommend BMI-for-age to identify the increasing number of children and adolescents at the distribution's upper end who are either overweight (≥95th percentile) or at risk for becoming overweight (≥85th percentile and ≤95th percentile; see Chapter 30). Less specific recommendations exist for the extreme lower distributions, but BMIs in this lower range may indicate underweight or at risk for underweight.[38,51,190]

BMI Limitations

Current classification for overweight and obesity assumes the relationship between BMI and percentage body fat and disease risk remains separate from age, sex, ethnicity, fitness status, and race, but this is not the case.[39,54,78,278] For example, Asians have a higher body fat content at a given BMI than Caucasians and thus show greater risk for obesity-related illness. A higher body fat percentage for a given BMI also exists among Hispanic American women compared with European American and African American women.[46] Failure to consider this bias alters individuals defined as obese by validated body fat assessments.[78,125] BMI accuracy in diagnosing obesity is limited for individuals in the intermediate BMI ranges, particularly in males and older adults.[153]

The BMI, similar to the weight-for-height tables, fails to consider the body's proportional composition or the body's **fat patterning** distribution.[250,251] Factors other than excess body fat—bone, muscle mass, and even increased plasma volume induced by exercise training—affect the BMI equation's numerator. A high BMI could lead to an incorrect overfatness interpretation in lean individuals with excessive muscle mass from genetic makeup or exercise training.[142]

BMI Limitations in Athletes

Misclassifying someone as overweight or obese by applying BMI standards pertains particularly to large-size field athletes, bodybuilders, weightlifters, heavier wrestlers, and most professional American football players. In Chapter 29, we present body size differences for the 2021 Super Bowl Kansas City Chiefs and Tampa Bay Buccaneers offensive and defensive linemen, including comparative data by position for over 53,000 NFL roster players from 1920 through 1996, including body composition measurements from our studies in exceptionally large NFL offensive and defensive linemen. The most recent data from 2021 revealed there were 427 NFL players among the 1700 NFL players representing about 25% from all NFL team rosters who exceeded 140-kg/300-lb body weight! Each of these players would be classified in the high or very high mortality risk categories, and each player would be graded as obese.

In the modern era, one of the largest current NFL players Trenton Brown, currently offensive tackle for the Las Vegas Raiders, weighs 162.8 kg/359 lb (203 cm/80 in. tall), with a 39.4 BMI, placing him as expected into the

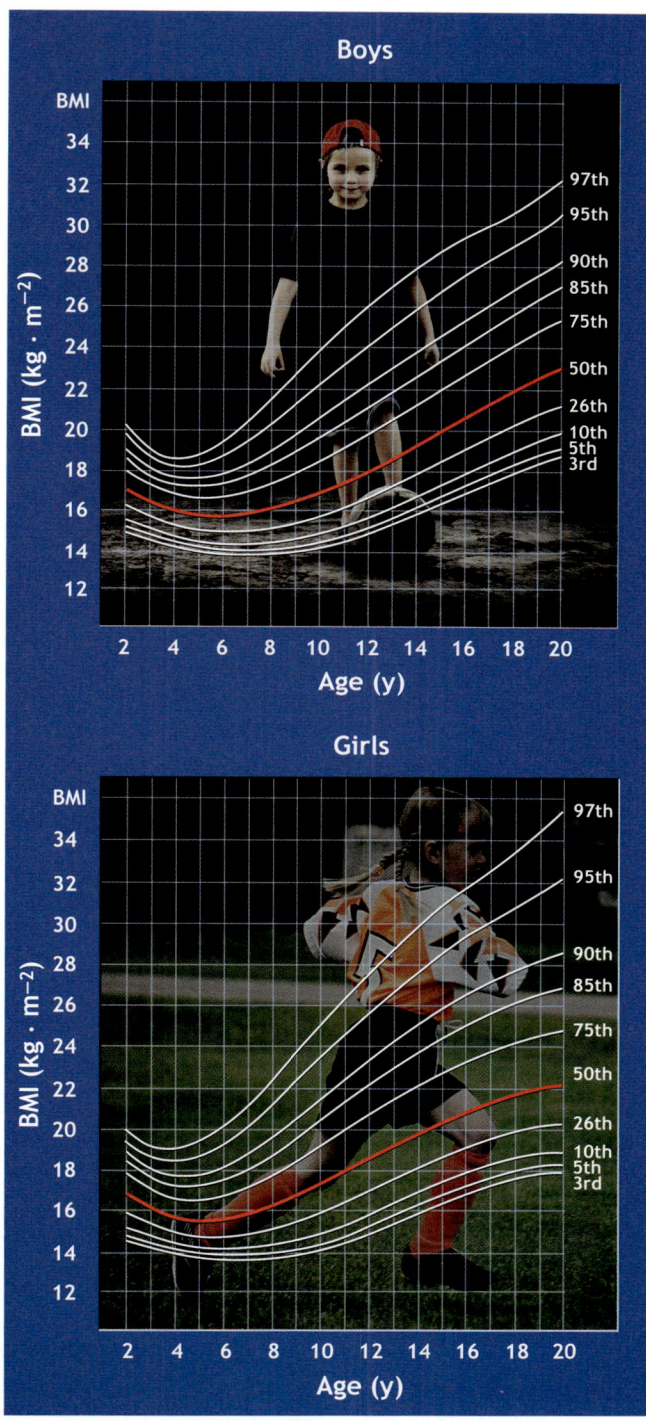

FIGURE 28.2. Body mass index-for-age percentiles for boys and girls ages 2 to 20 years. Developed by the National Center for Health Statistics in collaboration with the National Center for Chronic Disease Prevention and Health Promotion (2000).
(Shutterstock photos: Andrey Yurlov (boy), Maria Dryfhout (girl).)

From F. Katch

obese category. But the clear team objective when selecting Brown as an NFL lineman was not simply to capitalize only on his extremely large size but also for his phenomenal football skills and speed—40-yd dash in 5.29 s with a 71.1-cm standing vertical jump! As a frame of comparison, NFL running backs who achieved the most success in the 2020–2021 season ran the 40-yd dash between 4:40 and 4:49 s, an expected speed for relatively small athletes with large muscularity and minimal body fat. Usain Bolt, the fastest sprinter in recorded history, ran a 4.22-s 40-yd dash, faster than any NFL running back since records were kept (current NFL record is 4.29 s by Tyreek Hill, Kansas City Chiefs wide-receiver who weighs 83.9 kg/185 lb and is 177.8 cm/70 in. tall).

Another frame of comparison highlights the changes in overall body size among NFL players over nearly a century. A New York Giants offensive and defensive lineman's height in 1927 averaged 183 cm/72 in., whereas 40 years later in 1967, defensive linemen averaged 193 cm/76 in., and a half century later, a typical NFL lineman's height approached 200 cm/80 in.!

Beauty Pageant Contestants Should Not Be Considered Role Models

Many consider beauty pageant contestants to possess the ideal combination embracing beauty, grace, and talent. Each competitor survives the rigors in local and state contests, satisfying judges that finalists have "ideal qualities" worthy of role-model status. The consummate image of the beauty pageant physique to some extent shapes society's generalized "ideal" for female size and shape. Unfortunately, this ideal has permeated into almost every realm in girls' sports, particularly in dance, ice skating, and gymnastics, beginning in grade school.

The Barbie Doll Influence. Contributing to the myth that most young girls could achieve the Teenage Barbie look (http://fortune.com/2016/03/09/barbie-doll-body-photos/), a diet book was packaged with the doll beginning in 1959. The original Teenage Barbie included a typical bathroom scale preset to her ideal 110 lb. Over the ensuing six decades, the evolution of Barbie's physique and what it now attempts to achieve has changed considerably with updated clothes and a new look (and a Ken doll playmate), but the body dimensions remain essentially unchanged. If a Barbie doll were a real female, she would be 175.3 cm/69 in. tall, weigh 50 kg/110 lb, and have a BMI of 16.24—the weight criteria for anorexia and disturbed body image.[291,292] An important question concerns whether such images, televised worldwide to millions of viewers and ever present on social media, reinforce an unhealthful message to young girls and women who aspire to emulate such "ideal" physiques.

Beauty Pageant Physique Status. In 1967, only an 8% difference in body weight existed between professional fashion models and the average American female. Today, a beauty contestant's body weight averages about 20 to 23% lower than the national average. Similarly, elite gymnasts 20 years ago weighed about 9.1 kg/20 lb more than their contemporary counterparts. For example, gymnast Simone Biles, a multi-Olympic Gold medalist and 2013, 2014, and 2015 World Games champion, is very short by athletic standards (142.2 cm/4 ft 8 in.) and slightly more than 47.6 kg/105 lb, yet still highly muscled. It should come as little surprise that preoccupation with eating patterns and unrealistic, target weight goals (and general dissatisfaction with one's physique and pressure to appear "lean") still remain so prevalent among girls and women of *all* ages, regardless

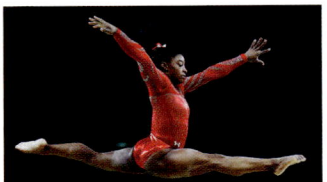
Salty View/Shutterstock

Fashion Model Physique: Not the Ideal

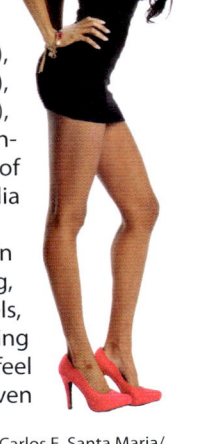
Carlos E. Santa Maria/Shutterstock

In 2021, a professional fashion model's body weight averaged 20 to 25% lower than the national average weight for similar-age females. Tremendous commercial pressure dominates the top modeling agencies worldwide to still recruit models in the lower body weight range of what most would consider "thin." The typical female acknowledged via interview that fashion/bikini models made them feel worse about their total weight (56%), stomachs (64%), waist (56%), overall appearance (56%), muscle tone (52%), legs (48%), thighs (49%), buttocks (43%), and hips (46%). In open-ended responses, approximately a third of females explicitly described negative media effects on their body image.

Female athletes who elect to compete in gymnastics, ballet, diving, sprint swimming, and cheerleading at all competitive levels, beginning in grade school and continuing through college and up to the elite levels, feel the pressure to "look thin to compete." Even the most well-intentioned female and male coaches and trainers have a difficult time convincing competitors to avoid extreme weight loss and to adopt healthy eating strategies during their competitive years. Disordered eating patterns and setting unrealistic weight goals remain a concern in sports that continues to foster a premium on physique status.

Sources:
Anixiadis F, et al. Effects of thin-ideal Instagram images: the roles of appearance comparisons, internalization of the thin ideal and critical media processing. *Body Image*. 2019;31:181.
Kwon H, et al. Incidence of cardiovascular disease and mortality in underweight individuals. *J Cachexia Sarcopenia Muscle*. 2021;12:331.
Ssentongo P, et al. Global, regional and national epidemiology and prevalence of child stunting, wasting and underweight in low- and middle-income countries, 2006-2018. *Sci Rep*. 2021;11:5204.
Zancu SA, et al. Alexithymia, body image and disordered eating in fashion models and student athletes. *Eat Weight Disord*. 2021.

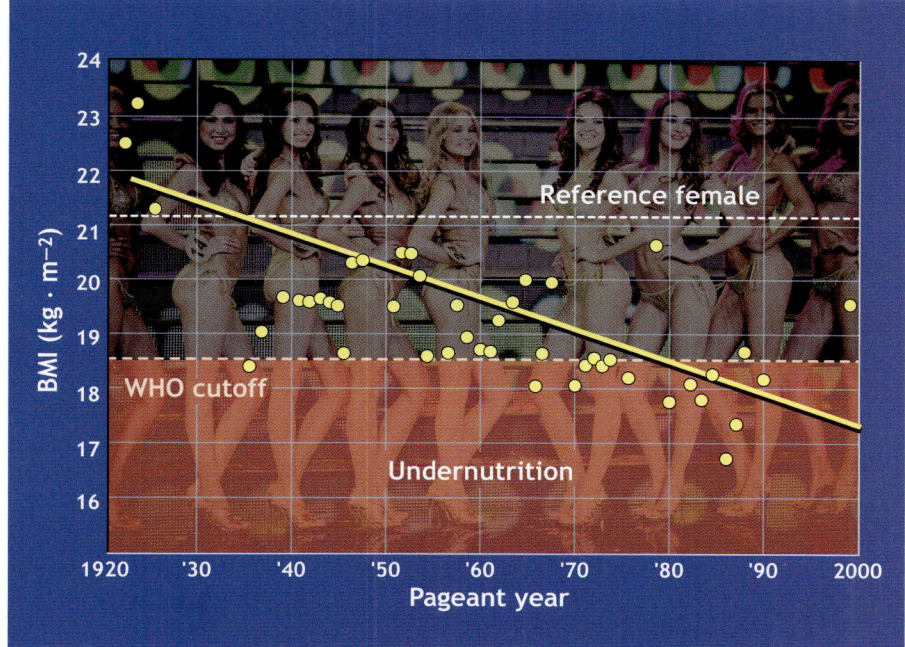

Andrey Bayda/Shutterstock. Data from F. Katch and V. Katch.

of athletic talent. To emphasize this point, consider the body size data for former Miss America contestants, discussed in the next section.

There currently are 29 different beauty pageants with participants from over 100 countries worldwide (https://en.wikipedia.org/wiki/List_of_beauty_pageants). The "Big Four" contests, in addition to hundreds of regional and local competitions, include Miss Earth, Miss International, Miss Universe, and Miss World. Similar events for men or boys carry other names and are sponsored events some would categorize as "bodybuilding contests." There also are female and male "fitness and figure" competitions. In these events, the competitors are judged solely on muscular symmetry and definition without requirements for height or weight (and thus BMI).

A unique data set includes the BMIs and accompanying anthropometric data for Miss America contestants between 1922 and 1999 (excluding 1927–1933, when the pageant was not held, and from 2000 on, when data were not readily available). The results were revealing. The *bottom horizontal white dashed line* shown in this unnumbered figure designates the World Health Organization (WHO) cutoff for **undernutrition** established at an 18.5 BMI.[206] The *top horizontal white dashed line* represents the BMI for the reference female (see Fig. 28.5; stature: 1.638 m/64.5 in.; body mass: 56.7 kg/126.7 lb; BMI: 21.1). The regression line's downward slope plotted from 1922 to 1999 shows a clear tendency for relative undernutrition from the mid-1960s to approximately 1990. Using the WHO cutoff, 14 of the 47 Miss America winners fell below BMI 18.5. Raising the BMI cutoff to 19.0 adds another 18 women, or almost 50% of the winners with undesirable BMI scores. Approximately 24% of contest winners had BMIs between 20.0 and 21.0, and no winner after 1924 had a BMI equaling that of the reference female!

Modeling Human Body Composition

In 1921, Czech anthropologist **Jindřich Matiegka** (1862–1941) described a four-component model consisting of skeletal weight (S), skin plus subcutaneous tissue (Sk + St), skeletal muscle (M), and a remainder (R).[119] The sum of the four components equaled the body mass, with water occupying 60%, protein 10%, and skeletal mass and body fat 15%.

The Matiegka concept has been updated to a five-level model to more completely identify the human body's different components. Each model level becomes more elaborate (atoms, molecules, cells, tissue systems, and whole body) as the body's complex biologic organization increases in accord with advanced assessment techniques. Note that subdivisions exist within each of the five levels. The model attempts to identify and then quantify each level's various components. An essential feature provides separate and distinct levels, each with directly or indirectly measurable characteristics. In Level 3, for example, the cellular component now uses state-of-art photomicrographic technology to reveal a cell's highly complex integrated structures, not simply a round, marble-like structure with a central nucleus, mitochondria, and other unpretentious organelles. This detailed look opens up new possibilities to explore here-to-fore unknown structures to help explain subcellular component functions.

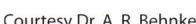

Courtesy Dr. A. R. Behnke

Measuring the Body's Intricate Components

Over the past 100 years, researchers have focused on how best to measure the body's intricate component parts. In the Civil War era and earlier in some colleges and universities, only body mass and stature would characterize overall body size. Individuals were considered thin, medium, and large size, with further descriptions as thin or underweight, muscular, and portly or too fat. A nonintricate, relatively unsophisticated method applied to many athletes was a visual "somatotype system" with three categories, ectomorph (thin), mesomorph (muscular), and endomorph fat or overweight).[236–238]

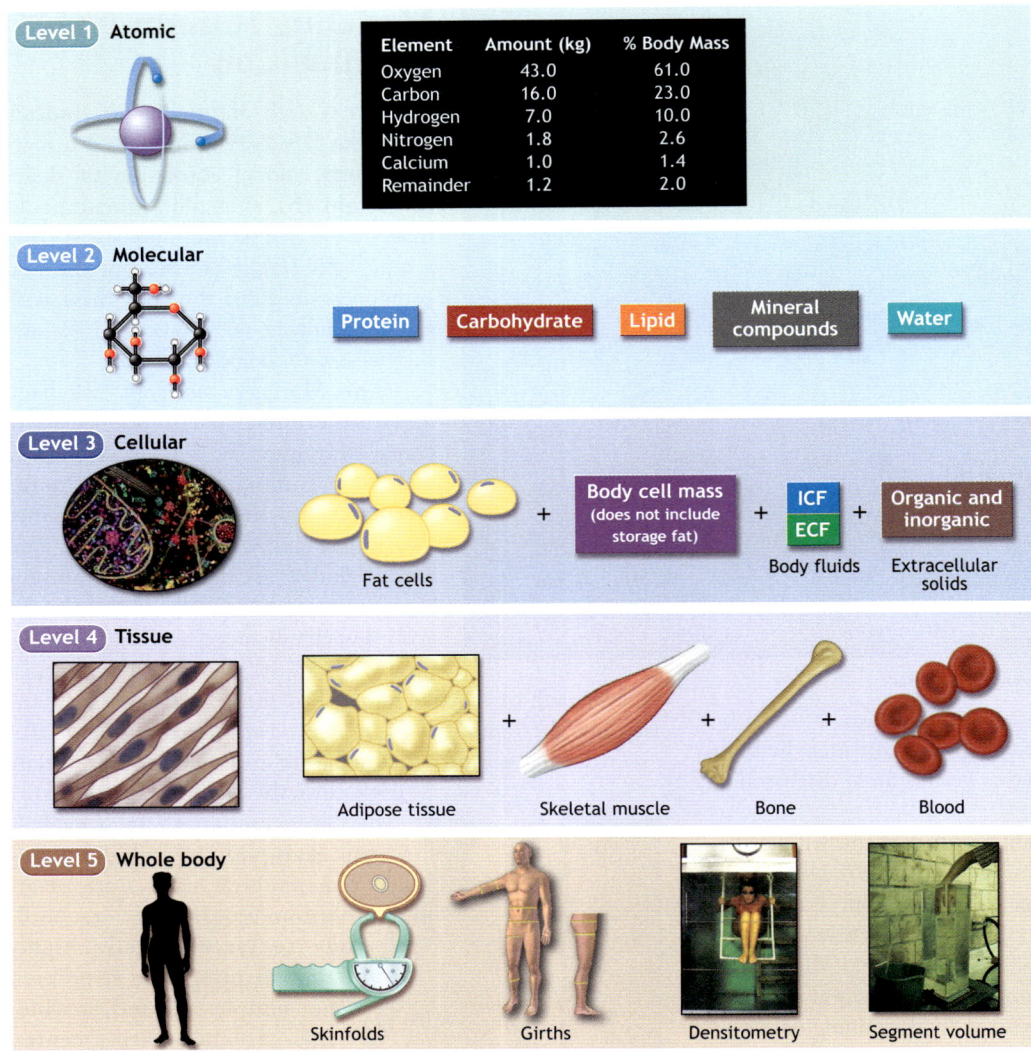

Adapted from Wang ZM, et al. The five-level model. A new approach to organizing body-composition research. *Am J Clin Nutr.* 1992;56(1):19. By permission of the American Society for Nutrition.

Somatotyping and Sheldon's Visual Taxonomic Approach

The visual classification taxonomic approach was based on front, side, and rear photographic views termed *somatotyping* in the early 1940s by American psychologist **William H. Sheldon**, PhD, MD (1898–1977; www.age-of-the-sage.org/psychology/sheldon.html). Sheldon described body shape by grouping individuals into one of the three broad categories described previously (thin, muscular, or fat).[264,265,268] Regrettably, visual appraisal does not quantify body dimensions such as chest or shoulder size, or how biceps development compares with thighs or calves or shoulders with hips; height also is not considered in the somatotype evaluation.

Despite these limitations, somatotyping provided a convenient way for coaches, trainers, and researchers to assess body size characteristics among top athletes in different sports as shown by the visual scoring method to classify individuals on a seven point scale to compare one athlete's body type with that of other athletes. No one pure body type existed, but rather combinations of the three main components, some more prominent than others. Sheldon argued that his reason for developing the somatographic method was to correlate human biologic traits and physique with future social and behavioral traits.

When the method became popular in the athletic community for its ease in categorizing athletes from thin to overweight on its own merits,[265,268] it became obvious that the variability in visual categorization in different sports showed considerable leeway within a category. This was particularly the case among endomorphs and ectomorphs seen in the composite representing four sports within one of the three primary categories. Athlete's placed into a particular A, B, or C physique category by either a coach or researcher could profoundly impact the athlete, who began to question whether their body shape and size was indeed "normal" or required an adjustment through dieting or advanced training to bring them more in accord with their rival performers.

Sheldon's Body Shape Taxonomy Draws Sharp Criticism. Sheldon's "scientific" approach to resolving questions about physique status based on a visual taxonomy garnered criticism for his theoretical premise

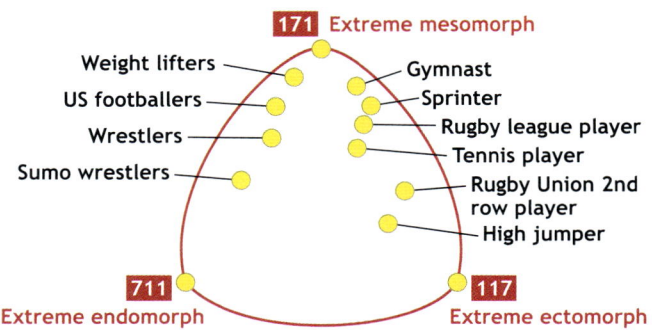

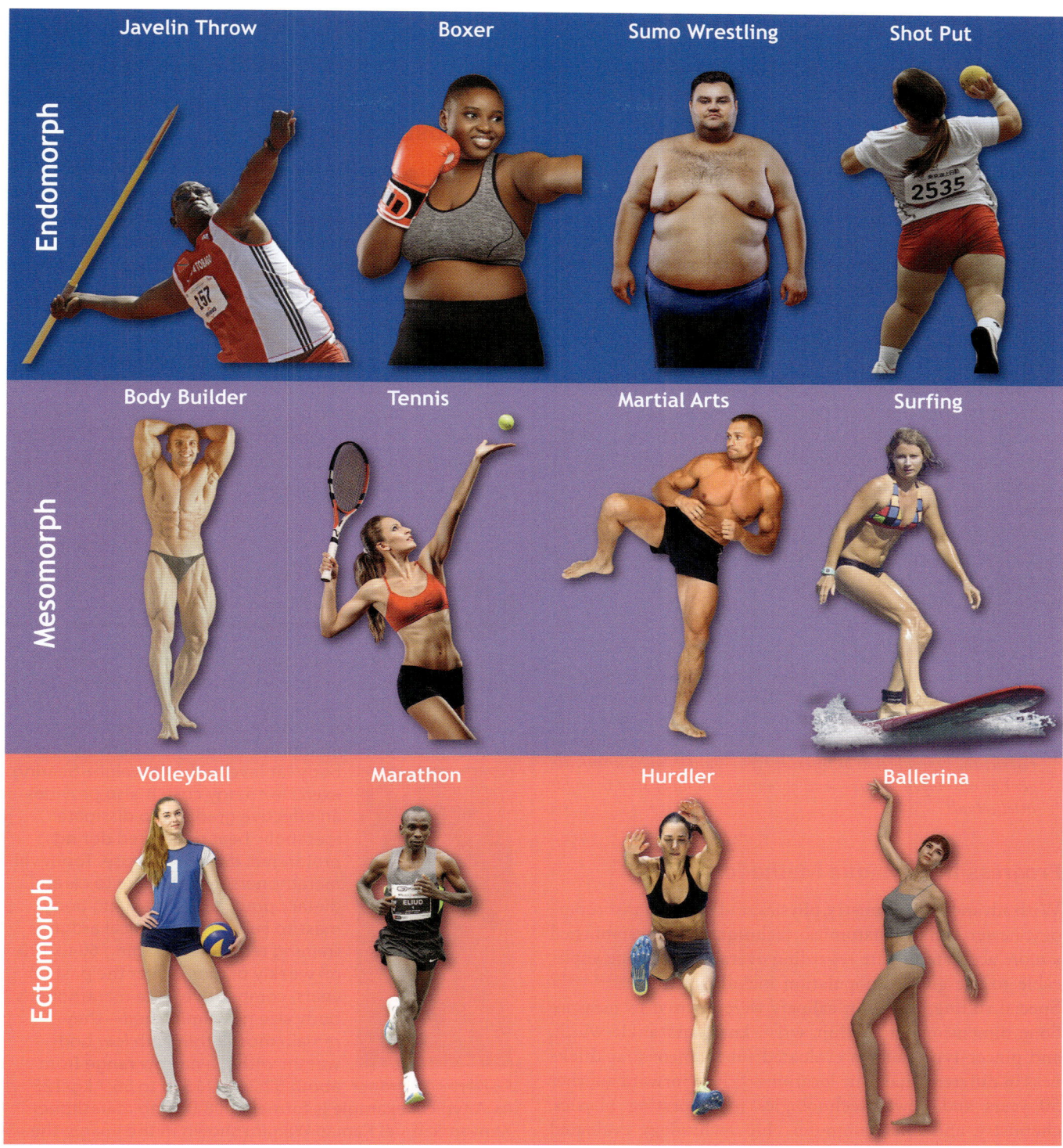

Shutterstock: Jamie Roach (javelin), Prostock-studio (boxer), Mike Orlov (sumo), hairul_nizam (shot put), Alexander Lukatskiy (body builder), NotarYES (tennis), Dumulena (martial arts), trubavin (surfing), Boris Ryaposov (volleyball), Maxisport (marathon), vectorfusionart (hurdler), TreesTons (ballerina)

regarding body shape's importance and its fundamental link to important "societal questions." Thirty years after his death, researchers worldwide became concerned that Sheldon's "unorthodox" methodology was grounded on explicitly racist eugenic views intended to discriminate against non-white Americans! Based on an evaluation of Sheldon's earlier writings, it became clear that Sheldon held the belief that his somatotyping science had partially evolved from the pseudoscience of "good" and "bad" posture, intended to identify "superior" and "inferior" human physiques tied to personality and intellectual characteristics.

In essence, Sheldon's early thinking had closely linked physical appearance (*attractiveness*) to particular character traits related to morality, temperament, gender characteristics and behaviors, and academic and professional relationships between "masculinity" and success supposedly achieved in later life.[264,266,267] Sheldon promoted the idea that knowledge about an individual's body type would provide important clues regarding various disease and disability treatments. His easily implemented methodology enticed many innocent followers to believe that physique status, identified through somatotyping (and unknown to most), determined one's world destiny with a final solution to rid society from degenerating and disabled bodies (www.utpjournals.press/doi/pdf/10.3138/cbmh.24.2.291)!

Sheldon's taxonomic approach became further mired in controversy with the investigative discovery that he relied on nude "photo-for-posture" photographs from many prestigious colleges and universities taken in required physical education classes. Sheldon's controversial procedures were exposed in an explosive 1995 article (www.nytimes.com/1995/01/15/magazine/the-great-ivy-league-nude-posture-photo-scandal.html) that confirmed the legitimacy that thousands of nude images had been taken over decades. According to Vertinsky[269]:

> The inspiration for such views came from the founder of social Darwinism and father of eugenics, Francis Galton, who, in the late 19th century, had proposed a photo archive and beauty map for the whole British population which could serve as a guide for selective breeding. Galton's idea was to use his archives to restrict the reproduction of inferior types—unfit, ugly, unintelligent or misshapen people—and encourage a kind of stud farm for intellectuals.

Progress in Physique Methodology

With advances in chemistry, physics, and physical anthropology, newer surface anatomical techniques have established a more accurate picture regarding overall body shape applicable to the general population including athletes.[239,240,282] Special sliding, precision calipers were devised to measure bone dimensions at the hip, wrist, knee, and ankle width, and pincer-type calipers evaluated subcutaneous fat thickness in different anatomic locations.[241] Fast forward another 50 years and newer technologies incorporating physics, chemistry, and microcomputer chip technology evaluated the body's internal and surface external dimensions. Anyone with access to a computer and the Internet can purchase clothing tailor-made to fit their particular body frame from tall to short, stout to thin, and everything in between. The latest smart wrist watches and beneath-the-skin patches containing hundreds of micro-needles embedded into the patch can detect interstitial water content and estimate total muscle and fat mass. These newer technologies partition the body into two distinct compartments—fat-free body mass (i.e., theoretically the body without fat) and the **fat mass** remainder—a four-component model with distinct compartments for water, protein, skeletal mass, and total body fat.

Chemical Methods Provide Basic Body Composition Insights

Homogenized fat-free tissue samples in small mammals is $1.100 \text{ g} \cdot \text{cm}^{-3}$ at $37°C/98.6°F$ value for tissue density.[152] Fat-free tissue contains about 73.2%[134] water content with 60 to 70 $\text{mmol} \cdot \text{kg}^{-1}$ potassium in males and 50 to 60 $\text{mmol} \cdot \text{kg}^{-1}$ in females.[20] In contrast, fat stored in adipose tissue has a $0.900 \text{ g} \cdot \text{cm}^{-3}$ density at $37°C$.[126]

Subsequent body composition studies expanded the two-component model to account for biologic variability in three (water, protein, lipid) or four (water, protein, bone mineral, lipid) distinct components specific to males.[202,204] Consequently, gender-specific reference standards provide a framework to evaluate what constitutes a "normal" body composition. Behnke's model reference male and reference female provide a useful comparison to assess an individual's various structural components.[16,245,259–261]

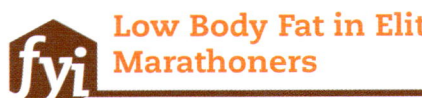

Low Body Fat in Elite Marathoners

The low body fat levels in marathon runners, ranging from 1 to 8% body mass, probably reflect self-selection in these individuals and an adaptation to long-term training for distance running and a reduced energy intake relative to energy output from intense training. A relatively low body fat level reduces weight-bearing exercise energy cost; it also provides an effective gradient to dissipate metabolic heat generated during prolonged, intense exercise. Top-level marathoners must adhere to careful dietary practices to maintain body mass to support the typical arduous training regimen averaging 60 to 120 mi weekly or more. Over the past 60 years, competitive, elite marathoner's body size has diminished—they remain mostly thin with low body weight within a narrow range from about 52.2 kg/115 lb to 56.7 kg/125 lb. A typical example is former 2008 Beijing marathoner Kenyan Samuel Kamau Wanjiru shown in the image; the former Olympic record holder (2:06:32) weighed only 52.2 kg/115 lb, the same weight as current Kenyan marathon world record holder Eliud Kipchoge (2:01:39; 2018 Berlin Marathon).

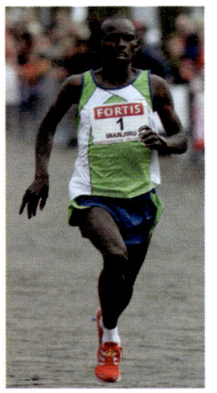

Bas Rabeling/Shutterstock

Sources:
Knechtle B, Nikolaidis PT. Physiology and pathophysiology in ultra-marathon running. *Front Physiol*. 2018;9:634.
Sengeis M, et al. Competitive performance of Kenyan runners compared to their relative body weight and fat. *Int J Sports Med*. 2021;42:323.
Stellingwerff T. Contemporary nutrition approaches to optimize elite marathon performance. *Int J Sports Physiol Perform*. 2013;8:573.

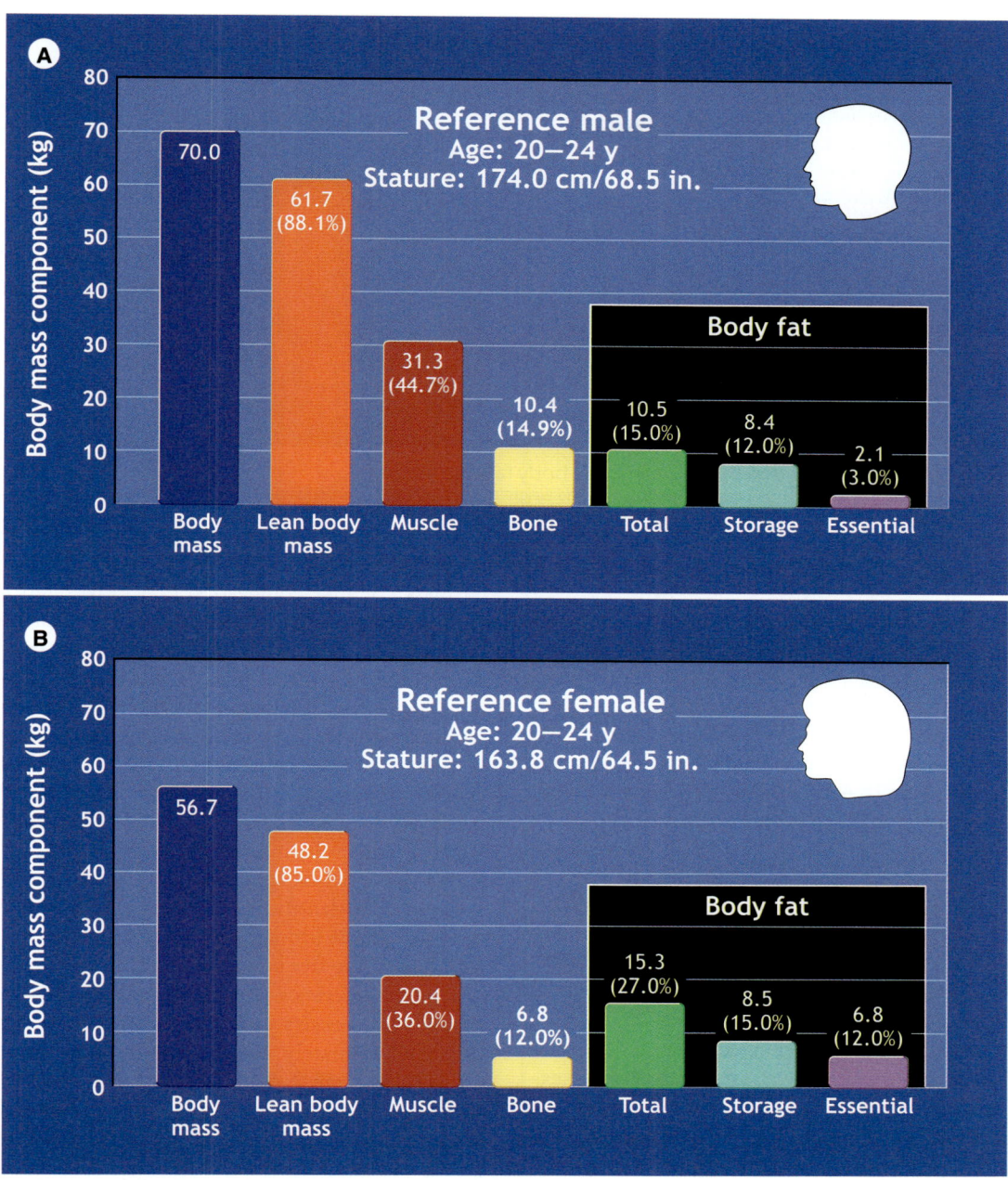

FIGURE 28.3. Behnke's theoretical body composition model for the reference male **(A)** and reference female **(B)**. Values in parentheses express percentage of total body mass for lean body mass, muscle, and bone, and the partition of body fat into total, storage, and essential fat components.

Reference Male and Reference Female

FIGURE 28.3 displays the body composition compartments for Behnke's **reference male and reference female**.[230] The different color schema partitions body mass into lean body mass, muscle, and bone, with total body fat subdivided into storage and essential fat components. This model integrates the average physical dimensions from thousands of individuals measured in large-scale civilian and military anthropometric surveys with data from laboratory studies including tissue composition and structure.[16,24,230,245]

The reference male is taller and heavier, his skeleton weighs more, and he possesses a larger muscle mass and lower body fat content than the reference female. These differences exist even when expressing fat, muscle, and bone as a percentage of body mass. Just how much of gender differences in body fat relate to biologic and behavioral factors, perhaps from lifestyle differences, remains unclear. Undoubtedly, hormonal differences play an important role. This reference model proves useful for statistical comparisons and interpretations of data from other studies of elite athletes, individuals involved in exercise training, different racial and ethnic groups, and the underweight and the obese.

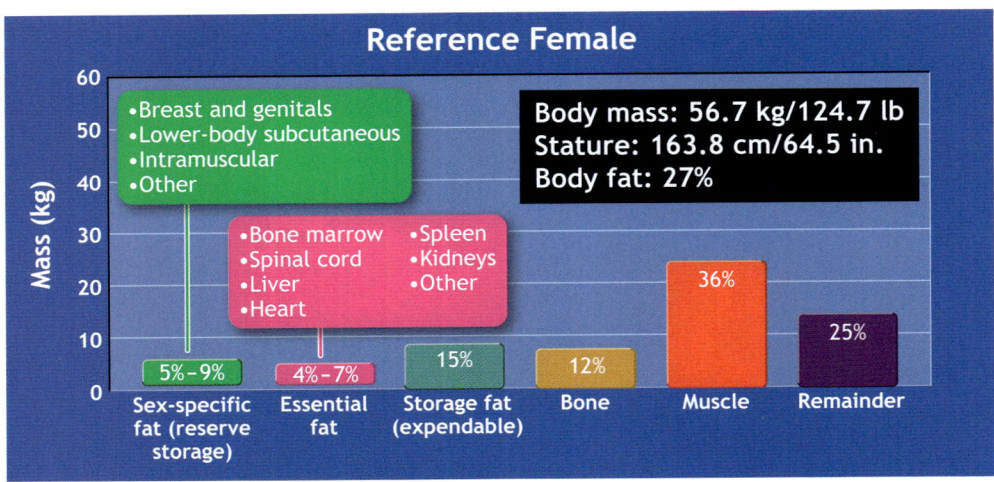

FIGURE 28.4. Theoretical model for the reference female's body fat distribution. (Adapted with permission from Katch VL, et al. Contribution of breast volume and weight to body fat distribution in females. *Am J Phys Anthropol.* 1980;53:93.)

Essential and Storage Fat

In the reference model, total body fat exists in two storage sites or depots: essential fat and storage fat. **Essential fat** consists of the lipid in the heart, lungs, liver, spleen, kidneys, intestines, muscles, and lipid-rich tissues of the central nervous system and bone marrow. *Normal physiologic functioning requires this lipid.* In the heart, for example, dissectible lipid from cadavers represents approximately 18.4 g/0.65 oz or 5.3% for an average heart weighing 349 g/12.3 oz in males and 22.7 g/0.80 oz or 8.6% weighing 256 g/9.03 oz in females.[205] Importantly, essential fat in the female includes additional **sex-specific essential fat**.[234,242] Whether this fat provides reserve storage for metabolic fuel is unclear.

FIGURE 28.4 partitions body fat for the reference female. As part of the 5 to 9% sex-specific fat reserves, breast fat probably contributes no more than 4% to total body mass, whereas total body fat content ranges between 14 and 35%.[90,256] We interpret this to mean other substantial sex-specific fat depots in the pelvic, buttock, and thigh regions primarily contribute to the female's body fat stores. The adipose tissue energy reserve contains approximately 83% pure lipid, 2% protein, and 15% water within its supporting structures. Storage fat includes the visceral fatty tissues that protect the organs within the thoracic and abdominal cavities from trauma, and the larger adipose tissue volume deposited beneath the skin's surface. A similar proportional storage fat distribution occurs in males and females (12% of body mass in males and 15% in females), but total essential fat percentage in females with the sex-specific fat averages four times males' value.

The additional essential fat in females most likely serves biologically important functions for childbearing and other hormone-related functions. Considering the reference female's approximately 8.5 kg/18.7 lb storage fat, this depot theoretically represents 63,500 kcal available energy to power the body's multifaceted functions throughout the day.[89]

Fat-Free Body Mass Versus Lean Body Mass

The terms **fat-free body mass (FFM)** and **lean body mass** refer to specific entities. Lean body mass contains the small percentage of non–sex-specific essential fat equivalent to approximately 3% body mass. In contrast, FFM represents the body mass excluding *all* extractable fat (FFM = body mass − fat mass). Behnke emphasized that FFM refers to an *in vitro* entity appropriate to carcass analysis. He considered lean body mass as an *in vivo* entity relatively constant in water, organic matter, and mineral content throughout the active adult's life span. *In normally hydrated, healthy adults, the FFM and lean body mass differ only in the essential fat component.*

Lean body mass in males and **minimal body mass** in females consist chiefly of essential fat (plus sex-specific essential fat in females), muscle, water, and bone (see **FIG. 28.4**). The whole-body density in the reference male with 12% **storage fat** and 3% essential fat approximates $1.070 \text{ g} \cdot \text{cm}^{-3}$, with a $1.094 \text{ g} \cdot \text{cm}^{-3}$ FFM density. If the reference male's body fat percentage totals 15.0% (storage fat plus essential fat), the density for a hypothetical fat-free body attains the $1.100 \text{ g} \cdot \text{cm}^{-3}$ upper limit.

In the reference female, the average $1.040 \text{ g} \cdot \text{cm}^{-3}$ for whole-body density represents a 27% body fat percentage, with approximately 12% essential body fat. For females, a $1.072 \text{ g} \cdot \text{cm}^{-3}$ density value represents the minimal 48.5-kg/106.7-lb body mass. In actual practice, density values exceeding 1.068 in females (14.8% body fat) and 1.088 $\text{g} \cdot \text{cm}^{-3}$ in males (5% body fat) rarely occur except in young, lean competitive athletes.

Minimal Leanness Standards *A biologic lower limit exists beyond which a person's body mass cannot decrease without impairing health status or altering normal physiologic functions.* To estimate the lower body fat limit in males (i.e., lean body mass), subtract storage fat from body mass. For the reference male, the lean body mass (61.7 kg/136 lb) includes approximately 3% (2.1 kg/4.6 lb) essential body fat. Encroachment into this reserve may impair optimal health and capacity for vigorous physical activity.

Low body fat values exist for male world-class endurance athletes and some conscientious objectors to military service who voluntarily reduced body fat stores during a prolonged semistarvation experiment. The low fat levels in marathon runners, which ranges from 1 to 8% of body mass, probably reflect adaptation to intense distance run training over many years,[105] but not to a common DNA variant.[280] A low body

ilusmedical/Shutterstock

fat level reduces the weight-bearing physical activity energy cost and also provides an effective gradient to rapidly dissipate metabolic heat generated in intense workouts several hours daily.

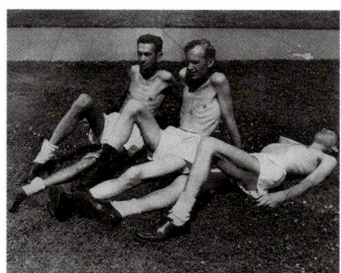
J. Henning Buchholz/Shutterstock

Considerable variation exists in different athlete's FFM, with values ranging from a low of about 48.1 kg/106 lb for some jockeys to over 177 kg/390 lb for American football defensive and offensive linemen and shot-put field-event athletes. Seven elite **sumo wrestlers** (*sekitori*, ranked in one of the top two professional sumo divisions) possessed an average 109-kg/240-lb FFM.[95]

Minnesota Semi-Starvation Experiments The **Minnesota semi-starvation experiments** identified low body fat values in experiments with conscientious objectors—but also apply to male world-class endurance athletes, jockeys, dancers, gymnasts, and wrestlers in the low body weight categories—who voluntarily reduced body fat stores with semistarvation during a yearlong nutritional experiment near the end of World War II. From November 1944 through October 1945, University of Minnesota physiologist Ancel Keys (1904–2004; http://www.nytimes.com/2004/11/23/obituaries/23keys.html?_r=0) conducted nutrition experiments on body wasting and physiologic functioning sponsored by the U.S. Army (www.mnopedia.org/event/starvation-experiment-dr-ancel-keys-1944-1945).

Courtesy Hennepin County Library

In 1941, Keys created the famous "**K rations**," compact nutritional packets for breakfast, lunch, and dinner meals used by the military during World War II. A subsequent experiment at the opposite spectrum explored the best way to "re-feed" millions of "starving" war victims, prisoners, and refugees worldwide. The government had speculated that starvation during the war could pose serious re-feeding challenges after the war ended. A two-volume report of the experiment, *The Biology of Human Starvation*, can be accessed at www.ncbi.nlm.nih.gov/pmc/articles/PMC1526048/ and is recommended reading regarding body composition changes during starvation, food consumption patterns, dietary practices, and psychological ramifications including physiological effects from wasting disease that occurs concurrently with suboptimal dietary intakes.

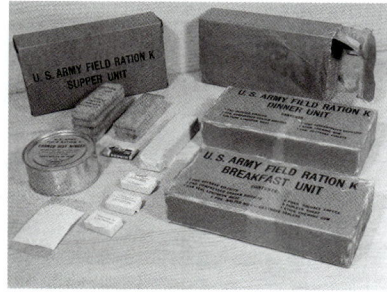
Photo: Howard Hollem, March 1943

Minimal Body Mass for Females

In comparison to the lower body mass limit for the reference male (with 3% essential fat), the reference female's lower limit includes approximately 12% essential fat. This theoretical lower limit termed *minimal body mass* is 48.5 kg/107 lb for Behnke's reference female. Generally, the leanest females in the population do not possess less than 10 to 12% body fat, a narrow range at the lower limit for most females in good health. *Behnke's theoretical minimal body mass concept in females that incorporates 12% essential fat corresponds to the lean body mass in males with 3% essential fat.*

Leanness, Regular Physical Activity, and Menstrual Irregularity

Physically active female participants in the "low weight" or "appearance" sports increase their likelihood for one of three maladies:

1. Delayed menstruation onset
2. Irregular menstrual cycle (**oligomenorrhea**)
3. Complete menses cessation (**amenorrhea**)

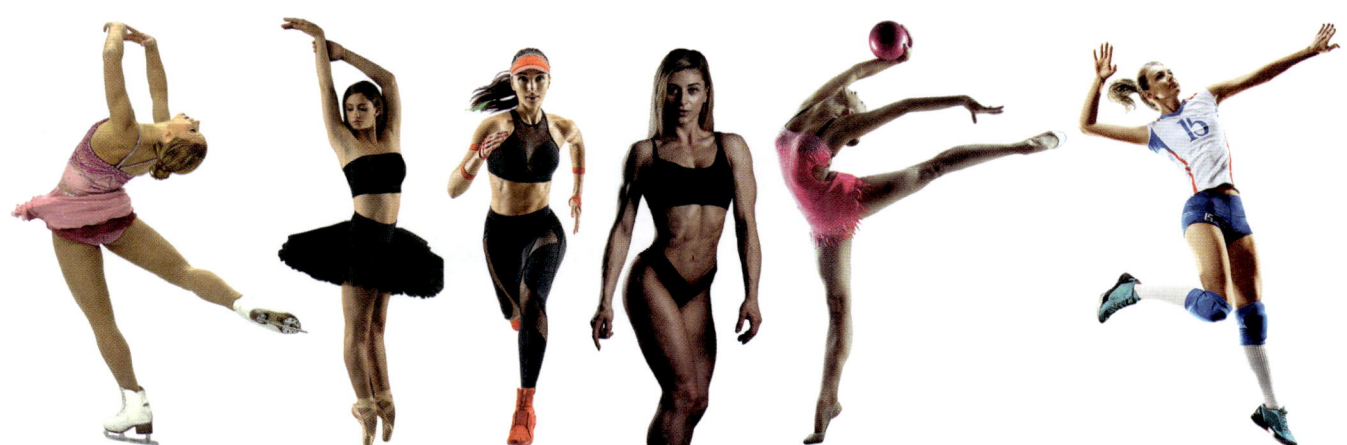
Shutterstock: Paolo Bona (ice skater), Sinisa Lucic (ballet dancer), Romariolen (runner), Romvy (body builder), Artur Didyk (rhythmic gymnast), Eugene Onischenko (volleyball player)

Menstrual and ovarian dysfunction results largely from changes in the pituitary gland's normal pulsatile luteinizing hormone secretion regulated by the hypothalamic gonadotropin-releasing hormone (www.ncbi.nlm.nih.gov/books/NBK279070/).

Within the general population, amenorrhea occurs in 2 to 5% in reproductive age females but can attain 40% in some athletic groups.[154,178] As a group, ballet dancers remain lean, with a greater incidence of menstrual dysfunction and eating disorders and a higher mean age at menarche than age-matched, nondance counterparts.[52] A third to half of female endurance athletes exhibit some menstrual irregularity. Premenopausal irregularity or absence in menstrual function accelerates bone loss and increases musculoskeletal injury risk during exercise and causes a longer interruption during training (see Chapter 2).[15,137]

Prolonged physical stress may disrupt the hypothalamic-pituitary-adrenal axis and modify **gonadotropin-releasing hormone** output, interrupting regular menstruation referred to as the **exercise stress hypothesis**. A competing hypothesis maintains that an inadequate energy reserve to sustain pregnancy induces cessation in ovulation (**energy availability hypothesis**).

Lean-to-Fat Ratio

An optimal **lean-to-fat ratio** supports normal menstrual function, perhaps through peripheral fat's role that converts androgens to estrogens or through adipose tissue's leptin production, a hormone intimately linked to body fat levels and appetite control (see Chapter 30) and puberty.[175] A linkage exists among hormonal regulating sexual maturity onset and stored energy from accumulated body fat.

Some researchers assert that 17% body fat represents a lower-end critical level to trigger menstruation onset, with 22% fat needed to sustain normal menses.[52,53] Objective data indicate that physically active females who are below a supposedly critical 17% body fat level have normal menstrual cycles without compromising physiologic and exercise capacity. Conversely, some amenorrheic athletes maintain body fat levels considered average for the population. One of our laboratories compared 30 athletes and 30 nonathletes, all with less than 20% body fat, for menstrual cycle regularity.[87] Four athletes and three nonathletes ranging from 11 to 15% body fat maintained regular cycles, whereas seven athletes and two nonathletes had irregular cycles or were amenorrheic. For the total sample, 14 athletes and 21 nonathletes maintained regular menstrual cycles. These data indicate that normal menstrual function does not require a critical 17 to 22% body fat level.

The complex interplay involving seven potential causes can impact normal menstrual cycle functions[94]:

- Physical
- Nutritional
- Genetic
- Hormonal
- Regional fat distribution
- Psychological
- Environmental

An intense physical activity session triggers the release for an array of hormones, some of which disrupt normal reproductive function.[61,199] Intense and/or prolonged exertion releases cortisol and other stress-related hormones that can alter ovarian function via the hypothalamic-pituitary-adrenal axis.[36,115]

Consuming well-balanced, nutritious meals on a regular basis helps to prevent or reverse **athletic amenorrhea** without requiring the athlete to reduce training volume or intensity.[114] The approach may take up to 1 year involving nonpharmacologic intervention to promote weight gain with continuation in physical activity.[7] When injuries to young amenorrheic ballet dancers[209] prevent them from exercising regularly, normal menstruation resumes even though body weight remains low.[81] Proponents of this "energy deficit" explanation maintain that physical exertion *per se* exerts no deleterious effect on the reproductive system other than the potential impact of its additional energy cost on creating a negative energy balance.[6,112,113,116]

The risks of sustained amenorrhea on the reproductive system remain unknown. A gynecologist/endocrinologist should evaluate failure to menstruate or cessation of the normal cycle because it may reflect pituitary or thyroid gland malfunction or premature menopause,[14,111] perhaps from ovarian failure related to a genetic aberration in the X chromosome.[12] As we point out in Chapter 2, prolonged menstrual dysfunction negatively changes normal bone mass and its function.

Delayed Onset Menstruation and Cancer Risk Delayed onset menarche in chronically active young females may actually confer positive health benefits. Female athletes who start training in high school or earlier show a lower lifetime occurrence of breast and reproductive organ cancers, and non–reproductive-system cancers than less-active counterparts.[53] Even among older women, regular activity protects against reproductive cancers. Swedish researchers studied the country's entire female population ages 50 to 74 years in 1994–1995.[133] Higher levels of occupational and leisure-time physical activity in normal-weight nonsmokers during ages 18 to 30 years related to lower postmenopausal endometrial cancer risk. Females who exercise an average of 4 hr weekly following menarche reduce breast cancer risk by 50% compared with age-matched inactive females.[18] One proposed mechanism for reduced cancer risk links lower total estrogen production or a less potent estrogen form over the athlete's lifetime with fewer ovulatory cycles from delayed menstruation onset.[106,195] Lower body fat levels in physically active individuals also may contribute to lowered cancer risk because peripheral fatty tissues convert androgens to estrogen.

Common Techniques to Assess Body Composition

Two procedures evaluate body composition:

1. *Direct* measurement by chemical analysis of the animal carcass or human cadaver
2. *Indirect* estimation by hydrostatic weighing, skinfold and girth anthropometric measurements, and other clinical and laboratory procedures

Direct Assessment

Two approaches directly assess body composition. One technique dissolves a cadaver in a chemical solution to determine its lipid and lipid-free component mixture. Such analyses involve ethical questions and legal hurdles in obtaining cadavers for research.[30–32,270]

A competing approach relies on anatomists and forensic specialists to dissect the total fat mass, muscles, bones, and separate cadaver organ tissues to determine their chemical composition, including detailed chemical breakdown depicted in the inset image showing the percentages for the different elemental substances present in those tissues. The outer ring shows 12 separately colored elemental substances by their chemical symbol expressed as a percentage compared with the five most common components—water (62%), protein, (16%), lipid (16%), minerals (6%), and carbohydrate (1%)—accounting for more than 96% of the body's total elemental substances. Few studies with humans have been analyzed because they are labor-intensive and require tedious analyses using expensive and highly specialized laboratory equipment.

Direct body composition assessment suggests that while considerable individual differences exist in total body fatness, the compositions of skeletal mass and the fat-free and fat tissues remain relatively stable. *The relative constancy among these tissues allows researchers to develop mathematical equations to indirectly predict the body's total fat percentage.*

Indirect Assessment

Diverse indirect procedures assess body composition. One process utilizes **Archimedes' principle** applied to **densitometry** (also referred to as hydrodensitometry, underwater weighing, or hydrostatic weighing). This method computes percentage body fat from body density (body mass to body volume ratio). Other procedures predict body fat from skinfold thickness and girth measurements (**anthropometry**), x-ray, total body electrical conductivity or bioimpedance (including segmental impedance), near-infrared interactance, ultrasound, computed tomography, air plethysmography, and magnetic resonance imaging.

A less often used anthropometric technique developed in 1959 by Behnke assesses body build with a sliding caliper to measure skeletal distance between two bony landmarks at eight sites (biacromial, bi-iliac, bitrochanters, chest, wrists, elbows, knees, and ankles).[259] The inset image at the bottom of this page identifies two common trunk diameter locations—biacromial diameter in the shoulder region and bitrochanteric diameter in the hip region. A strong $r = 0.90$ correlation was obtained between lean body mass calculated from skeletal diameters (lean body mass = $D^2 \times h$), where D is the average of the eight diameters using established constants based on reference male and female data. Lean body mass was calculated from total body water determined by the deuterium oxide method[153,257] and body density by hydrodensitometry.[211] The relationship was made possible by the nearly constant ratio existing between mean bone diameter size throughout the growth period beginning about age four and continuing to maturity.[245,259] The Behnke skeletal method determined what any person should weigh relative to their skeletal build based on selected diameters combined with an accurate measurement for stature to within 0.5 cm/0.2 in.[260–262]

Hydrostatic Weighing: Archimedes' Principle

The Greek mathematician, engineer, researcher, and inventor **Archimedes** (287–212 BC) discovered a fundamental principle currently applied to evaluate human body composition. Legend has it that an itinerant scholar from that era described the circumstances surrounding the event (https://ed.ted.com/lessons/mark-salata-how-taking-a-bath-led-to-archimedes-principle):

> King Hieron in the ancient Greek city Syracuse on Sicily's east coast suspected that his pure gold crown had been altered by the substitution of silver for gold. The King directed Archimedes to devise a method to test the crown for its gold content without dismantling it. Archimedes pondered over this problem for many weeks without success, until one day, he stepped into his bath filled to the top with water and observed the overflow. He thought about this for a moment, and then, wild with joy,

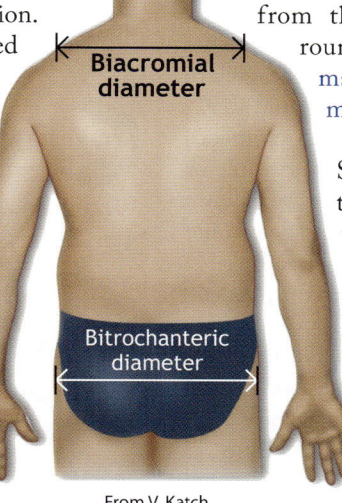

From V. Katch

Michal Sanca/Shutterstock

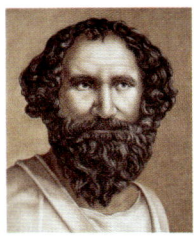
A.Sych/Shutterstock

jumped from the bath and ran naked through the streets of Syracuse shouting, "Eureka, Eureka, I have solved the mystery about the King's gold crown."

Archimedes reasoned that a substance such as gold must have a volume proportional to its mass, so measuring the volume of an irregularly shaped object would require submerging the crown in a water-filled container and collecting the overflow. Archimedes took lumps of gold and silver of the same mass as the crown and submerged each in the container. He discovered the crown displaced more water than the lump of gold and less than the lump of silver. He repeated his experiment by combining an equal weight of silver with the gold to create the same shaped crown. If the crown weighed less when submerged because both densities differed, he would conclude the crown consisted of both silver *and* gold, confirming the King's belief the crown was adulterated and not constructed from pure gold.

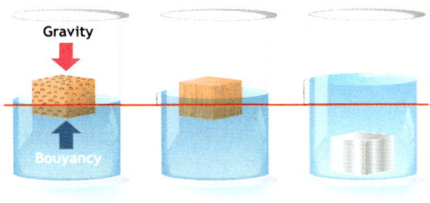
Designua/Shutterstock

Essentially, Archimedes compared the crown's **specific gravity** with the specific gravities for the gold and silver metals. As the inset image shows, he also reasoned that an object submerged or floating in water becomes buoyed up by a counterforce that equals the weight of the volume it displaces. This buoyant force supports an immersed object against gravity's downward pull so an object loses weight in water. *The loss of weight in water equals the weight of the water volume it displaces. In this case, specific gravity refers to an object's mass in air divided by its lower weight in water. Stated mathematically, the loss equals the weight measured in air minus its weight submerged in water.*

> **Specific gravity = Weight in air ÷ Lost weight in water**

In practical terms, suppose a crown weighs 2.27 kg/5 lb in air and 0.13 kg/0.3 lb less, or 2.14 kg/4.7 lb, when weighed underwater. Dividing the crown's 2.27-kg/5-lb mass by its 0.13-kg/0.3-lb weight loss in water yields a specific gravity equal to 17.5. This ratio differs considerably from gold's 19.3 specific gravity, so we, too, can conclude what Archimedes said, "Eureka, the crown is a fraud!" The physical principle of hydrostatic water displacement Archimedes discovered allows us to apply the same water submersion technique to determine the body's volume. Dividing body mass by its volume yields **body density** (density = mass ÷ volume) and from this, an estimate of percentage body fat (see next section).

Within the framework relating to Archimedes' discovery, one can view specific gravity as an object's "heaviness" related to its volume. Objects with the same volume may vary considerably in density. For water, 1 g occupies exactly 1 cm³ at 4°C/39.2°F; the density equals 1 g · cm⁻³. Water achieves its greatest density at 4°C/39.2°F, so increasing water temperature

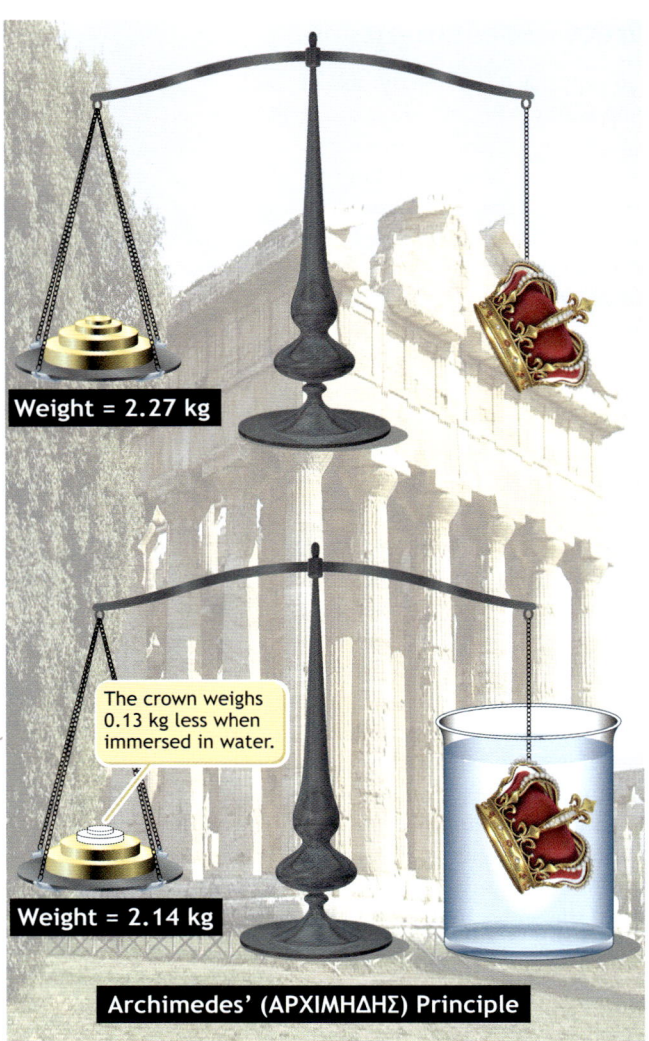

increases the volume it displaces per gram and thus decreases its density. Researchers "adjust" an object's volume weighed in water for its density at the weighing temperature.

 Appendix D, available online at Lippincott Connect, lists common metric system conversion constants in exercise physiology.

INTEGRATIVE QUESTION

Why does a solid steel object sink in water whereas the world's largest battleships float?

Body Volume Measurement

The principle discovered by Archimedes applies body volume measurement in one of two ways:

1. Water displacement
2. Hydrostatic weighing

Body volume requires accurate measurement. Small volume variations can substantially impact the density calculation for both body segments and the whole body—and for the latter, the computed percentage body fat and FFM from body density.

Water Displacement for Body Segments

An object's volume submerged in water equals the corresponding rise in the water level within a container fitted with a finely calibrated tube secured to its side to determine the water's rise. A smaller body segment's volume also can be determined using water displacement to measure limb volume or parts of limbs such as hands with appropriate methodology.[73] This technique has proved effective to assess segmental arm and leg volumes and their corresponding changes with exercise training, tissue changes with weight gain or loss, or changes in body dimensions from physical inactivity.[215]

Hydrostatic Weighing

Hydrostatic weighing applies Archimedes' principle to determine body volume, which computes the volume as the difference between body mass measured in air (M_a) and body weight measured during water submersion (W_w; the correct term because body mass remains unchanged under water). When weighing a submerged human, the air volume remaining in the lungs during full head submersion must be determined before, during, or following submersion.

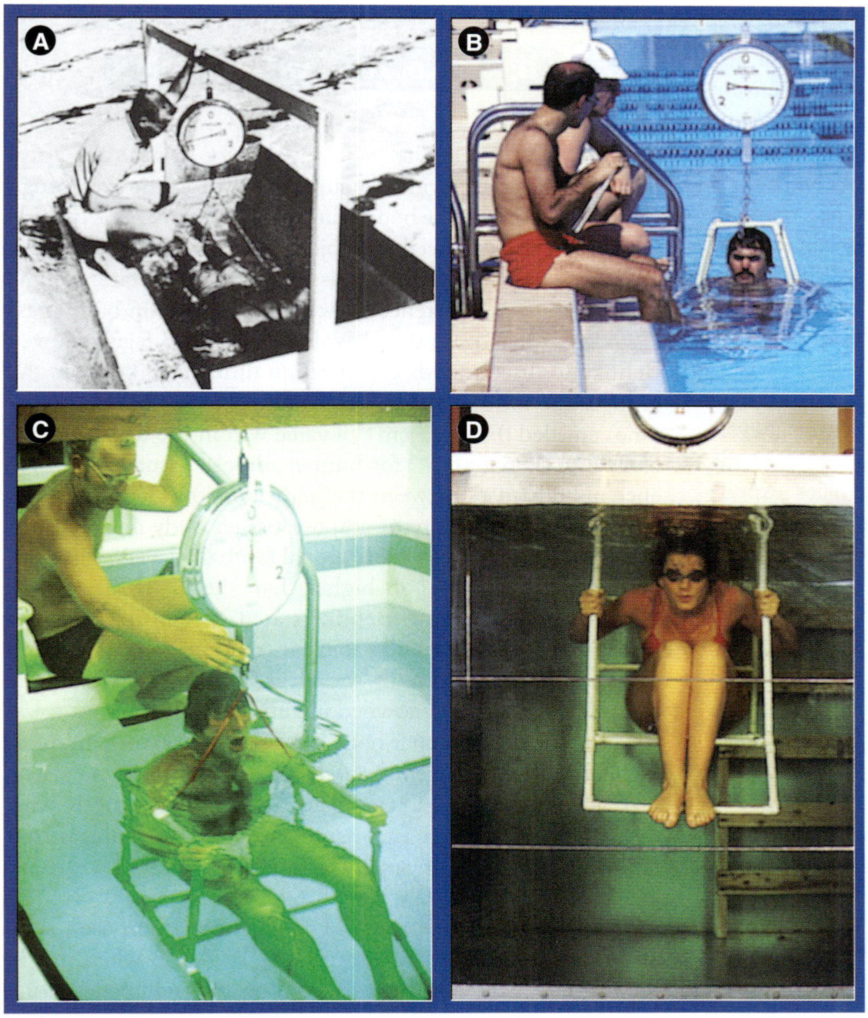

FIGURE 28.5 shows four hydrostatic weighing strategies to assess body volume. The first step before determining body volume accurately assesses the subject's body mass in air on a calibrated balance scale within ±50 g/1.8 oz. In image A, the subject wears a nylon swim suit and then lies across a lightweight frame suspended from the scale and submerged beneath the water's surface at a 1.2-m/4-ft depth, which keeps the water within the confined box area to remain still during lap swimming.[254] A swimming pool in image B serves the same purpose as the marine plywood box placed in the water, with the scale and chair assembly suspended from a support at the side of the pool (or suspended from the end of the pool diving board). Swimming pool temperature is maintained at a water temperature fairly close to skin temperature. Knowing the water temperature provides a correction factor to determine water density at the weighing temperature. In fatter subjects who tend to float and have difficulty submerging their head under water, a diver's belt secured around the waist (or placed across the lap) stabilizes the subject from floating toward the surface during submersion. The underwater weight for the belt and chair (tare weight) is then subtracted from the subject's total weight underwater. The final net underwater weight calculation must account for the underwater weight of these added objects. In images C and D, water temperature was ideal at about 35°C/95°F, particularly for subjects apprehensive about submerging their head underwater and holding their breath for about 10 s.

FIGURE 28.5. Measuring body volume by underwater weighing with residual lung volume measured before, during, or after the weighing. **(A)** In a swimming pool with subject lying prone across a metal frame suspended from the scale. **(B)** Seated in a tubular frame suspended from the scale hanging across a protruding wooden beam anchored to a water-filled metal drum at poolside during Boston Red Sox spring training. **(C)** Seated on a PVC pipe chair in a therapy pool (1976 New York Jets team training camp, Hofstra, NY.) **(D)** Seated inside a stainless steel underwater weighing tank with Plexiglas front (Exercise Physiology Laboratory, Kinesiology Department, UMass, Amherst, MA.)
(Photos from F. Katch)

Seated with the head above water, the subject makes a forced maximal exhalation while slowly lowering the head under the water. The breath is held for 5 to 8 s to allow the scale pointer to stabilize at the midpoint of the oscillations or rely on an electronic readout with appropriate instrumentation. The subject repeats the procedure 8 to 12 times to obtain a dependable underwater weight score.[255] Even when achieving a full exhalation, a small volume of air, the residual lung volume, remains in the lungs. Body volume calculation requires subtracting the residual lung volume's buoyant effect measured before, during, or following the underwater weighing.[271] Failure to subtract the residual lung volume *underestimates* whole-body density because the lungs' air volume contributes to buoyancy. This omission literally creates a "fatter" person when converting body density to body fat percentage. Assessing residual volume must not be neglected even at sports training sites shown in **FIGURE 28.5B AND C**. For any of the methods, a snorkel with nose clip eases apprehension about head submersion. In the authors' experience with thousands of subjects, allowing them three to five "practice" trials at pool side or in the tank in which they hold their breath for 5 s while remaining still substantially reduces the measurement time for the "real trials." With all of the methods, an autopsy scale accurate to within ± 10 g was used to record the underwater weight. This accuracy level compares to scale accuracy in most grocery stores to weigh produce and meat products.

Variations With Menstruation. Normal fluctuations in body mass (chiefly body water) related to the menstrual cycle generally do not impact body density and subsequent body fat assessed by hydrostatic weighing. Some females experience noticeable increases in body water (≥1.0 kg/2.2 lb) during menstruation. Water retention can affect the body density and introduce a small error when computing body fat percentage.[25]

Calculating Body Composition From Body Mass, Body Volume, and Residual Lung Volume. Data for two professional football players, an offensive guard and a quarterback, illustrate the sequence of steps in computing body density, percentage fat, fat mass, and FFM (**TABLE 28.1**).

TABLE 28.1 Sequential steps to compute body density, percentage fat, fat mass, and fat-free mass in two American professional football players

Mass ÷ volume is the equation to compute density, with density expressed in grams per cubic centimeter (g · cm⁻³), mass in kilograms, and volume in liters. The difference between M_a and W_w equals body volume after applying the appropriate water temperature correction (D_w). Air remaining in the lungs and other body "spaces" (e.g., abdominal viscera, sinuses) contributes some buoyancy to the underwater weight. In the extreme, consuming an 800-mL/27-oz carbonated beverage increases gastric gas volume by approximately 600 mL/20 oz. This *underestimates* body density by hydrostatic weighing by 0.7% and *overestimates* percentage body fat by 11% compared with measures made before drinking the beverage.[136] In most subjects, abdominal gas and sinus air volume remain small (<100 mL) and inconsequential. *This contrasts with the relatively large and variable residual lung volume and its subsequent subtraction from total body volume.*

Whereas the residual lung volume decreases slightly in a person immersed in water compared with residual volume in air (from water's compressive force against the thoracic cavity), the difference exerts only a small effect on computed percentage body fat.[71]

The following formula computes body density (D_b) from underwater weighing variables:

$$D_b = \text{Mass} \div \text{Volume} = M_a \div [(M_a - W_w) \div D_w] - RLV$$

For ease in computation, the following formula can be used to compute body density:

$$D_b = M_a \times D_w / (M_a - W_w - RLV \times D_w)$$

Hydrostatic Weighing Validity to Estimate Body Fat. Experimental evidence supports hydrostatic weighing's validity to estimate the body's fat content. Behnke's early studies of Navy divers placed 64 subjects into two groups based on their measured body density assessed by hydrostatic weighing.[16] The mean difference between the groups in body mass (12.4 kg/27 lb 5 oz) and body volume (13.3 L/3.5 gal) allowed Behnke to discern body composition differences between the groups. The ratio of the average differences (Δ mass ÷ Δ volume) equaled 0.933 g · cm⁻³, a value within the density range of 0.92 to 0.96 g · cm⁻³ for human adipose tissue. The difference in body mass between the high- and low-density groups represented the density of adipose tissue. Body density for a group of heavy but lean professional football players, with lean body mass 20 kg/44.1 lb higher than the Navy divers who averaged 1.080 g · cm⁻³. Behnke stated, "Here indeed was a presumptive demonstration that fat could be 'separated' from bone and muscle *in vivo* or 'the silver from the gold' by application of a principle renowned in antiquity."

The lower and upper body density limits among humans range from 0.93 g · cm⁻³ in the massively obese to nearly 1.10 g · cm⁻³ in the leanest males. This coincides nicely with the 1.10 density of fat-free tissue and 0.90 for homogenized fat tissue samples from small mammals.

Computing Body Density. For illustrative purposes, suppose a 50-kg/110-lb female weighs 2 kg/4.5 lb when totally submerged under the water. According to Archimedes' principle, a loss of 48 kg/106 lb of weight in water equals the displaced water's weight. In this example, 48 kg/106 lb of water equals 48 L, or 48,000 cm³ (1 g of water = 1 cm³ by volume at 4°C/39.2°F). In practice, researchers use warmer water and apply the appropriate density water correction factor at the weighing temperature (http://butane.chem.uiuc.edu/pshapley/GenChem1/L21/2.html).

The density for this person, computed as body mass divided by body volume, equals 50,000 g (50 kg) ÷ 48,000 cm³ or 1.0417 g · cm⁻³. The next step incorporating body volume estimates percentage body fat and the fat and fat-free tissue masses.

Computing Percentage Body Fat. An equation that incorporates whole-body density estimates the body's fat percentage. The simplified equation, derived by UC Berkeley biophysicist William Siri (1919–1998), substitutes 0.90 g · cm^{-3} for fat density and 1.10 g · cm^{-3} for fat-free tissue density.[164] The final derivation referred to as the **Siri equation** computes percentage body fat from body density:

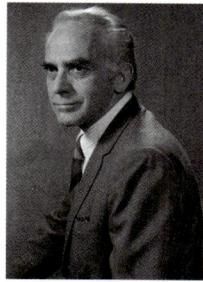
Photo from F. Katch

> **Percentage body fat = (495 ÷ body density) − 450**

This equation assumes the body composition **two-component model**; the density of fat extracted from adipose tissue equals 0.90 g · cm^{-3} and 1.10 g · cm^{-3} for fat-free tissue at 37°C/98.6°F. The early pioneer researchers maintained that each of these densities remains relatively constant among individuals despite large individual variations in total fat and FFM. They also assumed, although incorrectly, that the lean tissue component densities for bone and muscle remained the same among individuals. In this model, body fat percentage represents 15% of the total body mass, while the fat-free component represents an 85% value.

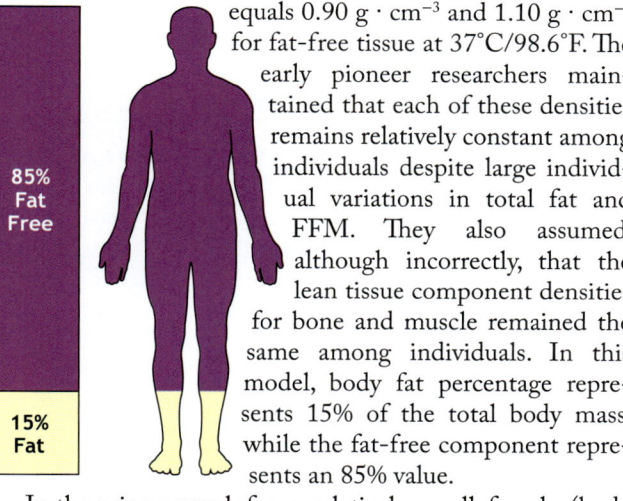

In the prior example for a relatively small female (body mass: 50 kg/110 lb; body volume: 48 L/12.7 gal), 1.0417 g · cm^{-3} for whole-body density converts to 25.2% percentage fat by the Siri equation.

> **Percentage body fat = (495 ÷ 1.0417) − 450**
> **= 25.2%**

Several formulae other than Siri's equation also estimate percentage body fat from body density.[24,92] The basic difference among them in calculating body fat generally averages less than 1% body fat units for body fat levels ranging between 4 and 30%.

Density Assumption Limitations

The generalized density values for the fat-free (1.10 g · cm^{-3}) and fat (0.90 g · cm^{-3}) tissue compartments represent averages for young and middle-aged adults. These "constants" vary among individuals and groups, particularly the FFM density and its chemical composition. Such variation places some limitation in partitioning body mass into fat and fat-free components and percentage body fat prediction from whole-body density.[55] Specifically, the average FFM density is greater for Blacks and Hispanics than for Whites (1.113 g · cm^{-3} Blacks, 1.105 g · cm^{-3} Hispanics, 1.100 g · cm^{-3} Whites).[143,159,170] Racial differences also exist among adolescents.[177] The existing equations based on the assumptions for Whites to calculate body composition from body density for Blacks or Hispanics *overestimates* FFM and *underestimates* percentage body fat. Modifying the Siri equation for Blacks more accurately computes percentage body fat from body density:

> **Percentage body fat = (437.4 ÷ body density) − 392.8**

Other Error Considerations. Applying constant density values for the different tissues in growing children or aging adults also introduces errors to predict body composition.[272] For example, FFM's water and mineral content continually changes during the growth period, including in osteoporosis with aging. Reduced bone density makes the fat-free tissue density in young children and older adults lower than the assumed 1.10 g · cm^{-3} constant. This invalidates assumptions about the constant densities for the fat and fat-free masses in the two-compartment model and *overestimates* **relative body fat** expressed as a percentage calculated from densitometry. For this reason, many researchers do not convert body density to percentage body fat in children and aging adults. Applying a four-component model adjusts body density in prepubertal children to compute percentage body fat.[165,197] **TABLE 28.2** lists equations adjusted to maturation level to predict percentage body fat in boys and girls ages 7 to 17 from whole-body density.[74]

> **TABLE 28.2** Body composition prediction equations for boys and girls ages 7 to 17

Adjust for Large Musculoskeletal Development

Chronic resistance training affects FFM density, altering body fat estimation based on whole-body density. Caucasian male weightlifters with considerable muscular development and nontrained controls were assessed for body density, total body water, and bone mineral content.[131] Comparisons included body fat percentage with both the two-compartment model shown previously and a four-compartment model incorporating the body's lipid, water, mineral, and protein content and their corresponding density values. In contrast to the two-compartment model, the four-compartment model as pointed out in a prior section includes 60% water, 10% protein, 15% skeletal mass, and the same 15% body fat percentage. The body fat component applying the Siri equation produced higher body fat percentage values than the body fat percentage from the four-compartment model for the weight trainers but not for untrained controls. A *lower* FFM density in weight trainers than in controls, 1.089 versus 1.099 g · cm^{-3},

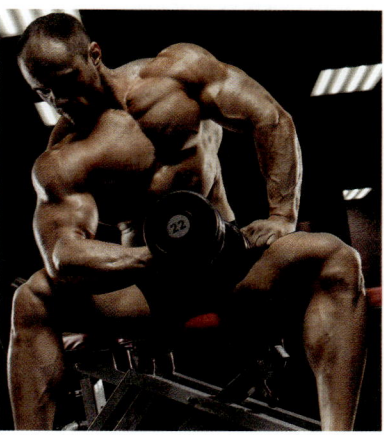
Lebedev Roman Olegovich/Shutterstock

explained this discrepancy; it resulted from larger water and smaller mineral and protein FFM fractions in the resistance-trained men. For them, incorrect assumptions underlying the Siri equation *overestimated* percentage body fat.

For the weightlifters, muscularity increased disproportionately to changes in bone mass. A lower FFM density occurred because the density of their fat-free muscle (1.066 g · cm^{-3}) was below the 1.1 g · cm^{-3} value the Siri equation assumes. Disproportionate increases in muscle mass relative to increases in bone mass accounted for the reduced density of the FFM below 1.1 g · cm^{-3}, *overpredicting* percentage body fat from the two-compartment model. If resistance training does progressively lower FFM density, then applying the Siri equation fails to accurately reflect true body composition changes from this training mode.

Based on revised densities for FFM (1.089 g · cm^{-3}) and fat mass (0.9007 g · cm^{-3}), a modified equation more accurately describes resistance-trained White males[131]:

$$\text{Percentage body fat} = (521 \div \text{body density}) - 478$$

Computing Fat Mass. Using data from the previous example, fat mass computes by multiplying body mass by percentage body fat with this equation:

$$\begin{aligned}\text{Fat mass} &= \text{body mass} \times (\% \text{ fat}/100) \\ &= 50 \text{ kg} \times 0.252 \\ &= 12.5 \text{ kg}\end{aligned}$$

Further computations subdivide this person's fat mass into essential and storage fat. A female with 25.2% body fat has approximately 12% essential fat, or 6.0 kg (0.12 × 50 kg); the remaining 13.2% (6.6 kg/14.5 lb) exists as storage fat (0.132 × 50 kg). For a male with 3% essential fat and 22.2% storage fat (based on 25.2% total body fat), the corresponding values equal 1.5 kg/3.4 lb for essential fat and 11.1 kg/24.6 lb for storage fat. Clearly, for a male and female with identical percentage body fat, the male rates "fatter" because storage fat represents a larger total body fat percentage. Each gram of body fat (83% pure lipid) contains approximately 7.5 kcal (7500 kcal per kg). Thus, for the total storage fat depot, the values are 49,500 kcal for the female and 83,260 kcal for the male. For essential fat, including female sex-specific fat, the values are 45,000 kcal for the female and 11,250 kcal for the male.

Computing FFM. Compute FFM by subtracting fat mass from body mass.

$$\begin{aligned}\text{FFM} &= \text{Body mass} - \text{Fat mass} \\ &= 50 \text{ kg} - 12.5 \text{ kg} \\ &= 37.5 \text{ kg}\end{aligned}$$

BOD POD Measures Body Volume

An alternate procedure assesses body volume and its changes for groups that range from infants to older adults, to collegiate wrestlers and exceptionally large athletes like American professional football and basketball players.[50,182,208] The **BOD POD** method has adapted helium-displacement plethysmography first reported in the late 1800s. With this method, the person sits inside a small chamber for 3 to 5 min as shown in **FIGURE 28.6**. The technique exhibits high

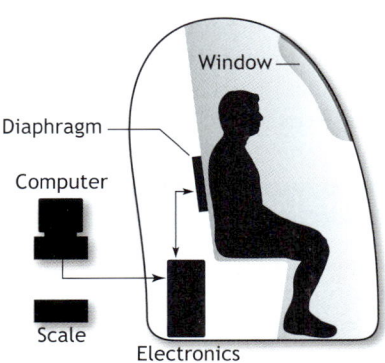

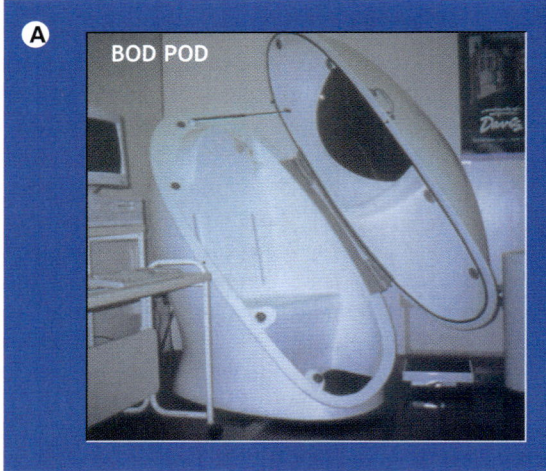

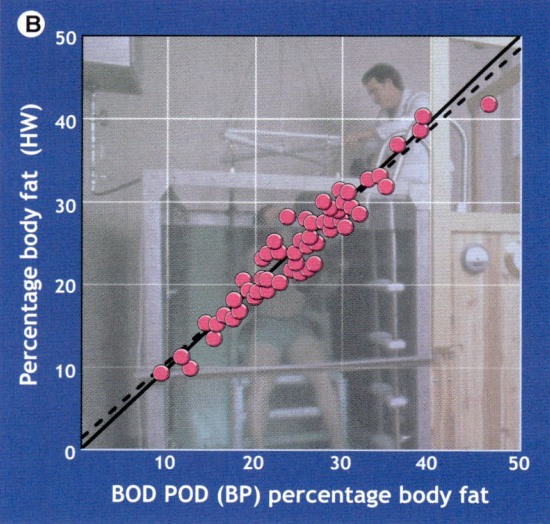

FIGURE 28.6. **(A)** BOD POD for body volume measurement. **(B)** Regression statistics with percentage body fat by hydrostatic weighing (HW) versus percentage body fat by BOD POD (BP).
(Data from McCrory MA, et al. Evaluation of a new air displacement plethysmograph for measuring human body composition. *Med Sci Sports Exerc*. 1995;27:1686. Photo in **A** courtesy Dr. Megan McCrory, Purdue University, West Lafayette, IN.)

test score reproducibility ($r \geq 0.90$) within and across days. After being weighed to the nearest ±5 g on an electronic scale (*bottom left* in the BOD POD apparatus), the person sits in the 750 L/198 gal volume, dual-chamber fiberglass shell. The molded front seat separates the unit into front and rear chambers. The electronics housed in the rear chamber contain pressure transducers, breathing circuit, and air circulation system.

The BOD POD determines body volume by measuring the empty chamber's initial volume and then the volume with the person inside.[193] To ensure measurement reliability and accuracy, the person wears a tight-fitting swimsuit.[188] Body volume represents the initial volume minus the reduced chamber air volume with the person inside. The person breathes several breaths into an air circuit to assess pulmonary gas volume, which when subtracted from measured body volume yields the true body volume. Body density computes as body mass (measured in air) divided by body volume (measured in BOD POD, including a correction for a small negative volume caused by isothermal effects related to skin surface area). The Siri equation converts body density to percentage body fat.

Literature Discrepancies

FIGURE 28.6B shows the regression for percentage body fat assessed by hydrostatic weighing versus BOD POD (www.cosmed.com/en/products/body-composition/bod-pod) in ethnically diverse adult males and females. A difference of only ±0.3% (±0.2% fat units) occurred between hydrostatic weighing and BOD POD body fat ($r = 0.96$ validity coefficient). In contrast to these findings, BOD POD assessment of body fat in collegiate football players and other athletes,[11,17] though producing reliable scores, *underpredicted* body fat compared with hydrostatic weighing and **dual-energy x-ray absorptiometry (DXA)**, described later in the chapter.[93] Underpredicting body fat also occurred in Black males who varied in age, stature, body mass, body fat percentage, and self-reported physical activity level and socioeconomic status.[194] The method underpredicted body fat percentage compared with densitometry (−1.9% fat units) and DXA (−1.6% fat units). Similar underpredictions compared with DXA-derived body fat (−2.9% fat units) occurred in 54 boys and girls ages 10 to 18.[109] BOD POD also underestimated young adults' body fat compared with body fat predicted from the four-compartment model.[49,129] The method overestimated body fat percentage among lean adults.[187] A BOD POD validation study in children ages 9 to 14 concluded that, compared with DXA, total body water, and densitometry, BOD POD precisely and accurately estimated fat mass without introducing bias estimates.[47] The method also accurately detected body composition changes from a small-to-moderate weight loss in overweight females and males.[124,198,216] Many studies have assessed BOD POD efficacy compared with other body composition methods in infants and children; young, middle-aged, and older adults; and obese persons and athletes.[5,8,33,48,148,189,217,287] The PEA POD, a similar system, estimates fat and fat-free mass in infants weighing from 1 kg/2.2 lb to 8 kg/17.7 lb.[288]

Skinfold and Girth Measurements

In field situations, two anthropometric procedures that measure either subcutaneous fat (skinfolds) or circumferences (girths) predict body fatness with reasonable accuracy.[231] Eleven girths representing total body shape also separates the body's muscular from nonmuscular components to provide a visual "profile" about body proportionality for individuals and athletes of both sexes and similar ages.[232,252]

Subcutaneous Fat Measurement With Skinfolds

The rationale for using skinfolds to estimate body fat comes from the interrelationships among three factors:

1. Adipose tissue directly beneath the skin (**subcutaneous fat**)
2. Internal fat
3. Whole-body density

The Skinfold Caliper. By 1930, a special pincer-type caliper developed in research laboratories devoted to body composition assessment accurately measured subcutaneous fat at selected body sites. Pioneering scientist and physical anthropologist William M. Cobb (1906–1990; BA, Amherst College, 1925; MD, Howard University College of Medicine, 1929; PhD, Case Western Reserve University, 1932) used various spreading metal sliding calipers[290] and x-ray to

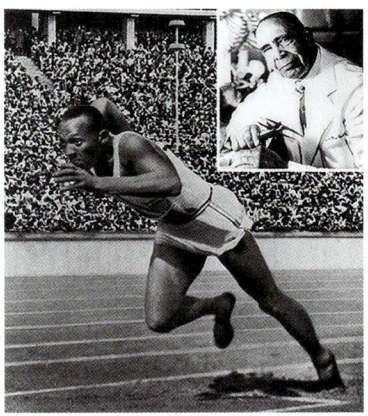

assess 1936 Olympian Jesse Owens' (1930–1980) physical dimensions (www.tandfonline.com/doi/full/10.1080/09523360701740349). Photos of his calipers are on display at the Smithsonian National Museum of African American History and Culture, Washington, DC. Dr. Cobb was the first African American to earn a PhD in anthropology, subsequently publishing over 1100 articles and books integrating race and athletics, skeletal biodiversity, and societal concerns. He was first in a scientific publication to debunk the idea that the success of Black sprinters and broad jumpers was due to supposedly racially determined characteristics such as "a longer heel bone," "a long Achilles tendon," and a "short-bellied calf" (https://dh.howard.edu/cgi/viewcontent.cgi?article=1489&context=newdirections). Cobb compared x-rays of 1936 Olympic champion Jesse Owens' heel with those of a randomly selected White male of the same age and reported that Owens' heel bone was shorter and did not support the supposed racial characteristic. Cobb then compared Owens' legs to the White world record co-holder in the 100-yd dash; he discovered the White runner had "Black" calve characteristics and vice versa. Cobb concluded:

The physiques of champion Negro and white sprinters in general and Jesse Owens in particular reveal nothing to indicate Negroid physical character or anatomy concerned with the present dominance of Negro athletes in national competition in the short dashes and the broad jump. There is not a single physical characteristic which all the Negro stars in question have in common, which would definitely identify them as Negroes.[289]

In 1990, William Cobb received the American Medical Association's prestigious Distinguished Service Award (among over 100 other prestigious honors) for helping to transform modern medicine into a new era.

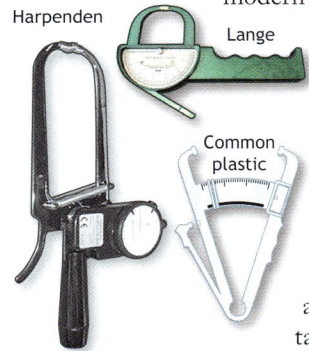

From F. Katch

The Harpenden pincer-type **skinfold caliper** accurately measured subcutaneous fat at selected anatomic sites. The three calipers shown in the insert image (more modern Lange, Harpenden, and inexpensive plastic versions) operate on a principle similar to a micrometer that measures distance between two points. Measuring **skinfold** thickness requires firmly grasping a fold of skin and its underlying subcutaneous fat with the thumb and forefingers and pulling it away from the muscle tissue while following the skinfold's natural contour. When calibrated with a precision force-measuring instrument, the pincer jaws exert a relatively constant 10 g · mm^{-2} tension at the point of contact with a double skin plus subcutaneous adipose tissue layer as shown in the inset image. The caliper dial records skinfold thickness in millimeters within 2 s after applying the caliper's full force and remains essentially constant for up to 60 s thereafter. Thus, to achieve a "true" thickness, apply the caliper for no longer than 2 s. Keeping the caliper on the skin for longer periods displaces fluid under the skin layer and produces a lower score. This time limitation avoids skinfold compression when taking measurements at different sites. Achieving measurement consistency requires duplicate or triplicate practice measurements on approximately 50 individuals who vary in body fat from relatively thin to clearly overfat. This minimum practice strategy conquers the "learning curve" for taking skinfold measurements and ensures high measurement score reproducibility.[253]

Measurement Sites. Common anatomic sites for skinfold measurement include triceps, subscapular, suprailiac, abdominal, and upper thigh. The investigator should take a minimum of two or three measurements in rotational order at each site on the right side of the body with the subject standing. The average value represents the skinfold score. **FIGURE 28.7** shows the anatomic location for five frequently measured sites:

1. *Triceps*: Vertical fold at the right upper arm's posterior midline, halfway between the shoulder tip and the elbow in an extended, relaxed position
2. *Subscapular*: Oblique fold, just below the bottom tip of the right scapula
3. *Iliac* (iliac crest): Slightly oblique fold, just above the right hipbone (crest of ileum); the fold follows the natural diagonal line
4. *Abdominal*: Vertical fold 1 in. left of the umbilicus facing the person
5. *Thigh*: Vertical fold at the right thigh's midline, two thirds the distance from the middle of the patella (kneecap) to the iliac crest

Other measurement sites include the *chest* (diagonal fold with long axis directed toward the right nipple; on the anterior axillary fold as high as possible) and *biceps* (vertical fold along the right upper arm's posterior midline).

Usefulness of Skinfold Scores

Skinfold measurements provide meaningful information about body fat and its distribution. We recommend two ways to use skinfolds. The first sums the skinfold scores to indicate relative fatness among individuals. For example, if the sum of five skinfolds equals 82 mm for a young male athlete and 135 mm for the same age nonathlete, then the young athlete clearly has less subcutaneous fat assessed at five sites and would have less total body fat assessed by densitometry than the nonathlete. The sum of skinfolds and/or individual values also can therefore reflect either absolute or percentage skinfold changes before and after an activity and/or dietary intervention program.

One can draw the following three conclusions from the skinfold data in **TABLE 28.3** for a female college student before and following a 16-wk aerobic conditioning program:

1. The largest changes in skinfold thickness occurred at the iliac and abdomen sites.
2. Triceps showed the largest percentage decrease and the subscapular the smallest percentage decrease.
3. Total reduction in subcutaneous skinfolds at the five sites was 16.6 mm, or 12.6% lower than the "before" condition.

TABLE 28.3 Changes in selected skinfolds of a young female during a 16-week exercise program

A second way to use skinfolds incorporates population-specific mathematical equations to predict body density or percentage body fat from different skinfold sites either alone

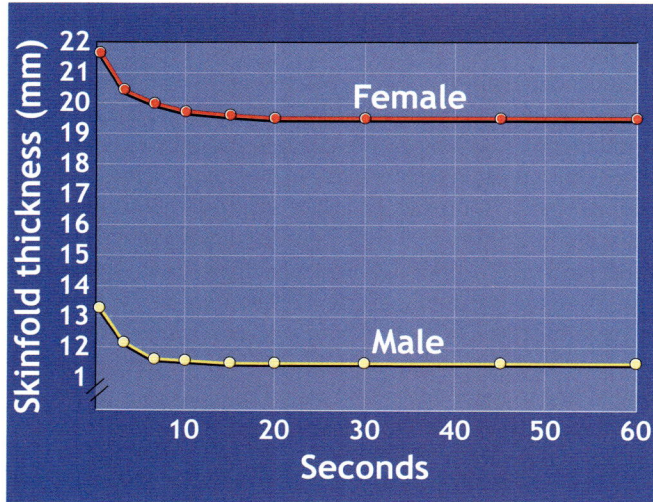

Adapted from Becque DM, et al. Time course of skin-plus-fat compression in males and females. Hum Biol. 1986;58(1):33. Copyright © 1986 Wayne State University Press, with the permission of Wayne State University Press.

Our laboratories have developed validated equations to predict percentage body fat from triceps and subscapular skinfolds in young females and males[84–86]:

Young females ages 17 to 26

$$\% \text{Body fat} = 0.55A + 0.31B + 6.13$$

Young males ages 17 to 26

$$\% \text{Body fat} = 0.43A + 0.58B + 1.47$$

In both equations, A is triceps skinfold (mm) and B is subscapular skinfold (mm). We computed the "before" and "after" body fat percentage for the female who participated in the 16-wk physical conditioning program (Table 28.3). Percentage body fat equaled 24.4% by substituting the pretraining values for triceps (22.5 mm) and subscapular (19.0 mm) into the equation.

$$\begin{aligned}\% \text{Body fat} &= 0.55A + 0.31B + 6.13 \\ &= 0.55(22.5) + 0.31(19.0) \\ &\quad + 6.13 \\ &= 12.38 + 5.89 + 6.13 \\ &= 24.4\%\end{aligned}$$

Substituting the posttraining values for triceps (19.4 mm) and for subscapular (17.0 mm) skinfolds produced a 22.1% body fat value.

$$\begin{aligned}\% \text{Body fat} &= 0.55(19.4) + 0.31(17.0) \\ &\quad + 6.13 \\ &= 10.67 + 5.27 + 6.13 \\ &= 22.1\%\end{aligned}$$

Body fat percentage determined before and after a physical conditioning or weight-loss program can assess body composition adaptations independently from body weight changes.

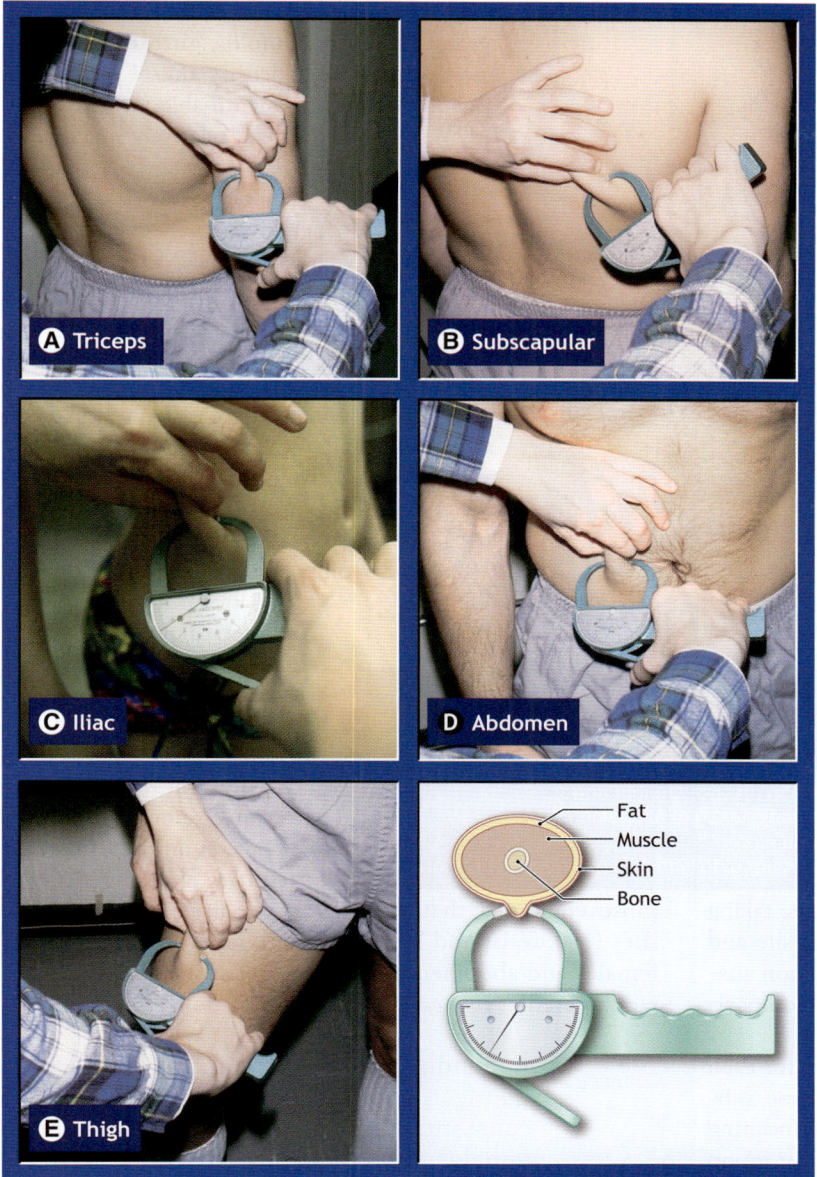

FIGURE 28.7. Five common skinfold anatomic sites: **(A)** Triceps. **(B)** Subscapular. **(C)** Iliac. **(D)** Abdomen. **(E)** Thigh. Measurements taken with a Lange caliper on the body's right side in the vertical plane except diagonally at subscapular and iliac sites.
(Images A through E from F. Katch.)

or in combination with other variables, such as body weight and stature. The equations prove accurate for subjects similar in age, gender, training status, fatness, and race to the group from which they were derived.[22,44,67,136,139,147] *When meeting these criteria, predicted body fat for an individual usually ranges between ±3 and ±5% body fat units computed from body density measured hydrostatically.* The ±3 to ±5% range in body fat units represents an average "error" from a theoretical average body fat percentage value. If the predicted body fat is 12%, then the "true" body fat, assuming it could accurately be determined, would fall between 9 and 15% from the predicted 12% value in 67 of 100 determinations (equivalent to ±1 standard deviation) among different individuals from the same population cohort.[263]

Skinfolds and Age

In young adults, approximately half the total fat contains subcutaneous fat with the remainder visceral and organ fat. With advancing age, proportionately more fat accumulates internally than subcutaneously. *For this reason, use age-adjusted generalized equations to predict body fat from skinfolds or girths in older males and females.*[76,77,151,175] The unfortunate acceleration of the "obesity epidemic" may require new generalized equations to predict body fat in subjects whose skinfold sum exceeds 120 mm, typically measured at seven sites—chest, axilla, triceps, subscapular, abdominal, iliac, and thigh.[138]

User Beware. Skinfold assessment requires expertise with proper measurement techniques. The particular caliper, whether metal, spring-loaded, plastic, electronic, or with wide and thin pincer pads, contributes to measurement errors.[58,218]

Another error source occurs when trying to measure skinfolds in obese individuals because skinfold thickness often exceeds the width of the caliper's jaws! For these reasons, we advocate taking girth rather than skinfolds as the preferred assessment technique in obese persons (see next section).

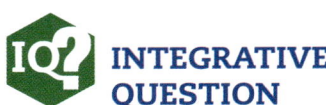

INTEGRATIVE QUESTION

A friend complains that three different fitness centers determined her percentage body fat from skinfolds as follows: 21, 25, and 29%. How would you explain these differences?

Girth Measurements

Lightly applying a linen or plastic (but not metal) measuring tape to the skin surface allows the tape to remain taut but not tight. This avoids skin compression, which produces below-normal scores. We advocate taking a minimum of two duplicate measurements at each site and averaging the scores. The inset image shows six common anatomic landmarks by anthropometry to assess body composition.

Equations to predict body fat from girths exist for each gender and age group.[84,128,181] The equations for these subgroups show considerable population specificity—meaning that a particular equation only applies to the particular group upon which the equations were developed.

For example, equations developed on younger subjects should not be applied to predict percentage body fat in older age groups, but unanimity is not universal on this point.[102] We believe that this same specificity approach should apply to males and females and particular athletic groups. The equations should not be used with individuals who:

1. Are overly thin or excessively fat
2. Regularly train in strenuous endurance sports or activities with substantial resistance training designed to enhance muscular enlargement
3. Or belong to a racial group different from the specific group used to derive the original equations (i.e., do not use equations derived from Caucasian groups to predict body fat in African Americans or Asians, and vice versa)

Usefulness of Girth Scores

Girths prove most useful in ranking individuals within a group according to relative fatness, as for example, the lowest measured body fat to the greatest body fat within the group. As with skinfolds, girth-based equations predict body density and/or percentage body fat with a quantifiable error component, albeit relatively small.

On average for about 70 of every 100 people measured, the equations will predict body fat within the 2.5 to 4.0% body fat units compared with the person's body fat had it been assessed by a more valid criterion such as hydrostatic weighing, DXA, or BOD POD. The prediction error depends on whether the individual portrays physical characteristics similar to the original validation group. Such relatively small errors make girth predictions particularly useful in nonlaboratory settings. Specific equations based on girths also estimate body composition in obese adult males and females.[21,180,196,219,220]

Along with predicting percentage body fat, girth scores can analyze body fat distribution patterns to uncover changes in fat patterning during weight loss.[63,192] Fat patterning refers to body fat distribution on the trunk and extremities. Not surprisingly, those equations that use the more labile fat deposition sites (e.g., waist and hips instead of upper arm or thigh in females and abdomen in males) provide the greatest accuracy to predict *changes* in body composition.[51]

1. **Abdomen:** 1 in. above umbilicus
2. **Buttocks:** Maximum protrusion with heels together
3. **Right thigh:** Upper thigh, just below buttocks
4. **Right calf:** Widest girth midway between ankle and knee
5. **Right upper arm:** Palm up, arm straight and extended in front of body; taken at midpoint between shoulder and elbow
6. **Right forearm:** Maximum girth with arm extended in front of body

Lippincott® Connect — Appendix L, available online at Lippincott Connect, presents equations and constants for young and older males and females to predict body fat within ±2.5 to 4.0% body fat units from an actual or "true" value.

Body Fat Predictions from Girths

From the appropriate tables in Appendix L (Lippincott Connect), substitute the corresponding constants A, B, and C in the formula shown at the bottom of each table. This requires one addition and two subtraction steps. The following five-step example shows how to compute percentage fat, fat mass, and FFM for a 2-year-old male who weighs 79.1 kg/174 lb:

Step 1. Measure upper arm, abdomen, and right forearm girths with a cloth tape to the nearest 0.25 in./0.6 cm: upper arm = 11.5 in./29.21 cm; abdomen = 31.0 in./74 cm; right forearm = 10.75 in./27.30 cm

Step 2. Determine the three constants A, B, and C corresponding to the three girths from the table: A, corresponding to 11.5 in. = 42.56; B, corresponding to 31.0 in. = 40.68; and C, corresponding to 10.75 in. = 58.37.

Increased Body Mass Index and Obesity Associate with Poor Sleep

Lack of nightly sleep may associate with an increased body mass index (BMI) and obesity.[100] This seems paradoxical because sleep remains the quintessential sedentary behavior, and people with minimal physical activity patterns do indeed have higher BMIs than more active counterparts. The National Sleep Foundation (www.sleepfoundation.org) points out that sleep duration has steadily decreased over the past century. Individuals who slept 5 to 6 hr nightly gained an average 2 kg/4.4 lb more over 6 years than those who slept 7 to 8 hr nightly. In one study, an inverse relationship occurred between sleep duration and BMI in 1024 participants who slept less than 8 hr nightly. In a large study involving 22,281 adults, those who slept more (with significantly lower BMIs) reported fewer cardiovascular problems. In young obese females, sleep disorders were linked to a specific central-abdominal phenotype rather than a typical body profile pattern. It seems safe to conclude that longer sleep duration associates with better health in children and adults, which in turn associates with desirable body composition and anthropometric characteristics, particularly neck girth.

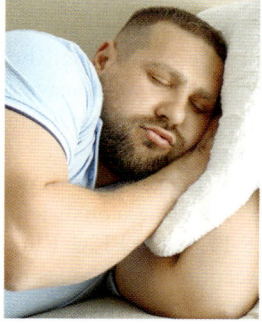
New Africa/Shutterstock

Sources:
Gasa M, et al. Anthropometrical phenotypes are important when explaining obstructive sleep apnea in female bariatric cohorts. *J Sleep Res*. 2019;28: e12830.
Katz SL, et al.; Canadian Sleep and Circadian Network. Does neck circumference predict obstructive sleep apnea in children with obesity? *Sleep Med*. 2021;78:88.
Santos RB, et al. Accuracy of global and/or regional anthropometric measurements of adiposity in screening sleep apnea: the ELSA-Brasil cohort. *Sleep Med*. 2019;63:115.

Step 3. Compute percentage body fat by substituting the constants from step 2 in the formula for young men as follows:

$$\begin{aligned}\text{Percentage fat} &= A + B - C - 10.2\\ &= 42.56 + 40.68 - 58.37 - 10.2\\ &= 83.24 - 58.37 - 10.2\\ &= 24.87 - 10.2\\ &= 14.7\%\end{aligned}$$

Step 4. Determine fat mass

$$\begin{aligned}\text{Fat mass} &= \text{body mass} \times (\%\text{ fat} \div 100)\\ &= 79.1\text{ kg} \times (14.7 \div 100)\\ &= 79.1\text{ kg} \times 0.147\\ &= 11.6\text{ kg}\end{aligned}$$

Step 5. Determine FFM

$$\begin{aligned}\text{FFM} &= \text{body mass} - \text{fat mass}\\ &= 79.1\text{ kg} - 11.6\text{ kg}\\ &= 67.5\text{ kg}\end{aligned}$$

Application of Surface Anthropometry: The Body Profile from Girths

In the early 1960s, Dr. Albert Behnke created a method to visually represent body shape based on a grid system using deviations in body dimensions from normative reference male and female data. The black vertical line shown in the inset figure for females applies for ages 4 to 64 plotted in 5-year intervals. Behnke originally named the method "Somatogram,"[245] but in later publications, it took the name Ponderal Somatogram[243,258] and subsequently Body Profile.[232,244,252] The six girths for the reference female at age 20 to 24 plot directly on the vertical line to represent ideal proportionality for the different body girths, hence these plots are in fact the standard by which to compare girth proportionality among different females. Unfortunately, there are no comparable age-related longitudinal or cross-sectional changes in males for these same girth measurements.

If a female's girths plotted within ±2 deviation units on either side of the black line to account for individual variation, that individual would indeed reflect body dimensions that mimics reference standard proportionality. In essence, this is exactly what physique competitions try to assess—the most perfectly proportioned male or female contestant. The chest girth would be in proportion to the waist girth, the waist girth would be in proportion to the hip girth, and so on. If for example, the calf girth plots to the left of the line, this would mean that anatomic region would reflect "underdevelopment" relative to the other body areas. *And that is exactly what happens in females from ages 30 to 34 and 60 to 63—the waist girth in the mid-trunk region indicated by the red dot continues to increase in size compared with the other body areas.* This region is the one body area where fat continues to accumulate despite efforts through dietary restraint and seriously increased physical activity duration and intensity. This "fact of life" for the abdominal region causes the other areas to plot relatively smaller because the waist region continues to increase disproportionately to the other body regions.

The plots from age 20 to 24 onward reveal what most adults in Western societies experience—waist girth continues to plot to the right of the vertical line, indicating this single measurement reflects increased fat accretion in that body sector. Stated another way, the waist girth continues to increase out of proportion *relative* to the other girth sites. Note that none of the other girths plots to the right or positive side of the vertical, not even the hip girth, which many believe also increases with waist enlargement. Hip girth most likely increases, but not proportionally to waist enlargement. A desired body fat level also can be estimated from changes in abdominal girth, where body weight loss remains proportional to percentage changes in total fat loss.[247] In essence, these relationships permit extrapolation to

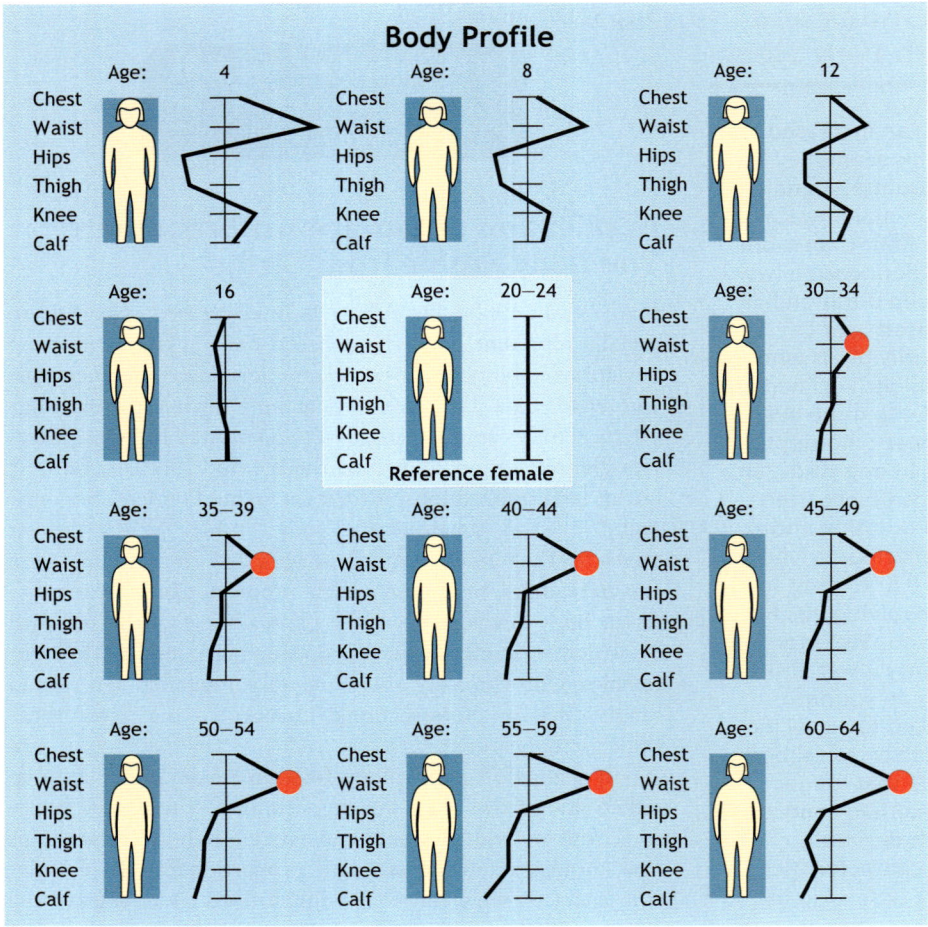

From F. Katch and V. Katch

a projected target abdominal girth that corresponds to a desired body fat percentage.[246,279]

Body Profile Analysis in Athletes

Behnke's Body Profile has been applied to athletes to indicate how body proportionality changes when individuals reduce body mass with dieting or increase body size with serious (and prolonged) resistance training. Of all body areas, the biceps in our experience produces the most significant muscle hypertrophy with overload weight training. In contrast, some body regions are designated as nonmuscular areas (abdomen, hips, knees, wrist, and ankles). These areas do not hypertrophy compared with the more muscular sites (shoulders and quadriceps). In a comparison between Division 1 university baseball pitchers (UMass, Amherst) and baseball roster Boston Red Sox pitchers assessed for body composition during early spring training, the patterns in body proportionality were fairly similar when 11 girths were placed into muscular and nonmuscular categories.

The contracted biceps girth in the college players plotted more than −5 deviation units to the left of the vertical line compared with the expected greater developed +2 deviation for the biceps in the professionals. Note that the abdominal girth in both groups had already plotted to the right, more so for the professionals as they are for the elderly as an expected finding. The major league players also were heavier and taller, yet their absolute and relative body fat values determined by densitometry were the same as those of the amateurs; the professionals had about a 4-kg/8.8-lb greater FFM. Elite athletes have exceptional physiques to match their sport requirements.

One would not expect a professional baseball pitcher to achieve success with "underdeveloped" biceps in their pitching arm, nor an Olympic discus or shot put athlete to have underdeveloped upper body characteristics or poorly developed calves and thighs required for maximum power output for success in their event.[243] At the opposite body size extreme, elite female dancers are diminutive for body mass and stature, an entirely different body profile described in the next section.

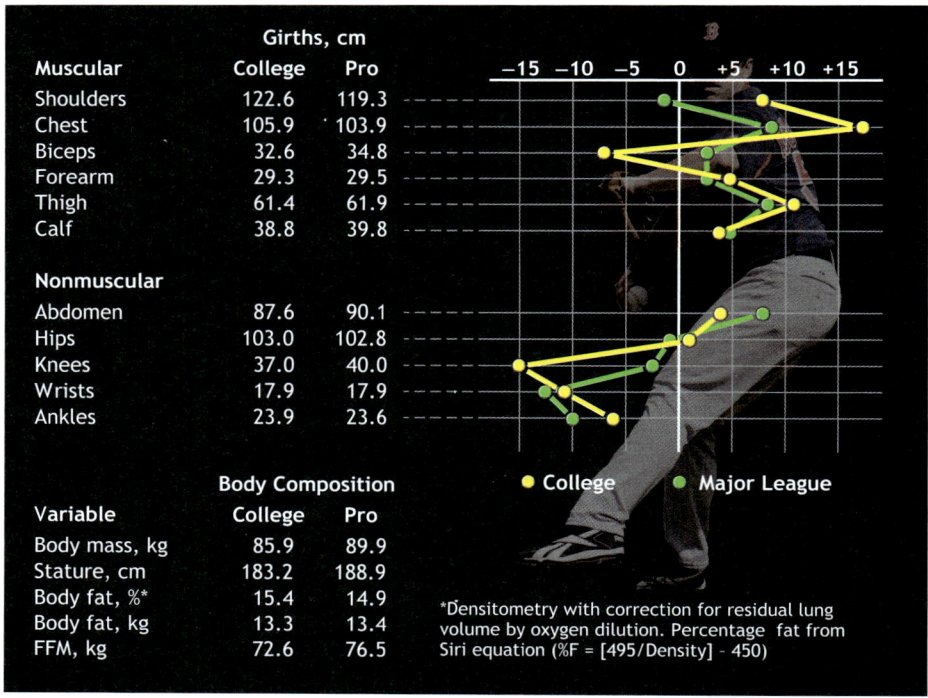

Girths, cm		
Muscular	College	Pro
Shoulders	122.6	119.3
Chest	105.9	103.9
Biceps	32.6	34.8
Forearm	29.3	29.5
Thigh	61.4	61.9
Calf	38.8	39.8
Nonmuscular		
Abdomen	87.6	90.1
Hips	103.0	102.8
Knees	37.0	40.0
Wrists	17.9	17.9
Ankles	23.9	23.6

Body Composition		
Variable	College	Pro
Body mass, kg	85.9	89.9
Stature, cm	183.2	188.9
Body fat, %*	15.4	14.9
Body fat, kg	13.3	13.4
FFM, kg	72.6	76.5

*Densitometry with correction for residual lung volume by oxygen dilution. Percentage fat from Siri equation (%F = [495/Density] − 450)

Background photo: Matt Trommer/Shutterstock. Data from V. Katch and F. Katch

Body Profile for Ballet Dancers. A unique data set representing 10 elite professional ballet dancers illustrates how their body profile resembles the reference female profile but unfortunately not for relative health status established by WHO standards.[252] At a 51-kg/112-lb body mass and 166.4-cm/65.2-in. stature, their low 18.4 BMI clearly categorizes these elite female athletes not only underweight but also in a wasting, undernourished, and precarious health state. As pointed out in a prior section, participants in the "low weight" or "appearance" sports (e.g., bodybuilding, figure skating, diving, ballet, and gymnastics) physically increase their likelihood for many health-related maladies such as delayed menstruation onset, oligomenorrhea, amenorrhea, and other endocrine-related dysfunction.

Bioelectrical Impedance Analysis

In single low-frequency mode **bioelectrical impedance analysis (BIA)**, a small alternating current flowing between two electrodes passes more rapidly through hydrated fat-free body tissues and extracellular water than through fat or bone tissues because the fat-free component exhibits greater electrolyte content and consequently lower electrical resistance. In essence, the body's water content helps to conduct electrical charge flow through the fluid medium, and sensitive instrumentation detects the water's impedance or resistance to the current flow. Impedance to electric current flow, calculated by measuring current and voltage, is based on Ohm law ($R = V/I$, where R = resistance, V = voltage, and I = current; https://ohmslawcalculator.com/ohms-law-calculator). These relationships quantify the water volume within the body and subsequent estimate for percentage body fat and FFM.

FIGURE 28.8A AND B shows an example for single-frequency BIA. A person lies on a flat, nonconducting surface with injector (source) electrodes attached on the foot and wrist dorsal surfaces, and detector electrodes attached between the radius and ulna (styloid process) and ankle between medial and lateral malleoli. A painless, localized electrical current (800 μA at 50 kHz) is introduced, and the impedance to current flow is determined between the source and detector electrodes. Converting the impedance value to body density and including additional input variables to the equation—body mass and stature gender, age, sometimes race, fatness level, and several girths—computes percentage body fat with proprietary BIA equations. Any data input unreliability produces different prediction results, becoming more pronounced for individuals at the body composition extremes.[281] For example, only a 5-mm difference in a girth measurement from different measurement times can produce up to ≥2% change in an output variable—unrelated to any "true" change in a computed fat mass or FFM body composition variable.

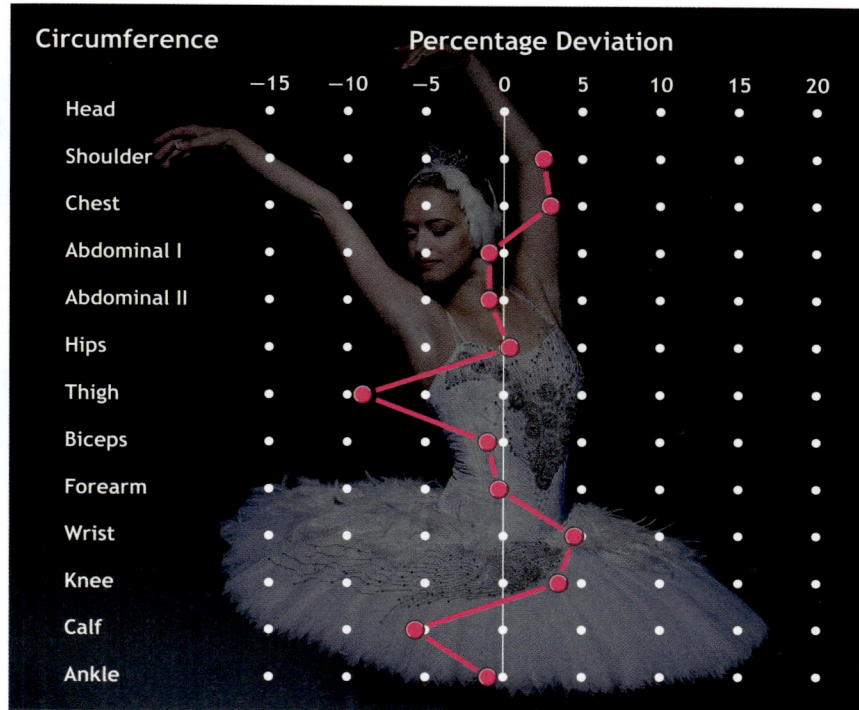

Background photo: True Touch Lifestyle/Shutterstock

FIGURE 28.8C illustrates the segmental measurement approach including electrode configuration and how electric current (I) and voltage (V) are assessed for the right arm, trunk, and right leg.

Spurious Correlations with BIA Can Be Misleading

Adding multiple inputs that themselves co-relate (e.g., body mass co-relates highly with height, body mass can co-relate highly with non–weight-supported fitness tests) will "generate" a specious or "bogus" density value and thus becomes a **spurious correlation**. Including fewer input variables into the final body fat output value considerably reduces contaminating the true relation among the BIA input variables and thus the percentage body fat from the BIA computed output value. A well-known example in the fitness domain involved a spurious correlation between distance run during a 12-min track run and maximum oxygen uptake ($\dot{V}O_{2max}$; greater distance covered was reported as correlating highly [$r = 0.90$] with treadmill-determined $\dot{V}O_{2max}$). Upon closer inspection, it turned out that distance covered and body weight *both* correlated substantially with $\dot{V}O_{2max}$, introducing an essentially severely diminished co-relation between the intended variables (originally $r = 0.90$ to $r = 0.20$)![273] This example shows clearly that relying on relationships that violate statistically proper analysis can lead to erroneous conclusions. A correlation $r = 0.90$ would warrant a meaningful interpretation, a correlation $r = 0.20$ would not. *BIA prediction equations that add multiple co-founding variables into the prediction will reduce their validity to predict FFM and percentage body fat accurately and thus will confer an inauthentic interpretation about the true relationship.*

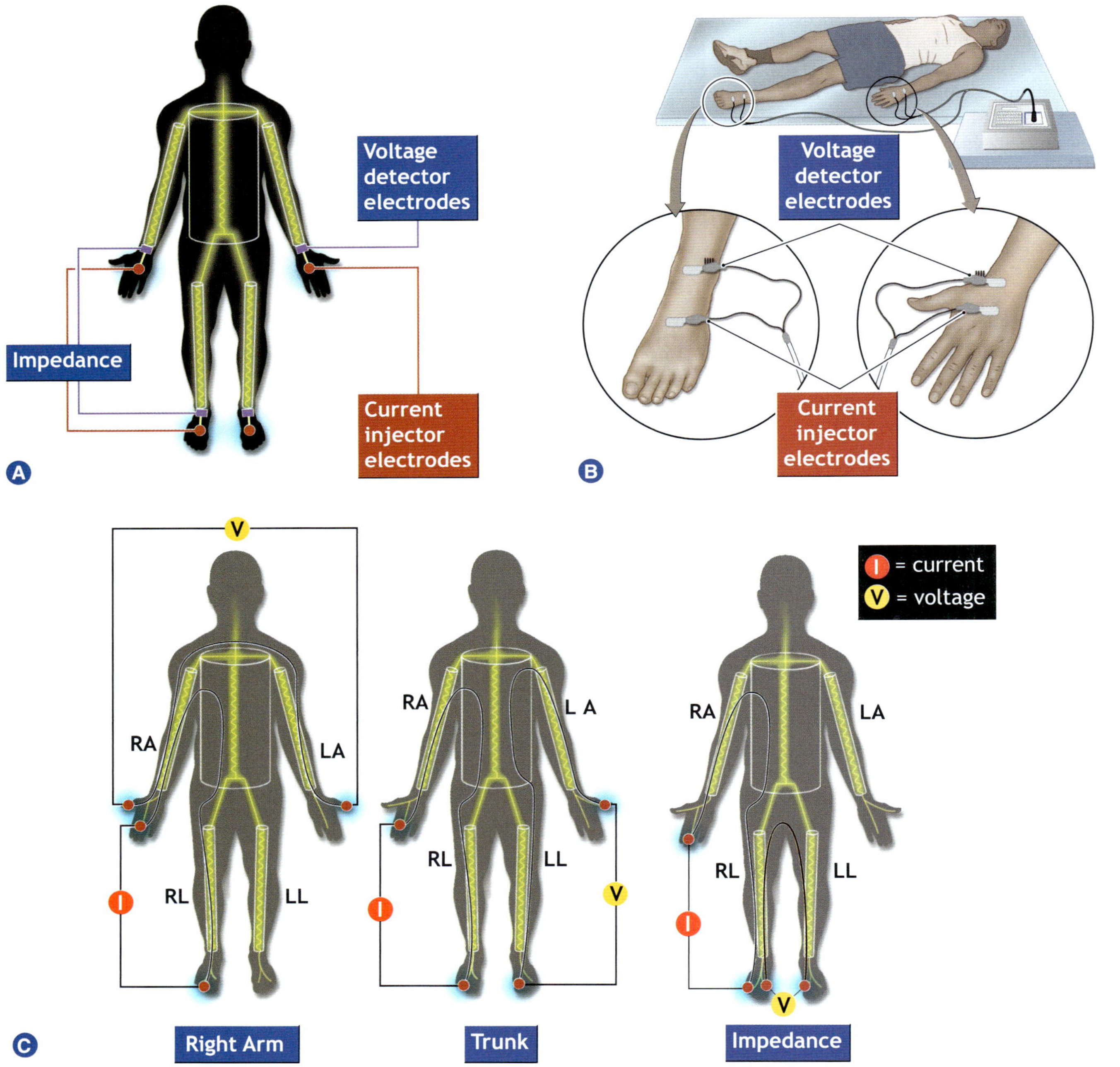

FIGURE 28.8. Method to assess body composition by bioelectrical impedance analysis. **(A)** Four-surface electrode technique (whole-body impedance) applies current via one pair of distal injector electrodes, while the proximal detector electrode pair measures electrical potential across the conducting segment. **(B)** Standard electrode and body position placement during whole-body assessment. **(C)** Segmental measurement illustrates current (*I*) path and voltage (*V*) for the right arm, trunk, and right leg.

Hydration Level Impacts BIA Accuracy

Hydration level affects BIA accuracy by incorrectly estimating body fat content.[97,141] Hypohydration and hyperhydration alter the body's normal electrolyte concentrations; this in turn affects current flow independently from real body composition changes. Skin temperature, influenced by ambient conditions, also lowers whole-body resistance and BIA predicted body fat because moist skin from any reason produces less impedance to electrical flow than normal temperature skin. Body fat predictions with BIA prove less valid than with hydrostatic weighing as the established criterion. BIA tends to overpredict body fat in lean and athletic subjects and underpredict body fat in obese subjects.[117,160] BIA often predicts body fat less accurately than do girths and

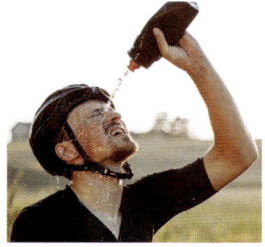

LovetheLifeyouLive/Shutterstock

skinfolds.[23,42,88,171] Whether BIA detects small changes in body composition during weight loss remains unclear.[99,149]

At best, BIA represents a noninvasive, safe, relatively easy, and generally consistent means to assess total body water. The technique requires that experienced personnel make measurements under standardized conditions. Particularly important factors include electrode placement and the subject's body position, hydration status, plasma osmolality and sodium concentration, skin temperature, recent physical activity, and previous food and beverage intake.[19,98,99,194] For example, eating several successive meals within a short time interval progressively decreases electrical impedance, possibly from the combined effects from increased electrolytes and extracellular fluid redistribution to decrease computed percentage body fat.[166] Body fatness and racial characteristics also influence BIA's predictive accuracy.[4,144,172] The tendency to overestimate percentage body fat increases among Black athletes[68,160] and lean subjects.[173] Fatness-specific BIA equations exist to predict body fat in obese and nonobese American Indian, Hispanic, White males and females,[192] and diverse population groups.[43,158,162,207] With proper measurement standardization, the menstrual cycle does not affect BIA-assessed body composition.[122]

Use Caution When Using BIA with Athletes

Coaches and athletes require a safe, easily administered, and valid tool to assess body composition and detect changes with caloric restriction and physical conditioning. A major limitation in achieving these goals concerns BIA's poor sensitivity to detect small body composition changes, particularly without appropriate control over factors affecting measurement accuracy and reliability. These factors include sweat loss dehydration from prior physical activity or reduced glycogen reserves (and associated glycogen-bound water loss) from an intense training session that reduces body resistance to electrical current flow.

This chapter's "In a Practical Sense" includes waist-to-hip girth ratio equations to estimate body fat distribution and associated disease risk. Without sport-specific equations, population-based generalized equations that account for age and gender usually provide an acceptable alternative to estimate percentage body fat.[77,163,176]

Near-Infrared Interactance Spectroscopy

Near-infrared interactance (NIR) spectroscopy applies technologies developed by the U.S. Department of Agriculture to assess body composition and lipid content in oil-bearing grains and animal tissues (https://naldc.nal.usda.gov/download/CAT89919964/PDF), and organic materials in the chemical and pharmaceutical industry (https://pubmed.ncbi.nlm.nih.gov/22469433/). This technology uses the NIR light region in the electromagnetic spectrum (800–2500 nm; wavelength 10^{-4} m), which ranges from radiation and x-ray wavelength (10^{-10} to 10^{-9} m) to radio wavelength (10^{-2} to 10^{-3} m). The commercial versions designed to assess human body composition rely on established principles relating to light absorption and reflection (www.futrex.com). The insert image shows a fiber optic probe emits a low-energy infrared light beam into a single measuring site on an arm or leg limb extremity along the anterior midline skin surface. A detector within the same probe measures the reemitted light's intensity expressed as optical density. Shifts in the reflected beam's wavelength as it interacts with organic material in an arm (or leg) muscle interfaces with a manufacturer's prediction equation to compute percentage body fat and FFM by including adjustments for body mass and stature, estimated frame size, gender, and physical activity level. The safe, portable, lightweight equipment requires minimal training to use and necessitates little physical contact with the person during measurement. These test administration aspects make NIR popular for body composition assessment in health clubs, hospitals, and weight loss centers. The important question about NIR concerns its validity in body composition assessment among different age and sex groups including athletes.

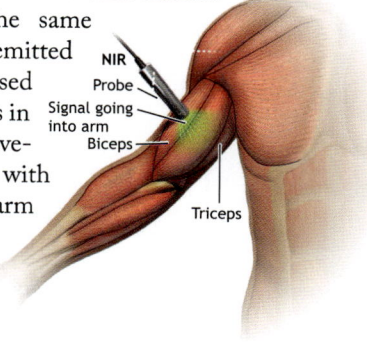

Questionable NIR Validity

Early research indicated a positive relationship among spectrophotometric measures with light interactance at various body sites and total body water to evaluate body composition.[37] Subsequent studies with humans have not supported NIR's validity versus hydrostatic weighing or skinfold measurements. NIR does not accurately predict body fat across a broad range or in body fat levels in nonathletes and athletes, and only fair accuracy compared with skinfolds.[23,66,80,186,274] In general, NIR overestimates body fat in lean males and females and underestimates it in fatter subjects.[123]

The data in **FIGURE 28.9** show the inadequacy when using NIR measurements compared to skinfold measurements versus hydrodensitometry to predict body fat percentage. In more than 47% of subjects, an error greater than 4% body fat units occurred with NIR, with the largest errors at the body fatness extremes. NIR produced relatively large errors when estimating body fat in children[28] and youth wrestlers[70] and underestimated body fat in collegiate football players[69] and elite rowers.[274] NIR also did not accurately assess body composition changes from resistance training.[23] In general, research does not support NIR as a robust, valid criterion method to assess human body composition across a broad range of ages, sexes, and racial and athletic categories.[235]

Ultrasonography, Computed Tomography, Magnetic Resonance Imaging, and DXA

Ultrasonography with A-Mode and B-Mode Imaging

Ultrasound technology can image fat and muscle thickness in deeper muscle tissues, including the abdominal region for fetal

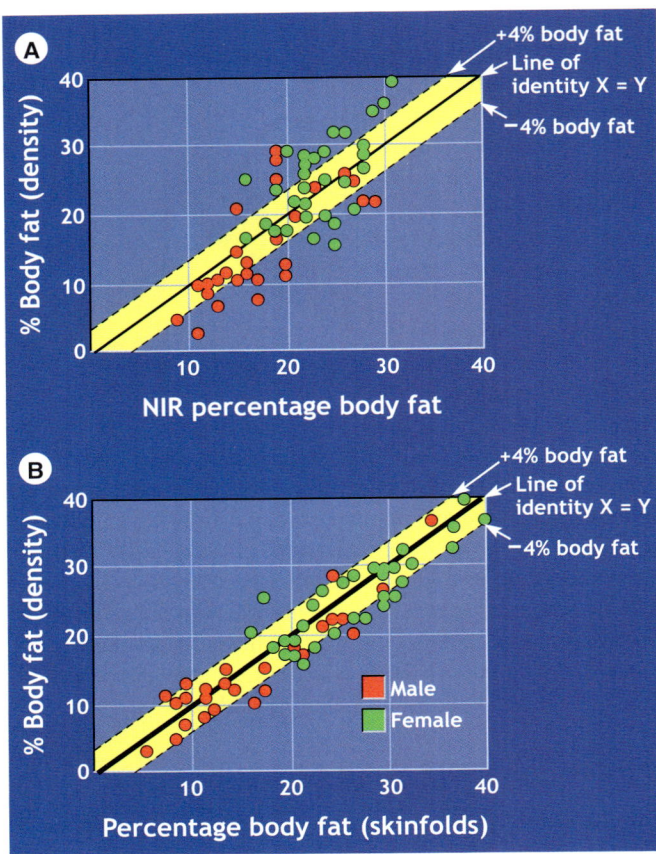

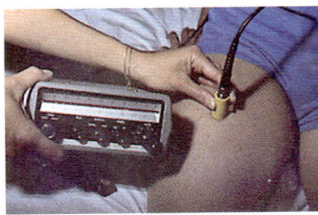

Photo: F. Katch

FIGURE 28.9 Comparison of near-infrared interactance **(A)** and skinfolds **(B)** for assessing percentage body fat. *Yellow shaded area* around black "best-fit" line incorporates 64% body fat units.
(Adapted with permission from McLean K, Skinner JS. Validity of Futrex-5000 for body composition determination. *Med Sci Sports Exerc.* 1992;24:253.)

monitoring during pregnancy (www.criticalecho.com/content/tutorial-2-modes-ultrasound). This method converts electrical energy through a probe into high-frequency pulsed sound waves that penetrate skin's surface into underlying tissues. The sound waves pass through adipose tissue and penetrate the muscle layer. The waves then reflect against the bone to the fat-muscle interface to produce an echo, which returns to a receiver within the probe. The simplest *A-mode* ultrasound does not produce an image in the underlying tissues. Rather, the time required for sound wave transmission through the tissues and back to the transducer converts to a distance score that indicates fat or muscle thickness. Color and multiple-frequency imaging allow clinicians to trace blood flow through organs and tissues, and with miniaturized probes, identify internal tissues, vessels, and organs. In consumer-oriented research, ultrasonically imaging thigh fat depth provided evidence that treatments using two topical cream applications to the thighs and buttocks to reduce "cellulite" (so-called dimpled fat) failed to reduce local fat thickness compared with control conditions.[35] With the more expensive and technically demanding *B-mode* ultrasound, a two-dimensional image shows considerable detail and tissue differentiation.

Ultrasonography exhibits high reliability for repeated measurements at multiple sites in the lying and standing positions on the same day and different days.[75,83] The technique can determine total and segmental subcutaneous adipose tissue volume.[2] It has also shown high validity to assess FFM in high school wrestlers, which may prove useful as a field-based body composition assessment method,[183] and other athletic groups employing a multicomponent model that considers variability in the density of the body's fat mass.[3] Ultrasound proves particularly useful with obese persons who show considerable variation when compressing subcutaneous body fat using skinfold methods.

Ultrasonography to map muscle and fat thickness at different body regions can quantify changes in the topographic fat pattern as a valuable adjunct to whole-body composition assessment. In hospitalized patients, ultrasound fat and muscle thickness determinations assist in nutritional evaluation during weight loss and weight gain. Other noninvasive technologies are evaluating treatment strategies to reduce excess fat deposition (cellulite), with several studies providing encouraging results but further confirmation studies are needed.[221–223]

Computed Tomography

Computed tomography (CT) scanning revolutionized medicine when first introduced in the mid-1970s as organs and bones became visible with clarity in anatomy textbooks. With built-in x-ray emitters and detectors, the CT scan generates detailed cross-sectional, two-dimensional radiographic body segment images when an x-ray ionizing radiation beam passes through different density tissues. The CT scan produces pictorial and quantitative information about total tissue area, total fat and muscle area, and tissue thickness and volume within an organ.[57,130,191]

The inset image in **(A)** plots pixel element frequency from a CT scan, illustrating bilateral adipose and muscle tissue in cross-section views at mid-thigh level. View **(B)** shows a mid-thigh cross-section in the upper legs in a professional walker who trekked 42.2 km/26.2 mi daily (a marathon distance) for 52 consecutive wks across the United States, with planned 3-month breaks for routine cardiovascular, pulmonary, muscular strength, hematologic, and CT testing and nutritional analysis at the University of Massachusetts Medical School, Worcester, and Department of Exercise Science, Amherst. Total mid-thigh and muscle cross-section increased by 3 to 4%, and subcutaneous fat in those regions decreased by about the same amount in post-race scans (not shown). Studies have demonstrated CT scan efficacy to establish the relationship among simple skinfold and girth measures at the abdomen and total **abdominal fat** volume measured from single or multiple pictorial "slices" through this region.[161] A single cut through the L4 to L5 region minimizes radiation dose, providing the best view of visceral and subcutaneous fat.

CT Radiation Dose Risk. According to the FDA (www.fda.gov/radiation-emitting-products/medical-x-ray-imaging/what-are-radiation-risks-ct), the quantity most relevant to

In a Practical Sense

Waist-to-Hip Girth Ratio to Determine Disease Risk

The waist-to-hip girth ratio (WHR) indicates relative fat distribution in adults and disease risk. A higher ratio reflects a greater proportion of abdominal fat with greater risk for hyperinsulinemia, insulin resistance, type 2 diabetes, endometrial cancer, hypercholesterolemia, hypertension, and atherosclerosis. The girth technique is straight-forward and easily mastered. WHR computes as abdominal girth (centimeters or inches) ÷ hip girth (centimeters or inches). The figure shows the two girths' anatomical landmarks. The waist girth represents the smallest girth around the abdomen (the "natural") waist) measured with a plastic retractable anthropometric or sewing kit cloth but not metal tape. The hip girth reflects the girth measured around the widest part of the buttocks.

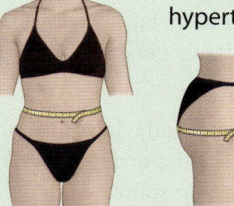

Abdomen: Minimum girth *Hips:* Maximum girth

TAKING MEASUREMENTS

Record the waist girth with the subject standing, feet placed normally apart and looking straight ahead; record the girth score following a normal exhalation. Verify the tape remains in a horizontal position and is not higher in the front or back. Keep the tape snug but not tight around the waist without compressing the skin. The subject should take 3 or 4 breaths while the tape remains around the waist so they become comfortable with the procedure. If a subject looks down to view the process, they will contract their abdominal muscles and obscure a true reading. Take duplicate measurements 30 s to 1 min apart and use an average score as the final girth. For the buttocks measurement, place the feet together, standing relaxed with legs straight, eyes focused straight ahead without looking down at the waist, and arms crossing the chest or out to the side to avoid contact with the tape. Take duplicate measurements 30 s to 1 min apart and use an average score as the final buttocks measurements; both scores should agree to within 0.5 cm/0.2 in.

CALCULATING WHR

Example 1

Man: age, 21 years; abdominal girth, 101.6 cm; hip girth, 93.5 cm

$$\text{WHR} = \text{abdominal girth (cm)} \div \text{hip girth (cm)}$$
$$= 101.6 \div 93.5$$
$$= 1.08 \text{ (very high disease risk)}$$

Example 2

Woman: age, 41 years; abdominal girth, 83.2 cm; hip girth, 101 cm

$$\text{WHR} = \text{abdomen girth (cm)} \div \text{hip girth (cm)}$$
$$= 83.2 \div 101$$
$$= 0.82 \text{ (high disease risk)}$$

Waist-to-Hip Girth Ratio and Disease Risk

	Age, y	Risk level			
		Low	Moderate	High	Very high
Males	20—29	<0.83	0.83—0.88	0.89—0.94	>0.94
	30—39	<0.84	0.84—0.91	0.92—0.96	>0.96
	40—49	<0.88	0.88—0.95	0.96—1.00	>1.00
	50—59	<0.90	0.90—0.96	0.97—1.02	>1.02
	60—69	<0.81	0.91—0.98	0.99—1.03	>1.03
Females	20—29	<0.71	0.71—0.77	0.78—0.82	>0.82
	30—39	<0.72	0.72—0.78	0.79—0.84	>0.84
	40—49	<0.73	0.73—0.79	0.80—0.87	>0.87
	50—59	<0.74	0.74—0.81	0.82—0.88	>0.88
	60—69	<0.76	0.76—0.83	0.84—0.90	>0.90

Sources:

Cameron AJ, et al. Combined influence of waist and hip circumference on risk of death in a large cohort of European and Australian adults. *J Am Heart Assoc*. 2020;9:e015189.

Duan X, et al. Association of healthy lifestyle with risk of obstructive sleep apnea: a cross-sectional study. *BMC Pulm Med*. 2022;22:33.

Hsuan CF, et al. The waist-to-body mass index ratio as an anthropometric predictor for cardiovascular outcome in subjects with established atherosclerotic cardiovascular disease. *Sci Rep*. 2022;12:804.

Ke JF, et al. Waist-to-height ratio has a stronger association with cardiovascular risks than waist circumference, waist-hip ratio and body mass index in type 2 diabetes. *Diabetes Res Clin Pract*. 2022;183:109151.

Li K, et al. Causal associations of waist circumference and waist-to-hip ratio with type II diabetes mellitus: new evidence from Mendelian randomization. *Mol Genet Genomics*. 2021;296:605.

Naudin S, et al. Healthy lifestyle and the risk of pancreatic cancer in the EPIC study. *Eur J Epidemiol*. 2020;35:975.

---

assess cancer risk from a CT procedure is the "effective dose" expressed in millisieverts (mSv), similar to that determined on short and longer space flight missions (Chapter 27). The effective dose compares the risk estimates associated with partial or whole-body radiation exposures, and incorporates different radiation sensitivities in various body organs depending on the patient, the body part examined, and particular CT equipment. In general, CT radiation dosage is relatively trivial and the CT scanning benefits far exceed the risks. For example, scans in the abdominal and pelvic regions emit mSv equal

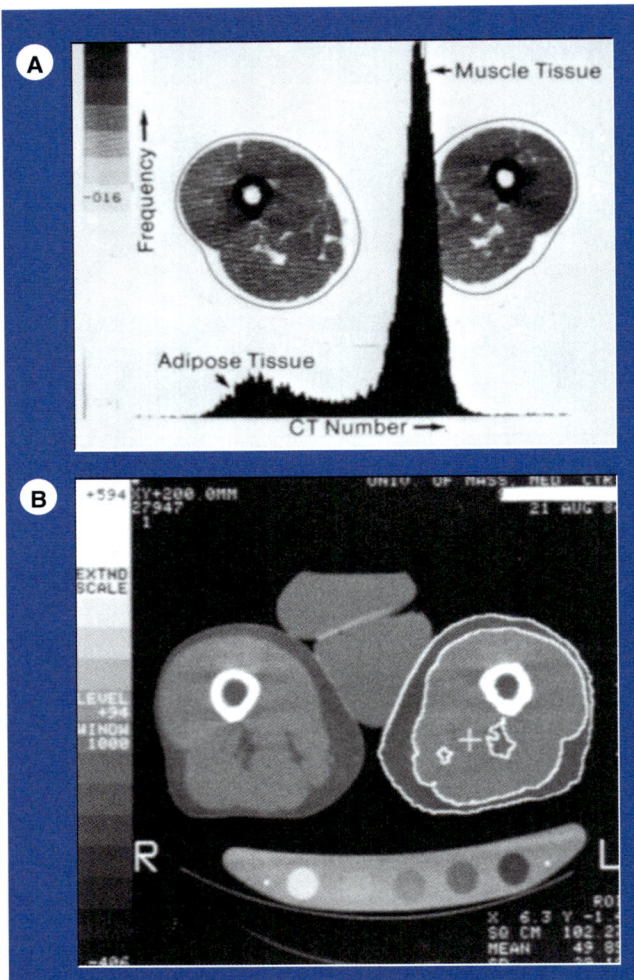

Scans courtesy Dr. Steven Heymsfeld

discusses lipodystrophy, a subtle but often underappreciated disease.

Lipodystrophy: An Underappreciated Disease. Lipodystrophies (LDs; Greek "lipo" = fat and "dystrophy" = derangement) represent metabolic disorders affecting white adipose tissue (WAT) characterized by a loss and/or functional disorder in this tissue mass in two ways[277]:

1. A restricted region under the skin related to medical injections, regional subcutaneous fat loss in the lower limbs, and generalized loss in total body fat
2. Familial or acquired from underlying genetic mutation susceptibility

The inset figure shows the general body locations for White (WAT) and brown (BAT) adipose tissue depots. WAT stores the excess fat as a potential energy source under the skin or internal organ/visceral regions (visceral WAT), or as visceral WAT around the heart (pericardial) and peritoneal organ omental cavity (stomach), mesenteric (gut), and retroperitoneal depots. BAT contains fat stored in cervical, clavicular, paravertebral, and perirenal regions exploited for thermogenesis.

LDs historically are considered rare diseases, with an estimated prevalence between 1 in 7000 in the general population for the inherited type,[275] and between 1.3 and 4.7 per 1 million people for all LDs.[276]

Most patients with LD are advised to remain moderately physical active most days in the week (approximately 200 kcal to about 3 years in naturally, yearly accumulated 1- to 3.5-mSV background radiation. The United States Environmental Protection Agency operates 140 radiation air monitors in 50 states 24 hr daily collecting near-real-time background gamma radiation measurements (www.epa.gov/radnet). For most people, radon in the environment is the single greatest environmental radiation exposure source, which significantly increases lung cancer risk from combined radon and smoking effects (www.epa.gov/radiation/calculate-your-radiation-dose).

Deep Visceral Adipose Tissue. FIGURE 28.10 illustrates the strong association ($r = 0.82$) between deep **visceral adipose tissue** (**VAT**) area and waist circumference. The strength in this robust relationship means that males with larger waist girth also possess greater VAT (but not that one variable *caused* the other). The relationship exceeded the association between subcutaneous fat thickness (skinfolds) and VAT. Chapter 30 discusses regional fat distribution (android vs. gynoid-type obesity) relating to undesirable cardiometabolic problems—type 2 diabetes risk, blood lipid profile disorders, lung disease, hypertension, and other cardiometabolic factors and cardiovascular disease factors.[29,62,74,108] The next section

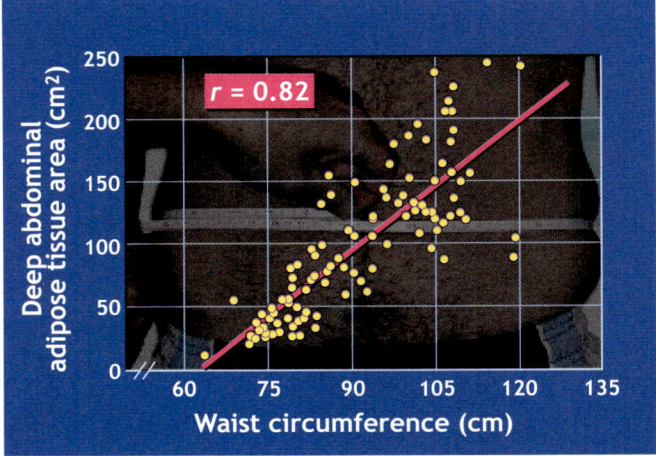

FIGURE 28.10 Relationship between deep visceral adipose tissue (VAT) by computed tomography scanning and waist girth in 110 males aged 18 to 42 years who differed in percentage body fat assessed by densitometry. The VAT best predictors included abdominal skinfold in mm (*a*), waist girth in cm (*b*), and the waist-to-hip ratio (*c*). VAT (cm^2) = $-363.12 + (-1.113a) + 3.478b + 186.7c$. As an example, if abdominal skinfold = 23.0 mm, waist girth = 92.0 cm, and the waist-to-hip ratio = 0.929, then by substitution in the equation, VAT = 104.7 cm^2.

(Adapted from Dépres J-P, et al. Estimation of deep abdominal adipose-tissue accumulation from simple anthropometric measurements in men. *Am J Clin Nutr*. 1991;54(3):471. By permission of the American Society for Nutrition. Photo: from F. Katch)

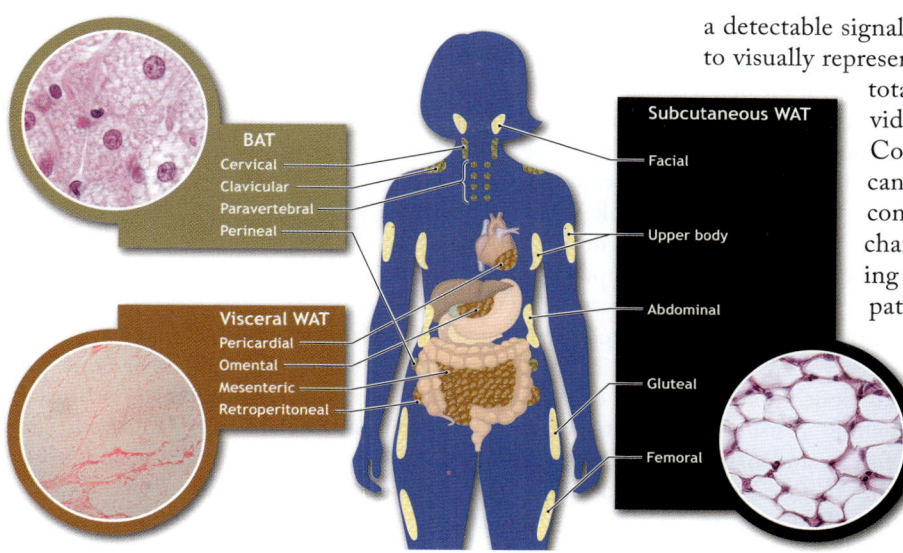

Shutterstock: Jose Luis Calvo (subcutaneous WAT, BAT), Choksawatdikorn (visceral WAT), kubicka (heart), logika600 (gastrointestinal system), Pikovit (woman)

a detectable signal that rearranges under computer software to visually represent various body tissues. MRI can quantify total and subcutaneous adipose tissue in individuals with different body fat percentages.[150] Combined with muscle mass analysis, MRI can assess changes in a muscle's lean and fat components following resistance training, changes in muscle volume before and following training, as a diagnostic tool for various pathologies (e.g., ligamentous knee damage or femoral condyle necrosis), or during different growth stages in youth and adolescence and different life stages with aging.[79,179] MRI analysis has assessed postflight changes in muscle volume and other tissues following a 17-d space mission and 16- to 28-wk duration Space Shuttle/Mir missions[103] and other space voyages.[224,226]

MRI has wide acceptance for diagnosis in almost all medicine and related disciplines, as for example in muscular

energy expenditure) and adhere to a strict dietary regimen to improve overall metabolic health and manage the dyslipidemia.[40,277] Nevertheless, adhering to an active lifestyle may be difficult with musculoskeletal pain, fatigue, or psychological stress. Current clinical management involving bariatric surgery to thwart the genetic-based mutations involved in adipocyte dysfunctional differentiation helps some patients, but less intrusive methods and therapies are being investigated by 54 international groups from 25 countries (eclip-web.org). In Chapter 30, we examine other more common health risks from excessive stored fat.

Magnetic Resonance Imaging

Physician and research scientist and Nobel prize winner Raymond Damadian (1936–) first proposed **magnetic resonance imaging (MRI)** in a grant application in 1969 dealing with soft tissue cancer imaging. The first published article on his novel idea appeared in 1971.[210] MRI, patented in 1974 and first constructed at the Downstate Medical Center in Brooklyn, NY, in 1976, provided noninvasive detailed, high-resolution contrasts in the body's tissue compartments without ionizing radiation risks in x-ray and CT scanning.[1,82,104] The schematic inset part A shows the arrangement for different muscular structures, with the light yellow areas that surround the thigh corresponding to both subcutaneous and internal fat. Note the minimal fat intrusion located among and within the different muscles. The femur bone appears at the center of the cross-section. The bottom B image view shows an MRI transaxial midthigh section in a 30-year-old male middle-distance runner. Computer software subtracts fat and bony tissues (white areas) to compute thigh muscle cross-sectional area. With MRI, electromagnetic radiation in a strong magnetic field excites the hydrogen nuclei in the body's water and lipid molecules. These nuclei are more concentrated in lipid and less so in water and blood, and least in bone. The nuclei then project

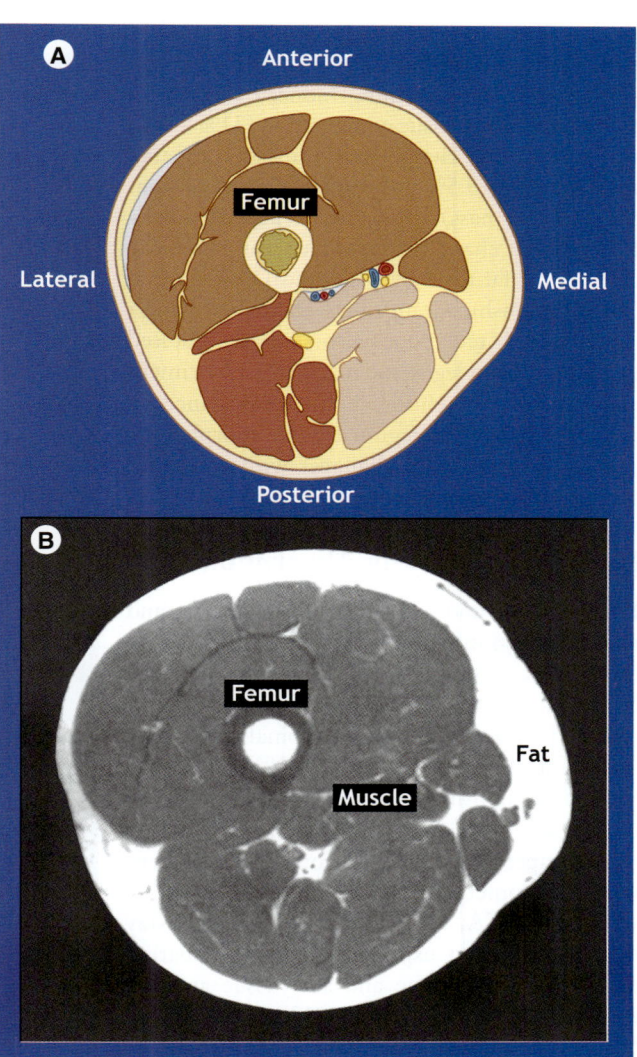

Adapted with permission from Moore KL, et al. *Clinically Oriented Anatomy*. 8th ed. Baltimore: Wolters Kluwer Health; 2018, p. 730.

dystrophy care and spaceflight applications.[56,224,225] The latest MRI technologies allow pacemaker imaging with fiber optic leads rather than wire leads, using MRI compatible defibrillators. Stand-up MRI developed by Dr. Damadian scans patients in weight-bearing standing, sitting, and flexion and extension positions, and the conventional lie-down position (www.fonar.com).

MRI and Resistance Training Effects.

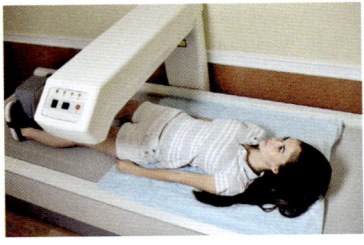
Evgeniy Kalinovskiy/Shutterstock

MRI and DXA (discussed in the next section) assessed changes in regional trunk and extremities and whole-body fat mass, lean body mass, and bone mineral content while resistance training for 3- and 6-mo intervals in 31 females.[140] MRI measured changes in thigh muscle morphology in a subset with 11 female exercisers.

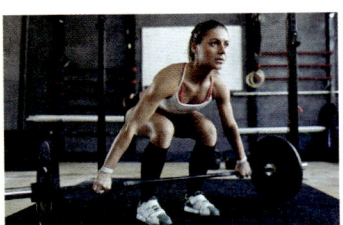
Pressmaster/Shutterstock

Fat mass decreased by 10% and body mass and soft tissue lean mass by 2.2%, but bone mineral content did not change compared with nontraining male and female groups. Soft tissue lean mass was distributed less in females' arms compared with males' both before and after training. The most striking training-induced differences occurred in the females' arms tissue composition (31% loss in fat mass without change in lean mass) compared with the legs (5.5% gain in lean mass without change in fat mass). Fat decreased in the trunk by 12% without change in soft tissue lean mass. The changes for fat mass by MRI and DXA showed close relationships (range between $r = 0.72$ and $r = 0.92$). Both techniques also similarly assessed increases in lean leg tissue mass. This experiment and others[227,228] reinforces the importance to appraise changes in regional tissue morphology (including total body changes) with resistance training as an experimental treatment.[229]

Dual-Energy X-Ray Absorptiometry

DXA reliably and accurately quantifies fat and nonbone regional lean body mass, including the mineral content within the body's deeper bony structures.[34,91,94,110,146,155] It has become the accepted clinical tool to assess spinal osteoporosis and related bone disorders.[45,101] When used for body composition assessment, DXA does not require assumptions concerning the fat and fat-free components' biologic constancy inherent with densitometry.[14,233]

With DXA, two distinct low-energy x-ray beams with short exposure with low radiation dosage penetrate bone and soft tissue areas to a depth approximately 30 cm/12 in. The subject lies supine on a table so the source and detector probes slowly pass across the body over a 10- to 20-min period (www.radiologyinfo.org/en/info/dexa). Computer software reconstructs the attenuated x-ray beams to image the underlying tissues and quantify bone mineral content, total fat mass, and FFM. Analysis can include selected trunk and limb regions for details about tissue composition related to disease risk, injury, and exercise training and detraining effects.[107,118,203]

DXA shows excellent agreement with other bone mineral content independent estimates. Strong relationships also exist between DXA-determined total body fat and body fat by either densitometry,[64,120] segmental body composition (upper- and lower-extremity mass), total body potassium, or total body nitrogen[121] and abdominal adiposity.[55] Studies have focused on body fat estimation by DXA with other methods in young children,[40] prepubertal children,[27,72,168,174] younger and older males[10] and females,[9,132] older adults,[59,167] and intense resistance training changes.[60,156,185]

The inset image shows DXA scans for an anorexic woman (two left images) and a typical woman (two right images) with 25% body fat percentage (56.7-kg/125-lb total body mass). The average anorexic subject weighed 44.4-kg/97.9-lb with

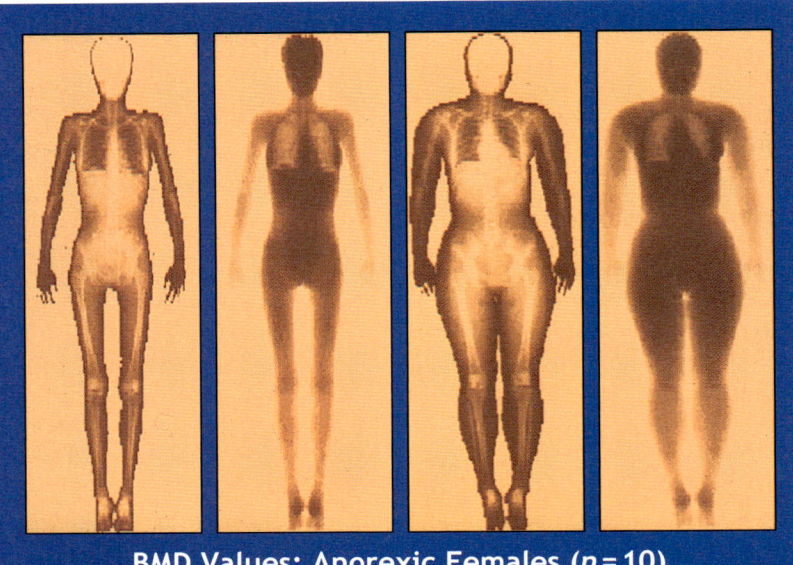

	BMD Values: Anorexic Females ($n = 10$)			
	BMD (g · cm⁻²)		Percentage of normals	
	$\bar{X}$	SD	$\bar{X}$	SD
Head	1.97	.26	—	—
Arms	0.74	.04	99.5	5.9
Legs	1.03	.09	94.1	8.2
Trunk	0.77	.05	76.8	4.6
Spine	0.83	.06	72.8	5.1
Total	0.99	.06	90.3	5.0
L2-L4	0.99	.08	78.5	6.6
Neck	0.87	.09	86.9	9.8

Images courtesy Dr. R. B. Mazess and Lunar Radiation Corporation

DXA-estimated 7.5% body fat from the fat percentages at the arms, legs, and trunk regions. The values in the inset table's right column show the average percentage values for bone mineral density (BMD) for different regional body areas in the anorexic group compared with the 287 normal weight women ages 20 to 40.

FIGURE 28.11 depicts the strong association between percentage body fat estimates by DXA and hydrostatic weighing over a broad age range in males and females. Note that prediction strength decreases for older and fatter subjects but remains within the typical range for comparisons among discrete methodologies. Using a more robust body composition assessment model, the error accounts for less than 2% body fat units between DXA and densitometry in the heterogeneous age group of adults shown in the figure.[65]

Average Percentage Body Fat

In general, percentage body fat for young adult males averages between 12 and 15% and 25 and 28% for females. The general trend for males and females across the age spectrum based on available body composition data reveals percentage body fat steadily and invariably increases with aging. The mechanisms for the increases are not clearly explained. Increased fatness does not imply that such increases represent a desirable and/or expected aging progression, chiefly because vigorous physical activity participation throughout life can minimize the accumulation.[184,200,201] Regular physical activity maintains or increases bone mass while preserving muscle mass. A mostly sedentary lifestyle increases storage fat particularly in the abdominal region while concomitantly reducing muscle mass even if daily caloric intake remains unchanged.

Statistical Confirmation

When discussing the typical body fat percentage for young college-age males and females, statistics reveal that for every 68 people in a group of 100 similar people in a group measured for body composition, the variability from the "average" or mean body fat percentage approximates ±5% body fat units about the average value. This means that for a typical college-age male living in the United States, his body fat will range from 20% (+5% body fat units above the 15% body fat average) to 10% (−5% body fat units below the 15% average). For the remaining 32 males from the 100-person male group, 16 would have a 20 to 25% body fat percentage, whereas 16 others would range from 10 to 5% body fat. Stated somewhat differently, in any distribution of college-age males with 100 similar males per group, 95 will have a body fat percentage ranging between 5 and 25%. The same reasoning applies to females—every 68 females in a 100 person group will have a body fat percentage within 5% above the 26% average and 5% below that average (range 21 to 31%). This too means that in groups of 100 randomly selected college-age females, 95 females will range in body fat from 16 to 36%. A ±15% body fat unit value (equivalent to ±3 standard deviations) includes 98% of the 100 females, which means 98 females range in body fat between 15 and 36%. Statistically, very few females would have a body fat percentage at the low end 15%—the same minimal essential fat in prolonged starvation indicating a life-threatening eating disorder.

No absolute "average" percentage body fat level applies to all individuals, just a probability reference point related to a specific population and age group. Genetic factors greatly influence body fat distribution (and associated health risk) and play an important role in programming body size *in utero* and its ultimate link with disease risk throughout life. Individuals should be evaluated for body composition with a valid

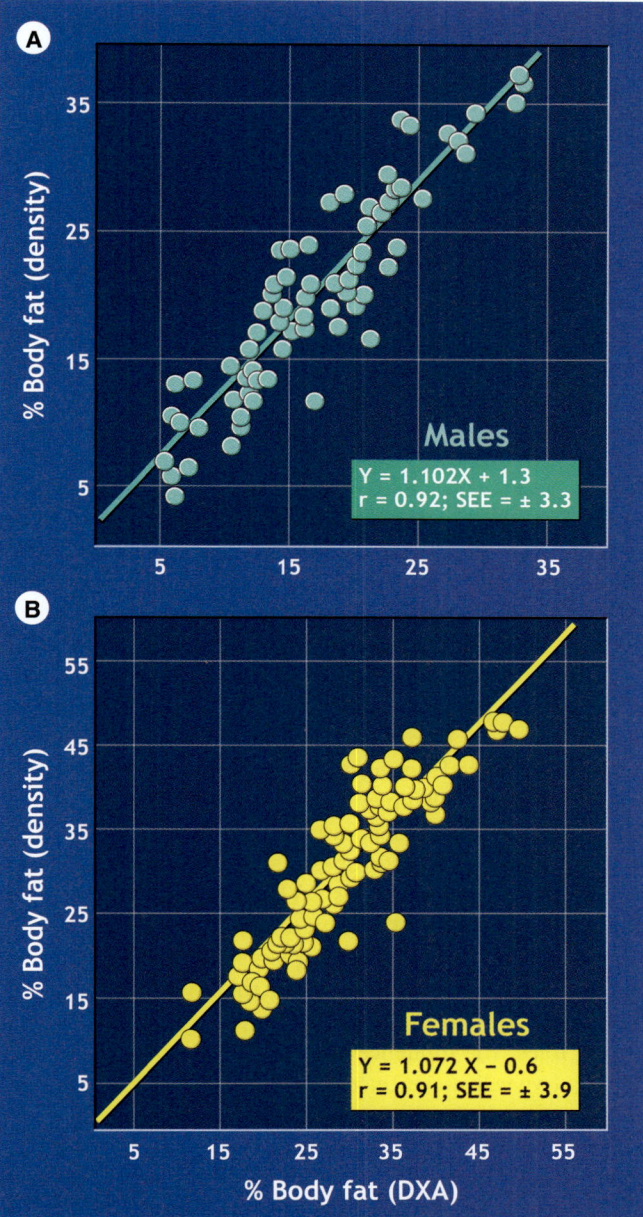

FIGURE 28.11 Strong relationships between total body fat determined by hydrostatic weighing versus dual-energy x-ray absorptiometry (DXA) in males **(A)** and females **(B)**.
(Adapted with permission from Snead DB, et al. Age-related differences in body composition by hydrodensitometry and dual-energy absorptiometry. *J Appl Physiol.* 1993;74:770. ©The American Physiological Society (APS). All rights reserved.)

method to understand their place along the low-fat to high-fat continuum. Armed with this information about "*How fat am I*", allows health care professionals (particularly the person's primary care physician) to take the next step—prioritizing a prudent and individualized body mass goal centered on aesthetic and/or medical considerations.

How to Determine Goal Body Mass

In contact sports and activities that require high muscular power (e.g., football, sprint swimming and running, field-events in track and field), successful performance typically requires a large FFM with average or below-average body fat established for specific sports. Successful athletes in endurance and ultra-endurance activities possess a relatively low body mass and low body fat percentage. *Proper body composition assessment, not simply body mass measurement, should determine a person's ideal body mass. For athletes, goal body mass must coincide with optimizing sport-specific measures related to physiologic functional capacity and performance.* The following equation computes goal body mass based on a new, desired percentage body fat level:

> Goal body mass = FFM ÷ (1.00 − desired %fat)

Consider a 91-kg/201-lb college-age male currently with 24% body fat determined by hydrostatic weighing who wants to know how much fat mass he must lose to attain a new body fat level equal to the 15% "average" for young males. Follow these computational steps for the solution:

> Fat mass = 91 kg / 201 lb × 0.20
> = 18.2 kg / 40.1 lb
> FFM = 91 kg / 201 lb − 18.2 kg / 40.1 lb
> = 72.8 kg / 161 lb
> Goal body mass = 72.8 kg / 161 lb (1.00 − 0.10)
> = 72.8 kg / 161 lb ÷ 0.90
> = 80.9 kg / 178 lb
> Goal fat loss = current body mass − goal body mass
> = 91 kg / 201 lb − 80.9 kg / 178 lb
> = 10.1 kg / 22.2 lb

If this athlete reduced body fat by 10.1 kg/22.2 lb, his new 80.9-kg/178.0-lb body mass would now contain fat equal to 10% body mass. *These calculations assume no change in FFM during body mass loss.* Moderate caloric restriction plus increased daily energy expenditure through physical activity generates fat loss and conserves FFM. Chapter 30 discusses effective approaches to alter body fat percentage.

Looking to a Brighter Future

In the first edition of this textbook published over 40 years ago, we had not expected the "obesity epidemic" to expand so rapidly into such a serious problem, nor did we envision how important body composition assessment procedures would become to the fitness industry and exercise and weight management programs. It now is crystal clear that obesity is a primary risk factor for many cardiometabolic diseases, particularly diabetes, hypertension, and heart failure in coronary artery disease in males and females as they age.[284–286]

In this chapter, we have emphasized that adipose tissue *location* particularly in the visceral region, including its *composition* as white versus brown fat, significantly accelerates serious medical conditions and their secondary connections. WAT correlates with energy excess as stored triacylglycerol and thus links strongly with obesity, while brown adipose tissue (BAT) associates with increased thermogenesis by reducing inflammatory responses throughout the body and possibly creating more favorable cardiometabolic conditions to promote greater proinflammatory gene expression. We are encouraged that future research among many cooperating disciplines will make this come to fruition, which revitalizes our outlook for a brighter future and happier ending.

The inset schematic above presents twelve known interrelated conditions tied to obesity and disease dysregulation placed into three categories. While our own bias targets physical activity as an important driver in the overall environmental category, so do two other large category influences—epigenetics (gene expression rather than manipulate genetic code alterations) and hereditary factors (genetics) also play pivotal roles. The influence of CRISPR-Cas9's unique technology (www.livescience.com/58790-crispr-explained.html) offers expectations as an exceptionally versatile new tool with two other CRISPR molecule types in molecular biology research discussed in Chapter 33. Our hope is for future graduates in exercise physiology to join the legion of scientists and researchers looking to strangle obesity's accelerating advances. The field needs to unlock more secrets about the body's compositional structures and discover underlying mechanisms to minimize debilitating diseases, hospitalizations, and morbidity and mortality statistics to improve the human condition.[190]

Shutterstock: Razym (physical activity), nobeastsofierce (mutations), Alila Medical Media (risk alleles), Dotted Yeti (infections), ronstik (light), DisobeyArt (family history), nadianb (food), Mitar Vidakovic (temperature)

Summary

1. Standard weight-for-height tables reveal little about the body's composition—overweight does not necessarily coincide with excessive body fat.
2. BMI relates more closely to body fat and health risk than simply body mass and stature. BMI still fails to consider the body's proportional composition.
3. For the first time in the United States, overweight (BMI 25 to 29) and obese individuals (BMI ≥ 30) outnumber persons who maintain a desirable weight.
4. Sheldon's taxonomic visual approach to establish body size and shape standards based on somatotyping falls short as a valid approach to quantitatively assess body composition.
5. Total body fat consists of essential fat and storage fat.
6. Essential fat contains fat present in bone marrow, nerve tissue, and organs; it is not a labile energy reserve, but instead an important component for normal biologic functions.
7. Storage fat represents the energy reserve that accumulates mainly as adipose tissue beneath the skin and in visceral depots.
8. Storage fat averages 12% of body mass for males and 15% for females.
9. The greater essential fat for females probably relates to childbearing and hormonal functions.
10. An individual probably cannot reduce body fat below the essential fat level and still maintain optimal health and physical performance.
11. A sumo wrestler has the largest fat-free body mass (FFM) reported in the literature (121.3 kg/267 lb); this value likely represents an approximate upper limit for male athletes (80 kg/176 lb for athletic females) assessed by a valid body composition procedure.
12. Menstrual dysfunction in athletes who train assiduously to maintain low body fat levels relates to the interaction between the physiologic and psychologic stress inherent with regular intense training, hormonal balance, energy and nutrient intake, and low body fat.
13. Delayed menarche onset in chronically active young females may confer health benefits because they show a lower lifetime reproductive organ and other cancer occurrences.
14. Popular indirect body composition assessments include hydrostatic weighing and anthropometric prediction methods based on skinfold and girth measurements.
15. Hydrostatic weighing determines body density with subsequent estimation of percentage body fat.
16. The average young adult male has 15% body fat, whereas females average 26% body fat.
17. Subtracting fat mass from body mass yields FFM.
18. The air displacement BOD POD method provides a reasonable alternative to hydrostatic weighing for body volume determination and body composition assessment.
19. The built-in error to predict body fat from whole-body density depends on the correct assumptions concerning the densities in the body's fat and fat-free components that rely on assumed race and age constants and athletic experience.
20. Hydrostatic weighing and BOD POD represent "gold standards" to assess body density and percentage body fat among different male and female populations.
21. Specific skinfold and girth equations to predict body composition exhibit population specificity and are most valid with subjects similar to those who participated in the equations' original derivation.
22. Behnke's body profile analysis represents a visual representation for body shape expressed as deviations in body dimensions from normative girth reference male and female data and different athletic groups for comparison in 5-year increments with aging.
23. Hydrated fat-free body tissues and extracellular water facilitate electrical flow in bioelectrical impedance analysis compared with fat tissue from the greater electrolyte content in the fat-free component.
24. Ultrasound, CT, MRI, and DXA indirectly assess body composition.
25. The valid, indirect methods to assess body composition each have a unique application to expand current knowledge about the separate but linked components related to human body composition and performance assessment.
26. Goal body mass computes as FFM ÷ (1 − desired %fat).
27. Twelve well-known interrelated conditions link to obesity and disease dysregulation, with physical activity playing an important driver as an environmental influence, epigenetics (gene expression influences rather than genetic code alterations), and hereditary factors (genetics).

Key Terms

Abdominal fat: Subcutaneous and visceral fat in the abdominal region

Amenorrhea: Complete cessation of menses

Anthropometry: Standardized techniques with calipers and cloth tape to predict body size, proportion, shape, and composition

Archimedes: Mathematician and inventor in ancient Greece who described the relation between a sphere's surface and volume and its circumscribing cylinder

Archimedes' principle: Formulated by the Greek mathematician Archimedes who determined that an object's loss of weight in water equals the weight of water volume it displaces

Athletic amenorrhea: Serious athletes who experience amenorrhea attributed to stress imposed by regular, hard training over many months and inadequate food intake to sustain normal metabolic functions

Behnke, Albert: Navy physician and research scientist who pioneered body composition research including hydrodensitometry and surface anthropometric measurements to quantify percentage body fat and fat-free body mass and the framework for the reference male and reference female

Bioelectrical impedance analysis (BIA): Device that passes alternating current between two electrodes more rapidly through hydrated fat-free body tissues and extracellular water than fat or bone tissue, in accordance with Ohm law ($R = V/I$, where R = resistance, V = voltage, and I = current)

BOD POD (air plethysmography): Plethysmographic device to assess body volume and its changes by measuring initial air volume of the empty chamber minus the air volume with the person inside

Body density (D_b): Body mass expressed per unit of body volume (D_b = body mass ÷ body volume)

Body mass index (BMI): Ratio of body mass to stature squared (body mass, kg ÷ stature, m^2)

Computed tomography (CT): An array of x-ray emitters and detectors that generate detailed cross-sectional, two-dimensional images of body segments when an ionizing radiation beam passes through tissues of different densities; scan produces pictorial and quantitative information about total tissue area, total fat and muscle area, and thickness and volume of tissues within an organ

Densitometry: Archimedes' principle of water displacement to estimate whole-body volume and body density; also known as hydrodensitometry, underwater weighing, and hydrostatic weighing

Dual-energy x-ray absorptiometry (DXA): Clinical device that emits two distinct low-energy x-ray beams with short exposure radiation dosage that penetrate bone and soft tissue areas and quantifies fat and nonbone regional lean body mass, and mineral content in deeper bony structures

Energy availability hypothesis: Inadequate energy reserve to sustain pregnancy that induces ovulation cessation

Essential fat: Fat in heart, lungs, liver, spleen, kidneys, intestines, muscles, and lipid-rich tissues of the central nervous system and bone marrow; required for normal physiologic functioning

Exercise stress hypothesis: Prolonged chronic physical stress disrupt the hypothalamic-pituitary adrenal axis and gonadotropin-releasing hormone output to produce irregular menstrual cycles

Fat-free body mass (FFM): All residual lipid-free chemicals and tissues, including water, muscle, bone, connective tissue, and internal organs

Fat mass: All extractable lipids from adipose and other body tissues

Fat patterning: Distribution pattern of trunk and extremity body fat

Goal body weight: fat-free mass ÷ (1.00 − %fat desired)

Gonadotropin-releasing hormone: Controls the menstrual cycle

K rations: Compact nutritional packets for breakfast, lunch, and dinner meals used by the military in World War II

Lean body mass: Theoretical entity that includes fat-free body mass plus essential body fat

Lean-to-fat ratio: Lean body mass ÷ fat mass

Lipodystrophies (LDs): Abnormal or degenerative conditions affecting the body's adipose tissue regions

Magnetic resonance imaging (MRI): Electromagnetic radiation in a strong magnetic field excites hydrogen nuclei in body's water and lipid molecules to quantify total and subcutaneous adipose tissue

Matiegka, Jindřich: Czech anthropologist who described a four-component body composition model consisting of skeletal weight (S), skin plus subcutaneous tissue (Sk + St), skeletal muscle (M), and a remainder (R)

Minimal body mass: Body mass plus essential body fat (includes sex-specific essential fat) that equals 48.5 kg/106.9 lb for the reference female; computed from bone diameters, stature, and other constants

Minnesota semi-starvation experiments: Classic nutrition experiments on body wasting and physiologic functions with prolonged caloric restriction

Near-infrared interactance (NIR): Body fat measurement that uses the principles of light absorption and reflection to measure body fat; applies technology originally developed by the U.S. Department of Agriculture to assess body composition of livestock and lipid content of various grains

Obese syndrome: Constellation of nine comorbidities: glucose intolerance, insulin resistance, dyslipidemia, type 2 diabetes, hypertension, elevated plasma leptin concentrations, increased visceral adipose tissue, increased coronary heart disease risk, and some cancers

Obesity: For young males, percentage body fat content that exceeds 20%; in older males, body fat content that exceeds 30%. In young females, body fat content that exceeds 30%; in older females, body fat content that exceeds 35%

Oligomenorrhea: Infrequent or light menstrual cycles

Overfat: Excess body fat above a predefined limit based on age and gender

Overweight: Excess body weight relative to other individuals of the same gender, age, or height without accompanying body fat measures

Quetelet Index: Ratio of body weight in kg divided by the square of height in meters

Reference male and reference female: Behnke's reference standards for body dimensions developed from military and anthropometric surveys for males and females that partition body mass into lean body mass, muscle, and bone, with fat subdivided into storage and essential fat

Relative body fat: Fat mass expressed as a percentage of total body mass

Sex-specific essential fat: Fat in females, mainly in breast and tissues, related to childbearing and selected hormonal functions

Sheldon, William H.: Developed a visual classification taxonomic approach based on front, side, and rear photographic views to assess body size characteristics among individuals based on a seven-point scale to compare thin, muscular, and overweight body-type characteristics

Siri equation: Represents the most popular equation to convert body density to percentage body fat (percentage body fat = (495 ÷ body density) − 450)

Skinfold caliper: Pincer jaws exert a constant tension of 10 g · mm^{-2} at the point of contact

Skinfold: The double layer of skin plus subcutaneous fat at selected anatomic sites (e.g., triceps, subscapula, iliac, abdomen, thigh)

Somatotyping: Taxonomy developed by W. H. Sheldon to categorize human physique according to the relative contribution of three fundamental elements and classified as ectomorphic (lean and slender), mesomorphic (muscular and husky), and endomorphic (round with increased body fat)

Specific gravity: Object's mass in air divided by loss of weight in water (body mass ÷ [body mass − body weight in water])

Spurious correlation: The co-relation between two variables that wrongly implies a cause and effect between the two variables because the variables of immediate interest are themselves influenced by co-related variables

Stature: Height expressed in metric units; for example, 72 in. = 182.88 cm or 1.829 m

Storage fat: Fat or triacylglycerols packed primarily in adipose tissue that contains approximately 83% pure lipid, 2% protein, and 15% water within its supporting structures

Subcutaneous fat: Adipose tissue located beneath the skin's surface

Sumo wrestlers: Wrestler attempts to force opponent out of a circular ring or into touching the ground with a body part other than the soles of the feet (usually by throwing, shoving, or pushing him down)

Two-component model: Views the body containing fat-free tissues and fat tissue

Ultrasound: Converts electrical energy into high-frequency pulsed sound waves that penetrate skin surfaces into the underlying tissues to produce an echo and image of underlying tissues

Undernutrition: According to the World Health Organization, there are four broad subtypes of undernutrition—wasting, stunting, underweight, and deficiencies in vitamins and minerals, with wasting signifying low weight for height (body mass index ≤18.5)

Visceral adipose tissue (VAT): Adipose tissue within and surrounding thoracic (e.g., heart, liver, lungs) and abdominal (e.g., liver, kidneys, intestines) cavities

References are available online at Lippincott Connect.

Additional References

Agalliu I, et al. Overall and central obesity and prostate cancer risk in African men. *Cancer Causes Control.* 2022;33:223.

Alkutbe RB, et al. Fat mass prediction equations and reference ranges for Saudi Arabian Children aged 8-12 years using machine technique method. *PeerJ.* 2021;9:e10734.

Aragón-Vela J, et al. Impact of exercise on gut microbiota in obesity. *Nutrients.* 2021;13:3999.

Atakan MM, et al. The role of exercise, diet, and cytokines in preventing obesity and improving adipose tissue. *Nutrients.* 2021;13:1459.

Barber JL, et al. Regular exercise and patterns of response across multiple cardiometabolic traits: the HERITAGE family study. *Br J Sports Med.* 2022;56:95.

Beck D, et al. Adipose tissue distribution from body MRI is associated with cross-sectional and longitudinal brain age in adults. *Neuroimage Clin.* 2022;33:102949.

Bellafronte NT, et al. Comparison between dual-energy x-ray absorptiometry and bioelectrical impedance for body composition measurements in adults with chronic kidney disease: a cross-sectional, longitudinal, multi-treatment analysis. *Nutrition.* 2021;82:111059.

Blue MNM, et al. Validity of body-composition methods across racial and ethnic populations. *Adv Nutr.* 2021;12:1854.

Bouchard C. Genetics of obesity: what we have learned over decades of research. *Obesity (Silver Spring).* 2021;29:802.

Bouchard C. The study of human variability became a passion. *Eur J Clin Nutr.* 2021. doi: 10.1038/s41430-021-00871-z.

Brener A, et al. The heritability of body composition. *BMC Pediatr.* 2021;21:225.

Brotman SM, et al. Subcutaneous adipose tissue splice quantitative trait loci reveal differences in isoform usage associated with cardiometabolic traits. *Am J Hum Genet.* 2022;109:66.

Choi YS, et al. Prevalence of optimal metabolic health in U.S. adolescents, NHANES 2007-2016. *Metab Syndr Relat Disord.* 2021;19:56.

Colleluori G, Villareal DT. Aging, obesity, sarcopenia and the effect of diet and exercise intervention. *Exp Gerontol.* 2021;155:111561.

Corrêa CR, et al. Relative fat mass is a better tool to diagnose high adiposity when compared to body mass index in young male adults: a cross-section study. *Clin Nutr ESPEN.* 2021;41:225.

Cullin JM. Implicit and explicit fat bias among adolescents from two US populations varying by obesity prevalence. *Pediatr Obes.* 2021;16:e12747.

da Silva JSM, et al. Estimations of body fat by anthropometry or bioelectrical impedance differ from those by dual-energy X-ray absorptiometry in prefrail community-dwelling older women. *Nutr Res.* 2021;86:1.

Dechenaud ME, et al. Total body and regional surface area: quantification with low-cost three-dimensional optical imaging systems. *Am J Phys Anthropol.* 2021;175:865.

De Sousa RAL, et al. Physical exercise consequences on memory in obesity: a systematic review. *Obes Rev.* 2021;22:e13298.

Enríquez Guerrero A, et al. Effectiveness of an intermittent fasting diet versus continuous energy restriction on anthropometric measurements, body composition and lipid profile in overweight and obese adults: a meta-analysis. *Eur J Clin Nutr.* 2021;75:1024.

Faulkner MS, Michalisyn SF. Exercise Adherence in Hispanic adolescents with obesity or Type 2 diabetes. *J Pediatr Nurs.* 2021;56:7.

Francisco R, et al. Validity of water compartments estimated using bioimpedance spectroscopy in athletes differing in hydration status. *Scand J Med Sci Sports.* 2021;31:1612.

Frank AP, et al. Determinants of body fat distribution in humans may provide insight about obesity-related health risks. *J Lipid Res.* 2019;60:1710.

Galmes-Panades AM, et al. Targeting body composition in an older population: do changes in movement behaviours matter? Longitudinal analyses in the PREDIMED-Plus trial. *BMC Med.* 2021;9:3.

González-Arellanes R, et al. Agreement between laboratory methods and the 4-compartment model in assessing fat mass in obese older Hispanic-American adults. *Clin Nutr.* 2021;40:3592.

Gonzalez MC, et al. Calf circumference: cutoff values from the NHANES 1999-2006. *Am J Clin Nutr.* 2021;113:1679.

Guo Y, et al. Intermittent fasting improves cardiometabolic risk factors and alters gut microbiota in metabolic syndrome patients. *J Clin Endocrinol Metab.* 2021;106:64.

Hall ME, Kipchumba R. HuR brings the heat: linking adipose tissue to cardiac dysfunction. *Am J Physiol Heart Circ Physiol.* 2021;321:H214.

Harty PS, et al. Novel body fat estimation using machine learning and 3-dimensional optical imaging. *Eur J Clin Nutr*. 2020; 74:842.

Heymsfield SB, et al. Phenotypic differences between people varying in muscularity. *J Cachexia Sarcopenia Muscle*. 2022:35170220.

Ishaq M, et al. Key signaling networks are dysregulated in patients with the adipose tissue disorder, lipedema. *Int J Obes (Lond)*. 2021;35:101511.

Jarraya M, Bredella MA. Clinical imaging of marrow adiposity. *Best Pract Res Clin Endocrinol Metab*. 2021;35:101511.

Kalenga CZ, et al. Sex influences the effect of adiposity on arterial stiffness and renin-angiotensin aldosterone system activity in young adults. *Endocrinol Diabetes Metab*. 2022;5:e00317.

Katta N, et al. Obesity and coronary heart disease: epidemiology, pathology, and coronary artery imaging. *Curr Probl Cardiol*. 2021;46:100655.

Kennedy S, et al. Digital anthropometric evaluation of young children: comparison to results acquired with conventional anthropometry. *Eur J Clin Nutr*. 2022;76:251.

Kirk B, et al. Body composition reference ranges in community-dwelling adults using dual-energy X-ray absorptiometry: the Australian Body Composition (ABC) Study. *J Cachexia Sarcopenia Muscle*. 2021;12:880.

Kompaniyets L, et al. Body mass index and risk for covid-19–related hospitalization, intensive care unit admission, invasive mechanical ventilation, and death United States, March–December 2020. *MMWR*. 2021;70:355.

Lee G, et al. Development and validation of prediction equations for the assessment of muscle or fat mass using anthropometric measurements, serum creatinine level, and lifestyle factors among Korean adults. *Nutr Res Pract*. 2021;15:95.

Lee MR, et al. Obesity-related indices and its association with kidney stone disease: a cross-sectional and longitudinal cohort study. *Urolithiasis*. 2022;50:55.

Lim K, et al. Lipodistrophy: a paradigm for understanding the consequences of "overloading" adipose tissue. *Physiol Rev*. 2021; 101:907.

Maguire S, Wilson F, Gallagher P, O'Shea F. Central obesity in axial spondyloarthropathy: the missing link to understanding worse outcomes in women? *J Rheumatol*. 2022:35232810.

Mao T, et al. Short-term fasting reshapes fat tissue. *Endocr J*. 2021;68:387.

Mazahery H, et al. Air displacement plethysmography (Pea Pod) in full-term and pre-term infants: a comprehensive review of accuracy, reproducibility, and practical challenges. *Matern Health Neonatol Perinatol*. 2018;4:12.

Miller-Matero LR, et al. The Influence of health literacy and health numeracy on weight loss outcomes following bariatric surgery. *Surg Obes Relat Dis*. 2021;17:384.

Moazzam-Jazi M, et al. Diverse effect of MC4R risk alleles on obesity-related traits over a lifetime: evidence from a well-designed cohort study. *Gene*. 2022;807:145950.

O'Donoghue G, et al. What exercise prescription is optimal to improve body composition and cardiorespiratory fitness in adults living with obesity? A network meta-analysis. *Obes Rev*. 2021;22:e13137.

Pflanz CP, et al. Central obesity is selectively associated with cerebral gray matter atrophy in 15,634 subjects in the UK Biobank. *Int J Obes (Lond)*. 2022:10.1038/s41366-021-00992-2.

Pillon NJ, et al. Metabolic consequences of obesity and type 2 diabetes: balancing genes and environment for personalized care. *Cell*. 2021;184:15302.

Pulit SL, et al. Meta-analysis of genome-wide association studies for body fat distribution in 694,649 individuals of European ancestry. *Hum Mol Genet*. 2019;28:166.

Qian YT, et al. The adiposity indicators in relation to diabetes among adults in China: a cross-sectional study from China Health and Nutrition Survey. *Ann Palliat Med*. 2022;35073720.

Rojo-Tirado MA, et al. Body composition changes after a weight loss intervention: a 3-year follow-up study. *Nutrients*. 2021;13:164.

Rosberg V, et al. Simple cardiovascular risk stratification by replacing total serum cholesterol with anthropometric measures: The MORGAM prospective cohort project. *Prev Med Rep*. 2022;26:101700.

Sarzynski AR, Bouchard C. World-class athletic performance and genetic endowment. *Nature Metab*. 2020;2:796.

Shuey MM, et al. Exploration of an alternative to body mass index to characterize the relationship between height and weight for prediction of metabolic phenotypes and cardiovascular outcomes. *Obes Sci Pract*. 2021;8:124.

Sobhiyeh S, et al. Digital anthropometric volumes: toward the development and validation of a universal software. *Med Phys*. 2021;48:3654.

Steele CC St, et al. The relationship between dietary fat intake, impulsive choice, and metabolic health. *Appetite*. 2021 165:105292.

Strack C, et al. Gender differences in cardiometabolic health and disease in a cross-sectional observational obesity study. *Biol Sex Differ*. 2022;13:8.

Suthahar N, et al. Relative fat mass, a new index of adiposity, is strongly associated with incident heart failure: data from PREVEND. *Sci Rep*. 2022;12:147.

Świątkiewicz I, et al. Time-restricted eating and metabolic syndrome: current status and future perspectives. *Nutrients*. 2021;13:221.

Tchang BG, et al. Best practices in the management of overweight and obesity. *Med Clin North Am*. 2021;105:149.

Tinsley GM, et al. Resting metabolic rate in muscular physique athletes: validity of existing methods and development of new prediction equations. *Appl Physiol Nutr Metab*. 2019;44:397.

Tinsley GM. Five-component model validation of reference, laboratory and field methods of body composition assessment. *Br J Nutr*. 2021;125:1246.

Trinschek J, et al. Maximal oxygen uptake adjusted for skeletal muscle mass in competitive speed-power and endurance male athletes: changes in a one-year training cycle. *Int J Environ Res Public Health*. 2020;17:6226.

Urlacher SS, et al. Childhood daily energy expenditure does not decrease with market integration and is not related to adiposity in Amazonia. *J Nutr*. 2021;151:695.

Verboven K, Hansen D. Critical reappraisal of the role and importance of exercise intervention in the treatment of obesity in adults. *Sports Med*. 2021;51:379.

Versic S, et al. Differential effects of resistance- and endurance-based exercise programs on muscular fitness, body composition, and cardiovascular variables in young adult women: contextualizing the efficacy of self-selected exercise modalities. *Medicina (Kaunas)*. 2021;57:654.

Vidal Pérez D, et al. Relationship of limb lengths and body composition to lifting in weightlifting. *Int J Environ Res Public Health*. 2021;18:756.

Westbury LD, et al. Relationships between level and change in sarcopenia and other body composition components and adverse health outcomes: findings from the health, aging, and body composition study. *Calcif Tissue Int*. 2021;108:302.

Wilson OWA, et al. Freshmen weight and body composition change determinants: a scoping review. *J Am Coll Health*. 2021;69:298.

Wong HS, et al. Genome-wide association study identifies genetic risk loci for adiposity in a Taiwanese population. *PLoS Genet*. 2022;18:e1009952.

Wood AC, et al. Identification of genetic loci simultaneously associated with multiple cardiometabolic traits. *Nutr Metab Cardiovasc Dis*. 2022:35168826.

Table 28.1 Body Density, Percentage Fat, Fat Mass, and Fat-Free Body Mass in Two American Professional Football Players

Variable	Symbol	Defensive Lineman	Running Back
Body mass (kg)	M_a	121.73	97.37
Net underwater weight (kg)	W_w	7.30	6.52
Water temperature correction	D_w	0.99336	0.99336
Residual lung volume (L)	RLV	1.213	1.374
Total body volume (L)	TBV	113.89	90.08
Body density (g · cm^{-3})	D_b	1.0688	1.0809
Body Composition			
Relative percentage body fat (%)	%Fat	13.1	8.0
Absolute body fat (kg)	FM	15.9	7.2
Fat-free body mass (kg)	FFM	105.8	90.2

Table 28.2 Body Composition Prediction Equations for Boys and Girls Ages 7 to 17

Age, y	Boys	Girls
7–9	%Fat = (5.38/D_b − 4.97) × 100	%Fat = (5.43/D_b − 5.03) × 100
9–11	%Fat = (5.30/D_b − 4.86) × 100	%Fat = (5.35/D_b − 4.95) × 100
11–13	%Fat = (5.23/D_b − 4.81) × 100	%Fat = (5.25/D_b − 4.84) × 100
13–15	%Fat = (5.08/D_b − 4.64) × 100	%Fat = (5.12/D_b − 4.69) × 100
15–17	%Fat = (5.03/D_b − 4.59) × 100	%Fat = (5.07/D_b − 4.64) × 100

D_b, body density; %Fat, percentage body fat.
Data from Lohman T. Applicability of body composition techniques and constants for children and youth. *Exerc Sports Sci Rev*. 1986;14:325.

Table 28.3 Changes in Selected Skinfolds of a Young Female During a 16-Week Exercise Program

Skinfolds (mm)	Before	After	Absolute Change	Percentage Change
Triceps	22.5	19.4	−3.1	−13.8
Subscapular	19.0	17.0	−2.0	−10.5
Suprailiac	34.5	30.2	−4.3	−12.8
Abdomen	33.7	29.4	−4.3	−12.8
Thigh	21.6	18.7	−2.9	−13.4
Sum	131.3	114.7	−16.6	−12.6

CHAPTER 29
Physique, Performance, and Physical Activity

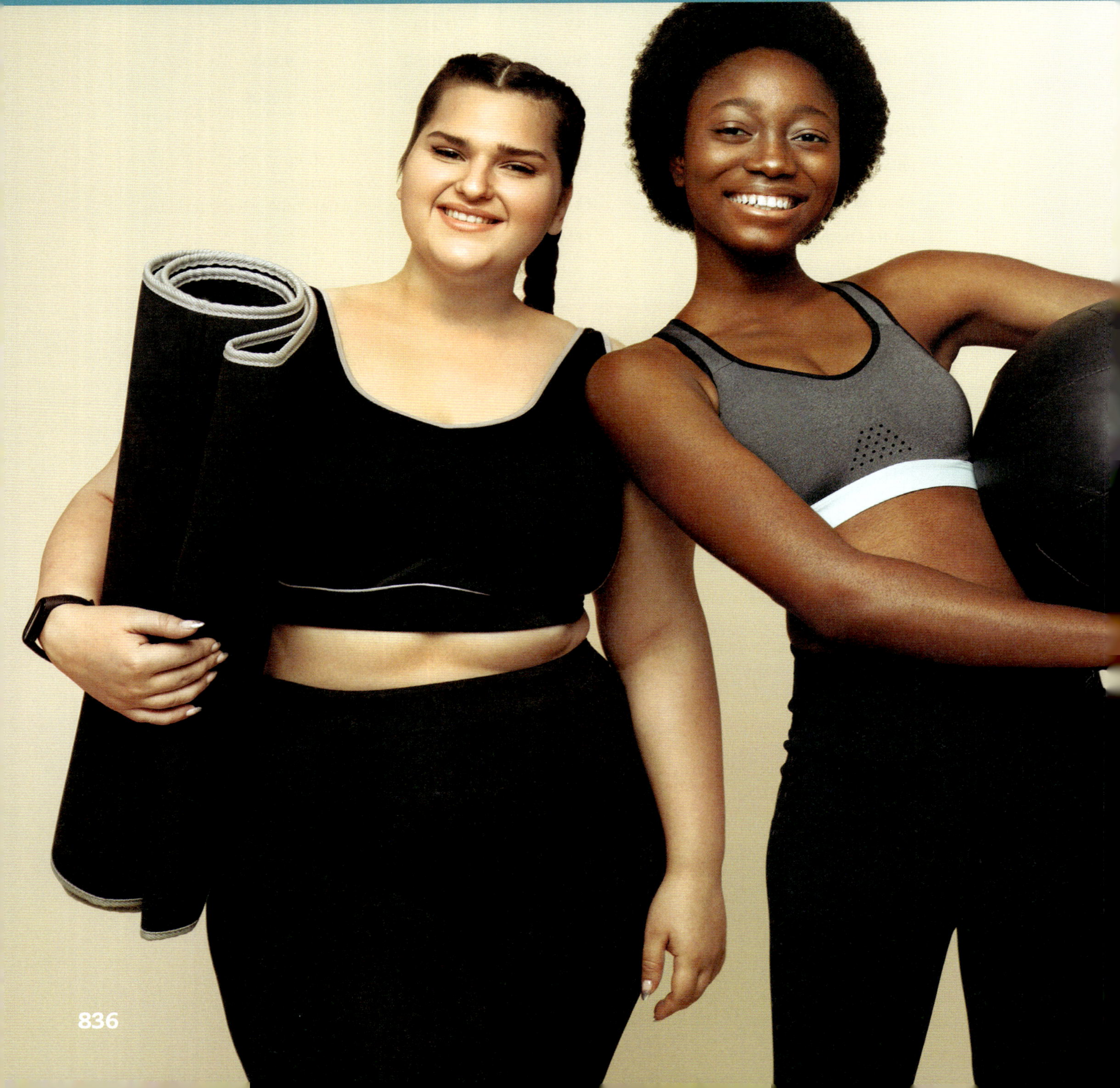

Chapter Objectives

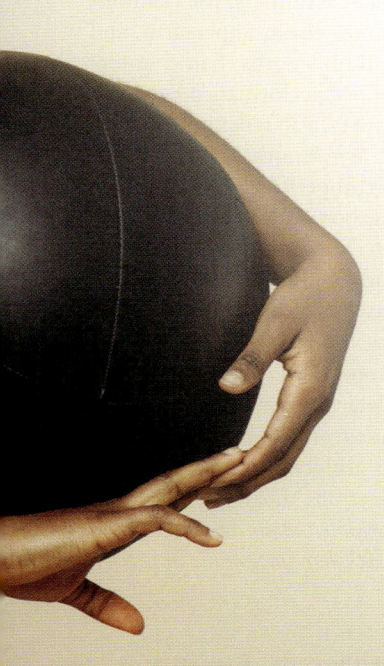

- Compare body composition characteristics among average young males and females with elite competitors in endurance running, wrestling, triathlon, professional golf, and weightlifting and bodybuilding
- Contrast body fat values for male and female competitive swimmers with runners and give plausible reasons for any differences
- Summarize body composition characteristics between early American professional football players and modern day counterparts
- Summarize body composition characteristics between modern American professional football players with current collegiate Division I and III players
- Contrast body composition characteristics between elite high school wrestlers and less successful counterparts
- Contrast body composition, girths, and excess muscle mass between male and female bodybuilders
- Contrast female bodybuilders with other elite female athletes for fat-free body mass (FFM) to fat mass ratio
- Discuss the upper limit for FFM in "large-sized" male and female athletes
- Discuss three main differences in body composition and anthropometry between male and female centenarians

Ancillaries at-a-Glance

Visit Lippincott Connect to access these resources.

- References: Chapter 29
- Appendix H: Links for Supplemental Animations and Videos
- Focus on Research: Body Composition Analysis by Dissection

Introduction

Body composition evaluation partitions gross body mass into two major structural components—body fat and fat-free body mass (FFM). In Chapter 28, we characterized the major physique differences between males and females from childhood through older age. Pronounced physique differences also exist among same gender participants in most high-skill sports.

Different anthropometric methodologies quantify physique status. Visual appraisal often describes individuals as small, medium, and large, or as thin (**ectomorphic**), muscular (**mesomorphic**), or fat (**endomorphic**). The latter older approach somatotyping, proposed by psychologist/physician William H. Sheldon (1898–1977) and profiled in Chapter 28, describes body shape by placing a person into categories and grading them on a 1-to-7 scale for the three somatotype components often accompanied by nude photographs! Sheldon's work was turned over to the Smithsonian Institution, which has sealed all public access to the photos (www.nytimes.com/1995/01/21/us/nude-photos-are-sealed-at-smithsonian.html) due to concerns about his appraisal methods, namely attempting to correlate body type differences (relying on photographs) with social hierarchy (and even intelligence; www.ncbi.nlm.nih.gov/pubmed/18447308). Nonetheless, somatotyping quantifies neither body dimensions (e.g., abdominal size related to hip size) nor how biceps development compares with thigh or calf development. Somatotyping served previously as a simple yet ineffective methodology to analyze meaningful differences in world-class athletes' physique status[5–9,13] and familial heritability.[39,58]

In this chapter, we focus on objectively determined body fat and FFM components in champion athletes in different sport and competition categories. Specifically, we consider differences in physique among Olympic competitors, endurance runners, collegiate and professional American football players, triathletes, high school wrestlers, champion male and female bodybuilders, collegiate gymnasts, PGA golfers, and NBA basketball players. Highly skilled male and female competitors train to perfect their competitive performance skills featuring other high-achieving and dedicated rivals. At the opposite end of the athleticism scale, we consider the unique anthropometric characteristics for individuals well past their athletic days—100-year-old males and females.

Physique Status in Champion Athletes

Body composition differs considerably between athletes and nonathletes, particularly among same-sex participants. Research may eventually discover how body size and composition contribute to and are a prerequisite for elite performance in specific sports. In fact, considerable debate continues on whether the newer molecular biology CRISPR cas-9 breakthroughs (which we feature in Chapter 33) eventually will edit the gene line to create tomorrows "super athletes."[81,84] Scientists already have demonstrated that genetic engineering can manipulate a muscle's delicate internal cellular architecture. Such desirable traits would be expressed as increased muscle size and shape by "turning on" and "turning off" crucial genes by "editing" them to positively contribute to physical performance excellance.[82,83,85] An ethical debate focuses on the future use with gene editing to determine small height to taller height or vice versa, aerobic enzyme functioning to enhance fitness status, facilitate muscle strength potential, and more efficient neural function to improve dysfunctional muscle coordination patterns to improve the human condition by eradicating horrible, incurable diseases (e.g., Huntington disease, sickle cell anemia, muscular dystrophy, and many neurodegenerative disorders).[90,91]

Olympic Competitor Research

Research from the 1964 Tokyo and 1968 Mexico City summer Olympic games[13,14,27] also have included Australian elite judo, wrestling, taekwondo, and boxing combatants; elite male and female collegiate athletes competing in soccer, swimming, track and field, lacrosse (females), volleyball (females), and baseball (males)[88]; and elite Greek female basketball, volleyball, and handball players.[89] Such studies have successfully linked physique characteristics to high-level achievement across sport types.[43,61] The best male swimmers, for example, were heavier and taller and had larger chest, upper-arm, and thigh girths and upper- and lower-limb lengths than counterparts not ranked in a particular sport performance category. The best female breaststroke swimmers, also taller and heavier, possessed larger arm span, foot and arm lengths, and hand and wrist breadths than less successful competitors.

The different sport governing bodies should encourage scientific cooperation among exercise physiology and sports medicine researchers to assess body composition. The measurement process should begin early in developing the most promising young athletes and systematically follow them as they train for higher-level competition. This would provide longitudinal data as the athlete progresses in skill level throughout their competitive endeavors. Subtle differences in physique characteristics among athletes in the same sport may help to unravel an age-old question: "*What physique characteristics and other performance variables about an athlete make them achieve excellence compared with less successful competitors in the same sport?*"

Michael Phelps: World Champion Swimmer Superstar

An anomaly in body proportions seems apparent in world and Olympic champion swimmer Michael Phelps (1985–), winner of a total of 28 medals (23 gold, 3 silver, 2 bronze), with 13 of the gold medals, 2 silver, and 1 bronze being in individual events. This equates to more medals won by any previous athletes who won medals in different Games (Carl Lewis, track; Mark Spitz, swimming; Paavo Nurmi, running; and Larisa Latynina, gymnastics). Latynina, a gymnast from the Soviet Union, competed between 1956 and 1964, amassing 18 total medals (9 gold), second-most behind Phelps. Consider Phelps' physical characteristics: height 193 cm/76 in., weight 89.8 kg/198 lb, "wingspan" that exceeded his stature (2.03 m/79.9 in.), and a size 14 foot. Exercise physiologists and fans worldwide wanted to know, *"What made Michael Phelps achieve such extraordinarily consistent performances when he competed in his first Olympiad at age 15 (2000 Melbourne Games) over five consecutive Olympic Games through the Rio 2016 Games?"*

Salty View/Shutterstock

Limited body composition data are available to shed light on this question. Phelps' arm span—measured 203 cm/79.9 in. (see inset image during his butterfly 200-m swim in the 2016 Rio Olympics)—exceeds the nearly perfect arm-to-leg-to-torso ratios in Leonardo da Vinci's Vitruvian Man (refer to "Notable Achievements by European Scientists" in the book's Introduction). A typical male in his early 20s has an arm span equal to his stature, with arm span measured outstretched fingertip-to-fingertip with arms horizontal (as in the swim image) while standing against a wall. This, coupled with his large foot size and reported ability to bend his foot 15° farther at the ankle than other swimmers, turns his feet into virtual "dolphin-like flippers." The added flexibility also applies to his knees and elbows, which should theoretically increase propulsive efficiency characteristics on each complete stroke cycle. Phelps' larger upper body length compared with his relatively smaller-proportioned lower body helps to explain his superior thrust through the water at about 4.7 mph/7.56 km · h^{-1}, equivalent to a brisk walking speed.

Even if one considers the Beijing Games Water Cube (www.chinahighlights.com/beijing/attraction/water-cube.htm) the world's fastest pool (the 3-m/9.8-ft depth is the deepest allowed, and the 10 lanes apparently reduce speed-robbing turbulence), it is difficult to argue that pool characteristics explain how Phelps so convincingly demolished existing world records. A counterargument that the swimsuit Phelps wore during the Games provided the "edge" to crush these records because he wore the full-length LZR suit in only three of his eight races (200-m freestyle, the 4 × 100-m, and 4 × 200-m freestyle relays) does not seem logical. He swam without this suit in his five butterfly and individual medley contests. Phelps and his counterparts did not wear the LZR suit in the 2012 London Games because that equipment was banned from competition by the Fédération Internationale de Natation (FINA; https://abcnews.go.com/Politics/full-body-swimsuit-now-banned-professional-swimmers/story?id=9437780). Thereafter, redesigned suits were mandated to comply with new Olympic swimsuit requirements. Phelps' unique physical dimensions undoubtedly played an essential role in his extraordinary athletic achievements. His incomparable stroke mechanics were honed after practicing for thousands of hours and nearly two decades during carefully supervised, 3-hr daily in-pool workouts over 6 days weekly cumulatively covering 80 km/50 mi each week in training.

In Chapter 10, we noted that a swimmer's morphology alters the swim's horizontal lift and drag components. Selected anthropometric variables influence to what extent propulsive and resistive forces affect the swimmer's forward movement.[10,11,92] In well-trained freestyle swimmers, arm length, leg length, and hand and foot size—factors governed largely by genetic makeup—influence stroke length and stroke frequency.[23,91]

Fat-Free-to-Fat Ratio

FIGURE 29.1 compares the FFM to fat mass (FM) ratio derived from the world literature for male and female competitors in specific sports. The ratio components are based on the average body mass and percentage body fat assessed by densitometry established for each sport from world literature data. Values in the *inset tables* represent averages for body composition if the literature contained two or more citations for the sport. Male marathon runners and gymnasts have the largest FFM:FM ratios; American football offensive and defensive linemen and shot

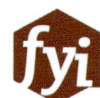

Can Genetics Predict Elite Marathon Running Performance?

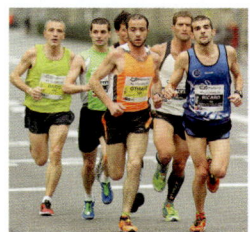

Maxisport/Shutterstock

In the last decade, researchers have sharpened their focus using new molecular techniques to better recognize the multiple genetic contributions to elite sports performance. Competitors in most sports have a well-defined physique that draws them to the sport, as for example, thinner individuals gravitate to sports that require a sustained, high rate of energy output, and larger-size competitors are drawn to sports that reward extreme power generation (i.e., weight lifting, football, discus, and shot put). Identifying the genes most likely coupled with sport success may offer advantages to training and nutritional strategies during adolescence or even earlier. A recent study assessed genomic data from 3889 elite endurance athletes (2984 marathon runners) to determine the contribution from genetic variation (polymorphisms) and genes (heredity unit transferred from a parent to offspring) that determine an offspring's characteristics to differentiate elite marathon performance from the performance of 6109 nonelite, power athletes and nonathletic controls. The researchers identified 16 possible variations in a single DNA sequence in 14 separate genes to help distinguish performance differences among the elite performers and the other athletic comparison groups. The authors concluded that this analytic strategy helps to better focus research affecting multiple gene interactions with complex endurance-related traits, particularly genes implicated in elite marathon running success.

Sources:
Bouchard C. DNA sequence variations contribute to variability in fitness and trainability. *Med Sci Sports Exerc*. 2019;51:1781.
Del Ginevičienė V, et al. Perspectives in sports genomics. *Biomedicines*. 2022; 10:298.
Lightfoot JT, et al. Systems exercise genetics research design standards. *Med Sci Sports Exerc*. 2021;53:883.
Moir HJ, et al. Genes and elite marathon running performance: a systematic review. *J Sports Sci Med*. 2019;18:559.

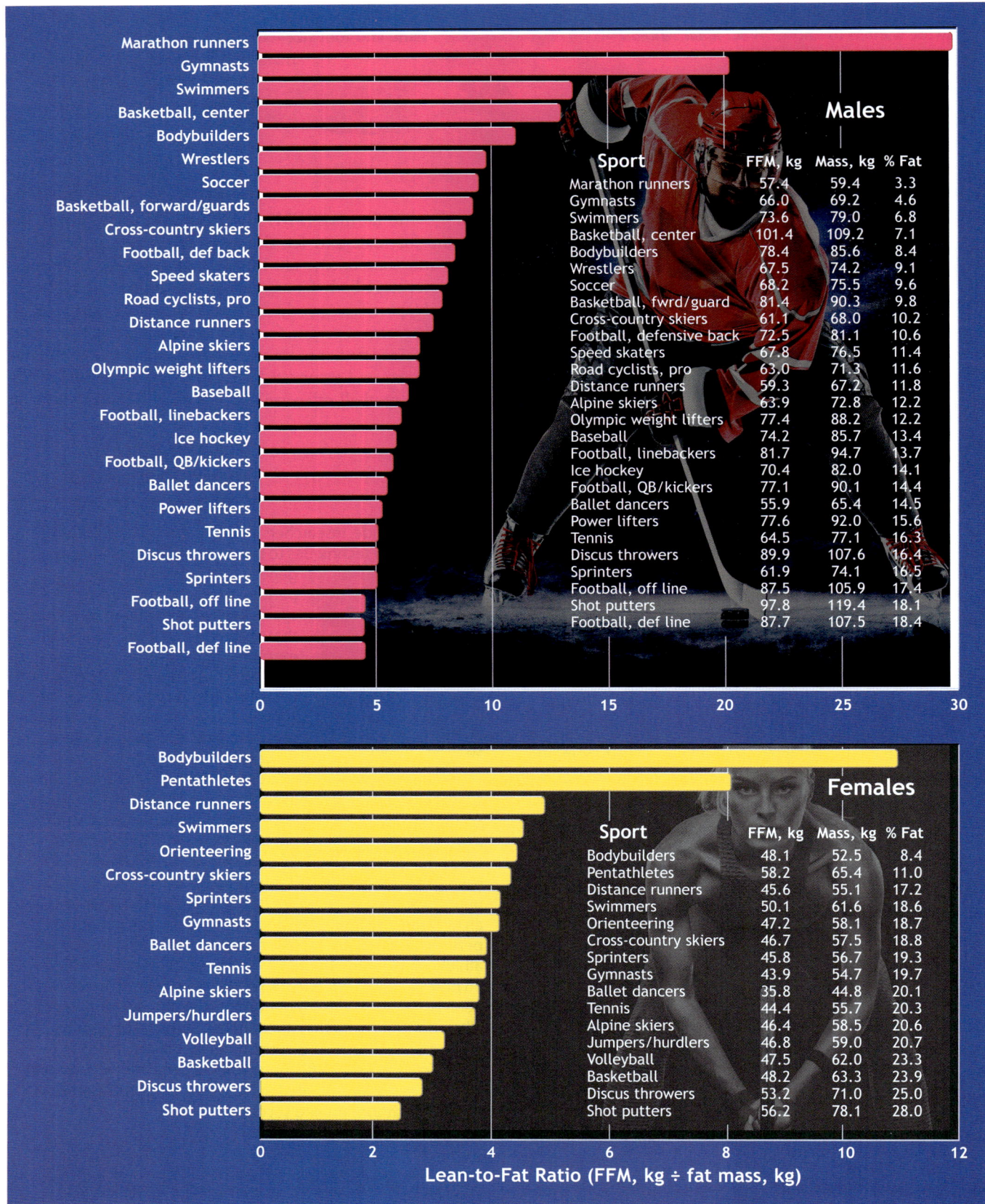

FIGURE 29.1. Fat-free mass (FFM) to fat mass (FM) ratio (FFM [kg] ÷ FM [kg]) among male and female competitors in diverse sports.
(Shutterstock background images: Mike Orlov [female], Eugene Onischenko [male])

putters show the smallest ratios. Among females, bodybuilders have the largest FFM:FM values, equal to male values, whereas the smallest FFM:FM ratios emerge for field-event participants. Female gymnasts and ballet dancers rank in the middle compared with other female sport participants.

Racial Differences

Racial differences in physique may affect athletic performance.[65,72,93] Black sprinters and high jumpers, for example, have longer limbs and narrower hips than White counterparts, but this does not mean a "true" racial advantage exists. From a mechanical perspective, a Black sprinter with leg and arm size identical to a White sprinter has a lighter, shorter, and slimmer body to propel through water. This may help to equalize a more favorable power:body mass ratio at any given body size among different racial groups and assist in establishing optimal movement-connected neural patterns coupled with well-coached training regimens involving 3- to 5-hr workouts during macrocycles lasting approximately 14 to 15 wk over a 20-year period, coupled with substantial training volume monitored by blood lactate measurements ≤ 4 mmol $\cdot$ L^{-1} and ≥ 6 mmol $\cdot$ L^{-1} at different workout intensities.[143]

Greater power output relative to body mass affords an advantage in jumping and sprint-running events, in which success depends on generating energy rapidly over brief durations, sometimes measured in seconds. The advantage diminishes in the throwing events that require propelling an absolute mass with maximum technical accuracy. Compared with Whites and Blacks, Asian athletes have short legs relative to upper torso components, a dimensional characteristic beneficial in short- and longer-distance races and in weightlifting. Successful weightlifters representing all races compared with other athletic groups have relatively short arms and legs for their stature.

The 1988 Seoul Olympics were a focal point to begin serious discussions about the obvious racial disparities evident in endurance running events because Kenya's top male runners won gold in the 800-, 1500-, and 5000-m runs and 3000-m steeplechase races.[54,75] These East African athletes from a population of 500,000 located in a highland region above the Great Rift Valley (the continuous geographic trench, approximately 6000 km/3700 mi in length that runs from northern Syria to central Mozambique in South East Africa) won almost 40% of international distance running competitions—with three times more top finishes than any other country worldwide. The Kenyans won 14 medals in the 2008 Beijing Olympic Games; in 2011, they achieved the 20 fastest marathon times. Ironically, Patrick Makau set a new 2:03:38 world record at the Berlin Marathon in September 2011 but did not make the 2012 London Olympic Games Kenyan team! From that initial "awakening" in Seoul, considerable research has focused on individual differences in physiological factors (muscle fiber type,[96] maximum oxygen uptake, fractional $\dot{V}O_{2max}$ utilization, running economy[3,24,46,51,63,76]) including genetic factors,[12,15,34,66,68,69,80] discussed in Chapter 14 to explain superior athletic accomplishments among some African and non-African groups.[94,95]

Anthropometry and Percentage Total Body Fat

Considerable literature describes anthropometric characteristics and percentage body fat levels, as well as body mass index (BMI), in male and female elite athletes in diverse sports, and also from population studies involving relationships among

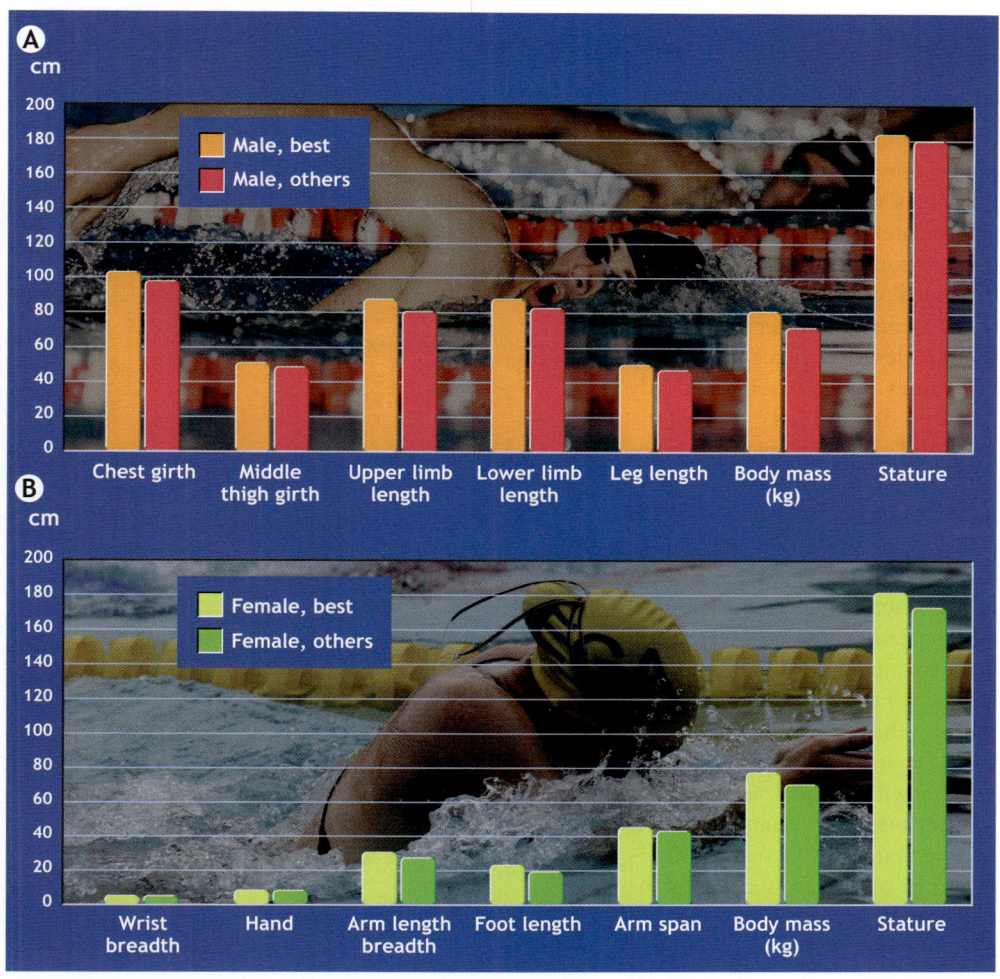

Adapted with permission from Mazza JC, et al. Absolute body size. In: Carter JE, Ackland TR, eds. *Kinanthropometry in Aquatic Sports. A Study of World-Class Athletes.* Champaign: Human Kinetics; 1994. Shutterstock background photos: Dean Drobot (male), Gert Very (female).

BMI and skinfolds and anthropometric variables reflecting variation in lean body frame size.[139–142] Body frame dimensions reflect largely trunk volume and trunk-to-limb proportions, with larger lean trunk size generally associating with greater total body fatness.

Inset image A on the previous page compares body mass, stature (last two columns), girths for the chest, upper- and lower-limbs, and leg length for 12 male swimmers rated "best" in the 200- and 400-m freestyle with less successful counterparts.[97] The measurement units in the upper and lower figures are given in cm for stature and girths and kg for body mass (multiply kg by 2.205 to convert to lb). The data in B compares selected body size variables between the 12 "best" 50-, 100-, and 200-m female breaststroke swimmers with other competitors. It is evident that the best male swimmers are heavier and taller and have larger chest, upper-arm, and thigh girths and upper- and lower-limb lengths than counterparts not ranking among the top 12. The best female breaststroke swimmers, also taller and heavier, possess larger arm span, foot and arm lengths, and hand and wrist breadths than less successful competitors.

Percentage Body Fat by Sport Category

The unnumbered figure below presents six sport activity classifications based on common characteristics and performance requirements, with percentage body fat rankings within each category for male and female participants (https://pubmed.ncbi.nlm.nih.gov/6650717/). This compendium provides percentage body fat values within a broad reasonably related sport grouping. The comparison red value for males is displayed within the yellow bars when a corresponding value exists for females. The percentage body fat values were based on body density determined hydrostatically and represent averages from the literature. The elite male athletes in the high-skill sports with the lowest body fat percentage are in alpine skiing, golf, and long jump, whereas marathon runners, as expected, have the lowest body fat percentage in the endurance category. Female power lifters and discus athletes have the highest body fat percentage, yet these values are within the "average" 25 ± 5% body fat for noncompetitive, college females (20 to 30% body fat range by densitometry). In the endurance group, female triathletes averaged 12.7% body fat, still less than the average 15% body fat (±5%) for male noncompetitive, college students.[35]

Field Event Athletes

FIGURE 29.2 displays body composition obtained by hydrostatic weighing and anthropometry—percentage body fat, FM, FFM, and lean-to-fat ratio—for the 10 top American athletes in the hammer throw, shot put, discus, javelin, and running 2 years before the 1980 Moscow Olympics. The figure includes comparative data for runners (international elite middle- and long-distance competitors with average $\dot{V}O_{2max}$ 76.9 mL·kg^{-1}·min^{-1}) and body composition data (Ref man represents values for Behnke's reference man; see Chapter 28).

Among these elite power athletes, shot putters clearly possessed the largest overall body size (body mass and girths), followed by discus, hammer, and javelin throw athletes. When these vintage data are compared with the body size for the 2000 to 2012 Olympic shot put champions and essentially the same competitors during the 2000 to 2015 World Championships, the increase in overall body size is remarkable. For example, in comparison with the 1978 shot putters, their modern Gold medal counterparts were taller by 6 cm/2.4 in. and heavier by 19 kg/41.1 lb! The current world record, established on Jan 21, 2021, by Ryan Crowser (1992–) during his 2016 Rio Olympics Gold medal–winning throw was even larger in body size (weight 145 kg/320 lb and height 200.7 cm/79 in.) compared with his competitors. These large differences in physique size over the past decades have been matched by huge 1.77-m/70-in. increases in shot put performance—essentially the equivalent for the current competitors' height!

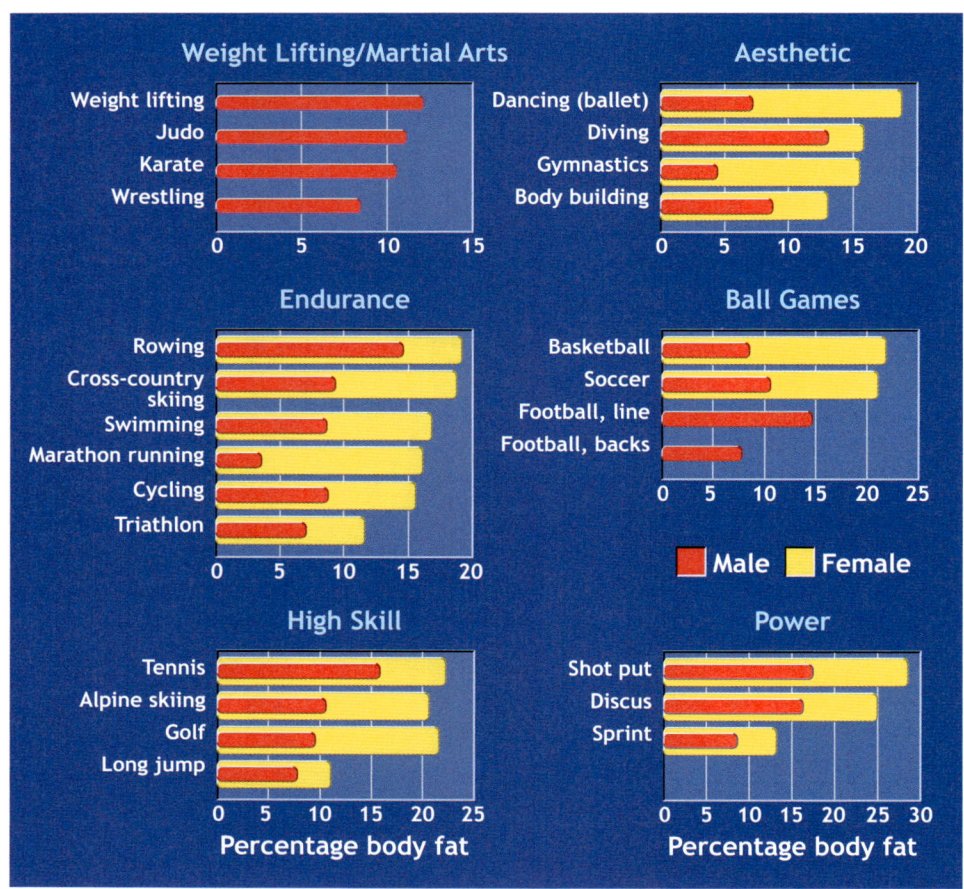

CHAPTER 29 • Physique, Performance, and Physical Activity

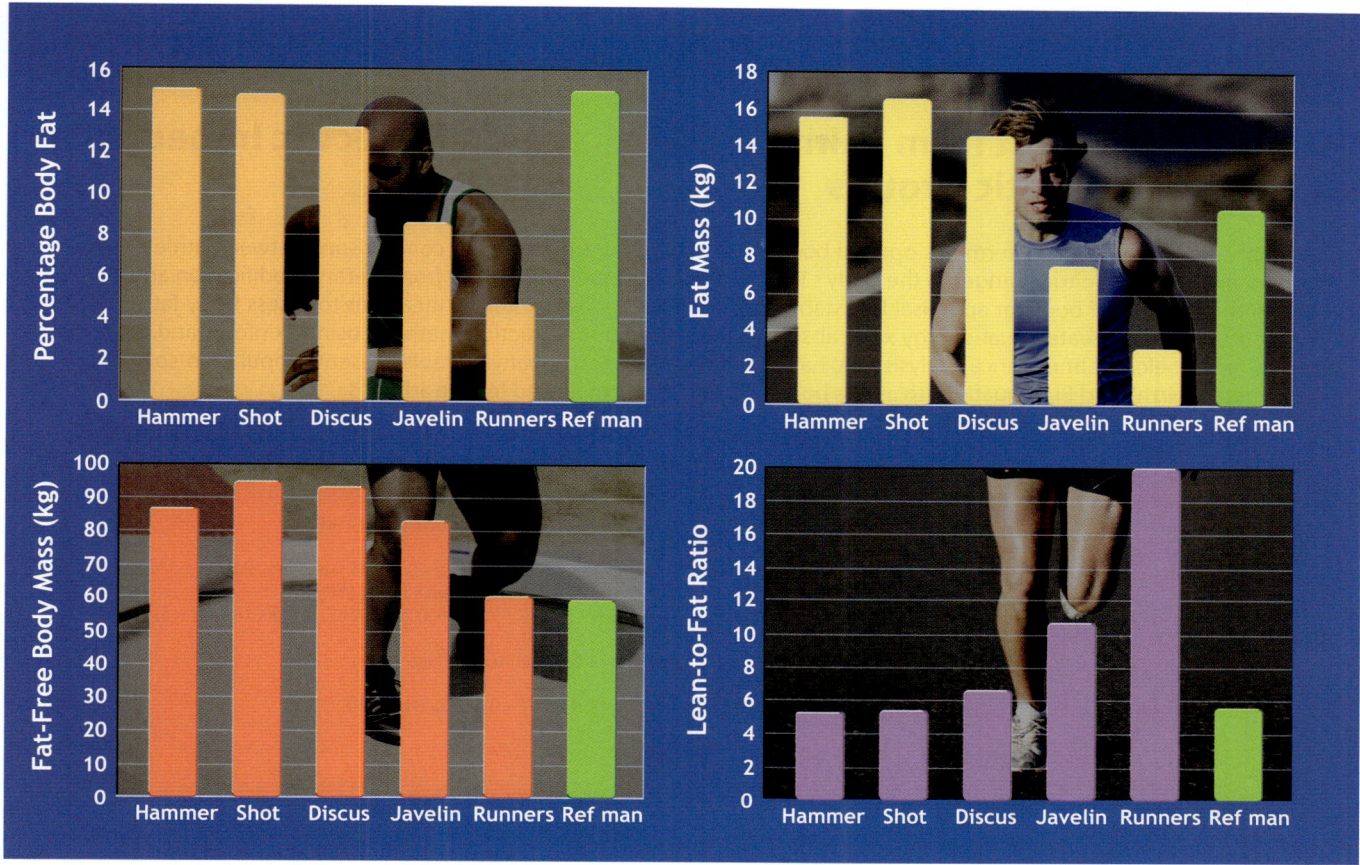

FIGURE 29.2. Body composition for the top 10 American male athletes in the hammer throw, shot put, discus, javelin, and running determined by hydrostatic weighing. (Shutterstock background images: sirtravelalot [discus thrower], Maridav [runner])

When East German Udo Beyer (1955–) won the shot put in the 1976 Montreal Olympics, he weighed "only" 135.2 kg/298 lb at 195.6 cm/77 in tall. His winning 21.05-m/69.1-ft performance would not even have placed among the top 15 competitors at the men's 2020 outdoor world championships (www.worldathletics.org/records/toplists/throws/shot-put/outdoor/men/senior)!

Mac Wilkins (1950–), an elite discus throw athlete who participated in the 1978 Olympic mini-camp (Fig. 29.2), was the first American to break the 70-m/230-ft barrier and won the 1976 Montréal Olympic Gold medal with a 67.51-m/221.5-ft throw (www.youtube.com/watch?v=8VQ8uy1Vsa4). By today's standards, Wilkins was relatively short at 1.93 m/76 in. and weighed "only" 115 kg/254 lb. His throwing competitor, John Powell (1947–), also participated in the mini-camp study and was a discus superstar. He finished fourth at the 1972 Munich Olympics and won bronze at both the 1976 Montreal and 1984 Los Angeles Olympics. When he established the world record in 1975 (69.08 m/227 ft), he weighed 110 kg/243 lb and was 188 cm/74 in. tall. Clearly, Wilkins, Powell, and Dr. Tom Fahey, four-time discus gold medal winner in consecutive Master's World Games, were relatively large in body size with low body fat for that era, but they and their contemporaries pale in comparative size to today's elite power field-event athletes. **TABLE 29.1** presents skinfold and girth data for the mini-camp athletes described in Figure 29.2. The next-generation exercise scientist will include genomic mapping to track superstar-athletes' progress to determine the key underlying physiological and neuromuscular factors that explain their elite performance accomplishments.

TABLE 29.1 Skinfold and girth data for the mini-camp athletes and world-class runners and Behnke's reference man

Unique Body Composition Comparisons Among Olympic Male Sprint, Distance, Marathon, and Decathlon Olympians

The 2012 London Olympics presented a unique research opportunity to measure physique status among elite male sprint, distance, marathon, and decathlon competitors for BMI, calculated lean body mass (LBM), and percentage body fat. We have made several comparisons for weight

Photo: F. Katch

In a Practical Sense

Predicting Body Fat from Skinfolds, Girths, and Bioelectric Impedance for Different Athletic Groups

Body composition assessment determines optimal body weight for competition, allows comparisons between athletes within the same sport, and helps monitor changes in the body's lean and fat components resulting from dietary modification and/or exercise training. In the absence of body fat appraisal by established, valid noncadaver criterion measures to assess body fat content (e.g., densitometry, total body water, dual-energy x-ray absorptiometry), various prediction methods using skinfolds and/or girth measurements, and bioelectric impedance analysis (BIA) have been used. The accompanying table presents population-specific skinfold, anthropometric (girth), and BIA equations to assess body composition in male and female athletes.

Method	Sport	Gender	Equation	Reference
Skinfolds	All	Females (18–29 yr)	D_b (g · cm^{-3})^a = 1.096095 − 0.0006952 (Σ4SKF)^b + 0.0000011 (Σ4SKF)^2 − 0.0000714 (age)	32
	All	Males (14–19 yr)	D_b (g · cm^{-3})^a = 1.10647 − 0.00162 (subscapular SKF) − 0.00144 (abdomen SKF) − 0.00077 (triceps SKF) + 0.00071 (midaxillary SKF)	20
	All	Males (18–29 yr)	D_b (g · cm^{-3})^a = 1.112 − 0.00043499 (Σ7SKF)^c + 0.00000055 (Σ7SKF) − 0.00028826 (age)	31
	All	Males and females	%BF = 10.566 + 0.12077 (7SKF)^d − 8.057 (gender) − 2.545 (race)	16
	Wrestling	Males (HS)	D_b (g · cm^{-3})^a = 1.0982 − 0.000815 (Σ3SKF) − 0.00000084 (Σ3SKF)^2	67
BIA	All	Females (NR)	FFM (kg) = 0.73 (HT^2/R) + 0.23 (X_c) + 0.16 (BW) + 2.0	30
	All	Females (college)	FFM (kg) = 0.73 (HT^2/R) + 0.116 (BW) + 0.096 (X_c) − 4.03	49
	All	Males (college)	FFM (kg) = 0.734 (HT^2/R) + 0.116 (BW) + 0.096 (X_c) − 3.152	49
	All	Males (19–40 yr)	FFM (kg) = 1.949 + 0.701 (BW) + 0.186 (HT^2/R)	55
Girths	All	Females (18–23 yr)	FFM (kg) = 0.757 (BW) + 0.981 (neck C) − 0.516 (thigh C) + 0.79	53
	Ballet	Females (11–25 yr)	FFM (kg) = 0.73 (BW) + 3.0	26
	Wrestling	Males (13–18 yr)	D_b (g · cm^{-3})^a = 1.12691 − 0.00357 (arm C) − 0.00127 (AB C) + 0.00524 (forearm C)	35
	Football	White males (18–23 yr)	%BF = 55.2 + 0.481 (BW) − 0.468 (HT)	29

^{a}Use the following formulas to convert body density (D_b) to % body fat (BF): Males %BF = [(4.95/D_b) − 4.50] × 100; Females %BF = [(5.01/D_b) − 4.57] × 100; Males (7–12 yr) %BF = [(5.30/D_b) − 4.89] × 100; Males (13–16 yr) %BF = [(5.07/D_b) − 4.64] × 100; Males (17–19 yr) %BF = [(4.99/D_b) − 4.55] × 100.
^{b}4SKF (mm) = sum of four skinfolds: triceps + anterior suprailiac + abdomen + thigh.
^{c}7SKF (mm) = sum of seven skinfolds: chest + midaxillary + triceps + subscapular + abdomen + anterior suprailiac + thigh.
^{d}7SKF (mm) = subscapular + triceps + chest + midaxillary + suprailiac + abdominal + thigh; gender = 0 for female, 1 for male; race = 0 for White, 1 for Black.
^{e}HT, height (cm); BIA, bioelectric impedance analysis; R, resistance (Ω); X_c, reactance (Ω); BW, body weight (kg); FFM, fat-free mass; C, girth (cm) [measured for the thigh at the gluteal fold]; AB C (cm), average abdominal girth [(AB1 + AB2)/2], where AB1 (cm), abdominal girth anteriorly midway between the xyphoid process of the sternum and umbilicus, and laterally between the lower end of the rib cage and iliac crests, and AB2 (cm), abdominal girth at the umbilicus level; NR, age not reported; HS, high school.

Adapted with permission Heyward VH, Stolarczyk LM. *Applied Body Composition Assessment*. Champaign: Human Kinetics, 1996.

CALCULATION EXAMPLE

Boy Athlete (age 18)

Data: Subscapular (SS) skinfold (SKF): 10 mm; abdominal (AB) SKF: 18 mm; triceps (TRI) SKF: 10 mm; midaxillary (MA) SKF: 8 mm; %BF = percent body fat

D_b = 1.10647 − (0.00162 × SS$_{SKF}$) − (0.00144 × AB$_{SKF}$) − (0.00077 × TRI$_{SKF}$) + (0.00071 × MA$_{SKF}$)
= 1.10647 − (0.00162 × 10) − (0.00144 × 18) − (0.00077 × 10) + (0.00071 × 8)
= 1.10647 − 0.0162 − 0.02592 − 0.0077 + 0.00568
= 1.06233

%BF = [(499 ÷ D_b) − 455]
= [(499 ÷ 1.06233) − 455]
= 14.7%

Event[a]	Height (cm)	Weight (kg)	BMI	LBM[b] (kg)	% Body Fat[c]
Sprint[d]					
London	184.9	79.3	23.20	69.7	12.1
Tokyo, Mexico City	176.9	70.3	22.46	63.8	9.2
Distance[e]					
London	171.9	62.8	20.17	60.3	4.0
Tokyo, Mexico City	172.8	61.1	20.47	60.9	3.3
Marathon					
London	172.2	58.3	19.66	60.5	NA[f]
Tokyo, Mexico City	169.5	58.7	20.43	58.6	1.7
Decathlon					
London	188.0	87.0	24.62	72.1	7.5
Tokyo, Mexico City	182.3	80.5	24.23	67.8	15.8

[a]Top 8 finishers, 2012 London Olympics.
[b]Calculated by Behnke's method: LBM = $h^2 \times 0.204$, where h = stature, dm (from reference 2).
[c]Body fat (%) = (body mass − LBM)/body mass × 100.
[d]Sprint athletes included 100 m, 200 m, 4 × 100 m, 110-m hurdles.
[e]Distance athletes included 3000 steeplechase, 5000 m, 10,000 m.
[f]Could not compute because average body mass lower than calculated LBM.
BMI, body mass index; LBM, lean body mass; NA, not applicable.

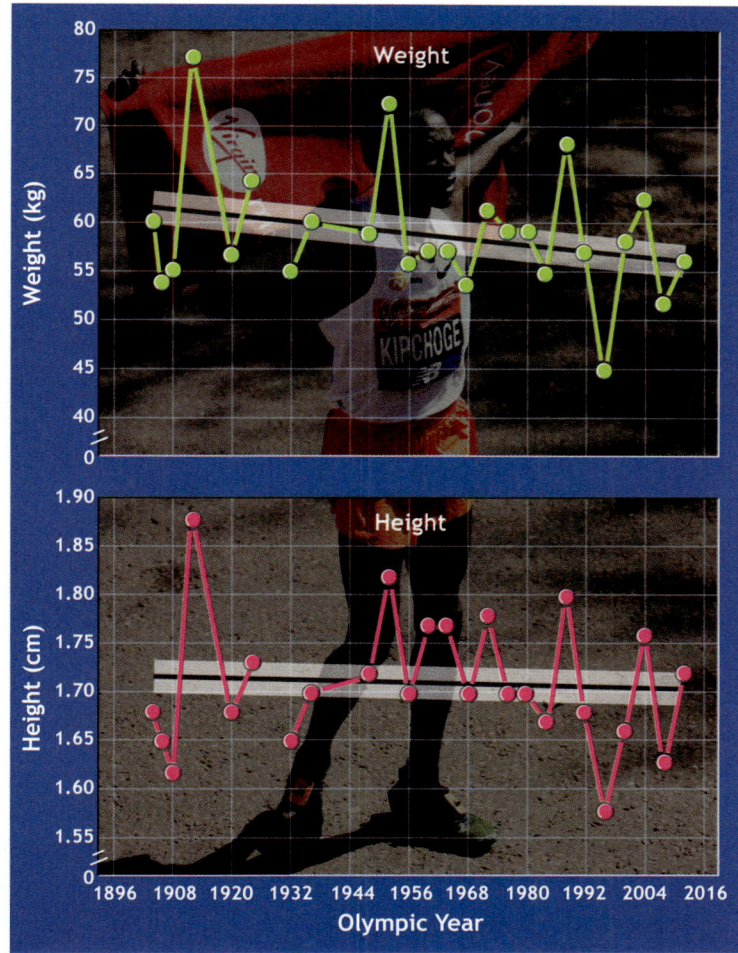

Background photo: Keith Larby/Shutterstock

and height between an Olympic marathoner from 1904 and the latest 2016 Rio Olympic gold medalist from numerous data sets in the literature.[14,99–104] As shown in the inset table, the London, Tokyo, and Mexico City comparisons, Behnke's method was used to compute LBM using the equation, $h^2 \times 0.204$, where h = stature, dm, and body fat (%) = (body mass − LBM) ÷ body mass × 100. The remarkable findings include the extremely low BMIs (19.7 to 20.2) for distance and marathon runners and the similarity in BMI among the 1964 to 1968 and 2012 athletes.

The 2012 sprint athletes were slightly more than 8 cm/3 in. taller and almost 9 kg/22 lb heavier than the prior year Olympians (and 5.9 kg/13 lb heavier in LBM). Marathoners from both eras were nearly identical in all body size comparisons. The most apparent differences in physique among the 2012 decathletes versus sprinters and earlier counterparts were the 2012 sprinters' larger body mass, stature, and LBM. The London 2012 distance runners, for example, were the shortest athletes (171.9 cm/67.7 in.), whereas marathoners had the lowest (58.3-kg/128.6-lb) body mass.

As a further comparison among elite competitors, the 1904 USA marathon champion, who was the first marathoner with documented height and weight measurements (Thomas Hicks [time 3:28:53], 168-cm/66.1-in. height; 60-kg/132-lb weight), was about the same height but weighed more than the 2016 Rio Olympic gold medal winner Kenyan Eliud Kipchoge (1984–), who weighed 56 kg/124 lb and was 166 cm/65.4 in. tall (winning time, 2:08:44). The two inset figures show the trends in body weight and height for Olympic marathon champions from 1904 through 2016. The 1996 gold medalist from South Africa, Josia Thugwane, had the lowest body weight (45 kg/99 lb) among all gold medal marathoners, about 14 kg/30 lb less than the average weight for Olympic first-place finishers over nearly the last century.

Female Endurance Athletes

The unnumbered figure and table on the next page present the body mass, stature, and body composition for 11 female long-distance runners who had achieved national and international status.[78] The first three runners had established records for the marathon and 50-mi endurance runs, including National championships in cross-country running. The runners averaged 15.2% body fat (hydrostatic weighing), similar to reported data for high school cross-country runners but considerably lower than the 26% body fat for the same age sedentary females.[2,35] Compared with other athletic groups internationally,[104,106] female endurance runners are relatively

Subject	Age (y)	Sature (cm)	Mass(kg)	FFM (kg)	Body fat kg	Body fat %
1	24	172.7	52.6	49.5	3.1	5.9
2	26	159.8	71.5	46.2	25.3	35.4
3	28	162.6	50.7	47.6	3.1	6.1
4	31	171.5	52.0	47.3	4.7	9.0
5	33	176.5	61.2	50.8	10.4	17.0
6	34	166.4	52.9	44.8	8.1	15.2
7	35	168.4	55.0	48.7	6.3	11.6
8	36	164.5	53.1	44.3	8.8	16.6
9	36	182.9	61.5	50.4	11.1	18.1
10	36	182.9	65.4	55.7	9.7	14.8
11	37	154.9	53.6	44.0	9.6	18.0
Average	32.4	169.4	57.2	48.1	9.1	15.2

Adapted with permission from Wilmore JH, Brown CH. Physiological profiles of women distance runners. *Med Sci Sports.* 1974;6:178. Background photo: Hans Christiansson/Shutterstock.

lean and with less body fat than female collegiate basketball players (20.9%),[67] gymnasts (15.5%),[62] younger distance runners (18%),[43] swimmers (20.1%),[37] tennis players (22.8%),[37] or triathletes.[28,107]

In this research, the runners' average body fat equaled the 15% value generally reported for nonathletic males. The 6 to 9% body fat levels for several apparently healthy runners fall within the range for topflight male endurance athletes. The leanest females in the population based on Behnke's reference standard[2] have essential fat equal to 12 to 14% body mass. This apparent discrepancy between estimated fat content for distance runners and the theoretical lower limit for female's body fat requires further study. Note the relatively high 35.4% body fat for a top runner, suggesting that at least for this runner, other factors override the "dead weight" and thermoregulatory limitations to distance running excess fat imposes.

Male Endurance Athletes

TABLE 29.2 presents body composition data for 10 male elite middle- and long-distance runners and eight elite marathoners.[98] The group included Steve Prefontaine, former American record holder in the 800- and 1500-m runs, and Frank Shorter, the 1976 Olympic marathon gold medalist. A representative sample for 95 untrained college-age males provides the comparison as controls. Both groups of runners have extremely low body fat values considering that essential fat theoretically constitutes about 3% body mass. Clearly, these competitors represent the lowest end along the lean-to-fat continuum representing topflight endurance athletes. These remarkable data mirrored by more recent studies based on anthropometry[108] confirm the importance for heat dissipation and low body fat during endurance runs, from marathons to multiple-day 100-mi challenges.[41,42,109]

TABLE 29.2 Body composition for male elite middle- and long-distance runners

For body dimensions and structure, male distance runners generally have smaller girths and bone diameters than untrained males.[13] Structural differences, particularly bone diameters, reflect a genetic influence similar to the distinct anthropometric characteristics typical in world-class aquatic athletes.[5] The best long-distance runners inherit a slight build with well-proportioned skeletal dimensions. *The prime ingredients for a champion include a genetically optimal physique profile blended with a lean body composition, highly developed aerobic system, optimal distribution in muscle fiber architecture, and proper psychologic mindset for protracted intense training.* Interestingly, the body size and composition (lower limb lengths, skinfold thicknesses, extremity circumference, skeletal muscle mass, BMI, and percentage body fat) and training volume (weekly training hours, running years, completed marathons) in male Caucasian ultraendurance runners are not as important to predict performance in a 24-hr endurance race as their personal best marathon time.[25,40,105]

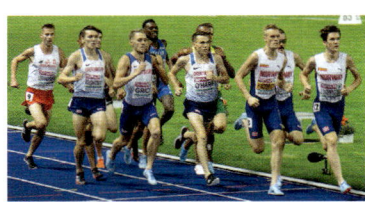

Alfaguarilla/Shutterstock

IQ? INTEGRATIVE QUESTION

What are the physiologic and anthropometric characteristics necessary for successful endurance running performance?

Triathletes. The triathlon combines continuous endurance swimming, bicycling, and running. The extreme triathlon, the ultra-endurance Ironman competition, requires competitors to first swim 3.9 km/2.4 mi, then bicycle 180.2 km/112 mi, and finish with a standard 42.2-km/26.2-mi marathon run. The 2021 Kona Ironman Hawaii current course record was set in 2019 by German Jan Frodeno (1981–; body mass 74.8 kg/165 lb; stature 193 cm/76 in.), whose winning time was 7 hr:51 min:13 s.

In 2021, the women's course record was 8 hr:26 min:18 s, set in 2018 by four-time Swiss National Triathlon Champion, two-time 2008 and 2012 Olympic triathlon competitor, and 2021 Dubai Ironman champion Daniela Ryf (1987–; 63-kg/139-lb weight; 175.3-cm/69-in. height). Ryf, a leader in laboratory sports training and testing, utilizes velodrome and wind-tunnel modeling to optimize racing bicycle performance, which includes attention to helmet, racing suit, and water bottle design (www.youtube.com/watch?v=SZD7zkov6tA). Sophisticated wind tunnel experiments provide an ideal testing venue also used by

fyi Serial Body Composition Changes by Densitometry on Dr. A.R. Behnke with Aging (1940–1977)

Dr. A. R. Behnke was a pioneer researcher who made fundamental contributions in body composition measurement: he created the Reference Male and Female (see Chapter 28), determined that overweight does not correlate with obesity for those with large lean body weight, and developed the Body Profile system we discuss in this chapter. He was measured four times during 1940 at ages 36 and 37 as a young Naval medical physician. He then volunteered for long-term densitometry (specific gravity) measurements over the next 37 years through age 74. This paved the way as preparation to measure NFL football players by the underwater weighing technique using a similar experimental procedure shown in the background figure. Although his body weight fluctuated somewhat from ages 36 to 37 through age 64, it returned to about the same initial weight range at ages 69 to 74. During his younger years, he was able to maintain his lean body weight until it steadily declined (with accompanying increases in percentage body fat). At age 55, his type 2 diabetes diagnosis coincided with a large increase in body weight and body fat. Thereafter, it began to stabilize, partly from his meticulous adherence to a 7-day weekly activity program he called "arm aerobics" by walking 2 to 4 city blocks near his home in San Francisco scooping up gutter trash with a large shovel!

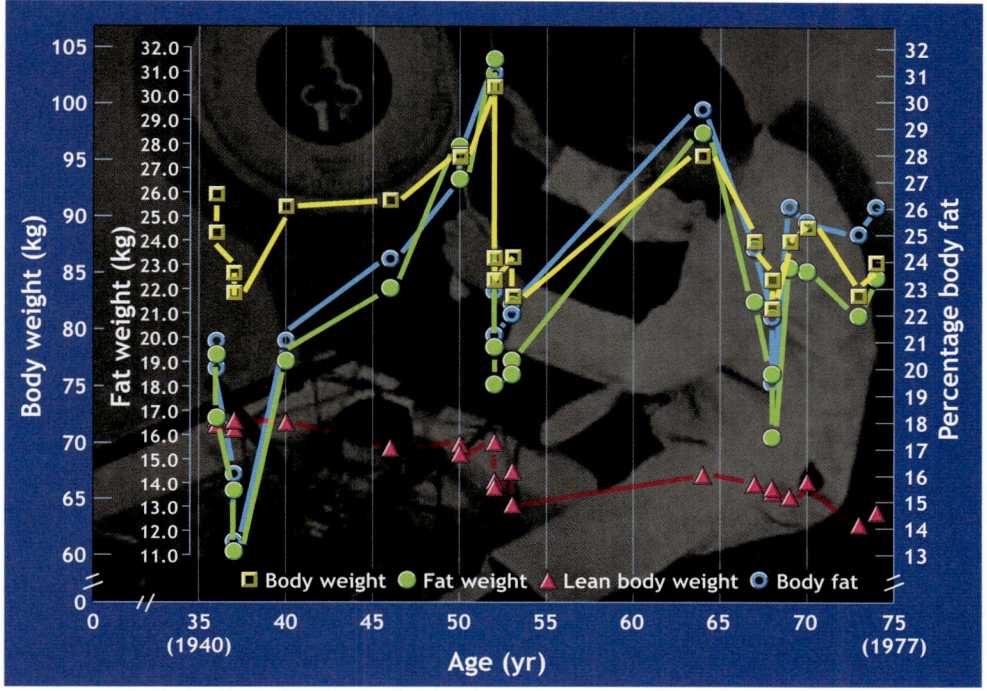

Data courtesy Dr. Tom Fahey (fortiuspress.com), provided by Dr. Behnke.

automobile manufacturers and NASA (www.grc.nasa.gov/www/k-12/WindTunnel/Activities/Drgstr_cars_inwndtun.html). Air is pushed over the object inside the tunnel at various speeds and intervals. Specialized instrumentation captures the pressures impacting the object, gathers crucial information about surface airflow over the object to determine the least and maximum resistance to airflow, and directly measures forces, torques, center of pressure, and moments on the rider with the equipment inside the tunnel. The serious triathlete's daily training averages over 4 hr (30 hr weekly), covering 451 km·wk^{-1}/280 mi·wk^{-1} by swimming 11.6 km/7.2 mi, equal to about a 30:00 min/km/pace, bicycling 227 mi/365.3km(18.6mph), and running 72.4 km/45 mi (a 7:42 min/km/pace).[55] Percentage body fat for six male and three female participants in the 1982 Ironman triathlon ranged between 5.0 and 11.3% for males and 7.4 and 17.2% for females. Body fat averaged 7.1% for the top 15 male finishers, with corresponding 72.0 mL·kg^{-1}·min^{-1} $\dot{V}O_{2max}$. In subsequent research, body fat was unrelated to training volume for both males (14.4% fat) and females (22.8% fat).[41] The authors concluded that a runner's body fat correlated poorly to total triathlon race time. A follow-up study showed that low body fat levels and large training volume benefited ultra-endurance triathletes in cycling and running, whereas cycling speed in training benefited total race time.[42] Triathletes' body fat content and aerobic capacity are comparable to other athletes in single endurance sports,[57] with a physique most closely resembling elite cyclists[56] or swimmers[47] but not runners. Their aerobic capacity

Rocksweeper/Shutterstock

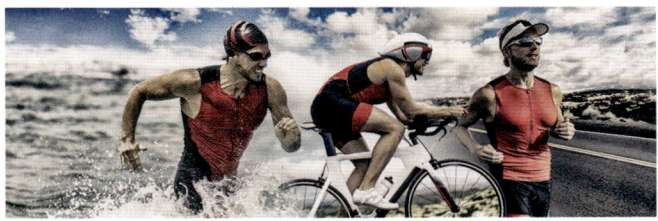

Maridav/Shutterstock

during swimming consistently averaged below treadmill running or stationary cycling values.[44,110,111] Significant reductions occurred in percentage body fat and skeletal muscle mass[1] following one ultraendurance event completed within 58 hr, in which athletes swam 11.6 km/7.2 mi, cycled 540 km/336 mi, and ran 126.6 km/78.7 mi.

A longitudinal study evaluated how a triathlon season affected bone dynamics and hormonal status in seven male competitive triathletes at the beginning and 32 wk after training.[50] Dual-energy x-ray absorptiometry assessed total and regional bone mineral density (BMD) and specific biochemical markers assessed bone turnover. The triathlon season had a small but favorable effect on BMD at the lumbar spine and skull, but no effect on total body or proximal femur BMD; no changes occurred in hormonal levels. For nine professional cyclists who participated in the Italian Giro d'Italia 3-wk stage race (www.giroditalia.it/en/), markers of bone activity measured 1 day pre-race and 12 and 22 days during the race indicated bone resorption had occurred.[48]

Swimmers Versus Runners

Male and female competitive swimmers generally have higher body fat levels than distance runners, despite swim training's considerable energy requirement. The training environment's cool water generally produces lower core temperatures than equivalent land exercise. Speculation exists that a lower core temperature in swim training may prevent depressed appetite often accompanying intense land training.

Limited evidence indicates similar daily energy intake for male collegiate swimmers (3380 kcal) and distance runners (3460 kcal), which balances training energy expenditure. In contrast, female swimmers averaged a higher daily energy intake (2490 kcal) compared with that of running counterparts (2040 kcal).[33] Swimmers had higher estimated daily energy expenditure than runners. The swimmers' energy expenditure surpassed energy intake, placing them in a slightly *negative* energy balance. A *positive* energy balance with intake greater than output cannot explain typically higher body fat levels in male (12% fat) and female (20% fat) swimmers than in male (7% fat) and female (15% fat) runners. Subsequent research from the same laboratory evaluated swimmers' and runners' energy expenditure and fuel use during their training (45 min at 75 to 80% $\dot{V}O_{2max}$ and 2 hr of recovery).[19] The hypothesis assumed that differences between the two activity modes in hormonal response and substrate catabolism accounted for the body fat differences between groups. The small between-group differences in energy expenditure, substrate use, and hormone levels could not explain differences in body fat levels.

American Football Players

The first detailed body composition analyses in American professional football players from the early 1940s demonstrated the inadequacy to determine a player's optimal body mass from height-weight standards.[74] The player's body fat content averaged only 10.4% body mass, whereas FFM averaged 81.3 kg/179 lb. These males certainly were heavy but not "fat." The heaviest lineman weighed 118 kg/260 lb (17.4% body fat; 97.7 kg FFM), whereas the lineman with the most body fat (23.2%) weighed 115.4 kg/254 lb. Body mass in a defensive back with the least fat (3.3%) was 82.3 kg/181 lb, with FFM of 79.6 kg/175 lb.

Collegiate Versus Professional Players

TABLE 29.3 presents average values for body mass, stature, percentage body fat, and FFM in college and professional football players grouped by position.[77,79]

> **TABLE 29.3** Body composition compared among collegiate and professional American football players grouped by position

The *Pro, older* group included 25 players from the 1942 Washington Redskins, the first professional players as a group measured hydrostatically for body composition.[2,74] The *Pro, modern* group represented 164 players from 14 teams in the National Football League (NFL; 69% veterans, 31% rookies). One hundred and seven 1976 to 1978 Dallas Cowboys and New York Jets players were in the third group. Four collegiate player groups included candidates for spring practice at St. Cloud State College in Minnesota, the University of Massachusetts (U Mass), Division III Gettysburg College, and teams from 1973 to 1977 University of Southern California (USC) national champion participants in two Rose Bowls. These data were selected because the body composition measurements among the different player groups all featured the criterion hydrostatic weighing with residual lung volume correction to obtain the most valid body fat percentage and FFM determinations deemed essential, as explained in Chapter 28. The body composition comparisons are unique because they were constrained to a single sport and sex, where variability among the collegiate players is relatively large due mainly to body size differences,[112,113] segmental body parameter differences,[114] and ponderal Somatogram analysis by position.[64,115,116] In contrast, professional players represented a highly targeted group with superior physical performance abilities that selected them into the professional level.

One would generally expect modern-day professional players to have a larger body size at each position than a representative collegiate group. This occurred for comparisons with St. Cloud and U Mass players, but the USC players exhibited physique's similar to modern professional players. Except for defensive linemen, the USC players at each position showed nearly the same body fat content as current professionals but they weighed less. For FFM, the USC players weighed no more than 4.4 kg/9.6 lb less than professionals at each position. The average defensive lineman in the NFL outweighed his USC counterpart in FFM by only 1.8 kg/4 lb. Total body mass for the professional linemen exceeded the USC players, primarily because the professionals possessed 18.2% body fat versus the collegians' 14.7%. These data suggest that in general, elite college and professional players have similar body size and body composition.

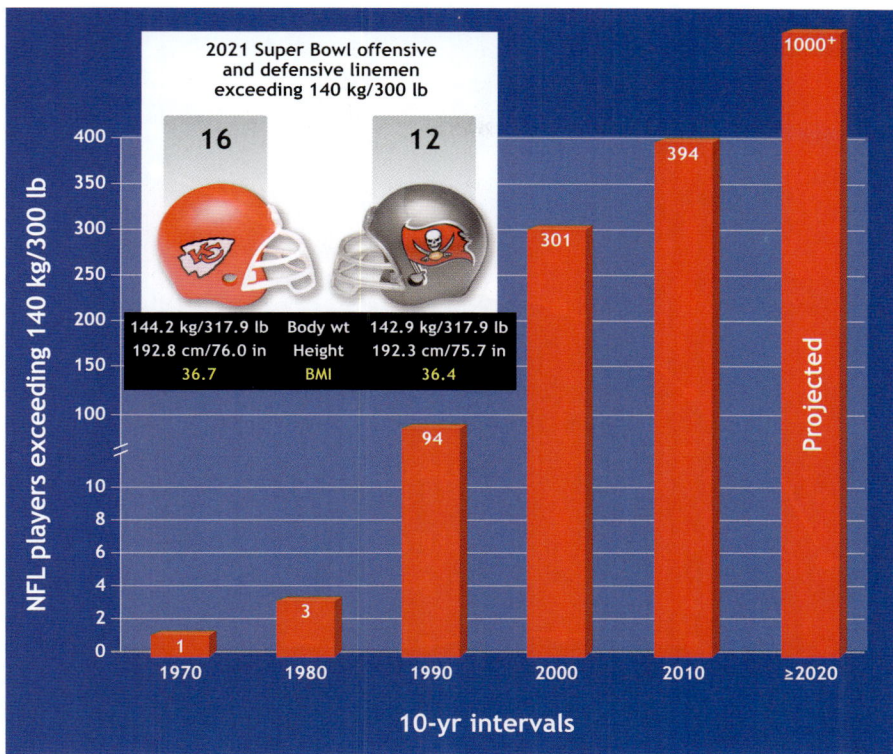

As a group, professional players from almost 80 years ago were lower in body fat and shorter and had lower total body mass and FFM than professionals four decades ago compared to today's players. The exceptions, defensive and offensive backs and receivers, were almost identical to 2021 players in body size and composition. The biggest differences in physique emerged for the defensive linemen; modern players were 6.7 cm/2.6 in. taller, 20 kg/44 lb heavier, and fatter by 4.2 percentage points and had 12.3 kg/27.1 lb more FFM. Obviously, "bigness" was not as important a factor in line play during the 1940s as it became 50 years later.

FIGURE 29.3 shows the average body weights for all roster players in the NFL (n = 51,333) over a 76-year period.[36] From 1920 to 1985, offensive linemen were the heaviest, but this changed beginning with the 1990 season, when defensive linemen achieved the same body weight as offensive linemen and then surpassed them in subsequent years. Whereas the body weight for offensive linemen appeared to level off at nearly 127 kg/280 lb, defensive linemen continued to increase in body weight, particularly from 1990 through 1996. At this time, they weighed an average 7.3 kg/16 lb more, or double the weight gain for offensive linemen in the comparable period. On average, offensive linemen were 0.6 kg/1.3 lb heavier yearly from 1920 to 1996. In Figure 29.3B, the body weight for the offensive and defensive linemen on each NFL team during the 1994 season ranged from heaviest (Kansas City Chiefs; Super Bowl 1970) to lightest (San Francisco 49ers; Super Bowls 1990 and 1995). For the 1994 season, the average body weight for the winning Dallas Cowboys Super Bowl offensive line ranked fifth highest among 28 teams. In the year's prior Super Bowl, 36 players exceeded 300 lb (20 for the 49er's and 20 for the victorious Ravens). These examples project that the typical lineman will weigh 152 kg/335 lb by the year 2025 (at an average 205.7-cm/6 ft 9-in. height) if the weight gain trend continues through this decade! The prediction almost occurred 3 years earlier than expected for the 2021 Super Bowl contestants (see next section). The BMI surely will soon exceed 36.0 for the first time, catapulting every 300-lb NFL offensive and defensive lineman into the *very high* disease risk obesity II category (www.ncbi.nlm.nih.gov/books/NBK541070/).

Body Size Differences Between the 2021 Super Bowl Kansas City Chiefs and Tampa Bay Buccaneers. The inset image depicts the body size differences for offensive and defensive linemen between the 2021 Super Bowl Kansas City Chiefs and Tampa Bay Buccaneers. For the Chiefs, BMI averaged 36.7 (body mass 144.2 kg/317.9 lb; stature 192.8 cm/76 in.). Eight Chiefs' linemen exceeded 145 kg/320 lb; for the Buccaneers, four players weighed more than 145 kg/320 lb. There is no reason to believe that these results for body weight will be curtailed in the near future. Research must determine whether such relatively homogeneous elite, "*overweight*" athletes experience greater morbidity and mortality than normal-weight, non-pro football peers. This was evident by players exceeding 300 lb in 10-yr intervals from 1970 to 2021 (numbers at the top in each column in the figure); the extreme right column predicts that if the increase in the number of 136.1-kg/300-lb players continues as it did from 1970 to 2021 (there were 497 players on 32 teams who exceeded 145 kg/320 lb in 2021), then players who exceed 145 kg/320 lb should increase by 3 to 5% in each of the four seasons to Super Bowl LIX in 2025! This would bring the total to between 560 and 604 players who exceed 145 kg/320 lb with two top 2022 draft players near 400 lb!

Worrisome Trend Even Among Less Skilled and Younger Players. Exceptionally high BMIs also occur at less elite collegiate-level competition. The average 33.1 BMI for the Division III 1999 Gettysburg College offensive line (n = 15; BMI 29.9 for year 2000 offensive line, n = 13)[64] and 31.7 BMI for other NCAA Division III American football linemen[129] (n = 26; 1994–1995) raise similar concern about potential health risks (e.g., high blood pressure, insulin resistance, and type 2 diabetes) for such large young males (stature 1.84 m/72.4 in.; body mass 107.2 kg/236 lb), and longer-term medical outlook remains undetermined but not encouraging.[59,127] At the high school level, the BMI for *Parade* magazine's All-American football teams increased dramatically beginning in the early 1970s

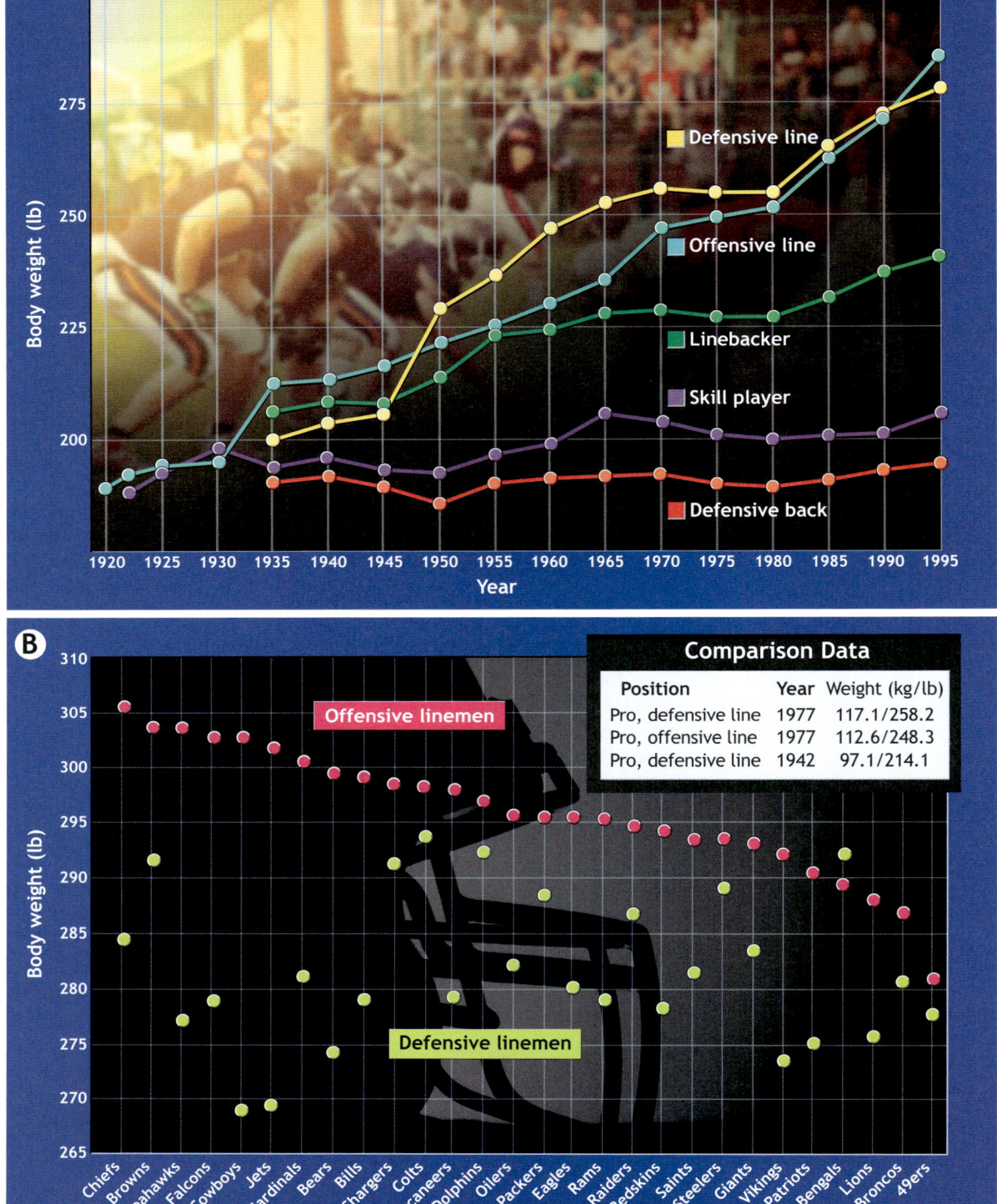

FIGURE 29.3. **(A)** Average body weight by position for all roster players in the NFL between 1920 and 1995. **(B)** Average body weight for all NFL 1994 roster offensive and defensive linemen.
(Data for Pro offensive and defensive line shown in the *inset box* are combined for the New York Jets and Dallas Cowboys football teams (measured by textbook authors FK and VK), and 1942 data are from the NFL Washington Redskins team, as discussed in Welham WC, Behnke AR. The specific gravity of healthy men. *JAMA*. 1942;118:498. Shutterstock background images: Melinda Nagy **[A]**, RONORMANJR **[B]**.)

through 1989 and then further increased through the year 2020.[73,117] A plot at 5-year intervals in the image below shows a clear shift at 1972 in the regression line slope (first *yellow line*) relating BMI to competition year compared with age-matched individuals from large-scale epidemiologic normative data (*red line*). This shift toward a higher BMI coincided with either improved nutrition and training and/or the emerging prevalence among high school athletes and performance-enhancing drugs (chiefly anabolic steroids).[4] Particularly disturbing are the 2016 data for nine high-school offensive and defensive linemen who on average increased BMI to 36.3 in 2010 (stature 194.7 cm/72.5 in.; body mass 137.6 kg/304.4 lb). While stature remained essentially unchanged over this 6-year period, body mass increased by 7.7 kg/17 lb. During that approximately 20-year time interval, the BMI for the elite high school players has increased dramatically and now is approaching the BMI values for the 2021 Kansas City Chiefs and Tampa Bay Buccaneer Super Bowl teams previously displayed.

Research has confirmed that stature, body mass, and BMI continue to increase as students' progress through their high school years,[118] as confirmed with worldwide BMI data from 200 countries comprising 19.2 million youth.[124] As seniors, offensive and defensive linemen are the tallest and heaviest among their football peers with the greatest BMI, which places them into the obese category 1 guidelines from the WHO (www.who.int/health-topics/obesity#tab=tab_1). In fact, approximately 95% of offensive and 78% of defensive high school linemen have greater BMIs than players at all other positions, which characterizes American high school football linemen as obese. At this young age, they already carry the burden of unhealthy body fat accumulation as they grow older.

INTEGRATIVE QUESTION

A football coach wishes to field a team whose players are not overly fat, so he uses body mass index to screen out any players who might be. Did he make the right decision—why or why not?

Long-Term Health Risk Outlook. The huge body mass and exceptionally high BMI for American football and other large athletes pose future health risks with troublesome long-term prognosis. Many population studies demonstrate that early-life weight gain and obesity predict adverse health characteristics including maladaptive cardiac remodeling, atherosclerosis, cardiometabolic disease, diminished quality of life, and overall mortality.[122] Underreported but important health risks in large athletes also concern disordered breathing problems and obstructive sleep apnea beginning in high school and college and continuing into retirement for professional football players.[22,119–121]

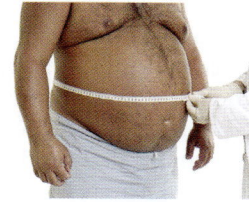
Luis Louro/Shutterstock

The average neck girth (45.2 cm/17.7 in.) and BMI elevated above 31.5 predicts increased sleep-disordered breathing and apnea with accompanying snoring and future health risks.[123] As we emphasize in Chapter 28, BMI to classify individuals as overfat can mislead, as confirmed in 85 collegiate American football players.[52] The BMI overestimated obesity

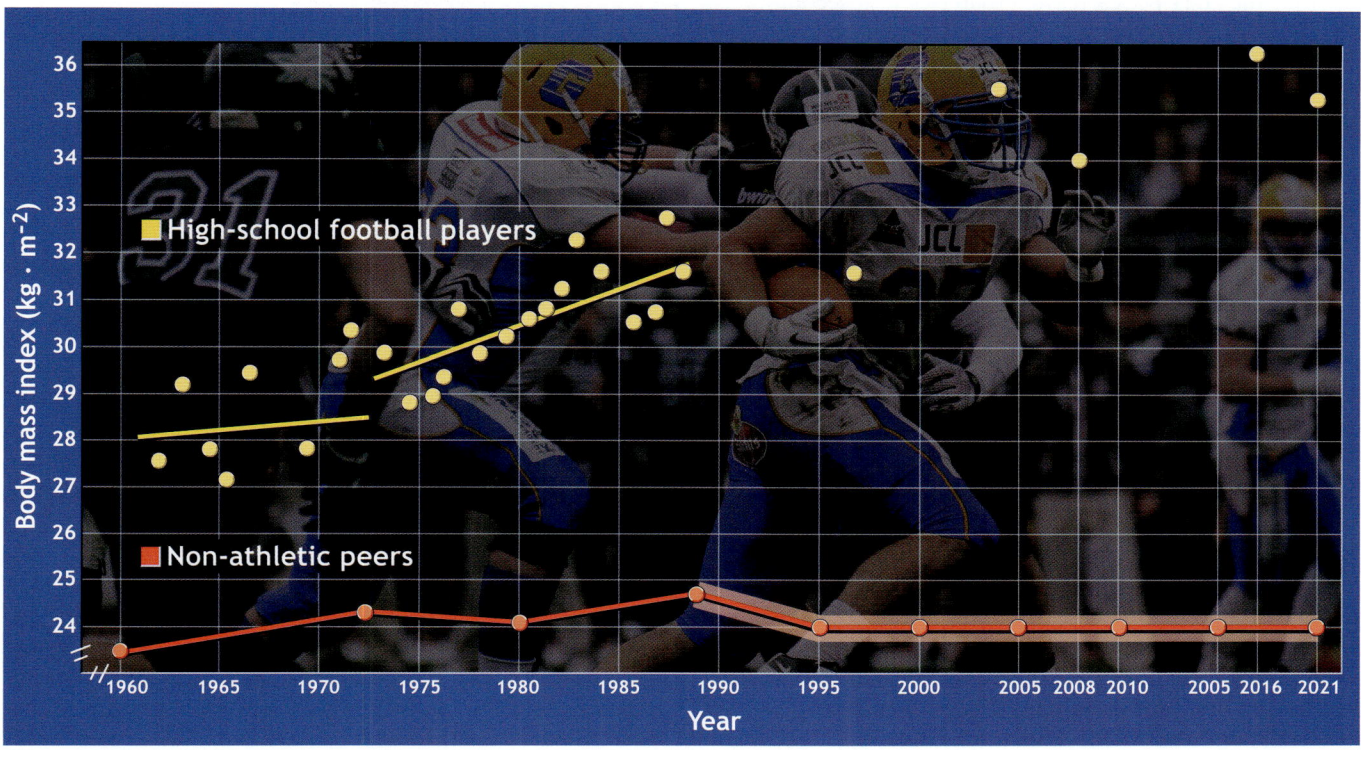

Background photo: Herbert Kratky/Shutterstock

prevalence in 51% of players, with only 14 players qualified as obese using valid body composition assessment techniques. Nonetheless, the offensive linemen exceeded the at-risk BMI criteria (≥30), neck girth (≥43 cm/16.9 in.), waist girth (≥102 cm/40.2 in.), and percentage body fat (≥25%). Despite these findings, it seems fair to say that exceptionally large high school football players about to enter college and their collegiate contemporaries will exhibit multiple, worrisome obesity-related health conditions throughout their lives.

Professional Golfers

Limited data exist for professional golfers in percentage body fat and LBM, although height and weight 2020 to 2021 data for tour Professional Golfers' Association (PGA) players can be compiled from a popular Internet source (www.foxsports.com/golf/golfers?association=1&season=2016&grouping=0&page=1&sort=2016&sequence=0). We were unable to capture similar data for the Ladies Professional Golf Association (LPGA) players because only stature, not body mass, data are available for these players. In a prior text edition, we obtained data for height, weight, and BMI for the male Champions Tour and PGA Tour champions, including 19 of the 2011 top 20 PGA competitors. A PubMed search did not return updated body composition data for PGA or other professional golfers. Consequently, we updated the available height, weight, and BMI for the top 15 golfers based on 2021 FedEx rankings (July 11, 2021; **TABLE 29.4**). Data for Behnke's reference man is included as a contrast among the different player groups. Interestingly, relatively small differences existed in the physical characteristics and BMI for three PGA player groups, but a dramatic downward shift occurred in the height, weight, and BMI for the 2021 FedEx player group (see next section).

TABLE 29.4 Comparing height, weight, and body mass index among top professional golfers

Mortality Ratio for Highly Skilled Golfers. The mortality ratio for the highly skilled golf athletes in Table 29.4 based on BMI would rate as very low as discussed in Chapter 28. The Swedish Golf Federation's membership registry and the nationwide Mortality Registry corroborates this classification for health status based on standardized mortality ratios for 300,818 Swedish golfers (203,778 males and 97,040 females) with stratification for age, sex, and socioeconomic status.[18] Swedish golfers had mortality rates about 60% of those in the general population for both sexes and in all age groups after adjusting for socioeconomic status. In a comparison study with 257 golfers stratified by proficiency levels based on handicap index, the BMI index was only marginally higher than the two pro groups. All three golf groups were still taller, heavier, and had a larger BMI compared to Behnke's reference man. When comparing these players' BMIs with the 2020 to 2021 FedEx Cup standings on July 11, 2021, there was a major shift in overall body size—BMI dramatically decreased (essentially 5 BMI points or 20%), as did average body weight (about 11 kg/24 lb), whereas players were substantially taller by about 6 cm/2.4 in. compared with the prior and FedEx 2021 data. This contrasts with high school and professional football players who classify as obese and fall in the high range for mortality risk. For obese NFL players, half place in the severely obese range (BMI ≥ 35), and those with a BMI ≥ 40 classify as morbidly obese.[25]

Stature and Golf Driving Distance. In the golf world, a premium accrues to players who drive the ball the farthest. Longer, successful drives off the tee translate to shorter next shots to the green. This, as expected, gives the player who can consistently drive the ball 350 yd/1050 ft a distinct advantage over a competitor who can drive the same shot "only" 300 yd/900 ft from the tee. One might surmise that taller

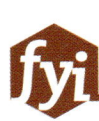

Medical Concern for Overweight and Obese High School, College, and Professional Athletes

Large-sized high school and college athletes tend to remain large-sized throughout adulthood. Former high school, college, and retired professional athletes—particularly American football players—have major medical issues dealing with excess central fat deposition in the abdominal region. Being large size combined with good athletic skills in football or wrestling in the higher weight categories in high school sets the groundwork for a future that unfortunately can alter the metabolic profile to increase risk for at least seven medical conditions:

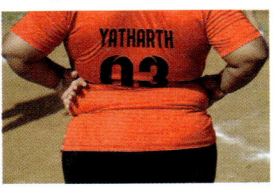
RAMNIKLAL MODI/Shutterstock

1. Hyperinsulinemia (insulin resistance)
2. Glucose intolerance
3. Type 2 diabetes
4. Hypertriglyceridemia
5. Hypercholesterolemia and a negatively altered lipoprotein profile
6. Hypertension
7. Atherosclerosis

In addition to assessing the deleterious impact of an altered metabolic profile from excess abdominal fat, research also has focused on neuropeptide–adipose tissue linkages and how such interactions bear upon intra-abdominal fat tissue physiology, chronic inflammation, and disease state associate with that anatomical region (e.g., Crohn disease and other gastrointestinal tract conditions; www.ncbi.nlm.nih.gov/pmc/articles/PMC5609829/), including quality of life and life satisfaction concerns with aging.

Sources:
Filbay S, et al. Quality of life and life satisfaction in former athletes: a systematic review and meta-analysis. *Sports Med.* 2019;49:1723.
Girard R, et al. The transcription factor hepatocyte nuclear factor 4A acts in the intestine to promote white adipose tissue energy storage. *Nat Commun.* 2022;13:224.
Lee SW, et al. Body fat distribution is more predictive of all-cause mortality than overall adiposity. *Diabetes Obes Metab.* 2018;20:141.

players would generally achieve the longest drives. This intuitively makes sense when comparing two top PGA golfers, one a foot taller than the other. Yet the graphic below shows this is not the case—some shorter golfers (note the red dot for the 1.7-m/67-in. pro golfer) can drive the ball about the same distance as the tallest, established pro players (see green dot). To accomplish this task, biomechanical and neural factors other than stature must play a dominant role in achieving long distance drives.[60] Perfecting the golf swing requires precise, coordinated neuromuscular and highly specific movement patterns developed over many years of purposeful practice—not simply clubhead speed, arm, back, leg, and torso muscle strength activated in the swing. Training *movements* rather than training muscles to become "stronger" pays greater dividends in striking the ball consistently with accuracy and driving it long distances (see Chapter 19).

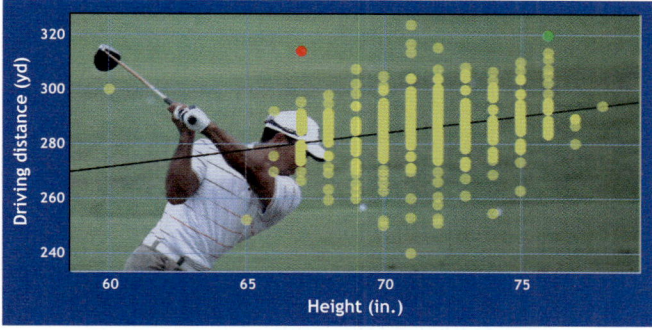

The three longest drives on the PGA tour since such statistics have been recorded were achieved for non–wind-aided, and no out-of-bounds roll to another fairway:

1. Louis Oosthuizen (1982–); 500 yd/1500 ft, 1st hole Blackstone Golf Club, Incheon, South Korea at the 2013 Ballantine's Championship; height, 178 cm/70 in.; weight, 82 kg/180 lb
2. Tiger Woods (1975–); 498 yd/1494 ft, 18th hole Plantation Course, Kapalua, Hawaii, 2002 Mercedes Championship; height, 185.4 cm/73 in.; weight, 83.9 kg/185 lb
3. Dustin Johnson (1984–); 489 yd/1467 ft, 12th hole, Austin Country Club, Texas, 2018 WGC Dell Technologies Match Play; height, 193 cm/76 in.; weight, 86 kg/190 lb

Although not set by LPGA or PGA tour professionals, world records for the longest drive for a female include a 413-yd/1239-ft drive (127-mph club head speed, 182-mph ball speed, 117-foot height apex) achieved in 2021 by World Champion Phillis Meti (1987–). Kyle Berkshire (1996–), the 2021 male World record Long Drive Champion, has not attained the same driving distance as the top 3 PGA tour players (492-yd/1476-ft drive; 229-mph ball speed; height 190.5 cm/75 in.; weight 97.5 kg/215 lb).

Weightlifters and Bodybuilders

Males. Resistance-trained bodybuilders, Olympic weightlifters, and power weightlifters exhibit remarkable muscular development and FFM combined with a relatively lean physique.[38] Percentage body fat computed from body density by underwater weighing averaged 9.3% in bodybuilders, 9.1% in power weightlifters, and 10.8% in Olympic weightlifters. Considerable leanness exists for each athlete group, even though height-weight tables classify up to 19% of these males as overweight, despite the groups not differing in skeletal frame size, FFM, skinfolds, and bone diameters. The only differences occurred for shoulders, chest, biceps, and forearm girths; bodybuilders were larger at each anatomic site. The bodybuilders exhibited nearly 16 kg/35.2 lb more muscle than predicted for their size compared with power weightlifters and Olympic weightlifters. The three- or four-compartment model is useful to assess body composition changes in male bodybuilders during training.[70] Attempting to determine the genetic basis to help explain the large LBM from "*sumo wrestler loci*" associated with an adverse metabolic profile may be useful in the future to identify "*body builder*" loci associated with metabolic protection.[125]

Females. During the late 1970s, bodybuilding gained widespread popularity among females in the United States. They enthusiastically accepted the vigorous resistance training demands, making competition become more intense, with achievement levels increasing considerably. Bodybuilding success depends on a slim and lean appearance, with a well-defined workout-specific enlarged musculature. These requirements raise interesting questions about females' body composition. How lean do competitors become, and does a larger muscle mass accompany their low body fat levels?

Scarce data exist about the body composition in "lean" competitive or professional female athletes. Ten competitive female bodybuilders averaged 13.2% body fat (range 8.0 to 18.3%) with 46.6 kg/103 lb of FFM.[21] Except for champion gymnasts, who also average about 13% body fat, bodybuilders were 3 to 4% shorter in stature, weighed 4 to 5% less, and had 7 to 10% less total FM than competitive female athletes in other sports. The bodybuilders' most striking physique characteristic was a dramatically large 7:1 FFM:FM ratio, nearly double the 4.3:1 ratio for other female athletic groups.[126] This difference presumably occurred without steroid use. Interestingly, 8 in 10 body builders reported normal menstrual function with concurrent relatively low body fat. When female bodybuilders trained for competition during a 12-wk preparation period, the major portion in their total weight lost (−5.8 kg/12.8 lb; from 18.3 to 12.7% body fat) occurred primarily from reduced FM, not FFM (−1.4-kg/−3.1-lb decline).[71] A 25.5-mm/1-in. decrease occurred in an eight skinfold sum besides the total body composition changes. These data reveal that healthy females at the lower end along the body fat continuum can still reduce FM over a 3-month training duration to a level that approaches the theoretical boundary for storage fat without inducing apparent deleterious, acute health effects. *Females*

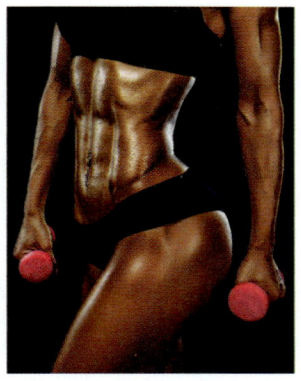

ladie_c/Shutterstock

probably can alter muscle size to the same relative extent as males, at least when scaled to body size. The larger hip size in females probably relates to greater fat stores in this anatomic region.

Collegiate Wrestlers

Collegiate wrestlers represent a unique athletic group who train intensely and attempt to keep a low body weight with a large FFM. The NCAA has introduced rule changes in response to three collegiate wrestlers in 1997 who died from excessive weight loss (largely from dehydration) to discourage dangerous weight-cutting practices and thereby increase safe participation. Another rule change required determining urine specific gravity (ratio in urine's density compared to water density) to ensure euhydration at weight certification. Athletes with a urine specific gravity ≤1.020 are considered euhydrated, whereas wrestlers'

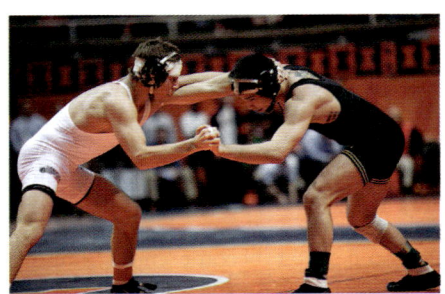
Ahturner/Shutterstock

urine specific gravity ≥1.020 cannot have their body fat assessed to determine minimum competitive wrestling weight for the upcoming season. Urine specific gravity reflects hydration status, but lags behind true hydration status in periods with rapid body fluid turnover during acute dehydration.

Sumo Wrestlers

The FFM for Japanese elite sumo wrestlers (*seki-tori*—top-ranked, salaried sumo wrestler who compete in the highest sumo divisions http://www.youtube.com/watch?v=gGJe42jSTYc) average 109 kg/240 lb.[45] These athletes share the distinction of being among the world's largest athletes, along with American professional football players, with some exceeding 172 kg/380 lb. It seems unlikely that athletes in this weight range would possess less than 15% body fat; the FFMs for the largest football players at 15% body fat theoretically corresponds to 135 kg/298 lb. In reality, a football player with a 159-kg/351-lb body mass would more likely have 20 to 25% body fat, similar to 198 large Japanese athletes based on BMI.[128] At 20% body fat, the FFM would be about 127 kg/280 lb, certainly the highest value ever measured hydrostatically. But this value remains hypothetical without published data. Even for an exceptionally large professional basketball player (body mass, 138.3 kg/305 lb; stature, 210.8 cm/83 in.) assessed when all draft players attended pre-screening physicals, percentage body fat is unlikely to be less than 10% body mass. Thus, FM at 13.8 kg/30.5 lb and FFM at 114.2 kg/252 lb perhaps push toward an upper limit FFM value for an athlete with such outsized body size dimensions.

Lippincott® Connect Appendix H, available on Lippincott Connect, provides a supplemental animation and video list, including a video about sumo wrestling.

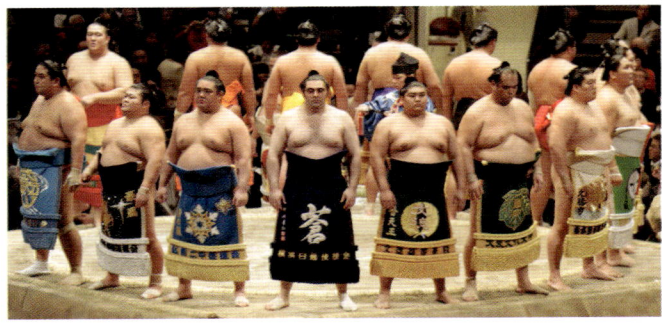
J. Henning Buchholz/Shutterstock

Upper FFM Limits

To gain additional insight into the question concerning an upper FFM limit among "large" athletes, we reviewed more than 40 years of data on body composition from our laboratories and other field studies to determine the largest FFM values determined densitometrically (with correction for residual lung volume). We reviewed data with 1467 determinations from five professional NFL teams, Major League Baseball Boston Red Sox, Mr. Universe Bodybuilding contestants representing 13 countries, all NBA basketball draft choices from a minicamp postdraft selection, and USA Olympic field event athletes (shot, discus, javelin, hammer) prior to an Olympic Games. From this extraordinary group of exceptional athletes, 35 elite competitors exceeded an FFM of 100 kg/220 lb; the top five values were 114.3 kg/252 lb, 109.7 kg/242 lb, 108.4 kg/239 lb, 107.6 kg/237 lb, and 105.6 kg/233 lb. The three top values were larger than the two 106.5-kg/235-lb values reported for defensive football linemen from 1969 to 1971 data[2] and other resistance-trained athletes.[17,86–88]

IAKIMCHUK IAROSLAV/Shutterstock

Exceptionally Large NFL Player

The body composition of an exceptionally large professional football player (NFL Oakland Raiders; unpublished data, Dr. R. Girandola, Department of Kinesiology, University of Southern California) determined by repeated underwater weighing trials exceeded published FFM values. The former defensive player (deceased, 2005 car accident), with a 11.3% body fat content (body mass: 141.4 kg/312 lb; stature: 193 cm/76 in.; BMI: 38.4), had a 125.4-kg/276-lb FFM, surely an uppermost value. With the continuing increase in professional football player's body size, this collegiate player's large FFM determined in 1997 before he turned professional will probably not remain the ultimate peak FFM value. Published body composition data on other large athletes using criterion body composition assessment techniques will unquestionably reveal a new ceiling. Until then, we assume that 125.4 kg/276 lb represents the current upper boundary for this body composition component in an elite "power" athlete.

Current studies with male athletes have quantified the proportional relationships among regional upper and lower body fat and fat-free tissue components and body size.[128] This novel research avenue has documented a "breakpoint" in the slope for whole-body FFM versus total body mass at a body mass approximating 85 kg/187 lb. At higher body mass levels, total FFM tends to increase at a much slower rate than do increases in FM, which then increases percentage body fat.

Body Composition in 100-Year-Old Males and Females

It is no simple feat to attain age 100. At precisely 10:22 PM on February 27, 2022, sec-by-sec statistics captured in real time established the world population as 7,930,184,889 (www.worldometers.info/world-population/). Considering the 7.9 billion people on the planet, only about 575,000 were alive at age ≥100 living in 195 countries on the five continents (0.007% of the population). Longevity projections to live to age 100 by 2050 will increase to more than 3 million people, with exponential increases at 10-year intervals through the end of the century (www.worldatlas.com). This has elevated the urgency to better understand factors related to body composition changes (including nutritional support and pharmacologic treatment scenarios) as the centenarians begin to exceed their metabolically predicted life spans—as was the case for an observational cross-sectional study in Portuguese male and female **centenarians** described in the next sections.

Background

The study on male and female centenarians is the only research to quantify body composition for this age group.[130] It was conducted during 2012 to 2014 throughout Portugal and focused on 196 females (77.8%) and 56 males (22.2%). Most centenarians were observed in nursing homes (72.2%), 19.8% at their residence with family, and 8% in either religious congregations or living with host families or alone, or in hospitals. Most centenarians were widowed (82.9%), with the remainder single (13.5%), married (2.4%), or divorced (1.2%).

Body Composition and Anthropometry Compared by Gender

TABLE 29.5 compares the results by gender for the anthropometric and body composition characteristics. Measurements included body weight, height, BMI, waist circumference, hip and waist-to-hip ratio using standard methods described in Chapter 28, and body fat percentage, FFM, muscle and bone mass, total body water, and resting metabolism by tetrapolar bioimpedance analysis (BIA).

TABLE 29.5 How male and female Portuguese centenarians compare on 24 anthropometric and body composition measurements

For the group, the average median age was 100.3 (range 97 to 109 years). There were significant differences among males and females in body weight, height, and BMI (females 20.7; males 22.4) Underweight prevalence in both groups was about the same (25.5%), with only five subjects classified obese by WHO criteria (Chapter 28). Males had significantly greater visceral fat, body FM, and FFM. Hypohydration prevalence was larger in females (15.4%) than in males (5%). There were gender differences in almost all anthropometric and body composition variables, notably larger values for localized fat regions (waist, waist-to-hip ratio, and visceral abdominal fat) in males compared with females. Osteoporosis was identified in 72% females and 95% males. In another study with "younger" older men average age 87, reduced muscle strength (with 73% suspected sarcopenia) was common and associated with mortality and stay during hospitalization.[138] In the Portuguese study for males aged 100, resting metabolic rate (RMR, kcal) was significantly different between genders (females = 1123 total daily kcal vs. 1350 kcal for males). Also, the overall mean 83.5-year metabolic age was significantly below the centenarian's chronologic age 100.

The research with centenarians supports prior aging studies with the "older-elderly" documenting changes in body composition, body fat distribution, RMR, decline in FFM, increased abdominal (visceral) fat in the trunk region, and diminished immune suppression (Chapters 28 and 32) and total body muscle strength.[131,132,136,137] Prior research has shown that FFM has functional significance related to aging, helping to explain the FFM decline responsible for the corresponding decline in RMR,[133–135] with relative thinness likely contributing to longevity rather than overweight reducing life expectancy. It also is plausible that excess abdominal (visceral) obesity links positively to noncommunicable diseases, eventually outpacing the FFM and RMR declines to hasten the dramatic body composition and fat patterning changes in the centenarians.[144]

Summary

1. Athletes generally have physique characteristics unique to their specific sport. Field-event athletes have a relatively large FFM and a high percentage body fat, whereas distance runners possess the least lean tissue and FM.
2. Champion performance blends unique physique characteristics and highly developed physiologic support systems.
3. Male and female triathletes possess a body composition and aerobic capacity most similar to elite competitive cyclists.
4. Body composition analyses for American football players reveal they are among the heaviest athletes, yet maintain a relatively lean body composition compared to nonplayer counterparts. At the highest competition levels, Division I American collegiate and professional NFL football players show remarkable body size and body composition similarity.
5. Top-rated high school football linemen are comparable in stature and body mass (and BMI) to former 2007–2021 NFL Super Bowl participants.

6. Competitive male and female swimmers generally have higher body fat levels than distance runners.
7. Female bodybuilders can alter muscle size by the same relative amount as male bodybuilders.
8. Competitive female bodybuilders have an FFM:FM ratio exceeding the FFM:FM ratio in other elite female athletes.
9. A value of 125.4 kg/276.5 lb represents the current, directly measured upper FFM limit in elite power athletes.
10. Quantifying the proportional relationships among the regional upper and lower body fat and fat-free tissue components provides a new research area to assess a "breakpoint" in the relationship between FFM and body mass.
11. Research with centenarians documents gender differences in almost all anthropometric and body composition variables, notably larger values for localized fat regions (waist, waist-to-hip ratio, and visceral abdominal fat) in males compared with females.
12. Significantly lower BMI in centenarians reflects relative thinness, which contributes to their longevity rather than significant overweight, which in non-centenarians, reduces longevity.

Key Terms

Centenarians: People 100 years old or older

Ectomorphic: Body type characterized by the degree of slenderness, angularity, and fragility—often a lean, slender body build with slight muscular development

Endomorphic: Body type characterized by a wider body shape than an ectomorph or mesomorph, with a thick ribcage, wide hips, and shorter limbs—often with significant body fat

Mesomorphic: Body type characterized by muscularity and large bone development—often with a muscular body build

References are available online at Lippincott Connect.

Additional References

Al-Ghadban S, et al. Adipose stem cells in regenerative medicine: looking forward. *Front Bioeng Biotechnol*. 2022;9:837464.

Aliberti SM, et al. Extreme longevity: analysis of the direct or indirect influence of environmental factors on old, nonagenarians, and centenarians in Cilento, Italy. *Int J Environ Res Public Health*. 2022;19:1589.

Campa F, et al. Assessment of body composition in athletes: a narrative review of available methods with special reference to quantitative and qualitative bioimpedance analysis. *Nutrients*. 2021;13:1620.

Carlsen EMM, Rasmussen RN. More than meets the eye: the metabolic state of the body shapes visual sensations. *Cell Metab*. 2022;34:9.

Chen GC, et al. Body fat distribution, cardiometabolic traits, and risk of major lower-extremity arterial disease in postmenopausal women. *Diabetes Care*. 2022;45:222.

Citarella R, et al. Association between dietary practice, body composition, training volume and sport performance in 100-Km elite ultramarathon runners. *Clin Nutr ESPEN*. 2021;42:239.

Collings PJ. Independent associations of sleep timing, duration and quality with adiposity and weight status in a national sample of adolescents: the UK Millennium Cohort Study. *J Sleep Res*. 2022;31:e13436.

Czeck MA, et al. Body composition and on-ice skate times for National Collegiate Athletic Association Division 1 collegiate male and female ice hockey athletes. *J Strength Cond Res*. 2022;36:187.

de Macêdo Cesário T, et al. Evaluation of the body adiposity index against dual-energy X-ray absorptiometry for assessing body composition in children and adolescents. *Am J Hum Biol*. 2021;33:e23503.

Gao M, et al. Associations between body composition, fat distribution and metabolic consequences of excess adiposity with severe COVID-19 outcomes: observational study and Mendelian randomisation analysis. *Int J Obes (Lond)*. 2022:1. doi:10.1038/s41366-021-01054-3.

Hai PC, et al. BMI, Blood pressure, and plasma lipids among centenarians and their offspring. *Evid Based Complement Alternat Med*. 2022;2022:3836247.

Jagim AR, et al. The influence of sport nutrition knowledge on body composition and perceptions of dietary requirements in collegiate athletes. *Nutrients*. 2021;13:2239.

Kasper AM, et al. Assessment of activity energy expenditure during competitive golf: the effects of bag carrying, electric or manual trolleys. *Eur J Sport Sci*. 2022:1. doi:10.1080/17461391.2022.2036817

Kitamura E, et al. The relationship between body composition and sleep architecture in athletes. *Sleep Med*. 2021;87:92.

Krajnik W, et al. sSfS: Segmented shape from silhouette reconstruction of the human body. *Sensors (Basel)*. 2022;22:925.

Lahav Y, et al. Comparison of body composition assessment across body mass index categories by two multifrequency bioelectrical impedance analysis devices and dual-energy X-ray absorptiometry in clinical settings. *Eur J Clin Nutr*. 2021;75:1275.

Lukaski H, et al. New frontiers of body composition in sport. *Int J Sports Med*. 2021;42:588.

Marra M, et al. Bioimpedance phase angle in elite male athletes: a segmental approach. *Physiol Meas*. 2021;41:125007.

Mascherini G, et al. Lifestyle and resulting body composition in young athletes. *Minerva Pediatr (Torino)*. 2021;73:391.

McGuire A, et al. Energy availability and macronutrient intake in elite male Gaelic football players. *Sci Med Footb*. 2022. doi:10.1080/24733938.2022.2029551.

Miranda KA, et al. Effects of gradual weight loss on strength levels and body composition in wrestler athletes. *J Sports Med Phys Fitness*. 2021;61:401.

Muros-Molina JJ, et al. Anthropometric differences between world-class professional track cyclists according to specialty (endurance vs. sprint). *J Sports Med Phys Fitness*. 2022. doi: 0.23736/S0022-4707.22.13280-9.

Nobari H, et al. The effects of 14-week betaine supplementation on endocrine markers, body composition and anthropometrics in professional youth soccer players: a double blind, randomized, placebo-controlled trial. *J Int Soc Sports Nutr*. 2021;18:20.

O'Donoghue G, et al. What exercise prescription is optimal to improve body composition and cardiorespiratory fitness in adults living with obesity? A network meta-analysis. *Obes Rev*. 2021;22:e13137.

Paoli A, et al. Effects of two months of very low carbohydrate ketogenic diet on body composition, muscle strength, muscle area, and blood parameters in competitive natural body builders. *Nutrients*. 2021;13:374.

Pepłońska B, et al. Common myelin regulatory factor gene variants predisposing to excellence in sports. *Genes (Basel)*. 2021;12:262.

Perera RS, et al. Effects of body weight and fat mass on back pain-direct mechanical or indirect through inflammatory and metabolic parameters? *Semin Arthritis Rheum*. 2022;52:151935.

Puccinelli P, et al. Distribution of body fat is associated with physical performance of male amateur triathlon athletes. *J Sports Med Phys Fitness*. 2022;62:215:33666075.

Rojo-Tirado MA, et al. Body composition changes after a weight loss intervention: a 3-year follow-up study. *Nutrients*. 2021;13:164.

Rubio-Arias JÁ, et al. Effects of whole-body vibration training on body composition, cardiometabolic risk, and strength in the population who are overweight and obese: a systematic review with meta-analysis. *Arch Phys Med Rehabil*. 2021;102:2442.

Sanchez-Lastra MA, et al. Physical activity and mortality across levels of adiposity: a prospective cohort study from the UK Biobank. *Mayo Clin Proc*. 2021;96:105.

Scantlebury S, et al. The anthropometric and physical qualities of women's rugby league Super League and international players; identifying differences in playing position and level. *PLoS One*. 2022;17:e0249803.

Seo MW, et al. Effects of 16 weeks of resistance training on muscle quality and muscle growth factors in older adult women with sarcopenia: a randomized controlled trial. *Int J Environ Res Public Health*. 2021;18:6762.

Severin AC, et al. Three-dimensional kinematics in healthy older adult males during golf swings. *Sports Biomech*. 2022;21:165.

Sheehan WB, et al. Physical Determinants of golf swing performance: a review. *J Strength Cond Res*. 2022;36:289.

Silveira A, et al. MicroRNAs in obesity-associated disorders: the role of exercise training. *Obes Facts*. 2022:1. doi: 0.1159/000517849.

Tatarczuk J, et al. Somatotypological structure of university students in the sex groups of equal body heights. *Anthropol Anz*. 2022;79:11.

Wagner R, et al. Metabolic implications of pancreatic fat accumulation. *Nat Rev Endocrinol*. 2022;18:43.

Walker EJ, et al. Seasonal change in body composition and physique of team sport athletes. *J Strength Cond Res*. 2022;36:565.

Wiecha S, et al. Transferability of cardiopulmonary parameters between treadmill and cycle ergometer testing in male triathletes-prediction formulae. *Int J Environ Res Public Health*. 2022;19:1830.

Table 29.1 Skinfold and Girth Anthropometry for the Top 10 American Athletes in the Discus, Shot Put, Javelin, and Hammer Throw

Measurement[a]	Discus	Shot Put	Javelin	Hammer	Runners	Ref Man
Body mass (kg)	108.2	112.3	90.6	104.2	63.1	70.0
Stature (cm)	191.7	187.0	186.0	187.3	177.0	174.0
Skinfolds (mm)						
Triceps	13.0	15.0	11.9	12.7	5.0	—
Scapular	18.0	23.8	12.5	21.5	6.4	—
Iliac	24.5	29.6	17.0	27.4	4.6	—
Abdomen	25.6	31.4	18.4	29.1	7.1	—
Thigh	16.4	15.7	13.3	17.3	6.1	—
Girths (cm)						
Shoulders	129.8	133.3	121.5	127.4	106.1	110.8
Chest	113.5	118.5	104.6	111.3	91.1	91.8
Waist	94.1	99.1	86.6	94.8	74.6	77.0
Abdomen	97.5	101.5	87.8	98.0	74.2	79.8
Hips	110.4	112.3	102.0	108.7	87.8	93.4
Thighs	66.3	69.4	61.5	67.3	51.9	54.8
Knees	41.5	42.9	40.0	41.0	36.2[b]	36.6
Calves	42.6	43.6	39.5	41.5	35.4	35.8
Ankles	25.4	24.9	24.1	24.3	21.0	22.5
Biceps	41.8	42.2	37.7	39.9	28.2	31.7
Forearms	33.1	33.7	30.8	32.4	26.4	26.4
Wrists	18.7	18.9	18.2	18.4	16.0	17.3
Diameters (cm)						
Biacromial	44.5	43.8	43.2	44.8	39.5	40.6
Chest	33.1	33.7	30.8	32.6	31.3	30.0
Bi-iliac	31.3	31.2	29.6	30.4	28.0	28.6
Bitrochanter	35.5	34.9	33.7	34.8	32.2	32.8
Knee	10.2	10.5	10.0	10.2	9.5	9.3
Wrist	6.3	6.2	6.0	6.2	5.6	5.6
Ankle	7.6	7.6	7.5	7.4	—	7.0
Elbow	7.6	7.6	7.6	7.2	—	7.0

[a]Measurement procedure details from Katch FI, Katch VL. The body composition profile: techniques of measurement and applications. *Clin Sports Med*. 1984;3:31. Data correspond to the athletic groups presented in Figure 29.2.
[b]Not measured; value computed for the reference man calf-to-knee ratio.
Ref, reference.

Table 29.2 Body Composition Characteristics of Elite Male Middle- and Long-Distance Runners and Marathoners

Group	Stature (cm)	Mass (kg)	Density (g·cm⁻³)	Body Fat (%)	FFM (kg)	Fat Mass (kg)	Sum 7 Skinfolds (mm)
Distance Runners							
Brown	187.3	72.10	1.07428	10.8	64.31	7.79	53.0
Castaneda	178.6	63.34	1.09102	3.7	61.00	2.34	32.5
Crawford	171.8	58.01	1.09702	1.2	57.31	0.70	32.5
Geis	179.1	66.28	1.07551	10.2	59.52	6.76	49.0
Johnson	174.6	61.79	1.08963	4.3	59.13	2.66	35.5
Manley	177.8	69.10	1.09642	1.5	68.06	1.04	32.0
Ndoo	169.3	53.97	1.08379	6.7	50.35	3.62	33.5
Prefontaine	174.2	68.00	1.08842	4.8	64.74	3.26	38.0
Rose	175.6	59.15	1.08248	7.3	54.83	4.32	31.5
Tuttle	176.8	61.44	1.09960	0.2	61.32	0.12	31.5
Mean	170.5	60.92	1.08916	4.5	58.18	2.74	34.5
Marathon Runners							
Cusack	174.6	64.19	1.08096	7.9	59.12	5.07	45.5
Galloway	180.9	65.76	1.08419	6.6	61.42	4.34	43.0
Kennedy	167.0	56.52	1.09348	2.7	54.99	1.53	37.0
Moore	184.1	64.24	1.09193	3.3	62.12	2.12	37.0
Pate	179.6	57.28	1.09676	1.3	56.54	0.74	32.5
Shorter	178.4	61.17	1.09475	2.2	59.82	1.35	45.0
Wayne	172.1	61.61	1.07859	8.9	56.13	5.48	42.5
Williams	177.2	66.07	1.09569	1.8	64.88	1.19	41.5
Mean	176.8	62.11	1.08954	4.3	59.38	2.73	40.5

FFM, fat-free mass.
Data from Pollock ML, et al. Body composition of elite class distance runners. *Ann NY Acad Sci.* 1977;301:361.

Table 29.3 Body Composition of Collegiate and Professional Football Players Grouped by Position

Position[a]	Level	N	Stature (cm)	Mass (kg)	Body Fat (%)	FFM (kg)
Defensive backs	St. Cloud[b]	15	178.3	77.3	11.5	68.4
	U Mass[c]	12	179.9	83.1	8.8	76.8
	USC[d]	15	183.0	83.7	9.6	75.7
	Gettysburg[e]	16	175.9	79.8	13.6	68.9
	Pro, modern[f]	26	182.5	84.8	9.6	76.7
	Pro, older[g]	25	183.0	91.2	10.7	81.4
Offensive backs and receivers	St. Cloud	15	179.7	79.8	12.4	69.6
	U Mass	29	181.8	84.1	9.5	76.4
	USC	18	185.6	86.1	9.9	77.6
	Gettysburg	18	176.0	78.3	12.9	68.2
	Pro, modern	40	183.8	90.7	9.4	81.9
	Pro, older	25	183.0	91.7	10.0	87.5
Linebackers	St. Cloud	7	180.1	87.2	13.4	75.4
	U Mass	17	186.1	97.1	13.1	84.2
	USC	17	185.6	98.8	13.2	85.8
	Gettysburg	—	—	—	—	—
	Pro, modern	28	188.6	102.2	14.0	87.6
Offensive linemen and tight ends	St. Cloud	13	186.0	99.2	19.1	79.8
	U Mass	23	187.5	107.6	19.5	86.6
	Gettysburg	15	182.6	110.4	26.2	81.0
	USC	25	191.1	106.5	15.3	90.3
	Pro, modern	38	193.0	112.6	15.6	94.7
Defensive linemen	St. Cloud	15	186.6	97.8	18.5	79.3
	U Mass	8	188.8	114.3	19.5	91.9
	USC	13	191.1	109.3	14.7	93.2
	Gettysburg	11	178.0	99.4	21.9	77.6
	Pro, modern	32	192.4	117.1	18.2	95.8
	Pro, older	25	185.7	97.1	14.0	83.5
All positions	St. Cloud	65	182.5	88.0	15.0	74.2
	U Mass	91	184.9	97.3	13.9	83.2
	USC	88	186.6	96.6	11.4	84.6
	Gettysburg	60	178.0	90.6	18.1	73.3
	Pro, modern	164	188.1	101.5	13.4	87.3
	Pro, older	25	183.1	91.2	10.4	81.3
	Dallas-Jets[h]	107	188.2	100.4	12.6	87.7

[a]Grouping according to Wilmore JH, Haskel WL. Body composition and endurance capacity of professional football players. *J Appl Physiol*. 1972;33:564.
[b]Data from Wickkiser JD, Kelly JM. The body composition of a college football team. *Med Sci Sports*. 1975;7:199.
[c]UMass data from Coach Robert Stull and F Katch, University of Massachusetts. Data collected during spring practice, 1985; %fat by densitometry.
[d]USC data from Dr. Robert Girandola, University of Southern California, Los Angeles, 1978, 1993.
[e]Data courtesy Dr. Kristin Steumple, Department of Exercise and Sport Science, Gettysburg College, Gettysburg, PA, 2000.
[f]Data from Wilmore JH, et al. Football pros' strengths—and CV weakness—charted. *Phys Sportsmed*. 1976;4:45.
[g]Data from Dr. A. R. Behnke.
[h]Data from Katch FI, Katch, VL. Body composition of the Dallas Cowboys and New York Jets football teams, unpublished, 1978.
FFM, fat-free mass.

Table 29.4 Height, body weight, and body mass index for 2005 Champions Tour Players, PGA Golf Tour Champion Players, 2011 Top 20 PGA Players, and 2021 Top-Ranked FedEx Players

Group[a]	Height (cm)	Weight (kg)	BMI
PGA Tour 2005 (N = 33)	182.0	84.1	25.4
Champions Tour 2011 (N = 18)	181.0	85.8	26.2
PGA Tour 2011[b] (N = 19)	184.0	81.2	24.0
PGA FedEx leaders 2021[c] (N=15)	188.6	72.4	20.0
Behnke reference man	174.0	70.0	23.1

[a]PGA and Champions Tour 2011 Annual report published by Boston Hannah International (filed for bankruptcy 2012).
[b]2011 players: Casey, Donald, Els, Fowler, Furyk, D. Johnson, Kuchar, McDonwell, Michelson, Oglivy, Poulter, Rose, Schwartzel, Scott, Stricker, Watney, Watson, Wilson, Woods.
[c]2021 FedEx Cup players (1 to 15 rank): Cantlay, English, Rahm, DeChambeau, Spieth, J. Thomas, Hovland, Schauffele, Kokrak, Morikawa, Burns, Koepka, Oosthuizen, Niemann, Cink.
BMI, body mass index.

Table 29.5 Anthropometric and Body Composition Characteristics in Portuguese Centenarians Compared by Gender

Variable	N	Min, max; M F	M F Combined; $\bar{X} \pm SD$	N	Female	N	Male	$p > .001$
Age (yr)	252	97, 109	100.3 ± 1.99	196	100.3 ± 1.95	56	100.1 ± 2.12	
Weight (kg)	241	29.3, 89.3	51.0 ± 11.03	188	48.7 ± 9.83	53	59.3 ± 11.18	*
Height (m)	252	1.38, 1.78	1.55 ± 0.07	196	1.53 ± 0.06	56	1.62 ± 0.07	*
BMI (kg/m^2)	241	12.29, 34.03	21.07 ± 3.69	188	20.70 ± 3.55	53	22.41 ± 3.88	
Waist (cm)	227	56, 120	85.3 ± 10.85	177	83.0 ± 9.66	50	93.5 ± 10.98	*
Hip (cm)	199	76, 137	97.4 ± 9.24	153	97.5 ± 9.42	46	97.2 ± 8.74	
Waist/hip	199	0.68, 1.09	0.88 ± 0.08	153	0.86 ± 0.06	46	0.96 ± 0.06	*
Fat mass (kg)	166	0.9, 40.9	10.7 ± 6.50	126	10.6 ± 6.90	40	11.1 ± 5.07	
Fat mass (%)	166	3.0, 45.8	19.6 ± 9.50	126	20.1 ± 10.39	40	18.2 ± 5.71	
Muscle mass (kg)	166	24.5, 59.8	38.8 ± 7.23	126	36.8 ± 6.27	40	45.1 ± 6.40	*
Muscle mass index (kg/m^2)	166	10.75, 23.1	15.910 ± 2.35	126	15.6 ± 2.29	40	17.0 ± 2.20	*
Fat-free mass (kg)	166	25.8, 63.0	40.9 ± 7.60	126	38.8 ± 6.60	40	47.5 ± 6.40	*
Lean mass index (kg/m^2)	166	11.36–24.30	16.8 ± 2.47	126	16.4 ± 2.41	40	17.9 ± 2.31	*
Fat mass index (kg/m^2)	166	0.37, 15.58	4.4 ± 2.64	126	4.4 ± 2.81	40	4.2 ± 2.03	
Bone mass (kg)	166	1.3, 3.2	2.1 ± 0.37	126	1.98 ± 0.32	40	2.4 ± 0.32	*
Bone mass index (kg/m^2)	166	0.61, 1.23	0.86 ± 0.12	126	0.84 ± 0.12	40	0.92 ± 0.11	*
Total water (%)	163	38, 84.6	53.8 ± 7.96	123	52.4 ± 7.75	40	58.1 ± 7.12	*
Total water (kg)	163	15.4, 44.7	27.5 ± 6.25	123	25.5 ± 5.07	40	33.7 ± 5.20	*
TBW/FFM (%)	163	59.7, 88.4	67.0 ± 4.38	123	65.8 ± 3.23	40	70.8 ± 5.24	*
RMR (kcal)	166	793–1776	1178 ± 202.01	126	1123 ± 173.9	40	1350 ± 188.88	*
RMR (KJ)	166	3318, 7431	4929 ± 845.18	126	4700 ± 727.6	40	5649 ± 790.30	*
Harris & Benedict (kcal/d) (RMR)	241	678, 1437	954 ± 125.7	188	935 ± 102.6	53	1018 ± 171.68	*
Visceral fat score	166	6–22	10.8 ± 3.56	126	9.3 ± 2.05	40	15.8 ± 2.73	*†
Metabolic age (yr)	166	80–90	83.5 ± 1.11	126	83.5 ± 1.17	40	83.5 ± 0.88	

Note: Min, max, minimum and maximum values in M (male) and F (female) groups; BMI, body mass index; TBW, total body water; FFM, fat-free mass; RMR, resting metabolic rate; SD, standard deviation; * = $p \leq .001$, independent samples t-test and Mann-Whitney test compared differences between genders.
Reprinted with permission from Pereira da Silva A, et al. Body composition assessment and nutritional status evaluation in men and women Portuguese centenarians. J Nutr Health Aging. 2016;20:256. Reprinted with permission from Springer Nature.

CHAPTER 30
Overweight, Overfatness (Obesity), and Weight Control

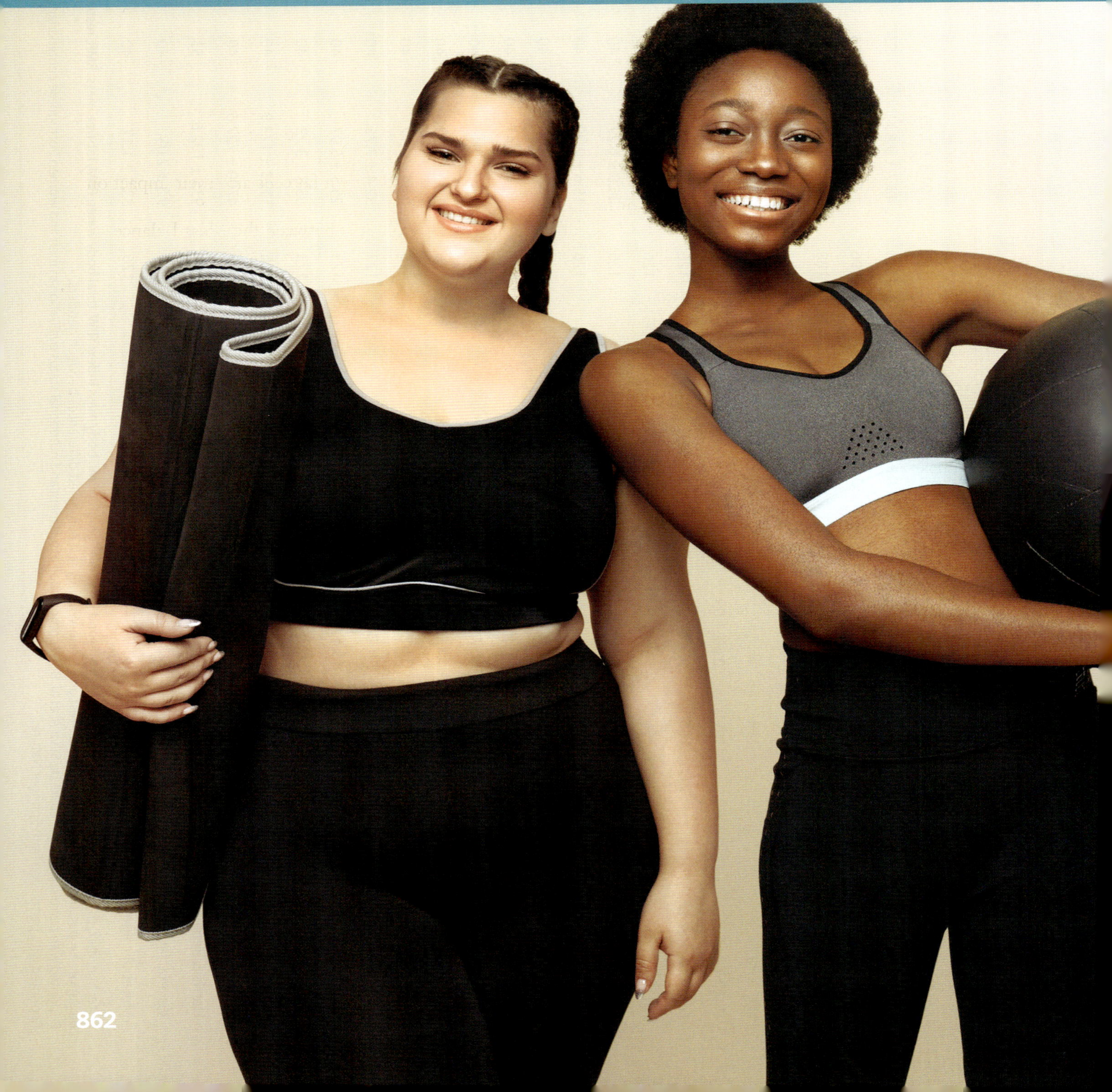

Chapter Objectives

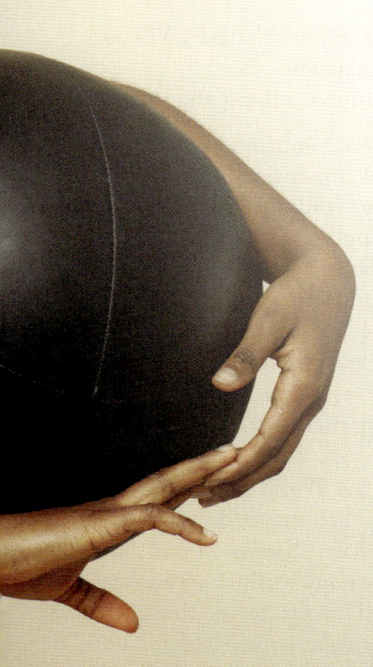

- Discuss the general economic impact from the worldwide obesity epidemic
- Describe how excess body fat in childhood and adolescence relates to adult risk for overfatness and poor health
- List 10 key health risks associated with excessive body weight and body fat
- Discuss three criteria to assess the overfat condition: body fat percentage, regional fat distribution, and fat cell size and number
- Explain how genetic factors create white and brown fat cells and their impact on the tendency for fat gain.
- Explain the main difference to explain weight loss between the Mass Balance Model and traditional energy balance equation, "calories-out" exceeding "calories-in"
- Outline three approaches to "unbalance" the energy balance equation to trigger weight loss
- Summarize two proposed advantages and disadvantages for ketogenic diets, high-protein diets, and very low-calorie diets
- Explain why combining regular physical activity with moderate food restriction provides an effective option for successful weight loss
- Summarize how two different physical activity modes affect body composition during resistance and aerobic training
- Give two diet and increased physical activity recommendations to gain body weight to improve appearance and/or enhance sports performance
- Explain how to determine minimal wrestling weight in wrestling

Ancillaries at-a-Glance

Visit Lippincott Connect to access the following resources.

- References: Chapter 30
- Appendix F: Energy Expenditure in Household, Occupational, Recreational, and Sports Activities
- Focus on Research: Genetic Tendency to Gain Weight

Part 1 Obesity

Historical Perspective

Biblical scholars throughout history have preached about personal misfortunes regarding excessive food intake and sedentary living. The 12th-century Jewish sage Rabbi Moses ben Maimon (also known as Maimonides; 1138–1204) quotes the Greek physician Galen (AD 129–201) in one of his numerous essays by writing that "*excess fat was harmful to the body and makes it sluggish, disturbs its functions, and hinders its movements.*" Maimonides also taught that everyone who practices a sedentary lifestyle and does not exercise will live a "*painful life.*" He posited that excessive eating mimics a deadly poison in the body that precipitates all illnesses.

Hippocrates (460–377 BC), the ancient Greek physician regarded as the "Father of Medicine," opined that obesity represented a major health risk that led to death from many diseases. The Hippocratic texts conveyed the overarching belief that obesity deviated from the norm so essential for maintaining a healthy balance throughout life. Galen and other contemporary physicians penned essays that promoted walking, running, wrestling, rope climbing, and vigorous, physically active pursuits in addition to baths, massage, rest, and an "*appropriate*" lifestyle as ways to rebalance one's health. Interestingly, Hippocrates believed that obese individuals should undertake physical activity (e.g., walking and jogging among city structures often used by athletes for training) before eating and to eat while still breathing hard from the previous exercise as a viable strategy to reduce excess weight.

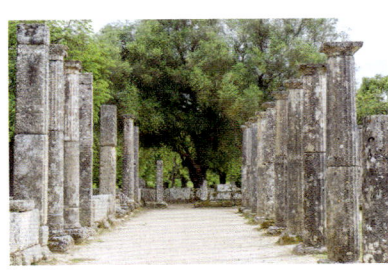
Alberto Loyo/Shutterstock

The ancient Assyrian physician Yuhanna ibn Masawayh (known in the Western world as Jean Mesue; CE 777–857; https://doi.org/10.1017/S0035869X0015868X) promoted modulating food intake to minimize disease conditions. This prolific early medical writer practiced medicine in Baghdad and served as personal physician to four Muslim religious and civil leaders (caliphs). Known for his medical aphorisms, Mesue produced the first known treatise concerning dietetics, incorporating ideas from Galen's earlier writings. This first ancient "medical nutritionist" described the essential properties in 140 foodstuffs from plants and animals and their subsequent effects on the human body. He and succeeding Persian anatomists also performed anatomical dissections on apes, exploring how to better comprehend bodily functions (www.ncbi.nlm.nih.gov/pmc/articles/PMC2100290/).

For the past 20 centuries, medical practitioners, writers, philosophers, scientists, and theologians throughout the world have advocated a sensible approach to healthy living, but ostensibly without lasting impact. From the ancient period to current times, general concepts about obesity focus on its molecular basis in childhood and perhaps even earlier.[15,190,238–240]

Obesity Remains a Global Epidemic

Today, no clear answer exists to explain why so many people gain so much extra weight and fat. An excessive gain in body fat occurs from complex interactions involving genetic, environmental, metabolic, physiologic, behavioral, social, and perhaps racial influences (refer to Chapter 28).[22,68,289,308] Individual differences predispose gains in body fat from at least 10 factors:

1. Disordered eating patterns and eating environment
2. Food packaging promoting spontaneous food purchases
3. Distorted body image
4. Reduced resting metabolic rate
5. Reduced diet-induced thermogenesis
6. Reduced spontaneous **nonexercise activity thermogenesis**[296,297]
7. Reduced basal body temperature
8. Susceptibility to viral infections
9. Diminished cellular adenosine triphosphatase (ATPase), lipoprotein lipase, and other enzymes
10. Reduced metabolically active brown adipose tissue

Obesity represents a complex condition with serious medical, social, and psychological dimensions that impacts all age and socioeconomic groups and threatens to overwhelm both developed and developing countries. Notwithstanding the upswing in attempts to lose weight, people throughout the industrialized nations are considerably more overweight and obese (with type 2 diabetes) than people even a decade ago. Unfortunately, obesity remains an equal-opportunity affliction, with the epidemic continuing to increase on all continents,[242,292] particularly so throughout the United States.[2,140,243]

FIGURE 30.1 illustrates what the World Health Organization (www.who.int/news-room/fact-sheets/detail/obesity-and-overweight) and International Obesity Task Force (http://s3-eu-west-1.amazonaws.com/wof-files/Physical_Activity_-_Position_Statement.pdf) refer to as the **global obesity epidemic**.[59,219] Six regions were considered for both males and females; the map reveals the data for adult females in the top five countries in each region identified with the highest obesity percentage. In almost all 200 countries surveyed in 2021, females had a higher obesity prevalence than males. We selected the female results to represent the uppermost in the range for percentage obesity by country. The red shaded region includes the Americas, with the United States at 41.8% and Mexico 40.2%. Canada, shaded in dark green, has a 27% obesity prevalence. The countries shaded blue have the lowest obesity prevalence (<10%) and include Timor-Leste (0.7%; north of Australia in Maritime Southeast Asia on half the Timor Island), Vietnam (1.7%), Cambodia (2.8%), Japan (3.4%), Nepal (5.3%), India (6.3%), China (6.8%), and Bangladesh (8.6%).

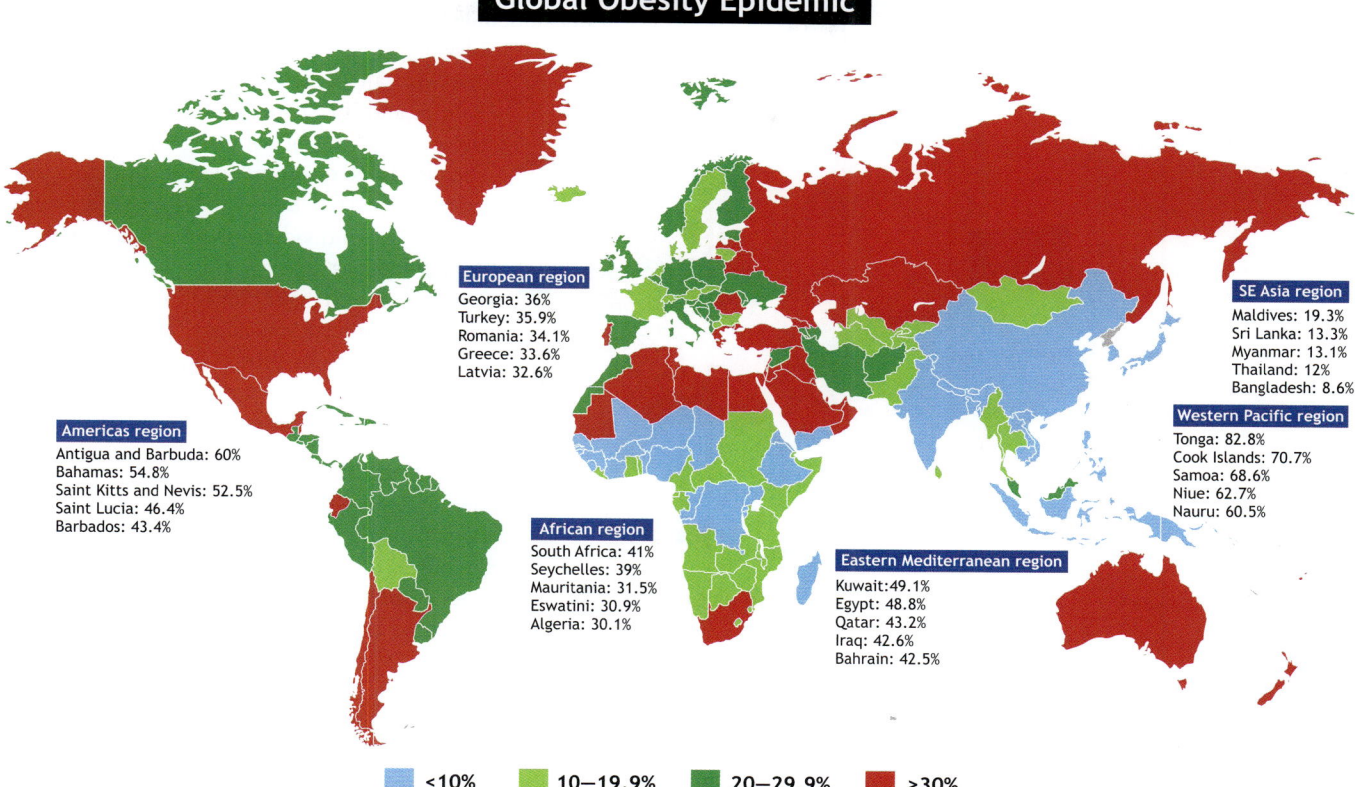

FIGURE 30.1. Global obesity epidemic. The map colors correspond to the obesity prevalence rate in women grouped into six regions with the top five countries in each group. The largest obesity percentage regions (≥30%) are depicted in *red shade* and lowest obesity prevalence region (<10%) in *blue shade*.
(Data for the country rankings within each region were summarized from data in the world literature from 2018 to 2021 and from the World Health Organization (www.who.int/news-room/fact-sheets/detail/obesity-and-overweight; www.worldobesity.org/news/global-obesity-observatory-updates). Map outline: Andrei Minsk/Shutterstock.)

Many countries in the world in 2021 had an astonishingly large obesity prevalence, assessed as body mass index (BMI) ≥ 30, with nine countries exceeding 50%: Tonga (82.8), Cook Islands (70.7%), American Samoa (68.6%), Niue (62.7), Nauru (60.5%), Kiribati (55.6%), Antigua and Barbuda (60%), Bahamas (54.8%), and Saint Kitts and Nevis (52.5%). Considered in total, worldwide obesity has nearly tripled since 1975, currently surpassing 750 million adults and another 400 million overweight and obese children and adolescents![244–246] Furthermore, most of the world's population live in countries where overweight and obesity kill more people than those who die from being underweight or malnourished.[176]

United States Obesity Epidemic: A National Disaster

FIGURE 30.2 presents the most recent 2020 data from the CDC for obesity prevalence percentage among U.S. adults by states and territories (www.cdc.gov/obesity/data/prevalence-maps.html). These findings reveal the following in comparison to 2011 data:

- No state or territory had an obesity prevalence less than 20%.
- Only one state, Colorado (CO), and the District of Columbia (DC) had an obesity prevalence from 20% to less than 25%, whereas in 2011, 10 states plus DC were in this category.
- Eleven states had an obesity prevalence from 25% to less than 30%, compared with 28 states plus Guam and Puerto Rico in 2011.
- Twenty-one states plus Guam and Puerto Rico have an obesity prevalence from 30% to less than 35%.
- Unfortunately, 15 states have the largest obesity prevalence ≥35% ever reported in the United States (AL, AR, IA, IN, KS, KY, LA, MI, MS, OH, OK, SC, TN, TX, and WV), whereas no state in 2011 exceeded 35%!

The 2021 estimates place the combined number for overweight and obese Americans at nearly 140 million (69% of the population), including 35% of college students,[130] an unprecedented increase from "only" 56% in 1982. If current trends continue, more than half of adult Americans in almost every state will classify as obese by 2030, with 56 million projected diabetes cases in the United States and 758 million worldwide![295] The expanding obesity epidemic has continued to strain the nation's medical burden, with more than 10 million additional diabetes cases and more than 15 million additional heart disease and stroke patients. The situation would become so unbridled that the obesity rate in Colorado, one of only two regions with the *lowest* obesity rates in 2019 at between 20 and

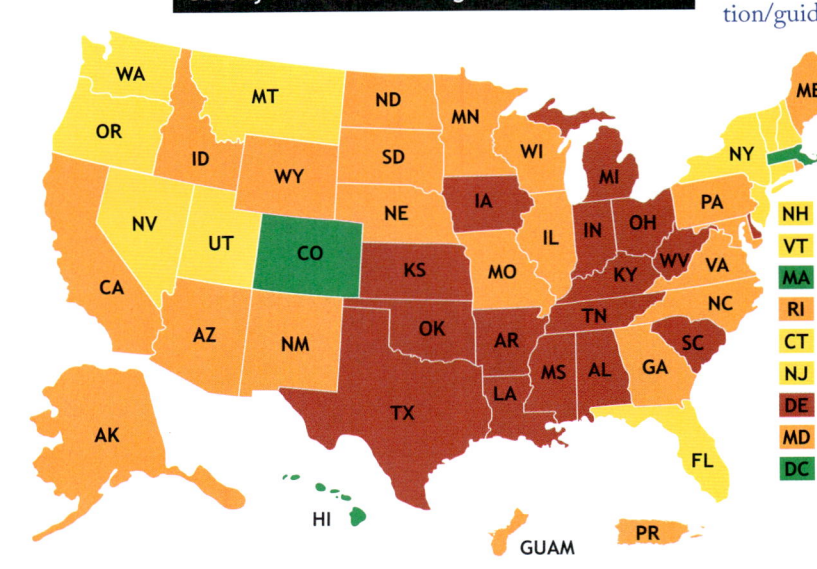

FIGURE 30.2. Prevalence of self-reported obesity among U.S. adults by state and territory.
(Source: www.cdc.gov/obesity/data/prevalence-maps.html.)

30% (formerly 20.7% in 2012), would more than double to 44.8%. In fact, obesity prevalence will be higher than 50% in 29 states and not below 35% in any state.[247] If the predictive models prove accurate, then 1 in 4 adults will be severely obese by 2030, with prevalence rates increasing by 25% in 25 states. For the entire United States, severe obesity will become the most common BMI category among females (27.6%), low-income adults (31.7%), and non-Hispanic Black adults (31.7%).

Milestone in Obesity Treatment

A milestone in American governmental action regarding obesity took place on December 1, 2003. The United States Preventive Services Task Force (www.ahrq.gov/prevention/guidelines/index.html), a government medical expert advisory group, urged physicians to weigh and measure all patients and recommend counseling and behavior therapy strategies for those classifying obese using BMI standards. The task force recommended that doctors prescribe intensive behavior therapy at least twice monthly (in individual or group sessions) for up to 3 months supervised by a health-professional team with psychologists, registered dietitians, and exercise specialists. These guidelines represented a major shift in how the health care system believes how to deal with the out-of-control obesity epidemic.

Impact on Children. Children experience an equally depressing situation because the overweight prevalence in children (BMI ≥ 95th percentile for age and sex) has attained grim proportions, with the total reaching almost 13 million or 17% of American youth ages 2 to 19 classified as obese.[26,149,198,247,248] A comprehensive report released about 20 years ago by the National Academies of Medicine (https://nam.edu/health-horizon/?gclid=CjwKCAiAvOeQ BhBkEiwAxutUVH3Q2i1u7qCpHCR9mOLFt7C3BslKm V0Dw17eNXiFPhQuygv-Bti1ERoCS84QAvD_BwE) on the causes and solutions for childhood obesity in the United States indicated that from 1970 to 2000, obesity had tripled among children ages 6 to 11, particularly in rural America, to nearly 15%. The rates had doubled for those ages 2 to 5 (>10%) and from age 12 to 19 to more than 15% as shown in the accompanying image. Pediatric obesity represents childhood's most common chronic disorder, particularly prevalent among poor and minority children.[54,211] About 70% of obese youth possess multiple risk factors for diabetes, elevated cholesterol, hypertension, bone and joint disorders, and social and psychological problems including stigmatization and poor self-esteem.

The rise in body weight was partially related to the nearly 300% increase between 1977 and 1996 from foods children consume at restaurants and fast food outlets.[197] Soft drink consumption in young consumers accounts for an additional 188 kcal each day above the energy intakes of children who do not consume these beverages. Excessive fatness in youth represents an even greater adult health risk than obesity begun in adulthood. Overweight children and adolescents, particularly young girls regardless of final body weight in adulthood, exhibit higher illness risks than normal-weight adolescents.[293]

The most recent data, from January 2021, may be compared with data from 1963 for children and adolescents ages 2 to 19. The results reveal a

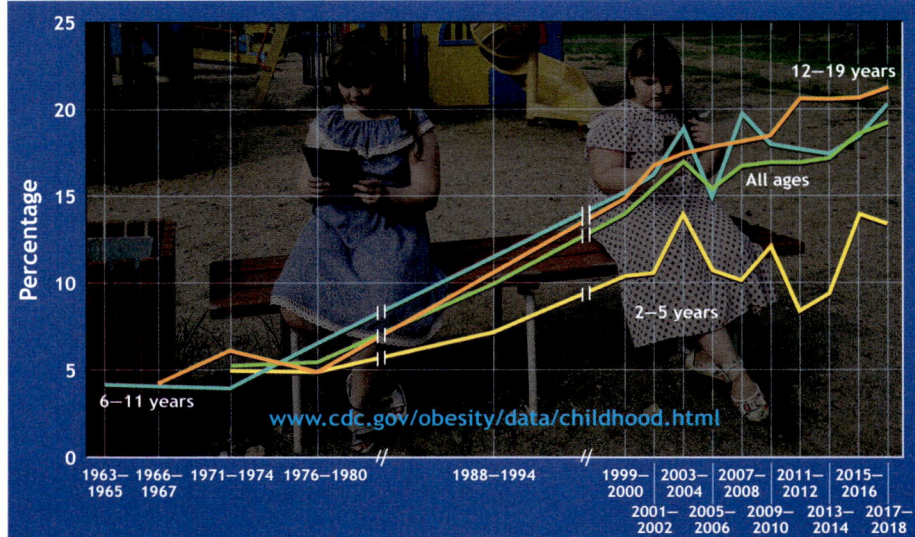

Data from www.cdc.gov/obesity/data/childhood.html. Background photo: Vlarvixof/Shutterstock

dire trend. There are four major findings related to the 2021 data:

- Obesity prevalence was 19.3%, impacting approximately 14.4 million U.S. children and adolescents.
- Childhood obesity was more common among certain populations. Age, sex, and race and Hispanic origin influence a given BMI category.
- Obesity prevalence was 13.4% among 2- to 5-year-olds, 20.3% among 6- to 11-year-olds, and 21.2% among 12- to 19-year-olds. Health risks may begin at a lower BMI among Asians.
- Obesity prevalence was 25.6% among Hispanic children, 24.2% among non-Hispanic Black children, 16.1% among non-Hispanic White children, and 8.7% among non-Hispanic Asian children.

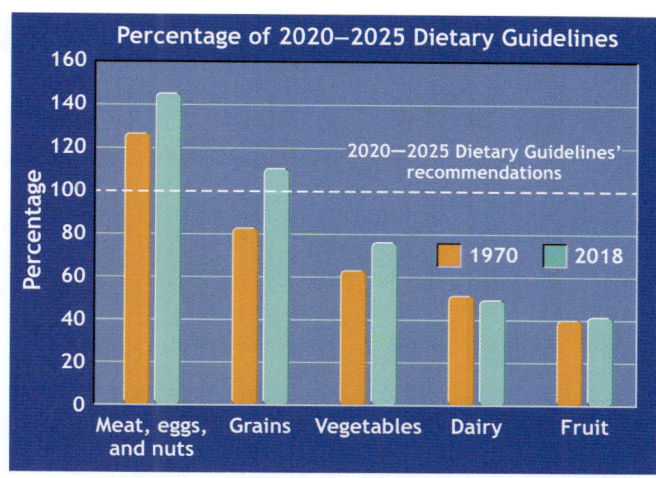

Source: USDA, Economic Research Service, Loss-Adjusted Food Availability Data and 2020–2025 Dietary Guidelines

Increased Body Fat: A Progressive Long-Term Process

Excess body fat accumulation or overfatness represents a heterogeneous disorder in which energy intake chronically exceeds energy expenditure.[290] The disruption in energy balance often begins in childhood to profoundly affect the likelihood for reaching the obesity category as one moves into adulthood. For example, obese children at ages 6 to 9 have a 55% chance of becoming obese as adults—a risk 10 times that of normal-weight children. Simply stated, a child or adolescent generally does not "outgrow" the overly fat condition.[294]

Ages 25 to 44 are the "danger" years when adults develop excessive fatness.[31] Middle-aged males and females invariably weigh more than college-aged counterparts at the same stature. Beginning between ages 20 and 40 and then on into their sixth decade, the typical relatively sedentary American gains about 1 kg/2.2l lb yearly for an 18-kg/40-lb gain in body weight. Females tend to gain the most weight; about 14% add more than 14 kg/30 lb between ages 25 and 34. It remains unclear as to whether "creeping obesity" in adulthood reflects a normal biologic pattern or a disruption in normal energy balance homeostasis related to elevated oxidative stressors from an accumulating adipose tissue mass.[249]

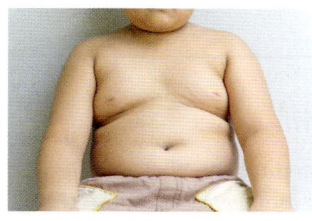

kwanchai.c/Shutterstock

Changing Dietary Patterns Play a Role

Mismatches in daily food consumption and daily energy expenditure patterns are particularly troublesome for overweight and obese individuals, who must dramatically upgrade daily dietary and physical activity behavior patterns (www.ers.usda.gov/data-products/chart-gallery/gallery/chart-detail/?chartId=58334).

U.S. Diets and Federal Recommendations

Individuals living in the United States typically consume more vegetables and fruit than in 1970, yet the average U.S. diet still falls short of the *2020–2025 Dietary Guidelines for Americans* for the five major food categories shown in the above image. On average, consumption of meat, eggs, nuts, and grains exceeded the recommended Guideline amounts. Expressed as a percentage of total food intake, Americans overconsume meats by about 42% and grains by about 8%, while substantially under-consuming fruits by 60%, vegetables by about 20%, and dairy products by approximately 55%.

The most disturbing dramatic increase in food consumption has occurred in added sugar intake. According to the USDA Farm Service Agency, in 1970, the average daily per capita calorie intake from added sugars (adjusted for spoilage and other waste) amounted to 332 kcal, with raw tonnage under 7000 tons (www.usda.gov/oce/commodity-markets/waob). In 2011, the amount jumped 11% to about 370 kcal daily per person, with an annual sugar production above 8000 tons! Most increases come from high-fructose corn syrup, glucose, and other corn sweeteners. The most current data from various sugar production sources (2011–2021; see the inset figure on the next page) reveal how the typical American diet has not declined in sugar consumption from 2011; in fact, raw sugar production was the highest during the last half century.

Genetics Influence Body Fat Accumulation

The notable interaction between genetics and environment makes it difficult to quantify their role in obesity development.[280] Research with twins, adopted children, and specific segments in the population attributes up to an 80% risk of becoming obese to genetic factors. For example, heavier than normal newborns become fat adolescents only when the father or particularly the mother is overweight.[61] Little risk exists for an overweight toddler to grow into an obese adult if both parents are not overweight. If one or both parents are obese, then a child under age 10 has more than twice the normal risk of becoming an obese adult.[209,227] Even for normal-weight prepubertal girls, body composition and regional fat distribution relate to both parents' body composition characteristics.[208]

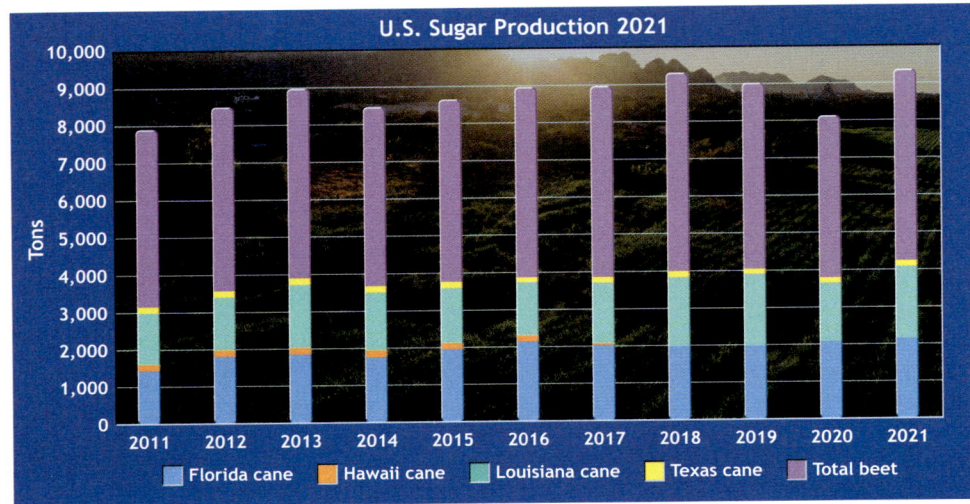

Altering the Threshold and Inherited Factors

One's genetic makeup does not necessarily cause obesity but instead lowers the *threshold* for its development from susceptibility genes.[160] Researchers have identified key genes and specific DNA sequence variants that relate to the molecular causes in appetite and satiety factors that predispose a person to gain excessive body fat. A more complete understanding about the genetic role in body fat accretion requires identifying key genes and their mutations including the relevant proteins that contribute to chronic energy imbalance.[241,279,281,296]

Inherited factors contribute to variability in weight gain among individuals fed an identical daily caloric excess and can contribute to the tendency to regain lost weight. Individuals who represent nine different kinds of relatives indicate that genetic factors that affect metabolism and appetite determine about 25% related to the total transmissible variation among persons in percentage body fat and total fat mass (**FIGURE 30.3**). A larger percentage variation in body fat status relates to a 30% transmissible cultural effect—an unhealthy expression in preexisting gene patterns. The remaining 45% nontransmissible effect may change as new research explores the multidimensional aspect regarding obesity. *In an obesity-producing environment—sedentary and stressful, with ready access to inexpensive, large-portion, high-calorie, good-tasting food—the genetically susceptible obesity-prone individual gains weight and possibly lots of it.* Athletes in weight-related sports with a genetic propensity for obesity must constantly battle to maintain optimal body weight and composition for competitive performance.

INTEGRATIVE QUESTION

What evidence documents that body fat accumulation among children and adults does not necessarily result from excessive food intake?

A Mutant Gene and Leptin

Human obesity links to a mutant gene that synthesizes **leptin** (derived from the Greek root *leptos*, meaning "thin"), a crucial satiety hormone released into the bloodstream with a primary function to regulate body weight and obesity.[309] Leptin acts on the hypothalamus to affect how much one eats, how much energy one expends, and ultimately how much one weighs.

The genetic model in **FIGURE 30.4** proposes that the **obese (*ob*) gene** normally becomes activated in adipose tissue and perhaps muscle tissue, where it encodes and stimulates leptin production, which then enters the bloodstream. This satiety-signaling molecule travels to the arcuate nucleus, a collection including specialized neurons in the mediobasal hypothalamus that develops soon after birth to control appetite and metabolism. Normally, leptin blunts the urge to eat when caloric intake maintains ideal body lipid stores. Leptin may affect specific hypothalamic neurons that suppress appetite control factors and/or reduce neurochemical levels that stimulate appetite.[76,119,142] Such mechanisms would explain how body fat remains intimately "connected"

FIGURE 30.3. Total transmissible variance for total body fat and percentage body fat determined by hydrostatic weighing.
(Data from Bouchard C, et al. Inheritance of the amount and distribution of human body fat. *Int J Obes*. 1988;12:205. Photo: Flotsam/Shutterstock.)

CHAPTER 30 • Overweight, Overfatness (Obesity), and Weight Control 869

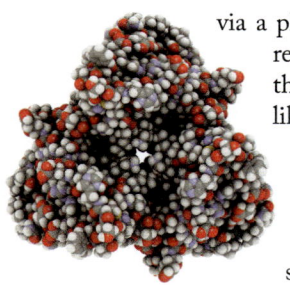

StudioMolekuul/Shutterstock

via a physiologic pathway to the brain to regulate energy balance. In a way, the adipocyte serves an endocrine-like function. With a gene defective for either adipocyte leptin production and/or hypothalamic leptin sensitivity, the brain inadequately assesses the body's adipose tissue status to further enable eating urges. In essence, leptin availability or lack thereof impacts appetite and the brain's dynamic "wiring," leading to appetite control dysregulation and obesity promotion throughout adulthood.

fyi When Reality Meets the Road

The inset image illustrates the reality faced by millions of Americans daily when they go out to eat—it reinforces the extreme difficulty in combating overeating and the obesity epidemic—the portion sizes are enormous! This hit home when two of the textbook authors stopped for breakfast at Tony's roadside diner about 20 mi north of Flint, Michigan while traveling to an American College of Sports Medicine National Convention. What a surprise when the scrambled eggs, toast, hash browns, and a side of bacon arrived. When asked if a mistake had been made in the bacon side order, the waiter confirmed that all bacon sides weigh in at 1 lb of cooked weight (we verified 58 pieces, about 2418 kcal with 184 g/6.5 oz of lipid—more than seven times the recommended daily intake just for the bacon!). The restaurant proudly advertises its specialty—*the United States of Bacon*—and advertise that they use up to 11,000 lb of bacon weekly!

Inability to Sustain Weight Loss

The hormone-hypothalamic biologic control mechanism helps to explain the extreme difficulty overfat persons have in sustaining fat loss. In children and adults, when energy balance remains in steady state, plasma leptin circulates in direct proportion to adipose tissue mass in the inset figure, with four times more leptin in obese compared with lean individuals. Consequently, human obesity may resemble a relative leptin resistance state similar to obesity-related insulin resistance.[70] High blood leptin concentrations shown in the brain scan by the green luminescence associate strongly with four core metabolic disturbances in the insulin-resistant metabolic syndrome—upper-body obesity, glucose intolerance, and hypertension. These unique metabolic disturbances ultimately act as a conduit to trigger higher incidence for heart disease, stroke, and type 2 diabetes.[199] Weight

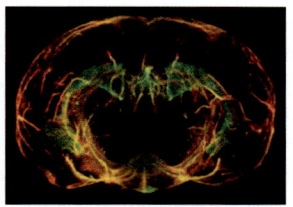

Reprinted with permission from Izquierdo AG, et al. Leptin, obesity, and leptin resistance: where are we 25 years later? *Nutrients*. 2019;11:2704.

loss reduces serum leptin concentration, while weight gain increases serum leptin.[113] Four additional factors—gender, hormones, pharmacologic agents, and the body's current energy requirements—also trigger leptin production. Neither short- nor long-term physical activity meaningfully affects leptin, independent from the activity's effects on total adipose tissue mass.[42,150] Subcutaneous recombinant leptin injections produced a dose-response effect with body weight and body fat loss in lean and obese males and females with elevated endogenous serum leptin concentrations.[80] This suggests a potential role for leptin and related hormones in treating

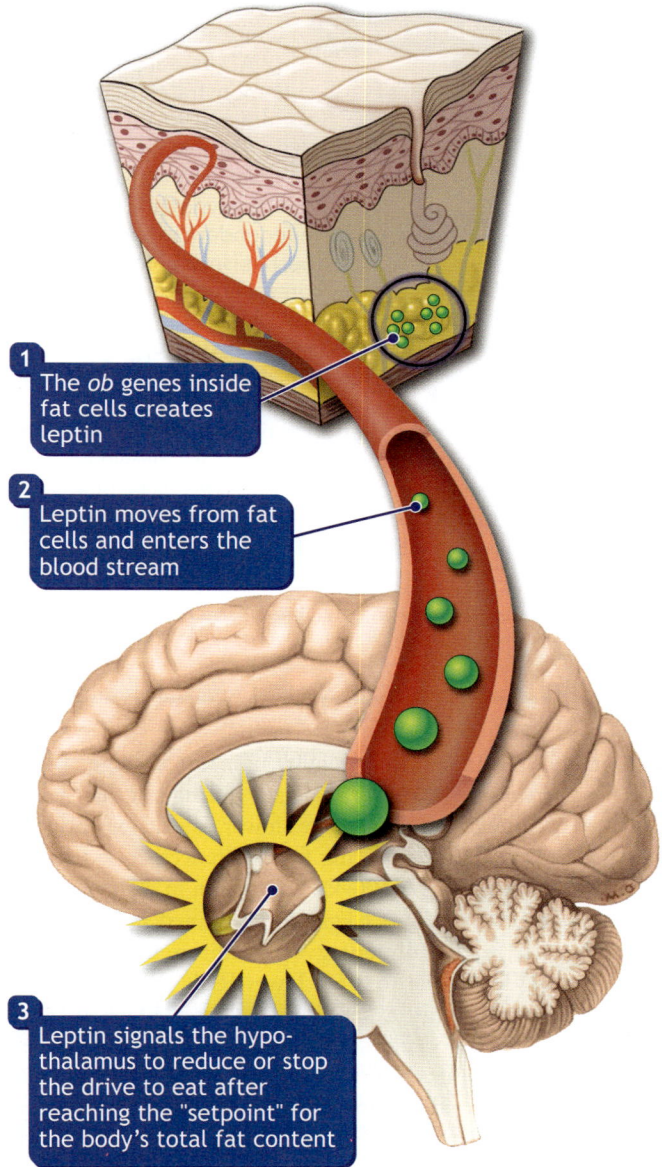

1. The *ob* genes inside fat cells creates leptin
2. Leptin moves from fat cells and enters the blood stream
3. Leptin signals the hypothalamus to reduce or stop the drive to eat after reaching the "setpoint" for the body's total fat content

FIGURE 30.4. A genetic model for obesity. A malfunctioning satiety gene markedly blunts satiety hormone leptin production by disrupting events in the hypothalamus from adjusting the body's fat storage levels.

obesity,[163] as proposed in a schematic overview showing the interrelationships among obesity, leptin resistance, and disrupted leptin signaling in the brain (where specific brain hormone analogs to leptin and receptor expressive molecules reside), all potentiating the need to increase food intake and thereby contribute to the obese condition.[250]

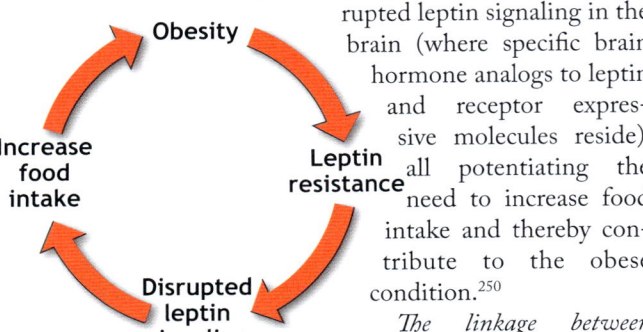

Reprinted with permission from Izquierdo AG, et al. Leptin, obesity, and leptin resistance: where are we 25 years later? *Nutrients*. 2019;11:2704.

The linkage between genetic and molecular abnormalities to obesity allows researchers to view overfatness as a disease rather than a psychologic flaw. Identifying genetic predisposition toward obesity early in life would make it possible to begin diet and physical activity interventions before obesity sets in and fat loss becomes exceedingly difficult if not highly improbable.

Leptin alone does not determine body fatness nor explain why some people seemingly eat whatever they want and gain little weight, while others become overfat with the same caloric intake. Besides *defective leptin production*, defective receptor action increases resistance to endogenous satiety chemicals. A specific gene, the **uncoupling Protein-2 (*UCP2*) gene**,[251] adds another piece to the complex obesity puzzle. The gene activates a specific protein that burns excess calories as heat energy without coupling to other energy-consuming processes. This **futile metabolism** blunts excess fat storage. Individual differences in gene activation and alterations in metabolic activity lend credence to a common mantra, *"Every little bit of excess food I eat seems to change to fat."* A drug that turns on the *UCP2* gene to synthesize more heat-generating protein could potentially provide a pharmacologic windfall to shed excess body fat. Other newly discovered molecules that control eating include agouti-related protein (AGRP), a protein controlled by leptin that may affect hypothalamic cells to increase caloric intake.[252,253] The brain also synthesizes melanin-concentrating hormone when leptin levels increase.[134] An excess in this protein molecule increases an animal's appetite, causing it to eat and gain weight. Future drugs that inhibit or "destabilize" brain chemicals may ultimately provide a novel long-term resolution to help control eating and excess fat accumulation.

Racial Differences

Racial differences in food consumption, physical activity patterns, and cultural attitudes toward body weight help to explain the greater prevalence of obesity in Black women (nearly 50%) than White women (33%).[57] Small differences in resting energy expenditure (REE), related to racial differences in lean body mass,[18] contribute to racial differences in obesity.[81,93] The "racial" effect, which also exists among children and adolescents,[201,207] predisposes a Black female to gain

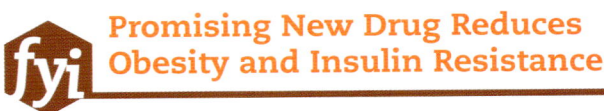

Promising New Drug Reduces Obesity and Insulin Resistance

Psoralea corylifolia L is a medicinal plant used in Chinese medicine since antiquity to treat various infirmities including excessive body fat. Researchers have now demonstrated that corylin ($C_{20}H_{16}O_4$), a flavonoid extract from this medicinal, exerts anti-inflammatory, anticancer, and antiatherosclerotic effects by reducing hyperlipidemia and insulin resistance. In a novel approach involving white adipose tissue (WAT), researchers demonstrated that corylin induced WAT to increase a browning effect in mice by activating lipolysis through independent molecular mechanisms. Compared with control groups, mice fed a high-fat diet with and without corylin significantly reduced body weight and fat accumulation (with hypertrophied adipocytes) by increasing insulin sensitivity, mitochondrial biogenesis, and β-oxidation pathways. The research demonstrated that corylin exerted antiobesity effects through the browning of white adipocytes by activating brown adipose tissue to promote increased lipid metabolism (via facultative thermogenesis, Chapter 9)—a promising future therapeutic approach to help combat the worldwide obesity epidemic.

Mice photo: Janson George/Shutterstock

Source:
Chen CC, et al. Corylin reduces obesity and insulin resistance and promotes adipose tissue browning through SIRT-1 and β3-AR activation. *Pharmacol Res*. 2021;164:105291.

weight and regain it after weight loss. On average, Black females burn nearly 100 fewer kcal daily during rest than aged-matched White counterparts. The slower caloric expenditure rate persists even after adjusting for differences in body mass and body composition. A 100-kcal reduction in daily metabolism translates to nearly 2.2 kg/1 lb fat gained monthly. For Black females, total daily energy expenditure averages 10% lower than Whites, due to a 5% lower REE and 19% lower physical activity energy expenditure.[22] Obese Black females also showed greater decreases in REE than White females following energy restriction and weight loss,[66] enhancing the racial divide among Black and White females. The combined lower initial REE and more profound REE depression with weight loss suggest that overweight Black females, including many younger athletes,[254] experience greater difficulty achieving and maintaining goal body weight than overweight White females. School lunch and home food environmental variables accounted for racial but not gender differences in obesity prevalence. Such childhood disparities have an enormous economic impact—$14 billion in direct medical costs. Moreover, obesity-related illnesses account for a staggering $190.2 billion or nearly 21% for annual medical spending in the United States (www.healthycommunitieshealthyfuture.org/learn-the-facts/economic-costs-of-obesity/). Childhood obesity also is commonplace in Australia, but with proportionately less economic impact due to aggressive intervention strategies.[255]

Remain Cautious About Racial Differences

One must carefully evaluate methods to explore purported racial differences in body composition characteristics and how these implicate health and physical performance.[32,218] For example, interethnic and interracial differences in body size, structure, and body fat distribution often mask true differences in body fat at a given BMI. A single generalized BMI-health risk model that combines all ethnic and racial groups obscures the potential to document chronic disease risks among different ethnically and racially diverse population groups.[63,188] As discussed in Chapter 28, the inherent relationship between BMI and health risk varies among racial and ethnic groups; these are real differences and cannot ascribed to measurement errors.

Physical Inactivity: A Crucial Component for Excessive Fat Accumulation

Regular physical activity, through either recreation or occupation, can help to minimize weight and fat gain. This effect thwarts the tendency to regain lost weight and counters a common genetic variation that makes people more likely to gain excess weight.[84,91,92,160,194] Maintaining a physically active lifestyle contributes positively to obesity-related health prevention and treatment outcomes independently from weight loss effect.[75]

Individuals who maintain weight loss show greater muscle strength and engage in more physical activity than counterparts who regained lost weight.[221] Variations in physical activity alone accounted for more than 75% regained body weight. Such findings highlight the need to identify and promote strategies that increase regular physical activity. Current guidelines by the Surgeon General and Institute of Medicine recommend a minimum 30 to 60 min moderate physical activity daily. *We endorse an increase to 80 to 90 min physical activity daily, 6 to 7 days a week (preferably seven) over and above regular routines, to try and dent the on-going U.S. obesity epidemic.* We believe individuals must increase daily whole-body movement behaviors rather than remain trapped year after year into duplicating daily sedentary behaviors.

Physical Activity and Body Fat Accumulation Throughout Life

From age 3 months to 1 year, the total energy expenditure of infants who later became overweight averaged 21% lower than

Regained Lost Weight Promotes More Fat and Less Muscle

Typically, weight regained after weight loss represents more fat and less muscle compared with the composition of weight lost. An experiment was conducted to determine whether the composition of body weight regained after intentional weight loss corresponded to the composition of body weight lost. Seventy-eight obese, sedentary, postmenopausal women reduced weight an average of 11.8 kg/26 lb over 5 months by reducing daily energy intake by 400 kcal 3 d · wk^{-1}. On average, 67% of the weight lost was fat and 33% lean body tissue. After 1 year, 54 women regained at least 2.0 kg/4.4 lb. For them, 81% of regained weight was body fat and 19% lean tissue.

Specifically, for every 1 kg/2.2 lb of body fat lost during weight-loss intervention, 0.2 kg/0.6 lb of lean tissue was lost; for every 1 kg/2.2 lb of body fat regained over the following year, only 0.12 kg/0.03 lb of lean tissue was regained.

Nina Buday/Shutterstock

Sources:
Beavers KM, et al. Is lost lean mass from intentional weight loss recovered during weight regain in postmenopausal women? *Am J Clin Nutr.* 2011;94:767.
Beavers KM, et al. Effect of exercise type during intentional weight loss on body composition in older adults with obesity. *Obesity (Silver Spring).* 2017;25:1823.
Beavers KM, et al. Association of sex or race with the effect of weight loss on physical function: a secondary analysis of 8 randomized clinical trials. *JAMA Netw Open.* 2020;3(8):e2014631. Erratum in: *JAMA Netw Open.* 2020;3(9):e2023164.

---

that of infants with normal weight gain.[166] For children ages 6 to 9 years, percentage body fat inversely related to physical activity level in boys but not girls.[8] Obese preadolescent and adolescent children generally spend less time in physical activity or engage in less intense physical activity than normal-weight peers.[35,125,216] By the time young girls attain adolescence, many do not engage in any leisure-time physical activity. The decline in time spent in physical activity averaged nearly 100% among Black and 64% among White girls between ages 9 and 10 and 15 and 16.[109] By age 16, 56% of Black girls and 31% of White girls reported no leisure-time physical activity.

Physically active lifestyles lessen the expected pattern to accumulate excess body fat throughout adulthood. For young and middle-aged men who engage in regular physical activity, activity level relates inversely to body fat level.[136] Not surprisingly, middle-aged long-distance runners remain leaner than sedentary counterparts. No relationship emerges between the runners' body fat level and caloric intake. Perhaps the relatively greater body fat among middle-aged runners results from less vigorous training, not greater food intake.[112]

Increasing Energy Output During Aging Modulates Weight Gain

Maintaining a lifestyle that prioritizes moderate physical activity can diminish but probably will not forestall the tendency to add weight through middle age. Sedentary males and females who undertake physical activity regimens (and moderate food intake) tend to reduce body weight and fat compared with those who remain sedentary. Moreover, a proportionality exists between weight loss and activity dose.[229,230]

FIGURE 30.5 displays the inverse association among distance run, BMI, and waist circumference for males in all age categories. Physically active men typically remained leaner than sedentary counterparts for each age group; men who ran longer distance each week weighed less than those who ran shorter distance. The typical male who maintained a constant weekly running distance through middle age gained 1.5 kg/3.3 lb and increased waist size about 1.1 cm/0.75 in. despite distance run. Such findings suggest that by age 50, a physically active man can expect to weigh about 4.5 kg/10 lb more with a 5.1-cm/3-in. larger waist than he weighed at age 20 despite maintaining a constantly increased physical activity level. This proclivity to gain weight and girth may relate to reduced testosterone and growth hormone levels that induce age-related changes in physique and increase abdominal and visceral fat. To counter weight gain in middle age, one should gradually increase weekly physical activity the equivalent compared with fast walking, jogging, or running 2.3 km/1.4 mi for each year beginning about age 30.

INTEGRATIVE QUESTION

Among physically active males and females, how can individuals who consume the most calories weigh less than those who consume fewer calories?

Excessive Body Fat's Health Risks

Obesity represents an unfortunate *cause* of preventable death in America. The combined effects from poor diet and decreased physical activity link closely to the year-over-year increase in death rate. One in five health care dollars spent on middle-aged Americans result from excessive body fat. Impaired glucose tolerance and overall diminished life quality emerge even among obese children, adolescents, and adults.[24,78,175,183] Hypertension, elevated blood sugar, 13 different cancers shown in the image, elevated total cholesterol, and decreased high-density lipoprotein (HDL) cholesterol heighten an overweight individual's poor health risk at any given excess weight level. Increased loads on the major joints can lead to pain and discomfort, complications from osteoarthritis, inefficient body mechanics, and reduced mobility.[82]

Staying healthy and maintaining a normal body weight also may reduce the risk from mental decline and impaired cognitive function with aging.[182] Obesity prevalence has counteracted the decline over previous years in coronary artery disease among middle-aged women.[87] Obese and overweight individuals with two or more heart disease risk factors should reduce weight, while overweight persons without any other risk factors should at least maintain current body weight. Even a modest weight reduction improves insulin sensitivity and the blood lipid profile, and prevents or delays diabetes onset in high-risk individuals.[39,66]

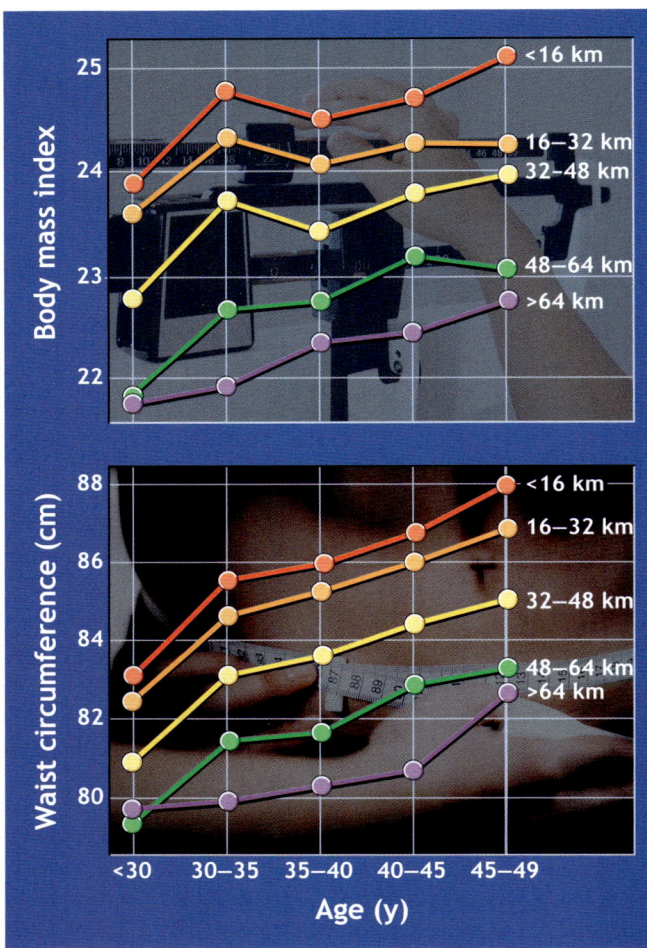

FIGURE 30.5. Relationship among average body mass index (*top*) and waist circumference (*bottom*) and age for men who maintained constant weekly running for varying distances (<16 to >64 km · wk^{-1}). Men who annually increase their running distance by 2.24 km/1.39 mi per wk compensate for the anticipated weight gain during middle age.
(Adapted with permission from Williams PT. Evidence for the incompatibility of age-neutral overweight and age-neutral physical activity standards from runners. *Am J Clin Nutr.* 1997;65:1391. With permission from the American Society for Nutrition, https://nutrition.org/. Background photos: Shutterstock—forestpath (scale), Microgen (waist).)

Designincolor/Shutterstock

Excessive Fatness in Childhood and Adolescence Predicts Adverse Adulthood Health Effects

Adverse health consequences relating to obesity often begin in childhood. Children who gain more weight than peers tend to

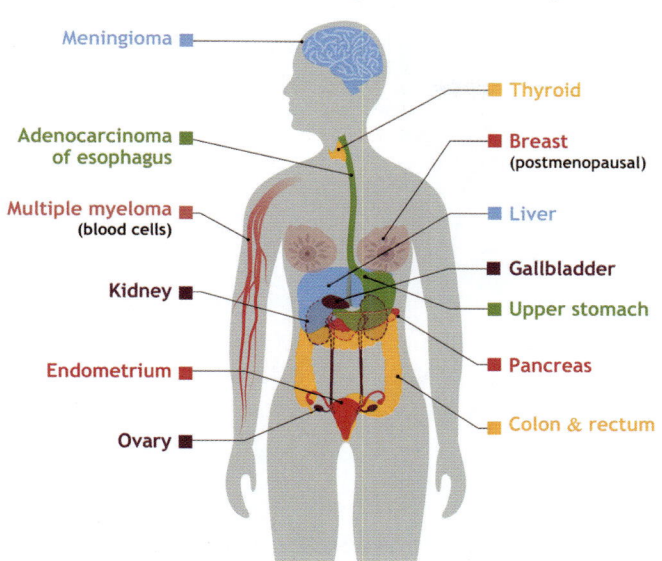

Source: cancer.gov/obesity-fact-sheet

become overweight adults with increased risk for hypertension, elevated insulin, hypercholesterolemia, and heart disease.[40] Being overweight during adolescence links to adverse health effects 55 years later. The Harvard Growth Study from 1922 to 1935 evaluated 3000 schoolchildren annually on different health variables, including triplicate body mass and stature measures, at the same time each year until they left or graduated high school.[34] From the initial group, the researchers studied 1857 subjects for an additional 8 years. Subjects were classified according to BMI as either lean (25th to 50th percentile) or overweight (>75th percentile). Compared with leaner subjects, overweight children as adults showed a greater mortality risk from all causes and a twofold higher coronary heart disease risk.[223] Women overweight during adolescence were eight times more likely to report problems with personal care and routine living tasks, such as walking, stair climbing, and lifting, and a 1.6-fold increase in arthritis than women rated lean in adolescence.

The alarming rise in obesity during childhood and adolescence requires immediate interventions to prevent subsequent risk for disease as these children grow into adulthood. **FIGURE 30.6A AND B** indicates the percentile cutoffs for a two-level procedure to identify overweight boys and girls (BMI ≥ 95th percentile, requiring in-depth medical assessment) versus those at risk for becoming overweight (BMI = 85th–95th percentile, requiring second-level screening including family history and risk factor assessment).

Defined Health Risks

Considerable evidence confirms that an increase in body fat levels leads to well-defined health risks in children, adolescents, and adults. Excessive body fat relates closely to the alarming increase in type 2 diabetes among children. For adults with diabetes, 70% are overweight and nearly 35% are obese. A moderate 4 to 10% increase in body weight after

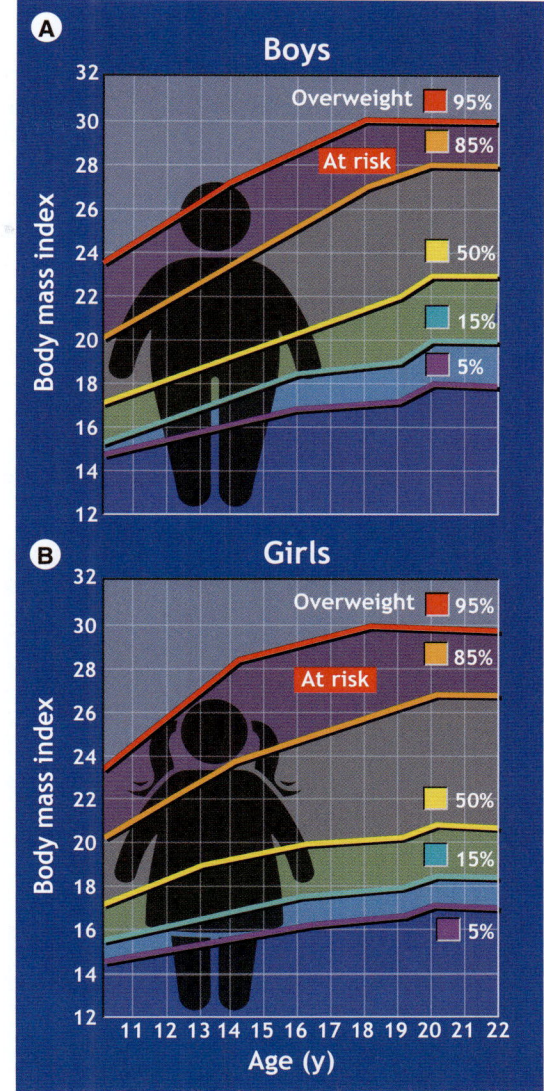

FIGURE 30.6. Two-level procedure using body mass index identifies overweight adolescents and those at risk for becoming overweight.
(Adapted with permission from Green M, ed. *Bright Futures: Guidelines for Health Supervision of Infants, Children and Adolescents*. Arlington: National Center for Education in Maternal and Child Health; 1994. Permission conveyed through Copyright Clearance Center, Inc. Background images: Cherstva/Shutterstock.)

age 20 associates with a 1.5-times greater risk for death from coronary artery disease and nonfatal myocardial infarction.[168] Even maintaining body weight at the high end of the normal range increases heart disease risk. An 8-year study with about 116,000 female nurses observed that all but the thinnest women showed increased risk for heart attack and chest pains.[131] Nurses with average body weight experienced 30% more heart attacks than thinner counterparts, whereas moderately overweight nurses had an 80% higher risk on average. This means that a woman who gains 9 kg/19.8 lb from her late teens to middle age doubles her heart attack risk. Epidemiologic evidence reveals that excess body weight serves as an independent yet powerful risk factor for congestive heart failure.[107] Weight gain also increases risk for breast, colon, esophagus, prostate, kidney, and uterine cancers.[19,200,234] Maintaining a

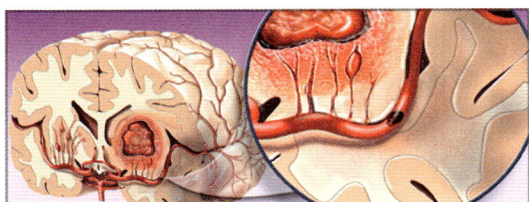

Stroke: Impairs neurologic function, leads to numbness, weakness, speech difficulty, coordination, or walking

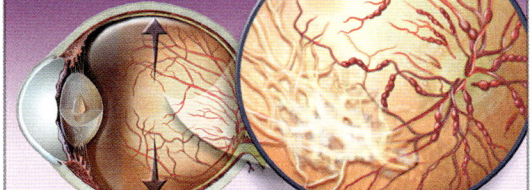

Eye disease: Causes blind spots and possibly blindness

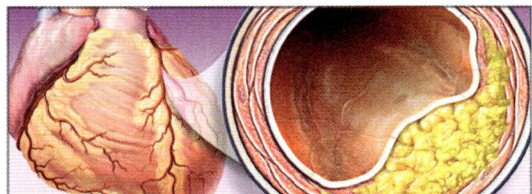

Heart disease: Causes heart attacks and congestive heart failure

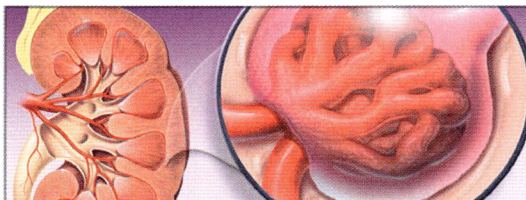

Kidney disease: Causes kidney failure

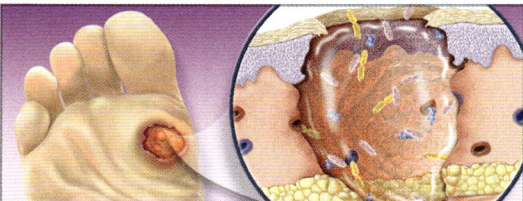

Circulatory problems: Causes sores that heal poorly; gangrene can lead to amputations

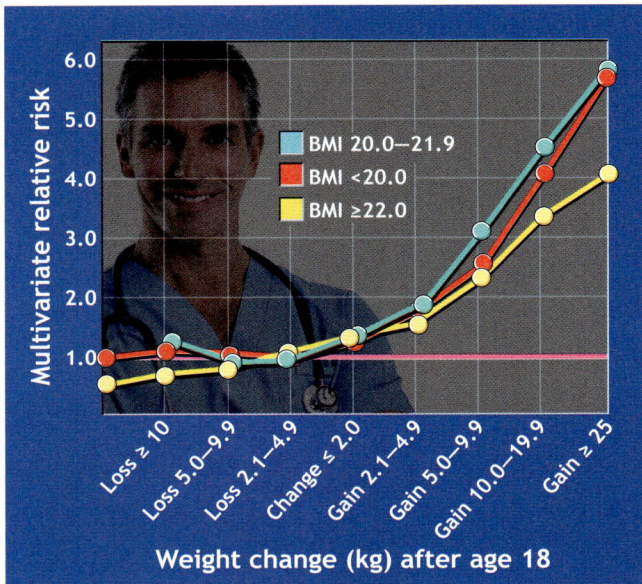

FIGURE 30.7. Multivariate relative hypertension risk according to weight change after age 18. BMI strata (horizontal pink line) indicates normal risk.
(From Huang Z, et al. Body weight, weight change, and risk for hypertension in women. *Ann Intern Med.* 1998;128(2):81. Copyright © 1998 American College of Physicians. All Rights Reserved. Reprinted with the permission of American College of Physicians, Inc. Background photo: kurhan/Shutterstock.)

BMI ≤25 could prevent one in six cancer deaths linked to overweightness in the United States, or about 90,000 deaths yearly,[19] including 33% of deaths from colon, endometrial, and breast cancer, as well as 50% of cardiovascular deaths linked to overweightness.

Researchers studied 82,000 female nurses ages 30 to 55 every 2 years from 1976 to determine whether initial BMI modifies the relationship between long-term weight gain or weight loss and hypertension risk. **FIGURE 30.7** reveals the adjusted hypertension multiple factor risk linked to hypertension in three groups stratified for BMI at age 18. The 1.0 horizontal pink line indicates normal risk. For females in the first and second BMI tertiles at age 18 (BMI ≥ 22.0), weight loss in later years did not reduce hypertension risk. Weight gain after age 18 markedly increased hypertension risk compared to females who maintained a stable body weight. For females with BMIs greater than 22.0, subsequent weight loss dramatically decreased hypertension risk. Weight gains increased hypertension risk similarly to the lighter female group. Obesity now ranks with the four other major heart attack risk factors—high cholesterol, hypertension, cigarette smoking, and sedentary lifestyle—in contrast to its former status formally listed only as a *contributing* risk factor.

Criteria for Excessive Body Fat: How Fat Is Too Fat?

In Chapter 28, we discussed limitations in using the weight-for-height tables and BMI to assess body composition. In this chapter, we present three valid approaches to assessing an individual's total body fat content:

1. Total body mass expressed as a percentage
2. Body fat patterning in distinctive anatomic regions
3. Adipose tissue fat cell size and number

Establishing Valid Standards for Body Fat Percentage

What determines the demarcation between a normal and excess body fat level? In our schema explained in Chapter 28, we suggested that a "normal" and reasonable body fat range for adult males and females should encompass an "average" literature-based percentage body fat value ±1 standard deviation. For males and females ages 17 to 50 years, this variation equals ±5% body fat units. Using this statistical boundary, overfatness then would correspond to a body fat level exceeding the average value +5% body fat. For example, in young males whose body fat averages 15%,

Excessive Obesity's Specific Health Risks

A Brain: Enormous psychologic burden and social stigmatization and discrimination, depression, low self-esteem

B Esophagus: Gastroesophageal reflux disease (GERD), heartburn

C Arteries: Impaired cardiac function from increased mechanical work and autonomic and left-ventricular dysfunction, abnormal plasma lipid and lipoprotein levels, hypertension, stroke, deep-vein thrombosis

D Lungs: Asthma. Sleep apnea, mechanical ventilatory constraints during exercise, and pulmonary disease from impaired function and added chest wall effort

E Heart: Coronary heart disease, heart attack

F Gallbladder: Gallstones, gallbladder inflammation, gallbladder disease

G Pancreas: Increased insulin resistance in children and adults, type 2 diabetes (80% of these children and adults are overweight)

H Kidneys: Renal cancer, uric acid nephrolithiasis (kidney stones)

I Colon: Colon cancer (also endometrial, breast, prostate cancers)

J Bladder: Cancer, bladder control problems (stress incontinence)

K Bones: Osteoarthritis (degeneration of cartilage and bone in the joints), gout (arthritis type deposits uric acid in joints)

Other: Menstrual irregularities, irregular ovulation, infertility, anesthetics problematic during surgery and other pregnancy complications, premature death

---

the borderline for excessive fatness becomes 20% body fat. For older males whose fat averages 25%, overfatness would include body fat in excess of 30%. For young females, overfatness corresponds to body fat greater than 30%, and for older females, borderline obesity corresponds to about 37% body fat. We emphasize that just because the average value for percentage body fat increases with age, this does not dictate that people should strive to gain body fat as they age! To the contrary, one criterion to determine a boundary for "too fat" emerges from data for the younger male and female groups—above 20% for males and above 30% for females. With a single gender-specific standard, average age-related population values do not become the reference standard and hence the accepted criterion. We also recognize that this classification standard based on an average for young adults becomes overly rigorous when applied to older populations. It probably places more than 50% of all adults in the overly fat category, a value below the current 69% value for overweight and obese Americans using BMI as the standard.[126] It also closely corresponds to proposed gender-based body fat standards computed for young adults from the relationship between BMI and the four- and five-component models to estimate Black and White percentage body fat.[62]

We posit that overfatness exists along a continuum from the upper limit for normal (≥20% body fat for males and ≥30% for females) to as high as 50% and a theoretical maximum of nearly 70% body mass in the massively obese. This latter group's weight ranges from 249 to 370 kg/375 to 550 lb or higher. This weight range has potential to create a life-threatening condition because in such extreme cases, the body's total fat content can exceed their lean body mass!

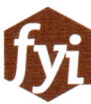

Exercise with Weight Loss Reduces Knee Osteoarthritis

Osteoarthritis (OA), the most common degenerative joint disease and once expected in older age adults, now occurs with increasing frequency due to increased obesity in younger individuals and those with traumatic sports injuries (e.g., anterior cruciate ligament rupture and/or meniscal tear). OA presents when the cushioning cartilage between the joints deteriorates. It affects more than 32 million people in the U.S. population (21 million ≥age 25), including more than 10% of males and 13% of females older than 60. Current medical advice recommends combining resistance exercise with regular low-impact aquatic exercise, cycling, swimming, or level walking/hiking to strengthen structures surrounding the knees, particularly the quadriceps and hamstrings, and with weight loss rather than just long-term pharmacologic treatment. A small 4.5-kg/10-lb weight loss can help mitigate persistent OA knee pain. Arthroscopic knee procedures cannot "cure" OA, and no published clinical trials advocate for arthroscopy to treat OA pain.

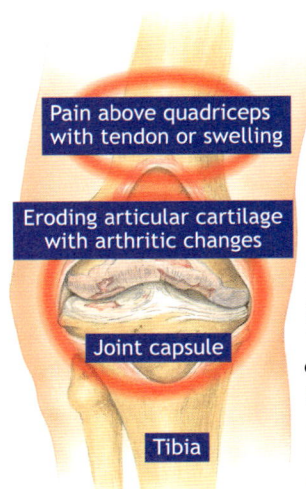

Sources:
Ackerman IN, et al. Hip and knee osteoarthritis affects younger people, too. *J Orthop Sports Phys Ther.* 2017;4:67.
Kolasinski SL, et al. 2019 American College of Rheumatology/Arthritis Foundation Guideline for the management of osteoarthritis of the hand, hip, and knee. *Arthritis Care Res (Hoboken).* 2020;72:149. Erratum in: *Arthritis Care Res (Hoboken)* 2021 May;73:764.

Fat Patterning in Different Anatomic Regions

The body's adipose tissue patterning in specific body regions, independent from the body's total body fat content, alters health risks in children, adolescents, and adults.[33,60,210,235,237]

FIGURE 30.8 depicts two regional fat distribution categories. Increased health risk from excessive fat deposition in the abdominal area (**central obesity** or android-type obesity), particularly internal visceral deposits, invariably results from this tissue's active lipolysis with catecholamine stimulation. Fat stored in this region shows greater metabolic responsiveness than fat in the gluteal and femoral regions, which, when excessive, is known as **peripheral obesity** or gynoid-type obesity. To help remember the differences, consider android or "apple" shape as fat accumulation above the waist and gynoid or "pear" shape as fat accumulation below the waist. Increases in central, android-type fat more readily support processes associated with heart disease[186] and metabolic syndrome.[165]

In males, the fat located inside the abdominal cavity (intra-abdominal or *visceral adipose tissue*) is twice as large compared with that in females.[12] In males, visceral fat

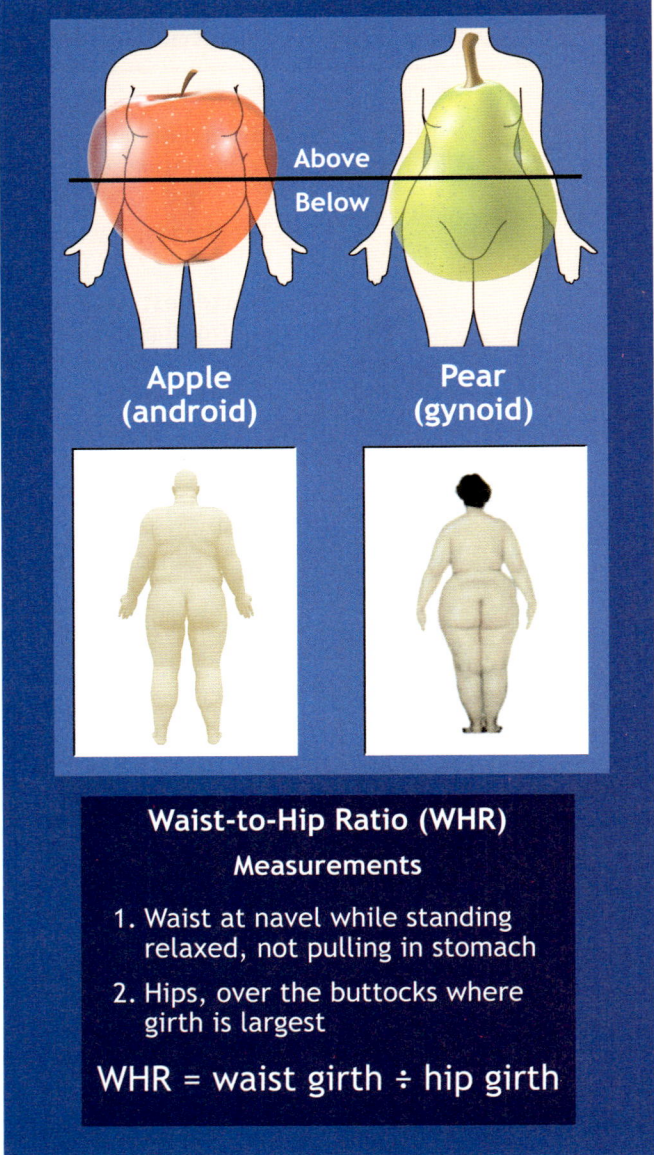

FIGURE 30.8. Male (android pattern) and female (gynoid pattern) fat patterning including the waist-to-hip girth ratio. (Shutterstock images: decade3d—anatomy online (male posterior), Orlov_Art (apple, pear).)

percentage increases progressively with age, whereas in females this regional fat deposition begins to increase at menopause onset.[115] Central fat deposition, particularly in the abdominal region, with increasing fatness levels shown in the figure, independent from fat storage in other anatomic areas, reflects an altered metabolic profile that increases health risk.

As a general guideline, a waist-to-hip girth ratio exceeding 0.80 for females or 0.95 for males increases death risk even after adjusting for BMI.[37,164] One limitation concerning the ratio is it poorly captures each girth measure's specific influence. Waist and hip girths reflect different body composition and fat distribution characteristics. Each has an independent and often opposite effect on cardiovascular disease risk. An increased waist girth represents the so-called malignant obesity form characterized by central fat deposition that may cripple the body's ability to mobilize and/or utilize insulin, setting the stage for type 2 diabetes and heart disease. This fat deposition region provides a reasonable indicator that intra-abdominal (visceral) adipose tissue predominates compared with fat deposition in other body regions. This makes abdominal girth a practical way to evaluate the metabolic and health risks and accelerated mortality with obesity.[101,144,178,196] *Over a broad BMI range, males and females with larger abdominal girth values possess greater relative risk for cardiovascular disease, type 2 diabetes, cancer, dementia, and cataracts (the leading cause of blindness worldwide) than individuals with small waist circumference or peripheral obesity.*[96,214,228]

Excess weight distribution in the abdominal area (and correspondingly high blood insulin levels) also increases colorectal cancer risk.[83,103] A waist girth that exceeds 91 cm/36 in. in males and 82 cm/32 in. in females nearly doubles this cancer's risk.[174] The inset figure below shows how to apply three BMI categories and waist girth measurements above and below 102 cm/40 in. for males and 87.8 cm/34.6 in. for females to assess a person's risk for health problems ranked from least risk to very high risk. To establish these standards, researchers examined the risk among BMI (measured without shoes), waist girth (narrowest torso girth), and waist-to-hip ratio versus death risk in 359,387 participants without prior cancer, heart disease, or stroke history at baseline from nine countries in the European Prospective Investigation into Cancer and Nutrition (EPIC; http://epic.iarc.fr/). The mean age at baseline was 51.5 ± 10.4 years, and 65.4% were females. After 9.7 years, 4% or 14,723 participants had died. The lowest death risk occurred at BMI ≤ 25.3 for males and ≤ 24.3 for females. As the researchers defined, BMI less than 18.5 refers to *underweight*, 18.5 to less than 25.0 refers to *normal weight*, 25.0 to less than 30 refers to *overweight*, and ≥30.0 refers to *obesity*. After adjustment for BMI, waist girth and waist-to-hip ratio also moderately to strongly associated with death risk. BMI remained significantly associated with death risk when the statistical analysis included either waist girth or waist-to-hip ratio.

Waist girth	BMI category		
	Normal 18.5–24.9 kg·m⁻²	Overweight 25–29.9 kg·m⁻²	Obese class I 30–34.9 kg·m⁻²
Men: < 102 cm Women: < 88 cm	Least risk	Increased risk	High risk
Men: ≥ 102 cm Women: ≥ 88 cm	Increased risk	High risk	Very high risk

Data from the world literature, including Douketis JD. Body weight classification. *Can Med Assoc J.* 2005;172:995.

Adipocyte Size and Number: Hypertrophy Versus Hyperplasia

Adipocyte size and number provide another way to assess and classify obesity. Adipose tissue mass increases in two ways:

1. **Fat cell hypertrophy**: Existing adipocytes enlarge or fill with lipid
2. **Fat cell hyperplasia**: Total adipocyte number increases

One technique to study adipose cellularity extracts small subcutaneous tissue fragments usually from the triceps, subscapular, buttocks, and/or lower abdomen into a syringe through a needle inserted directly into the fat depot. Chemically treating the tissue sample isolates the individual adipocytes to determine their average diameter and number. Dividing fat mass in the tissue sample by adipocyte number determines the average lipid quantity per cell. Total adipocyte number is determined by the body's total fat mass (densitometry, dual x-ray absorptiometry, or total body water by radioactive tracer methods[256,262]). For example, a person who weighs 88 kg/194 lb with 13% body fat has a 11.4 kg (0.13 × 88 kg) total fat mass. Dividing 11.4 kg by the average lipid content per cell estimates total adipocyte number. If the average adipocyte contains 0.60 μg of lipid, then this person's body contains 19 billion adipocytes (11.4 kg ÷ 0.60 μg).

> **Total adipocyte number = body fat mass ÷ fat content per cell**

Biopsy Method

In one of our laboratories, we used needle biopsy and photomicrographic techniques to extract lipid samples and measured the adipocyte's lipid content in the upper buttocks region (along with abdominal and subscapular sites not shown). The left panel of the inset figure on the next page illustrates the needle biopsy procedure to extract adipocytes from the upper buttock region, illustrating an adipocyte with greater internal lipid organelles. After sterilizing and anesthetizing a small area in the particular body region, the biopsy needle is inserted beneath the skin surface to literally "suck" a fluid and tissue sample into the attached syringe. Photomicrographs of the adipocytes were then prepared from 200 individual cell images and projected onto a computer screen to determine each cell's diameter with an electronic pencil to calculate cell radius needed in the formula to calculate volume (diameter/2 = radius); volume = 4/3 × π (pi = [3.14159] × radius³), and total cell number. The subjects, one of the textbook authors and several graduate students, were preparing to train for a marathon run, so it was serendipitous to obtain pre and post fat cell samples from the abdomen measured 1 inch to the right of the umbilicus, inferior right scapular border, and upper right buttocks quadrant to quantify changes in cell size and number over a 6-month training period.[285]

The center image shows adipocyte size for numerous cells, which look like semi-flattened marbles. In the right panel, cell diameter and volume post endurance marathon training averaged about 9 to 42% smaller than pre cellularity measurements.

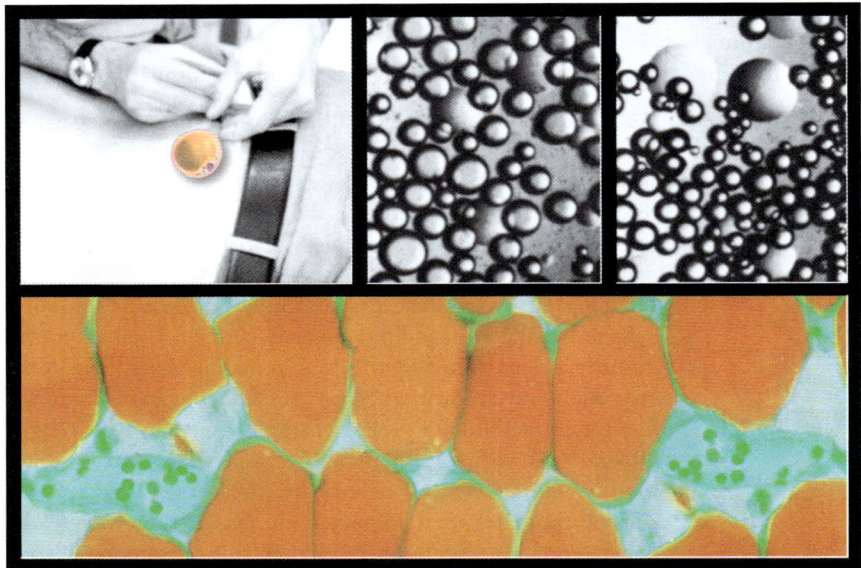

Photomicrographs courtesy P. M. Clarkson Kinesiology, UMass, Amherst, MA. Fat cell image: SciePro/Shutterstock

Calculating Adipocyte Number.
Densitometry determines total fat mass (Chapter 28) and, from this, adipose cell number. Fat mass was 17.02 kg/37.5 lb based on a 89.1-kg/196-lb body mass and 19.1% body fat. Adipose quantity per cell averaged 0.73 µg fat, and total estimated adipocyte number was 23.3 billion (17.02 kg ÷ 0.73 µg). The spherical structures in the background of the right inset figure are large lipid droplets.

At the extreme for adipose cell number, a morbidly obese male at age 30 can have between 200 and 250 billion fat cells at almost 60% body fat percentage! As expected, there is a curvilinear relationship between adipose cell volume and body fat mass.[298] Over the next 30 years, by age 60, he will likely gain another 11.3 kg/25 lb, presumably by increases in total fat mass at the expense of fat-free body mass (FFM) and muscle strength decline with aging.[300,301] In this case, the expected additional fat mass will reflect further increases in adipose cell enlargement (hypertrophy) *and* fat cell number (hyperplasia) due to further proliferation and differentiation in preadipocyte cells, perhaps by another 50 billion fat cells.[299]

Fat Cell Development and Adipocytes

Pioneering research in the early 1980s began to search for a molecular trigger to explain the link between newly developing **preadipocyte cells**, the precursors to mature fat cells and subsequent obesity. Researchers studied cellular differentiation to determine why some fat cells became excessively large and abundant and others remained normal in size without increasing their number. It had been determined that either the conservation of energy or energy expenditure differed in adult white adipose tissue and infant brown adipose tissue development. Specific genes were first expressed in preadipocytes compared to mature lipid cells. Once identified, attention focused on what transcription factors and enhancers "turned on" those genes. From hundreds of turned-on genes during fat cell differentiation, the **adipocyte protein 2 (*aP2*) gene** became a good candidate as an appropriate model to study differentiation between brown fat cell versus white fat cell growth and development.[67]

Research in the 1990s originally identified the **peroxisome proliferator-activated receptor gamma (PPARγ) gene** as the "master gene" in white fat cell development. Subsequent research has demonstrated that this gene also serves the following three functions[53,179,206]:

1. Serves as a receptor for antidiabetic drugs (TZD drug class or thiazolidinediones)
2. Triggers cellular metabolic effects to decrease adiposity
3. Functions to control cell proliferation, atherosclerosis, macrophage function, and overall immunity

The brown fat present in infants but not usually in adults has one main function—to serve as a heat source for the baby's survival. Heat production occurs metabolically by leaking

 Low Body Fat in Marathoners

World-class marathon runners typically have low body fat levels ranging from 1 to 8%, reflecting long-term training distance running adaptations coupled with reduced energy intake relative to energy output. Most top-level marathoners

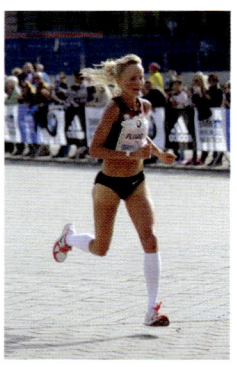

360b/Shutterstock

adhere to careful dietary practices to maintain sufficient body weight and energy reserves to support the typical 80 to 120 mi · wk^{-1} of arduous training. From 1986 to 2019, more than 100 million marathon race results were available from about 70,000 races worldwide (https://runrepeat.com/research-marathon-performance-across-nations). In 2018, there were 1,298,725 runners from 30 countries who competed, with 443,878 racers recorded in the U.S. with 196,586 female runners (43%) across the age span. For the most competitive female runners over the past three decades, their body size has decreased—remaining mostly thin-appearing with low body fat levels. The female winner of the 2017 New York City Marathon (2:26:53), 36-year-old American Shalane Flanagan, weighed 48.1 kg/106 lb, with a stature of 165.1 cm/65 in.

Sources:
Clemente-Suarez VJ, Nikolaidis PT. Use of bioimpedianciometer as predictor of mountain marathon performance. *J Med Syst*. 2017;41:73.
Czajkowska A, et al. The Effect of the ultra-marathon run at a distance of 100 kilometers on the concentration of selected adipokines in adult men. *Int J Environ Res Public Health*. 2020;17:4289.
Knechtle B, Nikolaidis PT. Physiology and pathophysiology in ultra-marathon running. *Front Physiol*. 2018;9:634.

hydrogen ions across the mitochondrion's inner membrane, generating futile metabolic heat rather than converting it into ATP in white fat cells as potential energy for other metabolic processes. **FIGURE 30.9** shows basic metabolic differences between how the mitochondria in brown fat convert food into the end product *heat* and what occurs in white fat to produce the end product *ATP* to power cellular functions.[51,177,189] In the figure, note the main structural differences between the white adipose cells at the left and the brown adipose cell structure at the right; the latter also contain a nucleus (shown in purple) and, in addition, numerous mitochondria and many small, separated lipid droplets. The bottom part in the figure spotlights the science behind the observation that white adipose cells produce ATP, while brown adipose cells produce heat as the end-product.

Molecular Switches. Specialized molecular switches govern fat cell differentiation. Two master regulator genes, PPARgamma with RXR (a cofactor retinoic acid receptor), initiates white fat development (left side Fig. 30.9); when PRDM16 switches on, the preadipocyte activates PGC-1, playing a central role in regulating cellular energy metabolism with other genes to define the brown fat phenotype (right side Fig. 30.9).[73] The evidence reveals that adipocytes simply are not inert globs of fat. Rather, they are dynamic and influential in exchanging chemical signals with the brain and reproductive and immune systems.

Existing adipocytes enlarge and shrink, and absorb and release energy-rich lipids as needed depending on substrate availability and utilization. When overloaded with surplus calories, lipid cells initiate cell division to absorb the oversupply;

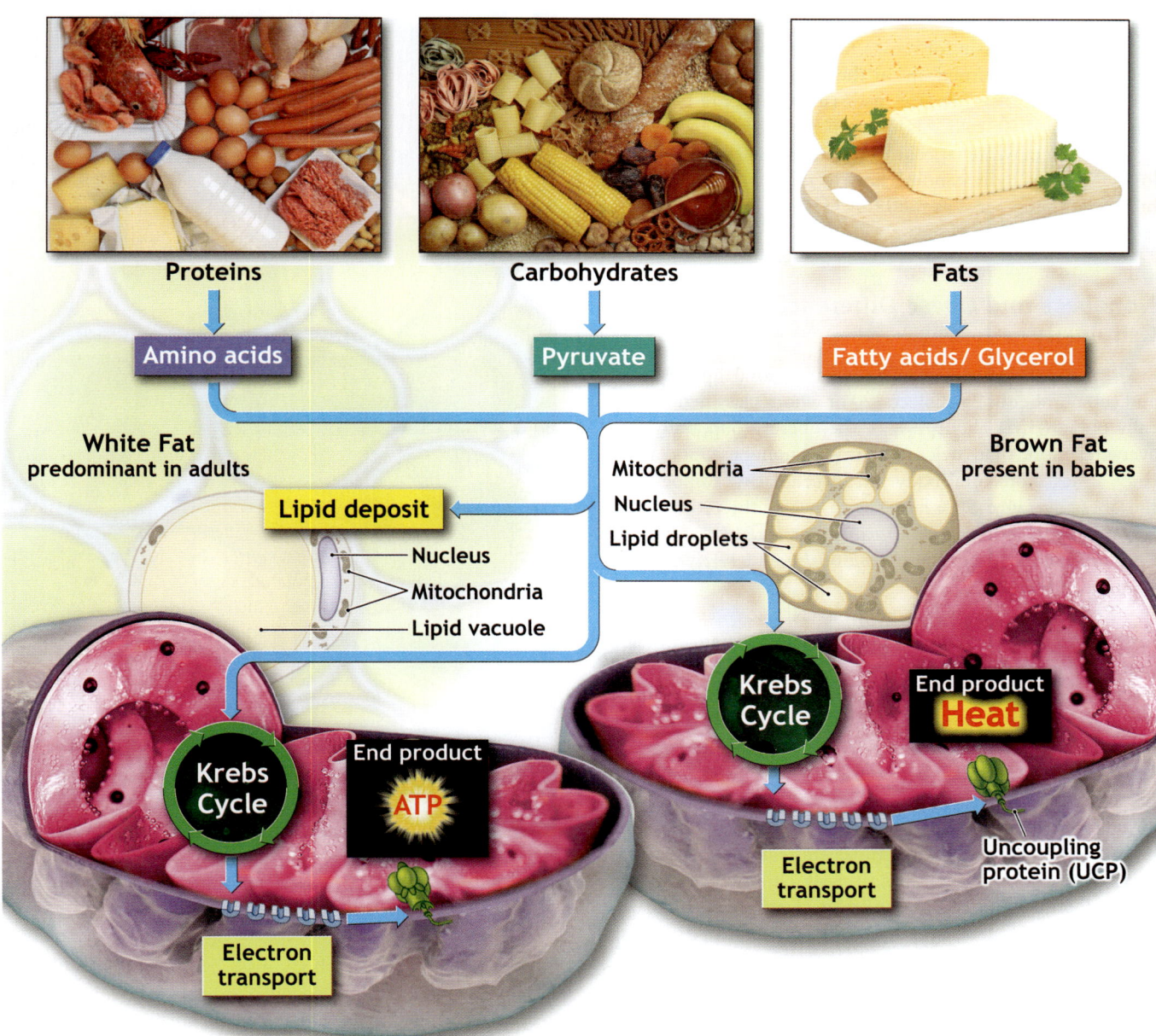

FIGURE 30.9. Unique molecular switches govern fat cell differentiation from energy in proteins, carbohydrates, and lipids. ATP, adenosine triphosphate.
(Shutterstock images: Elena Schweitzer (proteins, carbohydrates), SeDmi (fats).)

once they hypertrophy as they fill with excess lipid, they remain in a state of flux until a shift occurs in the energy balance equation. Molecular adipocyte remodeling has the potential to shift the balance to favor calorie expenditure rather than calorie storage. Research is continuing to explore what is reliably known about brown fat and its functions in humans. Three general conclusions have emerged as a prelude to a rapidly expanding knowledge base involving molecular biology techniques to further understand the role different adipose tissue cells play in obesity development and future treatment options[286–288]:

1. Lean individuals have more brown fat than overweight counterparts.
2. Brown fat accelerates its energy release in cooler environments.
3. Females tend to have more brown fat than males, with larger and more active deposits.

If the mechanism for brown fat heat production could be determined and "turned on" in the obese (as both cell types originate from the same precursor cells), the extra futile heat energy from these cells might compete with the energy storage function in white fat cells to tilt energy balance to favor fat loss.[30,224,257,258] Understanding how to fully activate the body's brown fat might serve as the Holy Grail in treating the obese condition.

Nonobese and Obese Differences in Cellularity

FIGURE 30.10 compares the body mass, total lipid per cell, and cell number in 25 subjects, 20 of whom classified as clinically obese (BMI about 40). In the obese group, body mass averaged more than twice that in the nonobese, and nearly three times more total body fat. In cellularity, adipocytes in the obese averaged 50% larger with nearly three times more cells (75 vs. 27 billion). *Cell number represents the major structural difference in adipose tissue mass between severely obese and nonobese individuals.*[23]

Relating total body fat content to cell size and cell number further demonstrates adipocyte number's important contribution to obesity. As body fat increases, adipocytes eventually reach a biologic upper size limit. Once this occurs, cell number becomes the key factor determining any further fat increase. Even doubling adipocyte size does not explain the large difference in total fat mass between obese and average persons. For comparison, an average-size person has between 25 and 30 billion adipocytes, whereas the clinically severe obese may have more than three to five times this number, particularly when excessive fatness occurs in early childhood or adolescence. Compositional differences in fatty acids also exist among overweight/obese males and females in perivisceral, omental, and subcutaneous adipose tissue regions.[64]

Weight Loss Effects

FIGURE 30.11 illustrates the results from a classic weight loss experiment on adipose tissue characteristics among 19 obese adults who participated in two weight loss stages strategies. In

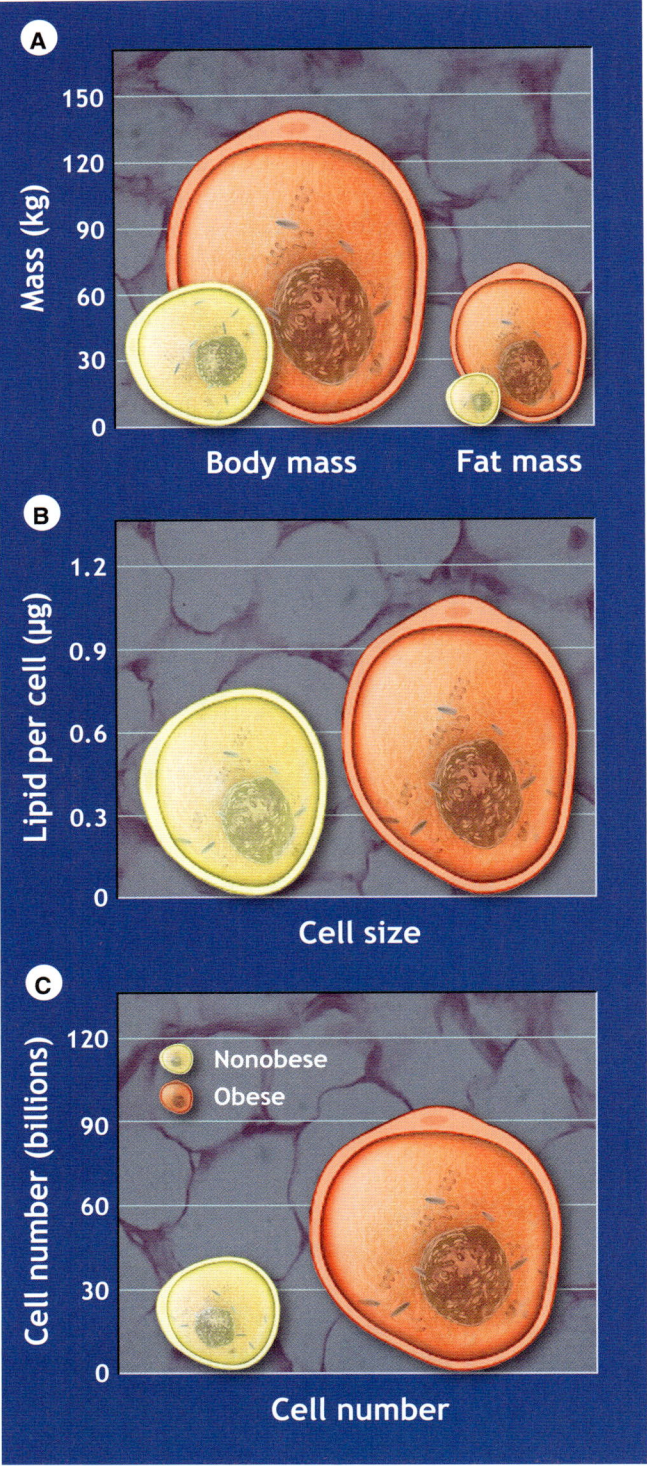

FIGURE 30.10. Body mass, total lipid per cell, and cell number in 20 clinically obese patients and five nonobese controls. (Shutterstock images: Choksawatdikorn (adipose tissue), Spectral-Design (fat cells).)

Stage 1, subjects reduced body mass by 46 kg/101 lb (149 to 103 kg/329 to 227 lb). Adipocyte number before weight reduction averaged 75 billion and remained unchanged even after the 46-kg/101-lb weight reduction. In contrast, adipocyte size decreased by 33% from 0.9 to 0.6 μg of lipid per cell. When subjects attained a normal 75-kg/165-lb body mass by losing an additional 28 kg/61.6 lb, cell number remained unchanged,

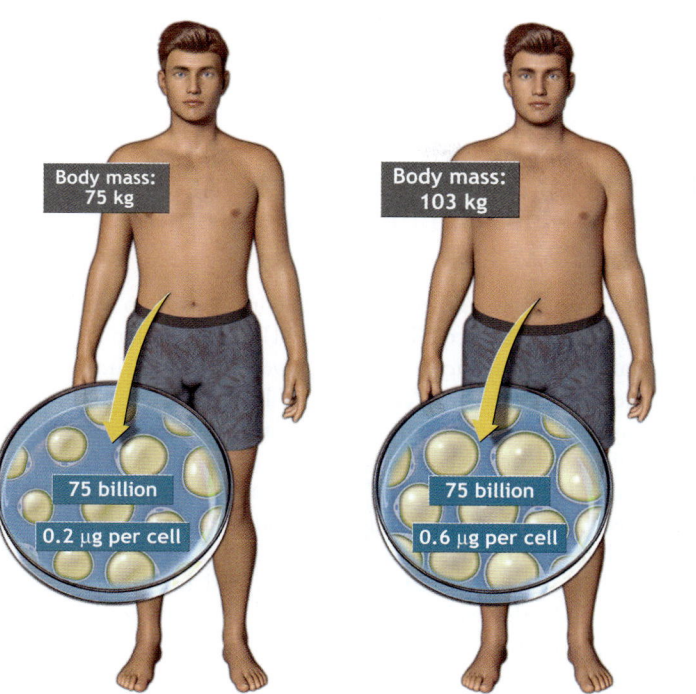

FIGURE 30.11. Changes in adipose cellularity with weight reduction in obese subjects. (Data from Hirsch J. Adipose cellularity in relation to human obesity. In: Stollerman GH, ed. *Advances in Internal Medicine*, Vol. 17. Chicago: Year-Book; 1971.)

Possible New Adipocyte Formation Possibility

Extreme body fat accumulation in adults stimulates increased adipose cellularity because adipocyte size reaches an upper 1.0 µg fat limit beyond which no further hypertrophy occurs. At extremes in morbid obesity, almost all adipocytes attain their hypertrophic limit. In this situation, the preadipocyte pool provides additional adipocytes to increase cell number, with a concomitant increase in lipid stored within the liver and between muscle fibers. *In maturity-onset severe obesity, in which the already obese adult gains even more body fat, hypercellularity may accompany existing adipocytes to increase their size!* This indeed is bad news, because increased cell number would indicate failure in adipocyte regulation, unfortunately leading to further fat accumulation.

but cell size continued to shrink to about a third compared to a nonobese comparison group. When the patients achieved their "normal" body mass and body fat level, adipocytes had become considerably smaller than in the nonobese controls, who showed no weight loss. *In adults, the major change in adipose cellularity in weight loss involves adipocyte shrinkage without changes in cell number.* These robust findings send a clear message about fat cellularity—formerly obese individuals who reduce body weight do not really "cure" their obesity based on fat cell hyperplasia.

Weight Gain Effects

Studies in the late 1960s and early 1970s evaluated weight gain dynamics on adipose tissue cellularity. In one study, adult male volunteers with an initial average 15% body fat content deliberately increased daily caloric intake by three times normal to about 7000 kcal for 40 wk.[184] For a typical subject, body mass increased 25% and percentage body fat nearly doubled from 14.6 to 28.2%. Fat deposition represented 10.5 kg/23.1 lb of the 12.7-kg/28-lb weight gained during the overfeeding period. In a similar experiment with subjects with no personal or family history of obesity, voluntary overeating increased body mass by 16.4 kg/36.2 lb.[171] In both experiments, adipocytes increased substantially in size with *no change* in cell number. When caloric intake decreased and subjects attained normal weight, total body fat declined and the adipocytes reverted to their original size. *In general, moderate weight gain from overeating in adults enlarges existing adipocytes rather than stimulating new adipocyte development.*

Summary

1. Obesity or excess body fat accumulation represents a heterogeneous disorder with a final common pathway where energy intake chronically overshadows energy expenditure.
2. Worldwide obesity currently surpasses 750 million individuals, many of whom live in countries where overweight and obesity kill more people than who die from being underweight or malnourished.
3. Approximately 400 million children and adolescents throughout the world age 5 to 19 are overweight or obese.
4. Over the past 40 years, Americans body weight continues to increase, with more than 140 million Americans or about 69% in the population either overweight (BMI 25 to <30) or obese (BMI ≥ 30).
5. Fifteen to 20% of American children and 12% adolescents classify as overweight, with excessive body fatness most prevalent among poor and minority children.
6. Genetic factors account for 25 to 30% excessive body fat accumulation, yet genetic predisposition does not necessarily cause excessive fatness, but in the right environment, the genetically susceptible individual gains body fat.
7. A defective gene for adipocyte leptin production and/or hypothalamic leptin insensitivity causes the brain to assess adipose tissue status improperly, creating a chronic positive energy balance.
8. Excessive body fat is a leading cause of preventable deaths in the United States.
9. Comorbid hypertension, elevated blood sugar level, postmenopausal breast cancer, and elevated total cholesterol and low HDL cholesterol levels increase an overweight person's poor health risk at any excess weight level.

10. The overfatness threshold for adult males and females should more closely reflect the body fat percentage levels in younger adults—males above 20% body fat and females exceeding 30% body fat.
11. Body fat patterning impacts health risks independently from total body fat. Fat distributed in the abdominal region (central or android-type obesity) poses a greater risk than fat deposited at the thighs and buttocks (peripheral or gynoid-type obesity).
12. Body fat increases in two ways before adulthood: enlarged individual adipocytes (*fat cell hypertrophy*) and increased total adipocite number (*fat cell hyperplasia*).
13. Modest adult weight gain and loss changes adipocyte size with little change in cell number, except in extreme body weight and fat gain, where adipocyte number increases once cell size reaches its hypertrophic limit.

Part 2 > Weight Control Primary Principles Involve Diet and Physical Activity

For many adults, body weight fluctuates only slightly during the year. This represents an impressive constancy considering that slight increases in daily food intake translate to substantial weight gain over time, if unaccompanied by compensatory increases in energy expenditure. *The human body functions in accord with thermodynamic laws. If total food calories exceed daily energy expenditure, excess calories accumulate and stockpile in adipose tissue as lipid.*

Energy Balance: Input Versus Output

German physician Julius Robert Mayer (1814–1878; www.uh.edu/engines/epi722.htm), discovered the *first law of thermodynamics* often called the law of conservation of energy. Mayer posited that energy transferred from one system to another in many forms but could not be created nor destroyed. In human terms, this meant that the energy balance equation dictated that body weight would remain constant when total caloric intake from food equaled total caloric expenditure. The latter included foods thermic effect, physical activity, and energy metabolism. **FIGURE 30.12** illustrates how any chronic imbalance on the energy output or input side of the equation impacts changes in body weight. In nutritional terms, this explanation is known as the **energy balance model (EBM)**. In this approach, body weight can decrease only when total calories consumed are less than total calories attributed to metabolism and physical activity.

The Mass Balance Model Versus the EBM

An alternative and competing theory to explain weight loss, the Mass Balance Model (MBM),[259–261] challenges EBM's validity to satisfactorily explain weight loss as simply "calories-out" exceeding "calories-in." In the MBM, accumulating either 1 g protein, lipid, or carbohydrate in the body's cells will increases body mass by exactly 1 g independent from the nutrient's per gram energy content (i.e., "calories-in"). Thus, oxidizing 1 g in any stored macronutrient reduces body mass by oxidating 1 g of its end-products, which when eliminated are considered inconsequential as "burned calories." In essence, the MBM predicts that with weight reduction interventions with identical energy isocaloric content, low-carbohydrate diets will produce greater body weight and body fat loss than low-fat diets because *less* food consumption occurs as the energy proportion from fat increases—a consequence from fats higher caloric density compared to carbohydrate or protein.[291]

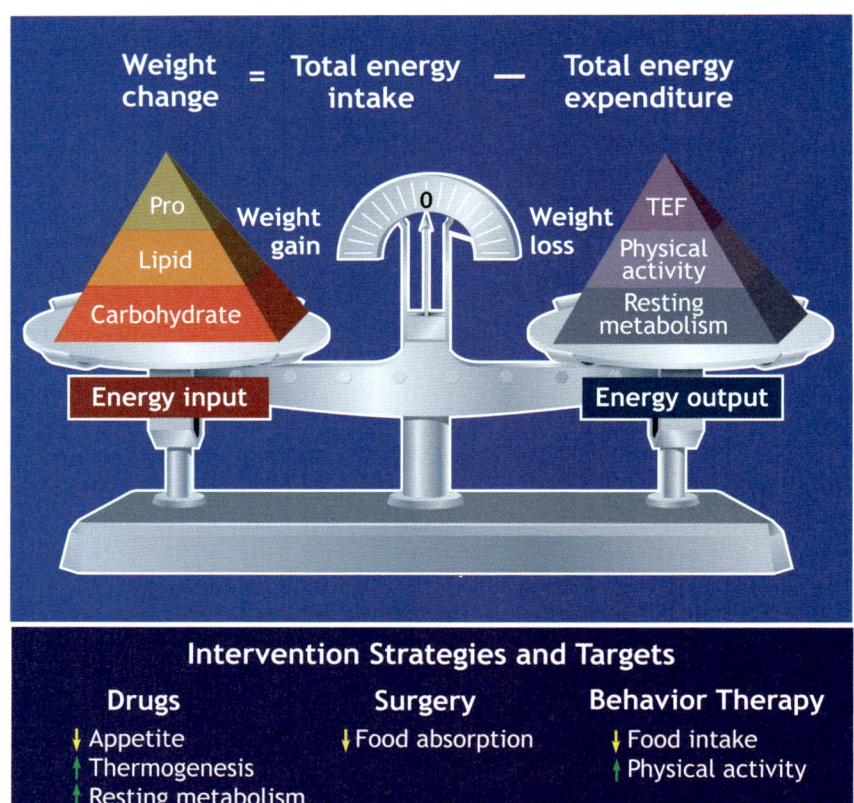

FIGURE 30.12. The energy balance equation plus intervention strategies and specific targets to alter energy balance toward weight loss. Pro, protein; TEF, thermic effect of food.

In the standard EBM, weight loss can occur in three ways:

1. Reduce caloric intake below daily energy requirements.
2. Maintain caloric intake and increase energy expenditure through additional physical activity above daily energy requirements.
3. Decrease daily caloric intake and increase daily energy expenditure.

When considering EBM's sensitivity but not challenging its validity, if caloric intake exceeds output by only 100 kcal daily, the surplus calories consumed in a year equal 36,500 kcal (365 d × 100 kcal). Because 0.45-kg/1.0-lb body fat contains about 3500 kcal (each 1-lb/454-g adipose tissue contains about 86% fat or 390.4 g/13.8 oz; therefore, 390.4 g × 9 kcal · g^{-1} = 3514 kcal per lb), this caloric excess causes a yearly 4.7-kg/10.3-lb body fat gain. These same calculations and conclusions would not apply in the MBM because their assumptions differ. Further comparative experiments between MBM versus EBM will help to explain several theoretical questions posed by the EBM.

A Prudent Recommendation

The main objective of weight-loss programs has changed dramatically over past decades. The previous approach assigned a **goal body weight** that coincided with an "ideal" weight based on body mass and stature. Achieving a goal body weight heralded the weight-loss program's success. Currently, the World Health Organization (www.who.int/en), the Institute of Medicine of the National Academy of Sciences (https://nam.edu/about-the-nam/), and the National Heart, Lung and Blood Institute (www.nhlbi.nih.gov/health-topics/overweight-and-obesity) recommend that an overweight/obese person reduce initial body weight by 5 to 15%. Setting the initial weight loss goal beyond the 5 to 15% recommendation often gives patients an unrealistic and potentially unattainable target.

Dieting for Weight Control

The first law of thermodynamics predicts that weight loss should occur whenever energy output exceeds energy input without considering the diet's macronutrient mixture. Advantages for consuming unrefined complex carbohydrates in a reduced-calorie diet include their moderate-to-low glycemic index; high vitamin, mineral, and phytochemical content; low energy density; and low saturated fatty acid levels. For most individuals, a prudent dietary approach to weight loss attempts to disrupt the energy balance equation by lessening energy intake by 300 to 1000 kcal below daily total energy expenditure. Moderately reduced energy intake (300 to 500 kcal daily) promotes greater fat loss relative to an energy deficit than more severe energy restriction. Individuals who create larger daily deficits to lose weight more rapidly tend to regain weight compared to those who lose weight at a slower rate.

Classic Approach

Consider the classic approach for an overfat person who normally consumes 2800 kcal daily and maintains a 79.4-kg/175-lb body mass and wishes to reduce weight mainly by caloric restriction ("dieting"). They maintain regular daily energy expenditure but reduce food intake to 1800 kcal to create a 1000 kcal daily deficit. In 7 days, the accumulated deficit would equal 7000 kcal or 0.9 kg/2.0 lb equivalent for body fat. Considerably more than this amount would realistically occur during the first week because the energy deficit initially accounts for a large percentage in the body's stored glycogen. Stored glycogen compared to stored lipid contains fewer kcal per g and considerably more water. For this reason, short-duration caloric restriction often encourages the dieter but produces a large water and carbohydrate percentage loss per unit weight loss with only a small decrease in body fat. As weight loss continues, a larger proportion of body fat supports the energy deficit created by food restriction (see Fig. 30.14). To reduce body fat by an additional 1.4 kg/3.1 lb, the dieter must maintain the reduced 1800 kcal caloric intake for another 10.5 days; at this point, body fat theoretically decreases at a rate equal to about 0.45 kg/1 lb every 3.5 days.

Long-Term Success

The potential for successful long-term weight loss maintenance generally varies inversely with one's initial fatness level. Note in the accompanying image that as obesity increases four stages from overweight to morbidly obese, the potential for success strikingly diminishes. For most individuals, the initial weight loss success unfortunately relates poorly to longer-term success. Participants in supervised weight-loss programs that include pharmacologic or behavioral interventions generally lose about 8 to 12% their original body mass. Regrettably, typically one to two thirds of the lost weight returns within a year, and almost all within 5 years.[108,138,146]

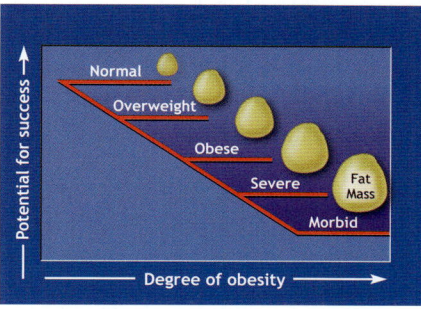

FIGURE 30.13 illustrates clearly that over a 9-year follow-up in over 120 patients, the return to original weight

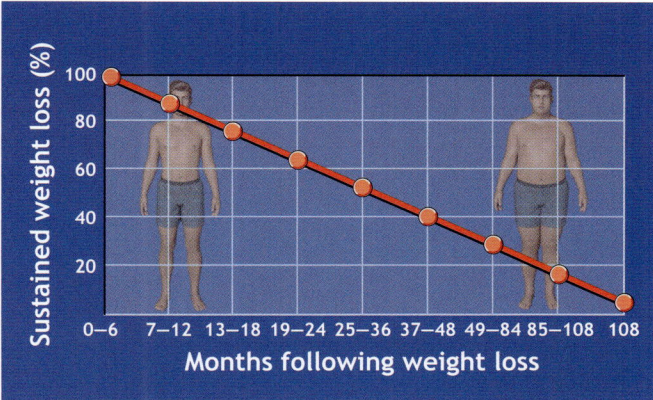

FIGURE 30.13. Percentage of patients able to sustain weight loss over a 9-year period.

occurred in 50% of the individuals within 2 to 3 years, with only seven people remaining at their reduced body weights by the end of the follow-up. These discouraging but typical statistics highlight the extreme difficulty in long-term weight-loss maintenance on a low-calorie diet even with initially successful weight loss.[152] It becomes particularly difficult long term in the relaxed atmosphere in one's home with ready access to food, often without much needed emotional support, and little willingness to participate in daily community-based or private health, wellness, and fitness classes at sufficient intensity to impact continued body weight and body fat losses.

National Weight Control Registry: Clues to Long-Term Success

Among lifetime members in a commercial weight-loss organization that promotes prudent caloric restriction, behavior modification, group support, and moderate physical activity, more than half maintained their original weight loss goal after 2 years, and more than a third after 5 years.[25,79,139,263] Behavior modification, a common intervention in weight loss programs, provides basic principles and techniques to change physical activity and eating habits. The therapy increases skills for replacing existing habits with new, more healthful habits. Behavior therapy characteristics include eating well-balanced meals with reduced portion size, restricting daily caloric intake by 500 to 700 kcal, keeping meticulous food intake and physical activity records, and increasing daily physical activity by at least 200 to 300 kcal.

One project recruited 629 females and 155 males in the 10,000-member National Weight Control Registry (NWCR; www.nwcr.ws), the largest subject database who achieved prolonged weight loss. Criteria for NWCR membership included being 18 years or older and maintaining a minimum 13.6-kg/30-lb weight loss for at least 1 year.

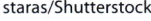
staras/Shutterstock

Participants averaged 30-kg/66-lb weight loss, while 14% lost more than 45.4 kg/100 lb. Members maintained the required 14-kg/30-lb weight loss over 5.5 years, and 16% maintained the lost weight for 10 years or longer. Most participants had been overweight since childhood; nearly half had one overweight parent, and about 25% reported both parents overweight. A new organization, the International Weight Control Registry, is attempting to explore the many global obesity challenges by supporting prospective weight control research projects (https://internationalweightcontrolregistry.org).

Lose Weight Successfully with Structured Assistance

The increasing overweight and obesity prevalence in primary medical care and community settings requires effective approaches to weight loss solutions. Commercial weight loss service providers (e.g., Weight Watchers; www.weightwatchers.com/us/) versus standard treatment primary care practices in Australia, Germany, and the United Kingdom evaluated 772 overweight and obese adults in a randomized controlled trial.[97] Participants received either 12 months standard care defined by national treatment guidelines, or 1-year free membership to a commercial program. Two hundred and thirty (61%) participants completed the commercial program and 214 (54%) participants completed standard care. Weight loss after 1 year averaged 5.1 kg/11.4 lb for commercial program participants versus 2.3 kg/5 lb for standard care. Providing regular weighing, diet, and physical activity advice, motivational strategies, and group support on a large scale proved a clinically useful early intervention for weight management in overweight and obese individuals. Not all research is conclusive. Another study confirmed greater weight loss after 3 months but not after 1 year when participants were tracking their weight changes online using an activity tracking device.[264] In both the experimental and control groups without logger activity, participants lost ≥5% body weight at both 3 and 12 months, but activity tracking *did not* achieve greater weight loss or physical activity increases compared to the control condition.

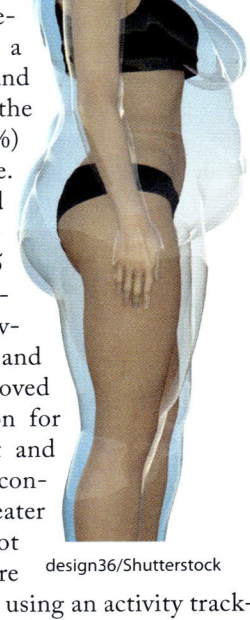
design36/Shutterstock

Weight Loss Improves Disease Risk Biomarkers

Weight loss in obese individuals often exerts a profound effect on biologic factors related to disease risk.[43,137] **FIGURE 30.14** displays the percentage changes from initial body weight and disease risk biomarkers in 100 male and female obese patients over a 27-month period using two energy-restricting meal plans. In Phase 1 during the first 3 months, Group A ($n = 50$) attempted to consume an energy-restricted 1200 to 1500 kcal daily diet with self-selected prepared meals; Group B ($n = 50$) consumed the same kcal amount by substituting two meals and two snack-replacement shakes, soups, hot chocolate, and snack bars for self-selected foods. In Phase 2 (4 to 27 months), all subjects consumed self-selected diets with equal caloric value with one meal and one shake replacement. Unequivocal results emerged from both study phases. Group B's greater weight loss during the 3-month phase occurred by a larger caloric deficit created with the eating plan. Thereafter, both groups reduced an additional 0.1% initial body weight each month (4.2 kg/9.3 lb for Group A and 3.0 kg/6.6 lb for Group B). Figure 30.14B shows absolute changes in eight disease biomarkers during Phases 1 and 2 over the 27-month weight-loss interval. Both groups

CHAPTER 30 • Overweight, Overfatness (Obesity), and Weight Control

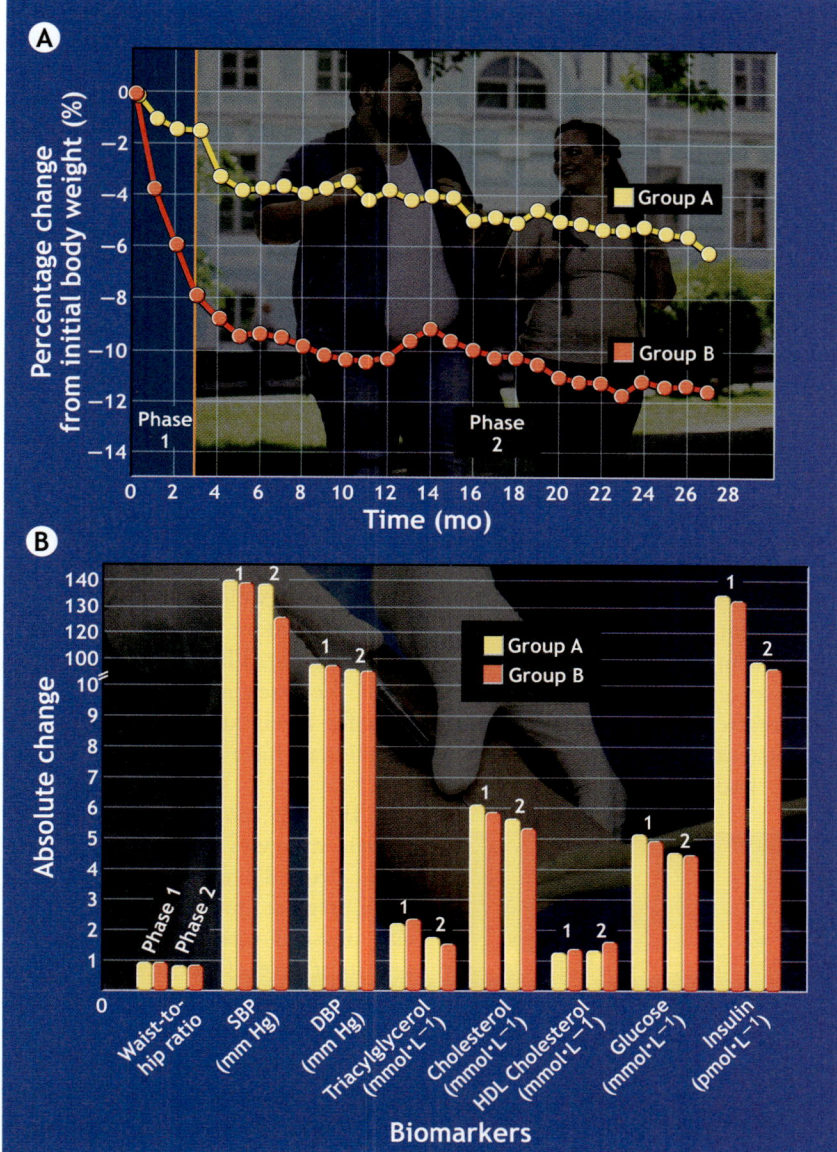

FIGURE 30.14. **(A)** Average percentage change from initial body weight in 100 obese male and female patients during 27-month treatment with daily energy intake restricted to 1200 to 1500 kcal. **(B)** Absolute changes in biomarkers for *Group A* (energy-restricted, self-selected, self-prepared meals) and *B* (Slim-Fast replacement meals) from baseline in Phase 1 to Phase 2 for 27-month energy restriction. DBP, diastolic blood pressure; HDL, high-density lipoprotein; SBP, systolic blood pressure.
(Adapted with permission from Detschuneit HH, et al. Metabolic and weight-loss effects of a long-term dietary intervention in obese patients. *Am J Clin Nutr.* 1999;69:198. With permission from the American Society for Nutrition, https://nutrition.org/.Shutterstock background images: **A**—Motortion Films; **B**—THALERNGSAK MONGKOLSIN.)

Set Point Theory: A Case Against Dieting

One can shed weight relatively quickly by simply not eating for several days, but unfortunately, success is always short-lived, and the urge to consume food wins out and the lost weight returns. Some argue that this failure to maintain weight loss represents a genetically determined "set point" for body weight or body fat that differs from what the person would like to achieve. **Set point theory** proponents maintain that individuals within the middle body weight spectrum along the continuum from thin to obese have a well-regulated internal control mechanism. This important regulating center located deep within the lateral hypothalamus helps to maintain a preset body weight and/or body fat level within a small range.

In a practical sense, the set point ensures that a person's body weight remains relatively constant when not counting intake calories. Physical activity may lower a person's set point, whereas dieting literally exerts little or no effect. Each time body weight decreases below one's preestablished set point, internal adjustments "automatically" adjust the individuals' customary food intake (and regulatory thermogenesis) to resist the change and conserve and/or replenish body fat stores.[36] For example, a slowdown resting metabolism conserves total energy output, and then making the individual obsess about food, literally making them unable to control spontaneous eating urges. At the spectrum's opposite end, when an individual overeats and gain body fat above their usual level, the set point resists this change by increasing resting metabolism and causing the person to become disinterested in food.[265]

Resting Metabolism Decreases

Resting metabolism often decreases when dieting progressively produces weight loss.[141,226] Hypometabolism with caloric deficit often exceeds the decrease attributable to body mass loss or FFM independently from weight status or prior dieting history. Depressed metabolism conserves energy, causing the diet to become progressively less effective even with restricted caloric intake. This produces a weight-loss plateau, where further weight loss occurs at a slower pace than predicted from restricted energy intake mathematics.

A close coupling exists between daily total energy expenditure required to maintain a constant FFM in obese significantly reduced systolic blood pressure but not diastolic blood pressure or plasma insulin, glucose, and triacylglycerol concentrations. A modest but sustained weight loss produced long-term health benefits by improving verifiable and documented risk factors.

and nonobese subjects at their usual body weights. When body weight decreased by 10% below the usual weight, total energy expenditure declined more than explained by the normal relation between energy expenditure and FFM. Both obese and normal-weight subjects became more energy efficient, requiring disproportionately lower energy intake to maintain the lower body weight. Conversely, increasing body weight by 10% above the person's usual weight produced a 15 to 20% unanticipated *increase* in energy expenditure that countered the gain in body fat. These data support the set point concept, or "high-level command signal," that modulates metabolism to defend a specific body fat level. Regrettably in obese individuals, hypothalamic regulation occurs at a higher body fat level,[86] which makes it even more difficult to lose weight. In adolescents and adults, recurring weight-loss cycles often lead to disappointment and depressive behaviors.[266,267]

FIGURE 30.15 shows further evidence regarding the body's basic "defense" against even moderate body weight fluctuations. This classic research carefully monitored body mass, resting oxygen uptake (minimal energy requirement), and caloric intake in six obese men for 31 days. During the prediet period (*red*), body weight and resting oxygen uptake stabilized at 3500 kcal daily food intake. Thereafter, daily caloric intake (bottom *yellow*) decreased to 450 kcal. When subjects switched to the low-calorie diet, body weight and resting metabolism decreased, but the percentage decline in metabolism exceeded the body weight decrease. The dashed line in the upper figure represents the expected weight loss for the 450-kcal diet. The decline in resting metabolism (*middle figure*) conserved energy to make the diet progressively less effective. More than half the total weight loss occurred over the first 8 dieting days. The remaining weight loss occurred during the final 16 days. A plateau in the theoretical weight-loss curve often frustrates and discourages dieters, causing them to forsake attempts at weight loss.

Biologic Feedback Mechanism

Further disconcerting news awaits those who anticipate permanent weight loss. When overfat people lose weight, adipocytes increase their fat-storing enzyme **lipoprotein lipase (LPL)** levels.[108] This adaptation facilitates body fat synthesis, and the fatter the person before weight loss, the greater the LPL production with weight loss. In essence, the fatter one is at the start, the more vigorously the body attempts to regain the lost weight. This observation supports a dedicated biologic feedback mechanism between the brain and the body's fat levels and helps to explain the difficulty overfat individuals have maintaining weight loss.

The set point theory delivers unwelcome news for those with a set point "tuned" too high; encouragingly, regular moderate-level intensity physical activity may lower the set point level. Concurrently, regular physical activity conserves and even increases FFM, raises resting metabolism if FFM increases, and induces metabolic changes that facilitate lipid catabolism. Each healthful adaptation augments the weight-loss effort. In the section "Misconception 1: Increased Physical Activity Increases Food Intake," we discuss how food intake tends to decline initially, despite the increase in energy output, for overly fat males and females who begin to exercise regularly. As a physically active lifestyle continues and body fat decreases, caloric intake balances daily energy requirements to stabilize body mass at a new, lower level.

Challenge to Set Point Proponents. Some research challenges the argument that individuals who lose weight necessarily *maintain* the initial depressed metabolism that predisposes them to weight regain.[220] Undoubtedly, energy restriction produces a *transient hypometabolic state* if

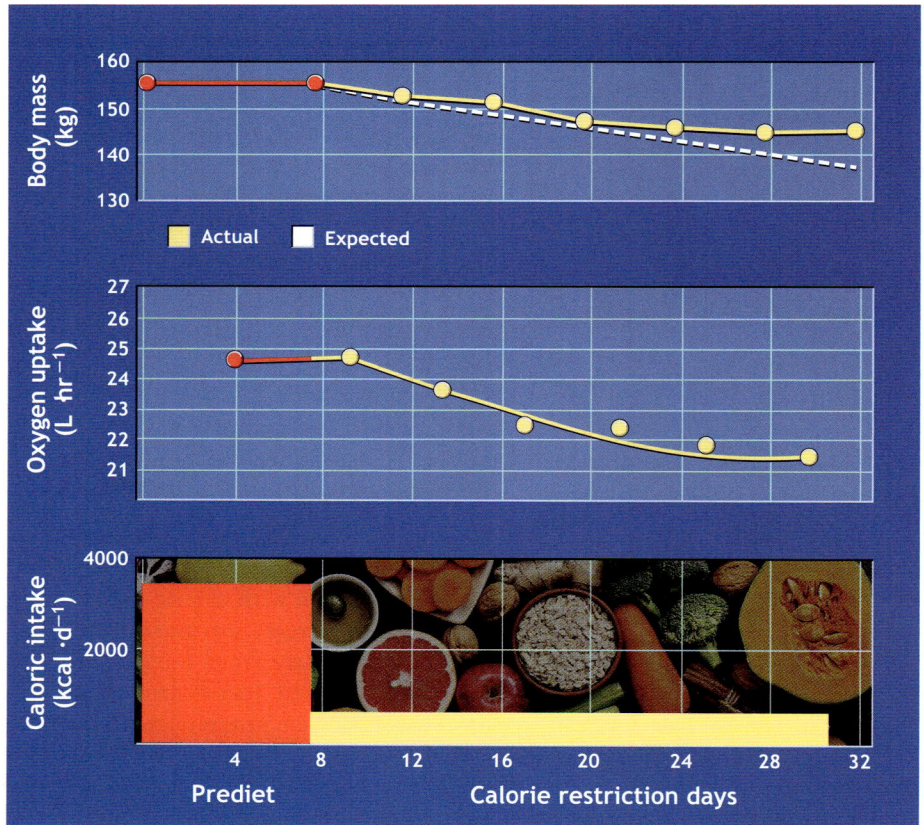

FIGURE 30.15. Classic study demonstrating how a reduced caloric intake impacts body weight and resting oxygen uptake. Weight loss does not keep pace with that predicted by food restriction (*top dashed white line*).
(Adapted with permission from Bray G. Effect of caloric restriction on energy expenditure in obese subjects. *Lancet.* 1969;2:397. With permission from Elsevier. Background photo: Yulia Gust/Shutterstock.)

High-Intensity Exercise Boosts Recovery Metabolism in Adults but not Overweight and Obese Adolescents

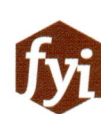

Vigorous physical activity in adults may increase recovery oxygen uptake for up to 14 hr postworkout. Ten males cycled vigorously for 45 min at a 73% maximum oxygen uptake ($\dot{V}O_{2max}$) cycling pace, with energy expenditure in recovery measured for 24 hr, where they expended 190 more kcal than when they remained sedentary (refer to EPOC in Chapter 6). The 37% recovery energy-expending bonus occurred in addition to 520 kcal expended during cycling. In contrast, for overweight and obese adolescents who trained for 3 to 6 months with aerobic training (AT), resistance training (RT), and combined AT and RT and some dietary restriction, resting metabolic rate (RMR; indirect calorimetry after a 10- to 12-hr overnight fast) and body composition (magnetic resonance imaging and dual x-ray absorptiometry) did not change with the different exercise modalities and dietary restriction.

Radu Razvan/Shutterstock

Sources:
Knab AM, et al. A 45-minute vigorous exercise bout increases metabolic rate for 14 hours. *Med Sci Sports Exerc.* 2011;43:1643.
Woods AL, et al. The effects of intensified training on resting metabolic rate (RMR), body composition and performance in trained cyclists. *PLoS One.* 2018;13:e0191644.
Yu WW, et al. Effects of exercise on resting metabolic rate in adolescents with overweight and obesity. *Child Obes.* 2021;17:249.

---

the dieter maintains a negative energy intake. This adaptive downregulation in resting metabolism does not persist when individuals lose weight but then reestablish balance where energy intake equals energy expenditure at their lower body weight. Consequently, research that fails to establish energy balance following weight loss gives the inaccurate impression that individuals who lose weight necessarily battle a prolonged overcompensating reduction in REE until they return to their original body weight.

Dieting Extremes

Professional organizations have voiced strong opposition to some dietary practices, particularly fasting and low-carbohydrate, high-fat, and high-protein diet extremes. Dietary extremes raise concern about athletes and other adolescents and young adults who routinely engage in bizarre and often pathogenic weight-control behaviors (see "In a Practical Sense: Recognizing Disordered Eating Warning Signs"). Researchers also studied a bulimic subgroup who abandoned binging.[105,106] These individuals do not binge eat. Instead, they generally maintain a normal body weight yet feel compelled to purge usually by vomiting, even after eating only a small or normal food amount. Dangers for this eating disorder subset mimic classic bulimic characteristics—dehydration; electrolyte imbalance; potential dental problems from self-induced vomiting; emotional and psychological problems; and body image dysphoria, anxiety, and depression.

Low-Carbohydrate Ketogenic Diets

Ketogenic diets emphasize carbohydrate restriction while generally ignoring total calories and the diet's cholesterol and saturated fat content. Billed as a "diet revolution" and championed by the late Robert C. Atkins, MD (1930–2003),[7] a diet first promoted in the late 1800s and since advocated in many forms. Long disparaged by the medical establishment, believers maintain that restricting daily carbohydrate intake to 20 g/0.7 oz or less for the initial 2 wk causes considerable lipid mobilization for energy. This strategy generates excess plasma ketone bodies (principally acetoacetic, acetone, and β-hydroxybutyric acids) produced by the liver and used peripherally as an energy source from incomplete carbohydrate catabolism. Theoretically, ketones lost in urine represent unused energy that should further facilitate weight loss. Some advocates claim that urinary energy loss becomes so large that dieters can eat all they want if they just restrict carbohydrates.

The singular focus in the low-carbohydrate diet craze may eventually reduce caloric intake, despite claims that dieters need not consider calorie intake if lipid represents the excess. Initial weight loss also may result largely from dehydration caused by an extra solute load on the kidneys that increases water excretion. Water loss does not reduce body fat. Low-carbohydrate intake also sets the stage for lean tissue loss because the body recruits amino acids from muscle to maintain blood glucose via gluconeogenesis—an undesirable side effect for a diet designed to induce fat loss.

Three clinical trials compared the ketogenic diet (i.e., Atkins-type, low-carbohydrate diet) with traditional low-fat diets for weight loss.[58,172,236] The low-carbohydrate diet was more effective for achieving a modest weight loss in severely overweight persons. Some measures relating to heart health also improved reflected by a more favorable lipid profile and glycemic control in those who followed the low-carbohydrate diet for up to 1 year.[193] Such findings lend credibility to low-carbohydrate diets and challenge conventional wisdom concerning potential dangers from consuming a high-fat diet.

Pitfalls. Atkins-type, high-fat, low-carbohydrate dietary plans, which place no limit on the amount of meat (bacon), fats and oils, and eggs combined with cheese a person consumes, pose nine potential health hazards:

1. Raise serum uric acid levels
2. Potentiate kidney stone development
3. Can initiate cardiac arrhythmias by altering electrolyte concentrations

In a Practical Sense

Recognizing Disordered Eating Warning Signs

Disordered eating includes a broad spectrum of complex behaviors, core attitudes, coping strategies, and conditions that share an emotionally based, inordinate and often pathologic focus on body weight, size, and shape.

ANOREXIA ATHLETICA

A cluster of personality traits exists in about 15 to 60% of athletes depending on their sport, often sharing commonality with patients who exhibit clinical eating disorders. The same traits that help an athlete excel in sports—compulsiveness, driven, dichotomous thinker, perfectionist, competitive, compliant and eager to please ("coachable"), and self-motivated—increase risks for developing disordered eating patterns. The

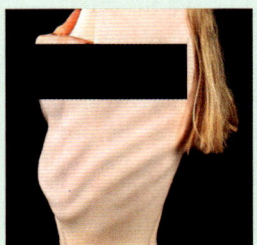

risk increases for individuals whose normal, genetically determined body size and shape deviate from an "ideal" imposed by the sport. The term *anorexia athletica* describes the subclinical eating behaviors continuum among athletes who do not meet established criteria for a true eating disorder. They exhibit at least one unhealthy weight control strategy, which includes fasting, vomiting, or use of diet pills, laxatives, or diuretics ("water pills").

For many athletes, disordered eating patterns coincide with the competitive season and abate when the season ends. Preoccupation with body weight may not reflect a true underlying pathology but a desire to achieve optimum physiologic function and competitive performance. For some competitors, the season never seems to end, and the athlete develops anorexia nervosa and bulimia. A third category, binge-eating disorder, does not include purging behavior.

ANOREXIA NERVOSA

Originally described in ancient writings, *anorexia nervosa* is an unhealthy physical and mental state characterized by a crippling obsession with body size. A "nervous loss of appetite" reflects a preoccupation with dieting and thinness and refusal to eat enough food to maintain normal body weight. The relentless pursuit toward thinness present in about 1 to 2% of the general population includes an intense fear they will gain weight and become too fat, despite an alarmingly low body weight, accompanied by amenorrhea. The true anorectic has a distorted body image, and truly believes they are "fat" despite their obvious. The image is the first published photo of an anorectic female (*N Engl J Med*. 1932;207(5)).

Anorexia nervosa usually begins with a normal attempt to lose weight through dieting, despite early warning signs for the disorder (**TABLE 1**). With prolonged dieting, the individual continues to eat less until they consume hardly any food. Eventually, food restriction becomes an obsession, and the person with anorexia achieves little satisfaction even with continued weight loss.

TABLE 1   COMMON ANOREXIA WARNING SIGNS

Preoccupation with dieting, counting calories, cooking, and eating
Amenorrhea
Significant body weight loss
Severe mood shifts
Guilt about eating
Multiple bingeing and purging

BULIMIA NERVOSA

The term *bulimia*, literally meaning "ox hunger," refers to "gorging" or "insatiable appetite." Purging and intense guilt and shame almost always follow binge eating episodes (**TABLE 2**). Approximately 2 to 4% of all female adolescents and adults, including 5% of college females, experience bulimia nervosa. Binge eating characterizes bulimia nervosa, unlike continual semistarvation in anorexia nervosa. The bulimic person regularly consumes calorically dense foods (often at night and privately), containing between 1000 and 10,000 kcal. This is repeated by fasting, self-induced vomiting, laxatives or diuretic use, or compulsively exercising to avoid weight gain.

TABLE 2   COMMON BULIMIA NERVOSA WARNING SIGNS

Excessive interest in body weight, size, and fatness
Frequent body weight gains and losses
Bathroom visits following meals
Compulsive dieting after binging
Depression, anxiety, severe mood shifts
Irregular menstrual cycle (oligomenorrhea)

BINGE-EATING DISORDER

Episodic bingeing, often without subsequent purging behavior common to bulimia, characterizes binge eating disorder. Food is consumed more rapidly than normal, and often food intake exceeds that determined by the physiologic hunger drive. Binge eating occurs with guilt, depression, or self-disgust. Individuals suffer greater self-anger, shame, lack of control, and frustration than nonbingeing overfat individuals. The diagnosis of binge-eating disorder requires that the individual experiences a lack of control over eating and marked psychologic distress when it occurs. The person binges at least 2 d·wk^{-1} for 6 months. Binge eating differs from obesity because the same self-anger, shame, lack of control, and frustration about binge eating does not necessarily accompany obesity. Little factual information exists about the prevalence of binge-eating disorder, but it may occur in about 2% of the U.S. population.

Sources:
Hosseini SA, Padhy RK. Body image distortion. In: *StatPearls* [Internet]. Treasure Island: StatPearls Publishing; 2021.
Mitchell JE, Peterson CB. Anorexia nervosa. *N Engl J Med*. 2020;382:1343.
Neale J, Hudson LD. Anorexia nervosa in adolescents. *Br J Hosp Med (Lond)*. 2020;81:1.

4. Cause acidosis
5. Aggravate existing kidney disorders from the extra solute burden in the renal filtrate
6. Deplete glycogen reserves contributing to fatigue
7. Decrease calcium balance and can increase bone loss risk
8. Cause dehydration
9. Can retard fetal development from inadequate carbohydrate intake

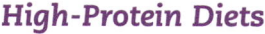
Elena Shashkina/Shutterstock

For high-performance endurance athletes who train at or above 70% maximum effort, switching to a high-fat diet is misguided because the body must maintain adequate blood glucose and glycogen packed into the active muscles and liver storage depots. Fatigue during intense physical activity exceeding 60 min occurs more rapidly when consuming higher fat rather than carbohydrate-richer meals.

High-Protein Diets

Low-carbohydrate, high-protein diets may shed pounds in the near term, but their long-term success remains questionable and may even pose health risks.[50] Advertising campaigns promoted the low-carbohydrate, high-protein diets as "last-chance diets." Earlier versions included protein in liquid form advertised as "miracle liquid." Unknown to the consumer, the liquid protein mixture often contained blended ground-up animal hooves and horns, with pigskin mixed in a broth with enzymes and tenderizers to "predigest" it. Collagen-based blends produced from gelatin hydrolysis supplemented with trace essential amino acids did not contain the highest-quality amino acid mixture and lacked required vitamins and minerals, particularly copper. A negative copper balance coincides with electrocardiographic abnormalities and rapid heart rate.[52] Protein-rich foods often contain high saturated fat levels, which increase the risk for heart disease and type 2 diabetes. Diets excessively high in animal protein increase urinary oxalate excretion, a compound that combines primarily with calcium to form kidney stones.[161] The diet's safety improves if it contains high-quality protein with ample carbohydrate, essential fatty acids, and micronutrients.[157]

Medical Pitfalls. Israeli researchers have posited that extremely high protein intake suppresses appetite through reliance on lipid mobilization and subsequent excess ketone formation.[268] The elevated thermic effect of dietary protein, with its relatively low digestibility coefficient (particularly plant protein), reduces the net calories available from ingested protein compared with a well-balanced meal with equivalent caloric value. This point has some validity, but one must consider additional factors when formulating a sound weight-loss program, particularly for physically active individuals. A high-protein diet has the potential for these four deleterious outcomes:

1. Strain on liver and kidney function and accompanying dehydration
2. Electrolyte imbalance
3. Glycogen depletion
4. Lean tissue loss

Semistarvation Diets

Therapeutic fasting or **very low-calorie diets (VLCDs)** may benefit severe clinical obesity when body fat exceeds 40 to 50% body mass. The diet provides between 400 and 1000 kcal daily as high-quality protein foods or liquid meal replacements. Dietary prescriptions usually last up to 3 months but only as a "last resort" before undertaking more-extreme medical approaches for morbid obesity that include various surgical treatments (collectively called *bariatric surgery*; https://asmbs.org/patients/wls-patient-videos). Surgical treatments that considerably reduce stomach size and reconfigure the small intestine induce a sustained weight loss, but are only prescribed for eligible patients with a BMI at least 40, or a 35 BMI when accompanied by other comorbidities.

Medical Concerns About Therapeutic Fasting. Dieting with VLCD requires close supervision, usually in a hospital setting. Proponents maintain that severe food restriction breaks established dietary habits, which in turn improves long-term prospects for success. These diets also may depress appetite to help compliance. Daily medications that accompany a VLCD include calcium carbonate for nausea, bicarbonate of soda and potassium chloride to maintain body fluid consistency, mouthwash, and sugar-free chewing gum for bad breath from a high ketone levels from fatty acid catabolism, and bath oils for dry skin. *For most individuals, semistarvation does not compose an "ultimate diet" or proper approach to weight control.* A VLCD provides inadequate carbohydrate, with the glycogen storage depots in the liver and muscles depleting rapidly. This impairs physical tasks that require either intense aerobic effort or shorter-duration anaerobic power output. The continuous nitrogen loss with fasting and weight loss reflects an exacerbated lean tissue loss, which may occur disproportionately from critical organs like the heart. The success rate remains poor for prolonged fasting.[145]

Most diets produce weight loss during the first several weeks, although body water represents the predominant initial lost weight. In addition, lean tissue loss occurs with dieting alone, particularly when beginning a VLCD. An individual can reduce weight through dieting alone, but few persons achieve long-term success to favorably alter body size and tissue composition.

Factors That Impact Weight Loss

Hydration level and energy deficit duration impact weight loss amount and composition.

Water Loss Predominates During Early Weight Loss Stages

When dieting, water loss predominates during the initial 4 wk as the major daily percentage composition in the lost weight.

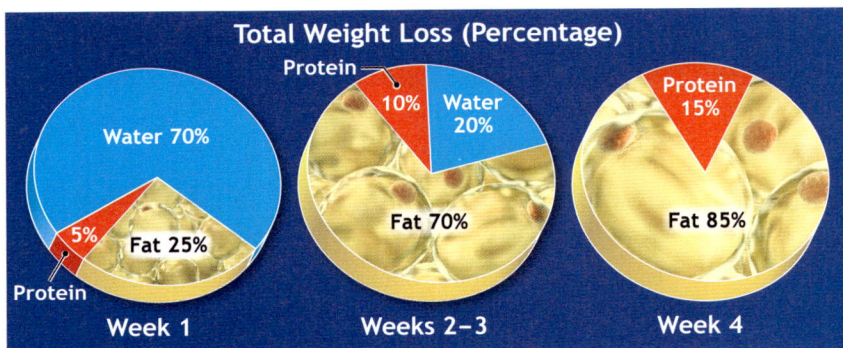

Background images: Kateryna Kon/Shutterstock

It progressively lessens thereafter, shown in the image above, amounting to about 20% weight loss in the 2nd and 3rd wk. Concurrently during this time frame, body fat loss accelerates from 25 to 70%. During the fourth dieting week, reductions in body fat produce about 85% of the weight loss without further increase in water loss. Protein's contribution to weight loss increases from 5% initially to about 15% after the 4th wk. In practical terms, counseling efforts should emphasize that the weight lost during the initial attempts to reduce weight, when successful, consists chiefly of water and not fat; it takes approximately 4 wk to establish the desired fat loss pattern for each pound in lost weight.

Hydration Level's Impact

Restricting water during the first several days with a caloric deficit increases the proportion for losing body water and and reducing body fat loss. There is some evidence that more total weight loss occurred by consuming additional water during a 1-year duration weight loss program.[269] Absolute and relative increases in drinking water occurred concurrently with decreases in body weight, waist circumference, and percent body fat (dual-energy x-ray absorptiometry) in overweight women assigned to four popular weight loss diets. Interestingly, an absolute increase in drinking water to greater than once daily occurred with a significantly greater 2-kg/5-lb weight loss over 12 months was consistent with prior experimental data showing that 500 mL drinking water increased energy expenditure by 100 kJ.[270] Weight loss attributable to drinking water acted independently from sociodemographic variables, baseline status, food composition changes, food's energy intake, and physical activity.

Longer-Term Deficit Promotes Fat Loss

A key dieting principle for weight loss underscores the caloric equivalent from lost weight increases as caloric restriction duration progresses. After about 8 wk, the weight loss caloric equivalent exceeds twice that in the first week and continues to increase throughout a 25-wk duration. *The ascending yellow data line in the inset graphic at right illustrates the need to maintain a caloric deficit for extended durations, at least 16 wk (indicated by the yellow arrow).* Shorter caloric restriction periods produce larger water and carbohydrate losses per unit weight reduction with only a minimal body fat decrease.

Increase Physical Activity for Weight Control

Conventional wisdom views excessive food intake as the prime cause for creating the overfat condition. Many believe the only way to reduce unwanted body fat requires caloric restriction by dieting. This overly simplistic strategy partly accounts for the dismal success in maintaining weight loss over the long term, refocusing debate on food intake's contribution to obesity.[75,180] A lifestyle characterized predominantly by reduced physical activity consistently emerges as a crucial factor in childhood, adolescent, and adult weight gain.[17,169,204]

Metabolic Inflexibility

The novel concept **metabolic inflexibility** helps to explain a potential underlying reason leading to sedentary behaviors, even among individuals who meet physical activity recommendations.[271,303] Sedentary behaviors refer to any waking behavior with an energy expenditure ≤1.5 metabolic equivalents while in a sitting or reclining posture. To explain "metabolic inflexibility," experiments determined that human skeletal muscle in insulin resistance accompanied *increased* rather than decreased muscle glucose oxidation under basal conditions, yet *decreased* glucose oxidation under insulin-stimulated circumstances.[305]

The major downside in sliding into metabolic inflexibility is cellular response inability to switch between lipid and carbohydrate oxidation (dysregulation in energy and fuel homeostasis), thereby promoting obesity, type 2 diabetes, and cardiovascular diseases.[102,304] On the upside, high physical activity levels promote sufficient cellular metabolic flexibility to create "safe" functional adaptations to mitigate severe medical consequences.

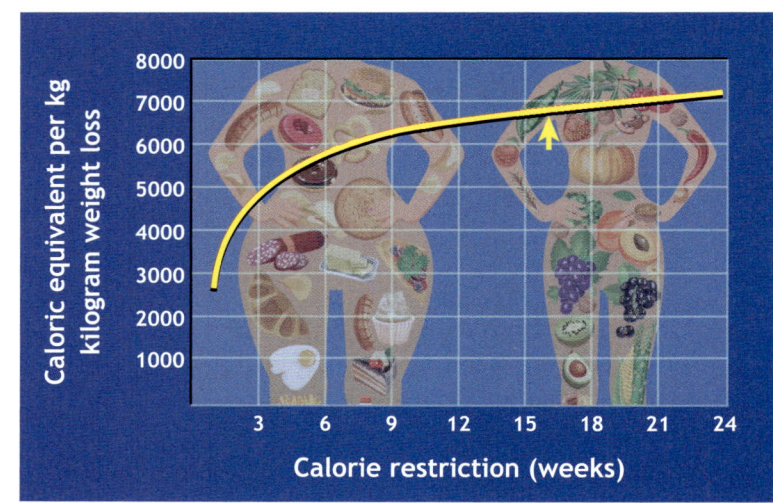

Background images: Tatsiana Tsyhanova/Shutterstock

Sedentarism may account for up to a shocking 6 million of the 60 million annual deaths around the world.[272] This means that when physical inactivity and sedentary behaviors predominate to define an adult's behavioral lifestyle profile,[302] variation in metabolic inflexibility becomes a key driver leading to adult deaths. Researchers in this new area hope to refine the guidelines on physical activity by better understanding how manipulating daily physical activity disparity in frequency, duration, intensity, and volume effects the metabolic flexibility concept.[271,306,307]

Not Simply Gluttony

Excess weight gain often parallels reduced physical activity rather than increased caloric intake. Physically active individuals who eat the most often weigh the least and maintain the highest physiologic fitness levels.

Obese Infants, Children, and Adolescents

Obese infants do not characteristically ingest more calories than recommended dietary standards. For children ages 4 to 6 years, daily energy expenditure averaged 25% below the current recommendation for energy intake for this age. A low daily physical activity level primarily produced the depressed energy output.[21] More specifically, 50% of boys and 75% of girls in the United States fail to engage in even moderate physical activity three or more times weekly.[1] Physically active children tend to be leaner than less active counterparts. For preschool children, no relationship emerged between total energy intake, or the lipid, carbohydrate, and protein composition for the diet and percentage body fat.[8] Excessive fatness relates directly to the hours spent watching television (a consistent marker for inactivity) among children, adolescents, and adults.[5,6,89] For example, viewing television 3-hr per day led to a twofold increase in obesity and a 50% increase in diabetes.[65,88] Each 2-hr daily increment in TV watching matches a 23% increase in obesity and a 14% rise in diabetes risk. Excessive television watching, playing video games, and otherwise remaining inactive characterizes overweight minority teens. Reducing the time spent watching television, playing video games, or using a computer would substantially reduce metabolic syndrome incidence.[69] Minimizing time devoted to such behaviors can help combat childhood fat gain.[56,167]

The observation that overfat children often eat the same or even less than average body weight peers also relate to less physically active adults as they slowly, progressively gain weight. *Overweight individuals often do not eat more on average than normal weight persons.* Consequently, it remains neither prudent nor justifiable to emphasize dieting alone to effectively induce long-term weight loss.

The Most Desirable Solution: Increase Energy Output

Physically active males and females throughout youth and adulthood usually maintain a desirable body composition within constraints in the normal aging process. An increased regular physical activity level combined with dietary restraint maintains weight loss more effectively than long-term caloric restriction alone.[3,213] A negative energy balance induced by increased caloric expenditure, through either lifestyle activities or formal physical activity programs, unbalances the energy balance equation for weight loss, improves physical fitness and the health risk profile, and favorably alters body composition and body fat distribution for children and adults.[49,151,169,185,218] Regular physical activity produces less central adipose tissue accumulation associated with aging.[100,170,212] Overweight women show a dose-response relationship between physical activity dosage and long-term weight loss.[94] Obese adolescents and adults improve body composition and visceral fat distribution using both moderate physical activity and more vigorous activity that improves cardiovascular fitness, with more intense physical activity being most effective.[90] For obese boys and girls, the most favorable body composition changes occur with long duration aerobic exercise and high-repetition resistance training, combined with a behavior modification component.[71,129,135,162] Additional spin-off benefits from regular physical activity include slowing age-related muscle mass loss, possibly preventing adult-onset obesity and improved obesity-related comorbidities, decreased mortality, and greater beneficial outcomes to existing chronic diseases.[14,74,127,132,195]

Two Physical Activity Misconceptions

Two arguments attempt to counter the increased physical activity approach to weight loss. One maintains that physical activity inevitably increases appetite to produce a proportionate increase in food intake that negates the caloric deficit that increased physical activity produces. The second argument claims that the relatively small calorie-burning effect with a normal exercise workout does not "dent" the body's lipid reserves as effectively as food restriction.

Misconception 1: Increased Physical Activity Increases Food Intake

Sedentary persons have difficulty balancing energy intake with energy expenditure. Failure to accurately regulate energy balance at the lower end along the physical activity spectrum contributes to the "creeping obesity" observed in highly mechanized and technically advanced societies. In contrast, regular participation in physical activity maintains appetite control within a reactive zone where food intake more readily matches daily energy expenditure.[173] As the inset image on the next page shows for six common snack foods, the calories in an extra cookie or cheese pizza slice quickly add up to many minutes required in different physical activities to match the food item's "extra" caloric content. For a single cheese pizza slice, it requires continuous swimming for about 1 hr to "burn-up" the same number of calories in the pizza slice! Appendix F presents the calories expended each min for household, occupational, recreational, and sport activities.

In considering physical activity's effects on appetite and food intake, a distinction must clarify activity type and duration versus the participant's body fat status. Lumberjacks, farm laborers, and endurance athletes consume about twice as many daily calories as sedentary individuals. Elite marathon runners, cross-country skiers, gymnasts, and cyclists consume about 4000 to 5000 kcal daily, yet are the leanest individuals in the population.

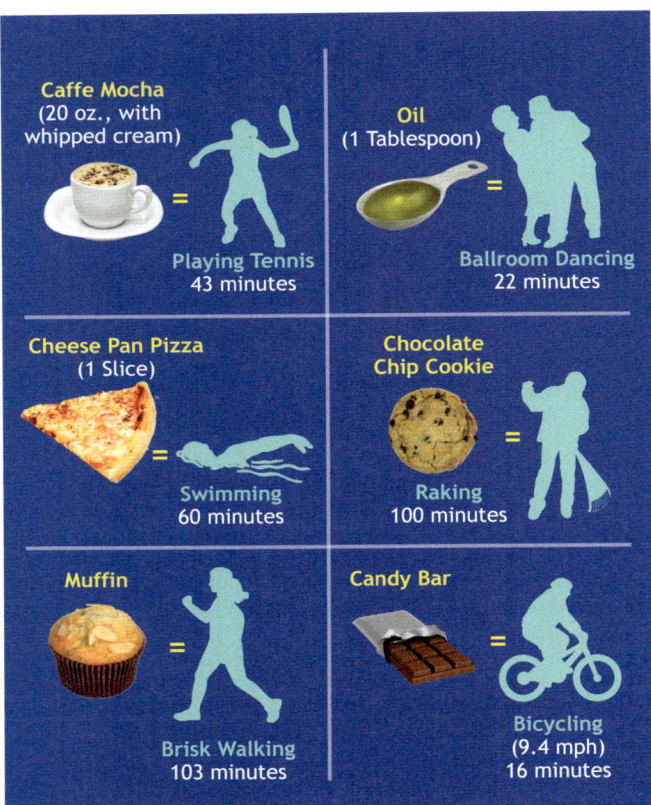

Shutterstock: marekuliasz (oil), Esteban De Armas (candy bar), M. Unal Ozmen (mocha), OLOS (muffin), Sergey Mironov (pizza), BW Folsom (cookie)

Obviously, their large caloric intake meets trainings' energy requirements while maintaining a lean body composition.

For the overweight or obese person, the extra energy required for increased physical activity more than offsets moderate physical activity's small compensatory appetite-stimulating effect. To some extent, the large energy reserve in the overfat person makes it easier to tolerate weight loss and physical activity without the obligatory increase in caloric intake typically observed for leaner counterparts.[110,175] No difference emerged in lipid, carbohydrate, or protein intake or total calories consumed for overweight males and females during 16 months supervised, moderate-intensity exercise training compared with a sedentary control group.[46] In essence, a weak coupling exists between the short-term energy deficit induced by physical activity and energy intake. Increased physical activity by overweight, sedentary individuals does not necessarily alter physiologic needs to automatically produce compensatory increases in food intake to balance additional energy expenditure.

Misconception 2: Physical Activity Does Not Burn Many Calories

A common misconception concerns the supposed negligible contribution to weight loss from the calories expended in typical physical activities. Some argue correctly that it requires an inordinate output involving short-term activity to lose just 0.45-kg/1-lb body fat; for example, chopping wood for 10 hr, playing golf for 20 hr, performing mild calisthenics for 22 hr, playing ping-pong for 28 hr, or volleyball for 32 hr. Consequently, a 2- or 3-month physical activity regimen can produce only a small fat loss in an overfat person. From a different perspective, if one played golf (no cart) for 2-hr daily (350 kcal) 2-d·wk^{-1} (700 kcal), it would take about 5 wk to reduce 0.45 kg/1 lb body fat. Assuming the person plays year-round, golfing 2-d·wk^{-1} produces a 4.5-kg/10-lb yearly fat loss if food intake remains constant. Even an activity as innocuous as chewing gum burns an extra 11 kcal·h^{-1}, a 20% increase over normal resting metabolism. Stepping in place or doing simple back and forth dance moves while watching television commercials during a 1-hr broadcast would produce an additional 25-min increased energy expenditure and 4.3 kcal liberated.[191] *Stated simply, the calorie-expending effects of increased physical activity during each minute of stepping add up over time. A 3500-kcal caloric deficit equals 0.45-kg/1-lb body fat loss, whether the deficit occurs rapidly or systematically over time.*

When estimating the energy cost to perform various physical activities, one assumes that exercise energy expenditure remains constant among similar size individuals. In Chapter 8, we noted that energy cost data for most physical activities represent averages, often based on observing only a few subjects. A wide range in energy expenditure values exists due to individual differences in performance style and technique; terrain, temperature, and wind resistance (environmental factors) and participation intensity. Consequently, energy expenditure values for the physical activities presented in Appendix F (available online at Lippincott Connect) do not represent constants. Rather, they reflect "average" values applicable under "average" conditions when applied to the "average" person at a given body weight. Nevertheless, the data provide useful approximations to establish the energy cost for diverse physical activities.

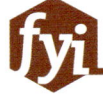 Appendix F, available on Lippincott Connect, presents energy expenditure values for household, occupational, recreational, and sports activities.

Eight Benefits to Adding Exercise to Dietary Restriction for Weight Loss

1. Increases the energy deficit
2. Facilitates visceral lipid mobilization from adipose tissue
3. Increases body fat loss while preserving fat-free body mass
4. Blunts a decline in resting metabolism with weight loss
5. Creates an energy deficit with fewer calorie restrictions
6. Contributes to longer duration weight loss success
7. Substantially improves overall health
8. Moderately suppresses appetite

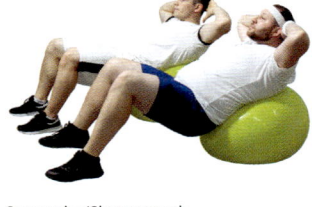

Satyrenko/Shutterstock

The Recovery "Afterglow." Controversy exists about the excess postexercise oxygen uptake contribution to the total energy expended.[111] With low-to-moderate exercise, as performed by most persons who exercise for weight control, the contribution from recovery metabolism—the **recovery afterglow**—to total energy expenditure remains small relative to exercise energy expenditure, ranging up to 75 kcal for 80-min exercise durations.[159] Exercise training induces faster adjustments in postexercise energetics to reduce the total recovery oxygen uptake. Calories expended during physical activity represent the most important factor in total exercise energy expenditure, *not* calories expended in recovery.[273]

Regular Physical Activity's Effectiveness

Adding physical activity to a weight-loss program favorably modifies the composition of the weight lost in the direction favoring greater fat loss, less lean tissue loss, and the maintenance or even physical capacity enhancement.[9,222] **FIGURE 30.16** clearly illustrates muscle-sparing effects with regular physical activity, which equates to about a 4.5-kg/10-lb weight loss over 12 months, induced by either *only* caloric restriction (*pink* data points) or *only* physical activity (*orange* data points) on thigh muscle volume in both legs as assessed on magnetic resonance imaging in 50- to 60-year-old males and females. Decreases in thigh muscle volume (6.8%) and composite knee flexion strength (27%), and $\dot{V}O_{2max}$ (27%) occurred only in the caloric restriction group, whereas $\dot{V}O_{2max}$ increased 15.5% in the exercise only group attempting to lose weight. Clearly, decreases in muscle mass, muscle strength, and aerobic capacity occurred during 12-month weight loss by caloric restriction, but not to an exercise-only–induced weight loss.

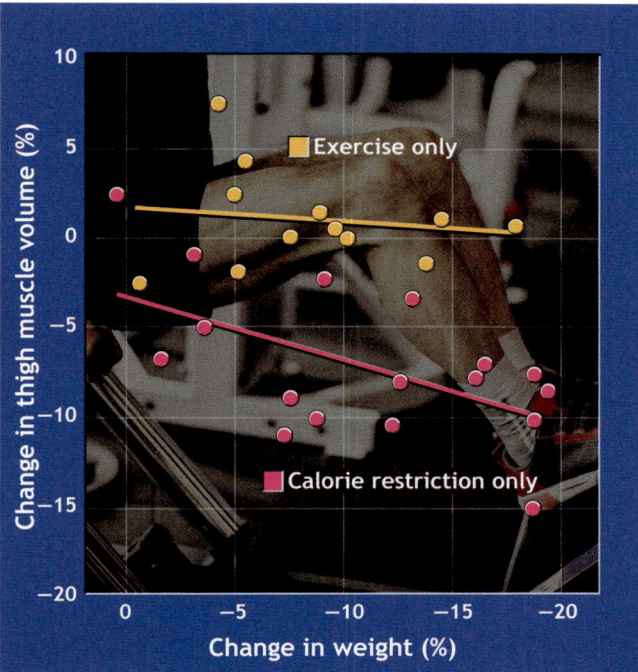

FIGURE 30.16. Relationship between weight loss magnitude with change in thigh muscle volume when losing weight by caloric restriction only versus weight loss by exercise only.
(Adapted with permission from Weiss EP, et al. Lower extremity muscle size and strength and aerobic capacity decrease with caloric restriction but not with exercise-induced weight loss. *J Appl Physiol.* 2007;102:634. ©The American Physiological Society (APS). All rights reserved. Background photo: Mladen Zivkovic/Shutterstock.)

Physical Activity Effectiveness and Excess Body Fat

Regular physical activity effectiveness for weight loss relates closely to excess body fat. Obese persons generally lose weight and fat more readily with increased physical activity than normal-weight individuals.[169] Aerobic physical activity and resistance training, even without dietary restriction, provide positive spin-off to any weight loss effort. They alter body composition favorably (reduced body fat and small FFM increase) for the otherwise healthy overweight person, postmenopausal woman, cardiac patient, and physically challenged individual.[116,181,203] Adolescent males who engaged regularly in vigorous activities showed less abdominal fat than sedentary counterparts.[41] This indicates that regular physical activity and improved aerobic fitness may target excess fat accumulation in the abdominal-visceral area to a greater extent than peripheral fat deposits. Even when an activity program produces no weight loss, substantial reductions occur in abdominal subcutaneous and visceral fat.[170] This outcome certainly diminishes the tendency toward insulin resistance and resulting predisposition to type 2 diabetes. **TABLE 30.1** lists typical results for weight loss from regular physical activity in overfat young men who exercised by walking 90 min in each session, 5 days a week for 16 wk. The men lost nearly 6 kg/13 lb of body fat, and decreased percentage body fat from 23.5 to 18.6% over the experimental sessions. Exercise capacity also improved as did HDL cholesterol (↑15.6%) and the HDL-to-low-density lipoprotein (LDL) cholesterol ratio (↑26%).

> **TABLE 30.1** Daily 90-min walking sessions for 16 wk alters body weight, body fat, HDL cholesterol concentration, and HDL-to-LDL ratio

Most health-related metabolic improvements in the obese with regular physical activity relate to total activity volume and quantity of fat loss rather than enhanced cardiorespiratory fitness.[37,38] Ideal physical activity involves continuous, large muscle activities with moderate-to-high caloric cost, such as circuit resistance training, walking, running, rope skipping, stair stepping, cycling, and swimming. Many recreational sports and games also are effective in promoting weight control, but precisely quantifying and regulating energy expenditure becomes difficult. Aerobic physical activity stimulates lipid catabolism, establishes favorable blood pressure responses, and generally promotes cardiovascular fitness. Interestingly, aerobic exercise training may elevate resting metabolism independently from FFM change.[233] No selective effect exists for running, walking, or bicycling; each promotes fat loss with equal effectiveness.[154] Expending 300 additional kcal daily (e.g., jogging 30-min) should produce 0.45 kg/1 lb fat loss in about 12 days. This represents a yearly caloric deficit equivalent to the energy in 13.6 kg/30 lb body fat.

Resistance Training

Resistance training provides an important adjunct to aerobic training for weight loss and weight maintenance, and overall decreased cardiovascular disease risk. The energy expended in circuit resistance training—continuous exercise using low resistance and high repetitions—averages about 9 kcal·min⁻¹ and yields substantial calorie output during a typical 30- to 60-min workout. Even conventional resistance training that involves less total energy expenditure positively affects muscular strength and FFM during weight loss compared with programs that rely solely on food restriction.[10,215] Individuals who maintain high muscular strength levels tend to gain less weight than weaker counterparts.[124] In addition to reducing coronary heart disease risk, resistance training performed regularly also improves glycemic control, favorably modifies the lipoprotein profile, and increases resting metabolic rate when FFM increases.[85,157,202]

Comparing conventional resistance training with endurance training illustrates unique resistance training benefits on body composition.[16,153,215] **TABLE 30.2** summarizes 12 wk of either endurance exercise or resistance training on nondieting, untrained young men. Endurance training reduced percentage body fat (hydrostatic weighing) from reduced fat mass (1.6 kg/3.5 lb; no change in FFM), while resistance training decreased body fat mass by 2.4 kg/5.4 lb and increased FFM by 2.4 kg/5.4 lb. As FFM remains metabolically more active than body fat, conserving or increasing this tissue depot with exercise training maintains a higher resting metabolism level, average daily metabolic rate, and possibly lipid oxidation during rest—factors that counteract age-related increased adiposity.[20,44,187]

> **TABLE 30.2** Effects on body composition of either endurance exercise or resistance training

FIGURE 30.17 depicts body composition changes in 40 obese women placed into four groups: (1) control, no exercise and no diet; (2) diet only (DO) without exercise; (3) diet plus resistance exercise (D + E), and (4) resistance exercise only (EO) without diet. The women trained 3-day weekly for 8 wk, and completed 10 repetitions for eight strength exercises and three sets. Body mass decreased 4.5 kg/10 lb for DO, and 3.9 kg/8.6 lb for D + E compared with +0.5 kg/1.2 lb for EO and +0.4 kg/1 lb for controls. Importantly, FFM increased for EO (+1.1 kg/2.5 lb), whereas the DO group lost 0.9 kg/2 lb. The data revealed that augmenting a calorie restriction program with resistance exercise training preserves FFM better than dietary restriction alone.

Dose-Response Relationship for Energy Expended and Weight Lost

The total energy expended in physical activity relates in a dose-response manner as a tool to effectively produce weight loss.[9,95] A reasonable goal progressively increases moderate activity to between 60 and 90 min daily or 2100 to 2800 kcal weekly.[55,98] To combat the worldwide obesity epidemic, the public health perspective must promote a population's need to substantially increase *total* daily energy expenditure on a daily basis rather than increase effort intensity solely to induce a training response. An overly fat person who begins with easily tolerated light physical activity, like slow walking, still accrues a considerable caloric expenditure simply by extending exercise duration. The focus on duration offsets the inadvisability in having a sedentary, obese individual begin a program with more strenuous physical activity. Also, the weight-bearing physical activity energy cost relates directly to body weight; the overweight person expends considerably more calories in such activities than an average weight person.

Walking-Running for Different Durations

Physical activity duration impacts fat loss. **TABLE 30.3** lists changes in body fat for three male groups who exercised by walking and running for 15-, 30-, or 45-min each workout session over a 20-wk period. The results also present distance covered and total weekly workout duration, training heart rate, body mass, six skinfold sum, and waist girth.

> **TABLE 30.3** How training duration by walking and running for 5 months impacts body composition

The three exercise groups decreased body fat, skinfolds, and waist girth compared with sedentary controls. Body weight also decreased with exercise, except in the 15-min group whose weight remained stable. Comparing the three groups, the 45-min group lost significantly more body fat than either the 30- or 15-min groups. This difference was closely linked to the greater caloric expenditure with longer activity, a salient example emphasizing the dose-response relationship.

Exercise Frequency

A now classic experiment published 47 years ago set a standard on how best to determine an optimal exercise frequency to elicit body composition changes.[155] To determine optimal

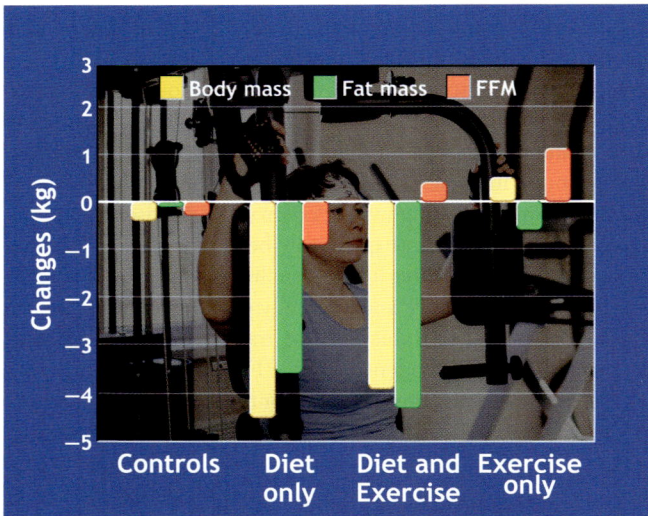

FIGURE 30.17. Changes in obese female's body composition by resistance exercise only, diet only, or resistance exercise plus diet. FFM, fat-free body mass.
(Adapted with permission from Ballor DL, et al. Resistance weight training during caloric restriction enhances lean body weight maintenance. *Am J Clin Nutr.* 1988;47:19. With permission from the American Society for Nutrition, https://nutrition.org/ Background photo: NatalyaBond/Shutterstock.)

exercise frequency for weight loss, subjects exercised for 30 to 47-min for 20 wk by either running or walking, with activity intensity maintained between 80 and 95% maximum heart rate. Training twice weekly produced no changes in body weight, skinfolds, or percentage body fat, but training 3 and 4 days weekly did. Subjects who trained 4 days a week reduced body weight and skinfolds more than subjects who trained 3 days a week. Percentage body fat decreased similarly in both groups. Individuals should participate in physical activity a *minimum* 3 days a week to favorably alter body composition; the additional caloric expenditure with more frequent activity produces even greater results. The threshold energy expenditure for weight loss probably remains highly individualized. The calorie burning effect for each activity session should eventually attain *at least* 300 kcal whenever possible. This generally occurs with 30 min in moderate-to-vigorous running, swimming, bicycling, circuit resistance training or 60 min of walking briskly for healthy people and those with disease but cleared medically to exercise.[274–276]

Start Slowly and Progress Gradually

The initial stage for a physical activity weight-loss program in previously sedentary, overly fat person should be developmental with moderate intensity demands. The individual should adopt long-term goals and personal discipline and restructure eating and physical activity behaviors. Unduly rapid training progressions prove counterproductive because most overfat individuals initially resist increasing their physical activity. During the first few months, faster-paced interval walking can replace walking at a slow, continuous pace. Meaningful changes in body weight and body composition require a minimum 12-wk commitment. Most overfat persons can realistically expect to reduce body weight by 5 to 15% with programs that focus on simultaneously modifying eating and exercise behaviors. Behavioral approaches should foster lifestyle changes in daily physical activity.[205] For example, walking or bicycling can replace the auto, stair climbing can replace the elevator, and manual tools can replace power tools.[4,47] Eating less and moving more proves more effective in a group situation than going it alone. Persons who joined a weight-loss program with several friends or family members lost more weight than individuals who participated alone.[232] This also applies to individuals who receive face-to-face behavioral support or participation with Web and social media technologies that offer virtual world weight loss engagement.[99,277,278]

Self-Selected Energy Expenditures and Physical Activity Mode

No selective effect exists among diverse big muscle aerobic activity modes with equivalent energy expenditures to favorably reduce body weight, body fat, skinfold thickness, and girths, yet other differences may emerge. For example, males and females generally self-select a higher energy expenditure level (with accompanying higher heart rates) when running for 20 min or longer on a treadmill compared with simulated cross-country skiing (NordicTrack; www.nordictrack.com), cycle ergometry, or aerobic riding (HealthRider; www.pro-form.com).[117] Males select a higher absolute exercise intensity and oxygen uptake level than females in each exercise mode; not surprisingly, treadmill running generates the greatest total oxygen uptake and energy expended. For individuals without physical activity limitations, rapid walking, jogging, and running at a moderate ≤9 min per mi pace usually provides the most suitable activity mode to maximize energy expenditure during self-selected continuous activities.

The Ideal Combination: Caloric Restraint Plus Physical Activity

Combining increased physical activity and caloric restraint offer considerably more flexibility for achieving a negative caloric imbalance than either exercise alone or diet alone.[48,123,231] Dietary restraint plus increased physical activity through lifestyle changes offer health and weight-loss benefits similar to those from combining dietary restraint and a vigorous structured physical activity program.[4] Adding physical activity to a weight-control program facilitates longer-term body fat loss maintenance than total reliance on either food restriction alone or increased activity alone.[95,158] **TABLE 30.4** summarizes the benefits by adding physical activity to a weight-loss regimen.

> **TABLE 30.4** Benefits of adding physical activity to a weight-loss program

How can an overfat person using increased physical activity and dietary restraint maintain a 0.45-kg/1-lb weight loss weekly to reduce body weight by 9.1 kg/20 lb? A prudent 1-kg/2.2-lb weekly fat loss requires approximately 20 wk. The weekly energy deficit to achieve this goal must average 3500 kcal with a daily 500 kcal deficit. A half-hour moderate physical activity (about 350 "extra" kcal) performed 3 days weekly adds 1050 kcal to the weekly deficit. Consequently, the weekly caloric intake need only decrease by 2400 kcal or about 350 kcal each day rather than 3500 kcal to lose the desired pound body fat each week. If activity days increase from 3 to 5, daily food intake requires a 250-kcal decrease. Extending the 5-day weekly workout duration from 30 min to 1 hr produces the desired weight loss without reducing food intake. In this case, extra physical activity creates the entire 3500 kcal deficit. If the 1-hr session intensity performed 5-day weekly increases by only 10% (cycling at 22 mph rather than 20 mph; running at 6.6 mph than 6.0 mph), the calories expended weekly with physical activity increases by an additional 350 kcal (3500 kcal × 0.10). This new 3850 kcal (550 kcal-d) weekly deficit allows the dieter to *increase* daily food intake by 50 kcal and still maintain a 1-lb weekly fat loss.

Clearly, physical activity combined with mild dietary restriction effectively *unbalances* the energy balance equation to favor weight loss. This approach produces a less intense need to eat and less psychologic stress than relying exclusively on caloric restriction. Furthermore, both aerobic and resistance activities protect against FFM loss that occurs with weight loss by diet alone. This occurs partly from the regular exercise effects on fatty acid reliance from adipose tissue.[133] Combining physical activity with weight loss produces desirable reductions in blood pressure at rest and in situations that typically elevate blood pressure such as intense physical activity and emotional distress.[192] Physical activity also facilitates protein retention in skeletal muscle and retards its breakdown rate. *In a weight-loss program, regular physical activity's fat-burning, protein-sparing benefits contribute to facilitated fat loss.*

INTEGRATIVE QUESTION

Give four specific examples of how small adjustments in daily energy expenditure and daily food intake can alter body fat content over time.

Reality Check

Despite the weight loss strategy, national and international organizations have raised concerns about the extreme difficulty in trying to solve the obesity epidemic on a long-term basis. Over 20 years ago, the influential National Task Force on the Prevention and Treatment of Obesity stated, "Obese individuals who undertake weight loss efforts should be ready to commit to lifelong changes in their behavioral patterns, diet, and physical activity."[147] Regrettably, fewer than half the people trying to lose or maintain weight pursue a more active lifestyle during their leisure time.[121,122]

The benefits for including regular physical activity for weight loss and weight maintenance outlined in Table 30.4 come primarily from highly structured experimental research on relatively few subjects who significantly increased physical activity with high compliance. In contrast, large-scale intervention studies (randomized control clinical trials) that compare diet only when combining diet and regular physical activity produce generally less remarkable results. In some cases, adding physical activity did not augment weight loss substantially; when a benefit did occur, the extra weight loss remained small. Clearly, the relatively modest extra physical activity in the exercise group combined with high noncompliance to the exercise regimen in large-scale studies accounts for helping to blunt the exercise effect. *The key to unlocking regular physical activity benefits for weight control in the general population lies in effectively implementing increased regular physical activity most days in the week by reducing the time spent sedentary.*

Spot Reduction Does Not Work to Selectively Reduce Local Fat Deposits

The popularity for advocating "spot reduction" comes from a belief rooted in antiquity that some exercises can reduce excess fat in a targeted area. More modern beliefs posit that an increase in a muscle's metabolic activity will stimulate relatively greater fat mobilization from the adipose tissue in proximity to the active muscle. As such, exercising a specific body area should "sculpt" it by selectively catabolizing more fat from that area than from a more distant area at the same metabolic intensity.

As an example, spot reduction advocates recommend performing an excessive number of sit-ups or side-bends ad nauseum to reduce excessive abdominal and hip fat. The promise to spot reduce fat in a particular body area seems attractive from an aesthetic standpoint because feeling "trim and firm" in the abdomen with a "six-pack" look certainly is an appealing goal. Unfortunately, critically evaluating the research evidence confirms that spot-reducing exercise targeting specific anatomical areas does not deliver on its promises.[114,120,148]

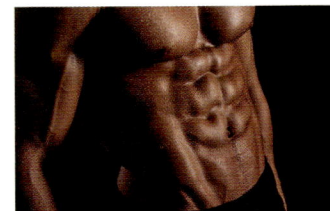
vishstudio/Shutterstock

For example, to examine spot reduction claims, researchers compared the girths and subcutaneous fat stores in high-caliber tennis players right and left forearms.[72] As expected, the girth in the dominant or playing arm exceeded the non-dominant arm from a modest muscular hypertrophy from the tennis activity overload. Measuring skinfold thickness revealed that regular and prolonged tennis training did *not* reduce subcutaneous fat in the dominant playing arm.

Another study evaluated fat biopsy specimens from abdominal, subscapular, and buttock sites before and after 27 days of training with repetitive, carefully monitored full sit-ups with knees bent in training.[104] Day 1 included 10 bouts of 10-s exercise, 7 sit-ups/bout, with 10-s rest intervals; on day 27, 14 bouts of 30-s exercise were performed, 24 sit-ups/bout, with 10-s rest intervals. The total sit-up number over the 27-day period was 5004. Lipid was extracted subcutaneously by needle biopsy, and the tissue was incubated in collagenase to release individual cells, which were then photographed immediately under a microscope. All cells were digitized electronically from the three body regions to determine cell diameter and to compute cell volume. Using sequential estimation analysis, adipose cell diameters in the abdominal, gluteal, and subscapular regions were reliably estimated with fewer than 100 cells.[284] Despite the considerable localized sit-up physical activity, adipocytes in the abdominal region were no smaller in size or volume than adipocytes in the unexercised buttock's or subscapular control regions. The expectation was that quantifying fat cell size from the abdominal region exercised over 27 days while performing 5000 sit-ups would show reduced cell size in the abdominal exercised region compared to two control areas without direct muscular involvement to stimulate lipolysis.

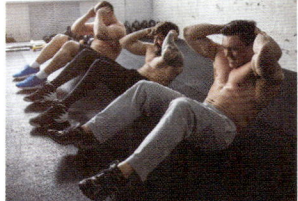
UfaBizPhoto/Shutterstock

The negative energy balance created through regular physical activity contributes to reducing total body fat. Physical activity stimulates fatty acid mobilization via hormones and enzymes that act on lipid depots throughout the body. The areas with the greatest fat concentration and/or lipid-mobilizing enzymes supply the greatest energy sources for physical activity. *The energy expenditure from selective activity does not cause greater fatty acid release from the fat pads directly over the active muscle.*

Possible Gender Difference in Physical Activity Responsiveness

An interesting question concerns gender differences in weight loss responsiveness from regular physical activity. A meta-analysis based on 53 research studies concluded that males generally respond more favorably than females to physical activity effects on weight loss.[9,283] One possible explanation involves the gender difference in body fat distribution. As discussed previously, fat distributed in the upper body and abdominal regions (central fat) shows active lipolysis to sympathetic nervous system stimulation and becomes preferentially mobilized for energy during physical activity.[6,217] Consequently, the greater upper-body fat distribution in men may contribute to a greater sensitivity for fat loss in the abdominal region with regular physical activity. Females also may more effectively preserve energy balance with increased physical activity.[45,47,225] Males often reduce energy intake with training, whereas depressed food intake with exercise may be less for females.

INTEGRATIVE QUESTION

Outline a prudent, effective three-stage strategy for a middle-aged woman who wants to shed 10 kg/22 lb of excess weight. Provide the rationale for each recommendation.

Weight Loss Recommendations for Wrestlers and Power Athletes

Weightlifters, gymnasts, and other athletes in sports that require greater muscular strength and power per unit body mass must reduce body fat without compromising FFM and athletic performance. Any increase in relative muscular strength and short-term power output capacity should improve competitive performance. The following discussion focuses on wrestlers but applies to all physically active individuals who desire to reduce body fat without negatively affecting health, safety, or physical capacity.

Determining Minimal Wrestling Weight

To reduce injury and medical complications from short- and longer-term weight loss and dehydration periods, the ACSM, NCAA, and AMA recommend assessing each wrestler's body composition. The National Federation of State High School Associations required adopting weight certification beginning with the 2005 season. This assessment takes place several weeks prior to the competitive season to determine a **minimal wrestling weight (MWW)** based on percentage body fat, *which represents the lowest acceptable level for safe wrestling competition.*[27,28] Importantly, percentage body fat must be determined in the euhydrated state because between 2 and 5% body dehydration through fluid restriction and exercise in a hot environment (techniques commonly used by wrestlers) violates the assumptions necessary to accurately and precisely predict MMW.[11,282]

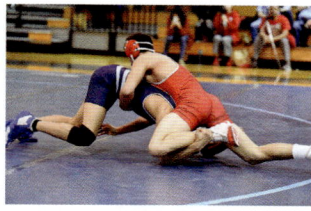
JoeSAPhotos/Shutterstock

Validating MWW

To achieve standards applicable to NCAA collegiate wrestlers in 7 conferences (EIWA, ACC, Big 12, MAC, SoCon, Pac-12, Big Ten), the first step must validate each wrestler's minimal weight. This requirement attempts to severely cripple undesirable dehydration practices wrestlers use to purge as much body water as possible before competition to "make weight" and compete in the lowest wrestling weight category. These methods included 24- to 48-hr starvation, wearing rubberized total body coverings to create excessive sweating while sitting or exercising inside a sauna maintained at high temperatures, laxatives, and **diuretics**. Supervising urine testing is the first step to determine **euhydration**, which also eliminates "switching" urine samples or adulterating specimens.

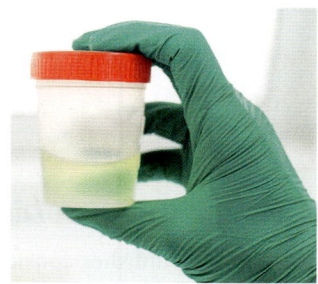
Near D. Krasaesom/Shutterstock

The color chart on the next page characterizes urine samples along a continuum from *good* to *very good* (normal) to *very* or *severely dehydrated* status. An electronic refractometer determines urine's specific gravity and where along the continuum, the required urine sample would fail the euhydration criterion before body fat percentage can be reassessed to establish a minimum wrestling weight.

The Basic 1.5% Week Rule

The 1.5% per week rule states that a competing wrestler should not lose more than 1.5% body weight weekly during the competitive season and through the ending season tournament championships. For example, a 74.8-kg/165-lb male athlete trying to "make-weight" to wrestle at the 157-lb weight class cannot lose body weight by more than 0.9 kg/2 lb or 1.2% weekly. This rule helps to minimize dehydration effects when attempting to lose too much body water too rapidly. Even a 1% dehydration effect decreases thermoregulatory control, blunts optimal muscle endurance, interferes with normal muscle firing patterns, and thus negatively impacts overall physical performance excellence.[29,156]

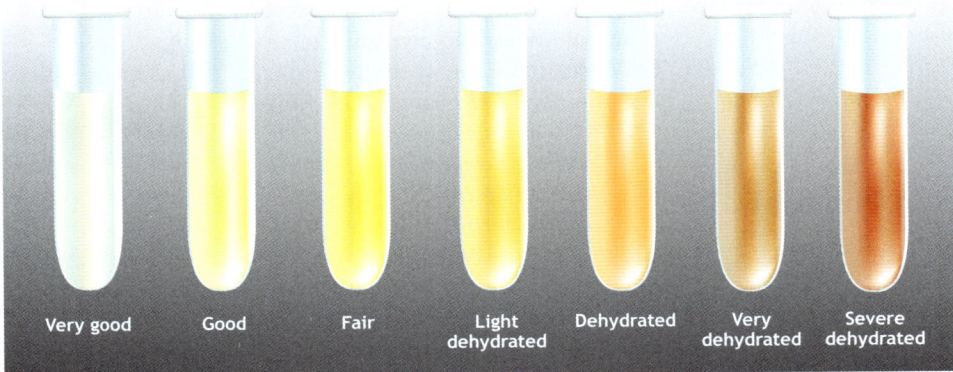

Akarat Phasura/Shutterstock

TABLE 30.5 outlines a practical application to determine MWW and an appropriate competitive minimum weight category (MWC). Four high-validity body fat percentage prediction equations based on underwater weighing as the criterion standard can compute body density and body fat percentage, fat-free weight to identify MWW, and provide a method to allow for a 2% error in determining the MWC.

TABLE 30.5 Examples of anthropometric equations to predict a minimal wrestling weight and to select a competitive weight class

NCAA Information Dissemination

The NCAA publishes considerable free, downloadable brochures and information booklets in various formats about sport and competition (www.ncaapublications.com), with topics ranging from rules and regulations covering male and female sanctioned sports, to research reports dealing with race and gender equity in intercollegiate athletics, substance use and abuse, and ethnicity. Useful information exists about wrestling in general and more specific statistical summaries regarding body fat percentages and MWWs covering over 8000 wrestlers in seven different conferences rostered by 298 NCAA and NAIA wrestling programs: www.levelchanger.com/blog/2021/3/6/how-fat-are-college-wrestlers-2020-2021.

Updated ACSM Guidelines Regarding Weight-Category Sports

In April 2021, the ACSM released new guidelines that support safer practices and more equitable competitions for athletes in weight-category sports (www.acsm.org/news-detail/2021/04/26/acsm-publishes-new-guidance-for-safer-practices-in-weight-category-sports). The expert consensus statement updates and replaces previous ACSM guidelines released in 1996. The new guidance will assist athletes and coaches establish practical and long-term approaches to body weight management for health and performance related to multiple weight-category sports. The latest guidance aligns with ACSM's mission to integrate scientific research to improve education and practical exercise science and sports medicine applications targeted at seven topic areas:

1. Differences in weight-category sports that influence weight making practices and a summary for weight categories, weigh-in procedures, and competition characteristics in specific sports
2. Common factors in weight-making practices and their associated potential benefits and disadvantages
3. Strategies for fluid and carbohydrate stores recovery between weigh-in and the event
4. Concerns associated with "making weight"
5. Rapid weight loss effects on performance
6. Strategies and rule changes to minimize harmful weight-making practices involving specific positive and negative intervention effects
7. Specific recommendations for sporting organizations, clinicians, coaches, and athletes to support safer weight making practices

Gaining Weight: The Competitive Athlete's Dilemma

Gaining weight to enhance body composition and physical performance in activities that require muscular strength and power or aesthetic appearance poses a unique problem not easily resolved. Most persons focus on weight loss to reduce excess body fat and improve overall health and appearance. Body weight and fat gain *per se* occurs all too readily by tilting the body's energy balance to favor greater caloric intake. Weight gain for athletes should target increases in muscle mass and accompanying connective tissue. Generally, such weight gain will occur if increased caloric intake—carbohydrate for adequate energy and protein sparing, plus the amino acid protein building blocks for tissue synthesis—accompanies a balanced, progressive resistance training regimen.

Unsupported Hype

Athletes attempting to increase muscle mass often fall easy prey to health food and diet supplement manufacturers who market "high-potency, tissue-building" substances—chromium, boron, vanadyl sulfate, β-hydroxy-methyl butyrate, and various protein and amino acid mixtures—none of which reliably increases muscle mass. Concerning protein supplementation, no evidence indicates that commercially prepared powdered protein, predigested amino acids, or special

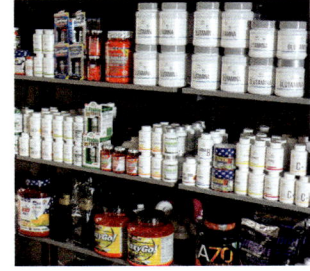

Iakov Filimonov/Shutterstock

high-protein "cocktail" mixtures promote muscle growth any more effectively than protein consumed in a well-balanced diet.[118]

Increase Lean Not Fat

Endurance training only increases FFM slightly, but the overall effect reduces body weight and fat loss from the calorie-burning and possible appetite-depressing effects from this training mode. In contrast, muscular overload through resistance training, supported by adequate energy and protein intake with sufficient recovery, increases muscle mass and strength. Adequate energy intake ensures that no protein catabolism available for muscle growth occurs due to an energy deficit. *Thus, intense aerobic training should not coincide with resistance training to increase muscle mass.*[77] More than likely, the added energy and perhaps protein demands from concurrent resistance and aerobic exercise training impose a limit on muscle growth and responsiveness to resistance training. In addition, on the molecular level, aerobic training may inhibit signaling to skeletal muscle protein synthesis machinery to negatively impact the muscle's adaptive response to resistance training.[13,143] A prudent recommendation increases daily protein intake to about 1.6 to 2.0 g · kg^{-1} body mass during resistance training.[128] The individual should select assorted plant and animal proteins; relying solely on animal protein (high in saturated fatty acids and cholesterol) potentially increases heart disease risk.

If all calories consumed in excess of the energy requirement during resistance training sustained muscle growth, then 2000 to 2500 extra kcal could supply each 0.5-kg/1.2-lb increase in lean tissue. In practical terms, 700 to 1000 kcal added to the well-balanced daily meal plan supports a weekly 0.5- to 1.0-kg/1.2- to 2.2-lb gain in lean tissue and additional training energy needs. This ideal situation presupposes that all extra calories synthesize lean tissue. Chapter 23 provided specific recommendations for nutrient timing to optimize muscle responsiveness to resistance training.

Expected Gains in Lean Tissue

A 1-year heavy resistance training program for young, athletic males increases body mass by about 20%, mostly from gains in lean tissue. The rate in lean tissue gain rapidly plateaus as training progresses beyond the first training year. For athletic females, first-year gains in lean tissue mass average 50 to 75% of the absolute male values, probably from female's smaller initial lean body mass. Individual differences in the daily nitrogen quantity incorporated into body protein (and protein incorporated into muscle) also help to explain differences among individuals in muscle mass increases with resistance training. **FIGURE 30.18** lists eight specific factors that affect lean tissue synthesis responsiveness to resistance training.

Confirming Evidence to Reduce Dietary Animal Fat

Males and females in northern Sweden in the 1970s had among the highest prevalence of cardiovascular diseases worldwide. These sobering statistics initiated Swedish epidemiological studies, begun in 1985, to examine trends in food and nutrient intake, serum cholesterol, and BMI for 25 years from 1985 to 2010. Individuals who switched from a lower fat diet to one higher in fat and lower in carbohydrate saw blood cholesterol levels increase—despite increased use of cholesterol-lowering medication. Although low-carbohydrate/high-fat diets may have provided short-term weight loss, long-term weight loss was not maintained, while at the same time this dietary strategy increased blood cholesterol and its potential negative impact on cardiovascular disease risk. Additional studies also have attempted to quantify how cancer and heart disease risk associates with red and processed meat consumption and the dairy products of yogurt, cheese, and eggs.

Tatsiana Tsyhanova/Shutterstock

Sources:
Johansson I, et al. Associations among 25-year trends in diet, cholesterol and BMI from 140,000 observations in men and women in Northern Sweden. *Nutr J*. 2012;11:40.

Key TJ, et al. Consumption of meat, fish, dairy products, and eggs and risk of ischemic heart disease. *Circulation*. 2019;139:2835.

Winkvist A, et al. Longitudinal 10-year changes in dietary intake and associations with cardio-metabolic risk factors in the Northern Sweden Health and Disease Study. *Nutr J*. 2017;16:20.

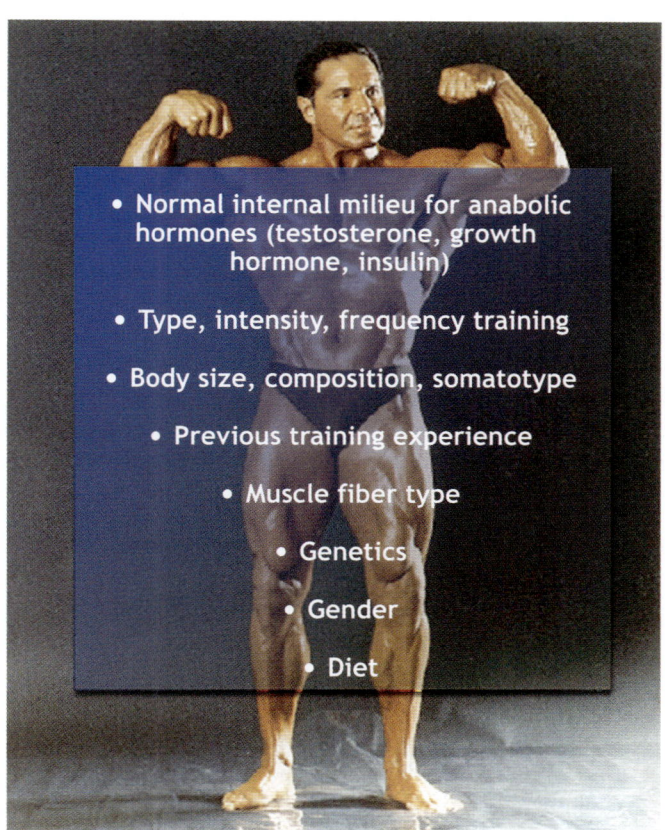

FIGURE 30.18. Specific factors influencing lean tissue synthesis with resistance training.
(Photo courtesy Bill Pearl [pictured], five-time professional Mr. Universe.)

Individuals with relatively high androgen-estrogen ratios and greater fast-twitch muscle fiber percentages probably increase lean tissue to the greatest extent. Muscle mass increases most when training begins in individuals with the largest relative FFM (FFM corrected for stature and body fat).[215] Regularly monitoring body mass and body fat verifies whether the training and additional food intake combination increases lean tissue and not body fat. This requires an accurate (valid) body composition appraisal at regular intervals throughout the training period.

Summary

1. Three ways to unbalance the energy balance equation to produce weight loss are reducing energy intake below energy expenditure, maintaining normal energy intake and increasing energy expenditure, and decreasing energy intake and increasing energy expenditure.
2. Long-term weight loss maintenance through dietary restriction has a success rate of less than 20%.
3. One to two thirds of reduced weight returns within a year and almost all the lost weight within 5 years.
4. A 3500-kcal caloric deficit, created through either diet or physical activity, represents the equivalent calories in 0.45 kg/1.0 lb of adipose tissue.
5. The Mass Balance Model predicts that weight reduction interventions with identical energy isocaloric content produces greater body weight and body fat loss than low-fat diets because *less* food consumption as a mass amount occurs as the energy proportion from fat increases.
6. Prudent dieting effectively promotes weight loss. Extremes in caloric restriction include FFM loss, lethargy, malnutrition, and depressed resting metabolism.
7. Reduced resting metabolism represents a well-documented response to weight loss through dieting.
8. Rapid weight loss during the initial caloric deficit mainly reflects body water and stored glycogen loss; greater fat loss occurs per unit weight lost as caloric restriction continues.
9. The calories burned during physical activity accumulate. Over time, regular extra physical activity creates a considerable energy deficit.
10. Physical activity's precise role in appetite suppression or stimulation remains unclear, but moderate increases in physical activity may depress appetite and energy intake in previously sedentary, overweight individuals.
11. Physical activity combined with caloric restriction offers a flexible and effective way to achieve weight loss.
12. Physical activity enhances lipid mobilization and catabolism to accelerate body fat loss.
13. Regular aerobic activity retards lean tissue loss, whereas resistance training increases FFM.
14. Selectively activating specific body regions by "spot exercise" is not more effective for localized fat loss than general physical activity at equivalent caloric expenditure.
15. Differences in body fat distribution partially explain gender difference in responsiveness to physical activity–induced weight loss.
16. Ideally, consuming 700 to 1000 extra kcal per day supports a weekly 0.5- to 1.0-kg/1.2- to 2.2-lb gain in lean tissue and meets resistance training energy requirements.

Key Terms

Adipocyte Protein 2 (*aP2*) gene: Gene for a fatty acid protein carrier primarily expressed in adipocytes and macrophages; also known as fatty acid–binding protein 4 (*FABP4*)

Bariatric surgery: Surgical procedure reduces stomach size by reconfiguring the small intestine

Central obesity: Fat deposited in the deep internal visceral abdominal region; also known as android-type obesity

Diuretics: Drugs that cause kidneys to produce more urine and void additional fluid and salt

Energy balance model (EBM): Body weight decreases only when total calories consumed are less than total calories expended by metabolism and physical activity

Euhydration: Water balance without hyperhydration (positive water balance or excess) and hypohydration (negative water balance or water deficit)

Fat cell hyperplasia: Increased total fat cell number

Fat cell hypertrophy: Existing adipose cells enlarge or fill with lipid

Futile metabolism: Genes activate a specific protein that burns excess calories as heat energy without coupling to other energy-consuming processes to blunt excess body fat storage

Global obesity epidemic: Rapid increase in worldwide obesity rate that represents a world health care crisis

Goal body weight: Fat-free body mass ÷ (1.00 − % fat desired)

Ketogenic diets: Emphasizes carbohydrate restriction while generally ignoring total calories ingested; examples: Atkins-type diet, low-carbohydrate diet

Leptin: Satiety hormone released from fat cells in adipose tissue to modulate body weight and obesity

Lipoprotein lipase (LPL): Fat-storing water soluble enzyme hydrolyzes triacylglycerols transported in lipoproteins

Metabolic inflexibility: Capacity to modulate daily fuel oxidation level to changes in fuel availability

Minimal wrestling weight (MWW): Lowest acceptable body weight for safe wrestling competition

Nonexercise activity thermogenesis: Energy expended for everything not related to sleeping, eating, or sport-like activities

Obese (*ob*) gene: Obese gene encodes a secreted protein in adipose tissue signaling pathway associated with early-onset obesity

Peripheral obesity: Excess fat deposition in the gluteal and femoral body regions known as gynoid-type obesity

Peroxisome proliferator-activated receptor gamma (*PPARγ*) gene: Master gene for white adipose cell development by reducing adipose tissue capacity to store fat in nonadipose tissue (lipotoxicity)

Preadipocyte cells: Lipid cells derived from mesenchymal stem cells create adipocytes through adipogenesis

Recovery afterglow: Elevated recovery metabolism related to any activity's total energy expenditure

Sedentarism: Personal habits and routines associated with low physical activity levels leading to health-related problems

Set point theory: Well-regulated internal control mechanism located in the lateral hypothalamus maintains a preset body weight and/or body fat level within a limited range

Uncoupling Protein 2 (*UCP2*) gene: Mitochondrial protein that uncouples oxidative phosphorylation from ATP synthesis and reduces the mitochondrial membrane potential to reduce reactive oxygen species production

Very low-calorie diets (VLCDs): Provide between 400 and 1000 kcal daily

Waist-to-hip girth ratio: Waist girth ÷ hip girth values exceed 0.80 for females and 0.95 for males indicate increased total body fatness and death risk

> References are available online at Lippincott Connect.

Additional References

Apperley LJ, et al. Childhood obesity: a review of current and future management options. *Clin Endocrinol (Oxf)*. 2022;96:288.

Ardavani A, et al. The effects of very low energy diets and low energy diets with exercise training on skeletal muscle mass: a narrative review. *Adv Ther*. 2021;38:149.

Arencibia-Albite F. Serious analytical inconsistencies challenge the validity of the energy balance theory. *Heliyon*. 2020;6:e04204; Erratum in: *Heliyon*. 2020;6:e04609.

Berge J, et al. Effect of aerobic exercise intensity on energy expenditure and weight loss in severe obesity—a randomized controlled trial. *Obesity (Silver Spring)*. 2021;29:359.

Berthoud HR, et al. Physiology of energy intake in the weight reduced state. *Obesity (Silver Spring)*. 2021;29:S25.

Bhattacharya S, et al. Prevention of childhood obesity through appropriate food labeling. *Clin Nutr ESPEN*. 2022;47:418.

Blüher M. Obesity: global epidemiology and pathogenesis. *Nat Rev Endocrinol*. 2019;15:288.

Bragg AE, et al. Changes in cardiometabolic risk among older adults with obesity: an ancillary analysis of a randomized controlled trial investigating exercise plus weight maintenance and exercise plus intentional weight loss by caloric restriction. *J Acad Nutr Diet*. 2022;122:354.

Brunelli DT, et al. Obesity increases gene expression of markers associated with immunosenescence in obese middle-aged individuals. *Front Immunol*. 2022;12:806400.

Buresh R, et al. Steps expressed relative to body fat mass predicts body composition and cardiometabolic risk in adults eating ad libitum. *J Sports Med Phys Fitness*. 2022;62:65.

Chen CC, et al. Corylin reduces obesity and insulin resistance and promotes adipose tissue browning through SIRT-1 and β3-AR activation. *Pharmacol Res*. 2021;164:105291.

Cichosz SL, et al. Body Composition Prediction-BOMP: a new tool for assessing fat and lean body mass. *J Diabetes Sci Technol*. 2022:19322968221076560.

Cicone ZS, et al. Generalized equations for predicting percent body fat from anthropometric measures using a criterion five-compartment model. *Med Sci Sports Exerc*. 2021;53:2675.

de Cuevillas B, et al. Fecal microbiota relationships with childhood obesity: a scoping comprehensive review. *Obes Rev*. 2022;23:e13394.

de Lara Perez B, Delgado-Rios M. Mindfulness-based programs for the prevention of childhood obesity: a systematic review. *Appetite*. 2022;168:105725.

Desdentado L, et al. Are peripheral biomarkers determinants of eating styles in childhood and adolescence obesity? A cross-sectional study. *Nutrients*. 2022;14:305.

Dunne A, et al. Body composition and bone health status of jockeys: current findings, assessment methods and classification criteria. *Sports Med Open*. 2022;8:23.

Dupuit M, et al. Effect of concurrent training on body composition and gut microbiota in postmenopausal women with overweight or obesity. *Med Sci Sports Exerc*. 2022;54:517.

Ehtesham N, et al. Modulations of obesity-related microRNAs after exercise intervention: a systematic review and bioinformatics analysis. *Mol Biol Rep*. 2021;48:2817.

Fan Z, et al. Body fat prediction through feature extraction based on anthropometric and laboratory measurements. *PLoS One*. 2022;17:e0263333.

Gaspar RC, et al. An update on brown adipose tissue biology: a discussion of recent findings. *Am J Physiol Endocrinol Metab*. 2021;320:E488.

Gutiérrez-Cuevas J, et al. Molecular mechanisms of obesity-linked cardiac dysfunction: an up-date on current knowledge. *Cells*. 2021;10:629.

Headid Iii RJ, Park SY. The impacts of exercise on pediatric obesity. *Clin Exp Pediatr*. 2021;64:196.

Hendrie GA, et al. Weight loss and usage of an online commercial weight loss program (the CSIRO Total Wellbeing Diet Online) delivered in an everyday context: five-year evaluation in a community cohort. *J Med Internet Res*. 2021;23:e20981.

Huebner M, Perperoglou A. Sex differences and impact of body mass on performance from childhood to senior athletes in Olympic weightlifting. *PLoS One*. 2020;15:e0238369.

Izquierdo AG, et al. Weight loss normalizes enhanced expression of the oncogene survivin in visceral adipose tissue and blood leukocytes from individuals with obesity. *Int J Obes (Lond)*. 2021;45:206.

Khoshnaw DM, Ghadge AA. Yoga as a complementary therapy for metabolic syndrome: a narrative review. *J Integr Med*. 2021;19:6.

Kotarsky CJ, et al. Time-restricted eating and concurrent exercise training reduces fat mass and increases lean mass in overweight and obese adults. *Physiol Rep*. 2021;9:e14868.

Lagou V, et al. Meta-analyses of glucose and insulin-related traits consortium (MAGIC). Sex-dimorphic genetic effects and novel loci for fasting glucose and insulin variability. *Nat Commun*. 2021;12:24.

Lee CK, et al. The relationship between body composition and physical fitness and the effect of exercise according to the level of childhood obesity using the MGPA model. *Int J Environ Res Public Health*. 2022;1:487.

Lee Y, Shin S. The effect of body composition on gait variability varies with age: interaction by hierarchical moderated regression analysis. *Int J Environ Res Public Health*. 2022;19:1171.

Li JB, et al. Adults who were overweight or obese: a population-based cohort study. *Obes Facts*. 2021;14:108.

Nana A, et al. Agreement of anthropometric and body composition measures predicted from 2D smartphone images and body impedance scales with criterion methods. *Obes Res Clin Pract*. 2022;16:37.

Ravelli MN, Schoeller DA. An objective measure of energy intake using the principle of energy balance. *Int J Obes (Lond)*. 2021;45:725.

Romanello V, Sandri M. The connection between the dynamic remodeling of the mitochondrial network and the regulation of muscle mass. *Cell Mol Life Sci*. 2021;78:1305.

Santos AL, Sinha S. Obesity and aging: molecular mechanisms and therapeutic approaches. *Ageing Res Rev*. 2021;67:101268.

Sárvári AK, et al. Plasticity of epididymal adipose tissue in response to diet-induced obesity at single-nucleus resolution. *Cell Metab*. 2021;33:437.

Siu PM, et al. Effects of Tai Chi or conventional exercise on central obesity in middle-aged and older adults: a three-group randomized controlled trial. *Ann Intern Med*. 2021;174:1050.

Stefan N, et al. Global pandemics interconnected—obesity, impaired metabolic health and COVID-19. *Nat Rev Endocrinol*. 2021;17:135.

Straight CR, et al. Current perspectives on obesity and skeletal muscle contractile function in older adults. *J Appl Physiol (1985)*. 2021;130:10.

Templeman I, et al. A randomized controlled trial to isolate the effects of fasting and energy restriction on weight loss and metabolic health in lean adults. *Sci Transl Med*. 2021;13:eabd8034.

Tirosh A, et al. Intercellular transmission of hepatic ER stress in obesity disrupts systemic metabolism. *Cell Metab*. 2021;33:319.

Tur JA, Martinez JA. Guide and advances on childhood obesity determinants: setting the research agenda. *Obes Rev*. 2022;23:e13379.

Vargas-Molina S, et al. Effects of a low-carbohydrate ketogenic diet on health parameters in resistance-trained women. *Eur J Appl Physiol*. 2021;121:2349.

Vliora M, et al. Irisin regulates thermogenesis and lipolysis in 3T3-L1 adipocytes. *Biochim Biophys Acta Gen Subj*. 2022;1866:130085.

Warner ET, et al. Genome-wide association study of childhood body fatness. *Obesity (Silver Spring)*. 2021;29:446.

Waseem R, et al. FNDC5/Irisin: physiology and pathophysiology. *Molecules*. 2022;27:1118.

Whiting S, et al. Physical activity, screen time, and sleep duration of children aged 6–9 years in 25 countries: an analysis within the who European childhood obesity surveillance initiative (COSI) 2015–2017. *Obes Facts*. 2021;14:32.

Wu T, et al. Urban sprawl and childhood obesity. *Obes Rev*. 2021;22:e13091.

Yarizadeh H, et al. The effect of aerobic and resistance training and combined exercise modalities on subcutaneous abdominal fat: a systematic review and meta-analysis of randomized clinical trials. *Adv Nutr*. 2021;12:179.

Zhang H, et al. Exercise training-induced visceral fat loss in obese women: the role of training intensity and modality. *Scand J Med Sci Sports*. 2021;31:30.

Table 30.1 Daily 90-min Walking Sessions for 16 wk Alters Body Mass, Body Fat, HDL Cholesterol Concentration, and HDL-to-LDL Ratio

Variable	Pretraining[a]	Posttraining[a]	Difference
Body mass (kg)	99.1	93.4	−5.7[b]
Body density (g · mL^{-1})	1.044	1.056	+0.012[b]
Body fat (%)	23.5	18.6	−4.9[b]
Fat mass (kg)	23.3	17.4	−5.9[b]
Fat-free body mass (kg)	75.8	76.0	+0.2
Sum of skinfolds (mm)	142.9	104.8	−38.1[b]
HDL cholesterol (mg · dL^{-1})	32	37	5.0[b]
HDL/LDL cholesterol	0.27	0.34	+0.07[b]

[a]Values are means.
[b]Statistically significant.
HDL, high-density lipoprotein; LDL, low-density lipoprotein.
Reprinted with permission from Leon AS, et al. Effects of a vigorous walking program on body composition, and carbohydrate and lipid metabolism of obese young men. *Am J Clin Nutr*. 1979;33:1776. With permission from the American Society for Nutrition, https://nutrition.org/.

Table 30.2 Effects on Body Composition of Either Endurance or Resistance Training

Variable	Controls		Resistance Trained		Endurance Trained	
	Pretreatment	Posttreatment	Pretreatment	Posttreatment	Pretreatment	Posttreatment
Relative body fat (%)	20.1 ± 8.5	20.2 ± 8.5	21.8 ± 6.2	18.7 ± 6.6[a]	18.4 ± 7.9	16.5 ± 6.4[a]
Fat mass (kg)	16.2 ± 10.8	16.3 ± 10.5	17.2 ± 7.6	14.8 ± 6.2[a]	14.4 ± 7.9	12.8 ± 7.1[a]
Fat-free body mass (kg)	64.3 ± 5.4	64.4 ± 6.6	61.9 ± 8.3	64.4 ± 9.0[a]	64.1 ± 8.2	64.7 ± 8.6
Total body mass (kg)	80.5 ± 8.1	80.7 ± 8.5	79.4 ± 8.3	79.2 ± 7.6	78.5 ± 8.2	77.5 ± 7.9

[a]Significant difference between pretest and posttest measurements ($p < .05$).
All values means ± SD.
Reprinted with permission from Broeder CE, et al. Assessing body composition before and after resistance or endurance training. *Med Sci Sports Exerc*. 1997;29:705.

Table 30.3 How Training Duration by Walking and Running for 5 Months Impacts Body Composition								
	\multicolumn{8}{c}{Training Group}
	Control (n = 16)		15-min (n = 14)		30-min (n = 17)		45-min (n = 12)	
Variable	Pre	Post	Pre	Post	Pre	Post	Pre	Post
Body mass (kg)	72.1	73.2	76.9	76.3	80.6	78.9	70.9	69.9
Body fat (%)	12.5	13.0	13.7	13.2	14.2	13.6	13.2	12.0
Sum skinfolds (mm)	73.8	79.6	83.0	77.0	90.0	83.8	77.5	67.0
Waist girth (cm)	82.7	84.9	84.3	82.8	88.2	86.1	83.6	81.8
Distance covered per workout (mi)			Week 4		1.56		2.89	4.13
			8		1.54		2.95	4.46
			13		1.79		3.19	4.82
			17		1.75		3.24	5.06
Total time of exercise (min:s)			Week 4		14:58		30:25	41:18
			8		14:11		28:40	42:48
			13		15:51		29:43	43:19
			17		14:53		30:12	42:27
Training heart rate (b·min^{-1})			Week 4		179		175	174
			8		179		174	169
			13		182		175	177
			17		180		175	175
Intensity (%max HR)			Week 4		89.4		83.8	84.5
			8		89.8		73.4	81.0
			13		94.0		90.1	89.5
			17		92.5		90.2	88.1

%max HR, percent of maximum heart rate.
Reprinted with permission from Milesis CA, et al. Effects of different durations of physical training on cardiorespiratory function, body composition, and serum lipids. *Res Q*. 1976;47:716. Copyright © Cardiovascular Research Foundation, http://www.crf.org/, reprinted by permission of Taylor & Francis Ltd, http://www.tandfonline.com on behalf of Cardiovascular Research Foundation, http://www.crf.org/

Table 30.4 Benefits of Adding Physical Activity to a Weight-Loss Program

- Increases overall size of the energy deficit
- Facilitates lipid mobilization and oxidation, especially from visceral adipose tissue depots
- Increases relative body fat loss by preserving fat-free body mass
- Blunts the drop in resting metabolism that accompanies weight loss by conserving and even increasing fat-free body mass
- Requires less reliance on caloric restriction to create an energy deficit
- Contributes to long-term success of the weight-loss effort
- Provides significant health-related benefits
- Offsets the deterioration in immune system function that often accompanies weight loss

Table 30.5 — Examples of Anthropometric Equations to Predict a Minimal Wrestling Weight and to Select a Competitive Weight Class

A. To predict body density (BD), use one of the following equations. (For each skinfold, record the average of at least three trials in mm.)
   1. Lohman equation[a]
      BD = 1.0982 − (0.00815 × [triceps + subscapular + abdominal skinfolds])
      + (0.00000084 × [triceps + subscapular + abdominal skinfolds]^2)
   2. Katch and McArdle equation[b]
      BD = 1.09448 − (0.00103 × triceps skinfold) − (0.00056 × subscapular skinfold) − (0.00054 × abdominal skinfold)
   3. Behnke and Wilmore equation[c]
      BD = 1.05721 − (0.00052 × abdominal skinfold) + (0.00168 × iliac diameter) + (0.00114 × neck circumference)
      + (0.00048 × chest circumference) + (0.00145 × abdominal circumference)
   4. Thorland equation[d]
      BD = 1.0982 − (0.000815 × [triceps + abdominal skinfolds])^2 + (0.00000084 × [triceps + abdominal skinfolds])

B. To determine fat percentage, use the Brožek equation:
% Fat = [4.570 + BD − 4.142] × 100

C. To determine fat-free weight and to identify a minimum weight class, follow the examples below:
   5. Fifteen-year-old wrestler who weighs 132 lb has a body density of 1.075 g·cc^{-1} and hopes to compete in the 119-lb weight class.
   6. Percentage fat is (4.570 + 1.075 − 4.142) × 100 = 10.9%
   7. Fat weight and fat-free weight are:
      a. 132.0 lb × 0.109 = 14.4 lb fat
      b. 132.0 lb − 14.4 lb fat = 117.6 lb fat-free weight

D. To calculate a minimal wrestling weight:
   8. Realize that the recommended minimum body weight for those 15-y and younger contains 93% (0.93) fat-free weight and 7% fat (0.07)
   9. Divide the wrestler's calculated fat-free weight by the greatest allowable fraction of fat-free weight to estimate minimal wrestling weight: 117.6 ÷ (93/100) = 117.6 ÷ 0.93 = 126.5 lb

E. To allow for a 2% error, perform the following calculations:
   10. 126.5 minimal weight × 0.02 = 2.5 lb error allowance
   11. 126.5 lb − 2.5 lb = 124.0 lb minimum wrestling weight

F. Conclusion: This wrestler cannot compete in the 119-lb weight class; instead, he must compete in the 125-lb class.

[a]Lohman TG. Skinfolds and body density and their relationship to body frames: a review. *Hum Biol.* 1981;53:181.
[b]Katch FI, McArdle WD. Prediction of body density from simple anthropometric measurements in college-age men and women. *Hum Biol.* 1973;l45:445.
[c]Behnke AR, Wilmore JH. *Evaluation and Regulation of Body Build and Composition.* Englewood Cliffs: Prentice Hall; 1974.
[d]Thorland W, et al. New equations for prediction of a minimal weight in high school wrestlers. *Med Sci Sports Exerc.* 1989;21:S72.

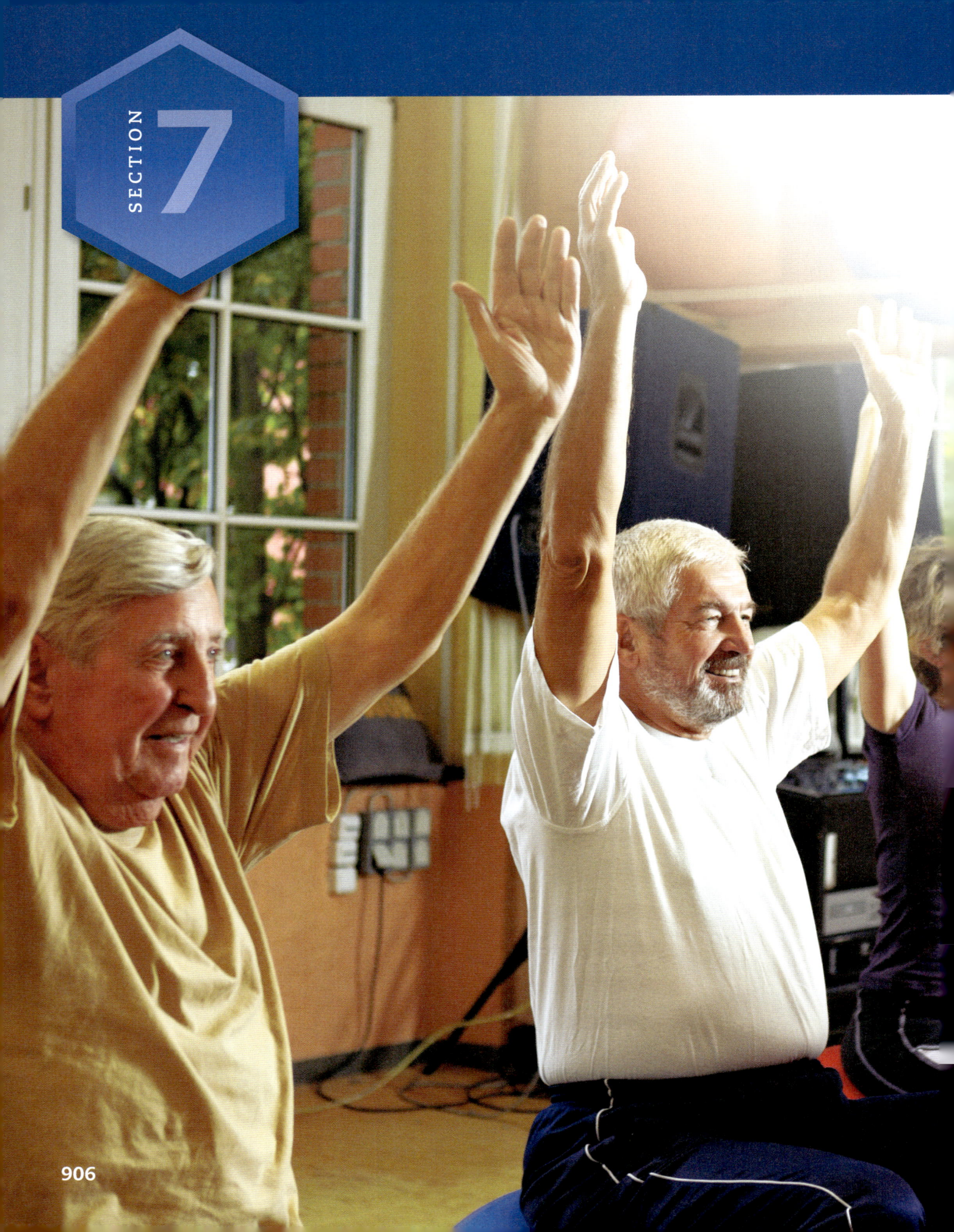

SECTION 7

Exercise, Successful Aging, and Disease Prevention

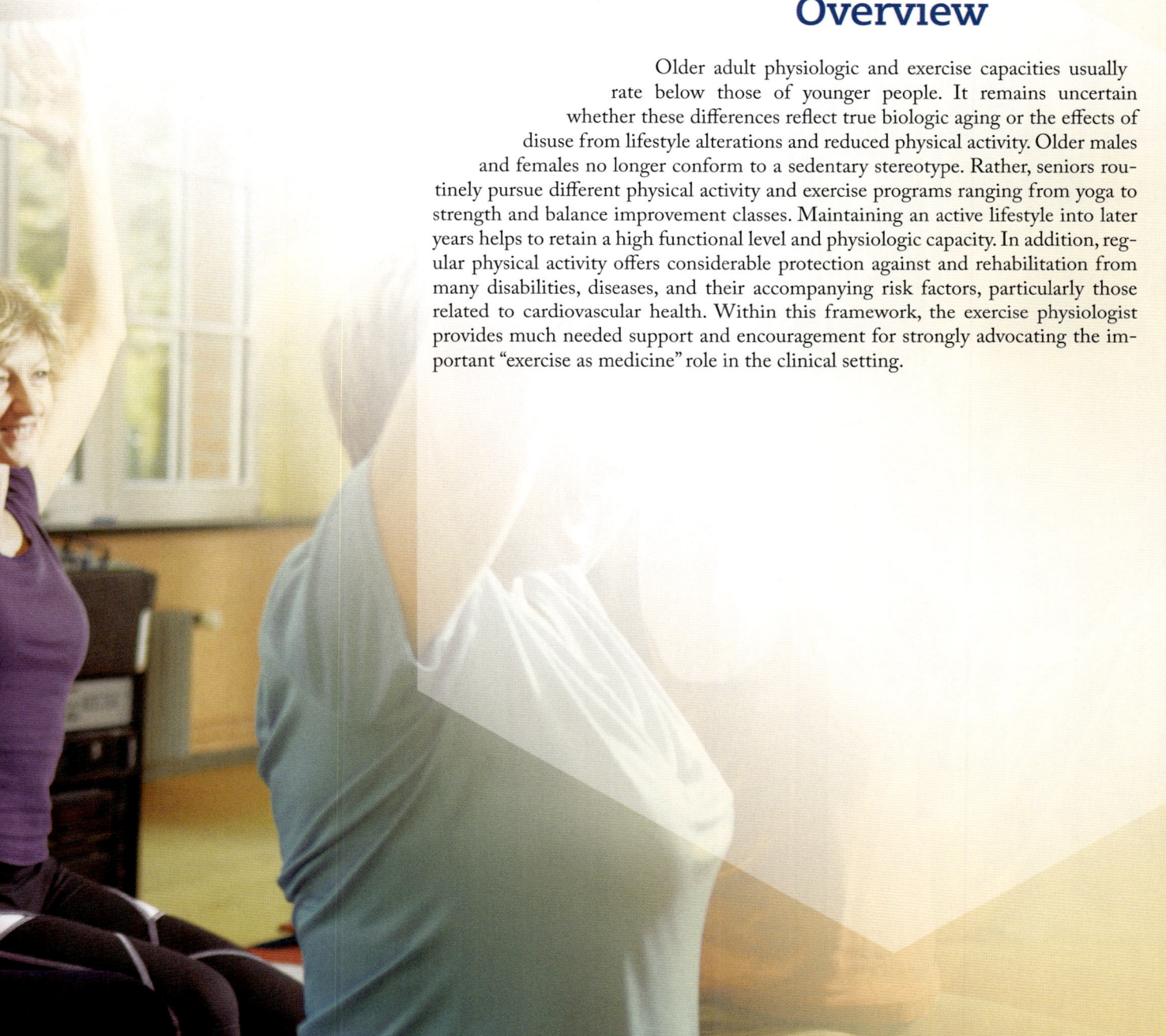

Overview

Older adult physiologic and exercise capacities usually rate below those of younger people. It remains uncertain whether these differences reflect true biologic aging or the effects of disuse from lifestyle alterations and reduced physical activity. Older males and females no longer conform to a sedentary stereotype. Rather, seniors routinely pursue different physical activity and exercise programs ranging from yoga to strength and balance improvement classes. Maintaining an active lifestyle into later years helps to retain a high functional level and physiologic capacity. In addition, regular physical activity offers considerable protection against and rehabilitation from many disabilities, diseases, and their accompanying risk factors, particularly those related to cardiovascular health. Within this framework, the exercise physiologist provides much needed support and encouragement for strongly advocating the important "exercise as medicine" role in the clinical setting.

CHAPTER 31
Physical Activity, Health, and Aging

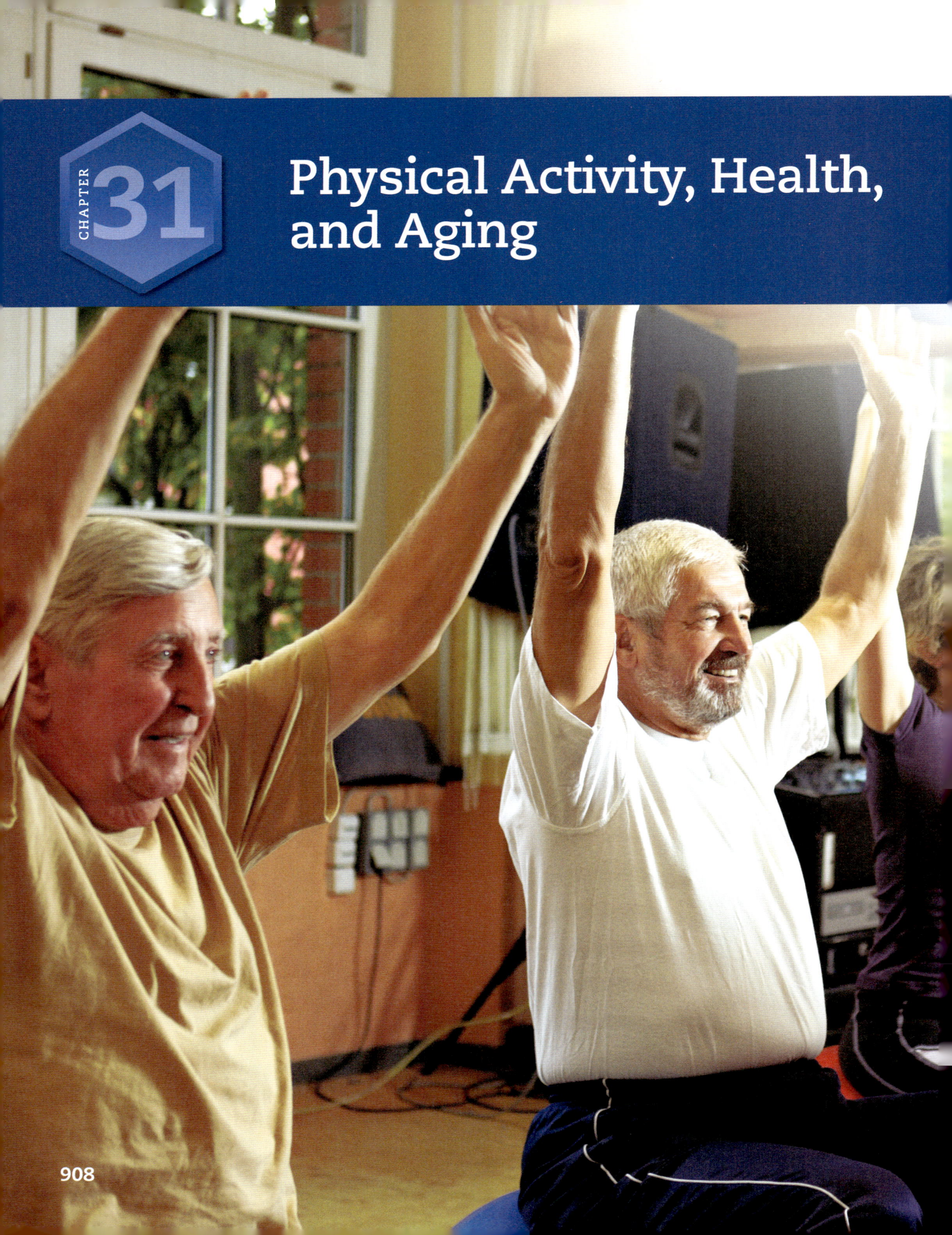

Chapter Objectives

- Summarize aging trends in the American population
- Describe physical activity levels for the typical adult American male and female
- Discuss the latest physical activity participation rates for Americans
- Answer the question: How safe is exercise?
- List factors that increase the likelihood of experiencing an exercise catastrophe
- Contrast children and adults' physiologic responses to physical activity and their implications for evaluating physiologic function and exercise performance
- List important age-related changes in the muscular, nervous, cardiovascular, and pulmonary system functions and body composition components
- Summarize the potential benefits of moderate resistance training for older adults
- Discuss the following statement: "A sedentary lifestyle causes losses in functional capacity at least as great as the effects of aging itself"
- Describe research about the role of regular physical activity in coronary heart disease prevention and life extension
- Indicate the types and levels of physical activity that induce the greatest improvement in the risk factor profile and overall health
- Describe vulnerable plaque and its proposed role in sudden death
- List the five major modifiable heart disease risk factors and how regular physical activity impacts each
- Outline the normal dynamics of homocysteine, its proposed role in coronary heart disease, and factors that affect plasma levels
- Discuss heart disease risk prevalence in children

Ancillaries at-a-Glance

Visit Lippincott Connect to access these following resources.

- References: Chapter 31
- Animation: Acute Inflammation
- Focus on Research: Physical Inactivity: A Significant Coronary Heart Disease Risk

The Graying of America

Older adults—those age 85 and older—make up the fastest growing segment of American society. Forty years ago, age 65 represented the onset of old age. **Gerontologists** now consider 85 the demarcation between "**oldest-old**" and age 75, "**young-old**." Based on 2019 statistics (www.census.gov/library/stories/2018/03/graying-america.html), nearly 15.2% of the country's population, or 49.2 million U.S. citizens, exceed age 65. From 2015 onward, the rate of increase in the population 65+ years is increasing about twice the rate as the total U.S. population, and this trend is projected to continue unabated. While the number of middle-age adults now outnumber children, the United States will reach a new milestone in 2034 where the U.S. Census Bureau projects that older adults will edge out children in population size. People age 65 and older are expected to number 77.0 million while children under age 18 will number a projected 76.5 million.

For perspective, Japan has the world's oldest population, where more than one in four people are at least 65 years old. Already, its total population has started to decline and, by 2050, it is projected to shrink by 20 million. Europe appears headed down the same aging path with some western European countries having populations older than the United States. Within 5 years, many of these populations are projected to shrink.

The image below from the U.S. Census Bureau (www.census.gov/content/dam/Census/library/stories/2018/03/graying-america-aging-nation.jpg) shows the projected number of U.S. children and older adults from 2016 through 2060.

No longer viewed as a quirk of nature, 2 in every 10,000 Americans now live to age 100, and by the middle of this century, more than 800,000 Americans will exceed age 100 with many maintaining relatively good **health**. Disease prevention, water purification and better sanitation, improved nutrition and healthcare, and more effective treatment of age-related heart disease and osteoporosis help people to live longer.

Physical inactivity relates causally to nearly 30% of all deaths from heart disease, colon cancer, and diabetes. Lifestyle changes could reduce mortality from these ailments and greatly improve cardiovascular and functional capacities, quality of life, and independent living.[34,85,89,174,201] Research confirms that aerobic and resistance training are important for maintaining cognitive and brain health in old age, an effect produced, in part, by vascular-mediated mechanisms related to increases in brain perfusion and the ability of cerebral blood vessels to respond to blood flow demands.[49,129,143,233] The equivalent of a daily brisk 30-min walk associates with a lower risk of cognitive impairment—as physical activity levels increase, the rate of cognitive decline decreases.[228] The greatest health benefits come from strategies that promote regular physical activity throughout one's lifetime.[2,3,77,148]

At any age, behavioral changes—becoming more physically active, quitting cigarette smoking, and controlling body weight and blood pressure—act independently to delay all-cause mortality and aging effects caused by diseases and environmental factors.[31,164,193] Individuals with more healthful lifestyles survive longer, and the risk of disability and the necessity to seek home healthcare is postponed and compressed into fewer years at life's end.[230,231]

The New Gerontology

Gerontologists maintain that research on older adults should focus on improving "**healthspan**," or the total years a person remains in excellent health, not simply increased lifespan. Healthspan addresses areas beyond age-related diseases and prevention to recognize that *successful aging* requires maintaining enhanced physiologic function and physical fitness.[249,251] *Vitality, not just longevity per se, remains the primary goal.* Researchers now view much of the physiologic deterioration previously considered "normal aging" as dependent on lifestyle and environmental influences subject to considerable modification with proper diet and regular physical activity.[35,61] For those who achieve older age, low muscular strength, diminished cardiovascular function, poor joint range of motion, and sleep disturbances, relate directly to functional limitations, independent from disease status.[94,144,189,246–248]

Successful aging includes four main components:

1. Physical health
2. Spirituality
3. Emotional and educational health
4. Social satisfaction

Maintaining and even enhancing physical and cognitive functions, fully engaging in life, and participating in productive activities and interpersonal relations contribute to achieving these goals.

Aging Science

The concept of successful aging as part of aging-science research is not new.[246,250] A Web search of the term "successful aging" produced more than 301 million entries (*Google*—March 22, 2022). Beginning in the 1950s and 1960s, gerontology and developmental science researchers began advancing the concept of "satisfaction with life" during the aging process as a metric to measure successful aging.[252–254]

Currently six models describe successful aging.

1. **Maintaining subjective well-being during aging**: This model uses individual *subjective* estimates, as opposed to *objective* health and well-being conditions. Subjective health has been shown to develop differently from objective health conditions. Whereas objective loss in functional capacity and any existing clinical manifestations clearly increase with age, subjective health evaluations remain stable over time.[255]

2. **Successful aging as achievement of objective criteria**: This model relies on objectively measurable criteria for successful aging, not subjective interpretations and evaluations of the quality of the aging process and its outcomes. The objective successful-aging criteria include (1) low probability of illness and related disability, (2) high level of cognitive and physical functioning, and (3) active engagement with life. This model claims that achieving these three criteria as fully as possible allows for the best life possible in the later period of the lifespan.[256,257]

3. **Successful aging as fulfilment of fundamental norms/values leads to a good life**: This model assumes that qualifying individuals as successfully aging requires reference to normatively framed ideal states or value judgments based on an agreed-upon index termed the "good life." Successful aging includes six dimensions:

   1. Self-acceptance
   2. Autonomy
   3. Personal growth
   4. Purpose in life
   5. Environment mastery
   6. Positive relationships

   The World Health Organization (WHO) has adopted this model to reflect the construct for "healthy aging," and the long-time established construct health-related quality of life (www.ncbi.nlm.nih.gov/pmc/articles/PMC6776218/).

4. **Successful aging incorporates efficient adaptation strategies**: This model states that three core processes needed to be coordinated throughout life to achieve the best possible gain-loss balance and optimal age adaptation. Aging optimization requires the reciprocal and dynamic interplay of selection and compensation among social, psychological, and physical domains.[258]

5. **Successful aging is what older adults themselves value important in their life**: This model relies on research of how people view their own aging processes. For most individuals, successful aging encompasses good health and diverse physical activities, social relations, finances and psychological resources, and attitudes and life-management skills.[259]

6. **Successful aging as slowing or abandoning biological aging**: The model argues that it may be more effective to proceed in a slower and more general manner and change the biological aging process *per se* by reducing the speed of aging and prolonging an individual's healthy lifespan. This research centers on efforts in biogerontological research that include antiaging drugs, caloric reduction, or transmitting blood from younger mammals into older counterparts.[260]

Chronological Versus Biological Age

The observation that individuals do not all age at the same rate introduces the **biological aging** concept, also called functional or physiological aging.[261,262] Whereas chronological aging refers only to the passage of time, biological aging relates to decline in function and increase in disease over time. Increased **longevity** (chronological aging) represents the main risk factor for vascular disease and the ensuing cardiovascular and cerebrovascular events, the leading causes of death worldwide (www.cdc.gov/nchs/fastats/death.htm). Vascular aging entails arterial degeneration and hardening that impairs vascular function and ultimately causes end-organ damage, predominantly of the heart, brain, and kidneys (refer to Chapter 32). Age-dependent arterial injury typically manifests clinically after the fifth or sixth decade of life, but with high inter-individual variability and associated mortality. For example, at one extreme are individuals aged 50 or older with vascular disease (diagnosed and undiagnosed); at the other extreme are centenarians/supercentenarians with no expression of vascular disease.

The image below illustrates the biological versus chronological aging relationships for individuals with dif-

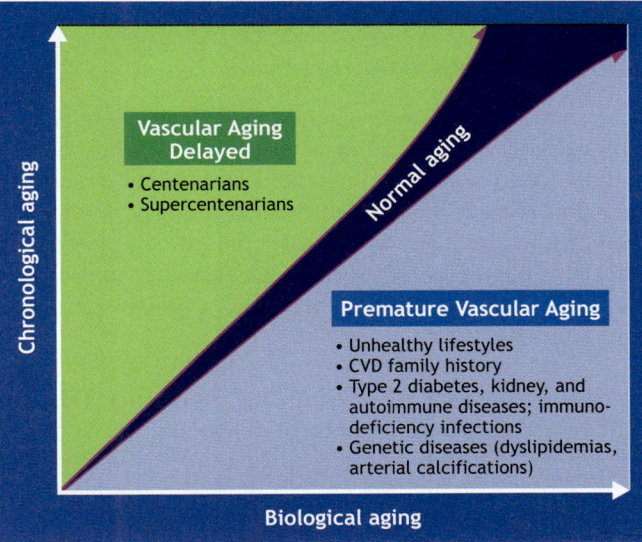

fering levels of **delayed vascular aging** (centenarians and supercentenarians with no disease) versus those with **premature vascular aging** (individuals with disease, genetic and acquired).

Biological-Vascular Aging Biomarkers

Biomarkers that reflect the state of vascular aging (termed biological aging) include the following molecular/cellular and functional/structural variables[64,263]:

Molecular/Cellular Biological Aging Markers

- Telomere length DNA methylation (DNAm) age (age based on DNA methylation levels measured from a DNA source such as a tissue sample)
- Somatic mutations
- Inflammatory variables (e.g., interleukin 6, C-reactive protein)
- Insulin-like growth factor 1 (IGF-1), growth hormone (GH), low-density lipoprotein-cholesterol
- Transcriptomic-based biomarker
- Proteomic-based biomarkers
- Metabolomics-based biomarkers
- Gut dysbiosis

Functional/Structural Biological Aging Markers

- Arterial wall stiffness
- Elevated blood pressure
- Endothelial dysfunction
- Arterial intima-media thickness
- Atherosclerosis
- Coronary artery calcification

Ideal biological-age biomarkers should correlate with chronological age yet outperform the latter as a major determinant for age-related morbidity and mortality. One advantage of biological age markers is that individuals of the same chronological age could possess different risks for age-associated diseases not revealed by chronological age separately.

Healthy Life Expectancy

The Centers for Disease Control and Prevention (CDC; www.cdc.gov) report that about one third of people age 65 or older report functional limitations of one kind or another; among people age 85 or older, about two thirds report functional limitations. Current estimates indicate that more than two thirds of 65 year olds will require assistance to deal with functional losses at some point as they age (www.cbo.gov/publication/44363).[264]

To estimate healthful longevity, the WHO has introduced the concept of **healthy life expectancy (HALE, HLE)**—the expected number of remaining years of life spent in good health from a particular age (typically birth or 65 years), assuming the rates of mortality and morbidity remain unchanged. These data are often expressed by gender and race.

In essence, HALE combines country or world mortality and morbidity data to estimate the expected years of life in good health for the average person in that area. The WHO began compiling these data into tables in 1999 using estimates of patterns and trends in all-cause and cause-specific mortality. Working in conjunction with the United Nations Population Division, the WHO releases updated HALE tables for its 180-plus member-states about every 2 years or so. Individual countries often break down HALE into regions, states, and communities.[265]

HALE Around the World

Recent HALE data indicate that global average HALE for someone age 60 was 75.8 years in 2016 (males: 74.8 years; females: 76.8 years). Regionally, people living in North, South, and Central America have the longest HALE at 77.6 years, whereas those living in Africa have the shortest expectancy at 72.5 years.[266,267]

The table below presents the latest HALE data, in years, by global region. In the United States, the average life expectancy is 84.1 years and the average HALE equals 78.9 years. On average, females live 2.6 years longer than males (85.3 vs. 82.7 years) and enjoy good health for about 2 years longer (79.8 vs. 77.9 years). Race and levels of poverty also contribute to decreased healthy longevity; Native Americans, rural African Americans, and inner-city poor experience health characteristics similar to those living in underdeveloped countries. Whites live an average of 84.2 years, 79.3 years of which represent good health; Blacks live an average of 83.1 years, but only 76.1 years in good health. The HIV/AIDS epidemic, tobacco-related diseases, violent deaths, lack of adequate and affordable healthcare, and prevalence of coronary heart disease all contribute to the U.S.'s lower overall health ranking among industrialized nations.

HALE by Global Region (y)

Region	All	Males	Females
Americas	77.6	76.4	78.7
Europe	77.4	75.9	78.7
Western Pacific	76.6	75.6	77.6
Eastern Mediterranean	73.3	73.0	73.6
South-East Asia	73.3	72.7	73.9
Africa	72.5	72.0	73.0

From: www.who.int/gho/mortality_burden_disease/life_tables/hale_text/en/

Background photo: ixpert/Shutterstock

Marital Status Positively Influences Total Life Expectancy

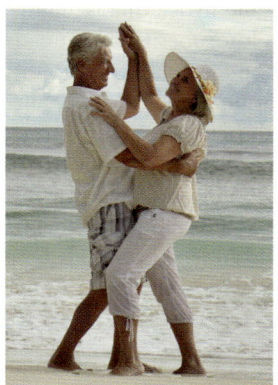
Ruslan Huzau/Shutterstock

Estimated total life expectancy (TLE) and active life expectancy (ALE) for 164,597 U.S. community-dwelling respondents aged ≥65 years at baseline and 2 years later were determined by marital status. Between ages 65 and 85, married males and females had a longer TLE and ALE than those who were unmarried. At 65 years, TLE for married males was 18.6 years, 2.2 years longer than unmarried males, and ALE for married males was 12.3 years, 2.4 years longer than unmarried males. Similarly, at 65 years, TLE for married females averaged 21.1 years, 1.5 years longer than unmarried females, and ALE for married females was 13.0 years, 2.0 years longer than unmarried females. Unmarried and never-married persons had the shortest TLE and ALE among males, and never-married, divorced, and widowed persons had a similar and shorter TLE and ALE among females. Marriage's protective effect is significant considering TLE and ALE, with protection greater in younger individuals.

Source:
Jia H, Lubetkin EI. Life expectancy and active life expectancy by marital status among older U.S. adults: results from the U.S. Medicare Health Outcome Survey (HOS). *SSM Popul Health*. 2020;12:100642.

Part 1: Physical Activity in the Population

Physical Activity Epidemiology

Epidemiology involves quantifying factors that influence the occurrence of illness to better understand, modify, and/or control a disease pattern in the general population. **Physical activity epidemiology** applies the general research strategies from epidemiology to study physical activity as a health-related behavior linked mainly to disease.

Physical Activity Terminology

Physical activity epidemiology applies specific definitions to characterize group behavioral patterns and outcomes under investigation. Relevant terminology includes the following:

- **Physical activity**: Body movement produced by muscle action that increases energy expenditure
- **Exercise**: Planned, structured, repetitive, and purposeful physical activity
- **Physical fitness**: Attributes related to how well one performs physical activity
- **Health**: Physical, mental, and social well-being, not simply disease absence
- **Health-related physical fitness**: Physical fitness components associated with good health and/or disease prevention
- **Longevity**: Length of life

Within this framework, *physical activity* becomes a generic term, with *exercise* its major component. Similarly, the definition of *health* focuses on the broad spectrum of well-being that ranges from complete absence of health (near death) to the highest levels of physiologic function. Such definitions often challenge how we objectively measure and quantify health and physical activity. They provide a broad perspective to study the role of physical activity in health and disease.

The trend in physical fitness assessment during the past 50 years deemphasizes tests that stress motor performance and athletic fitness (i.e., speed, power, balance, and agility). Instead, assessments now focus on functional capacities related to overall health and disease prevention. The four most common components of health-related physical fitness are aerobic and/or cardiovascular fitness, body composition, abdominal muscular strength and endurance, and lower-back and hamstring flexibility (see **FIGURE 31.1** and In a Practical Sense in this chapter).

Physical Activity Participation

More than 30 different methods have been used to assess physical activity. They include direct and indirect calorimetry, self-reports and questionnaires, job classifications, physiologic markers, behavioral observations, mechanical or electronic monitors, and activity surveys. Each approach offers unique advantages but also has disadvantages depending on the situation and population studied. Obtaining valid physical activity estimates in large groups is difficult because such studies, by necessity, apply self-reports of daily activity and exercise participation rather than direct monitoring or objective measurement. Efforts to develop tools to study physical activity behavior have produced insights about the positive role physical activity plays in promoting healthful outcomes.

FIGURE 31.1. Health-related physical fitness components.

Sedentary Behaviors

A new research area that complements and adds insights to understanding physical activity participation centers on **sedentary behavior physiology**—the flip side of physical activity physiology—a discipline that determines links between excessive sedentary behavior and adverse health-related indicators or outcomes primarily linked to cardiovascular morbidity and mortality.[268–272]

FIGURE 31.2 illustrates a conceptual model of movement-based terminology arranged around a 24-hr period, which forms the basis for studying sedentary behaviors. The figure organizes the movements that take place throughout the day into two components.[268] The inner ring represents the main behavior categories using energy expenditure as the defining variable, whereas the outer ring provides general categories using posture as the defining variable. (Note: the proportion of space occupied by each behavior in Figure 31.2 is *not* prescriptive about the time that should be devoted to these behaviors each day.)

Sedentary Environmental Death Syndrome

A review of the world literature over the last 50 years concludes that inactivity alone results in a constellation of problems and conditions eventually leading to premature death.[270,273–277]

The term **sedentary environmental death syndrome (SeDS)**, coined by Frank W. Booth, Professor of Biomedical Sciences at the University of Missouri, Columbia, aptly identifies this deteriorating condition.[30] Research evidence reveals the following about SeDS:

- SeDS will cause approximately 2.5 million Americans to die prematurely in the next decade.
- SeDS will cost $2 to $3 trillion in healthcare expenses in the United States in the next decade.
- Chronic diseases have increased because of physical inactivity. In the United States, type 2 diabetes has increased ninefold since 1958, obesity has doubled since 1980, and heart disease remains the number-one cause of death.
- U.S. children are now contracting SeDS-related diseases—they are increasingly overweight, showing fatty streaks in their arteries, and developing type 2 diabetes (a disease formerly restricted to adults).
- SeDS relates to the following conditions: high blood triacylglycerol, high blood cholesterol, high blood glucose, type 2 diabetes, hypertension, myocardial ischemia, arrhythmias, congestive heart failure, obesity, breast cancer, depression, chronic back pain, spinal cord injury, stroke, disease cachexia, debilitating illnesses, fall resulting in broken hips, and vertebral/femoral fractures.
- Efforts to lessen time watching television or videos or using a computer, if coupled with increases in physical activity above daily routines, could substantially decrease the prevalence of metabolic syndrome. Individuals who do not engage in any moderate or vigorous physical activity during leisure time have about twice the odds of having metabolic syndrome as those who exercise up to 150 min a week or more.

U.S. Adult Population: Physical Activity and Inactivity

The latest statistics on physical activity and inactivity participation of Americans (www.cdc.gov/physicalactivity/data/inactivity-prevalence-maps/) can be summarized as follows:

- Only about 15% of the population engages in vigorous physical activity during leisure time three times weekly for at least 30 min.
- More than 60% *do not* engage in physical activity regularly.
- Twenty-five percent lead sedentary lives (i.e., little or no exercise).
- Walking, gardening, and yard work are the most popular leisure-time activities.
- Twenty-two percent engage in light-to-moderate physical activity regularly during leisure time (five times weekly for ≥30 min).
- Physical inactivity occurs among females more than males, Blacks and Hispanics more than Whites, older more than younger adults, and less-affluent more than wealthier persons.

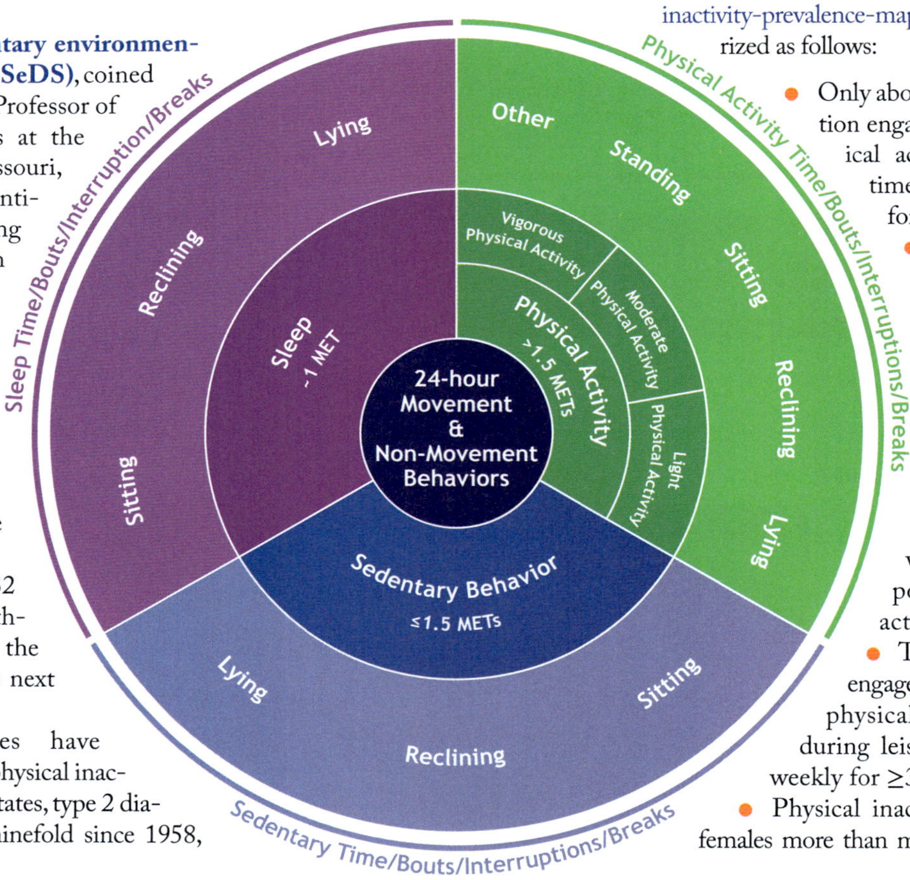

FIGURE 31.2. Conceptual model of movement-based terminology arranged around a 24-hr period. Inner ring represents the main behavior categories using energy expenditure. The outer ring provides general categories related to posture.
(Adapted with permission from Tremblay MS, et al. Sedentary behavior research network (SBRN)–Terminology consensus project process and outcome. *Int J Behav Nutr and Phys Act.* 2017;14:75. www.researchgate.net/publication/318460410_Sedentary_Behavior_Research_Network_SBRN_-_Terminology_Consensus_Project_process_and_outcome)

- Participation in fitness activities declines with age; a large number of older citizens have such poor functional capacity they cannot rise from a chair or bed, walk to the bathroom, or climb a single stair without assistance.
- At best no more than 20% and possibly fewer than 10% of adults in the United States, Australia, Canada, and England obtain sufficient regular physical activity at an intensity that conveys discernible health and fitness benefits.

U.S. Children and Teenagers

Physical activity data from a longitudinal study of boys and girls between ages 9 and 15 indicate that moderate-to-vigorous physical activity declined with age over the study period.[146] By age 15, daily physical activity decreased to just 49 min on weekdays and about 30 min per weekend day, well below the government's recommended 60-min duration. Overall, boys were only slightly more active than girls, moving an average of 18 more min daily. The percentage of children who met the government's 1-hr recommendation of moderate daily activity shifted markedly over time. Between ages 9 and 11, almost every child in the study was moving at least 1 hour daily. But by age 15, only 31% met the weekly guideline and just 17% on weekends.

Other data on the physical activity patterns of children, adolescents, and teenagers indicate the following:

- Nearly half of those between ages 12 and 21 do not exercise vigorously on a regular basis; a sharp decline in physical activity occurs during adolescence regardless of gender.
- Fourteen percent report no recent physical activity; this lack of activity occurs more frequently among females, particularly Black females.
- Twenty-five percent engage in light-to-moderate physical activity (e.g., walk or bicycle) nearly every day.
- Participation in all types of physical activity declines strikingly with increasing age and school grade.
- More males than females participate in vigorous physical activity, strengthening activities, and walking or bicycling.

Changing Fitness Trends

Beginning in 1996, the American College of Sports Medicine (ACSM) began an annual survey of worldwide fitness trends.[278] Electronic surveys sent to thousands of health and exercise professionals worldwide requested feedback on health and fitness trends for the following year. Responses to these surveys helped to guide health and fitness programming for the commercial (usually for-profit companies), clinical (including medical fitness programs), community (not-for-profit), and corporate divisions of the health/fitness industry.

The survey applies a Likert-type scale ranging from a low score of 1 (least likely to be a trend) to a high score of 10 (most likely to be a trend). Out of the 56,746 surveys sent, only 5.4% were returned.[279] **TABLE 31.1** presents the top 10 fitness trends for 2015 to 2020.[279]

TABLE 31.1 Top 10 worldwide fitness trends, 2015 to 2020

 Americans' Most Popular Physical Activities Practiced Daily

Of the relatively small number of people in the United States aged 15 years and older who engage in sports or exercise activities on a typical day, walking is the most popular activity (30%) compared among 25 different sports and exercise activities.

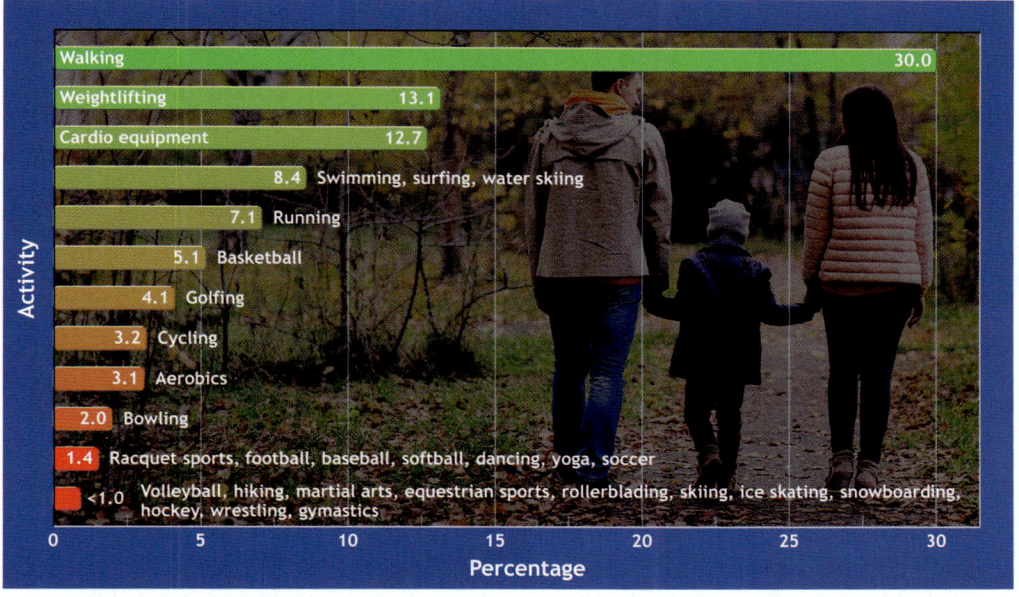

Background photo: Elena Nichizhenova/Shutterstock

Source: www.bls.gov/spotlight/2008/sports/#:~:text=Walking%20is%20Most%20Popular%20Exercise,popular%20form%20of%20exercise%20overall

In a Practical Sense

Assessing Joint Flexibility in Common Body Areas

Two types of flexibility include (1) *static*—full range of motion (ROM) of a specific joint, and (2) *dynamic*—torque or resistance encountered as the joint moves through its ROM. Improper vertebral column alignment accounts for more than 80% of all lower back and pelvic girdle ailments; this often results from poor flexibility in regions of the lower back, trunk, hip, and posterior thigh and weak abdominal and erector spinae muscles.

SPECIFICITY AND FLEXIBILITY

Considerable specificity exists for joint ROM depending on level of use and joint structure. Triaxial ball-and-socket hip and shoulder joints afford a greater degree of movement than either uniaxial or biaxial wrist, knee, elbow, and ankle joints. "Tightness" of soft tissue structures of the joint capsule and muscle and its fascia, tendons, ligaments, and skin constitute major factors that influence static and dynamic flexibility. Other influences include a well-developed musculature and excess fatty tissue of adjacent body segments. Flexibility progressively decreases with advancing age, mainly from decreased soft tissue extensibility, largely influenced by decreased levels of physical activity. On average, females remain more flexible than males at any age.

FIVE COMMON FIELD TESTS OF STATIC FLEXIBILITY

Field tests assess static flexibility indirectly through linear ROM measurement. A minimum of three trials should be administered following a warm-up.

Test 1: Hip and Trunk Flexibility (Modified Sit-and-Reach Test)

Starting position: Sit on the floor with the back and head against a wall with the legs fully extended with the bottom of the feet against the sit-and-reach box. Place hands on top of each other, stretching the arms forward while keeping the head and back against the wall **(A)**. Measure distance from the fingertips to the box edge with a yardstick. This becomes the zero or starting point.

Movement: Slowly bend and reach forward maximally (the head and back move away from the wall), sliding the fingers along the yardstick; hold the final position for 2 seconds **(B)**.

Score: Total distance reached to the nearest one-tenth inch.

Test 1: Hip-and-trunk flexibility (modified sit-and-reach test)

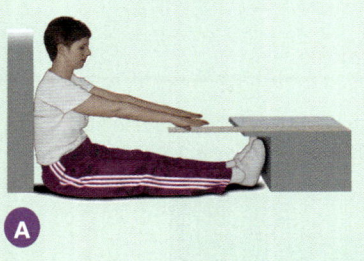
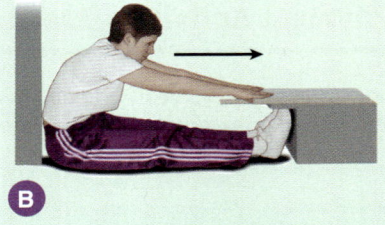

Test 2: Shoulder-wrist flexibility (shoulder-and-wrist elevation test)

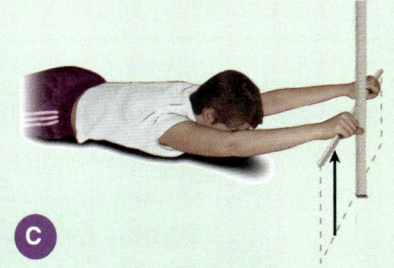

MODIFIED SIT AND REACH (IN INCHES), AGE RANGE

Performance Rating	Males		Females	
	Age <35 y	Age 36–49 y	Age <35 y	Age 36–49 y
Excellent	>17.9	>16.1	>17.9	>17.4
Good	17.0–17.9	14.6–16.1	16.7–17.9	16.2–17.4
Average	15.8–17.0	13.9–14.6	16.2–16.7	15.2–16.2
Fair	15.0–15.8	13.4–13.9	15.8–16.2	14.5–15.2
Poor	<15.0	<13.4	<15.4	<14.5

Data from Johnson BL, Nelson JK. *Practical Measurements for Evaluation in Physical Education.* 4th ed. New York: Macmillan Publishing; 1986.

Test 2: Shoulder-Wrist Flexibility (Shoulder and Wrist Elevation Test)

Starting position: Lie prone on the floor with arms fully extended overhead; grasp a yardstick with the hands shoulder width apart.

Movement: Raise the stick maximally (C).

- Measure the vertical distance (nearest 1/4 in./0.635 cm) the yardstick rises from the floor.
- Measure arm length from the acromial process to the tip of longest finger.
- Subtract the best vertical score from arm length.

Score: Arm length − best vertical score (nearest 1/4 in.).

SHOULDER AND WRIST ELEVATION (IN INCHES)

Performance Rating	Males	Females
Excellent	≥12.75	≥12.00
Good	12.50–11.75	11.75–11.00
Average	11.50–8.50	10.75–7.75
Fair	8.25–6.25	7.50–5.75
Poor	≤6.00	≤5.50

Data from Johnson BL, Nelson JK. *Practical Measurements for Evaluation in Physical Education*. 4th ed. New York: Macmillan Publishing; 1986.

Test 3: Trunk and Neck Flexibility (Trunk and Neck Extension Test)

Starting position: Lie prone on the floor with the hands clasped together behind the head.

Movement: Raise the trunk maximally while keeping the hips in contact with the floor. An assistant can stabilize the legs.

Score: Vertical distance (nearest 1/4 in.) from the nose tip to the floor.

TRUNK AND NECK EXTENSION (IN INCHES)

Performance Rating	Males	Females
Excellent	≥10.25	≥10.00
Good	10.00–8.25	9.75–8.00
Average	8.00–6.25	7.75–6.00
Fair	6.00–3.25	5.75–2.25
Poor	≤3.00	≤2.00

Data from Johnson BL, Nelson JK. *Practical Measurements for Evaluation in Physical Education*. 4th ed. New York: Macmillan Publishing; 1986.

Test 4: Shoulder Flexibility (Shoulder Rotation Test)

Starting position: Grasp one end of a rope with the left hand; 4 in. away, grasp the rope with the right hand.

Movement: Extend both arms in front of the chest and rotate the arms overhead and behind the back; as resistance occurs, slide the right hand farther from the left hand along the rope until the rope touches against the back.

- Measure the distance on the rope between the thumb of each hand after successfully rotating overhead with the rope against the back.
- Measure shoulder width from deltoid to deltoid. Subtract the rope distance from shoulder width distance.

Score: Shoulder-width distance—rope distance (nearest 1/4 in.).

SHOULDER ROTATION (IN INCHES)

Performance Rating	Males	Females
Excellent	≥20.00	≥18.00
Good	19.75–14.75	17.75–13.25
Average	14.50–11.75	13.00–10.00
Fair	11.50–7.25	9.75–5.25
Poor	≤7.00	≤5.00

Data from Johnson BL, Nelson JK. *Practical Measurements for Evaluation in Physical Education*. 4th ed. New York: Macmillan Publishing; 1986.

Test 5: Ankle Flexibility (Ankle Flexion Test)

Starting position: Stand facing a wall. With feet flat on the floor, lean into the wall.

Movement: Slowly slide back from the wall as far as possible while keeping the feet flat on the floor, body and knees fully extended, and chest in contact with the wall.

Score: Distance between the toe line and wall (nearest 1/4 in.).

ANKLE FLEXION (IN INCHES)

Performance Rating	Males	Females
Excellent	≥35.50	≥32.00
Good	35.25–32.75	31.75–30.50
Average	32.50–29.75	30.25–26.75
Fair	29.50–26.75	26.50–24.50
Poor	≤26.50	≤24.25

Data from Johnson BL, Nelson JK. *Practical Measurements for Evaluation in Physical Education*. 4th ed. New York: Macmillan Publishing; 1986.

2020 Top 10 Fitness Trends

1. **Wearable technology:** Estimated to be about a $95 billion industry
2. **High-intensity interval training (HIIT):** Short bursts of intense physical activity followed by a short rest period
3. **Group training:** More than five participants; group exercise instructors teaching, leading, and motivating individuals through intentionally designed larger in-person group movement classes
4. **Free weight training:** Free weights, barbells, kettlebells, dumbbells, and medicine ball classes or individual instructions
5. **Personal training:** One-on-one training including online, in health clubs, in the home, and in worksites with fitness facilities
6. **Exercise is medicine:** A global health initiative that focuses on encouraging primary care physicians and other healthcare providers to include physical activity assessment and associated treatment recommendations as part of every patient visit and refer their patients to exercise professionals
7. **Body weight training:** Combined variable resistance body weight training and neuromotor movements employing multiple movement planes with body weight as the training modality
8. **Older adult programs:** Individual and group programs for "baby boomers" and other older individuals (≥65 years)
9. **Health/wellness coaching:** Integrating behavioral science into health promotion and lifestyle programs using one-on-one and group activities; focuses on the client's values, needs, vision, and short-term and long-term goals using behavior change intervention strategies
10. **Employing certified fitness professionals:** Hiring certified health fitness professionals through educational and certification programs that are fully accredited for fitness professionals

Fitness Trend Comparisons: U.S. versus Europe, Latin America, and China. ACSM's Worldwide Survey of Fitness Trends includes respondents' data from Europe, but the targeted sample size was too small to produce Europe-specific conclusions. The *EuropeActive* (www.europeactive.eu/) and the *European Register of Exercise Professionals* (*EREPS*; www.ereps.eu/) in collaboration with ACSM conducted a separate fitness survey exclusively focused on the European region.[280] These data provide more focused insights about international trends, while supporting future comparisons at regional and international levels.[281,282]

Survey responses were received from 40 European countries, with the top five fitness trends in 2020 as follows:

1. Personal training
2. HIIT training
3. Body weight training
4. Functional fitness
5. Small group personal training

Healthy People 2030

A widespread erosion of physical activity patterns becomes particularly apparent with increasing age among American adolescents and adults.[38] Notwithstanding the cause for progressive inactivity with aging, *increased* physical activity levels predict *decreased* levels of all-cause morbidity and mortality, and the relationship appears to be graded.[30,95]

The Healthy People initiative is a national effort that sets goals and objectives to promote, strengthen, and evaluate the nation's efforts to improve the health and well-being of its citizens. **Healthy People 2030** focuses on new challenges and builds on lessons learned from its first four decades. The initiative began in 1979, when the U.S. Surgeon General issued a landmark report entitled, *Healthy People: The Surgeon General's Report on Health Promotion and Disease Prevention* (https://profiles.nlm.nih.gov/spotlight/nn/catalog/nlm:nlmuid-101584932X94-doc). This report focused on reducing preventable death and injury. It included ambitious, quantifiable goals and objectives to achieve national health promotion and disease prevention for the United States within a 10-year period to be achieved by 1990. This report was followed in later decades by the updated, 10-year Healthy People goals and objectives (*Healthy People 2000*, *Healthy People 2010*, and *Healthy People 2020*).

Since the Healthy People initiative was first launched, the United States has made significant progress in achieving its goals—which include reducing major death causes for heart disease and cancer; reducing infant and maternal mortality; reducing tobacco smoking, hypertension, and elevated cholesterol risk factors; and increasing childhood vaccinations.

The importance of collaborating across agencies at the national, state, local, and tribal levels with the private and public health sectors became clear. An important lesson learned was that a widely accessible plan over a 40-year time period containing achievable goals and objectives can guide the action of individuals, communities, and stakeholders to improve health.

Healthy People 2030's main components include four action areas listed below and displayed in **FIGURE 31.3** (www.healthypeople.gov/sites/default/files/Report%208_Implementation%20and%20Graphic_Formatted_%20EO_508c-final_0.pdf):

1. Closing gaps
2. Cultivating healthier environments
3. Increasing knowledge and action
4. Health and well-being across the lifespan

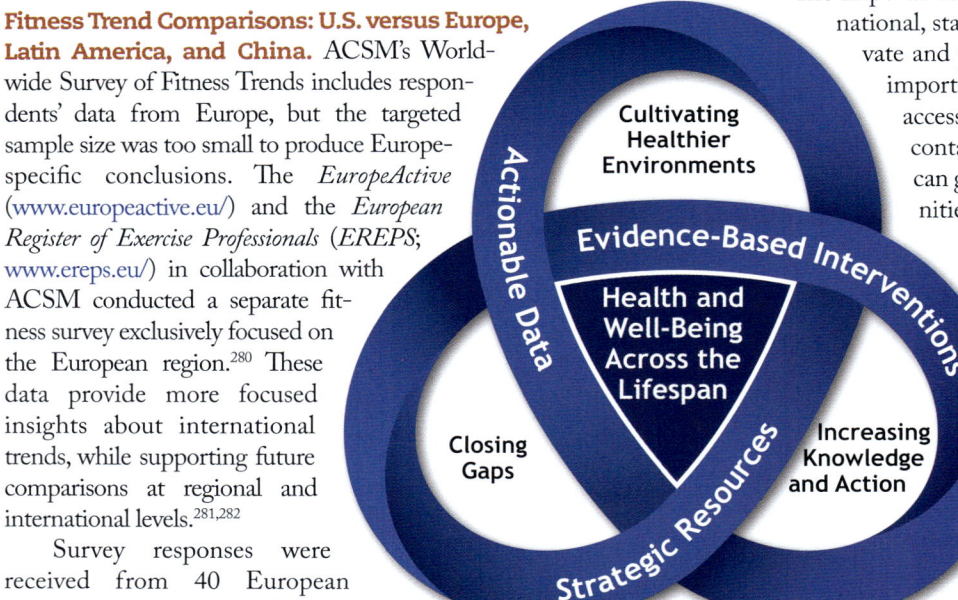

FIGURE 31.3. Proposed framework for *Healthy People 2030* to visually communicate the main components of the Healthy People 2030 Initiative.

The U.S. Department of Health and Human Services (www.hhs.gov) maintains a comprehensive, interactive online presence that includes the ability to search the extensive database of the U.S. government's efforts in developing the Healthy People 2030 program (www.healthypeople.gov/2020/tools-resources; www.healthypeople.gov/2020/About-Healthy-People/How-To-Use-HealthyPeople.gov).

The "*physical activity pyramid*" illustrated in FIGURE 31.4 summarizes major goals for increasing regular physical activity pursuits in the general population and emphasizing diverse behavioral and lifestyle options.

Is Physical Activity Safe?

Several well-publicized reports of sudden cardiac death during physical activity have raised the question of physical activity safety.[114,192]

Despite an overall increase in physical activity participation, the **death rate** during physical activity declined over the past 40 years. In one report of cardiovascular episodes over a 65-month period, 2935 exercisers recorded 374,798 activity hours that included 2,726,272 km/1 billion, 694 mi for running and walking. No deaths occurred during this time, with only two nonfatal cardiovascular complications. This amounted to two complications per 100,000 hours of physical activity for females and three complications for males. For individuals involved in marathon running, estimates place sudden **cardiac arrest** at approximately 1 in 57,000 runners, with the event most common among older runners, which occurs over the last 4 mi of the run.[236]

Intense physical exertion raises a small sudden death risk during the activity (e.g., one sudden death per 1.51 million episodes of exertion) compared with resting an equivalent time, particularly in sedentary persons as FIGURE 31.5 demonstrates.[10] The yellow horizontal solid line shows myocardial infarction risk without exertion compared with increasing weekly habitual vigorous physical activity frequency. The longer-term reduction in overall death risk for those who regularly engage in physical activity outweighs any small potential for acute cardiovascular complications.

Regular exercisers have considerably less risk of death *during* physical activity.[6] A 12-year follow-up of more than 21,000 male physicians showed that males who exercised at least five times a week had a much lower sudden death risk during vigorous exertion—about sevenfold less—than those who exercised only once weekly.[9] The likelihood of an exercise catastrophe—cerebrovascular accident, aortic dissection and rupture, lethal arrhythmias, myocardial infarction—increases under the following eight conditions:

1. Genetic predisposition (family history of sudden death at a young age)
2. Fainting history or chest pain with physical activity
3. Unaccustomed vigorous activity
4. Physical activity performed with accompanying and often undetected psychological stress
5. Environmental temperature extremes
6. Straining-type activities involving a static muscle-action component (e.g., shoveling wet snow without prior physical activity)
7. Physical activity during viral infection or when feeling ill
8. Comingling prescription drugs with dietary supplements (e.g., ephedra with different proteins)

Musculoskeletal injuries represent the most prevalent of the exercise complications. A longitudinal study of aerobic dance injuries in 351 participants and 60 instructors during nearly 30,000 hr of activity reported 327 medical complaints.[68] Only 84 of the injuries caused disability (2.8 per 1000 person-hr of participation) and only 2.1% required medical

Physical Activity Pyramid

FIGURE 31.4. Physical Activity Pyramid. Prudent goals to increase daily physical activity.
(Shutterstock photos: ESB Professional (aerobics), Andrey Burmakin (tennis), Robin Craig (mowing), Monkey Business Images (walking), Erick Santoz (golf), Syda Productions (stretching).)

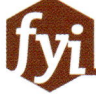

Should Children's Cholesterol Be Measured?

Guidelines issued by the National Cholesterol Education Program (www.americanheart.org) conclude that children should have their cholesterol measured if a family history of high cholesterol or heart disease exists, particularly if a parent had a heart attack before age 50. Shockingly, this parental "cardiac proneness" includes up to 25% of the United States adult population! Research with children ages 10 to 15 indicates that encouraging lifestyle habits of regular physical activity, improved cardiovascular fitness, and a prudent nutritional profile contribute to favorable lipid profiles similar to the association seen with adults.

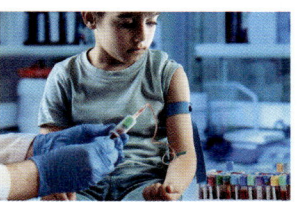
angellodeco/Shutterstock

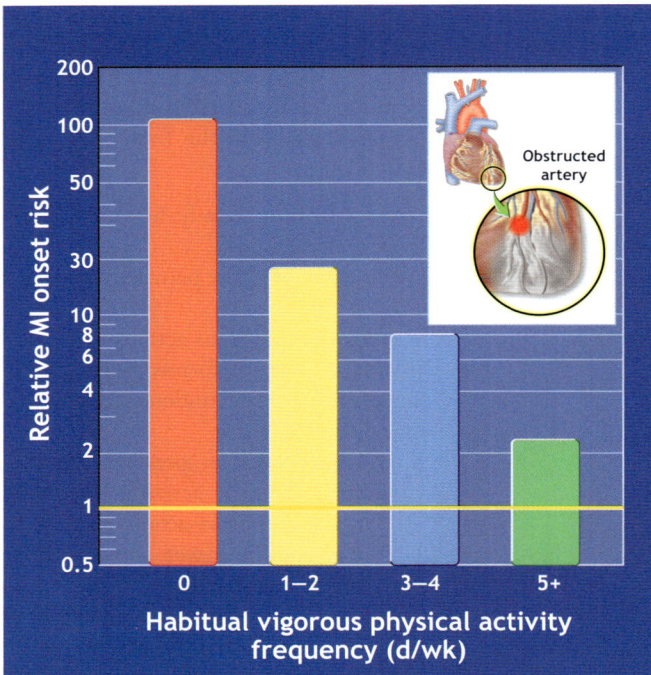

FIGURE 31.5. Triggering acute cardiac events. Relative risk of myocardial infarction (MI) associated with vigorous exertion (≥6 metabolic equivalents [METs]) according to habitual weekly vigorous physical activity frequency.
(From Mittleman MA et al. Triggering of acute myocardial infarction by heavy physical exertion—protection against triggering by regular exertion. *N Engl J Med*. 1993; 329:1680. Copyright © 1993 Massachusetts Medical Society. Reprinted with permission from Massachusetts Medical Society.)

attention. National estimates from self-reported injury frequency and severity in five common physical activities—walking, gardening, weightlifting, outdoor bicycling, and aerobics—reported minimal injury rates.[123,168] Most injuries required no treatment or reduced physical activity. Age does not affect orthopedic-required incidents for moderate intensity and duration activities. For activities that involve running, the greatest orthopedic injury risk occurs in those who run for prolonged durations exceeding 1 hr.[11]

Prospective epidemiologic research evaluated clinically significant medical incidents and emergencies for 7725 low-risk, apparently healthy corporate fitness enrollees in a supervised facility at a major medical center.[145] Almost 3 years of surveillance reported 15 medically significant events (0.048 per 1000 participant-hr) and two medical emergencies (both recovered), which equaled a rate of less than 0.01 per 1000 participant-hr. This illustrates convincingly that the health-related fitness benefits outweigh the relatively low participation risk.

Prehabilitation Reduces Sports and Recreational Injuries

For most individuals, participation in sports/athletic/recreational activities poses little risk, particularly in younger individuals. For those older than age 40, and particularly those above age 60, a carefully planned and systematic **prehabilitation program** can ensure readiness for participation and further reduce exercise-induced disability. Prehabilitation conditioning emphasizes joint stretching, muscle activation, core stability and strength, balance, and muscle coordination to ensure maximum motor unit recruitment and joint stability.[283,284]

fyi Risks Develop at an Early Age

A dismal picture emerges for selected cardiovascular health markers for U.S. adolescents, suggesting that the current generation of teenagers will increase their risk for heart disease later in life. The Centers for Disease Control and Prevention reported that 5450 adolescents between ages 12 and 19 performed poorly overall on the criteria set by the American Heart Association for ideal cardiovascular health. The poor quality of their diet was particularly noteworthy. Not one adolescent reported meeting recommended targets on five different nutritional categories, which included consuming at least 4 to 5 servings of fruits and vegetables daily, 3 whole-grain servings daily, 2 or more servings of fish weekly, consuming less than 1500 mg of sodium daily, and drinking less than 3 oz of sugar-sweetened drinks a week. Just 16.4% of boys and 11.3% of girls rated ideal on all of the other six criteria. For the physical activity category, disappointingly 50% of boys and 60% of girls failed to achieve the optimal 60-min daily exercise goal. Shamefully, between 10% and 20% reported engaging in no physical activity at all!

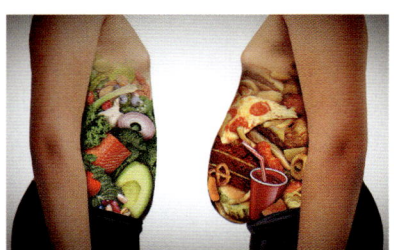

Lightspring/Shutterstock

Summary

1. Physical activity epidemiology evaluates the nature, extent, and demographics for physical activity participation in large populations, which often reflect disease occurrence and other undesirable health-related outcomes.
2. A discouraging picture has emerged over the decades about physical activity participation by adult Americans who do not obtain enough regular physical activity of adequate intensity to achieve health and fitness benefits.
3. Health benefits increase as a function of increased moderate physical activity mostly every day during the week.
4. Intense physical effort raises a low sudden death risk during the activity compared with resting for an equivalent time in sedentary people. However, the longer-term health benefits from regular physical activity outweigh the risk from acute cardiovascular complications.
5. The Healthy People 2030 initiative attempts to achieve four primary goals: closing gaps, cultivating healthier

environments, increasing knowledge and action, and health and well-being across the lifespan.

6. For activities that involve running, the greatest orthopedic injury potential exists among individuals who run for extended durations that exceed 1 hour.
7. Prehabilitation, particularly among older individuals using core-strengthening training, reduces injury potential.
8. Physical inactivity promotes unhealthy lifestyle habits; so increasing regular physical activity in a population must become a top public health priority.

Part 2 — Aging and Physiologic Function

Age Trends

FIGURE 31.6 illustrates that physiologic and performance measures improve rapidly during childhood and achieve a maximum between late adolescence and age 30. Functional capacity declines thereafter, with deterioration varying at any age depending on lifestyle and genetic characteristics. A similar age trend exists for physically active persons, yet physiologic function averages about 25% higher compared with sedentary counterparts at each age category. For example, an active 50-year old man or woman often maintains the functional level of his or her 30-year-old counterpart. All physiologic measures eventually decline with age, but not at the same rate. Nerve conduction velocity, for example, declines only 10% to 15% from age 30 to 80, but the resting cardiac index (ratio of cardiac output to body surface area) and joint flexibility decline 20 to 30%; maximum breathing capacity at age 80 averages 40% compared to 30-year-old. Brain cells die at a fairly constant rate until age 60, but the liver and kidneys lose 40 to 50% of their function between ages 30 and 70. By the seventh decade of life, the average female has lost 30% of her bone mass, while males lose only 15%.

Differences in Exercise Physiology Between Children and Adults

One must consider the interaction between physical activity and aging when evaluating physiologic responses and exercise performance across a broad age span. The distinct differences between children and adults can be summarized as follows:

- During weight-bearing walking and running, children's oxygen uptake ($mL \cdot kg^{-1} \cdot min^{-1}$) averages 10 to 30% higher than adults' at a designated submaximal pace.[235] The lower exercise economy from children's lower ventilatory efficiency, shorter stride length, and greater stride frequency make a standard walking or running pace physiologically more stressful and performance scores poorer than those of adult counterparts.
- Performance disadvantages exist even though children typically maintain equal or somewhat higher aerobic powers than adults. Also, walking and running economy and percentage of maximum oxygen uptake ($\dot{V}O_{2max}$) sustainable during activity at the lactate threshold continually improve as children age, independent of aerobic power changes. This limits the usefulness of a single walking or running performance test to predict $\dot{V}O_{2max}$ throughout childhood and adolescence.[47]
- Children exhibit lower absolute $\dot{V}O_{2max}$ values ($L \cdot min^{-1}$) than adults from a smaller fat-free body mass (FFM; see Fig. 11.11 in Chapter 11). Consequently, children are disadvantaged when exercising against a standard external resistance (unadjusted for body size) in stationary cycling and arm cranking. The fixed oxygen cost ($L \cdot min^{-1}$) of this activity represents a greater percentage of children's smaller absolute aerobic power. During weight-bearing activity, energy expenditure relates directly to body mass, so children are not disadvantaged by a smaller body size.
- Children score lower than adults on anaerobic power tests because they cannot generate a high level of blood lactate during maximal effort. Lower intramuscular levels of the glycolytic enzyme phosphofructokinase may contribute to children's poorer anaerobic performance.
- Children breathe larger air volumes (greater ventilatory equivalent) than adults at any submaximal $\dot{V}O_2$ level.
- Children score higher than adults on perception of effort (rating of perceived exertion) when both exercise at equivalent percentages of aerobic power. Greater pulmonary discomfort owing to the higher respiratory rate and ventilatory equivalent of children may produce this effect.[215,226]
- Children and adults increase muscle strength with resistance training. Prepubescent children, unlike pubescent children and adults, have limited ability to increase muscle mass, presumably because their androgen levels are relatively low.

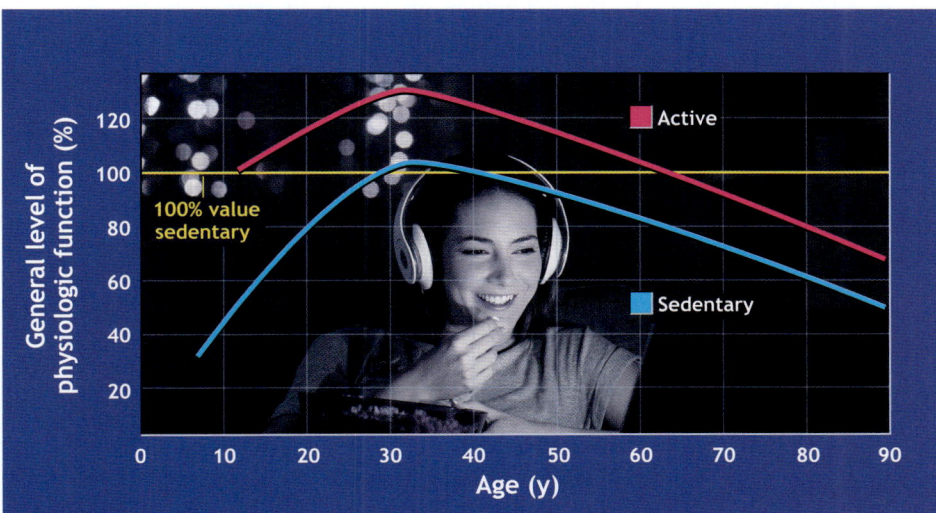

FIGURE 31.6. Generalized curve for age-related changes in physiologic function. All comparisons are against the 100% value achieved by a 20- to 30-year-old sedentary person. (Background photo: Antonio Guillem/Shutterstock.)

INTEGRATIVE QUESTION

What factors explain the relatively poor performances of children during a 10-km run compared with adults with equal aerobic power?

Muscular Strength

Age and gender affect muscular strength and power, with the magnitude of each effect influenced by the muscle group studied and the type of muscle action. The following summarizes general trends in muscular strength and power of adults with increasing age:

- Males and females attain their highest strength levels between ages 20 and 40, the time when muscle cross-sectional area is largest. Thereafter, concentric strength of most muscle groups declines, slowly at first and then more rapidly after middle age.
- Accelerated strength loss during middle age coincides with weight loss and the loss increases in chronic diseases such as stroke, diabetes, arthritis, and coronary heart disease.
- Older adult's muscles act with less maximum force, have slower relaxation rates, and show a downward shift in their force-velocity relationship.[36]
- The capacity for power generation with age declines faster than that for maximal strength.[91]
- Declines in eccentric strength begin at a later age and progress more slowly than for concentric strength. Strength loss begins at a later age for females than for males.[127]
- Arm strength for males and females deteriorates more slowly than leg strength.[133]
- Rate of decline in muscular power with aging is similar among male and female weightlifters including world record holders, elite master athletes, and healthy, untrained individuals.[210]
- Strength loss among older adults directly relates to limited mobility and fitness status and potential for increased incidence of accidents from muscle weakness, fatigue, and poor balance.[99,209]

Age Trends Among Elite Weightlifters and Powerlifters

Master athletes more accurately reflect the effects of physiologic aging because such healthy, motivated athletes maintain a rigorous training schedule to compete at the highest level. FIGURE 31.7 illustrates age trends for weightlifting and powerlifting records of the U.S. weightlifting and U.S. powerlifting organizations (www.usawa.com; www.usapowerlifting.com). There were four key findings:

1. Peak lifting performance declines for males and females with aging. Weightlifting performance (shown in **A**) follows a downward curvilinear trend, whereas powerlifting performance (shown in **B**) declines linearly with increasing age.[285]
2. The rate and overall magnitude of decline in performance with age are markedly greater in weightlifting than powerlifting.

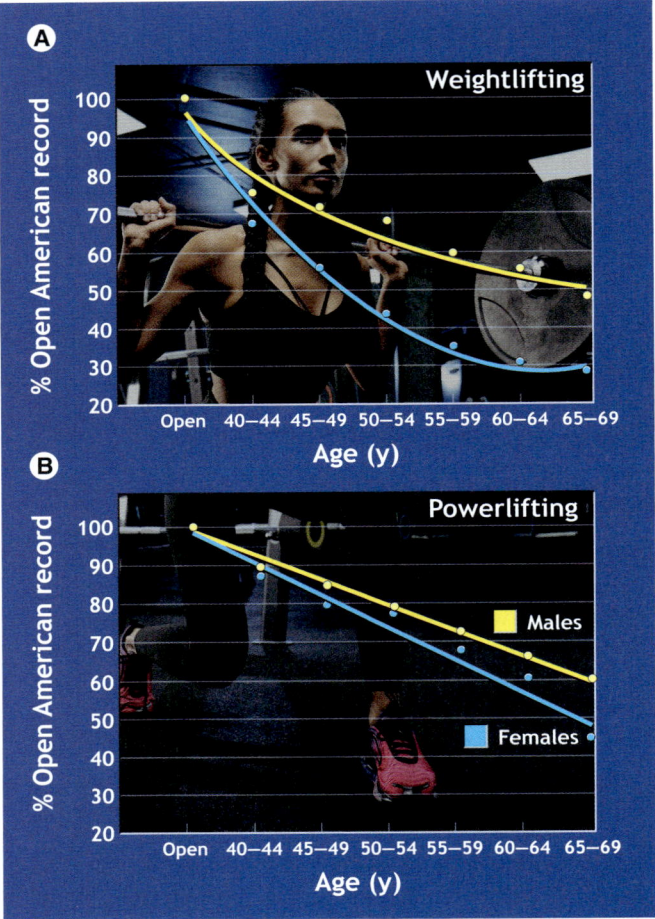

FIGURE 31.7. Age-related sex differences in **(A)** weightlifting (average snatch and clean and jerk scores) and **(B)** powerlifting (average deadlift, squat, and bench press scores) based on analysis of top age-group records of the U.S. Weightlifting and U.S. Powerlifting Organizations.
(From Anton MA, et al. Age-related declines in anaerobic muscular performance: weightlifting and powerlifting. *Med Sci Sports Exerc.* 2004;36:143. Background photo: Serhii Bobyk/Shutterstock.)

3. The magnitude of decline in peak muscular power is greater in weightlifting tasks that require more complex and explosive power movements.
4. Sex differences in age-related performance decrements emerge only in events that require more complex and explosive power movements, with performance decrements greater in females than in males.

The above list indicates a gender-specific and task-specific influence of age on muscular performance among elite resistance-trained athletes. More powerful and complex tasks undergo greater decline with age than tasks that require simpler movement patterns; females experience greater age-related declines in such tasks.

Muscle Mass Decrease

Motor unit remodeling represents a normal, continuous process that involves motor endplate repair and reconstruction. Remodeling progresses by selective muscle fiber denervation, followed by terminal axon sprouting from adjacent motor units. Motor unit remodeling gradually deteriorates in old age. This leads to **denervation muscle atrophy**, irreversible muscle fiber degeneration, particularly type II fibers. The condition associates with chronic inflammation and reduced circulating GH, IGF-1, muscle-specific isoforms of IGF, mitochondria number and capacity, cell nuclei, and endplate structures.[12,43,74,75,286,287]

Age-associated muscle wasting, termed **sarcopenia**, magnifies by reduced physical activity, which progressively reduces muscle cross section, and muscle mass and function, even after adjusting for body mass and stature changes.[28,32,96,286] Moreover, increased muscle loss associates with sleep quality and duration, particularly with increasing age.[288]

Muscle fibers tend to "*type group*" because fast-twitch and slow-twitch fibers lose their typical chessboard distribution and cluster within groups of similar type—perhaps from denervation and subsequent fiber necrosis. Older adults have more than twice the noncontractile content in locomotor muscles as younger adults.[103] Impaired neural drive does not explain the decline in muscle strength with age because older adults can still achieve full muscle activation during a maximal voluntary muscle action.[50]

The primary cause of reduced strength between ages 25 and 80 relates to a 40 to 50% reduction in muscle mass from muscle fiber atrophy and motor unit loss, even among healthy, physically active adults. **FIGURE 31.8A** shows that muscle-fiber size begins to decrease at approximately age 30, decreasing 10% by age 50. Reduction in total muscle area (Fig. 31.6B) usually parallels reduced fiber size, particularly fast-twitch fibers in the lower extremities. This proportionately increases the area occupied by slow-twitch (type I) muscle fibers. Note that after age 60, muscle area declines more precipitously largely from decreased total muscle fiber number.

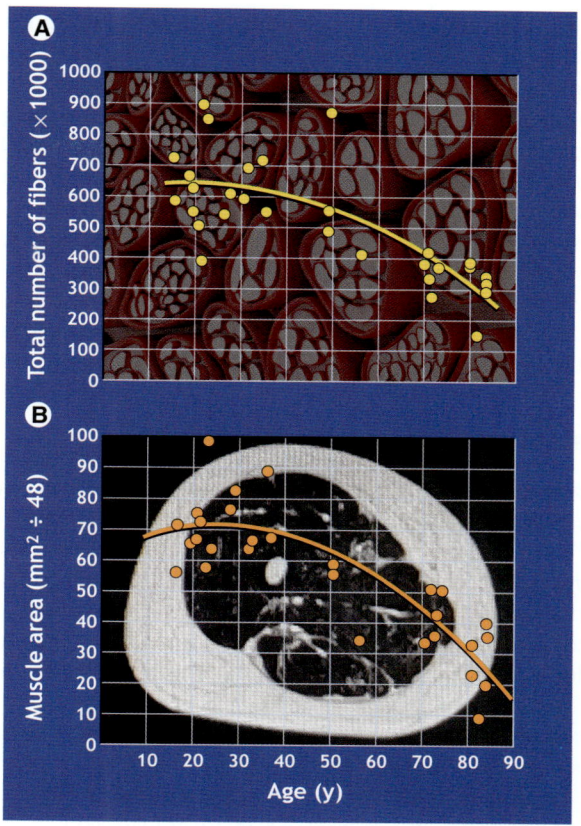

FIGURE 31.8. Relationship between age and total number of muscle fibers **(A)** and muscle cross-sectional area **(B)** as a function of age.
(From Lexell J, et al. What is the cause of the ageing atrophy? Total number, size, and proportion of different fiber types studied in whole vastus lateralis muscle from 15- to 83-year-old men. *J Neurol Sci*. 1988;84:275. Background Shutterstock images: Anton Nalivayko (A-fibers), Tossaporn Buttabut (B-area).)

 ### Sleep Disorders: An Underdiagnosed and Undertreated Coronary Heart Disease Risk Factor

The prevalence of sleep disorders, primarily obstructive sleep apnea (OSA), continues to increase worldwide. Adult OSA prevalence rates from different countries include 3 to 7% in adult males and 2 to 5% in adult females. OSA incidence is higher in overweight or obese subjects, older adults, and those of different ethnic origins. In the United States, approximately one in six individuals (43 million) suffer from sleep loss and an additional 20 to 30 million experience intermittent sleep-related problems that directly or indirectly impact coronary heart disease in the form of insulin resistance and hypertension, obesity and diabetes, increased carotid wall thickness, and nocturnal myocardial ischemia from apnea-associated oxygen desaturation. The National Commission on Sleep Disorders Research (www.nhlbi.nih.gov/about/divisions/division-lung-diseases/national-center-sleep-disorders-research) attributes $15.9 billion as the direct cost of disordered sleep, with an estimated $50 to $100 billion in indirect and related costs. The following institutes of the National Institutes of Health (NIH) provide excellent resources about sleep disorders:

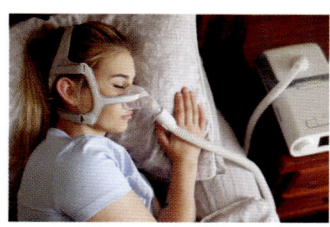
Independence_Project/Shutterstock

- National Institute of Neurological Disorders and Stroke (www.ninds.nih.gov)
- National Heart, Lung and Blood Institute (www.nhlbi.nih.gov/health-topics/education-and-awareness/sleep-health)
- National Center on Sleep Disorders Research (www.nhlbi.nih.gov/about/ncsdr/index.htm)
- National Sleep Foundation (www.sleepfoundation.org)
- Patient Education Institute (www.patient-education.com/)

Sources:
Brauer AA, et al. Sleep and health among collegiate student athletes. *Chest*. 2019;156:1234.
Petrovic D, et al. The contribution of sleep to social inequalities in cardiovascular disorders: a multi-cohort study. *Cardiovasc Res*. 2020;116:1514.

In longitudinal research studying age-related declines in muscular strength, nine males initially evaluated for muscular strength and muscle fiber composition were remeasured 12 years later.[67] Knee and elbow extensor and flexor strengths tested at slow and fast angular velocities decreased by 20 to 30%. CT scans for muscle cross-sectional area in the same muscle groups decreased between 13 and 16%. Muscle biopsies from the vastus lateralis muscle were reduced 42% in type I fibers without changing mean fiber type area. The capillary-to-fiber ratio decreased by 0.31 units after 12 years. The researchers concluded that changes in muscle cross-sectional area largely contributed to the strength decline from ages 65 to 77.

Resistance Training for Older Adults

Moderate resistance training provides a remarkably safe way to stimulate protein synthesis and retention while slowing the "normal" and somewhat inevitable loss of muscle mass and strength with aging.[3,66,90,134] Muscle fiber size and mechanical performance, particularly rate of force development, were consistently elevated in older adults exposed to lifelong resistance training.[1] Older males who resistance-train demonstrate greater absolute gains in muscle size and strength than females, but the percentage improvement is similar between genders, yet gains are somewhat less than those of younger counterparts.[109,218]

Healthy males between ages 60 and 72 who trained for 12 wk using standard-resistance exercise at loads equivalent to 80% of 1-RM demonstrate how well older adults respond to resistance training. **FIGURE 31.9** showed that muscle strength increased progressively throughout training. At week 12, knee-extension strength increased by 107% and knee-flexion strength by 227%. An improvement rate of 5% per training session matched similar increases in young adults. Fast-twitch and slow-twitch muscle fiber hypertrophy accompanied dramatic strength improvements. In other research, muscle cross-sectional area and strength in 70 year olds who had resistance-trained since age 50 equaled values for a group of 28-year-old university students.[106] Older individuals possess impressive plasticity in physiologic, structural, and performance characteristics despite the fact that the capacity to respond to muscle growth cues—mechanical load, nutrition, neural activity, hormones, and growth factors—declines with age.[175]

Muscle responds to vigorous training with rapid improvement into the ninth decade of life. **FIGURE 31.10** illustrates plasticity in physiologic response to resistance training among older adults. Shown are magnetic resonance images taken at the mid-thigh region of a male subject 92 years of age before (**A**) and after (**B**) 112 wk of resistance training of the knee extensor and flexor muscles. Quadriceps lean cross-sectional area increased by 44% in this individual. Improved muscle strength, bone density, dynamic balance, and overall functional status with regular physical activity can minimize or reverse the syndrome of physical frailty. For males and females ages 70 to 89, a regular program of aerobic, strength, flexibility, and balance training prevented both loss of muscle strength and increase in muscle fat infiltration associated with advancing age.[69] Regular strengthening and balance movements provide the most effective way to reduce orthopedic injury from high prevalence of falls in older males and females.[172]

For older persons disabled with knee osteoarthritis, regular aerobic

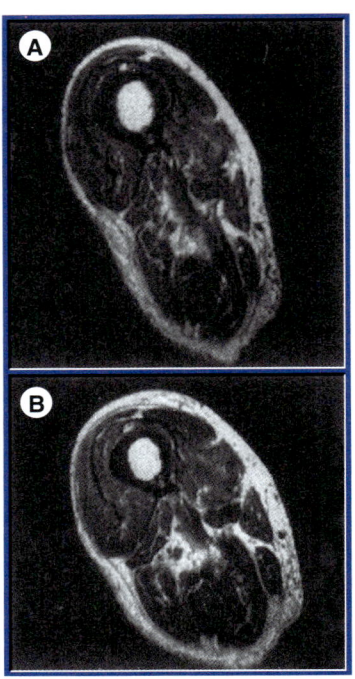

FIGURE 31.10. Magnetic resonance mid-thigh images in a 92-year-old male before (**A**) and after (**B**) 112 wk of resistance training for knee extensor and flexor thigh muscles.
(From Harridge SD, et al. Knee extensor strength, activation, and size in very elderly people following strength training. *Muscle Nerve*. 1999;22:831.)

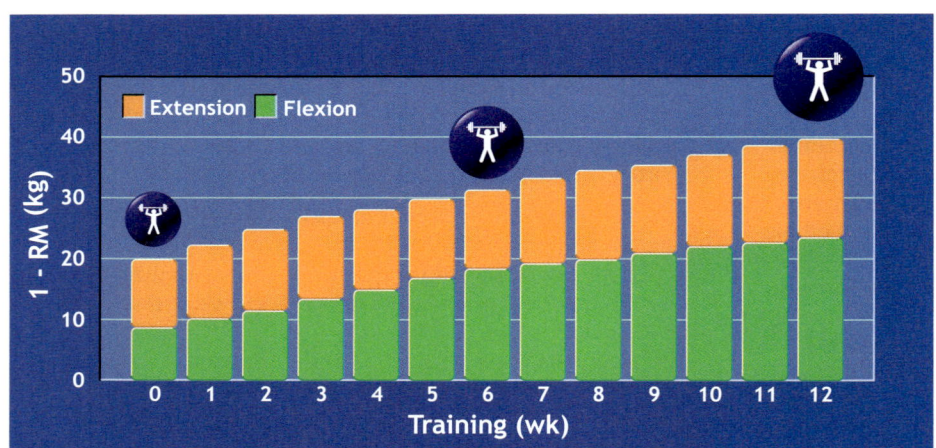

FIGURE 31.9. Dynamic 1-repetition maximum (1-RM) muscle strength in left knee extension (*orange*) and flexion (*green*) assessed weekly during resistance training in older males.
(Data from Frontera WR, et al. Strength conditioning in older men: skeletal muscle hypertrophy and improved function. *J Appl Physiol*. 1988;64:1038.)

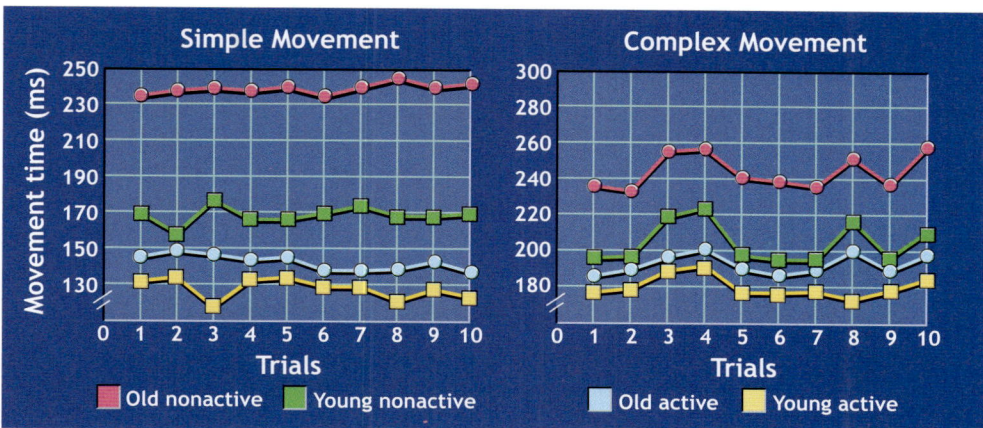

FIGURE 31.11. Simple and complex movement time in subjects classified as young active (*yellow*), old active (*light blue*), young nonactive (*green*), and old nonactive (*pink*). Note the slower movement times (higher scores) in simple and complex tasks for the old and young nonactive subjects compared with their active counterparts.
(From Spirduso WW. Reaction and movement time as a function of age and physical activity level. *J Gerontol.* 1975;30:435. With permission from the Gerontological Society of America, https://www.geron.org/)

or resistance exercises induce beneficial effects on measures of disability, pain, and physical performance.[57] For disabled older female cardiac patients, a 6-month program of resistance training improved muscular strength and physical capacity in a wide range of household physical activities and also improved endurance, balance, coordination, and flexibility.[7] This relative preservation in muscle structure and function may provide an important physical reserve capacity to retain muscle mass and function above a critical threshold for independent living.

Mechanisms that explain how middle-age and older adults respond to resistance training include enhanced motor unit recruitment and innervation patterns and muscular hypertrophy (see Chapter 22). Adaptations in muscle strength depend on the number of sets and repetitions, and intensity, duration, and frequency of training as in younger individuals.

Neural Function

A nearly 40% decline in the number of spinal cord axons and a 10% decline in nerve conduction velocity reflect the cumulative effects of aging on central nervous system function. These changes likely contribute to the age-related decrement in neuromuscular performance assessed by simple and complex reaction and movement times. Partitioning reaction time into central processing time and muscle action time, aging most adversely affects the time to detect a stimulus and process the information to produce the response. Knee-jerk reflexes do not involve neural processing in the brain, so aging affects them less than voluntary responses that involve reaction and movement. Physical inactivity may also be responsible for a large portion of the loss of neuromuscular function seen in older adults. Highly active versus low-active older females achieve greater peak torque, faster rate of torque development, shorter motor time, faster rate of electromyographic rise, and greater onset of electromyographic magnitude.[117,289] **FIGURE 31.11** shows slower movement times for simple and complex tasks by older subjects compared with younger subjects with similar physical activity levels. In all instances, the young or old active groups moved considerably faster than the less-active age group. A physically active lifestyle and specific training, combined with aerobic, balance, coordination, and strength training, influence neuromuscular functions positively to slow the age-related decline in cognitive performance associated with information processing speed.[225,289]

Physically active older adults who have relatively high cardiorespiratory fitness are less likely to experience cognitive decline and dementia with a lower risk of mortality from dementia.[4,128] Biologic mechanisms for such protection include reduced vascular risk, body fat, and levels of inflammatory markers and enhanced neuronal health and function (**FIG. 31.12**). Regular physical activity also increases mitochondrial biogenesis in the brain, which may have important implications for age-related dementia (often characterized by mitochondrial dysfunction).[196,202]

Exercise interventions associate with short-term improvements in cognitive function in sedentary elders.[17,21,39] Older individuals who remain physically active for 20 years or longer show reaction speeds that equal or exceed inactive younger adults and endorse regular physical activity to slow biologic aging in select neuromuscular functions. The potential magnitude of these changes and the amount of physical activity required to induce meaningful responses remain controversial.[191]

Endocrine Changes

Endocrine function changes with age. Approximately 40% of individuals ages 65 to 75 years and 50% of those older than

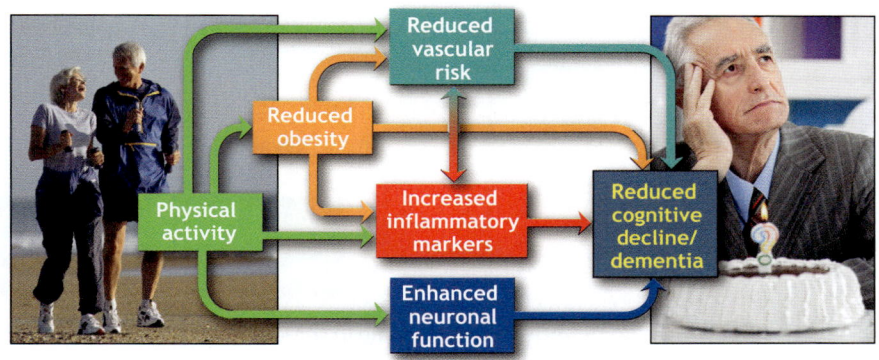

FIGURE 31.12. Potential mechanisms that underlie the association between physical activity and reduced cognitive decline and dementia risk in older adults.
(Photo of man with cake: Lucky Business/Shutterstock.)

age 80 have impaired glucose tolerance that leads to type 2 diabetes (see Chapter 20). Increased disease prevalence among older adults largely relates to the controllable factors of poor diet quality, inadequate physical activity, and increased body fat, particularly in the visceral-abdominal region.[4]

Advancing age lowers pituitary gland release of the thyroid-stimulating hormone thyrotropin, including reduced thyroxine output. Thyroid dysfunction directly impacts metabolic function, with resultant decreases in metabolic rate, glucose metabolism, and protein synthesis.

FIGURE 31.13 depicts the age-related decline in three hormone systems that impact biologic aging rate:

1. Hypothalamic-pituitary-gonadal axis
2. Adrenal cortex
3. GH/IGF axis

Decreased GH (Fig. 31.13, left) release by the anterior pituitary depresses IGF-1 production by the liver and other tissues, which inhibits cellular growth (a condition of aging termed **somatopause**). Decreased gonadotropic luteinizing hormone and follicle-stimulating hormone output by the anterior pituitary (Fig. 31.13, center), coupled with reduced estradiol secretion from the ovaries and testosterone from the testes, causes menopause (females) and **andropause** (males). Adrenocortical cells responsible for dehydroepiandrosterone production decrease their activity (termed adrenopause) without clinically evident changes in this gland's corticotropin and cortisol secretion (Fig. 31.13, right). A central pacemaker in the hypothalamus and/or higher brain areas mediates these processes to produce aging-related changes in peripheral organs (ovaries, testicles, and adrenal cortex).

Hypothalamic-Pituitary-Gonadal Axis

In females, alteration in the interaction between stimulating hormones from the hypothalamus and anterior pituitary gland and gonads decreases ovarian estradiol output. This effect probably initiates permanent cessation of menses (**menopause**). Changes in hypothalamic-pituitary-gonadal axis activity in males occur more slowly than in females. Serum total and free testosterone, for example, gradually decline with aging in males. Decreased gonadotropic secretions from the anterior pituitary gland characterize male andropause.

Adrenal Cortex

Adrenopause refers to reduced adrenal cortex output of dehydroepiandrosterone (DHEA) and its sulfated ester DHEAS. DHEA exhibits a long, progressive decline after age 30, in contrast to glucocorticoid and mineralocorticoid

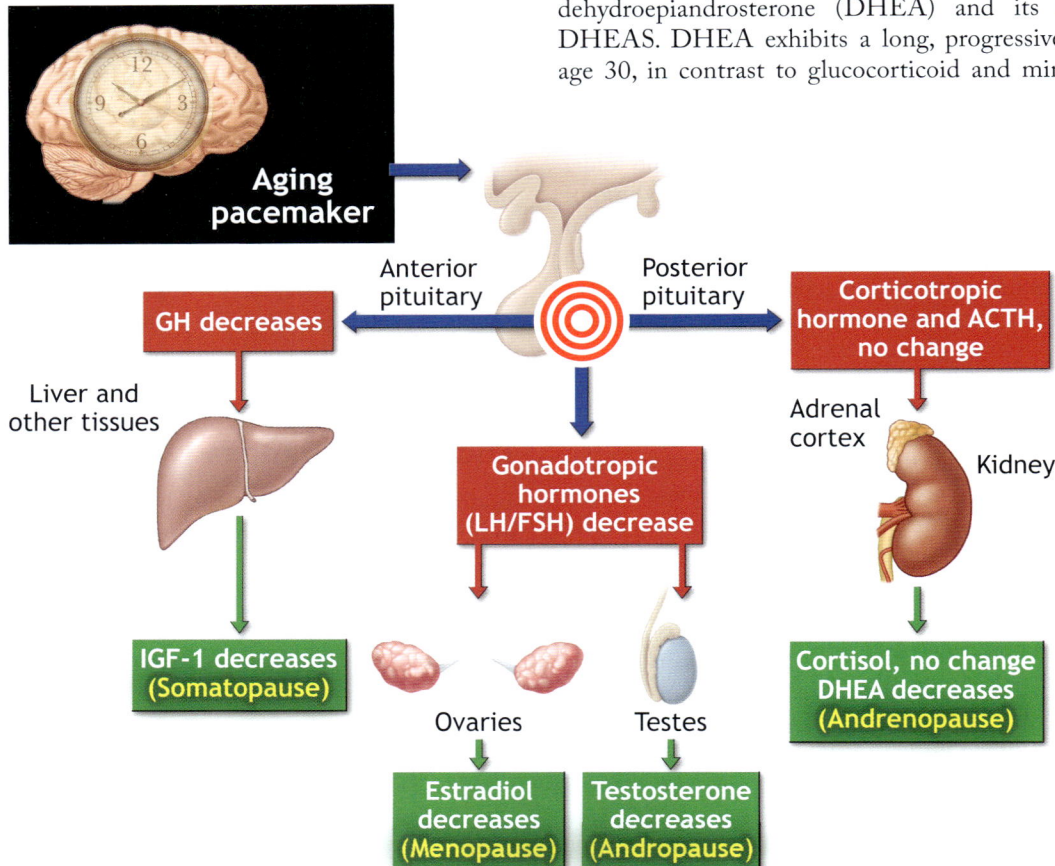

FIGURE 31.13. Age-related decline in three hormone systems that impact the rate of biologic aging. ACTH, adrenocorticotropic hormone; DHEA, dehydroepiandrosterone; FSH, follicle-stimulating hormone; GH, growth hormone; IGF-1, insulin-like growth factor 1; LH, luteinizing hormone.
(Brain, liver, and ovary images adapted from Moore KL, et al. *Clinically Oriented Anatomy*. 8th Ed. Philadelphia: Wolters Kluwer, 2018.)

adrenal steroids, whose plasma levels remain relatively high with aging. By age 75, DHEA plasma levels achieve only 20 to 30% of young adult value. This has evoked speculation that plasma DHEA levels might serve as biochemical markers of biologic aging and disease susceptibility. Animal research suggests that exogenous DHEA protects against cancer, atherosclerosis, viral infections, obesity, and diabetes; enhances immune function; and even extends life. Despite its quantitative significance as a hormone in humans, researchers know little about DHEA's role in the following four areas:

1. Health and aging
2. Cellular or molecular action mechanism(s)
3. Possible receptor sites
4. Potential for adverse effects from supplemental use among young adults with normal DHEA levels

Chapter 23 discusses the case for ergogenic effects of DHEA supplements (and potential risks) on adult males and females.

GH/IGF Axis

Mean pulse amplitude, duration, and fraction of secreted GH gradually decrease with aging, a condition termed *somatopause*. A parallel decrease also occurs in circulating levels of IGF-1, which stimulates tissue growth and protein synthesis. The interaction between the hypothalamus and anterior pituitary gland probably triggers the age-related GH decrease.

The extent to which changes in gonadal function (menopause and andropause) contribute to adrenopause and somatopause (present in both sexes) remains uncertain. Evidence indicates that muscle size and strength, body composition and bone mass alterations, and progression of atherosclerosis relate directly to hormonal changes with aging. Hormone replacement therapy, nutritional supplementation, and regular physical activity can delay or even prevent aspects of immune function deterioration and hormone-related aging dysfunctions.[163]

Pulmonary Function

Mechanical constraints on the pulmonary system progress with age to cause deterioration in static and dynamic lung function. Pulmonary ventilation and gas exchange kinetics during the transition from rest to submaximal exercise also slow substantially.[46] In older males, aerobic training increases gas exchange kinetics to levels that approach values for fit young adults.[16] Likewise, older endurance-trained athletes demonstrate greater pulmonary functional capacity than their sedentary peers. Values for vital capacity, total lung capacity, residual lung volume, maximum voluntary ventilation, forced expiratory volume in 1 second ($FEV_{1.0}$), and $FEV_{1.0}$/forced vital capacity in athletes above age 60 remain higher than predicted from body size and higher than values for sedentary, healthy individuals.[70] *Such findings indicate that regular physical activity retards pulmonary function decline with aging.*

Cardiovascular Function

Cardiovascular function and aerobic power do not escape age-related decrements.

Aerobic Power

The precise effect of regular aerobic training on the age-related decline in aerobic power remains unresolved. Cross-sectional data reveal that $\dot{V}O_{2max}$ declines between 0.4 and 0.5 mL · kg^{-1} · min^{-1} each year (approximately 1% per year) in adult males and females, although the rate of decline accelerates in advancing age, particularly for males.[64,93,239,290] Extrapolating this average rate of decline, reduces aerobic power by age 100 to a level that equals the resting oxygen uptake. This represents a severe and unrealistic estimate because differences exist in the age-related rate of $\dot{V}O_{2max}$ decline in sedentary and active individuals.[180] The decline in $\dot{V}O_{2max}$ with advancing age occurs nearly twice as fast in sedentary compared with physically active males and females. Studies of males who varied considerably in age, aerobic power, body composition, and lifestyle revealed that maintaining relatively stable physical activity and body composition levels over time produced an average yearly decline in $\dot{V}O_{2max}$ of 0.25 mL · kg^{-1} · min^{-1}. No decline in aerobic power occurred in individuals who maintained constant training during a 10-year period.[102,165]

For most individuals, regular aerobic physical activity cannot fully prevent the age-related decline in aerobic power with aging.[62,206,219] For example, the aerobic power of 50-year-old endurance athletes decreased between 8 and 15% per decade despite continued physical activity over a 20-year period.[166] *Even with this decline, research consistently shows that physically active older males and females maintain a 10 to 50% higher aerobic power than sedentary counterparts.*

Factors other than physical activity level influence the age-related decline in $\dot{V}O_{2max}$. Heredity undoubtedly plays a crucial role, as does increased body fat and decreased skeletal muscle mass.[180] In the later decades of life, declines in maximal cardiac output and $\dot{V}O_{2max}$ contribute equally to age-related decreases in $\dot{V}O_{2max}$.[227] Aging also relates to a decline in a muscle's oxidative function from reduced synthesis of mitochondrial and other proteins.[190] Analyzing aerobic power for young and older endurance-trained males and females (**FIG. 31.14**) indicates an average 0.5 L · min^{-1} lower $\dot{V}O_{2max}$ per kg of appendicular limb muscle mass for older athletes, independent of age-associated decreases in muscle and increases in fat. No clear answer exists as to how much the lower aerobic power per kg of limb muscle mass in the older subjects reflects reduced oxygen extraction by active muscles and/or reduced oxygen delivery via decreased cardiac output and/or active muscle blood flow. Leg blood flow and vascular conductance during cycle ergometer exercise averaged 20 to 30% lower in older endurance-trained males than in younger peers at similar submaximal oxygen uptake.[169] Consequently, older athletes achieve an equivalent submaximal oxygen uptake at reduced leg blood flows by increased local oxygen extraction (arterio–mixed venous oxygen difference

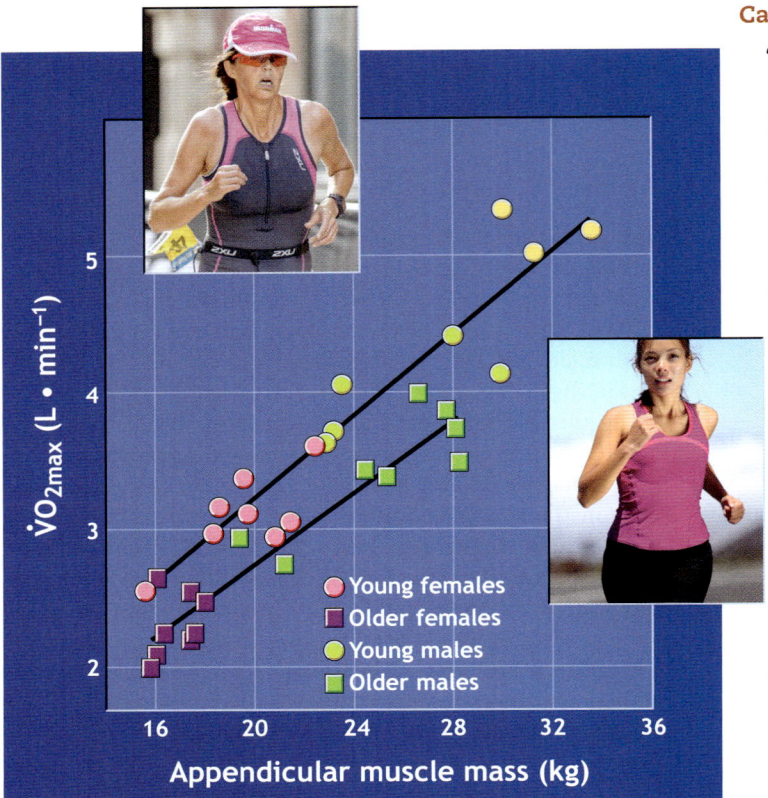

FIGURE 31.14. Relationship between appendicular muscle mass and maximum oxygen uptake ($\dot{V}O_{2max}$) for young and older trained males and females shows that aerobic power per kilogram appendicular muscle mass decreases with age in highly trained females and males. (Adapted with permission from Procter DN, Joyner MJ. Skeletal muscle mass and the reduction of $\dot{V}O_2$ in trained older subjects. *J Appl Physiol*. 1997;82:1411. ©The American Physiological Society (APS). All rights reserved. Shutterstock photos: Maridav (young female), Stefan Holm (older female).)

Cardiac Output. *Maximum cardiac output decreases with age in trained and untrained males and females because of a lower maximum heart rate and stroke volume.* The stroke volume decline reflects the combined effects of reduced left-ventricular systolic and diastolic myocardial performance. Healthy older adults often compensate for a diminished maximum heart rate with increased cardiac filling (end-diastolic volume preload), which subsequently increases stroke volume by the Frank-Starling mechanism.[63,239]

Large Artery Compliance. *Compliance of large arteries in the cardiothoracic circulation declines with age due to changes in the arterial wall's structural and nonstructural properties.*[162,186] The inability of the internal diameter of an artery to expand and recoil in response to fluctuations in intravascular pressure during the cardiac cycle associates with impaired cardiovascular function and hypertension, stroke, atherosclerosis, thrombosis, myocardial infarction, and congestive heart failure. Regular endurance activities slow or prevent the "stiffening" of the large arteries with advancing age and slow the decline in limb vasodilator capacity during healthy aging.[171,203,207,213]

Peripheral Factors. *Reduced peripheral blood flow capacity accompanies age-related decreases in muscle mass.* Decreased capillary-to-muscle fiber ratio and reduced arterial cross-sectional area produced lower blood flow to active muscle.[197]

[a-$\bar{v}O_2$ diff]) from the available blood supply. For a group of older untrained females, a diminished leg blood flow during peak exercise contributed considerably to their lower $\dot{V}O_{2peak}$ than untrained younger counterparts. The diminished leg blood flow occurred from both central (cardiac output) and peripheral (reduced vascular conductance) limitations.[170,177]

Central and Peripheral Cardiovascular Functions

Decrements in central and peripheral functions linked to oxygen transport and use influence the age-related decline in aerobic power.

Heart Rate. *A decline in maximum exercise heart rate represents a well-documented change with aging.* This age effect reflects reduced medullary sympathetic activity (depressed β-adrenergic stimulation) outflow that occurs similarly in males and females. Several longitudinal studies of elite athletes reveal that decreases in maximum heart rate from ages 50 to 70 years are smaller than typically predicted and indicative of a training response.[166,208]

Physiologic Loss with Aging: Lifestyle or Chronologic Age?

Sedentary living and unhealthy behaviors produce losses in functional capacity at least as great as the effects of aging. A high degree of trainability exists among older males and females and may not only slow but even reverse the decline in functional capacity with aging.[188] Positive training-induced adaptations in skeletal muscle structure and function, substrate metabolism, and cardiovascular function often equal those for younger individuals. Both low-intensity and higher-intensity physical activity enable older individuals to retain cardiovascular functions at a higher level than age-paired sedentary counterparts. Active middle-aged males who endurance trained over a 10-year period forestalled the usual 9 to 15% decline in aerobic power.[101] At age 55, the males maintained the same values for blood pressure, body mass, and $\dot{V}O_{2max}$ as 10 years earlier.

Endurance Performance

Comparing endurance performance of athletes of different ages provides further evidence for the impressive effects

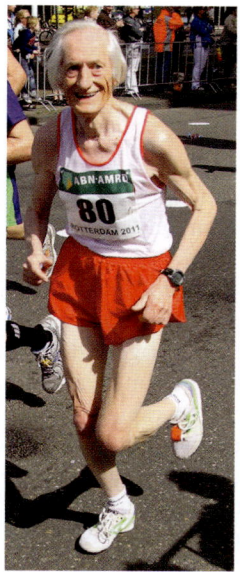

Repelsteeltje/Shutterstock

of regular physical activity on preservation of cardiovascular function throughout life. Age-group, world-record times for 50-, 100-, and 200-km runs for males and females are always recorded by the youngest athletes. For longer runs, however, older runners often excel. For example, data for the 70- to 74-year-old group marathon record is 2:54:23 (6:39 per mile pace), set in October 2018 by a 70-year-old retired computer programmer. This was the first time anyone above age 70 ran a sub–3-hr marathon (https://blog.strava.com/gene-dykes-marathon-world-record-run-17459/). In February 2013, at age 81, international track and field superstar Ed Whitlock (pictured above) obliterated the age-group world record at the Toronto Marathon with a time of 3:30:28. This was nearly 15 min faster than the previous world record for that age group, and roughly 45 min faster than that day's average marathon finisher—regardless of age. He also crushed the world record in the half-marathon, despite coming back from serious injuries. That individuals in their eighth and ninth decades of life successfully run for 12 to 14 hr affirms the tremendous cardiovascular potential in persons who continue vigorous training as they age.

Sprint Performance

FIGURE 31.15 illustrates the relationship between age and 100-m sprint performance in male and female master sprinters ages 35 to 88 years. Performance declined in both athlete groups with age, the decreases becoming more evident after age 60. Remarkable similarities exist for age-related decrements in running velocity between sexes. Running velocity during the different phases of the run declined from 5 to 6% per decade in males and 5 to 7% per decade in females. Reduced stride length and increase in contact time of the foot with the ground primarily accounted for the overall performance deterioration with age.

Body Composition

Cross-sectional studies indicate that after age 18, males and females progressively gain body weight and fat until the fifth or sixth decade of life, when total body mass decreases despite increasing body fat. This results partly from a disproportionately greater death rate among the obese in the upper age group, leaving fewer of these individuals to measure.

Most age-trend studies do not track the same subjects over time; instead, they evaluate different subjects in different age categories at the same time. From such **cross-sectional data**, one attempts to generalize about a specific individual's

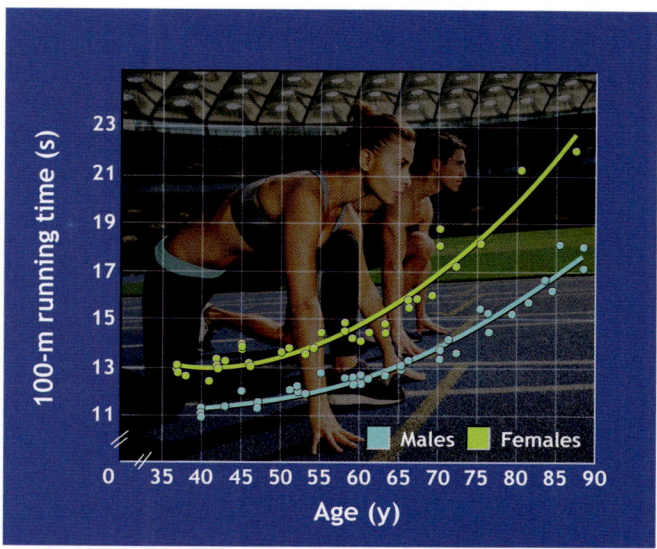

FIGURE 31.15. Individual values for 100-m sprint running by age in male and female sprinters.
(From Korhonen MT, et al. Age-related differences in 100-m sprint performance in male and female master runners. *Med Sci Sports Exerc*. 2003;35:1419. Background photo: Friends Stock/Shutterstock.)

expected age-related changes, but sometimes this creates misleading generalizations. For example, today's 70 and 80 year olds typically are shorter than 20-year-old college students. This observation does not necessarily mean that individuals become shorter with age (although this does happen to some extent).

The limited **longitudinal data** collected on the same subjects over time show trends in body fat changes similar to data from cross-sectional studies. It is not known whether body fat increases during adulthood represent a normal biologic pattern or simply reflect age-related sedentary lifestyle choices.

Longitudinal observations of individuals who maintain a physically active lifestyle support a tendency to gain fat with age. **FIGURE 31.16** shows body composition changes for 21 endurance athletes who continued to train over a 20-year period beginning at age 50. Despite maintaining a relatively constant body mass during the prolonged period of training, gains occurred in body fat and abdominal obesity while FFM declined. The roughly 3% body fat unit increase per decade paralleled increases in waist girth. The magnitude of increase in body fat and decrease in FFM, while discouraging to some, averages at least 20% less than reported for nonathletes. Habitual endurance physical activity confers at least some "protection" from the effects of aging on body composition.

Bone Mass

Osteoporosis poses a major problem with aging, particularly among postmenopausal females. This condition produces bone mass loss as the aging skeleton demineralizes and becomes

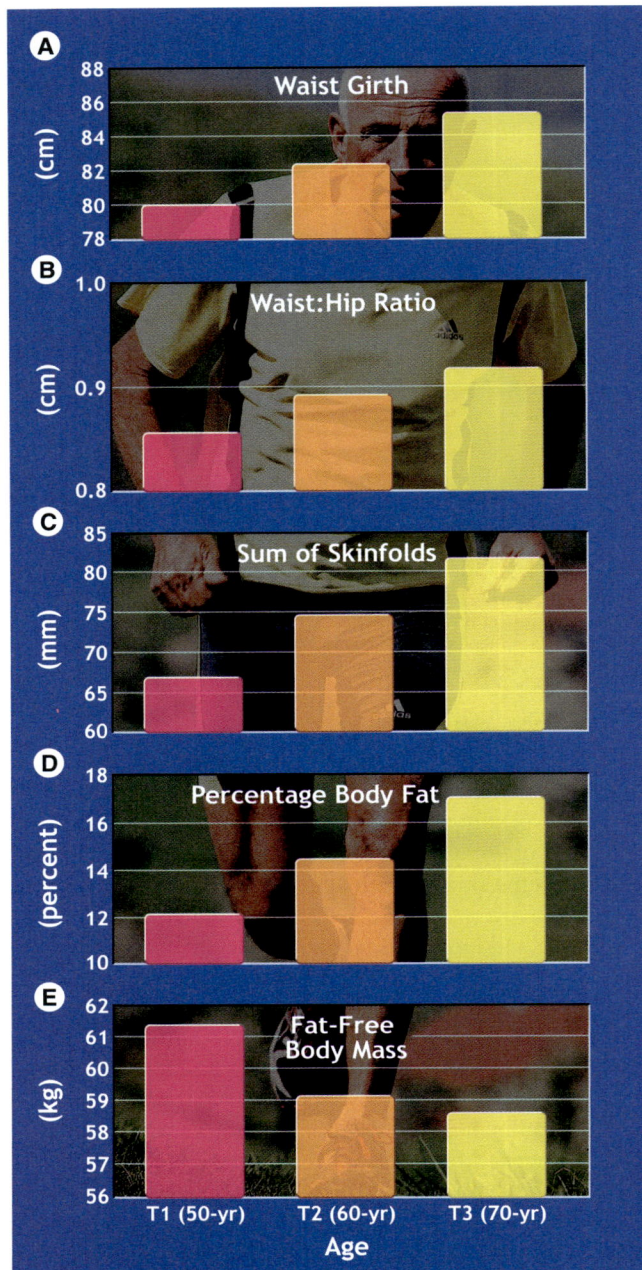

FIGURE 31.16. Changes in **(A)** waist girth, **(B)** waist-hip girth ratio, **(C)** sum of skinfolds, **(D)** percentage body fat, and **(E)** fat-free body mass for 21 endurance athletes who continued to train over a 20-year period, starting at age 50.
(From Pollock ML, et al. Twenty-year follow-up of aerobic power and body composition of older track athletes. *J Appl Physiol*. 1997;82:1508. ©The American Physiological Society (APS). All rights reserved. Background photo: Lisa-S/Shutterstock.)

porous. Bone mass can decrease by 30 to 50% in persons above age 60. As emphasized in Chapter 2, regimens of weight-bearing activity and resistance exercise not only retard bone loss but also often increase bone mass in older males and females.[5] In postmenopausal females, regular physical activity augments hormone replacement therapy to increase total bone mineral density and preserve these gains.[71,108]

Trainability and Age

Exercise training improves physiologic responses at any age. Several factors affect the magnitude of the training response, including initial fitness status, genetics, and specific type of training.

Research over the past 50 years has modified the classic view relating diminished improvements from physical activity with aging (**FIG. 31.17**).

The current view maintains that over a broad age range, improvements in physiologic function result from an appropriate training stimulus, often at a rate and magnitude free from age effects. Older males and females and younger adults show similar adaptations in muscle fiber size, capillarization, and glycolytic and respiratory enzymes to specific endurance or resistance-training exercise. These adaptations emerge most readily with relatively intense but even, short-duration bouts that continuously adjust to training improvements (see Chapter 22).

Aerobic Training: Gender Difference Among Older Adults

Aerobic exercise training for healthy older males enhances the heart's systolic and diastolic properties and increases aerobic power to the same relative extent (15 to 30%) as in younger adults.[33,55,185] Research has evaluated the contribution of training-induced increases in stroke volume and a-$\bar{v}O_2$ differences to aerobic fitness improvements in healthy older males and females. Nine months of endurance training increased $\dot{V}O_{2max}$ by 19% in males and 22% in females (**TABLE 31.2**). These values represent the higher-end improvement typically observed for younger adults. Gender differences emerged in certain aspects about the training response. For males, improved

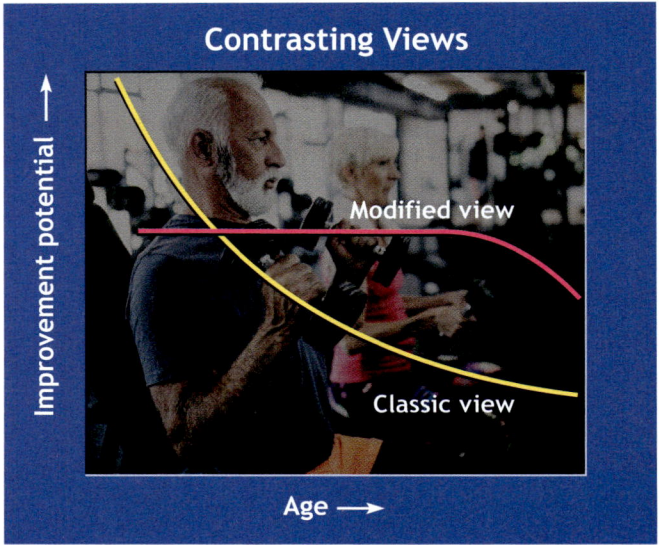

FIGURE 31.17. Contrasting traditional (classic) versus current (modified) views relating diminished improvements from physical activity with aging.
(Background photo: NDAB Creativity/Shutterstock.)

aerobic power was associated with a 15% larger maximum stroke volume (corresponding cardiac output increase represented two thirds of the $\dot{V}O_{2max}$ increase) and 7% greater maximum a-$\bar{v}O_2$ diff (representing one third of the $\dot{V}O_{2max}$).

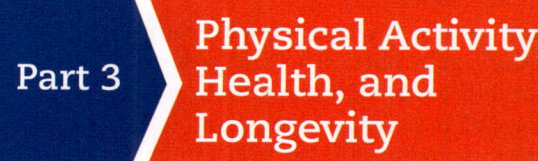

TABLE 31.2 Effects of 9 months of endurance training on $\dot{V}O_{2max}$ in older males and females

For the females, the a-$\bar{v}O_2$ diff explained the total $\dot{V}O_{2max}$ increase, with no change in left-ventricular performance at maximal exercise. This indicates that training-induced increases in aerobic power for older females depend on peripheral adaptations in trained muscle and suggests that sex hormones influence gender-related adaptations to endurance training.[105] The lack of a stroke volume increase among older females with training may result from three factors[197–199]:

1. Blunting of the normal plasma volume increase
2. Decreasing cardiopulmonary baroreflex sensitivity
3. Estrogen deficiency–related decrease in vascular compliance (i.e., increased vascular stiffness)

These apparent gender differences in physiology do not impair endurance performance in older females, as reflected by a relative consistency in male-female differences in ultra-distance running performance over a broad age range.

Summary

1. Physiologic and performance capabilities usually decline after age 30. Many factors, including diminished physical activity level, affect the rate of decline.
2. Regular physical activity and training enable older persons to retain higher levels of functional capacity, notably cardiovascular and muscular function.
3. Biologic aging relates to changes in three hormonal systems: hypothalamic-pituitary-gonadal axis, adrenal cortex, and GH-IGF axis.
4. Four factors are crucial when evaluating physiologic and performance differences between children and adults: exercise economy, FFM, anaerobic power, and anabolic hormone levels.
5. The primary cause of age-associated reduction in muscle strength between ages 25 and 80 is a 40 to 50% reduction in muscle mass from a loss of motor units and muscle fiber atrophy.
6. Considerable plasticity exists in physiologic, structural, and performance characteristics among older individuals; this plasticity enables marked and rapid strength improvement with training into the ninth decade of life.
7. A physically active lifestyle affects neuromuscular functions positively at any age and possibly slows the age-related decline in cognitive performance associated with speed of information processing.
8. Adult male and female $\dot{V}O_{2max}$ declines approximately 1% per year.
9. Physically active older males and females maintain a higher aerobic power than their sedentary peers at any age.
10. Sedentary living causes losses in functional capacity at least as great as aging itself.
11. Regular physical activity improves physiologic function at any age; initial fitness, genetics, and the type and amount of training control the magnitude of change.
12. Active older athletes average at least 20% less body fat and 20% more FFM than their nonathletic peers; this suggests that habitual physical activity confers some protection from the negative effects of aging on body composition.

Part 3 — Physical Activity, Health, and Longevity

Physical activity may not necessarily represent a "fountain of youth," yet the preponderance of evidence shows that regular physical activity retards the decline in functional capacity associated with typical aging and accompanying disuse.

Physical Activity, Health, and Longevity

In one of the first studies suggesting that sport and regular physical activity prolong life, former Harvard University oarsmen exceeded their predicted longevity by 5.1 years per man.[77] Other early studies showed similar but more modest lifespan extensions.[13] Methodologic problems in this research included inadequate record keeping, small sample size, improper statistical procedures to estimate expected longevity, and no accounting for socioeconomic status, body type, tobacco use, and family background.

Subsequent research contradicted these findings and showed that participation in athletics as a young adult did *not* ensure good health and longevity later in life.[173] *Overall, the overwhelming current scientific evidence maintains that increased physical activity and fitness throughout life confers significant health and longevity benefits.*[25,183,214,232,243] A continuing longitudinal study of the health consequences of different fitness levels in 25,341 males and 7080 females revealed that low aerobic fitness was a more important predictor of all-cause mortality than any other risk factors.[26] In addition, inverse risk gradients emerged across categories of low, moderate, and high fitness, with a lower death rate among moderately fit individuals compared to the low-fitness group. The least fit males and females were nearly twice as likely to die from all causes as most fit counterparts during an 8-year follow-up. *Low fitness emerged as a more powerful risk factor for death than high blood pressure, elevated cholesterol, obesity, and family history.*

Enhanced Quality of Life: The Harvard Alumni Study

The lifestyles and physical activity habits of 17,000 Harvard alumni who entered college between 1916 and 1950 provide evidence that *moderate* aerobic physical activity equivalent to jogging 3 mi daily at a pace slightly faster than fast walking promotes good health and adds several years to life. The results of long-term studies show four direct benefits from regular physical activity:

1. Counters the life-shortening effects of cigarette smoking and excess body weight
2. Reduces death rate by one half in individuals with hypertension who exercise regularly
3. Counters genetic tendencies toward early death with a lifestyle of regular physical activity; reduces death risk by 25% for individuals with one or both parents who died before age 65 (a significant health risk)
4. Decreases mortality rate by 50% for physically active males whose parents live beyond age 65

Persons who do more physical activity further reduce their risk of dying from any cause.[44,158] Males who walked nine or more miles each week, for example, had a 21% lower mortality rate than males who walked three miles or less. Life expectancy was higher for males who exercised at the equivalent of light sport activity than sedentary males. Life expectancy of Harvard alumni increased steadily from a weekly activity energy expenditure of 500 kcal up to 3500 kcal, a value equivalent to 6 to 8 hr of strenuous physical effort. The active males lived an average of 1 to 2 years longer than their sedentary classmates. Weekly activity beyond 3500 kcal conferred no additional health or longevity benefits.

Vigorous Physical Activity and Longevity

The Harvard alumni study examined only the total amount of weekly physical activity, not its intensity, in relation to heart disease and mortality. Further research from the same population revealed that vigorous regular activity exerts the greatest effect on extending life[117] and reducing major chronic disease risk, including cardiovascular disease.[41,142] Males who expended at least 1500 kcal weekly in vigorous activity during the 20-year study—equivalent to 6 metabolic equivalents (METs) or more (e.g., jogging or walking briskly, lap swimming, singles tennis, fast cycling, or intense yard chores for 1 hr, performed three or four times weekly)—had a 25% lower death rate than the most sedentary males. The most active males showed the greatest life expectancies, largely from reduced deaths from cardiovascular disease. The benefits of vigorous activity also extended to overweight smokers. Risk associated with a sedentary lifestyle equaled the risk of smoking one pack of cigarettes daily or being 20% overweight. Subsequent research with these males and others[8] showed that the activity equivalent of a 1-hr brisk walk 5 days weekly or a vigorous workout at least once weekly cut stroke risk almost in half; brisk walking for 30 min 5 days weekly reduced stroke risk by 24%.[121,122] Other stroke-protective activities included stair climbing or participating in moderate activities such as gardening, dancing, and bicycling. An intensive poststroke conditioning program also facilitates the stroke survivor's recovery of motor skills.

Epidemiologic Evidence

A critique of 43 studies examining the relationship between physical inactivity and coronary heart disease concluded that reduced regular activity contributes to heart disease in a cause-and-effect manner; the sedentary person has about twice the risk of developing heart disease as the most active individual.[167] The strength of the association between lack of physical activity and heart disease risk equals that for hypertension, cigarette smoking, and high serum cholesterol. This makes physical inactivity the greater heart disease risk because more people lead sedentary lifestyles than possess one or more of the other primary risk factors. *The life-protecting benefits of regular physical activity link more with preventing early mortality than extending life span.* Surprisingly, only light-to-moderate regular walking, gardening, stair climbing, and household chores produce health benefits for previously sedentary middle-age and older males and females.[22,107,123,179] These sedentary individuals represent the largest percentage of the population at greatest risk for chronic disease.

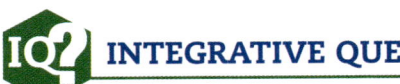

INTEGRATIVE QUESTION

Discuss when physical activity benefits a person's health profile even if the intensity does not produce a training effect?

Regular Moderate Physical Activity Benefits

A sedentary lifestyle represents an independent and powerful predictor of coronary heart disease risk and mortality, so encouraging the most sedentary 25% of the American adult population to become only moderately active would yield substantial public health benefits.[23,37,81,115,176,220] Even moderate activity such as walking reduces the level of diabetic, hypertensive, and cholesterol medication required by patients.[242] For postmenopausal females, walking briskly for 2.5 hr weekly (about 30 min per day 5 days per week) reduced heart disease risk by 30%—a reduction comparable to that achieved with cholesterol-lowering drugs—regardless of race, age, or how much the females weighed.[138] Females who did the most activity reduced risk by 63%. To further assess the health-related benefits of regular physical activity, research assessed the effect of miles walked daily on overall mortality rate in 707 non-smoking males ages 61 to 81 years.[73] An inverse relationship between distance walked and mortality emerged after adjusting for overall physical activity and other risk factors. Males who walked less than 1 mi daily had a cumulative death incidence in 7 years that required 12 years for the most active males who walked at least 2 mi daily. Over 7 years, 43.1% of the less active males died compared with 21.5% of the most active walkers.

Corroborative research compared the leisure-time physical activity in 333 patients ages 25 to 74 years who had a first heart attack and 503 control subjects without a heart attack selected randomly and matched for age and gender.[125] After adjustments for the heart disease risks of age, smoking, diabetes, and hypertension, regular walkers reduced cardiac arrest risk by 73%. Those who gardened regularly reduced risk by 66% compared with sedentary peers. Walking or gardening for more than 60 min·wk^{-1} reduced risk similarly to intense leisure-time physical activity. The benefits of walking also applied to females who regularly walked 3 mph or faster for at least 3 hr weekly; cardiac arrest risk decreased up to 40% below the risk for sedentary females. Risk was reduced by one half for females who walked briskly (≥3.0 mph) for 5 hr weekly.[137] These findings complement and further support physical activity recommendations from the CDC (www.cdc.gov/physicalactivity/) and ACSM (greatist.com/fitness/acsm-releases-new-exercise-guidelines) to accumulate 30 min or more of moderate-intensity activity on most days of the week.

Influence of Physiologic Factors

In addition to simple physical activity data, physiologic measures like low cardiorespiratory fitness level (including low exercise capacity, low $\dot{V}O_{2max}$, low heart rate recovery, and failure to achieve target heart rate) provide a strong independent predictor of increased risk for cardiovascular disease and all-cause mortality.[40,58,241]

One study directly examined aerobic fitness, rather than verbal or written reports of physical activity habits, and heart disease risk in more than 13,000 males and females observed over an average of 8 years.[24] To isolate the effect of physical fitness, the study accounted for cigarette smoking, high cholesterol and blood sugar levels, hypertension, and family history of heart disease. Based on age-adjusted death rates per 10,000 person-year, the least-fit group averaged more than three times the death rate of the most-fit individuals. The greatest health benefits emerged for the group rated just above the most sedentary category. For men, the decrease in death rate from the least-fit category to the next category exceeded 38 (64.0 vs. 25.5) deaths per 10,000 person-year. Enhanced aerobic fitness benefits females to a similar if not greater extent.[153] For every increased score of 1 MET in exercise capacity, the risk of death from all causes decreased by 17%.[138] To move from the most sedentary category to the next highest group—the change that produced the greatest health benefits—requires only such moderate-intensity effort as walking briskly for 30 min twice weekly.

Studies of Finnish males complement the above findings.[100] Aerobic power and leisure-time physical activity showed an inverse, graded, independent association with risk for acute myocardial infarction. After adjusting for genetic effects and other familial factors that predict mortality, current aerobic fitness and physical activity level still conferred significant protection from death.[113] Physical fitness also counters the negative impact of existing disease. For example, an inverse and independent relationship emerges between aerobic power and incidence of fatal and nonfatal cardiovascular events and all-cause mortality in male and female hypertensives followed over 16.5 years.[160]

TABLE 31.3 summarizes 30 years of research relating physical activity level or physical fitness to chronic disease or medical conditions. Clearly, a strong inverse association exists between regular physical activity and level of aerobic fitness and all causes of death. *Moderate-intensity regular activity substantially reduces the risk of dying from heart disease, cancer, and other causes.*

TABLE 31.3 Effects of regular physical activity and/or increased physical fitness on risk for chronic disease conditions

Structured Physical Activity Unnecessary

Researchers monitored two groups of 116 sedentary males and 119 females ages 35 to 60 years during a 2-year randomized clinical trial.[54] One group spent 20 to 60 min vigorously swimming, stair stepping, walking, or biking at a fitness center up to 5 d·wk^{-1}. The other group incorporated 30 min a day of "lifestyle" activities such as extra walking, raking leaves, stair climbing, walking around the airport while waiting for a plane, most days of the week. The lifestyle participants also learned cognitive and behavioral strategies to increase daily physical activity. For each program, intervention included 6 months intensive activity followed by an 18-month maintenance period. After 24 months, *both* groups showed similar improvements in physical activity level, cardiorespiratory fitness, systolic and diastolic blood pressure, and body fat percentage. These findings reinforce the conclusion that the health-derived benefits from regular physical activity do not require highly structured or vigorous exercise participation.

Summary

1. Vigorous physical activity early in life contributes little to increased longevity or health in later life. A physically active lifestyle throughout life confers significant health benefits.
2. Regular, moderate physical activity counters the life-shortening effects of coronary heart disease risks that include cigarette smoking and excess body weight.

3. A sedentary person runs almost twice the risk of developing heart disease as the most active individuals.
4. Coronary heart disease risk from sedentary living equals that for hypertension, cigarette smoking, and high serum cholesterol.
5. The life-protecting benefits of regular physical activity relate more to preventing early mortality than to extending overall lifespan.
6. A moderate amount of regular physical activity substantially reduces risk of dying from heart disease, cancer, and other medically related maladies.
7. The greatest health benefits emerge when a person alters a sedentary lifestyle and becomes just moderately physically active.
8. Strategies that modify lifestyle toward increased daily physical activity beneficially alter factors associated with coronary heart disease risk.

Deaths (%) from Heart Disease by Ethnicity, Race, and Sex

Race or Ethnic Group	Deaths	Males	Females
American Indian or Alaskan Native	18.3	19.4	17.0
Asian American or Pacific Islander	21.4	22.9	19.9
Black (Non-Hispanic)	23.5	23.9	23.1
White (Non-Hispanic)	23.7	24.9	22.5
Hispanic	20.3	20.6	19.9
All	23.4	24.4	22.3

Background photo: Peto Laszlo/Shutterstock

Part 4 — Cardiovascular Diseases

Cardiovascular diseases (CVDs) constitute a group of heart and blood vessel disorders and include the following related conditions:

- **Coronary heart disease (CHD; also known as atherosclerosis):** Disease of blood vessels supplying the myocardium
- **Cerebrovascular disease:** Disease of blood vessels supplying the brain
- **Peripheral artery disease**: Disease of blood vessels supplying the arms and legs
- **Rheumatic heart disease**: Damage to the myocardium and heart valves from rheumatic fever, caused by streptococcal bacteria
- **Congenital heart disease**: Malformations of heart structure existing at birth
- **Deep vein thrombosis and pulmonary embolism**: Blood clots in the leg veins, which can dislodge and precipitate serious life-threatening conditions when they travel to the heart and lungs

Heart attacks and strokes are usually acute events caused mainly by a vascular blockage that prevents blood from flowing to the heart or brain. The most common reason for a heart attack or stroke includes a fatty deposit build-up on the inner walls of the blood vessels that supply these tissues. Strokes can also be caused by bleeding from a blood vessel in the brain or from blood clots. The major causes of heart attacks and strokes usually involve the presence of a combination of risk factors such as tobacco use, unhealthy diet and obesity, physical inactivity and hypertension, diabetes and hyperlipidemia, and excessive use of alcohol.

CHD represents the number-one cause of death globally; more people die annually from this malady than from all other causes. Globally, estimates indicate that 18 million people died from CHD in 2019, representing 31% of all adult deaths. Over three quarters of these deaths occurred in low-income and middle-income countries. The United States records the most CHD-related deaths—roughly 48% of all deaths, of which 85% were from heart attack and stroke. This accounts for 1 in 4 deaths. Someone has a heart attack every 36 s. Moreover, every 60 s, at least one person in the United States dies from a heart disease–related event (https://theheartfoundation.org/heart-disease-facts-2/).

The average age at the first heart attack is 65.6 years for males and 72.0 years for females. For every American who dies from cancer, almost two die from CHD.

Death rates for females lag about 10 years behind men, but the gap has rapidly closed for females who smoke; for them, heart disease is now the leading cause of death.

Heart Attack Warning Signs: Males versus Females

Males and females often experience an impending heart attack differently. Whereas heart attack symptoms such as crushing chest pain that radiates down an arm are often similar for females and males, many females report vague or even silent symptoms that are often ignored and not recognized as heart attack warning signs. The list below presents common heart attack symptoms for males and females.

1. **Males and females:** Uncomfortable pressure, fullness, squeezing, or pain in the center of the chest lasting more than a few minutes; sensation of a vise being tightened through the chest
2. **More common in females but also experienced by men:** Pain spreading to the shoulders, neck, or arms, ranging from mild to intense; described as pressure, tightness, burning, or a heavy weight; located in the chest, upper abdomen, neck, jaw, or inside the arms or shoulders;

gradual or sudden, and may wax and wane before becoming more intense

3. **Mostly females:** Stomach pain often mistaken as heartburn, the flu, a stomach ulcer, or menstrual discomfort
4. **Males and females:** Chest discomfort with lightheadedness, fainting, stress-related or anxiety-related sweating (more common in females), nausea, or shortness of breath
5. **Males and females:** Anxiety, nervousness, or cold, sweaty skin
6. **Females:** Fatigue and feeling extreme "tiredness in the chest," even when sitting or lying down
7. **Males and females:** Paleness or pallor often in the late afternoon
8. **Males and females:** Increased or irregular heart rate
9. **Males and females:** Extreme anxiety, fear or feelings of impending doom

Heart Attack versus Cardiac Arrest

Heart attack's precipitating factors include the following:

1. Blockage in one or more arteries supplying the heart, thus restricting myocardial blood supply
2. Sudden spasms or constriction in one of the coronary vessels, causing part of the heart muscle to die (necrosis) from lack of oxygen (anoxia)

In contrast to a heart attack, cardiac arrest is characterized by irregular neural-electrical transmission within the myocardium, which produces chaotic, unregulated beating or fibrillation in the heart's ventricular chambers. The survival rate statistics are not encouraging for an out-of-hospital cardiac arrest.

CHD Links to Cellular Level Alterations

CHD involves degenerative changes in the intima, or inner lining, of the larger myocardial arteries. Damage to arterial walls begins as a multifactorial, largely immunologically mediated, **inflammatory response** to injury, primarily due to hypertension, cigarette smoking, infection, homocysteine, elevated cholesterol, or free radical action. One response triggers the chemical modification of various compounds, which includes the oxidation of low-density lipoprotein cholesterol (LDL-C). This initiates a complex series of changes that produce lesions that bulge into the vessel lumen or protrude outward into the arterial wall. Lesions initially take the form of fatty streaks, the first signs of atherosclerosis. With further inflammatory damage from continued lipid deposition and proliferation of smooth muscle cells and connective tissue, the vessel congests with lipid-filled plaques, fibrous scar tissue, or both. Progressive occlusion gradually reduces blood flow capacity, with ensuing myocardial ischemia (reduced oxygen supply).

Toll-like Receptor 2

In 2009, a team of English scientists identified the trigger for arterial plaque inflammation and tissue breakdown.[291] The specialized molecule, **toll-like receptor 2 (TLR-2)**, resides on the surface of an immune cell. When TLR-2 recognizes harmful molecules and cells, its role switches the immune cell into "attack mode" to protect the body. TLR-2 also can switch on immune cells when the body encounters stress. In addition, bacteria may activate the TLR-2 molecule, increasing the risk of plaques bursting to precipitate a stroke and heart attack.

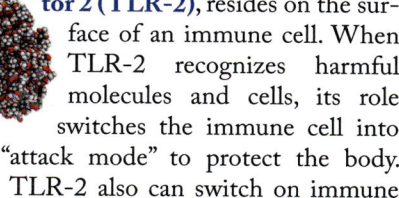
StudioMolekuul/Shutterstock

The research breakthrough about TLR-2 also demonstrated that antibodies could block its trigger mechanism. Sections of atherosclerotic carotid arteries were sampled from 58 patients following their stroke. The arterial tissues, decomposed with enzymes, formed a suspension of single cells in liquid. The researchers analyzed the liquid after 4 days and observed that the cells had produced an unusually large amounts of inflammatory molecules and enzymes known to damage arterial structures. The cells were then grown with several different antibodies to block different receptors and other molecules involved in the inflammation process. Blocking TLR-2 using an antibody dramatically reduced production of inflammation-derived molecules and enzymes.

 See the animation "Acute Inflammation" at Lippincott Connect.

C-Reactive Protein and Arterial Inflammation

About half of persons with heart disease have normal or just moderately elevated cholesterol levels, which has led researchers to consider other factors in the heart disease process. Guidelines from major health agencies propose an important role for inflammation testing to judge whether persons need aggressive treatment to protect their hearts and vascular system. Mounting evidence indicates that painless chronic low-grade arterial inflammation, including that in the coronary arteries, is central to every stage of atherosclerotic disease and a major trigger for heart attack—more substantial even than high blood cholesterol. The inflammation produces a heart attack by weakening blood vessel walls, making plaque burst, and interfering with substances that increase myocardial circulation. **C-reactive protein (CRP)**, a plasma protein discovered in 1930 by American internist and microbiologist William Smith Tillett (1892–1974) and American virologist and epidemiologist Thomas Francis (1900–1969) (www.clinchem.org/content/55/2/209.long), is produced by the liver and adipocytes to help fight vascular injury, inflammation, and infection. Levels of this protein rise dramatically during both acute and more chronic inflammatory reactions in the body. This compound may be just as important an independent coronary artery disease risk factor as elevated LDL cholesterol. Numerous causes of an elevated CRP include acute and chronic conditions and can be infectious or noninfectious in etiology. However, markedly elevated CRP levels most often associate with an infectious cause. Trauma also can cause elevations in CRP (alarm response). More modest elevations tend to be associated with a broader spectrum of etiologies, ranging from sleep disturbances to periodontal disease.

CRP values are reported in either $mg \cdot dL^{-1}$ or $mg \cdot L^{-1}$. When used for cardiac risk stratification, CRP levels ≤ 1 $mg \cdot dL^{-1}$ are considered low risk; levels between 1 and 3 $mg \cdot dL^{-1}$ are considered moderate risk; and a level ≥ 3 $mg \cdot dL^{-1}$ is considered high risk for CVD.[292]

CRP Interpretation Levels

1. **Less than 0.3 $mg \cdot dL^{-1}$**: Normal (level seen in most healthy adults)
2. **0.3 to 1 $mg \cdot dL^{-1}$**: Normal or minor elevation (seen in obesity, pregnancy, depression, diabetes, common cold, gingivitis, periodontitis, sedentary lifestyle, cigarette smoking, and genetic polymorphisms)
3. **1.0 to 10.0 $mg \cdot dL^{-1}$**: Moderate elevation (systemic inflammation such as rheumatoid arthritis, systemic lupus erythematosus or other autoimmune diseases, malignancies, myocardial infarction, pancreatitis, bronchitis)
4. **≥ 10.0 $mg \cdot dL^{-1}$**: Marked elevation (acute bacterial infections, viral infections, systemic vasculitis, major trauma)
5. **≥ 50.0 $mg \cdot dL^{-1}$**: Severe elevation (acute bacterial infections)

Certain medications, such as nonsteroidal anti-inflammatory drugs (NSAIDs), will falsely decrease CRP levels. Statins, as well, have falsely reduced CRP levels. Recent injury or illness can elevate levels, particularly when using this test for cardiac risk stratification. Magnesium supplementation can decrease CRP levels.

In chronic CVDs, CRP frequently rises when arteries begin to accumulate plaque. High CRP levels also associate with the development of hypertension,[187] a finding that suggests that hypertension is part of an inflammatory disorder. Individuals with high CRP levels (3.0 to 4.0 $mg \cdot dL^{-1}$) are four times more likely to experience impaired blood flow to the heart. They also are twice as likely to die from heart attacks and strokes as individuals with high cholesterol—a finding that explains why some persons with low cholesterol develop heart disease or why lowering cholesterol can fail to prevent serious heart problems. Strategies to lower CRP include weight loss, abstinence from cigarette smoking, consuming a healthful diet, and regular physical activity (e.g., combined aerobics with resistance training).[204]

Medications That Positively Impact Blood Lipids

StudioMolekuul/Shutterstock

Medications affect blood lipids, with the statin category the most prescribed drug worldwide:

1. Bile acid sequestrants (e.g., cholestyramine resin and colestipol hydrochloride), which bind or sequester cholesterol-rich bile in the gastrointestinal tract and prevent its gut resorption.
2. Fibric acid derivatives (e.g., gemfibrozil, probucol, clofibrate), which lower triacylglycerols and LDL-C 5 to 20%, and elevate HDL-C an average 6% yearly.
3. Popular statins include the most prescribed simvastatin (see inset illustration), followed by atorvastatin, pravastatin, rosuvastatin, and lovastatin, which inhibit the HMG-CoA reductase enzyme to control cholesterol synthesis by cells and increase liver's LDL-C receptors to remove 18 to 55% LDL-C from serum. The good news—raising HDL-C by 34 $mg \cdot dL^{-1}$ during a 5-year gemfibrozil therapy trial reduced heart attacks, strokes, and death by 24% in patients with initially low HDL-C levels.

Vulnerable Plaque: Difficult to Detect Yet Lethal

Vulnerable plaque, a soft type of metabolically active, unstable plaque, does not necessarily produce significant coronary artery narrowing but tends to fissure and burst. The rupture of unstable fatty plaques exposes blood to thrombogenic compounds. This triggers a cascade of chemical events that culminate in a clot formation or **thrombus**, leading to a myocardial infarction and possible death. A sudden, complete obstruction in a coronary vessel frequently occurs in arteries that previously had only mild-to-moderate obstructions (approximately 70% blockage). Arterial blockage often occurs before the vessel has narrowed enough to produce symptoms of angina or electrocardiogram (ECG) abnormalities or to require revascularization procedures (e.g., coronary bypass surgery or balloon angioplasty). Acute disruption and rupture of arterial plaque provides a plausible explanation for sudden death from acute physical exertion or emotional stress in middle-aged males with coronary artery disease who may not have experienced prior symptoms compared with sudden death under resting conditions. The beneficial effects of cholesterol-lowering strategies on heart disease risk do not always improve coronary blood flow.[126] A reduction in overall blood cholesterol may, however, improve vulnerable plaque stability and reduce the likelihood of future arterial plaque rupture.

The Vulnerable Patient

Recognizing the role of vulnerable plaque has introduced a new way of looking at cardiovascular medicine and risk assessment. Rupture-prone plaques are not the only vulnerable plaque forms. All types of atherosclerotic plaque with high likelihood of rapid progression and thrombotic complications are now considered vulnerable. Vulnerable blood (prone to thrombosis) and a vulnerable myocardium (prone to fatal arrhythmia) also play a role in future outcomes. Consequently, the term "*vulnerable patient*" may be more appropriate for identifying individuals with high likelihood of developing a traumatic cardiac event. Researchers have quantified methods for cumulative risk assessment to identify the vulnerable patient, which may include variables based on plaque type, blood characteristics, and myocardial vulnerability. Recently developed assays, imaging techniques (e.g., computed tomography [CT] and magnetic resonance imaging), noninvasive electrophysiological tests (for vulnerable myocardium), and specialized catheters (to localize and characterize vulnerable plaque) in combination with future genomic and proteomic techniques will guide the search to identify the vulnerable patient.

Vascular Degeneration Begins Early in Life

Landmark studies of atherosclerosis in young American soldiers killed in Korea in the 1950s showed advanced heart lesions in males whose ages averaged 22 years.[56] These surprising findings focused attention on the possible childhood origins of atherosclerosis. Researchers now know that fatty streaks and clinically significant fibrous plaques develop rapidly during adolescence through the third decade of life. In children and adolescents with metabolic syndrome, CRP levels are also elevated.[65] Autopsies of 93 young people aged 2 to 39 years, most of whom died from trauma, revealed that fatty streaks and fibrous plaques in the aorta and coronary arteries appear early and progress in severity with aging.[19] Body mass index, systolic and diastolic blood pressure, total serum cholesterol, triacylglycerols, and LDL-C were strongly and positively related to the extent of vascular lesions in the deceased young people (high-density lipoprotein cholesterol [HDL-C] related negatively). History of cigarette smoking magnified the vascular damage.[178] As the number of risk factors increased, so did the severity of atherosclerosis in these asymptomatic individuals. Analyses of microscopic qualities of coronary atherosclerosis in 760 teenagers and young adults who died from accidents, suicide, and murder indicated that many had arteries so clogged that they could have had a myocardial infarction.[141] Two percent of those ages 15 to 19 and 20% of those 30 to 34 had advanced plaque formation, the blockages considered most likely to break off and precipitate a heart attack or stroke. Collectively, the autopsy findings support the wisdom of primary prevention of atherosclerosis through risk factor identification and intervention early in childhood or adolescence.

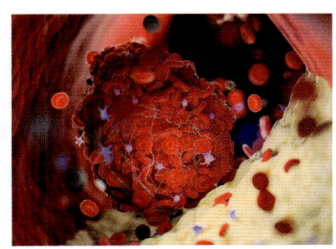
SciePro/Shutterstock

FIGURE 31.18 shows the progressive occlusion of an artery from a buildup of calcified fatty substances in atherosclerosis. The first overt sign of atherosclerotic change occurs when lipid-laden macrophage cells cluster under the endothelial lining in the artery to form a bulge or fatty streak (Fig. 31.18A). Over time, proliferating smooth muscle cells migrate to the inner endothelial layer and accumulate to narrow the lumen (center) of the artery. A thrombus forms and plugs the artery, depriving the myocardium of normal blood flow and oxygen supply. When the thrombus blocks one of the smaller coronary vessels, a portion of the heart muscle dies (**necrosis**) and the person has a heart attack (**myocardial infarction [MI]**).

The saphenous vein from the leg is the most commonly used bypass vessel during the **coronary artery bypass procedure (CABP)** to repair damaged vessels. CABP involves sewing the graft vessel to the coronary artery beyond the narrowing or blockage, with the other end of the vein attached to the aorta. Medications (statins) lower total and LDL cholesterol, and daily low-dose aspirin (81 mg) can reduce post-CABP artery narrowing beyond the insertion site of the graft. CABP surgical mortality averages 5 to 10%. MIs are caused by blockage in one or more arteries that supply the heart, throttling myocardial blood supply or causing sudden spasms (constrictions) of a coronary vessel that triggers necrosis from oxygen deprivation. MI contrasts with cardiac arrest from irregular neural-electrical transmission within the myocardium. The latter results from chaotic, unregulated beating in the heart's upper (atrial fibrillation) or lower chambers (ventricular fibrillation).

If coronary artery narrowing progresses to produce brief periods of inadequate myocardial perfusion, the person may experience temporary chest pains, termed **angina pectoris** (see Chapter 32). These pains usually appear during exertion because physical activity increases myocardial blood flow demand. Anginal attacks provide painful, dramatic evidence of the importance of adequate myocardial oxygen supply.

CHD Risk Factors

Research over the past 60 to 70 years has identified various personal characteristics, behaviors, and environmental factors linked to increased CHD susceptibility. Many of these factors relate strongly to CHD risk, but the associations do not necessarily imply a causal relationship (e.g., male-pattern baldness).[131] In some instances, it remains unclear whether risk-factor modification offers effective disease protection.

Until definite proof emerges, it seems prudent to assume that either elimination or reduction of one or more of the modifiable risk factors will reduce the likelihood of developing CHD and cumulative disability during later years.

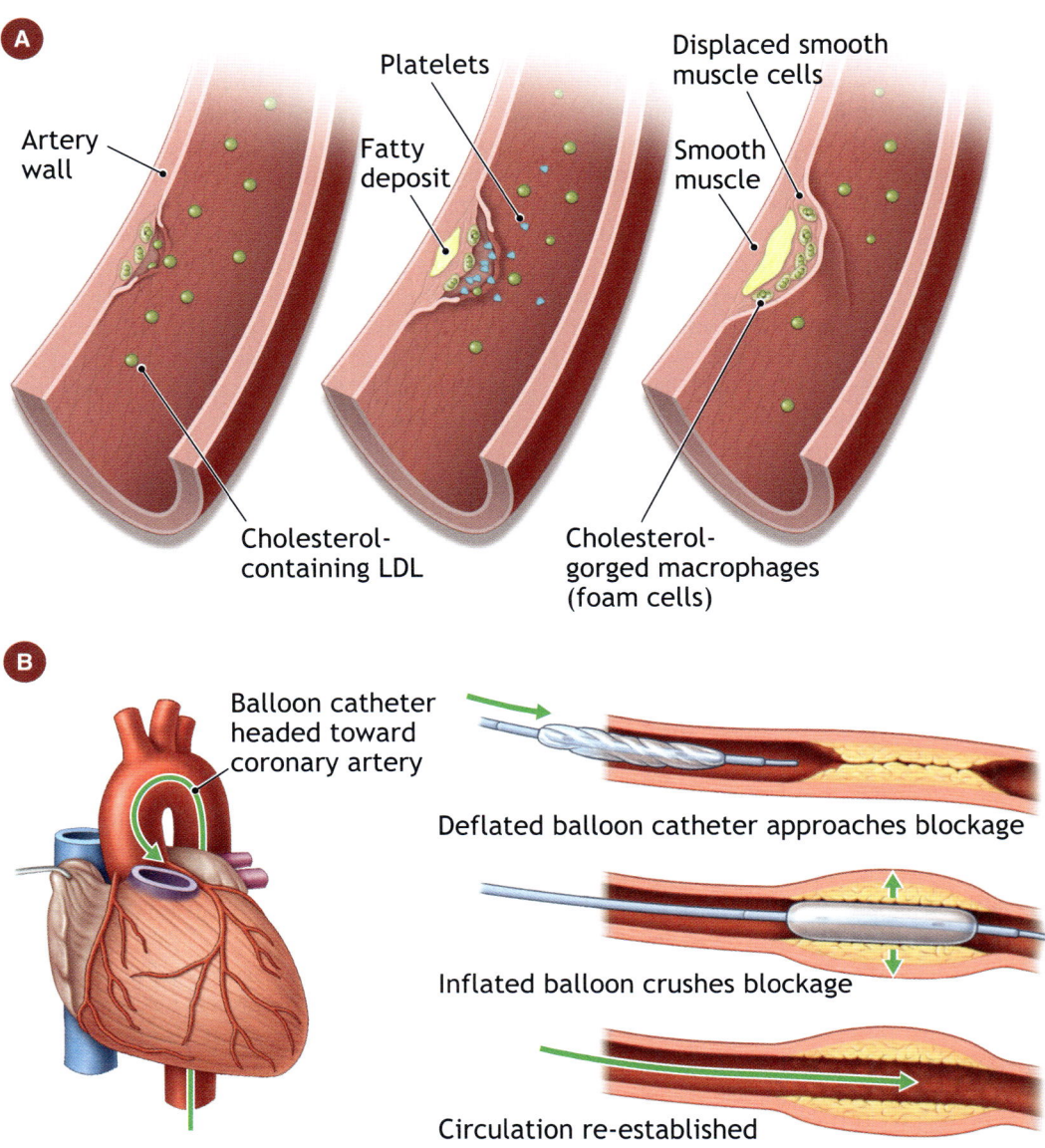

FIGURE 31.18. (A) Stages in coronary artery deterioration from fatty substances that roughen the vessel's lumen, eventually forming a thrombus above the plaque and blocking blood flow through the artery, often producing a myocardial infarction, or heart attack. **(B)** Coronary artery bypass graft creates a new "transportation route" during an angioplasty procedure around the blocked region to allow blood flow delivery of oxygen and nutrients to the heart muscle. LDL, low-density lipoprotein. (B: Reprinted with permission from Moore KL, et al. *Clinically Oriented Anatomy*. 8th Ed. Philadelphia: Wolters Kluwer, 2018.)

For example, a radical heart risk–reduction program that includes a plant-based diet, limiting lipid intake to no more than 10% of total calories, and including regular physical activity, stress-management training, and support meetings substantially reduces subsequent heart attack rate and other adverse heart events such as bypass operations and angioplasty procedures.[156] In contrast, patients in conventional care steadily worsened over the same 5-year period. The inset table on the next page lists both modifiable and unmodifiable risk factors most frequently implicated in CHD.

Age, Gender, and Heredity

Age represents a CHD risk factor largely from its association with hypertension, elevated blood lipid levels, and glucose intolerance. After age 35 for males and age 45 for females, the chances of dying from CHD increase progressively and dramatically.

Modifiable Risk Factors	Unmodifiable Risk Factors
• Cigarette smoking • Diabetes mellitus • Non-nutritious diet • ECG abnormalities • Elevated blood lipids • Elevated homocysteine • Excessive body fat • High serum uric acid • Hypertension • Personality and behavior patterns • Poor education • Pulmonary dysfunction • Sedentary lifestyle • Sleep apnea • Tension and stress	• Age • Family history • Gender • Ethnic background • Male-pattern baldness from high androgen levels

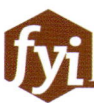

Congenital Heart Disease Causes and Effects

Congenital heart disease includes heart defects present at birth. An estimated 1% of babies born in the United States each year have these congenital defects:

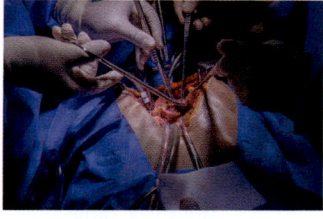

Peerayut Chan/Shutterstock

- Heart valve disorders, which include aortic valve narrowing (restricts blood flow)
- Hypoplastic (underdeveloped) left heart syndrome
- Openings found in the walls between the chambers and between major blood vessels leaving the heart (e.g., including ventricular and atrial septal defects, patent ductus arteriosus), and other serious ventricular septum, compromised pulmonary artery blood flow, and aortic abnormalities

Congenital heart disease in infants can be successfully treated with surgery, catheter procedures, medications, and in the most severe cases heart transplant. Cardiovascular specialists advocate an optimal strategy to provide for immediate and long-term cardiovascular benefits to those who survive early-onset birth defects and acquired potential heart failure and future cardiovascular disease— this also includes much needed early intervention physical activity programs in children and adolescents.

Source:
van Deutekom AW, Lewandowski AJ. Physical activity modification in youth with congenital heart disease: a comprehensive narrative review. *Pediatr Res*. 2021;89:1650.

In contrast to the beliefs of some who still adhere to the antiquated notion that CVD is primarily a man's illness, the following facts indicate otherwise (www.cdc.gov/heart disease/women.htm)[83,139,223]:

- Heart disease is the leading cause of death for females in the United States.
- The same number of females and males die each year of heart disease in the United States.
- Heart disease is the leading cause of death for African American and White females in the United States. Among Hispanic females, heart disease and cancer cause roughly the same number of deaths each year. For American Indian or Alaska Native and Asian or Pacific Islander females, heart disease occurrence is second only to cancer.
- About 5.8% of all White females, 7.6% of Black females, and 5.6% of Mexican American females have CHD.
- Almost two thirds of females who die suddenly of CHD have no previous symptoms.

Females account for about half of the coronary artery disease deaths in the United States, yet they receive only about one third of the nearly 1 million annual intervention procedures. To close this gap, the American Heart Association (AHA) recommends gender-specific guidelines that encourage doctors to make greater use of cardiac imaging tests in females, which include single photon emission CT and stress echocardiography[92] (see Chapter 32). The AHA also recommends special attention to females with diabetes, who have a particularly high heart disease risk, as do females with metabolic syndrome and polycystic ovary syndrome (a hormonal disorder among females of reproductive age). The pattern of coronary artery blockage may also differ between sexes. Males exhibit discrete blockages at distinct focal points, making them more amenable to stenting, while females show a more diffuse blockage that occupies a longer segment of the vessel. Heart attacks that strike at an early age tend to run in families. Familial predisposition relates to a genetic role in determining heart disease risk.

The following sections examine (1) cigarette smoking, (2) hypertension, (3) diabetes, (4) blood lipid abnormalities, (5) obesity, and (6) physical inactivity related to CHD. These modifiable factors represent the "big six" heart disease risks proposed by the AHA. Each exists as a potent, independent CHD risk that can improve considerably with lifestyle modification.

INTEGRATIVE QUESTION

How can risk factor modification affect changes in CHD risk?

Cigarette Smoking

Cigarette smoking, either active or passive through environmental exposure, directly increases CHD risk. Smokers experience twice the risk of death from heart disease as nonsmokers. Smokers with diabetes and hypertension experience even greater risk than individuals without these conditions. The CDC estimates that every cigarette smoked shortens a smoker's life by 7 min. CHD risk increases the more one smokes or receives passive exposure, the deeper one inhales, and the stronger the cigarette's tar and noxious byproduct content. The increasing death rate from heart disease among females in the United States almost parallels their increased cigarette use.[293]

Smokers between ages 30 and 40 years have five times as many heart attacks as nonsmokers in the same age range. Moreover, smokers run a five times greater risk for stroke than nonsmokers, and those who smoke one pack or more per day are 11 times more likely to experience a specific type of a sudden, deadly stroke most common in younger males and females. Surprisingly, more smokers die from CHD than from lung cancer.

Smoking risk usually remains independent of other risk factors. If additional risk factors exist, then smoking accentuates their influence. Cigarette smoking facilitates heart disease through its potentiating effect on serum **lipoproteins**; individuals who smoke have lower levels of HDL-C than nonsmokers. When smokers quit, the HDL-C and heart disease risk return to nonsmoker levels over time. A frightening statistic predicts that by the year 2030, smoking will become the world's single leading cause of death and disability, notwithstanding obesity's continuing its meteoric increase.

Hypertension

The American College of Cardiology and the AHA define two levels of hypertension: Stage 1 is defined as a pressure at or above 130/80 mm Hg, and stage 2 is defined as a blood pressure at or above 140/90 mm Hg. In Chapter 32, we discuss blood pressure classification levels and behavioral factors responsible for increasing hypertension levels around the world.

One of every four or five people experiences chronic, abnormally high blood pressure sometime during life. Uncorrected hypertension can precipitate heart failure, heart attack, stroke, and kidney failure. High blood pressure is often called the "silent killer" as it progresses without any overt symptoms or warning signs. Modification of lifestyle behaviors can lower high blood pressure; these modifications include weight loss, regular physical activity, cessation of smoking, and reducing salt intake. *On a population level, lowering systolic blood pressure just 2 mm Hg reduces death from stroke by 6% and heart disease by 4%.*

Unfortunately, in more than 90% of individuals, hypertension's underlying cause(s) remain unknown. Prescription drugs that either reduce fluid volume or decrease peripheral resistance to blood flow effectively treat high blood pressure.

Diabetes

Diabetics are up to four times more likely to develop CVD from multiple risk factors usually coincident with the diabetic condition. These risk factors include four conditions:

1. **Obesity:** Represents a major risk factor for CVD that strongly associates with insulin resistance, which may provide the mechanism by which obesity leads to CVD.
2. **Physical inactivity:** A modifiable risk factor for insulin resistance and CVD.
3. **Hypertension:** Positively correlates with insulin resistance in diabetes. For a person with both hypertension and diabetes the CVD risk doubles.
4. **Atherogenic dyslipidemia:** Often-called **diabetic dyslipidemia** in type 2 diabetes, relates to insulin resistance characterized by high triacylglycerol levels (hypertriglyceridemia) and high levels of small LDL particles and low HDL levels (see next section).

Blood Lipid Abnormalities

Serum cholesterol levels in adults have declined substantially in the United States over the past 50 years, a decline that coincides with a decreased national incidence of CHD. Despite this support for the effectiveness of public health programs geared to lowering heart disease risks, nearly 30% of adults still require intervention for high cholesterol levels.[98] Unfortunately, data from the CDC indicate that approximately 60% of persons with high cholesterol levels did not know those levels were high. Of those who knew, only 14% were taking a cholesterol-lowering drug. An abnormally high blood lipid level, or **hyperlipidemia**, plays an important role in atherosclerosis genesis.

Cholesterol and Triacylglycerol Recommendations

FIGURE 31.19 shows the rate of increase in death risk from CHD related to total serum cholesterol. The inset table presents the AHA (www.heart.org/) serum cholesterol and lipoprotein and triacylglycerol level classifications for adults. Recommendations also include that individuals above age 20 have a fasting "lipoprotein profile" every 5 years (9 to 12 hr following the last meal and without liquids or pills).

Cholesterol guidelines focus both on total cholesterol and its lipoprotein components based on findings concerning effects of the powerful cholesterol-lowering statin drugs on heart health (i.e., reduced risk of heart attack, bypass surgery, plaque growth in coronary vessels, angioplasty).[27,118,151,184]

Early treatment becomes crucial because of a strong association between high serum cholesterol as a young adult and CVD in middle age. A cholesterol level of 200 mg·dL^{-1} or lower is usually deemed desirable, although risk for a fatal heart attack begins to rise at 150 mg·dL^{-1}. A cholesterol level of 230 mg·dL^{-1} increases heart attack risk to about twice that of 180 mg·dL^{-1}, and 300 mg·dL^{-1} increases the risk fourfold. For triacylglycerol, 150 to 199 mg·dL^{-1} is considered as

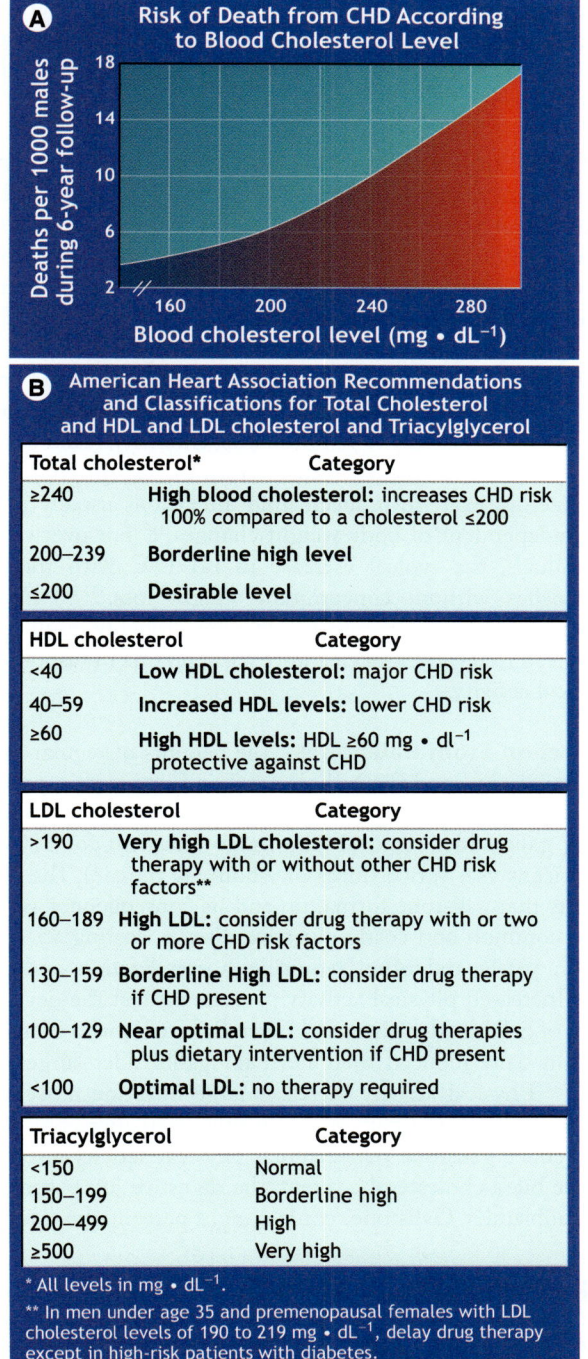

FIGURE 31.19. (A) Death risk from coronary heart disease (CHD) related to total serum cholesterol level in middle-aged males. (B) The American Heart Association recommendations and adult classifications for serum cholesterol, lipoproteins, and triacylglycerol levels. HDL, high-density lipoprotein; LDL, low-density lipoprotein.

an upper-limit normal level, with 200 to 499 considered high. The latter requires modifications in physical activity, diet, and possibly drug intervention if accompanied by other CHD risk factors.

Lipids do not circulate freely in blood plasma; they combine with a carrier protein to form lipoproteins. Lipoproteins are composed of a hydrophobic cholesterol core and a coat of free cholesterol, phospholipid, and regulatory protein (**apolipoprotein [Apo]**). **TABLE 31.4** lists the four different lipoproteins, their approximate gravitational densities, and percentage composition in the blood. *Serum cholesterol consists of a composite of the total cholesterol contained in each of the different lipoproteins.* Discussions commonly refer to hyperlipidemia, but the more meaningful focus addresses the different types of hyperlipoproteinemia.

TABLE 31.4 Approximate composition of serum lipoproteins

Cholesterol distribution among various lipoproteins provides a more powerful heart disease risk predictor than total blood cholesterol. Specifically, elevated HDL-C levels relate causally with a lower heart disease risk even among individuals with total cholesterol below 200 mg · dL^{-1}. Overwhelming evidence links high LDL-C and apolipoprotein (B) levels with increased CHD risk.[116] A more effective evaluation of heart disease risk than either total cholesterol or LDL-C levels divides total cholesterol by HDL-C. *A ratio greater than 4.5 indicates high heart disease risk; a ratio of 3.5 or lower represents a more desirable risk level.*

LDL-C, synthesized in the liver, and very low-density lipoprotein cholesterol (VLDL-C) transport lipids to cells, including the smooth muscle walls of arteries. Upon oxidation, LDL-C participates in artery-clogging, plaque-forming atherosclerosis by stimulating monocyte-macrophage infiltration and lipoprotein deposition.[194] LDL-C's surface coat contains the specific apolipoprotein (Apo B) that facilitates cholesterol removal from the LDL-C molecule by binding to LDL-C receptors of specific cells. Prevention of LDL-C oxidation, in contrast, slows CHD progression. In this case, any potential benefit of dietary antioxidants such as vitamins C and E and β-carotene, within a food matrix and not as isolated dietary supplements, on heart disease risk may lie in their ability to blunt LDL-C oxidation (see Chapter 2).[48,51,76,112,152]

LDL-C targets peripheral tissue and contributes to arterial damage. HDL-C is also produced in the liver. Its levels relate to genetic factors.[93] HDL-C facilitates reverse cholesterol transport: it promotes surplus cholesterol removal from peripheral tissues, including arterial walls, for transport to the liver for bile synthesis and subsequent excretion. The apolipoprotein A-1 (Apo A-1) in HDL-C activates **lecithin acetyl transferase**. This enzyme converts free cholesterol into cholesterol esters, facilitating cholesterol removal from lipoproteins.[157]

Importance of LDL Particle Size Assessment

Clinicians employ various tests to assess heart disease risk, in particular LDL particle size. A blood sample containing a larger proportion with small LDL particles with high density is more atherogenic (up to 300% greater heart disease risk) than larger particles that appear less dense or "fluffy" for any given level of LDL. This risk may relate to increased deposition in the plaque-forming subendothelial arterial space, an increased uptake by macrophages, and increased susceptibility to oxidation, both early steps in plaque formation; it also may result from decreased clearance from reduced affinity for the LDL receptor. Small dense LDL particles associate with high triacylglycerol levels, so the assessment of this blood lipid (value ≥ 140 mg $\cdot$ dL^{-1} represents increased risk) may prove useful in targeting individuals with small, dense LDL particles. Effective treatments include physical activity, weight loss, niacin supplements, and **fibrates** (medication class that lowers blood triacylglycerol levels).

Factors That Affect Blood Lipids

Six behaviors that favorably affect cholesterol and lipoprotein levels include the following six variables:

1. Weight loss
2. Regular aerobic physical activity (independent of weight loss)
3. Increased dietary intake of water-soluble fibers (fibers in beans, legumes, and oat bran)
4. Increased dietary intake of polyunsaturated-to-saturated fatty acid ratio and of monounsaturated fatty acids
5. Increased dietary intake of unique polyunsaturated fatty acids in fish oils (omega-3 fatty acids) and eliminating *trans*-fatty acids
6. Reduced alcohol consumption

Four variables that adversely affect cholesterol and lipoprotein levels include the following:

1. Cigarette smoking
2. Diet high in saturated fatty acids and preformed cholesterol and *trans*-fatty acids
3. Emotionally stressful situations
4. Oral contraceptives

Specific Effects of Physical Activity

Short-Term Effects. Reaching the threshold that changes blood lipid and lipoprotein levels in a single physical activity session requires considerable physical activity. For example, healthy trained males needed to expend 1100 kcal in one physical activity bout to elevate HDL-C, 1300 kcal of physical activity to lower LDL-C, and 800 kcal physical activity to decrease triacylglycerol levels.[59]

Long-Term Effects. A single physical activity session produces only transient favorable changes in lipid and apolipoprotein concentrations, yet the change persists with exercising at least every other day.[45]

Low-Density Lipoprotein Cholesterol. Exercising regularly usually produces only small reductions in LDL-C level when controlling for serum cholesterol-related factors of body fat and dietary lipid and cholesterol intake. Regular physical activity may improve the quality of this circulating lipoprotein by promoting a less oxidized form of LDL-C to reduce atherosclerosis risk.[218] In addition, regular aerobic activity increases the success of dietary efforts to favorably alter high-risk lipoprotein profiles.[200]

High-Density Lipoprotein Cholesterol. Endurance athletes usually maintain relatively high HDL-C levels, while favorable alterations occur for sedentary males and females of all ages who engage in regular moderate-to-vigorous aerobic activity.[52] To some extent, physical activity intensity and duration exert independent effects in modifying specific CHD risk factors. In general, duration exerts the greatest effect on HDL-C, while intensity most favorably modifies blood pressure and waist girth.[240] A favorable change in lipoprotein profile does not necessarily require effort intensity reach a level to improve cardiovascular fitness. With the exception of triacylglycerols, exercise-induced lipid alterations usually progress independent of body weight changes.[119] For overweight individuals, the typical increase in HDL-C with training diminishes without concomitant weight loss.[149,212] Favorable activity-related lipoprotein changes probably result from enhanced triacylglycerol clearance from plasma in response to physical activity.

Protection From Gallstones. The benefits of regular aerobic activity on modifying cholesterol and lipoprotein profiles extend to protection against painful gallstones and accompanying gallbladder removal (the usual treatment for 500,000 Americans yearly, two thirds of whom are female). The NIH reports that gallstone formation and its consequences are the most common and costly digestive disease, costing $5 to $7 billion yearly and often requiring hospitalization and surgery. Increased physical activity protects against the development of gall bladder disease.[111] Overall, females who exercised 30 min daily reduced their need for gallbladder surgery by 31%.[124] Physical activity increases large intestine movement and improves blood glucose and insulin regulation; both factors reduce gallstone risk. Regular physical activity also may reduce bile's cholesterol content, the digestive juice stored in the gallbladder. Gallstones contain eight percent cholesterol.

Other Influences

Even trained endurance athletes exhibit considerable variability in HDL-C levels, with some elite runners' values approaching the median value for the general population. No single factor—nutrition, body composition, or training status—distinguishes runners with high HDL-C values from runners with lower values. This suggests that genetic factors exert a strong influence on the blood lipid profile. In fact, a specific gene produces **endothelial lipase (EL)**, an enzyme that may affect HDL-C production.[97,101] Activating this gene increases EL synthesis, which may lower HDL-C and subsequently increase cardiovascular risk.

Standard resistance training exerts little or no effect on serum triacylglycerol, cholesterol, or lipoprotein levels. From a dietary perspective, substituting soy-derived protein (and other plant-based protein) for animal protein sources improves the cholesterol and lipoprotein profile, particularly in persons with high blood cholesterol levels.[14] A moderate daily alcohol intake—2 oz/59.1 mL of 90-proof alcohol, three 6 oz/177.4 mL glasses of wine, or slightly less than three 12 oz/355 mL beers—reduces an otherwise healthy person's risk of heart attack and stroke independent of their physical activity level.[42,86,182] The heart-protective benefit of alcohol consumption also applies to individuals with type 2 diabetes.[224] The mechanism for the benefit remains elusive, yet a moderate alcohol intake increases HDL-C and its subfractions HDL_2 and HDL_3. The polyphenols in red wine may inhibit LDL-C oxidation, thus blunting a critical step in plaque formation.[150] Moderate wine intake also associates with more heart-healthy dietary choices, with a positive impact on plasma lipids. Excessive alcohol consumption offers no lipoprotein benefit and increases liver disease and cancer risk.

Lipoprotein(a). Lipoprotein(a) [Lp(a)] represents a protein particles formed in the liver when two distinct apolipoproteins unite. Lp(a) structurally resembles LDL-C but contains an additional unique apolipoprotein(a) coat. Heredity determines elevated Lp(a) levels, which occur in approximately 20% of the population. The independent risk for atherosclerosis, thrombosis, and acute MI increases when Lp(a) levels exceed 25 to 30 mg·dL^{-1} with raised LDL-C levels.[20] Dietary changes and either short-term or long-term physical activity exert little or no effect on serum Lp(a) concentrations.[82,87,88,135]

Dietary Fiber, Insulin, and CHD Risk. *Insulin resistance and consequent hyperinsulinemia act as independent CHD risk factors.*[181]

The combined effects of CHD risk factors account for approximately 50% of the observed variability in insulin resistance and hyperinsulinemia within the population. The question then is what other factors might contribute to excessive insulin output and, by implication, increased CHD risk. Perhaps total lipid or saturated fatty acid intake and dietary carbohydrates are causal factors. Dietary fiber also may play a key role in optimizing insulin response.[132] For example, dietary fiber reduces insulin secretion by slowing the rate of nutrient digestion and glucose absorption following a meal.

A low-fiber meal with its inherently high glycemic index stimulates more insulin secretion than a high-fiber meal of equivalent carbohydrate content. Dietary fiber can serve a dual role in heart disease prevention by attenuating the insulin response to a carbohydrate-containing meal and reducing the tendency to accumulate body fat from insulin's facilitatory role in lipid synthesis. Excessive body fat increases insulin resistance, which ultimately leads to hyperinsulinemia.

Immunologic Factors. An immune response likely triggers plaque development within arterial walls. During this process, mononuclear immune cells produce proteins called **cytokines**, some of which stimulate plaque buildup whereas others inhibit plaque formation. Regular physical activity can stimulate the immune system to inhibit agents that facilitate arterial disease. For example, 2.5 hr of weekly physical activity for 6 months decreased cytokine production that aids in plaque development by 58%, while cytokines that inhibit plaque formation increased by nearly 36%.[195]

Hyperhomocysteinemia

Homocysteine, a highly reactive, sulfur-containing amino acid, forms as a by-product of methionine metabolism found in high protein-rich animal products. Researchers in the 1960s and 1970s described three different inborn errors of homocysteine metabolism that involved B-vitamin enzymes. High blood and urine levels of homocysteine are common to all three disorders of the afflicted individuals, and half of these persons developed arterial or venous thrombosis by age 30. Researchers postulated that moderate elevation of homocysteine in the general population predisposes individuals to atherosclerosis in a manner similar to elevated cholesterol concentration. A near lockstep association occurs between plasma homocysteine levels and heart attack and mortality in males and females.[72,84,130,161,227,234,238,244]

High homocysteine levels help explain why some persons with low-to-normal cholesterol levels contract heart disease. In the presence of other conventional CHD risks such as smoking and hypertension, synergistic effects magnify

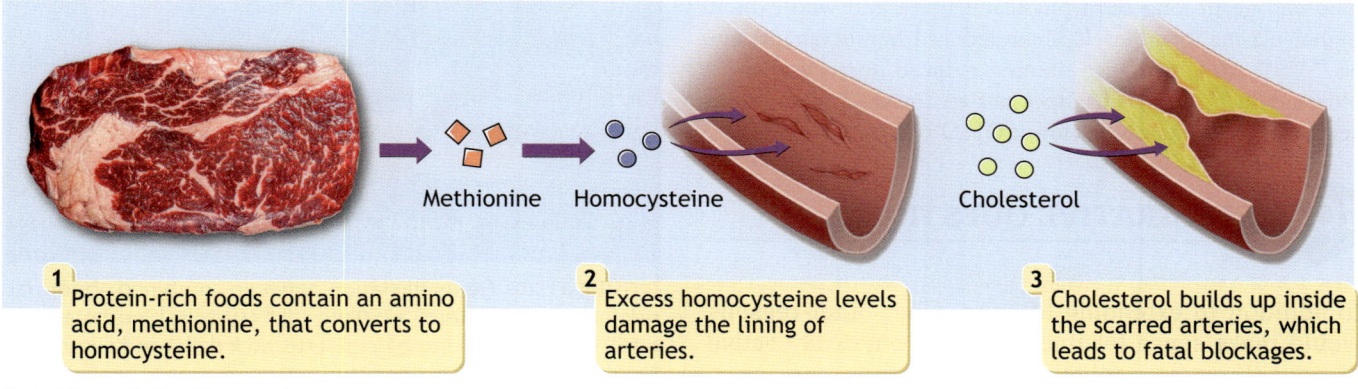

1. Protein-rich foods contain an amino acid, methionine, that converts to homocysteine.
2. Excess homocysteine levels damage the lining of arteries.
3. Cholesterol builds up inside the scarred arteries, which leads to fatal blockages.

Photo: Mironov Vladimir/Shutterstock

the negative impact of homocysteine.[136,221,245] This metabolic abnormality occurs in nearly 30% of CHD patients and 40% of patients with cerebrovascular disease. Excessive homocysteine causes blood platelets to clump, fostering blood clots and deterioration of smooth muscle cells that line the arterial wall, as depicted in the illustration on the previous page. Chronic homocysteine exposure eventually scars and thickens arteries and provides a fertile medium for circulating LDL-C to initiate damage. Resting homocysteine levels exert an independent increased risk on a continuum for vascular disease similar to that of smoking and hyperlipidemia. A powerful multiplicative interaction effect also emerges in the presence of other risks, particularly cigarette smoking and hypertension. Persons in the highest quartile for homocysteine levels experience nearly twice the risk of heart attack or stroke of those in the lowest quartile. Why some persons accumulate homocysteine remains uncertain, but evidence points to a deficiency of B vitamins (B_6, B_{12}, and particularly folic acid); lifestyle factors of cigarette smoking and coffee and high meat intake also associate with elevated homocysteine concentrations.[147,155,194,205,211]

No clear standard currently exists for normal or desirable homocysteine levels. Most evidence indicates that the current "normal range" of 8 to 20 $mmol \cdot L^{-1}$ of plasma is too high. Evidence suggests as little as 12 $mmol \cdot L^{-1}$ can double heart disease risk. Until recently, debate has focused on whether normalizing homocysteine reduces risk of arterial occlusive disease that precipitates heart attack and stroke. Consequently, little is known regarding whether an elevated homocysteine level is simply a CHD risk factor or an actual CHD cause (not an effect).[140,154] A double-blind, randomized, controlled trial determined whether once-daily high doses of folic acid (2.5 mg), vitamin B_6 (25 mg), and vitamin B_{12} (0.4 mg) over a 2-year period lowered homocysteine levels and reduced recurrent stroke risk in patients with ischemic stroke.[217] Reduction of total homocysteine averaged 2.0 $mmol \cdot L^{-1}$ greater in the group that received the high-dose supplement than in the group receiving lower doses. The moderate homocysteine reduction produced no effect on vascular outcomes during a 2-year follow-up.

Research on the effects of physical activity on homocysteine levels remains inconclusive. Intense training may increase homocysteine levels accompanied by changes in vitamin B_{12} and folate status.[53,79,80] Other data indicate that individuals who engage in long-term physical activity, and who exhibit higher plasma folate levels, show reduced homocysteine levels.[78,110,159] Also, resistance training reduced homocysteine in older adults.[229] The AHA does not recommend taking folic acid or other B vitamins to lower CHD risk.

IQ? INTEGRATIVE QUESTION

In addition to extending lifespan, what other reasons would make sense for maintaining a physically active lifestyle throughout middle and older age?

CHD Risk Factor Interactions

Many risk factors interact with each other and with CHD. **FIGURE 31.20** shows that the presence of three primary CHD risk factors in the same person magnify individual effects. With one risk factor, a 45-year-old man's chance of CHD during the year averages twice the risk for a man without risk factors. With three risk factors, this man's chance for angina, heart attack, or sudden death increases to nearly 10 times the level for those without risk factors.

Some researchers posit that the five major modifiable cardiovascular risk factors—cigarette smoking, physical inactivity, **diabetes mellitus**, hypertension, and hypercholesterolemia—account for only about 50% of individuals who subsequently develop CHD. Other novel markers and nontraditional risk factor candidates have been investigated to increase cardiovascular risk predictability (**TABLE 31.5**).[29,230]

TABLE 31.5 Novel risk factors that independently associate with atherosclerotic vascular disease

Several reports directly challenge the "only 50%" claim for the aforementioned five risk factors.[295] Analysis of data from 14 randomized clinical trials (N = 122,458) and three observational studies (N = 386,915) showed that 80 to 90% of patients who developed clinically significant CHD and more than 95% of patients who experienced a fatal CHD event had at least one of the five traditional major risk factors, including overweight/obesity. These findings may even underestimate the true extent of the relationship, given the self-report design of the observational studies and number of patients unaware or not diagnosed as having risk factors at the time of evaluation. Such findings have enormous public health implications for targeting a large segment of the population at risk

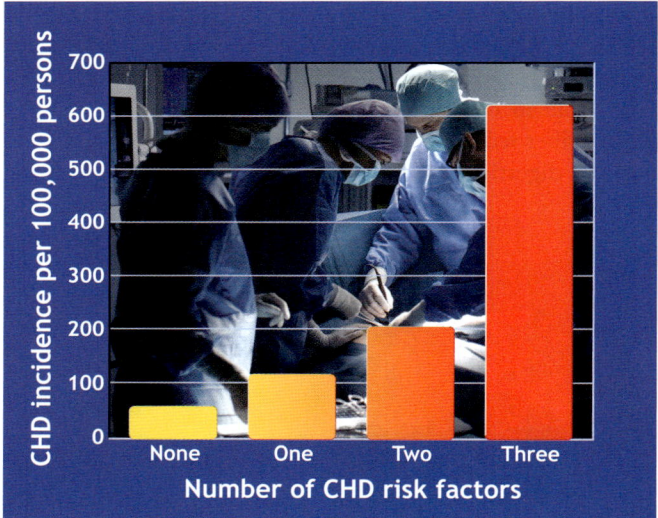

FIGURE 31.20. General relation between combined abnormal risk factors (cholesterol ≥250 $mg \cdot dL^{-1}$; systolic blood pressure ≥160 mm Hg; smoking ≥1 cigarette pack daily) and coronary heart disease (CHD) incidence.
(Background photo: Gorodenkoff/Shutterstock.)

of developing CHD. Smoking is arguably the single most important modifiable and preventable CVD risk factor and one of the strongest predictors of premature CHD. Equally important CHD predictors include obesity and physical inactivity.

Many CHD risks link in common to behavioral patterns; they become influenced by similar and identical interventions. For example, regular physical activity exerts a positive influence on obesity, hypertension, type 2 diabetes, stress, and elevated blood lipid profile. *No other modifiable behavior exerts such a potent positive effect for the greatest number of persons, causing many to argue that regular physical activity constitutes the most important behavioral intervention to reduce CHD.*

Risk Factors in Children

The frequent occurrence of multiple CHD risk factors in young children emphasizes the need for early CHD interventions to reduce atherosclerosis risk later in life.[216,241] Risk factors assessed in childhood and adolescence associate with carotid artery thickness with aging. As with adults, the association between body fat and serum lipid levels becomes readily apparent in overfat children; the fattest children usually have higher serum cholesterol and triacylglycerols levels. General adiposity and visceral adipose tissue also relate to unfavorable hemostatic factors that increase CHD morbidity and mortality in adulthood.[60] Of 62 overfat children ages 10 to 15 years, only one child had just one CHD risk factor.[18] Of the remaining children, 14% had two risk factors, 30% three, 29% four, 18% had five, and the remaining five children, or 8% had six. A subsample then enrolled in a 20-wk program to evaluate the effects on the risk profile from either a program of diet plus behavior change therapy (A) or regular physical activity plus diet plus behavior change therapy (B). No changes resulted in multiple risk reduction in either the control group (C) or the group receiving only diet plus behavior treatment. In contrast, children undergoing exercise plus diet plus behavior therapy dramatically reduced multiple risks (**FIG. 31.21**). Clearly, a supervised program of moderate food restriction and increased physical activity with behavior modification reduces CHD risk factors in obese adolescents. A growing body of research supports the addition of regular physical activity to augment risk factor intervention effectiveness.[294]

Autopsy evidence and prevalence of CHD risk factors among preadolescents and adolescents indicate that heart disease origins begin in childhood. Usually, the most sedentary children who watch the most TV have more body fat and a higher BMI than more physically active peers.[15] School-based programs that increase the level of daily physical activity, reduce risk factors, and increase students' knowledge about risk factors and benefits of physical activity can produce a long-term positive effects on activity habits and overall health.[104,222] Regular physical activity upgrades (or stabilizes) a poor risk factor profile. School curricula at all grade levels (especially kindergarten and elementary grades) should encourage more physically active lifestyles.

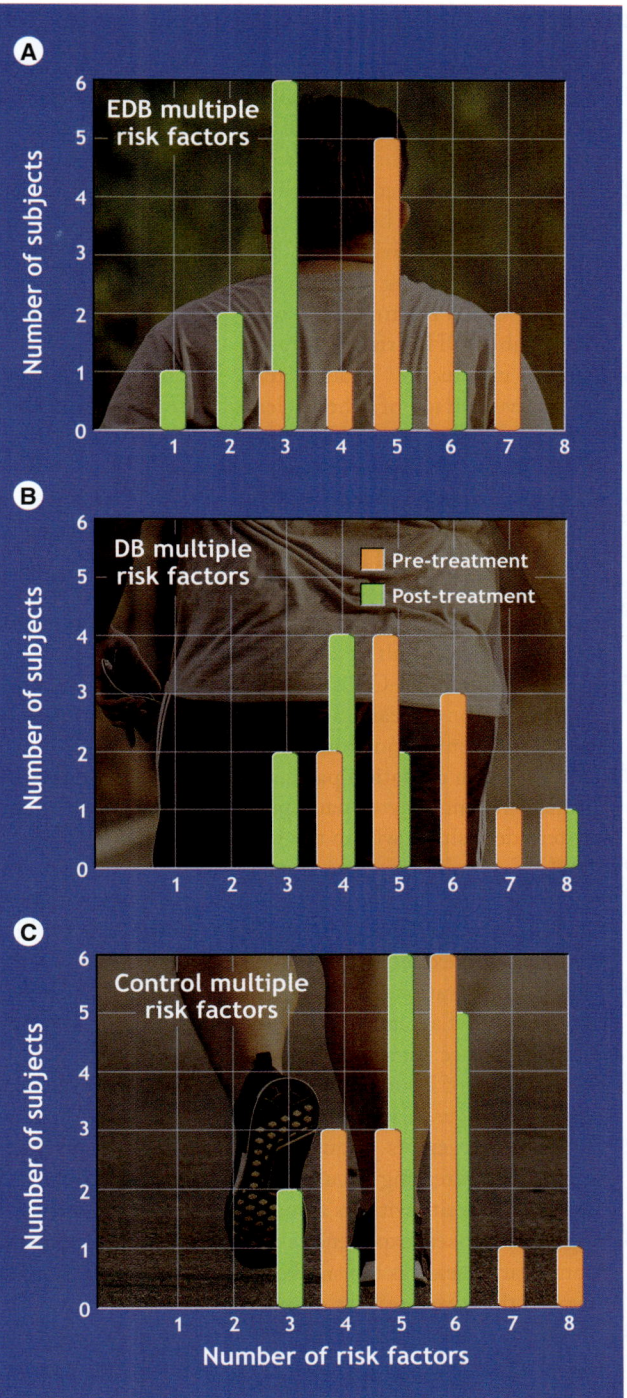

FIGURE 31.21. Multiple coronary heart disease risk factors in obese adolescents before and after treatment. DB, diet + behavior change group; EDB, exercise + diet + behavior change group.
(Reproduced with permission from Becque DB, et al. Coronary risk incidence of obese adolescents: reduction by exercise plus diet intervention. *Pediatrics.* 1988;81:605. Copyright 1988 by the American Academy of Pediatrics. Background photo: Piyawat Nandeenopparit/Shutterstock.)

Not implementing required daily physical education in the school curriculum at all grade levels, especially in elementary school, is counterproductive from a public health policy standpoint.

Summary

1. CHD represents the most prevalent cause of death in the Western world. Its pathogenesis involves degenerative changes in the inner lining of the arterial wall that progressively occlude the blood vessel.
2. Major CHD risk factors include age and gender, blood lipid abnormalities, hypertension, cigarette smoking, obesity, physical inactivity, diet, family history, and ECG abnormalities during rest and exercise.
3. Prudent CHD treatment attempts to eliminate or reduce "modifiable" CHD risk factors.
4. Painless chronic low-grade arterial inflammation is central to every stage of atherosclerotic disease and a major trigger for heart attack. High levels of C-reactive protein (CRP) reflect the inflammatory process.
5. A serum cholesterol level of 200 $mg \cdot dL^{-1}$ or lower is desirable, but experts recommend even lower values to achieve the lowest CHD risk.
6. Treating elevated cholesterol should begin early in life because of a strong association between serum cholesterol level as a young adult and CVD in middle age.
7. HDL-C and LDL-C distribution provides a more powerful predictor of heart disease risk than total serum cholesterol concentration alone.
8. LDL-C upon oxidation participates in atherosclerosis by stimulating monocyte-macrophage infiltration and lipoprotein deposition within the vessel's lumen.
9. HDL-C facilitates reverse cholesterol transport by removing surplus cholesterol from peripheral tissues (including arterial walls) for transport to the liver for bile synthesis and excretion via the small intestine.
10. Favorable alterations in HDL-C occur in sedentary males and females of all ages who regularly participate in moderate to intense aerobic exercise.
11. A high level of homocysteine exerts a powerful independent risk for vascular disease.
12. Dietary fiber exerts a dual role to prevent hyperinsulinemia by decreasing circulating insulin levels directly and thwarting obesity with its associated insulin resistance.
13. Cigarette smokers experience almost twice the risk of death from heart disease as nonsmokers. One mechanism for risk involves the adverse effects of smoking on lipoprotein levels.
14. Sedentary males and females face approximately twice the risk of a fatal heart attack than more physically active counterparts.
15. Maintenance of a physically active lifestyle throughout life lowers CHD risk factors and disease occurrence.
16. The interaction among CHD risk factors magnifies their individual effects on overall disease risk.
17. Nutrition, physical activity, and weight control programs favorably alter CHD risk factors to improve the overall health profile.

Key Terms

Andropause: Male menopause characterized by age-related decreases in gonadotropic secretions from the anterior pituitary gland

Adrenopause: Reduced adrenal cortex output of DHEA and its sulfated ester DHEAS

Angina pectoris: Temporary chest pains from inadequate myocardial blood (oxygen) perfusion

Apolipoprotein (Apo): High-density lipoprotein that plays a key role in cholesterol transport

Biological aging: Relates to decline in function and increase in disease states with increasing chronological aging

Cardiac arrest: Unexpected loss of heart function, breathing, and consciousness resulting from disruption of the heart's pumping action with blood flow cessation throughout the body

Cardiovascular diseases (CVDs): Heart and blood vessel disorders that include coronary heart disease, cerebrovascular disease, rheumatic heart disease, and other conditions

Cerebrovascular disease: Disease of blood vessels to the brain

Congenital heart disease: Malformations of heart structure existing at birth

Coronary artery bypass procedure (CABP): Procedure to bypass a damaged coronary vessel; involves sewing a graft vessel to the coronary artery beyond the narrowing or blocked area with the lower end of the vein attached to the aorta

Coronary heart disease (CHD): Disease of blood vessels supplying the myocardium; also known as atherosclerosis

C-reactive protein (CRP): Plasma protein that increases during inflammation to tissue injury or infection

Cross-sectional data: Data collected by observing subjects at one point or period of time

Cytokines: Proteins secreted by immune cells, that stimulate plaque buildup while others inhibit plaque formation

Death rate: Number of deaths per 100 individuals over a particular time period

Deep vein thrombosis and pulmonary embolism: Blood clots in the leg veins which can dislodge and move to the heart and lungs

Delayed vascular aging: Centenarians and supercentenarians with no noticeable vascular disease

Denervation muscle atrophy: Irreversible degeneration of muscle fibers, particularly type II fibers, that associates with chronic inflammation and reduction in circulating growth hormone (GH), insulin-like growth factor-1 (IGF-1), muscle-specific isoforms of IGF, and decreased mitochondria number and capacity, cell nuclei, and endplate structure

Diabetes mellitus: Group of metabolic diseases resulting in higher than normal blood sugar levels

Diabetic dyslipidemia: Insulin resistance characterized by high levels of triacylglycerols (hypertriacylglycerolemia), high levels of small LDL particles, and low levels of HDL

Endothelial lipase (EL): Enzyme that affects HDL-C production

Exercise: Planned, structured, repetitive, and purposeful physical activity

Fibrates: Medication that lowers blood triacylglycerol levels

Gerontologists: Researchers who study aging and related problems

Health: Physical, mental, and social well-being, not simply absence of disease

Health-related physical fitness: Physical fitness components associated with good health and/or disease prevention

Healthspan: Total number of years a person remains in excellent health

Healthy life expectancy (HALE, HLE): Number of years a person can expect to live in "full health"

Healthy People 2030: Fifth-generation established goals and objectives with a 10-year target to guide national health promotion and disease prevention efforts

Homocysteine: Highly reactive, sulfur-containing amino acid formed as a byproduct of methionine metabolism; high levels constitute significant health risk

Hyperlipidemia: Abnormal blood lipid level that plays an important role in the genesis of atherosclerosis

Inflammatory response: Complex vascular biological responses to harmful pathogens, damaged cells, or irritants, with classical signs of pain, heat, redness, swelling, and functional losses

Lecithin acetyl transferase: Endoplasmic reticulum intracellular protein that forms cholesterol esters from cholesterol

Lipoprotein(a) [Lp(a)]: Protein particles formed in the liver when two distinct apolipoproteins unite

Lipoproteins: Biochemical structures containing protein and lipid that allow lipids to move through intracellular and extracellular fluids

Longevity: Length of life (chronological aging)

Longitudinal data: Data tracking the same subjects at different points in time

Menopause: Cessation of menses resulting from factors that decrease ovarian estradiol output

Myocardial infarction (MI): Another term for heart attack

Necrosis: Tissue or cell death

Oldest-old: People age 80 to 85 years and older

Peripheral artery disease: Disease of arterial blood vessel supplying the arms and legs

Physical activity: Body movement produced by muscle action that increases energy expenditure

Physical activity epidemiology: Field of study that uses general research strategies of epidemiology to study physical activity as a health-related behavior linked to disease and other outcomes

Physical activity pyramid: Major goals to increase the level of regular physical activity in the general population emphasizing diverse behavioral and lifestyle options

Physical fitness: Attributes related to how well one performs physical activity

Prehabilitation program: Activities that help patients build strength prior to surgery and shorten postoperative recovery time

Premature vascular aging: Individuals with early-onset blood-vessel disease, both genetic and acquired

Rheumatic heart disease: Damage to the heart muscle and heart valves from rheumatic fever, caused by streptococcal bacteria

Sarcopenia: Age-associated muscle wasting

Sedentary behavior physiology: A discipline that studies links between excessive sedentary behavior and adverse health indicators or outcomes, primarily cardiovascular morbidity and mortality

Sedentary environmental death syndrome (SeDS): Denotes a collection of disorders directly caused by or worsened by physical inactivity

Somatopause: Mean pulse amplitude, duration, and fraction of secreted growth hormone that gradually decrease with aging

Successful aging: Optimal physical, spiritual, emotional, educational, and social satisfaction

Thrombus: Blood clot that forms inside a blood vessel and obstructs blood flow

Toll-like receptor 2 (TLR-2): Protein encoded by the *TLR2* gene, which is expressed on the surface of certain cells and recognizes foreign substances and passes on appropriate signals to the immune system cells

Vulnerable patient: High likelihood of developing a traumatic cardiac event

Vulnerable plaque: Soft metabolically active unstable plaque (macrophages and lipids) that accumulates in arterial walls

Young-old: People ages 65 to 74

> References are available online at Lippincott Connect.

Additional References

Ahmad Rahman F, Quadrilatero J. Mitochondrial-apoptotic signaling involvement in remodeling during myogenesis and skeletal muscle atrophy. *Semin Cell Dev Biol*. 2022:S1084-9521(22)00039-8.

Alizadeh Pahlavani H. Exercise therapy for people with sarcopenic obesity: myokines and adipokines as effective actors. *Front Endocrinol (Lausanne)*. 2022;13:811751.

Bilski J, et al. Multifactorial mechanism of sarcopenia and sarcopenic obesity. Role of physical exercise, microbiota and myokines. *Cells*. 2022;11:160.

Blackburn H. Early contributions to the design and conduct of clinical trials from a largely unknown 1960s pilot trial of physical activity and a well-known diet-heart feasibility study for the primary prevention of coronary heart disease (CHD). *Am J Epidemiol*. 2022:kwab296. doi:10.1093/aje/kwab296.

Bosnes I, et al. Processing speed and working memory are predicted by components of successful aging: a HUNT study. *BMC Psychol*. 2022;10:16.

Chen W, et al. DHA alleviates diet-induced skeletal muscle fiber remodeling via FTO/m^{6}A/DDIT4/PGC1α signaling. *BMC Biol*. 2022;20:39.

Chow LS, et al. Exerkines in health, resilience and disease. *Nat Rev Endocrinol*. 2022. doi:10.1038/s41574-022-00641-2.

Dawson LP, et al. Coronary atherosclerotic plaque regression: JACC state-of-the-art review. *J Am Coll Cardiol*. 2022;79:66.

De Bacquer D, et al. Poor adherence to lifestyle recommendations in patients with coronary heart disease: results from the EUROASPIRE surveys. *Eur J Prev Cardiol*. 2022;29:383.

Del Pozo Cruz B, et al. Prospective associations of accelerometer-assessed physical activity with mortality and incidence of cardiovascular disease among adults with hypertension: the UK Biobank Study. *J Am Heart Assoc*. 2022;11:e023290.

Forbes SC, et al. Meta-analysis examining the importance of creatine ingestion strategies on lean tissue mass and strength in older adults. *Nutrients*. 2021;13:1912.

Foyster JM, et al. "If they can do it, I can do it": experiences of older women who engage in powerlifting training. *J Women Aging*. 2022;34:54.

Franco AC, et al. Skin senescence: mechanisms and impact on whole-body aging. *Trends Mol Med*. 2022;28:97.

Gardner AW, et al. Association between daily steps at moderate cadence and vascular outcomes in patients with claudication. *J Cardiopulm Rehabil Prev*. 2022;42:52.

Global Burden of Disease 2019 Cancer Collaboration. Cancer incidence, mortality, years of life lost, years lived with disability, and disability-adjusted life years for 29 cancer groups from 2010 to 2019: a systematic analysis for the global burden of disease study 2019. *JAMA Oncol*. 2022;8:420.

Gómez-Sánchez L, et al. The Association of dietary intake with arterial stiffness and vascular ageing in a population with intermediate cardiovascular risk: a MARK study. *Nutrients*. 2022;14:244.

Gries KJ, et al. Muscle-derived factors influencing bone metabolism. *Semin Cell Dev Biol*. 2022;123:57.

Hsiu H, et al. Discrimination of vascular aging using the arterial pulse spectrum and machine-learning analysis. *Microvasc Res*. 2022;139:104240.

Hsu CC, et al. Supervised cycling training improves erythrocyte rheology in individuals with peripheral arterial disease. *Front Physiol*. 2022;12:792398.

Infante MA, et al. One repetition maximum test-retest reliability and safety using Keiser pneumatic resistance training machines with older women. *J Strength Cond Res*. 2021;35:3513.

Joshi P, Tampi RR. Occupational factors of successful aging. *Int Psychogeriatr*. 2022;34:1.

Katzmarzyk PT, et al. Physical inactivity and non-communicable disease burden in low-income, middle-income and high-income countries. *Br J Sports Med*. 2022;56:101.

Lee J, et al. Influence of successful aging, quality of life, and factors related to potential stressors on older consumers' purchase of private health insurance in South Korea: an empirical study based on proactive coping theory. *J Appl Gerontol*. 2022;41:253.

Lee PHU, et al. Factors mediating spaceflight-induced skeletal muscle atrophy. *Am J Physiol Cell Physiol*. 2022;322:C567.

Lin K, et al. Exploring the relationships between four aging ideals: a bibliometric study. *Front Public Health*. 2022;9:762591.

Mao L, et al. The relationship between successful aging and all-cause mortality risk in older adults: a systematic review and meta-analysis of cohort studies. *Front Med (Lausanne)*. 2022;8:740559.

McDermott MM, et al. Effect of low-intensity vs high-intensity home-based walking exercise on walk distance in patients with peripheral artery disease: the LITE randomized clinical trial. *JAMA*. 2021;325:1266.

Moskalev A, et al. Targeting aging mechanisms: pharmacological perspectives. *Trends Endocrinol Metab*. 2022;33:266.

Özsungur F. A research on the effects of successful aging on the acceptance and use of technology of the elderly. *Assist Technol*. 2022;34:77.

Rehkopf DH, et al. A US State Index of successful aging: differences between states and over time. *Milbank Q*. 2022;100:102.

Renzini A, et al. Histone deacetylases as modulators of the crosstalk between skeletal muscle and other organs. *Front Physiol*. 2022;13:706003.

Saenz-Pipaon G, et al. The role of circulating biomarkers in peripheral arterial disease. *Int J Mol Sci*. 2021;22:3601.

Streit IA, et al. Body weight multicomponent program improves power and functional capacity responses in older adults: a quasi-experimental study. *Exp Gerontol*. 2021;155:111553.

Theret M, et al. Macrophages in skeletal muscle dystrophies, an entangled partner. *J Neuromuscul Dis*. 2022;9:1.

Thompson PD. The role of physical activity and exercise in preventive cardiology. *Med Clin North Am*. 2022;106:249.

Toth M, et al. Trends in the use of residential settings among older adults. *J Gerontol B Psychol Sci Soc Sci*. 2022;77:424.

van Deutekom AW, Lewandowski AJ. Physical activity modification in youth with congenital heart disease: a comprehensive narrative review. *Pediatr Res*. 2021;89:1650.

Vieira IP, et al. Effects of high-speed versus traditional resistance training in older adults. *Sports Health*. 2022;14:283.

Vints WAJ, et al. Exerkines and long-term synaptic potentiation: mechanisms of exercise-induced neuroplasticity. *Front Neuroendocrinol*. 2022;66:100993.

Volgman AS, et al. Management of atrial fibrillation in patients 75 years and older: JACC state-of-the-art review. *J Am Coll Cardiol*. 2022;79:166.

Wang T, et al. Protective effects of physical activity in colon cancer and underlying mechanisms: a review of epidemiological and biological evidence. *Crit Rev Oncol Hematol*. 2022;170:103578.

Zabransky DJ, et al. Shared genetic and epigenetic changes link aging and cancer. *Trends Cell Biol*. 2022;32:338.

Zerlotin R, et al. Irisin and secondary osteoporosis in humans. *Int J Mol Sci*. 2022;23:690.

Zouhal H, et al. Effects of exercise training on anabolic and catabolic hormones with advanced age: a systematic review. *Sports Med*. 2021. doi:10.1007/s40279-021-01612-9.

| Table 31.1 | Top 10 Worldwide Fitness Trends, 2015 to 2020 |

Rank	2015	2016	2017	2018	2019	2020
1	BW training	Wearable technology	Wearable technology	HIIT	Wearable Technology	Wearable technology
2	HIIT	BW training	BW training	Group training	Group training	HITT
3	Employing CFP	HIIT	HIIT	Wearable technology	HIIT	Group training
4	Strength training	Strength training	Employing CFP	BW training	Programs for older adults	Training with free weights
5	Personal training	Employing CFP	Strength training	Strength training	BW training	Personal training
6	Exercise and BW loss	Personal training	Group training	Employing CFP	Employing CFP	EIM
7	Yoga	Functional fitness	EIM	Yoga	Yoga	BW training
8	Employing CFP	Employing CFP	Yoga	Personal training	Personal training	Programs for older adults
9	Functional fitness	Exercise and BW loss	Personal training	Programs for older adults	Functional fitness	Health/wellness coaching
10	Group training	Yoga	Exercise and BW loss	Functional fitness	EIM	Employing CFP

HIIT, high-intensity interval training; BW, body weight; EIM, exercise is medicine; CFP, certified fitness professional.
Data from Thompson, WR. Worldwide survey of fitness trends for 2020. *ACSM Health Fit J.* 2019;23:10. www.elementssystem.com/wp-content/uploads/2019/11/WORLDWIDE_SURVEY_OF_FITNESS_TRENDS_FOR_2020.6.pdf

| Table 31.2 | Nine Months' Endurance Training Effects on Maximum Oxygen Uptake and Cardiovascular Function in 15 Males Age 63 ± 3 years and 16 Females Age 64 ± 3 years |

	$\dot{V}O_{2max}$ L·min^{-1}	$\dot{Q}_{max}$ L·min^{-1}	HR$_{max}$ beats·min^{-1}	SV$_{max}$ mL	a-$\bar{v}O_2$ diff mL·dL^{-1}
Men					
Before	2.35	17	170	101	13.8
After	2.8[a]	19[a]	164[a]	116[a]	14.8[a]
Women					
Before	1.36	11.2	161	70	12.2
After	1.66[a]	11.5	164	70	14.4[a]

Note: Values are means; $\dot{V}O_{2max}$, maximum oxygen uptake; $\dot{Q}_{max}$, maximum cardiac output; HR$_{max}$, maximum heart rate; SV$_{max}$, stroke volume at maximal exercise; a-$\bar{v}O_2$ diff, arterio–mixed venous oxygen difference.
[a] $p \leq 0.01$ versus before training.
Reprinted from Spina RJ, et al. Differences in cardiovascular adaptations to endurance-exercise training between older men and women. *J Appl Physiol*. 1993;75:849. ©The American Physiological Society (APS). All rights reserved.

Table 31.3 General Trend for Effects of Regular Physical Activity and/or Increased Physical Fitness and Risk for Chronic Disease Conditions	
Disease or Condition	**Strength of Evidence**
All-cause mortality	↑↑↑
Coronary artery disease	↑↑↑
Hypertension	↑↑
Obesity	↑↑↑
Stroke	↑
Peripheral vascular disease	→
Cancers	
Colon	↑↑
Rectum	→
Stomach	→
Breast	↑
Prostate	↑
Lung	↑
Pancreas	→
Type 2 diabetes	↑↑↑
Osteoarthritis	→
Osteoporosis	↑↑

Strength of evidence: →, *No apparent difference* in disease rates; ↑, *some* evidence of reduced disease rates; ↑↑, *good* evidence of reduced disease rates; ↑↑↑, *excellent* evidence of reduced disease rates.

Table 31.4 Approximate Composition of Serum Lipoproteins				
	Chylomicrons	Very Low-Density Lipoproteins (VLDL:Prebeta)	Low-Density Lipoproteins (LDL:Beta)	High-Density Lipoproteins (HDL:Alpha)
Density (g·cm^{-3})	0.95	0.95–1.006	1.006–1.019	1.063–1.210
Protein (%)	05–1.0	5–15	25	45–55
Lipid (%)	99	95	75	50
Cholesterol (%)	2–5	10–20	40–45	18
Triacylglycerol (%)	85	50–70	5–10	2
Phospholipid (%)	3–6	10–20	20–25	30

Table 31.5 Novel Risk Factors for Atherosclerotic Vascular Disease

Inflammatory Markers	Hemostatic/Thrombosis Markers	Platelet-Related Factors	Lipid-Related Factors	Other Factors
C-reactive protein	Fibrinogen	Platelet aggregation	Low-density lipoprotein (LDL)	Homocysteine
Interleukins (e.g., IL-6)	von Willebrand antigen factor	Platelet activity	Lipoprotein (a)	Lipoprotein-associated phospholipase A(2)
Serum amyloid A	Plasminogen activator inhibitor 1 (PAI-1)	Platelet size and volume	Remnant lipoproteins	Microalbuminuria
Vascular and cellular adhesion molecules	Tissue-plasminogen activator		Apolipoproteins A1 and B	Insulin resistance
Soluble CD40 ligand	Factors V, VII, VIII		High-density lipoprotein subtypes	PAT-1 genotype
Leukocyte count	• D-Dimer • Fibrinopeptide A • Prothrombin fragment 1+2		Oxidized LDL	• Angiotensin-converting enzyme genotype • ApoE genotype • Infectious agents: cytomegalovirus, *Chlamydia pneumonia*, *Helicobacter pylori*, herpes simplex virus • Psychosocial factors

Source: Hackam DG, Anand SS. Emerging risk factors for atherosclerotic vascular disease: a critical review of the evidence. *JAMA*. 2003;290:932.

CHAPTER 32
Clinical Exercise Physiology for Cancer, Cardiovascular, and Pulmonary Rehabilitation

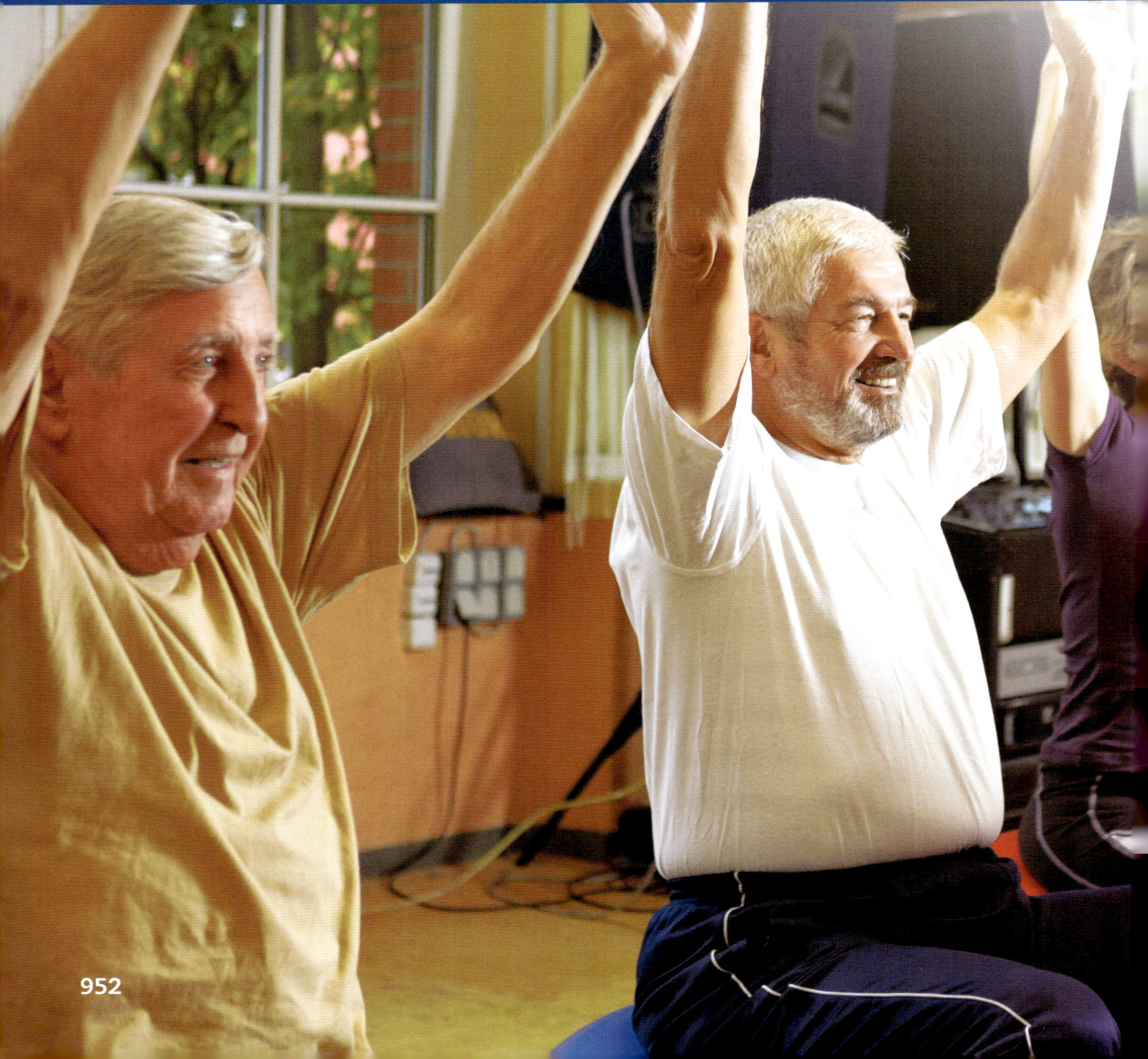

Chapter Objectives

- Discuss the exercise physiologist and health and fitness professional's role in the clinical setting
- Summarize the physical activity's benefits for cancer prevention and rehabilitation and make physical activity recommendations for persons with cancer
- Discuss physical activity's benefits for treating moderate hypertension and congestive heart failure
- Discuss the general components to clinically assess cardiac disease
- Summarize noninvasive and invasive procedures to identify specific cardiac dysfunctions
- Describe three cardiac rehabilitation phases, including objectives, required supervision levels, and prudent physical activity recommendations
- Give three reasons to include graded exercise stress testing for coronary heart disease screening
- Describe five objective coronary heart disease indicators during an exercise stress test
- Categorize and describe five diseases that affect the pulmonary system
- Outline two proposed mechanisms for exercise-induced bronchospasm and factors that modify its severity
- Describe the role of physical activity in rehabilitation from three different neuromuscular diseases
- Describe the major classifications of cognitive/emotional diseases and physical activity's potential as adjunctive therapy

Ancillaries at-a-Glance

Visit Lippincott Connect to access the following resources.

- References: Chapter 32
- Appendix H: Links for Supplemental Animations and Videos
- Animations: Asthma, Congestive Heart Failure, Coronary Angiography: Left Coronary System—Parts A and B, Edema, Stroke
- Focus on Research: Physical Fitness Protects Against Death

The Exercise Physiologist in the Clinical Setting

Regular physical activity (PA) plays an increasingly important role in the global prevention of disease, in rehabilitation from injury, and as adjunctive therapy for medically related disorders. Attention now focuses on understanding the mechanisms by which PA improves health, physical fitness, and rehabilitation potential of patients challenged by chronic disease and disability.[179]

The clinical exercise physiologist has become an integral component in the team approach to health and total patient care. In the clinical setting, the exercise physiologist focuses primarily on restoring patient mobility and functional capacity while working closely with physical therapists, occupational therapists, and physicians.

The Clinical Exercise Physiologist's Responsibilities

Assess exercise tolerance	Evaluate adverse signs/symptoms Consider medical history and health status Assess barriers to exercise
Establish treatment goals	Collaborate with referring physician and other licensed professionals Assist in identifying patient short-term and long-term objectives
Individualize exercise-based interventions	Determine "readiness to change" Promote safety and effectiveness Counsel patient on lapses or setbacks
Monitor progress	Conduct outcome evaluations Provide updates to the patient and referring physician Encourage pleasurable activities in a supportive environment

Background photo: Photographee.eu/Shutterstock

The exercise physiologist has an expanded role in clinical practice because of fundamental relationships among measures of functional capacity, physical fitness, and overall good health. *The World Health Organization (WHO; www.who.int) defines health as "a state of complete physical, mental and social well-being, not merely the absence of disease and infirmity."* This definition considers good health as an ability to complete physical tasks successfully and maintain functional independence.

Vital Link Between Sports Medicine and Exercise Physiology

One traditional view about **sports medicine** concerns rehabilitating athletes from sports-related injuries. In its broader context, sports medicine relates to scientific and medical aspects dealing with PA, physical fitness, health, and sports performance. The WHO defines physical fitness as the ability to perform muscular work satisfactorily. This definition encompasses one's capacity to perform PA at work, at home, or on the athletic field. Sports medicine closely links to clinical exercise physiology because the sports medicine profession treats a broad spectrum of individuals. Individuals with low functional capacity recovering from injury, disease, and medical interventions comprise one end of the continuum; the other extreme encompasses healthy, able-bodied, and disabled athletes with well-developed levels of total body fitness. Carefully prescribed PA contributes to just about all individuals' overall good health and quality of life. **TABLE 32.1** presents the health benefits of regular physical activity to improve aerobic and musculoskeletal fitness.

TABLE 32.1 Health benefits of regular physical activity to improve aerobic and musculoskeletal fitness

Training and Certification Programs for Professional Exercise Physiologists

Regular PA continues to gain widespread acceptance as an integral part of rehabilitative programs dealing with the care and health maintenance for a growing list of chronic diseases and disabling conditions. Likewise, expanding public interest in PA for health promotion has stimulated a parallel need to certify qualified professionals to provide sound advice and supervision regarding physical activities for preventative and rehabilitative purposes.

Educational Requirements

A practicing **clinical exercise physiologist (CEP)** requires an earned bachelor's degree at minimum but is encouraged to pursue advanced degrees in exercise science, physiology, or a closely related field. In most educational curricula, a clinical internship experience is required, and desirable. Locations of student internships depend on the chosen area of expertise (e.g., cardiology, sports medicine, wellness). Ample opportunities exist for CEPs in cardiology practices to conduct stress tests and work in programs of preventive cardiology and cardiac rehabilitation. In addition, students who have attained a master's degree may be certified as a registered CEP (RCEP), which requires a broad expertise range designated for those interested in working with high-risk or diseased individuals as well as the healthy population.

The table on the top of the next page lists different CEP levels of education and associated clinical roles.

Certifications

In 1975, the **American College of Sports Medicine (ACSM; www.acsm.org)** initiated the first ACSM Clinical and Health/Fitness Certification program. The ACSM continues as the preeminent organization to offer certification programs, newsletters, and continuing education credits (CEUs or CECs) to support the professional growth of health and fitness professionals.

Levels of Education and Associated Clinical Roles of the CEP

Education/Certifications	Clinical Roles/ & Responsibilities
Bachelor degree; ACSM Certified Clinical Exercise Specialist; Certified Health Fitness Specialist; National Strength & Conditioning Association certified Strength and Conditioning Specialist	Cardiac rehabilitation (clinical coordinator/ supervisor); diagnostic stress testing (personal trainer); clinical weight management (wellness specialist); chronic disease exercise prescription (corporate fitness specialists, research coordinator/leader; manuscript preparation)
Master's degree; ACSM Registered Clinical Exercise Physiologist	Registered Clinical Exercise Physiologist; Cardiac rehabilitation (college/university teaching); Diagnostic stress testing (director, research coordinator); Pulmonary rehabilitation (administrator, research coordinator, authorship); Metabolic disease management (administrator; research; authorship); Cancer recovery (administrator, research, authorship); Support grant writing
Doctorate degree; ACSM Registered Clinical Exercise Physiologist	Registered Clinical Exercise Physiologist; Clinical program director; college university professor/lecturer; Manuscript authorship; Grant writing; Research and development; Student/intern supervision

ACSM, The American College of Sports Medicine; CEP, Clinical Exercise Physiologist

Background photo: G-Stock Studio/Shutterstock

Clinical certifications are often required by many hospitals, medical centers, and private physician practices. Perhaps the most widely recognized and longstanding clinically oriented certification is the ACSM's **Certified Clinical Exercise Specialist (CES)**. This level requires a baccalaureate degree in exercise or health-related studies, 600 hr of relevant clinical experience, current cardiopulmonary resuscitation certification (CPR; basic life support), and successful completion of a computer-based comprehensive examination.

The ACSM publishes a list of current knowledge, skills, and abilities that comprise the foundations in the various certification exams, and minimum requirements for experience, education level, and competencies (www.acsm.org/get-stay-certified/get-certified). The inset figure below shows the content for these clinical certifications:

ACSM certifications consist of three different tracks:

1. **Health/Fitness Track** includes ACSM Certified Personal Trainer (ACSM-CPT), ACSM Certified Exercise Physiologist (ACSM-EP), or ACSM Certified Group Exercise Instructor (ACSM-GEI). These certifications target those wanting to train individuals on a one-on-one basis or to instruct groups and develop and implement safe, effective exercise programs, and modify them to meet clients' specific needs.
2. **Clinical Track** for professionals who desire to become part of a healthcare team dedicated to improving the quality of life of patient groups at high risk or with existing disease as well as apparently healthy individuals. CEPs help to increase the likelihood of long-term physical, social, and economic independence of patients through individualized patient education, behavior change, and primary and secondary prevention strategies.
3. **Specialty Credentials** are intended for those who already have an accredited certification and want to add a specialty credential to broaden their expertise. Specialty credentials consist of the Exercise is Medicine Credential, ACSM/ACS Certified Cancer Exercise Trainer (CET), ACSM/NCHPAD Certified Inclusive Fitness Trainer (CIFT), and ACSM/NPAS Physical Activity in Public Health Specialist (PAPHS).

Content Matter for American College of Sports Medicine Certification

- Exercise physiology and related exercise science
- Pathophysiology and risk factors
- Health appraisal, fitness and clinical exercise testing
- Electrocardiography and diagnostic techniques
- Patient management and medications
- Medical and surgical management
- Exercise prescription and programming
- Nutrition and weight management
- Human behavior and counseling
- Safety, injury prevention, and emergency procedures
- Program administration, quality assurance, and outcome assessment

Background photo: Jacob Lund/Shutterstock

Competency-based certification at a given level requires a knowledge and skills base commensurate with a specific certification. Each level has a minimum experience requirement, education level, or other ACSM certifications. Certification programs continually undergo review and revision to ensure the highest level of professionalism. Numerous groups and organizations offer different "certifications," some without undergraduate degree requirements and some requiring a short examination or "experience" to replace objective core knowledge. These so-called "*certifications*," without approved standards and exclusions, confuse the public about the competence level or care provided by a "certified" exercise professional.

Clinical Applications of Exercise Physiology to Diverse Diseases and Disorders

The following sections present clinical applications of exercise physiology for the major areas of oncology, cardiovascular diseases, pulmonary system disabilities, neuromuscular diseases and disorders, renal disease, and psychologic disorders. We focus on these disabilities because the CEP deals mostly with these conditions.

Estimated Number of New Cancer Cases and Deaths by Sex, United States, 2020

Sites	Male New Cases	Male Deaths	Female New Cases	Female Deaths
All sites	893,660	321,160	912,930	285,360
Digestive system	187,620	97,560	146,060	70,230
Respiratory system	130,340	76,370	116.93	64,360
Bones and joints	2120	10,000	1480	720
Skin	65,350	8030	43,070	3450
Breast	2620	520	276,480	42,170
Urinary system	110,230	23,540	48,890	10,280
Endocrine system	14,160	1600	41,510	1660
Lymphoma	47,070	12,030	38,650	8880
Leukemia	25,470	12,420	25,060	9680

Background image: Martial Red/Shutterstock

Oncology

Cancer represents a group of diseases collectively characterized by uncontrolled abnormal cell growth. More than 100 different cancer types exist, mostly in adults. **Carcinomas** develop from epithelial cells that line body surfaces, glands, and internal organs. They account for 80 to 90% of all cancers that include prostate, colon, lung, cervical, and breast cancer. Cancers also can arise from blood cells of the cardiovascular system (**leukemias**) and the immune system (**lymphomas**) and connective tissues such as bones, tendons, cartilage, fat, and muscle (**sarcomas**).

The current population of more than 17 million Americans with a history of cancer (as of March 2022) projects to rise to 18 million by 2022 (www.cancer.org/content/dam/cancer-org/research/cancer-facts-and-statistics/annual-cancer-facts-and-figures/2022/2022-cancer-facts-and-figures.pdf). This illustrates the ongoing need for rehabilitative and maintenance options for health professionals in this area. The most serious outcomes for current cancer patients and survivors include body mass and functional status loss. Depressed functional status includes difficulty walking even short distances and serious fatigue that limits completing simple household chores. Approximately 75% of cancer survivors report extreme fatigue during and following radiotherapy or chemotherapy treatment. Weight loss, decreased muscular strength, and suboptimal cardiovascular endurance characterize these decrements. Maintaining and restoring functional capacity challenges the cancer survivor, even those considered "cured." Sufficient rationale now justifies PA intervention for cancer patients during and following different treatment modalities to not only facilitate the recovery process but also prevent the disease recurrence. Guidelines established by the American Cancer Society (www.cancer.org) urge doctors to talk to their cancer patients about eating healthfully, exercising, and reducing body weight to satisfy desirable weight for age and gender.

Cancer Statistics

The estimated number of new United States cancer cases in 2021 is 1.9 million, with over 608,000 total cancer deaths. This translates to about 1667 deaths each day—cancer is the second most common cause of death in the United States, exceeded only by cardiovascular diseases (see Chapter 31). New methodologies and increased surveillance and reporting techniques now allow the American Cancer Society to update cancer statistics yearly (www.cancer.org/research/cancer-facts-statistics.html). The unnumbered table presents the latest estimated number of new cancer cases and deaths by gender in the United States in 2020.

Clinical Features

Clinical features regarding cancer relate to the effects of three primary cancer treatment modalities: surgery, radiation, and systemic (pharmacologic) therapy, which includes **proteomics**, which relies on proteins as biomarkers for clinical diagnosis.

1. **Surgical operations** that remove high-risk tissues to prevent cancer development, biopsies from abnormal tissue to diagnose cancer, tumor excision of with curative intent, inserting central venous catheters to support chemotherapy infusions, reconstruction procedures following definitive surgery, and palliative or symptom relief for incurable disease such as partial bowel removal or resection.
2. **Radiation** involves photon penetration into a specific tissue to produce an ionized (electrically charged) particle that damages DNA to inhibit cell replication and produce cell death. Daily radiation treatment typically lasts between 5 and 8 wk. Pharmacologic therapy is prescribed for many advanced solid tumors if cancer cells metastasize beyond the primary site and infiltrate regional lymph nodes.
3. **Chemotherapy**, endocrine therapy, and biologic therapy represent the three major systemic therapy types.

TABLE 32.2 presents common clinical symptoms, effects, and outcome from surgery, radiation therapy, and systemic therapy interventions.

TABLE 32.2 Cancer therapies and their complications

Cancer Rehabilitation and Physical Activity

Regular physical activity (PA) helps cancer patients recuperate and return to a normal lifestyle with greater independence and functional capacity.[21,62,81] The most serious health outcomes for most cancer survivors include body mass loss and decreased energy level and functional status. This occurs predominantly following surgery and during chemotherapy and radiation therapy.[29,31,52] Loss of functional status includes difficulty walking more than one block and chronic fatigue that limits completing routine household chores, insomnia, pain, appetite loss, coughing, anxiety, and depression.

Most cancer survivors report extreme fatigue during radiation therapy and/or chemotherapy, probably from weight loss and muscle atrophy and loss of cardiovascular endurance. Home-based activity regimens reduce feelings of fatigue and enhance life quality and other biosocial outcomes following cancer diagnosis.[26,150,180]

Maintaining and restoring function present distinct challenges to the cancer survivor. Evidence justifies PA intervention for breast cancer survivors,[69,87,137,151] and nutrition intervention plus regular PA reduces risk of contracting additional cancers.[144,164,167]

Ten general preventive and intervention goals for patients who face sustained periods of inactivity, disuse, and bed rest include the following:

1. Improve overall functional status.
2. Improve active motion for nonrestrictive segments and joints.
3. Prevent flexibility loss by active motion and passive movements.
4. Stimulate peripheral and central circulation through active motion PA based on current functional level.
5. Increase ventilatory function with systematic breathing exercises.
6. Prevent thrombosis through physical activities.
7. Prevent motor control and muscle strength and endurance loss with resistance exercises.
8. Reduce bone loss rate through weight-bearing aerobic and muscle-strengthening exercises.
9. Through active aerobic and resistance exercise, slow fat-free body mass loss and subsequent basal metabolic rate reduction that accompany deconditioning.
10. Monitor signs of increased fatigue or weakness, lethargy, dyspnea, pallor, dizziness, claudication, or cramping during or following PA.

The healthcare team's overall goal is to rehabilitate the patient to a functional level that allows them to return to work and pursue normal recreational activities. Results of a meta-analysis on the effects of home-based PA programs related to physical capacity, disease symptoms, and quality of life in lung cancer patients, the most prevalent type of cancer, are encouraging.[180] Fourteen random controlled trials and quasi-experimental trials involving 694 patients at all lung cancer stages revealed the following about the effects of home-based PA compared to nonexercise control groups:

1. **Exercise capacity**: significant improvements in the intervention group after the intervention
2. **Cancer-related fatigue**: lower in the intervention group after the intervention
3. **Insomnia**: greater improvements in the intervention group after the intervention
4. **Pain**: no significant improvement in pain in the intervention group
5. **Appetite loss**: Home-based PA did not significantly reduce coughing in lung cancer patients
6. **Depression**: levels lower after intervention
7. **Quality of life**: significantly improved after intervention

PA: Protective Effects on Cancer Occurrence

Firm epidemiologic evidence confirms an inverse relation between amount of occupational or leisure-time PA and reduction in *all-cause* cancer risk. One review concluded, "*the magnitude of the protective effect of PA on estrogen-dependent cancer warrants including low-to-moderate activity as a prudent preventive strategy.*"[93] Other large-scale, community-based studies of colorectal, breast, and prostatic hyperplasia revealed increased PA-reduced cancer risk and mortality.[34,75,104,134,163,183] A study involving 122,000 females found that exercising at least 1 hr daily reduced breast cancer risk by 20%.[144] The benefits may differ depending on menopausal status, with a greater risk reduction for postmenopausal females.[50] The proportion of males at high colon cancer risk would decrease considerably if males eliminated the modifiable risk of physical inactivity and excessive red meat consumption, obesity, alcohol intake, cigarette smoking, and low folic acid intake.[135]

PA-Induced Reductions in Tumor Growth

PA is known to impact immune cell function by altering the immune response, which researchers believe may help to explain the underlying positive effects of PA on cancer risk and disease progression. The metabolic demands of strenuous physical exertion generally induce significant changes in nutrient use via enhanced aerobic metabolism. These PA-induced nutrient metabolism alterations positively shift intramuscular metabolite profiles to promote tumor growth reductions.

The immune system's cytotoxic T cells primarily keep tumor growth under control. By recognizing mutation-derived neoantigens (antigens encoded by tumor-specific mutated genes) during **immunosurveillance**, T cells target and eliminate malignant cells.[181] Lack of immune control permits progressive cancer growth (www.cancer.gov/types/metastatic-cancer). Tumors maintain control in a number of ways, primarily by dampening antitumor T-cell responses.[182]

One study investigated the association between exercise, tumor growth, and function of the **CD8+ T cell** (also called cytotoxic T cell, cytotoxic T lymphocyte, cytolytic T cell,

T-killer cell, or killer T cell).[74] The researchers studied exercise-induced changes in tumor progression to discover whether exercise releases metabolites and whether they would alter cytotoxic T-cell function. The result was clear—exercise alone modified cytotoxic T-cell metabolism, and the exercise-induced effects on tumor growth depended on the cells cytotoxic activity. In essence, intense PA altered the intrinsic metabolic machinery and antitumoral cytotoxic T-cell effector functions. Exercise-derived metabolites, whether systemically delivered or draining into an adjacent lymph node, can boost a nascent T-cell response and suppress tumor development.[84,184–186]

PA Effects on Cancer: Strong Evidence

PA plays an important role in cancer rehabilitation. Both strong and moderate evidence provides a basis for establishing activity guidelines, yet insufficient evidence also should be considered. Regular PA confers these 10 cancer-related health benefits:

- **Reduces anxiety:** Moderate-intensity aerobic PA three times per week for 12 wk or twice weekly combined aerobic plus resistance training for 6 to 12 wk reduces anxiety in cancer survivors during and after treatment.[187] It does not appear that resistance training alone reduces anxiety. Anxiety improvements appear greater in supervised PA programs or in programs with a larger supervised component than those that are predominantly unsupervised or home-based.
- **Reduces depressive symptoms:** Moderate-intensity aerobic PA 3 times per week for at least 12 wk or twice weekly combined aerobic plus resistance training lasting 6 to 12 wk reduces depressive symptoms in cancer survivors during and after treatment.[188]
- **Reduces fatigue:** For PA programs that last at least 12 wk, moderate-intensity aerobic PA three 3 times per week can reduce cancer-related fatigue both during and after treatment.[189] Moderate-intensity combined aerobic plus resistance training sessions performed 2 to 3 times per week or twice weekly moderate-intensity resistance training is effective, with the latter particularly effective during prostate cancer therapy.[190] Whether or not more PA translates to less cancer-related fatigue remains unclear, although suggestive evidence indicates that fatigue reductions are greater with PA sessions longer than 30 min and programs longer than 12 wk compared with less or no PA.
- **Improves health-related quality of life:** Combined moderate-intensity aerobic and resistance exercise performed 2 to 3 times weekly for at least 12 wk results in improvements in health-related quality of life both during and after disease treatment.[191]
- **Improves physical function:** Moderate-intensity aerobic PA, resistance training, or combined training performed 3 times per week for 8 to 12 wk improves self-reported physical functions.[192]

PA Effects on Cancer: Moderate Evidence

- **Bone health:** Two recent systematic reviews of cancer survivors concluded that across all trials, the evidence for PA to improve bone health is inconclusive.[193,194]
- **Sleep:** Reviews of cancer survivors provided mixed evidence for exercise effects on overall sleep quality, indicating either a positive effect of regular walking or no effect.[195,196] Other research has shown consistent evidence of a small-to-moderate effect of aerobic PA on overall sleep quality.[197]

PA Effects on Cancer: Insufficient Evidence

Insufficient evidence for a specific outcome does not mean that cancer survivors would not benefit in other ways from engaging in regular PA or should remain sedentary.

- **Cardiotoxicity:** The ability of regular PA to prevent or ameliorate **cardiotoxicity** is an emerging field of research. Promising results exists for a protective effect of PA in animal models and some novel evidence in humans for cardiac function, including measures of left ventricular and vascular endothelial functions.[198]
- **Chemotherapy-induced peripheral neuropathy:** To date, too few high-quality trials exist to support the benefits of PA for preventing and/or managing chemotherapy-induced peripheral neuropathy and related side effects such as balance impairment and falls.[199]
- **Cognitive functions:** Although promising results from animal studies are emerging for a protective effect of aerobic activity on cancer treatment–related changes in cognitive function, the current evidence for humans is limited.[200]
- **Nausea**: Reduction in nausea is a commonly reported benefit of regular PA during chemotherapy, but only limited data exist from high-quality trials with nausea as a primary end point.

Regular Physical Activity Reduces Breast Cancer Risk

Strong evidence exists that regular physical activity (PA) reduces breast cancer risk from long-term regulation of circulating sex and metabolic hormones, inflammatory factors, adipokines, and myokines. Chronic PA substantially alters whole body homeostasis by altering plasma metabolites, reactive oxygen species, microRNAs, and the gut microbiota profile. In principle, every cell and organ might ultimately be positively impacted by biological perturbations induced by regular PA, which should be considered an efficacious nonpharmacologic medical therapy. Emphasizing PA as an effective strategy in primary cancer prevention supports the claim, "Exercise is Medicine."

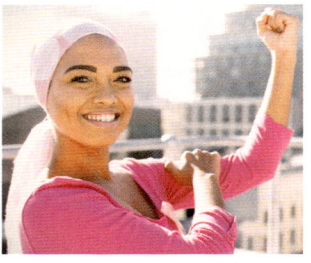

vectorfusionart/Shutterstock

Sources:
Cheung AT, et al. Physical activity for pediatric cancer survivors: a systematic review of randomized controlled trials. *J Cancer Surviv*. 2021;15:876.
Hong BS, Lee KP. A systematic review of the biological mechanisms linking physical activity and breast cancer. *Phys Act Nutr*. 2020;24:25.

- **Pain:** Most controlled trials with cancer survivors have examined nonspecific pain and/or included pain as a secondary outcome, which limits data interpretation. There is, however, evidence from controlled trials where pain was the primary outcome that a combined home-based aerobic plus supervised resistance training intervention in females with breast cancer reduced arthralgia associated with aromatase inhibitor therapy.[201]
- **Sexual function:** Insufficient evidence exists on the effect of PA on sexual function during or after cancer therapy. Promising early results for a positive effect on sexual functions among prostate cancer patients treated with androgen deprivation therapy have been reported.[202,203]

PA Prescription and Cancer

Limited research exists regarding the proper PA prescription for different cancer types, including the proper timing of PA relative to various treatment phases. Determining the best time to initiate PA intervention in cancer recovery remains problematic, but not without encouraging signs.[204,205]

In light of limited information, PA prescription recommendations for cancer rehabilitation generally include symptom-limited, progressive, and individualized physical activities.[88,116,175] Ambulation of any kind as soon as practical becomes important for the most sedentary and deconditioned patients. Emphasis should focus on intervals of low-to-moderate aerobic activity performed several times daily rather than in one relatively strenuous bout. A dose–response relationship seems to emerge between increased PA and improved health and functional capacity.[69] Most sedentary patients derive clinically significant benefits by accumulating up to 30 min of daily walking or equivalent energy expenditure in other activities. Health benefits accrue whether PA takes the form of structured PA, home-based programs, or sport, household, occupational, or recreational activities.

Cancer patients initially receive a symptom-limited, graded exercise stress test on a treadmill or cycle ergometer to form their PA prescription. Testing procedures remain the same as for healthy individuals except the patient receives greater attention about their sensations of fatigue and/or pain. Generally, patients should *not* exercise to maximum. The PA prescription initially aims to produce ambulation if no specific contraindications exist. The prescription also provides for range-of-motion movements and other activities to improve muscular strength, augment fat-free body mass (FFM), and improve overall mobility (e.g., submaximal static exercises of the antigravity muscles, deep breathing exercises, and dynamic trunk rotation movements). Progression and intensity of activity are individualized, with initial work–rest ratios of 1:1 increasing to 2:1. Eventually, continuous activity for up to 15 min replaces the intermittent bouts.[206]

Breast Cancer Rehabilitation and PA

Carcinoma of the breast, the most common form of cancer in white females ages 40 years and older, causes the greatest number of deaths in females between 40 and 55 years of age. By age 30, the chance of being diagnosed with breast cancer remains just 1 in 2000; by age 40, the chances increase considerably to 1 in 233, and by age 60, 1 in 22. Ten common breast cancer risk factors include:

1. Family history: especially a mother, sister, or daughter who had breast or ovarian cancer
2. Age: above age 60
3. Personal history of cancer
4. First menstrual period started before age 12
5. Menopause started after age 55
6. Hormones: prior history of estrogen plus progestin following menopause
7. Breast density: dense breast tissue verified by mammogram
8. Abnormal breast cells: atypical hyperplasia or carcinoma *in situ*
9. First child born after age 30 or no childbirth
10. High-fat diet and excess body weight

Most studies of PA involve only aerobic training for cancer patients and have demonstrated its physiologic and psychologic benefits.[36,78,80,157,170,207–209] Unfortunately, most of this research remains limited because it did not involve randomized controlled trials and/or used small sample sizes. High levels of estrogens have been implicated in the development and growth of breast cancer. One postulated mechanism for the beneficial effects of aerobic activity for females at high risk for breast cancer relates to the estrogen-lowering effects of this activity form and the concurrent reduction in breast cancer recurrence or new diagnosis.[91] Following menopause, fat cells, not the ovaries, are the main source of estrogen, and regular aerobic activity provides a potent means to control body fat levels. Breast cancer patients who are physically active and less overweight have a greater chance of surviving the disease.[62,80,167]

Resistance exercise during cancer management can also effectively counteract disease and treatment side effects and contribute to the maintenance of a positive body image.[113,158] In a study from one of our laboratories, 28 patients recovering from breast cancer surgery enrolled in a 10-wk program of circuit-resistance training to evaluate the effects of PA on depression, self-esteem, and anxiety.[152] Patients performed hydraulic resistance exercises in a 14-station aerobic exercise circuit 4 days weekly with a self-paced, individualized program adjusted to their needs and fitness levels. **FIGURE 32.1** shows that exercisers decreased depression by 38% compared with a 13% increase

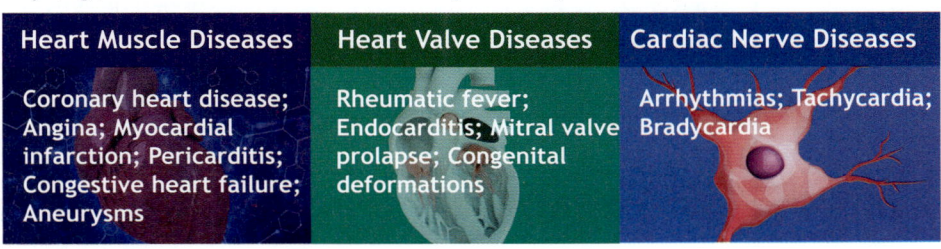

Shutterstock background image: jijomathaidesigners (muscle), SciePro (valve), BlueRingMedia (nerve)

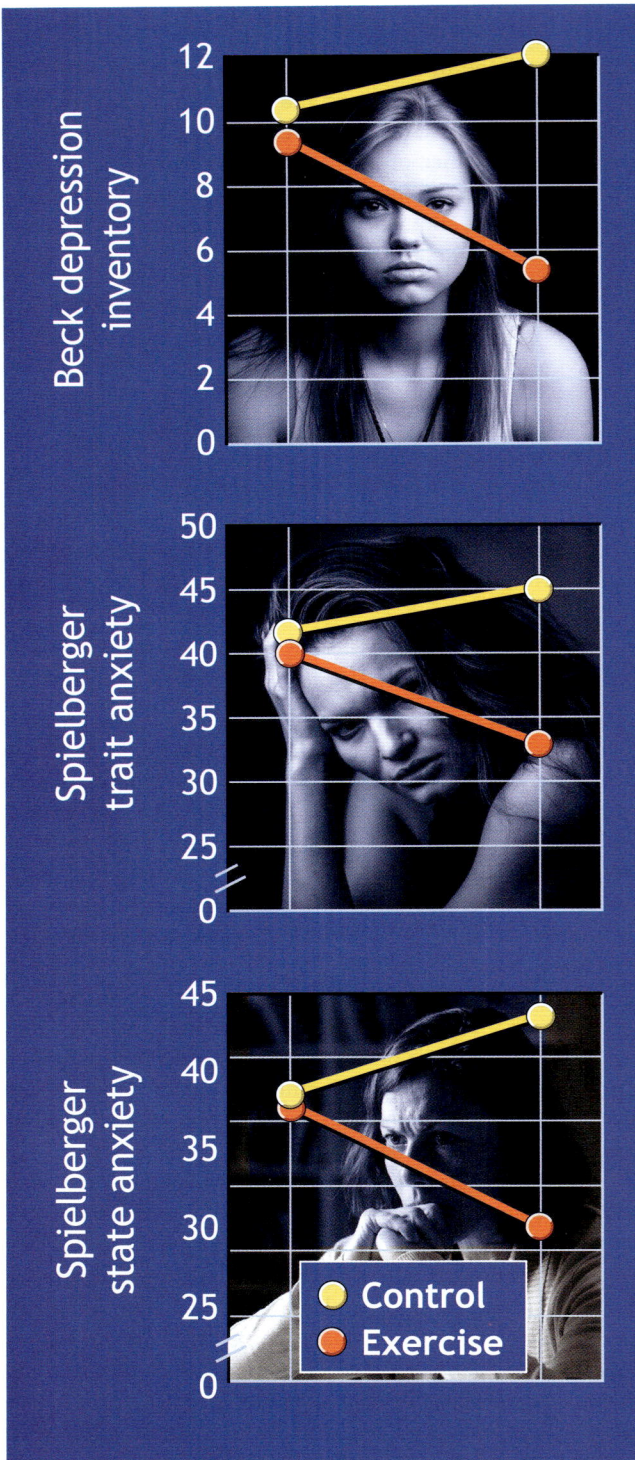

FIGURE 32.1. Effects of 10 weeks of moderate aerobic circuit resistance exercise on depression in females recovering from breast cancer surgery **(top)** and two trait anxiety test results **(middle and lower)**.
(Data courtesy M. Segar, Applied Physiology Laboratory, University of Michigan, Ann Arbor, MI. Shutterstock background photos: iatlo [top], restyler [middle], Pheelings media [bottom]).

for nonexercising counterparts recovering from breast cancer surgery. The exercisers also decreased trait anxiety by 16% and state anxiety by 20%, whereas nonexercising patients increased in both variables. These potent exercise effects on psychosocial variables during breast cancer rehabilitation bode well for advocating structured, comprehensive activity programs.

Cardiovascular Diseases

This section examines the prevalence of different cardiovascular system diseases, their possible causes and diagnosis, and specific PA applications for rehabilitation.

Diseases of the cardiovascular system account for the largest number of deaths in industrialized nations (see Chapter 31). Because increased PA represents a prudent first-line defense to combat these diseases, exercise physiologists should be familiar with all aspects of this disease category. Heart diseases generally may be categorized into three main areas: those affecting the myocardium, those affecting heart valves, and those affecting the cardiac nervous system, as shown in the figure on the previous page.

Heart Muscle Diseases

Diseases of the myocardium become prevalent with advancing age. These conditions are known as **degenerative heart disease**, atherosclerotic cardiovascular disease, arteriosclerotic cardiovascular disease, coronary artery disease (CAD), and coronary heart disease (CHD).

Advances in molecular biology have isolated possible genetic links to CHD. One of these genes (on chromosome 19 near the gene related to low-density lipoprotein cholesterol [LDL-C] receptor function), called the **atherosclerosis susceptibility gene,** accounts for about 50% of all CHD cases. This gene triples the risk of myocardial infarction. These characteristics include abdominal obesity and low levels of high-density lipoprotein cholesterol (HDL-C) and high LDL-C levels.[122]

Lippincott® Connect — Appendix H, available online at Lippincott Connect, provides a list of supplemental animations and videos on this topic.

Symptoms rarely present in the early CHD stages. As the disease progresses and coronary arteries narrow, clinical symptoms become evident and advance with increasing severity. The first sign of CHD is often slight angina pain accompanied by decreased functional capacity. This eventually leads to **ischemia** and possible myocardial tissue necrosis. In severe cases, the person experiences persistent chest pain, anxiety, nausea, vomiting, and dyspnea. Chronic, untreated angina weakens the myocardium and eventually produces heart failure as cardiac output fails to meet metabolic demands. Pulmonary congestion with a persistent cough often accompanies heart failure. At this stage, the patient becomes dyspneic even when sitting at rest and can have a sudden myocardial infarction. CHD pathogenesis progresses in five stages:

1. Injury to coronary artery endothelial cell walls
2. Fibroblastic proliferation of the artery's inner lining (intima)
3. Further blood flow obstruction as lipid accumulates at the arterial intima and middle lining junction

Similarity of Angina and Heartburn Symptoms

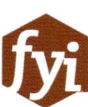

The sensation of angina pectoris includes squeezing, burning, and pressing or choking in the chest region, sensations that often go ignored because they mimic benign heartburn discomfort.[132]

Angina Pectoris	Heartburn
• Gripping, viselike-pain feelings or pressure behind breast bone	• Frequent heartburn feeling
• Radiating pain to neck, jaw, back, shoulders, or arms (mainly left arm)	• Antacids' frequent use to relieve pain
• Toothache	• Heartburn that awakens person during sleep
• Burning indigestion	• Acid or bitter taste in mouth
• Shortness of breath	• Burning chest sensation
• Nausea	• Discomfort after eating spicy foods
• Frequent belching	• Difficulty swallowing

Comparison of Symptoms of Angina Pectoris and Heartburn

Shutterstock background photos: Monster e (left), namtipStudio (right)

---

4. Cellular degeneration and subsequent hyalin formation (a translucent, homogeneous substance produced in degeneration) within the arterial intima
5. Calcium deposition at hyalinated area edges

The major disorders caused by reduced myocardial blood supply in CHD include angina pectoris, myocardial infarction, and congestive heart failure.

Angina Pectoris

Chest-related pain, called angina pectoris, occurs in approximately 30% of initial CHD manifestations. This temporary but painful condition indicates that coronary blood flow and oxygen supply momentarily reach inadequate levels. Current theory suggests that metabolites within an ischemic segment of the heart muscle stimulate myocardial pain receptors. Anginal pain usually lasts 1 to 3 min. Approximately one third of individuals who experience recurring anginal episodes die suddenly from a myocardial infarction. Chronic stable angina (often called *walk-through angina*) occurs at a predictable physical exertion level. Drugs that promote coronary artery vasodilation and reduce systemic peripheral vascular resistance (e.g., **nitroglycerin**) commonly treat this condition. FIGURE 32.2 illustrates the usual pain pattern with an acute episode of angina pectoris. Pain generally appears in the left shoulder along the arm to the elbow or occasionally in the midback region near the left scapula along the spinal cord.

Myocardial Infarction

A myocardial infarction (MI) results from sudden insufficiency in myocardial blood flow, usually from coronary artery occlusion. A prior clot or thrombus formed from plaque accumulation in one or more coronary vessels (see Chapter 31) can trigger sudden occlusion. Severe fatigue for several days without specific pain frequently precedes the MI onset. FIGURE 32.3 shows the varied locations for pain and discomfort that represent an early MI warning. During the infarction, severe, unrelenting chest pain can persist for more than 1 hr.

Congestive Heart Failure

More than 6.2 million Americans and 22 million people globally experience **congestive heart failure (CHF)**, also known as chronic decompensation or heart failure, in which the heart fails to adequately pump to meet other organ needs (www.cdc.gov/heartdisease/heart_failure.htm). This causes fluid to flow back into the lungs, which can leave the person struggling to breathe. CHF results from one or several of these seven factors:

1. Narrowed arteries from CHD that limit myocardial blood supply
2. Past MI with accompanying scar tissue (necrosis) that diminishes myocardial pumping efficiency
3. Chronic hypertension
4. Heart valve disease from past rheumatic fever or other pathology
5. Primary myocardial disease, called **cardiomyopathy**
6. Defects present in the heart at birth (congenital heart disease)
7. Heart valves and/or myocardium infection (endocarditis or **myocarditis**)

A "failing" heart keeps pumping, but inefficiently. Heart failure produces shortness of breath and fatigue with only minimal exertion. As blood flowing from the heart slows, blood returning to the heart

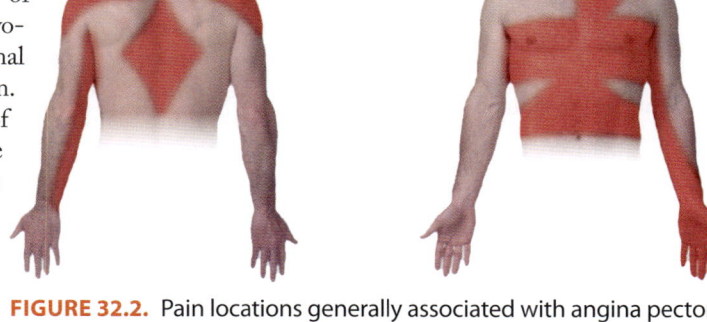

FIGURE 32.2. Pain locations generally associated with angina pectoris. Cardiac pain can refer to the left side, right side, both sides, or midback. (Reprinted with permission from Moore KL, et al. *Clinically Oriented Anatomy*. 8th ed. Baltimore: Wolters Kluwer; 2018. Anterior and posterior images: CLIPAREA | Custom media/Shutterstock.)

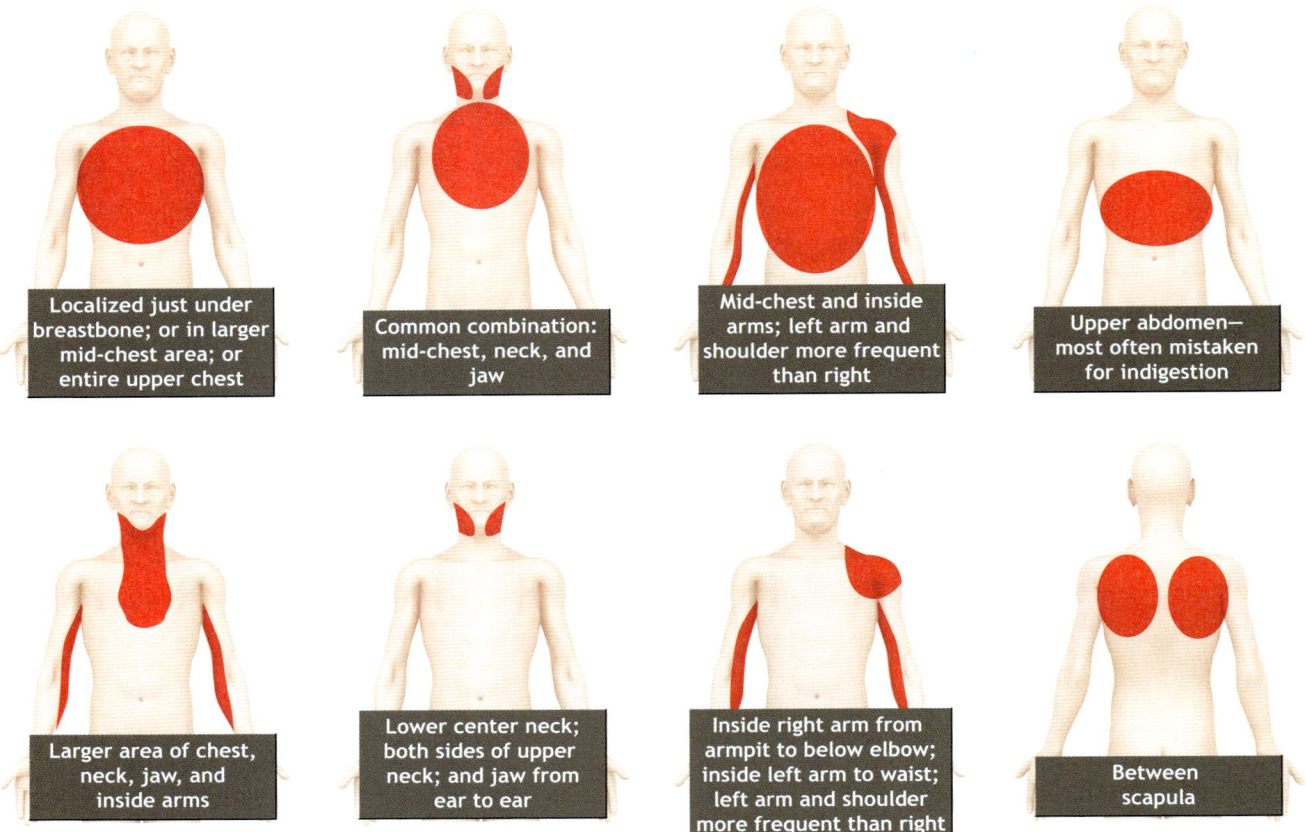

FIGURE 32.3. Anatomic locations for myocardial infarction's early warning signs. Note the diverse pain locations. (Anterior and posterior images: CLIPAREA | Custom media/Shutterstock.)

through the veins backs up, causing fluid to accumulate in the lungs with accompanying leg and ankle edema. Fluid in the lungs interferes with breathing to cause shortness of breath, especially when lying supine. CHF also affects the kidneys' disposal of sodium and water to further accentuate edema.

 See the animation "Edema" on Lippincott Connect for a demonstration of this process.

CHF represents the leading cause for hospitalization in persons older than age 65, accounting for 28.4% of all hospital stays in the United States, and affecting at least 26 million people worldwide. Estimates place the annual incidence of CHF in the United States at 10 per 1000 person-years in those aged 65 and older.[210] For individuals who contract the disease before age 60, about 20% die within 1 year of diagnosis and nearly half die within 5 years.[211]

CHF usually develops slowly as the heart gradually weakens and performs less effectively. Three primary CHF causes include:

1. Chronic hypertension
2. Intrinsic myocardial disease
3. Structural defects (e.g., diseased heart valves)

These three conditions produce an oversized, misshapen heart with inadequate pump performance and low resting **left-ventricular ejection fraction (LVEF)**. This marker of life-threatening heart dysfunction reflects a failure to increase heart rate during exercise.[6,43,82] Associated CHF risk factors include diabetes, alcoholism, and chronic lung diseases such as emphysema. Disease symptoms produce extreme disability, but symptom intensity frequently bears little relation to disease severity.[5,129] Patients with a low LVEF may not exhibit symptoms, whereas individuals whose hearts demonstrate normal pump function can experience severe disability. Heart disease and chronic hypertension contribute to CHF-disease progression. At the extreme stage, cardiac output from the left and/or right ventricles decreases to an extent that blood accumulates in the abdomen and lungs and sometimes in legs and feet. This stage of CHF produces fatigue, shortness of breath, and eventual flooding of the alveoli with blood, a condition termed **pulmonary congestion**. Impaired blood flow may also damage other organs, particularly the kidneys, resulting in renal failure.

 See the animation "Congestive Heart Failure" on Lippincott Connect for a demonstration of this process.

CHF Treatment and Rehabilitation. Before the 1980s, rest was advocated for all stages of CHF as the immediate treatment to reduce stress on the compromised cardiovascular

Congestive Heart Failure Growing at an Alarming Rate

By 2030, more than 8 million people will experience congestive heart failure (CHF), accounting for a 46% increase in prevalence. Each year in the United States, there are about 915,000 new CHF cases accounting for an incidence approaching 10 per 1000 people in the population aged 65 years and older. At age 40, the lifetime CHF risk is one in five, and at age 80, the remaining lifetime CHF risk stays at 20% despite a shorter life expectancy.

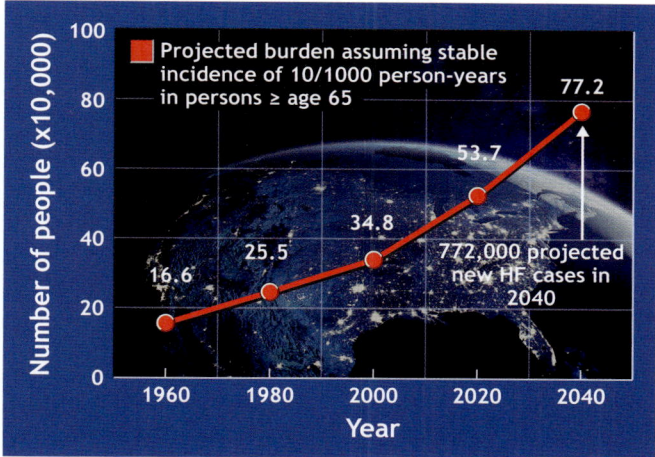

Data from Savarese G, Lund LH. Global public health burden of heart failure. *Card Fail Rev*. 2017;3:7. Background photo: NicoElNino/Shutterstock

Source:
Tsao CW, et al. Heart disease and stroke statistics-2022 update: a report from the American Heart Association. *Circulation*. 2022;145:e153-e639.

---

system. Patients also routinely received drugs aimed primarily at easing symptoms (e.g., digitalis to increase the heart's pumping function, called the inotropic effect). Current recommendations promote a four-drug regimen with two traditional drugs, digitalis and a diuretic to increase fluid excretion by kidneys, with newer angiotensin-converting enzyme inhibitors and β-blockers. Sixty years ago, Sir James Whyte Black (1924–2010), Scottish physician and pharmacologist who established the physiology department at the University of Glasgow, reported the first clinically significant β-blockers—*propranolol* and *pronethalol*—for medical management of angina pectoris.

Surgical treatment can replace damaged heart valves or repair myocardial aneurysms. Cardiac transplantation represents the extreme treatment of progressive disability from CHF, yet the shortage of donor organs persists. For patients awaiting a transplant, electrically powered pump implants placed in the abdomen below the heart mechanically assist ventricular function.

CHF and Regular PA. Clinicians have reevaluated the role of regular PA in heart disease treatment because many of the functional deteriorations in CHF duplicate extreme physical deconditioning. Reduced physical fitness and intrinsic skeletal muscle changes exacerbate the patient's physical incapacity.[55] *Current therapy advocates regular activity as an effective adjunct in CHF rehabilitation.*[6,61,101,120]

Clinical practice indicates that regular, moderate PA formulated from a symptom-limited graded exercise stress test with medications benefits relatively low-risk, stable, compensated patients.[33,112,142,176] Even intense endurance and resistance exercise training increases cardiac function, physical capacity, and peripheral muscle function and quality of life in these patients.[38,212]

PA benefits often accrue independent of the degree of baseline left ventricular dysfunction.[2] These benefits include improvements in functional capacity, exercise tolerance, muscle metabolism, level for dyspnea and the ventilatory response to exertion, risk for arrhythmias, left ventricular function, quality of life, and a shift toward greater vagal dominance.

It remains controversial whether the benefits of exercise rehabilitation for CHF link directly to enhanced central circulatory function—either improved myocardial performance per se or disease reversal reflected by reduced heart size.[10,43,61] To a large extent, peripheral adaptations accompanying regular physical activity enhance function and foster symptomatic improvements.

The clinician supervises the PA program for compensated patients. The graded exercise stress test provides the basis for the exercise prescription. For patients with marked exercise intolerance, relatively brief intervals of 2 to 5 min of light activity with a 1- to 3-min recovery afford benefits. The prescription also includes multiple PA sessions interspersed throughout the day. Abnormal heart rate response in CHF patients who exercise between 40 and 60% of maximum oxygen uptake ($\dot{V}O_{2max}$) provides a more objective standard to establish initial PA intensity. Alternatively, a rating of perceived exertion (RPE) on the Borg scale of "light" to "somewhat hard" (see Fig. 21.19, Chapter 21) and/or 2 on the dyspnea scale ("mild, some difficulty"; see Fig. 32.13) proves effective. Supervisory personnel should recognize the following six cardiac decompensation warning symptoms:

1. Dyspnea
2. Hypotension
3. Cough
4. Angina
5. Lightheadedness
6. Arrhythmias

After the patient begins to increase PA, duration can increase to 20 to 40 min at least three times weekly. Following 6 to 12 wk of supervised activity, patients usually can undertake an unsupervised home PA program.

Aneurysm

Aneurysm describes an abnormal dilation in the wall of an artery, vein, or cardiac chamber. Vascular aneurysms develop when a vessel wall weakens from trauma, congenital vascular disease, infection, or atherosclerosis. Aneurysms are either arterial or venous according to their specific region of origin (e.g., thoracic aneurysm). Most aneurysms develop without symptoms and often are discovered during a routine x-ray. The most common symptoms include chest pain with a specific palpable, pulsating mass in the chest, abdomen, or lower back mostly occurring near the skin's surface; they may be painful with swelling and a visible throbbing mass.

The most common areas for occurrence include the following:

1. Aortic aneurysm—major heart artery
2. Cerebral aneurysm—brain
3. Popliteal artery aneurysm—leg behind the knee
4. Mesenteric artery aneurysm—intestine
5. Splenic artery aneurysm—a spleen artery

Pericarditis

Pericarditis, an inflammation of the heart's outer lining, classifies as either acute or chronic (recurring or constrictive). Acute pericarditis symptoms vary but usually include chest pain, shortness of breath or dyspnea, and an elevated resting heart rate and body temperature. The prognosis for acute pericarditis remains excellent, but chronic pericarditis from bacterial origin presents a persistent serious pathology. Coxsackievirus B virus and echovirus are the more common viral causes (https://my.clevelandclinic.org/health/diseases/17353-pericarditis). Chronic pericardial inflammation creates extreme chest pain caused by fluid accumulation in the pericardial sac, which prevents the heart from fully expanding during diastole.

Heart Valve Diseases

Three medical conditions relate to heart valve abnormalities:

1. **Stenosis**: Narrowing or constriction that prevents heart valves from opening fully; may result from growths, scars, or abnormal calcified deposits.
2. **Insufficiency** (also known as regurgitation): Occurs when a heart valve closes improperly and blood moves back into a heart chamber.
3. Prolapse: Enlarged mitral valve leaflets bulge backward into the left atrium during ventricular systole.

Valvular abnormalities increase the heart's workload, causing it to pump harder to propel blood through a stenosed valve or to maintain cardiac output if blood seeps backward into one of its chambers during diastole. **Rheumatic fever** (www.webmd.com/a-to-z-guides/understanding-rheumatic-fever-directory), a serious group A streptococcal bacterial infection, scars and deforms heart valves. The most common symptoms include fever and joint pain. Penicillin and other antibiotics treat this inflammatory condition, which typically occurs in children ages 5 to 15 years.

Endocarditis

Endocarditis, usually of bacterial origin, represents an inflammation of the innermost layer of the heart or endocardium (https://medlineplus.gov/ency/article/001098.htm). The disease damages the tricuspid, aortic, or mitral valves from direct bacteria tissue invasion. Patients initially have musculoskeletal symptoms that include arthritis, lower back pain, and general weakness in one or more joints. Antibiotics can treat endocarditis before it become fatal.

Congenital Malformations

Congenital heart defects appear in 1 of every 100 births and include heart valve defects such as ventricular or atrial **septal defects** (hole between ventricles and atria) and **patent ductus arteriosus** (shunt caused by an opening between the aorta and pulmonary artery). For most infants, septal defects normally resolve within the first year of life or can be corrected with surgical repair.

Mitral Valve Prolapse

Mitral valve prolapse (MVP) occurs in about 10% of Americans involving variations in either the mitral valve's shape or structure. This defect has been called "floppy valve syndrome," "Barlow syndrome," and the "click-murmur syndrome." MVP diagnosis has increased over the past decade secondary to endocarditis, atherosclerosis, and muscular dystrophy. MVP most likely results from connective tissue abnormalities in mitral valve leaflets. Sixty percent of patients have no symptoms—the remainder experience profound fatigue during PA.

Cardiac Nervous System Diseases

Cardiac diseases that affect the heart's electrical conduction system include the following: **dysrhythmias** (also known as arrhythmias) that cause the heart to beat too rapidly (tachycardia), too slowly (bradycardia), or with extra contractions (**ectopic, extrasystole,** or **premature ventricular contractions [PVCs]**) that possibly lead to **fibrillation** (fine, rapid contractions or twitching of myocardial fibers). Dysrhythmias can produce changes in circulatory dynamics that can cause hypotension, heart failure, and shock. They often occur following a stroke induced by increased physical exertion or other stressors.

Sinus tachycardia describes a resting heart rate *above* 100 bpm; bradycardia describes a resting heart rate *below* 60 bpm. **Sinus bradycardia** occurs frequently in endurance athletes and young adults, generally representing a benign dysrhythmia. This may benefit cardiac function by producing a longer cardiac cycle ventricular filling time.

Cardiac Disease Assessment

Before initiating an intervention program of PA, the healthcare team decides on the health screening necessary. This always

PREPARTICIPATION HEALTH SCREENING

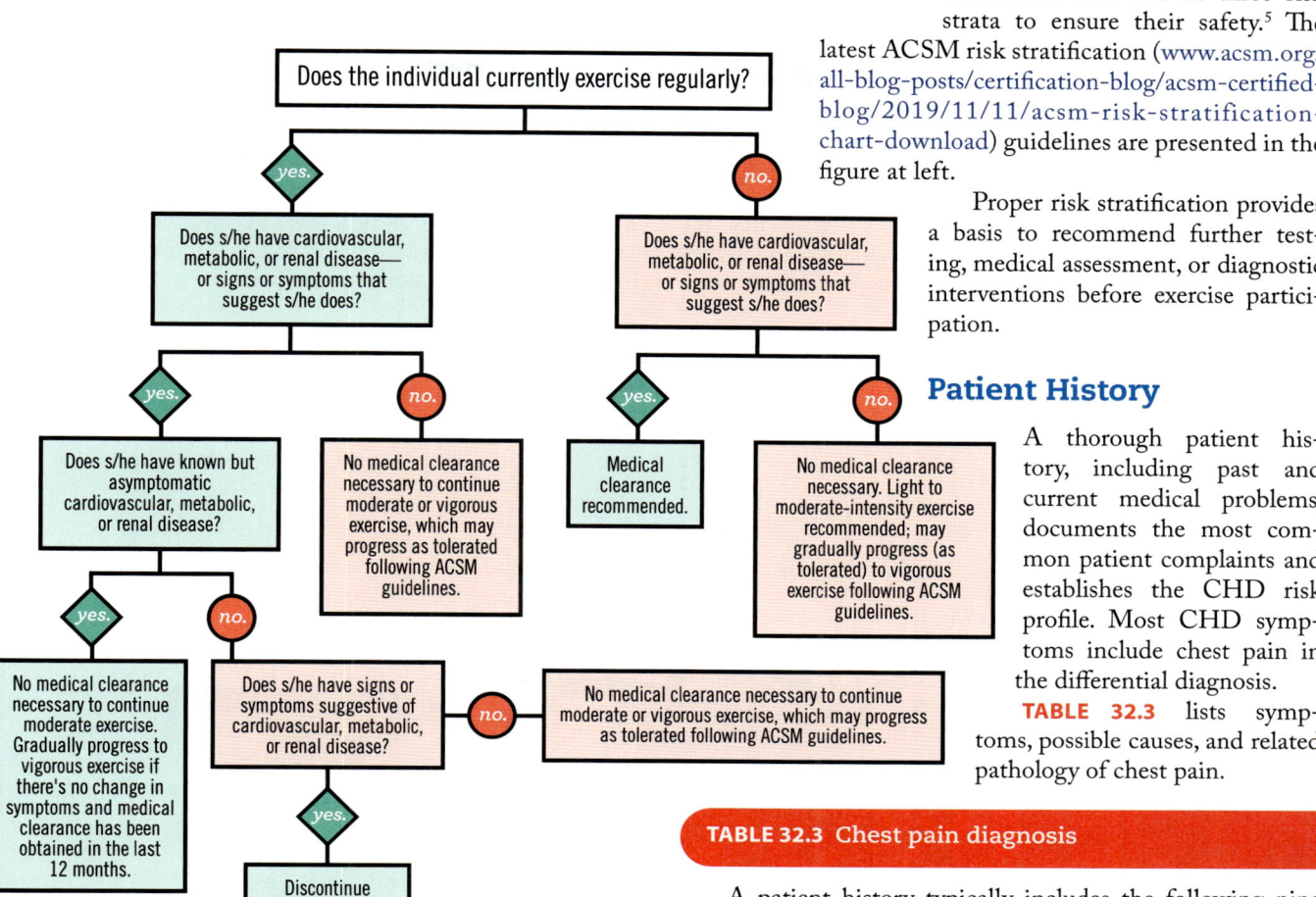

Reprinted with permission from American College of Sports Medicine. *Exercise Preparticipation Health Screening Resource.* Available at: www.acsm.org/all-blog-posts/certification-blog/acsm-certified-blog/2019/11/11/acsm-risk-stratification-chart-download.

includes a medical history, physical examination, and various laboratory assessments, and pertinent physiologic testing.

Health Screening and Risk Stratification

Assessing specific risk factors and/or symptoms for chronic cardiovascular, pulmonary, and metabolic diseases optimizes safety during exercise testing and program participation. Proper preparticipation screening accomplishes the following three goals:

1. Identifies and excludes persons with medical contraindications to PA
2. Identifies persons who require in-depth medical evaluation due to age, symptoms, and/or risk factors
3. Identifies persons with clinically significant disease who require medical supervision during exercise

Before beginning a physical conditioning program, the ACSM recommends using age, health status, symptoms, and risk factor information to classify individuals into one of three risk strata to ensure their safety.[5] The latest ACSM risk stratification (www.acsm.org/all-blog-posts/certification-blog/acsm-certified-blog/2019/11/11/acsm-risk-stratification-chart-download) guidelines are presented in the figure at left.

Proper risk stratification provides a basis to recommend further testing, medical assessment, or diagnostic interventions before exercise participation.

Patient History

A thorough patient history, including past and current medical problems, documents the most common patient complaints and establishes the CHD risk profile. Most CHD symptoms include chest pain in the differential diagnosis. **TABLE 32.3** lists symptoms, possible causes, and related pathology of chest pain.

TABLE 32.3 Chest pain diagnosis

A patient history typically includes the following nine entries:

1. Medical diagnosis of diseases
2. Previous physical examination findings to uncover abnormalities
3. Recent illnesses, hospitalizations, or surgical procedures
4. History of significant symptoms
5. Orthopedic concerns
6. Medications
7. Work record
8. Family background
9. Psychologic record

Physical Examination

The physical examination includes vital signs (body temperature, heart rate, breathing rate, and blood pressure) and other problem indicators. Assessments encompass auscultation of lungs; palpation and inspection of lower extremities for edema; neurologic function tests (reflexes and cognition); and inspection of the skin, especially of lower extremities in diabetics. Resting cardiorespiratory variables sometimes provide indirect, noninvasive clues to cardiovascular dysfunction. For example, sinus tachycardia or abnormal bradycardia and increased breathing rate and systolic blood pressure can contraindicate exercise without further evaluation.

In a Practical Sense

Determining Heart Rate from an Electrographic Tracing

The electrocardiogram (ECG) depicts the pattern of electrical activity across the myocardium. As the wave of depolarization travels throughout the heart, electrical currents spread through the highly conductive body fluids for monitoring by electrodes placed on the skin's surface. Standard markings on the ECG paper allow time interval and voltage measurements during ECG propagation.

STANDARD ECG TRACING

FIGURE 1 shows a standard ECG tracing with time recorded on the horizontal axis. The paper normally moves at 25 mm · s^{-1}.

A repeating grid marks the ECG paper; major grid lines occur 5 mm apart (at 25 mm · s^{-1} paper speed, 5 mm = 0.20 s), minor grid lines occur 1 mm apart (at 25 mm · s^{-1} paper speed, 1 mm = 0.04 s). The graph's vertical axis indicates electrical voltage. The standard calibration factor equals 0.1 mV (millivolt) per mm of vertical deflection.

DETERMINING HEART RATE

Three methods are used to determine heart rate from the standard ECG tracing.

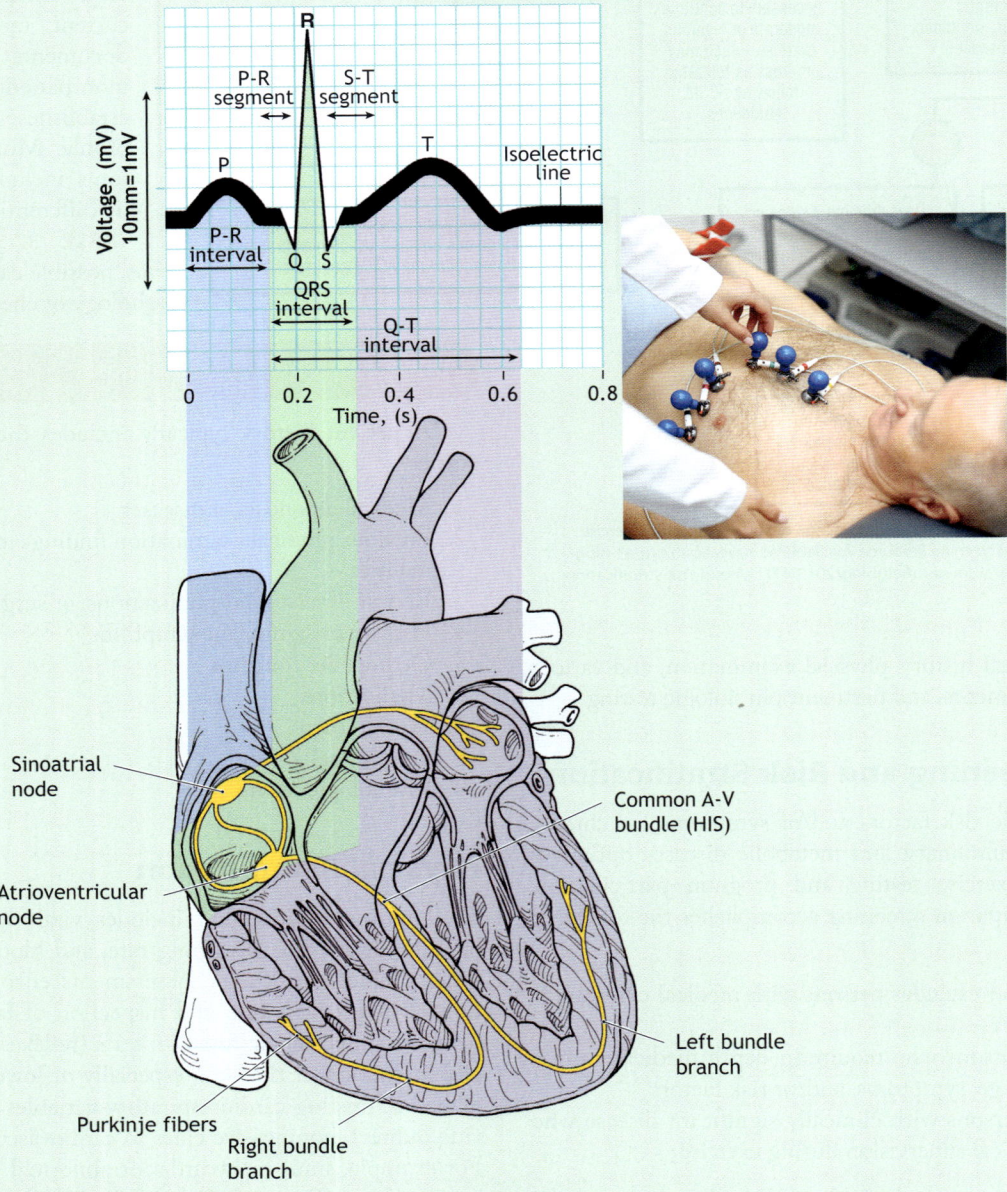

FIGURE 1. Normal electrocardiographic tracing.
(Photo: Pressmaster/Shutterstock)

Method 1

FIGURE 2A shows the standard R-R method. The R-R interval indicates the time between successive R waves. An approximate heart rate in beats per minute (bpm) can be determined by dividing 1500 (60 s × 25 mm · s^{-1}) by the number of mm between adjacent R waves. In the example, heart rate equals 125 bpm because 12 mm occurs between two successive R waves.

Method 2

This method begins with an R wave that falls on a thick blue line of the tracing (Fig. 2B). Moving to the right, the next six thick lines represent heart rates of 300, 150, 100, 75, 60, and 50 mm · s^{-1} (these numbers need to be memorized). If the next R wave (after the first one falling on the thick line) falls on either the first through sixth subsequent thick lines, the corresponding number (300 to 50) indicates heart rate in mm · s^{-1}. Interpolation becomes necessary if the next R wave falls between two thick lines. In this instance, the first R wave falls between points 60 and 75 at 70 mm · s^{-1}.

Method 3

This method (Fig. 2C), often used with irregular heart rates, counts the number of complete R-R intervals in a 6-s ECG strip multiplied by 10. In this example, six complete R-to-R intervals occur in 6 s; this equals a heart rate of 60 bpm (6 × 10 = 60).

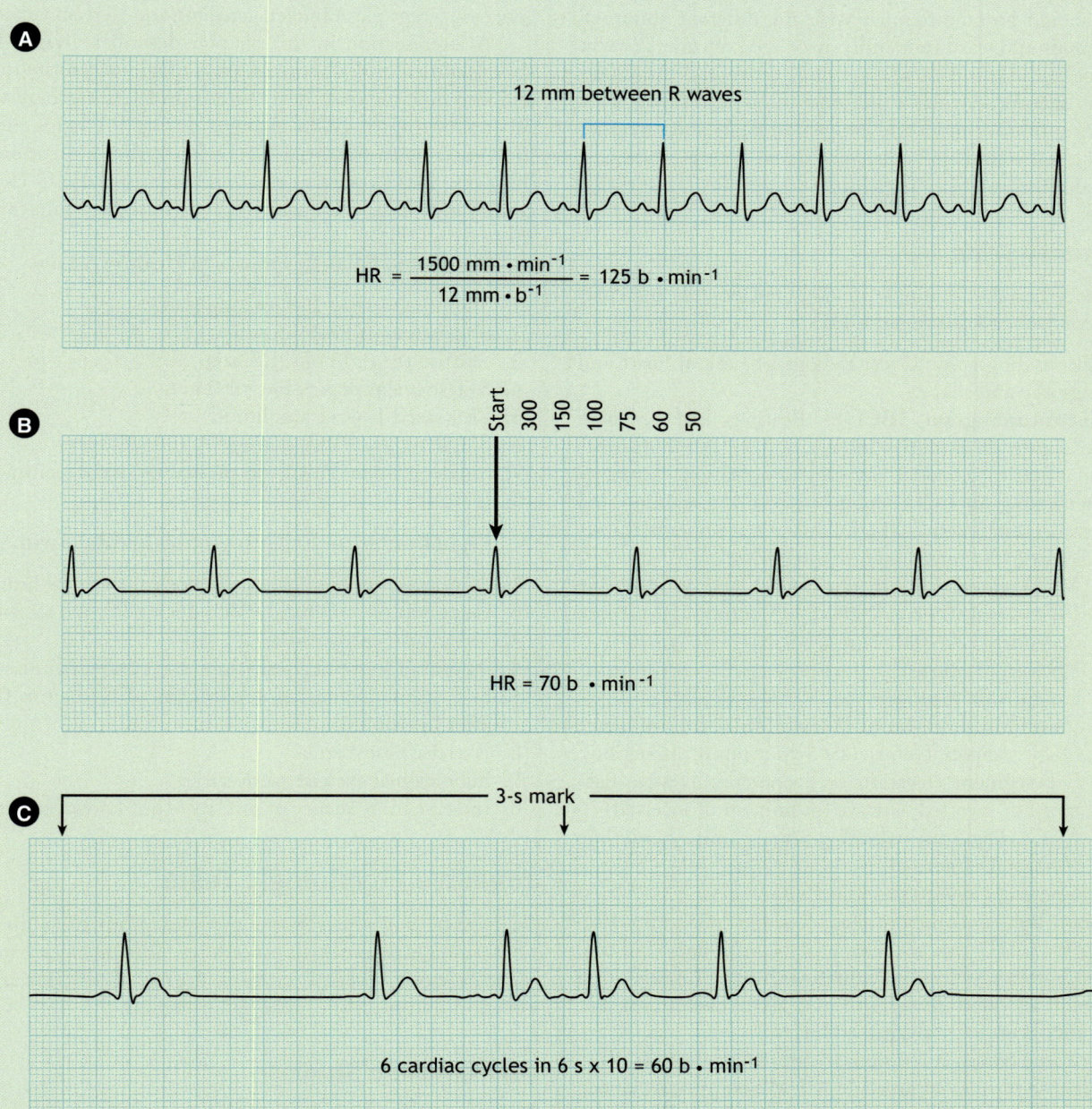

FIGURE 2. Three methods to determine heart rate from electrocardiographic tracings.

The CEP assesses the patient's heart rate and blood pressure response to graded exercise to prescribe PA and identify potential warning signs. For example, an increase in systolic blood pressure of 20 mm Hg or more with 2 to 4 metabolic equivalents (METs) of low-intensity PA often reflects abnormal myocardial oxygen demand that signals cardiovascular impairment. Similarly, failure of systolic blood pressure to increase (hypotensive response) can indicate blunted ventricular function; a depressed response in intense activity (e.g., failure to achieve systolic blood pressures above 140 mm Hg in near-maximal effort) frequently indicates dormant cardiac disease.

Heart Auscultation

Listening to heart sounds (**auscultation**) during the cardiac cycle helps to assess cardiac performance. The exercise physiologist should become familiar with the different abnormal heart sounds and learn to identify associated murmurs (www.practicalclinicalskills.com/heart-sounds-murmurs). Auscultation can uncover valvular conditions (e.g., MVP, diagnosed by click-murmur sounds) and congenital heart abnormalities (regurgitation sounds in ventricular septal defects; www.cdc.gov/ncbddd/heartdefects/facts.html).

Laboratory Tests

Laboratory-based screenings provide considerable information to confirm and document CHD.

- Chest radiography: Chest radiographs reveal heart and lungs size and shape.
- **Electrocardiogram (ECG)**: Resting and exercise ECG provide essential information to assess myocardial electrical conductivity and oxygenation. Correctly interpreting an ECG requires specialized training and considerable practice. The following list presents the six different ECG interpretation categories:
  1. Measurements: heart rate (atrial and ventricular); PR interval (0.12 to 0.20 s); QT interval (heart rate dependent); frontal plane QRS axis (−30° to 90°)
  2. Rhythm diagnosis
  3. Conduction diagnosis
  4. Waveform description: P wave (atrial enlargement); QRS complex (ventricular hypertrophy, infarction); S-T segment elevation or depression; T wave flattened or inverted; U wave (prominent or inverted)
  5. ECG diagnosis: within normal limits–borderline abnormal; abnormal
  6. Comparison with previous ECG
- Blood lipid and lipoproteins: Routine laboratory testing for CHD risk includes analysis of blood lipid and lipoprotein profiles. Individuals with heart disease often exhibit elevated cholesterol and LDL cholesterol, but neither is useful to diagnose CHD.
- Serum enzymes: Alterations in serum enzymes can often diagnose or rule out an acute MI. When myocardial cell death (necrosis) or prolonged lack of blood flow (ischemia) occurs, specific enzymes from the damaged muscle leak into the blood because of the plasma membrane's increased permeability. This leakage increases serum levels of these three enzymes:
  1. **Creatine phosphokinase (CPK)**
  2. Lactate dehydrogenase (LDH)
  3. **Serum glutamic oxaloacetic transaminase (SGOT)**

Elevated CPK levels reflect either skeletal or cardiac muscle fiber damage. To pinpoint the enzyme leak source, electrophoresis or radioimmunoassay analysis separates CPK into three different isoenzymes: MM-isoenzyme, unique to skeletal muscle; BB-isoenzyme, specific to brain tissue; and MB-isoenzyme, specific for cardiac muscle necrosis. LDH fractionates into different isoenzymes (as does CPK), one of which increases during an infarction. An acute MI also raises SGOT levels. Additional blood tests for CHD diagnosis include serum homocysteine (see Chapter 31), lipoprotein(a), fibrinogen, tissue-type plasminogen activator, and C-reactive protein.

A later section in this chapter describes various ECG abnormalities and abnormal physiologic responses to PA and also how to count heart rate from ECG tracings. Careful monitoring of ECG changes during PA helps identify individuals with potential CHD for further evaluation. The following lists present normal and abnormal ECG changes commonly observed during PA in healthy adults and in those with CHD.

Prominent ECG Responses in Healthy Adults

1. Slight increase in P wave amplitude
2. Shortening of P–R interval
3. Shift to the right of QRS axis
4. S–T segment depression <1.0 mm
5. Decreased T-wave amplitude
6. Single or rare PVCs during PA and recovery
7. Single or rare PVCs or premature atrial contractions (PACs)

Eight Prominent ECG Responses in Adults with CHD

1. Appearance of bundle branch block at a critical heart rate
2. Recurrent or multifocal PVCs during PA and recovery
3. Ventricular tachycardia
4. Appearance of bradyarrhythmias, tachyarrhythmias
5. S–T segment depression/elevation of >1.0 mm 0.08 s after J point
6. Exercise bradycardia
7. Submaximal exercise tachycardia
8. Increase in frequency or severity of any known arrhythmia

Invasive Physiologic Tests

Invasive cardiovascular testing provides information unattainable through noninvasive procedures. This includes coronary atherosclerosis severity, location, degree of ventricular dysfunction, and specific cardiac abnormalities.

Radionuclide Studies

Radionuclide studies require injecting a radioactive isotope (e.g., mostly technetium-99) into the circulation during rest and PA (https://my.clevelandclinic.org/health/diagnostics/4902-nuclear-medicine-imaging). Two examples include the following:

1. **Thallium imaging**: Evaluates myocardial blood flow areas and tissue perfusion to differentiate between a true-positive and false-positive S–T segment depression obtained by ECG evaluation during a graded exercise stress test
2. **Nuclear ventriculography**: Radiographic imaging that analyzes regional left ventricular contractility following injection of a radioactive isotope contrast material

Pharmacologic Stress Testing. A **pharmacologic stress test** benefits individuals unable to undergo routine stress testing because of extreme deconditioning, peripheral vascular disease, orthopedic disabilities, neurologic disease, or other health problems (www.drugs.com/cg/pharmacologic-stress-testing.html).

This test involves systematic intravenous drug infusion (e.g., dobutamine, dipyridamole, or adenosine) every 3 min to attain the desired dosage. Echocardiography and/or thallium scanning then monitor for changes in wall motion abnormalities or coronary perfusion limitations, respectively. Heart rate response, arrhythmias, angina symptoms, S–T segment depression, and blood pressure dynamics also reflect myocardial viability during the test.

Cardiac Catheterization

Cardiac catheterization (www.nhlbi.nih.gov/health-topics/cardiac-catheterization) involves threading a small-diameter, flexible tube (**catheter**), guided by x-ray, directly into an arm or leg vein or artery up into the heart's right or left side. Sensors on the catheter tip accurately measure pressure gradients at various locations within the heart's chambers or large vessels; they also assess the heart's electrical patterns to determine coronary artery blockage. The oxygen content in arterial and mixed venous blood is determined from blood sampled from the atria or ventricles. Catheterization takes place under local anesthesia, depending on the point of catheter entry into the arm or leg. The patient remains awake during the procedure, and test results usually become available on the same day (www.youtube.com/watch?v=A0UvHQcfavE).

 See the animations "Coronary Angiography: Left Coronary System-Part A" and "Coronary Angiography: Left Coronary System-Part B" on **Lippincott Connect** for a demonstration of this process.

Coronary Angiography. Radiography images the coronary circulation by injecting a contrast medium, essentially a dye that flows into the coronary vasculature. The highly effective technique evaluates coronary atherosclerosis and represents the gold standard to assess coronary blood flow for baseline and future test comparisons. Unlike thallium imaging, angiography cannot determine how easily blood flows within portions of the myocardium and cannot be utilized during exercise. The angiogram depicted in **FIGURE 32.4** pinpoints impaired blood flow represented by the circle around

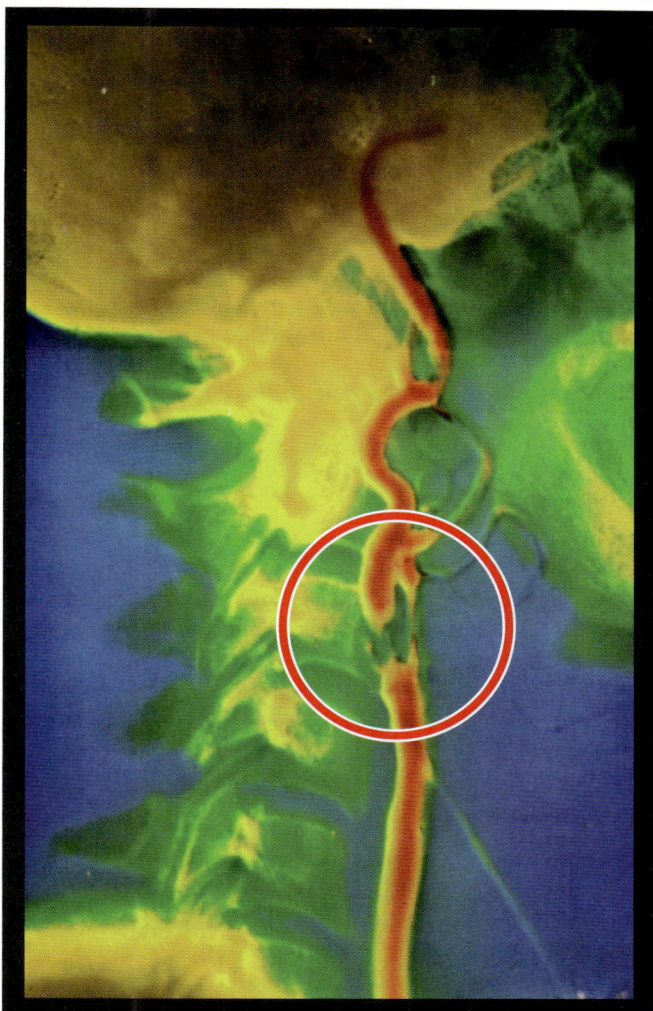

FIGURE 32.4. Angiogram showing constriction and absence of blood flow through the right carotid artery (in *red*).
(Courtesy Dr. Barry Franklin, Beaumont Hospital, Birmingham, MI.)

the occluded vessel in the carotid artery. Resectioning a vessel or removing its atherosclerotic plaques significantly improves blood flow to reduce stroke occurrence.

Lippincott® Connect Appendix H, available online at **Lippincott Connect**, provides a list of supplemental animations and videos on this subject, including an animation of angiography.

Noninvasive Physiologic Screening and Assessment

Echocardiography

Echocardiography uses reflected ultrasound pulses to evaluate heart function and morphology to identify the heart's structural components and measure distances within the myocardial chambers (http://asecho.org). Estimating various chamber sizes or volumes includes blood vessel dimensions and myocardial component thickness. The echocardiogram has surpassed the ECG in recognizing chamber enlargement, myocardial hypertrophy, and other structural abnormalities. Echocardiograms

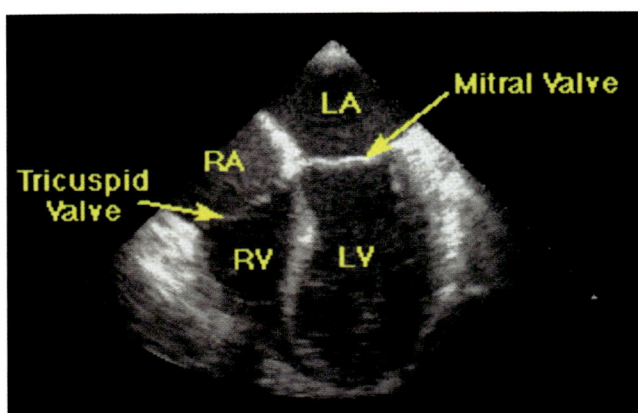

FIGURE 32.5. Grey-scale mode echocardiogram shows right and left ventricles (RV, LV) and atria (RA, LA) and mitral and tricuspid valves.

can diagnose heart murmurs, evaluate valvular lesions, and determine congenital heart diseases and myopathies.

FIGURE 32.5 presents a typical echocardiographic image showing the left and right atrium, left and right ventricle, and tricuspid and mitral valves. The echocardiogram can provide different size and function diagnostic parameters in the heart's chambers. The advent of three-dimensional echocardiograms has enhanced echocardiography as a valuable diagnostic tool (depts.washington.edu/cvrtc/ocarinas.html).

Ultrafast Computed Tomography Scan

This 10-min noninvasive test uses an **ultrafast electron beam computed tomography (EBCT) scan** to assess calcium deposition within the plaque in coronary artery linings (www.medicinenet.com/ebct_electron_beam_computerized_tomography/definition.htm). Test results determine how aggressively to treat blood lipid abnormalities (e.g., diet and PA vs. drug therapy) and additional CHD risk factors. Testing to detect coronary calcium deposition with EBCT is highly sensitive for males and females with coronary disease validated by coronary angiography.[56] Exclusion of coronary calcium buildup can identify individuals with a low probability for significant vascular stenosis.

Graded Exercise Stress Testing

A **graded exercise stress test (GXT)** systematically uses exercise for four purposes:

1. Observe cardiac rhythm abnormalities.
2. Assess overall physiologic adjustments to increased PA metabolic demands.
3. Objectify functional capacity of patients with known disease.
4. Evaluate progress following surgery or other therapeutic interventions.

TABLE 32.4 presents subjective and objective information obtained during a GXT used to diagnose and formulate an exercise prescription. The cardiologist and exercise physiologist supervise the exercise test, interpret the data, and prescribe the appropriate PA intervention.

TABLE 32.4 Exercise stress test results: diagnose and formulate exercise prescriptions

Multistage bicycle and treadmill tests represent the most common stress testing modes. These tests graded for intensity, usually include several 3- to 5-min submaximal intervals to bring the person to a self-imposed fatigue end point. Graded testing allows intensity to increase in small increments to isolate ischemic symptom and rhythm disorders related to anginal pain and ECG abnormalities. With heart disease, exercise testing provides a reliable, quantitative index about a person's functional impairment to objectify the diagnosis and subsequent exercise prescription.[45,133] Testing generally does not require maximal effort, but the person should attain at least 85% of age-predicted maximum heart rate.

Exercise stress testing cannot identify CHD extent or its specific location. Twenty-five to 40% of people with advanced CHD with significant blockage in one or more coronary arteries achieve a normal GXT evaluation. Interestingly, an abnormal heart rate recovery (i.e., failure of heart rate to decrease by more than 12 bpm in the first min after peak exercise) predicts subsequent mortality in patients referred specifically for exercise electrocardiography independently from ECG assessment.[121] Thus, recovery heart rate provides additional prognostic information to complement exercise stress test interpretations.

Stress Testing for CHD Evaluation

Stress testing serves the following six functions to evaluate CHD:

1. **Diagnoses overt heart disease and screens for "silent" coronary disease in apparently healthy adults.** Approximately 30% of persons with confirmed CHD have a normal resting ECG. Graded exercise testing generally uncovers 70% of the abnormalities.
2. **Assesses exercise-related chest symptoms.** For individuals older than age 40 who have chest or related pain in the left shoulder or arm during physical exertion, ECG analysis identifies myocardial abnormalities and more precisely diagnoses exercise-induced pain.
3. **Screens candidates for entry into preventative and cardiac rehabilitative programs.** Test results provide an objective framework to design a program based on current functional capacity and health status. Repeat testing assesses progress and adaptations to regular PA and provides a basis for program modification.
4. **Uncovers abnormal blood pressure responses.** Individuals with normal resting blood pressure sometimes show greater than normal increases in systolic blood pressure during mild-to-moderate PA, which may signify developing cardiovascular complications.
5. **Monitors therapeutic intervention effectiveness (drugs, surgery, nutrition) to improve heart disease status and cardiovascular function.** A patient's capacity to achieve a target heart rate without complications often confirms successful coronary bypass surgery.
6. **Quantifies functional aerobic capacity ($\dot{V}O_{2\,max}$) to evaluate its deviation from normal standards**

Who Requires Stress Testing? TABLE 32.5 presents screening and supervisory procedures for exercise testing that conform to policies and practices of the ACSM.

TABLE 32.5 Medical examination, exercise testing, and supervision of exercise testing pre-participation recommendations

Informed Consent. All testing and exercise training must be performed on "informed" volunteers. **Informed consent** should raise a subject's awareness about potential participation risks. It must include a written statement about the opportunity to ask questions about any procedures, with sufficient information clearly stated so that consent occurs with an informed (knowledgeable) perspective. A legal guardian or parent must sign a consent form for minors. Individuals require assurance that test results remain confidential, and they can terminate testing or training at any time and for any reason. TABLE 32.6 shows a sample exercise stress testing informed consent document.

TABLE 32.6 Sample graded exercise stress test informed consent

Stress Testing Contraindications

Certain conditions preclude administering a stress test (absolute contraindications), while other conditions require the GXT be more closely monitored (relative contraindications).

Absolute Contraindications. A stress test should *not* take place without direct medical supervision under the following contraindications:

- Resting ECG suggestive of acute cardiac disease
- Recent complicated MI
- Unstable angina pectoris
- Uncontrolled ventricular arrhythmias
- Uncontrolled atrial arrhythmias that compromise cardiac function
- **Third-degree atrioventricular (AV) heart block** without pacemaker
- Acute heart failure
- Severe **aortic stenosis**
- Active or suspected myocarditis or pericarditis
- Recent systemic or pulmonary embolism
- Acute infection
- Acute emotional distress

Relative Contraindications. A GXT can be administered with caution and with medical personnel in the test area under the following conditions:

- Resting diastolic blood pressure ≤115 mm Hg or systolic blood pressure ≤200 mm Hg
- Moderate valvular disease
- Electrolyte abnormalities
- Frequent or complex **ventricular ectopy**
- Ventricular aneurysm
- Uncontrolled metabolic disease (e.g., diabetes, thyrotoxicosis)
- Chronic infectious disease (e.g., hepatitis, mononucleosis, acquired immunodeficiency syndrome)
- Neuromuscular or musculoskeletal disorders
- Pregnancy (complicated or in the last trimester)
- Psychologic distress and/or apprehension concerning test participation

GXT Termination. Graded exercise testing is generally safe when following recognized guidelines and taking proper precautions. At least 12 reasons exist for terminating a GXT before the person attains maximum volitional fatigue.

1. Angina onset or angina-like symptoms
2. Significant 20-mm Hg drop in systolic blood pressure or failure of systolic blood pressure to rise as PA intensity increases
3. Excessive rise in blood pressure: systolic pressure ≥260 mm Hg or diastolic pressure ≥115 mm Hg
4. Signs of poor vascular perfusion characterized by light-headedness, confusion, ataxia, pallor, cyanosis, nausea, or cold and clammy skin
5. Heart rate failure to increase with increasing PA intensity
6. Noticeable change in heart rhythm
7. Patient requests to stop
8. Physical or verbal manifestations of severe fatigue
9. Testing equipment failure
10. Early-onset horizontal or downsloping S–T segment depression or ≥4 mm elevation
11. Increasing ventricular ectopy; multiform PVCs
12. Sustained supraventricular tachycardia

Stress Test Outcomes

A clinically successful GXT depends on its predictive outcome, which means how effectively the test correctly diagnoses a person with heart disease.

Four possible GXT outcomes include the following:

1. **True positive** (successful test): GXT correctly identifies a person with heart disease.
2. **True negative** (successful test): GXT correctly identifies a person without heart disease.
3. **False positive** (unsuccessful test): GXT incorrectly identifies a normal person as having heart disease.
4. **False negative** (unsuccessful test): GXT incorrectly identifies a person with heart disease as normal.

Test sensitivity refers to the percentage of persons whose test detects an abnormal (positive) response. This represents a true-positive condition that only subsequent follow-up can verify. False-negative results (unsuccessful test) occur 25% of the time, and false-positive results (unsuccessful test) occur approximately 15% of the time. Factors that contribute to false-negative results include the patient's failure to reach an ischemic threshold, failure to recognize non-ECG signs and symptoms associated with underlying CHD, and technical or

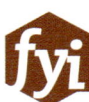

False-Positive Versus False-Negative Test Results

The differences between false-positive and false-negative test results often seem confusing. When test results indicate "Yes" or "No," such as for coronary heart disease (CHD) screening, it is important to consider whether the test could be wrong. The terms True and False refer to the truth; the terms Positive and Negative refer to the test results.

Possible outcomes include the following:

True Positive	The <u>truth</u> is positive: The person has CHD. The test accurately confirms CHD
True Negative	The <u>truth</u> is negative: The person does not have CHD. The test accurately confirms the person does not have CHD
False Negative	The <u>truth</u> is positive: The person has CHD. The test inaccurately reports the person does not have CHD
False Positive	The <u>truth</u> is negative: The person does not have CHD. The test inaccurately reports they have CHD

Background images: JY FotoStock/Shutterstock

observer errors. Various drugs and conditions also increase the probability of false-negative results, particularly if the person takes β-blockers, nitrates, or calcium channel blocker agents.

Test specificity refers to the number of true-negative test results—correctly identifying someone without CHD. More false-positive results occur when the individual takes the drug digitalis and has hypokalemia (low blood potassium levels), MVP, pericardial disorders, or anemia.

Stress Testing the "Oldest-Old". The stress testing guidelines in Table 32.4 do not apply to individuals ≥75 years, those considered among the "*oldest-old*."[59] Only a small, highly select subgroup of these individuals participates in vigorous PA or can successfully complete a stress test. For example, approximately 30% of persons age 75 to 79 can achieve a maximal physical effort, 25% of those ages 80 to 84 years, and only 9% ≥85 years.[75] The oldest-old differ markedly from persons ≤70 years in the following two key areas relative to stress testing:

1. High asymptomatic CHD prevalence
2. Coexistence with other chronic conditions and physical limitations

Older, asymptomatic males and females exhibit increased ECG abnormalities, many of which diminish GXT diagnostic accuracy. Asymptomatic ischemic episodes uncovered by the exercise ECG increases dramatically among older adults with no history of MI or ECG abnormalities. Given the large asymptomatic CHD prevalence among older persons, routine exercise stress testing would likely initiate follow-up invasive cardiac procedures.[54,169] Lacking strong evidence to support aggressive evaluations, this practice in older adults would subject many persons to unnecessary complications from invasive assessment. For this reason, empirical screening for older adults prescribes PA based on the person's previous activity experiences and overall sense of well-being. This approach to exercise testing, training, and safety monitoring observes the widely accepted geriatric dictum "*start low and go slow.*"

Exercise-Induced CHD Indicators

PA creates the greatest demand for coronary blood flow, making exercise testing an effective way to probe for existing CHD.

Angina Pectoris

Myocardial ischemia—usually from restricted coronary circulation induced by atherosclerosis—stimulates sensory nerves in coronary artery and myocardial walls. Pain or discomfort generally manifests in the upper chest region, yet frequently presents as increased pressure or constriction in the left shoulder or arm, neck, or jaw (see Figs. 32.2 and 32.3). Impaired cardiac performance—reduced stroke volume and cardiac output— also accompanies angina. The pain usually subsides after 2 to 3 min without PA and no permanent myocardial damage. PA frequently triggers an angina episode, yet angina also can occur at rest (**Prinzmetal angina** or variant angina), with attacks typically occurring in the late evening through early morning. Approximately two thirds of people with variant angina caused by a coronary artery spasm have severe blockage in at least one major coronary vessel. **Stable angina** signals predictable chest pain on exertion or mental and/or emotional stress.

Electrocardiographic Abnormalities

Alterations in the heart's normal electrical activity pattern signify insufficient myocardial oxygen supply. Such electrical "cues" seldom emerge unless myocardial metabolic and blood flow requirements exceed resting conditions.

FIGURE 32.6A traces the dynamic electrical activity in the myocardium throughout the cardiac cycle. Standard ECG paper contains 1- and 5-mm squares. Horizontally, each small square represents 0.04 s (with normal paper speed 25 mm · s^{-1}); each large square represents 0.2 s. On the vertical axis, a small square indicates a 0.1-mV deflection with a 10-mm · mV^{-1} calibration. One normal heartbeat in a cardiac cycle consists of five major electrical waves labeled P, Q, R, S, and T. The P wave reveals an electrical impulse or depolarization wave before atrial contraction. The Q, R, and S waves, collectively known as the QRS complex, represent ventricle depolarization immediately before their contraction.

Ventricular repolarization generates the T wave. The cause of **S–T segment depression** (Fig. 32.6B) remains unknown, yet this abnormal deviation correlates with other CHD indicators that include coronary artery narrowing. *Individuals with significant S–T segment depression usually have severe, extensive obstruction in one or more coronary arteries.* Unfortunately, a consistently large S–T segment depression directly relates to future CHD death. Generally, a 1- to 2-mm S–T segment depression during exercise coincides with a nearly fivefold increase in CHD mortality. The death risk increases approximately 20-fold for those with a depression of more than 2 mm. Current opinion advocates including nonspecific ECG findings in the overall heart disease risk assessment.[27] Even nonspecific minor S–T segment or T-wave abnormalities or both (termed ST–T abnormalities) provide a disquieting hint to increased long-term mortality risk from cardiovascular disease.

During a standard ECG-monitored treadmill test, special electrodes can identify extremely subtle electrical patterns to predict a patient's risk for ventricular fibrillation. The test, termed the alternans test, identifies electrical alternation of the heart. Specifically, it uses a device to analyze T-wave alternans, which represent beat-to-beat electrical fluctuations of just one-millionth of a volt. T-wave alternans reflect abnormalities in the way myocardial cells recover after transmitting the heart's electrical impulse. Oscillation of the cells' impulse can initiate a chain reaction that produces arrhythmias, fibrillation, and subsequent sudden cardiac arrest; in more than 356,000 out-of-hospital cardiac arrests in the United States, nearly 90% are fatal.[213]

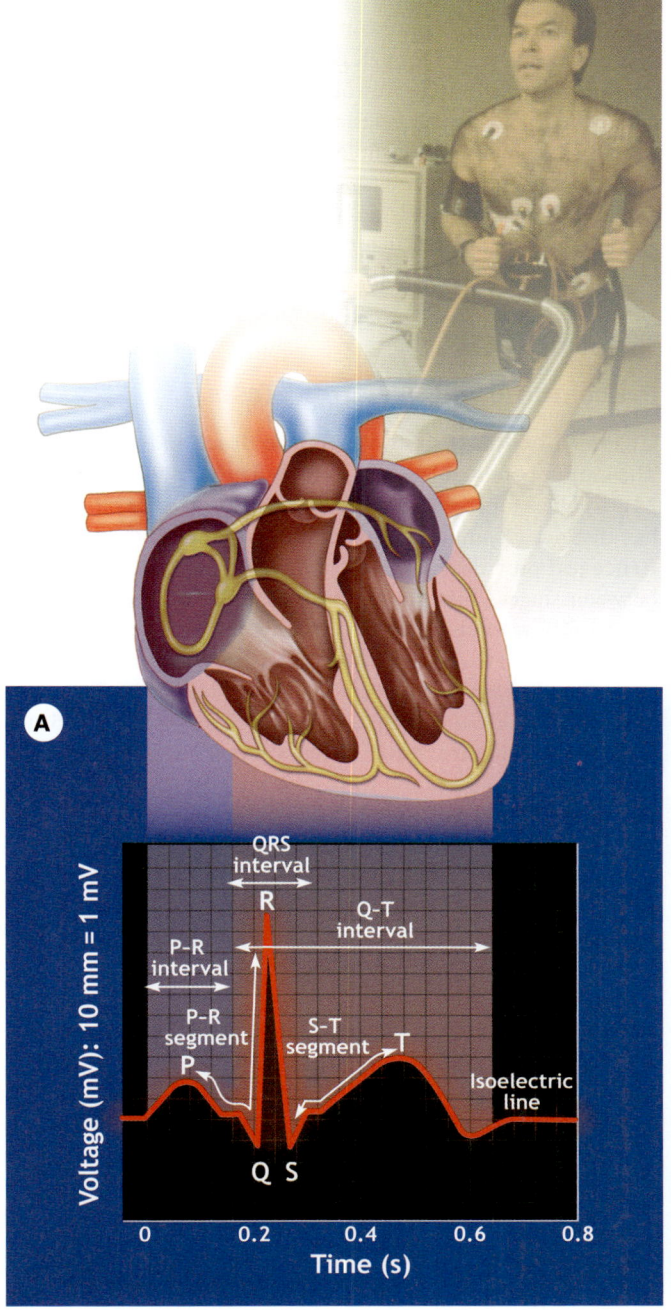
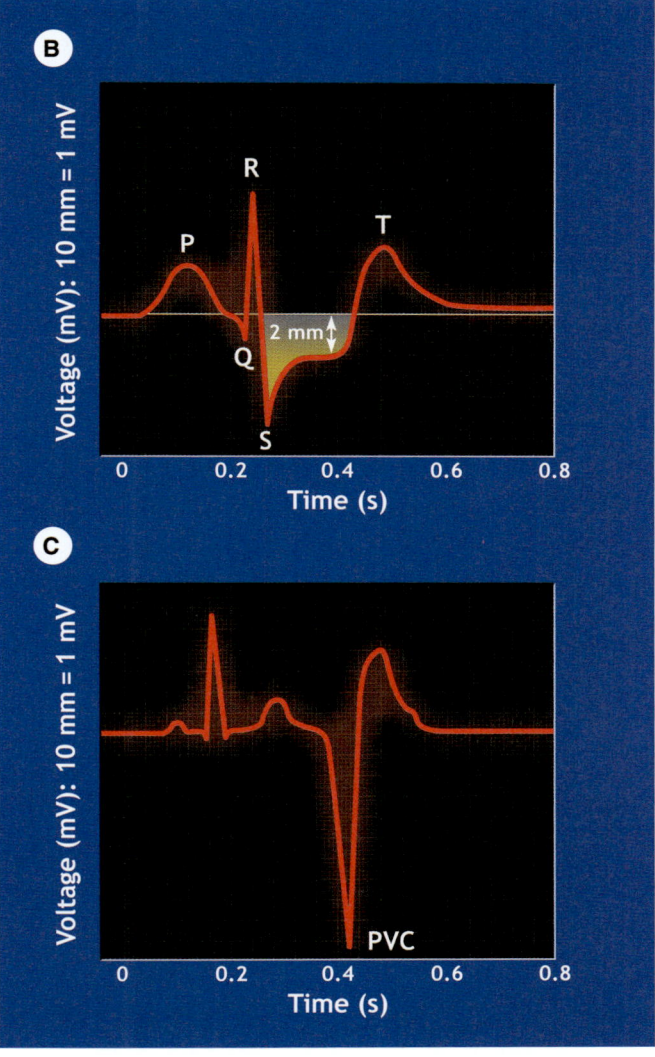

FIGURE 32.6. **(A)** Normal electrocardiogram (ECG) tracing with an upward-sloping S–T segment. **(B)** Abnormal horizontal S–T segment 2 mm depression (*shaded area*) measured from a stable baseline. **(C)** Premature ventricular contraction (PVC).

Predicting risk for sudden death via T-wave alterations gives high-risk patients medical protection that might include an implanted defibrillator (placed beneath the skin of the chest) to automatically correct deviant cardiac electrical activity. The defibrillator activates a built-in pacemaker to restabilize the heart's normal rhythm when it detects minor arrhythmias. If that fails, the pacemaker delivers a small defibrillating electrical jolt that resets to the rhythm.

Cardiac Rhythm Abnormalities

Graded exercise testing uncovers abnormalities in the heart's electrical activity pattern. A PVC (Fig. 32.11C) during PA often reflects abnormal alteration in cardiac rhythm, or **arrhythmia**. In this case, the normal depolarization wave through the AV node does not stimulate the ventricles. Instead, portions of the ventricle spontaneously depolarize to produce an "extra" ventricular beat without the P wave (atrial depolarization) that normally precedes it.

PVCs during PA generally herald severe ischemic atherosclerotic heart disease often involving two or more major coronary vessels. This specific myocardial electrical instability with PA has greater predictive value than S–T segment depression for CHD diagnosis. Patients with exercise-induced PVCs have a 6 to 10 times greater sudden death risk from abnormal ventricular movements (**ventricular fibrillation**) than patients without such instability. Fibrillation risk becomes more prevalent in individuals with familial history of fibrillation occurrence. With fibrillation, the ventricles do not contract in a unified manner, allowing cardiac output to decrease dramatically. Sudden death without a return to normal ventricular rhythm is almost a certainty without mitigating this risk. One successful strategy involves implanting an electrical stimulator to adjust abnormal myocardial electrical conductance patterns.

Other Exercise-Induced CHD Indicators

Blood pressure and heart rate responses to PA provide three useful non-ECG indices of possible CHD:

1. **Hypertensive exercise response**: Normally, systolic blood pressure progressively increases during graded exercise from approximately 120 mm Hg at rest to 160 to 190 mm Hg during peak-intensity of effort. The change in diastolic pressure generally is less than ±10 mm Hg. During PA, systolic blood pressure can rise to well above 200 mm Hg, whereas diastolic pressure can approach 150 mm Hg. This abnormal hypertensive response provides a significant clue to a cardiovascular disease state.
2. **Hypotensive exercise response**: Inability for blood pressure to increase during graded exercise reflects cardiovascular malfunction. When systolic blood pressure does not increase by at least 20 or 30 mm Hg, it often indicates diminished cardiac reserve.
3. **Heart rate response**: A rapid, large increase in heart rate (tachycardia) early in graded exercise often indicates cardiac dysfunction. Likewise, abnormally low exercise heart rates (bradycardia) in non–endurance-trained individuals

may reflect unhealthy sinoatrial node function. Inability of heart rate to increase during graded exercise (**chronotropic incompetence**), particularly when accompanied by extreme fatigue, indicates cardiac strain and CHD. Reduced maximal exercise heart rate in apparently healthy males and females raises cardiovascular disease mortality risk.[89,97] Failure to achieve at least 85% of age-predicted maximum heart rate during PA predicts an eventual all-cause mortality risk, independent of exercise-induced myocardial perfusion defects.[98]

Stress Test Protocols

Test duration, initial exercise intensity level, and intensity increments between stages for GXT protocols dictate a "best" test to administer. A national survey of 1400 exercise stress test centers, based on 75,828 exercise tests performed at Veterans Affairs Medical Centers with cardiology divisions, reported that 78% used the treadmill, with 82% of these preferring the Bruce or Modified Bruce protocols. In all of this testing, only three MIs and one sustained ventricular tachycardia cardiac event occurred, representing a 1.2 per 10,000 event rate from exercise testing.[115]

Treadmill GXTs

Bruce and Balke Treadmill Tests

Chapter 11 outlines protocols for the Bruce and Balke GXTs. The unnumbered table on the top of the next page displays the MET values for the Bruce and Modified Balke tests. Each test has distinct advantages and disadvantages. For example, the **Bruce test** provides more abrupt increases in exercise intensity between stages. This may improve sensitivity to detect ischemic ECG responses, but the patient must possess adequate fitness to tolerate the increased exercise levels. Both protocols begin at relatively high levels of PA for cardiac patients and older individuals and often require modification.[70] The Bruce protocol incorporates lower initial exercise levels, whereas the **Balke test** includes a preliminary 2- to 3-min initial stage at 2 mph and 0% grade.

Choice of a specific exercise test considers overall health, age, and the person's fitness status. A stress test generally begins at a low level, with increments in intensity every several minutes. A warm-up, either separately or incorporated within the test protocol, eases the patient into exercise. Total exercise duration should average at least 8 min. A test much longer than 15 min adds little additional information because the most meaningful cardiac and physiologic data emerge within this time interval. Specifics of the Bruce and Balke test protocols were presented in Chapter 11.

Bicycle Ergometer GXTs

Bicycle ergometers have distinct advantages for exercise stress testing. In contrast to the treadmill, power output on the ergometer is readily computed and remains independent of the person's body mass. Most bicycle ergometers are portable, safe, and relatively inexpensive. Generally,

Stage	Treadmill (MPH)	Treadmill (%Grade)	Time (Min)	O_2 Cost ($mL \cdot kg^{-1} \cdot min^{-1}$)	METs
Bruce Test (Normally Used for Young Active Adults)					
1	1.7	10	3	14.0-17.5	4-5
2	2.5	12	3	24.5-28.0	7
3	3.4	14	3	31.5-35.0	9.5
4	4.2	16	3	45.5-49.0	13.5
5	5.0	18	3	59.5-63.0	17
6	5.5	20	3	70.0-73.5	20.5
Modified Balke Test (Normally Used for Normal Sedentary Adults)					
1	2	0	2	8.75	2.5
2	3	2.5	2	12.25	3.5
3	3	5	2	15.75	4.5
4	3	7.5	2	19.25	5.5
5	3	10	2	22.75	6.5
6	3	12.5	2	26.26	7.5
7	3	15	2	29.75	8.5
8	3	17.5	2	33.25	9.5
9	3	20	2	36.75	10.5
10	3	22.5	2	40.25	11.5
11	3	22.5	2	43.75	12.5
12	3	25	2	47.25	13.5

MET, metabolic equivalent; MPH, miles per hour.

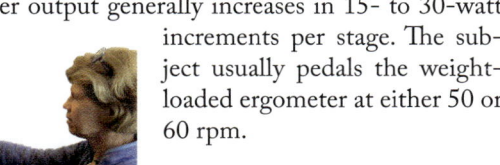

Data from Figure 5.3 in Pescatello LS, et al., eds. *ACSM's Guidelines for Exercise Testing and Prescription*. 9th ed. Baltimore: Lippincott Williams & Wilkins; 2014:124. Background photo: Photographee.eu/Shutterstock

assessment during upper-body effort) and for lower body-disabled individuals. Chapters 15 and 17 point out that arm exercise lowers $\dot{V}O_{2max}$ up to 30%, and maximum heart rate generally averages 10 to 15 bpm lower than with treadmill or bicycle exercise. Blood pressure is also difficult to measure during arm crank exercise. Furthermore, submaximal arm cranking produces higher blood pressure, heart rate, and oxygen uptake values than the same power output during leg exercise. Nevertheless, graded exercise protocols similar to those developed for leg cycling tests apply to evaluating the upper-body exercise response. The initial frictional resistance remains lower in arm exercise, with smaller increments in power output adjusted accordingly.

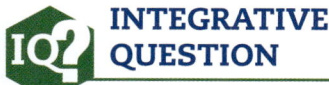

INTEGRATIVE QUESTION

Which type of exercise prescription (and why) most benefits a patient with coronary heart disease who experiences angina during upper-body work in their job as a plasterer or paperhanger?

---

two types of ergometers have application for graded exercise testing:

1. Electrically braked ergometers
2. Weight-loaded, friction-type ergometers

With electrically braked ergometers, preselected power output remains fixed within a range of pedaling frequencies. With weight-loaded ergometers, power output, usually expressed in $kg\text{-}m \cdot min^{-1}$ or watts (1 W = 6.12 $kg\text{-}m \cdot min^{-1}$), relates directly to frictional resistance and pedaling rate.

The general guidelines for treadmill testing also apply to bicycle ergometer testing. Test protocols provide 2- to 4-min graded stages with an initial resistance between 0 and 15 or 30 watts; power output generally increases in 15- to 30-watt increments per stage. The subject usually pedals the weight-loaded ergometer at either 50 or 60 rpm.

Arm-Crank Ergometer Tests

Arm cranking has application for graded exercise testing in special situations (e.g., cardiac

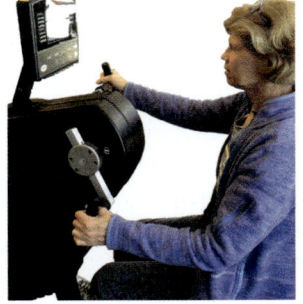

From F. Katch

Stress Testing Safety

*Stress testing safety largely depends on knowing who **not** to test (prescreening health histories reveal noncandidates for testing), knowing when to terminate a test, and preparing for emergencies.*

Research indicates that during submaximal and maximal stress testing about 1 person per 10,000, or approximately 0.01%, will exhibit positive test episodes (https://cdnsciencepub.com/doi/pdf/10.1139/h11-048). This represents about 1 person per 10,000, or approximately 0.01% of the total group tested. In more than 9000 stress tests, no cardiovascular episodes occurred for subjects with increased heart disease risk. In other reports, the risks of coronary episodes for healthy, middle-aged adults during a maximum stress test equaled about 1 in 3000.[18,47,82,161] In most middle-aged individuals, test risk generally increases about 6 to 12 times higher than for young adults. For patients with documented CHD, including previous MI or angina episodes, the cardiovascular incidents during stress testing increase 30 to 60 times above normal. Based on total risk analyses, however, many experts believe that a lower "overall risk" exists for those who take a GXT and then initiate a regular PA program than those who refrain from testing and remain sedentary.

Despite differences in testing techniques, purposes, safety precautions, type, and testing mode, three conclusions about GXT risk appear warranted:

1. Low death risk (≤0.01%)
2. Low acute MI risk (≤0.04%)
3. Low complication risk that requires hospitalization, including acute MI or serious arrhythmias (≤0.2%)

Clearly, the risk–benefit ratio favors GXT testing as part of the medical evaluation process.

Cardiovascular Disease and Exercise Capacity

When designing aerobic activity programs for cardiac patients, three factors are considered:

1. Specific disease pathophysiology
2. Mechanisms that limit exercise performance
3. Individual differences in functional capacity

In Chapter 11, we presented the current blood pressure classifications and risk stratifications. The five classifications comprise the following:

1. Normal: ≤120/80 mm Hg
2. Elevated: 120 to 129 systolic and ≤80 mm Hg diastolic
3. Hypertension stage 1: ≥130 to 139 systolic or 80 to 89 mm Hg diastolic
4. Hypertension stage 2: ≥140/90 mm Hg
5. Hypertensive crisis: ≥180/120 mm Hg

TABLE 32.7 presents the risk stratification and recommended treatment options for individuals within a specific hypertension classification.

TABLE 32.7 Risk stratification and recommended treatment for hypertension

Regular PA and Hypertension

With aerobic training, systolic and diastolic blood pressures decrease by 6 to 10 mm Hg in previously sedentary males and females independent of age. Beneficial results occur with normotensive and hypertensive individuals during rest and PA.[30,46,57,92,173,214,215]

Regular PA, as preventative therapy, also controls the tendency for blood pressure to increase over time in individuals at risk for hypertension.[130] Patients with mild hypertension respond favorably to exercise training, a response also noted among children and adolescents.[4,83,90,103,119,216] Physical activity overall has also shown to improve academic performance.[155] Hypertension medication may even be reduced by progressively increasing effort intensity by walking faster each week.[174]

In one study, the average resting systolic blood pressure decreased from 139 to 133 mm Hg in seven middle-aged male patients following 4 to 6 wk of interval training.[217] During submaximal exertion, systolic pressure decreased from 173 to 155 mm Hg, whereas diastolic pressure decreased from 92 to

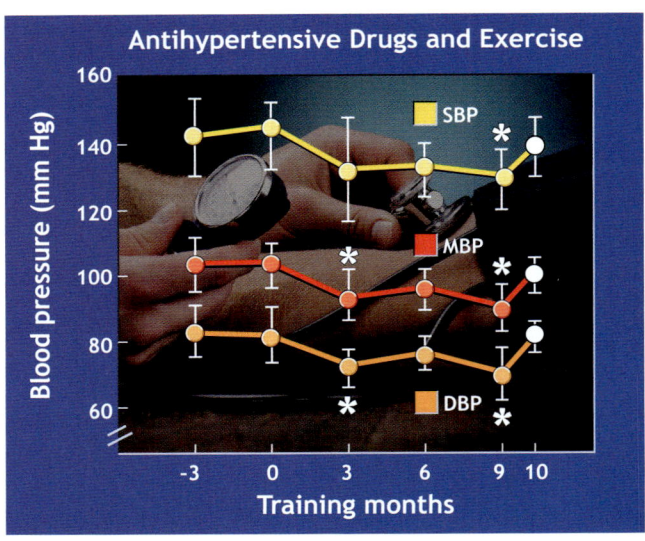

FIGURE 32.7. Blood pressure changes in older hypertensive patients receiving hypertensive medication following 9-month exercise training at the lactate threshold and after detraining for 1 month. SBP, systolic blood pressure; MBP, mean blood pressure; DBP, diastolic blood pressure. *Statistically significant from baseline value.
(Reprinted with permission from Motoyama M, et al. Blood pressure lowering effect of low intensity aerobic training in elderly hypertensive patients. *Med Sci Sports Exerc.* 1998;30:818. Background photo: Andrey_Popov/Shutterstock)

79 mm Hg. Training produced approximately a 14% decrease in mean arterial exercise blood pressure. Similar results occurred for an apparently healthy yet borderline hypertensive group of 37 middle-aged males following regular aerobic training for 6 months.[20] For hypertensive older males and females, low-intensity aerobic activity for 9 months lowered systolic blood pressure by 20 mm Hg and diastolic pressure by 12 mm Hg.[59]

FIGURE 32.7 illustrates changes in resting blood pressure with aerobic training and 1 month of detraining in hypertensive older adults who trained at the lactate threshold three to six times per week for 36 wk. Baseline values 3 months prior to training (−3 in the figure) indicate subjects' blood pressures with normal antihypertensive drug therapy. Regular exercise with continued medication produced a 15-mm Hg decreases in systolic blood pressure, an 11-mm Hg decrease in mean arterial pressure, and a 9-mm Hg decrease in diastolic blood pressure. Blood pressure returned to pretraining levels within 1 month for the five subjects who discontinued training. The ACSM's "Position Stand on Exercise and Hypertension" can be accessed at https://journals.lww.com/acsm-msse/Fulltext/2004/03000/Exercise_and_Hypertension.25.aspx.

The precise mechanism(s) remains unclear for how regular PA lowers blood pressure, but two contributing factors include:

1. Reduced sympathetic nervous system activity with possible arteriole morphology normalization, resulting in a decrease in peripheral resistance to blood flow[3,128]
2. Altered renal function facilitating sodium elimination from the kidneys, which subsequently reduces fluid volume and hence blood pressure

Not all research supports PA as a strategy to treat hypertension.[25,49] Even when research shows that regular PA lowers blood pressure, the studies often have methodologic shortcomings and inadequate design, particularly a lack of appropriate controls who have their blood pressure measured but do not exercise. *Despite these limitations, regular aerobic activity (and proper diet to induce weight loss when necessary) is recommended as a first-line strategy to manage borderline hypertension.*[4,84,159]

Improved fitness often neutralizes increased mortality associated with elevated blood pressure. Even if regular PA does not return elevated blood pressure to a normal range, aerobic training confers important independent health benefits. Aerobically fit individuals with hypertension achieved a 60% lower mortality rate than unfit normotensive peers.[13] More severe elevations in blood pressure require pharmacologic interventions.

Chronic Resistance Training Effects on Blood Pressure

Despite the relatively large rise in blood pressure during resistance exercise, long-term resistance training does not elevate resting blood pressure.[24,40,60] Resistance training reduces the typical short-term blood pressure increases during this exercise mode. Trained bodybuilders, for example, show smaller increases in systolic and diastolic blood pressures with resistance exercise than novice bodybuilders and untrained individuals.[40,147] The diminished blood pressure response posttraining becomes most evident when a person exercises at the same absolute load during pretraining and posttraining.[106] Some resistance training protocols even lower resting blood pressure,[58,172] but aerobic exercise training (not standard resistance training) confers the greater blood pressure–lowering benefits for hypertensive individuals.[84,85,127] *As a general guideline, resistance training should not serve as the sole activity mode to lower blood pressure in hypertensive individuals.*

Prescribing PA and Exercise

An exercise prescription should improve fitness, promote overall health by reducing risk factors, and ensure a safe and enjoyable activity experience. *Prescribing PA involves successful integration of exercise science with behavioral objectives to enhance patient compliance and goal attainment.*

Heart rate and oxygen uptake (or exercise intensity) measured during the stress test provide the basis for the exercise prescription. The prescription individualizes exercise based on current fitness and health status, with emphasis on intensity, frequency, duration, and exercise type.

Initiating a PA program at the proper level takes on added importance for CHD patients because beginners do not often recognize their exercise limitations.

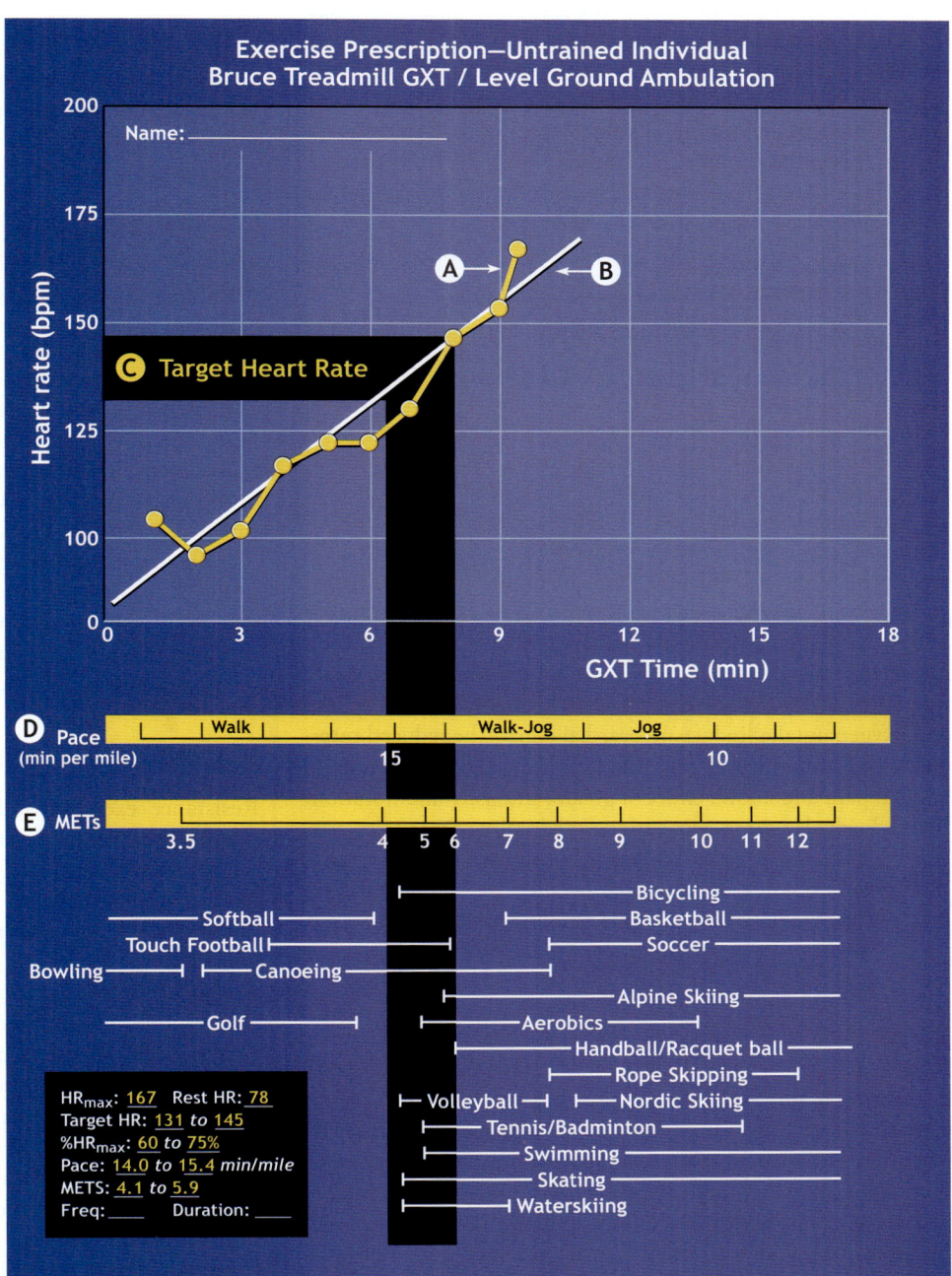

FIGURE 32.8. Exercise prescription based on functional translation algorithm for level-ground ambulation. Letters in figure identified in text. Freq, frequency; GXT, graded exercise stress test; HR, heart rate; Max, maximum; METs, metabolic equivalents; Rest, resting. (Courtesy Dr. Carl Foster, University of Wisconsin–LaCrosse.)

Practical Illustration

FIGURE 32.8 illustrates a practical approach that permits functional translation of treadmill or bicycle exercise test responses to the exercise prescription. The figure depicts data for a male cardiac patient generated from an algorithm of responses from the Bruce treadmill protocol for level-ground ambulation. Heart rate (*A*) was plotted as a function of time, with a mathematical best-fit line (*B*) applied to the data points. A target zone for heart rate (*shaded portion, C*) represents approximately 75 to 85% maximum heart rate (170 bpm). The individualized prescription is then detailed for pace (13.8 to 15.4 min · mi^{-1}, *D*) and/or METs (4.1 to 5.9, *E*). The acceptable intensity range in area C, based on heart rate response during the exercise test, includes the following recreational activities: aerobics, bicycling, canoeing, light-to-moderate volleyball, skating, skiing, tennis and badminton, swimming, skating, touch football, and waterskiing. This practical approach to prescribing PA may improve the prescription's effectiveness and adherence for healthy, previously sedentary individuals and CHD patients.

Improvements in CHD Patients

A properly prescribed and monitored PA program safely improves a cardiac patient's functional capacity. Exercise training post-MI may also favorably modulate deleterious changes in the myocardium's connective tissue metabolism in response to the MI, which may negate the deleterious effects of increased cardiac stiffness characteristics and associated diastolic function abnormalities seen after an MI.[177] Clinical symptoms (e.g., ECG abnormalities) often improve or disappear. This occurs partly from structural and functional myocardium changes. Cardiac patients and healthy individuals respond to exercise training with physiologic adjustments that reduce cardiac work at any given external exercise load. For example, reduced exercise heart rate and BP (two major determinants of myocardial workload and oxygen uptake) reduce myocardial effort. The reduced **rate–pressure product** (heart rate × systolic BP) delays the onset of anginal pain and allows effort of greater intensity and duration. For individuals whose occupations predominantly require arm activities, training (and testing) should emphasize this musculature because physical conditioning benefits are highly task specific and generally not transferable among muscle groups.

The Program

The most effective preventive and rehabilitative PA programs focus on individual needs. Low-to-moderate–intensity regimens evoke greater adherence than intense PA programs. Prescribed activities usually include rhythmic big-muscle movements that stimulate cardiovascular improvement; examples include walking, jogging, cycling, rope skipping, swimming, stair-climbing and cross-country ski simulation, dynamic calisthenics, and higher-intensity interval training, even among older adults and patients with CHF.[1,109,110] On an outpatient basis, less restricted activities such as mountain biking serve as a recreational adjunct to rehabilitate regularly active MI patients with stable CHD.[77]

Chapter 21 discussed guidelines for decision making concerning training frequency, duration, and intensity. Ideally, the personalized exercise prescription should include a recommendation for weight loss and dietary modification (if necessary), warm-up and cool-down exercises, and a developmental flexibility and strength enhancement program. Some heart disease patients exhibit a reduced exercise heart rate response with correspondingly reduced maximum heart rate. In such cases, target heart rates based on age-predicted maximum for the general, healthy population grossly overestimate the appropriate training intensity. *This supports the wisdom of exercise stress testing each patient to symptom–limited maximum and then formulating the exercise prescription from the subjects' heart rate data.*

Supervision Level

TABLE 32.8 presents suggested categories for entry into different cardiac rehabilitation programs depending on patient symptoms and maximum functional capacity (MET level) achieved on a bicycle or treadmill symptom-limited exercise test.

TABLE 32.8 Suggested categories for exercise programs related to patient symptoms

Depending on entry level, different cardiac rehabilitation programs require different supervision levels—either unsupervised or supervised. Within the supervised category there are four different levels of supervision, inpatient, outpatient, in-home, or community. Unsupervised programs meet the needs of most asymptomatic participants of any age with an 8-MET functional capacity and without known major risk factors.

The supervised programs focus on patients with specific needs. These include asymptomatic physically active or inactive persons of any age with CHD risk factors but no known disease and symptomatic individuals, including individuals with recent onset of CHD and those with a changed disease status.

Resistance Exercise Provides Benefits

Resistance exercises added to a cardiac rehabilitation program restore muscular strength, promote FFM preservation, improve psychologic status and quality of life, and increase glucose tolerance and insulin sensitivity.[48,106,107] Combining resistance and aerobic training yields more pronounced physiologic adaptations (improved aerobic capacity, muscle strength, and lean body mass) in patients with CAD than aerobic training alone.[105] For patients with advanced heart disease, no adverse effects occur while performing weightlifting arm exercise at 50, 65, and 85% of 1-repetition maximum.[86] In comparing resting and exercise responses, no changes occurred in pulmonary wedge pressures, S–T segment of the ECG, or incidence of dysrhythmias. Contraindications to resistance training for cardiac patients parallel those for aerobic training.[136] The following six conditions preclude cardiac patients from participating in resistance training:

1. Unstable angina
2. Uncontrolled arrhythmias
3. Left ventricular outflow obstruction (e.g., hypertrophic cardiomyopathy with obstruction)

4. CHF recent history without follow-up and treatment
5. Severe valvular disease, hypertension (systolic blood pressure ≥160 mm Hg and/or diastolic blood pressure ≥105 mm Hg)
6. Poor left ventricular function and exercise capacity below 5 METs with anginal symptoms or ischemic S–T segment depression

Resistance Training Prescription. Cardiac patients should exercise with light resistance in the range of 30 to 50% of 1-RM because of the exaggerated blood pressure responses with straining-type exercise. Elastic bands, light (1 to 5 lb) cuff and hand weights, light free weights, and wall pulleys can be applied at entrance to an outpatient resistance training program. Do not initiate low-level resistance training until 2 to 3 wk post-MI. Introduce barbells and/or weight machines after a 4- to 6-wk convalescence.

Most cardiac patients begin range-of-motion movements using relatively light weight for the lower and upper extremities. In accordance with AHA recommendations, start with one set of 10 to 15 repetitions to moderate fatigue, using 8 to 10 different exercises such as chest press, shoulder press, triceps extension, biceps curl, lat pull-down, lower back extension, abdominal crunch/curl-up, quadriceps extension or leg press, leg curl, and calf raise. Exercises performed 2 to 3 days weekly produce favorable adaptations.[136] The RPE should range from 11 to 14 on the original Borg scale (*"fairly light"* to *"somewhat hard"*).

To minimize dramatic blood pressure fluctuations during lifting, patients should be warned to avoid straining, performing the Valsalva maneuver, and gripping weight handles or bars tightly.

Cardiac Medications and Exercise Response

Knowledge of the physiologic effects of drug intervention allows the CEP to properly assess patient response during PA. **TABLE 32.9** presents six common cardiac drug classifications along with trade names, side effects, and possible effects on exercise responses.

TABLE 32.9 Cardiac medications: Their use, side effects, and exercise response effects

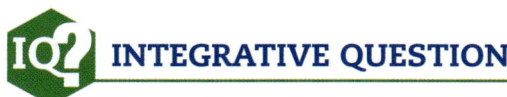

INTEGRATIVE QUESTION

Why would participating in a weightlifting competition pose a risk to a person with advanced CHD?

Cardiac Rehabilitation

A comprehensive cardiac rehabilitation program focuses on improving longevity and quality of life, in addition to risk factor modification.[35,126] After diagnosis and intervention (e.g., aggressive risk factor reduction, bypass surgery, angioplasty), the exercise physiologist evaluates the cardiac patient for functional capacity and ensuing classification and rehabilitation.[37]

Patients differ greatly in symptoms, functional capacities, and rehabilitation strategies. The rehabilitation program incorporates stringent guidelines to promote low-risk treatment.[41,64,165] CHD patients with mild ischemia tolerate steady-rate exercise at intensities consistent for aerobic training, without progressive deterioration in left ventricular function. For patients without ischemia, left ventricular function in prolonged physical effort remains similar to healthy control individuals.[42] Five important aspects for a successful cardiac rehabilitation program include the following:

1. Appropriate patient selection
2. Concurrent medical, surgical, and pharmacologic therapies
3. Comprehensive patient education
4. Appropriate exercise prescription
5. Careful patient monitoring during rehabilitation

Traditional cardiac rehabilitation programs consist of three distinct phases with different objectives, physical activities, and required supervision. More contemporary programs have changed on the basis of new theories about risk stratification, exercise safety data, and changes in the healthcare industry. Current programs recognize individual differences in rehabilitation when determining program length, degree of supervision, and required ECG monitoring.

Contemporary cardiac rehabilitation includes inpatient and outpatient programs and services, with emphasis on outcome measures. Almost all postsurgery patients benefit from inpatient activity intervention, risk factor assessment, lifestyle activity and dietary counseling, and patient and family education. Patient's stay at the hospital averages 3 to 5 days before release.

Inpatient Programs

Inpatient cardiac rehabilitation focuses on the following four objectives:

1. Medical surveillance
2. Patient's identification with significant impairments before discharge
3. Rapid patient return to daily activities
4. Patient and family preparation to optimize recovery

In-hospital PA during the first 48 hr following an MI and/or cardiac surgery is restricted to self-care movements, including arm and leg range of motion and intermittent sitting and standing to maintain cardiovascular reflexes. After several days, patients usually sit and stand without assistance, perform self-care activities, and walk independently up to six times daily, provided none of the following contraindications exist:

- Unstable angina
- Elevated resting blood pressure

- Orthostatic systolic blood pressure above 200 mm Hg with symptoms
- Critical aortic stenosis
- Acute systemic illness or fever
- Uncontrolled atrial or ventricular arrhythmias
- Uncontrolled sinus tachycardia above 120 bpm
- Uncompensated heart failure
- Active pericarditis or myocarditis
- Recent embolism or thrombophlebitis
- Resting S–T segment displacement of ≥2 mm
- Severe orthopedic conditions

Outpatient Programs

Upon discharge, the cardiac patient should know appropriate and inappropriate physical activities and dietary guidelines and have a prudent and progressive plan of risk reduction with a specific exercise prescription. Enrollment in an outpatient activity program is the ideal. Four goals for outpatient cardiac rehabilitation include:

1. Monitoring and supervising patient to detect changes in clinical status
2. Returning patient to premorbid/vocational/recreational activities
3. Assisting patient to implement an at-home, unsupervised activity program
4. Providing family support and education

Most outpatient programs encourage multiple physical activities that include resistance exercise and walking, cycling, and swimming. Supervision should include personnel trained in CPR and advanced life support, and in some cases, a home defibrillator (known as an **automated external defibrillator**; https://nhcps.com/lesson/bls-how-to-use-automated-external-defibrillator-aed/).

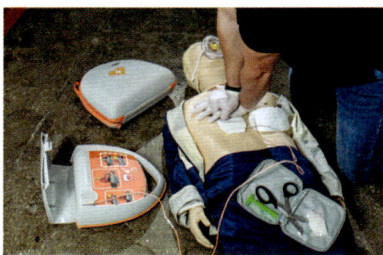
Egor_Kulinich/Shutterstock

Pulmonary Diseases

The CEP's involvement in treating patients with pulmonary disease focuses on improving ventilatory capacity, decreasing the energy cost of breathing, and increasing overall physiologic function. The personal history, physical examination, pertinent laboratory data, and imaging studies provide important background information. Cardiovascular system disorders almost always affect pulmonary function, which eventually leads to varying degrees of pulmonary disability. Conversely, pulmonary disease intimately relates to cardiovascular complications. Patients with pulmonary disease and disabilities often benefit from exercise rehabilitation. Pulmonary abnormalities classify as either obstructive (normal airflow impeded) or restrictive (lung volume dimensions reduced). Despite the convenience of this classification system, pulmonary disorders often reflect both restrictive and obstructive impairment.

Restrictive Lung Dysfunction

Abnormal reduction in pulmonary ventilation, along with diminished lung expansion, decreased tidal volume, and loss of functioning alveolar–capillary units, characterize a large and diverse group of pulmonary disorders, collectively termed **restrictive lung disease (RLD)**.

RLD involves three aspects of pulmonary ventilation pathophysiology:

1. Lung compliance
2. Lung volumes and capacities
3. Breathing energy cost

In RLD, the chest and lung tissues stiffen and resist expansion under breathing's normal pressure differentials. The additional resistance to lung expansion requires greater pulmonary force to maintain adequate alveolar ventilation.[63] This increases normal ventilation's energy cost and accounts for up to 50% of the total oxygen requirement during PA.[74] Eventually, RLD progression negatively affects all lung volumes and capacities. Diminished inspiratory and expiratory reserve volumes occur consistently under all conditions.

TABLE 32.10 lists major RLD conditions, along with their causes, signs and symptoms, and suggested treatment options.

TABLE 32.10 Restrictive lung diseases

RLD known causes include rheumatoid arthritis, immunologic pathology, massive obesity, diabetes mellitus, trauma from injury, penetrating wounds, radiation, burns, other inhalation injuries, poisoning, and complications from drug therapy, including reactions to antibiotics and anti-inflammatory drugs.

Chronic Obstructive Pulmonary Disease

Chronic obstructive pulmonary disease (COPD), also termed chronic airflow limitations, comprises several respiratory tract diseases that obstruct airflow (e.g., emphysema, **asthma**, and **chronic bronchitis**). COPD destroys the lung parenchyma, causing a mismatch between regional alveolar air and blood flow. This ultimately affects the lung's mechanical function to compromise gas exchange (ventilation–perfusion ratio) at the alveolar level. *A dramatic decrease in exercise tolerance almost always accompanies COPD.* The natural history of COPD spans 20 to 50 years and closely parallels a chronic cigarette smoking history.

Changes in pulmonary function measures, most notably decreased expiratory flow rate and increased residual lung volume, usually form the diagnosis of COPD. The classic disease symptoms include spontaneous bronchial smooth muscle spasms that produce a chronic cough, increased mucus production, inflammation and mucosal lining of the

Differences Among Major COPD Diseases

Name	Area Affected	Pathology
Bronchitis	Membrane lining bronchial tubes	Inflammation of bronchial lining
Bronchiectasis	Bronchial tubes (bronchi or air passages)	Breakdown of alveolar walls with enlarged air spaces
Emphysema	Air spaces beyond terminal bronchioles (alveoli)	Bronchial dilation with inflammation
Asthma	Bronchioles (small airways)	Bronchioles obstructed by muscle spasm; swelling of mucosa; thick secretions
Cystic fibrosis	Bronchioles	Bronchioles become obstructed and obliterated; mucus clings to airway walls, leading to bronchitis, atelectasis, pneumonia, pulmonary abscess

Background photo: pathdoc/Shutterstock

The following sections focus on four major COPD diseases:

1. Chronic bronchitis
2. Emphysema
3. Cystic fibrosis
4. Asthma and exercise-induced bronchospasm

Chronic Bronchitis

Acute bronchitis—trachea and bronchi inflammation—usually is short duration and self-limiting. In contrast, prolonged exposure to nonspecific irritants produces chronic bronchitis. Over time, the swollen mucous membranes and increased mucus production obstruct airways, causing wheezing and chronic coughing. Partial or complete airway blockage from mucus secretion produces inadequate arterial oxygen saturation, diminished carbon dioxide elimination, and pulmonary edema. Eventually, the patient develops the characteristic look of a *"blue bloater"* (**FIG. 32.9**). Chronic bronchitis develops slowly and worsens over time. Patients usually have a decade's history of cigarette smoking. Functional capacity decreases considerably, and fatigue occurs readily with mild exertion. If left untreated, this disease leads to premature death.

bronchi and bronchioles thickening, wheezing, and exertional dyspnea.

Factors predisposing to COPD include chronic cigarette smoking (greater effect in females than males; particularly on the increase among college students),[143] air pollution, occupational exposure to irritating dusts or gases, heredity, infection, allergies, aging, and drugs. *COPD rarely occurs in nonsmokers.* The airways narrow to obstruct pulmonary airflow in all forms of COPD. Airway narrowing hinders ventilation by trapping air in the bronchioles and alveoli; in essence, the disease increases pulmonary physiologic dead space. The obstruction also increases resistance to airflow (chiefly in expiration), hinders normal gas exchange, and reduces exercise performance by increasing the energy cost of breathing. The latter reduces ventilatory capacity to hinder full **arterial oxygen saturation** and carbon dioxide elimination. Patients with severe COPD exhibit decreased whole-body mechanical efficiency during PA.[141] This suggests that factors associated with the respiratory effort also magnify the whole-body activity energy requirements to further negatively impact physical capacity. Exercise intervention can sometimes reverse peripheral COPD-induced abnormalities.[171]

Emphysema

An abnormal, permanent air space enlargement distal to the terminal bronchioles characterizes **emphysema**. The disease occurs most frequently among chronic

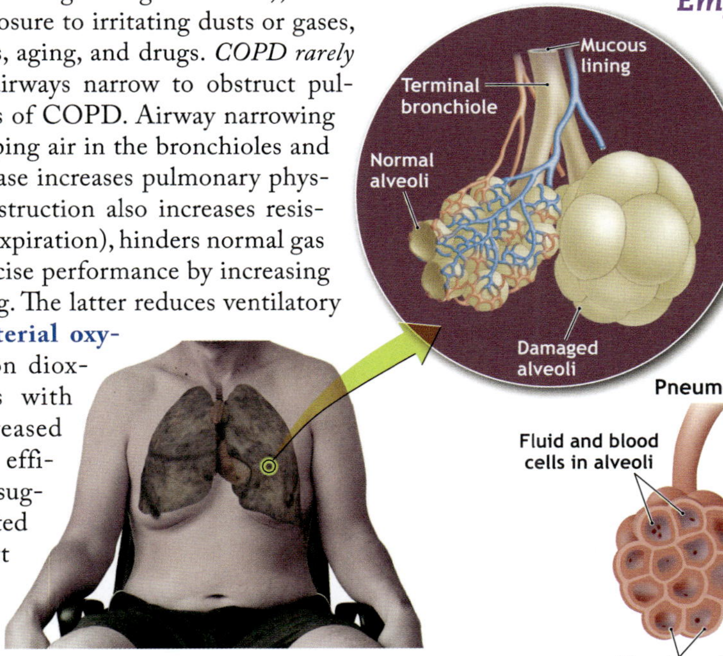

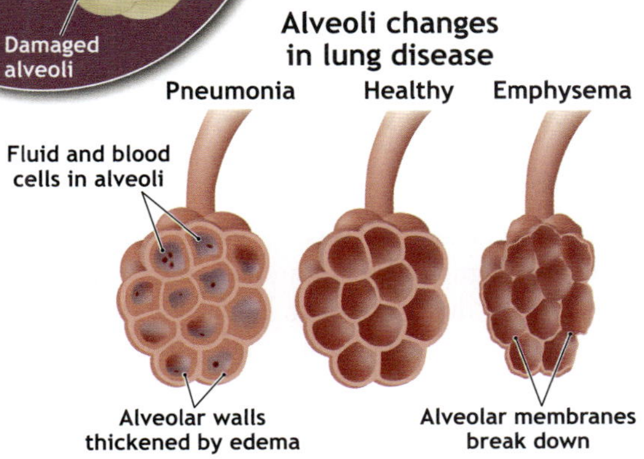

FIGURE 32.9. A person with chronic bronchitis usually develops cyanosis and pulmonary edema with a characteristic appearance known as "blue bloater." Bottom right image shows the cumulative chronic bronchitis effects: misshapen and/or large alveolar sacs with reduced surface for oxygen and carbon dioxide gas exchange.
(Shutterstock images: PRASAN MAKSAEN [background photo], Alila Medical Media [alveoli changes].)

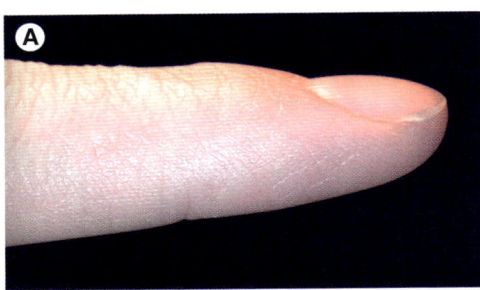
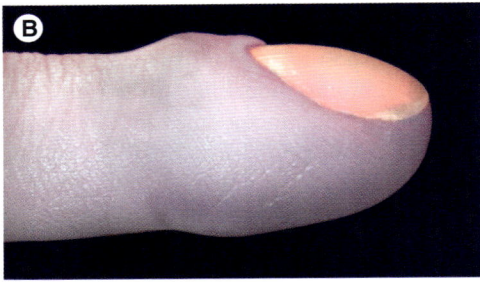

FIGURE 32.10. **(A)** Normal digit configuration. **(B)** Digital clubbing. Club fingers and toes reflect a common diagnosis in emphysema due to tissue hypoxia.

cigarette smokers. It develops consequent to chronic bronchitis; its symptoms include dyspnea, **hypercapnia**, persistent cough, **cyanosis**, and **digital clubbing** (evidence of chronic hypoxemia; **FIG. 32.10**). Patients with emphysema consistently demonstrate low physical capacity and extreme dyspnea with exertion; patients appear thin and often lean forward with arms braced on the knees to support the shoulders and chest to ease the cost of breathing. The chronic effects of trapped air and alveolar distension change chest size and shape causing the characteristic emphysemic "barrel chest" appearance (**FIG. 32.11**). Regular PA does not improve pulmonary function of individuals with emphysema, but it enhances cardiovascular fitness, strengthens both respiratory and nonrespiratory musculature, and improves psychologic status.[11,226]

In selected patients with severe emphysema, lung volume reduction surgery has improved pulmonary function, physical capacity, and quality of life. Its effects on longevity remain uncertain.[53]

Cystic Fibrosis

The term **cystic fibrosis (CF**; www.cff.org) originates from the diagnosis of cysts and scar tissue observed on the pancreas during autopsy. Pancreatic cysts and scar tissue often exist but do not reflect the primary disease characteristics. The following represent the clinical signs and symptoms of CF and related pulmonary involvement:

- **Early-stage CF**: persistent cough and wheezing, recurring pneumonia, excessive appetite but poor weight gain, salty skin or sweat, and bulky, foul-smelling stools (from undigested lipids)

- **Later-stage CF**: **tachypnea** (rapid breathing), sustained chronic cough with mucus production on vomiting, barrel chest, cyanosis and digital clubbing, exertional dyspnea with decreased exercise capacity, pneumothorax, and right heart failure secondary to pulmonary hypertension

CF is characterized by thickening secretions of all exocrine glands (e.g., pancreatic, pulmonic, gastrointestinal). These secretions plug the lung's bronchioles and ultimately lead to a chronic cough, difficulty breathing, and lung tissue obstruction. CF, the most common inherited disease (both parents must carry the recessive trait) in Whites, affects approximately 1 in 2500 to 3500 Caucasian infants in the United States. It is less common in other ethnic groups, affecting about 1 in 17,000 African Americans and 1 in 31,000 Asian Americans. More than 30,000 Americans are currently living with CF (more than 70,000 worldwide). Approximately 1000 new cases are diagnosed each year and more than 75% diagnose by age 2 years; the median age of survival for a person with CF is 47 years. Approximately 5% (12 million) of Americans carry the gene for CF located on chromosome 7, first identified in 1985. This produces defective or missing CF transmembrane conductor regulator proteins, which results in poor ion flow across cell membranes, including the lung.

A positive sweat electrolyte (chloride) test confirms diagnosis of CF. Patients possess a faulty copy of the gene that

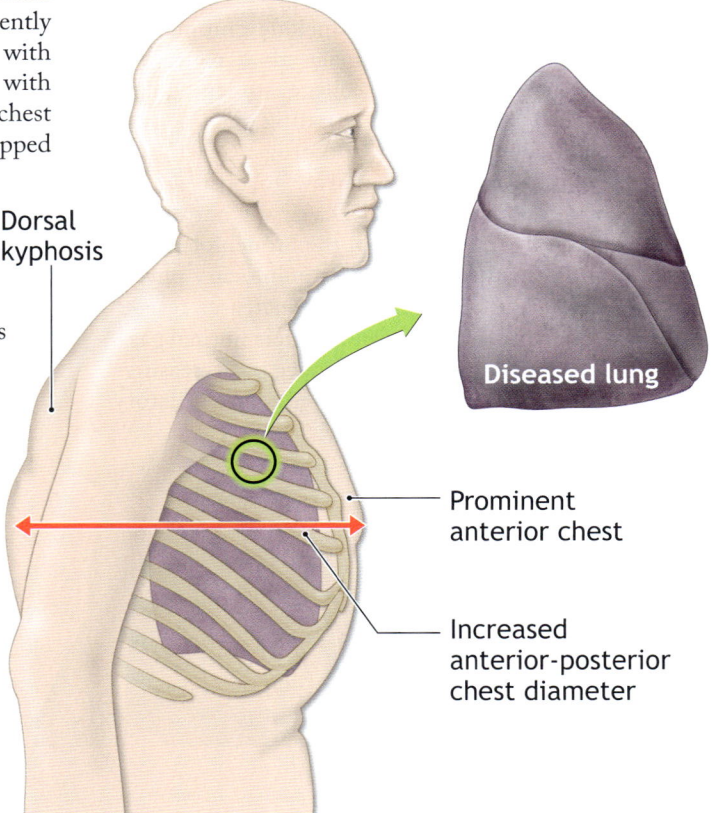

FIGURE 32.11. Emphysema traps air in the lungs making exhalation difficult. With time, the patient's physical features change, they have difficulty catching their breath, and their faces redden while gasping for air, leading to such patients being known as "pink puffers."

allows cells to construct a channel for the passage of chloride ions. Consequently, the resulting poor ion flow across cell membranes causes salt to accumulate in cells that line the lungs and digestive tissues, making the surrounding mucus thicker and salty. These mucous secretions, the critical feature of CF, obstruct ducts and passages in the pancreas, liver, and lungs. Pulmonary impairment represents the most common and severe manifestation of CF. Airway obstruction leads to chronic lung hyperinflation.

Over time, RLD superimposes on the obstructive disease that leads to chronic hypoxia, hypercapnia, and acidosis. These three maladies increase the risk of arterial desaturation during exercise. The disease progresses to pneumothorax and pulmonary hypertension and eventually death.

Treatment of CF includes antibiotics, the FDA-approved mucus-thinning drug Pulmozyme, TOBI (tobramycin) solution for inhalation, high dosages of ibuprofen, enzyme supplements, nutritional intervention, and frequent mucous secretion removal. In most instances, regular PA is recommended for patients with CF as it delays pulmonary disease development in patients via mechanisms that improve airway hydration and mucociliary clearance and reduce markers of inflammation.[19] For children with CF, aerobic fitness correlates inversely with 8-year mortality.[123] The anaerobic power of children with CF records lower than healthy counterparts, although CF patients rely more on anaerobic pathways during strenuous activity.[14,15] Oxygen uptake kinetics slow in patients with CF.[66] Aerobic activity helps to clear airways of excessive secretions, with increasing minute ventilation.[148,178] For example, aerobic exercise for 20 to 30 min can replace one session of secretion removal for some children with CF. Thus, increasing physical fitness can delay CF's crippling effects. An abnormally high NaCl loss in the sweat increases plasma hypoosmolality and a concomitant reduction in thirst drive. A flavored drink with relatively high salt content (e.g., 50 mmol · L^{-1}) enhances drinking and reduces exercise dehydration risk in these CF patients.[94]

Pulmonary Assessments

Exercise physiologists do not diagnose pulmonary disease, but they must understand the different tests and their results to assists in planning and implementing exercise interventions. *Pulmonary disease diagnosis involves several different objective measures that include chest imaging, flow and volume tests, blood gas analyses, and cytologic and hematologic evaluations.*

Lippincott® Connect — Appendix H, available online at Lippincott Connect, provides a list of supplemental animations and videos on this subject, including a discussion of working with dyspnea.

X-Ray

Chest and lung imaging continue as the most prevalent pulmonary assessment technique. These include the conventional medical x-ray in which roentgen rays, named in honor of 1901 Physics Nobel Laureate Wilhelm Conrad Röntgen (1845–1923, who took the first x-ray of his wife's hand [see image]), penetrate human tissues to provide an image (known as a **radiograph** or roentgenogram). This standard diagnostic tool screens for abnormalities, provides a baseline for subsequent assessments, and monitors disease progression.

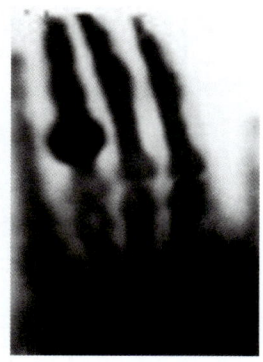

A chest radiograph shows body fat, water, tissue, bone, and air space. The low density of air in the lungs allows greater roentgen ray penetration, which produces a dark image. Relatively dense bone represents the other extreme; it allows fewer roentgen rays to penetrate its tissue, thus producing a white image. **FIGURE 32.12A** illustrates a normal chest radiograph taken in the posteroanterior position. Figure 32.12B shows the same radiograph with the normal anatomic structures labeled. Abnormal radiographic densities identify specific lung lesions.

Computed Tomography

Most clinical radiologists consider computed tomography (CT) scanning, invented in 1972, the single greatest advance in radiography of anatomic structures since the 1895 discovery of roentgen rays. This coveted discovery earned the 1979 Nobel Prize in Physiology or Medicine to Godfrey N. Hounsfield (1919–2004) and Allan M. Cormack (1924–1998; www.nobelprize.org/prizes/medicine/1979/cormack/facts/). CT scans use a narrow x-ray beam that moves across the body to define adjacent cross-sectional columns of tissue known as a translation. Another pass of the beam progresses at a different angle or rotation. Repeated translations and rotations in different directions in a given plane with subsequent digitization produce a clear computer-summated image of x-ray transmission data for diagnostic interpretation.

Other Measures

Chapter 12 discussed static and dynamic lung function tests with simple spirometry. Carefully collected data on forced vital capacity (FVC), forced expiratory volume in 1 s ($FEV_{1.0}$), maximum voluntary ventilation, peak expiratory flow, and lung compliance provide crucial diagnostic information. To measure compliance, the patient swallows a balloon catheter; the technician positions the catheter in the lower third of the esophagus and connects it to a manometer to measure esophageal pressure. The relation of lung volume change to any change in pressure within the catheter then establishes the curve for lung compliance.

Other useful functional tests include **pulmonary diffusing capacity**, expressed in mL · min^{-1} · mm Hg^{-1}, which measures how much gas enters pulmonary blood per unit time per unit pressure differential across the alveolar–capillary membrane. Flow-volume loops provide graphic

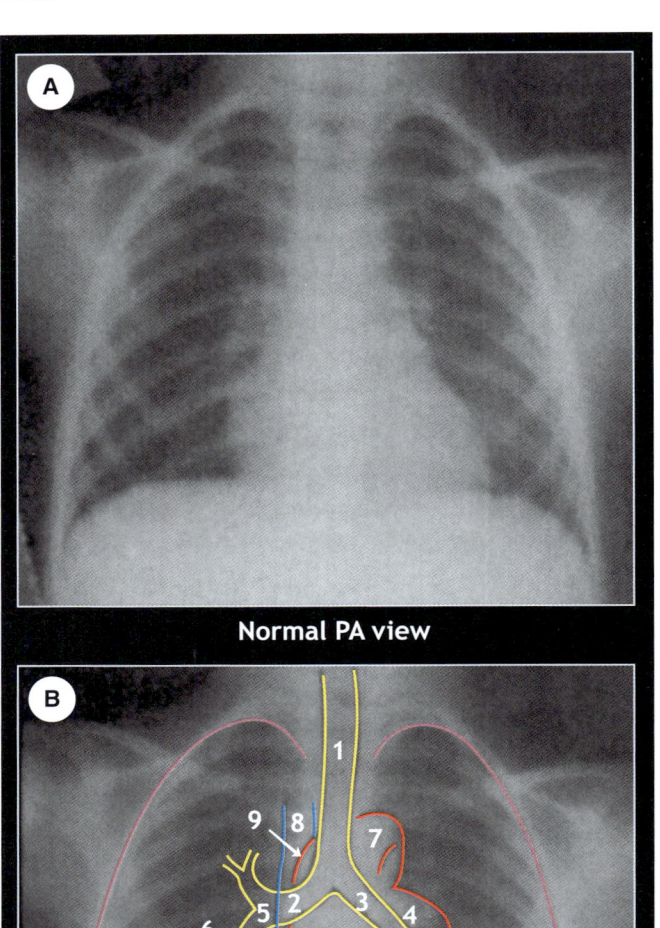

FIGURE 32.12. X-ray chest image. **(A)** Radiograph showing a normal human x-ray in the posterior-anterior (PA) view. **(B)** Radiograph showing nine normal anatomic structures, where *1*, trachea; *2*, right mainstem bronchus; *3*, left mainstem bronchus; *4*, left pulmonary artery; *5*, pulmonary vein to the right upper lobe; *6*, right interlobular artery; *7*, aortic knob; *8*, superior vena cava; *9*, ascending aorta.

Pulmonary Rehabilitation and PA Prescription

Pulmonary rehabilitation programs receive less attention than programs for cardiovascular and musculoskeletal diseases. The lack of emphasis on pulmonary rehabilitation stems from a failure of rehabilitation to improve pulmonary function significantly or "cure" these potentially deadly diseases.

Lippincott® Connect: Appendix H, available online at Lippincott Connect, provides a list of supplemental animations and videos on this subject, including a discussion of ongoing research about dyspnea.

Nevertheless, successful pulmonary rehabilitation places central focus on increased PA because of its positive impact on respiratory and nonrespiratory muscle functions, ventilatory equivalents for oxygen, psychologic status, quality-of-life variables (e.g., self-esteem and self-efficacy), frequency of hospitalization, and disease progression.[11,23,125] The spiral of progressive physical deconditioning from a sedentary lifestyle (as patients attempt to avoid dyspnea) is not simply the direct effect of COPD.[138,154] Peripheral and respiratory muscle weakness frequently contribute to the poor exercise and physiologic performance of patients with COPD.[65,153] Within this framework, the eight major goals for pulmonary rehabilitation include the following:

1. Improve health status.
2. Improve respiratory symptoms (shortness of breath and cough).
3. Recognize early signs that require medical intervention.
4. Decrease respiratory problems' frequency and severity.
5. Maximize arterial oxygen saturation and carbon dioxide elimination.
6. Enhance daily functional capacity through improved muscular strength, joint flexibility, and cardiorespiratory endurance.
7. Modify body composition to enhance functional capacity.
8. Optimize nutritional status.

The overall pulmonary rehabilitation program emphasizes general patient care, pulmonary respiratory care, exercise and functional training, disease education, and psychosocial management.

Since breathlessness is the primary determinant of exertional tolerance for the COPD individual, *ratings of shortness of breath* can be used to monitor activity intensity. Intensity should not be limited by shortness of breath before patients experience moderate exertion levels. Intermittent exercise, comprising short activity intervals alternating with regular rest periods, usually allows for improvement in exercise exertion. After accommodating to a regular PA schedule, the individual may be able to sustain a higher percentage of peak capacity for 30 to 40 min per training session. Some may even participate in high-intensity exercise training.[114] Regular PA benefits typically increase as the training load gradually progresses. For most COPD patients, 15 min moderate PA 3 days a week represents the minimum amount to ensure appropriate benefits.

representations of events occurring during forced inspiration and expiration. Recording the flow versus volume in an X–Y presentation helps to diagnose central or peripheral airway obstructions.

Blood gas analyses provide important information to assess problems related to acid–base balance, alveolar ventilation, and level of arterial oxygen saturation and carbon dioxide elimination. Cytologic and hematologic tests identify microorganisms that cause pulmonary disease.

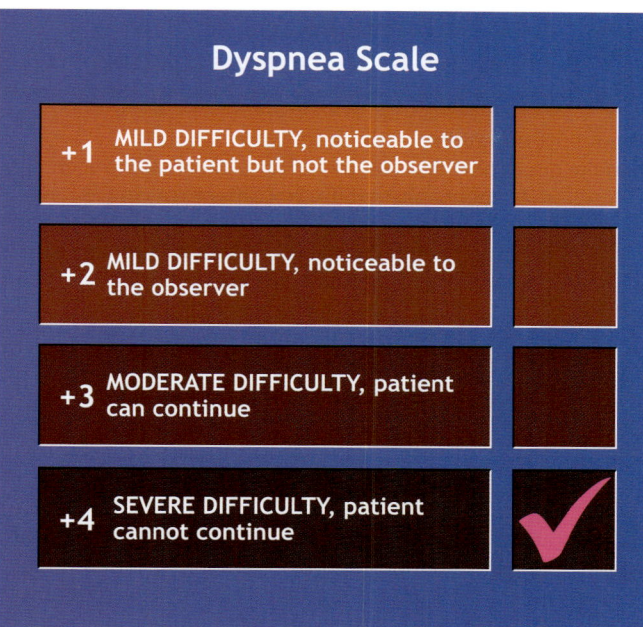

FIGURE 32.13. Dyspnea scale. Subjective ratings of dyspnea on a 1-to-4 scale during graded exercise testing. Dyspnea usually accompanies poor exercise capacity and impaired systolic blood pressure responses.

Physiologic monitoring during exercise rehabilitation typically includes heart rate, blood pressure, respiratory rate, arterial oxygen saturation by pulse oximetry, and dyspnea ratings. Dyspnea monitoring as a target for physical training involves a perceived **dyspnea scale** (**FIG. 32.13**) similar to the ratings on the perceived exertion scale.[44,73] The dyspnea scale emphasizes symptoms of breathing difficulty rather than perceptions of whole-body physical distress, which the RPE measures. Self-monitoring of effort intensity in this manner is advised for two reasons:

1. Respiratory disease usually impairs pulmonary function rather than cardiovascular response.
2. Healthy individual's training heart rate usually exceeds the peak heart rate achieved when stress testing pulmonary patients.

The most common reasons for stopping activity include extreme shortness of breath, fatigue, palpitations, chest discomfort, and a 3 to 5% decrease in pulse oximetry.

The pretraining GXT and spirometric analyses form the basis for the exercise prescription.[28] Interpretation of the exercise stress test includes examining three factors:

1. Whether the test terminated due to cardiovascular or ventilatory end points
2. The difference between preexercise and postexercise pulmonary function (e.g., a 10% decrease in $FEV_{1.0}$ indicates the need for bronchodilator therapy before exercise)
3. Need for supplemental oxygen during activity (e.g., a pretest to posttest decrease in Pao_2 of more than 20 mm Hg, or a Pao_2 below 55 mm Hg)

Exercise prescriptions based on cycling, walking, treadmill exercise, and stair climbing for patients with mild lung disease—shortness of breath with intense exercise—remains similar to requirements for healthy persons. Exercise for patients with moderate lung disease—shortness of breath with normal daily activities or clinical symptoms of RLD or COPD—typically achieves an intensity no greater than 75% of the ventilatory reserve, or the point where the patient becomes noticeably dyspneic. For most patients, this exercise intensity usually falls in the middle of the calculated training heart rate range—50 to 70% of age-predicted maximum with a goal that corresponds to 40 to 85% of maximum MET level on the GXT. In this case, exercise duration averages 20 min, three times weekly. If the patient can exercise only for a shorter duration (e.g., 5 to 15 min per session), exercise frequency can increase to 5 to 7 days weekly.

Patients with severe lung disease—shortness of breath during most daily activities and FVC and $FEV_{1.0}$ below 55% of predicted values—require a modified approach to exercise testing and prescription. Low-level, discontinuous testing usually begins at 2 to 3 METs with increments every 2 to 3 min. Exercise prescription relies on symptom-limited walking speeds and distances. Brief bouts of interval exercise also provide an option. The low level of the initial training prescription means that patients should exercise a minimum of once daily. Even small gains in physical tolerance add to improving daily function and quality of life.

General activities and specific expiratory muscle training effectively improve respiratory muscle function and reduce sensations of respiratory effort during PA in nearly all pulmonary disease patients.[22,96,162] Two training approaches achieve this goal:

1. Specific ventilatory musculature resistance training with a **continuous positive airway pressure (CPAP) device**, which specifically overloads the respiratory muscles similarly to progressive resistance exercise for nonrespiratory skeletal muscles
2. Increasing respiratory muscle force and endurance capacity through regular aerobic training

Pulmonary Medications

Pulmonary medications include bronchodilators, anti-inflammatory agents, decongestants, antihistamines, mucokinetic agents, respiratory stimulants, depressants, and paralyzing and antimicrobial agents. The drugs promote **bronchodilation**, facilitate removal of lung secretions, improve alveolar ventilation and arterial oxygenation, and optimize breathing patterns. **TABLE 32.11** lists the most commonly administered pulmonary drugs, their uses, and possible side effects.

TABLE 32.11 Major pulmonary bronchodilator drugs: their uses and side effects

PA and Asthma

Asthma causes a swelling and narrowing of the airways that carry air from the nose and mouth to the lungs. Hyperirritability of the pulmonary airways followed by bronchial spasm, edema, and mucus secretion characterize this obstructive pulmonary disease. Allergens or irritating substances entering the lungs trigger asthma symptoms that include trouble breathing, wheezing, coughing, and chest tightness. There is currently no cure for this potentially deadly disease, but it can be managed with prevention and proper treatment if an asthma attack arises.

 See the animation "Asthma" on Lippincott Connect for a description and explanation of this condition.

A high level of physical fitness does not confer immunity from asthma.[39,76,100,124,131,166] The recreational road runner is more likely to report symptoms of allergy and/or asthma but less likely to have prescription medication than the Olympic athlete.[111,139] Based on data from five Olympic games, a study by the University of Western Australia identified those athletes with asthma and airway hyperresponsiveness. With an 8% prevalence, these are the most common chronic conditions among Olympic athletes and could be related to the nature of their intense training.[39] Studies of Finnish elite track and field athletes report physician-diagnosed asthma in 17% of long-distance runners, 8% of power athletes, and 3% of nonathletic controls, while 35% of figure skaters showed a significant increase in airway resistance following skating routines.[68,102]

For nearly 90% of people with asthma and 30 to 50% of those with allergic rhinitis and hay fever, PA provides a potent stimulus for bronchoconstriction, termed **exercise-induced bronchospasm (EIB)** (https://acaai.org/asthma/types-of-asthma/exercise-induced-bronchoconstriction-eib/). Reduced vagal tone and increased catecholamine release from the sympathetic nervous system during exertion *normally* relax pulmonary airway smooth muscle.[9] Initial bronchodilation with activity occurs in healthy persons and those with asthma. For the person with asthma, however, bronchospasm accompanied by excessive mucus secretion follows initial bronchodilation. An acute episode of airway obstruction often occurs within 5 to 15 min postexercise; recovery usually occurs spontaneously within 30 to 90 min. One useful technique to detect an exercise-induced asthmatic response applies progressive exercise increments. A spirometric FVC and $FEV_{1.0}$ evaluation takes place after each exercise period and during 10 to 20 min into recovery. *A 10 to 15% reduction in pre-exercise $FEV_{1.0}$/FVC confirms an EIB diagnosis.*[71,95,108] For elite athletes who perform in cold weather sports (e.g., biathlon, canoeing/kayaking, Nordic and Alpine skiing, ice hockey, and speed skating), combining pulmonary function testing with near-maximal sport-specific exercise testing, preferably in a cold, dry environment, provides greater sensitivity for screening than laboratory-based warm air environmental challenges or self-reported symptoms.[74,145,146]

Sex Differences in Exercise-Induced Bronchoconstriction

About 90% of patients with underlying asthma (a sexually dimorphic disease) experience exercise-induced bronchospasm (EIB). Sex differences in EIB have not been extensively studied, but a study using a meta-analysis evaluated sex differences in EIB and atopy (immediate hypersensitivity reaction associated with immunoglobulin E (IgE) in athletes. The literature review identified 60 studies in 7591 postpubertal athletes with EIB and/or atopy. Collectively, these studies reported 23% prevalence of EIB in athletes, higher atopy prevalence in males versus females, a higher atopy prevalence in athletes with EIB, and higher atopic EIB rate in males versus females. Physiological changes during exercise may differentially impact male and female athletes differently, and an interaction among males, exercise, and atopy status in EIB.

Source:
Rodriquez Bauza ED, Silveyra P. Asthma, atopy, and exercise: sex differences in exercise-induced bronchoconstriction. *Exp Biol Med (Maywood)*. 2021;246:1400.

Duplass/Shutterstock

Sensitivity to Thermal Gradients and Fluid Loss

Several mechanisms help to explain bronchospastic responses to PA. An attractive theory relates to how ventilation during PA and recovery alters the rate and magnitude of heat and water exchange in the tracheobronchial tree. As the incoming breath of air moves down the respiratory tract, heat and water move away from the airway lining as the air warms and humidifies. The conditioning of inspired air ultimately cools and dries the respiratory mucosa. Drying increases mucosal lining osmolality, with accompanying mast cell degranulation. This in turn releases powerful proinflammatory mediators that trigger bronchoconstriction (e.g., leukotrienes, histamine, and prostaglandins). Rewarming the airways following PA dilates the bronchial microcirculation to increase blood flow. Bronchial vasculature engorgement precipitates edema that constricts the airways, independent of any constrictive action of bronchial smooth muscle. Bronchial cooling during activity and rewarming during recovery also stimulate chemical mediator release that induces bronchoconstriction.

Regardless of the precise mechanism, the large incompletely conditioned inspired air volume taxes the tracheobronchial tree's smaller airways, causing a decrease in mucosal temperature. Airway heat loss during PA relates directly to the degree of bronchoconstriction. In susceptible individuals, the thermal gradient generated by the combination of airway cooling during exercise and subsequent rewarming during recovery intensifies bronchospastic processes.

Environmental Impact

A warm–humid (summer) environment suppresses the magnitude of EIB regardless of air temperature. Inhaling ambient air fully saturated with water vapor limits airway epithelial cell disruption and injury and often abolishes the bronchospastic exercise response in those with asthma.[16] This explains why persons with asthma tolerate walking or jogging on a warm, humid day or swimming in an indoor pool, in contrast to outdoor winter sports that typically trigger an asthmatic attack.[79,149]

Benefits of Warm-Up and Medication

Light-to-moderate, continuous warm-up for 15 to 30 min or a strategy that includes at least some repeat high-intensity warm-up intervals initiate a refractory period where subsequent intense activity does not trigger as severe as a bronchoconstrictive response.[9,12,140,160] The warm-up benefit continues for up to 2 hr, perhaps from prostaglandin release. Prolonging the cooldown period also reduces the postexercise bronchoconstriction severity; this could occur by slowing airway rewarming and subsequent bronchiole vascular dilation and edema.

Effective pre-exercise medications limit bronchoconstriction for those desiring to exercise regularly without adversely affecting performance. Medications include bronchodilators such as theophylline or the leukotriene receptor antagonist montelukast or β2-agonists (salmeterol) and inhaled heparin therapy or anti-inflammatory corticosteroids or cromolyn sodium.[17,32,118]

Exercise training does not eliminate or cure an asthmatic condition; instead, it increases pulmonary airflow reserve and reduces ventilatory work by potentiating exercise bronchodilation. This response permits persons with asthma to maintain a higher airflow and sustain relatively intense effort despite impaired pulmonary function. For children with asthma, aerobic training, primarily swimming and cycle ergometry, improves $\dot{V}O_{2max}$ and suppresses asthmatic symptoms.

Neuromuscular Diseases, Disabilities, and Disorders

Neuromuscular diseases and disabilities affect the brain in specific ways. Progressive degeneration or trauma to specific brain neurons induces distinct impairment that ranges from simple to complex.

Stroke

Stroke refers to a potentially fatal reduction in the brain's blood flow from ischemia (restricted blood flow) or **hemorrhage** (bleeding). The resulting brain injury affects multiple systems depending on injury site and sustained damage amount. Effects include motor and sensory impairment and language, perception, and affective and cognitive dysfunction. Strokes can cause severe limitations in mobility and cognition or can be less severe with short-term, nonpermanent consequences (www.stroke.org/en/about-stroke).

 See the animation "Stroke" on Lippincott Connect to learn more about the different types of strokes.

Clinical Features

Strokes' clinical features depend on location and severity of injury. Hemorrhagic stroke signs include altered levels of consciousness, severe headache, elevated blood pressure, and extreme fatigue.[218] Cerebellar hemorrhage usually occurs unilaterally and associates with disequilibrium, nausea, and vomiting. **Cerebral blood flow (CBF)** represents the primary marker to assess ischemic strokes (www.youtube.com/watch?v=hfG8J_X1D5Q). When CBF drops below 10 mL per 100 g · min^{-1} brain tissue (normal CBF = 50 to 55 mL per 100 g · min^{-1}), synaptic transmission failure occurs; cell death results at a CBF of ≤8 mL per 100 g · min^{-1}.

Stroke produces physical and cognitive damage. Left hemisphere lesions typically associate with expressive and receptive language deficits compared with right hemisphere lesions. Motor impairment from a stroke usually triggers **hemiplegia** (paralysis of one side of the body) or **hemiparesis** (weakness on one side of the body). Damage to descending neural pathways produces abnormal spinal motor neuron regulation. This adversely changes postural and stretch reflexes and produces difficulty with voluntary movement. Deficits in motor control involve muscle weakness, abnormal synergistic movement organization, impaired force regulation, decreased reaction times, abnormal muscle tone, and active range of joint motion loss.

Exercise Prescription

The emphasis for stroke survivors centers on movement (passive and active-assisted flexibility and muscle strength) rehabilitation during the first 6 months of recovery. The few exercise training studies with stroke patients support PA to improve mobility and functional independence and prevent or reduce further disease progression and functional impairment.[8,99,168] While resistance training may be beneficial in supporting the recovery of stroke patients, the current objective evidence is weak.[219] Stroke survivors vary widely in age, degree of disability, motivational level, and number and severity of comorbidities, secondary conditions, and associated circumstances. Specific exercise prescription focuses on reducing these conditions and improving functional capacity.

Multiple Sclerosis

Multiple sclerosis (MS) represents a chronic, often disabling disease characterized by destruction of the myelin sheath or demyelination that surrounds central nervous system fibers (www.nationalmssociety.org/index.aspx). Inflammatory demyelination lesions can be present in any part of the brain and spinal cord.

Clinical Features

Two or more areas of demyelination confirm the MS diagnosis. This disease usually develops between ages 20 and 40. Frequently, a transient neurologic deficit history emerges that include extremity numbness, weakness, blurred vision, and diplopia (double vision) in childhood or adolescence prior to more persistent neurologic deficits that lead to the definitive diagnosis. Fatigue is the most common MS symptom. MS occurs worldwide at a higher frequency in latitudes farther from the equator (40°). For as yet unknown reasons, MS prevalence in the United States below the 37th parallel is 57 to 78 cases per 100,000, whereas the prevalence rate above the 37th parallel averages 140 cases per 100,000. Patients with a definite MS diagnosis often have a variety of other autoimmune illnesses such as systemic lupus erythematosus, rheumatoid arthritis, polymyositis, and myasthenia gravis. A person who has a first-degree relative with MS has a 12- to 20-fold increased chance of developing MS.

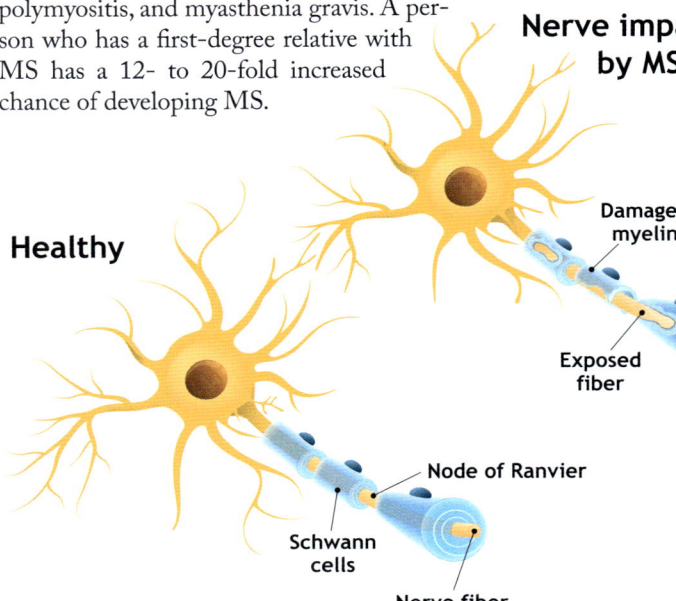

Designua/Shutterstock

Exercise Prescription

MS patients benefit from a comprehensive health prescription that involves aerobic, strength, balance, coordination, and flexibility exercises. About 80% of MS patients report adverse effects to heat exposure. This occurs whether generated environmentally by outside climatic changes or internally via fever or exercise-induced thermogenesis. This effect makes continuous exercise training difficult and not well tolerated. Nevertheless, MS patients and others with autoimmune illness still can improve their cardiovascular function.[51] Stationary cycling, walking, and low-impact chair or water aerobics provide excellent training choices depending on personal interest and physical impairment level. Ideal activity includes walking in a climate-controlled area that provides stable temperatures, a level surface, and opportunity to rest frequently. Controlling body temperature is a primary consideration in the exercise prescription. A realistic and achievable goal for structured activity provides training three times a week for 30 min minimum per session divided into three 10-min periods.

Parkinson Disease

Parkinson disease (PD) belongs to a group of conditions called motor system disorders, which are the result of the loss of dopamine-producing brain cells (www.parkinson.org).

Clinical Features

The four clinical PD symptoms include the following:

1. Varying degrees of tremor
2. Decrease in spontaneity and movement (**bradykinesia**)
3. Rigidity
4. Impaired postural reflexes

These conditions produce extreme gait and postural instability that increase falling episodes and difficulty walking. Some patients exhibit a complete lack of movement (**akinesia**). Functional problems hinder getting out of bed or a car and rising from a chair. Other problems include difficulties dressing, writing, talking, and swallowing. A person with PD generally experiences difficulty with more than one task at a time. As the disease progresses, these problems become more pronounced, and the person eventually loses ability to perform activities of daily living. In the last disease stage, the person becomes wheelchair and/or bed bound.

Exercise Prescription

Most exercise prescriptions for PD patients are individualized and directed toward interventions that affect motor control problems. They emphasize slow, controlled movements for specific tasks through various ranges of motion while lying, sitting, standing, and walking. Treatment protocols include range-of-motion activities that emphasize slow static stretches for all major muscle–joint areas, balance and gait training, mobility, and/or coordination exercises.

Exercise training, as adjunctive treatment and complementary therapy, can improve the plasticity of cortical striatum and increase the release of dopamine. Exercise training has been proven to effectively improve motor disorders (including balance, gait, risk of falls, and physical function) and nonmotor disorders (sleep impairments, cognitive function, and quality of life) in PD patients.[220,221]

Renal Disease

Treatment modalities for the major metabolic diseases of diabetes (see Chapter 20), obesity (see Chapter 30), and renal dysfunction use regular PA as adjunctive therapy. This section reviews aspects of renal disease related to exercise physiology.

Chronic renal disease occurs when kidneys no longer adequately carry out their filtering functions. **Acute renal failure** occurs from a toxin (e.g., drug allergy or poison) or severe blood loss or trauma. Diabetes represents the primary cause of kidney disease, responsible for ≥40% of all kidney failures. Hypertension is the second major cause of renal failure, responsible for about 25%. Genetic diseases, autoimmune diseases, and birth defects also commonly cause kidney ailments.

Clinical Features

Common symptoms of **chronic kidney disease (CKD)**, sometimes referred to as uremia (retention in the blood of waste products normally excreted in urine), include the following 10 characteristics:

1. *Changes in urination*: Producing more or less urine than usual, feeling pressure when urinating, changes in urine color, foamy or bubbly urine, or having to get up frequently at night to urinate
2. *Feet, ankles, hands, or face swelling*: excess tissue fluid accumulation due to kidney failure
3. *Fatigue or weakness*: caused by waste buildup or a shortage of red blood cells (anemia)
4. *Shortness of breath*: due to lung fluid buildup
5. *Ammonia breath or an ammonia or metal mouth taste*: bad breath, changes in taste, or an aversion to protein foods such as meat due to waste buildup
6. *Back or flank pain*: due to kidney inflammation
7. *Itching*: severe itching, especially in the legs due to waste accumulation
8. *Appetite loss*
9. *Nausea and vomiting*
10. *Increased hypoglycemic episodes*

Chronic uremia eventually progresses to **end-stage renal disease** that requires life-long dialysis (see image of patients monitored during dialysis) or kidney transplant (www.youtube.com/watch?v=UQ6qFg4oy1w). Nearly 80% of transplant patients function at or near normal levels compared with 40 to 60% who were treated with dialysis. Almost 75% of transplant patients resume work compared with 50 to 60% of patients receiving dialysis.

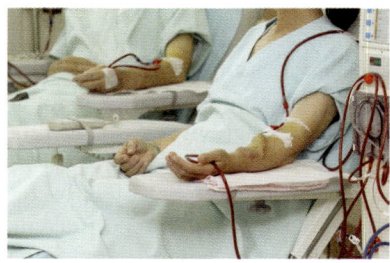
Picsfive/Shutterstock

Exercise Prescription

Regular PA is important in rehabilitating dialysis and transplant patients to better adapt to their illness. The rehabilitation program should begin prior to the start of dialysis to optimize its beneficial effects. Normal low-level endurance training (following ACSM guidelines) reduces muscle protein degradation in moderate renal insufficiency, reduces resting blood pressure in some hemodialysis patients, and modestly improves aerobic capacity in patients who undergo hemodialysis.

Aerobic exercise training could benefit adult chronic kidney disease patients by improving cardiorespiratory function, exercise duration, HDL-C level, and overall quality of life.

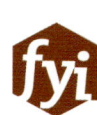

Critical Care Dialysis System Spin-off from the Groundbreaking Apollo Space Program

The highly successful NASA Apollo space program produced many practical "spinoffs"—partnerships created between NASA and private industry to commercialize technologies developed from cooperative space missions, including health and medicine (www.youtube.com/watch?v=iWSewFlU6o8). Work in the late 1960s involved purifying and recycling water during different duration space missions (usually <18 days), and another experiment focused on seawater desalinization. NASA researchers discovered that chemical processes could remove toxic waste from dialysis fluids. This discovery sparked another project, which evolved into the kidney dialysis machine. The discovery marked the birth of "sorbent" dialysis, a method to remove urea from human blood by treating a dialysate solution—the fluid and solutes in a dialysis process that flow through the dialyzer. Dialysis treatment currently provides a lifesaving bridge for patients awaiting a kidney transplant now performed routinely in major medical centers (https://spinoff.nasa.gov).

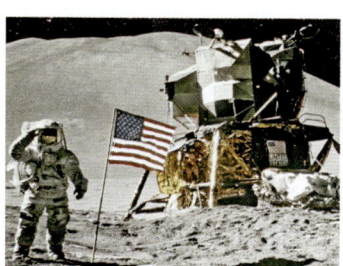
Castleski/Shutterstock

In adult kidney transplant patients, a structured exercise program improved aerobic capacity, muscle performance, and quality of life.[222,223] No deleterious effects were observed in the short-term, but, longer-term randomized controlled trials are needed. Overall, for middle age kidney transplant patients without major comorbidities, a supervised aerobic or resistance training program lasting 3 to 6 months could be part of a comprehensive treatment program. Uremic patients who maintain diverse PA report enhanced quality of life, increased physical capacity, improved muscle strength and function, decreased blood pressure, and improved biomarkers of inflammation and oxidative stress.[67,72]

Cognitive/Emotional Diseases and Disorders

The National Institute of Mental Health (www.nimh.nih.gov) estimates that about 26% of Americans ages 18 and older—about 1 in 4 adults—have a diagnosable mental disorder in a given year. In addition, 4 of the 10 leading causes of disability in the United States and other developed countries are mental disorders—major depression, bipolar disorder, schizophrenia, and obsessive–compulsive disorder. Suicide, closely linked to depression, represents the third-leading cause of death among

10- to 24-year-olds. Also, 6 to 8% of all outpatients in primary care settings suffer from major depression. Despite the large numbers of depressed patients, mental disorders remain underdiagnosed; only about one third of those diagnosed receive treatment.

The five major classifications of cognitive/emotional diseases include the following:

1. **Major depressive disorder**—commonly referred to as "depression"
2. **Dysthymia**—mildly depressed on most days over a period of at least 2 years
3. **Seasonal affective disorder**—recurrence of the depressive symptoms during certain seasons (e.g., winter)
4. **Postpartum depression**—in females who have recently given birth; typically occurs in the first few months after delivery but can happen within the first year after giving birth
5. **Bipolar disorder** (previously known as manic-depressive illness)—characterized by extremes in mood and behavior that last for at least 2 wk

Clinical Features

Depression has no single cause but often results from a combination of factors or events. Whatever its cause, depression is not just a "state of mind." Depression relates to physical changes in the brain and a chemical imbalance of neurotransmitters.

Females are almost twice as likely to suffer from depression as males, partly because of hormonal changes from puberty, menstruation, menopause, pregnancy, and discrimination. Males are more likely to go undiagnosed and less likely to seek help. Males may show the typical symptoms of depression—they tend to be angry and hostile or mask their condition with alcohol or drug abuse. Suicide remains a serious risk for depressed males, who are four times more likely than females to commit suicide. Depression among older adults poses a unique situation. Older persons often lose loved ones and have to adjust to living alone. Physical illness depresses normal levels of PA, further contributing to depression. Loved ones may attribute signs of depression to normal aging, and many older persons are reluctant to talk about their symptoms. Consequently, older persons may not receive proper treatment for depression. Common depression signs and symptoms include:

1. Loss of enjoyment from things that were once pleasurable
2. Loss of energy
3. Feelings of hopelessness or worthlessness
4. Difficulty concentrating
5. Difficulty making decisions
6. Insomnia or excessive sleep
7. Stomachache and digestive problems
8. Decreased sex drive
9. Aches and pains (e.g., recurrent headaches)
10. Appetite change causing weight loss or gain
11. Thoughts of death or suicide
12. Attempting suicide

Four common underlying causes/factors for depression include the following:

1. **Family situation**—childhood trauma, financial stress, ending a relationship, family member death, other major life changes
2. **Pessimistic personality**—higher risk for individuals who have low self-esteem and a negative outlook
3. **Health status**—medical conditions such as heart disease, cancer, and human immunodeficiency virus
4. **Other psychologic disorders**—anxiety disorders, eating disorders, schizophrenia, and substance abuse that often appear with depression

Exercise Prescription

Exercise studies in clinically depressed populations include both hospitalized and ambulatory patients. Overall, the data support regular PA's (aerobic and resistance training) positive effects on depressive symptoms.[7,117,156] In most cases, physically active patients have decreased depression scores.[224,225]

Most studies have used running or other aerobic-type activities when studying depression. Such fitness-related indicators as lower blood pressure and increased aerobic capacity frequently improve in depressed patients undergoing programs of regular PA.

The exercise prescription for patients with depression considers the following eight factors:

1. **Anticipate barriers**. Common depression symptoms—fatigue, lack of energy, and psychomotor retardation—pose formidable barriers to PA. Hopelessness and worthlessness feelings interfere with exercise motivation.
2. **Keep expectations realistic**. Make PA recommendations with caution. Depressed patients often self-blame and may view exercise as another occasion for failure. Do not raise false expectations that can arouse anxiety and guilt. Explain that PA provides an adjunct but not a substitute for primary psychologic treatment.
3. **Design a feasible plan**. Make the exercise prescription realistic and practical, not an additional burden to compound the patient's sense of futility. Consider the individual's background and history. For severely depressed patients, postpone exercise until medication and psychotherapy alleviate symptoms. Previously sedentary patients should start with a light activity schedule; for example, just a few minutes of walking each day.
4. **Accentuate pleasurable aspects**. Guide the PA choice by the patient's preferences and circumstances. Use pleasurable activities that are easily added to the patient's schedule.
5. **Include group activities**. Depressed, isolated, and withdrawn patients are most likely to benefit from increased social involvement. The stimulation of being outdoors in a pleasant setting may enhance mood; exposure to light exerts therapeutic effects for seasonal depression.
6. **State specifics**. Walking is almost universally acceptable, carries minimal risk of injury, and benefits mood

enhancement. In keeping with ACSM recommendations for healthy adults, a 20 to 60 min walking goal or other aerobic activity, three to five times a week, remains reasonable. The ACSM also recommends resistance and flexibility conditioning 2 to 3 days weekly.

7. **Encourage compliance**. Improved fitness may be a valuable consequence of exercise participation but is not necessary to produce an antidepressant effect. Compliance increases with less physically demanding programs.
8. **Integrate PA with other treatments**. The primary treatments for depression should not present obstacles to increasing PA. Antidepressant medication can improve a patient's well-being when depression impairs their ability to function.

Summary

1. In the clinical setting, the exercise physiologist focuses on total patient care and restoring patient mobility and functional capacity.
2. Disability refers to diminished functional capacity compounded by an inactive lifestyle; handicapped denotes a physical performance frame of reference defined by society.
3. Exercise plays an important role in cancer risk reduction by increasing levels of anti-inflammatory cytokines.
4. The exercise prescription for cancer patients is symptom-limited, progressive, and individualized, with improved ambulation the primary goal.
5. A carefully planned, circuit resistance exercise program decreases depression and state and trait anxieties for females recovering from breast cancer surgery.
6. Cardiovascular disease affects the heart muscle directly, the heart valves, or neural regulation of cardiac function each with a specific pathogenesis and intervention strategy.
7. Myocardial pathologies include angina pectoris, MI, pericarditis, CHF, and aneurysm.
8. Moderate-intensity PA and prescribed medications provide benefits with relatively low risk for stable, compensated CHF patients.
9. Heart valve diseases include stenosis, insufficiency (regurgitation), prolapse, and endocarditis. Congenital malformations include ventricular or atrial septal defects and patent ductus arteriosus.
10. Dysrhythmias (bradycardia, tachycardia, and PVCs) are diseases of the heart's nervous system.
11. Cardiac patient assessment includes medical history, physical examination, heart auscultation to uncover murmurs and valvular problems, and laboratory tests (chest x-ray, ECG, blood lipid analyses, serum enzyme testing).
12. Physiologic assessments for CHD include noninvasive tests (echocardiography, exercise stress testing, and ECG analysis).
13. Invasive testing includes radionuclide thallium imaging, cardiac catheterization, and coronary angiography.
14. Resistance exercise in cardiac rehabilitation restores and maintains muscular strength, promotes preservation of FFM, improves psychologic status and quality of life, and increases glucose tolerance and insulin sensitivity.
15. Graded exercise stress testing provides low-risk screening for CHD preventative and rehabilitative PA programs.
16. Multistage bicycle and treadmill tests usually include several levels of 3 to 5 min of submaximal exercise to self-imposed fatigue.
17. Alterations in the heart's normal electrical activity pattern often indicate insufficient myocardial oxygen supply.
18. Significant S–T segment depression heralds extensive obstruction in one or more coronary arteries.
19. PVCs in exercise generally indicate severe atherosclerotic heart disease, often involving two or more major coronary vessels.
20. Sudden death from ventricular fibrillation averages 6 to 10 times higher in patients with frequent PVCs.
21. Significant deviations from normal blood pressure and heart rate responses during graded exercise testing often indicate underlying cardiovascular pathology.
22. Stress tests have four possible outcomes: true positive (test successful); false negative (person with CHD misdiagnosed); true negative (test successful); false positive (healthy person misdiagnosed).
23. Cardiac patients improve functional capacity to the same extent as healthy counterparts with a properly prescribed and monitored exercise program.
24. RLD and COPD represent the two major categories of pulmonary disease.
25. Regular PA effectively manages pulmonary disease if guidelines are followed for exercise intensity, patient monitoring, and exercise progression.
26. EIB associates with low ambient temperature and humidity and their drying effects on the respiratory mucosa.
27. Drying increases mucosal lining osmolality, which stimulates release of powerful mediators that trigger bronchoconstriction.
28. Physical training does not "cure" asthma but can increase airflow reserve and reduce breathing work during PA.
29. The few exercise training studies with stroke patients support PA as a strategy to improve mobility and functional independence and reduce further disease and functional impairment.
30. Fatigue represents the most common MS symptom; other symptoms include muscle weakness in the extremities, clumsiness, and numbness and tingling.
31. Patients benefit from a comprehensive health prescription that involves aerobic, strength, balance, and flexibility activities.
32. Clinical symptoms of PD include varying degrees of tremor, decreased spontaneity and movement (bradykinesia), rigidity, and impaired postural reflexes.
33. Individualized exercise prescriptions for PD provide interventions that affect associated motor control problems. They emphasize slow, controlled movements for specific tasks through various ranges of motion while lying, sitting, standing, and walking.
34. Overall, research supports the positive effects on depressive symptoms of regular PA, including resistance training.

Key Terms

Acute bronchitis: Self-limiting and short-duration inflammation of the trachea and bronchial tree

Acute renal failure: Sudden renal dysfunction from severe blood loss or trauma

Akinesia: Loss or impairment in spontaneous movement (e.g., in facial expression) or associated movement (e.g., arm swing during walking)

American College of Sports Medicine (ACSM): Largest sports medicine and exercise science organization in the world; promotes and integrates scientific research, education, and practical applications to sports medicine and exercise science

Aneurysm: Abnormal dilatation of arterial or venous wall

Aortic stenosis: Aortic valve narrowing that restricts blood flow from the left ventricle to the aorta; also affects atrial pressure in the left atrium

Arrhythmia: Irregular or abnormal heart rhythm

Arterial oxygen saturation: Relative oxygen amount dissolved or transported in arterial blood

Asthma: Pulmonary airways hyperirritability followed by bronchial spasm, edema, and mucus secretion

Atherosclerosis susceptibility gene: Located on chromosome 19; regulates the receptor that removes low-density lipoprotein cholesterol from blood

Auscultation: Listening to heart sounds

Automated external defibrillator: Portable electronic device that automatically diagnoses and treats life-threatening cardiac arrhythmias

Balke test: Treadmill graded exercise protocol to assess maximum oxygen uptake that uses a 1% per minute treadmill elevation at a constant 3.3 mph

Bipolar disorder: Behavior characterized by extremes in mood and behavior that last ≥2 wk

Bradykinesia: Decrease (slowness) in spontaneity of movement; major Parkinson disease symptom

Bronchodilation: Expansion of bronchial air passages

Bruce test: Treadmill graded exercise protocol to monitor cardiac function with large increases in grade and/or speed every 3 min

Carcinomas: Cancers arising in skin epithelial tissue or lining of internal organs

Cardiac catheterization: Procedure to diagnose and treat certain cardiovascular conditions; involves insertion of a long thin tube (catheter) into an artery or vein and into the heart

Cardiomyopathy: Primary disease of the myocardium

Cardiotoxicity: Cancer drugs and treatments that damage the myocardium

Catheter: Flexible tube inserted through a narrow opening into a body cavity

CD8+ T cell: White blood cell type that kills intracellular pathogens, viruses, bacteria, and cancer cells

Cerebral blood flow (CBF): Blood supply to the brain in a given time period; typically averages about 15% of an adult's cardiac output

Certified Clinical Exercise Specialist (CES): Requires a baccalaureate degree in exercise or health-related studies, 600 hr of relevant clinical experience, current cardiopulmonary resuscitation certification (basic life support), and the successful completion of a comprehensive examination

Chronic bronchitis: Obstructive lung disease characterized by long-term breathing problems and poor airflow

Chronic kidney disease (CKD): Gradual loss of kidney function over time

Chronic obstructive pulmonary disease (COPD): Several respiratory tract diseases that obstruct airflow including emphysema, asthma, and chronic bronchitis; also known as chronic airflow limitations

Chronotropic incompetence: Heart rate does not increase during graded exercise

Clinical exercise physiologist (CEP): Certified health professional who designs, implements, and supervises exercise testing and programming

Congenital heart defects: Heart defects present at birth appear in one of every 100 births

Congestive heart failure (CHF): The heart fails to adequately pump sufficient blood to meet the body's needs; also known as chronic decompensation or heart failure

Continuous positive airway pressure (CPAP) device: External machine that sends air or oxygen into the nose and mouth to keep the airways open

Creatine phosphokinase (CPK): Enzyme that catalyzes the creatine plus adenosine triphosphate reaction to phosphocreatine plus adenosine diphosphate

Cyanosis: Bluish or purplish skin or mucous membrane discoloration due to low oxygen saturation

Cystic fibrosis (CF): Inherited autosomal recessive disease that affects the lungs, pancreas, liver, kidneys, and intestines

Degenerative heart disease: Vascular diseases affecting the myocardium

Digital clubbing: Finger or toenail deformity associated with heart and lung diseases

Dyspnea scale: Subjective dyspnea ratings on a 1-to-4 scale during graded exercise

Dysrhythmias: Diseases of the heart's nervous system that include bradycardia, tachycardia, and premature ventricular contractions; also known as arrhythmias

Dysthymia: Mild depression on most days over a period ≥2 years

Echocardiography: Sound waves that produce heart images

Ectopic: Cardiac rhythm disturbance frequently related to the heart's electrical conduction system where beats arise from stimulus outside the normal myocardial pathway

Electrocardiogram (ECG): Graphic representation of heart's electrical activity

Emphysema: Damage to alveoli causing inadequate blood oxygenation and shortness of breath

Endocarditis: Endocardium inflammation usually bacterial in origin

End-stage renal disease: Permanent kidney dysfunction

Exercise-induced bronchospasm (EIB): Airway constriction during exercise

Extrasystole: Heart rhythm disorder from a premature myocardial contraction

Fibrillation: Repetitive rapid myocardial fiber contractions or twitchings of atria or ventricles

Graded exercise stress test (GXT): Exercise testing methods designed to be increasingly more difficult as the test progresses up to a submaximum or maximum termination point

Hemiparesis: Weakness on one side of the body

Hemiplegia: Paralysis on one side of the body

Hemorrhage: Bleeding

Hypercapnia: Elevated blood carbon dioxide levels

Immunosurveillance: Immune system cells recognize foreign pathogens, such as bacteria and viruses or precancerous and cancerous cells

Informed consent: Obtaining an individual's permission before conducting a healthcare intervention or disclosing personal information

Insufficiency: Improper heart valve closure resulting in blood flowing back into a myocardial chamber, also known as regurgitation

Ischemia: Restricted blood flow causing inadequate oxygen supply

Left ventricular ejection fraction (LVEF): Percentage of left ventricle blood volume ejected with each heartbeat

Leukemias: Cancers that arise from blood cells

Lymphomas: Cancers that arise from immune system cells

Major depressive disorder: Depression

Mitral valve prolapse (MVP): Bulging of the leaflets of the mitral valve (prolapse) into the left atrium during systole causing blood to leak back into the atria; also known as floppy valve syndrome, Barlow syndrome, click-murmur syndrome

Multiple sclerosis (MS): Disabling disease characterized by myelin sheath destruction or central nervous system nerve fiber demyelination

Myocardial ischemia: Reduced blood flow to the heart from a partial or complete coronary artery blockage

Myocarditis: Myocardium infection causing inflammation

Nitroglycerin: Drug that promotes coronary artery dilation and reduces systemic peripheral vascular resistance

Nuclear ventriculography: Radiographic imaging procedure to analyze regional left ventricular contractility following radioactive isotope contrast injection

Parkinson disease (PD): Progressive nervous system disorder that affects body movement

Patent ductus arteriosus: Vascular shunt caused by an opening between the aorta and pulmonary artery

Pericarditis: Inflammation of the heart's pericardial lining

Pharmacologic stress test: Systematic intravenous drug infusion during echocardiography and/or thallium scanning to monitor wall motion abnormalities or coronary perfusion limitations

Postpartum depression: Depression following birth; typically occurs within the first few months or first year after delivery

Premature ventricular contractions (PVCs): Extra contractions that originate in the ventricles and disrupt the heart's normal rhythm

Prinzmetal angina: Syndrome consisting of angina during rest or sleep, in contrast to stable angina triggered by exertion

Proteomics: Study of proteins produced or modified by an organism or body system

Pulmonary congestion: Heart failure stage that produces fatigue, shortness of breath, and flooding of the alveoli with blood

Pulmonary diffusing capacity: How much gas enters pulmonary blood per unit time

Radiograph: Image produced on a sensitive plate or film by x-rays, gamma rays

Radionuclide studies: Imaging technique that uses a small radioactive chemical (isotope) dose injected or swallowed that can detect cancer, trauma, infection, or other disorders

Rate–pressure product: Myocardial work estimate; calculated as heart rate × systolic blood pressure

Restrictive lung disease (RLD): Extrapulmonary, pleural, or parenchymal respiratory disease category with a decreased lung volume, increased work of breathing, and inadequate ventilation and/or oxygenation

Rheumatic fever: Disease after an infection with group A streptococcus bacteria

Sarcomas: Cancers from connective tissues (bones, tendons, cartilage, fat, and muscle)

Seasonal affective disorder: Recurring depressive symptoms during certain seasons (e.g., winter)

Septal defects: Holes between ventricles and atria

Serum glutamic oxaloacetic transaminase (SGOT): Enzyme in liver and myocardial cells released into blood, with liver or heart damage

Sinus bradycardia: Slow, regular heart rhythm characterized by a decrease in the electrical rate impulses arising from the sinoatrial node

Sinus tachycardia: Elevated heart rhythm increases the electrical rate impulses from the sinoatrial node; (resting heart rate ≥100 bpm)

Sports medicine: Field of study that relates scientific and medical aspects particular to physical activity, physical fitness, health, and sports performance

Stable angina: Brief episodes of pain, squeezing, pressure, or chest tightness

Stenosis: Constriction that prevents heart valves from opening fully

Stroke: Potentially fatal reduction in the brain's blood supply

S–T segment depression: ST segment abnormally below the baseline; signifies myocardial ischemia

Tachypnea: Rapid breathing

Test sensitivity: Percentage of persons whose tests detect an abnormal (positive) response; represents a true-positive condition

Test specificity: Number of true-negative test results (e.g., rate of correct identification of people without coronary heart disease)

Thallium imaging: Method to determine myocardial blood supply while a radioactive tracer flows into the coronary circulation

Third-degree atrioventricular (AV) heart block: Nerve impulse generated in the sinoatrial node in the heart's atrium cannot properly propagate into the ventricles

Ultrafast electron beam computed tomography (EBCT) scan: Fast and sensitive x-ray test for detecting calcium build-up in coronary arteries

Ventricular ectopy: Common clinical presentation in patients suffering idiopathic ventricular outflow tract arrhythmias

Ventricular fibrillation: A serious heart rhythm dysfunction in which the ventricles beat excessively fast

> References are available online at Lippincott Connect.

Additional References

Abbasi F, et al. The effects of exercise training on inflammatory biomarkers in patients with breast cancer: a systematic review and meta-analysis. *Cytokine*. 2022;149:155712.

Braz de Oliveira MP, et al. Effect of resistance exercise on body structure and function, activity, and participation in individuals with Parkinson disease: a systematic review. *Arch Phys Med Rehabil*. 2021;102:1998.

Buras AL, et al. The association of resistance training with risk of ovarian cancer. *Cancer Med*. 2021;10:2489.

Cannioto RA, et al. Physical activity before, during and after chemotherapy for high-risk breast cancer: relationships with survival. *J Natl Cancer Inst*. 2021;113:54.

Cerexhe L, et al. Blood lactate concentrations during rest and exercise in people with multiple sclerosis: a systematic review and meta-analysis. *Mult Scler Relat Disord*. 2022;57:103454.

Dauwan M, et al. Physical exercise improves quality of life, depressive symptoms, and cognition across chronic brain disorders: a transdiagnostic systematic review and meta-analysis of randomized controlled trials. *J Neurol*. 2021;268:1222.

Fan B, et al. What and how can physical activity prevention function on Parkinson's disease? *Oxid Med Cell Longev*. 2020;2020:4293071.

Fraser SF, et al. The effect of exercise training on lean body mass in breast cancer patients: a systematic review and meta-analysis. *Med Sci Sports Exerc*. 2022;54:211.

Galán-Arroyo C, et al. Depression and exercise in older adults: exercise looks after you program, user profile. *Healthcare (Basel)*. 2022;10:181.

Gamborg M, et al. Parkinson's disease and intensive exercise therapy: an updated systematic review and meta-analysis. *Acta Neurol Scand*. 2022; doi: 10.1111/ane.13579.

Heimark S, et al. Blood pressure altering method affects correlation with pulse arrival time. *Blood Press Monit*. 2022;27:139.

Hortobágyi T, et al. Functional relevance of resistance training induced neuroplasticity in health and disease. *Neurosci Biobehav Rev*. 2021;122:79.

Hoshino J. Renal rehabilitation: exercise intervention and nutritional support in dialysis patients. *Nutrients*. 2021;13:1444.

Iwai K, et al. Usefulness of aerobic exercise for home blood pressure control in patients with diabetes: randomized crossover trial. *J Clin Med*. 2022;11:650.

Jang MK, et al. Does the association between fatigue and fatigue self-management preference vary by breast cancer stage? *Cancer Nurs*. 2022;45:43.

Langeskov-Christensen M, et al. Efficacy of high-intensity aerobic exercise on common multiple sclerosis symptoms. *Acta Neurol Scand*. 2022;145:229.

Lemogne C, et al. Management of cardiovascular health in people with severe mental disorders. *Curr Cardiol Rep*. 2021;23:7.

Lindgren M, Börjesson M. The importance of physical activity and cardiorespiratory fitness for patients with heart failure. *Diabetes Res Clin Pract*. 2021;176:108833.

Liu Y, et al. Relationship between serum 25-hydroxyvitamin D and target organ damage in children with essential hypertension. *J Hum Hypertens*. 2022. doi:10.1038/s41371-021-00622-4.

Moraes RF, et al. Resistance Training, fatigue, quality of life, anxiety in breast cancer survivors. *J Strength Cond Res*. 2021;35:1350.

Mudalige NL, et al. The clinical and radiological cerebrovascular abnormalities associated with renovascular hypertension in children: a systematic review. *Pediatr Nephrol*. 2022;37:49.

Nielsen RE, et al. Cardiovascular disease in patients with severe mental illness. *Nat Rev Cardiol*. 2021;18:136.

O'Neil A, et al. How does mental health impact women's heart health? *Heart Lung Circ.* 2021;30:59.

Palma S, et al. High-intensity interval training in the prehabilitation of cancer patients: a systematic review and meta-analysis. *Support Care Cancer.* 2021;29:1781.

Park C, et al. The effects of lower extremity cross-training on gait and balance in stroke patients: a double-blinded randomized controlled trial. *Eur J Phys Rehabil Med.* 2021;57:4.

Pedersen ES, et al. Diagnosis in children with exercise-induced respiratory symptoms: a multi-centre study. *Pediatr Pulmonol.* 2021;56:217.

Prieto-Gómez V, et al. Effectiveness of therapeutic exercise and patient education on cancer-related fatigue in breast cancer survivors: a randomised, single-blind, controlled trial with a 6-month follow-up. *J Clin Med.* 2022;11:269.

Roldán-Jiménez C, et al. Design and implementation of a standard care programme of therapeutic exercise and education for breast cancer survivors. *Support Care Cancer.* 2022;30:1243.

Ruiz-González D, et al. Effects of physical exercise on plasma brain-derived neurotrophic factor in neurodegenerative disorders: a systematic review and meta-analysis of randomized controlled trials. *Neurosci Biobehav Rev.* 2021;128:394.

Salam A, et al. Effect of post-diagnosis exercise on depression symptoms, physical functioning and mortality in breast cancer survivors: a systematic review and meta-analysis of randomized control trials. *Cancer Epidemiol.* 2022;77:102111.

Salari N, et al. The effect of exercise on balance in patients with stroke, Parkinson, and multiple sclerosis: a systematic review and meta-analysis of clinical trials. *Neurol Sci.* 2022;43:167.

Schultz MG, et al. The identification and management of high blood pressure using exercise blood pressure: current evidence and practical guidance. *Int J Environ Res Public Health.* 2022;19:2819.

Shen YL, et al. Timing theory continuous nursing, resistance training: rehabilitation and mental health of caregivers and stroke patients with traumatic fractures. *World J Clin Cases.* 2022;10:1508.

Singh B, Toohey K. The effect of exercise for improving bone health in cancer survivors—a systematic review and meta-analysis. *J Sci Med Sport.* 2022;25:31.

Streja E, et al. The quest for cardiovascular disease risk prediction models in patients with nondialysis chronic kidney disease. *Curr Opin Nephrol Hypertens.* 2021;30:38.

Syed-Abdul MM. Benefits of resistance training in older adults. *Curr Aging Sci.* 2021;14:5.

Teles GO, et al. HIIE protocols promote better acute effects on blood glucose and pressure control in people with type 2 diabetes than continuous exercise. *Int J Environ Res Public Health.* 2022;19:2601.

Tsao CW, et al. Heart disease and stroke statistics–2022 update: a report from the American Heart Association. *Circulation.* 2022;145:e153.

Wang X, et al. Systematic review and meta-analysis of the effects of exercise on depression in adolescents. *Child Adolesc Psychiatry Ment Health.* 2022;16:16.

Winters-Stone KM, et al. A randomized-controlled trial comparing supervised aerobic training to resistance training followed by unsupervised exercise on physical functioning in older breast cancer survivors. *J Geriatr Oncol.* 2022;13:152.

Yoshimura Y, et al. Chair-stand exercise improves sarcopenia in rehabilitation patients after stroke. *Nutrients.* 2022;14:461.

Zambolin F, et al. The association of elevated blood pressure during ischaemic exercise with sport performance in master athletes with and without morbidity. *Eur J Appl Physiol.* 2022;122:211.

Table 32.1 Health Benefits of Regular Physical Activity to Improve Aerobic and Musculoskeletal Fitness

Physical Activity Benefit	Surety Rating	Physical Activity Benefit	Surety Rating
Body Fitness		**Cigarette Smoking**	
Improves heart and lung function	****	Improves success in quitting	**
Improves muscular strength/size	****	**Diabetes**	
Cardiovascular Disease		Prevents type 2	****
Prevents coronary heart disease	****	Treats type 2	***
Causes atherosclerosis regression	**	Treats type 1	*
Treats heart disease	***	Improves life quality	***
Prevents stroke	**	**Infection and Immunity**	
Cancer		Prevents the common cold	**
Prevents colon cancer	****	Improves overall immunity	**
Prevents breast cancer	**	Slows progression of HIV to AIDS	*
Prevents uterine cancer	**	Improves life quality of persons with HIV	****
Prevents prostate cancer	**	**Arthritis**	
Prevents other cancers	*	Prevents arthritis	*
Treats cancer	*	Treats/cures arthritis	*
Osteoporosis		Improves life quality/fitness	****
Increases bone mass and density	****	**High Blood Pressure**	
Prevents osteoporosis	***	Prevents high blood pressure	****
Treats osteoporosis	**	Treats high blood pressure	****
Blood Cholesterol/Lipoproteins		**Asthma**	
Lowers blood total cholesterol	*	Prevents/treats asthma	*
Lowers LDL cholesterol	*	Improves life quality	***
Lowers triacylglycerols	***	**Sleep**	
Raises HDL cholesterol	***	Improves sleep quality	***
Low Back Pain		**Psychologic Well-Being**	
Prevents low back pain	**	Elevates mood	****
Treats low back pain	**	Buffers effects of mental stress	***
Nutrition and Diet Quality		Alleviates/prevents depression	****
Improves diet quality	**	Reduces anxiety	****
Increases total energy intake	***	Improves self-esteem	****
Weight Management		**Special Issues for Women**	
Prevents weight gain	****	Improves total body fitness	****
Treats obesity	**	Improves fitness while pregnant	****
Helps maintain weight loss	***	Improves birthing experience	**
Children and Youth		Improves fetal health	**
Prevents obesity	***	Improves health during menopause	***
Controls disease risk factors	***		
Reduces unhealthy habits	**		
Improves odds of adult activity	**		
Older Adults and the Aging Process			
Improves physical fitness	****		
Counters loss in heart/lung fitness	**		
Counters loss of muscle	***		
Counters gain in fat	***		
Improves life expectancy	****		
Improves life quality	****		

****	Strong consensus without conflicting data
***	Most supportive data; more research required
**	Some supportive data; more research required
*	Little or no supporting data

AIDS, acquired immunodeficiency syndrome; HDL, high-density lipoprotein; HIV, human immunodeficiency virus; LDL, low-density lipoprotein.
From Nieman DC. The human body: designed for action. *ACSM's Health Fitness J.* 1998;2(3):30 (Table 1).

Table 32.2 Cancer Therapies and Their Complications

Treatment Type	Description and Effects/Outcome
Surgery	**Lung:** reduced lung capacity, dyspnea, deconditioning **Neck:** reduced range of motion, muscle weakness, some cranial nerve palsy **Pelvic region:** urinary incontinence, erectile dysfunction, deconditioning **Abdomen:** deconditioning, diarrhea **Limb amputation:** chronic pain, deconditioning
Radiation therapy	**Skin:** redness, pain, dryness, peeling, sloughing, reduced elasticity **Brain:** nausea, vomiting, fatigue, memory loss **Thorax:** some irreversible lung fibrosis, pericardial inflammation or fibrosis resulting from radiation to the heart, premature atherosclerosis, cardiomyopathy **Abdomen:** vomiting, diarrhea **Pelvis:** diarrhea, pelvic pain, bladder scarring, occasional incontinence, sexual dysfunction **Joints:** connective tissue and joint capsule fibrosis; possible decreased range of motion
Systemic therapy	**Chemotherapies** (depending on type and amount): extreme fatigue, anorexia, nausea, anemia, neutropenia, muscle pain, sensory and motor peripheral neuropathy, ataxia, anemia, vomiting, muscle mass loss, deconditioning, infection **Endocrine therapies** (highly specific to type): fat redistribution (truncal and facial obesity), proximal muscle weakness, osteoporosis, edema, infection, weight gain, extreme fatigue, hot flashes, muscle mass loss **Biologic therapies** (depending on type and amount): fevers or allergic reactions, chills, fever, headache, extreme fatigue, low blood pressure, skin rash, anemia

Reprinted from Courneya KS, et al. In: Myers J, ed. *ACSM's Resources for Clinical Exercise Physiology: Musculoskeletal, Neoplastic, Immunologic, and Hematologic Conditions.* 2nd ed. Baltimore: Lippincott Williams & Wilkins; 2009.

Table 32.3 Chest Pain Diagnosis

Pain/Complaint/Findings	Possible Causes	Stimuli	Possible Pathology
Pressure, ache, tightness or burning in midsternum, left shoulder, arm; sweating; nausea; vomiting; S–T segment changes	MI	Exertion; cold; smoking; heavy meal; fluid overload	CHD
Sharp pain worsens with inspiration, improves with sitting	Inflammation	Acute MI	Pericarditis
Chest tightness with breathlessness; low-grade fever	Infection	IV drug use; microbes	Myocarditis; endocarditis
Sharp, stabbing pain; breathlessness; cough; loss of consciousness	Pulmonary	Recent surgery	Pulmonary embolism
Burning pain; indigestion relieved by antacids	Referred pain	Heavy meal, spicy food	Esophageal reflux
Angina pain; breathlessness; wide pulse pressure; ventricular hypertrophy on ECG	Ventricular outflow tract obstruction	Exertion; CHD	Aortic stenosis; mitral valve prolapse

CHD, coronary heart disease; ECG, electrocardiogram; IV, intravenous; MI, myocardial infarction.

Table 32.4 Exercise Stress Test Results: Diagnose and Formulate Exercise Prescriptions

Subjective data
- Angina pain
- Dyspnea ratings
- Fatigue and weakness
- Leg discomfort
- Dizziness
- Rating of perceived exertion

Objective data
- **Physical examination data**
  - Breathing sounds
  - Murmurs and gallops
  - Blood pressure
  - Pulmonary function tests (before or after exercise)
  - Heart rate response
  - Blood gas parameters
  - Rate–pressure product (heart rate × systolic blood pressure)
- **Physical performance data**
  - Time on treadmill/cycle ergometer
  - Maximum work or power output
- **Electrocardiogram data**
  - S–T segment changes
  - Rate responses
  - Dysrhythmias
  - Conduction abnormalities
- **Cardiorespiratory data**
  - Lactate threshold
  - Carbon dioxide output
  - Minute ventilation
  - Oxygen uptake
  - Respiratory exchange ratio

Table 32.5 Exercise Preparticipation Health Screening Logic Model for Aerobic Exercise Participation

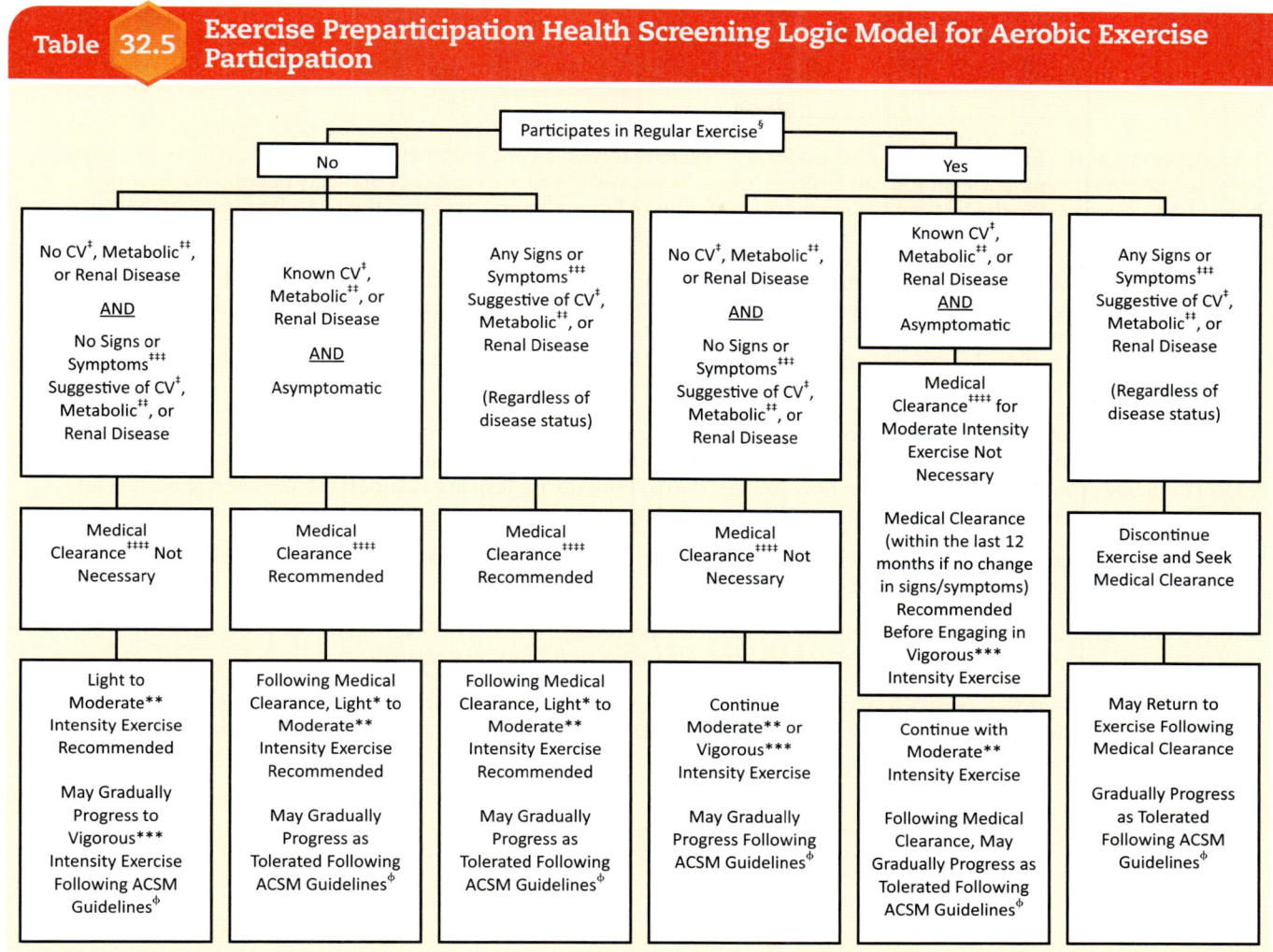

§Exercise participation, performing planned, structured physical activity at least 30 min at moderate intensity on at least 3 d · wk−1 for at least the last 3 months.
*Light-intensity exercise, 30% to <40% HRR or $\dot{V}O_2R$, 2 to <3 METs, 9–11 RPE, an intensity that causes slight increases in HR and breathing.
**Moderate-intensity exercise, 40% to <60% HRR or $\dot{V}O_2R$, 3 to <6 METs, 12–13 RPE, an intensity that causes noticeable increases in HR and breathing.
***Vigorous-intensity exercise ≥60% HRR or $\dot{V}O_2R$, ≥6 METs, ≥14 RPE, an intensity that causes substantial increases in HR and breathing.
†CVD, cardiac, peripheral vascular, or cerebrovascular disease.
‡‡Metabolic disease, type 1 and 2 diabetes mellitus.
‡‡‡Signs and symptoms, at rest or during activity; includes pain, discomfort in the chest, neck, jaw, arms, or other areas that may result from ischemia; shortness of breath at rest or with mild exertion; dizziness or syncope; orthopnea or paroxysmal nocturnal dyspnea; ankle edema; palpitations or tachycardia; intermittent claudication; known heart murmur; or unusual fatigue or shortness of breath with usual activities.
‡‡‡‡Medical clearance, approval from a health care professional to engage in exercise.
ΦACSM Guidelines, see *ACSM's Guidelines for Exercise Testing and Prescription, 9th edition*, 2014.
Adapted with permission from Riebe D, et al. Updating ACSM's recommendations for exercise preparticipation health screening. *Med Sci Sports Exerc*. 2015;47(8):2477 (Fig. 2).

Table 32.6 Sample Graded Exercise Stress Test Informed Consent

Name _____

1. **Explanation of the Exercise Test** You will perform an exercise test on a cycle ergometer or a motor-driven treadmill. The exercise intensity begins at a level you can easily accomplish and will advance in stages of difficulty depending on your fitness level. We may stop the test at any time because of signs of fatigue, or you may stop the test when you wish because of fatigue or discomfort that you feel, particularly at the higher exercise levels.

2. **Risks and Discomforts** The possibility exists that certain abnormal changes can occur during the test. These include abnormal blood pressure, fainting, disorder of heart beat, and in rare instances, heart attack, stroke, or death. Every effort will be made to minimize these risks by evaluating preliminary information related to your health and fitness and by observations during testing. Emergency equipment and available trained personnel can deal with unusual situations that may arise.

3. **Responsibilities of the Participant** Information you possess about your health status or previous experiences of unusual feelings with physical effort may affect the safety and value of your exercise test and you should report this information now. Your prompt reporting of how you feel during the exercise test also is important. You are responsible for fully disclosing such information when requested to do so by the testing staff.

4. **Expected Benefits from the Test** The results obtained from the exercise test may assist in diagnosing your illness, or evaluating what type of physical activities you might do with low risk.

5. **Inquires** We encourage you to ask any questions about the procedures used in the exercise test or in the estimation of your functional capacity. If you have doubts or questions, please ask us for further explanations.

6. **Freedom of Consent** Your permission to perform this exercise test is voluntary. You are free to deny consent or stop the test at any point. I have read this form and understand the test procedures. I voluntarily consent to participate in this test.

Date: _____

Signature of Patient: _____

Signature of Witness: _____

Questions: _____

_____

Responses: _____

Signature of Physician or Delegate: _____

Table 32.7 Risk Stratification and Recommended Treatment for Hypertension

Blood Pressure Stages (mm Hg)	Risk Group A (No Risk Factors; No TOD[a] or CCD[b])	Risk Group B (One Risk Factor excluding Diabetes; No TOD or CCD)	Risk Group C (TOD and/or CCD and/or Diabetes, with or Without Other Risk Factors
High-normal: 130–139/85–89	Lifestyle modification	Lifestyle modification	Drug therapy
Stage 1: 140–159/90–99	Lifestyle modification	Lifestyle modification	Drug therapy
Stages 2 and 3: >160/>100	Drug therapy	Drug therapy	Drug therapy

A person with diabetes, 142/94 mm Hg blood pressure, and left ventricular hypertrophy is classified as stage 1 hypertension with target organ disease (left ventricular hypertrophy) and another major risk factor (e.g., diabetes). This patient would be classified as stage 1, risk group C and recommended for immediate drug therapy.

[a]TOD, target organ disease.
[b]CCD, clinical cardiovascular disease.

From the sixth report of the Joint Committee on Prevention, Detection, Evaluation, and Treatment of High Blood Pressure (JNVI), Public Health Service, National Institutes of Health, National Heart, Lung and Blood Institute, NIH Publication No. 98-4080, November 1997.

Table 32.8 Suggested Categories for Exercise Programs Related to Patient Symptoms

Program Type	Participants	Functional Capacity (MET Level)	Supervision
Unsupervised	Asymptomatic	8+	None
Supervised			
1. Inpatient	All symptomatic (post-MI, postoperative, pulmonary disease)	3	Supervised ambulatory therapy
2. Outpatient	All symptomatic (post-MI, postoperative, pulmonary disease)	3+	Exercise specialist, physician on call
3. In-home	Symptomatic + asymptomatic	>3–5	Unsupervised; periodic hospital reevaluation
4. Community	Symptomatic + asymptomatic, (6–8 wk post-MI; 4–8 wk postoperative)	>5	Exercise program director + exercise specialist

MI, myocardial infarction.

Table 32.9 Cardiac Medications: Their Use, Side Effects, and Exercise Response Effects

Type/Trade Name	Use	Side Effects	Exercise Response Effects
I. Antianginal Agents			
A. Nitroglycerin compounds (Amyl nitrate; Isordil; Nitrostat)	Smooth muscle relaxation; decrease cardiac output	Headache, dizziness, hypotension	Hypotension; increase exercise capacity
B. β-Blockers (Inderal; propranolol; Lopressor; Corgard; Blocadren)	Block β receptors; decrease sympathetic tone; decrease HR, myocardial contractility, BP	Bradycardia, heart block, insomnia, weakness, nausea, fatigue, increased cholesterol and blood sugar	Decrease HR; hypotension; decrease cardiac contractility
C. Calcium antagonists (Verapamil; nifedipine; Procardia)	Block influx of calcium; dilate coronary arteries; suppress dysrhythmias	Dizziness, syncope, flushing, hypotension, headache, fluid retention	Hypotension
II. Antihypertensive Agents			
A. Diuretics (Thiazides, Lasix, Aldactone)	Inhibit Na$^+$ and Cl$^-$ in kidney; increase excretion of sodium and water, and control high BP and fluid retention	Drowsiness, dehydration, electrolyte imbalance; gout, nausea, pain, hearing loss, elevated cholesterol and lipoproteins	Hypotension
B. Vasodilators (Hydralazine, Captopril, Apresoline, Loniten, Minoxidil)	Dilate peripheral blood vessels; used with diuretics; decrease BP	Increase HR and contractility; headache, drowsiness, nausea, vomiting, diarrhea	
C. Drugs interfering with sympathetic nervous system (Reserpine, Propranolol, Aldomet, Catapres, Minipress)	Decrease BP, HR, and cardiac output by dilating blood vessels	Drowsiness, depression, sexual dysfunction, fatigue, dry mouth, stuffy nose, fever, upset stomach, fluid retention, weight gain	Hypotension
III. Digitalis Glycosides, Derivatives			
Digoxin, Lonoxin, digitoxin	Strengthen heart's pumping force and decrease electrical conduction	Arrhythmias, heart block, altered ECG, fatigue, weakness, headache, nausea, vomiting	Increase exercise capacity; increase myocardial contractility

(Continued)

Table 32.9 Cardiac Medications: Their Use, Side Effects, and Exercise Response Effects (Continued)

Type/Trade Name	Use	Side Effects	Exercise Response Effects
IV. Anticoagulant Agents Coumadin, sodium heparin, aspirin, Persantine	Prevent blood clot formation	Easy bruising, stomach irritation, joint or abdominal pain, difficulty swallowing, unexplained swelling, uncontrolled bleeding	
V. Antilipidemic Agents Cholestyramine, Lopid, Niacin, Atromid-S, Mevacor, Questran, Zocor, Lipitor	Interfere with lipid metabolism and lower cholesterol and low-density lipoproteins	Nausea, vomiting, diarrhea, constipation, flatulence, abdominal discomfort, glucose intolerance, myalgia, liver dysfunction, muscle fatigue	
VI. Antiarrhythmic Agents Cardioquin, procaine, quinidine, lidocaine, Dilantin, propranolol, bretylium tosylate, verapamil	Alter conduction patterns throughout the myocardium	Nausea, palpitations, vomiting, rash, insomnia, dizziness, shortness of breath, swollen ankles, coughing up blood, fever, psychosis, impotence	Hypotension; decrease HR; decrease cardiac contractility

BP, blood pressure; ECG, electrocardiogram; HR, heart rate.

Table 32.10 Restrictive Lung Diseases[a]

Causes/Type	Etiology	Signs and Symptoms	Treatment
I. Maturational A. Abnormal fetal lung development B. Respiratory distress syndrome (hyaline membrane disease)	Premature birth (hypoplasia-reduced lung tissue) Insufficient maturation of lungs due to premature birth	Asymptomatic; pulmonary insufficiency ↑ Respiration rate; ↓ lung volumes; ↓ P_{AO_2}; acidemia; rapid and labored respiration pressure	No specific treatment Treat mother prior to birth (corticosteroids); hyperalimentation; continuous positive airway pressure
C. Aging	Aging and cumulative effects of pollution, noxious gas, inhaled drug use, cigarette smoking	↑ Residual volume; ↓ vital capacity; repetitive periodic apnea	No specific treatment; increase physical activity
II. Pulmonary A. Idiopathic pulmonary fibrosis	Unknown origin (perhaps viral or genetic)	↓ Lung volumes; pulmonary hypertension; dyspnea; cough; weight loss, fatigue	Corticosteroids; maintain adequate nutrition and ventilation
B. Coal workers' pneumoconiosis	Repeated coal dust inhalation (10–12 yr)	↓ TLC, VC, FRC; ↓ lung compliance; dyspnea; ↓ P_{AO_2}; pulmonary hypertension; cough	Nonreversible, no known cure
C. Asbestosis	Long-term exposure to asbestos	↓ Lung volumes; abnormal x-ray; ↓ P_{AO_2}; dyspnea on exertion, shortness of breath	Nonreversible, no known cure
D. Pneumonia	Inflammatory process caused by various bacteria microbes, viruses	↓ Lung volumes; abnormal x-ray; tachypneic dyspnea; high fever, chills, cough; pleuritic pain	Drug therapy (antibiotic)

Table 32.10 Restrictive Lung Diseases[a] (Continued)

Causes/Type	Etiology	Signs and Symptoms	Treatment
E. Adult respiratory distress syndrome	Acute lung injury (fat emboli, drowning, drug-induced, shock, blood transfusion, pneumonia)	Abnormal lung function tests; P_{AO_2} <60 mm Hg; extreme dyspnea; cyanotic; headache; anxiety	Intubation and mechanical ventilation
F. Bronchogenic carcinoma	Tobacco use	Variable, depending on type and location of growth	Surgery, radiation, chemotherapy; specific drainage
G. Pleural effusions	Accumulation of fluid within pleural space; heart failure; cirrhosis	Shortness of breath; pleuritic chest pain; ↓ P_{AO_2}	
III. Cardiovascular			
A. Pulmonary edema	↑ Pulmonary capillary hydrostatic pressure secondary to left ventricular failure	↑ Respiration rate; ↓ lung volumes; ↓ P_{AO_2}; arrhythmias; report feelings of suffocation, shortness of breath, cyanotic, cough	Drug therapy, diuretics; supplemental oxygen
B. Pulmonary emboli	Complications of venous thrombosis	↓ Lung volumes; ↓ P_{AO_2}; tachycardia; acute dyspnea, shortness of breath; syncope	Heparin therapy; mechanical ventilation
IV. Neuromuscular			
A. Spinal cord injury	Trauma paralysis of respiratory muscle	↓ Lung volumes; hypoxemia; fatigue; shortness of breath; inability to cough; ↓ voice volume	Active and passive chest wall stretching
B. Amyotrophic lateral sclerosis	Degenerative disease of nervous system	↓ Lung volumes; ↓ maximum voluntary volume	No treatment except supportive therapy
C. Poliomyelitis	Viral infectious disease that attacks motor nerves	Paralysis of diaphragm; shortness of breath	No treatment except supportive therapy
D. Guillain-Barré syndrome	Demyelinating disease of motor neurons	Profound muscular weakness; ↓ lung volumes	Passive range-of-motion exercises; active exercise
E. Neuromuscular diseases (myasthenia gravis, tetanus, muscular dystrophy)	Diseases of neuromuscular system, genetic or other cause resulting in chronic muscular weakness and wasting	Weakness, fatigue, muscle function and strength loss, paralysis affects pulmonary system with eventual functional loss	Drugs; passive and active exercise; supportive therapy
V. Musculoskeletal			
A. Diaphragmatic paralysis	Loss or impaired diaphragm muscle motor function from a specific lesion	↓ Lung volumes; dyspnea, shortness of breath	Not needed
B. Kyphoscoliosis	Excessive anteroposterior and lateral curvature of thoracic spine (cause unknown)	↓ Lung volumes; exertional dyspnea	Use orthotic devices; active exercise
C. Ankylosing spondylitis	Chronic, inherited inflammatory spine disease	Exertional dyspnea	No treatment

[a]www.nlm.nih.gov/medlineplus/
FRC, functional residual capacity; P_{AO_2}, partial pressure of oxygen in the alveoli; TLC, total lung capacity; VC, vital capacity.

Table 32.11 Major Pulmonary Bronchodilator Drugs: Their Uses and Side Effects

Drug/Name	Action and Clinical Uses	Side Effects
Sympathomimetics Isoproterenol, ephedrine, Bronkosol, Alupent, Brethine, Proventil, Ventolin (Albuterol inhaler)	Decrease intracellular calcium; smooth muscle relaxation; bronchodilation	Tachycardia, palpitations, GI distress, nervousness, headache, dizziness
Methylxanthines Amnodur, Elixophyllin, Theophylline, Choladril, Dylix	Increase cAMP; block cAMP decrease	Agitation, hypotension, chest pain, nausea, tachycardia, palpitations, GI distress, nervousness, headache, dizziness
α-Sympatholytics	Block cAMP decrease; bronchodilation	Agitation, hypotension, chest pain, nausea, tachycardia, palpitations, GI distress, nervousness, headache, dizziness
Parasympatholytics Atrovent, atropine sulfate	Block parasympathetic stimulation and prevent increases in cGMP; prevent bronchoconstriction	Central nervous system stimulation with low doses and depression with high doses; delirium, hallucinations, decreased GI activity
Glucocorticoids Prednisone, Cortisol, Azmacort, Vanceril	Decrease inflammatory response; bronchodilation	Obesity, growth suppression, hyperglycemia and diabetes, mood changes, irritability or depression, thinning of skin, muscle wasting
Cromolyn sodium Intal, Fivent	Prevents influx of calcium ions, thus blocking mast cell release of mediators responsible for bronchoconstriction; bronchodilation	Throat irritation, hoarseness, dry mouth, cough, chest tightness, bronchospasm

GI, gastrointestinal; cAMP, cyclic adenosine monophosphate; cGMP, cyclic guanosine monophosphate.

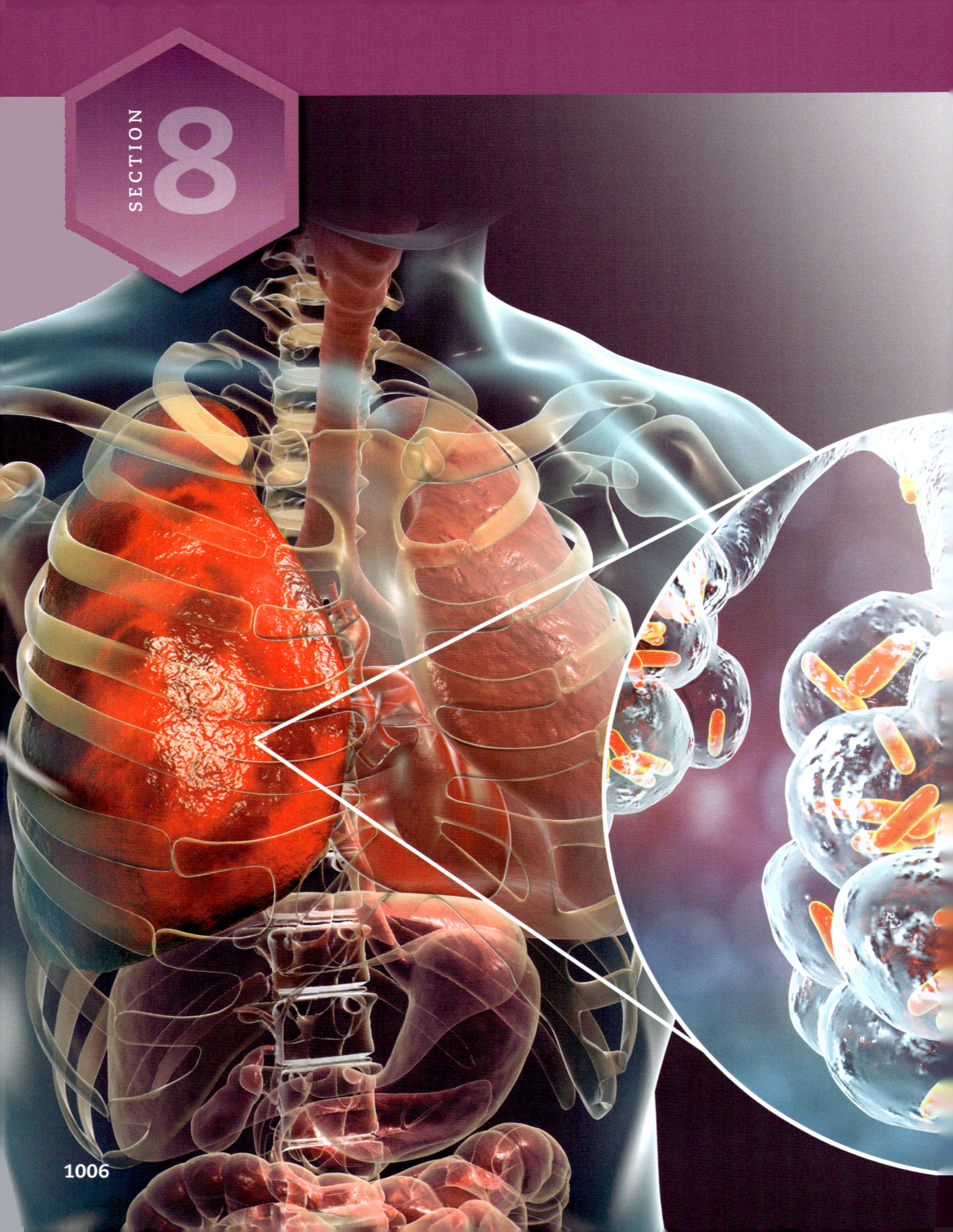

SECTION 8

On the Horizon

The most sensible way to prepare for the challenges and opportunities arising from progress in the identification of the genetic and molecular basis of health and disease is to become familiar with this field and to learn its tools.
—Bouchard C, Malina R, Pérusse L. *Genetics of Fitness and Physical Performance.* Champaign, IL: Human Kinetics, 1997.

Overview

The early 1950s ushered in the dawn of the modern age of molecular biology, and during the past 20 years exercise physiology research has embraced this opportune field. Techniques now available to study how genetic characteristics shape human behavior are revolutionizing almost every facet of human physical activity and sports medicine. The new generation of exercise physiologists has a fantastic opportunity to study the molecular world of genes and their role in human exercise performance and health and disease. This section traces the early historical origins of how the pioneers in the emerging field of basic biology, heredity, and genetics developed their views that eventually led to the modern study in their quest to understand life's molecular basis.

CHAPTER 33

Molecular Biology: New Vista for Exercise Physiology in Health, Disease, and Performance

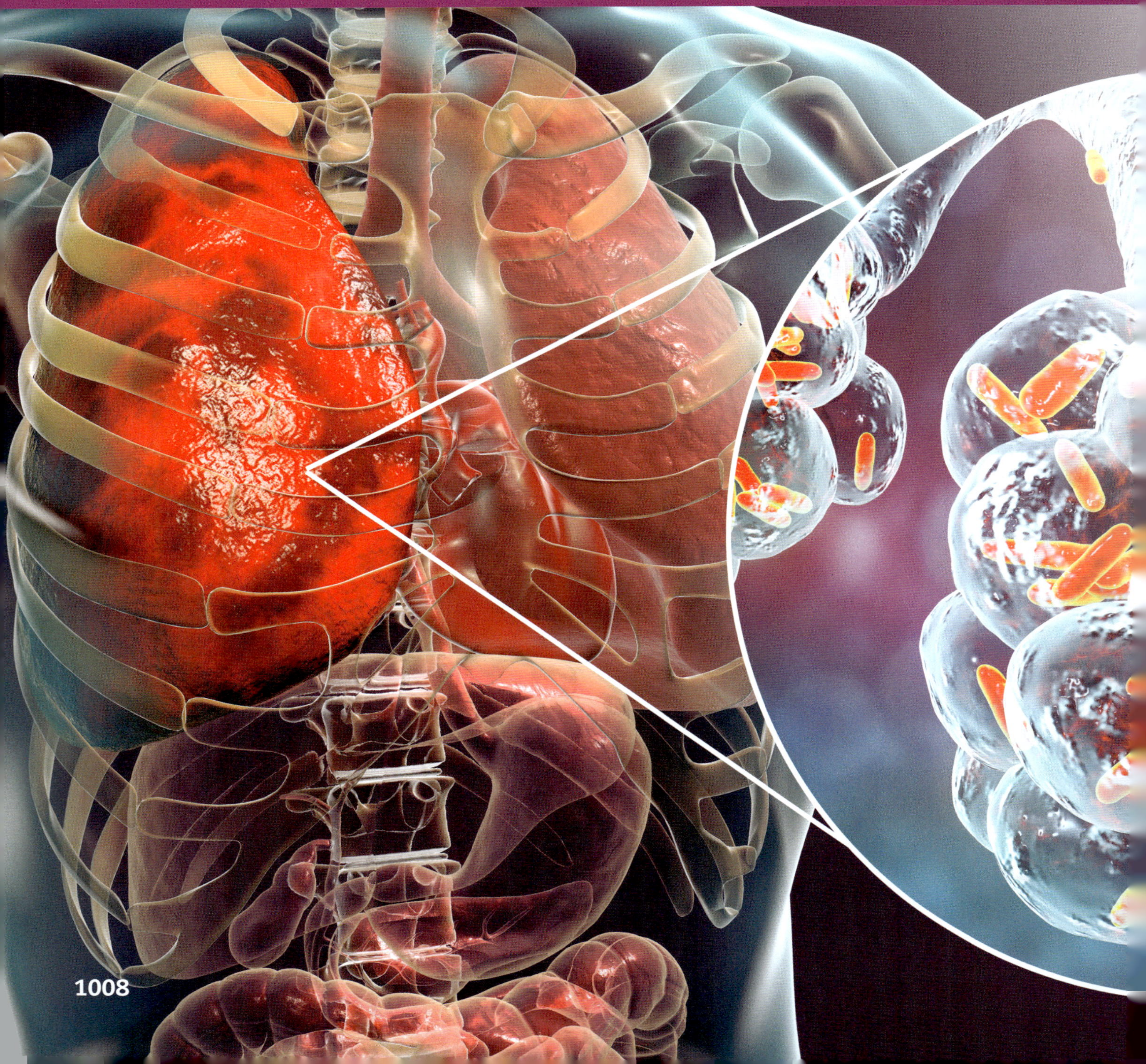

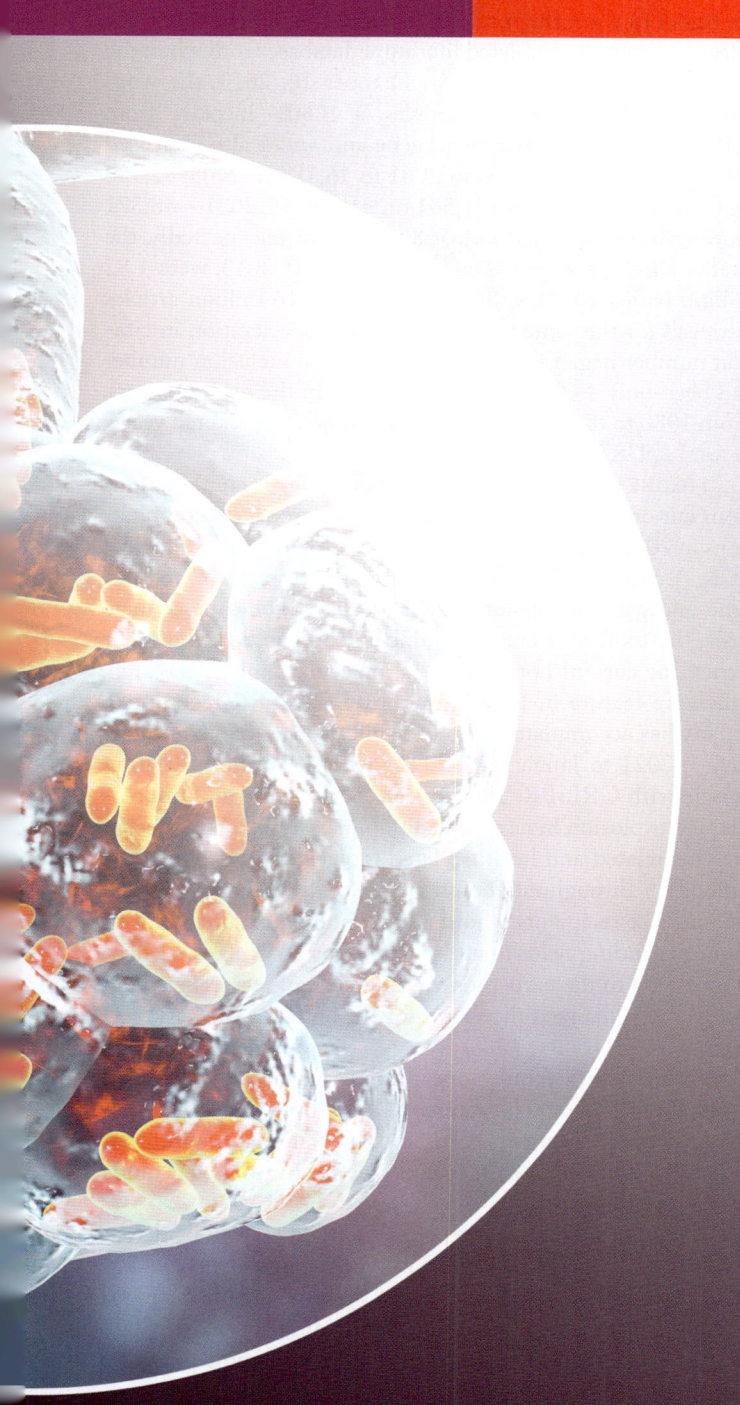

Ancillaries at-a-Glance

Visit Lippincott Connect to access the following resources.

- References: Chapter 33
- Appendix M: Selected References and Supplemental Materials: Human and Animal Research and Molecular Biology Grouped by Year (Pre-2012, 2012–2021)
- Appendix N: Selected References: CRISPR Technologies in Health, Disease, and Exercise—2013–2021
- Animations: ATPase, DNA Repair, DNA Synthesis, DNA Synthesis/Replication, Polymerase Chain Reaction (PCR), Protein Synthesis, Protein Synthesis Overview

Today's exercise physiology faculty and students cooperate in research projects with basic science, clinical and environmental medicine, chemistry, **molecular biology** and **molecular genetics**, **pharmacogenetics** (www.ncbi.nlm.nih.gov/), **epigenetics** (www.cdc.gov/genomics/disease/epigenetics.htm), **pharmacogenomics** (www.cdc.gov/genomics/disease/pharma.htm), **bioinformatics** (www.genome.gov/genetics-glossary/Bioinformatics), **metagenomics** (www.genome.gov/genetics-glossary/Metagenomics), and other emerging disciplines, many with their own specialty journals in the physical and life sciences.

Exercise physiology/kinesiology scientists and undergraduate and graduate program offerings now probe for answers about the molecular basis relating to physical activity and inactivity in promoting disease, physical dysfunction, and human performance[210] (e.g., https://mcip.ucdavis.edu/; www.bsu.edu/academics/collegesanddepartments/kinesiology; https://hlkn.tamu.edu/academics/). Research topics run the gamut from the role **genetics** plays in training and exercise performance to skeletal muscle and neurovestibular adaptations to microgravity. Occupational, physical, and rehabilitation medicine can apply the new **gene therapy** strategies to transfer genetic material to enhance a patient's specific growth factor production (e.g., www.ncmrr.org/). Small protein molecules stimulate cell proliferation, migration, and differentiation, and they promote matrix synthesis to facilitate healing injured or surgically repaired tissues with limited blood supply and slowed cell growth that impair normal tissue repair processes.[99]

In addition to delivering therapeutic proteins to injured tissues, molecular biology provides a way to engineer new tissues (https://bioeng.berkeley.edu/research/cell-tissue). Such biologic substitutes—exogenous structures and/or tissue scaffolding—can link gene therapy procedures to support tissue regeneration and healing from athletic trauma. Molecular biology also focuses on how short-term and ongoing physical activities interact to foster structural and functional adaptations that enhance exercise performance and desirable health outcomes.[49]

Booth and colleagues[15–18] assert that future exercise physiology research should emphasize primary disease prevention, with a focus on uncovering the environmental roots in modern chronic diseases notably type 2 diabetes, almost entirely preventable with increased regular physical activity.[88] Such maladies annually cause in excess of 350,000 premature deaths and play a role in $4 to $7 trillion in healthcare costs for conditions associated with sedentary living, not to mention the toll on human suffering. Booth coined the term *sedentary environmental death syndrome* to characterize sedentary lifestyle effects with unhealthy outcomes.[17,19–21,150]

Studying basic biology involving organisms at the molecular level offers novel ways to illuminate disease mechanisms and strategies that best combat them.[280] Research challenges also emerge in the exercise biology sciences. More than two decades ago, Baldwin made a compelling case that the membership of the American College of Sports Medicine should exploit new fields and technologies involved with "molecular exercise sciences."[8] Booth and Baldwin (and the authors of this text) maintain that exercise physiology and sports medicine have progressed over the past decades from an exercise biochemistry focus at the organ level to an emphasis on molecular biology at the cellular level. We posit that our field has already shifted to the molecular age, as evidenced by research emphasis in integrative biology and **proteomics**.[211] A literature search on PubMed for these terms reinforces the point (https://pubmed.ncbi.nlm.nih.gov/?term=integrative+biology+and+proteomics).

A tremendous proliferation has occurred in molecular biology interdisciplinary research through 2021 related to the exercise sciences. For example, in the prior sixth edition text, we began to track the total publication number generated for select terms in the PubMed literature database from when the term(s) were first indexed. On October 10, 2013, the word *genome* produced 873,331 articles, a 1260% increase from 2001. Citations with the terms gene and *muscle* also increased greatly, from 502 citations in 2001 to 16,184 in 2005, 82,930 on October 10, 2013, to 131,501 on August 15, 2021—48,571 more articles published in just 8 years. Not unexpectedly, the citations for "gene" recorded on October 10, 2013, were 1.82 million (since 2012), with an additional 1.16 million articles retrieved for the same word in 2021. The acceleration in citation number began in 1980, when the total inclusion number had been only 44,000 for the word gene in the prior 68 years. From 1980 to the present, the total number skyrocketed yearly to total 2,938,067 entries.

FIGURE 33.1 compares the different term combinations from our original 2013 analysis with the same term combinations in 2021 to reveal the phenomenal growth in these subject areas. A clear trend emerges—adding the term *health* to both gene and gene expression has far outpaced, on a percentage basis, the total new citation numbers compared to the other terms. The current hottest area in molecular biology research, which we feature in Part 2 (the novel **CRISPR** technique), already has accumulated 25,691 publications (7250 from January 1, 2021 to January 29, 2022), with 195 articles relating muscle with CRISPR. This indicates a bountiful and unprecedented explosion in new multidisciplinary research in specific exercise-related and health-related molecular biology investigations.[281] Throughout the chapter, we also acknowledge 28 Nobel Prize recipients who made monumental contributions to the expanding fields in molecular biology. We all owe a debt of gratitude to the early pioneers and current researchers who have forever changed the world for the better in the basic sciences.

As an historical milestone, funding for genomics reached its peak in 2003–2004, totaling $437 million (from the U.S. Department of Energy [DOE] and the National Institutes of Health). Unfortunately for science, the DOE no longer funds research in this area.

Future limits to athletic performance likely will be determined less by an athlete's innate physiology and anatomy (and commitment to training) and more by surgical enhancement (e.g., more flexible tendons) and genetic interventions (including banned drugs) engineered for faster-acting, more powerful

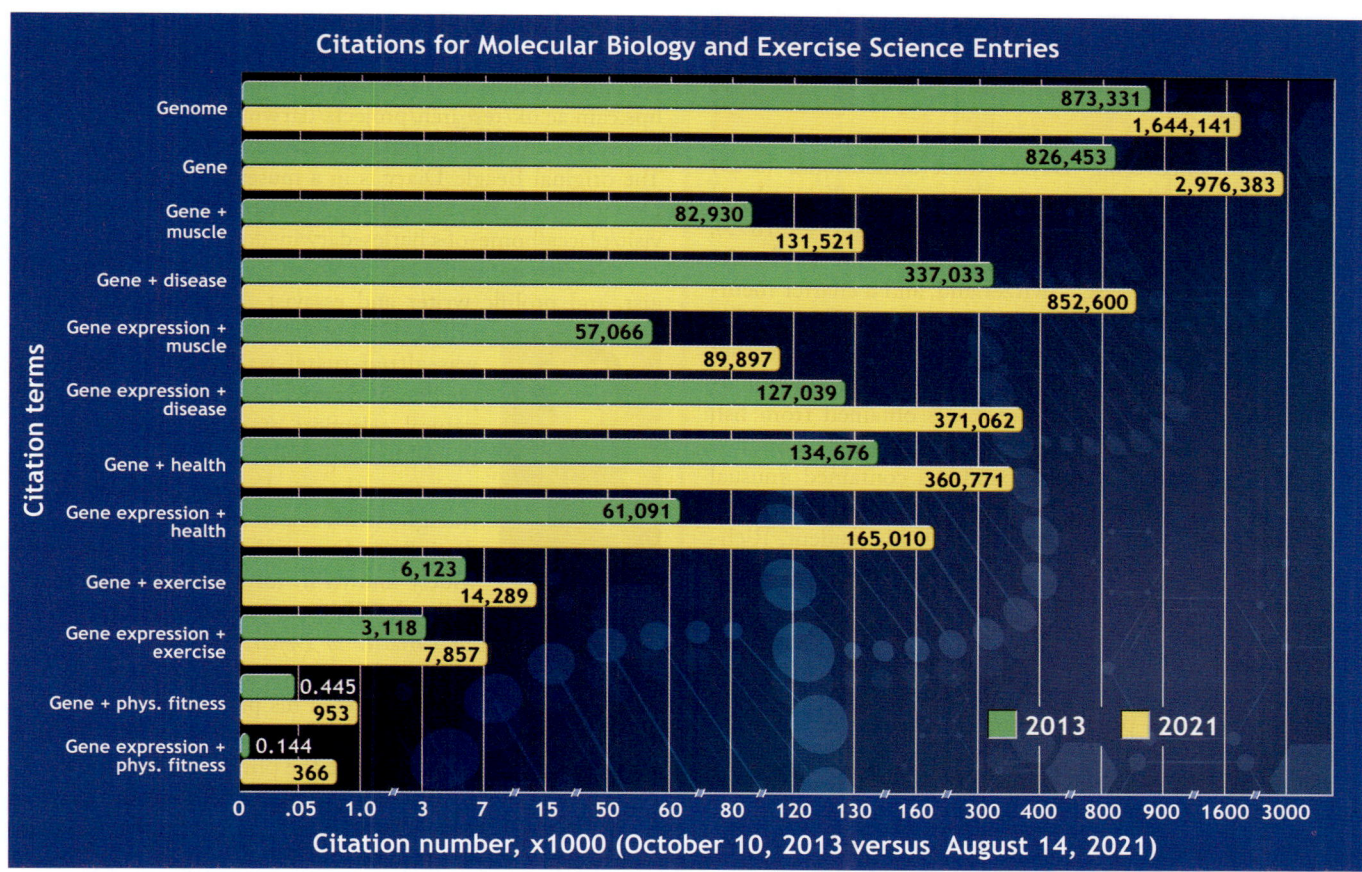

FIGURE 33.1. Comparing popular citation terms in molecular biology and exercise science for 2013 searched on PubMed. October 10, 2013 versus August 14, 2021).
(Background image: wanpatsorn/Shutterstock.)

muscles; greater oxygen transport and utilization; and more rapid circulation. The ongoing abuse by athletes exploiting banned substance use, uncovered at every international Olympiad since Tokyo 2021 (and the Tour de France for many years before that), highlights the challenges facing the World Anti-Doping Association (www.wada-ama.org/), the independent drug-testing agency charged with curbing continuing illegal drug use in Olympic Games. Breakthroughs in gene therapy techniques in the coming years will likely infiltrate the athlete's arsenal of "tricks" in Olympic and other world-class competitions. As increasing numbers of amateur and professional athletes in many sport disciplines cheat with advanced molecular biology techniques to gain a competitive edge, both athletes, governing organizations, and an educated general public will confront specialists in exercise physiology concerning new applications in molecular biology, gene therapy, and sport and exercise genetics.[172–174]

The chapter has three major parts:

Part 1. *Molecular Biology Historical Tour* chronicles the key leaders and associated events in DNA development and techniques leading up to a simple and versatile tool for genomic editing.[184–187]

Part 2. *New Horizons in Molecular Biology* traces Watson and Crick's pioneering achievements in deciphering DNA's molecular structure to successfully sequence the human genome, which at that time represented one of the most remarkable scientific achievements in medical science history. Within the last decade, **CRISPR gene editing** modified human genomes by delivering **Cas9 nuclease** complexed with a synthetic guide RNA into cells. The new technology evolved from discoveries that bacteria use an internal genetic coding system as an evolutionary protective mechanism to shred the DNA from invading viruses. This discovery opened-up another window in the molecular chemistry's technical toolbox to improve the human condition by battling many different disease states.[176,177,182]

Part 3. *Human Performance Research* investigates physical activity and exercise training, seeking to decipher signaling pathways by which genes transcribe mechanical stressor effects and resultant phenotypic expression.[178–181,183] For example, research has demonstrated that estrogen depletion in rodents and humans leads to physical inactivity, fat accumulation, and diabetes, particularly during menopause coincident with aging.[3,111,166] Manipulating neural-signaling control centers in the brain in rodents substantially alters physical activity output and causes the animal to pursue a more vigorous activity profile and alters negative physiological outcomes associated with prolonged physical inactivity. The implications seem clear—techniques gleaned from molecular biology research can rebalance the brain's energy allocation mechanisms to provide a better understanding of strategies to remain physically active throughout hormonal transitions with aging, particularly in women during menopause.[275]

SECTION 8 • On the Horizon

Part 1 — Molecular Biology Historical Tour

The road to uncovering DNA's three-dimensional (3-D) structure began with an innocent discovery by Swiss physiologist Friedrich Miescher (1844–1895), professor of physiology at the University of Basel, Switzerland, and a charter member to the 1889 First International Congress of Physiologists. In 1869, Miescher identified what he considered a new biologic substance. Cells obtained from fish sperm and human tissue cells obtained from pus in discarded surgical bandages contained unusual nitrogen and phosphorus proportions in their nuclei. Miescher called the substance *nuclein*, which his student, Richard Altman (1852–1900), later termed *nucleic acid* because it had slightly acidic properties. Altman, also remembered for creating an aniline-acid fuchsin histological pigment, stained mitochondria crimson against a yellow background (www.chemistryexplained.com/Ne-Nu/Nucleic-Acids.html). Ten years after Altman's primary experiments, Ludwig Albrecht Kossel 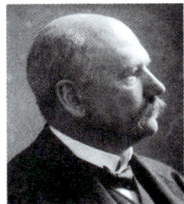 (1853–1927; www.nobelprize.org/nobel_prizes/medicine/laureates/1910/kossel-bio.html), a German physiological chemist, won the 1910 Nobel Prize in Physiology or Medicine for his pioneering work on proteins and the nucleic substances and their cleavage products.

Ludwig Albrecht Kossel

As late as the second half of the 19th century, chemists and biologists did not know what role, if any, genes played in transmitting hereditary information in plants or animals. This changed when English naturalist, geologist, avid anti-slavery advocate, and biologist Charles Robert Darwin (1809–1882) (www.nhm.ac.uk/discover/charles-darwin-most-famous-biologist.html) proposed an evolution theory based on **natural selection** of random variation.[40] Darwin developed his theory gradually after many years of insightful geologic and biologic observations on unspoiled lands, particularly along the western South American coast, including the Galapagos Islands (www.gct.org/darwin.html) and his 1835–1836 shore observations in New Zealand and Australia (www.mja.com.au/journal/2009/191/11/charles-darwin-s-impressions-new-zealand-and-australia-and-insights-his-illness). His ideas about evolution emerged mainly from observations in the subtle differences among plant and animal species during his 57-months, 2-day voyage around the world (www.aboutdarwin.com/voyage/voyage03.html), begun in 1831 aboard the British survey ship HMS Beagle (FIG. 33.2).[38] Darwin's careful observations about the distribution and continuation in animal and plant phenotypic traits were first published on November 26, 1859, 10 years before Miescher

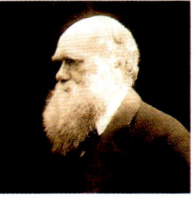

Charles Darwin

discovered nuclein. Further details about Darwin's travels and every letter written by and to Darwin between 1837 and 1859 are chronicled in the "*Darwin Correspondence Project*" (www.hps.cam.ac.uk/research/projects/darwin-correspondence and www.darwinproject.ac.uk/letters/darwins-letters-timeline). The original Beagle Diary is in a museum at Darwin's home, Down House, Kent, England (www.english-heritage.org.uk/visit/places/home-of-charles-darwin-down-house/).

English naturalist and explorer, evolutionist, anthropologist, and prolific writer and essayist Alfred Russel Wallace (1823–1913; www.nhm.ac.uk/discover/who-was-alfred-russel-wallace.html) had independently formed his own views regarding natural selection at about the same time Darwin completed his work dealing with evolution theory. Except for sharing his thoughts with selected colleagues in various disciplines, Darwin had not yet made them widely known in formal publications. Darwin's reading of Wallace's 1855 paper about natural selection, *On the Tendency of Varieties to Depart Indefinitely From the Original Type* (reprinted in *Contributions of the theory of natural selection*),[160] no doubt accelerated his pace to publish his single-volume discourse on evolutionary theory. It was Wallace who encouraged Darwin to use the phrase "*survival of the fittest*" (coined by British sociologist and philosopher Herbert Spencer [1820–1903]) to convey the basic idea about natural selection to the general public.

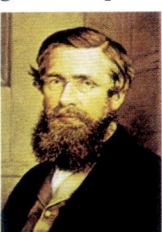

Alfred Russel Wallace

Darwin's carefully crafted, thought-provoking treatise, *On the Origin of the Species, by Means of Natural Selection, or the Preservation of Favoured Races in the Struggle for Life*,[39] indirectly provided empirical "data" on how environmental pressures selected a species' observable characteristics (traits)

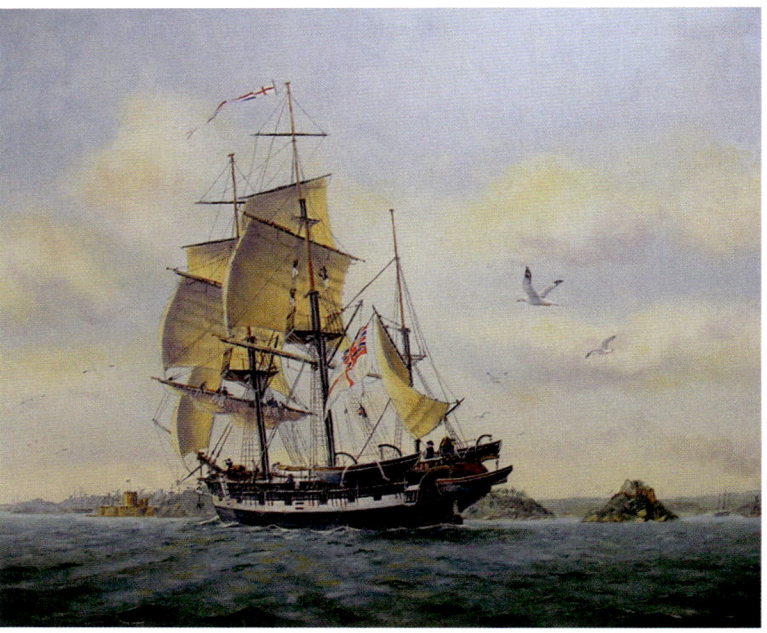

FIGURE 33.2. The HMS Beagle (235 tons, 27-m length, 7-m breadth, six canons) engaged in three survey missions from 1826 to 1843, with the naturalist Charles Darwin on the second survey.
(Image courtesy marine artist Ron Scobie, ASMA (https://ronscobie.webs.com).)

Discovering Darwin's Inherited Medical Malady

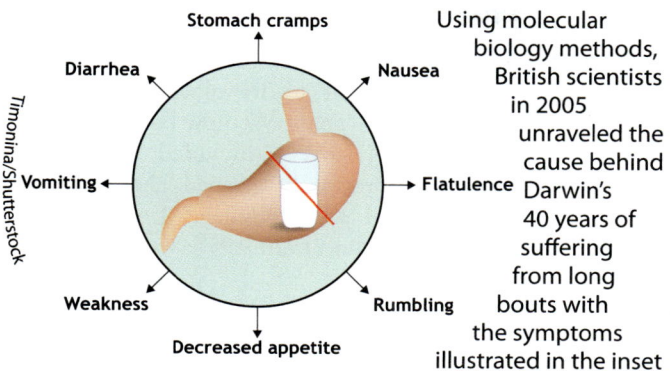

Using molecular biology methods, British scientists in 2005 unraveled the cause behind Darwin's 40 years of suffering from long bouts with the symptoms illustrated in the inset image.[28] Darwin's family history revealed a major inherited predisposition for hypolactasia (cream aversion from inability to digest milk and to metabolize milk sugar–producing lactase). The molecular basis associated with inherited hypolactasia and thus lactose intolerance may involve distinct polymorphisms in helicase molecules, enzymes involved in remodeling nucleic acid or nucleic acid protein complexes. Intolerance to some foods results from reduced lactase activity in the small bowel's mucosal brush border. The authors concluded that Darwin's multifold symptoms and illnesses (including long isolation from friends and colleagues) point to Crohn disease and highlight a missed observation—the importance of lactose in mammalian and human evolution. Darwin's malady is one of the most common food intolerances and occurs when individuals may be lactose intolerant to varying degrees. Gut microbiota are supposed to digest unfermented lactose, but if not, it can precipitate symptoms that include abdominal pain, bloating, flatulence, and diarrhea with considerable intraindividual and interindividual variability.

Sources:
Catanzaro R, et al. Lactose intolerance: an update on its pathogenesis, diagnosis, and treatment. *Nutr Res*. 2021;89:23.
Montoro-Huguet MA, et al. Small and large intestine (I): malabsorption of nutrients. *Nutrients*. 2021;13:1254.

---

to survive from one generation to the next. Darwin's theory explained how adaptive modifications to environmental stressors impacted the common descent in animal and plant species and how natural selection over time preserved a species' survival.

Interestingly, Miescher's discovery of nuclein came 4 years after Austrian monk Gregor Johann Mendel's (1822–1884) elegant 25-year breeding experiments with 10,000 varieties of edible pea plants, *Pisum sativum*. Mendel vigilantly tracked the peas' inherited characteristics and in 1865 submitted his findings, "Versuche über Pflanzen-Hybriden," to an obscure natural history society journal. The work appeared in 1866 and about 1902 was translated into English by William Bateson (1861–1926; www.dnalc.org/view/16206-Biography-5-William-Bateson-1861-1926-.html).[11] The pea genome was published in 2019, divulging the intricate genomic structures following Mendel's early descriptive genetic pairings chronicled in 1866.[244] Darwin's unifying evolution theory and Mendel's experiments on heredity formed "scientific pillars" to embrace a relatively new field—molecular biology—that would subsequently dominate fundamental discoveries in biology, chemistry, genetics, nutrition, and medicine through future decades.

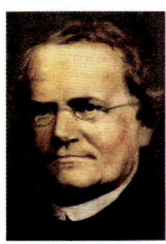

Gregor Johann Mendel

Mendel's meticulous scientific insights remained relatively obscure for nearly three decades until three scientists—German botanist Carl Correns (1864–1933; www.dnalc.org/view/16223-Biography-6-Carl-Correns-1864-1933-.html), Dutch botanist Hugo De Vries (1848–1935; www.britannica.com/EBchecked/topic/633337/Hugo-de-Vries; working with flowering plants), and Austrian agronomist Erich van Tschermak-Seysenegg (1871–1962; www.eucarpia.org/secretariate/honorary/tschermak.html; using peas)—rediscovered his research in about 1900. It would take nearly 65 years after Mendel's initial publication and enormous progress in biochemical techniques to unravel further secrets highlighting the mysteries relating to hereditary transmission in human cells.

In 1929, Phoebus A. T. Levene (1869–1940; www.jbc.org/content/277/22/e11) discovered that the essential components in the nucleic acids DNA and **ribonucleic acid (RNA)** were long chained repeating **nucleotides**. It remained unclear to Levene and others how these molecules assembled. If the **genes** indeed contained the hereditary information, scientists needed to understand the processes involved in gene transmission. Twenty-five years later, a major breakthrough occurred—Watson and Crick's discovery about DNA's structure delivered the biggest biologic thunderbolt since Darwin. This significant breakthrough impacted at least 10 other crucial scientific milestones through 2022:

1. 1966—cracking the DNA genetic code
2. 1972 to 1973—splicing DNA components together to form genes (called *recombinant molecules*) and then inserting them into bacteria to produce human proteins
3. 1977—revealing a microorganism's complete genetic information, paving the way for the historic **Human Genome Project**
4. 1981—creating the first transgenic animal by inserting a viral gene into mouse DNA, allowing such animals to serve as models to study human diseases
5. 1984—devising the polymerase chain reaction method to replicate DNA
6. 1997—cloning the first mammal, the lamb Dolly, from an adult sheep cell
7. 2000 to 2004—deciphering the **human genome**; sequencing the fruit fly *Drosophila melanogaster* genome; sequencing rice DNA (first crop decoding); initial sequencing and comparative analysis of mouse and brown Norway rat genomes; producing a single embryonic stem cell line from a human blastocyst through somatic cell **nuclear transfer** (SCNT) technology (representing the first published report involving cloned human stem cells)[278]

8. 2005 to 2009—creating human stem cell lines from human embryos by cloning, then extracting patient-specific, immune-matched human embryonic stem cells to create genetic matches in patients with disease or injury
9. 2009 to 2014—human and animal cloning, causing controversies to erupt; advancing research on human stem cells to better understand debilitating genetic malfunctions (e.g., amyotrophic lateral sclerosis [Lou Gehrig disease], Alzheimer disease, blindness, blood disorders, malfunctions in blood supply, cancers, cartilage damage, rheumatoid arthritis, diabetes, hearing loss, heart and circulatory disease, infertility, lung damage, memory loss due to brain tumor treatment, multiple sclerosis, muscular dystrophy, organ replacement, platelet transfusions, spinal cord injury); modifying crop genetics; gene analysis companies competing for cloud-based solutions for gene mapping[24]
10. 2009 to 2022—developing breakthrough CRISPR-CAS9 sophisticated cutting-edge genome editing and cell therapy development platforms to advance new pharmacologic strategies[286] to fight devastating human diseases[286]

Revolution in the Biologic Sciences

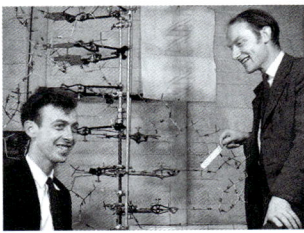
© Barrington Brown/Science Source

In 1953, James Dewey Watson (1928– ; www.nobelprize.org/nobel_prizes/medicine/laureates/1962/watson-bio.html), an American postdoctoral student who earned a PhD in genetics from Indiana University at age 22, teamed with English physicist Francis Harry Compton Crick (1916–2004; www.nobelprize.org/nobel_prizes/medicine/laureates/1962/crick-bio.html), who was pursuing a PhD in x-ray studies involving protein in the influential Cavendish Laboratory, Cambridge, England (www.phy.cam.ac.uk/history/). At Cavendish, Professor Sir Lawrence Bragg (1890–1971; British physicist and x-ray crystallographer and 1915 Nobel Prize winner in Physics; www.nobelprize.org/nobel_prizes/physics/laureates/1915/wl-bragg-bio.html) developed x-ray crystallography as a powerful tool to understand biological molecule structures. Bragg was instrumental in allowing Watson and Crick to pursue their model-building work at his laboratory (http://paulingblog.wordpress.com/2009/04/30/the-watson-and-crick-structure-of-dna/).

Watson and Crick's breakthrough, deduced from other scientists published and unpublished research, posited that the DNA molecule had two polynucleotide linear strands coiled around each other to form a **double helix**.[161]

The image shows Watson (left) and Crick (right) at the Cavendish Laboratory in May 1953 next to their DNA ball and wire model. They proposed that the two helical strands connected like spiral staircase steps by nucleotide base pairs held together by hydrogen bonds. Their eventual 1962 Nobel Prize rewarded their contribution about DNA's architecture and the 3-D fit to its molecular components. We now know this discovery included substantial theoretical contributions previously gleaned about DNA's helical structure from rival Kings College, London, colleague Rosalind Elsie Franklin (1920–1957; www.sdsc.edu/ScienceWomen/franklin.html).

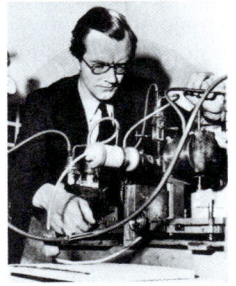
Maurice H. F. Wilkins

In their 1953 landmark publication in *Nature* describing DNA's molecular structure, Watson and Crick state that their research efforts were stimulated by "a knowledge of the general nature of the unpublished experimental results and ideas of Drs. M. H. F. Wilkins (1926–2004; www.nobelprize.org/nobel_prizes/medicine/laureates/1962/wilkins-bio.html; www.whatisbiotechnology.org/index.php/people/summary/Wilkins) and R. E. Franklin and coworkers at King's College, London." This statement, interpreted with the hindsight of investigative follow-up by historians and researchers, paints quite a different picture of Franklin's prior crucial discoveries about DNA's structure, which eventually led Watson and Crick to deduce DNA's final configuration correctly.

Franklin's sophisticated x-ray diffraction photo reflecting her expertise with x-ray crystallography (shown to Watson and Crick surreptitiously without Franklin's knowledge or permission) provided the missing piece about DNA's double helix, empowering them to correctly deduce that DNA must have originated from a twisted **helix** ladder-shaped molecule. Watson and Crick quickly deciphered the structural puzzle after viewing the photo (FIG. 33.3). Interestingly, unlike many biologists, Watson and Crick did not conduct experiments. Their technique involved thinking, arguing, and rethinking ideas and concepts about how to put together complicated puzzle pieces

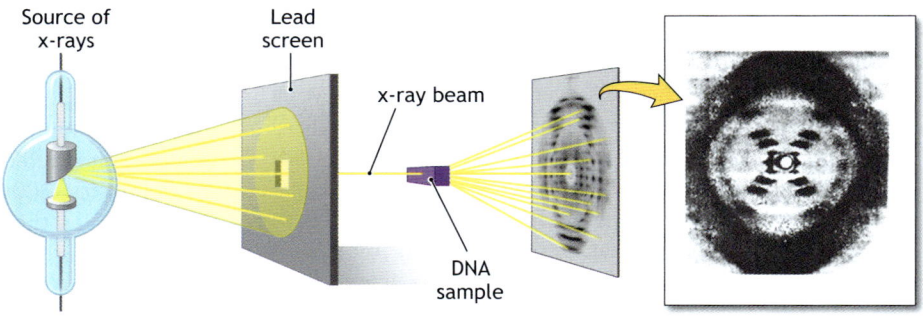

FIGURE 33.3. The x-ray crystallography technique bombards crystals with thin x-ray beams with single (monochromatic) wavelength to determine a substance's three-dimensional crystal structure. The *right* photo shows Franklin's DNA x-ray photograph; she focused the x-ray beam on extra-wet DNA fibers for a longer-than-usual time, with a 62-hr exposure to obtain the vivid photo revealing DNA's cruciform pattern.

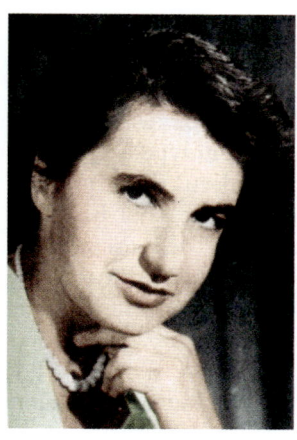

Dr. Rosalind Franklin. Courtesy National Library of Medicine

with many interconnected components. Undoubtedly, this discovery represented a major milestone in the history of science, which served as the cornerstone to modern molecular biology. A new era had begun, which quickly mushroomed to a better understanding about how genes control cells' chemical processes. The implications were direct and straight forward—understanding the genetic code could satisfactorily explain protein synthesis, the driving force behind millions of simultaneous chemical reactions continually operating among the body's 100 trillion cells from 80 known organs.

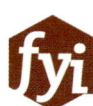 **Rosalind Franklin: An Unsung Hero in Discovering the Double Helix**

For an historical perspective, we recommend three books with different views about how the DNA puzzle was eventually solved. Watson's interpretation details one of the most important discoveries in all of science by one scientific team member who helped to solve DNA's final structural configuration.[163] His book, *The Double Helix,* makes only passing reference to DNA's helical structure from British Chemist Rosalind Franklin's unpublished discovery while surreptitiously reviewing her x-ray crystallography images of the now famous helix structure. Their book published *after* Franklin's life was cut short by ovarian cancer at age 37, before she had the opportunity to set the record straight about the true nature revealing DNA's dual helix structure.

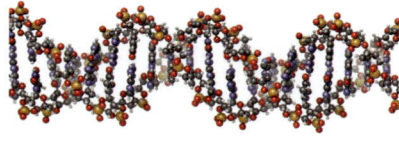

StudioMolekuul/Shutterstock

American writers Ann C. Sayre (1923–1998)[138] and Brenda Maddox (1932–2019; www.ncbi.nlm.nih.gov/pmc/articles/PMC1125153/)[209] provide compelling and insightful first full accounts about Rosalind Franklin's previously unacknowledged major contribution to discovering DNA's ultimate helical configuration (www.ncbi.nlm.nih.gov/pmc/articles/PMC1083834/). The Sayre and Maddox book revelations uncover an ugly side in the basic sciences—cutthroat ways and blind ambition ran roughshod over a female's research contributions without proper attribution (both authors strongly suggest sexism and jealousy in play), with only timid reference by Watson and Crick to the most important key component that helps to confirm DNA's discovery yet then claim credit for the discovery with scant reference to Franklin's contributions, even in their Nobel acceptance speech! In 1962, Maurice Wilkins, James Watson, and Francis Crick received the Nobel Prize, but it was Franklin's data and DNA x-ray photographs that truly clinched their ultimate prize.

From Watson's and Crick's decisive "discovery," we know definitively that DNA's helical structure carries the biologic blueprint for specifying the *order* in which the body's 20 amino acids assemble to create a protein. Each protein has its own unique amino acid sequence; this sequence ultimately dictates the protein molecule's final shape and distinctive chemical and functional characteristics. We also know that each double-helix strand provides a **template** for synthesizing a new strand, something Watson and Crick had hinted at in their seminal 1953 *Nature* publication. A **template strand** represents an original DNA strand. Once faithfully copied, each newly created double-helix strand represents a duplicate of its predecessor, with its genetic code sequence perfectly preserved. This self-replication mechanism preserves the genetic information flow to ensure that successive generations receive the same coded DNA "messages." In fact, all living things on Earth share their unique, basic molecular plan. Each human's 100 trillion cells rely on four basic molecular building blocks—nucleic acid, protein, lipid, and polysaccharide—along with other nano-sized biomolecules—to perform their functions efficiently. In addition, all living cells shuttle the information flow from DNA to RNA to protein. The full impact of what Watson and Crick deduced about DNA's structural configuration cannot be over stated: their contribution and subsequent investigations have impacted every facet involving biomedical science, from how primordial DNA formed and survived, to how deadly diseases begin and the all-out search for their eventual cure. Unraveling DNA's structure has profoundly impacted the sciences, particularly subsequent discoveries about human, viral, plant, and animal genomes (see next section).

In fact, molecular biology has shown such explosive growth during the past five decades, a Nobel Prize has been awarded for research related to this field. Since its 1901 inception, 4 of only 10 women awarded a Nobel Prize in science won for molecular biology–related research.[106]

The Human Genome

The human **genome** represents the full complement of genetic material in a human cell (www.genome.gov/About-Genomics/Introduction-to-Genomics). The December 1999 issue of *Nature* featured a milestone scientific achievement (www.nature.com/articles/990031)—the sequence or "genetic map" for 12 contiguous human chromosome 22 segments, the second smallest among the 23 chromosomes (chromosome 22 contains about 1.6 to 1.8% total genomic DNA).[44] On June 26, 2000, a private company, Celera Genomics, and the publicly funded National Human Genome Research Institute (www.genengnews.com/insights/the-human-genome-project-in-2020-hindsight/) announced completion of the first assembly draft of the human genome. By November 2000, more than half the genome classified, sequenced, and recorded in public databases (e.g., www.nature.com/scitable/topicpage/genomic-data-resources-challenges-and-promises-743721/). The Human Genome Project had achieved its major objective to produce a high-quality version involving the human genome, freely available in April 2003 in public databases.[193]

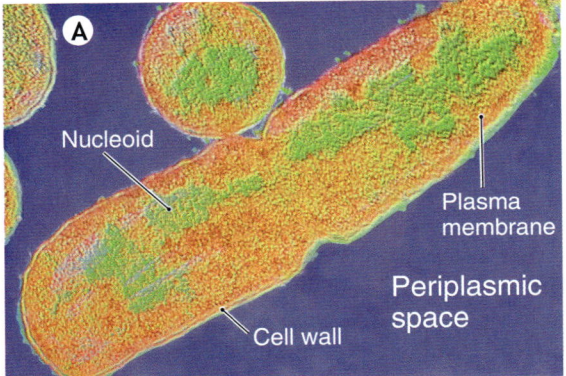
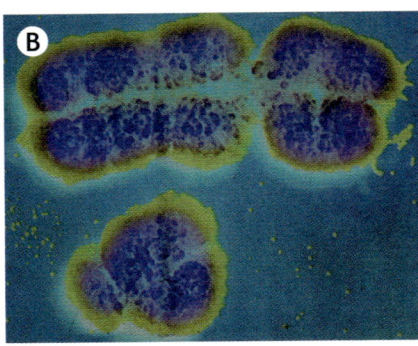

FIGURE 33.4. **(A)** The bacterium *Escherichia coli*. **(B)** The Y chromosome, one of the smallest human chromosomes, has an estimated average size of 60 million base pairs (Mb). Note the larger top chromosome compared with the smaller Y chromosome.

To unravel the submicroscopic secrets within genetic material, sophisticated detection techniques help scientists "decode" the human genome (https://genome.cshlp.org/content/genome/22/9/1599.full.html). Most decoded DNA sequences were not included in the final transcript that ultimately directs protein synthesis.

Genome size determines total base pair number. The human genome, distributed among 23 **chromosome** pairs that each repeat over and over like a genetic stutter without interruption, imparts our individual uniqueness. At conception, one complete chromosome set from the biological father's sperm (22 plus an **X chromosome** or **Y chromosome**) joins with one complete set from the biological mother's egg (22 plus an X sex chromosome) to give each human offspring 46 chromosomes.

The helical DNA structures (**genotype**) contain the genetic blueprint or "roadmap" for almost every aspect of our being (**phenotype**). The phenotype reflects the expression from our gene pool based on the physical dimensions, texture, color, composition, and shape for every internal and external body part to our personalities with all their idiosyncrasies. Human genome size greatly exceeds that of other organisms. For example, the bacterium *Escherichia coli* (*E. coli*) shown in **FIGURE 33.4A** (primary member of the large bacterial family *Enterobacteriaceae*) contains 4.6 million base pairs, while yeast contains 15 million base pairs. In contrast, the smallest human chromosome (the male or Y chromosome; Fig. 33.4B) has 58 million base pairs (www.genome.gov/27557513/the-y-chromosome-beyond-gender-determination) and occupies an estimated 20,000 to 25,000 total genes in the human genome. The largest human chromosome contains 250 million base pairs. For some idea about the enormity of the genetic structures, consider these four analogies:

Analogy 1. A double-spaced 8.5 × 11–in page of text using normal margins contains about 3000 letters, or roughly 250 words. Porting the human genome to pages would equal

The Future Holds Promise for an Eventual Cure for a Deadly Inherited Blood Disorder

Normal hemoglobin β-chain amino acids						
Valine	Histidine	Leucine	Threonine	Proline	Glutamic acid	Glutamic acid
Sickle cell anemia hemoglobin β-chain amino acids					↓	
Valine	Histidine	Leucine	Threonine	Proline	Valine	Glutamic acid

Sickle cell anemia, a form of sickle cell disease (www.cdc.gov/ncbddd/sicklecell/facts.html), provides a salient example when an abnormality occurs in the normal hemoglobin molecule with seven β-chain amino acids illustrated in the above inset table's second row. Sickle cell anemia is usually a fatal hereditary disease affecting hemoglobin; it develops when the amino acid valine substitutes for glutamic acid because of a change in its codon nucleotide sequence from G-A-A to G-U-A.[87] This blood disease occurs genetically when a person inherits two abnormal β-globin genes that make hemoglobin, one from each parent. The disease afflicts two of every 1000 African Americans; the erythrocyte becomes irregular, thin, elongated, and crescent-shaped, severely affecting its oxygen transport capacity.

In the sickle cell condition (circled in yellow), the amino acid valine shown in red substitutes for glutamic acid and alters hemoglobin's β chain from a codon change from G-A-A to G-U-A. Despite the lack of progress in eradicating sickle cell disorders worldwide, newer gene editing platforms such as CRISPR/Cas9 may provide future hope to correct the disease-causing mutation in hematopoietic stem cells in individuals with the condition.[208] The CRISPR technology is being extensively studied in pharmaceutical trials to "correct" diseases, including bone marrow cells in persons afflicted with the sickle cell trait by "turning on" desired genes to correct the DNA with bad gene sequences to positively alter and even halt disease progression (www.vrtx.com).

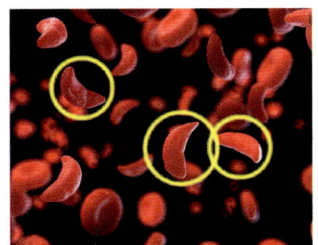

SciePro/Shutterstock

the number of letters in 1000 copies of the Sunday *New York Times* or about 1200 copies of this textbook.

Analogy 2. Reading one letter of code every second would take about 100 years without a break to peruse the entire genome!

Analogy 3. A single DNA strand in one **diploid** human cell with 23 chromosome pairs, if unwound and stacked end to end, would stretch to a person 60 in tall, yet it occupies a width only 50-trillionths of an inch!

Analogy 4. The DNA in a single human cell, if unfurled and stretched out, would become a six-foot long strand containing six billion letters from the DNA code playbook.

The human DNA sequence includes the longest DNA continuous stretch ever deciphered and assembled, with over 23 million letters. Sequencing chromosome 22 allowed scientists for the first time to view a chromosome's entire DNA. At least 27 human disorders link to chromosome 22 genes, including ovarian, colon, and breast cancers; cataracts; congenital heart disease; schizophrenia; **neurofibromatosis**; mental retardation; and nervous system and fetal development disorders (www.nature.com/articles/990031).

Scientists view sequencing of the human genome as somewhat analogous to completing an intricately detailed inaugural chapter in the human genetic instruction book, which in turn comprises many complex chapters. An international collaboration from eight laboratories in the United Kingdom, Japan, the United States, Canada, and Sweden helped to complete the analysis of the body's 23 chromosomes through 2006, and through June, 2013, over 70 leading healthcare, research, and disease advocacy organizations from more than 40 countries initiated a global alliance for genetic health[285] dedicated to enabling the secure genomic and clinical data sharing in a technical and regulatory effective and responsible manner (www.ornl.gov/sci/techresources/Human_Genome/project/timeline.shtml; www.broadinstitute.org/news/globalalliance). Knowing the identity and order in DNA's chemical components in the 23 human chromosome pairs has provided an important tool to evaluate health and disease status.

A relatively few discrete genetic instructions ultimately determine all the subtlety in the human species developed and transmitted over thousands of years in disparate fields from ancient architecture, language, mathematics, sculpture, and poetry, to medicine, computer science, chemistry, and virology. Anatomic and psychological differences between any two unrelated individuals really reflect relatively few differences in their genomic blueprint—perhaps one or two gene sequences in thousands. Examples include multiple Olympic gold medal gymnastics champion Simone Biles, NBA basketball greats Michael Jordan, Wilt Chamberlain, and Lebron James, to civil rights leaders Martin Luther King and John Lewis, and brilliant Austrian physicist Lise Meitner[142] (1878–1968, www.atomicarchive.com/Bios/Meitner.shtml; deprived a Nobel Prize for contributing to nuclear fission's discovery based on her religion and professional animosities). In fact, every person born from the earliest days in human existence to the present (except for about 10% of adults born with genetic mutations) are far more alike in their genetic makeup than they are different! The variety among individuals approaches infinity, even for the expressed traits in identical multiples (e.g., twins and triplets)!

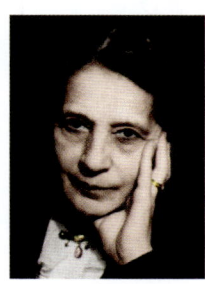
Dr. Lise Meitner

The Fight Against Chromosome 21 Mutations

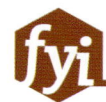

Chromosome 21, the second chromosome identified by the Human Genome project, is the smallest human chromosome with 48 million base pairs representing about 1.5 to 2% of a cell's total DNA. Unfortunately, mutations along a stretch of genes on chromosome 21 give rise to Alzheimer disease (www.alz.org/alzheimers-dementia/stages), amyotrophic lateral sclerosis (www.alsa.org), epilepsy, deafness, autoimmune disease, birth defects, and manic depression (www.genome.gov/about-genomics/fact-sheets/Chromosome-Abnormalities-Fact-Sheet). The inset image shows a neuron with amyloid plaques in an Alzheimer patient's brain. For Down syndrome (named after English physician John Langdon Down [1828–1896], who observed individuals in a British asylum in 1866 and published *Observations on an Ethnic Classification of Idiots*; www.ndss.org), researchers are on a quest to develop animal models for this genetic mental insufficiency variant and other genetic abnormalities using genetically engineered strategies to eradicate them. Gene testing also may prove useful for patients who respond differently to warfarin (Coumadin; www.drugs.com/coumadin.html), a widely prescribed anti–blood-clotting drug strategy to combat identified genetic variations.[74,80]

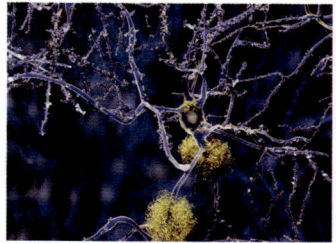
Juan Gaertner/Shutterstock

Sources:
Fockens MM, et al. Tracheal anomalies associated with Down syndrome: a systematic review. *Pediatr Pulmonol*. 2021;56:814.
Moreau M, et al. Metabolic diseases and Down Syndrome: how are they linked together? *Biomedicines*. 2021;9:221.
Moyer AJ, et al. All creatures great and small: new approaches for understanding Down Syndrome genetics. *Trends Genet*. 2021;37:444.

Nucleic Acids

FIGURE 33.5 shows the central configuration differences between the two **nucleic acids**, DNA and RNA; the three *yellow text boxes* highlight the important differences (www.nature.com/articles/1205996). Note that in RNA, **uracil** replaces thymine to pair with adenine. When cells divide, both DNA and RNA carry and then transmit the hereditary information, ensuring, for example, that liver cells produce liver cells, and from generation to generation through reproductive cells.

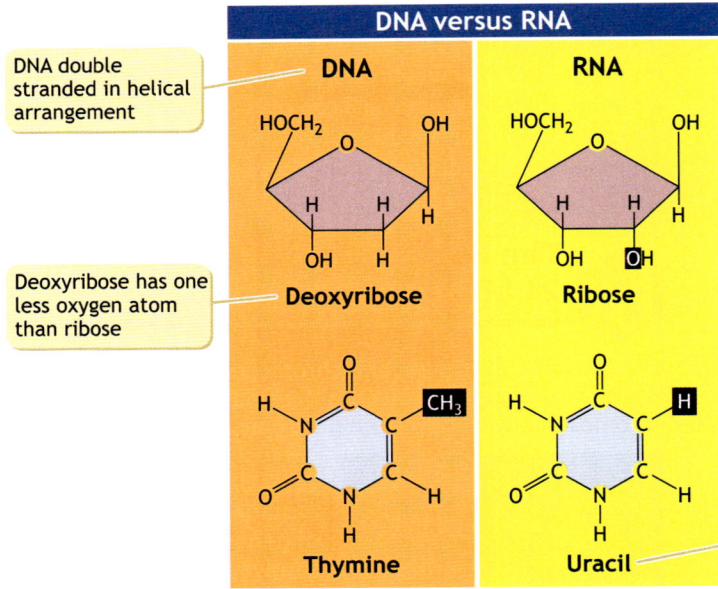

FIGURE 33.5. Differences in molecular configuration between DNA and RNA.

at specific carbon locations on the sugar molecule. These locations, numbered in the *red circles* from 1′ to 5′, begin with 1′ to the right of the oxygen (O) atom in the ring. The "prime" symbol (′) distinguishes the carbons in the sugar from carbons in the base. Note from **FIGURE 33.6** that RNA has one additional O atom in its sugar. Thus, the ribose sugar in RNA differs from the **deoxyribose** sugar in DNA. Nucleotides link when the phosphate at carbon 5′ on one sugar combines at the carbon 3′ position on another sugar. The phosphate group attaches to the 5′ carbon; the base attaches to the 1′ carbon. DNA and RNA synthesis always proceeds in the 5′ to 3′ direction.

The top in **FIGURE 33.7** shows the successive DNA packaging levels or stages in a chromosome, proceeding from condensed **metaphase** (*upper left*) to super-coiled (*middle right*), loosely condensed, and uncondensed chromatin fiber stages. The negatively charged DNA molecule encircles and binds to eight positively charged **histone** protein clusters (www.sciencedirect.com/topics/biochemistry-genetics-and-molecular-biology/histone-gene). The histone purple ball-like structure clamps the DNA to the molecule's core. The term **nucleosome** describes DNA wrapped around the puck-shaped histone proteins. Examining this region by electron microscopy reveals that one beadlike nucleosome contains 146 nucleotide base pairs wound twice like a rope around one eight histone cluster. The cluster contains two,

Within all living cells, genes encode the hereditary instructions that determine an organism's unique characteristics, from a simple bacterium such as *Streptococcus pneumoniae* to the tremendously complex multicellular human species, *Homo sapiens*. As organisms within a species increase in complexity, the total information stored within the genome also increases. In subsequent sections, we describe how much encoded information can be transcribed and then translated to ultimately create the proteins that characterize the unique cells, tissues, and organs that define the organism.

Think about DNA as the raw material or gene building blocks and RNA as the link or intermediary to protein synthesis. Articles began to highlight studies touting DNA and the revolution it spawned (www.nature.com/articles/nature01626; www.nature.com/articles/500028a) and animations to help to explain discrete molecular biology processes (www.dnalc.org/resources/animations/; https://dnalc.cshl.edu/resources/3d/23-dna-unzip.html).

DNA and RNA

The nucleic acids DNA and RNA include repeating polarized **polymer** subunit nucleotides. A nucleotide has a nitrogen-containing organic base having six carbon atoms, a 5-carbon sugar, and a phosphate molecule (**FIG. 33.6**). A nucleotide's main support structure or "backbone" includes sugar and phosphate molecules. The sugar-phosphate backbone lies on the outside the helix, with the amine bases on the inside. In this configuration, a base on one strand points at a base on the second strand. When nucleotides join to form **polynucleotides**, they link

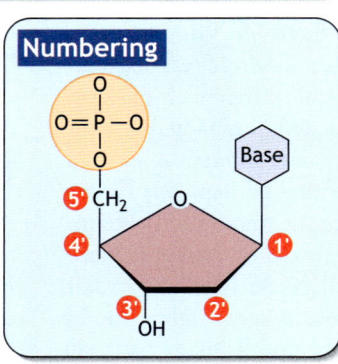

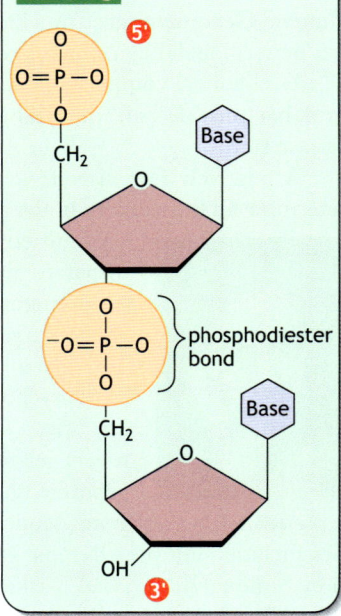

FIGURE 33.6. The components of a nucleotide, nucleotide-numbering nomenclature, and how nucleotides join together by phosphodiester bonding.

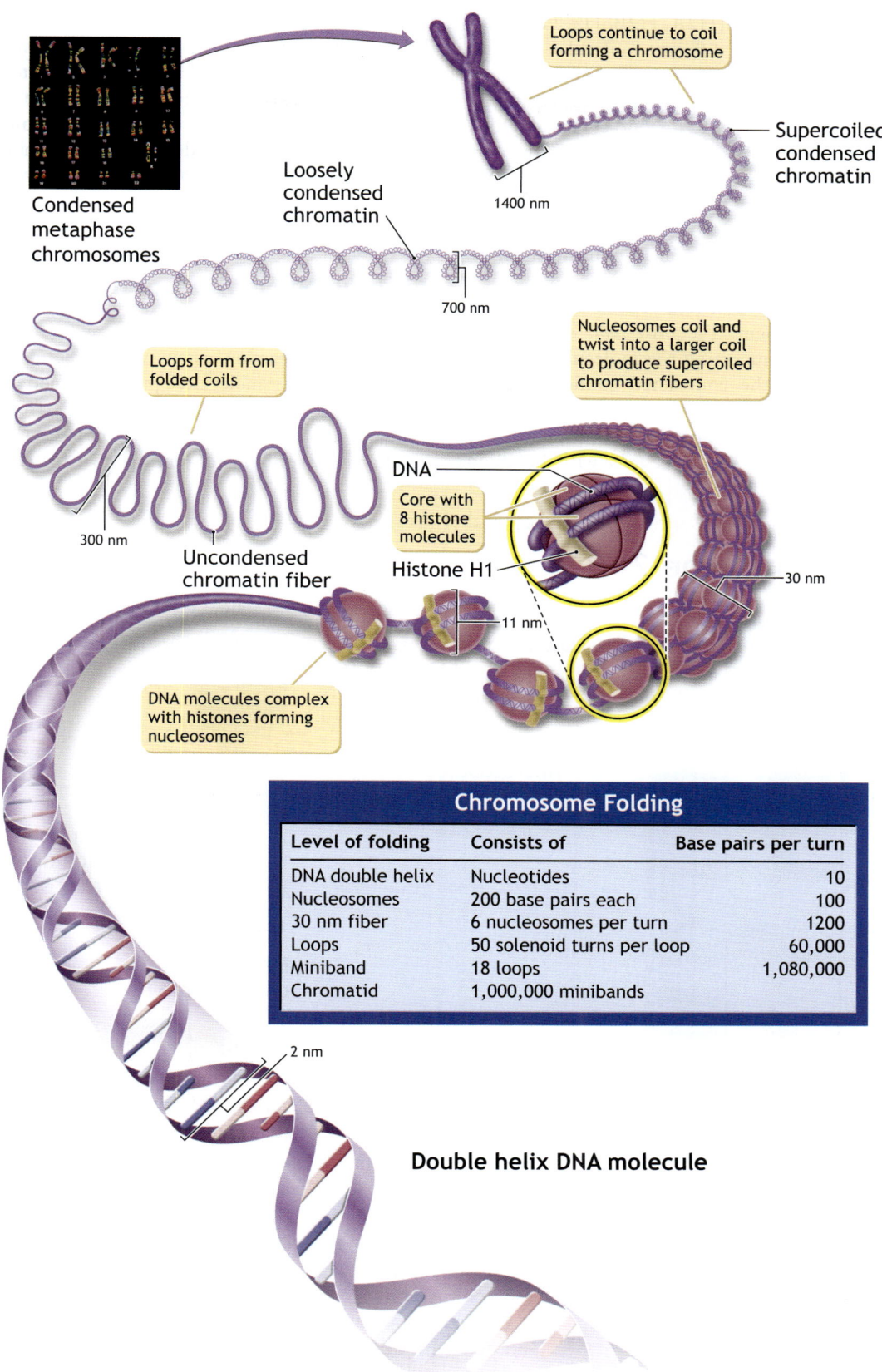

FIGURE 33.7. Double-helix DNA molecule packaged in a chromosome from the condensed metaphase stage, to supercoiled stage, to loosely condensed stage, and uncondensed chromatin fiber stage. The **inset table** provides summary details about chromosome folding from the DNA double helix to the chromatid in nm (nanometer units; 1 nm equal to one-millionth mm).

four different protein subunits (H2A, H2B, H3, H4), with each specific subunit having a different molecular mass. A DNA strand with about 60 base pairs and a ninth histone molecule links each cluster to the next one. During **replication**, the DNA uncoils from the histone core. The DNA molecule shown at the *bottom* in the figure eventually packs into the single metaphase chromosome displayed at the *top left* of the figure. The Figure 33.7 *inset table* provides relevant information about chromosome folding in the DNA double helix, nucleosomes, 30-nm fiber, loops, minibands, and chromatids.

The DNA packaging within cells reflects a remarkable architectural accomplishment. The *inset table* summarizes DNA folding and how compacting the molecule enhances replication efficiency. In the compacted configuration as chromosomes, no transcription takes place, to ensure that DNA remains intact to survive **mitosis** (cell division). The **chromatids** listed in the *last line in the table* with 1 million minibands represent duplicate DNA strands held together by a **centromere** just before the DNA separates into two **daughter chromosomes**. **FIGURE 33.8** shows the details for chromosome 2, and the general nomenclature to identify specific genes on the short p and long q chromosome arms. The image on the right side reveals the architectural details for a condensed metaphase chromosome with its kinetochore microtubules.

Linking Nucleotides: Phosphodiester Bonding

The chemical reaction when two nucleotides link together eliminates a water molecule, a process termed *dehydration synthesis*; it involves the phosphate molecule from one nucleotide and another nucleotide's hydroxyl (OH) molecule. The resultant **phosphodiester bond** shown for RNA and DNA

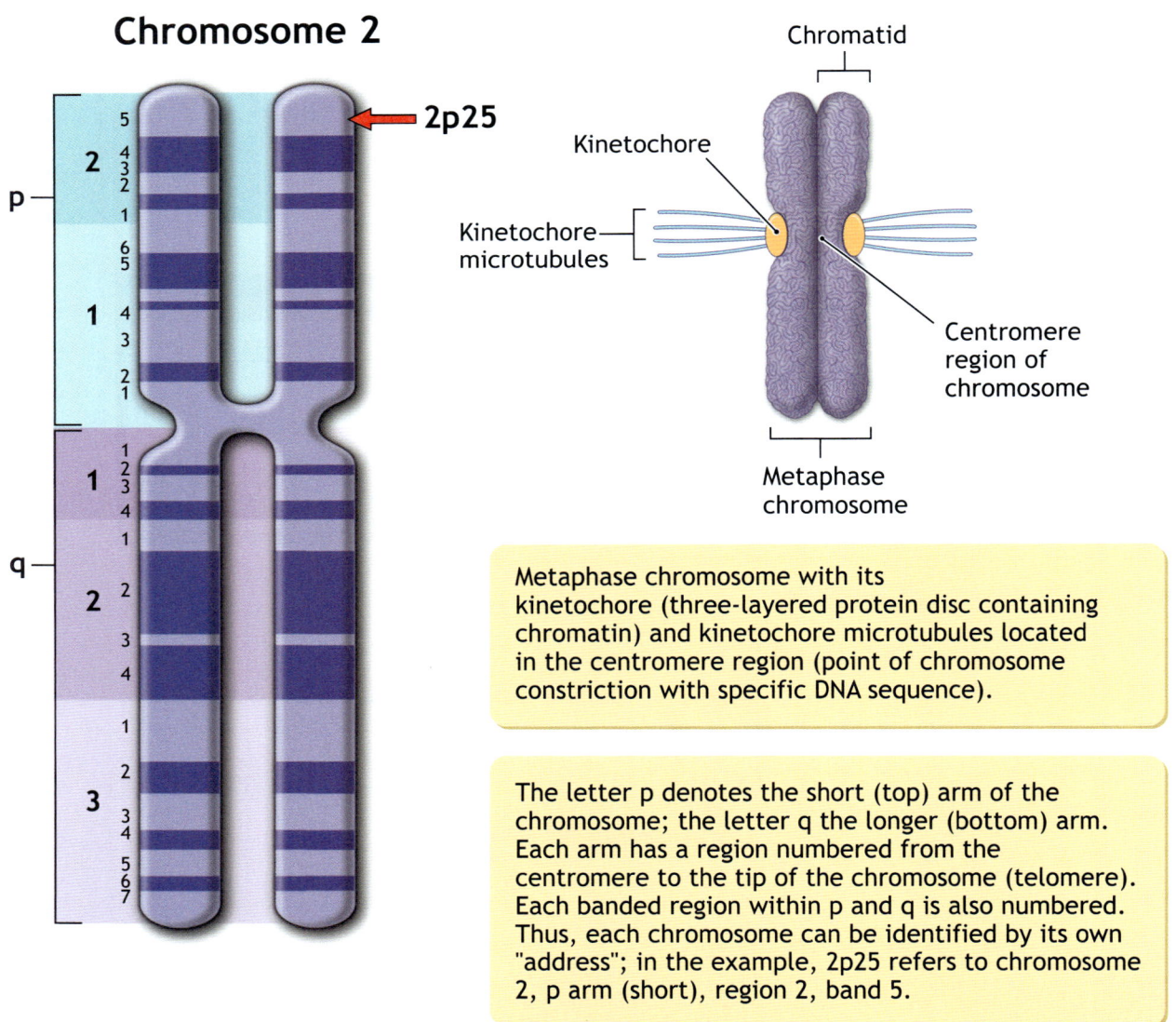

FIGURE 33.8. Chromosome 2. **(Left)** Gene 2p25 on chromosome 2. **(Right)** Metaphase chromosome.

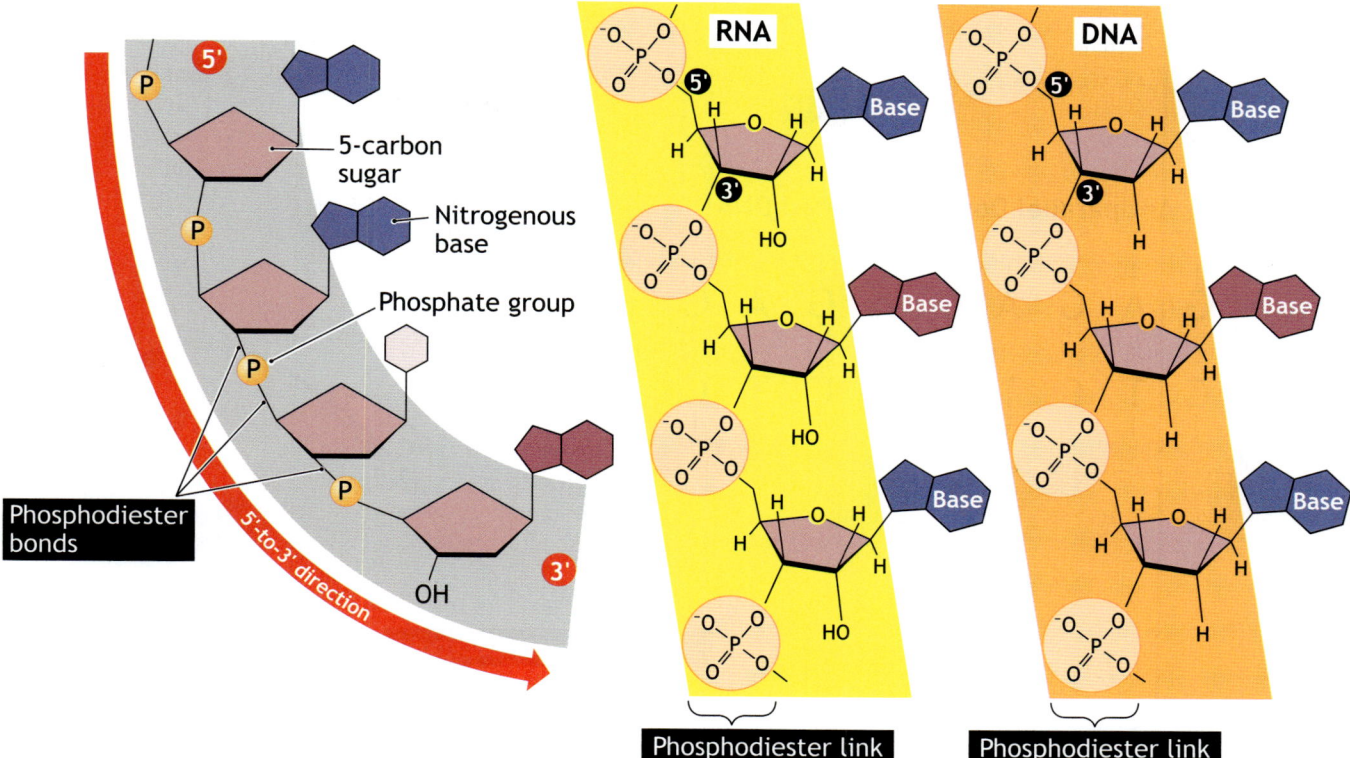

FIGURE 33.9. Linking nucleotides by phosphodiester bonding in RNA and DNA. The general schema shown at the *bottom left* illustrates the relative sugar, base, and phosphate group positions within a nucleotide along the 5′ to 3′ direction, including phosphodiester bonding.

(**FIG. 33.9**) represents a relatively strong **covalent bond**. The new polymer, now two units long, still has free phosphate and OH groups for linking to other nucleotides. This linkage forms an incredibly long chain with thousands of nucleotides, although the example shows only a few. In DNA measurement, the term **kilobase (kb)** represents a DNA unit fragment with a length equal to 1000 nucleotides. Another nucleic acid, adenosine triphosphate (ATP), contains a 5-carbon sugar base (adenine) and three phosphate groups. Unlike DNA and RNA, which transfer genetic information, ATP continually transfers chemical energy to power the body's cells throughout life discussed in Chapters 5, 6, and 7.

DNA Structure

FIGURE 33.10 shows a DNA molecule with a sugar phosphate chain sequence with hydrogen bonding between nitrogenous bases. In the double-stranded DNA molecule, the strands are not identical. They lie parallel but line up in opposite directions. One strand runs in the 5′ to 3′ direction, and its **complementary strand** runs from 3′ to 5′. The top left in the figure illustrates the double-stranded DNA strand **antiparallel** arrangement, including a close-up view with hydrogen bonding (shown as red dots) between the base pairs that hold the parallel spiral ribbons together. The deduction by Watson and Crick about the DNA strand's antiparallel nature resolved a remaining mystery about DNA's structure and ultimately how replication proceeds.

Base Pairing

One of DNA's "golden rules" regarding its molecular arrangement displayed in **FIGURE 33.11** relates to its four-base pairing, the letters representing the DNA alphabet. **Guanine** (**G**; shown in purple) always links with **cytosine** (**C**; shown in light blue) and **adenine** (A; shown in pink) always links with **thymine** (**T**; shown in gold) in the same proportions within all DNA molecules. Stated somewhat differently, whenever a G base occurs in one of the strands, a C base occurs opposite it in the opposing strand. Likewise, when an A base occurs in one strand, a T base occurs in the other strand. In 1950, Erwin Chargaff (1905–2002; www.famousscientists.org/erwin-chargaff/) of Columbia University confirmed the proportionality in the four bases and determined the relative amounts each base contributed to DNA. In essence, Chargaff discovered key "facts" required to determine DNA's basic chemical structure. Referred to as **"Chargaff's rule,"** his discoveries determined regularity among the four chemical DNA bases (www.nytimes.com/2002/06/30/nyregion/erwin-chargaff-96-pioneer-in-dna-chemical-research.html). The molar amount for thymine always equaled the molar amount for adenine, and similarly, molar amounts for guanine always equaled cytosine on one DNA strand ([T] with [A]; [G] with [C]).

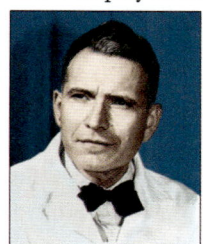
Erwin Chargaff

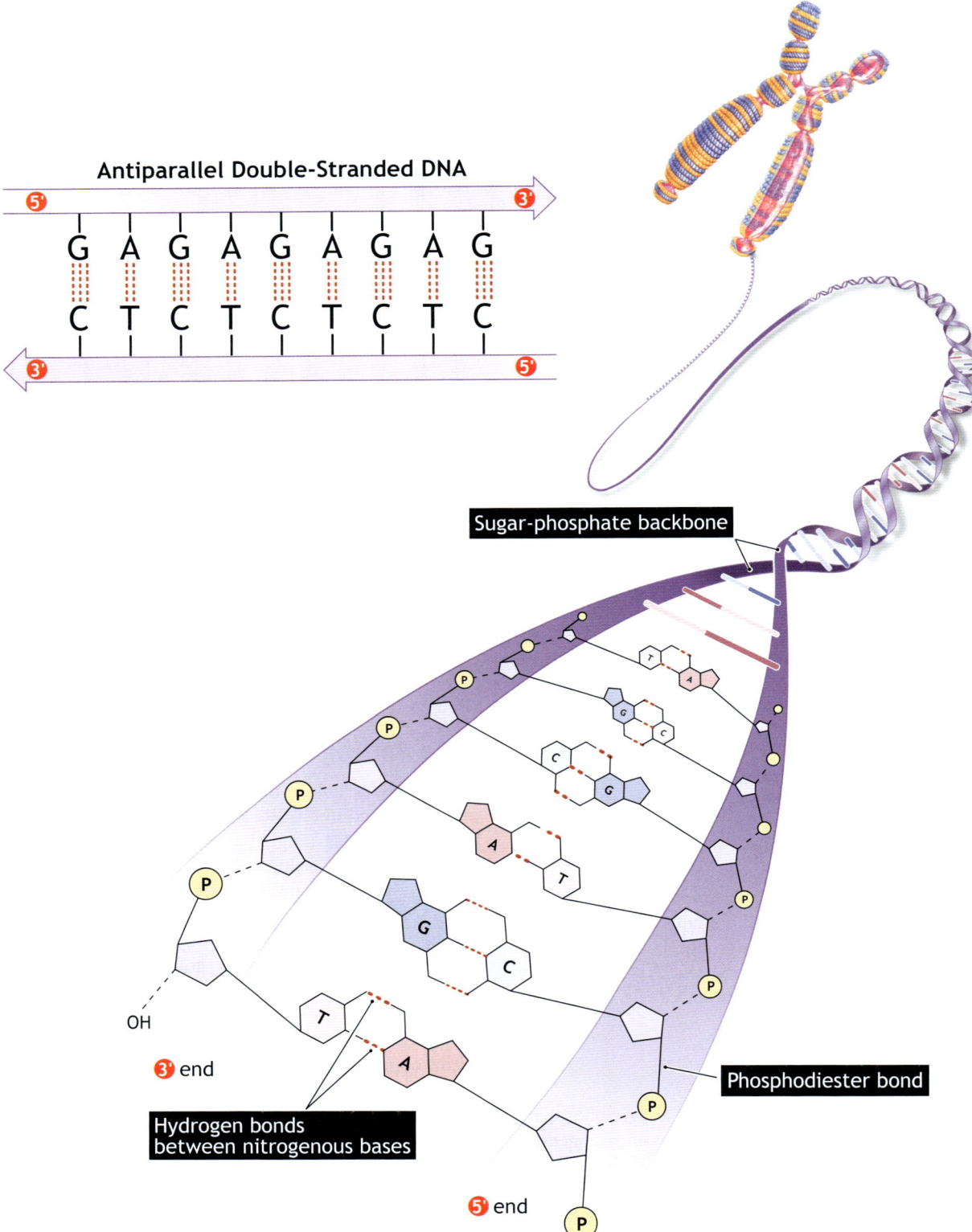

FIGURE 33.10. DNA molecule. **Top:** Antiparallel DNA double-strand arrangement from the 5′ to 3′ and 3′ to 5′ directions. Note the hydrogen bonding between G and C and A and T. **Bottom:** DNA molecule with its sugar-phosphate chain sequence and hydrogen bonding between nitrogenous bases. The specific base pair sequences ultimately determine every protein's specific characteristics. Adenine always binds with thymine.

Watson and Crick relied on this information to piece together DNA's molecular configuration. In their model, each rung in the DNA ladder has a purine connected to a pyrimidine. The term *base pairing* refers to the joining **complementary bases** (G with C, or A with T). The G and A nitrogenous bases have two rings (called a **purine**), whereas the two other bases, C and T, have a single ring (called a **pyrimidine**). Thus, each **base pair** has one larger purine base mated to a smaller pyrimidine base (http://library.med.utah.edu/NetBiochem/pupyr/pp.htm). Adenine and thymine form two strong **hydrogen bonds** between the base pairs but not with G or C. Similarly, G and C form three strong hydrogen bonds to keep the C–G base pair intact but not with A or T. The additive effect with millions of relatively weak hydrogen bonds within the DNA molecule keeps the helix from separating. Applying Chargaff's rule within an organism, the pyrimidine content (TC) equals the purine content (AG); however, the relative amounts of pyrimidines and purines differ among organisms.

Figure 33.11A illustrates the DNA double-helix molecule, with the base pairing and hydrogen bonding for A–T and G–C. Precise x-ray measurements have determined that the DNA double helix has a 2.0-nm width (nm = nanometers; 10^{-9} m [or 10 Å] one-millionth millimeter, or 1000 nm = 1 mm), with exactly 10 base pairs in each full turn, with the height in each turn equal to 3.4 nm. Figure 33.11B shows the five bases classified as either purine or pyrimidine bases. Note the pyrimidine base uracil (shown in grey). In RNA (next section), uracil replaces thymine, so that adenine pairs with uracil as A–U. Including uracil helps to distinguish RNA from DNA—besides RNA's extra oxygen atom in the ribose sugar and usually single-strand configuration. The simple mnemonic "*cut the pie*" helps to associate the pyrimidine or purine bases: CUT represents cytosine, uracil, and thymine, with the pyrimidines represented by pie.

The heat required to dissociate the H bonds between DNA's two strands determines the DNA molecule's **melting point**. Proportionality exists between bond number in the base pair and the energy required to break the bonds. Thus, the three hydrogen bonds that hold C and G together require more heat to break (higher melting point) than the two hydrogen bonds between A and T.

Different RNA Forms

The three RNA forms include the following:

1. **Messenger RNA (mRNA)** molecules, which serve as a template for protein synthesis, based on the molecular sequence from a small section in the DNA molecule
2. **Transfer RNA (tRNA)** molecules, which, as the name implies, transfer amino acids to the growing peptide chain on the ribosome
3. **Ribosomal RNA (rRNA)** molecules, which account for about 50% ribosomal mass whose structures aid in assembling amino acids into polypeptides

Each of the three RNA forms has its own **polymerase**, or complex enzyme: polymerase I associates with rRNA, polymerase II with mRNA, and polymerase III with tRNA. RNA polymerases, unlike their DNA counterparts, do not require a **primer** to initiate RNA chain synthesis. The term **primase** refers to the RNA polymerase that produces the primer for DNA synthesis. The three RNA polymerases have between 6 and 10 protein subunits that differ in molecular structure and regulatory function. About 97% in cellular RNA exists as rRNA, mRNA accounts for about 2%, and tRNA less than 1%. Compared with the DNA in a single chromosome that contains up to 250 million base pairs, RNA contains no more than a few thousand, which makes an RNA molecule considerably shorter. This makes sense because RNA carries only sparse information from one DNA molecule segment that it copied. Later in this chapter, we discuss how mRNA duplicates DNA's genetic information and the roles rRNA and tRNA play in protein synthesis.

Codons and Nature's Genetic Code

The coded message carried by the mRNA molecule exists as a three base series or **codon** (www.nobelprize.org/prizes/medicine/1968/nirenberg/biographical/). The codon was first presented by Marshall Nirenberg (1927–2010; 1968 Nobel Prize in Physiology or Medicine; interpreting the genetic code and its function in protein synthesis; www.nobelprize.org/nobel_prizes/medicine/laureates/1968/nirenberg-bio.html) with assistance from Johann Matthaei (1927–; www.ncbi.nlm.nih.gov/pmc/articles/PMC223177/; best known for discovering that the RNA sequence "UUU" directs joining phenylalanine to any growing protein chain) of the National Institutes of Health in 1961 at the International Congress of Biochemistry in Moscow (and 3 years later by Philip Leder (1934–) and Marshall Nirenberg; 1927–2010). Each DNA and RNA three-letter codon information block corresponds to one of the body's 20 amino acids. A codon codes for one amino acid, but most amino acids have more than one codon. If only one base coded for an amino acid, only four amino acids coded instead of 20. Even if two adjacent bases coded for an amino acid, there would still not be enough combinations to make 20 amino acids. Fortunately, scientists deduced that three bases coding for an amino acid (4^3 = 64 combinations) met the requirement to include all the amino acids. For example, the triplet sequence A-U-G on mRNA displayed in **FIGURE 33.12** (*green box within left yellow panel*) refers to a specific code for the sulfur-containing essential amino acid **methionine**. The A (adenine) is the first letter; U (uracil), the second letter; and G (guanine), the third letter. With only 20 amino acids and 64 codons, several codons code for more than one amino acid. In fact, most amino acids have more than one codon or letter sequence, with no intervening code disrupting the sequence.

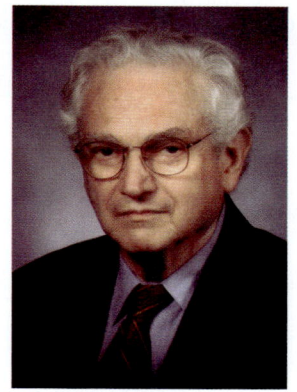

Marshall Nirenberg

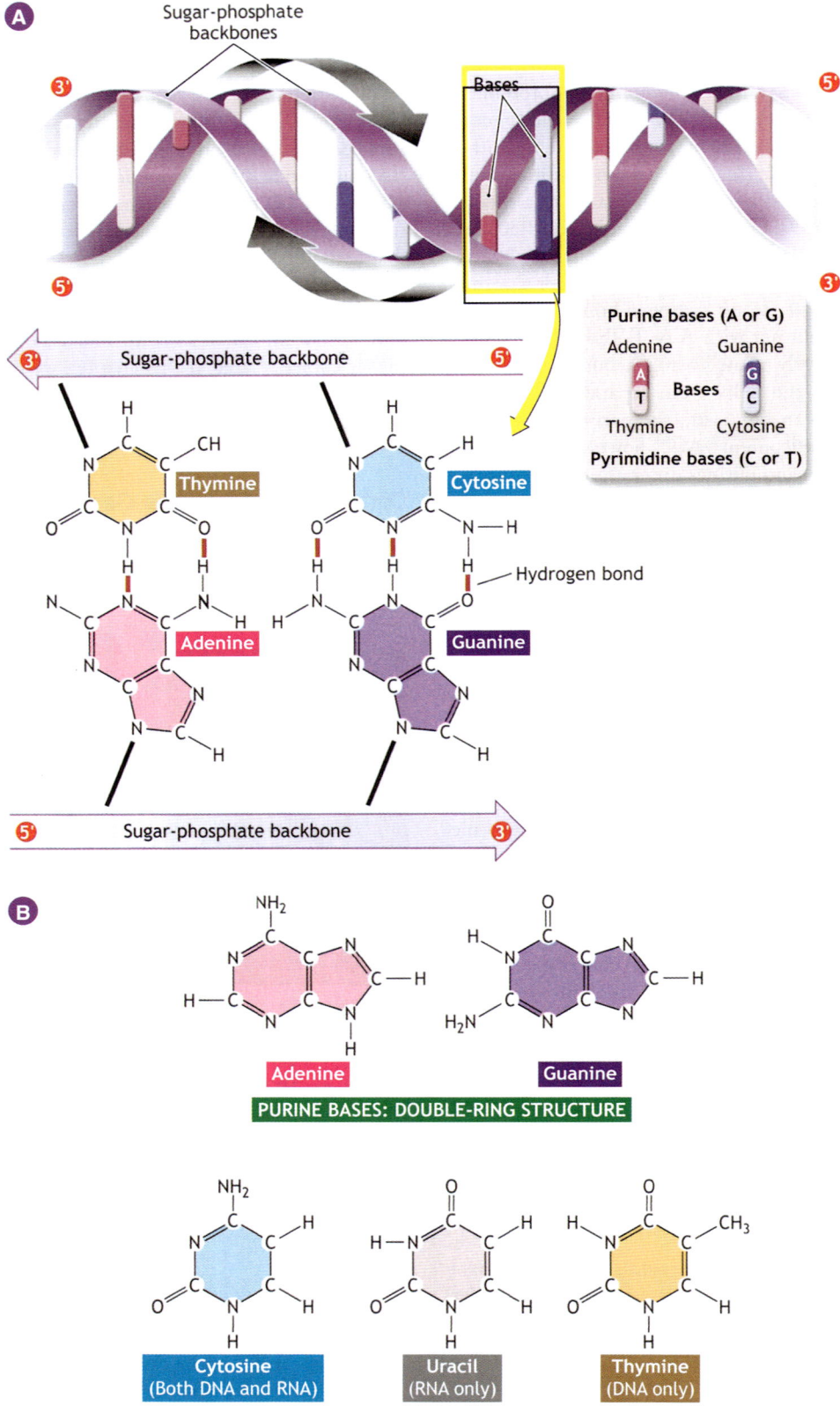

FIGURE 33.11. Base pairing. **(A)** Configuration details for the DNA double-helix molecule with base pairing and hydrogen bonding for adenine (A)–thymine (T) and guanine (G)–cytosine (C). The two spiral ribbons represent the sugar (deoxyribose)-phosphate DNA backbone. Note that two hydrogen bonds shown in *dark red* form between A and T and three form between G and C. This happens because the two polynucleotide chains that contain them lie antiparallel to each other. **(B)** The five bases are classified as purines (A and G) or pyrimidines (C, uracil, T).

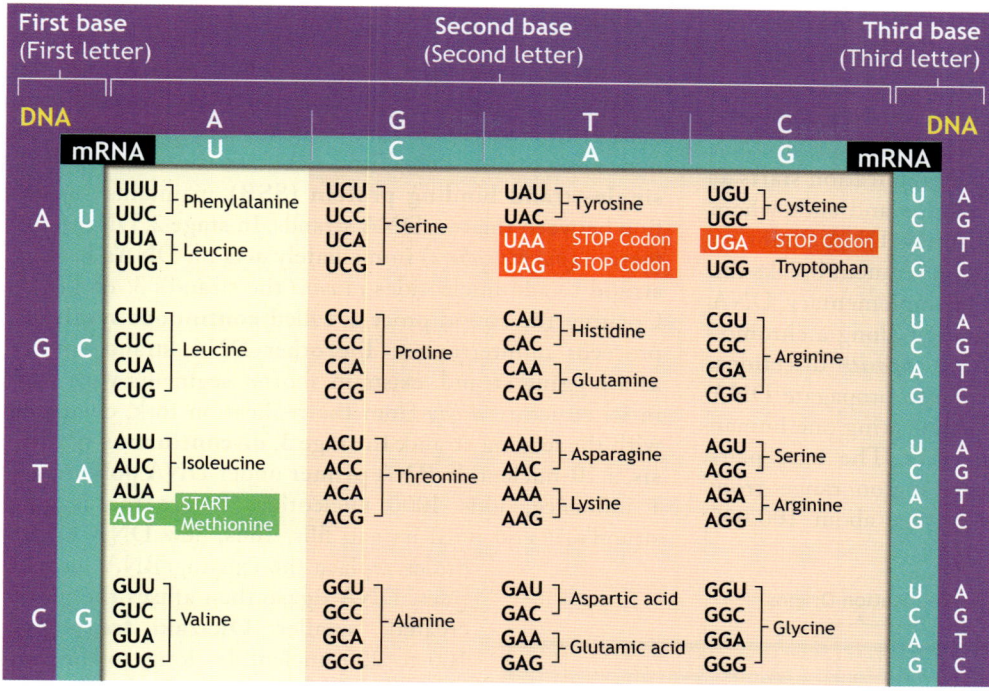

FIGURE 33.12. The codon table—the alphabet for the universal genetic code. From the time that Watson and Crick correctly deduced DNA's helical structure in 1953, different coding schemes attempted to explain DNA's alphabetic configuration (including imaginative proposals by physicists George Gamow, Richard Feynman, and Edward Teller); in 1964, Paul Leder and Marshall Nirenberg established the final code-breaking sequences for RNA synthesis.[79] The three-letter codon "word" in mRNA is complementary to the corresponding three-letter codon within DNA from which it was transcribed.

Codon Sequencing

The amino acid serine exemplifies a four-codon sequence that differs only in the base occupying the third nucleotide or letter. The sequence is U-C-U, U-C-C, U-C-A, and U-C-G, with identical first two letters. The first two bases are the defining letters in the codon sequence. Reading from the 5′ end in each codon, the first and second letters remain generally constant for each amino acid, while the base in the third position "wobbles." Thus, for example, the codon for phenylalanine contains a U or C as the third letter. Because both U-U-U and U-U-C code for phenylalanine, phenylalanine then merges into a newly synthesized polypeptide if U-U-U or U-U-C is "read" during translation or protein synthesis.

Similar to the English alphabet with its 26 letters, the *codon table* in Figure 33.12 provides the **genetic code** "alphabet," but with only four distinct letters—the code words in the analogy (https://bmcbioinformatics.biomedcentral.com/articles/10.1186/s12859-017-1793-7). When excluding the three **stop codons** (*red boxes*) that signal termination in the polypeptide chain linkages, the remaining 61 codons represent the useful information for protein synthesis. The stop codons, U-A-A, U-A-G, and U-G-A, signal the end of a genetic message (i.e., terminating protein synthesis), like periods at the end of a sentence.

Translation halts when the translation machinery encounters one of these chain terminators by releasing the polypeptide from the translation complex. Because the start codon for methionine (A-U-G) initiates polypeptide formation, it also codes for methionine within peptide chains. A *Codon Wheel* provides a visual alternative compared to the codon table in Figure 33.12 to translate DNA codons into amino acids. The start Met codon AUG begins in the black box at the wheel's outer left, reads as A (inner wheel), and then U (in blue) followed outward to G (red).

How DNA Replicates

A **DNA replication fork** refers to the Y-shaped region for replicating DNA molecules. As the double helix unwinds, nucleotide duplication occurs on both strands at a rate equal to about 50 nucleotide additions per second. Each strand serves as a template to create two new daughter strands by complementary base pairing. This mechanism provides each daughter helix with one intact strand from the parent (original strand) and one newly synthesized strand. Each strand, a complementary mirror image of the other, can serve as a template to reconstruct the other strand. **FIGURE 33.13** presents a schematic overview involving DNA replication presented in three stages. Replication begins with the untwisted, unzipped appearance of two DNA strands (the helicase unwinds a DNA segment) on the *top*, in stage 2, where replication starts at specific zones called **replication origins** and ends where RNA primers (*green*, in stage 3) start new DNA chains on the leading strand. Unwinding a DNA segment breaks the hydrogen bonds between the two complementary DNA strands. Several replication origins exist along a chromosome, replicating simultaneously in *opposite* directions. Multiple replications reduce the time to propagate DNA by an order of magnitude because duplicating one human DNA strand takes approximately 6 hr. The base pairs along the chromosome's replication region range from 10,000 up to 1 million, with an average about 100,000 base pairs.

Three DNA Replication Stages

FIGURE 33.14 amplifies the three DNA replication stages illustrated in Figure 33.13 referred to as a replication bubble. In **stage 1**, **helicase** enzymes (*orange*) unwind the molecule's double helix. This stabilizes the strands, while **single-strand binding protein (SSB)** maintains separation between the two DNA strands. In **stage 2**, DNA polymerase (*purple sphere*) immediately acts on DNA's **leading strand** to add nucleotides *toward* the strand's 3′ end (*red*). Creating the strand process, called **continuous synthesis**, proceeds uninterrupted. The other DNA strand, known as a **lagging strand**, exists in shorter segments with gaps in its structure *away* from the replication fork, compared with the leading strand. In **stage 3**, **discontinuous synthesis**, a 10-nucleotide **RNA primer** under **DNA polymerase I** influence, adds 1000 nucleotides before the lagging strand's 5′ end until its gap fills. Thus, new DNA nucleotides replace the existing RNA nucleotides. **DNA ligase** then affixes the newly created, smaller **Okazaki fragments**, 100 to 200 nucleotides long, to the lagging strand in the 5′ to 3′ direction to make a complete DNA strand.

 See the animation "DNA Synthesis/Replication" on Lippincott Connect to view this process.

Pivotal Role for DNA Polymerase

DNA polymerase plays the central role in life's processes because this enzyme consistently duplicates the genetic information from generation to generation. The rich instructional DNA information bank, modified and improved over more than 3 billion years, builds proteins and other molecules atom by atom according to selective molecular directions. For every cell that divides, DNA polymerase duplicates its entire DNA, so that cells transfer one copy to each daughter cell. DNA polymerase, among approximately 1300 enzymes in a human cell, is the most accurate because it creates an exact DNA copy, transmitting less than one "error" in a billion bases. Stated another way, an analogy would be the equivalent to only one grammatical mistake in a thousand novels! The excellent match for C to G and A to T provides much needed specificity needed for high accuracy, but DNA polymerase adds an extra step. After it copies each base, it "proofreads" it and then deletes any wrong base sequence from its grasp. Polymerases can vary in structure

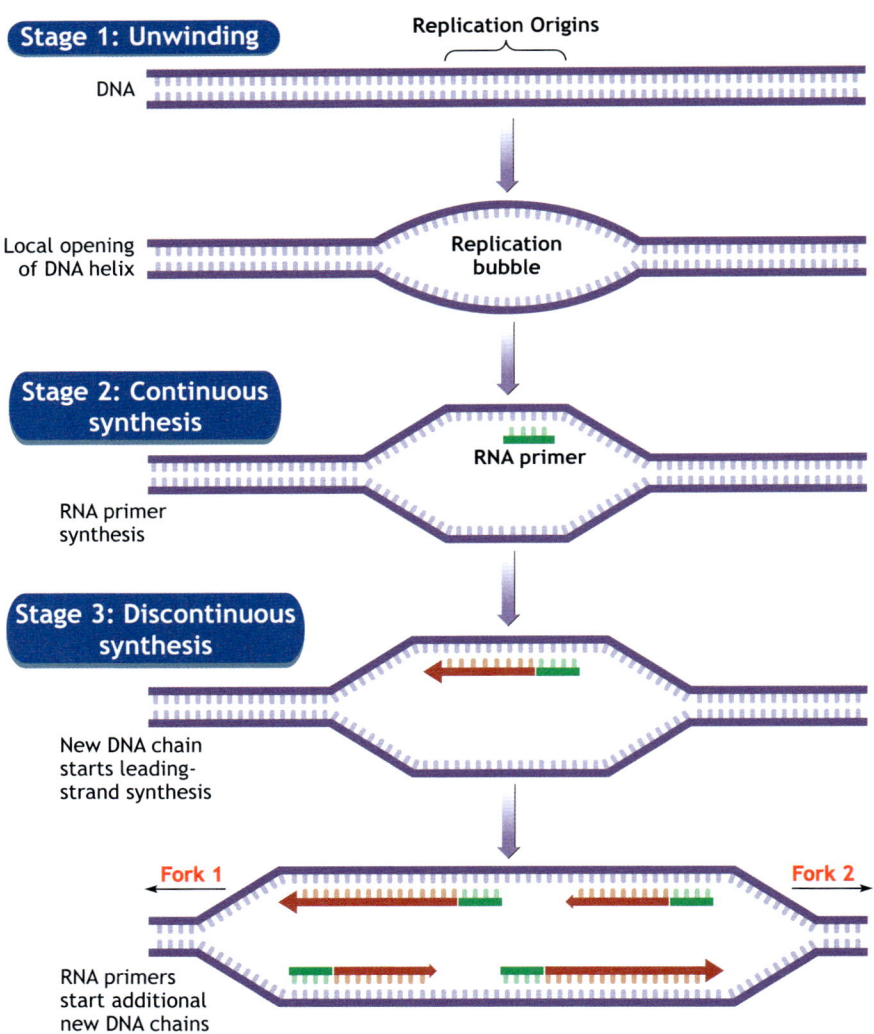

FIGURE 33.13. Replication bubble and DNA replication. Note the straight (not helical) double DNA strands in **stage 1** after untwisting by DNA gyrase and unwinding by helicase. The DNA represents an elongated bubble as the double strand opens and DNA begins to divide (**stage 2**, continuous synthesis). In **stage 3** (discontinuous synthesis), replication proceeds in opposite directions along each end in the Y-shaped replication forks.

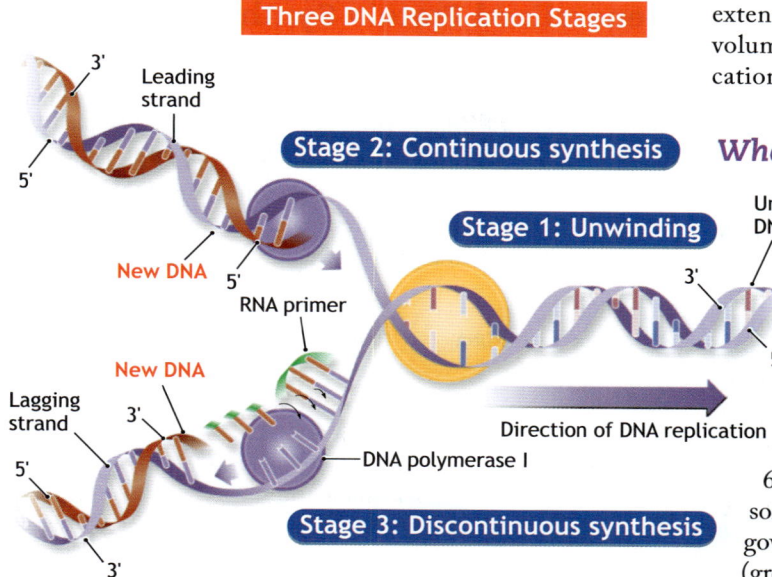

FIGURE 33.14. Three DNA replication stages. **Stage 1**, unwinding; **stage 2**, continuous synthesis; **stage 3**, discontinuous synthesis.

extensive identical DNA strands from a miniscule DNA volume amount from a crime scene or **paternity** identification case.

What Controls DNA Synthesis?

Several molecular control mechanisms trigger DNA synthesis in cells. The **cell cycle** illustrated in **FIGURE 33.15** depicts the four phases and accompanying three important checkpoints in cellular functions. Comparable to a clock or thermostat, each phase has defined "on" and "off" periods regulated by enzymes that start and terminate a particular stage. DNA replication (synthesis) occurs in the S phase (*yellow* arrow), which lasts approximately 6 hr. The three checkpoints serve as the thermostat's sensors, each with specific regulator enzymes called **cyclins** governing a specific function. Toward the end of the **G1** (growth) stage (*orange* arrow), cyclin enzymes achieve a critical activity level that triggers a response when the cell achieves adequate size within a favorable environment.[159]

If cell size and environment prove satisfactory, the cell proceeds to S phase for DNA synthesis. Following DNA synthesis, the G1 cyclins degrade as the cell prepares to enter mitosis (M phase). The next checkpoint occurs between the **G2** and M phases (*purple* arrow), a crucial time in the cell cycle. When the DNA replicates without error, the cell enters mitosis and then progresses to complete **telophase**. Mitosis produces two cells genetically identical to the original parent cell.

from relatively "simple" to complex. In humans, polymerases are complex structures that unwind the helix, build an RNA primer, and construct a new strand. Some even have a ring-shaped structure that clamps the polymerase to the DNA strand. Polymerase function varies from the day-to-day DNA repair and maintenance to DNA's complex replicating task when the cell divides. DNA polymerase plays an important role in **forensic medicine** in building

Cell Life Cycle Controllers

Figure 33.15 also provides insights about the cell life cycle controllers. Cyclin-dependent kinases (cdk1 and cdk2) activate specific cyclins. Once this occurs, the two protein **kinase** complexes regulate how the cell proceeds through its cycle. After each stage, cyclin degradation temporarily halts CDK activity. With mitosis complete, the process begins again, accumulating cyclins for the next initial G1 growth stage.

The cdk2 protein "turns on" in the transition between the G1 and S stages; cdk1 drives the cell cycle from stage G2 to M stage. In other words, the cyclin-dependent protein kinases phosphorylate their target cyclin proteins through the different cell cycle stages. Signaling proteins called growth factors operate in concert during the cycle. For example, mitosis-promoting factor governs the sequencing between the G1 and M cell cycle phases. Other growth factors also exert their effect. The hormone **erythropoietin**, produced by the kidneys (see Chapters 20, 23, and 24), initiates proliferating red blood cell precursors and their maturation to erythrocytes; nerve growth factor modulates

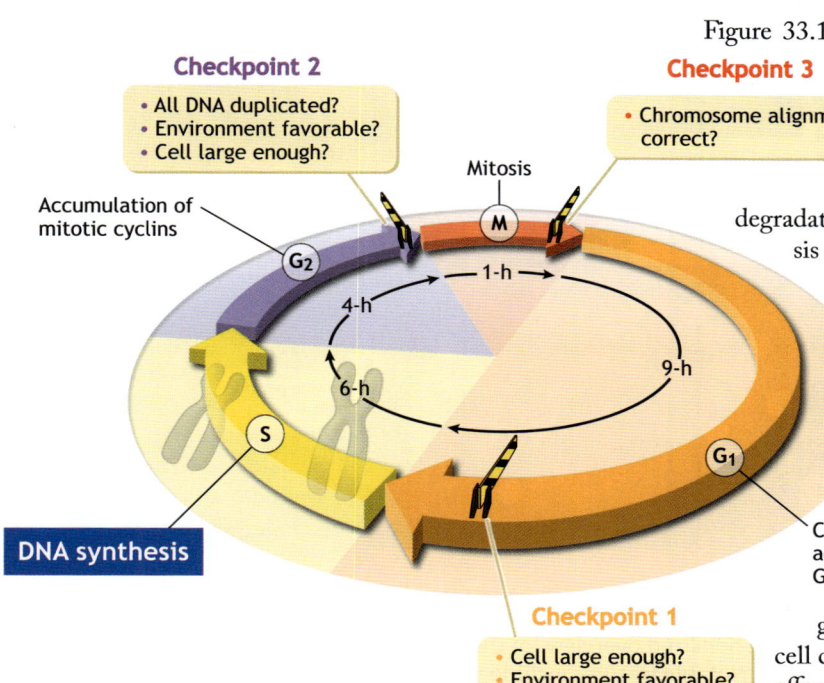

FIGURE 33.15. Four cell cycle stages and their molecular control mechanisms. Note the three checkpoints and the question(s) posed prior to DNA synthesis during the Ⓢ phase in DNA synthesis.

neuronal cell growth during nervous system development; interleukin-2 participates in immune cell proliferation; and insulinlike growth factor facilitates many metabolic events related to muscle cellular growth and development,[54,135] including a role in the brain's center for smell,[139] a role in muscle strength and aerobic training in older adults,[153] and a role in increased breast cancer risk and/or death.[71,283]

A unique feature about growth factors relates to how they control the transition stages during cellular growth and differentiation. Failure to work in concert with cyclins and kinases during cellular proliferation terminates cellular proliferation, causing cells to continue to divide unchecked, which may serve both positive and negative functions. Unchecked cell division can precipitate lethal effects because DNA synthesis may progress to the M stage by successfully reproducing a mutant cancer gene. If highly specialized genes called tumor suppressors (e.g., the *p53* gene) cannot halt the cell cycle long enough for DNA repair enzymes to function, then cell growth proceeds rapidly and unchecked to produce tumors. Deleterious mutations also can pass to progeny cells; the successive mutagen buildup likely develops into cancer.

Protein Synthesis: Transcription and Translation

Protein synthesis involves two prominent events:

1. **Transcription** in the cell **nucleus** that creates a single-stranded RNA copy with the genetic information stored in the double-stranded DNA molecule
2. RNA **translation** in the cell cytoplasm to form proteins

In essence, the DNA molecule's nucleotide base sequence defines the protein's ultimate 3-D shape.

Protein synthesis begins with a "roadmap" highlighting key events in assembling proteins from precursor biomolecules (i.e., lipids, carbohydrates, proteins, and nucleic acids). The process originates in the cell's ribosomes and ends with creating a fully **functional protein**—a unique molecule whose structure dictates its overall operational functions.

Generalized Protein Synthesis Overview

FIGURE 33.16 provides a generalized overview for six important stages in protein synthesis. Prior to stage 1, DNA, under enzyme control, "untwists" to expose its code. Before DNA's hydrogen bonds break, DNA topoisomerase enzymes (e.g., **DNA gyrase**; www.sciencedirect.com/topics/biochemistry-genetics-and-molecular-biology/dna-gyrase) "relax" the **supercoiled DNA**

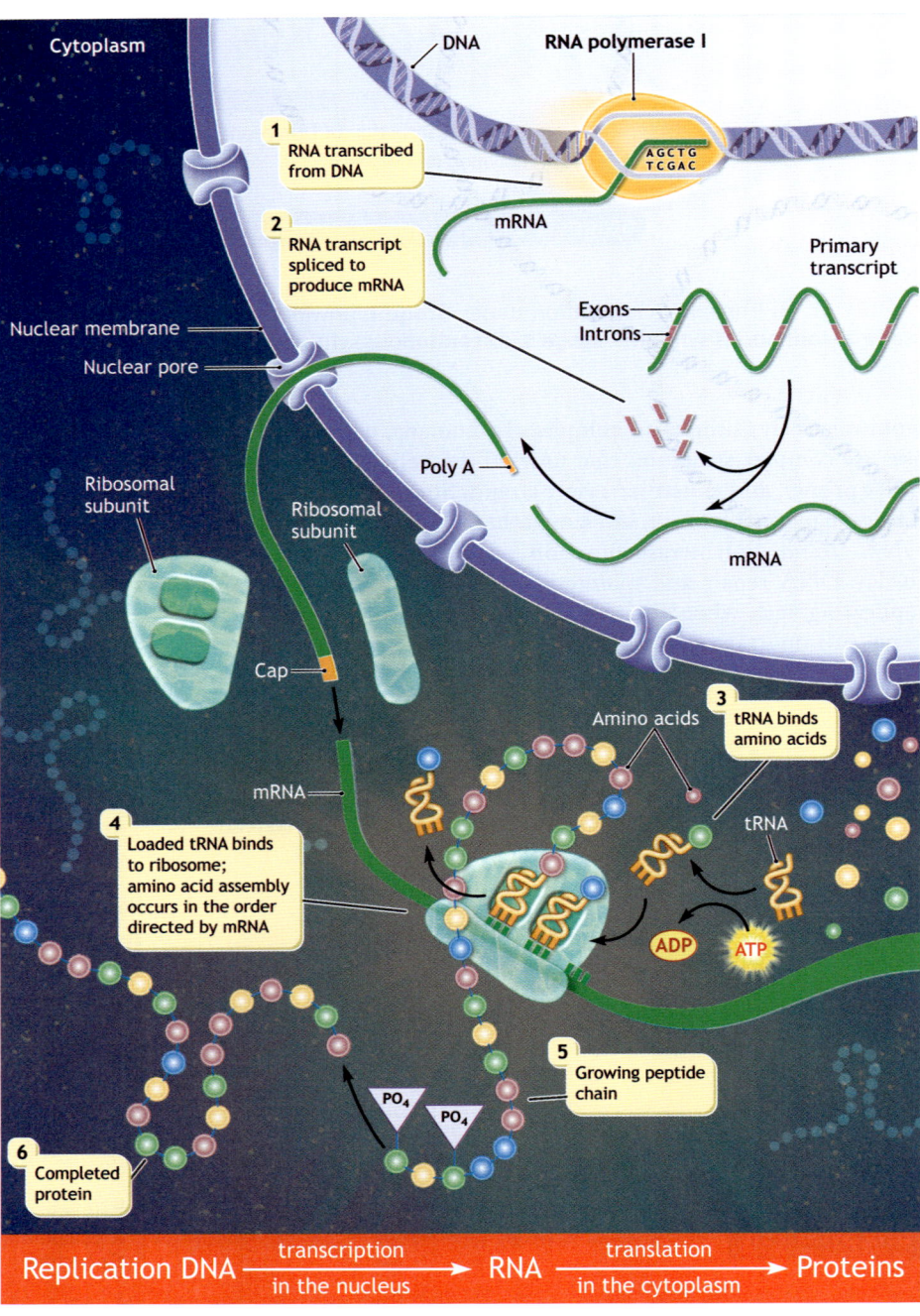

FIGURE 33.16. Generalized overview for the six stages (*numbered yellow boxes*) in protein synthesis. Notable features include the events during transcription (stages labeled 1 and 2 within the cell's nucleus) and translation (stages labeled 3 to 6 in the cell's cytoplasm). The **bottom red inset box** summarizes transcription and translation in protein synthesis following DNA molecule replication.
(Shutterstock images: The Biochemist Artist [background image], Mitar Vidakovic [ATP].)

by literally cutting the DNA to create a double-stranded break but maintain a hold on both ends of the DNA. The two halves in the molecule then rotate relative to each other (untwist) before rejoining. Once the strand untwists, **DNA helicase** unwinds the helical DNA molecule by separating the hydrogen bonds between the base pairs (https://pdb101.rcsb.org/motm/).[168] The SSB binds to one unpaired DNA strand to inhibit its reemerging with its neighbor (complementary) strand. This prevents the strands from recoiling and re-forming the double helix. **DNA polymerase III (Pol III)** serves as a "verifier" to ensure that the bases pair correctly. If they do, the enzyme joins the nucleotides together. If not, it rejects the mismatched base pair.

See the animation "ATPase" on Lippincott Connect to view this process.

Stage 1 signifies when transcription begins. This involves copying a discrete genetic sequence directly from the DNA template to the growing RNA strand. The enzyme **RNA polymerase I** (depicted in gold in Fig. 33.16 and referred to as "I" before discovering other polymerases) binds to the specific **promoter** (initiator) region on the gene.

Arthur Kornberg (1947–2007; www.nobelprize.org/prizes/medicine/1959/kornberg/biographical/; www.nytimes.com/2007/10/28/science/28kornberg.html) American biochemist from Stanford University, Palo Alto, California, shared the 1959 Nobel Prize in Physiology or Medicine with Severo Ochoa 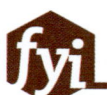 (1905–1993; www.nobelprize.org/prizes/medicine/1959/ochoa/facts/), distinguished Spanish physiologist and biochemist, for discovering the mechanisms in synthesizing RNA and **deoxyribonucleic acid (DNA**; www.ncbi.nlm.nih.gov/pmc/articles/PMC5778255/).

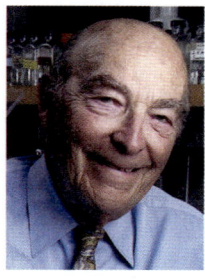
Arthur Kornberg

By studying bacteria, the scientists succeeded in isolating DNA polymerase in 1956, an active enzyme in DNA formation. Using a DNA molecule as a blueprint, the enzyme builds a DNA molecule copy from DNA's building block nucleotides.

Linking to a specific nitrogenous base sequence alerts transcription to initiate formation on the complementary RNA strand. When RNA polymerase arrives at the gene, it receives a "stop" signal from one of three nucleotide sequences (U-A-A, U-A-G, U-G-A; see Fig. 33.12) and disengages from the DNA. The newly assembled RNA strand, called the gene's **primary RNA transcript**, processed in (stage 2) to eventually exit the nucleus to the cytoplasm through the octagon disk-shaped **nuclear pore complex**. This complex selectively transports proteins across the nuclear envelope after specific protein receptors dock with the protein, allowing it to enter its channel and pass to the cytoplasm. Note that once mRNA leaves the nucleus in stage 2, it links to the ribosome's poly A site and waits to bind to the appropriately coded amino acid floating freely in the cytoplasm. A specific mRNA orientation on the ribosome exposes only one codon at a time to match and bind with its tRNA anticodon.

Within the cytoplasm, translation proceeds through stage 3 (tRNA binds amino acids), stage 4 (tRNA binds to a ribosome, signifying amino acid assembly), and stage 5 (the growing peptide chain increases in length), until stage 6, which forms a fully functional protein. The *red bar* (*bottom* in Fig. 33.16) summarizes protein synthesis in two crucial aspects following DNA molecule replication:

Chronic Jetlag Can Alter Diurnal Gene Expression

Nearly every cell and organ in the body operates under autonomous central circadian "clock" control to maintain diurnal homeostasis through complex chemically mediated molecular control mechanisms with four stage and three cycle checkpoints (see Fig. 33.15). Numerous experiments have verified the suprachiasmatic nucleus (SCN) in the hypothalamus as the master circadian clock regulator for core body temperature, autonomic and neuroendocrine functions, memory and psychomotor performance, and other behavioral and physiological processes.[206,207] The SCN plays a crucial role in neural control, particularly the circadian clock's timing system. Distracting stressful circumstances include jet lag or changes in a job shift work, and disrupted homeostasis to normal rhythmicity, can play havoc on circadian physiology mainly on expressed pancreatic genes. In mouse experiments, a precise jet lag protocol mimicked a 4-hr phase advancement for 12 hr:12 hr to simulate jet lag and a standard lighting condition cycle every 2 to 3 days for 4 wk before returning to standard lighting conditions. Twelve mice (6 males/6 females) were euthanized by cervical dislocation and the pancreas dissected for analysis every 4 hr for 48 hr to assess rhythmicity in pancreatic gene expression.

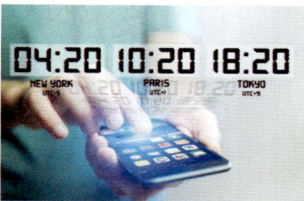
Production Perig/Shutterstock

Following chronic jet lag, transcript number rhythmicity decreased the transcriptome (total mRNA molecules expressed from the genes by 3.6%), and most core clock genes shifted peak gene expression timing called phase shift (www.genome.gov/about-genomics/fact-sheets/Transcriptome-Fact-Sheet). The pancreatic transcriptome's rhythmically expressed genes (95%) revealed the phase shift, many of these key genes controlling metabolic processes. These changes in the phase shift persisted for 9 days following normalizing light to dark cycles. This indicated a persistent failure in endocrine and exocrine cell pancreatic clock control and its' rhythmic gene expression to re-adapt to the prior light-dark cycle from jet lag perturbation influences. Future experiments will help to better understand how jet lag influences pancreatic function in normal and disease-prone states.

Source:
Schwartz PB, et al. Chronic jetlag-induced alterations in pancreatic diurnal gene expression. *Physiol Genomics.* 2021;53:319.

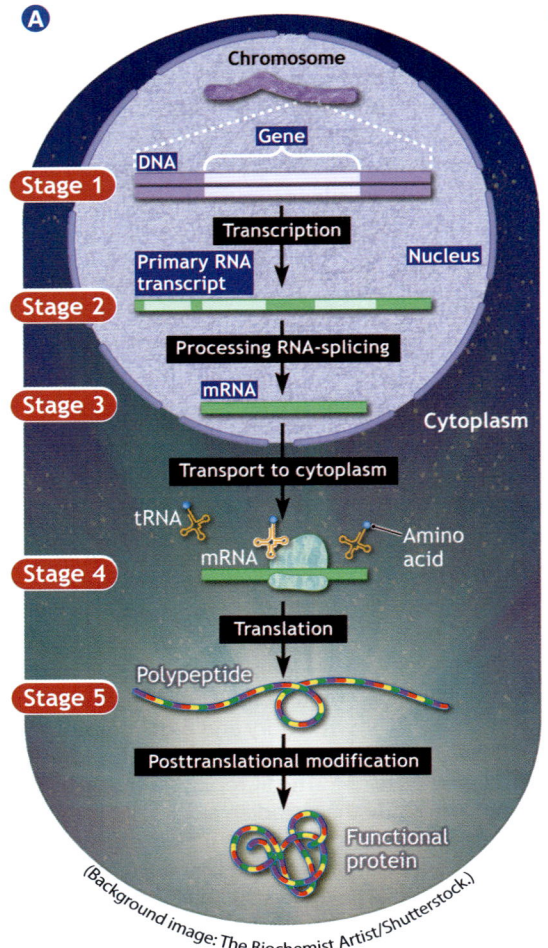
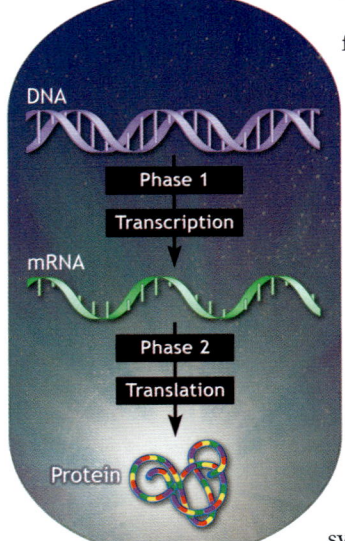

FIGURE 33.17 **(A)** Gene expression and translation. Transcription (**stages 1–3**) produces an mRNA copy of the gene. In translation (**stage 4**), the information in mRNA molecules "directs" which amino acid to produce and where to position the amino acids when the ribosomes synthesize polypeptides. Translation refers to a protein's creation on the ribosome; this copies the specific coded information from the DNA strand. Posttranslational modifications can alter polypeptides transitioning to functional proteins in **stage 5**. **(B)** Crick's 1956 working hypothesis called central dogma posits that two distinct phases play the defining role in expressing the genetic information encoded in DNA molecules. In **phase 1** (transcription), RNA polymerase enzyme assembles an mRNA molecule with its nucleotide sequence complementary to the gene's nucleotide sequence. In **phase 2** (translation), a ribosome assembles the polypeptide protein in which mRNA's nucleotide sequence specifies the final amino acid configuration.

a particular gene provides the driving force for many molecular biologists' passion for the field.

FIGURE 33.17A highlights the five stages for **gene expression** in human cells. The same two basic sequences occur whether in the simplest **bacteria** or **prokaryotes** (organisms without membrane-bound structures including a nucleus) that dominated Earth during its first 2 billion or so in evolution or for eukaryotes that evolved about 1.5 billion years ago. The **eukaryotes** include unicellular and multicellular organisms and humans, each with membrane-bound **organelles**. Their cells include a true nucleus with chromosomes. The DNA in prokaryotes remains single stranded and the main coupled events—transcription in the nucleus and translation in the cytoplasm. In eukaryotes, translating the protein synthesis code does not occur until the RNA strand exits the nucleus.

Figure 33.17B illustrates the proposed genetic information flow Francis Crick termed the *central dogma* (www.ncbi.nlm.nih.gov/pmc/articles/PMC5602739/). During a lecture to the Society for Experimental Biology held at University College London on September 19, 1957, Crick in his opening sentence, laid out the framework for what turned out to be an historic lecture—despite experimental evidence about how genes produced proteins. Crick boldly relied on what he excelled in—outlining general, bold concepts that pulled together many information strands into a compelling whole. Crick's main thesis for the central dogma posited that that once information had gone from DNA into the protein, it could not escape the protein and go back into the genetic code.[194] In fact, there was little direct experimental support for this mechanistic concept that RNA serves as DNA's template.

"I shall … argue that the main function of the genetic material is to control (not necessarily directly) the synthesis of proteins. There is a little direct evidence to support this, but to my mind the psychological drive behind this hypothesis is at the moment independent of such evidence." Francis Crick, 1957

The Watson and Crick hypothesis speculated that chromosomal DNA functions as the template for RNA molecules. These molecules then move to the cytoplasm to dictate a protein's amino acid arrangement. The first *down arrow* from the DNA strand at the top *in* Figure 33.17A emphasizes the proposition that DNA provides the template for self-replication. The next phase underscores that all cellular RNA molecules exist on (transcribed from) DNA templates. Concomitantly, RNA templates translated or formed the proteins. The two arrows unidirectionality between stage 3 (transport to cytoplasm) and stage 4 (translation) and between stages 4 (translation) and 5 (posttranslational modification) indicate that

1. Transcribing information in the genetic code from DNA molecules to RNA molecules in the nucleus for decoding (RNA synthesis)
2. Synthesizing proteins by translating genetic information in the cytoplasm

Genetic Code Transcription: RNA Synthesis and Gene Expression

A gene, located along a specific chromosome at a specific site, contains the sequence code or "plan" to synthesize protein. The gene within the DNA molecule ranges from several thousand to millions of bases. Unlocking the regulation mechanism in

protein templates would never determine RNA sequences, nor would RNA templates create DNA. With few exceptions, the central dogma has withstood critical challenges and remains essentially valid. Except in some instances in which the **retrovirus** reproductive cycle adds a step using a reverse transcriptase enzyme, proteins almost never serve as templates for RNA. If it did, the arrows would go bidirectionally between DNA and RNA.

Gene Expression Examples

Beginning with conception, gene expression lays the eventual groundwork for each person's diverse cells, tissues, organs, and systems. Gene expression explains why no two people match exactly in any outer or even inner physical traits. No two hearts, livers, kidneys, brains, vertebrae, adrenal glands, intra-abdominal fat distributions, teeth, nostrils, ears, or fingerprints ever match precisely. Even identical twins with the same starting genetic machinery have unique and subtle outward physical characteristics and often not-so-subtle distinctive personalities.

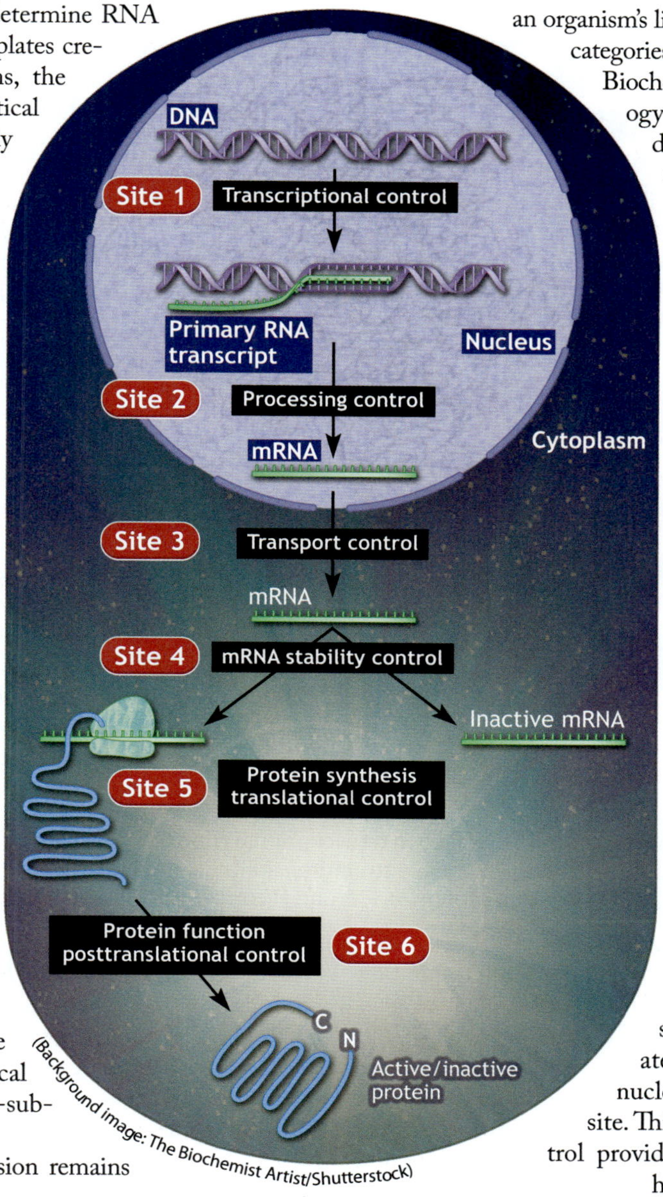

At times, some gene expression remains repressed or "off," no longer needing to remain active or "on." Gene expression "fits" or modulates to the body's current metabolic state, persisting throughout the individual's life span. The biologic catalysts—the enzymes containing a minimum 100 amino acid residues—effectively control the genetic machinery and subsequent transformation and control the different energy forms. **FIGURE 33.18** shows six sites within the nucleus and cytoplasm that regulate gene expression. When the mRNA travels to the cytoplasm from the nucleus, protein regulation via translation in the cytoplasm at site 3 (transport control) to site 6 (control posttranslational protein function) can begin with further modifications once a protein forms at site 6.

Protein Enzymes

Acting as biomolecular switches, enzymes selectively regulate numerous cellular activities simultaneously, coupling some and uncoupling others. They coordinate in milliseconds throughout an organism's life. To categorize different enzyme categories, the International Union of Biochemistry and Molecular Biology (IUBMB; www.iubmb.org/) devised a nomenclature and numbering system for six major enzyme classes, each with subgroups and sub-subgroups:

1. *Oxidoreductases*: catalyze oxidation-reduction reactions
2. *Transferases*: catalyze transfer functional groups between molecules
3. *Hydrolases*: catalyze hydrolytic cleavage
4. *Lyases*: catalyze removing a group or adding a group to a double bond, or other changes involving electron rearrangement
5. *Isomerases*: catalyze intramolecular rearrangement
6. *Ligases*: catalyze reactions that join two molecules

Transcription Control

Diverse "switches" or regulator enzyme activator proteins and repressor proteins affect gene expression during transcription. These switches operate at the active gene site and on nucleotides away from the starting site. This geography in operational control provides great regulatory freedom in how genes initially switch on and off prior to and during transcription. For example, some enzymes accelerate the RNA polymerase capture to enhance transcription, while others repress transcription by delaying different event sequences. In essence, activator and repressor proteins control transcription rate in the following two ways:

1. **Activator proteins** bind to DNA at sites called **enhancer sites**. **FIGURE 33.19** shows the transcription complex (proteins involved in transcription) correctly positioning RNA polymerase at the proper gene location. Folding DNA strands bring the enhancer site in proximity to the transcription complex. This increases communication between the activator proteins and the transcription complex. Other **coactivator proteins** transmit signals from activator proteins to other factors (called *basal factors*) close to the DNA strand, helping to position RNA polymerase correctly at the precise location in DNA's coding region.

FIGURE 33.18. Six potential sites regulate gene expression.

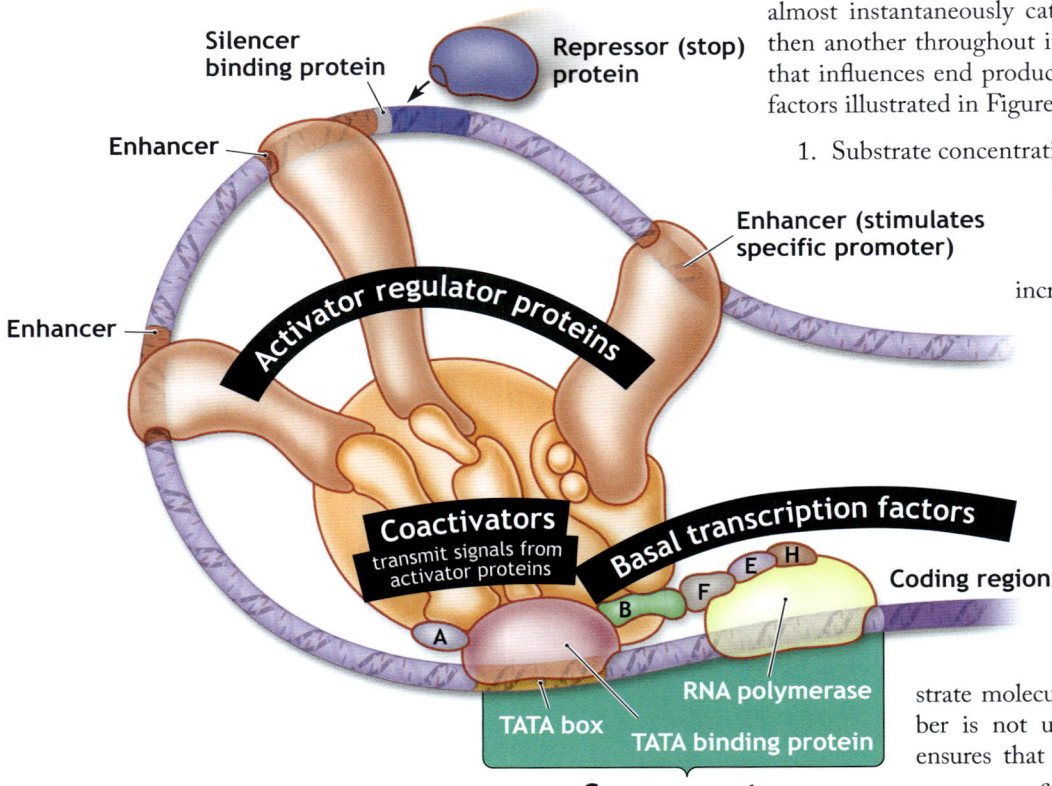

FIGURE 33.19. Transcription complex structure involved in transcriptional control. The coding sequence begins along DNA's double helix (*purple* ropelike structure), the basal (transcription) factors labeled (from left to right) A, TATA binding protein, B, F, E, and H correctly position RNA polymerase and then release it to transcribe mRNA.

2. **Repressor proteins** bind to "silencer" protein-binding sites along the DNA strand (the darker blue protein region under the larger repressor or stop protein). The silencer sequence, adjacent to or overlapping the enhancer region, can prevent an activator protein from binding to a neighboring enhancer site. This delays or cancels transcription from commencing their intended functions at a discrete mRNA coding sequence.

Enzyme Turnover Number

Some enzymes fulfill their functions more quickly than others. An important way to measure an enzyme's performance relates to how quickly it binds to and releases from its substrate(s) during biomolecular reactions or its turnover rate or number (www.nature.com/articles/s41467-018-03106-1). To encourage a reaction, an enzyme must correctly orient itself with its substrate. A substrate's electrical properties change depending in part on its correct spatial arrangement with the substrate. In essence, the enzyme's positive and negative charges align with the substrate's positive and negative charges to favorably continue a chemical reaction.

FIGURE 33.20A shows an enzyme arranging to link up with its intended substrate to create an enzyme-substrate complex. Once the enzyme fulfills its function, the complex breaks down to release its end product. The enzyme then almost instantaneously catalyzes another reaction and then another throughout its operational cycle. The rate that influences end product formation depends on two factors illustrated in Figure 33.20B:

1. Substrate concentration
2. Enzyme-substrate's reaction rate

As substrate concentration increases, the reaction rate moves toward its maximum (*yellow* line). At this point, all enzyme active sites fully engage the substrate's active sites. Continued new product formation now depends only on how rapidity the substrate engages referred to as turnover number. This can vary tremendously, from 1 to 10,000 molecules per second, but a 1000 substrate molecule per second turnover number is not uncommon. A high turnover ensures that enzymes remain "turned on" at their optimal concentration during gene expression. The enzyme's binding sites, while they remain in the "on" position with their substrate for extremely brief periods, can also do so more dynamically. Rather than remaining coupled for the entire period, other similar binding sites may switch places with the originally bound site (analogous to "hit-join-and-run"), suggesting that enzyme molecules maintain considerable mobility. The bottom red line shows a typical reaction rate without an enzyme present despite increasing substrate availability.

Gene Expression and Human Exercise Performance

The current and future exercise physiology research continues to build upon the rapidly developing knowledge base about gene expression and the human gene map for exercise performance and health-related phenotypes (see *Med Sci Sports Exerc* 2001;33:885, with annual updates through 2012, and the obesity gene map database [www.ncbi.nlm.nih.gov/pmc/articles/PMC4757102/] with access to recent publications from the HERITAGE Family study, Québec Family Study, Cardio Fitness Study, Swedish Obese Subjects Study, Genathlete, and Hypgene).[130]

Gene Edited Future Astronauts and Athletes

Currently, exercise scientists routinely incorporate molecular biologic techniques to assess an individual's potential for strength, speed, endurance, and other traits that can be "turned

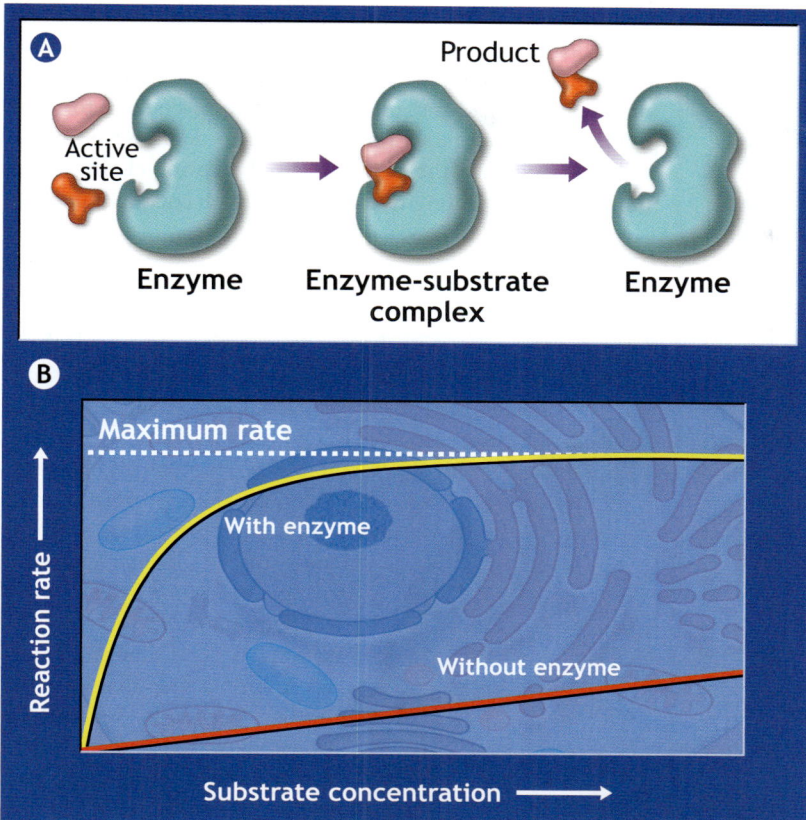

FIGURE 33.20. **(A)** Enzyme-substrate interaction. **(B)** Reaction rate versus substrate concentration with and without enzyme action.

myosin protein filament enlargement remains "on," while gene expression for generating new muscle cells remains "off" because cellular hypertrophy, not hyperplasia, usually prevails. These "on-off" genes are referred to as "**housekeeping genes.**" In body processes such as coding for the proteins involved in aerobic metabolism, gene expression does not shut down but remains continually on until death. The same applies to all cell and tissue metabolic activities controlled by enzymes that dominate cellular and subcellular events. Organisms from bacteria to humans incorporate the same two basic gene expression principles. First, an RNA duplicate from a particular gene with its unique coding sequence on a DNA template represents a combined sequence for the genetic letters G, C, T, A. Second, the RNA copy containing the genetic code on the ribosome sequence located outside the nucleus orchestrates the amino acid sequential construction into a protein possessing unique biomolecular characteristics.

Exons and Introns

The primary RNA transcript molecule contains the information required from the gene to create a protein. This molecule's structure discovered by Crick,[162] called a **coding region** or **exon** shown in the green primary transcript within the nucleus in **FIGURE 33.21**, also contains additional, unwanted nucleotide "spacers," or noncoding regions termed **introns** (introns shown within the primary RNA transcript in Fig. 33.21). The 1993 Nobel Prize in Physiology or Medicine was awarded to British biochemist and molecular biologist Sir Richard John Roberts (1943–; www.nobelprize.org/prizes/medicine/1993/roberts/biographical/) and American geneticist and microbiologist Phillip Allen Sharp (1944–; www.nobelprize.org/prizes/medicine/1993/sharp/biographical/) for discovering "split genes" or introns (http://nobelprize.org/nobel_prizes/medicine/laureates/1993/press.html). Introns account for approximately 97% in DNA's double helix. An example for three exons and two introns shows the individual numbering for the base pair sequences within each exon and intron. For example, the numbers 1 to 30 designate the base pairs for the first exon along the RNA strand, while 105 to 146 signify the base pairs for the last exon. The two introns with their

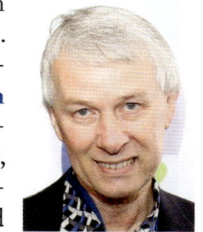

Sir John Roberts. (Licensed under Creative Commons Attribution Share-Alike 2.0 Generic license: https://creativecommons.org/licenses/by-sa/2.0/deed.en)

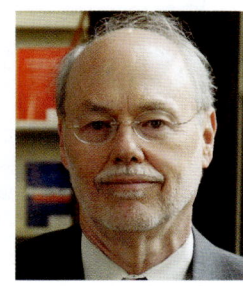

Phillip Allen Sharp. (Licensed under Creative Commons Attribution Share-Alike 3.0 Unported license: https://creativecommons.org/licenses/by-sa/3.0/deed.en)

on" to selectively enhance exercise performance.[175] It might seem far-fetched now, but choosing astronauts for extended-duration missions to other planets may rely on genomic data to "select" candidates who possess genes more resistant to bone loss or spatial disorientation with prolonged microgravity exposure (www.bbc.com/future/article/20171123-will-we-ever-have-genetically-modified-astronauts). Sometime in the future, coaches and trainers will undoubtedly apply technologies from molecular medicine to genetically screen young children for gene clusters that indicate potential for desirable athletic traits (https://interestingengineering.com/gene-editing-the-future-of-olymic-athletics-or-a-looming-crisis). This undoubtedly will include traits related to training responsiveness (e.g., specific muscle fiber types, aerobic enzyme predominance, muscle capillaries, or left ventricular cavity size).

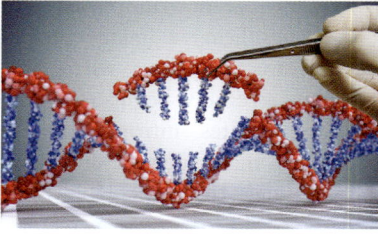

vchal/Shutterstock

Today, sports scientists use laboratory and field testing to screen athletes for performance and physiologic capacities, including the applying molecular genetics with the ACTN3 gene that encodes the protein actin in skeletal muscle to assess potential for sports and athletic performance.[2,103,115,120,125,128] When muscle tissue rebuilds, gene expression for actin and

base pairs have the numbers 30 to 31 and 104 to 105. During transcription, removing intron links 30 to 31 and 104 to 105, leaving the remaining three exons that splice together (their base pairs now numbered 1 to 146) creates the final mRNA transcript. This must occur before the mRNA strand leaves the nucleus and enters the cytosol.

The cytoplasm cannot receive partially processed transcripts. Intron removal likely occurs because these structures provide no known usable code for any sequence in the polypeptide initially specified by the gene. These repeated clusters, apparently nonfunctional and random DNA sequences scattered throughout the genome, exist as either short interspersed elements with 500 or fewer base pairs or long interspersed elements with more than 1000 base pairs in length. The mature mRNA transcript at the bottom in Figure 33.21 contains the correct code sequence to create proteins. The example shows the specified order for seven amino acids inserted into the elongating **polypeptide chain**, determined originally during translation based on codon sequence.

RNA Splicing

RNA splicing removes unwanted intron sequences from the primary transcript before translation to avoid those sequences. Introns usually occupy an area 10 to 30 times greater than exons. Small nuclear RNAs (snRNAs; proteins and RNA) play a contributing role in RNA splicing (www.pnas.org/content/113/4/801). Another protein (small nuclear ribonucleoprotein or snRNP) contains snRNA. This structure can bind to the intron's 5′ end, while a different snRNP binds to the intron's 3′ end. Introns interact to form a loop that joins the intron's free ends. An snRNP assembly collection is known as a spliceosome. Its function is to excise the intron, allowing the entron to join it but without the snRNPs. The final, matured mRNA strand is shorter than the primary transcript from excising approximately 90% of introns in the primary transcript before translation. Consider exon splicing a unique protein construction phase when protein assembly begins. Splicing manipulates intron sequencing in many ways to form polypeptides. The hemoglobin (Hb) molecule, for example, requires 432 nucleotides to encode its 144 amino acids, yet before intron excision, 1356 nucleotides exist in the *Hb* gene's primary mRNA transcript. Regulating gene expression occurs by changes in how splicing takes place during different stages in a cell's development and type.

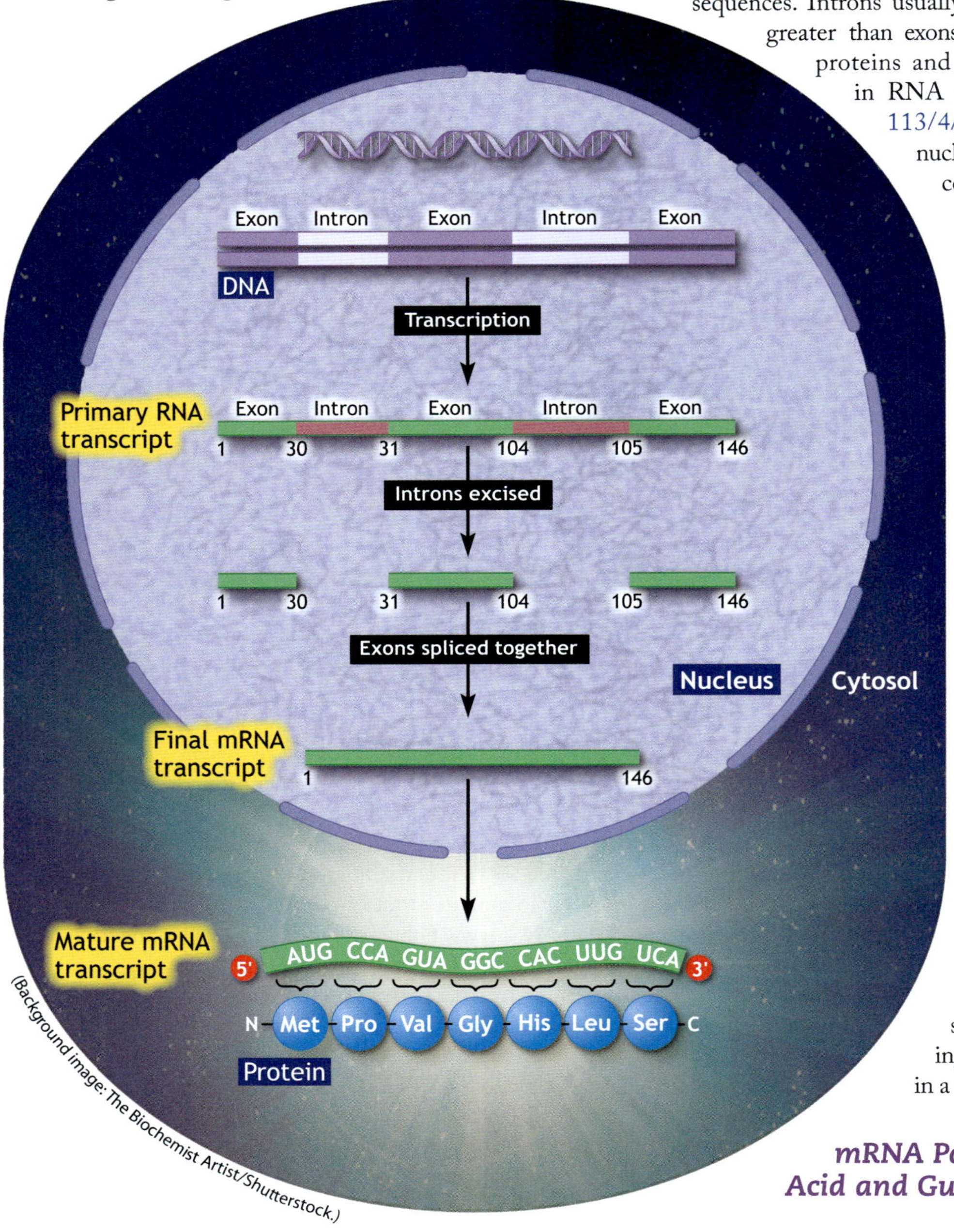

mRNA Packaging: Polyadenylic Acid and Guanosine Triphosphate Tails and Caps

Before the RNA transcript migrates through the nuclear pore as the final transcripted mRNA, a **polyadenylic acid**

FIGURE 33.21. Exon and intron individual numbering for base pair sequences, and intron excision and exon splicing to form the final (mature) mRNA transcript (structure bottom outside cell in *green*). For this structure, note the three-letter codons shown in *white* lettering along the mRNA strand, and the corresponding amino acids listed in the *blue circles* below (see the codon table in Fig. 33.12 for amino acid names).

[poly(A)] tail, 100 to 200 adenine nucleotides long, joins one end at the 3′ region by enzyme poly(A) polymerase action and a terminal portion or "cap" (methylated **guanosine triphosphate [GTP]**) joins near the 5′ end. Analogous to wearing a cap and gown during a graduation ceremony, mRNA must be "capped and tailed" to prepare the transcribed molecule for translation before it exits the nucleus to participate in subsequent protein synthesis. The newly formed cap initiates translation when it binds the mRNA to the smaller ribosome's two subunits.

FIGURE 33.22A shows how the GTP cap and poly(A) tail join to RNA. The capping enzyme (symbolized by the *shorter curved purple arrow*) cleaves two phosphates (*circles enclosed in red*) from GTP and one phosphate from the mRNA strand. In forming the cap, the GTP now attaches near the terminating end in the first mRNA base. Figure 33.22B illustrates adding the poly(A) tail when a specific endonuclease enzyme (*orange*) recognizes the sequence A-A-U-A-A-A on the mRNA and snips the strand near that point. This permits a 100- to 200-adenine residue tail to affix to the 3′ mRNA strand's end, thereby promoting mRNA stability. This allows the mRNA molecule to maintain translation for up to several weeks, sometimes producing 100,000 protein molecules. Recall that transcription that uses DNA occurs inside the cell's nucleus, whereas ribosomal assembly takes place in the cytoplasm. The capping and tailing function allow mRNA to exit the nucleus to begin the next protein synthesis phase.

Exiting the Nucleus

The mRNA contains a specific nucleotide sequence copy from the DNA gene. The mRNA then shuttles the "coded message" following the transcription stage through the nuclear membrane into the cytoplasm where protein synthesis (translation) begins. Translation includes three main stages:

1. Initiation
2. Elongation
3. Termination

Using high-resolution x-ray crystallography (www.ncbi.nlm.nih.gov/pmc/articles/PMC4491318/), researchers have determined that a tunnel-shaped groove runs through the larger 50S subunit's middle, providing the location that links amino acids together.[118] Thirty-one separate proteins affix to the subunit's outside where they also reach inside the ribosome. Because a protein needs to be within a 3-Å distance to induce any effect, and because the proteins on the surface and those that reach around the surface remain within 18 Å, RNA must be the source in any subsequent protein interaction. In this case, adenosine 2486 is the nucleotide in question, with an associated nitrogen atom. Consequently, the RNA gives the catalytic power to protein synthesis—in essence, ribosomes serving as ribozymes. This helps to explain why some bacteria remain resistant to antibiotics. A mutation on a single ribosomal protein within the ribosomal groove locks up within the antibiotic molecule, preventing the peptide from exiting the region, thus stopping further antibiotic binding and subsequent bacterial damage.

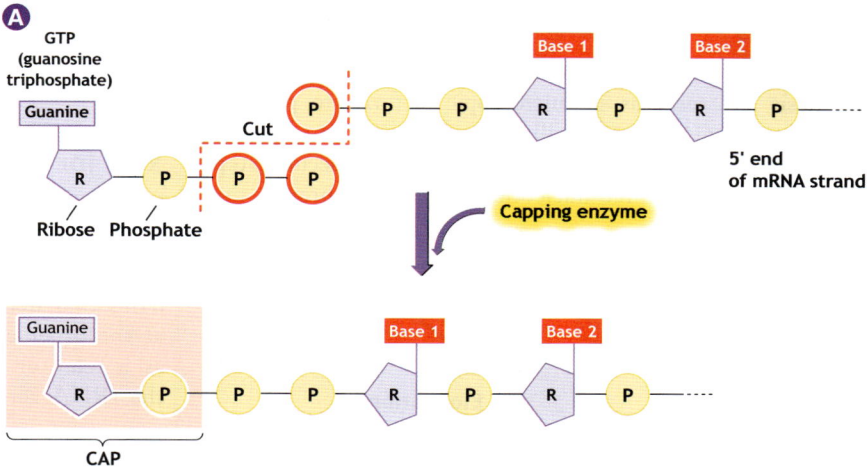

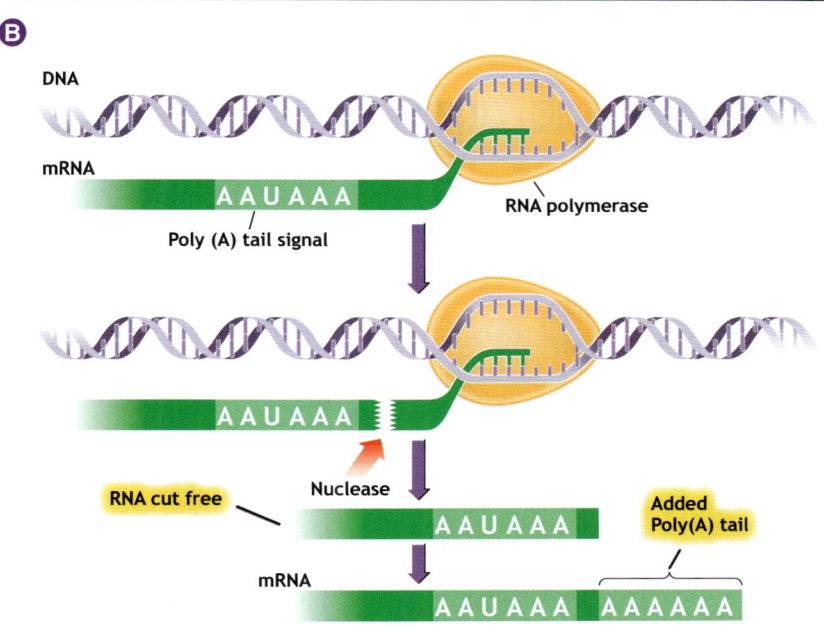

FIGURE 33.22. Caps and tails. **(A)** Adding a guanosine triphosphate (GTP) cap to mRNA. The *red dashes* indicate where the "cut" occurs by the capping enzyme. **(B)** Adding a poly(A) tail to mRNA. The mRNA molecule exits the nucleus once capping and tailing occurs, delivering the "coded message" to the protein synthesis translation phase.

Translating the Genetic Code: Polypeptide Ribosomal Assembly

Translation initiates protein construction. Once the mRNA enters the cytoplasm through the nuclear pore, it seeks out a ribosome and binds with it. The nucleus is the original source for the millions of ribosomes in the cell's cytoplasm. A ribosome contains a large and a small subunit, the latter fitting into a depression on the ribosome's larger surface. A ribosome has three sites that associate with mRNA:

1. A-site (A for attachment)
2. P-site (P for polypeptide)
3. E-site (E for exit)

Ribosomes and Polypeptide Synthesis: Initiating Protein Construction

The cell's **ribosomes** provide the catalysts to initiate protein synthesis and serve as submicroscopic factories to produce polypeptides. **FIGURE 33.23** illustrates a four-step sequence to bind a ribosome to one end of an mRNA molecule (**step 1**) and subsequent three-nucleotide increments through the mRNA molecule.

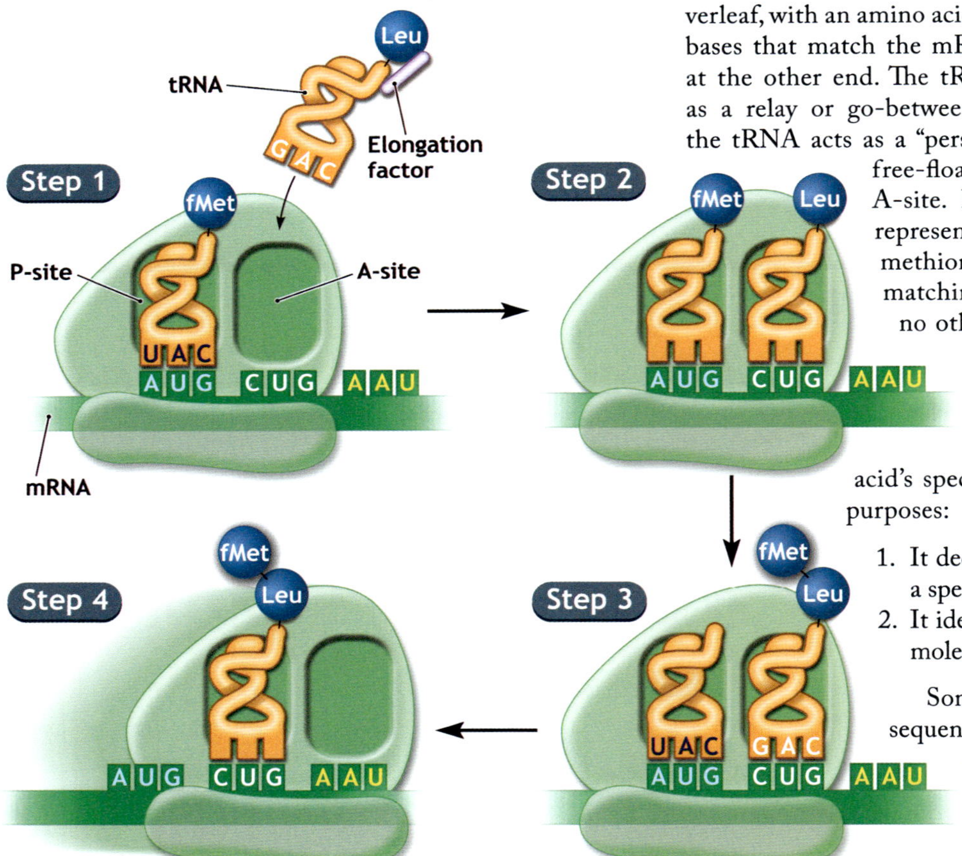

Polypeptide synthesis proceeds from the top in **step 1** with the tRNA anticodon complementary to the mRNA codon. The tRNA occupies the ribosome's A-site, with an anticodon complementary to the mRNA's codon at the opposite A-site. The ribosome translocates down the mRNA one codon at a time. In **step 2**, the lengthening polypeptide chain fMet (f, formyl-methionyl; Met, amino acid methionine) transfers to Leu (leucine), the incoming amino acid. The ribosome ejects the original tRNA (**step 3**) with its amino acid, exposing the next codon on the mRNA chain. When the tRNA molecule recognizes the next exposed codon, it binds to that codon, thus lengthening the growing peptide chain (**step 4**). fMet represents an addition to the lengthening polypeptide chain already occupied by Leu.

Decoding genetic information occurs when ribosomes bound to mRNA translate a genetic code sequence. The tRNA then interacts with a specific amino acid, adding one at a time to the end in the progressively elongating polypeptide chain.

Role for tRNA

The computer-generated tRNA molecule shown at the top left in **FIGURE 33.24** has a 3-D structure resembling a cloverleaf, with an amino acid at one end and three nitrogenous bases that match the mRNA's codon called an **anticodon** at the other end. The tRNA with matching codon serves as a relay or go-between in protein synthesis. In effect, the tRNA acts as a "personal shuttle" to deliver a specific free-floating amino acid to the ribosome's A-site. For example, the triplet U-A-C represents the codon for the amino acid methionine. When the tRNA with the matching U-A-C anticodon (it carries no other amino acid) interacts with the free-floating U-A-C amino acid, it binds to it by action with the activating enzyme **aminoacyl-tRNA synthetase**. Each amino acid's specific activating enzyme serves two purposes:

1. It deciphers and then binds (couples) to a specific amino acid.
2. It identifies the anticodon on the tRNA molecule.

Some activating enzymes decipher the sequence in one anticodon and thus only one tRNA, while others recognize multiple tRNA molecules. Thus, the activating enzyme "reads" the genetic code on both the essential amino acid tryptophan and its tRNA tryptophan anticodon sequence A-C-C. Figure 33.24 shows three tRNA views:

1. Computer-generated model

FIGURE 33.23. Ribosomes, the protein synthesis initiators. Sequentially linking amino acids by peptide bonding in the four-step process ultimately forms the specific protein with its unique genetically determined information to achieve its specific function(s). In this example, creating fMet in step 4 represents an addition to the lengthening polypeptide chain already occupied by Leu.

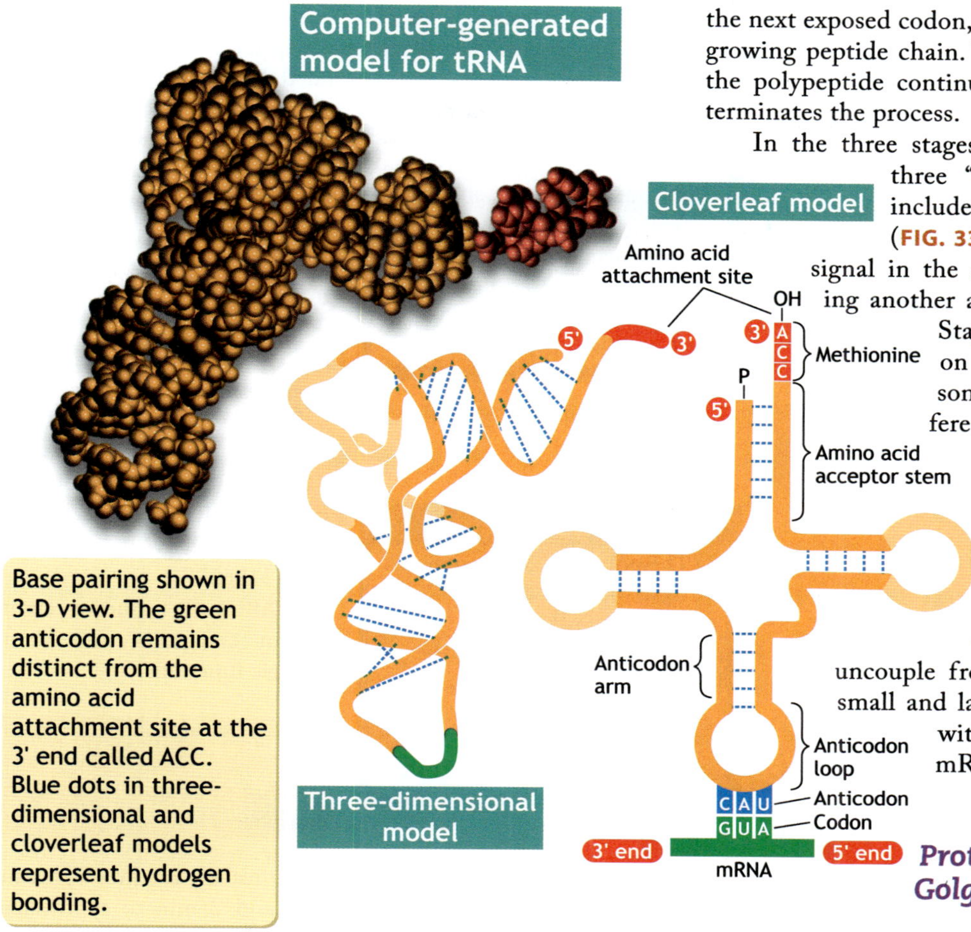

the next exposed codon, it binds to it, thus lengthening the growing peptide chain. The elongation procedure to build the polypeptide continues repeatedly until a stop codon terminates the process.

In the three stages in polypeptide termination, the three "stop" codons or base sequences include U-A-A, U-A-G, and U-G-A (FIG. 33.25). These codons "turn off" the signal in the mRNA message, preventing adding another amino acid sequence to the chain. Stage 1 shows the stop codon U-A-A on the mRNA strand within the ribosome's A-site, where one in three different releasing factors—eRF1, eRF2, or eRF3—locks into position to split apart the linking covalent bond. In stage 2, the polypeptide chain releases from tRNA at the ribosome's P site to effectively end protein synthesis. Once the polypeptide and tRNA uncouple from the termination complex, the small and large ribosomal units recycle along with mRNA in stage 3 for further mRNA translation.

FIGURE 33.24. Three tRNA views—computer-generated molecular model and three-dimensional and cloverleaf models depicting hydrogen bonding among the various molecular structures. Note that the anticodon displayed at the bottom in the cloverleaf model at the right (complementary three-nucleotide sequence) matches up with the mRNA codon using complementary (antiparallel) binding between the anticodon (*blue*, CAU) and codon (*green*, GUA).

2. Three-dimensional representation that highlights internal base pairing with hydrogen bonding
3. Two-dimensional cloverleaf model with the tRNA anticodon shown in *blue*

The example represents the complementary three-nucleotide sequence C-A-U matching mRNA's codon G-U-A.

Polypeptide Elongation and Termination

The polypeptide chain increases in length when an amino acid from tRNA translocates to it. The A-U-G codon shown in Figure 33.23 within the mRNA message initiates the "start" signal for peptide elongation. The same A-U-G sequence that encodes tryptophan also encodes methionine. The first A-U-G message "sensed" in the mRNA molecule initiates translation. The ribosome translocates down the mRNA three nucleotide blocks with one codon at a time. At each third nucleotide, the ribosome ejects the original tRNA with its amino acid to expose the next codon on the mRNA chain. When the tRNA molecule recognizes

Protein Delivery System: The Golgi Complex

Once the ribosome produces its polypeptide, newly formed strands can exit a cell through its outer membrane into the external interstitial fluid environment. The highly membranous **Golgi complex** structures within the cell provide the transfer mechanism for moving materials from the cell to its external environment. Italian physiologist and microscopist Camillo Golgi (1843–1926; www.nobelprize.org/prizes/medicine/1906/golgi/biographical/) who shared the 1906 Nobel Prize in Physiology or Medicine with Spanish researcher Santiago Ramón y Cajal (1852–1934; www.nobelprize.org/prizes/medicine/1906/cajal/facts/) for their work on nervous system anatomy structure. These scientists in 1898 first called attention to these minute intracellular structures using a light microscope (www.sciencedirect.com/topics/agricultural-and-biological-sciences/light-microscopes). Many biology colleagues doubted the existence of such structures; 60 years later, the **electron microscope** confirmed their existence in exquisite detail (www.explainthatstuff.com/electronmicroscopes.html).

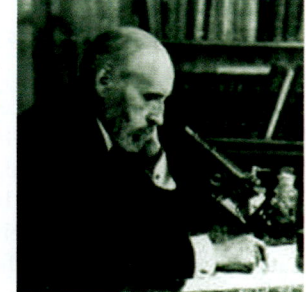

Santiago Ramón y Cajal

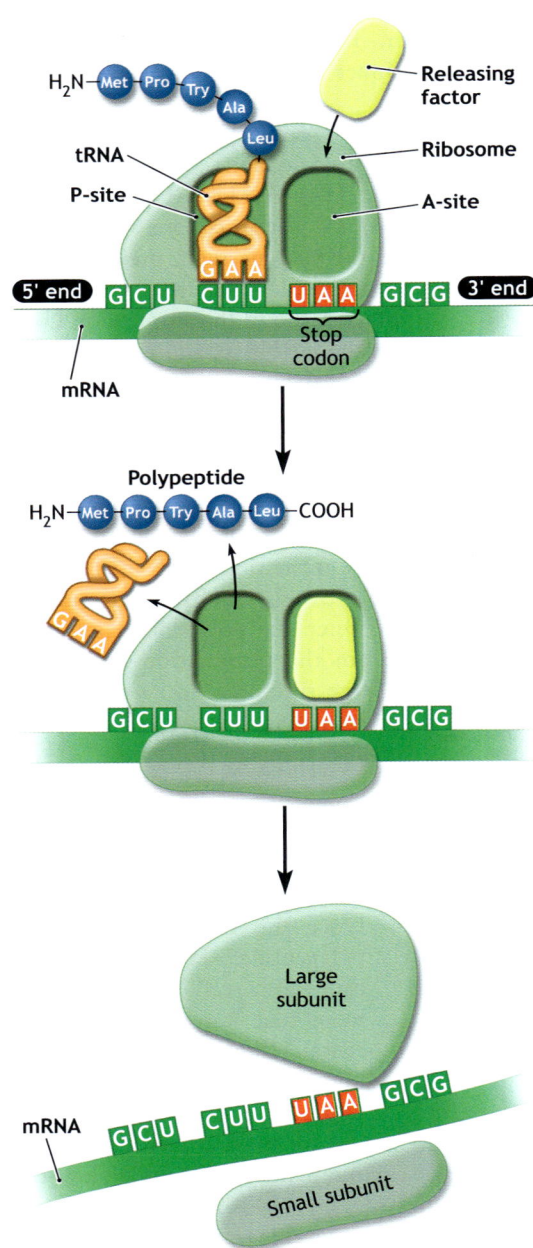

FIGURE 33.25. Three stages in polypeptide termination.

Stage 1
1. The stop codon U-A-A appears at the ribosome's A site
2. A releasing factor binds to the ribosome's A site at the stop codon (U-A-A) and locks into this position

Stage 2
1. The polypeptide disconnects from the tRNA at the ribosome's P site
2. A water molecule, not an amino acid, attaches to the polypeptide when the releasing factor disconnects the polypeptide from tRNA

Stage 3
1. The small and large ribosomal subunits separate
2. The mRNA remains free to initiate new mRNA translation

The Golgi complex receives a polypeptide from the cell's **endoplasmic reticulum**. **FIGURE 33.26** illustrates polypeptide transport into the Golgi complex, where this molecule depicted as blue dots may become a **glycoprotein** with carbohydrate as the nonprotein component. When a polysaccharide binds to a lipid, it forms a **glycolipid**. Glycoproteins or glycolipids then collect within the flattened, membranous sacs—the *cisternae region in the Golgi complex*—where specialized enzymes modify the protein component. The transport vesicles that hold proteins passing from the endoplasmic reticulum pinch off and break away from the roughened endoplasmic surfaces. The tiny vesicles attached to the cell's outer membrane expel their contents to the extracellular spaces via secretory vesicles. In essence, but not always, the Golgi complex takes up the polypeptide on the Golgi surface and then modifies and repackages it into molecules that leave the Golgi complex by a transport vesicle at its other membrane.

Terminating Protein Synthesis

The end point in protein synthesis collectively creates several thousand completed or functional proteins, each with a specific function depending in part on its structure (www.ncbi.nlm.nih.gov/pmc/articles/PMC3186377/).

TABLE 33.1 shows eight protein categories and their biologic functions.

TABLE 33.1 Eight protein categories and their biologic functions

It usually requires between 20 s and 2 min to synthesize most proteins, depending on the protein's complexity. The Hb molecule and its amino acid sequence serves as an excellent example representing four protein structure levels highlighted in **FIGURE 33.27** in black. This generalized example begins with the linear amino acid sequence from the amino acid at the amino-terminal end through to the carboxyl-terminal residue. The polypeptide strand formed when peptide linkages join amino acid monomers represent protein's **primary structure**. In a **secondary structure**, the protein can twist into a 3-D form known as an α helix. It can also fold back onto itself to give a flat look (β-pleated sheets), with regular repeating interactions using hydrogen bonding among closely linked residues in the primary sequence. Interactions among residues farther apart in the primary structure determine a **tertiary structure** such in disulfide bond formation between two cysteine residues. In this conformation, the protein literally folds up on itself, much like making dough strands twist into a pretzel. The topology in the α helices and β-pleated sheets plays important roles in determining the protein's final shape.[34] The complex Hb molecule contains two α subunits and two β subunits (tetramer). The term **quaternary structure** refers to protein's subunit structure, and Hb contains multiple subunits.

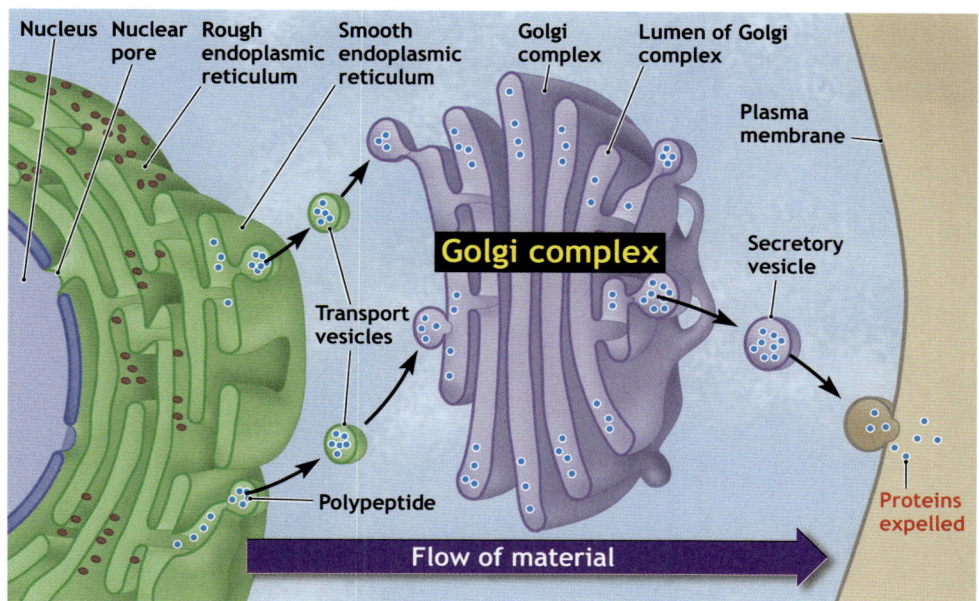

FIGURE 33.26. The Golgi complex accepts polypeptides depicted as *blue dots* on one of its surfaces after ribosomes release them through the cell's plasma membrane for repackaging as glycoproteins. They then are expelled from secretory vesicles for final expulsion through the plasma membrane or delivery to another cell area. The Golgi structures modify the proteins within their lumen for use within or outside cells once they pass through the plasma membrane.

Hb Evolutionary Tree

The Hb molecule illustrated in Figure 33.27 was deciphered first in 1960 by British molecular biologist Max Perutz 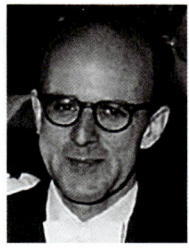 (1914–2002; shared 1962 Nobel Prize for Chemistry; www.nobelprize.org/nobel_prizes/chemistry/laureates/1962/perutz-bio.html) with John Kendrew (1917–1997; www.nobelprize.org/prizes/chemistry/1962/kendrew/biographical/) for their discoveries about the atomic structure in heme-containing globular proteins using x-ray crystallography—Perutz for Hb (www.mayoclinicproceedings.org/article/S0025-6196(15)00506-6/fulltext) and Kendrew for myoglobin (www.ncbi.nlm.nih.gov/pmc/articles/PMC5980623/). The purified Hb molecule's precise arrangement was based on the way its crystals diffracted x-ray beams. The molecule contains two α and two β chains, with the heme group associated with each chain. The central iron atom (shown in *red*) binds with one oxygen molecule and acts as a magnet to attract and hold it. Knowledge about protein structure configuration has increased exponentially since Perutz and Kendrew first discovered the details about the Hb and myoglobin structures. For example, the Protein Data Bank (www.rcsb.org) archives information about proteins, nucleic acids, and their complex 3-D shapes to help with understanding protein synthesis in health and disease related to biomedicine and agriculture.

The chimpanzee, our closest genetic relative, has an identical α chain. As a comparison, the Hb amino acid sequence in cows and pigs diverges from humans by about 12%, while for chickens, the divergence increases to 25%. Molecular biologists have constructed an evolutionary tree for many proteins (e.g., the iron-containing mitochondrial cytochromes) to track evolutionary change.[195]

Some proteins change relatively slowly, spanning millions of years to evolve. For example, histones change at a rate equal to about 0.25 mutations per 100 amino acids per 100 million years. In contrast, other neurotoxin and immunoglobulin proteins mutate more rapidly (rates 110 to 140 mutations per 100 million years). Variation in the resistance to change makes "sense" because crucial cellular functions like energy generation in the citric acid cycle or correct DNA folding requires that gene sequences remain almost invariant. Proteins sensitive to relatively large variations in their operational properties sustain faster evolutionary changes (www.nature.com/scitable/topicpage/reading-a-phylogenetic-tree-the-meaning-of-41956/).

Proteolysis: Proteins' Ultimate Fate

Protein synthesis from amino acids and degradation into amino acid constituents progress unabated throughout life. The rates of protein synthesis and degradation, a process called **proteolysis**, regulate the organism's total protein content at any given time independently from the proteins' structural configurations (bone or muscle) or functions (metabolic and intracellular enzymes). The highly sophisticated protease complex provides for highly selective and efficient protein hydrolysis by controlling cellular activities to catalyze biological reactions (www.sciencedirect.com/topics/neuroscience/proteolysis).

As an example, the structural protein in bone may not decay significantly for months or years, while enzyme proteins in intermediary metabolism or those that regulate cell growth may survive only for minutes, milliseconds (hundredths), microseconds (millionths), or nanoseconds (billionths) fractions. The enzymes that control proteolysis (proteases) hydrolyze the amino acids' **peptide bonds**, splitting them into the constituent molecules. **FIGURE 33.28** illustrates how a relatively large rounded trash-can–shaped **proteasome** formed from protease enzymes degrades the unwanted proteins in the cell's highly dense, crowded cytoplasm (https://jasn.asnjournals.org/content/17/7/1807). These cylindrical structures capture proteins destined for destruction by recognizing

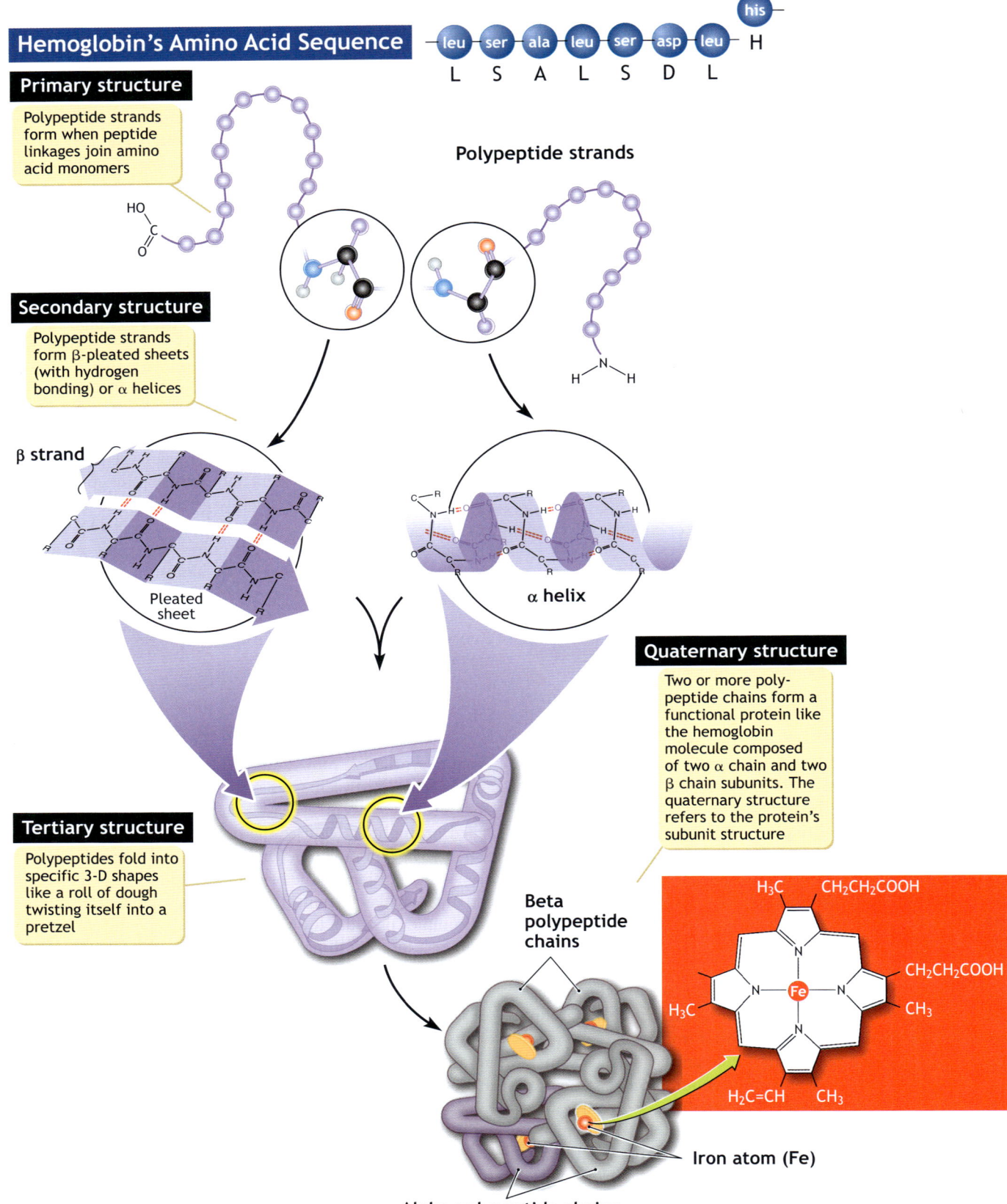

FIGURE 33.27. Four protein structures (primary, secondary, tertiary, and quaternary) synthesize the complex hemoglobin molecule. Hemoglobin's tertiary structure contains eight helical regions, and the quaternary structure has two α and two β chains. Note the isolated central iron (Fe) atom attached to four N atoms within the ring (https://pdb101.rcsb.org/motm/41).

a small marker or tag protein (**ubiquitin**) that attaches by covalent bonding to an active protein site. Once tagged, the ubiquitinated protein enters the proteasome, which degrades it to small peptide units before expelling it along with the ubiquitin red tag in the figure. Proteasomes degrade many protein types, from denatured or misfolded ones to misformed or oxidized amino acids.

Most Plentiful Structural Protein. Collagen, the most plentiful structural protein, accounts for about a fourth the body's protein. In essence, it forms molecular cables that strengthen the tendons with plentiful, resilient sheets that support the skin and internal organs. This simple protein has three chains wound together in a tight triple helix, with more than 1400 amino acids in each chain. Collagen forms from a repeated three amino acid sequence; every third amino acid is glycine, a small amino acid fitting perfectly inside the helix. Many remaining positions along the chain fill with proline and hydroxyproline amino acids, the latter a modified proline version. Hydroxyproline formation involves modifying normal proline amino acids after collagen construction. The reaction requires vitamin C to assist in adding oxygen. Vitamin C deficiency slows hydroxyproline production and stops new collagen creation, ultimately causing scurvy (https://journals.physiology.org/doi/full/10.1152/ajpgi.00369.2016). When heated, collagen triple helix unwinds and the chains separate. When the denatured tangled chains cool, they soak up surrounding water like a sponge to form gelatin commonly used in cooking.

Summarizing Protein Synthesis

TABLE 33.2 charts the key events sequences in the genetic information flow in living cells from DNA → RNA → protein.

Mutations

The slightest aberration in the 3 billion letter genome sequence can escalate to irreversible effects on health and well-being. Fortunately, exquisite internal repair mechanisms or specialized protein complexes correct mismatches along the double helix, thus avoiding dreadful, life-altering genetic disorders. Daily factors in the external environment continually threaten the brain's DNA from cosmic and ultraviolet radiation bombardment, to radioactive decay and galactic cosmic radiation,[276,277] and dangerously reactive **free radical** species discussed later in this chapter.

A **mutation** results from a minor alteration or "misspelling" in the DNA sequence that cripples the corresponding RNA or protein. Many human diseases generally form from protein abnormalities caused by a change in the sequence in only one of the 3×10^9 or more DNA nucleotide pairs in the human genome. Not all coding sequences in amino acids make "sense." The term **junk DNA** (also called *noncoding DNA*) describes such DNA sequences. Junk DNA replicates inside a cell the same way any other DNA molecules replicate but without gene expression. Scientists had believed inherited sequences performed no known "genetically useful" purpose,[12,156] yet recent data confirm the opposite (www.medicalnewstoday.com/articles/250006.php).

TABLE 33.2 Essential concepts and sequences in protein synthesis

Junk DNA Is Not Junk

Many papers published in prestigious journals have rejected the notion that most DNA is "junk," as accumulated over time during routine evolutionary development.[81,104,119] Project ENCODE (www.genome.gov/12513456/encode-project-background) was developed based on the accumulated work from diverse research groups across the United States, United Kingdom, Spain, Singapore, and Japan. The database relied on more than 1600 experiments on 147 tissue types with technologies standardized across the consortium. The research from Project ENCODE determined that 80% of the human genome serves a biochemically active purpose. The inset image shows a vial with purified DNA fluorescing orange under ultraviolet light. The experiments

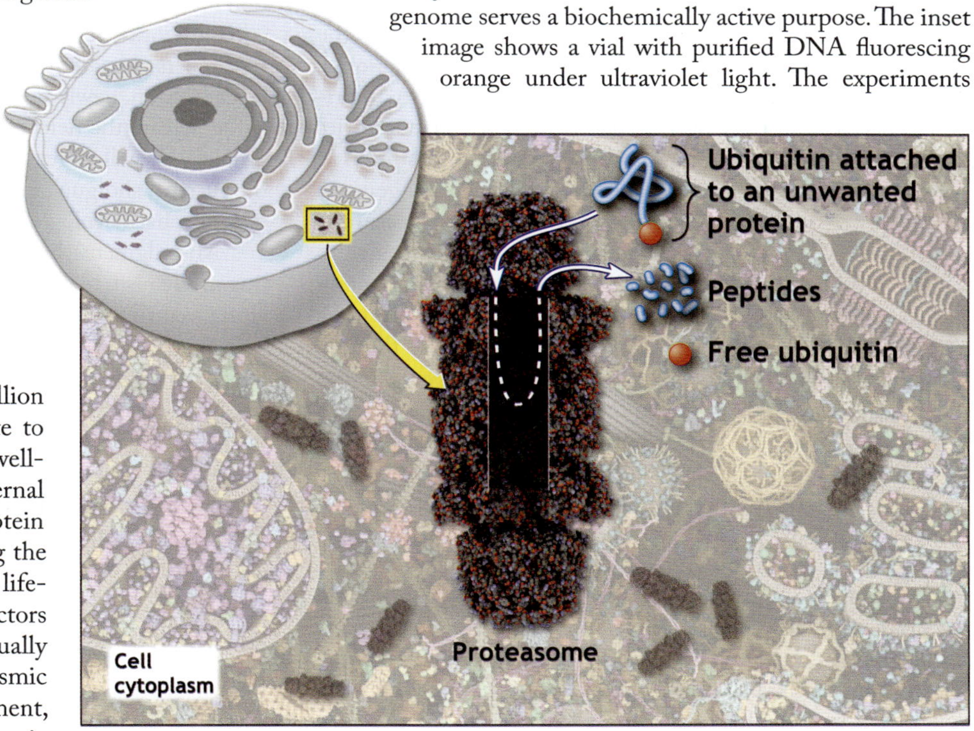

FIGURE 33.28. Proteasomes in the cell cytoplasm maintain a balance between protein synthesis and protein degradation. The free ubiquitin tag (displayed in *red*) attaches to an active site on the designated protein, identifying it for degradation to its peptide components within the proteasome's cylindrical structure. Once ejected, the ubiquitin recycles to another unwanted protein.
(Proteasome image: StudioMolekuul/Shutterstock.)

FYI: Supercharged Carrots and Lettuce

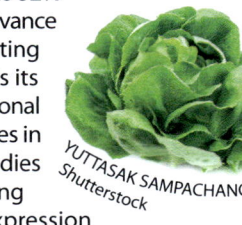
Sunwand24/Shutterstock

Researchers have uncovered a way to tweak a gene to increase calcium transport —a mineral nutrient relatively low in foods from the plant-based foods. The scientists loaded their super-vegetables with a modified calcium-proton antiporter (known as short cation exchanger 1), which pumps calcium into plant cells. For carrots, volunteers absorbed 41% more calcium compared to a group that consumed the "typical" carrot. The supercharged lettuce contained 25 to 32% more calcium than controls. The relevance of this tinkering and nutrient-boosting enhancement of a dietary staple is its potential to impact prevalent nutritional disorders (e.g., building strong bones in osteoporosis prevention). Such studies highlight the possibility of increasing plant nutrient content through expression of high-capacity molecular biology transporters.

YUTTASAK SAMPACHANO/Shutterstock

Sources:
Bæksted Holme I, et al. A roadmap to modulated anthocyanin compositions in carrots. *Plants (Basel)*. 2021;10:472.
Wang YH, et al. Transcript profiling of genes involved in carotenoid biosynthesis among three carrot cultivars with various taproot colors. *Protoplasma*. 2020;257:949.

---

relied on innovative next-generation DNA sequencing technologies, mainly attributed to advances enabled by the National Human Genome Research Institute (www.genome.gov) sequencing technology development program. A multi-year concerted effort by over 40 researchers in 32 laboratories worldwide produced the first holistic view about how the human genome functions. ENCODE researchers used up-to-date technologies to assess DNA and its variations among different population groups. In total, ENCODE generated more than 15 trillion raw data bytes, consuming the equivalent equal to 300 years in computing time in the analyses.

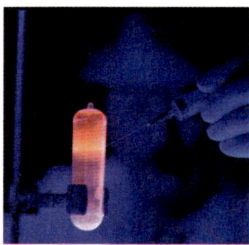
Purified DNA. (Image courtesy www.genome.gov)

Mutation Varieties

The guiding central dogma principle discussed previously implicitly stated that any change in the inherited genetic material produces a ripple effect on replication, transcription, and translation. A mutation in the original daughter chromosomes passes these characteristics to the next generation so the offspring inherits the mutation. The new CRISPR-CAS9 genetic engineering system can replace the defective sequences or arrest their development by clipping out single or multiple unwanted sequences in targeted specific genes. For example, short-circuiting bases away from a particular gene (*PAX6*) can alter the gene's expression and cause a mutation in which a typical characteristic (e.g., iris in the eye) fails to develop, producing a developmental syndrome called aniridia (https://rarediseases.org/rare-diseases/aniridia/). Poorly understood processes can *silence* genes up to 90 million bases down the chromosome. Once transcription uses the DNA template to make an RNA copy for an inherited mutated sequence, the altered RNA translates the defective code during protein synthesis. The body's vital processes depend on proteins for their intended functions, even if mutated genes pose a health hazard.

The doggerel in **TABLE 33.3** provides eight examples for different mutation types and what can happen to disrupt the orderly genetic code sequence.

TABLE 33.3 Genetic mutation types

A graphic example points out how the probability for "errors" can creep into a DNA sequence. If the total DNA compacted in the body's 10 trillion cells were laid end to end like long sausage links, it would stretch from Earth to the sun 667 times—not a trivial length, 93 million miles! Consequently, a single genetic code mismatch can wreak havoc on the "normal" DNA nucleotide sequence and hence genes. A defect in code sequence often remains **quiescent** for nearly a lifetime before it emerges. For example, it may take 60 y before a seemingly minor misalignment in a receptor gene devastates heart function, causing congestive heart failure within a few months (www.sciencedaily.com/releases/2021/03/210302150016.htm) or an errant mutation for type 2 diabetes emerges in middle or older ages (https://jamanetwork.com/journals/jama/fullarticle/645914). When researchers can identify this human gene variant years before its expression, newly developed, highly specific drugs hopefully will eradicate the defect. Within the next several decades, new drug classes will target specific mutated cells instead rather than the current "shotgun" approach used to cripple most cells with a massive pharmacologic overdose.

Misjudgments in drug doses can critically affect the clotting mechanism to potentially cause fatal bleeding (https://psnet.ahrq.gov/primer/medication-errors-and-adverse-drug-events). The gene *VKORC*, known as vitamin K epoxide reductase, makes the enzyme involved in blood clotting mechanisms to stop excessive bleeding from unexplained nosebleeds (epistaxis), prolonged menstrual blood flow (menorrhagia), blood disorders, minor cuts, tooth brushing or flossing, trauma, or gastrointestinal or genitourinary tract disease. DNA variations responsible for changing the gene's activity and the protein yield account for 25% in the overall drug dosage variation to prevent bleeding episodes.

Single-Nucleotide Polymorphisms

Pharmaceutical and computer chip manufacturers have partnered to develop techniques to identify specific molecular markers called single-nucleotide polymorphisms or SNPs (pronounced *snips*), thousands which reside within each person's genetic code (www.ncbi.nlm.nih.gov/snp). Most tiny nucleotide genetic code "snippets" normally configure with no deviant code. Some, however, have a single "mismatch" in the nucleotide sequence that predisposes an individual to a particular disease or injury (e.g., knee ligament tear in football or gymnastics), which may be identified in the future with multiple genetic probing to identify the risk or render the immune system resistant to drug treatment[26] (www.sciencedirect.com/science/article/pii/S2405579421000437).

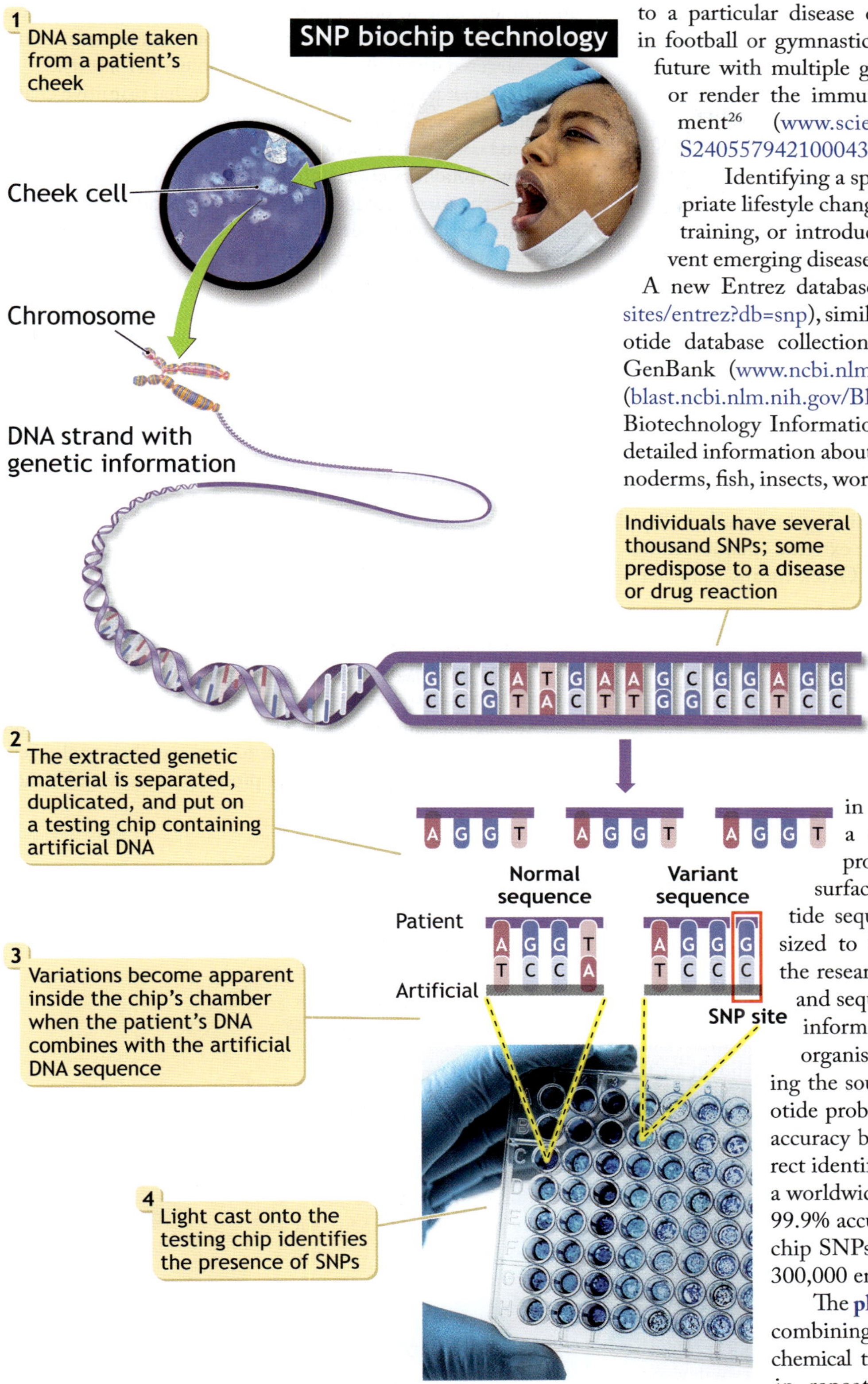

Identifying a specific gene variant will allow appropriate lifestyle changes in nutrition, weight loss, exercise training, or introducing a particular drug class to prevent emerging diseases or disabilities, or delay their onset. A new Entrez database, dbSNP (www.ncbi.nlm.nih.gov/sites/entrez?db=snp), similar in operation to the Entrez nucleotide database collection (www.ncbi.nlm.nih.gov) includes GenBank (www.ncbi.nlm.nih.gov/Genbank/) and BLAST (blast.ncbi.nlm.nih.gov/Blast.cgi). These National Center for Biotechnology Information genome resource guides include detailed information about mammals, birds, amphibians, echinoderms, fish, insects, worms, plants, fungi, and protozoa.

SNP assessment (**FIG. 33.29**) uses microarray biochips or a "library" with artificial DNA to compare the individual's DNA sample with the chips' existing gene sequences. SNP identification (explained in the yellow text boxes) has current application to identify and differentiate different ancestral lines.[124]

A microarray DNA chip shown in the inset image below represents a spatial array with oligonucleotide probes arranged on a tiny supporting surface. The probe, representing nucleotide sequences in known genes, is synthesized to the support surface, which allows the researcher to know each probe's position and sequence with high accuracy. With this information, the DNA chip can identify organisms and select genes by hybridizing the source DNA to the chips' oligonucleotide probes. This process must achieve 100% accuracy because even a small error or incorrect identification could prove disastrous from a worldwide health standpoint.[30] For example, 99.9% accuracy in matching the 300,000 biochip SNPs for only 1000 people would create 300,000 errors!

The **photolithography** technique involves combining etching, chemical deposition, and chemical treatments in repeated steps on an initially flat substrate or nanoscale device[85] (www.youtube.com/watch?v=9x3Lh1ZfggM). Nanoscale is extremely small—

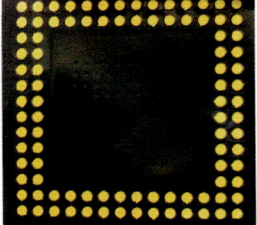
Elpisterra/Shutterstock

FIGURE 33.29. Four main stages in single-nucleotide polymorphism (SNP) biochip technology assess multiple genes simultaneously to determine expression in specific cell types. A single square-inch slide can contain thousands of individual genes, which barcode-scanning facilitates on the biochip. Identifying specific SNPs allows reference links to genes, probe samples, reagents, and experimental protocols.
(Shutterstock images: Dragana Gordic (cheek swab), TiffanyRobyn (cheek cell micrograph), angellodeco (testing chip photo).)

the page you are reading is about 100,000 nanometers (nm) thick (1×10^{-9} m or 1/1,000,000,000 m). Etching microcircuits on a silicon chip could also encode a single biochip containing the entire human genome. Figure 33.29 illustrates the four main stages to identify SNPs and their specific genetic sequences or anomalies. The challenge is to map as many SNP genotypes as possible to analyze an individual's genome (www.mitomap.org/MITOMAP) to discover susceptibility to debilitating diseases.[91,98,107,154,196,197]

Cancer

The body's defense mechanisms include "error-correcting" proteins that literally "erase" an apparent aberration in DNA sequencing. Unfortunately, external ionizing and ultraviolet radiation and chemical and pharmacologic **mutagens** exert catastrophic effects on the body's genetic machinery, specifically DNA's code sequences. In extreme mutations, structural defects in embryos produce gross missing limb and multiple organ deformities. In these cases, the extreme chemical mutagen known as a **teratogen** (*teras* in Greek means "monster") produces the effect.

The term **carcinogen** refers to any agent that causes cancer (www.osha.gov/SLTC/carcinogens/). In **cancer**, cell growth proceeds unchecked, forming larger than normal cell clusters called a **tumor**. A **benign tumor** remains in one location; cells from a malignant tumor migrate to invade other tissues and form secondary cancers. Cancers that form from connective tissue, muscle, or bone are known as **sarcomas**; the most prevalent breast and lung cancers, called carcinomas, originate from epithelial

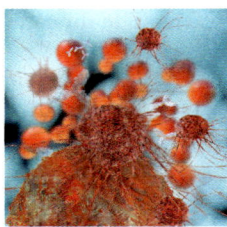
xrender/Shutterstock

tissue. **Malignant tumors** tend to **metastasize** or spawn cells that invade healthy tissue when they travel via the lymphatic or vascular circulation to form new secondary cancers termed *metastases*. A mutated gene into an **oncogene** or cancer-causing gene often produces numerous cancers as shown in the inset 3-D rendered spidery looking cancer cells, many not eradicated by surgery and/or drugs that target specific cells or tissues. Cancer occurs from a failure to "turn on" specific genes that code nucleotide sequences to repress uncontrolled cell division. A tumor cell can develop from a mutation in any stage that regulates cell growth and differentiation. In colon cancer, for example, silencing the *APC* gene (adenomatous polyposis coli) on chromosome 5q alters the gut's normal epithelial tissue lining. Abnormally altered DNA can induce malignant colon carcinoma and metastasis. Cell-imaging technology (https://anatomypubs.onlinelibrary.wiley.com/doi/full/10.1002/ar.22554) pinpoints the exact location in tissues that produce high levels in the β-4 protein thymosin, which triggers tumor growth.[144,169] Digital computer images that locate specific tissue proteins determine when new proteins invade tumor cells or when normally produced proteins disappear. Protein imaging has opened new vistas in cancer screening to search for specific molecule comparisons between normal and disease states and developing strategies to arrest existing cancers (www.cancer.gov/about-cancer/treatment/types/targeted-therapies/targeted-therapies-fact-sheet).

Some cancerous cells become more lethal primitive channels because they create blood vessels in a process called **vasculogenesis** (www.ncbi.nlm.nih.gov/books/NBK53252/). The new blood vessels eventually connect with pre-existing vessels at the tumor's edge. This process, separate from **angiogenesis**, may explain why therapies that attack angiogenesis may not treat some cancers effectively. **FIGURE 33.30** shows angiogenesis and subsequent tumor vascularization. First, the tumor proliferates as it forms small cell masses (note no blood vessels in Fig. 33.30A). Without blood vessels, a tumor remains small. Second, protein factors stimulate the endothelial cells in nearby blood vessels to grow toward the tumor cells (Fig. 33.30B). Third, blood vessels proliferate, creating almost unlimited tumor growth. Note the approximate quadrupling in tumor cells (Fig. 33.30C).

Gene therapy strategies in clinical trials (www.cancer.gov/CLINICALTRIALS) attack tumor growth (e.g., angiogenesis inhibitors). For example, in an older 2003 trial, a pharmaceutical company in cooperation with the National Cancer Institute received Food and Drug Administration (FDA) approval to market bortezomib (Velcade) to treat multiple myeloma in patients who previously received at least two prior therapies and demonstrated disease progression on the last therapy (www.drugs.com/history/velcade.html). This new, successful drug class targets the proteasome to remove abnormal, aged, or damaged proteins. By blocking proteasome activity, Velcade

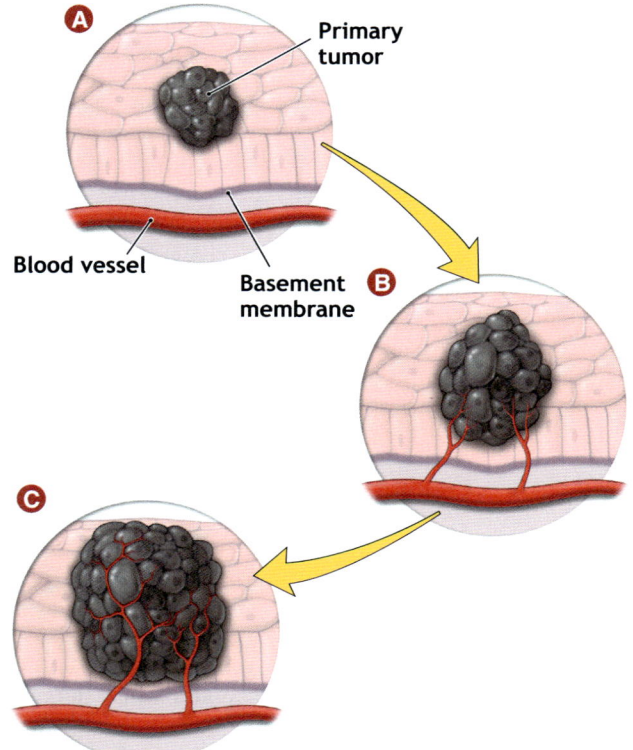

FIGURE 33.30. Angiogenesis and subsequent tumor vascularization.

increased the protein concentration within the cell. The protein BAX promotes cell suicide or programmed cell death known as **apoptosis**[22] (*apopt*, "falling off"; *osis*, "process"), by blocking antiapoptosis protein activity (www.ncbi.nlm.nih.gov/pmc/articles/PMC2117903/). As BAX levels increase in response to Velcade, BAX inhibition in *bcl-2* also increases, and the cell ultimately undergoes apoptosis.[35]

The newer anticancer approaches use a peptide that targets tumor blood vessels, invades cells, and literally "tricks" cancer cells into obliterating themselves. The peptide contains two domains: one that seeks out tumor blood vessels and one that triggers apoptosis. This normally occurring process in invertebrate and vertebrate biology exemplifies nature's numerous defense mechanisms to purge cells damaged by mutation, viral invasion, external radiation, malignancy, and other deleterious cellular events (not always abnormalities).

Researchers studied four main apoptosis areas[1,121,123]:

1. Molecular mechanisms involved in apoptosis induction
2. Control intracellular protease pathways responsible for induction
3. Biochemical events during apoptosis, particularly events that mediate cell death
4. Mechanisms involved in normal development and disease

Anticancer drugs attempt to eradicate specific cancers once SNPs or related technology identifies them. A later section discusses the fight against mutation-caused diseases with new genetically engineered vaccines.

Mitochondrial DNA Mutations and Diseases

Scientists normally view the chromosomes as the sole DNA repository, but it also exists in the mitochondria. The MITO-MAP database (www.mitomap.org/) reports published and unpublished data on human mitochondrial DNA (mtDNA) variation. The complete human mitochondrial genome, including the human mitochondrial sequence published in 2008 identified 16,569 base pairs, with the genetic blueprint for 37 molecules, which produce about 90% of the body's energy requirements.

Chapters 5 and 6 described energy release during cellular respiration, when electron transfer ultimately produces water by uniting oxygen and hydrogen in synthesizing significant energy-rich ATP. Researchers have determined the mtDNA codes for 13 proteins that regulate respiratory chain oxidation and for 24 RNA molecules (2 tRNAs, 22 rRNAs) that manufacture subunit respiratory chain proteins. A mutation in mtDNA can induce devastating and unpredictable effects on basic cellular metabolic processes to devastate neural, muscular, renal, and endocrine tissues.

FIGURE 33.31 lists 12 diseases associated with mtDNA mutations. The DNA ring displayed in the schematic view shows different mtDNA base pairs, numbered counterclockwise from the top center position labeled O_H in *white*. mtDNA mutations are implicated in aging and impact free radical intrusion in cardiovascular system tissues. Other mtDNA functions fall into two categories: forensic medicine and molecular anthropology. In forensic medicine, mtDNA analysis proves useful because many nucleotide polymorphisms called *sequence variants* allow discrimination among individuals and/or biologic samples. Even when degraded by environmental insult or time, minute samples in body fluids or fragments in hair, skin, muscle, bone, and blood may yield enough material for typing the mtDNA locus.[7,73,93,145] The likelihood to recover mtDNA in small or degraded biologic samples exceeds that for nuclear DNA. mtDNA molecules exist in thousands of copies per cell compared with only two nuclear copies per cell. Also, since mtDNA inherits only one copy from the mother, any maternally related individual can provide a reference sample in situations where an individual's DNA cannot directly compare with a biologic sample. In molecular anthropology, mtDNA analysis examines genetic variation in humans and the relatedness in world populations including other mammals.[27,62,78,110,112,127,133,134]

mtDNA also reveals ancient population histories and delineates migration patterns, expansion dates, and geographic homelands (www.talkorigins.org/faqs/homs/mtDNA.html). mtDNA, extracted and sequenced from Neanderthal skeletons, provides evidence that modern humans do not share a close relationship with Neanderthals in the human evolutionary tree. The Neanderthal mtDNA studies strengthen the arguments that Neanderthals should be a separate species that did not contribute significantly to the modern gene pool.[57,122,129]

Federal Bureau of Investigation Laboratory mtDNA Casework Unit

The DNA Casework Unit (DCU) provides forensic DNA examinations to the Federal Bureau of Investigation (FBI) and other law enforcement agencies to support criminal, missing persons, and intelligence cases through evidence testing using forensic serological, mtDNA, and nuclear DNA methodologies (www.fbi.gov/services/laboratory/biometric-analysis/dna-casework) conduct millions of examinations annually from skin, fabric, hair, bones, and teeth involved is suspected crimes. Another special unit, Terrorist Explosive Device Analytical Center (TEDAC), is a multi-agency center that coordinates bomb-related evidence and intelligence collection for the U.S. government. TEDAC's experts analyze bombs. They also support law enforcement, the intelligence community, military border protection, and science and technology partners. Created in 2003 and located in Huntsville, Alabama, TEDAC directly supports these five main activities, in addition to providing expert witness testimony in court regarding the examination results.

- Bombing crime scene investigations
- Searching bomb factories and safe houses
- Deploying to major bombings, both in the United States and internationally
- Providing expertise on major bombing scenes
- Training FBI and law enforcement personnel

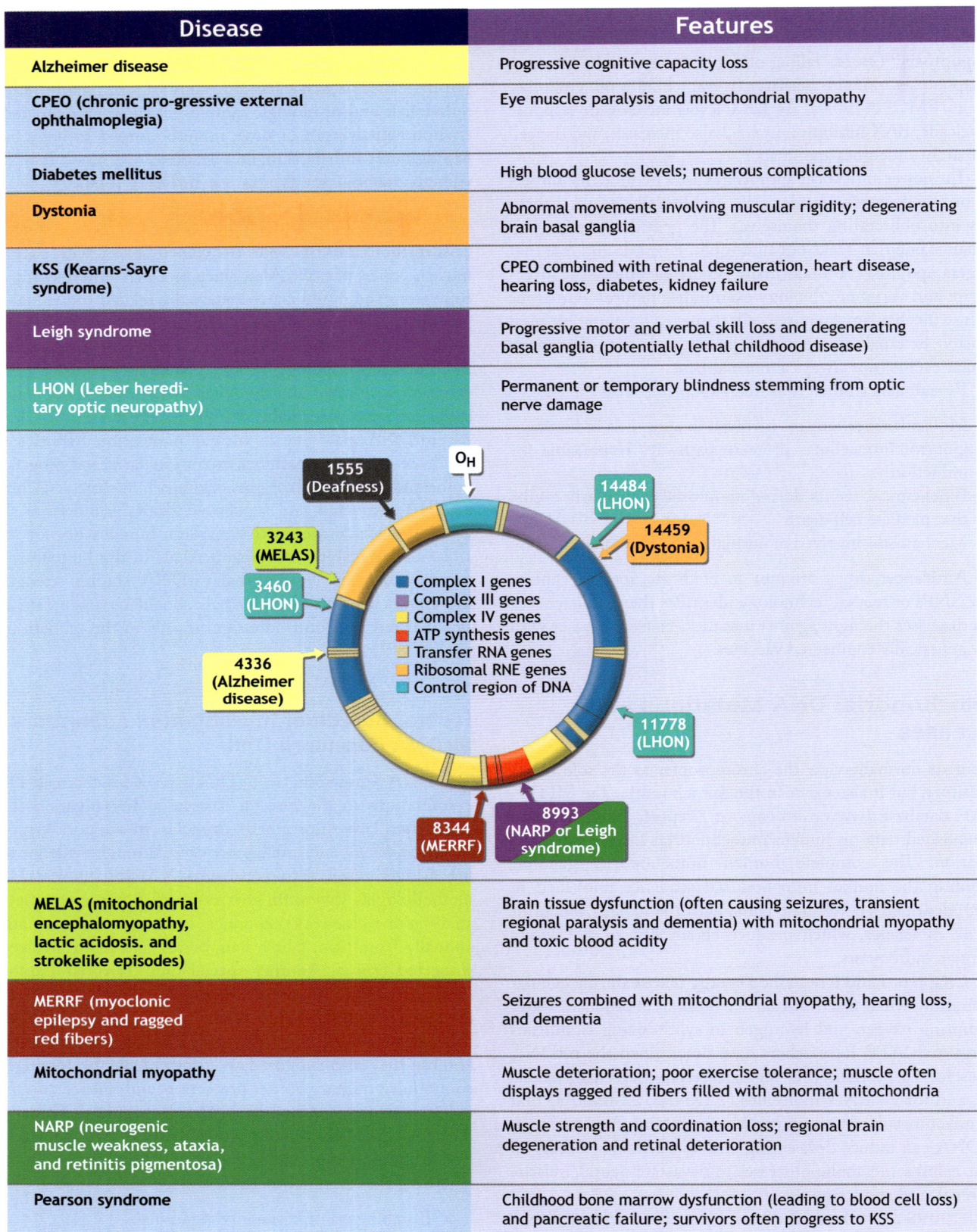

Disease	Features
Alzheimer disease	Progressive cognitive capacity loss
CPEO (chronic pro-gressive external ophthalmoplegia)	Eye muscles paralysis and mitochondrial myopathy
Diabetes mellitus	High blood glucose levels; numerous complications
Dystonia	Abnormal movements involving muscular rigidity; degenerating brain basal ganglia
KSS (Kearns-Sayre syndrome)	CPEO combined with retinal degeneration, heart disease, hearing loss, diabetes, kidney failure
Leigh syndrome	Progressive motor and verbal skill loss and degenerating basal ganglia (potentially lethal childhood disease)
LHON (Leber heredi-tary optic neuropathy)	Permanent or temporary blindness stemming from optic nerve damage
MELAS (mitochondrial encephalomyopathy, lactic acidosis. and strokelike episodes)	Brain tissue dysfunction (often causing seizures, transient regional paralysis and dementia) with mitochondrial myopathy and toxic blood acidity
MERRF (myoclonic epilepsy and ragged red fibers)	Seizures combined with mitochondrial myopathy, hearing loss, and dementia
Mitochondrial myopathy	Muscle deterioration; poor exercise tolerance; muscle often displays ragged red fibers filled with abnormal mitochondria
NARP (neurogenic muscle weakness, ataxia, and retinitis pigmentosa)	Muscle strength and coordination loss; regional brain degeneration and retinal deterioration
Pearson syndrome	Childhood bone marrow dysfunction (leading to blood cell loss) and pancreatic failure; survivors often progress to KSS

FIGURE 33.31. Mitochondrial DNA disease ring shows the genes associated with a particular disorder. Many mitochondrial DNA diseases are inherited but also can occur spontaneously in developing embryos and become widespread during fetal development. The mutations also can form in different tissues at different times during the life span, often taking years for full expression and potentially lethal or severely debilitating.
(Adapted with permission from Wallace DC, et al. Report of the Committee on Human Mitochondrial DNA. In: Cuticchia, A. Jamie, Michael A. Chipperfield, Patricia A. Foster, and the Genome Database, eds. *Human Gene Mapping, 1995: A Compendium*. pp. 1284, Fig. 1. © 1996 The Johns Hopkins University Press. Adapted with permission of The Johns Hopkins University Press.)

Part 2 — New Horizons in Molecular Biology

Watson and Crick's pioneering achievements in deciphering DNA's molecular structure ushered in a new era in medically related science research.[31,82,141] Advanced genetic engineering techniques also shape strategies to improve food's nutrient content and in human exercise performance.[14,69,149] Successful human genome sequencing has achieved remarkable scientific success. Understanding humans' genetic blueprint has transformed the quest to discover innovative new drugs to battle existing medical-related diseases and genetic disorders (www.genome.gov/For-Patients-and-Families/Genetic-Disorders).

Medically Related Research

All allied medical professions have benefitted from molecular biology/molecular genetics research.[89,95,108,255] Within the past 40 years, researchers in many fields have created new strategies to fight cancer, acquired immunodeficiency syndrome (AIDS), asthma, coronavirus disease 2019 (COVID-19), diabetes, influenza, heart and vascular disease, rheumatic fever,[94] and malaria. The new disease fighters use genetic engineering to improve the immunologic antigen defense machinery against viral, bacterial, fungal, or parasitic **pathogens**. All pathogens contain antigens in their structure, so the new genetically engineered vaccines severely blunt their destructive effects, including the virus known as severe acute respiratory syndrome coronavirus 2 (SARS-CoV-2), which is the virus that causes COVID-19,[188,189] and the more virulent delta variant (www.cdc.gov/coronavirus/2019-ncov/variants/delta-variant.html). The traditional vaccines use components from whole viruses or bacteria (e.g., proteins or sugars), whereas the new RNA and DNA vaccines incorporate genetic material from the **virus** or bacteria to manufacture specific foreign proteins. The body then integrates the new substances to identify and fight the invaders during the immune process.[279] The DNA vaccines send instructions for creating the protein as DNA, while the mRNA vaccines incorporate RNA pathways.

FIGURE 33.32 provides a capsule view in four disease-fighting approaches with vaccine techniques that manipulate the genetic code.

1. *Live vector vaccines* (www.niaid.nih.gov/research/vaccine-types). Genes from a dangerous virus such as HIV are placed into a harmless human virus. When injected, the altered virus prompts a strong **immune response** to combat the pathogen.
2. *Reassortment virus vaccines* (virology-online.com/viruses/Influenza.htm). Combining genes from different pathogenic strains creates a decoy virus that looks dangerous to the pathogen but remains harmless while triggering an appropriate immune response.
3. *Naked DNA vaccines* (www.pbs.org/wgbh/nova/bioterror/vacc_hiv.html). A pathogen's DNA is injected directly into the body. The cells incorporate the DNA, using the preprogrammed specific genetic "instructions" to create antigens to fight offending pathogens or existing tumors.
4. *Recombinant subunit vaccines* (www.ncbi.nlm.nih.gov/pmc/articles/PMC4927204/). Culturing a pathogen's genetic code or genes produces massive specific antigen quantities. The disease-fighting vaccine consists of cultured antigens rather than the whole pathogen.

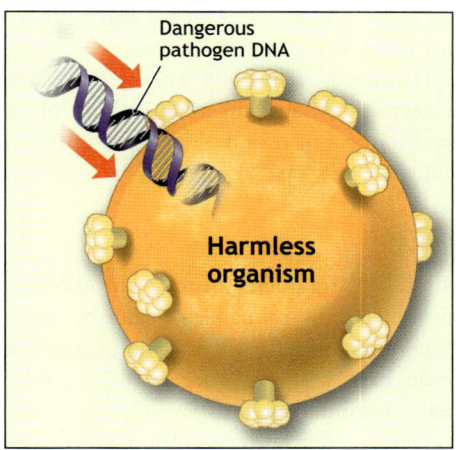
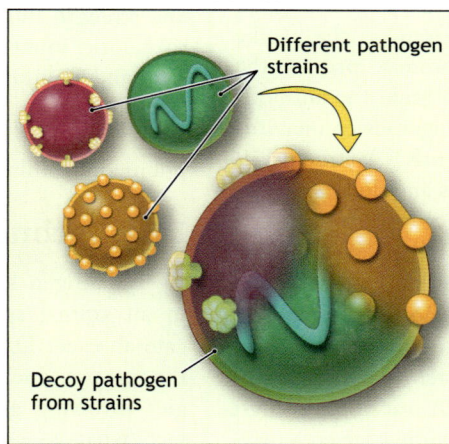
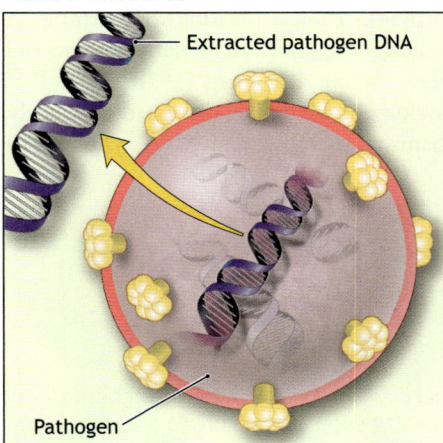
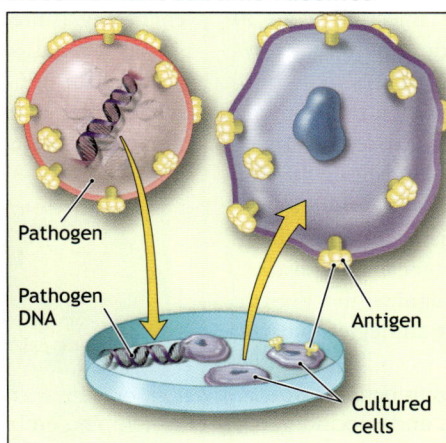

FIGURE 33.32. Genetic engineering a new generation of four vaccine types to fight human diseases.

mRNA Vaccines

mRNA vaccines are single-stranded nucleic acid molecules that transport DNA inside a cell's nucleus to ribosomes located in the cytoplasm outside the nucleus. The mRNA molecule's primary function is to transport detailed instructions from the DNA template to the ribosomes to assemble proteins. With this "built-in" technical instructional set, researchers can reconfigure specific genetic sequences to encode for proteins novel to the invading virus. A breakthrough in vaccine development occurred when a modified laboratory-derived mRNA-containing lipid nanoparticles incorporated in early vaccine development led to the Pfizer-BioNTech and Moderna COVID-19 vaccines in battling the 2019–2022 worldwide coronavirus pandemic.[256–258]

To combat the infectious coronavirus SARS-CoV-2, the injected mRNA vaccine stimulates cells near the injection site to produce the ubiquitous spike S protein (yellow), and the other proteins (HE, M, and E) appear in different colors on the red-stained coronavirus cell insert image. In essence, the spike protein primes the immune system to build the antibodies and T cells to diminish the real but dangerous coronavirus infection when it invades the body. The mRNA structure is enclosed in "nano-sized" **plasmid** particles and does not enter the individual's genome because it is physically separated from chromosomal DNA and can replicate independently. This approach to the 2020–2022 coronavirus worldwide epidemic was a departure from other traditional vaccine approaches. Rather than injecting a weakened live or killed virus, the novel mRNA approach trains the immune system directly with a single protein. The efficacy with mRNA vaccines is high (≥90%) in nonimmunocompromised individuals given a two-dose regimen separated by 30 days, but the immune response weakens for moderate to highly immunocompromised individuals. This ultimately requires a "booster" injection about 30 days following a second mRNA vaccine dose (www.cdc.gov/coronavirus/2019-ncov/vaccines/booster-shot.html).

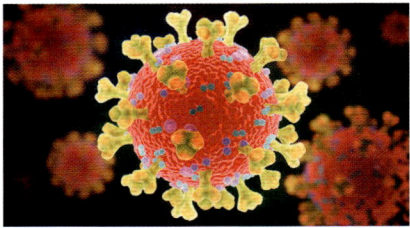
Dotted Yeti/Shutterstock

Some genetically engineered vaccines trick the immune system into creating antibodies to seek out and destroy undesirable molecules before they cross the blood-brain barrier. For example, small cocaine molecules escape the body's protein antibody defenses without mechanisms to stop them. Engineered vaccines can create a larger cocaine derivative, which the immune system can then recognize and disarm. This genetic design aspect offers innovative strategies to battle addictive diseases.

FIGURE 33.33A lists the body's 22 numbered chromosomes, including X and Y chromosomes, and specific genes on each chromosome linked to many cancers and metabolic-endocrine,[233] neurologic-psychiatric, and cardiovascular disorders. Figure 33.33A profiles chromosome 17 on which seven deadly cancers exist. Researchers estimate that chromosome 17 contains from 1200 to 1300 genes (depending assessment technique), which includes about 81 million DNA building blocks or 2.5 to 3.0% the body's total DNA (http://ghr.nlm.nih.gov/chromosome/17; www.genome.gov/11508982). Figure 33.33B shows the mechanism underlying two different chemical carcinogens (smoking and food contamination) on tumor suppressor gene *p53* nucleotide sequence. Inactivating this gene accounts for approximately 50% of human cancers. Each carcinogen produces a distinctive nucleotide substitution. Note the C or G substitution that displaces six T nucleotides.

Many areas in medicine other than cancer benefit from new findings in molecular biology.[157] Individuals with advanced sleep-phase syndrome (ASPS) cannot resist the urge either to sleep or to wake up early.[45] Research indicates that ASPS does not reflect a learned behavior or some other factor but follows a specific inherited pattern (https://sleepeducation.org/sleep-disorders/advanced-sleep-wake-phase/). Eventually, researchers may tie disorders to a single gene, opening new vistas to human biologic clock genetics,[47,64,77] with applications applied to human exercise performance (www.ncbi.nlm.nih.gov/pmc/articles/PMC6545246/). Several research strategies have provided insights concerning blood pressure control, endurance and strength training adaptations, maturational shifts related to caloric input and output, hormonal balance with exercise, and pulmonary, cardiovascular, body weight regulation (including anorexia nervosa[56,113] and circadian rhythm phase shifts impacting exercise in younger and older adults; https://pubmed.ncbi.nlm.nih.gov/30784068/).

DNA Technologies

By isolating a small DNA fragment from a chromosome in an animal species including humans, researcher duplicate an exact DNA segment copy in a test tube to preserve the precise nucleotide base pair sequence with technologies involving **genetic engineering** (www.yourgenome.org/facts/what-is-genetic-engineering), **gene splicing** (https://genomebiology.biomedcentral.com/articles/10.1186/s13059-018-1482-5, and **recombinant DNA** (www.rpi.edu/dept/chem-eng/Biotech-Environ/Projects00/rdna/rdna.html).

A crucial step along the path to genetic engineering occurred in 1967 when Arthur Kornberg (1918–2007; 1959 Nobel Prize in Physiology or Medicine; discussed previously) discovered the mechanisms in DNA and RNA synthesis for

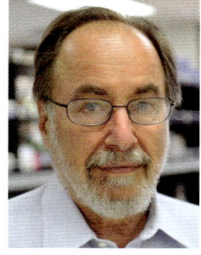 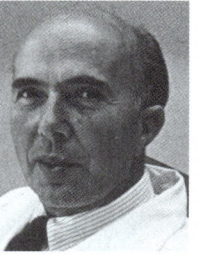 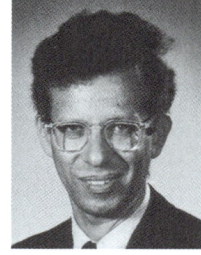

David Baltimore, Renato Dulbecco, and Howard Temin. (Baltimore image licensed under Creative Commons Attribution Share-Alike 3.0 Unported license: https://creativecommons.org/licenses/by-sa/3.0/deed.en)

Chromosome 1
- Malignant melanoma
- Prostate cancer
- Deafness

Chromosome 2
- Congenital hypothyroidism
- Colorectal cancer

Chromosome 3
- Susceptibility to HIV infection
- Small cell lung cancer
- Dementia

Chromosome 4
- Huntington disease
- Polycystic kidney disease

Chromosome 5
- Spinal muscular atrophy
- Endometrial carcinoma

Chromosome 6
- Hemochromatosis
- Dyslexia
- Schizophrenia
- Myoclonus epilepsy

Chromosome 7
- Growth hormone deficient dwarfism
- Pregnancy-induced hypertension
- Cystic fibrosis
- Severe obesity

Chromosome 8
- Hemolytic anemia
- Burkitt lymphoma

Chromosome 9
- Dilated cardiomyopathy
- Fructose intolerance

Chromosome 10
- Congenital cataracts
- Late-onset Cockayne syndrome

Chromosome 11
- Sickle cell anemia
- Albinism

Chromosome 12
- Inflammatory bowel disease
- Rickets

Chromosome 13
- Breast cancer, early onset
- Retinoblastoma
- Pancreatic cancer

Chromosome 14
- Lukemia/T-cell lymphoma
- Goiter

Chromosome 15
- Marfan syndrome
- Juvenile epilepsy

Chromosome 16
- Polycystic kidney disease
- Familial gastric cancer
- Tuberous sclerosis-2

Chromosome 17 (shown at right)

Chromosome 18
- Diabetes mellitus
- Familial carpal tunnel syndrome

Chromosome 19
- Myotonic dystrophy
- Malignant hyperthermia

Chromosome 20
- Isolated growth hormone deficiency
- Fatal familial insomnia

Chromosome 21
- Autoimmune polyglandular disease
- Amyotrophic lateral sclerosis

Chromosome 22
- Ewing sarcoma
- Giant cell fibroblastoma

X chromosome
- Colorblindness
- Mental retardation
- Gout
- Hemophilia
- Male pseudo-hermaphroditism

Y chromosome
- Gonadal dysgenesis

Mitochondrial DNA
- Leber hereditary optic neuropathy
- Diabetes and deafness
- Myopathy and cardiomyopathy
- Dystonia

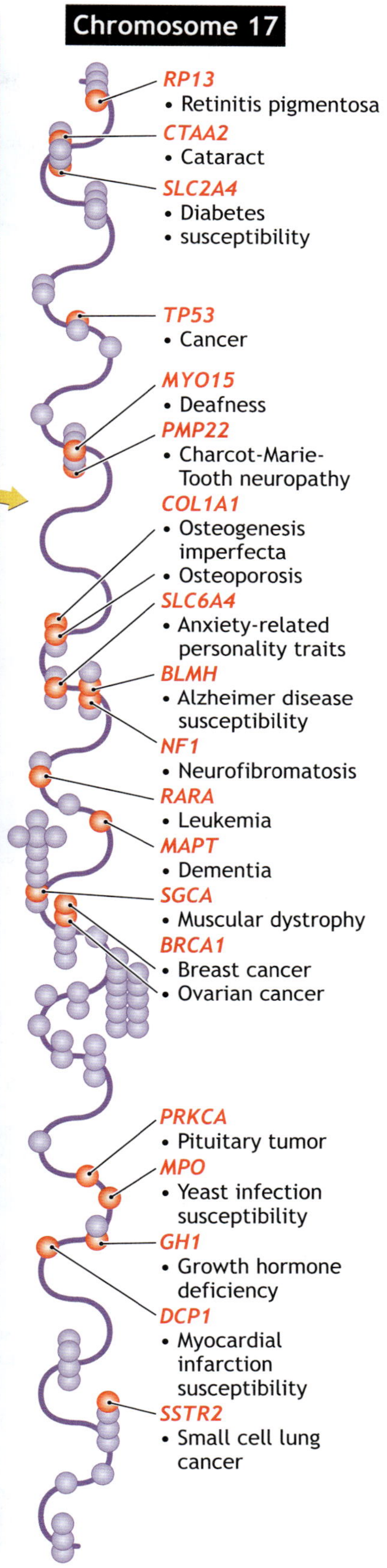

Chromosome 17

- *RP13* — Retinitis pigmentosa
- *CTAA2* — Cataract
- *SLC2A4* — Diabetes susceptibility
- *TP53* — Cancer
- *MYO15* — Deafness
- *PMP22* — Charcot-Marie-Tooth neuropathy
- *COL1A1* — Osteogenesis imperfecta; Osteoporosis
- *SLC6A4* — Anxiety-related personality traits
- *BLMH* — Alzheimer disease susceptibility
- *NF1* — Neurofibromatosis
- *RARA* — Leukemia
- *MAPT* — Dementia
- *SGCA* — Muscular dystrophy
- *BRCA1* — Breast cancer; Ovarian cancer
- *PRKCA* — Pituitary tumor
- *MPO* — Yeast infection susceptibility
- *GH1* — Growth hormone deficiency
- *DCP1* — Myocardial infarction susceptibility
- *SSTR2* — Small cell lung cancer

FIGURE 33.33. Links on the body's chromosomes to specific cancer, metabolic-endocrine, neurologic-psychiatric, and cardiovascular disorders. **(A)** Chromosome 17 designates the specific gene name and specific location in *red*.

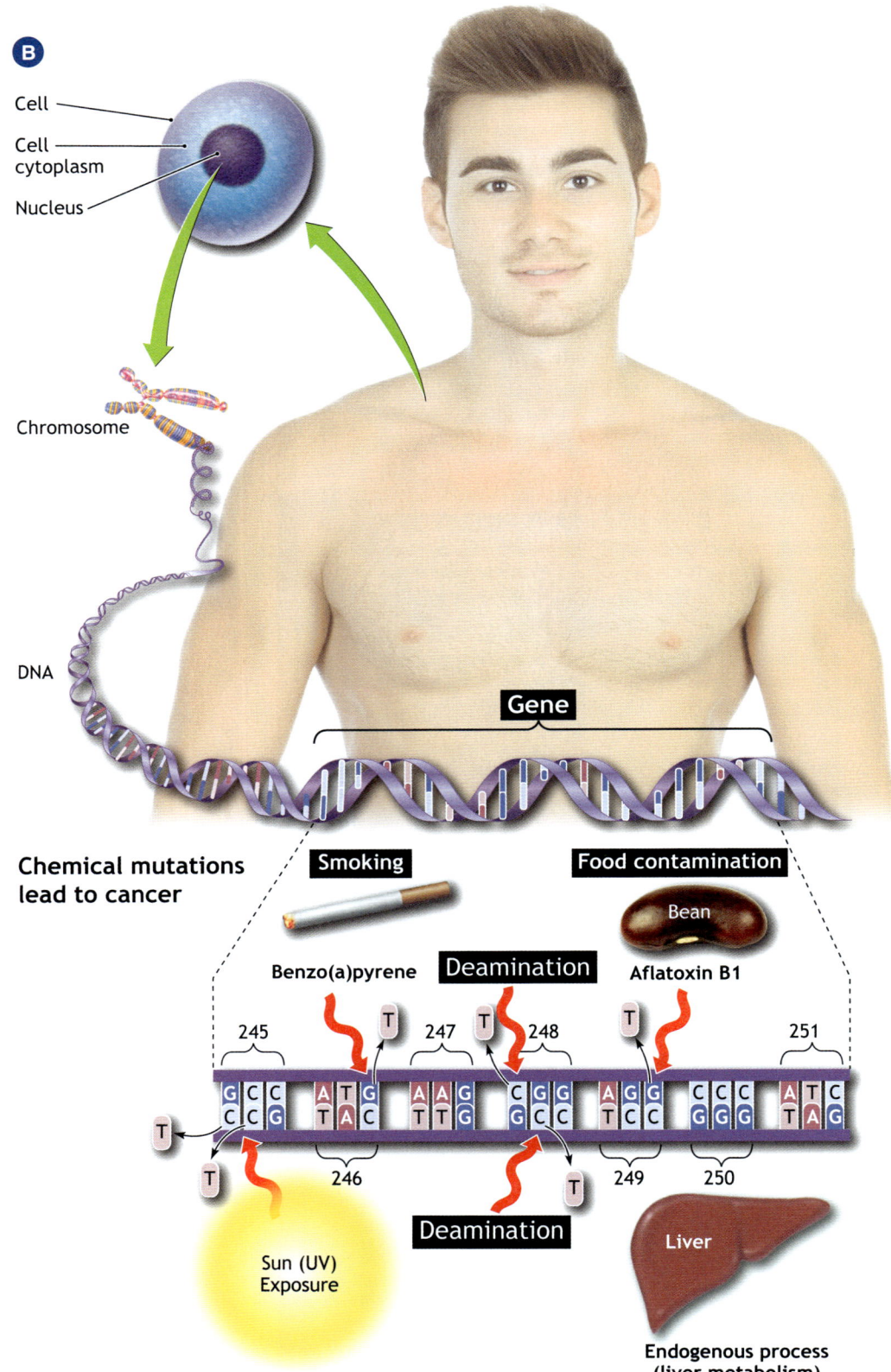

FIGURE 33.33. *(continued)* **(B)** How different carcinogens impact the p53 gene nucleotide sequence responsible for about 50% of human cancers. The p53 gene's name comes from the product it encodes, a polypeptide with a molecular mass of 53,000 daltons (Da), where 1 Da equals 1/12th the mass for carbon-12; for comparison, a water molecule weighs 18 Da and hemoglobin weighs 64,500 Da. In chemical terms, one hydrogen molecular atom has molecular mass = 1 Da, so 1 Da = 1 g · mole^{-1} (mol). To convert mol to g, multiply the mole value for the substance by its molar mass, where mol = g · molar mass^{-1}.
(Shutterstock images: Ninetechno [bean], Gelpi [man].)

biologically active DNA (www.nobelprize.org/nobel_prizes/medicine/laureates/1959). Three years later in 1970, David Baltimore 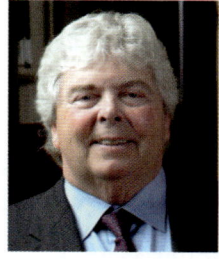 (1938–; www.nasonline.org/member-directory/members/58030.html), Renato Dulbecco 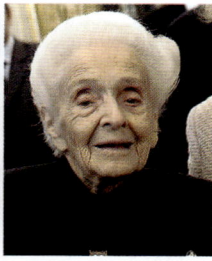 (1914–2012; www.nobelprize.org/prizes/medicine/1975/dulbecco/biographical/), and Howard Temin 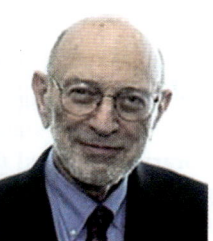 (1934–1994; www.nobelprize.org/prizes/medicine/1975/temin/biographical/) won the 1975 Nobel Prize in Physiology or Medicine for their discoveries concerning the interaction between tumor viruses and a cell's genetic material (www.nobelprize.org/nobel_prizes/medicine/laureates/1975/). They discovered that a specific enzyme tumor virus enzyme called reverse transcriptase made a DNA copy from RNA. The researchers used purified mRNA from muscle or liver tissue to show that this enzyme interacts with the mRNA. **Reverse transcriptase** duplicates the mRNA to the specific **complementary DNA (cDNA)** sequence. DNA polymerase then converts the single-stranded DNA to a double strand for eventual cloning into a bacteriophage or other vector. These experiments proved transfer in the genetic material's content stored in DNA. Subsequent experiments proved that purified DNA from one cell introduced into other cells produce new RNA tumor virus particles.

In 1973, two American researchers introduced the recombinant DNA technique shown schematically in **FIGURE 33.34**;

Stanley Cohen, Rita Levi-Montalcini, and Herbert Boyer. (Boyer photo attribution: Science History Institute; licensed under Creative Commons Attribution Share-Alike 3.0 Unported license: https://creativecommons.org/licenses/by-sa/3.0/deed.en. Stanley photo courtesy NICHD-NIH. Levi-Montalcini photo attribution: Presidenza della Repubblica Italiana.)

they were Stanford University's (Palo Alto, California) Stanley Cohen (1922–2020; www.nobelprize.org/prizes/medicine/1986/cohen/biographical/; https://circulatingnow.nlm.nih.gov/2019/01/24/stanley-n-cohen-papers-open-for-research/), a cofounder of Genentech (www.gene.com/), a pioneering biotechnology corporation, and Herbert Boyer (1916–2020; www.ncbi.nlm.nih.gov/pmc/articles/PMC2741595/), recipient of the 1986 Nobel Prize in Physiology or Medicine with Rita Levi-Montalcini (1909–2012; www.nobelprize.org/prizes/medicine/1986/levi-montalcini/biographical/) for discoveries to understand mechanisms regulating cell and organ growth (www.nobelprize.org/nobel_prizes/medicine/laureates/1986/). They cut DNA from an amphibian gene (primitive frog *Xenopus*) into segments, using a restriction endonuclease enzyme (*Eco*RI) to cut the plasmid (FIGURE 33.34). They then rejoined the 9000-nucleotide segment to form a circular plasmid called pSC101, so named by Cohen because it was the 101st plasmid he isolated.

Their experimental procedure, explained further in the section on RNA cloning, produced the first plasmid to clone a vertebrate gene. In essence, the frog-bacterial molecule represented recombinant DNA using gene splicing to rejoin plasmid pSC101 two ends. Consider this technique as "cutting" and "pasting" text or images from one document section to another into a computer word processing program. The endonuclease first cleaves the amphibian DNA to set it free. The two ends in the rRNA gene now join the pSC101 plasmid cleaved by *Eco*RI. Fundamentally, gene splicing creates a new genetic blueprint in a test tube that leapfrogs nature's own genetic engineering methods based on natural selection, a process that has commingled genes within Earth's plant and animal species over millions of millennia. Scientists can now short-circuit nature's process in hours and produce thousands of DNA's exact nucleotide sequence from a particular gene in a genome. By manipulating DNA's configuration, a newly created gene can insert into plant and animal cells to create new cells or species with unique characteristics expressed by the newly created genetic instructions.

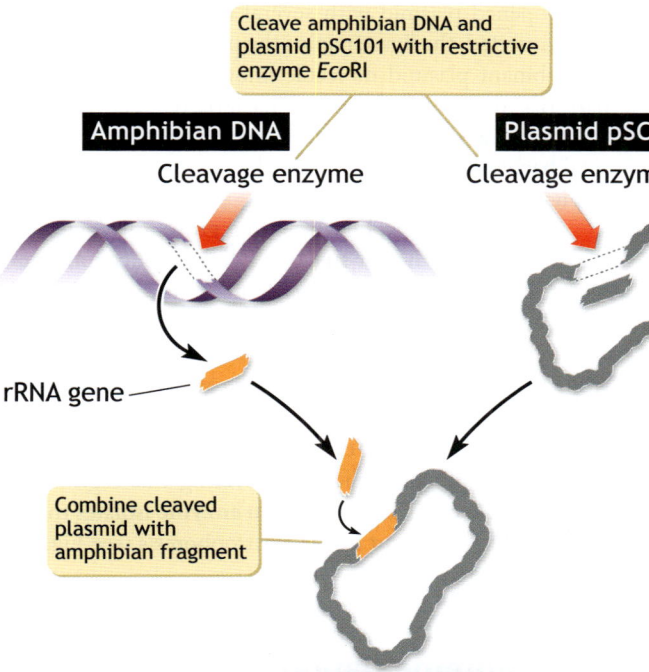

FIGURE 33.34. In 1973, Drs. Stanley Cohen and Herbert Boyer, genetic engineering pioneers, produced the first recombinant DNA organism using the restriction endonuclease enzyme (*Eco*RI). Their pioneering experiment combined the cleaved plasmid vector (pSC101 shown at the *right*) with an amphibian DNA fragment (shown at the *top left*) using restriction endonuclease enzyme (*Eco*RI) to produce the recombinant plasmid shown at the *bottom*. The cells that contained the plasmid that carried the tetracycline gene grew and formed a cell colony containing the frog ribosomal RNA gene.

DNA Cloning Isolates Human Genes

DNA **cloning** progresses in several stages. The first involves mechanically breaking the genetic material within a DNA sample or, alternatively, using restriction endonucleases that precisely cut the nucleotide sequence along DNA's double helix into smaller segments to facilitate manipulation. The collecting DNA pieces formed by endonuclease cleavage represent single, random DNA segments, which represent all the organism's genetic material. The term **genomic library** describes the cloned fragment collection. Many genomic libraries exist in the public domain (e.g., https://musagenomics.org), so researchers can use them without having to reduplicate a DNA sequence. **FIGURE 33.35** shows forming a genomic library from human DNA. This basic strategy led to tremendous advances in the role such techniques play in the medical sciences.[10,68,165]

A **restriction endonuclease** cleaves a short human double helix chromosomal DNA strand, usually four to six base pairs in length, into millions of fragments. Restriction endonucleases have become a fundamental tool in molecular biology research because DNA treatment with the same restriction endonuclease allows any two DNA fragments to join together—providing an essentially endless DNA supply for further experimentation. A widely used chemical techniques, **gel electrophoresis** (Greek *phoresis*, "to be carried"), was perfected by Arne Wilhelm Tiselius 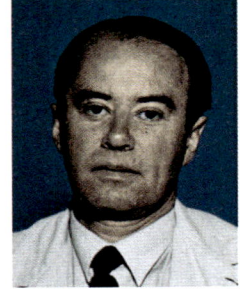 (1902–1971; www.nobelprize.org/nobel_prizes/chemistry/laureates/1948/tiselius-bio.html), recipient of the 1948 Nobel prize in Chemistry for research on electrophoresis and adsorption analysis and discoveries concerning separating DNA fragments within an electric field. The DNA strands inserted into a circular plasmid carrier molecule recombine the DNA (hence the term *recombinant DNA*). This occurs when the enzyme DNA ligase, by adding ATP, covalently links the DNA fragment to the previously opened plasmid with several thousand nucleotide pairs. Once inserted, the ligase rejoins the plasmid to produce the new recombinant plasmid molecule known as a **vector**. Recombinant plasmids are inserted into bacteria (e.g., *E. coli*) to ensure that only one bacterium receives one plasmid. At this stage, the total bacterial culture represents the genomic library illustrated in Figure 33.35.

Arne Wilhelm Tiselius

The next stage in DNA cloning grows the bacterium in a nutrient-rich broth that sustains cell multiplication that doubles its number every hour. This doubles the recombinant DNA copies. By simple multiplication, doubling the DNA copies each hour over 24 hr produces almost 17 million new copies from a single bacterium! The bacteria are destroyed (lysed) and the millions of DNA copies culled from the larger bacterial chromosome, and other cellular contents provide pure original DNA segment replicas. Recovering this segment occurs after the specific **restriction enzyme** isolates the plasma DNA segment by gel electrophoresis (see Fig. 33.38).

FIGURE 33.35. Creating a genomic library from human DNA. The library includes bacteria with specific DNA fragments contained in plasmid carrier-type substances. Note how four different-colored DNA segments (*red, blue, purple, green*) from the original human DNA shown at the top end up within the bacterial host. The remaining DNA fragments also can make clones.

Practical Application in Bioremediation

Implementing bacterial cloning has practical applications in **bioremediation** (http://ei.cornell.edu/biodeg/bioremed/), which uses bacteria to degrade dangerous environmental pollutants.[96,170] For example, the pink-colored bacteria that smell like rotten cabbage, *Deinococcus radiodurans*, shown in **FIGURE 33.36**, have been genetically cloned from *E. coli* strains previously made resistant to toxic wastes (www.genomenewsnetwork.org/articles/07_02/deinococcus.shtml). *D. radiodurans* was isolated in 1956 from ground beef that had been "sterilized" by gamma radiation but

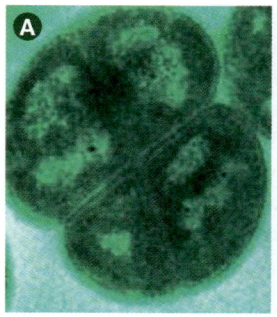 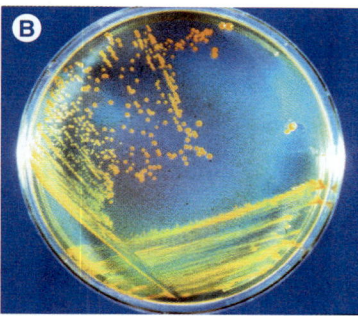

FIGURE 33.36. Bioremediation. **(A)** *Deinococcus radiodurans* electron photomicrograph sequenced in the Department of Energy Microbial Genome Program[4] as a cluster of four cells or tetrad. *D. radiodurans* and related species have been identified worldwide, 77 including in Antarctic granite and in tanks with powerful cobalt-60 irradiators in Denmark. **(B)** Nutrient agar plate growing *D. radiodurans*; the *orange color* is from carotenoid pigment.
(Images from the Uniformed Services University of the Health Sciences, Bethesda, MD; www.usuhs.mil.)

still spoiled. Researchers determined that *D. radiodurans* survived approximately 17 kGy (1.7 million rads), a value equal to 3000 times the lethal human radiation dose. The *D. radiodurans* economic value is straightforward. Producing trillions of the new bacterium has the potential to save close to a trillion dollars in biohazard cleanup. For example, *D. radiodurans* consumes heavy metals and radioactive waste and thus has an ability to scavenge toxic wastes buried at more than 1300 toxic waste sites throughout the United States (www.statista.com/statistics/1147665/number-of-hazardous-waste-sites-in-the-united-states/). Across the United States, New Jersey has the most hazardous waste sites (114), followed by California (97) and Pennsylvania (91). The fewest sites are in Nevada, District of Columbia, and Wyoming (1).

Researchers have also fused a gene that encodes toluene dioxygenase (the enzyme that decomposes toluene) to a *D. radiodurans* promoter (site activating the gene) and then inserted it into a bacterium chromosome. The resulting recombinant bacterium "upgraded" *D. radiodurans* for degrading toluene and other organic compounds at levels that exceed those at radioactive waste sites. *D. radiodurans* not only survives high radiation doses but also long dehydration and ultraviolet irradiation periods. *D. radiodurans* apparently repairs its radiation-damaged DNA base pairs by redundant genetic "signals." The 2-billion-year-old microbe has from 4 to 10 DNA molecules. The protein RecA matches the damaged DNA base pairs and splices them together. During the repair process, cell-building activities shut down, and the broken DNA pieces remain in place. The complete decoded *D. radiodurans* genome can be retrieved from the J. Craig Venter Institute Web site (www.jcvi.org/). The DNA in *D. radiodurans* has 3.3 million chemical base units. The genome contains two circular chromosomes, one about 2.6 million and the other 400,000 base pairs, and two smaller circular molecules (megaplasmid with 177,000 base pairs and 45,000 base pair plasmids). Despite its high tolerance for radioactivity, *D. radiodurans* decomposes at 45°C/113°F.

In addition to unraveling *D. radiodurans's* secrets, the Institute published the first diploid human genome[190] and ongoing Sorcerer II Global Ocean Sampling Expedition (www.jcvi.org/research/gos). The quest was to unlock ocean secrets by sampling, sequencing, and analyzing the ocean microorganism's DNA.[212] Thus far, scientists have uncovered more than 60 million new genes from the Sorcerer II Global Expedition (www.jcvi.org/research/gos) and nearly 1000 novel protein families from the seawater organisms during global circumnavigation experiments. The ongoing research efforts include sampling water off the California and United States western coastlines and sampling with other collaborators in Antarctica and deep-sea ocean vents.[192,265,266] In addition, researchers sequenced the microbial flora found in human environments (www.jcvi.org/about/overview/; microbiome, oral cavity, vagina, digestive tract).

Locating Specific Genes with Plasmids

Creating cloned DNA involves locating a specific gene within the plasmid or viral culture. Consider the analogy when entering a five-story department store that lacks signs or a computer database to search for a single unmarked item. One could begin searching on the first floor, proceeding to every shelf and cupboard on every floor until finding the item, but the inefficiency in this strategy seems obvious. To facilitate locating a specific gene, a specific **DNA probe** with known nucleotide sequence, labeled with colored fluorescent markers or **radioisotopes**, searches the genomic library for identifiable DNA fragments among millions of existing gene sequences. This process continues until the probe locates a matching code on a specific chromosomal gene or a specific RNA sequence in cells or tissues.

The Search Becomes Complicated

Searching for a single gene remains complicated because the gene can contain both coding exons and noncoding introns. If the clone with its isolated sequences contains only exons (i.e., only the uninterrupted coding sequences), then the new genomic library is known as a **cDNA library** (the *c* refers to a copy or complementary DNA). Different cDNA libraries reflect different tissues because the libraries contain the specifically transcribed mRNA from the original source tissue. A cDNA library contains the gene's coding regions, often including the leading and trailing mRNA sequences.[191] Non-functioning chromosomal DNA creates **cDNA** clone's most distinguishing characteristic. The reverse transcriptase enzyme uses the source cell or tissue mRNA to construct DNA. Cloning cDNA molecules is comparable to cloning genomic DNA fragments. Each different tissue type (e.g., heart, liver, kidney) has a different cDNA library associated with it. Cloned DNA makes it possible to manufacture exact and "pure" genetic copies relatively quickly from among millions of nucleotide sequences. The uninterrupted coding sequence for a particular gene gives the cDNA clone a clear advantage for duplicating the gene in bulk or deducing a protein's amino acid sequence. Like genomic libraries, cDNA libraries exist in the public domain for sharing among researchers; commercial vendors also make them available for purchase. Many Internet sites provide valuable links to

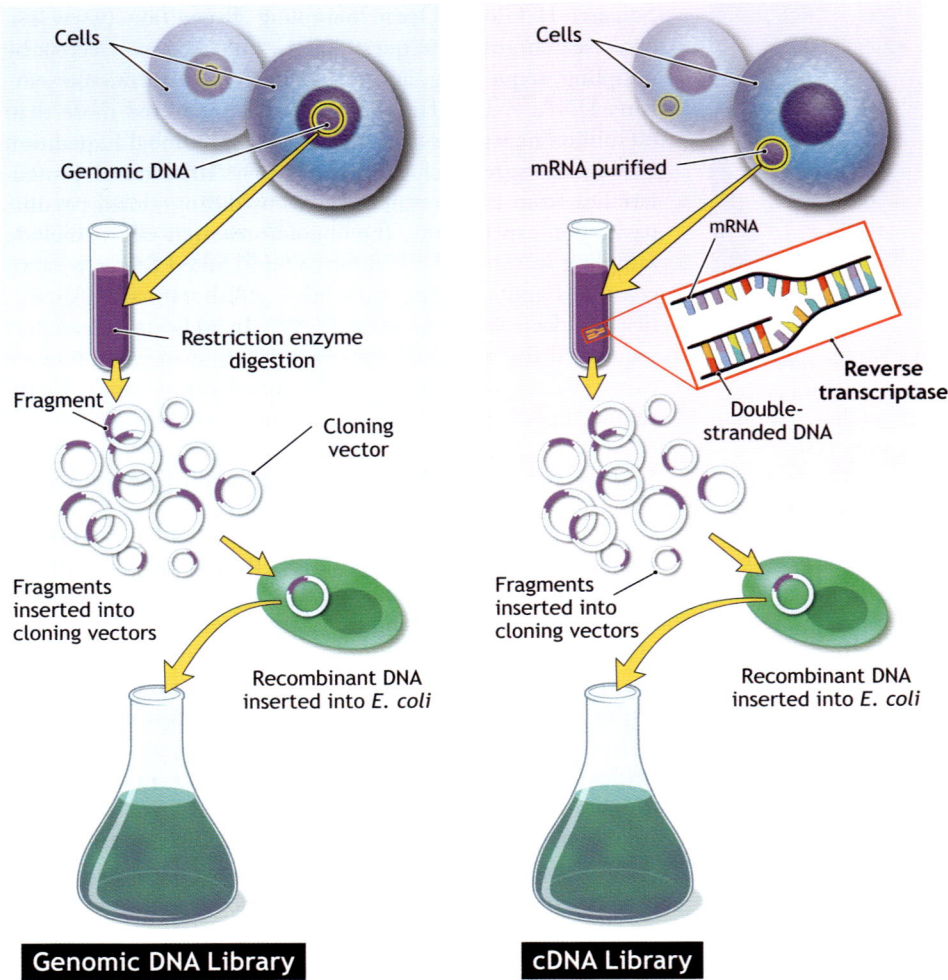

FIGURE 33.37. Basic differences in creating genomic DNA and cDNA libraries.

they pass through the electric field from top (negative) to bottom (positive) through an agarose gel slab. Heating the gel causes its protein fibers to congeal and form a grid through which DNA fragments pass. Separating DNA fragments by size in an electric field allows for distinguishing them among DNA segments. Note the bands at the gel's *lower right panel*. These represent smaller DNA fragments than the upper longer fragments. The DNA shows up clearly because soaking the medium with a DNA-specific or RNA-specific dye (ethidium bromide) stains DNA orange (purplish in photo) under **ultraviolet light**. DNA extraction provides pure DNA fragments used in cloning experiments or for matching to other DNA fragments.[79,151]

Figure 33.38B shows an alternative **autoradiography** technique using the labeled radioisotope ^{32}P to expose DNA bands when photographic paper placed over the gel reveals particles emitted from the isotope. **FIGURE 33.39** illustrates three gel transfer methods to separate genetic material fragments and proteins—**Southern blot**, **Northern blot**, and **Western blot** (www.youtube.com/watch?v=Pt_NaNExry8).

databases for mammals and other vertebrates, fungi, plants, eukaryotes, prokaryotes, viruses, specific gene groups, and large-scale genome sequencing centers (e.g., www.ddbj.nig.ac.jp/index-e.html). **FIGURE 33.37** illustrates the basic difference in creating genomic DNA and cDNA libraries. In both cases, fragments representing digested DNA (shown as *purple* fragments) insert into cloning vectors such as a **bacteriophage** or phage (from the Greek "to devour"), a virus that invades and then replicates within bacteria. These structures populate the biosphere and are omnipresent in seawater, soils, and animal intestinal flora.[192]

Electrophoresis and Gel Transfer Methods

The electrophoresis technique moves proteins through an electrically charged supporting medium. The negatively charged phosphate groups in DNA molecules migrate to the apparatus positive pole (anode). **FIGURE 33.38A** shows two ways to separate DNA fragments. The top example (A) shows cutting the same DNA molecule from the one (bacteriophage) genome with two different restriction endonucleases, *Eco*RI and *Hin*dIII (numerous other enzymes with distinct isolated specificity). Small fragments migrate faster than large fragments when

DNA Amplification with the Polymerase Chain Reaction

The **polymerase chain reaction (PCR)** method, developed in 1987 by American biochemist Kary Banks Mullis (1944–; 1993 Nobel Prize in Chemistry [www.nobelprize.org/prizes/chemistry/1993/mullis/biographical/]; PCR method inventor), represents a milestone in molecular biology[114] (http://siarchives.si.edu/research/videohistory_catalog9577.html). The PCR method, carried out *in vitro* without prior transfer in living cells, artificially amplifies an extremely small DNA amount and rapidly creates billions of copies in a single molecule's specific DNA region.

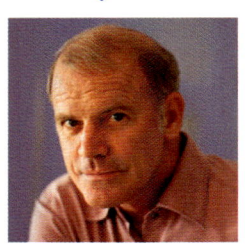

Kary Banks Mullis

FIGURE 33.40 illustrates the basic PCR concept in which purified DNA polymerase copies a DNA template in three replication cycles. In the first initial cycle step, a tiny double-stranded DNA sample then is heated to about 94°C/201.2°F for several min to denature (separate) the strands. Each strand has a known nucleotide sequence on the target nucleotides. Next, two specifically designed synthetic primers with known DNA

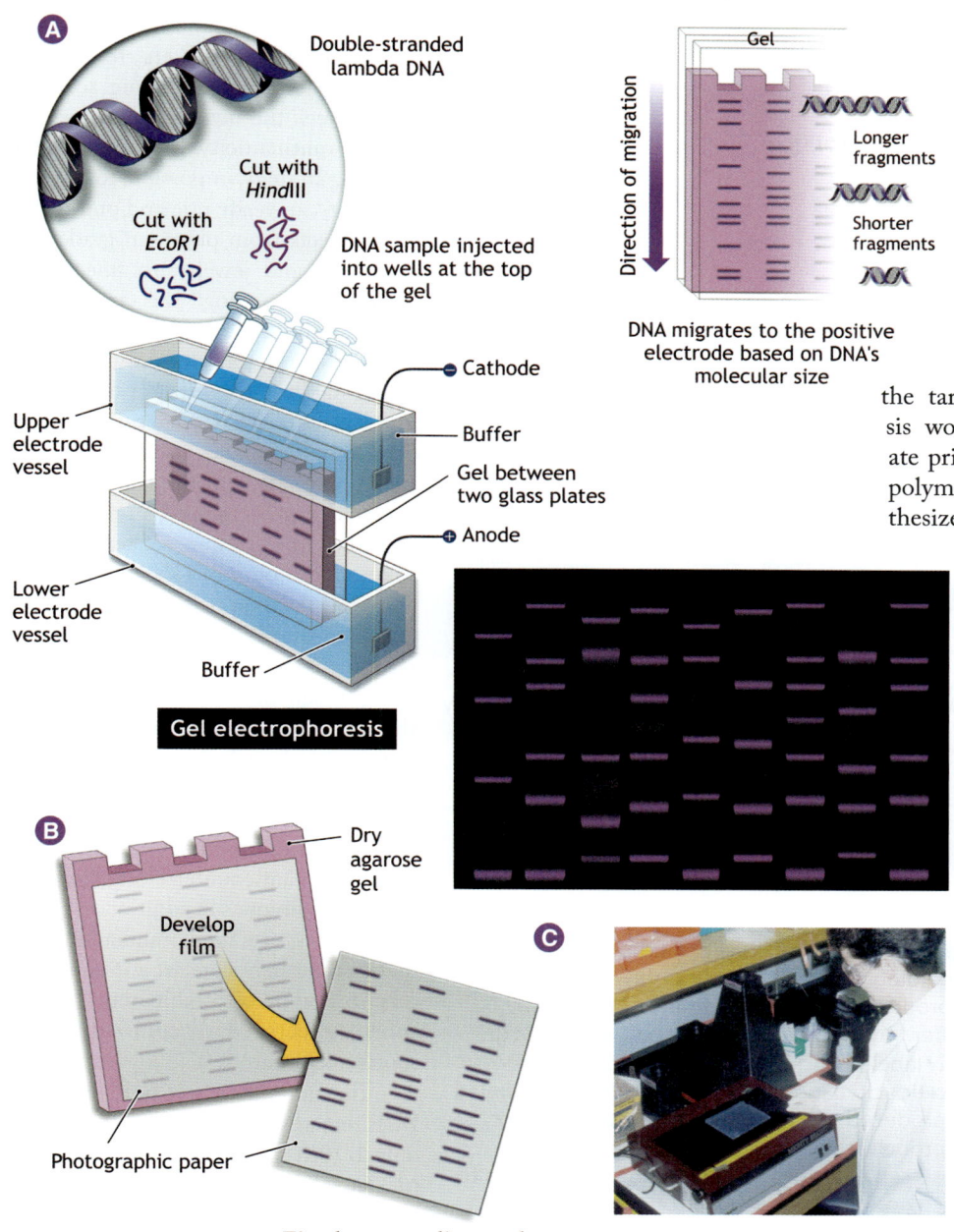

FIGURE 33.38. Gel electrophoresis: separating DNA fragments by molecular size. **(A)** Two restriction endonucleases cleave DNA into two segments to place atop a thin agarose gel slab supported in a vertical position. An electric current separates the DNA fragments as they pass through the hydrated gel according to their mobility; small fragments move more quickly through the electric current and fixate at the bottom of the gel at the positive electrode. Larger fragments settle nearer to the top. The *top right photo* reveals the DNA bands fluoresced under ultraviolet light. Note: The restriction enzyme takes the initials of the bacterial type and strain from its source; *Eco*RI refers to *Escherichia coli* strain RY13, and the 1 means this restriction enzyme was found first in the strain. The cleavage site is 5–GAATTC–3 and 3CTTAAG–5; the *Hind*III source is *Haemophilus influenzae* Rd. The cleavage site is 5–AAGCTT–3 and 3–TTCGAA–5. **(B)** Autoradiography technique displays radioisotope 32P-labeled DNA bands on exposed photographic paper placed over the agarose gel. **(C)** Dr. Kristin Stuempfle, Department of Health and Exercise Sciences, Gettysburg College, reviews a sequencing gel film on a light box. (Gel micrograph image: extender_01/Shutterstock.)

words, only the target sequence, bracketed by the primers, duplicates because no primers attach elsewhere along the DNA fragment.

The annealing process cannot withstand the initial high temperature required to separate the double helix, so it occurs at a lower 54°C/129.2°F. At this temperature, the single-stranded DNA fragments match complementary nucleotide sequences at the ends in the target DNA sequence. DNA synthesis would not proceed without appropriate primers. Adding a heat-resistant DNA polymerase to the reaction in cycle 3 synthesizes a new DNA strand to create two strands. The most widely used thermostable DNA polymerase (Taq) then separates from the heat-resistant bacterium *Thermus aquaticus*. The temperature, now increased to 70°C/158°F, lets the polymerase elongate new DNA strands that begin at the primers. The PCR technique requires that reactants cycle through a varied temperature profile during incubation, and the PCR apparatus (thermocycler) automatically progresses through a preset thermal sequence. The first cycle, repeated 20 to 40 times, doubles the DNA amount synthesized in each succeeding cycle. After 30 cycles, what began as a single DNA molecule increases dramatically into more than a billion new copies ($2^{30} = 1.02 \times 10^9$).

The PCR method only clones DNA fragments with known beginning and ending sequences. With prior knowledge about the code, it takes only 20 repeat cycles to duplicate enough target DNA to produce 1,048,536 original sequence copies (2^{20}). The second and third cycles displayed in Figure 33.40 show how the three different PCR cycles eventually copy millions or billions original DNA sequences. Note the example for three cycles at the right of the figure. The second cycle repeats the first cycle. It progresses through each temperature change, first to separate strands at about 94°C/201.2°F, then to anneal the primers at a cooler 54°C/129.2°F, and finally through polymerase action to make two additional DNA strands at 72°C/161.6°F. Note that the

sequences (shown in *green* and *red*) hybridize or **anneal** to one of the two separated strands at the exact beginning and ending position along the target DNA nucleotide sequence. In other

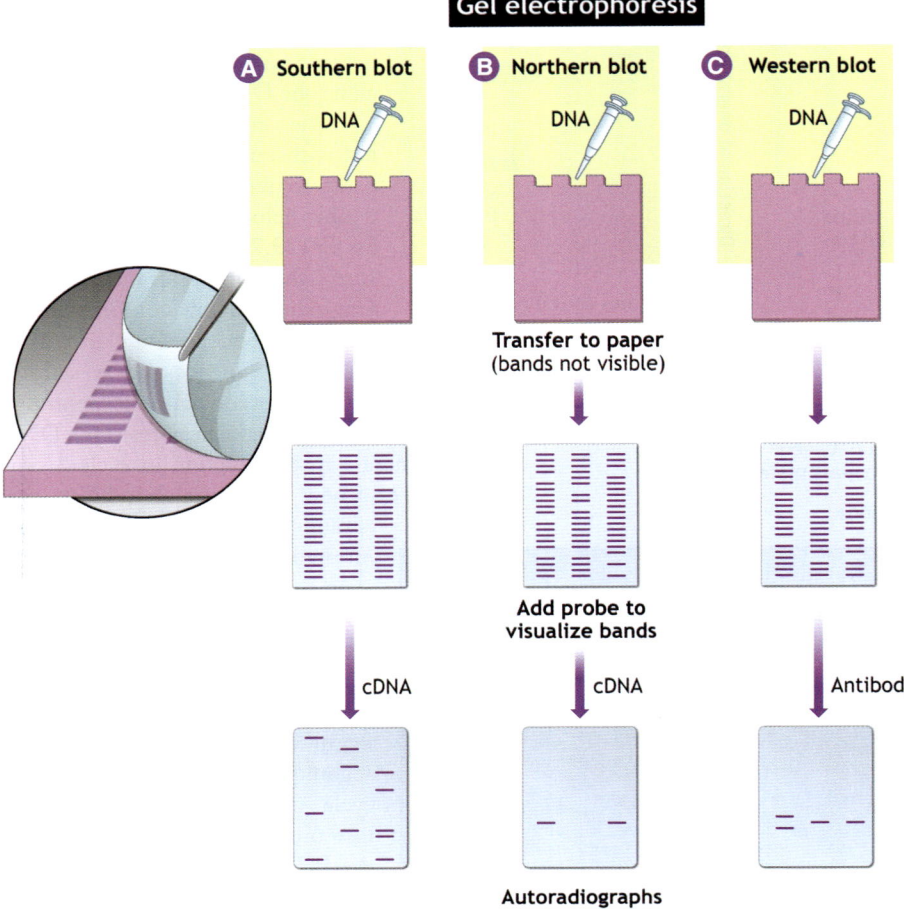

FIGURE 33.39. Identifying DNA sequences by three gel transfer methods. **(A)** Southern blot (named to honor British molecular biologist Dr. E. M. Southern; www.genome.gov/genetics-glossary/Southern-Blot) produced when single-stranded DNA on a sheet of nitrocellulose is placed in a buffer tray atop a sponge. The pattern on the gel is copied or "blotted" to the radioactively labeled nucleic acids. This process produces radioactive bands, which allows the nucleic acid bands to hybridize with bands labeled by radioactivity. **(B)** Northern blots are produced when RNA on a nitrocellulose blot hybridizes with a single-stranded DNA probe without using alkali (alkali hydrolyzes RNA). **(C)** Western blot gel electrophoresis separates proteins using antibody probes to target specific proteins.

third cycle produces eight double-stranded DNA molecules. After seven cycles, the newly created DNA double strands with flush ends (same length) uniquely identical to the original target sequence. The next 17 cycles produce the additional 1,048,528 copies, and just 10 more cycles produce 1000 million more target molecules!

PCR Applications

The PCR technique has impacted numerous fields besides molecular biology[69]; they include biotechnology, entomology and the environmental sciences, molecular epidemiology, forensic science, genetic engineering, most medical specialties, microbiology, proteomics, the food industry, and even apparel manufacturing. At the 2000 Sydney Olympic Games, for example, a special ink containing a small DNA snippet from a saliva swab from two Australian athletes was attached to labels, tags, pins, and official Olympic merchandise stickers to thwart counterfeiters. An electronic scanner could check the invisible ink to verify an item's authenticity. The same DNA-marking strategy, impossible to reverse engineer, can verify rare and one-of-a-kind objects from premium grade oil, diamonds and jewelry, to fine wine. The DNA "tagging" was applied to items at the 2013 Super Bowl game (see "DNA Tagging to Thwart Counterfeit Collectables at Major Sporting Events"). PCR also can identify diverse viruses and bacteria or any DNA extracted from a current or ancient plant or animal organism. It identifies the unique sequence in a miniscule amount of DNA nucleotide material, even in substances formed early in the Earth's creation. More recent guidance from the Center for Drug Evaluation and Research from the FDA (www.fda.gov/regulatory-information) includes new physical-chemical identifiers to track and then authenticate legitimate drug products through the pharmaceutical supply chain as an anticounterfeiting strategy. Similar techniques in addition to those applied to sports memorabilia now are routinely authenticate art antiques and other precious collectable items (www.sportscollectorsdaily.com/category/sports-memorabilia/).

The amplification potential for PCR remains truly awesome. It requires only 1/10th to one-millionth liter (0.1 µL) in saliva or another body fluid or tissue to prove that the genetic sample's sequence originated from a specific person or species. The PCR method can easily produce 1 g of substance (about 500 base pairs long), equal to one-millionth gram (10^6), enough to completely sequence or clone DNA. In fact, beginning with less than a picogram (0.000 000 000 001 or 10^{12} g) DNA with 10,000 nucleotides (about 100,000 molecules) chain length, PCR will produce several micrograms in DNA (10^{11} molecules). The applications seem right out of science fiction movies. Scientists have identified the genetic blueprint in insects trapped within 80-million-year-old amber (fossilized pine resin) from a miniscule DNA sample using present-day insects to "match" the DNA sequences. In a controversial report published in *Nature*,[275] scientists reported reviving a bacterium spore from a drop of fluid trapped for 250 million years in a crystal from rock salt excavated 1850 ft below the Earth's surface. In some extinct fossils, not enough DNA sequences exist for cloning because the DNA decomposes significantly every 5000 years. Although some gene fragments may survive, clon-

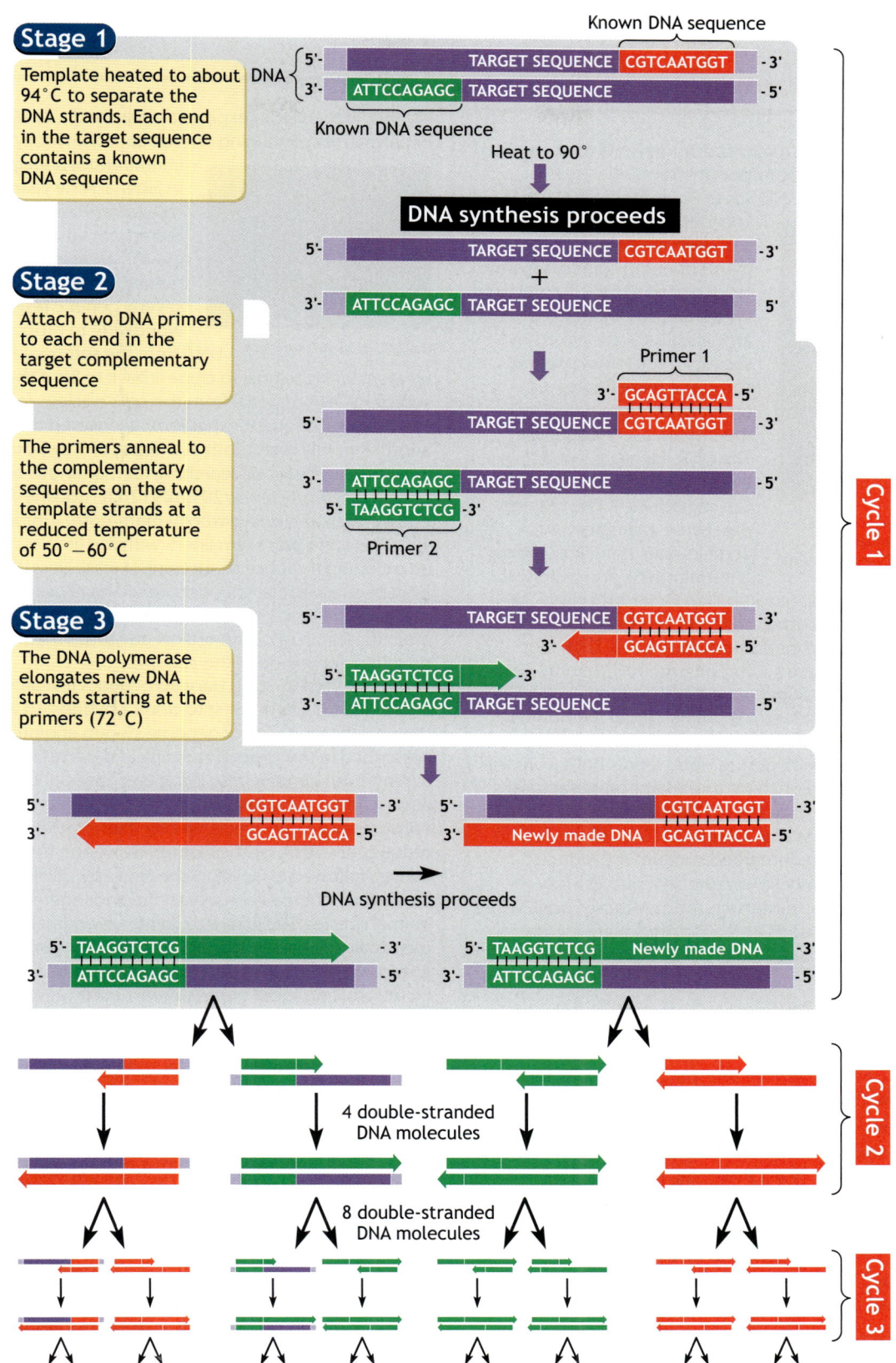

FIGURE 33.40. Artificial DNA amplification using the polymerase chain reaction (PCR). **Cycle 1.** Three stages during the first PCR cycle. **Cycle 2.** Produces four double DNA strands. **Cycle 3.** Produces eight double-stranded DNA molecules. Each succeeding cycle produces twice as much DNA as in the prior cycle. Thirty cycles produce more than 1 billion DNA fragments, and in several hours, hundreds of billions more exact copies. The thermocycler PCR apparatus controls reaction temperature to ensure that repeated replication cycles and separation occur systematically on a preset schedule.

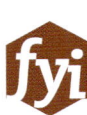

DNA Tagging to Thwart Counterfeit Collectables at Major Sporting Events

DNA tagging continues at major sporting events to uncover fraudulent claims regarding important items related to important events. At the 2013 Super Bowl, for example, over 100 footballs, sideline pylons, and even the coin used for the game-opening coin toss were tagged with a specially prepared synthetic DNA ink that leaves an invisible-to-the-naked-eye security mark (www.psadna.com). The mark fluoresces green when illuminated by the proper laser frequency. The DNA ink has a 1-in-33 trillion chance counterfeiters can reproduce it. The tagging procedure examines and certifies over 18 million sports, entertainment, and historical collectibles with a combined $1 billion value, including the world's most valuable football card, the certified 1935 Bronko Nagurski National Chicle card sold for $350,000. DNA tags also include Mark McGuire's 70th homerun ball, Sammy Sosa autographed baseballs, Super Bowl XXXV artifacts, well-known sports artists' paintings, Warner Brothers Studio memorabilia, counterfeit military electronic tracking parts, pellets filled with DNA in police surveillance during riots, tennis balls from the US Open Tennis Championships, and major manufacturer's apparel. A 2020 report from the US Department of Homeland Security (DHS) estimates that losses to U.S. businesses from the counterfeiting of trademarked consumer products exceed $509 billion yearly (www.dhs.gov/publication/combating-trafficking-counterfeit-and-pirated-goods), while seizures of infringing goods at U.S. borders have increased 10-fold between 2000 and 2018 from 3244 seizures yearly to 33,810.

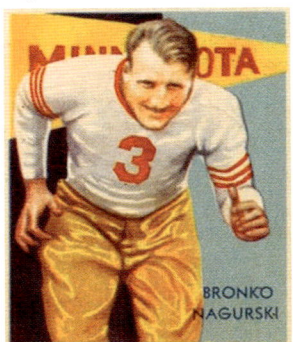

Bronco Nagurski. (Image of card courtesy Vintage Football Card Gallery, www.footballcardgallery.com)

---

ing a "Jurassic Park" prehistoric monster falls outside the realm of possibility with today's available molecular paleoarcheology technologies. While cloning may never occur for prehistoric animals, animals from the Pleistocene era may become candidates for cloning (e.g., Pyrenean ibex, Tasmanian tiger, woolly mammoth, and saber-toothed cats; www.treehugger.com/extinct-animals-that-could-be-resurrected-4869339). Advocates for cloning prehistoric or extinct animals believe that the time will come when biomolecular systems involving gene editing will be sufficiently advanced to accomplish what today is not possible (www.the-scientist.com/news-opinion/the-booming-call-of-de-extinction-68057).

In forensic medicine, a single hair salvaged from a crime scene compares for its DNA sequence to hair samples from a suspect or victim (www.ncjrs.gov/pdffiles1/nij/bc000614.pdf). When a PCR-generated DNA sequence matches the original DNA template strand sequence, misidentifying the true suspect becomes almost infinitesimal against a coinciden-

Is Cloning an Extinct Mammal Possible?

In 1999, French polar explorers unearthed a 23,000-lb block of permafrost containing the remains of a woolly mammoth (*Mammuthus primigenius*) in Siberia. Nine years later, researchers sequenced this extinct mammoth's nuclear genome (www.nature.com/articles/nature07446). This finding led to several genetic research facilities worldwide to propose extracting DNA from the soft tissues of the extinct creature with the goal to clone it back to life if they can extract sufficient DNA material from the cell's nucleus for cloning.[247–250] In 2012, a subsequent expedition uncovered the remains of another woolly mammoth at a depth of 5 to 6 m/16 to 20 ft in a tunnel dug by locals searching for mammoth bones (www.csmonitor.com/Science/2012/0912/Pleistocene-Park-Scientists-edge-closer-to-cloning-woolly-mammoth). Unfortunately, little soft tissue and bone remained (with too little quality DNA) to give cloning a chance to succeed. Nonetheless, had sufficient DNA been available, scientists would have used a cloning method similar to clone Dolly the sheep (see Fig. 33.44; www.animalresearch.info/en/medical-advances/medical-discovery-timeline/cloning-dolly-the-sheep/).

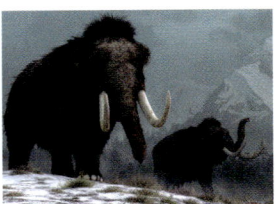

Daniel Eskridge/Shutterstock

Fast forward to 2021. Harvard genetics researchers have embarked on a new quest to clone a hybridized woolly mammoth using CRISPR genome system engineering (described in this chapter) to copy and paste DNA from a mammoth genome into living elephant cell cultures as described in the Revive and Restore project (https://reviverestore.org/projects/woolly-mammoth/). The method requires raw DNA synthesis, then delivering the DNA into a source, followed by splicing the genes by CRISPR gene editing to cut the DNA to eventually create endangered or extinct animal species. The idea is to create "re-engineered" hybrid mammals with many similar traits to the original mammoths to reconvert the permafrost tundra region back to grasslands by introducing these grazers even 10,000 years after their disappearance. The new species would create a nutrient cycle that allows grasses to out-compete the tundra flora, converting the ecosystem favoring grazers and grasses to a new landscape after their disappearance. The approximately 16-square-km/6-square-mile area in Siberia, Russia, currently supports bison, musk ox, moose, horses, and reindeer as explained in these videos, the summary from a TedxTalkDeExtinction by a geneticist involved in the new research project (https://reviverestore.org/projects/woolly-mammoth/; https://reviverestore.org/events/tedxdeextinction/).

Sources:
Clyde D. A new view of genome organization. *Nat Rev Genet*. 2021;22:134.
Novak BJ. De-Extinction. *Genes (Basel)*. 2018;9:548.
Payne AC, et al. In situ genome sequencing resolves DNA sequence and structure in intact biological samples. *Science*. 2021;371:eaay3446.

---

tal DNA match. In fact, if an individual's known DNA profile matches the DNA profile from the crime scene, the probability is 82 billion to 1 that the crime scene DNA comes from that person!

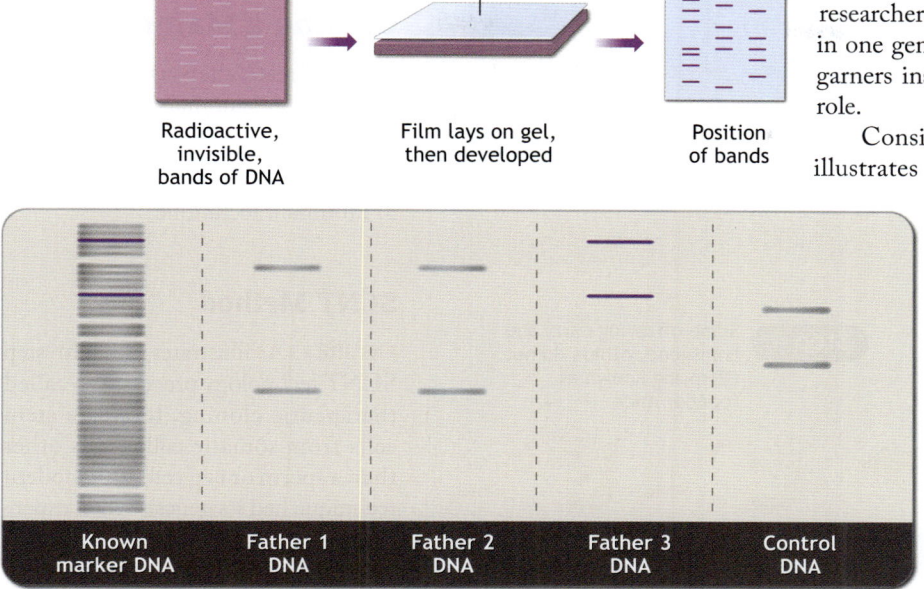

FIGURE 33.41. DNA fingerprinting autoradiography compares DNA fragments after their separation by gel electrophoresis to identify the child's father. Matched DNA banding patterns from different tissues or body fluids confirm the original DNA source. Specific restriction enzymes sever the DNA fragments at precise sites in the chain. Thus, DNA snippets, known as restriction fragment-length polymorphisms (RFLPs), have different lengths and hence different molecular weights. A match between the known marker DNA and the sample (e.g., father 3) provides prima facie direct evidence that father 3 is the biologic father. As of February 3, 2022, over 300 previously convicted criminals, averaging 13 years in prison, have been exonerated based on DNA forensic evidence (https://innocenceproject.org/exonerations-data/).

Paternity cases routinely involve DNA analysis using PCR techniques with DNA fingerprinting autoradiography to identify parental offspring correctly (**FIG. 33.41**). In the figure's example, the DNA from suspected fathers 1 and 2 did not match the known marker DNA from the child; thus father 3, with an exact banding match, was determined the biologic father. The control DNA from a known source verifies the test procedure validity. The many variations in PCR methodology allow researchers to produce hybrid genes with desirable (or undesirable) traits. Fusing DNA segments from different biologic specimens "transferred" to the gel opens an enormous avenue to study cell and tissue genetic variation. It also elucidates how "errors" in specific gene sequences relate to diseases and how genetic engineering can combat them.

Injection Experiments

Injection **transfection** performed in cultured cells refers to a microtechnique to introduce an outside (exogenous) DNA donor source into a recipient host. Injecting purified DNA with a known nucleotide sequence for a particular gene presents a potentially desirable strategy to express a host's outcome trait. Injection strategies have been useful in exercise physiology–related animal research. By injecting a gene with a particular trait into the mother's egg, the new trait in the offspring can be "turned on." This allows researchers to observe how "knocking out" a section in one gene and replacing it with another segment garners insight into that gene product's functional role.

Consider the example in **FIGURE 33.42** that illustrates the basic microinjection principle applied to a mouse model. Immediately after the **gametes** join (one egg and one sperm), a microinjection technique with a thin glass needle inserts a target gene or **transgene** into the larger male **pronucleus** just before the cells fuse into a single egg. The egg, surgically harvested, is then implanted into a female rodent's womb who serves as the "foster" mother. When the mother produces progeny, the newborns, referred to as **founder mice**, should contain a transgene copy on a single chromosome (i.e., **heterozygous** for the transgene). When two founder mice breed, 25% of the progeny receive two transgene copies (i.e., **homozygous** for the transgene), 50% have one transgene, and 25% have no transgenes. These percentages follow basic inheritance laws discovered by geneticist Gregor Mendel (www.dnaftb.org/1/bio.html). Researchers have manipulated hundreds of genetically modified organism (GMO) traits in plants and animals to study metabolic and disease developmental characteristics (www.nature.com/scitable/topicpage/genetically-modified-organisms-gmos-transgenic-crops-and-732/).

Working with **transgenic** organisms has proved beneficial in experimenting with different genetic manipulations including mutated genes to shed light on possible disease mechanisms. Researchers apply four methods to conduct such experiments:

1. Replace a normal gene with a mutant gene ("trading places") and observe the effects on the offspring (**knockin animal model**).
2. Inactivate or interrupt a normal gene's function and observe the effects on the offspring (**knockout animal model**).
3. Add a mutant gene and observe the combined mutant gene and normal gene effects on the offspring.
4. Increase protein expression by increasing gene copy number.

For its relevance to exercise physiology, we take a closer look later in this chapter at strategies to disable genes related to obesity using the elegant "knockout" or gene-targeting

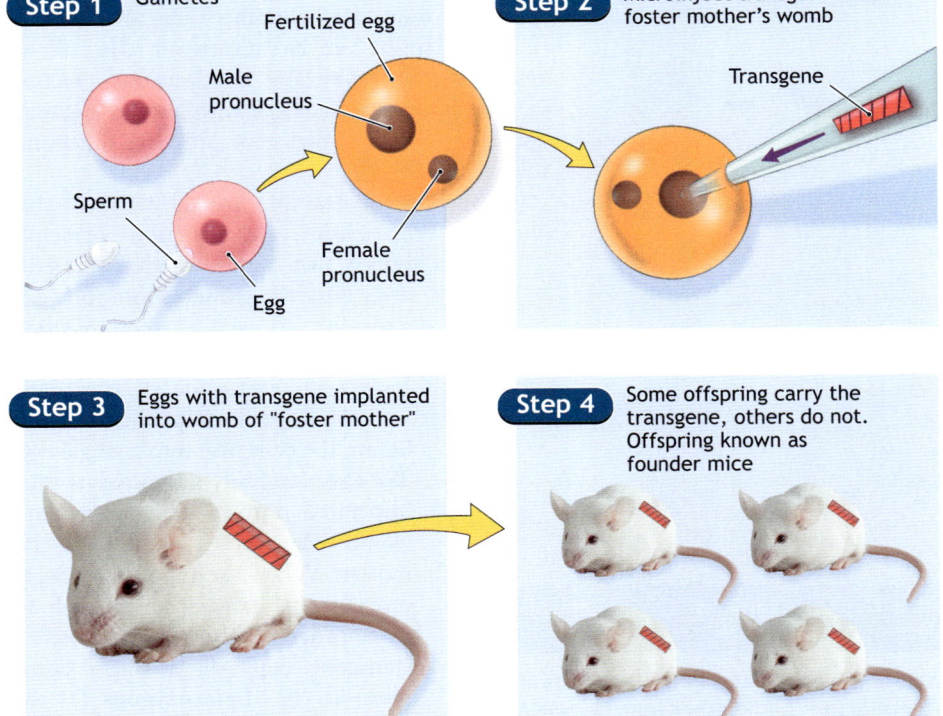

FIGURE 33.42. Generalized procedure to create transgenic offspring by injecting a target gene (transgene) into a fertilized egg. Several progeny called founder mice carry the transgene in their chromosomes.

techniques. Similar techniques led to the 2007 Nobel Prize in Physiology or Medicine awarded to researchers Mario R. Capecchi (1937–; www.nobelprize.org/prizes/medicine/2007/capecchi/biographical/; Nobel laureate James Watson was his doctoral advisor; www.nobelprize.org/nobel_prizes/medicine/laureates/1962/watson-bio.html), Sir Martin J. Evans (1941–; www.nobelprize.org/prizes/medicine/2007/evans/facts/), and Oliver Smithies (1925–2017; www.nobelprize.org/prizes/medicine/2007/smithies/facts/; www.ncbi.nlm.nih.gov/pmc/articles/PMC4639968/) for their groundbreaking advances related to powerful techniques for introducing specific gene modifications in mice by embryonic stem cells and mammal recombinant DNA

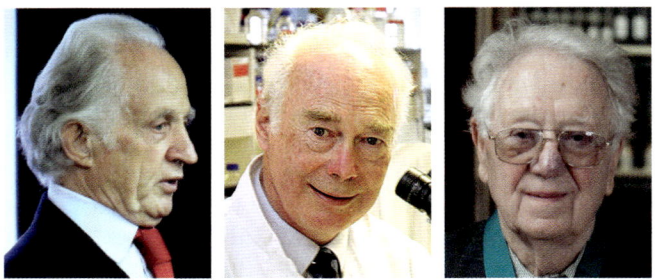

Mario R. Capecchi, Sir Martin J. Evans, and Oliver Smithies. (Capecchi photo licensed under Creative Commons Attribution Share-Alike 4.0 International license: https://creativecommons.org/licenses/by-sa/4.0/deed.en. Evans (attribution: Public Relations Office, Cardiff University); and Smithies (attribution: Science History Institute) photos licensed under Creative Commons Attribution Share-Alike 3.0 Unported license: https://creativecommons.org/licenses/by-sa/3.0/deed.en.)

(http://nobelprize.org/nobel_prizes/medicine/laureates/2007/press.html).

Cloning a Mammal

Genetics researchers use three methods to clone mammals:

1. SCNT
2. Roslin technique
3. Honolulu technique

SCNT Method

FIGURE 33.43 illustrates the eight-step SCNT technology process, also called therapeutic cloning, to create stem cells from somatic cells (cells other than a sperm or egg cell). This modern technique had its genesis when experimental embryologist Hans Spemann (1869–1938; www.nobelprize.org/prizes/medicine/1935/spemann/biographical/; 1935 Nobel Prize in Physiology or Medicine for discovering the "organizer effect" in embryonic development at the gastrula stage) with colleague experimental embryologist Hilde Mangold (1898–1924; she died before the Nobel Prize award and thus ineligible) pioneered microsurgical techniques while working with embryos (https://embryo.asu.edu/pages/hilde-mangold-1898-1924; https://embryo.asu.edu/pages/spemann-mangold-organizer). Spemann and Mangold's histologic evidence from experiments with five manipulated embryos proved the induction concept (interaction between two cell groups in which one group directly influences the other's developmental fate).[198]

The SCNT technique requires two cells—a donor cell and an oocyte (an unfertilized egg cell early in development). Somatic cells from the patient are prepared for the next step, transferring the nucleus in the cell with its DNA into an enucleated oocyte (not having a nucleus eliminates most genetic information). This process (step 3) prompts the cell to begin forming an embryo (a fertilized egg that can begin cell division). In step 4, the embryo undergoes cell division until it develops into the blastocyst stage (100 cell mass). At this developmental stage, the mass remains as undifferentiated cell group. Step 5 separates the inner cell mass (ICM) from the cell by a microchemical technique called immunosurgery (using different chemicals to dislodge the ICM from the cell wall). The cultured ICMs produce pluripotent stem cells (step 6), versatile cells with the potential to become different tissue types (e.g., skin, brain, heart, muscle,

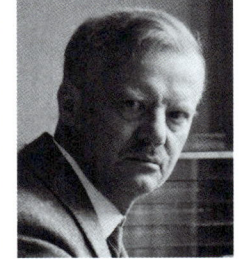

Hans Spemann. (Sueddeutsche Zeitung Photo/Alamy Stock Photo)

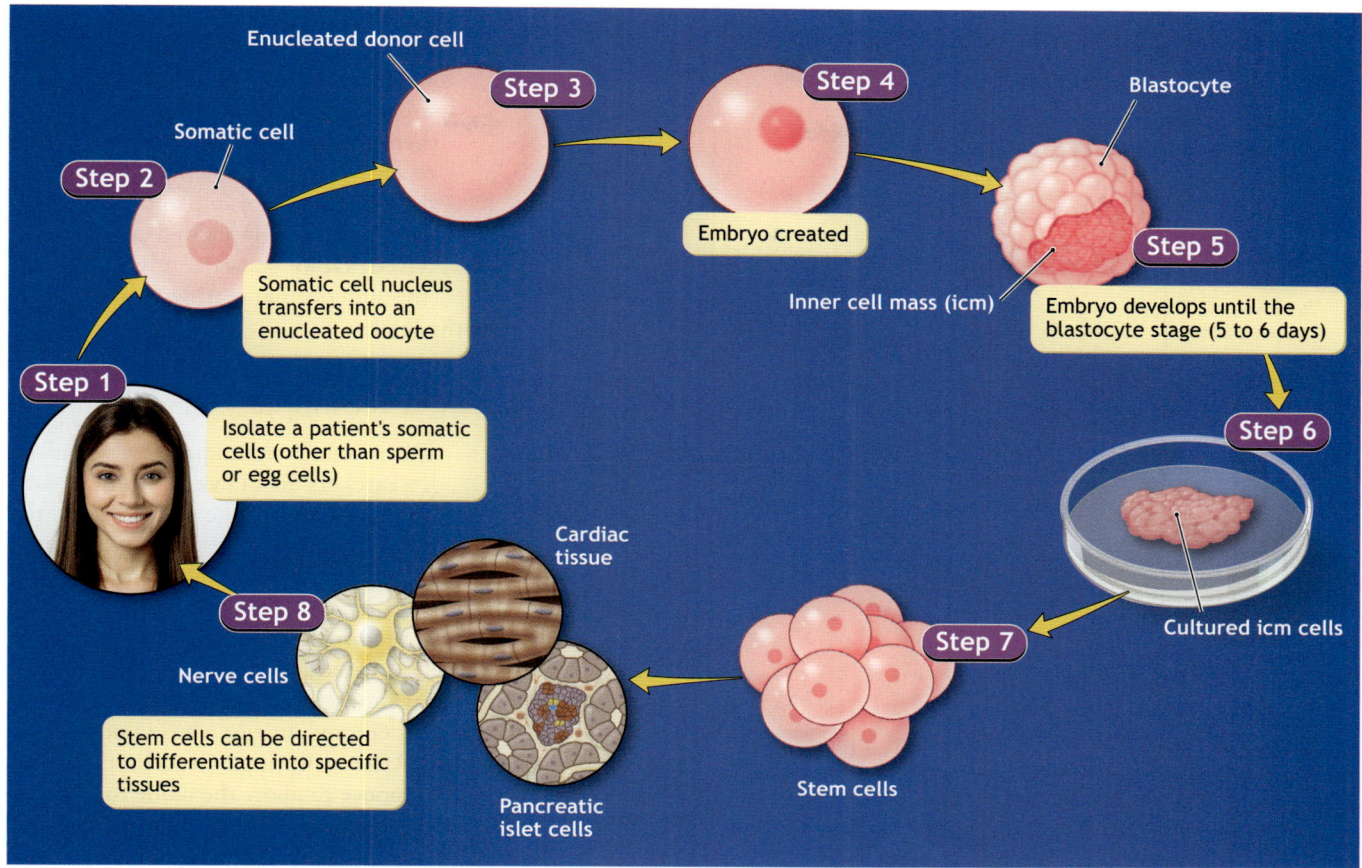

FIGURE 33.43. Eight-step somatic cell nuclear transfer (SCNT) technology to create stem cells from somatic cells (cells other than reproductive cells). SCNT eliminates tissue rejection because the new tissue grafts are autologous (donor and host are the same individual). SCNT is not reproductive cloning because it uses only unfertilized egg cells to generate stem cells.[82] The International Society for Stem Cell Research provides additional details about SCNT (www.isscr.org/; https://thestemcellreport.buzzsprout.com). (Shutterstock images: Medvedka (petri dish), Mix and Match Studio (woman).)

kidney, bone, pancreas, intestine). In essence, relatively unspecialized stem cells have not yet differentiated into any specific issue type. Once they differentiate (e.g., acquire a specialized cell features and develop into specific tissues in step 7), the new specialized cell types can be reintroduced into the patient to begin the process to replace or repopulate damaged or diseased tissues with newly created ones.

Roslin Method

In 1997, scientists at Edinburgh's Roslin Institute in Scotland (www.ed.ac.uk/roslin) tapped the complete genetic library contained within the zygote (cell **totipotent** potentiality) to clone the Dorset sheep "Dolly." This milestone represented the first such viable intact donor derived from adult mammalian cells.[164] Several clones produced in laboratories before Dolly the sheep including mice, sheep, and cows, but these clones were incorporated from DNA from *embryos*. For Dolly, the researchers removed an unfertilized oocyte from an adult ewe and replaced its nucleus with the nucleus from an adult sheep mammary gland cell.[105] They then implanted the egg in another ewe, producing the healthy offspring sheep. The idea behind the nuclear transfer experiment was to produce genetically engineered transgenic mammals inexpensively that could reliably produce large pharmaceutical components in their milk. A likely benefit would create human proteins for drug synthesis to treat cystic fibrosis, hemophilia, and emphysema, with potential benefits toward aging and cancer research. Milk produced from transgenic sheep, goats, and cattle can yield up to 40 g protein · L^{-1} at relatively low cost. This circumvents the need to use purified, expensive blood to harvest protein, with contamination risk from AIDS or hepatitis C. Proteins produced in human cell cultures have high cost and relatively low yields. Transgenetically produced proteins have application in the **nutraceutical** industry[267] and **xenotransplantation**, animal disease models, and cell therapy.[235]

The first Dolly experiments represented a milestone in cloning technology but not before unyielding criticism concerning ethical and scientific issues related to possible future experiments with human cloning. Similar concerns have emerged about future CRISPR-Cas9 gene editing systems, which we discuss later in this chapter. **FIGURE 33.44** shows that Dolly possesses the same genes as the cells from the ewe's udder. The reproductive cell cycle

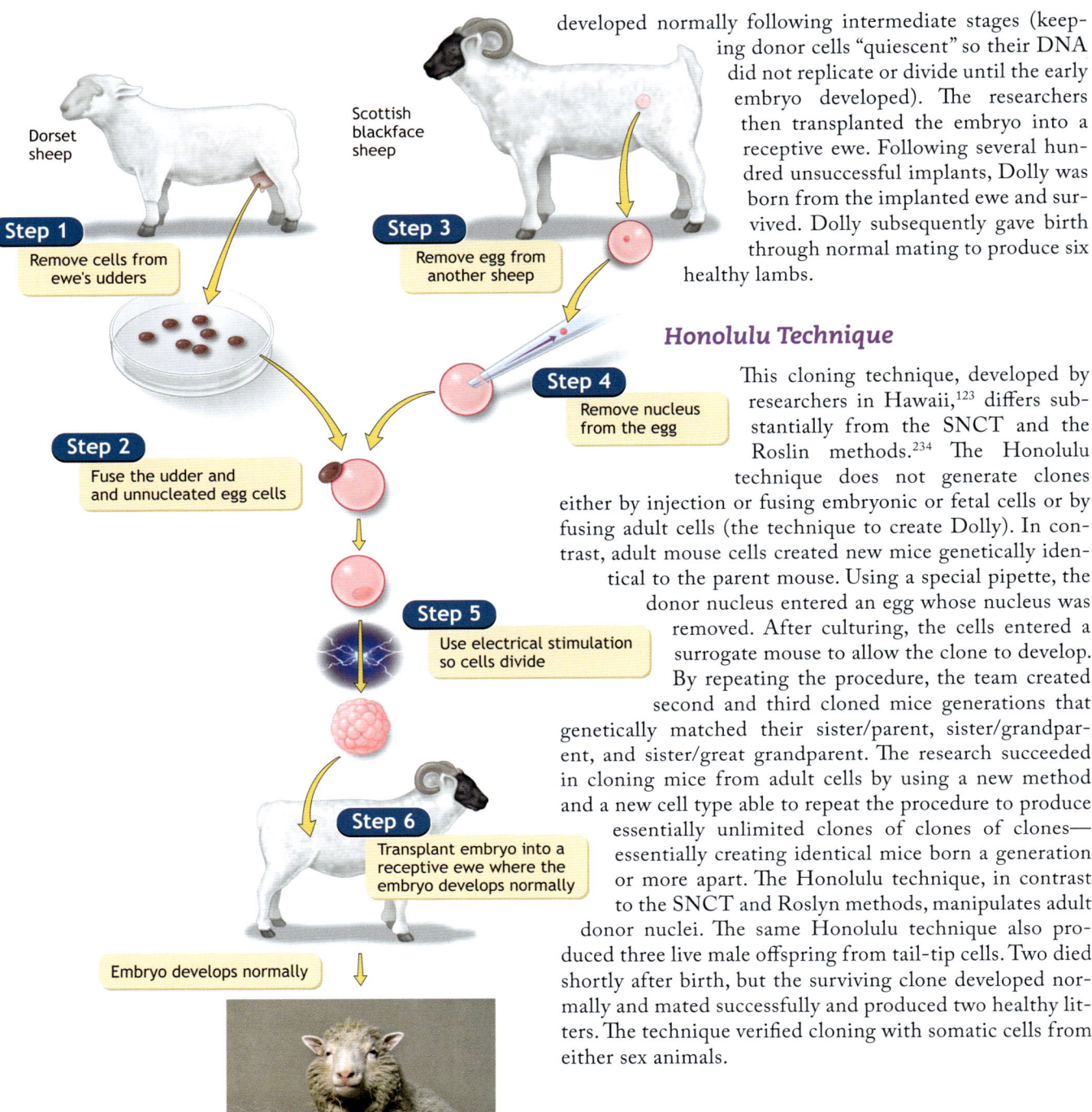

developed normally following intermediate stages (keeping donor cells "quiescent" so their DNA did not replicate or divide until the early embryo developed). The researchers then transplanted the embryo into a receptive ewe. Following several hundred unsuccessful implants, Dolly was born from the implanted ewe and survived. Dolly subsequently gave birth through normal mating to produce six healthy lambs.

Honolulu Technique

This cloning technique, developed by researchers in Hawaii,[123] differs substantially from the SNCT and the Roslin methods.[234] The Honolulu technique does not generate clones either by injection or fusing embryonic or fetal cells or by fusing adult cells (the technique to create Dolly). In contrast, adult mouse cells created new mice genetically identical to the parent mouse. Using a special pipette, the donor nucleus entered an egg whose nucleus was removed. After culturing, the cells entered a surrogate mouse to allow the clone to develop. By repeating the procedure, the team created second and third cloned mice generations that genetically matched their sister/parent, sister/grandparent, and sister/great grandparent. The research succeeded in cloning mice from adult cells by using a new method and a new cell type able to repeat the procedure to produce essentially unlimited clones of clones of clones—essentially creating identical mice born a generation or more apart. The Honolulu technique, in contrast to the SNCT and Roslyn methods, manipulates adult donor nuclei. The same Honolulu technique also produced three live male offspring from tail-tip cells. Two died shortly after birth, but the surviving clone developed normally and mated successfully and produced two healthy litters. The technique verified cloning with somatic cells from either sex animals.

Gene Knockout Technique

Mice provide a useful model to study genetic manipulations with the control afforded experimental subjects and the environment, and the animal's shorter life span. For example, researchers can study a normal-sized mice strain with black fur, obese mice with black fur, obese mice with white fur, and so on. Genetic "tampering" can verify whether the gene modulated the specific effect independently from fur color influence. Deactivating a gene(s) within the DNA known to produce an obese mice strain ordinarily produces normal-weight mice litters.

FIGURE 33.44. Six simplified steps in cloning a mammal. Dorset sheep Dolly (*bottom photo*) has genes identical to the ewe that donated the original genes (Dorset white sheep without horns, *upper left*). Dolly was the first mammal to be cloned from adult DNA (https://dolly.roslin.ed.ac.uk/facts/the-life-of-dolly/index.html). Dolly suffered from lung cancer and crippling arthritis. The unnamed sheep from which Dolly was cloned died several years prior to Dolly's creation.
(Photo of Dolly and her lamb, Bonnie, courtesy The Roslin Institute, The University of Edinburgh. Electrical stimulation image: Lane V. Erickson/Shutterstock.)

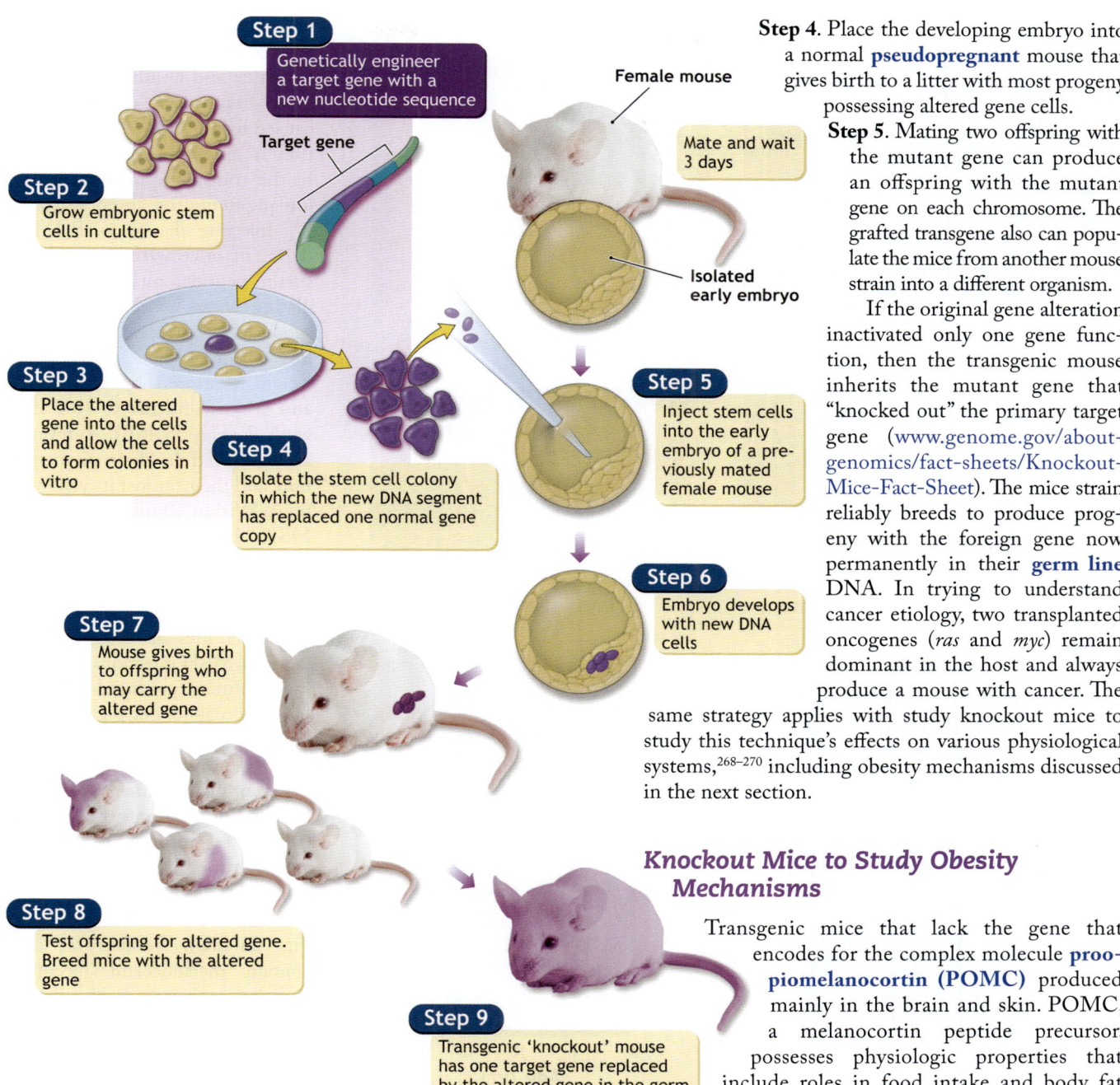

FIGURE 33.45 Nine-step procedure with a knockout gene to create a transgenic mouse. Transgenic mice represent a unique tool for understanding how interactions between individual genes and environmental stressors affect human health and disease.

FIGURE 33.45 illustrates the five-step experimental strategy to create a transgenic mouse with a knocked-out gene.[236]

Step 1. A DNA fragment receives a genetically modified gene (**gene cassette**, shown in purple), thus altering the target gene's usual nucleotide sequence.

Step 2. Cell culture growth produces one or more cell colonies containing the altered gene. Identifying a colony means the mutant gene altered the DNA fragment.

Step 3. Inject the genetically altered cells into the developing embryo in a previously mated female mouse.

Step 4. Place the developing embryo into a normal **pseudopregnant** mouse that gives birth to a litter with most progeny possessing altered gene cells.

Step 5. Mating two offspring with the mutant gene can produce an offspring with the mutant gene on each chromosome. The grafted transgene also can populate the mice from another mouse strain into a different organism.

If the original gene alteration inactivated only one gene function, then the transgenic mouse inherits the mutant gene that "knocked out" the primary target gene (www.genome.gov/about-genomics/fact-sheets/Knockout-Mice-Fact-Sheet). The mice strain reliably breeds to produce progeny with the foreign gene now permanently in their **germ line** DNA. In trying to understand cancer etiology, two transplanted oncogenes (*ras* and *myc*) remain dominant in the host and always produce a mouse with cancer. The same strategy applies with study knockout mice to study this technique's effects on various physiological systems,[268–270] including obesity mechanisms discussed in the next section.

Knockout Mice to Study Obesity Mechanisms

Transgenic mice that lack the gene that encodes for the complex molecule **proopiomelanocortin (POMC)** produced mainly in the brain and skin. POMC, a melanocortin peptide precursor, possesses physiologic properties that include roles in food intake and body fat accretion.[84,237,271–273] Researchers originally intended to study POMC-deficient mice to evaluate **neurohormone** signaling and central nervous system functioning. Unfortunately, their transgenic mutant mice overate and became obese, with altered pigmentation that produced yellowish fur on their abdomen rather than typical brownish-black fur. They also showed significantly less adrenal tissue than normal size littermates. **FIGURE 33.46A** shows that by age 2 mo, the body weight in the mutant mice steadily increased to twice the normal littermate weight and color.

These findings coincided with a previous report describing a rare genetic disease in two children caused by a mutant

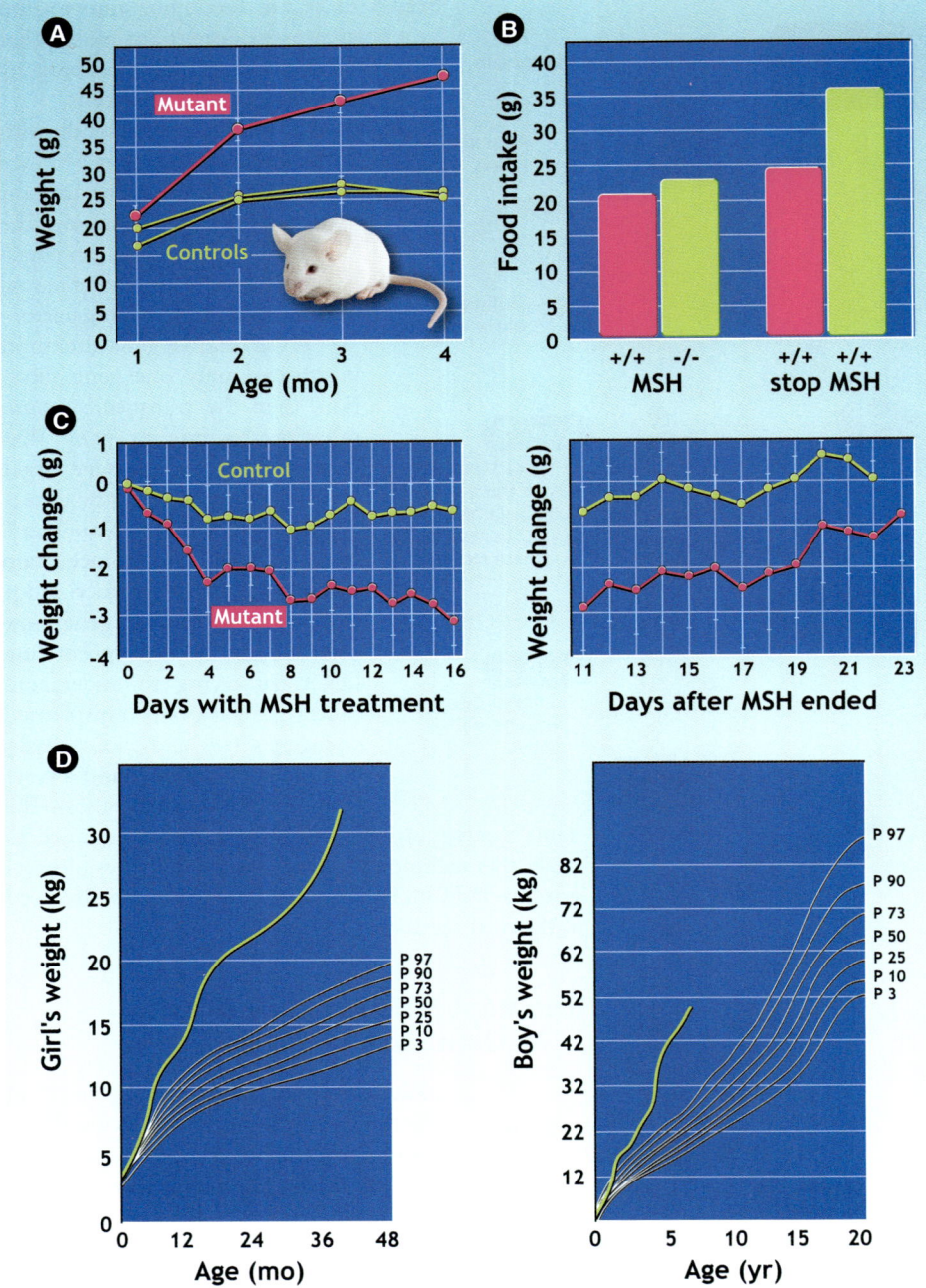

FIGURE 33.46. Proopiomelanocortin (POMC)-deficient transgenic mice provide new clues to obesity. **(A)** Body weight gain in mutant and control mice. **(B)** Change in body weight with and without treatment. **(C)** Differences in food intake with and without treatment. **(D)** Extreme weight gain in a young boy and girl with the POMC mutation. The *white lines* represent growth curves for children representing the 3rd through 97th percentile (p). (Data from A, B, and C modified from Yaswen L, et al. Obesity in the mouse model of proopiomelanocortin deficiency responds to peripheral melanocortin. *Nat Med.* 1999;5:1066.
(Data in D from Krude H, et al. Severe early-onset obesity, adrenal insufficiency and red hair pigmentation caused by POMC mutations in humans. *Nat Genet.* 1998;19:155.)

far exceeded typical age standards. The connection between the mice and children was striking; functional characteristics caused by the POMC gene mutation in humans paralleled those in the transgenic mice with yellow pigmentation and obesity.

Injecting the obese, POMC-deficient mice with the melanocortin peptide, melanocyte-stimulating hormone (MSH) agonist produced a significant body weight loss within 1 d; at 1 wk, body weight decreased by about 38% and declined further to 48% after week 2 (Fig. 33.46B). A reversal also occurred in their pigmentation, and their fur lost its yellowish tinge. Within 10 min to introduce MSH "therapy," the mice began to regain lost weight, reaching preinjection weight in another 14 days. Their yellow fur color in the ventral and dorsal sites also reappeared. In contrast, MSH injections and ceasing treatment produced no effect on body mass or fur pigmentation in normal control littermates. The researchers explained that weight loss during treatment exceeded expectations from the energy balance equation. This occurred although the mutant mice ate significantly more food daily than the control mice (35.7 vs. 24.2 g; Fig. 33.46C). Because fat cells contain melanocortin receptors, and these receptors induce lipolysis, melanocortin-based drugs may eventually prove helpful as therapeutic agents to combat obesity.[238]

Interestingly, MSH analogues injections also reduced excess body fat in another obese transgenic mice strain deficient in the hormone leptin.[63] In studies involving 87 unrelated Italian obese children and adolescents, three new mutations were identified within the POMC signal peptide (substituting Ser with Thr at codon 7; Ser with Leu at codon 9; Arg with Gly at codon 236).[41] The researchers believed mutations in codons 7 and 9 in the signal peptide altered pre-POMC **translocation** into the endoplasmic reticulum explained the linkage between POMC and the genetic predisposition to obesity. Further studies

POMC gene.[84] These red-haired children had no melanocortins, and they developed severe obesity soon after birth and suffered adrenal insufficiency. Figure 33.46D shows the rapid weight gain for this young girl and boy, whose weight

provided new insights concerning obesity etiology,[13,46] and ongoing experiments with transgenic animal and human models may someday help researchers to better understand obesity etiology and its treatment.[65,239]

Extremes in obesity have linked to DNA polymorphisms in the translated leptin (*LEP*) gene.[97] Leptin-regulated endocannabinoids (cannabislike substances naturally produced in the brain) stimulate appetite and play a role in food regulation as a component in the leptin-signaling cascades.[42] Excess body fat may provide a ready stem cell resource from which to create replacement tissues (e.g., bone, muscle, cartilage) for diseased or damaged ones.[171,240] Incorporating a person's own stem cells would avoid rejecting transplanted tissues and circumvent moral objections concerning human embryonic stem cell strategies. Consequently, genetic techniques using **antisense RNA** to suppress target gene expression can assess gene function, thereby selectively blocking targeted gene functions (www.nature.com/articles/nrd3625). This allowed researchers to add new editing tools to sequence altered genes to fight invading organisms that cause havoc in expressing devastating diseases.[58,148,166,241]

Ion Channel Nanopore. Scientists have developed selective ion channel nanopore techniques (www.sciencedirect.com/science/article/pii/S2590049819301213), which discriminate among almost identical DNA molecules that differ by only one base pair or one nucleotide.[155] Such differentiation allows highly accurate molecular identification to unscramble gene expression intricacies and ultimately develops strategies to target mutagens. Research with 380 Europeans with early-onset and morbid adult obesity and 1416 age-matched, normal weight controls identified three new genetic loci for obesity (*NPC1*, endosomal/lysosomal Niemann-Pick C1 gene; near *MAF*, encoding the transcription factor c-MAF; near *PTER*, phosphotriesterase-related gene).[109]

Gene Editing

In a living organism, four different nucleases can genetically engineer DNA's molecular pathways by inserting, deleting, or modifying specific locations along the DNA strand. The inset image graphically illustrates the most common gene-targeting platforms and their common end points (meganucleases, **zinc finger nucleases, transcription activator–like effector nucleases** specific DNA-binding proteins **(TALEN)**, and **CRISPR-Cas9**). They all share a common purpose—to create a split in DNA's double strand and then to edit a target gene to achieve a particular objective.[214–216] The thinner red to greener block at the top inset shows that CRISPR-Cas9 offers the greatest potential for breakthroughs in gene editing procedures.

Attribution: Mazhar Adii; licensed under Creative Commons Attribution Share-Alike 4.0 International license: https://creativecommons.org/licenses/by-sa/4.0/deed.en.

CRISPR Technology

Biochemists Jennifer Doudna (1964–) and Emmanuelle Charpentier (1968–) won the 2020 Nobel Prize in Chemistry for developing the gene editing system CRISPR Cas-9 that interprets DNA's genetic code. This was the first time two women have jointly won the Nobel Prize in Chemistry. Only five other women have been honored for their achievements in chemistry (www.nobelprize.org/prizes/lists/nobel-prize-awarded-women/; Marie Curie (1903; discovering radium and polonium), her daughter Irène Joliot-Curie (1935; synthesizing new radioactive elements), Dorothy Crowfoot Hodgkin (1964; discovering biological substances), Ada Yonath (2009; ribosome structure and function), and Frances H. Arnold (2018; directed enzyme evolution). The next section shows the CRISPR-Cas9 developmental timeline from 1987 to 2020.

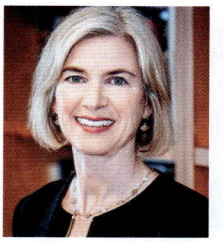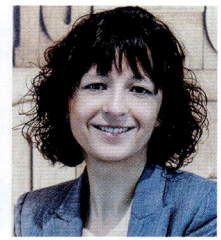

Jennifer Doudna and Emmanuelle Charpentier. (CHINE NOUVELLE/SIPA/Shutterstock)

CRISPR Timeline

The inset image (next page) shows the developmental timeline from 1987 to 2020 for CRISPR-Cas9 and related gene editing tools. Japanese scientists in 1987 had discovered unknown tandem repeats in the *E. coli* genome but had not explored their biological significance.[275] In 2002, an acronym defined the

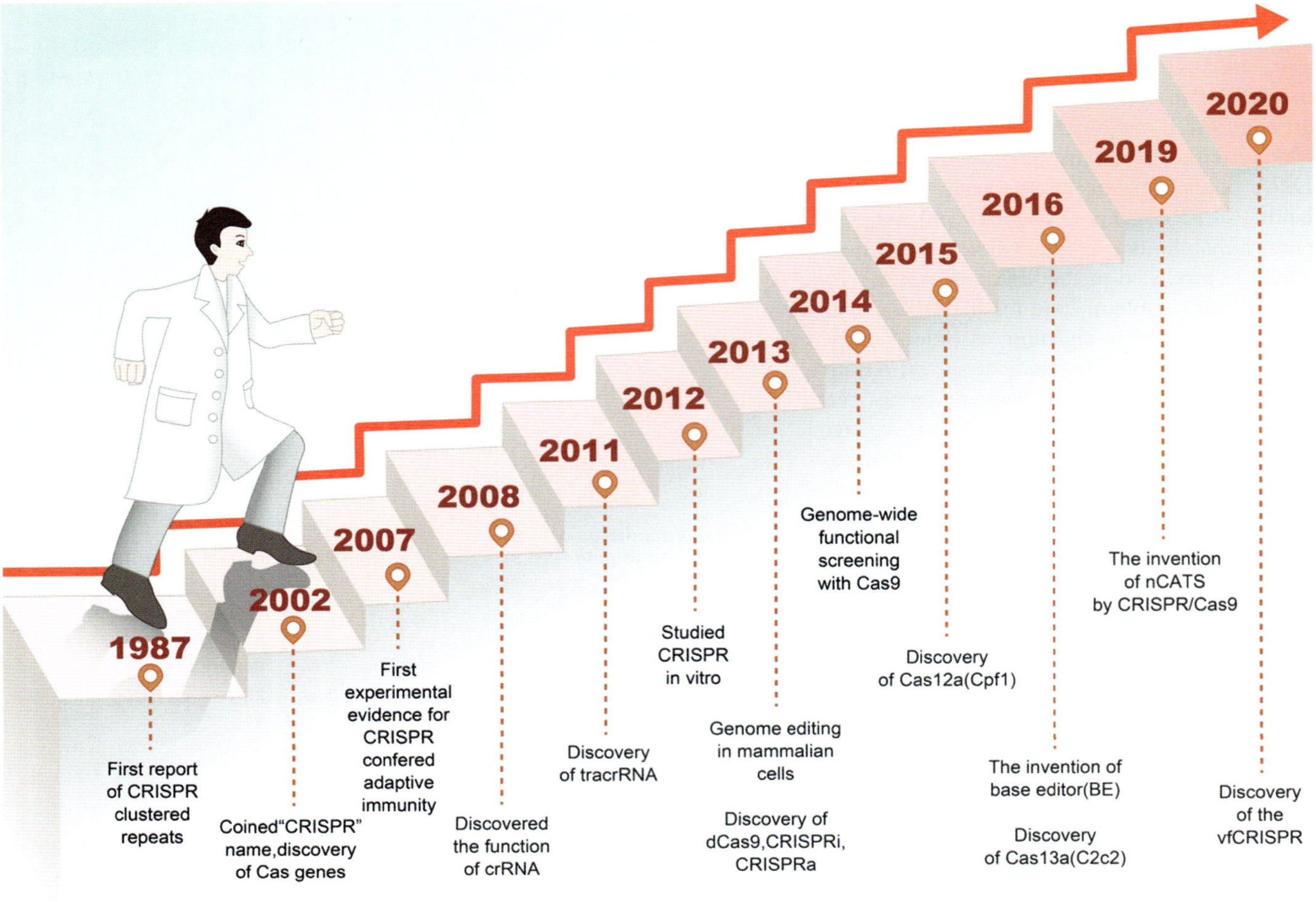

From Zhang H, et al. Application of the CRISPR/Cas9-based gene editing technique in basic research, diagnosis, and therapy of cancer. *Mol Cancer*. 2021;201:126. Licensed under Creative Commons Attribution Share-Alike 4.0 International license: https://creativecommons.org/licenses/by-sa/4.0/deed.en.

repeat sequences as Clustered Regularly Interspaced Short Palindromic Repeats **(CRISPR)**, yet their significance remained elusive.[276] By 2013, the Cas system and DNA gene editing was introduced in mammalian cells, and by 2020, its widespread implementation began for both DNA and RNA system level components. Further advancements with more precise CRISPR technologies followed and are continuing.

Doudna and Charpentier Breakthrough Experiments

The process Doudna and Charpentier pioneered slices the DNA at precise locations by guiding a small protein enzyme tracer that acts as a DNA "molecular scalpel" to clip out a targeted section along the DNA strand for eventual relocation with its replacement protein. In a Charpentier 2011 experiment targeting a destructive bacteria *Streptococcus pyogenes*,[223] a destructive gram-positive bacteria, which infects human hosts (she also discovered **transactivating CRISPR RNA [tracrRNA]** shown in red), a previously unknown molecule became a key component to unlock one of nature's closely guarded secrets—disarming harmful viruses contained within ancient bacteria with the small tracrRNA regulatory molecule by cleaving their DNA and ridding the virus from the host by destroying it (www.ncbi.nlm.nih.gov/books/NBK554528/). This elegant molecular mechanism signifies a "dead end" to the virus, which no longer can infect the host because the effect is lethal to the virus. A year later, Charpentier collaborated with Doudna to recreate the bacteria's "genetic scalpel" in the laboratory to streamline the scalpel's intricate molecular components.[184] The essence of their collaborative research in 2011 determined how the special programmable protein (Cas-9, formerly identified as endonuclease Csn1) present in ancient bacteria, directed the dual guided RNA protein to a specific region in a dual stranded DNA sequence.

The programmable aspect allows the protein to seek out and find sections in the DNA sequence. Their experiments had determined that the RNA CRISPR molecule in nature was a dual RNA-guided protein that uses a CRISPR RNA molecule to direct it to a DNA sequence that matches a CRISPR RNA sequence. This required a second RNA "tracer" molecule that provided the molecular interaction with CRISPR RNA to assemble and repurpose a Cas-9 complex. Together, the two RNAs guide the Cas-9 within the CRISPR complex to make a precise cut

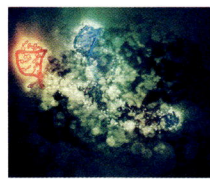

Wirestock Creators/ Shutterstock

CHAPTER 33 • Molecular Biology: New Vista for Exercise Physiology in Health, Disease, and Performance

in the double-stranded 1DNA helix. Deciding where to make the cut occurs because the CRISPR system preserves memories from prior infections by introducing short DNA foreign segments (termed spacers), into the CRISPR array.

The Doudna and Charpentier breakthrough experiments explained how these molecules were able to cut the DNA molecule at any predetermined location by creating a single guide RNA by matching with known DNA sequences,[186] thus expanding the genetic code within the molecule and literally rewriting it. Also, the newly engineered cell repairs the cut in the DNA, thereby turning off the gene's original function. This meant researchers could insert, repair, and edit the DNA template to literally decide where to slice the genome to change the gene sequence and thus reconfigure its genetic code.

The experiments with CRISPR-Cas9 revolutionized molecular biology, as did discovering DNA's helical structure more than a half century earlier.[194] The new, powerful but elegant genetic tool almost immediately triggered new scientific efforts in almost every biological science field by showing how nature uses the dual RNA system to guide Cas-9 DNA sequences and how to molecularly engineer the dual RNA guide as a single RNA guide to include the protein's target information and structural elements to ply apart the DNA molecule and match precise sequences in it along the chain with the RNA.

The breakthrough CRISPR genomic platform applications range from integrated pest management control (entomology),[226] creating disease-resistant fruits and vegetables (agriculture),[227] animal breeding (animal science),[224] implantable engineered tissues (regenerative medicine),[225] and the anticipated holy grail—better understanding and curtailing (and even curing) the most destructive inherited degenerative human disease mutations (e.g., muscular dystrophy, blindness, sickle cell, Parkinson's, diabetes, and inherited heart, liver, kidney, pancreas, and reproductive organ).[229,230]

How CRISPR Works

Over billions of years, bacteria,[117] eukaryotes (any cell or animal, plant, and fungi with a clearly defined nucleus), and archaea (primitive prokaryotes based on their distinct characteristics in a separate domain from bacteria and eukaryotes) relied on specialized repeating sections in their DNA as an adaptive protective mechanism against invading detrimental phage viruses that infect and replicate with bacteria and archaea. Each time an assaulting virus would enter a cell, these newly identified repeating DNA sections called CRISPRs pair with guide RNA (gRNA), an invader-fighting RNA molecule to track down the intruding DNA section located in specific gene sequences in the virus and destroy it. For CRISPR-Cas9, the palindromic sequence refers to the four letters in DNA's genetic code that reads the same in both directions, either from the molecule's 5′ or 3′ prime end as illustrated in the unnumbered image. The protospacer adjacent motif sequence shown in red (NGG) represents a 2- to 6-base pair DNA sequence usually in the DNA region, the CRISPR-Cas9 targets for cleavage.

To accomplish the mission, gRNA first teams up with specialized enzymes (Cas9) for transport to the virus and attaches to it. When gRNA and Cas9 infiltrate the target DNA, it slices into the molecule in the exact location along the organism's DNA strand. Consequently, the gRNA creates a perfect chemical match with the virus DNA's molecular sequence. Once connecting with the intended target invaders' specifically identified DNA sequence, Cas9 precisely cleaves the DNA and eliminates the undesirable DNA section (www.youtube.com/watch?v=UKbrwPL3wXE). The inset figure schematically

fyi CRISPR Genome Editing for Harmful DNA Ionizing Radiation on Space Flights

Over 100 different duration U.S. and Soyuz (Russian) space missions have ranged from weeks to over 1 yr, including more than 62 different International Space Station (ISS) missions. Ever since the first Project Mercury flights (1958–1963), legitimate concern has focused attention about harmful DNA damage caused by ionizing radiation (see Chapter 27). One strategy to

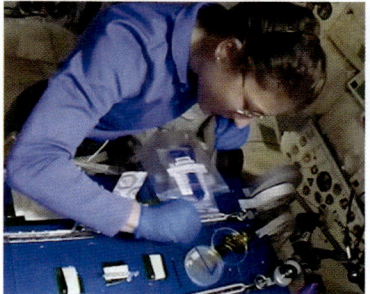
Credit: NASA

assess radiation's impact on ISS missions includes the CRISPR gene editing system described in this chapter. The image shows an astronaut placing different DNA repair template colony sequences grown in yeast extracts on an agar dish following a 6-day incubation. Prior research had determined that future space exploration with the upcoming Artemis Moon mission (www.nasa.gov/artemisprogram) and then sending astronauts from the moon to Mars within the next two decades (www.nasa.gov/topics/moon-to-mars/overview) would negatively impact DNA's molecular repair pathways during the 7-month flight to Mars (https://mars.nasa.gov/mars2020/timeline/cruise/) including planet colonization will significantly increase radiation exposure. These onboard experiments described the successful genetic transformation and genome editing to complement the astronaut's "medical toolkit" onboard ISS. The DSBs, in which the phosphate backbones in both DNA strands undergo hydrolysis, are particularly prone to harmful DNA lesions from galactic cosmic radiation exposure.[227] Altering "normal" DNA on Earth increases cancer risk from high linear energy transfer particle bombardment in space.[259] Studying DNA repair in space is advantageous because radiation or other metabolic reagents in spaceflight do not impact this genome's editing system by triggering nonspecific DNA damage. Second, polymerase chain reaction methods[260] and DNA sequencing[261] can validate changes to repaired, mutated undesirable DNA sequences.

Sources:
Stahl-Rommel S, et al. CRISPR-based assay for the study of eukaryotic DNA repair onboard the International Space Station. *PLoS One.* 2021;16:e0253403.
Stahl-Rommel S, et al. Real-time culture-independent microbial profiling onboard the International Space Station using nanopore sequencing. *Genes (Basal).* 2021;12:106.

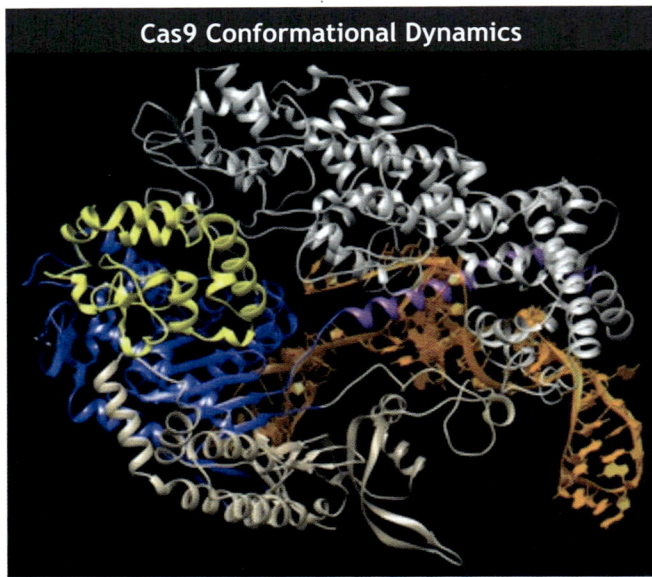

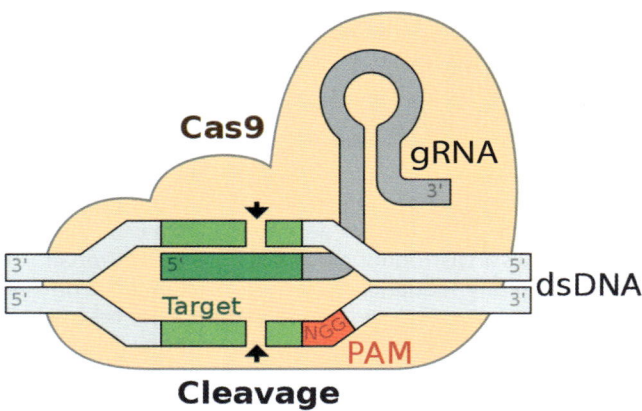

From Marius Walter; Licensed under Creative Commons Attribution Share-Alike 4.0 International license: https://creativecommons.org/licenses/by-sa/4.0/deed.en

illustrates the Cas9 protein intertwined with the gRNA and target DNA strand, creating the scissor cut at the exact NGG gene position. The black up and down arrows represent the cleavage location along the targeted molecule's double-stranded DNA sequence (2 white strands with opposite 3′ and 5′ DNA ending locations in the specific base pair sequence).

Closer Look at Cas9. The protein cascade (Cas) works with other proteins to construct the CRISPR archive in its fight to protect invading yet destructive viruses. The Cas protein group has two recruiting proteins (Cas1 and Cas2), which immediately confront the invader virus while at the same time saving bits for future identification, akin to taking a snapshot and capturing that coded sequence and later recognize it when another invading virus attacks the bacteria. Once detected, Cas3 finishes the mission by destroying the virus. In essence, the Cas3 protein serves as both a "secondary scout" and "executioner."

The major enzyme involved in gene editing, Cas9, mimics "molecular scalpel" pairs that slice through DNA's double strands, allowing it to fix broken genes, splice in new ones, or disable known target genes. The inset image shows the large Cas9 complex (blue) surrounding the virus (yellow) and single-stranded DNA (violet). When viruses invade a bacterium, Cas9 with specific gRNA coordinate and destroy the destructive intruder and render it inoperable within the cell. Retaining small bits in viral cell content remain within the genome to act as a future remembering system should the same virus reenter the cell. When it does, the same "cut and paste" approach remembers and then destroys the viral attacker. Almost immediately, the invaded cell repairs itself with its built-in restorative machinery, a novel strategy evolved over millennia to preserve the cell line.

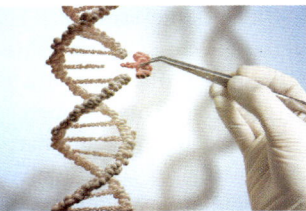

vchal/Shutterstock

Closer Look at gRNA. The gRNA strand illustrated in the inset 3-D image (orange strand) is a 20-base pair long RNA sequence within a longer RNA scaffold structure. It binds to a specified DNA (green section opened DNA sequence) and relocates or "guides" Cas9 (purple) to cut into the precise location complementary to the target's double-stranded DNA sequence where the "scissors" cut occurs. The new gRNA configuration only binds to the intended target sequence and not to any other regions along the DNA helix. The existing cut by the nuclease then repairs naturally by DNA's inherent ability to achieve homeostasis and "stitch" the two cut DNA strands back together. The small alteration in the DNA structure creates a mutation in the new DNA to alter its original function or to render the molecule inoperative. The cell uses the modified DNA piece as a template to repair future breaks, potentially creating unlimited new DNA copies in perpetuity from its creation.

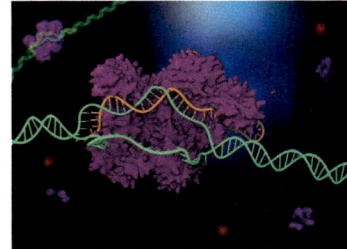

Meletios Verras/Shutterstock

CRISPR's Future

The CRISPR-Cas9 molecular components already play important and ground-breaking roles in the basic sciences to create transformative new medicines.[231,232] These include targeting existing disabling mutation-enabled genes in inherited diseases, changing a single nucleotide base (single letter A, T, C, G) in the double helix genetic code, adding a fluorescent protein to identify a particular region inside known DNA sequences, and using gene "knockout" and "knockin" methods with small animals to turn specific gene sequences "on" and "off" in experiments to create animal offspring with desirable or undesirable characteristics (see Figs. 33.42 and 33.45).

The CRISPR-Cas9 naturally occurring genome editing tool has become an affirming genetic breakthrough to treat human genetic diseases (e.g., cardiovascular diseases, neural disorders, eye diseases, and cancers among others). Several human genetically linked diseases account for a large proportion

CHAPTER 33 • Molecular Biology: New Vista for Exercise Physiology in Health, Disease, and Performance

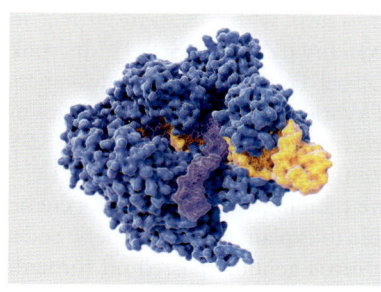
Juan Gaertner/Shutterstock

in deaths worldwide—1 in 200 people die from hypertrophic cardiomyopathy, the most common inherited disease altering heart functions, which leads to other heart-related conditions including sudden cardiac death.[263] Applying CRISPR-Cas9 methods, researchers have determined that 1 in a 1000 known mutations in a myosin gene (P710R) disrupted myosin hypercontractility and relaxed-state functions to impact traction forces that regulate "normal" contractility at the sarcomere level as this molecule's force patterns interact with the actin molecule.[262]

Each new finding helps to clear the path toward a better understanding about such catastrophic diseases and the possible strategies to reduce their mortality (disease death rate) and morbidity (disease incidence) risk. But such bright spots are not without future risks to individuals, which must consider toxicity and "off-target" consequences when the time comes to employ therapies to treat gene-mutated diseases in the clinical setting.

New advances in CRISPR delivery systems will not only impact the current CRISPR-Cas9 methodology but also limit the downstream, off-target impact.[217,228,243] New CRISPR-Cas9 highly specific hybrid RNA-DNA guides have developed mitigate techniques to off-target activity and improve specificity.[242] Pharmaceutical companies are actively searching to resolve such problems, and there is little doubt they will succeed—hopefully sooner rather than later.

Current CRISPR genome editing[218] employs biological tools to engineer DNA changes in living cells. The latest advances in type II CRISPR genome editing techniques now consider two basic components in newer type II CRISPR systems; first, the nuclease protein that precisely slices DNA, and second, the RNA molecule(s) that steer the nuclease to generate a site-specific, double-stranded break in a DNA segment by directing an edit at the specified genomic location. Newly developed chRDNAs (pronounced "chardonnays") represent more precise genome RNA-DNA hybrid guides compared with current all-RNA guides. The new chRDNA technology will deliver high efficiency multiple edits and multiplex gene insertions, which lead to anticipated CRISPR-edited therapies as a front-line strategy to fight existing diseases.

As author Walter Issacson points out in his highly acclaimed consumer book, "*The Code Breaker*,"[213] important moral questions require answers, "*Should we edit our species to make us less susceptible to deadly diseases such as Alzheimer's and blindness?*" Most people are likely to first answer "yes," but then perfectly reasonable fear and doubt turns into a slippery slope. If future gene editing technology were to become theoretically 100% fail-safe within the next few decades, should parents be able to "program" their child's IQ, or skin color, or muscular strength ability, or even their height and weight? Debilitating and life-threatening diseases are one thing, but where does society draw the line? Such perplexing moral and ethical questions have not escaped the very researchers who are working diligently to advance therapeutic gene editing.[219–222]

CRISPR Educational Videos Can Close the Knowledge Gap. Research with CRISPR-Cas9 technologies has accelerated so rapidly that it literally is impossible in a textbook to remain current about this new genomic tool. From inception to completion, a textbook takes more than a year to produce and publish. In that lag interval, thousands of articles advance new ideas and concepts to move the field forward. For example, we have pointed to the extremely rapid rise in "older" genomic research citations in the past four text editions (see Fig. 33.1). If we were to add CRISPR to the PubMed search, there would have been 2356 articles published between 2012 and 2015 when the CRISPR technique gained research momentum in research laboratories around the world before the 2020 Nobel Prize announcement. It almost triples the prior number (6428 publications) between 2015 and 2017, and a further 25,107 publications over the next 4-yr period when research in the area had truly ramped up. From January 1, 2001 to February 1, 2022, there "only" were about 7270 peer-reviewed articles! So how can this deficit in the new knowledge explosion be overcome, particularly to a public audience and college and university students so they can better understand the science underlying a particular technique?

We believe one approach is to rely on educational videos via streaming and other media methods to fill the gap between numerous monthly published peer-review articles important for researchers in their niche and the general public. To this end, we list videos, some with beautiful animations to the back of the chapter, which contains supplemental videos, animations, and podcast resources about how the sophisticated yet simple and versatile CRISPR-Cas9 system allows scientists to rewrite DNA sequences with high specificity in any cell. The list includes a lecture by Professor Doudna several years prior to her Nobel selection (https://innovativegenomics.org/education/digital-resources/what-is-crispr/), and her insightful Nobel 2020 lecture (www.nobelprize.org/prizes/chemistry/2020/doudna/lecture) and that of her co-laureate French biochemist Emmanuelle Charpentier (www.nobelprize.org/prizes/chemistry/2020/charpentier/lecture/), an influential TED talk by Doudna (www.ted.com/talks/jennifer_doudna_how_crispr_lets_us_edit_our_dna?language=en), and other elegantly produced videos about CRISPR-Cas9 functions (www.crisprtx.com/gene-editing/crispr-cas9; www.livescience.com/58790-crispr-explained.html; www.youtube.com/watch?v=4YKFw2KZA5o), and several longer productions from two workshops about CRISPR-Cas9 (www.youtube.com/watch?v=WZ6pVWvAd2M&t=1063s; www.youtube.com/watch?v=F03n34PZtzs).

Lippincott® Connect — Appendix N online at Lippincott Connect lists selected references to CRISPR technologies in health, disease, and exercise, 2013 to 2022.

Part 3: Human Performance Research

Molecular biologists studying physical activity and exercise training seek to decipher signaling pathways by which genes transcribe the effects of a mechanical stressor and resultant phenotypic expression. For example, resistance training applies muscular overload of the biceps as a mechanical stressor, while increasing upper-arm strength and size represent expression of a phenotype characteristic. Crucial, unanswered questions concern "where" and "how" skeletal overload translates into newly acquired "strength" and muscle hypertrophy. The answers likely reside within signal transduction pathways leading from cell surface receptors to the nucleus, resulting in gene transcription and subsequent protein synthesis. Scientists study the intricacies about how different signaling processes interact, integrate, and differentiate to execute a particular function and its consequences, and how they share common intermediates.[6]

Research Scope

Consider numerous highly complex, coordinated individual maneuvers at the start in a triple back somersault from a 10-m/32.8-ft diving platform. The movement components require precisely coordinating and integrating neural stimulation and muscular actions for dive success. Each movement pattern demands specific timing and muscular force requirements as in a well-tuned orchestra each instrument doing its designated task as a part of the whole movement to achieve a desired outcome.

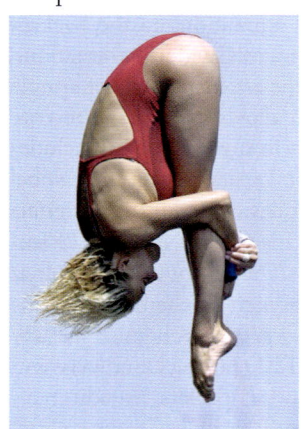
Paolo Bona/Shutterstock

At the molecular level, precision requirements are controlled by highly specific enzymes acting in concert with the specific muscle/nerve complex by turning "on" and "off" at precisely the right time and in the correct sequence to make the movement successful (or at times unfortunately unsuccessful). An unsuccessful attempt occurs when an essential component in muscle to nerve timing functions asynchronously to create mismatches among the different essential components as measured in microseconds! The very small disrupted intervals among the different timing patterns make the difference between a gold medal winning performance and a silver or bronze medal effort. A better understanding about signaling processes governing enzyme activity between stressors and genes may someday illuminate why individual differences in human movement capacities help to explain why some athletic achievements last for decades while in others, continual improvement regularly establishes new records previously thought impossible to achieve. As for enduring records, the world record in the men's long jump, for example, was achieved at the 1968 Mexico City Olympic Games by Robert Beamon (United States), with a 8.90-m/29-ft 2 in jump (www.youtube.com/watch?v=IZCzG_bS_9Q). It took another 23 years before Michael Powell (United States) shattered that record at the 1991 World Athletics Championships in Tokyo with the longest jump ever in track and field history (8.95 m/29 ft 4 in; www.youtube.com/watch?v=zuqNxHmtBD8).

To the future molecular biologist, the role of genetic makeup someday may be able to explain why the genetic code, deeply buried within an athlete's genome passed on through prior generations, makes it so exceedingly difficult to truly standout as the "best" in different sport competitions. Thankfully, a video record highlighting such achievements exists as a benchmark in future performance comparisons (www.youtube.com/watch?v=v3m_DlYSJOA). We hope the next-generation exercise and sport scientists will unravel the molecular level secrets waiting for discovery to explain why some athletes truly perform consistently at an extraordinarily high level and establish new records—but not very often.

Twin Studies

Studying identical twins attempts to explain why one twin participates regularly in sports and physical activities while the other twin shows little inclination to remain physically active (www.ncbi.nlm.nih.gov/pmc/articles/PMC4919929/). In the large-scale HERITAGE Family Study,[32,76] a search for genes related to body composition changes following exercise training for 20 wk in 364 sib-pairs from 99 Caucasian families provided evidence about a fat-free mass and insulinlike growth factor 1 gene linkage, including gene sites for body mass index and fat mass, and plasma **leptin** levels with the low-density lipoprotein receptor gene.

Research has attempted to explain why one identical twin performs better than the other twin in a particular activity. Identical twins come from the same genetic pool, so one would expect little difference in their performance, but this is not always the case. Even if the twins had identical experiences, from practice time to coaching, in mastering an activity's mechanics, their performance levels differ. Fractional seconds or tenths of a centimeter often mean the difference between victory and second place—whether the performers are twins or nonrelated Olympians.

Biochemical Individuality. Combined biochemical individuality and known allelic variations should serve as a backbone to determine optimal nutritional profiles (i.e., targeted vitamin, mineral, and other nutrient doses) to create personalized, comprehensive lifestyle prescriptions tailored to each person's needs.[48] A tremendous challenge also exists among disciplines to better understand the molecular basis involved in both monogenic disorders (defect in an inherited single gene; e.g., cystic fibrosis, sickle cell anemia, thalassemia, Huntington disease, Duchenne muscular dystrophy, hemophilia A, chronic granulomatous diseases) and multifactorial diseases—cancers (multiple genetic alterations), diabetes (influences all ages on all continents), and cardiovascular diseases (greatest morbidity and mortality worldwide).[3,59,86,111,152,245,263]

Turning Genes On and Off. When reduced to the most fundamental level, all physical activities (and literally all aspects of life), ultimately depend on multiple molecular events that regularly and systematically turn genes "on" and "off" to achieve desired functional outcomes. The new-generation exercise scientist who specializes in cross-disciplinary molecular biology research must expand the research horizons to uncover how different signaling mechanisms in the nerve-muscle connections regulate transcriptional, translational, and posttranslational events. Understanding the mechanisms about their interactions will go a long way to manipulate experimental variables to answer questions relevant to the field. For example, how does long-term exercise intensity and duration alter specific mRNA levels or an upstream signaling molecule such as Ca^{2+} to impact multiple signal transduction cascades downstream?[50] A simple, single muscle action corresponds to a 100-fold increase in intramuscular Ca^{2+} concentration (from 107 to 105 M). Some researchers believe that the huge Ca^{2+} influx, which coincides with myofilament cross-bridge cycling (see Chapter 18), serves as an important signaling messenger that links a muscle's function to transcriptional dynamics.[6] Other exercise-related physiologic transcription regulators include hypoxia and cellular oxidative stress (or redox).

The hypoxic state also affects erythropoietin (*EPO* gene) and **glucose transporter-1 (GLUT-1)** production. Consequently, understanding how these genes operate under hypoxic conditions will yield key information about oxygen delivery to cells and ultimately its use via citric acid cycle reactions, electron transport, and ATP synthesis associated with oxidative energy transformations.[66,246]

Oxygen Free Radicals and Antioxidant Agents. Reducing agents (antioxidants) modulate transcription.[143] In Chapter 6, we discuss how the mitochondrion reduces oxygen to form water, serving as the final common step in ATP synthesis. This pathways' imprecise coupling forms a **reactive oxygen species (ROS)**. The different antioxidants within skeletal muscle then scavenge and quench most ROS intruders.[25,132,136,140] Nevertheless, during high-intensity endurance exercise when aerobic metabolism increases 15- to 20-fold, ROS form in greater numbers to create damaging effects similarly produced by lipid peroxidation.[62,83,92,146]

The protein **thioredoxin** (reduces oxidized proteins) helping to balance a cell's redox state during energy metabolism also affects its transcriptional activity.[67] Determining how ROS influence transcription will pave the way for improved understanding about how aerobic-type activities affect long-term health effects (or potential risks) associated with ROS. Endurance training nearly doubles mitochondrial protein and mitochondrial mass.[51,116] This means that having a robust experimental model (e.g., endurance exercise/training) to study gene expression should lead to important new discoveries about endurance exercise effects and its many adaptations. Experiments have already described altered mRNA gene expression with long-term electrical stimulation,[167] including exercise effects related to muscle mitochondria,[16,75] and molecular-related alterations in skeletal muscle and muscle fiber type.[52] Microgravity's effects on gene expression in skeletal muscle also provide a fruitful area for further study.[9,43,60,67,72,100,102,137,146,168]

Gene Therapy Techniques

Three viable molecular biology research areas in the sport sciences involve different gene viral and nonviral delivery therapy techniques:

1. To treat acute and chronic musculoskeletal muscle tears, cartilage defects, and tendon ruptures
2. To reconstruct ligaments, osseous nonunions, and meniscus tears
3. To transplant tissue or genetic material for health and life enhancement

Inserting relevant genes directly into target tissues or systemically by vectors into the bloodstream should hopefully increase the probability for successful therapy and accelerated recuperation.[101,240] Researchers in the molecular biology sciences are now tracking flaws in human DNA that cause debilitating musculoskeletal disease, as for example, those involved with lumbar disks,[5,99] and other degenerative diseases[245] and other protein structures and functions related to chromosomal diseases.[55,219]

Lysosomes. The body's defense mechanisms involve lysozymes, membrane-bound, dense structures containing hydrolytic enzymes responsible for intracellular and extracellular digestion (https://microbenotes.com/lysosomes-structure-enzymes-types-functions/).

The 3-D structural model for the lysozyme enzyme shown in **FIGURE 33.47** is a relatively small but stable molecule generated by the Golgi apparatus to catalyze and then destroy protective cell walls chiefly in bacteria. These infectious structures have a tough outer layer with carbohydrate chains interlocked by short peptide strands that brace their delicate outer membrane against the cell's high osmotic pressure. Lysozymes break carbohydrate chains and destroy the bacterial cell's structural integrity. This action causes bacteria to burst spontaneously under their own increased internal osmotic pressure.

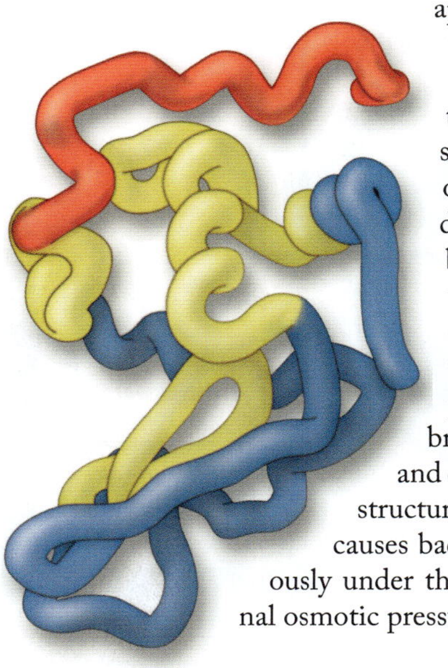

FIGURE 33.47. Computer-3-D-generated white lysozyme hen egg molecule, discovered in 1928 by Sir Alexander Fleming (1881–1955) 5 years before he discovered the first true antibiotic penicillin. Lysozymes protect against bacterial infection in egg whites and in human mucosal cavities (nasal cavity, eyelids, inside the mouth, trachea, lungs, lip, vagina, stomach and intestines, urethral opening, and anus).

Gene–Exercise Interactions

Crucial questions concern what "signals" control cooperation among different molecules and whether changes occur selectively in some regions within specific protein molecules and not others. This raises the question concerning how genetic and environmental factors affect the complex etiology in many common and debilitating diseases.[23] The model describing gene-exercise interaction in **FIGURE 33.48** can modify health status indirectly by altering gene expression that itself can temper intermediate phenotypes and disease outcome.[147] In addition, increased physical activity through formal exercise and training influence health.[70,158] Both indirect and direct evidence can link a particular disease state with an outcome physical activity variable.[199,200] The journal *Medicine & Science in Sports & Exercise* publishes updates about the human gene map related to performance-related and health-related fitness phenotypes.[201–205]

Lippincott® Connect — Appendix M online at **Lippincott Connect** lists selected references for human and animal molecular biology research from 2013 through 2021.

In the first comprehensive examination linking strenuous physical activity with Parkinson disease risk, Harvard researchers reported that males who exercised regularly and vigorously early in their adult life had a lower risk for developing Parkinson's than sedentary counterparts.[33] The most physically active males cut their risk for developing Parkinson's by 50% compared with males who were the least physically active. Men who regularly engaged in strenuous physical activity in early adult life cut their risk by 60% compared with those who did no physical activity. Among females, strenuous activity in the early adult years linked to Parkinson lower risk, but the relationship was not statistically significant, and no clear association existed between physical activity later in life and disease risk.

A recent randomized control trial assessed progressive resistance exercise (PRE) effects on Parkinson disease motor function scales.[37] The study compared 6-, 12-, 18-, and 24-mo outcomes in patients with Parkinson disease who received either PRE only or a modified program (MP) with stretching, balance, and strengthening exercise. Patients matched by sex and off-medication scores on the motor subscale Unified Parkinson Disease Rating Scale (UPDRS-III) assigned randomly into two interventions. Patients exercised 2 days weekly for 24 months at a gym. A personal trainer directed both weekly sessions for the first 6 months and 1 weekly session after 6 months. The primary outcome was the posttest off-medication UPDRS-III score. Of 51 patients, 20 in the PRE group and 18 in the MP group completed the trial. At 24 months, the mean off-medication UPDRS-III score decreased significantly more with PRE than with MP (mean difference, -7.3 points; 95% confidence interval, -11.3 to -3.6; $p < 0.001$). PRE training statistically and clinically reduced UPDRS-III scores compared with MP training was a useful adjunct therapy to improve parkinsonian motor signs.

A crucial challenge to information generated from this type of research requires resolution. Scientists must connect the evidence about the interaction with the genes involved in Parkinson's with physical inactivity throughout life.[29,126,251] This is true for all other major diseases and the increasingly suggestive role concerning one's physical activity level's genetic basis.[53] A content review posits that **dopamine receptor 1** (*Drd1*; five different research lines suggest *Drd1*'s involvement in physical activity regulation) and nescient helix loop helix (Nhlh2; through its effect on β-endorphin production and interaction with melanocortin-4 receptor) serve as excellent candidate genes to regulate physical activity level and the scientific rush to understand inactivity-induced diseases.[252] Research supports several other potential candidate genes that include myostatin (*Mstn*), glucose transporter 4 (*Slc2a4*), and 3-phosphoadenosine 5-phosphosulfate synthase (*Papss2*).[253,254]

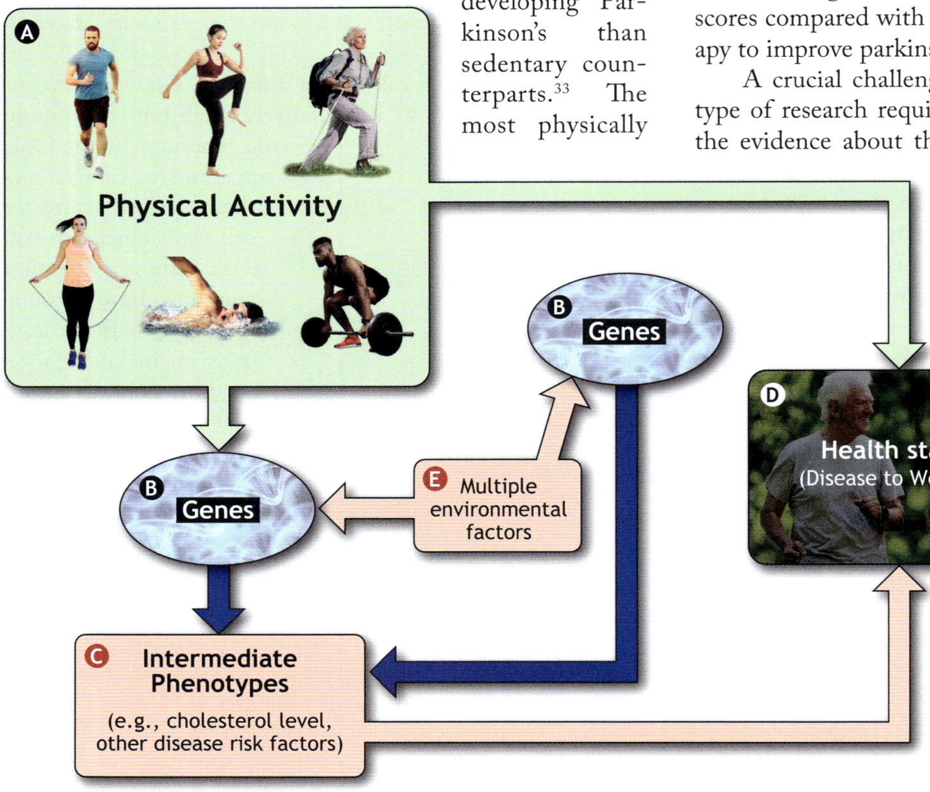

FIGURE 33.48 Model among gene-exercise interactions, intermediate phenotype, and multiple environmental factor interactions for health status along the disease-wellness continuum. (Adapted with permission from Bray MS. Genomics, genes, and environmental interaction: the role of exercise. *J Appl Physiol*. 2000;88:788. ©The American Physiological Society (APS). All rights reserved. Shutterstock images: Dejan Stanic Micko [runner], Nattakorn_Maneerat [yogi], Desizned [hiker], Maridav [swimmer], Iryna Inshyna [jump roper], Lightfield Studios [weight lifter], pikselstock [couple], Billion Photos [genes].).

Discoverer of Parkinson Disease

In 1817, British surgeon and accomplished paleontologist James Parkinson (1755–1824) was first to clinically describe a central nervous system degenerative disorder as the "shaking palsy or *Paralysis Agitans*," now referred to as Parkinson disease (PD) (https://archive.org/details/shaking_palsy_2004_librivox). His perceptive observations about this syndrome were not fully appreciated during his lifetime, which spanned the American Revolution, French Revolution, and Napoleonic Wars. He describes cases and strategies to provide relief to his patients, as did the physician Galen (AD 131–201) and other ancient medical practitioners before and following the Greek Golden ages (see History section). Parkinson described the affliction as follows: "Involuntary tremulous motion, with lessened muscular power, in parts not in action and even when supported; with a propensity to bend the trunk forwards, and to pass from a walking to a running pace: the senses and intellects being uninjured." Different strategic models to study PD now include experiments with rodents, nonhuman primates, and nonmammalian species. The basic experimental models include isolating transcription factors from pluripotent (immature) stem cells, neurotoxin-induced animal strategies, and genetic assessment to identify disease-causing gene interactions. The 3-D illustration depicts a degenerating dopaminergic neuron, a key stage in PD development leading to partial limb paralysis. The American Parkinson Association (www.apdaparkinson.org/resources-support/) has local chapter networks to deliver education, support, and offer patient services to people with PD and their families.

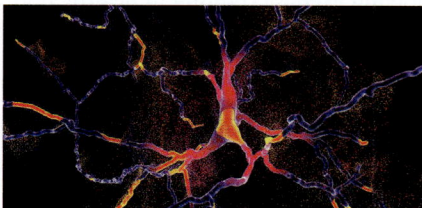

Kateryna Kon/Shutterstock

Sources:
Chia SJ, et al. Historical perspective: models of Parkinson's disease. *Int J Mol Sci*. 2020;21:2464.
Ludtmann MHR, Abramov AY. Mitochondrial calcium imbalance in Parkinson's disease. *Neurosci Lett*. 2018;663:86.
Weintraub D, et al. The neuropsychiatry of Parkinson's disease: advances and challenges. *Lancet Neurol*. 2022;21:89.

Snapshot: Strength-Related Studies and Genes

Studies have examined how different genetic variants relate to aerobic and exercise genomics,[177] and resistance-type activities,[178,180] muscle fiber type and handgrip strength,[179,181] and the skeletal genome.[172,264] On the other hand, controlled experiments have not yet validated the gene—to phenotype interactions among popular physical activity modes and their sport activity–related derivatives.[181]

The following examples briefly summarize the focus from selected studies and their main findings and/or future research directions dealing with resistance-type activities (including elite champion athletes) and mtDNA.[183,274] The citation sources follow each of the six summaries.

Mapping Robust Genetic Variants

Researchers have summarized robust and consistent genetic variants associated with aerobic-related and resistance-related phenotypes (12 single-nucleotide polymorphisms, 7 associated with aerobic-related and resistance-related phenotypes).[287] Few studies have investigated genes and environmental factors related to physiological trait development. Future experiments should include large-scale exercise studies to understand their functional relevance to known genomic markers, which allow more rigor and reproducible exercise genomic research.

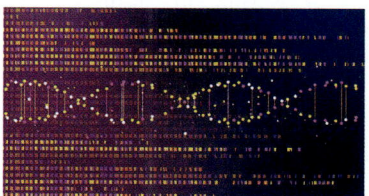

majcot/Shutterstock

Epigenetic Modifications in Skeletal Muscle with Exercise

Physical activity and sports play major roles in overall human health, particularly many molecular adaptations in muscle fibers in the skeletal muscle transcriptome.[288] The pathways that induce changes in gene expression patterns without altering the DNA base sequence may play an important role to control skeletal muscle transcriptional patterns. Epigenetic mechanisms include DNA and histone modifications and specific microRNA expression. Current knowledge about epigenetic changes induced in exercising skeletal muscle, their target genes, and resulting phenotypic changes suggests a practical application with known epigenetic modifications can help to design and manage, optimize, and individualize training protocols to predict training adaptations considering an individual's targeted genomic patterns known to play a role in skeletal muscle function.[131]

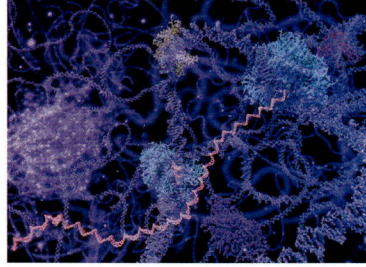

Juan Gaertner/Shutterstock

Alleles Associated with Fast-Twitch Fibers, Lean Body Mass, and Handgrip Strength

The brain-derived neurotrophic factor (BDNF) plays a role in neurogenesis and forming regenerated myofibers following injury or damage. Prior studies suggested that the BDNF overexpression increases their proportion in fast-twitch muscle fibers, while the BDNF deletion promotes a fast-to-slow twitch transition. This experiment with 164 physically active individuals (113 males, 51 females) evaluated the association between the BDNF gene rs10501089 polymorphism (associated with blood BDNF levels), muscle fiber composition, and power athlete status. BDNF genotype and allele frequencies compared 508 Russian power athletes, 178 endurance athletes, and 190 controls. Carriers of the minor A-allele (the BDNF-increasing g allele) had significantly greater percentage fast-twitch muscle fibers than individuals homozygous for the G-allele (males: 64.3% vs. females: 50.3%). The A-allele was associated with greater handgrip strength in a subgroup of 83 physically active subjects and overrepresented in power athletes compared with controls. The A-allele (i.e., AA + AG genotypes) rather than GG genotype increased the probability of being a power athlete compared with controls or endurance athletes. The authors concluded that the rs10501089 A-allele associated with an increased proportion in fast-twitch muscle fibers and greater handgrip strength, which may have accounted for the association between the AA/AG genotypes and power athlete group.

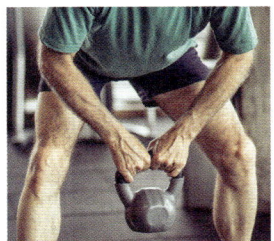
Mladen Zivkovic/Shutterstock

In a different but related experiment, targeted genotype analyses used in genome-wide association studies (GWAS) previously identified six, single-nucleotide polymorphisms (SNPs) associated with lean body mass (LBM) and handgrip strength (HGS). This follow-up study assessed 48 elite master athletes (MAs) and 48 age-matched controls with variable muscle mass and function. A significant association emerged in the ADAMTSL3 genotype with LBM. For the three HGS-linked SNPs, neither GBF1 nor GLIS1 associated with HGS, but there was a significant association with this genotype and HGS. Of the six SNPs analyzed, ADAMTSL3 and TGFA significantly associated with LBM and HGS. The authors concluded that the ADAMTSL3 SNP in body composition and TGFA in strength revealed significant genetic components in elite MA phenotypes. The authors cite 42 prior research studies (1997–2020) as background to their analyses. Genetic screening systems in mice and *Caenorhabditis elegans* also have causally linked GWAS gene candidates to potentially identify genes associated with human diseases.[289,290,291]

Epigenetic Changes in Skeletal Muscle Following Exercise

Complex environmental and genetic factors each guide adaptations to exercise training. The epigenetic factors help to foster gene expression; the factors include histone modifications (DNA coils around the histone protein shown in the image), epigenetic regulating noncoding RNAs (miRNA), and DNA methylation (modified cytosine base between cytosine and guanine separated by a phosphate). The term myomiRs applies to noncoding

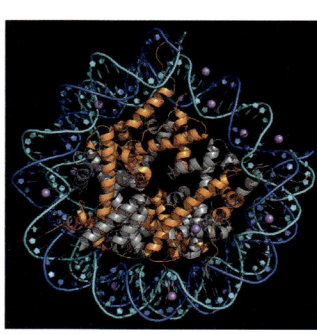
MoleculeQuest/Shutterstock

miRNA exclusively expressed in skeletal muscle. Ten miRNA studies involved these biomarkers and the others, which served as viable conduits between the genotype and common environment factors in specific tissues (e.g., diet, stress, drugs, toxins, smoking, and particularly muscle tissue).[292] The biomarkers in muscle tissue help to track "end-game" response patterns following an acute exercise bout, a pre/postexercise intervention design, or a case/control experiment. The researchers initially considered 454 published studies to identify skeletal muscle epigenetic changes following exercise training in healthy populations from five databases in 2018 (PubMed, MEDLINE, CINAHL, SCOPUS, and SPORTDiscus). Following a careful filtering process, 22 studies met the inclusion criteria. The authors carefully reviewed the clearly identified epigenetic marks altered in response to exercise and their potential influence on skeletal muscle metabolism. They cautioned not to ascribe these epigenetic marks as having a definite physiological impact due to exercise. They were cautiously optimistic that the emerging science of exercise epigenetics is still a young research field, with the newer advanced CRISPR-cas9 models unraveling the secrets within the epigenome.[284]

DNA Polymorphisms in Weightlifters

Many heritable traits totaling 196 SNPs associate with HGS identified in three GWASs. This study validated the association using 35 SNPs with strength in elite Russian and Polish weightlifters.[293] The researchers identified the rs12055409 G-allele near the MLN gene, the rs4626333 G-allele near the ZNF608 gene, and the rs2273555 A-allele in the GBF1 gene. These genes associated with greater total weight lifted in snatch and clean and jerk adjusted for sex and weight in 53 elite Russian weightlifters. In a replication study with 76 subelite Polish weightlifters, rs4626333 GG homozygotes also prominently expressed in the lifting competitions, and histones larger to relative

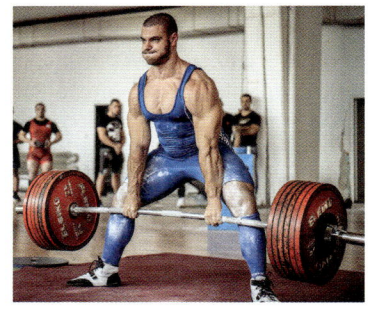
Jordan Jovkov/Shutterstock

muscle mass in the top performers adjusted for sex, weight, and age compared with the A-allele carriers. The results indicated the strength-associated allele number positively associated with fast-twitch muscle fiber cross-sectional area in 20 different male power athletes and with HGS in 87 physically active individuals. The authors concluded that by replicating previous findings in four independent studies, the rs12055409 G-allele, rs4626333 G-allele, and rs2273555 A-allele associate with higher strength levels, total muscle mass, and muscle fiber size.

mtDNA and Elite Athletic Performance

Aerobic ATP generation by the mitochondrial respiratory oxidative phosphorylation system (OXPHOS) plays a vital metabolic role in endurance exercise. mtDNA has codified 13 of 83 polypeptides within the respiratory chain. Consequently, a strong

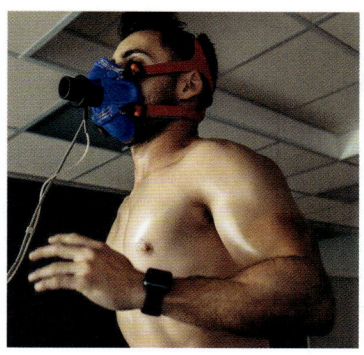
Jacob Lund/Shutterstock

association existed between mtDNA variants and "aerobic" (endurance) exercise phenotypes.[293] This study identified nuclear genes involved in mitochondrial genesis and elite endurance athletic status. Several studies in nonathletic people have demonstrated an association between certain mtDNA lineages and aerobic performance, characterized by maximal oxygen uptake ($\dot{V}O_{2max}$). Whether mtDNA haplogroups also are associated with elite endurance athlete status is more controversial, with differences between studies arising from the different ethnic backgrounds in the athletic cohorts with diverse genetic associations (Caucasians with mixed, Asiatic, or East African geographic origins).

The Future Is Now

A general systems genetics research design flow proposes to determine a phenotype's genetic basis.[90] Four key questions can help to shape the future in molecular genomics research in kinesiology and the other exercise sciences (**FIG. 33.49**). The left side of the figure presents four key questions to answer, with the right view offering bullet point choices related to each question. For question 1, for example, research with family and twin studies and mouse and human models remains robust—it supports research into exploring significant genetic influences on physical activity, which accounts for 20 to 92% in the genetic heritability relevant to a particular activity trait.

For question 2, prior research with genome mapping indicates where prior research has looked to discover what parts in the genome associate with a particular trait. Prior mapped genomic regions known as quantitative trait loci (QTL) have narrowed the research focus for possible gene candidates related to physical activity. Accordingly, the QTL approach categorizes a single effect where the genetic factors act individually to influence physical activity, or as epistatic, where the QTL genetic factors must work synergistically with genetic factors in other genomic locations before they can affect the phenotype. The answer to question 3, identifying the involved genes, has been more problematical. Only limited genes have been definitively associated with predisposing links that steer individuals into a lifetime devoted to exercise and fitness. Researchers may eventually discover inherited genetic sequences related to undesirable sedentary behaviors (and undesirable disease conditions), and through techniques akin to today's CRISPR-Cas9 techniques, genetically reduce these gene sequences with replacement "fitness and wellness"

gene sequences. The final two questions must continue to rely on cooperative research among many disciplines in the basic and applied sciences. This approach makes sense to us in order to move the ball forward to find answers to difficult questions and then develop appropriate solutions. Pharmaceutical solutions and new gene editing techniques are leading the way.

Focused Academic Preparation

To students with a keen interest in genetics and molecular biology related to physical activity and inactivity, the future academic path to discovery remains wide open and to be pursued. The decade ahead is rich with almost unlimited topics worthy of scientific investigation related to human movement, health, and physical fitness.[36] We believe that the kinesiological sciences have a shared responsibility with other basic and applied disciplines to contribute to a robust understanding in these developing new areas.

We anticipate that during the next decade, researchers from diverse disciplines will continue to cross boundaries to solve challenging questions within the exercise physiology domain we have covered in this text. From our experience spanning many decades, there comes a time when newly acquired knowledge takes new twists and turns in a students' life path after graduation. Our advice keeps the door wide

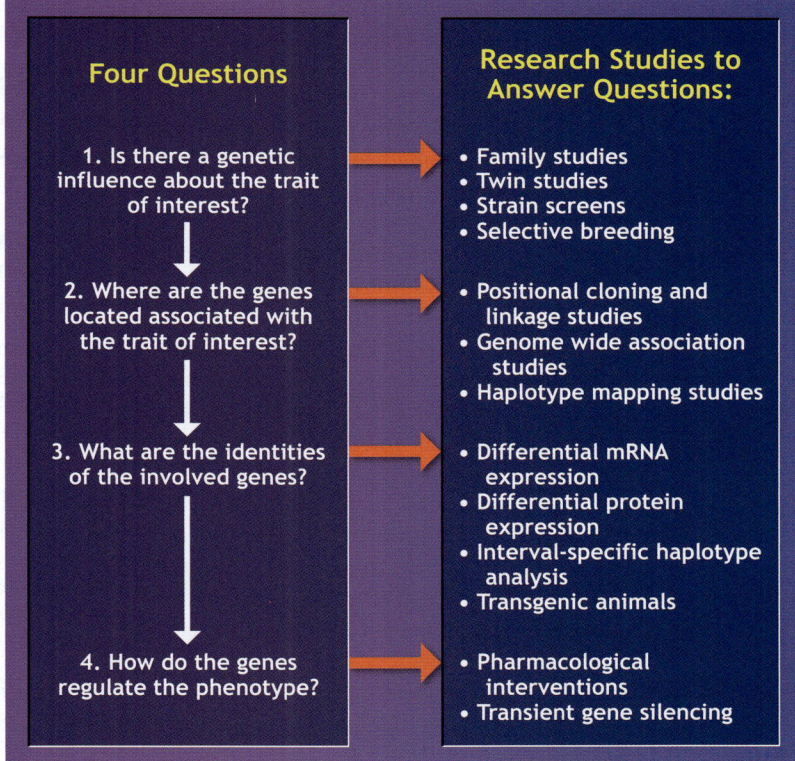

FIGURE 33.49. Proposed research schema to determine the genetic basis for physical activity. About 11 years ago, a research paper cited 49 animal and human studies related to the genetics of physical activity, presenting different evidence lines to support the first three questions posed in the figure.
(Modified with permission from Lightfoot JT. Current understanding of the genetic basis for physical activity. *J Nutr.* 2011;141(3):526. Copyright © 2011 American Society for Nutrition.)

open to new opportunities in the sciences, particularly connections between kinesiology and related disciplines. And one never knows when the door marked "molecular biology sciences" opens for opportunities in this relatively new and exciting field to pursue, as it did for 2020 Nobel laureate Jennifer Doudna as an inquisitive teenager attending school in Hawaii. She never dreamed her future in the sciences would someday lead to her CRISPR discoveries revolutionizing chemistry with far-reaching impact in most science fields today.

Unexpected Connections and Serendipity

Each of us can recall a time when students would tell us about an experience they had in a totally different field. A biology student was studying for an exam in an undergraduate entomology course (studying insects) and asked the kinesiology student roommate if the student knew why birds could fly such long distances during migration? The answer seemed straight forward to the kinesiology student—it probably had to do with what food types the birds consumed and metabolized during their migration. The biology student said some birds fly essentially nonstop during a 2000 mi migration and do not have time (nor need) during the flight to forage for food. The kinesiology student said she had walked on a treadmill in the exercise physiology laboratory class, with energy expenditure measured continually during a 2-hr walk that simulated mild hill climbing and without access to food. The student told the biology major that by analyzing her oxygen uptake and carbon dioxide production during the walk each minute and for a 30-min recovery period, the proportion of lipids and carbohydrates could be determined along with the total energy expended for the walk. Would the same approach apply to migrating birds?

The biology major was determined to find out and reported back the next day that the roommate was indeed correct. When the student asked the entomology course teaching assistant, he told the student that this project involved measuring the oxygen uptake and energy expenditure in hummingbirds using closed circuit spirometry! In fact, they both learned the same approach to answer the question by essentially employing similar equipment and methodology—one for humans and one for birds. The kinesiology student told the professor about the encounter, and later learned there were research collaborations between entomology and kinesiology professors to assess species differences in energy expenditure economy and nutrient consumption. Wow! We were not surprised that both undergraduate students continued their education and earned MS and PhD degrees, one in entomology and the other kinesiology, and today are productive scholars with academic appointments combining teaching undergraduate and graduate students, writing books, and conducting research in their laboratories. Before going on to graduate school, the kinesiology student took a year to attend meaningful courses in other disciplines by scouring university course catalogs—integrative physiology, computer animation science, cognitive motor neuroscience, neurobiology, space physiology, forensic anthropology, functional genomics, and many more available for study. Both students' initial encounters as roommates turned out to be a driving force for their eventual future scientific endeavors. This surely represented serendipity by design and not coincidence.

Working together, exercise physiologists trained in molecular biology (or molecular biologists with training in exercise physiology) can profit from the insights of biologists, geneticists, pharmacologists, and chemists who study human physical activity at the molecular level. Their shared explorations will benefit all humanity.

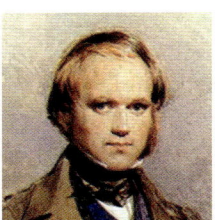

Each being at some period of life, during some season of the year, during each generation or at intervals, has to struggle for life, and to suggest great destruction. When we reflect on this struggle, we may console ourselves with the full belief that the war of nature is not incessant, that no fear is felt, that death is generally prompt, and that the vigorous, the healthy, and the happy survive and multiply.

Charles Darwin

Key Terms

Activator protein: Binds to DNA at enhancer sites to position RNA polymerase correctly on the gene

Adenine: One in four DNA bases always pairs with thymine adenosine triphosphate

Aminoacyl-tRNA synthetase: Activating enzyme that covalently links amino acids to their cognate transfer RNA 39 ends

Angiogenesis: New blood vessel formation during embryonic development and abnormally around malignant tumors

Anneal: Rejoining separated single complementary DNA strands to form a double helix

Anticodon: Three complementary bases at the tRNA molecule end that recognize and bind to a messenger RNA codon

Antiparallel: Arranged in parallel but with opposite orientation as in DNA

Antisense RNA: DNA transcript with 19 to 23 nucleotides complementary to messenger RNA to control gene expression in replication, transcription, and translation

Apoptosis: Cell death following preprogrammed "instructions" from caspase proteases to initiate the apoptotic death signal

Autoradiography: Process that produces an image on a photographic film (autoradiograph) placed flat on an electrophoresis gel that shows the radioactive molecule position on the gel

Bacteria: Large unicellular microorganisms (spherical, rod, spiral, and comma-shaped), with cell walls but lacking organelles and an organized nucleus

Bacteriophage: A bacterium infected by a virus

Base pairs: Two complementary nucleotide bases (G-C or A-T) in a double-stranded DNA molecule held together by hydrogen bonds

Benign tumor: Tumor that remains in one location, no longer responds to normal growth control, and lacks capacity to invade distant sites

Bioinformatics: Understanding organisms' underlying chemical codes by interpreting gene sequences, converting primary linear code into complex three-dimensional structures, managing automated screens, and running combinatorial chemistry syntheses

Bioremediation: Using microorganisms to consume and break down environmental pollutants

Cancer: Accelerated, unplanned mutant cell growth and division that forms larger-than-normal cell clusters that become tumors

Cas9 nuclease: RNA-guided endonuclease that catalyzes site-specific double-stranded DNA cleavage

cDNA: Single-stranded DNA complementary to an RNA and synthesized from it using reverse transcriptase to code exons

cDNA library: Contains the genes' coding regions with leading and trailing mRNA sequences

Cell cycle: Four stages comprising a cell's life

Central dogma: Crick's belief that the genetic information flow creates proteins from DNA (transcription in the nucleus) and RNA (translation in the cytoplasm) to protein

Centromere: Region in a mitotic chromosome before replication where two daughter chromatids join

Chargaff rule: Pyrimidine content (T C) equals purine content (A G), where ([T] [A]; [G] [C]); (A T)/(G C) varies between different organisms but remains constant within an organism

Chromatid: One in two double-stranded DNA daughter molecules from a duplicated, mitotic chromosome joined by a centromere

Chromosome: Threadlike DNA and protein strand in the cell nucleus with the genes that transmit hereditary information

Cloning: Creating a cell(s) or molecule(s) from a single ancestral cell or molecule

Coactivator protein: Transmits signals from activator proteins to basal factors

Coding region: Location on the DNA strand where transcription occurs

Codon: Sequence in three DNA or RNA bases (nucleotides) that encode a single amino acid

Complementary bases: Pairing in DNA between bases A–T or T–A and C–G or G–C

Complementary DNA (cDNA): Single-stranded DNA complementary to an RNA and synthesized from it using reverse transcriptase to code exons

Complementary DNA (cDNA) library: Contains the genes' coding regions with leading and trailing messenger RNA sequences

Complementary strand: DNA strand that runs opposite of another (i.e., from 3′ to 5′ compared with 5′ to 3′ direction)

Continuous synthesis: Creating a DNA strand

Covalent bond: Sharing one or more electron pairs between two atoms

CRISPR: Acronym for **C**lustered **R**egularly **I**nterspaced **S**hort **P**alindromic **R**epeats; DNA sequences used to edit a gene's base pairs

CRISPR gene editing: Genetic engineering technique to modify *in vivo* living organism's genomes by delivering Cas9 nuclease complexed with a synthetic guide RNA into a gene's base pairs

Cyclins: Specific cell regulator enzymes activate and deactivate protein kinases in the cell cycle aid progression from one stage in the cycle to the next until destroyed after their function by a ubiquitin-signaled process

Cytosine: One in DNA's four bases always pairs with guanine

Daughter chromosome: Descendent chromosome following the original (mother) chromosome replication

Dehydration synthesis: Removing a water molecule from two subunit molecules when forming a new, larger molecule

Deoxyribonucleic acid (DNA): Double-helix molecule with two complementary nucleotide chains containing an organism's total hereditary information

Deoxyribose: Sugar with five carbon atoms

Diploid: Having two representatives from every chromosome (i.e., two copies in each gene)

Discontinuous synthesis: Ten nucleotide RNA primer under DNA polymerase I influence, adding 1000 nucleotides situated before the lagging strand's 59 end until its gap fills

DNA gyrase: Enzyme that relaxes supercoiled DNA

DNA helicase: Enzyme that catalyzes unwinding double-helical DNA by using energy released from ATP hydrolysis

DNA ligase: Enzyme binds short Okazaki fragments in the lagging strand into a continuous strand in DNA replication during stage 3 discontinuous synthesis

DNA polymerase: Enzyme responsible for creating new DNA strands during replication or repair

DNA polymerase I: Enzyme that makes small DNA bits to fill gaps between Okazaki fragments during stage 3 discontinuous synthesis

DNA polymerase III (Pol III): Enzyme involved in making DNA when chromosomes replicate

DNA probe: Radioactive or fluorescent-labeled nucleotide that identifies, isolates, or binds to a gene or gene product

DNA replication fork: Y-shaped region in replicating DNA molecules where enzymes replicate a DNA molecule bound to an untwisted, single DNA strand

Dopamine receptor 1 (Drd1): Protein in humans encoded by the DRD1 gene

Double helix: Two DNA strands twisted in a spiral around each other

Electron microscope: Electron beams with wavelengths thousands of times shorter than visible light replace light, allowing significantly higher resolution and magnification

Endoplasmic reticulum: Tubules, vesicles, and flattened sac structures in a cell's endomembrane system

Enhancer site: Gene expression increases from contact with the transcription complex

Epigenetics: Changes in gene function without changes in DNA sequence

Erythropoietin: Kidney-produced hormone initiates red blood cell precursors and their maturation to erythrocytes

Escherichia coli (E. coli): Rodlike anaerobic bacterium with 4.6 million base pairs present in humans and other mammals

Eukaryotes: Multicellular animal, plant, and fungi organisms with membrane-bound organelles and a true nucleus containing multiple linear chromosomes (Greek; from eu-karyon, or "true nucleus")

Exon: Gene's protein-coding DNA sequence

Forensic medicine: Applying the law to medical and paramedical scientific knowledge

Founder mice: Original engineered mice (with one transgene copy) bred together to create transgenic animals

Free radical: Highly reactive ionized atom or molecule with a single unpaired electron in the outer orbit can cause mutation from its interaction with DNA

Functional protein: Protein with its own genetically determined information to carry out specific function(s)

G1: Period within the cell cycle preceding DNA synthesis

G2: Period within the cell cycle from DNA synthesis termination and M phase initiation

Gamete: Egg or sperm

Gel electrophoresis: Separating electrically charged substances (e.g., proteins) through a gel mesh according to substance size

Gene: DNA segment with an ordered nucleotide sequence to encode a specific functional substance (i.e., a protein or RNA molecule)

Gene cassette: Artificially constructed DNA segment containing a genetic restriction marker at the nucleotide segment's both ends

Gene expression: Converting a gene's coded information by transcription and translation into cellular structures, where expressed genes transcribe (copy) DNA nucleotide sequences into mRNA, then translated by ribosomes into specific nucleotide sequences to form protein

Gene splicing: Attaching a DNA fragment from one species (e.g., mammal) to another species (e.g., bacterium)

Gene therapy: Introducing genes into cells (genetic surgery) to alter phenotype (i.e., cure diseases like cystic fibrosis using engineered adenovirus carrying a "good" gene to replace the crippled cystic fibrosis gene)

Genetic code: Nucleotide sequence coded in triplets (codons) along the mRNA determines the amino acid sequence in protein synthesis

Genetic engineering: Laboratory-altered DNA that changes its characteristics through cleaving source DNA, creating recombinants, cloning recombinant copies, and locating desired gene cloned copies

Genetics: Science that studies inheritance patterns for specific traits in successive generations

Genome: Organism's complete genetic DNA and RNA information

Genome-wide association studies (GWAS): An approach in genetics research to associate specific genetic variations with known diseases

Genomic library: DNA fragments from an organism's genome includes noncoding DNA and cDNA

Genotype: Individual's genetic makeup at the molecular level comprising the entire gene set

Germ line: Cell lineage includes mature reproductive sperm and egg germ cells

Glucose transporter-1 (GLUT1): Facilitates glucose transport across the plasma membrane independently from insulin

Glycolipid: Polysaccharide bound to lipid

Glycoprotein: Protein complexed with polysaccharide

Golgi complex: Membrane-bound vesicles between the endoplasmic reticulum and plasma membrane involved in posttranslational protein modification to sort and deliver them to different intracellular compartments

Guanine: One in four DNA bases always pairs with cytosine

Guanosine triphosphate (GTP): Initiates translation when it binds mRNA at the molecule's 5′ end to the ribosome's two smaller subunits

Helicase: Enzymes catalyze and separate double-stranded DNA or RNA during its replication

Helix: One possible polypeptide secondary structure in a right-handed peptide chain maintained by hydrogen (H) bonds between carbon (C) and oxygen (O) atoms in every fifth amino acid along the chain

Heterozygous: Two different alleles in a particular gene

Histone: Positively charged small nuclear protein molecule cluster that binds to DNA winding around it before it uncoils at the replication site

Homozygous: Having two identical alleles in the same gene

Housekeeping genes: Genes automatically switched "on" to maintain essential cell functions

Human genome: Maximum genetic material in a human cell containing about 80,000 to 140,000 genes and from 3.12 to 3.15 billion nucleotide base pairs

Human Genome Project: Department of Energy and National Institutes of Health project created DNA segments from known chromosomal locations, developed new computational methods to analyze genetic maps and DNA sequence data, and developed new techniques and instruments to detect and analyze DNA

Hydrogen bonds: Weak, interactive bonding from simultaneous attraction with a positive hydrogen atom to other atoms with negative charges

Immune response: Immune system immediate defensive reaction when invaded by a foreign pathogen

Intron: DNA base noncoding sequence that interrupts a gene's protein-coding sequence that gets excised from the "message" before it translates into protein

Junk DNA: Noncoding DNA regions in chromosomes

Kilobase (kb): Unit of length for DNA fragments equal to 1000 nucleotides

Kinase: Enzyme that shuttles a phosphate group (PO_4) from ATP or another nucleoside triphosphate to a different molecule

Knockin animal model: Replacing a normal gene with a mutant gene (akin to "trading places" at a specific gene location or locus) and observing the effects on the offspring

Knockout animal model: Specific gene(s) inactivated (disabled) by inserting a gene cassette to disrupt the coding sequence linked to a specific target gene

Lagging strand: New shorter DNA strand formed during discontinuous synthesis joined end to end by DNA ligase away from the replication fork

Leading strand: New DNA daughter strand formed during continuous DNA synthesis

Leptin: Protein hormone involved with appetite and lipid storage

Locus: Specific gene location on a chromosome

Malignant tumor: Tumor that invades other tissues and forms secondary or tertiary cancers

Melting point: Temperature range for a solid where it changes state from solid to liquid, and the solid and liquid phases exist in equilibrium

Messenger RNA (mRNA): Molecule that carries genetic information (complementary copy for one of the two DNA strands) between a gene and the ribosomes, which translate the genetic information into proteins

Metagenomics: Studying genetic material from different organisms contained in an environmental sample

Metaphase: Step in mitosis (or meiosis) in which microtubules organize into a spindle and chromosomes move to the cell's equator to align in pairs but have not yet migrated to the poles

Metastasize: Cancerous cells spread from the original tumor mass to form secondary cancers (metastases) elsewhere in the body

Methionine: Nutritionally essential amino acid serves as the most natural source for active methyl groups in the body

Mitosis: Separating duplicated chromosomes to create identical daughter cells with mirror-image proceed in prophase, metaphase, anaphase, and telophase stages

Molecular anthropology: Applying molecular biology and genetics to contemporary populations and ancient specimen origins

Molecular biology: Deals with proteins and nucleic acid structures and functions essential to life

Molecular genetics: Subfield in biology that addresses how variation in DNA molecular structure differs among organisms

Mutagen: Ionizing radiation, ultraviolet radiation, or a chemical agent disrupts DNA code sequence and produces mutations

Mutation: Gene with permanently altered or defective genetic information initiates heritable changes

Natural selection: Darwin's basic idea that species survive because more favorable phenotypic traits pass down through successive generations

Neurofibromatosis: Hereditary disorder characterized clinically hyperpigmentation in cutaneous and subcutaneous tumors over the entire body

Neurohormone: Hormone formed by neurosecretory cells and liberated by nerve impulses (e.g., norepinephrine)

Northern blot: Binding a DNA probe in a specific RNA sequence in the RNA molecule

Nuclear DNA: DNA contained within each cell nucleus in a eukaryotic organism

Nuclear pore complex: Octagonal, disk-shaped structure allows proteins to cross the nuclear envelope into the cytoplasm after protein receptors dock with the protein

Nuclear transfer: DNA removed from an unfertilized egg and introduced into a specially prepared cell nucleus by an electrical pulse or chemical to fuse the two substances to initiate their development

Nucleic acid: Large molecule containing nucleotide subunits

Nucleosome: DNA coiled around clustered histone proteins

Nucleotide: Nucleic acid segment containing a 5-carbon sugar, phosphate group, and nitrogen-containing base

Nucleus: Structure that contains the cell's genetic chromosomal DNA material

Nutraceutical: Genetically engineered product that alters or modifies a product or by-product characteristics

Okazaki fragments: Short DNA segments 100 to 200 nucleotides long assembled by discontinuous replication in the 5′ to 3′ direction away from the replication fork to form the lagging strand

Oncogene: Mutant gene that promotes the loss in cellular growth control

Organelle: Intracellular structure within a cell that carries out specialized functions (e.g., mitochondrion)

Paternity: Father to a known child (fatherhood)

Pathogen: Any virus, microorganism, or other substance that causes disease (e.g., *Streptococcus* bacteria cause scarlet fever, rheumatic fever, and pneumonia in humans; in plants, and destructive blights, soft rots, and wilts)

Peptide bonds: Chemical linking binds amino acids in a protein when the carboxyl group in an amino acid reacts with the amino group in a second amino acid

Pharmacogenomics: Genetic engineering to design specific drugs to target specific disease conditions of an individual's genetic code, and investigate how genetic diversity affects targeted drug efficacy and side effects

Phenotype: Observable characteristics resulting from gene expression

Phosphodiester bond: Strong covalent bond formed when two nucleotides link together, eliminating a water molecule; bonding involves the phosphate molecule from one nucleotide and the hydroxyl (OH) molecule in another nucleotide

Photolithography: Technology to etch (transfer) electrical circuits on suitable media (silicon wafer with silicon dioxide)

Plasmid: Small, extrachromosomal DNA molecule within a cell physically separated from chromosomal DNA that can replicate independently; typically a small circular molecule in bacteria without chromosomal DNA that serves as a vector for transferring genes among cells

Polyadenylic acid [poly(A)] tail: Chain 100 to 200 adenine nucleotides long joins one end at the 39 region in the final transcripted mRNA before it migrates through the nuclear pore

Polymer: High molecular weight substance linked together by repeating similar or identical subunits (e.g., glucose polymer starch)

Polymerase: Enzyme catalyzes nucleic acid synthesis on preexisting nucleic acid templates for assembling RNA from ribonucleotides or DNA from deoxyribonucleotides

Polymerase chain reaction (PCR): Technique to artificially amplify a target DNA sequence usually by 106- to 109-fold during repeated denaturation cycles, annealing with primer, and extension with DNA polymerase

Polynucleotide: Two or more nucleotides joined together with the phosphate at carbon 59 in one sugar combined at the 39 position in another sugar

Polypeptide chain: Repeated, linked amino acid chains

Primary RNA transcript: mRNA molecule transcribed as an exact complement to a gene

Primary structure: Specific amino acid linear sequence determined by the gene's nucleotide sequence encoding the protein

Primase: Enzyme synthesizes the RNA primer to initiate DNA synthesis

Primer: Short nucleotide segment that pairs with a single DNA strand at a free 3-OH end (template strand) so DNA polymerase can synthesize a DNA chain

Prokaryote: Cell or organism lacking a structurally discrete nucleus or nuclear membrane containing a single circular chromosome

Promoter: Site on DNA where RNA polymerase binds and initiates transcription (promotes gene expression); required to express and regulate gene transcription

Pronucleus: Fertilized egg contains the haploid egg or sperm nucleus

Proopiomelanocortin (POMC): Neurotransmitter (endorphins) and hormones (melanocortin peptide) precursors whose roles include pigmentation, adrenocortical function, food intake and lipid storage, and immune and neural functions

Proteasome: Proteolytic enzyme degrades unwanted proteins in eukaryotic cell cytoplasm

Protein kinase: Enzyme that transfers phosphate groups to other proteins, changing their activity

Protein synthesis: Creating a protein from amino acid subunits

Proteolysis: Protein degradation

Proteomics: Systematically analyzing protein expression in healthy and unhealthy genomes at the molecular level by identifying, characterizing, and quantifying proteins

Pseudopregnant: Ovulation induced by sterile copulation

Purine: Nitrogen-containing, double-ring basic compound in nucleic acids—purines in DNA and RNA include adenine and guanine

Pyrimidine: Nitrogen-containing, single-ring basic compound in nucleic acids; include cytosine and thymine in DNA and cytosine and uracil in RNA

Quaternary structure: Complex, three-dimensional functional protein structure formed by joining two or more polypeptides

Quiescent: Stopping the fundamental functions in a cell

Radioisotope: More stable isotope when emitting radiation

Reactive oxygen species (ROS): Oxygen free radical formed from imprecise coupling during oxygen's reduction to water in the final electron transport-oxidative phosphorylation stage

Recombinant DNA: Hybrid DNA molecule by fusing DNA fragments by attaching a DNA segment from one species to another species, and then inserting the hybrid molecule into a host organism

Replication: DNA duplication prior to cell division

Replication origins: Sites on DNA where replication begins

Repressor protein: Blocks RNA polymerase action on DNA to turn genes "off"

Restriction endonuclease: Enzyme that cleaves a specific short DNA nucleotide sequence at a target site

Restriction enzyme: Cuts DNA at precise locations and reassembles the components into desired sequences

Retrovirus: RNA virus that can enter a cell using reverse transcriptase to reproduce its copy into the genome

Reverse transcriptase: Enzyme that allows a single-stranded RNA template to synthesize a double-stranded DNA copy for insertion in the genome

Ribonucleic acid (RNA): Usually a single-stranded nucleic acid that contains the sugar ribose

Ribosomal RNA (rRNA): Ribosome's structural part containing RNA molecules for assembling amino acids into polypeptides

Ribosome: Small cellular component (organelle) with specialized ribosomal RNA

RNA polymerase I: Enzyme that synthesizes RNA from a DNA template

RNA primer: Ten RNA nucleotides complementary to the parent DNA template that adds DNA nucleotides to it to synthesize a new DNA strand

RNA splicing: Excising unwanted intron sequence from the primary transcript, which fuses exons together

Sarcoma: Cancers forming from connective, muscle, or bone tissue

Secondary structure: Coiled protein similar to paired DNA strands or folded back onto itself to give a flat look

Sickle cell anemia: Potentially fatal hereditary disease affecting hemoglobin when the amino acid valine substitutes for glutamic acid because from changes in its codon nucleotide sequence from G-A-A to G-U-A

Single-nucleotide polymorphism (SNP): Polymorphism from variation at a single nucleotide

Single-strand binding protein (SSB): Protein that keeps separated DNA strands from rejoining

Southern blot: Detecting single-stranded DNA from transferring DNA fragments to nylon paper with a DNA-binding probe

Stop codon: Three of 64 codon combinations that terminate a polypeptide assembly

Supercoiled DNA: Twisted DNA packed into a cell prior to replication

TALEN: Acronym for Transcription Activator-Like Nuclease; cuts specific DNA sequences by fusing a TAL effector DNA-binding domain to a DNA cleavage domain

Telophase: Final stage in mitosis or meiosis where the spindle disappears and separated chromosomes daughter sets decondense, the cytoplasm splits, a nuclear envelope re-surrounds the chromosomes, and nucleoli appear

Template: Repeatable nucleotides sequences to form a complementary DNA or RNA strand

Template strand: Original DNA strand that synthesis a new DNA strand by complementary base pairing

Teratogen: Agent that causes extreme mutations

Tertiary structure: Final three-dimensional folded polymer chain

Thermus aquaticus: Thermally stable bacterium that survives at very high temperatures found in hot springs and geysers

Thioredoxin: Protein component in oxidation-reduction reactions to balance the cell's redox state

Thymine: One in four DNA bases always pairs with adenine

Totipotent: The cell possesses the required genetic information or "blueprint" to form an intact organism

Trans-activating CRISPR RNA (tracrRNA): Base pairs with crRNA to form a functional guide RNA

Transcription: RNA polymerase assembles an mRNA molecule complementary to the gene's nucleotide (making an RNA gene copy)

Transcription activator–like effector nucleases: Restriction enzymes that can cut specific DNA sequences by fusing a TAL effector DNA-binding domain to a DNA-cleavage domain

Transfection: Introducing an external donor DNA source into a recipient host

Transfer RNA (tRNA): RNA molecules that transport a specific amino acid to ribosomes, translating information in the mRNA nucleotide into the polypeptide amino acid sequence

Transgene: Genetic engineering technique places a foreign gene in different species' cells

Transgenic: Transforming genes from one species into another

Translation: Polypeptide formation (protein synthesis) on a ribosome using the amino acid sequence specified by an mRNA nucleotide sequence

Translocation: Movement along the ribosome by an mRNA molecule three nucleotide blocks (one codon) at a time

Tumor: Abnormal tissue growth

Ubiquitin: Small protein attaches by covalent bonding to a protein destroyed by proteasomes

Ultraviolet light: Higher-frequency electromagnetic rays than frequencies at the lower end in the visible violet spectrum

Uracil: Base that replaces thymine in RNA that pairs with the adenine base

Vasculogenesis: *In vivo* blood vessel formation by vascular precursor cell differentiation

Vector: Plasmid, retrovirus, or bacterial or yeast artificial chromosome used to transfer a foreign DNA segment among cells or species represents the genome that transports alien DNA into a host cell

Virus: Small adenovirus, retrovirus, and adeno-associated viral structures that infect other cells

Western blot: Antibody probe to separate genetic fragments to a target protein

X chromosome: Sex chromosome present in two copies in female animals

Xenotransplantation: Organ or tissue transfer from a donor in one species to a recipient in another species

Y chromosome: Sex chromosome present in one copy in male animals

Zinc finger nucleases: Artificial restriction enzymes generated by fusing a zinc finger DNA-binding domain to a DNA-cleavage domain to target specific DNA sequences

References are available online at Lippincott Connect.

Additional References

Aimo A, et al. RNA-targeting and gene editing therapies for transthyretin amyloidosis. *Nat Rev Cardiol*. 2022. doi:10.1038/s41569-022-00683-z.

Alvarez-Romero J, et al. Mapping robust genetic variants associated with exercise responses. *Int J Sports Med*. 2021;42:3.

Baena-Marín M, et al. Velocity-based resistance training on 1-RM, jump and sprint performance: a systematic review of clinical trials. *Sports (Basel)*. 2022;10:8.

Balon K, et al. Targeting cancer with CRISPR/Cas9-based therapy. *Int J Mol Sci*. 2022;23:573.

Barrangou R. CRISPR Rewrites the future of medicine. *CRISPR J*. 2022;5:1.

Barrangou R, Marraffini LA. Turning CRISPR on with antibiotics. *Cell Host Microbe*. 2022;30:12.

Bekaert B, et al. CRISPR/Cas gene editing in the human germline. *Semin Cell Dev Biol*. 2022;S1084-9521(22)00079-9.

Bharathkumar N, et al. CRISPR/Cas-based modifications for therapeutic applications: a review. *Mol Biotechnol*. 2022;64:355.

Bolsterlee B. A new framework for analysis of three-dimensional shape and architecture of human skeletal muscles from in vivo imaging data. *J Appl Physiol (1985)*. 2022;132:712.

Bouchard C. Genetics of obesity: what we have learned over decades of research. *Obesity (Silver Spring)*. 2021;29:802.

Bouchard C. The study of human variability became a passion. *Eur J Clin Nutr*. 2021. doi:10.1038/s41430-021-00871-z.

Brown B, et al. An economic evaluation of the whole genome sequencing source tracking program in the U.S. *PLoS One*. 2021;16:e0258262.

Charpentier E, et al. New Insights into blood circulating lymphocytes in human *Pneumocystis* pneumonia. *J Fungi (Basel)*. 2021;7:652.

Chaudhuri A, et al. Classification of CRISPR/Cas system and its application in tomato breeding. *Theor Appl Genet*. 2022;135:367.

Chavez-Granados PA, et al. CRISPR/Cas gene-editing technology and its advances in dentistry. *Biochimie*. 2022;194:96.

Chen S, et al. Modulating CRISPR/Cas9 genome-editing activity by small molecules. *Drug Discov Today*. 2022;27:951.

Chen Y, et al. Distinct genetic subtypes of adiposity and glycemic changes in response to weight-loss diet intervention: the POUNDS Lost trial. *Eur J Nutr*. 2021;60:249.

Díaz Ramírez J, et al. The GALNTL6 gene rs558129 polymorphism is associated with power performance. *J Strength Cond Res*. 2020;34:3031.

Donohoue PD, et al. Conformational control of Cas9 by CRISPR hybrid RNA-DNA guides mitigates off-target activity in T cells. *Mol Cell*. 2021;81:3637.

Doudna JA, Charpentier E. Genome editing. The new frontier of genome engineering with CRISPR-Cas9. *Science*. 2014;346:1258096.

Dragon-Durey MA, et al. Differential association between inflammatory cytokines and multiorgan dysfunction in COVID-19 patients with obesity. *PLoS One*. 2021;16:e0252026.

Erkut E, Yokota T. CRISPR therapeutics for Duchenne Muscular Dystrophy. *Int J Mol Sci*. 2022;23:1832.

Eynon N. The champions' mitochondria: Is it genetically determined? A review on mitochondrial DNA and elite athletic performance. *Physiol Genomics*. 2011;43:789.

Ferri Marini C, et al. HRR and VO$_2$ R fractions are not equivalent: is it time to rethink aerobic exercise prescription methods? *Med Sci Sports Exerc*. 2021;53:174.

Gao Y, et al. Maternal exercise before and during pregnancy facilitates embryonic myogenesis by enhancing thyroid hormone signaling. *Thyroid*. 2022; doi:10.1089/thy.2021.0639.

Giles JR, et al. Human epigenetic and transcriptional T cell differentiation atlas for identifying functional T cell-specific enhancers. *Immunity*. 2022;55:557.

Goh YJ, Barrangou R. Portable CRISPR-Cas9^N system for flexible genome engineering in *Lactobacillus acidophilus, Lactobacillus gasseri*, and *Lactobacillus paracasei*. *Appl Environ Microbiol*. 2021;87:e02669-20.

Guilherme JPLF, et al. The A-allele of the FTO gene rs9939609 polymorphism is associated with decreased proportion of slow oxidative muscle fibers and over-represented in heavier athletes. *J Strength Cond Res*. 2019;33:691.

Guilherme JPLF, et al. The BDNF-increasing allele is associated with increased proportion of fast-twitch muscle fibers, hand-grip strength, and power athlete status. *J Strength Cond Res*. 2020. doi:10.1519/JSC.0000000000003756.

Hagoort I, et al. Age- and muscle-specific reliability of muscle architecture measurements assessed by two-dimensional panoramic ultrasound. *Biomed Eng Online*. 2022;21:15.

Hall ECR, et al. Prediction of muscle fiber composition using multiple repetition testing. *Biol Sport*. 2021;38:277.

Hasanzadeh A, et al. Smart strategies for precise delivery of CRISPR/Cas9 in genome editing. *ACS Appl Bio Mater*. 2022;5:413.

Hopkins, W. Replacing statistical significance and non-significance with better approaches to sampling uncertainty. 2022. https://sportsci.org/2022/sampling.pdf

Hou Q, et al. Using metagenomic data to boost protein structure prediction and discovery. *Comput Struct Biotechnol J*. 2022;20:434.

Jabbar A, et al. Advances and perspectives in the application of CRISPR-Cas9 in livestock. *Mol Biotechnol*. 2021;63:757.

Jacques M, et al. Epigenetic changes in healthy human skeletal muscle following exercise—a systematic review. *Epigenetics*. 2019;14:633.

Jakhanwal S, et al. A CRISPR-Cas9-integrase complex generates precise DNA fragments for genome integration. *Nucleic Acids Res*. 2021;49:3546.

Johansen KH. How CRISPR/Cas9 gene editing is revolutionizing T cell research. *DNA Cell Biol*. 2022;41:53.

Katti A, et al. CRISPR in cancer biology and therapy. *Nat Rev Cancer*. 2022. doi:10.1038/s41568-022-00441-w.

Ke W, et al. Genes in human obesity loci are causal obesity genes in *C. elegans*. *PLoS Genet*. 2021;17:e1009736.

Kim DS, et al. The genetics of human performance. *Nat Rev Genet*. 2021. doi:10.1038/s41576-021-00400-5.

Knott GJ, Doudna JA. CRISPR-Cas guides the future of genetic engineering. *Science*. 2018;361:866.

Kocak DD, et al. Increasing the specificity of CRISPR systems with engineered RNA secondary structures. *Nat Biotechnol*. 2019;37:657.

Krukowski K, et al. The impact of deep space radiation on cognitive performance: from biological sex to biomarkers to countermeasures. *Sci Adv*. 2021;7:eabg6702.

Kumar P, et al. Artificial intelligence and synthetic biology approaches for human gut microbiome. *Crit Rev Food Sci Nutr*. 2022;62:2103.

Lapinaite A, et al. DNA capture by a CRISPR-Cas9-guided adenine base editor. *Science*. 2020;369:566.

Li X, et al. Blood DNA methylation at TXNIP and glycemic changes in response to weight-loss diet interventions: the POUNDS lost trial. *Int J Obes (Lond)*. 2022; doi:10.1038/s41366-022-01084-5.

Lin H, et al. Neurogranin as an important regulator in swimming training to improve the spatial memory dysfunction of mice with chronic cerebral hypoperfusion. *J Sport Health Sci*. 2022;S2095-2546(22)00023-0.

Lin-Shiao E, et al. CRISPR-Cas9-mediated nuclear transport and genomic integration of nanostructured genes in human primary cells. *Nucleic Acids Res*. 2022;50:1256.

Liu G, Lin Q, et al. The CRISPR-Cas toolbox and gene editing technologies. *Mol Cell*. 2022;82:333.

Liu H, et al. Novel strategies for immuno-oncology breakthroughs with cell therapy. *Biomark Res*. 2021;9:62. doi:10.1186/s40364021-00316-6.

Liu X, et al. Programmable biosensors based on RNA-guided CRISPR/Cas endonuclease. *Biol Proced Online*. 2022;24:2.

Marchetti M, et al. Enzyme replacement therapy for genetic disorders associated with enzyme deficiency. *Curr Med Chem*. 2022;29:489.

Martins-Dias P, Romão L. Nonsense suppression therapies in human genetic diseases. *Cell Mol Life Sci*. 2021;78:4677.

Miccio A, et al. Novel genome-editing-based approaches to treat motor neuron diseases: promises and challenges. *Mol Ther*. 2022;30:47.

Modell AE, et al. CRISPR-based therapeutics: current challenges and future applications. *Trends Pharmacol Sci*. 2022;43:151.

Moreland E, et al. Polygenic profile of elite strength athletes. *J Strength Cond Res*. 2020. doi:10.1519/JSC.0000000000003901.

Najafi S, et al. Therapeutic potentials of CRISPR-Cas genome editing technology in human viral infections. *Biomed Pharmacother*. 2022;148:112743.

Nambiar TS, et al. CRISPR-based genome editing through the lens of DNA repair. *Mol Cell*. 2022;82:348.

Nogueira JE, et al. Molecular hydrogen downregulates acute exhaustive exercise-induced skeletal muscle damage. *Can J Physiol Pharmacol*. 2021;99:812.

O'Hara V, et al. A highly prevalent SINE mutation in the myostatin (MSTN) gene promoter is associated with low circulating myostatin concentration in thoroughbred racehorses. *Sci Rep*. 2021;11:7916.

Park H, Kim J. Activation of melatonin receptor 1 by CRISPR-Cas9 activator ameliorates cognitive deficits in an Alzheimer's disease mouse model. *J Pineal Res*. 2022;72:e12787.

Pickering C, et al. A Genome-wide association study of sprint performance in elite youth football players. *J Strength Cond Res*. 2019;33:2344.

Poncumhak P, et al. Validity and feasibility of a seated push-up test to indicate skeletal muscle mass in well-functioning older adults. *Physiother Theory Pract*. 2022;1. doi:10.1080/09593985.2021.2023931.

Porika M, et al. CRISPR/Cas: a new tool in the research of telomeres and telomerase as well as a novel form of cancer therapy. *Int J Mol Sci*. 2022;23:3002.

Porter JJ, et al. Therapeutic promise of engineered nonsense suppressor tRNAs. *Wiley Interdiscip Rev RNA*. 2021;12:e1641.

Puig-Serra P, et al. CRISPR approaches for the diagnosis of human diseases. *Int J Mol Sci*. 2022;23:1757.

Ribeiro FM, et al. Is there an exercise-intensity threshold capable of avoiding the leaky gut? *Front Nutr*. 2021;8:627289.

Saha K, et al. The NIH somatic cell genome editing program. *Nature*. 2021;592:195.

Savadi S, et al. Advances in genomics and genome editing for breeding next generation of fruit and nut crops. *Genomics*. 2021;113:3718.

Schmidt R, et al. CRISPR activation and interference screens decode stimulation responses in primary human T cells. *Science*. 2022;375:eabj4008.

Schwarzer M, et al. Genetically determined exercise capacity affects systemic glucose response to insulin in rats. *Physiol Genomics*. 2021;53:395.

Sharma SK, et al. CRISPR-Cas-led revolution in diagnosis and management of emerging plant viruses: new avenues toward food and nutritional security. *Front Nutr*. 2021;8:751512. doi:10.3389/fnut.2021.751512.

Shin H, Kim J. Nanoparticle-based non-viral CRISPR delivery for enhanced immunotherapy. *Chem Commun (Camb)*. 2022;58:1860.

Shivram H, et al. Controlling and enhancing CRISPR systems. *Nat Chem Biol*. 2021;17:10.

Song X, et al. Delivery of CRISPR/Cas systems for cancer gene therapy and immunotherapy. *Adv Drug Deliv Rev*. 2021;168:158.

Sorrenti V, et al. Deciphering the role of polyphenols in sports performance: from nutritional genomics to the gut microbiota toward phytonutritional epigenomics. *Nutrients.* 2020;12:1265.

Srinivas US, et al. PLK1 inhibition selectively induces apoptosis in ARID1A deficient cells through uncoupling of oxygen consumption from ATP production. *Oncogene.* 2022. doi:10.1038/s41388-022-02219-8.

Tanisawa K, et al. Sport and exercise genomics: the FIMS 2019 consensus statement update. *Br J Sports Med.* 2020;54:969.

Van Guilder GP, et al. Impacts of circulating microRNAs in exercise-induced vascular remodeling. *Am J Physiol Heart Circ Physiol.* 2021;320:H2401.

Vellers HL, et al. Association between mitochondrial DNA sequence variants and VO_2 max trainability. *Med Sci Sports Exerc.* 2020;52:2303.

Wang X, et al. Inhibition mechanisms of CRISPR-Cas9 by AcrIIA17 and AcrIIA18. *Nucleic Acids Res.* 2022;50:512.

Xu K, et al. Glycolysis fuels phosphoinositide 3-kinase signaling to bolster T cell immunity. *Science.* 2021;371:405.

Yang Y, et al. CRISPR/Cas: advances, limitations, and applications for precision cancer research. *Front Med (Lausanne).* 2021;8:649896.

Yeh TK, et al. Bacteriophages and phage-delivered CRISPR-Cas system as antibacterial therapy. *Int J Antimicrob Agents.* 2022;59:106475.

Yi JY, et al. New application of the CRISPR-Cas9 system for site-specific exogenous gene doping analysis. *Drug Test Anal.* 2021;13:871.

Yilmaz SG. Genome editing technologies: CRISPR, LEAPER, RESTORE, ARCUT, SATI, and RESCUE. *EXCLI J.* 2021;20:19.

Zhang B. CRISPR/Cas gene therapy. *J Cell Physiol.* 2021;236:2459.

Zhang H, et al. Application of the CRISPR/Cas9-based gene editing technique in basic research, diagnosis, and therapy of cancer. *Mol Cancer.* 2021;20:126.

Zhou T, et al. Genetically determined SCFA concentration modifies the association of dietary fiber intake with changes in bone mineral density during weight loss: the preventing overweight using novel dietary strategies (POUNDS Lost) trial. *Am J Clin Nutr.* 2021;114:42.

Zhou Z, et al. An inducible CRISPR/Cas9 screen identifies DTX2 as a transcriptional regulator of human telomerase. *iScience.* 2022;25:25.

Supplemental Videos (CRISPR) and Podcasts

Supplemental Videos (CRISPR)

www.nobelprize.org/prizes/chemistry/2020/doudna/lecture/ (Nobel lecture: The Chemistry of CRISPR: Editing the Code of Life; Jennifer Doudna)

https://innovativegenomics.org/education/digital-resources/what-is-crispr/ (What is CRISPR? A brief introduction to CRISPR genome editing: technology, uses, and ethics; Innovative Genomics Institute)

www.pbs.org/wgbh/nova/video/gene-editing-reality-check (NOVA: CRISPR Gene-Editing Reality Check)

www.crisprtx.com/gene-editing/crispr-cas9 (Specific, efficient and versatile gene-editing technology to harness, modify, delete, or correct precise DNA regions)

www.youtube.com/watch?v=4YKFw2KZA5o (CRISPR: Gene editing and beyond; Nature video)

www.youtube.com/watch?v=2pp17E4E-O8 (McGovern Institute: Genome Editing with CRISPR-Cas9)

www.youtube.com/watch?v=WZ6pVWvAd2M&t=1063s NSTA 2021: CRISPR as an Adaptive Immune System in Bacteria)

www.youtube.com/watch?v=F03n34PZtzs (NSTA 2021: CRISPR Cas9: A Powerful new Tool for Editing the Human Genome)

www.youtube.com/watch?v=cKHuuALENZk Walter Isaacson & Jennifer Doudna join Washington Post Live to discuss CRISPR (Live, 3/12)

www.youtube.com/watch?v=TdBAHexVYzc (How CRISPR lets us edit our DNA | Jennifer Doudna)

www.youtube.com/watch?v=47pkFey3CZ0 (Innovative Genomic Institute: Jennifer Doudna: CRISPR Basics)

www.youtube.com/watch?v=Kh88cLtlclw (NYT: SciShow)

www.youtube.com/watch?v=VvvsyoFtP_c (Jennifer Doudna and Sid Mukherjee in Conversation)

www.youtube.com/watch?v=RKh2mi3tsmc (CRISPR: History of Discovery. NIE Singapore

www.youtube.com/watch?v=pVIVSpUgR44CRISPR :(What is the future of gene editing? |Start Here (Al Jazeera)

www.youtube.com/watch?v=dy4hfJR55W4 (Ark Invest: CRISPR Talk with Jennifer Doudna)

www.youtube.com/watch?v=jm5QqxN7Hkw (Wonder Collaborative. Discovery Story: Genome Engineering with CRISPR-Cas9 (Doudna, Jinek, Charpentier)

www.youtube.com/watch?v=cR5An16ifj0 (NIH (Q&A between 2020 Nobel Prize Winner Dr. Jennifer Doudna and NIH Director Dr. Francis Collins)

www.youtube.com/watch?v=cUe-cOgpDDw (Nierenberg Prize. Scripps. UCTV: Into the Future with CRISPR Technology with Jennifer Doudna)

www.youtube.com/watch?v=GMndqLvTqhA (Conversations in Science with Dan Rather & Jennifer Doudna: CRISPR)

www.youtube.com/watch?v=60mtV-OedrM (CBS Sunday Morning. Jennifer Doudna on the curiosity of a child)

www.youtube.com/watch?v=UtQkoW8yQ4A (The Magic of RNA: From CRISPR to Coronavirus Vaccines." presented by Tom Cech)

www.youtube.com/watch?v=MFXhhkv5UKs (UC Davis Research: Distinguished Speaker Series in Research and Innovation- Jennifer Doudna, PhD)

www.youtube.com/watch?v=ciAzW47o3kk (Chardan. CRISPR Gene Editing: State of the Tech and What's Next featuring Dr. Jennifer Doudna)

www.youtube.com/watch?v=85ZUjs-tY90 (Emmanuelle Charpentier—Alexander von Humboldt Professorship 2014)

Podcasts

Consult one of these channels for availability—Apple podcasts, Castbox, Google Play, iHeartradio, Amazon music, or wherever you get your podcasts, with several listed below available as Internet podcasts.

- *Genetics unzipped* (The Genetics Society podcast; 10 podcasts dealing with gene editing. "A brief history of CRISPR – how we learned to edit the genome," can be accessed at https://geneticsunzipped.com/blog/2021/4/8/s407-a-brief-history-of-crispr-how-we-learned-to-edit-the-genome) (36 min)
- *Crisper Cuts* (30 Podcasts covering gene editing topics from 2018–2021)
- *Genetics audio* from www.uctv.tv
- *StarTalk Podcast:* The Code of Life and CRISPR with Jennifer Doudna and Walter Isaacson (www.youtube.com/watch?v=u6tFWjXbOfw)
- GuidePost (A Podcast Series from The CRISPR Journal)
- Essentials of CRISPR-based Animal Models in Drug Discovery (Podcast miniseries available at www.listennotes.com/podcasts/essentials-of-crispr-based-animal-models-in-DvtnS5jVPmc/)

Table 33.1 Eight Protein Categories and Their Biologic Functions

Protein Category	Function	Example
1. Contractile	Form muscles	Actin, myosin
2. Enzyme	Catalyze biological processes	Protease
3. Hormone	Regulate body functions	Cortisol
4. Protective	Fight infection	Antibodies
5. Storage	Store nutrients	Calcium within bone
6. Structural	Form structures	Endoplasmic reticulum
7. Transport	Deliver substances among cells, tissues, and organs	Hemoglobin
8. Toxic	Act as defense mechanism	Snake venom (disintegrins)

Table 33.2 Essential Concepts and Sequences in Protein Synthesis

1. A nucleotide sequence from DNA provides the genetic information required to begin transcription into RNA.
2. The enzyme RNA polymerase binds to the specific gene's promoter region; nucleotide sequences in the DNA indicate beginning and ending transcription.
3. RNA polymerase manufactures messenger RNA (mRNA) molecules to mirror the DNA base sequence; transcription copies a genetic code sequence in the direction from DNA to an mRNA strand; this includes both coding and noncoding genetic information segments.[61]
4. The RNA transcript contains the information it needs to create a protein; RNA splicing removes random, intervening unwanted "junk" nucleotides sequences (introns) from mRNA.
5. The mRNA strand (linked entrons) carrying a genetic code duplicate copy shuttles the "coded message" (codon sequence), exiting the nucleus and entering the cytoplasm to begin protein synthesis.
6. Translation initiates protein construction; the A-U-G codon acts as the "start" signal.
7. In the cytoplasm, the mRNA molecule searches to bind with a ribosome (ribonucleoprotein, a "protein-manufacturing machine").
8. The transfer RNA (tRNA) anticodon positions itself to match up with a three-nucleotide codon sequence, each codon corresponding to one amino acid; the codon contains a copy or transcripted DNA code.
9. With the four RNA nucleotides, 64 different codons in the genetic code exist, with each amino acid having at least one (and usually more than one) codon.
10. Binding takes place at the ribosome's attachment site between the tRNA molecule (carrying the same genetic sequence on its anticodon) and the complementary base mRNA codon sequence (e.g., G-A-C with C-U-G).
11. The ribosome, coupled to the mRNA molecule at one end, shifts (translocates) over one codon (three nucleotide blocks) to the polypeptide site, allowing new codon exposure; a new incoming tRNA (with its amino acid) links to the ribosome's attachment site; the amino acid at the ribosome's polypeptide region releases and binds to a new amino acid on tRNA at the ribosome's attachment site; the tRNA with one amino acid now gains another amino acid, then another one, and so on; successively adding new amino acids elongates the peptide chain.
12. Protein synthesis terminates when a chain-terminating nonsense "stop" codon (UAA, UAG, UGA) turns off the signal to add more amino acids to the peptide chain.
13. A complete (fully assembled) protein exists in one of four geometric configurations (primary, secondary, tertiary, quaternary) shown in Figure 33.26.

Table 33.3 Genetic Mutation Types

Mutation Type	Example Disruption in the Coding Sequence
Wild type	The cat sat on the mat
Substitution	The rat sat on the mat
Insertion (single)	The cat spat on the mat
Insertion (multiple)	The cattle sat on the mat
Deletion (single)	The c-t sat on the mat
Deletion (multiple)	The cat—the mat
Inversion (small)	The tac sat on the mat
Inversion (large)	Tarn echt no tas tac echt

Index

Page numbers in italics denote figures. Those followed by (*t*) denote tables

A

A (adenine), 1021
A band, sarcomere, 396–397, 397*f*
AAS (anabolic adrenergic steroids), 595–596, 639
Abdomen
  fat, 824
  flexibility and strengthening exercises for, 584*b*
  muscles, 280
Abdominal fat, 824
Absolute muscle strength, gender differences in, 552–553, 553*f*
Absolute strength, 571*b*
Acclimation, 648
Acclimatization
  Acclimation *vs.*, 693*b*
  to altitude
    at home, 663–664, 664*f*
    immediate responses to exposure, 650–653
    longer-term adjustments, 652*b*, 653–658
    time required for, 658
  to cold, 693–694
  defined, 648
  to heat, 686–687, 699*t*
Acclimatization level, sodium loss, 73–74
Accommodating-resistance exercise, 562
Acetylcholine (ACh), 408*f*
Acetyl-CoA (acetyl-coenzyme A), 164–165
Acetyl-coenzyme A (acetyl-CoA), 164–165
ACh (acetylcholine), 408*f*
Acid metabolites, buffering of, 258
Acid-base balance
  average value for, 321
  readjustment at altitude, 653–656
  regulation of, 321
Acidosis, 322
Acini, 466
Acquired immunity system, 487
Acromegaly, 605, 639
ACSM. *see* American College of Sports Medicine (ACSM)
ACSM guidelines regarding weight category sports, 898
ACSM's Certified Clinical Exercise Specialist (CES), 955
ACTH (adrenocorticotropic hormone), 619
Actin
  function of, 419*t*
  link between myosin, ATP, 406–407
  overview, 395
  structural rearrangement of, 403*f*
Actin-myosin filaments
  interaction with Ca^{2+} and ATP, 407*f*
  orientation of, 401–402, 401*f*, 402*f*
Action potential, 432–433
Activation energy, 140
Activator protein, 1031, 1032*f*
Active glycogen turnover, 164
Active life expectancy (ALE), 913*b*
Active recovery, 190
Active transport, 139
Active vitamin D$_3$, 495*t*
Activities of daily living (ADL), 575
Activity. *see* Physical activity
Actomyosin, 402
  research tools, 404–405
Acute mountain sickness (AMS), 654*t*, 654*b*
Acute renal failure, 988–989
Added sugars, 9*b*
Adenine, 1021
Adenosine 3´,5´-cyclic monophosphate (cyclic AMP), 169
Adenosine diphosphate (ADP), 152
Adenosine monophosphate (AMP), 153
Adenosine triphosphatase (ATPase)
  energy-transforming activities, 152–154, 152*f*, 153*f*

and PCr, anaerobic phosphate-bond energy sources, 154, 154*f*
  stages of, 160, 160*f*
Adenosine triphosphate (ATP), 136, 879*f*
  muscle action, 406–407, 407*f*
  phosphodiester bonding, 1020–1021
Adenosine triphosphate-phosphocreatine (ATP-PCr) system, 180
Adenylate cyclase, 453
Adenylate kinase reaction, 154
Adequate hydration, 683
Adequate Intake (AI), 46
ADH (antidiuretic hormone), 458, 480
Adipocyte protein 2 (*a*P2) gene, 878
Adipocytes, 15
  lipid storage and mobilization, 168–169, 169*f*
  obesity, criteria for
    biopsy method, 877–878, 878*f*
    calculating number, 878
    fat cell development, 878–880, 879*f*
    new adipocyte formation, 881
    nonobese and obese differences in cellularity, 880, 880*f*
    weight gain, 881
    weight loss, 880–881, 881*f*
Adipose tissue, 496*t*–498*t*
  as endocrine organ, 477–478
Adjusted ATP accounting, 167
Adolescents. *see also* Children
  oxygen uptake and energy expenditure in, 238*f*
  RDA protein recommendations, 31
Adrenal cortex, 460, 462, 496*t*–498*t*, 926–927
Adrenal gland, 450, 451*f*, 460*f*
Adrenal hormones
  adrenal medullar, 460–462
  adrenocortical, 462–464
  aldosterone, 481
  cortisol, 482
  epinephrine, 481, 482*f*
  norepinephrine, 481, 482*f*
Adrenal medulla, 460–461, 496*t*–498*t*
Adrenal medullar hormones, 460–462
Adrenergic agonists, 603–604
  sympathomimetic β$_2$-adrenergic agonists, 605
  training status, difference in
    animals, 605
    humans, 605
Adrenergic fibers, 362
Adrenocortical hormones
  androgens, 464, 464*f*
  glucocorticoids, 463–464, 463*f*
  mineralocorticoids, 462–463, 462*f*
Adrenocorticotropic hormone (ACTH), 455*f*, 458, 463*f*, 480, 619, 926*f*
Adrenopause, 926–927
Adults
  effect of excessive fatness in childhood and adolescence, 872–873
  exercise physiology, 921–922
  oxygen consumption, 263–264
  physical activity and inactivity participation in, 914–915
  running economy, 236–237
Advanced resistive exercise device (ARED), 756*b*
Advice to students entering exercise science research, 114
  RDA protein recommendations, 31
Aerobic capacity
  prediction tests
    based on heart rate, 265–266, 265*f*
    endurance runs, 264–265
    from nonexercise data, 267
    overview, 263–267
    step test, 266–267

relative VO$_{2max}$, 263
  on return to sea level, 661
Aerobic energy
  effects of aging, 927–928, 928*f*
  maximal oxygen consumption
    assessment of, 258–263
    criteria for, 259, 260*f*
    tests, 259–260
  metabolism, 157, 165*f*, 188–189
    free radicals, 165*b*
  prediction tests
    based on heart rate, 265–266, 265*f*
    endurance runs, 264–265
    from nonexercise data, 267
    overview, 263–267
    step test, 266–267
Aerobic glycolysis, 161
Aerobic resynthesis, ATP, 154
Aerobic system, 182–185
Aerobic training
  absolute aerobic power, 921
  cancer patients, 959
  carbohydrate metabolism, 509
  cardiovascular adaptations with
    blood flow and distribution, 514–515
    blood pressure, 515
    cardiac hypertrophy, 509–511, 509*f*, 510*b*, 541*t*
    cardiac output, 513–514, 513*f*
    heart rate, 511–512, 511*f*
    oxygen extraction, 514, 514*f*
    plasma volume, 511
    stroke volume, 512–513
  factors affect aerobic responses, 518–525
    initial level of fitness, 518
    training duration, 524
    training frequency, 524
    training intensity, 518–524, 519*f*, 520*f*, 521*f*, 523*f*
    training mode, 524
    training progression, 524–525
    training volume, 524
  fatty acids, 27
  gender difference among older adults, 930–931, 949*t*
  heart rate-oxygen uptake, 519*f*
  improvements in fitness, 525–526, 525*f*
  lactate concentration, 516, 516*f*
  lipid metabolism, 508–509, 508*f*
  metabolic adaptations with
    carbohydrate metabolism, 509
    lipid metabolism, 508–509, 508*f*
    muscle fiber type and size, 509
    overview, 507
  methods
    best training, 530
    continuous training, 530
    factors, 528, 528*f*
    Fartlek training, 529–530
    high-intensity interval training, 528
    one-minute intense exercise, 528–529
  muscle fiber type and size, 509
  overview, 507–518, 507*f*
  pulmonary adaptations with
    maximal physical activity, 515
    submaximal physical activity, 515–516, 516*f*
    ventilatory endurance, 516
  resistance training plus, 559–560
  specificity, 505, 505*f*
  typical session, 530*b*, 530*f*
  well-rounded overall training program, 525
Aerogel material, 775*b*
Aerosinusitis, 722
Aerospace medicine, 736. *see also* Microgravity
Aerotitis (middle-ear squeeze), 722
AF (anaerobic fatigue), 254
Afferent neurons, 422, 429

1088 Index

Africa, life expectancy, 912f
African Americans, life expectancy, 912
Afterload, 377
Age/aging. see also Adults; Children
   Americans, 910
   benefits of increased energy output with, 871–872, 872f
   chronological vs. biological age, 911–912
   components, 910
   coronary heart disease
      cellular level alterations, 935–937
      risk factors, 937–945
   and gender comparisons, 214–216, 214f, 938–939
   gerontology, 910–913
   healthy life expectancy, 912–913, 912f
   heat stress tolerance, 687–688, 687f
   longevity, 911
      causes of death, 950t
      epidemiologic evidence, 932
      Harvard Alumni study, 932
      overview, 931
      regular moderate exercise, 932–933
   maximum heart rates, 520, 520f
   nation, 910f
   physical activity in population
      Healthy People 2030, 918–920, 918f
      prehabilitation program, 920
      terminology, 913
   physical activity participation
      advantages, 913
      assessment, 913
      disadvantages, 913
      sedentary behaviors, 914, 914f
   physiologic function
      age trends, 921–930
      body composition, 929, 930f
      bone mass, 929–930
      cardiovascular function, 927–929, 928f
      children and adults, 921–922
      endocrine function changes, 925–927, 926f
      generalized curve for age-related changes in, 921, 921f
      muscular strength, 922–925
      neural function, 925, 925f
      pulmonary function, 927
      sprint performance, 929, 929f
   positive muscle and tendon adaptations from, 575, 575f
   resistance training, 924–925, 924f
   science, 911
   sedentary environmental death syndrome, 914–918
      changing fitness trends, 915–918, 949t
      2020 top 10 fitness trends, 918
      U.S. adult population, 914–915
      U.S. children and teenagers, 915
   skinfold measurements, 817–818
   trainability and, 930–931, 930f
Aging
   skeletal muscle mass decline with, 412b
Aging muscle, plasticity of, 575, 575f
Agouti-related protein (AGRP), 870
AGRP (Agouti-related protein), 870
AHA (American Heart Association), 941
AI (Adequate Intake), 46
AIDA International (International Association for Development of Apnea), 714b
Air embolism, 720, 721f
Air resistance, 237–238, 238f
Airflow, 278–279
Airflow calorimeter, 197
Akinesia, 988
Alactic (alactacid) oxygen debt, 188
Alanine-glucose cycle, 36, 36f
Albert Project, 740
Albumin, 18
Alcohol intake, 942–943
Aldosterone, 66, 462–463, 481, 675
ALE (active life expectancy), 913b
Alkaline reserve, 323
Alkalosis, 322
Allometric scaling, 554–556
All-or-none law action, 437
Allosteric modulation, 453
Alpha (α) motor neurons, 425–427
Alpha blockers, 341
α motor neurons, 425–427
α-actinin, 419t
α-sympatholytics, 1004t

Altered protein dynamics, 763–764
Alternans test, 973
Altitude, 646–666
   acclimatization
      at home, 663–664, 664f
      immediate responses to exposure, 650–653
      longer-term adjustments, 653–658
      time required for, 658
   aerobic capacity on return to sea level, 661
   circulatory factors, 660–661
   combining altitude stay with low-altitude training, 662–664, 664f
   for endurance athletes, 662b
   exercise performance, 659f, 660
   maximal oxygen uptake, 659–660, 659f
   medical problems related to, 654b
   oxygen loading, 649–650
   possible negative effects, 661
   sea-level performance, 661–662, 661f
   stressors, 648, 649f
Altitude hypoxia, 650, 652b
Altman, Richard, 1012
Alveolar air, 295
Alveolar minute ventilation
   breathing rate vs. tidal volume, 286–287, 287f
   dead space vs. tidal volume, 284
   overview, 284, 291t
   physiologic dead space, 286, 286f
   ventilation-perfusion ratio, 284–286
Alveoli, 276–278
Alveoli rupture, 720, 721f
Ama (women divers), 693, 693f, 704
Ambient air, 295
Amenorrhea, 60–61, 807
American Cancer Society, recommended lipid intake, 22–23
American College of Sports Medicine (ACSM)
   anabolic steroids position statement, 600b
   pre-requisites to participation in exercise programs, 971, 999t
American Heart Association (AHA), 941
   lipid intake recommendations, 22–23
Americas, life expectancy, 912f
Amine group, 28–29
Amine hormones, 450, 494t
Amino acids
   after nitrogen removal, 35b
   branch-chain, 597, 620
   essential, 29
   metabolic pathways for, 33f
   nonessential, 29
   role of, 32
   supplementation, 609–613
Aminoacyl-tRNA synthetase, 1036
Amoros, Francis, 544
AMP protein kinase (AMPK), 478f
Amphetamines, 613, 613f, 639
AMS (acute mountain sickness), 654t, 654b
Amylin, 466
Amylopectin, 8
Amylose, 8
Anabolic adrenergic steroids (AAS), 595–596, 639.
   See also Anabolic steroids
Anabolic phase, nutrient intake, 610b
Anabolic steroids, 596
   abuse, 602b
   action of, 596–603
   administrating, 598, 598f
   dosage, 600
   effectiveness, 599–600
   following, 598–599
   hormone interactions, 596–600, 596f
   improving athletic performance, 601–603
   myelin's role in motor skills without, 598, 598f
   perfecting movement skills, 597
   risks, 600–601
      abuse and disease precursors, 600–601, 601f
      elite female competitors abuse, 601
      to females, 601, 601f
   sources, 599
   structure of, 596–603
Anabolism, 212
Anaerobic energy
   biologic indicators
      blood lactate levels, 256–257, 257f
      glycogen depletion, 257–258, 257f
   individual differences

      buffering of acid metabolites, 258
      motivation, 258
      training, 258
   maximally accumulated oxygen deficit, 256
   performance tests
      age differences, 256
      gender differences, 256
      interrelationships among, 253
      jumping-power tests, 252
      overview, 253–256
      stair-sprinting power tests, 253
      physiologic tests, 253–258
   short-term energy system assessing
      blood lactate levels, 256–257, 257f
      glycogen depletion, 257–258, 257f
Anaerobic fatigue (AF), 254
Anaerobic glycolysis, 161
Anaerobic glycolytic reactions, 164–165
Anaerobic resynthesis, ATP, 154
Anaerobic training
   intramuscular high-energy phosphates, 527
   lactate-generating capacity, 527
   system changes with, 506–507, 506f
Anaerobic work (AW), 255
Anatomic dead space, 278–279
Anderson, Michael, 771b
Androgens, 462, 464, 464f
Android-type obesity, 876
Andropause, 926
Androstenedione, 606f, 608–609, 639
Anemia, 62–63
   effect on oxygen transport, 299–300
   exercise-induced, 63
   functional, 65
Aneurysm, 963–964
Angina pectoris, 346, 937, 961, 961f
Angiogenesis, 514, 1044, 1044f
Angiotensin II, 463
Angiotensin II receptor blockers, 341
Angiotensin II type 1 receptors (AT1), 463
Angiotensin III, 463
Angiotensin-converting enzyme (ACE) inhibitors, 341
Animal polysaccharide, 10–11, 10f
Ankle flexibility, 916b, 917t
Ankle flexion test, 916b, 917t
Ankle weights, 232
Anneal, 1054–1055
Annulospiral nerve fiber, 439–440
Anorexia athletica, 888b
Anorexia nervosa, 888b
Anterior cardiac veins, 345
Anterior motor neuron
   excitation, 432–433
   facilitation, 433–435
   inhibition, 435
   neuromuscular junction, 432
   overview, 431–432
Anterior pituitary hormones
   adrenocorticotropic hormone, 458, 463f, 480, 619
   gonadotropic hormones, 458, 480
   growth hormone
      direct and indirect metabolic actions, 457f
      effects of aging, 922–923
      genetic engineering, 605–606
      insulin-like growth factors, 457
      overview, 456, 480
      physical activity and tissue synthesis, 456–457
   prolactin, 458, 480
   testosterone
      anabolic steroids, 596
      overview, 464–465, 464f, 465f, 480
   thyroid-stimulating hormone, 457
Anthropometry, 291t, 809
   body composition and compared by gender, 855, 861t
   and percentage total body fat, 841–854, 841f
   skinfold and girth, 843, 857t
Antianginal agents, 1001t–1002t
Antiarrhythmic agents, 1001t–1002t
Anticholinergics, 1004t
Anticodon, 1036
Anticortisol compounds, 619–620
Antidiuretic hormone (ADH), 458, 480, 675
Antihypertensive agents, 66, 976f, 1001t–1002t
Antilipidemic agents, 1001t–1002t
Antioxidant agents, 49–50, 52, 1071
Antiparallel arrangement, DNA strands, 1021

Antisense RNA, 1065
Aorta, 330–331
Aortic stenosis, 971
aP2 (adipocyte protein 2) gene, 878
Aphanizomenon flos-aquae, 608b
Apolipoprotein (Apo), 941
Apolipoprotein A-1 (Apo A-1), 941
Apollo 11, 742–743
Apollo and Space Shuttle Programs, 774, 789t–790t
Apoptosis, 392, 1044–1045
Apple-shaped body, 876f
AquaLung Cousteau-Gagnan unit, 707
Archimedes, 809–810
Archimedes' principle, 809
ARED (advanced resistive exercise device), 756b
Arginine, higher-dose supplementation, 633b
Arm exercise, 382, 382f
Arm-crank ergometer tests, 975
Armstrong, Neil, 737
Arnold, Frances H., 1065
Arrhythmia, 974
Artemis missions, 740
Arterial hypoxia, 648
Arterial inflammation, 935–937
Arterial system
  blood pressure
    cardiac output and total peripheral resistance, 333–334
    diastolic, 333
    mean arterial, 333
    systolic, 333
  overview, 330–334
Arteriogenesis, 514
Arterioles, 330–331
Arterio-mixed venous oxygen (a-vO$_2$) difference
  overview, 514, 514f
Arteriovenous oxygen difference, 303
Artificial gravity, 759
Ascending nerve tracts, 425
Asthma, 986–987
  area affected and results of, 981b
  environmental impact, 987
  exercise-induced, 302b
  fluid loss, 986
  medication, 987
  thermal gradients and fluid loss, sensitivity to, 986
  warm-up, 987
Åstrand protocol, 261f
Astrobiology, 775
Astronauts, 737
  African American, 771b
  Chinese, 748
Atherosclerosis, 22, 927, 934. *See also* Coronary heart disease (CHD)
Atherosclerosis oxidative modification hypothesis, 48
Atherosclerosis susceptibility gene, 960
Athletes, 45, 88
  chronic fatigue prevention, 91
  iron supplement for, 64
Athlete's heart (cardiac hypertrophy), 509–511, 509f, 510b, 541t
Athletic amenorrhea, 808
At-home altitude acclimatization, 663–664, 664f
Atkins, Robert C., 887
Atomic force microscope (AFM), 404
ATPase. *see* Adenosine triphosphatase (ATPase)
ATP-PCr (adenosine triphosphate-phosphocreatine), 180
Atrial depolarization, 357f
Atrial natriuretic hormone, 495t
Atrioventricular (AV) bundle, 354
Atrioventricular (AV) node, 354
Atrioventricular valves, 328–329
Atwater 4-9-4 kilocalorie rule, 128–129
Atwater general factors, 128
Atwater, Wilber Olin, 128, 196
Atwater-Rosa calorimeter, 196
Auscultation, 968
Auscultation method, 333
Autologous transfusion, 621, 639
Autolytic process, 580–581
Autonomic nerves, 429
Autonomic nervous system, 363f, 429
Autophagy, 392
Autoradiography, 1054
Autoregulatory mechanisms, 365
AV (atrioventricular) bundle, 354
AV (atrioventricular) node, 354

a-vO$_2$ difference (AU: Please check symbol)
  during physical activity, 381–382, 381f
  during rest, 381
AW (anaerobic work), 255
Axon, 431
Axons, spinal cord, 432f, 446t

B
Babbage, Charles, 548
Back crawl, 241, 241f
Back leg lift dynamometer, 548f
Bacteria, 1030
Bacteriophage, 1053–1054
Bag technique, 200–201, 201f
Balance dynamics, 764–765, 765f
Balke protocol, 261f
Ballard, Robert, 709
Ballistic resistance training, 564
Baltimore, David, 1048, 1051
Barbara, Santa, 710
Bariatric surgery, 889
Barometric pressure, 648, 649f
Baroreceptors, 365, 425
Barton, Otis, 706–707
Basal metabolic rate (BMR)
  determining from body mass, stature, age, 218b
  fat-free body mass, 212–214, 214f
  as function of age and gender, 214–216, 214f
  normalcy of, 215, 215f
  overview, 212, 214
  thyroid hormones, 459
Base pair(ing), 1021–1023, 1024f
Baseball pitching speed, 437b
Basedow, Johann, 544
Basketball players, 838, 845–846, 854
Bateson, William, 1013
Bayliss, William Maddock, 355, 450b
Bazett, H.C., 220
BCAAs (branch-chain amino acids), 597, 620
Beebe, William, 706–707
Beef Burger, nutrition facts, 24b
Behnke, Albert, 707, 711, 722, 727b, 796
Behnke, Dr. A.R., 847b
Behnke's method, 843–845
Behnke's theoretical model, 804, 805f
Beijing games water cube, 839
Bellows effect, 675
Bench press, one-repetition maximum for, 414b–415b
Bench stepping work calculation, 141b
Bends (decompression sickness)
  astronauts, 752
  consequences of inadequate decompression, 724
  higher prevalence with patent foramen ovale, 724–725
  nitrogen elimination, 723–724, 723f
  overview, 723, 723f
  treatment, 724, 724f
Benedict, Francis G., 218
Benign tumor, 1044
Bent-knee sit-up exercise, 584b
Bergstrom, Jonas, 409
Bert, Paul, 704–705
Beta blockers, 341
Beta (β)-oxidation, 170
β$_2$-adrenergic agonists, 603–604
β-Alanine, 618, 639
Beyond Burger, nutrition facts, 24b
Beyond Meat's, 24b
β-Hydroxy-β-methylbutyrate (HMB), 620–621, 620f, 639
BIA (bioelectrical impedance analysis), 821–823, 822f
Bicarbonate, 305–306, 618f
Bicarbonate buffer, 322–323
Bicuspid valve, 328–329
Bicycle ergometer tests, 269t, 974–975
Bicycling. *see* Cycling
Bile salts, 16
Binge-eating disorder, 888b
Bioastronautics, 739–740
Bioelectrical impedance analysis (BIA), 821–823, 822f
Bioenergetics
  coenzymes, 142–143
  defined, 136
  enzymes, 136
Bioinformatics, 1010
Biologic work, in humans, 139

Biological aging
  biological-vascular aging biomarkers, 912
  concept, 911
  vs. chronological aging, 911–912, 911f
Biopsy method, 877–878, 878f
Biosynthesis, 136
Bipennate muscle, 398–400
Bipolar configuration, ECG, 355
Bipolar disorder, 990
Blackout, 715
Blood boosting, 621
Blood clot (thrombus), 346, 936–937, 938f
Blood doping (red blood cell reinfusion), 621–622
Blood lactate, 182
Blood lactate threshold, 181–182
Blood lipid profile, 9b
Blood pressure
  cardiac output and total peripheral resistance, 333–334
  diastolic, 333
  heat, exercise in, 678
  lifestyle choices that lower, 341
  mean arterial, 333
  response to physical activity
    graded exercise, 343, 343f
    recovery, 343–345
    resistance exercise, 342–343
    steady-rate exercise, 343
    upper-body physical activity, 343
  systemic circulation, 336
  systolic, 333
Blood vessels, wall structure, 332f
Blood volume (BV), pre-to postflight changes in, 752–753, 752f
Blood-brain barrier, 72
Blue bloater appearance, 981f
Bluford, Guion S., 771b
BMD (bone mineral density), 577, 756, 848
BMI. *see* Body mass index (BMI)
BOD POD measurement, 814–815, 814f
BOD POD method, 814–815
Body composition, 229
  aging, 929, 930f
  at altitude, 658
  and anthropometry compared by gender, 855, 861t
  assessment, 794–834, 844b
    average percentage body fat, 829–830, 829f
    bioelectrical impedance analysis, 821–823, 822f
    body mass index, 797–801, 798f, 799f
    body volume measurement, 810–814
    computed tomography, 824–827, 826f
    determining goal body weight, 830
    direct assessment, 809
    dual-energy X-ray absorptiometry, 828–829, 829f
    girth measurements, 818
    height-weight tables, limitations of, 796
    hydrostatic weighing, 809–810
    indirect assessment, 809–810
    magnetic resonance imaging, 827–828, 827f, 828f
    menstruation, delayed onset of and cancer risk, 808
    minimal leanness standards, 806–807
    near-infrared interactance, 823
    obesity prevalence, 797
    overfat, 796–797
    overweight, 796–797
    reference man and reference woman, 805–807, 805f
    skinfold measurements, 815, 817f, 835t
    ultrasound assessment of fat, 823–824
  changes by densitometry, 847b
  comparisons among elite male sprint, distance, marathon, and decathlon competitors, 843–845, 845t, 845f
  effects of endurance training, 903t
  effects of microgravity, 766–767, 766f
  effects of resistance training, 903t
  effects of running, 904t
  effects of walking, 904t
  of football players, 859t
  hydrostatic weighing, 843f
  of runners and marathoners, 858t
  in 100-year-old males and females, 855
Body density (Db), 796, 810
  percentage body fat estimated from, 810

Body fat
  anthropometry and percentage total, 841–854, 841f
  average values by age, 829–830, 829f
  of bodybuilders, 853–854
  cold, exercise and, 692
  collegiate vs. professional players, 848–852, 849f, 850f, 851f, 859t
  creatine supplementation and, 635f
  distribution of, theoretical model for, 806, 806f
  of endurance athletes
    female, 845–846, 846f
    male, 846–848, 858t
  estimated from body density, 810
  of field event athletes, 842–843, 843f
  of football players, 848
  gender differences, 262
  of golfers, 852–853, 860t
  heat stress tolerance, 689
  loss, 638
  predicting, 844b
  of runners, 848
  by sports category, 842, 842f
  of swimmers, 848
  total transmissible variance for, 868f
  of weightlifters, 853–854
Body fluids, changes associated with microgravity, 752–753, 752f, 783t–784t
Body frame size (BFS), 796
Body mass (BM)
  allometric scaling, 554–556
  at altitude, 658
  of astronauts, 766, 766f
  creatine supplementation and, 635f
  effect of on energy cost of household, 222
  effects of walking, 230–231
  logarithmic plot of, 212, 212f
  in obese and nonobese subjects, 880f
  relationship between muscle strength expressions and, 555f
Body mass index (BMI)
  anthropometric characteristics and percentage body fat levels, 841–854, 841f
  category, 877f
  computation of, 797–798
  defined, 797
  football players, 851f
  of football players, 799
  of golfers, 852, 860t
  index-for-age percentiles, 799, 799f
  long-term health risk outlook, 851–852
  new standards for, c0028:f0005c0028:f0006, 798–801
  relationship between health risk, 871
  and waist circumference, 872, 872f
  weight classifications and health risks, 798–799, 798f
Body movements, 675
Body surface area-to-body mass ratio, 688
Body volume measurement
  BOD POD measurement, 814–815, 814f
  hydrostatic weighing, 811–814, 811f, 835t
  overview, 814–815, 814f
  water displacement, 811
Body weight
  of football players, by position, 850f
  of golfers, 860t
  microgravity, 763–767
Body weight training, 918
Body weight-loaded training, 565–567
Bodybuilders, 853–854
Bohr, Christian, 302–303
Bohr effect, 302–303
Bohr, Niels, 39, 303
Bolden, Charles F., 771b
Bolt, Usain, 180
Bomb calorimeter methodology, 125
Bone density, gender differences, 577
Bone health
  estrogen's role, 57b
  through physical activity, 59
Bone mass, aging, 929–930
Bone mass related to muscular strength, 58
Bone matrix increase, 58–59
Bone mineral density (BMD), 58, 577, 756, 848
Booth, Frank W., 914
Borg scale, 523, 523f
Boycott, Arthur, 706
Boyer, Herbert, 1051
Boyle, Robert, 705

Boyle's Law, 712, 713f–717f
Bradycardia, 364, 964
Bradykinesia, 988
Bragg, Lawrence, 1014
Brain
  blood flow to, 380, 987
  central nervous system, 422–425, 423f, 424f
  on cognitive function, 925
  complex motor pattern systems, 435
  image of, 424f
  training with transcranial magnetic stimulation, 435–436
Brain concussion, 422–423
Brain-derived neurotrophic factor (BDNF), 486–487, 1073–1074
Brainstem, 423–424, 424f
Branch-chain amino acids (BCAAs), 597, 620
Brazelton Neonatal Assessment Scales, 534, 534f
Breast cancer, 950t
  rehabilitation and physical activity, 959–960, 960f
Breaststroke, 241, 241f
Breaststroke swimmers, 838
Breath-hold diving, 704, 713–716
Breathing reserve, 320
British thermal unit (BTU), 122–123
Broca area, 425
Broca, Paul Pierre., 425
Bronchi, 276
Bronchiectasis, 981b
Bronchioles, 276
Bronchitis, 981b
Brown fat, 878–879, 879f
Bruce and Balke treadmill tests, 974
Bruce protocol, 261f
Buffering acid-base regulation
  chemical buffers, 322–323
  overview, 321–323
  physiologic buffers, 323
Buffering solutions, 618–619, 618f
Bulimia nervosa, 888b
Bundle of His, 354
Bundles, 446t
Buoyancy, swimming, 242
Burton, Alan, 220
Bushnell, David, 709b
Butenandt, Adolph, 594
BV (blood volume), pre-to postflight changes in, 752–753, 752f

C

C (cytosine), 1021
C protein, 397f, 419t
CABG (coronary artery bypass graft), 938f
Cable tensiometry, 548, 548f
CABP (coronary artery bypass procedure), 937
Caffeine, 613–616, 613f, 639
  effects on muscle, 615
  ergogenic effects, 614, 614f, 615f
  powdered, 616b
  warning about, 615–616
Caffeinism, 615–616, 639
Cagle, Yvonne Darlene, 771b
Cajal, Santiago Ramón y, 442, 1037
Cal Dive, 708–709
Calcitonin, 459
Calcium, 53–59
  bone health diagnostic criteria, 57b
  effect of microgravity, 753, 755f, 756, 787t
  food sources, 48
  muscle action, 407f
  osteopenia, 53
  osteoporosis, 54
  recommended daily intake, 44
Calcium channel blockers, 341
Calipers, 815–816
Caloric restraint, 895–896, 904t
Caloric value for oxygen, 198
Calories, 892–893
  conversion, 124b
  energy content of food, measurement of, 122
  versus kilocalories, 122b
Calorimetry, 125
  Bomb, 125
  Direct, 124
  direct, 196–197, 197f, 202
  indirect, 198–201

Cameron, James, 710
Cancer, 1028, 1044–1045, 1044f
  aerobic training, 959
  breast, 950t, 959–960, 960f
  chemotherapy, 956
  colon, 950t
  delayed onset of menstruation and risk of, 808
  effects of physical activity on, 950t
  lung, 950t
  number of deaths from, 956
  oncology
    overview, 956–960
    rehabilitation, 957–960
    statistics, 956
  pancreatic, 950t
  and physical activity, 490
  physical activity prescription, 959
  prostate, 950t
  protective effects, 957
  radiation, 956
  rectal, 950t
  stomach, 950t
  surgical operations, 956
  therapies and complications, 956b
  weight gain, 872–874
Capacitance vessels, 337
Capecchi, Mario R., 1060
Capillaries, 334–336, 334f
Capsule, 446t
Carbamino compounds, 306
Carbohydrate flame, 174
Carbohydrate loading, 627, 639
Carbohydrate-protein-creatine supplementation, 611–612, 611f
Carbohydrates, 6, 14–15, 97–98, 126
  combustion heat, 125
  creatine loading, 635–636, 636f
  depletion, 91
  diets effect on muscle glycogen, 14
  distribution of, 10–11, 11f
  dynamics in physical activity, 12–14
    intense exercise, 12–13, 13f
    moderate and prolonged exercise, 13–14, 13f
  energy release from, 160–168
  fatigue and glycogen availability, 14
  feedings during physical activity, 109–110
  intake modification
    classic loading procedure, 627–629, 628f
    gender differences in glycogen storage and catabolism, 629, 629f
    modified loading procedures, 629–630, 630f
    nutrient-related fatigue, 627, 627f
    overview, 627
  intake of, 89
    during physical activity, 108–110
    precompetition meal, 114
    prior to physical activity, 106–108
  kinds and sources of
    monosaccharides, 6
    oligosaccharides, 6–7
    polysaccharides, 8–9
  loading, 627–629
  low-carbohydrate ketogenic diets, 887–889
  metabolism, 509
  needs during intense training, 91
  physiological inequality, 9
  recommended intake of, 11
  replenishing glycogen reserves, 107–108
  respiratory quotient for, 203
  role of
    as energy source, 11
    as fuel for CNS, 12
    as metabolic primer/prevents ketosis, 12
    as protein-sparer, 11–12
Carbon dioxide (CO_2)
  production of, 202–203
  rebreathing method, 375
  transport of
    as bicarbonate, 305–306
    in Hb, 306
    in physical solution, 305
    plasma and red blood cells, 305, 305f
Carbon monoxide poisoning, 725
Carbonic acid, 322
Carbonic anhydrase, 305
Carcinogen, 1044
Carcinomas, 956

Cardiac arrest, 937
  during physical activity, 919
  vs. heart attack, 935
Cardiac catheterization, 969
Cardiac cells, 390
Cardiac dimensions, comparison of, 541t
Cardiac enlargement, 510
Cardiac hypertrophy (athlete's heart), 509–511, 509f, 510b, 541t
Cardiac impulse, 354f
Cardiac muscle, 328, 394b
Cardiac nervous system diseases, 964
Cardiac output (Q)
  aging, 928
  breath-hold divers, 717, 717f
  distribution
    blood flow at rest, 378, 379f
    blood flow during exercise, 379, 379f
  in endurance athletes, 513f
  measuring
    CO_2 rebreathing method, 375
    direct Fick method, 374
    indicator dilution method, 374
  oxygen transport
    a-vO_2 difference (AU: Please check symbol), 381–382
    physical activity, 380–381
    rest, 380
  during physical activity
    enhancing stroke volume, 376–378
    overview, 376–378
  at rest
    endurance athletes, 375–376
    overview, 375–376
    untrained individuals, 375
  and total peripheral resistance, 333–334
Cardiac rehabilitation program
  inpatient programs, 979–980
  outpatient programs, 980
Cardiac rhythm abnormalities, 974
Cardiac transplantation, exercising after, 368f, 369–370, 369f
Cardiometabolic disorders, 95
Cardiomyopathy, 961
Cardiotoxicity, 958
Cardiovascular adaptations with training
  blood flow and distribution, 514–515
  blood pressure, 515
  cardiac hypertrophy, 509–511, 509f, 510b, 541t
  cardiac output, 513–514, 513f
  heart rate, 511–512, 511f
  oxygen extraction, 514, 514f
  plasma volume, 511
  stroke volume, 512–513
Cardiovascular disease (CVD)
  cardiac nervous system diseases, 964
  chest pain, 965, 997t
  exercise-induced indicators
    angina pectoris, 972
    cardiac rhythm abnormalities, 974
    electrocardiographic abnormalities, 972–974, 973f
    heart rate response, 974
    hypertensive exercise response, 974
    hypotensive exercise response, 974
  health screening and risk stratification, 965
  heart muscle disease
    aneurysm, 963–964
    pericarditis, 964
  heart muscle diseases, 960–964
    angina pectoris, 961, 961f
    congestive heart failure, 961–963
    myocardial infarction (MI), 961, 962f
  heart valve diseases, 964
  hypertension, 976–977, 976f
  informed consent, 971, 1000t
  patient history, 965, 997t
  physical examination
    heart auscultation, 968
    invasive physiologic tests, 968–969
    laboratory tests, 968
    noninvasive physiologic tests, 969–972
  prescribing physical activity and exercise
    illustration, 978
    improvements, 978
    medications and exercise response, 979, 1001t–1002t
    program, 978–979, 1001t
  rehabilitation
    inpatient programs, 979–980
    outpatient programs, 980
  stress testing
    ACSM recommendations, 971, 999t
    contraindications, 971
    oldest-old, 972
    outcomes, 971–972
    protocols, 974–976
Cardiovascular drift, 377–378
Cardiovascular fitness categories, 186t, 186b
Cardiovascular function with aging
  aerobic power, 927–928, 928f
  central and peripheral cardiovascular functions, 928
  endurance performance, 928–929
  physiologic loss, 928
Cardiovascular overload, 528
Cardiovascular regulation and integration
  cardiac transplantation, exercising after, 369–370
  distribution of blood
    exercise effects, 366–367
    physical factors affecting blood flow, 365–366
  heart rate
    extrinsic regulation of heart rate and circulation, 360–365
    intrinsic regulation of heart rate, 354–360
  integrative exercise response, 367
Cardiovascular response, 651, 651f
Cardiovascular system
  blood pressure response to physical activity
    graded exercise, 343, 343f
    recovery, 343–345
    resistance exercise, 342–343
    steady-rate exercise, 343
    upper-body physical activity, 343
  cardiac output
    distribution, 378–380
    measuring, 374–375
    oxygen transport, 380–382
    during physical activity, 376–378
    at rest, 375–376
  components of
    arterial system, 330–334
    capillaries, 334–336, 334f
    heart, 328–330
    venous system, 336–338
  heart, 345–347
  hypertension, 338–341
  myocardial metabolism, 347
  neural regulation, 361f
  schematic view of, 329f
  upper-body exercise
    maximal oxygen consumption, 382
    physiologic response, 382–384
    submaximal oxygen consumption, 382–384, 382f
Carnitine acyltransferase, 168
Carotid arteries, 311f, 365
Carotid artery palpation, 365
Cas9 nuclease, 1011
CAT (computed axial tomography), 577
Catabolism, 212
Catecholamines, 362, 461–462, 461f, 494t, 651–652, 651f, 653f, 666t
CBF (cerebral blood flow), 987
CBF (cutaneous blood flow), 378, 378f
CD8+ T cell, 957–958
cDNA (complementary DNA), 1048–1051
cDNA clone's, 1053–1054
cDNA library, 1053–1054
Cell body, 431
Cell cycle, 1027, 1027f
Cell damage
  altered sarcoplasmic reticulum, 580–581
  current DOMS model, 581, 581f
  overview, 579–580
Cell life cycle controllers, 1027–1028
Cell-based protein meat, 24b
Cellular adaptations, at altitude, 657–658
Cellular energy transfer reactions, 137
Cellular glucose uptake, 111–112
Cellular oxidation
  electron transport, 155, 155f
  oxidative phosphorylation, 156–157, 157f
Cellular respiration, 139

Centenarians, 855
Central dogma, 1030, 1030f
Central nervous system (CNS), 422, 423f
  brain
    brainstem, 423–424, 424f
    cerebellum, 422, 424
    diencephalon, 424
    image of, 424f
    limbic system, 425
    telencephalon, 425
  diagram of, 423f
  spinal cord, 425–427
    ascending nerve tracts, 425
    descending nerve tracts, 425–427
    image of, 426f
    reticular formation, 427
Central obesity, 876
Centrifugal force, 738
Centromere, 1020
Cerebellum, 422, 424
Cerebral blood flow (CBF), 987
Cerebral cortex, 313, 422
Cerebrovascular diseases (CVDs)
  coronary heart disease (see Coronary heart disease (CHD))
  effects of physical activity, 950t
  overview, 987
Certification programs
  for exercise physiologists, 954–955
  organizations that offer, 954
Certifications, 954–955
Chargaff, Erwin, 1021
Chargaff's rule, 1021
Charpentier, Emmanuelle, 1065
Chemical buffers, 322–323, 323f
Chemical energy, 138f
Chemical work, 136, 139
Chemiosmotic coupling, 156
Chemoreceptors, 365, 425
Chemotherapy, 956
Chest pain, diagnosing causes of, 997t
Chest radiography, 968
Children
  anaerobic energy performance tests, 256
  cardiac output, 381
  cholesterol measurement in, 919b
  cold, exercise in, 692
  endurance runs, 264–265
  excessive fatness in, 872–873
  heat stress tolerance, 688
  maximal oxygen consumption tests, 263, 263f
  obesity impact on, 866–867
  physical activity population, 915
  physiologic function, 921–922
Chimney effect, 675
China Space Agency (CAST), 748
Chinese astronauts, 748
Chinese National Space Administration (CNSA), 736
Chloride shift, 306
Chlorine, 66–67, 83t
Cholecystokinin, 478, 495t
Cholesterol, 20, 943f
  and coronary heart disease risk, 22
  dynamics in body, 21f
  factors affecting, 942
  functions, 22
  LDL particle size assessment, 941–942
  recommendations for, 940–941
  reverse transport of, 20, 941
  risk of death from CHD, 941f
Cholinesterase, 433
Chromatids, 1020
Chromium
  beneficial effects, 630
  double-blind study, 632
  minimal benefits, 630–632
  overview, 630
Chromium chloride, 632
Chromium picolinate, 630, 639
Chromosome, 1016, 1016f
Chromosome 2, 1020, 1020f
Chromosome 21 mutations, 1017b
Chronic athletic fatigue, 91
Chronic kidney disease (CKD), 989
Chronic mountain sickness (CMS), 654b

Chronic obstructive pulmonary disease (COPD)
  asthma and exercise-induced bronchospasm (see Asthma)
  chronic bronchitis, 981, 981f
  cystic fibrosis, 981b, 982–983
  emphysema, 981–982, 981b, 982f
  major COPD diseases, 981b
  risk factors, 981
  smoking, 318–320
Chronic stable angina, 961
Chronotropic effect, 362
Chronotropic incompetence, 974
Chylomicrons, 20, 636–637, 639
Cigarette smoking
  acute effects of, 320b
  body mass index, 798
  coronary heart disease risk, 940
  heart rate response, 320b
  as vascular risk factor, 937
Circuit resistance training (CRT), 578–579
Circulation, as heat-dissipating mechanism, 675
Circulatory problems, 874f
Citrate, 165
Citric acid cycle, 161–162, 167
Clenbuterol, 603–604, 639
Climate
  cold
    acclimatization to, 693–694
    body fat, 692
    children, 692
    overview, 691–692
    respiratory tract during, 695–696
    wind-chill temperature index, 694–695, 695f
  effect on energy expenditure, 217–219
  heat
    circulatory adjustments, 679
    complications from excessive, 689–691
    core temperature, 679–680, 679f
    factors that modify tolerance, 686–689
    water loss, 680–683
  vs. weather, time as a factor, 670
  worldwide climate change, 673b
Clinical exercise physiologist (CEP), 954
Clinical track, ACSM, 955
Clo units (clothing insulations), 675, 697t–698t
Clo value, 675
Closed-circuit mixed-gas system, 727–728, 728f
Closed-circuit scuba system, 719–720, 719f
Closed-circuit spirometry, 198, 199f
Closed-kinetic chain exercise, 565
Clothing
  clothing insulations, 675, 697t–698t
  cold-weather, 677
  cycling helmet, 678
  football uniforms, 677–678, 677f
  overview, 675
  warm-weather, 677
Clustered Regularly Interspaced Short Palindromic Repeats (CRISPR), 1065–1066
CMS (chronic mountain sickness), 654b
CN (cranial nerves), 428f
Coactivator protein, 1031, 1032f
Cobb, Geraldine (Jerrie), 744
Coding region, 1031, 1032f, 1033–1034
Codons
  definition, 1023
  sequencing of, 1025
  table, 1023, 1025f
Coefficient of digestibility, 127
Coenzymes, 44, 142–143
Cognitive function, effects of strength training on, 925
Cognitive/emotional diseases and disorders
  clinical features, 990
  exercise prescription, 990–991
Cohen, Stanley, 1051
COLBERT (Combined Operational Load Bearing External Resistance Treadmill) treadmill, 746
Cold injuries, 694
Cold treatments, 685–686
Cold-weather clothing, 677
Cold-weather exercise
  acclimatization to, 693–694
  body fat, 692
  children, 692
  hormonal output, 672
  muscular activity, 672

overview, 691–692
respiratory tract during, 695–696
vascular adjustments, 672
wind-chill temperature index, 694–695, 695f
Collagen fibers, 391–392
Collegiate football players, 848–852, 849f, 850f, 851f, 859t
Collegiate wrestlers, 854, 854f
Colon cancer, effects of physical activity on, 950t
Combustion heat, 125–126
Commissure, 446t
Common plastic caliper, 816
Competition phase, strength training, 559
Competition walking, energy expenditure during, 232–233, 232f–233f
Competitive inhibitors, 143
Competitive maximum strength, 571b
Complementary bases, 1023
Complementary DNA (cDNA), 1048–1051
Complementary strand, 1021
Complete protein, 29
Complex carbohydrate, 8
Complex fusiform arrangement, skeletal muscle, 400
Compound lipids, 20
Computed axial tomography (CAT), 577
Computed tomography (CT)
  body composition assessment, 824–827, 826f
  cardiovascular disease, 970
  pulmonary diseases, 983
Computerized exercise-monitoring systems, 201, 202f
Concentric action, 557, 753–756
Concentric cardiac hypertrophy, 509
Concussions, 422–423
Condensation, 15
Condensation reactions, 143–144, 144f
Conducting zones, ventilatory system, 278, 279f–280f
Conduction, heat loss by, 673
Congenital heart defects, 964
Congestive heart failure
  at alarming rate, 963b
  causes, 962
  regular physical activity, 963
  and regular physical activity, 963
  risk factors, 961
  treatment and rehabilitation, 962–963
Congestive heart failure (CHF), 961–963
Conservation of energy principle, 136
Continuous oxygen consumption test protocol, 260
Continuous positive airway pressure (CPAP) device, 985
Continuous synthesis, 1026
Continuous training, 528, 530
Convection, heat loss by, 673
Conversational exercise, 519
Cooperative binding, 300
Copper, 44, 81t
Core stability and strength, 920
Core temperature
  Clo values required to maintain, 675, 697t
  heat, exercise in, 679–680, 679f
  overview, 670, 670f
  physiological changes with decrease in, 700t
Core training, 567–568, 568f
Cori cycle, biochemical reactions, liver synthesis, 164f
Cormack, Allan M., 983
Coronary angiography, 969, 969f
Coronary artery bypass graft (CABG), 938f
Coronary artery bypass procedure (CABP), 937
Coronary circulation, 345, 345f
Coronary heart disease (CHD), 476b
  causes and effects, 939b
  cellular level alternation
    arterial inflammation, 935–937
    C-reactive protein, 935–937
    toll-like receptor 2, 935
    vascular degeneration, 937, 938f
    vulnerable patient, 936–937
    vulnerable plaque, 936
  death from, risk of, 941f
  effects of physical activity on, 950t
  risk factor, 923b
    age, 938–939
    blood lipid abnormalities, 940–943
    in children, 945, 945f
    cigarette smoking, 940
    diabetes, 940

gender, 938–939
heredity, 938–939
homocysteine, 943–944, 943f
hypertension, 940
interactions between, 944–945, 944f, 951t
lifestyle changes, 934
obesity, 945f
physical inactivity, 932
sedentary lifestyles, 932–933
sleep disorders, 923b
Coronary sinus, 345
Corpus callosum, 422
Correns, Carl, 1013
Cortex
  adrenal, 460, 462, 496t–498t
  cerebral, 313, 424f
  defined, 446t
  motor, 425–427
Cortical bone, 53
Cortical influence, ventilatory control, 312
Cortical width, 53
Corticotropic releasing hormone (CRH), 463f
Corticotropin, 458
Corticotropin-releasing factor, 463
Cortisol, 463, 482, 619
Countermeasure strategies, 748
Countermeasure strategies, microgravity
  inflight space station daily exercise, 760, 760f, 761f
  lower-body negative pressure, 761–767, 762f, 763f
  overview, 759–767, 788t
  space pharmacology, 761, 788t
  spaceflight nutrition, 762–767, 765f, 766f
Cousteau, Jacques-Yves, 707, 717–718, 727b
Covalent bond, 1020–1021
CPAP (continuous positive airway pressure) device, 985
CPK (creatine phosphokinase), 968
Cranial nerves (CN), 428f
C-reactive protein (CRP), 935–937
Creatine
  age effects, 634
  benefits, 632–634, 633f
  body mass and composition, 634–635, 635f
  component in high-energy phosphates, 632, 632f
  creatine loading, 635–636, 636f
  overview, 632
Creatine kinase, 154
Creatine loading, 633f
Creatine monohydrate (CrH_2O), 632, 639
Creatine phosphokinase (CPK), 968
Creutzfeldt-Jakob disease, 606, 639
CRH (corticotropic releasing hormone), 463f
CrH_2O (creatine monohydrate), 632, 639
Crick, Francis Harry Compton, 1014
CRISPR gene editing, 1011
CRISPR technology, 1010, 1065–1069
  Doudna and Charpentier breakthrough experiments, 1066–1067
  educational videos, 1069
  future prospectives, 1068–1069
  genome editing, 1067b
  process, 1067–1068
    Cas9, 1068
    gRNA, 1068
  timeline, 1065–1066
CRISPR-Cas9, 595, 640, 1065–1066
Crohn disease, 1013b
Cromolyn sodium, 1004t
Crossbridge cycling, 399b
Crossbridges, 401–403
Cross-leg stretch, 584b
Cross-sectional data, body composition, 929
Crowser, Ryan, 842–843
CRP (C-reactive protein), 935–937
CRT (circuit resistance training), 578–579
Curbeam, Robert L., 771b
Curie, Marie, 1065, 45
Cutaneous blood flow (CBF), 378, 378f
Cycle ergometer work calculation, 141b
Cyclic adenosine monophosphate (cAMP), 614
3'5'-Cyclic adenosine monophosphate (cyclic AMP), 453, 453f, 454b
Cyclic AMP (3'5'-cyclic adenosine monophosphate), 453, 453f, 454b
Cycling, 91
  helmet, 678
  Tour de France, 99–100

Cyclins, 1027
Cytochrome oxidase, 155
Cytochromes, 62, 155
Cytokines, 943
Cytosine, 1021

D

Dalton law, 294
Damadian, Raymond, 827, 828
Damant, Guybon, 706
Darwin, Charles Robert, 1012
Darwin's inherited medical malady, 1013b
Dash (Dietary Approaches to Stop Hypertension) Diet, 68b
DASH diet to lower blood pressure with dietary intervention, 68b
Data resources, 775b
Daughter chromosome, 1020
Davis, Robert, 706
de Laplace, Pierre Simon, 196
De Vries, Hugo, 1013
Deamination, 32, 172
Deane, Charles Anthony, 705
Death rate, during physical activity, 919
Decompression sickness (DCS)
  astronauts, 752
  consequences of inadequate decompression, 724
  higher prevalence with patent foramen ovale, 724–725
  nitrogen elimination, 723–724, 723f
  overview, 723, 723f
  treatment, 724, 724f
Deconditioning syndrome, treatment goals for, 957
Deep veins, 336f
Degenerative heart disease (DHD), 960
Dehydration, 680
  diuretics, 683
  magnitude of, 680–681, 699t
  overview, 680
  physiologic and performance decrements, 683
  significant consequences of, 682, 682f
Dehydration synthesis, 8, 143–144, 1020–1021
Dehydroepiandrosterone (DHEA), 464, 606–608, 606f, 607f, 926–927, 926f
Dehydrogenase enzymes, 145, 155
Delayed vascular aging, 911–912
Delayed-onset muscle soreness (DOMS), 579, 591t
Delta efficiency, 229
Dementia, 925
Denayrouze, Auguste, 705
Dendrites, 431
Denervation muscle atrophy, 922–923
Denitrogenation, 752
Densitometry, 809
Deoxyribonucleic acid (DNA)
  amplification, 1054–1056, 1057f
  base pairing, 1021–1023, 1024f
  chromosome, 1020, 1020f
  cloning, 1051–1052, 1052f
  components of, 1018, 1018f
  defined, 1012, 1029
  fragment separation, 1054–1065, 1055f–1056f
  molecular control mechanisms, 1027–1028, 1027f
  overview, 1017–1025
  packaging in chromosome, 1019f
  phosphodiester bonding, 1020–1021, 1021f
  polymerase, pivotal role for, 1026–1027
  replication, 1025–1028, 1026f, 1027f
  replication fork, 1025–1026
  structure of, 1021, 1022f
  synthesis of, 1027
  technologies
    bioremediation, 1052–1053, 1053f
    DNA cloning, 1051–1052, 1052f
    history of, 1048–1052, 1051f
    plasmids, 1053–1054, 1054f
    recombinant DNA organism, 1051f
  vs. RNA, molecular configuration, 1017–1018, 1018f
Deoxyribose, 1018
Depleted carbohydrate, 91
Depolarization wave, 395
Depth–time limits breathing pure oxygen during diving, 712, 712b, 731t
Depth–time limits, diving, 719–720, 725, 731t–732t

Derived lipids, 20–22
Descending nerve tracts, 425–427
Desmin, 419t
Detraining, 506, 577–578
  durations, physiologic and metabolic function changes with various, 506, 539t
  and muscle fiber type changes, 508b
Dextroamphetamine sulfate, 613
DHD (degenerative heart disease), 960
DHEA (dehydroepiandrosterone), 464
DHT (dihydrotestosterone), 596–597
Diabetes mellitus, 468–470, 944
  classifications, 468–469
  diagnostic tests, 469–470
  effects of physical activity on, 475, 950t
  insulin actions and impaired glucose homeostasis, 470, 471f
  obesity, 873–874
  and physical activity, 475
  on rise, 470
  risk factor, 940
  in women, 939
Diabetic dyslipidemia, 940
Diaphragm, 279
Diastole, 328
Diastolic blood pressure, 333
Diastolic filling, 376–377
Diencephalon, 424
Diet, 44, 104–105. see also Nutrition
  bone loss prevention, 54–57
  carbohydrates, 8, 11, 14
  effect on blood lipids, 23
  effect on muscle glycogen, 14, 14f
  high-fat, 89–90
  low-fat, 90
  osteoporosis, prevention through, 53, 53b
  respiratory quotient for mixed, 205, 209t
  water intake through, 70–71
Diet induced thermogenesis (DIT), 216–217
Diet linked to mortality, 94b
Diet soda, 7b
Dietary Approaches to Stop Hypertension (DASH) diet, 68b
Dietary components, health outcomes, 95b
Dietary fiber, 943
Dietary Guidelines Advisory Committee (DGAC), 22
Dietary guidelines for Americans, 93–98
Dietary Guidelines Update: 2020–2025, 94–95, 98b
Dietary lipids, 18–20, 19f
Dietary Reference Intakes (DRIs), 31, 46–47
  minerals, 52, 81t
  vitamin, 44, 79t
Dietary Supplement Health and Education Act (DSHEA), 617b
Dietary supplement sales, 50
Dietary supplements, cardinal rule for purchasing, 617b
Dieting, for weight control
  classic approach, 883
  extremes in, 883–889, 883f–884f
  long-term success, 883–885, 883f–884f
  set point theory, 885–889, 886f
Diffusion, 139
Digestibility, 133t
  coefficient of, 127
Digital clubbing, 981–982
Digitalis glycosides, derivatives, 1001t–1002t
Dihydrotestosterone (DHT), 596–597
Dipeptide, 28
2,3-diphosphoglycerate (2,3-DPG), 303–304, 658
Diploid, 1017
Direct calorimetry, 124, 196–197, 197f
Direct Fick method, 374
Disaccharides, 6
Discontinuous oxygen consumption test protocol, 260
Discontinuous synthesis, 1026
Disease prevention, resistance training for, 559
Disinhibition, 435
Disuse syndrome, treatment goals for, 957
DIT (diet induced thermogenesis), 216–217
Diuretic-induced dehydration, 683
Diuretics, 897
Diurnal pattern (cycle), 463–464
Divers Alert Network, 709
Diving, 702–733
  Ama, 693, 693f, 704
  breath-hold, 713–716

depth–time limits breathing pure oxygen during, 712, 712b, 731t
diving reflex, 716–717
guidelines to avoid high-pressure nervous system injury during, 727b
history of, 704–711
mammals' adaptations to deep, 716b
mixed-gas
  helium-oxygen mixtures, 726, 732t
  overview, 725, 726f
  saturation diving, 726–727, 727f
  technical diving, 727–728, 728f
pressure-volume relationships and depth, 712
  diving depth and gas volume, 712, 713f–717f, 731t
  diving depth and pressure, 712, 731t
problems
  aerotitis, 722
  air embolism, 720, 721f
  carbon monoxide poisoning, 725
  decompression sickness, 723–725, 723f
  nitrogen narcosis, 722–723
  overview, 720–725, 721f
  oxygen poisoning, 725, 732t
  pneumothorax, 720
  risks for females, 725
scuba
  closed-circuit scuba, 719–720, 719f
  open-circuit scuba, 718–719, 718f, 719f
  overview, 717–720
snorkeling, 712–718
underwater swimming energy cost, 728, 728f
Diving bells, 704, 705f, 707
Diving reflex, 716–717
DLW (doubly labeled water), 764–765
DNA. See Deoxyribonucleic acid (DNA)
DNA Casework Unit (DCU), 1045
DNA fingerprinting autoradiography, 1059, 1059f
DNA gyrase, 1028–1029
DNA helicase, 1028–1029
DNA ligase, 1026
DNA polymerase, 1026–1027
DNA polymerase I, 1026
DNA polymerase III (Pol III), 1028–1029
DNA probe, 1053
DNA tagging, 1056, 1058b
Dolly, 1062f
DOMS (delayed-onset muscle soreness), 579, 591t
Dopamine receptor 1, 1072
Dorsal horn, spinal cord, 425
Dorsiflexors, muscle architectural properties, 400f
Dose-response relationship of energy expended, 894–895
  exercise frequency, 894–895
  gradually progress, 895
  physical activity mode, 895
  self-selected energy expenditures, 895
  walking-running for different durations, 894, 904t
Double helix, 1014, 1015b
Double-helix DNA molecule package, 1019f
Doubly labeled water (DLW) technique, 202, 764–765
Doudna, Jennifer, 1065, 1069, 1076
Douglas, C.G., 200–201, 648
Dowd, Daniel L., 547b
Down, John Langdon, 1017b
Down syndrome, 1017b
Downhill walking, energy expenditure during, 231, 231f
Down-regulation, 453
2,3-DPG (2,3-diphosphoglycerate), 303–304
Drafting, 238–239
Drag forces, 239–241
Drag, swimming, 240–241
Drew, Benjamin Alvin, 771b
DRIs (dietary reference intakes), 46–47, 46b, 52b
Drosophila melanogaster, 1013
Dry suit, 719
Dry-land swimming exercise, 584b
Dual-energy X-ray absorptiometry (DXA), 764–765, 815, 828–829, 829f
Dubois-Reymond, Emil, 355
Duchenne de Boulogne, Guillaume-Benjamin-Amand, 409
Dulbecco, Renato, 1048–1051
Dumas, Frederic, 707, 722
Duodenum, 451f

DXA (dual-energy X-ray absorptiometry), 764–765, 828–829, 829f
Dying bug exercise, 584b
Dynamic constant external resistance (DCER) training, 557
Dynamic flexibility, 916b
Dynamic lung volumes, 282–283
Dynamic muscle action, 556, 556f
Dynamometers, 548–549, 548f
Dynamometry, 548–549
Dyspnea, 287, 985, 985f
Dyspnea scale, 985, 985f
Dyspneic, 960
Dysrhythmias, 964
Dysthymia, 990
Dystonia, 1046f
Dystrophin protein, 409

E

Eagle, 742–743
Early strongmen popularized body building and strength training, 547b
Earplugs, 722
Eastern Mediterranean, life expectancy, 912f
Eat More and Weigh Less, 103
Eating disorders, 888b
EBCT (electron beam computed tomographic) scan, 970
Eccentric action, 557, 753–756
Eccentric cardiac hypertrophy, 509
Echocardiography (ECG), 356–360, 761–762, 969–970, 970f
ECRB (extensor carpi radialis brevis muscle), 405
Ectomorphic, 838
Edema, 338
Efferent neurons, 422, 425, 429
Efficiency, net mechanical, 228–229
EIH (exercise-induced arterial hypoxemia), 320–321
Einthoven, Wilhelm, 356
Eisenhower, Dwight D., 741
Ejection fraction, 376–377
EL (endothelial lipase), 942
Electrical energy, 138f
Electrocardiogram (ECG), 356–360
Electrocardiographic tracing, 966b, 966f
Electrolytes, 66, 84t, 112–113
  exercise, 112
  replacement of, 685, 685f, 686b
Electromyography (EMG), 394b
  integrated, 570
Electron beam computed tomographic (EBCT) scan, 970
Electron microscope, 1037
Electron microscopy, 1018–1020
Electron transport, 145, 167–168
Electron transport–oxidative phosphorylation efficiency, 157
Electron-dense cellular deoxyribonucleic acid (DNA), 47
Elite marathon performance, genetics prediction during, 839b
Ellestad protocol, 261f
Emboli, 720
Emotional disorders, 989–991
Employing certified fitness professionals, fitness trends, 918
EMU (extravehicular mobility unit), 745–746
End, Edgar, 707
End-diastolic volume, 376–377
Endergonic chemical reactions, 137, 137f
Endocarditis, 964
Endocrine glands, 450
Endocrine system, 448–498
  adipose tissue as
    leptin and ghrelin, 477–478
    leptin regulation, 478, 479f
    overview, 477
  endocrine gland stimulation, 455f
  exercise training
    adrenal hormones, 460–464, 460f, 481–482
    anterior pituitary hormones, 479–480
    pancreatic hormones, 482–485, 482f
    parathyroid hormone, 460, 481
    posterior pituitary hormones, 480
    thyroid hormones, 481
  function changes with aging
    adrenal cortex, 926–927
    age-related decline in three hormone systems, 926, 926f
    growth hormone/insulin-like growth factor axis, 927
    hypothalamic-pituitary-gonadal axis, 926
  gonadal hormones
    overview, 464–465
    testosterone, 464–465, 464f, 465f
  liver, gut, and hypothalamic hormones, 478
  metabolic syndrome, 475–477
  muscle tissue as, 477, 478f
  opioid peptides and physical activity, 486–487
  organ locations, 450, 451f
  organization
    hormone level factors, 454
    hormone-receptor binding, 453
    hormones types, 450–452
    hormone-target cell specificity, 452
    overview, 450–454, 494t
  overview, 450, 451f, 496t–498t
  pancreatic hormones, 466–468, 466f
    insulin, 466–468, 467f, 468f
  physical activity
    and cancer, 490
    upper respiratory tract infections, 488–490, 488f
  resistance training, 485–486, 486f
  resting and exercise-induced secretions
    adrenal hormones, 460–464, 460f
    anterior pituitary hormones, 455–458, 456f
    parathyroid hormones, 460
    posterior pituitary hormones, 458–459
    thyroid hormones, 459–460, 459f
Endogenous cholesterol, 22
Endogenous opioid peptide effects, 487
Endomorphic, 838
Endomysium, 392
Endoplasmic reticulum, 1038
Endorphins, 486–487
Endothelial lipase (EL), 942
Endplate potential, 432–433
End-stage heart disease, 369
End-stage renal disease (ESRD), 989
Endurance activities, 99–100, 100f
  aging, 928–929
  body composition, effects on, 903t
  body fat of athletes
    female, 845–846, 846f
    male, 846–848, 858t
  caffeine, 614
  exogenous pyruvate on, 638
  oxygen treatment, 627f
  swimming, 242–243
Energy and sports drinks, 105, 105b
Energy availability hypothesis, 808
Energy balance equation, 882, 882f
Energy balance model (EBM), 882–883
Energy capacities
  aerobic energy
    endurance runs, 264–265
    long-term energy system, 258–267
    prediction tests, 263–267
    step test, 266–267
  anaerobic energy
    biologic indicators, 256–257, 257f
    buffering of acid metabolites, 258
    maximally accumulated oxygen deficit, 256
    motivation, 258
    performance tests, 250–252
    physiologic tests, 254
    training, 258
    overview, 250
    specificity versus generality of, 250, 250f
Energy deficit explanation, 808
Energy expenditure, 228
  adults, 236–237, 237f
  children, 237, 237f
  effect of different terrain, 245t
  exercise efficiency, factors influencing, 229
  human movement economy, 230–233
  human movement efficiency
    delta efficiency, 229
    and economy, 228
    gross mechanical efficiency, 228
    net mechanical efficiency, 228–229
  measurement of
    direct calorimetry, 196–197, 197f
    doubly labeled water technique, 202
    indirect calorimetry, 198–201
    respiratory exchange ratio, 205–207
    respiratory quotient, 202–205
  during physical activity
    average energy expenditure, 221
    classification, 221
    energy cost, 222, 222f
    heart rate, 222–223, 223f
    MET, 221, 225t
  for resistance exercise modes, 591t
  at rest
    basal metabolic rate, 212, 214
    factors that affect energy expenditure, 216–219
    metabolic rates, 214–216, 214f
    metabolic size concept, 212–213, 213f, 214f
    resting metabolic rate, 212
  during running
    air resistance, 237–238, 238f
    competition walking, 236, 236f
    drafting, beneficial outcomes, 238–239
    economy of running fast or slow, 234
    marathon running, 239
    net energy expenditure, 234, 245t–246t
    running economy, 236–237
    speed, 234–236
    stride frequency, 234–236
    stride length, 234–236
    treadmill versus track running, 239, 246t
  during walking
    body mass, influence of, 230–231, 244t
    competition walking, 232–233, 232f–233f
    downhill walking at grades, 231, 231f
    footwear and other distal leg loads, 231–233
    on level surface, 230, 231f
    versus resistance exercise modes, 591t
    terrain and walking surface, 231, 245t
Energy intake, spaceflight, 765, 765f
Energy interconversions, 124, 137–139, 138f
Energy metabolism regulation, 167–168
Energy phase, nutrient intake, 610b
Energy release
  from lipid
    adipocytes, 168–169
    fatty acid, catabolism of, 170
    glycerol, catabolism of, 170
    hormonal effects, 169
    total energy transfer, 170
  from macronutrients
    carbohydrates, 160–168
    lipid, 168–170
    protein, 172, 172f
  processes, 136–137, 137f
  rate alteration, 137f, 139–143
Energy source, 35b
Energy transfer
  biologic work in humans
    chemical work, 136, 139
    mechanical work, 139
    transport work, 139
  in body
    lipid, 168–170
    macronutrients, 158–160
    phosphate bond energy, 152
    protein, 172
  coenzymes, 142–143
  condensation reactions, 143–144, 144f
  energy-conserving processes, 136–137, 137f
  energy-releasing processes, 136–137, 137f
  enzymes
    alter reaction rates, 140–142, 142f
    biologic catalysts, 140–142
    classification, 140, 140b
    inhibition, 143
    mode of action, 142, 142f
  during exercise
    adenosine triphosphate-phosphocreatine system, 180
    aerobic system, 182–185
    energy spectrum, 185–187, 185f, 193t
    lactate-forming energy system, 180–182
    oxygen consumption during recovery, 187–191
  hydrolysis reactions, 143, 144f
  interconversions of energy, 137–139

forms, 138–139, 138f
photosynthesis, 138, 139f
respiration, 139, 140f
kinetic energy, 136
measuring in humans, 146
oxidation and reduction reactions, 144–145
potential energy, 136, 136f
Energy value of food, measurement of, 124–126
calories, 122, 124b
challenges, 124–125
gross, 124–126
net, 126–127
Energy-conserving processes, 136–137, 137f
Energy-generating pathways, 504, 504f
Enhancer site, 1031, 1032f
Enterogastrin, 495t
Enthalpy, 137
Entropy, 137–138
Environment
 cold
  acclimatization to, 693–694
  body fat, 692
  children, 692
  overview, 691–692
  respiratory tract during, 695–696
  wind-chill temperature index, 694–695, 695f
 heat
  circulatory adjustments, 679
  complications from excessive, 689–691
  core temperature, 679–680, 679f
  factors that modify tolerance, 686–689
  water loss, 680–683
Enzyme turnover number, 1032, 1033f
Enzymes
 action, 142, 142f
 biologic catalysts, 140–142
 classification, 143
 inhibition, 143
 reaction rate alteration, 140–142, 142f
Enzyme-substrate complex, 142
Enzyme-substrate interaction, 1033f
Ephedra, 616–617
Ephedrine, 616–617, 640
Epigenetics, 1010
Epimysium, 392
Epinephrine, 162
 chemical structure of, 461f
 cold exposure, 672
 effect of altitude on excretion, 651f
 overview, 481
 release of, 362, 460–461
 role in mobilizing glucose, 461f
EPO (erythropoietin), 452, 495t, 622–623, 657, 1027–1028
EPOC. see Excess postexercise oxygen consumption (EPOC)
Epps, Jeanette J., 771b
EPSP (excitatory postsynaptic potential), 433–434, 434f
Ergogenic aid, 594, 640
 higher-dose arginine supplementation, 633b
 levels of evidence on research findings, 595, 642t
 proposed mechanisms for, 597b
Ergometer, 141b
ERV (expiratory reserve volume), 281
Erythrocythemia, 621
Erythropoietin (EPO), 452, 495t, 622–623, 657, 1027–1028
ESADDI (Estimated Safe and Adequate Daily Dietary Intake), 630
Escherichia coli, 1016, 1016f
Essential amino acids, 29
Essential fat, 806
Essential fatty acids, 16
Esterification, 17
Estimated average requirement (EAR), 46
Estimated Safe and Adequate Daily Dietary Intake (ESADDI), 630
Estimated Safe and Adequate Daily Dietary Intakes (ESADDIs), 31
Estradiol, 465
Estrogen, 53
Estrogen's role in bone health, 57b
Euglycemia, 111
Euhydration, 897
Eukaryotes, 1030

Europe, life expectancy, 912f
European Space Agency (ESA), 736
Eustachian tube, blockage of, 721f, 722
EVA (extravehicular activity), 745
Evans, Martin J., 1060
Evaporation, heat loss by, 674–675
Excess dietary protein accumulation, 172b
Excess postexercise oxygen consumption (EPOC)
 implications for physical activity and recovery, 189–190
 intermittent interval exercise, 191, 193t
 metabolic dynamics, 188–189
 non-steady-rate exercise, 190–191, 190f
 steady-rate exercise, 190
Exchangeable lactate pool, 164
Excitation, anterior motor neuron, 432–433
Excitation-contraction coupling, 407, 407f
Excitatory postsynaptic potential (EPSP), 433–434, 434f
Exercise
 acid-base regulation, effects on, 323
 aerobic system changes with, 507–518, 507f
  cardiovascular adaptations, 509–515, 509f
  lactate concentration, 516, 516f
  metabolic adaptations, 507–509
  pulmonary adaptations, 515–516, 516f
 after cardiac transplantation, 369–370
 anaerobic system changes with, 506–507, 506f
 defined, 913
 effect on distribution of blood, 366–367
 energy transfer during
  adenosine triphosphate-phosphocreatine system, 180
  aerobic system, 182–185
  energy spectrum, 185–187, 185f, 193t
  lactate-forming energy system, 180–182
  oxygen consumption during recovery, 187–191
 genetic background, 525–526, 526f
 improvements in fitness, 525–526, 525f
 maintenance of aerobic fitness gains, 526–527
 in medicine, 918
 methods
  aerobic training, 528–530
  anaerobic training, 527
 overtraining considerations, 531–533, 532f
 during pregnancy
  current opinion, 534–536
  fetal effects, 533–534
  maternal effects, 533
  prescription, 535b
 principles of
  individual differences, 506
  overload, 504
  reversibility, 506
  specificity, 504–506
 pulmonary ventilation during
  aerobic power and endurance, 320–321
  oxygen cost of breathing, 317–320
  regulation of, 313
  steady-rate exercise, 314
 special aids to, 592–643
  challenge to fair competition, 594–595
  future of, 595
  nonpharmacologic approaches, 621
  pharmacologic agents, 596
 training impacts the anaerobic system, 506, 540t
Exercise countermeasures, 756
Exercise high, 487
Exercise hyperpnea, 312
Exercise immunology, 487
Exercise interval, 529
Exercise metabolism, food's calorigenic effect on, 217
Exercise physiology
 clinical applications of, 956
 in clinical setting
  regular physical activity, 954, 954b
  sports medicine, 954
Exercise Physiology Laboratory Countermeasures Program (ExPC), 745–746
Exercise pressor reflex, 365
Exercise stress hypothesis, 808
Exercise stroke volume, 512, 512f
Exercise-induced asthma, 302c
Exercise-induced bronchospasm (EIB), 986
Exercise-related amenorrhea, 60
Exercise-related anemia, 63
Exergonic chemical reactions, 136–137, 137f, 140f

Exertional heat stroke, 690
Exhalation, 278f
Exhaustive exercise
 EPOC, 189, 189f
 short-term benefits, 488
Exocrine glands, 450
Exogenous anabolic steroids, 608
Exogenous erythropoietin, 657b
Exons, 1033–1035, 1034f
Exothermic combustion reaction, 123
Expiration, 280
Expiratory reserve volume (ERV), 281
Exploration extravehicular mobility unit (xEMU), 745
Extensor carpi radialis brevis muscle (ECRB), 405
External eye muscles, 394b
External intercostal muscle, 280
External pressure, depth in water, 712, 712b, 731t
External work output, 228
Extracellular compartment, 69
Extracellular fluid, 69
Extrafusal fibers, 439
Extrapolation procedure, 265
Extrapyramidal (ventromedial) tract, 427, 427f
Extravehicular activity (EVA), 745
Extravehicular mobility unit (EMU), 745–746
Extreme ultraendurance sports, food intake, 102–103
Extrinsic factors, 229
Extrinsic regulation of heart rate and circulation
 input from higher centers, 364
 parasympathetic influence, 364
 peripheral input, 365
 sympathetic influence, 362, 363f
Eye disease, 874f

F

Facemask squeeze, 720–722, 721f
Facilitation, anterior motor neuron, 433–435
Facilitative diffusion, 162–163, 466
Facultative thermogenesis, 216
FAD (flavin adenine dinucleotide), 155
Fahey, Dr. Tom, 843
Falco, Albert, 708
False Claims Act, 623b
Fartlek training, 528–530
Fasciculus, 392
Fast- and slow-twitch muscle fiber ratios, 574f
Fast component of recovery oxygen consumption, 188
Fast glycolytic (FG) fiber, 411
Fasting plasma glucose (FPG) test, 470
Fast-oxidative-glycolytic (FOG) fibers, 411
Fast-twitch muscle fiber, 438f
Fast-twitch (type II) muscle fibers
 aerobic system, 184–185
 overview, 411
Fat cell differentiation, 879f
Fat cell hyperplasia, 877
Fat cell hypertrophy, 877
Fat mass (FM), 804
Fat metabolism, 45
 water-soluble vitamins, 44
Fat patterning, 824
Fat, percentages for athletes, 930f
Fat-free body mass (FFM), 806, 838
 of astronauts, 766, 766f
 basal metabolic rate, 212–214, 214f
 body composition, 930f
 creatine supplementation and, 635f
 overview, 806–807
Fat-free-to-fat ratio, 839–841, 840f
Fatigue, 14
Fatigue resistance, 438–439
Fat-soluble vitamins, 44
Fatty acid carbon chains, 15–16
Fatty acids, 15, 170
 breakdown, 174
FDA (Food and Drug Administration), 17b, 18, 31b, 104–105, 617
Feces, water loss through, 72
Federal Bureau of Investigation Laboratory mtDNA Casework Unit, 1045
Feedback regulation, glycogen, 11
Female athlete triad, 59–61, 60b, 60f
Ferritin, 62
FES. see Functional electrostimulation (FES)
FEV (forced expiratory volume), 282–283, 927, 983

FEV-to-FVC ratio, 282–283, 282f
FFAs (free fatty acids), 614
FFM (fat-free body mass). see Fat-free body mass (FFM)
FG fiber. see Fast glycolytic (FG) fiber
Fiber, 8, 127
    coefficient of digestibility, 127
    content of common foods, 9b, 40t
    deficiency, health implications of, 8–9
    effect on lipids, 943
    recommended daily intake, 9f
Fiber hypertrophy, 563
Fiber length-Muscle length (FL:ML) ratio, 400–401, 400f
Fibrates, 941–942
Fibrils, 391–392
Fick, Adolf Eugen, 279
Fick, Adolf Gaston, 374
Fick equation, 374
Fick's law of diffusion, 279
Field event athletes, body fat, 842–843, 843f
Filaments, 396
First lady astronaut trainees (FLATS), 744
First law of thermodynamics, 123–124, 136
First messenger, 453
First transition phase, strength training, 558
Fischer, Emil, 142
Fitness, defined, 913
Fitness level, 229
Fitness trends
    comparisons, 918
    2020 top 10, 918
Fitzgerald, Mabel Purefoy, 648
Fitzgerald, M.P., 648
Fixed blood lactate concentration, 319
FLATS (first lady astronaut trainees), 744
Flavin adenine dinucleotide (FAD), 155
Fleuss, Henry A., 705
Flexibility, 916b
FL:ML ratio (fiber length-muscle length ratio), 400–401, 400f
Flower-spray ending, 439–440
Fluid compartments, 66, 69
Fluid loss, 652–653
Fluorescent probes, 405
Fluoride, 81t
FM (fat mass), 804
FOG (fast-oxidative-glycolytic) fibers, 411
Follicle-stimulating hormone (FSH), 458, 480, 926f
Food. see Diet; Nutrition
Food and Drug Administration (FDA), 17b, 18, 31b, 104–105, 617
Food and Nutrition Board of the National Academy of Sciences, 8, 31
Food items in picture portion size, 98, 99f
Food labels, 34b
Food macronutrients, 174
Food's calorigenic effect on exercise metabolism, 217
Foods' insulin index, 111–112
Food's net energy value, 126–127
    calculation, 127–130
    limitations of, 127
Football players
    body composition, 859t
    body fat, 848
    body mass index, 799, 851f
    body weight, 850f
    collegiate vs. professional players, 848–852, 849f, 850f, 851f, 859t
    exceptionally large professional, 854–855
    underwater weighing, 812, 835t
Football uniforms, 677–678, 677f
Footwear, 231–233
Force gradation, 437–438, 438f
Forced expiratory volume (FEV), 282–283, 927, 983
Forced vital capacity (FVC), 281, 983
Forensic medicine, 1026–1027
Founder mice, 1059
FPG (fasting plasma glucose) test, 470
Frank, Otto, 377
Franklin, Rosalind Elsie, 1014–1015, 1015f, 1015b
Frank-Starling law of the heart, 377
Frank-Starling mechanism, 928
FRC (functional residual capacity), 295
Free diving training, 714b
Free energy, 153
Free fatty acids (FFAs), 18, 614

Free radical, 1041
Free weight training, 918
Frog stretch, 584b
Front crawl, 241, 241f
Frostbite stages, 694b
Fructose, 6, 107–108
FSH (follicle-stimulating hormone), 458, 480, 926f
Functional anemia, 65
Functional electrostimulation (FES), 757
Functional genomics research, 411–412
Functional protein, 1028
Functional residual blood volume, 377
Functional residual capacity (FRC), 295
Functional strength training, 561–562
Furchgott, Robert F., 366
Fusiform fibers, 398, 398f
Futile metabolism, 870
FVC (forced vital capacity), 281, 983

G

G1 (growth) stage, 1027
G2 (growth) stage, 1027
Gagarin, Yuri, 747
Gagge, A. Pharo, 220
Gagnan, Emile, 707, 717–718
Gaining weight, 898–900
Galactose, 6
Galen, 337, 864
Galilei, Galileo., 390
Galileo, 294
Gallstones, protection from, 942
Galvani, Luigi, 355
Gama (γ)-efferent fiber, 440
Gametes, 1059
Gamow hypobaric chamber, 663
Ganglion, 446t
Gas exchange
    concentrations and partial pressures of respired gases
        alveolar air, 295
        ambient air, 295, 295f
        tracheal air, 295
    in lungs, 297–298
    movement of gas in air and fluids
        pressure differential, 296, 296f
        solubility, 295
    pressure gradients for, 297f
    surface, 276
    in tissues, 298
Gas pressure symbols, 295
Gas solubility coefficients, 296
Gastric emptying, 108, 112
Gastrin, 478, 495t
Gastrointestinal tract, 496t–498t
GDR (German Democratic Republic), 601
Gel electrophoresis, 1052, 1055f–1056f
Gender
    aging and trainability, 930–931, 949t
    cardiac output differences, 381
    coronary heart disease, 938–939
    differences in glycogen storage and catabolism, 629, 629f
    differences in lung volumes, 283
    differences in responsiveness to exercise, 897
    differences in training responses
        bone density, 577
        males vs. female muscle hypertrophy, 577
        muscular strength and hypertrophy, 576–577
        transgender athlete participation, 576–577
    heart attack warning signs, 934–935
    heat stress tolerance, 688–689
    minimal leanness standards, 806–807
    positive muscle and tendon adaptations from, 575, 575f
    sweating, 688
Gene, 870
Gene cassette, 1063
Gene doping, 595, 640
Gene editing, 1065–1069
Gene expression, 1010, 1011f, 1030, 1029b
    examples, 1031, 1031f
    and human exercise performance, 1032–1033
    and translation, 1030–1031, 1030f
Gene knockout technique, 1062–1063, 1063f
Gene splicing, 1048
Gene therapy

    in clinical trials, 1044–1045
    definition, 1010
    techniques, 1071
Gene-exercise interactions, 1072–1073, 1072f
General reentry syndrome (GRS), 759
General warm-up, 623, 640
Generalized equations, 817
Genes, defined, 1013
Genetic abnormality, 65
Genetic background, 525–526, 526f
Genetic code, 1023, 1025, 1025f
Genetic engineering, 1042, 1047f, 1048
Genetic model, for obesity, 868–869, 869f
Genetic variants, 1073
Genetics, 1010
Genome, 1010, 1015–1016
Genome-wide association studies (GWAS), 1074
Genomic library, 1051–1052, 1052f
Genotype, 261, 1016
Germ line, 1063
German Democratic Republic (GDR), 601
Gestational diabetes mellitus, 468
Ghrelin, 477–478
Gibbs, Willard, 137
Gigantism, 605, 640
Gilpatric, Guy, 706
Gimbal Rig, 744
Ginseng, 616, 640
Girandola, Robert, 854
Girth anthropometry
    athletes, 857t
    body fat predictions, 822–823
    bodybuilders, 857t
    overview, 818
    sites for, 818
    usefulness of, 818
Glenn, John, 744
Global obesity epidemic, 864–867, 865f
Glottis, 288
Glover, Victor J., 771b
Glucagon, 11, 475–477, 477f
Glucocorticoids, 462–464, 463f, 1004t
Glucogenic, 172
Gluconeogenesis, 6, 35b, 174
Glucose, 6, 7f, 112–113
    cellular uptake, 108
    controlling, 484f
    homeostasis, impaired, 470
    postexercise, 611–612, 611f, 612f
    transporters, 467
Glucose catabolism, total energy transfer from, 167–168, 167f
Glucose conversion to lipid, 174
Glucose feedings, 112–113
Glucose paradox, 163–164
Glucose synthesis from triacylglycerol components, 171b
Glucose to glycogen metabolism, 162–164
Glucose transporter-1 (GLUT-1), 1071
GLUT 4 (Glu T4), 162–163
GLUT-4 protein, 574
Glutamine, 489–490, 619–620, 640
Gluteus maximus, 394b
Glycated hemoglobin, 470
Glycemic control, 483–484
Glycemic index, 106–108, 107f, 111
Glycemic load, 106–107
Glycemic response, 106–107
Glycerol, 15, 170
    and fatty acid catabolism, 170
Glycerol-phosphate shuttle, 163
Glycogen, 10–11, 106
    concentrations of pre-and post-carbohydrate loading, 629f
    depletion of, 257–258, 257f
    gender differences in, 629
    replenishing reserves, 106
    storage
        capacity, 10–11, 11f
        dietary plan to increase, 628f
    supercompensation, 627, 629
Glycogen biosynthesis, 10, 10f
Glycogen, depletion of, 257f
Glycogen phosphorylase, 12–13
Glycogen replenishment, 111
Glycogen synthase, 10, 627–628

Glycogen to glucose metabolism, 162–164
Glycogenesis, 10, 162
Glycogenolysis, 10
Glycogenolysis cascade, 158b
Glycohemoglobin test, 470
Glycolipid, 1038
Glycolysis
  anaerobic energy release, 162
  anaerobic vs. aerobic, 161
  glycogen metabolism, regulation of, 162–164
  glycogenesis, 10
  glycogenolysis, 162
  hydrogen release, 163
  lactate, 163–164
  regulation of, 162–163
  substrate-level phosphorylation, 162
Glycolytic (Lactate-Forming) system, 180–182
Glycoprotein, 1038
Glycosuria, 469, 473–475
Goal body weight, 830, 883
Golfers, body composition, 852–853, 860t
Golgi, Camillo, 441, 442b, 1037
Golgi complex, 1037–1038, 1039f
Golgi tendon organs (GTO), 441–442, 442f
Gonadal hormones, 464–465
  estradiol, 465
  overview, 464–465
  pancreatic hormones, 466–468, 466f
  progesterone, 465
  testosterone, 464–465, 464f, 465f
Gonadocorticoids, 464
Gonadotropic hormones, 458
Gonadotropin-releasing hormone, 808
Graded exercise, 246t, 259, 343, 343f
Graded exercise stress test (GXT), 970–971, 998t
Gradient layer calorimetry, 197
Gravitational density, 20
Gravitational loading, 753, 755f
Gravity (g or G), 736–737, 736f
  on Moon and Mars, 737b
Gray matter, 422, 446t
Gregory, Frederick D., 771b
Grimek, John, 547b
Grimsey, Trent, 242
Gross energy value of foods, 124–126
  carbohydrates, 126
  comparing, 126–127
  lipids, 127
  proteins, 127
Gross mechanical efficiency, 228
Group training, 918
Growth hormone (GH)
  anabolic steroids, 597
  direct and indirect metabolic actions, 457, 457f
  effects of aging, 922–923, 926f
  genetic engineering, 605–606
  human, 605
  insulin-like growth factors, 457
  overview, 456, 479f, 480
  physical activity and tissue synthesis, 456–457
Growth hormone/insulin-like growth factor axis, 927
Growth phase, nutrient intake, 610b
GRS. see General reentry syndrome (GRS)
Gruener, John J., 708
GTO (Golgi tendon organs), 441–442, 442f
GTP (guanosine triphosphate), 1034–1035, 1035f
Guanine, 1021
Guanosine triphosphate (GTP), 1034–1035, 1035f
Gut, 478
GXT (graded exercise stress test), 970–971, 998t
Gymnasticon, 547
Gynecomastia, 600, 640
Gynoid-type obesity, 876

H

H band, sarcomere, 396–397, 397f
HACE (high-altitude cerebral edema), 654t, 654b
Haldane effect, 306
Haldane gas analysis method, 201
Haldane, John Scott, 201, 306, 704, 706
Haldane, J.S., 648
Haldane method, 201
Haldane transformation, 204
Half-life, 613–614, 640
Half-life, hormones, 450

Halley, Edmund, 705
Halteres, 544
Hamstring stretch, 584b
Hamstrings muscle architectural properties, 400f
Hand-grip dynamometer, 548f
Handheld weights, 232
HAPE (high-altitude pulmonary edema), 654t, 654b
Harbor protocol, 261f
HArH (high-altitude retinal hemorrhage), 654b
Harpenden caliper, 816
Harris, Bernard A., 771b
Harris, Jay Arthur, 218
Harvard Fatigue Laboratory, 188
Harvard School of Public Health (HSPH), 95–96
Harvey, William, 337
HbA1c (Hemoglobin A1c) test, 470
HDL (high-density lipoprotein), 20, 21f
  and cancer risk, 22b
Head-down bed rest, 762
Health, 910, 1010
  defined, 913
Health enhancement, resistance training for, 559
Health risks, obesity, 872–874, 873f, 875b
Health/fitness track, ACSM, 955
Health-related physical fitness, defined, 913
Healthspan, 910
Health/wellness coaching, 918
Healthy eating plate, 96–97, 96f
Healthy life expectancy (HALE), 912–913, 912f
Healthy People 2030, 918–920, 918f
Heart, 451f, 496f–498t
  blood flow to, 380
  blood supply, 345–347
  overview, 328–330
  schematic of, 328
Heart attacks, 346
  and strokes, 934
  vs. cardiac arrest, 935
  warning signs between males and females, 934–935
Heart auscultation, 968
Heart disease, effects of physical activity on, 873–874, 874f, 933
Heart muscle diseases
  aneurysm, 963–964
  angina pectoris, 961, 961f
  congestive heart failure, 961–963
  myocardial infarction, 961, 962f
  pericarditis, 964
Heart rate (HR), 374
  age-predicted maximum, 520, 520f
  age-related factors, 687f
  aging, 928
  β_1–adrenoceptor, 378f
  breath-hold divers, 717, 717f
  cardiovascular adaptations with training, 511–512
  computing lower-limit and upper-limit target training, 522b
  determination, 966b, 966f
  in endurance athletes, 511f
  oxygen consumption, 222–223, 223f
  in space, 760, 761f
  variability, 515b
Heart rate reserve (HRR), 522b
Heart rate variability (HRV), 512
Heart transplants, 368f, 369–370, 369f
Heart valve diseases, 964
Heartburn, 961b
Heartburn vs angina pectoris, 961b
Heat, 127
  acclimatization, 686–687, 699t
  defined, 127
  exhaustion, 689
  gain/loss factors, 670f, 672f
  illness, 689
Heat combustion, 125–126
Heat cramps, 689
Heat energy, 138f
Heat loss
  by conduction, 673
  by convection, 673
  by evaporation, 674–675
  heat-dissipating mechanisms, 675
  hormonal adjustments, 675
  overview, 672–673, 672f
  by radiation, 673
  during swimming, 242

Heat of combustion, 133t
Heat stroke, 690–691
Heat-related disorder, 690b
Heat-stress index, 676b
Heavy work, 221
Heavy-resistance exercise, blood pressure, 343f
Height, golfers, 860t
Height-weight tables, limitations of, 796
Helicase, 1026
Heliox, 719
Helium-neon laser procedure, 406f–407f
Helium-oxygen mixtures, 726, 732t
Helix, 1014–1015
Hematocrit, 303, 622–623, 657, 658f
Hematologic changes, longer-term adjustment to altitude exposure, 656–657
Heme, 64–65
Hemiparesis, 987
Hemiplegia, 987
Hemispheres, 422
Hemoconcentration, 382, 621–622, 640
Hemoglobin, 64
  at altitude, 649–650, 658f
  molecule, 299f
  oxygen-carrying capacity of, 299
  PO_2 and hemoglobin saturation, 300
  pre-to postflight changes in, 752–753, 752f
Hemoglobin A1c (HbA1c) test, 470
Hemorrhage, 987
Hemosiderin, 62
Henderson, Y., 648
Henry, William, 295, 720
Henry's law, 295, 720
Hepatic portal vein, 16
Hereditary hemochromatosis, 65
Herniated disk, 425
Herodotus, 704
Heterozygous, 1059
Higginbotham, Joan E., 771b
High altitude, 648
High-altitude cerebral edema (HACE), 654t, 654b
High-altitude pulmonary edema (HAPE), 654t, 654b
High-altitude retinal hemorrhage (HArH), 654b
High-carbohydrate diets, 14, 35
High-density lipoprotein cholesterol (HDL-C), 941–942
High-density lipoproteins (HDLs), 20, 21f
  and cancer risk, 22b
High-energy phosphate compound, 153–154
Higher-dose arginine supplementation, 633b
High-fat diets, 89–90
High-glycemic foods, obesity, 110–111
High-glycemic index (HGI) foods, 96, 103
High-intensity interval training (HIIT), 918
High-pressure nervous syndrome (HPNS), 726
High-protein diets, 889
High-risk sports, 103
High-risk sports for marginal nutrition, 103
Highway tubule system, muscle fiber, 402f
Hill, Archibald Vivian, 188
Hind-limb suspension technique, 757, 757f
Hip-and-trunk flexibility, 916b, 916f
Hippocrates, 864
Hips, flexibility of, 916
His, Wilhelm, Jr., 354
Histone, 1018–1020
Hitting the wall, 628b
Hlavacova, Yvetta, 242
HMB (β-hydroxy-β-methylbutyrate), 620–621, 620f, 639
HMS Beagle (British survey ship), 1012, 1012f
Hodgkin, Dorothy Crowfoot, 1065, 45
Homo sedentarius, 221
Homocysteine, 943–944, 943f
Homologous transfusion, 621, 640
Homozygous, 1059
Honolulu technique, 1062
Hopkins, Frederick Gowland, 42, 140
Hopkins, John, 384
Horizontal and grade running, 246t
Hormonal adjustments, as heat-dissipating mechanism, 675
Hormonal blood boosting, 622–623
Hormonal stimulation, endocrine gland, 454, 455f
Hormone level factors, 454
Hormone-receptor binding, 453

Hormones, 450
    effect on enzymes, 453–454
    nonsteroid action, 453f
    produced by endocrine system glands, 451f
    release patterns, 454
    terminology, 450b
    types, 450–452, 494t
Hormone-sensitive lipase, 168
Hormone-target cell specificity, 452
Hot-weather exercise
    circulatory adjustments, 679
    complications from excessive
        heat cramps, 689
        heat exhaustion, 689
        heat stroke, 690–691
    core temperature, 679–680, 679f
    factors that modify tolerance
        age, 687–688, 687f
        body fat level, 689
        gender, 688–689
        heat acclimatization, 686–687, 699t
        training status, 687
    physiologic adjustments, 686–687, 699t
    rectal temperature, 677f, 678
    water loss
        diuretics, 683
        fluid balance maintenance, 683–686
        magnitude of, 680–681, 699t
        overview, 680
        physiologic and performance decrements, 683
        significant consequences of, 682, 682f
Hounsfield, Godfrey N., 983
Housekeeping genes, 1033
HPNS (high-pressure nervous syndrome), 726
Hubble Space Telescope, 748
Hultman, Eric, 409
Human exercise performance, 1032–1033
Human genome, 1013, 1015–1017
Human Genome Project, 1013, 1015–1017, 1017b
Human growth hormone (hGH), 605, 640
Human vastus lateralis muscle, 410f–409f
Humidity, heat loss during high, 674–675
Humoral stimulation, endocrine gland, 454, 455f
Huxley, Andrew Fielding, 403
Huxley, Hugh, 403
Hydration recommendations, ultramarathon running events, 74b
Hydrocortisone (cortisol), 619
Hydrodensitometry, 809
Hydrogen bonds, 1021, 1022f, 1023
Hydrogen oxidation, 155–156
Hydrogen shuttle, 181
Hydrogenation, 17
Hydrolases, 148t, 1031
Hydrolysis reactions, 143, 144f
Hydrostatic gradient, 767, 769f
Hydrostatic weighing
    of athletes, 843f
    body density, 812
    fat mass, 814
    limitations of, 813
    menstruation, variations with, 812
    overview, 809–810
    percentage body fat, 813
    residual lung volume, 812, 835t
    validity of, 812
Hyperbaria, 712
Hyperbaric chamber, 724
Hyperhomocysteinemia, 943–944, 943f
Hyperhydration, 683–686
Hyperinsulinemia, 9
Hyperinsulinemic clamp, 470
Hyperlipidemia, 940
Hyperlipoproteinemia, 941
Hyperoxic gas mixtures, 625, 640
Hyperplasia
    fat cell, 877
    muscle, 575–576
Hyperpnea, exercise, 312
Hypertension, 67, 940
    by age, 339f
    blood pressure, 977
    chronic resistance training, 977
    C-reactive protein, 936
    defined, 335
    effects of physical activity on, 950t

by gender, 339f
overview, 338–341
by race, 339f
regular physical activity, 976–977, 976f
risk stratification and recommended treatment, 976
sodium-induced, 67
weight gain, 874f
Hyperthermia, 536, 670, 689, 700t
Hyperthyroidism, 460, 481
Hypertrophic response, 573
Hypertrophy
    adipocytes, 877–881
    gender differences in training responses, 576–577
    males vs. female muscle, 577
    overview, 572–573, 572f
Hypertrophy-induced adaptations, 569, 569f
Hyperventilation (HV)
    at altitude, 650–651
    breath-hold diving, 715
    overview, 287
    oxygen cost of, 318b
Hypoestrogenesis, 61
Hypoglycemia, 12, 468, 472b, 475, 485
Hypogonadism, 598, 640
Hyponatremia, 72–73
    predisposing factors, 74b
Hypophysis, 455–456
Hypotensive response to exercise, 343–345
Hypothalamic hormones, 478
Hypothalamic temperature regulation, 671, 671f
Hypothalamic-pituitary dysfunction, 65
Hypothalamic-pituitary-adrenal axis, 458
Hypothalamic-pituitary-gonadal axis, 926
Hypothalamus, 424, 451f, 496t–498t, 671
Hypothalamus-pituitary hormones, 479f
Hypothyroidism, 460
Hypotonic water, 72
Hypovolemia, 680
Hypoxia, 648, 652b
Hypoxico altitude tent, 663–664, 664f

I

I band, sarcomere, 396–397, 397f
Ibn Masawayh, Yuhanna (Jean Mesue), 864
Iditasport ultramarathon, 102
IGF (insulin-like growth factor), 456–457, 1027–1028
IGF-1 (insulin-like growth factor-1), 912
IIa fiber, 411
IIb fiber, 411
IIx fiber, 411
Immediate energy system, 250f
Immune function, physical activity and
    nutrition effects on
        glutamine, 489–490
        macronutrients, 489
        micronutrients, 489
        optimizing, 490
        relationship between stress, physical activity, illness, 488f
        resistance training on, 489
        upper respiratory tract infections, 488–490, 488f
Immune response, 1047
Immunologic factors, 943
Immunosurveillance, 957
Impaired alveolar gas transfer, 296b
Impaired glucose homeostasis
    type 1 diabetes, 470–473
    type 2 diabetes, 473–475
IMTG (intramuscular triacylglycerol), 27, 27f
Inactivity
    effect on life expectancy, 910, 931–932
    effects of physical activity on, 950t
    excessive fat accumulation, 871–872
Incomplete protein, 29
Indian Space Research Organization (ISRO), 736
Indicator dilution method, 374
Indirect calorimetry
    closed-circuit spirometry, 198, 199f
    open-circuit spirometry
        bag, 200–201, 201f
        computerized instrumentation, 201, 202f
        portable, 199–200, 200f
        ventilated Hood technique, 201, 201f
    vs. direct calorimetry, 202
Individual differences

aerobic energy
    endurance runs, 264–265
    long-term energy system, 258–267
    prediction tests, 263–267
    step test, 266–267
anaerobic energy
    biologic indicators, 256–257, 257f
    buffering of acid metabolites, 258
    maximally accumulated oxygen deficit, 256
    motivation, 258
    overview, 250
    performance tests, 250–252
    physiologic tests, 254
    specificity versus generality of, 250, 250f
    training, 258
Inducible nitric oxide synthase (iNOS) inhibitor, 761–762
Inferior vena cava, 336
Inflammatory response, 935
Inflight adaptations, physiologic responses to spaceflight, 767, 770f
Inflight space station daily exercise, long-duration missions, 760, 760f, 761f
Informed consent, 971
Ingested protein during endurance activity, 110b
Inherited blood disorder, 1016b
Inhibition, anterior motor neuron, 435
Inhibitory postsynaptic potential (IPSP), 434f, 435
Innate immunity system, 487
iNOS (inducible nitric oxide synthase) inhibitor, 761–762
Inotropic effect, 362
Inpatient cardiac programs, 979–980
Insensible perspiration, 71–72
Insertion, 395
Inspiration, 278f, 279–280
Inspiratory reserve volume (IRV), 281
Inspired gas pressures, depth in water, 712, 712b, 731t
Insufficiency, 964
Insufficiency/regurgitation, 964
Insulin, 453, 466–468
    actions and impaired glucose homeostasis, 470, 471f
    diabetes mellitus, 468–470
    glucose transporters, 467
    glucose-insulin interaction, 467–468
    impaired glucose homeostasis, 470, 471f
        type 2 diabetes, 473–475
    primary functions of, 467f
    resistance to, 473
    responsiveness, 470
    sensitivity to, 470
Insulin index, foods, 111–112
Insulin, protein intake during recovery, 111
Insulin resistance, 471f, 473, 943
Insulinemic response, 106–107
Insulin-glucose interaction, 473
Insulin-like growth factor (IGF), 456–457, 1027–1028
Insulin-like growth factor-1 (IGF-1), 912
Insulinotropic effect, 111
Interconversions of energy, 137–139, 138f
    forms, 138–139
    photosynthesis, 138, 139f
    respiration, 138–139, 140f
Interim resistive exercise device (iRED), 759–760, 760f
Interleukin (IL)-6, 478f
Intermittent interval physical activity, 191, 191b
Internal intercostal muscles, 280
International Association for Development of Apnea, 714b
International Cycling Union, 622–623
International Geophysical Year, 741
International Obesity Task Force, 864
International Space Station (ISS), 736, 738–740
    and body composition experiments, 765–766
    parabolic flights
        and astronaut training, 739
        simulate microgravity, 738–739, 739f
International System of Units (SI units), 123–124, 550, 590t
International Union of Biochemistry and Molecular Biology (IUBMB), 1031
Interneurons, 425, 429, 430f
Interstitial fluid, 69
Interval training, 191
    rationale for, 529
    sprint-type, 529
Intervertebral disks, 425
Intestinal fluid absorption, 103, 112
Intracellular compartment, 69

Intracellular cytoskeletal tubule systems, 402–403, 402f
Intracellular water (ICW), 766, 766f
Intrafusal fiber, 439
Intramuscular triacylglycerol (IMTG), 27, 27f
Intrapulmonic pressure, 279
Intrathoracic pressure, 288, 288f
Intrinsic regulation of heart rate, 354–360
Introns, 1033–1035, 1034f
Involuntary muscle, 429
Involuntary nerves, 429
Ion channel nanopore techniques, 1065
Ion channel regulators, 407
IPSP (inhibitory postsynaptic potential), 434f, 435
iRED (interim resistive exercise device), 759–760, 760f
Iron, 62–65, 63b
    absorption, 64b
    deficiency risk in females, 63
    exercise-induced anemia, 63
    females, risks for, 63
    functional anemia, 65
    real anemia/pseudoanemia, 63–64
    recommended dietary allowances, 44, 79t
    sources for, 62–65
Iron deficiency anemia, 62–63, 299–300
IRV (inspiratory reserve volume), 281
Ischemia, 960
Islets of Langerhans, 466
Isoforms, 409
Isokinetic dynamometer, 549–550
Isokinetic resistance training
    experiments, 563, 563f
    fast-versus slow-speed, 563
    overview, 562
    versus standard weightlifting, 562–563
Isokinetic training, 556
Isomerases, 148t, 1031
Isometric action, 405f, 556, 556f, 579
Isometric tension curve
    in human muscle fibers in vivo, 405–406, 406f–407f
    in isolated fibers, 405, 405f
Isometric training, 556
Isometric training response specificity, 561–562
Isovolumetric contraction period, 329–330
ISS. *see* International Space Station (ISS)

J
Jahn, Friedrich Ludwig, 544–545
James, William, 705
Japan Aerospace Exploration Agency (JAXA), 736
Jejunum, 451f
Jemison, Mae C., 771b
Jerky movement sequences, 435
Jogging, 233
Joint flexibility of, 916b
Joint stability, 920
Joliot-Curie, Irène, 1065, 45
Jones, Marion, 595
Joule, James Prescott, 123–124
Joules (J), 123–124
Jumping exercises, 564
Junk DNA, 1041–1042

K
K rations, 807
Karvonen method, 519, 522b
Kayaking, 241
KC-135 flights, 738–739, 739f
kCal (Kilocalorie), 122b, 123
Kendrew, John C., 304, 1039
Keplerian trajectory (parabolic) flights, 738–739, 739f
Ketogenic amino acids, 172
Ketogenic diets, 887–889
Ketone bodies, 12
Ketosis, 12, 464
KIAS (knots indicating air speed), 738–739, 739f
Kidney, 451f, 496t–498t
Kidney disease, effects of physical activity on, 873–874, 874f
Kilobase (kb), 1020–1021
Kilocalorie (kCal), 122b, 123
Kilojoule (kJ), 123
Kilopound (kp), 141b
Kinases, 1027
Kindling temperature, 152

Kinetic energy, 136, 136f
kJ (Kilojoule), 123
Knee-jerk reflex, 441
Knockin animal model, 1059
Knockout animal model, 1059
Knots indicating air speed (KIAS), 738–739, 739f
Kornberg, Arthur, 1048–1051, 1029
Korotkoff, Nikolai S, 335
Kossel, Ludwig Albrecht, 1012
Kouros, Yiannis, 100–101
Kramer, Erik, 709
Kreb cycle (citric acid cycle), 164–165
Krebs, Hans, 164–165, 44
Krebs, Hans Adolf, 164
Krogh, August, 36, 37, 39, 42, 44

L
Lactate, 164
    accumulation, 181–182, 181f
    anaerobic energy, 256–257, 257f
    concentration of
        aerobic training, 516, 516f
        during graded exercise to maximum, 314f
        relationship with blood pH, 324f
        producing capacity, 182
    shuttling, 164
    vs. lactic acid, 163b, 163f
Lactate dehydrogenase (LDH), 163, 968
Lactate flux, 180–181, 180f
Lactate paradox, 656, 656f
Lactate shuttle hypothesis, 180–181
Lactate shuttling, 164
Lactate threshold (LT), 315, 316b, 523–524, 523f
Lactate-generating capacity, 527
Lactic acid (lactacid) oxygen debt, 188
Lactic acid system, 186
Lactic acid theory of oxygen debt, 188
Lactose, 7
Lactovegetarian diet, 30
Lagging strand, 1026
Lange caliper, 816
Langerhans, Paul, 466
Laqueur, Ernst, 594
Large artery compliance, 928
Lashmanova, Elena, 232
Late-onset hypoglycemia, 472b
Lateral (pyramidal) tract, 425–427, 427f
Lavoisier, Antoine Laurent, 196
LBM (lean body mass), 806
LCAT (lecithin acetyl transferase), 941
LD_{50} (lethal oral caffeine dose), 616, 640
LDH (lactate dehydrogenase), 968
Le Prieur, Yves, 706–707
12-lead ECG configuration, 355
Leading strand, 1026
Lean body mass (LBM), 806, 843–845
Lean-to-fat ratio, 808, 842
Lecithin acetyl transferase (LCAT), 941
Left-ventricular ejection fraction (LVEF), 962
Left-ventricular end-diastolic cavity dimensions, 510
Leg exercise, 382
Leg press, one-repetition maximum for, 414b–415b
Lemniscus, 446t
Leptin, 868–869
    and ghrelin, 477–478
    regulation, 478, 479f
Lethal oral caffeine dose (LD_{50}), 616, 640
Lethbridge, John, 705
Leucine, 597, 640
Leukemias, 956
Levi-Montalcini, Rita, 45, 1051
LGI (low-glycemic index), 87b
LH (luteinizing hormone), 458
Life expectancy
    active, 913b
    effects of physical activity on, 950t
    effects of physical activity/inactivity on, 931–932
    healthy, 912–913, 912f
    total, 913b
Ligases, 148t, 1031
Light energy, 138f
Light work, 221
Limbic lobe, 425
Limbic system, 425
Ling, Pehr Henrik, 545

Linoleic acid, 16
Lipid
    glucose conversion to, 174
    protein conversion to, 174
    respiratory quotient for, 203
Lipid catabolism
    aerobic exercise, 508f
    energy sources, 168
Lipid metabolism
    hormonal effects on, 169
    metabolic adaptations with training, 508–509, 508f
Lipid peroxidation, 47–48
Lipid-rich cell membranes, 47
Lipids, 28, 127
    characteristics, 15
    combustion heat, 125
    compound, 20
    coronary heart disease, 940–941
    derived, 20–22
        cholesterol and coronary heart disease risk, 22
        cholesterol functions, 22
        U.S. Dietary Guidelines, 22
    diet *vs.* drugs to lower cholesterol, 23
    dynamics in physical activity, 25–27, 26f–27f
    energy release from
        adipocytes, 168–169
        fatty acid, catabolism of, 170
        glycerol, catabolism of, 170
        hormonal effects, 169
        total energy transfer, 170
    energy source and reserve, 23–24, 23f
    hormonal effects, 612–613, 642t
    kinds and sources of, 15–22
    recommended intake of, 22–24
    simple, 15–20, 16f
    slower energy release, 174
    supplementation, 636–637
    synthesis, 35b
    vital organs and thermal insulation, 24
    vitamin carrier and hunger depressor, 24
Lipodystrophies (LDs), 826–827
Lipogenesis, 174
Lipolysis, 17–18, 168
Lipoprotein(a) (Lp(a)), 943
Lipoprotein lipase (LPL), 18, 886
Lipoproteins, 600–601
    factors affecting, 942
Liquid meals, 104–106
Liquid, water intake through, 70–71
Live high-train low, 662–663
Live vector vaccines, 1047
Liver, 478, 496t–498t
Liver glycogenolysis, 10, 12, 461, 475
Lock-and-key mechanism, 142, 143f
Locus, 446t, 1045
Longevity
    age/aging
        causes of death, 950t
        epidemiologic evidence, 932
        Harvard Alumni study, 932
        overview, 931
        regular moderate exercise, 932–933
    defined, 913
Longitudinal data, body composition, 929
Longitudinal splitting, 575–576
Long-term energy system, 250f
Long-term exercise effects
    nutrition effects on immune function, 489–490
    resistance training, 489
Low nonheme iron bioavailability, 65
Low-carbohydrate ketogenic diets, 887–889
Low-density ipoprotein cholesterol (LDL-C), 941–942
Low-density lipoproteins, 20, 21f
Lower back
    flexibility, 913f
    and strengthening exercises for, 584b
    minimally invasive surgical techniques, 582b
    rationale for, 581–585
        high skill sport, 583
        improper technique, 583–585
        pain and inflammation, 582
        prevention and rehabilitation, 582
        resistance training and joint-flexibility exercise, 583
        resistance-training to prevent and reduce injury risk, 582–583
        workplace disability, 583

1100 Index

Lower-body negative pressure (LBNP)
   countermeasure combinations, 762
   device, 761, 762f
   orthostatic deconditioning effects, assessing, 762, 763f
   tilt test, 762, 763f
Low-fat diet, 90
Low-glycemic index (LGI), 87
Lowndes, Francis, 547
LPL (lipoprotein lipase), 18
LT (lactate threshold), 315, 316b, 523–524, 523f
Lumbar extension exercises, prone, 584b
Lung burst, 720
Lung cancer, 950t
Lung compliance, 282
Lung squeeze, 715
Lung volumes
   depth in water, 712, 712b, 731t
   dynamic, 282–283
   gender differences in, 283
   measurements and average values for, 281, 281f
   static, 281–282
Lungs
   anatomy of, 276–277
   gas exchange in, 297–298, 297f
   PO_2 in, 300–303
Luteinizing hormone (LH), 458, 479f, 480, 926f
LVEF (left ventricular ejection fraction), 962
Lyases, 148t, 1031
Lymphomas, 956
Lysosomes, 1071, 1071f

M

M band, sarcomeres, 397
M protein, 397, 397f, 419t
Mach, Ernst, 741
Mach numbers, 741
Macronutrients, 6, 122
   determining composition in foods, 124–125
   energy release from
     carbohydrates, 160–168
     lipid, 168–170
     protein, 172
   fuel sources, 160
   overview, 489
   pre-exercise testosterone concentrations, 613, 642t
Maddox, Brenda, 1015b
Magnesium, 62
Magnetic resonance imaging (MRI), 827–828, 827f, 828f
Major depressive disorder, 990
Major metabolic hormones, 459
Major minerals, 52
Malate-aspartate shuttle, 163
Male athlete triad, 61–62
Malignant tumor, 1044
Maltodextrin, 112
Maltose, 7
Mammalian target of rapamycin (mTOR), 596–597, 640
Manganese, 67
MAP (mean arterial pressure), 333
Marathon, 682b
Marathon running, energy expenditure during, 239
Marathoners, low body fat in, 878b
Marginal iron deficiency, 65
Marginal nutrition, high-risk sports, 103
Mariana Trench, 708, 710
Mask squeeze, 720–722, 721f
Mass action law, 306
Mass balance model (MBM), 129–130, 131f, 882–883
Masseter, 394b
Master gland, 455–456, 456b
Master's World Games, 843
Matiegka, Jindøich, 801
Matteuci, Carlo, 355
Maturity-onset severe obesity, 881
Matveyev, Leonid, 558
Maximal aerobic power, 184
Maximal cycling power (MCP), 757–758, 758f
Maximal exercise, at altitude, 660–661
Maximal explosive power (MEP), 757–758, 758f
Maximal oxygen uptake (VO_{2max}), 184, 184f
   aerobic power, 927–928, 928f
   in aerobic training, 525–526, 525f, 526f
   age differences, 263f
   in athletes of different sports, 413f
   criteria for, 259, 260f
   endurance training on, 930–931, 949t
   factors that affect tests of
     age, 263, 263f
     body size and composition, 262–263
     gender, 262
     heredity, 261–262, 262f
     mode of exercise, 261
     training, 262
   gender differences, 263f
   Olympic-caliber athletes compared to sedentary subjects, 259f
   relationship with maximum cardiac output, 380, 381f
   relationship with OBLA, 316
   specificity of, 505, 505f
   stroke volume, 513, 513f
   tests, 259–260
   in twins, 261–262
Maximal physical activity
   blood flow and distribution, 514–515
   pulmonary adaptations, 515
Maximal voluntary static contractions (MVCs), 65f
Maximal work, 221
Maximally accumulated oxygen deficit (MAOD), 256
Maximum strength, 571b
Maximum voluntary ventilation (MVV), 283, 983
McCann–Erickson Rescue Chamber, 707
MCFAs (medium-chain fatty acids), 637
M-CK protein, 419t
McNair, Ronald E., 771b
MCP (maximal cycling power), 757–758, 758f
MCSA (muscle cross-sectional area), 412b
MCTs (medium-chain triacylglycerols), 636–637, 637f, 640
Mean arterial pressure (MAP), 333
Mechanical efficiency (ME), 228
Mechanical loading through regular physical activity, 57
Mechanical work, 139
Mechanoreceptors, 365
Mediastinal emphysema, 721f
Mediterranean Diet Pyramid, 97–98, 97f
Medium-chain fatty acids (MCFAs), 637
Medium-chain triacylglycerols (MCTs), 636–637, 637f, 640
Medulla
   adrenal glands, 460–462
   respiratory center, 310
Medulla oblongata, 422
Megajoule (MJ), 124
Meitner, Lise, 1017
Melanocyte-stimulating-hormone (MSH) agonist, 1064
MELAS (Mitochondrial encephalomyopathy, lactic acidosis and strokelike episodes), 1046f
Melting point, 1023
Melvin, Leland D., 771b
Men
   anterior pituitary hormones, 480
   endurance athletes, 846–848, 858t
Mendel, Gregor Johann, 1013
Menopause, 926
Menstruation, 69
   bodybuilders, 853–854
   delayed onset of and cancer risk, 808
   iron loss during, 62–63
   osteoporosis, 53
   sweating, 688–689
   variations in hydrostatic weighing with, 812
MEP (maximal explosive power), 757–758, 758f
Mercury astronauts, 743
MERRF (myoclonic epilepsy and ragged red fibers), 1046f
Mesomorphic, 838
Messenger RNA (mRNA), 1023
Mesue, Jean (Yuhanna ibn Masawayh), 864
MET, 221, 225t
Metabolic adaptations
   carbohydrate metabolism, 509
   lipid metabolism, 508–509, 508f
   muscle fiber type and size, 509
   overview, 507
   during pregnancy, 533
Metabolic dynamics, 188–189
Metabolic inflexibility, 890–891
Metabolic mill, 173–174, 173f
Metabolic rates, 214–216, 214f
Metabolic size concept, 212–213, 213f, 214f
Metabolic syndrome, 475–477, 914, 937, 939
   definition, 475
   glucagon, 475–477, 477f
   indicators, 475
   prevalence, 475
   risk factor, 475
   in Western industrialized countries, 475
Metabolic water, 71
Metaboreflex, 365
Metagenomics, 1010
Metaphase, 1018–1020
Metarterioles, 334
Metastasize, 1044
Methionine, 943f, 1023
3-Methylhistidine excretion (3-MH), 612
Methylxanthines, 1004t
Meyerhof, Otto, 40, 44, 161
MI (myocardial infarction), 346, 937, 961, 962f
Microgravity
   countermeasure strategies
     inflight space station daily exercise, 760, 760f, 761f
     lower-body negative pressure, 761–767, 762f, 763f
     nutrition, 762–767, 765f, 766f
     overview, 759–767, 788t
     space pharmacology, 761, 788t
   future Mars missions, 773–775
   future of space exploration, 767–774
     exploring beyond earth, 770
   history of aerospace physiology and medicine, 740–748
     early Soviet human space program, 747–748
     early years, 740–741
     experimental aircraft, 742
     first astronauts, 743–745
     German rocket scientists strengthen NASA's efforts, 742–746
     high-altitude explorations, 741
     modern era, 741–742, 780t
     NASA rapid expansion, 741–742
     national aeronautics and space administration, 741
     Sputnik, 741
     suborbital flights, 740–741
     U.S. and Russian space programs, 742–746
     U.S. races into space, 742
   International Space Station (ISS)
     bioastronautics and space research, 739–740
     overview, 738–740, 739f
     parabolic flights and astronaut training, 739
   physiologic responses to spaceflight
     inflight adaptations, 767, 770f
     nutrition, 766, 766f
     overview, 767, 768f
     physical stressors, 767, 768f
     postflight readaptations, 767, 770f
     short-term and long-term responses, 767, 769f
   simulating, 738–739, 739f
   space biology research
     budget process for, 773–774
     dividends, 773
     practical benefits from, 774, 789t–790t
   spaceflight physiology
     body fluid, 752–753, 752f, 783t–784t
     cardiovascular, 751–752, 781t
     immune system changes, 758–759
     muscle ultrastructural changes, 757–758, 757f
     musculoskeletal, 753–756, 755f, 786t–787t
     overview, 748–749
     schema, 749, 750f
     sensory system, 753, 754f, 785t
     skeletal muscle, 756–757
   weightless environment, 736–738
     apparent sense of, 738
     associated with free fall, 738
     gravity, 736–737, 736f
Microgravity (μG), 736
Microneedles, 404
Micronutrients, 44, 489
Micro-Scholander method, 201
Midbrain, 423

Middle-ear squeeze (aerotitis), 722
Miescher, Friedrich, 1012–1014
Mild lung disease, 985
1.5-Mile Walk-Run Test, 383
Milk products and health, 55b
Mineralocorticoids, 462–463, 462f
Minerals, 52
  calcium
    bone health diagnostic criteria, 57b
    effect of microgravity, 753, 755f, 756, 787t
    food sources, 48
    muscle action, 407f
    osteoporosis, 54
    recommended daily intake, 45
  defense against mineral loss, 67
  dietary Approaches to Stop Hypertension (DASH) diet, 68b
  essentials, 52
  exercise performance and, 67–69
    defense against mineral loss, 67
    mineral loss in sweat, 67
    trace minerals and physical activity, 67–69
  female athlete triad, 59–61
  functions, 52–53, 52f
  iron
    exercise-induced anemia, 63
    females, risks for, 63
    functional anemia, 65
    real anemia/pseudoanemia, 63–64
    recommended dietary allowances, 44, 79t
    sources for, 62–65
  loss in sweat, 67
  magnesium, 62
  nature of, 52, 52b
  phosphorus, 62
  role of, 67–69, 82t
  sodium
    induced hypertension, 67
    optimal intake, 66
Mini-camp athletes, skinfold and girth data for, 843, 857t
Minimal body mass, 806
Minimal wrestling weight, 897–898, 905t
  1.5% per week rule, 897–898
  NCAA information dissemination, 898
  validating, 897
Minimum weight category (MWC), 898
Minnesota semi-starvation experiments, 807
12-Minute Swim Test, 383
Minute ventilation, 284
Mir Space Station, 756, 787t
Miss America, body mass index, 801
Mitochondria, 1045, 1046f
Mitochondrial DNA (mtDNA)
  and elite athletic performance, 1074–1075
  mutations and diseases, 1045, 1046f
Mitochondrial encephalomyopathy, lactic acidosis and strokelike episodes (MELAS), 1046f
Mitochondrial membranes, chemical events, 145f
Mitochondrial myopathy, 1046f
Mitochondrial oxygen shuttle, 156b, 157f
Mitophagy, 392
Mitosis, 1020, 1027
Mitosis-promoting factor (MPF), 1027–1028
Mitral valve, 328–329
Mitral valve prolapse (MVP), 964
Mixed-gas diving
  versus compressed air, 725, 726f
  helium-oxygen mixtures, 726, 732t
  overview, 725, 726f
  saturation diving, 726–727, 727f
  technical diving, 727–728, 728f
Mixed-venous blood, 336
MJ (Megajoule), 124
Moderate exercise, short-term benefits, 488
Moderate glycemic food, 88
Moderate lung disease, 985
Moderate-to-intense steady-rate exercise, 187, 187f
Modified loading procedure, 629–630, 630f, 640
Modified sit-and-reach test, 916t, 916b, 916f
Molecular anthropology, 1045
Molecular biology
  citations, 1010, 1011f
  defined, 1010
  DNA technologies
    bioremediation, 1052–1053, 1053f
    DNA cloning, 1051–1052, 1052f
    history of, 1048–1052, 1051f
    plasmids, 1053–1054, 1054f
    recombinant DNA organism, 1051f
  electrophoresis and gel transfer methods
    cloning a mammal, 1060–1065, 1061f, 1062f
    DNA amplification, 1054–1056, 1057f
    DNA fragment separation, 1054–1065, 1055f–1056f
    gene knockout technique, 1062–1063, 1063f
    injection experiments, 1059–1060, 1060f
    obesity, transgenic mice to, 1063–1065, 1064f
    PCR applications, 1056–1059, 1059f
  focused academic preparation, 1075–1076
  future perspectives, 1075–1076, 1075f
  history of, 1012–1014
  human genome, 1015–1017
  human performance research, 1070–1075
    research scope, 1070–1073
    strength-related studies and genes, 1073–1075
  medically related research
    body's chromosomes, 1048, 1049f–1050f
    cancer and metabolic disorders, 1048
    mRNA vaccines, 1047, 1047f
  mutations
    defined, 1041
    junk DNA, 1041–1042
    mitochondrial DNA, 1045, 1046f
    types, 1086t
    varieties of, 1042–1045, 1043f, 1044f, 1086t
  nucleic acids
    DNA, 1018–1020, 1019f
    molecular configuration between DNA and RNA, 1017–1018, 1018f
    RNA, 1018–1020, 1023
  protein synthesis
    enzyme turnover number, 1032, 1033f
    enzymes, 1031
    events, 1028
    gene expression, 1031, 1031f
    generalized overview, 1028–1030, 1028f
    human exercise performance, 1032–1033
    transcription control, 1031–1032, 1032f
    transcription of, 1030–1031, 1030f
    translation of, 1036–1041
  revolution, 1014–1015
  unexpected connections and serendipity, 1076
Molecular genetics, 1010
Molecular/cellular biological aging markers, 912
Monosaccharides, 6
Monosynaptic synapse, 441
Monounsaturated fatty acid, 16
Morganroth hypothesis, 509
Motoneurons, 429
Motor cortex, 425–427
Motor endplate, 431–435
Motor neuron pool, 430–431, 431f
Motor neurons (efferent), spinal cord, 425, 429
Motor sensory pathways, 429
Motor units, 430–431
  anatomy of, 430–436
  and muscle fiber types, 436, 447t
  recruitment, 437
Movement economy, 228
  physical activity oxygen uptake, 230, 230f
Movement speed, 229
Movement-based terminology, conceptual model of, 914, 914f
MPF (mitosis-promoting factor), 1027–1028
MRI. see Magnetic resonance imaging (MRI)
mRNA packaging, 1034–1035, 1035f
mRNA vaccines, 1048
MSH (melanocyte-stimulating-hormone) agonist, 1064
mTOR (mammalian target of rapamycin), 596–597, 640
Mullis, Kary Banks, 1054
Multicompartment model, 813f
Multipennate deltoid muscle, 398–400
Multiple sclerosis, 987–988
Muscle, 496t–498t
  action vs. muscle contraction, 390b
  aging, plasticity of, 575, 575f
  cell remodeling, 574–575, 574f
  composition, 395
  contraction and relaxation, 408f
  insertion location, 395
  nerve supply to, 430–439
  origin, 395
  PNF streching techniques, 440b
  ultrastructural changes, 757–758, 757f
Muscle biopsy, 409, 410f–409f
Muscle contraction, vs. muscle action, 390b
Muscle cross-sectional area (MCSA), 412b, 552, 552f
Muscle fiber, 391–392
  alignment, 398–401, 398f, 400f
  composition, 229
    in athletes of different sports, 413f
    training specificity, 412b
  type changes and detraining, 508b
  type differences among athletic groups, 412–413, 413f
  types of, 409–413, 410f–409f, 419t, 509, 576
Muscle glycogen, 10–11, 14, 88, 90b
Muscle hyperplasia, 575–576
Muscle hypertrophy, 597
Muscle oxidizes, 182
Muscle pump action, 337
Muscle spindles, 439–441, 439f, 441f
Muscle strength
  aging
    muscle mass decrease, 922–924, 923f
    powerlifters, 922, 922f
    resistance training, 924–925, 924f
    weightlifters, 922, 922f
  America's first athletic club, 545
  development in antiquity, 544
  educators to early strength science, 544–545
  forerunner to modern exercise machines, 547–548
  gender differences in
    absolute muscle strength, 552–553, 553f
    bone density, 577
    males vs. female muscle hypertrophy, 577
    muscle cross-sectional area, 552, 552f
    muscular strength and hypertrophy, 576–577
    overview, 552
    relative muscle strength, 553–554, 553f
    transgender athlete participation, 576–577
  international system (SI) units, 550, 590t
  measurement of
    cable tensiometry, 548, 548f
    computer-assisted, electromechanical, and isokinetic methods, 549–551, 550f
    considerations, 551–552, 551f
    dynamometry, 548–549
    learning factors affect, 551–552
    new generation technology, 550–551
    one-repetition maximum method, 549
    resistance-training equipment categories, 551
  muscle actions, 556, 556f, 579
  neural and muscular adaptations
    hypertrophic response specificity, 573
    muscular and psychologic factors, 572–573, 572f, 590t
    neural-psychologic factors, 570, 570f
    significant metabolic adaptations, 573–576, 574f, 575f
    in strength improvement with resistance training, 569, 569f
    training's impact at neuromuscular junction, 570–572
  resistance training objectives, 548
  weightlifting in early America, 545–547
  Zander mechanotherapy machines, late 19th century, 546, 546f
Muscle tissue, as endocrine organ, 477, 478f
Muscular endurance, 559
Muscular strength training
  body weight-loaded training, 565–567
  circuit resistance training, 578–579
  core training, 567–568, 568f
  detraining, 577–578
  isokinetic resistance training, 562–563, 562f, 563f
  isometric training response specificity, 561–562
  plyometric training, 563–565, 564f, 565f, 566f
  resistance training
    adaptations to, 569
    aerobic training plus, 559–560
    guidelines for health enhancement and disease prevention, 559
    and metabolic stress, 578
    progressive resistance exercise, 557–559, 558f
  sling suspension methods and performance improvements, 566–567

Muscular strength training (*Continued*)
  soreness and stiffness
    cell damage, 579–581, 580*f*, 581*f*
    eccentric actions, 579, 591*t*
    overview, 579
  static *versus* dynamic methods, 561–562
Musculoskeletal injuries, 919–920
Music therapy (MT), 515*b*
Mutagens, 1044
Muth, Johann Guts, 544
MVV (maximum voluntary ventilation), 283, 983
Myasthenia gravis, 548
Myelin sheath, 431
Myoblasts, 395
Myocardial blood flow, 515
Myocardial diseases. *see* Heart muscle diseases
Myocardial infarction (MI), 346, 937, 961, 962*f. see also* Heart muscle diseases
Myocardial ischemia, 935
Myocardial substrate, 347*f*
Myocarditis, 961
Myocardium
  definition, 328
  function at altitude, 653
  overview, 960
  oxygen supply, 346
Myofibrillar adenosine triphosphatase (myosin ATPase), 406
Myofibrils, 391–392, 396
Myofilaments, 396
Myogenic stem cells, 574
Myoglobin, 62, 304, 395, 509
Myomesin, 419*t*
Myosin
  crossbridge cycling, 399*b*
  function of, 419*t*
  link between actin, ATP, 406–407
  overview, 396
  structural rearrangement of, 403*f*
Myosin ATPase (myofibrillar adenosine triphosphatase), 406
Myotatic reflex, 563–564
MyPlate, 95–96, 95*f*
MyPyramid, 97–98

N
Nachtegall, Franz, 544
Naked DNA vaccines, 1047
Nandrolone decanoate toxicity, 598*b*
NARP (Neurogenic muscle weakness, ataxia and retinitis pigmentosa), 1046*f*
National Aeronautics and Space Administration (NASA), 736, 741, 776*f*
National Association of Underwater Instructors (NAUI), 708, 727*b*
National Cancer Institute, 48
National Federation of State High School Associations, 897
National Heart, Lung and Blood Institute (NHLBI), 595, 923*b*
National Institute of Neurological Disorders and Stroke, 923*b*
National Institutes of Health (NIH), 595
National Sleep Foundation, 923*b*
National Space Biomedical Research Institute (NSBRI), 739–740
National Space Biomedical Research Institute (NSBRI) Research Program, 746
National Weight Control Registry (NWCR), 884
Native Americans, life expectancy, 912
Natural killer (NK) cells, 488
Natural selection, 1012
Naughton protocol, 261*f*
NAUI (National Association of Underwater Instructors), 708
NCAA information dissemination, 898
Near-infrared interactance (NIR), 823
Near-Vegetarian Diet Pyramid, 97–98
Nebulin, 419*t*
Neck, flexibility of, 916*b*, 917*t*
Necrosis, 937
Negative nitrogen balance, 33
Negative work, 231
Nerve conduction velocity (NCV), 570
Nerve supply to muscle, 430–439

Nerve tracts
  ascending, 425
  descending, 425–427
Nerves, defined, 446*t*
Nerve-to-muscle signaling pattern, 435
Net energy, 126–127
  coefficient of digestibility, 127
  expenditure, 123, 234
  food, 126–127
  tabled values, 126–127
Net Mechanical efficiency, 228–229
Neural adaptations, 569*f*
Neural function, effects of aging, 925, 925*f*
Neural movement control
  motor unit functional characteristics
    and muscle fiber types, 436, 447*t*
    tension characteristics, 437, 438*f*
    twitch characteristics, 436–437, 436*f*
  nerve supply to muscle, 430–439, 431*f*, 432*f*, 433*f*
  neuromotor system organization
    brain, 422–425, 423*f*, 424*f*
    peripheral nervous system, 427–429, 428*f*
    reflex arc, 429–430, 430*f*
    spinal cord, 425–427, 426*f*, 427*f*
  proprioceptors
    Golgi tendon organs, 441–442, 442*f*
    muscle spindles, 439–441, 439*f*, 441*f*
    Pacinian corpuscles, 442
Neural stimulation, endocrine gland, 454, 455*f*
Neurilemma, 431
Neuroendocrine organ, 450
Neurofibromatosis, 1017
Neurogenic muscle weakness, ataxia and retinitis pigmentosa (NARP), 1046*f*
Neurohormone, 1063
Neurohypophysis, 458
Neuromotor system organization
  central nervous system
    brain, 422–425, 423*f*, 424*f*
    spinal cord, 425–427, 426*f*, 427*f*
  peripheral nervous system, 427–429, 428*f*
  reflex arc, 429–430, 430*f*
Neuromuscular diseases
  multiple sclerosis, 987–988
  Parkinson's disease, 988
  stroke
    clinical features, 987
    exercise prescription, 987
Neuromuscular junction (NMJ), 432–435, 433*f*, 570–572
Neurons, spinal cord, 446*t*
Newborn oxygen uptake, 158*b*
Newton, Isaac, 736
Newton third law, 737
Next-generation space suits, 745
NHLBI (National Heart, Lung and Blood Institute), 595, 923*b*
Nicotinamide adenine dinucleotide (NAD$^+$), 143, 155
NIH (National Institutes of Health), 595
NIR (Near-infrared interactance), 823
Nirenberg, Marshall, 1023, 1025
Nitric oxide, 366, 367*f*
Nitrogen balance, 764–765
Nitrogen exchange, 204
Nitrogen narcosis (rapture of the deep), 722–723
Nitroglycerin, 960
Nitrox, 719
Nitsch, Herbert, 709, 715–716
NK (natural killer) cells, 488
NMJ (neuromuscular junction), 432–435, 433*f*, 570–572
Nobel Prize recipients
  Arnold, Frances H., 1065
  Baltimore, David, 1048, 1051
  Bohr, Niels, 39, 303
  Boyer, Herbert, 1051
  Bragg, Lawrence, 1014
  Butenandt, Adolph, 594
  Cajal, Santiago Ramón y, 442, 1037
  Capecchi, Mario R., 1060
  Charpentier, Emmanuelle, 1065, 1066, 1067, 1069
  Cohen, Stanley, 1051
  Cormack, Allan M., 983
  Crick, Francis Harry Compton, 1014
  Curie, Marie, 45, 1065

  Damadian, Raymond, 827, 828
  Doudna, Jennifer, 1065, 1069, 1076
  Dulbecco, Renato, 1048, 1051
  Einthoven, Wilhelm, 356
  Evans, Martin J., 1060
  Fischer, Emil, 142
  Furchgott, Robert F., 366
  Golgi, Camillo, 441, 442, 1037
  Hill, Archibald Vivian, 188
  Hodgkin, Dorothy Crowfoot, 45, 1065
  Hopkins, Frederick Gowland, 42, 140
  Hounsfield, Godfrey N., 983
  Huxley, Andrew Fielding, 403
  Joliot-Curie, Irène, 45, 1065
  Kendrew, John C., 304, 1039
  Kornberg, Arthur, 1029, 1048
  Kossel, Ludwig Albrecht, 1012
  Krebs, Hans, 44
  Krebs, Hans Adolf, 164
  Krogh, August, 36, 37, 39, 42, 44
  Levi-Montalcini, Rita, 45, 1051
  Meyerhof, Otto, 40, 44, 161
  Mullis, Kary Banks, 1054
  Nirenberg, Marshall, 1023, 1025
  Ochoa, Severo, 1029
  Pauling, Linus Carl, 45
  Perutz, Max, 1039
  Roberts, Richard John, 1033
  Rohrer, Heinrich, 404
  Röntgen, Wilhelm Konrad, 983
  Ružička, Leopold, 594
  Sharp, Phillip Allen, 1033
  Smithies, Oliver, 1060
  Spemann, Hans, 1060
  Szent-Györgyi, Albert, 390
  Temin, Howard, 1048, 1051
  Tiselius, Arne Wilhelm, 1052
  Watson, James Dewey, 1014
  Wilkins, Maurice H. F., 44, 1014, 1015
  Yonath, Ada, 1065
Nodes of Ranvier, 431
Nohl, Max E., 707
Nomogram, 215
Noncompetitive inhibitors, 143
Nonepinephrine, cold exposure, 672
Nonessential amino acids, 29
Nonexercise activity thermogenesis, 864
Nonheme, 64–65
Nonpharmacologic training aids
  carbohydrate intake modification
    classic loading procedure, 627–629, 628*f*
    gender differences in glycogen storage and catabolism, 629, 629*f*
    modified loading procedures, 629–630, 630*f*
    nutrient-related fatigue, 627, 627*f*
    overview, 627
  chromium, 630–632
  creatine
    age effects, 634
    benefits, 632–634, 633*f*
    body mass ad body composition, 634–635, 635*f*
    creatine loading, 635–636, 636*f*
    important component in high-energy phosphates, 632
    overview, 632
  hormonal blood boosting, 622–623
  medium-chain triacylglycerols, 636–637, 637*f*
  oxygen inhalation
    overview, 625
    postexercise, 627, 627*f*
    pre-exercise, 625–626, 626*f*
  pyruvate, 637–638
  red blood cell reinfusion, 621–622, 622*f*
  warm-up, 623–625
Nonprotein, respiratory quotient for, 203–205, 209*t*
Non-steady-rate physical activity, optimal recovery, 190–191, 190*f*
Nonsteroid hormones, action of, 453*f*
Nonsteroidal anti-inflammatory drugs (NSAIDs), 395
Norepinephrine
  chemical structure of, 461*f*
  effect of altitude on excretion, 651*f*
  overview, 481
  release of, 362, 460–461
  role of, 461*f*
Northern blotting, 1054, 1056*f*

NSBRI (National Space Biomedical Research Institute), 739–740
NSBRI (National Space Biomedical Research Institute) Research Program, 746
Nuclear bag fiber, 439
Nuclear chain fiber, 439
Nuclear DNA, 1045
Nuclear energy, 138f
Nuclear fusion, 138
Nuclear pore complex, 1029
Nuclear transfer, 1013
Nuclear ventriculography, 969
Nucleic acids
  DNA
    bioremediation, 1052–1053, 1053f
    chromosome, 1020, 1020f
    cloning, 1051–1052, 1052f
    components of, 1018, 1018f
    history of, 1048–1052, 1051f
    molecular control mechanisms, 1027–1028, 1027f
    overview, 1017–1025
    packaging in chromosome, 1019f
    phosphodiester bonding, 1020–1021, 1021f
    plasmids, 1053–1054, 1053f
    polymerase, pivotal role for, 1026–1027
    recombinant DNA organism, 1051f
    replication, 1025–1028, 1026f, 1027f
    structure of, 1021, 1022f
    synthesis of, 1027
    vs. RNA, molecular configuration, 1017–1018, 1018f
  molecular configuration between DNA and RNA, 1017–1018, 1018f
  RNA
    forms of, 1023
    overview, 1018–1020
    splicing, 1034
    synthesis of, 1030–1031
Nucleosome, 1018–1020
Nucleotides, 1013
Nucleus, 446t, 1028
Nutraceutical, 1061
Nutrient deficiencies, 48b
Nutrient intake, 88–91
  among physically active, 88–91
Nutrient intake, pharmacologic training aids
  carbohydrate-protein-creatine supplementation, 611–612, 611f
  dietary lipid, 612–613, 642t
  optimize muscle response, 610b
  postexercise glucose ingestion, 612, 612f
Nutrient metabolism, 13f
Nutrition
  optimal for exercise, c0003
    athletic fatigue, 91
    carbohydrates, 90–91
    electrolytes, 105
    essentials of, 89
    food intake, 90
    glucose feedings, 112–113
    high-fat diets, 89–90
    lipid, 89–90
    low-fat diets, 90
    MyPlate, 95
    precompetition meal, 103–104
    prior to exercise, 104
    protein, 88–89
    water uptake, 112–113
  physical and mental performance, 108–110
  recovery from physical activity, 110
Nutrition bars, 104–106
Nutrition drinks, 104–106
Nutrition essentials, 93
Nutrition Facts label, 34b
Nutrition powders, 105
Nutrition Rainbow, 101b
Nutritional supplementation with herbal/botanical supplement, 608b
NWCR (National Weight Control Registry), 884

O

Obese (ob) gene, 868–869
Obese syndrome, defined, 797
Obesity, 797
  among United States, 865–867, 866f
  criteria for
    adipocytes, 877–881, 878f, 879f, 880f, 881f
    body fat percentage, 874–875
    overview, 874
    regional fat distribution, 876–877, 876f
  diabetes, 473, 873–874
  dietary patterns changes, 867
  duration and cardiometabolic health, 473b
  effects of physical activity on, 950t
  genetic influences
    altering threshold and inherited factors, 868, 868f
    genetic model, 869f
    inability to sustain weight loss, 869–870
    knockout mice for study of mechanisms of, 1062–1065
    mutant gene and leptin, 868–869, 869f
    overview, 867
    racial differences, 870–871
    transgenic mice to, 1063–1065, 1064f
  global epidemic, 864–867, 865f
  health risks of, 872–874, 873f, 874f
  historical perspective, 864
  impact on children, 866–867
  and insulin resistance, 870b
  milestone in treatment, 866–867
  physical inactivity, 871–872
  prevalence, 865
  progressive long-term process, 867–871, 868f
  risk factor
    for CHD, 875b
    for diabetes, 940
  U.S. Diets and Federal Recommendations, 867
Obligatory thermogenesis, 216
Obstructive sleep apnea (OSA), 923b
Ochoa, Severo, 1029, 1029
Okazaki fragments, 1026
Older adult programs, 918
Older adults
  protein intake and strength training in, 32b
  regular physical activity in, 217b
  resistance training guidelines for, 559
Oligodendrocytes (OL), 435–436
Oligomenorrhea, 807
Oligosaccharides, 6–7
Olympic competitor research, 838–839
Olympic-caliber walkers, 232
Omega-3 fatty acid, 19–20
Oncogene, 1044
Oncology
  rehabilitation and physical activity, 957–960
  statistics, 956
One-repetition maximum (1-RM) method, 549
Onset of blood lactate accumulation (OBLA)
  endurance performance, 316–317
  overview, 315–317
  racial differences, 317
  relationship with VO_{2max}, 316
  specificity of, 316
Open window hypothesis, 489
Open-circuit scuba system, 718–719, 718f, 719f
Open-circuit spirometry
  bag, 200–201, 201f
  computerized instrumentation, 201, 202f
  portable, 199–200, 200f
  ventilated Hood technique, 201, 201f
Opioid peptides, 486–487
Optical tweezers, 404
Oral glucose-tolerance test, 470
Oral rehydration beverages, 113
Oral rehydration solution, 112
Oral temperature, 691b
Organelle, 1030
Organic acid group, 28–29
Origin muscle, 395
Origins of replication, 1025–1026, 1026f
Orthostatic hypotension, 767
Orthostatic intolerance, 747
Orthotopic transplantation, 369
Osmolality, 112
Osteoarthritis (OA), 876b, 924–925, 950t
Osteoclast, 53
Osteopenia, 53
Osteoporosis, 53–54, 53b
  aging, 929–930
  diet, 54–57
  effects of physical activity on, 950t
  female athlete triad, 59–61
  physical activity, 45, 49–50
  risk factors, 53b
Outpatient cardiac programs, 980
Ovaries, 451f, 496t–498t
Overhydration risk during extended-duration activities, 74
Overload principle, 504
Overtraining, 487, 531–533, 532f
  forms, 531
Overtraining syndrome
  definitions, 531
  mechanisms underlying, 532f
Ovolactovegetarian diet, 30
Oxaloacetate, 165
Oxidation reactions, 144–145
Oxidative phosphorylation, 156–157, 157f
Oxidative stress, risk and antioxidant supplementation, 49–50
Oxidative-modification hypothesis of atherosclerosis, 48
Oxidizing agent, 145
Oxidoreductases, 148t, 1031
Oxygen debt, 188
Oxygen deficit, 182f, 183–184
Oxygen exposure limits, 726, 732t
Oxygen free radicals, 1071
Oxygen inhalation (hyperoxia)
  overview, 625
  postexercise, 627, 627f
  pre-exercise, 625–626, 626f
Oxygen loading, at altitude, 649–650
Oxygen poisoning, 725, 732t
Oxygen saturation of hemoglobin (S_aO_2), 651f
Oxygen transport
  a-vO_2 difference (Please insert symbol)
    overview, 514, 514f
    during physical activity, 381–382, 381f
    during rest, 381
  enhancing, 623
  hemoglobin, 299–300
  myoglobin, 304
  physical activity, 380–381
  in physical solution, 299
  PO_2
    in lungs, 300–303
    in tissues, 303–304
  variables that contribute to, 317f
Oxygen transport cascade, 300, 301f, 648, 649f
Oxygen uptake (VO_2)
  at altitude, 653f
  calculating using open-circuit spirometry, 204b
  in endurance athletes, 511f, 512f, 513f, 514f
  during exercise, 182–183, 182f
  expressing, 263t
  during graded exercise to maximum, 314f
  maximal, 184, 184f
  during recovery
    characteristics, 187
    EPOC, 187–188, 187f, 188f
    intermittent interval exercise, 191, 193t
    metabolic dynamics, 188–189
    non-steady-rate exercise, 190–191, 190f
    steady-rate exercise, 190
  relationship to heart rate, 222–223, 223f
  during running, 232f–233f
  during walking, 232f–233f
Oxygen uptake fast component, 182–183
Oxygen uptake kinetics, 183–184
Oxygen's role, in energy metabolism, 157–158
Oxyhemoglobin dissociation curve, 301f, 649–650
Oxytocin, 458

P

P wave, 356
Pacemakers, 354
Pacinian corpuscles, 442
Pancreas, 451f, 466f, 496t–498t
Pancreatic cancer, 950t
Pancreatic hormones, 466–468, 466f
  glucose transporters, 467
  insulin
    diabetes mellitus, 468–470
    glucose transporters, 467
    glucose-insulin interaction, 467–468

Pancreatic hormones (Continued)
  primary functions of, 467f
  regular physical activity and type 2 diabetes
    benefits, 483–485
    risk, 482–483
  regular physical activity and type 2 diabetes risk, 482–483
P$_a$O$_2$ (partial pressure of arterial oxygen), 649f
PAR (Physical activity ratio), 221
Parabolic flights, 739
Parabolic (Keplerian trajectory) flights
  and astronaut training, 739
  simulate microgravity, 738–739, 739f
Parasympathetic influence, 364
Parasympathetic nervous system, 363f, 429
Parasympathetic overtraining syndrome, 531
Parasympatholytics (anticholinergics), 1004t
Parathyroid glands, 451f, 496t–498t
Parathyroid hormone (PTH), 460, 481
Parkinson's disease, 988, 1072, 1073b
Partial pressure, 294
Partial pressure of arterial oxygen (P$_a$O$_2$), 649f
Partial pressure of oxygen in inspired air (P$_I$O$_2$), 649f
Passive recovery, 190
Patella tendon stretch reflex, 441f
Patent ductus arteriosus, 964
Patent foramen ovale (PFO), 724–725
Paternity, 1026–1027
Pathogens, 1047
Patient Education Institute, 923b
Pauling, Linus Carl, 45
PCR. see Polymerase chain reaction (PCR)
PCr (phosphocreatine), 632, 634f
PCSA (physiologic cross-sectional area), 398
Peak expiratory flow (PEF), 983
Peak oxygen uptake (VO$_2$), 259
Peak power output (PP), 528
Pear-shaped body, 876f
PEDs (performance-enhancing drugs), 595, 604b, 640
PEF (peak expiratory flow), 983
Peliosis hepatitis, 601, 640
Pelvic-flexion exercises, supine, 584b
Pennate fibers, 398, 398f
Peptide bonds, 28, 143–144, 1039–1041
Peptide hormones, 450, 494t
Perceived exertion, training at rating of, 521–523
Performance tests
  age differences, 256
  gender differences, 256
  interrelationships among, 253
  jumping-power tests, 252, 252f
  overview, 253–256
  stair-sprinting power tests, 253
Performance-enhancing drugs (PEDs), 595, 604b, 640
Pericarditis, 964
Perimysium, 392
Periosteum, 392
Peripheral factors, age-related decline in aerobic power, 928
Peripheral nervous system (PNS), 423f, 427–429, 428f
Peripheral obesity, 876, 876f
Peripheral resistance, 333–334
Peripheral thermal receptors, 671
Peripheral vascular disease, 950t
Permeation efficiency factor, 675
Peroxisome proliferator activated receptor gamma (PPARγ) gene, 878
Peroxisomes, 16
Personal training, 918
Personalized training assessments, 573b
Perutz, Max, 1039
PFO (patent foramen ovale), 724–725
PGC-1, regulating cellular energy metabolism, 879
PH, 322f
Pharmacogenetics, 1010
Pharmacogenomics, 1010
Pharmacologic stress testing, 969
Pharmacologic training aids
  amino acid supplementation, 609–613
  amphetamines, 613, 613f
  anabolic steroids
    abuse, taking a stand, 602b
    action of, 596–603
    administrating, 598, 598f
    dosage, 600
    effectiveness, 599–600
  following, 598–599
  hormone interactions, 596–600, 596f
  improving athletic performance, 601–603
  myelin's role in motor skills without, 598, 598f
  perfecting movement skills, 597
  risks, 600–601
  sources, 599
  structure of, 596–603
androstenedione, 606f, 608–609
β$_2$-adrenergic agonists, 603–604
β-hydroxy-β-methylbutyrate, 620–621, 620f
buffering solutions, 618–619, 618f
caffeine
  effects on muscle, 615
  ergogenic effects, 614, 614f, 615f
  powdered, 616b
  warning about, 615–616
clenbuterol, 603–604
dehydroepiandrosterone, 606–608, 606f, 607f
ephedrine, 616–617
ginseng, 616
glutamine, 619–620
growth hormone, 605–606
nutrient intake
  carbohydrate-protein-creatine supplementation, 611–612, 611f
  dietary lipid, 612–613, 642b
  optimize muscle response, 610b
  postexercise glucose ingestion, 612, 612f
phosphatidylserine, 620
Phasic motor neurons, 436, 436f
Phelps, Michael, 838–839
Phenotypes, 261, 1016
Phlebitis, 338
Phosphagens, 180
Phosphatase, 162
Phosphate bond energy
  adenosine triphosphate, 152–154
  cellular oxidation
    efficiency of, 157
    electron transport, 155, 155f, 156f
    oxidative phosphorylation, 156–157, 157f
    oxygen's role, in energy metabolism, 157–158
    phosphocreatine (PCr), 154
Phosphate bond formation to oxygen uptake (P/O ratio), 156
Phosphate buffer, 323
Phosphates, intramuscular high-energy, 527
Phosphatidylserine (PS), 620, 640
Phosphocreatine (PCr), 136, 154, 632, 634f
Phosphodiester bond, 1020–1021
Phosphofructokinase (PFK), 162
3-Phosphoglyceraldehyde, 170
Phosphoglycerate kinase, 161f
Phosphoglyceromutase, 161f
Phospholipid dipalmitoylphosphatidylcholine, 280–281
Phospholipids, 20
Phosphorus, 62
Photolithography technique, 1043–1044
Photomicrographic techniques, 877
Photosynthesis, 138
Physical activity, 88, 105b. see also Exercise
  at altitude, 646–666
    acclimatization, 650–658
    aerobic capacity on return to sea level, 661
    at-home altitude acclimatization, 663–664, 664f
    circulatory factors, 660–661
    combining altitude stay with low-altitude training, 662–664, 664f
    exercise performance, 659f, 660
    maximal oxygen uptake, 659–660, 659f
    possible negative effects, 661
    sea-level performance, 661–662, 661f
    stressors, 648, 649f
  a-vO2 difference (AU: Please check symbol), 381–382, 381f
  blood pressure response to
    graded exercise, 343, 343f
    recovery, 343–345
    resistance exercise, 342–343
    steady-rate exercise, 343
    upper-body physical activity, 343
  and cancer, 490
  cardiac output during
    enhancing stroke volume, 376–378
    overview, 376–378
  classification, 504, 504f
  cold stress during, 691, 700t
  core temperature during, 679–680, 679f
  defined, 913
  diabetes, 473–475, 482–485, 484f, 485b
  energy expenditure during
    average, 221
    classification, 221
    energy cost, 222, 222f
    heart rate, 222–223, 223f
    MET, 221, 225t
  fluid intake during, 683b
  and food intake, 98–103, 99f, 100f
  growth hormone and tissue synthesis, 456–457
  health benefits of, 954, 954b
  in heat, 678–683
  hypoglycemia, 472b
  nutrition, optimal for, 86–117
    carbohydrates, 88
    chronic athletic fatigue, 91
    electrolytes, 105
    essentials of, 89
    food intake, 90
    glucose feedings, 112–113
    high-fat diets, 89–90
    lipid, 89–90
    low-fat diets, 90
    MyPlate, 95.
    precompetition meal, 103–104
    prior to exercise, 106–110
    protein, 106
    water uptake, 112–113
  opioid peptides and, 486–487
    endogenous opioid peptide effects, 487
    exercise high, 487
    opioid effects, 486–487
  oxygen transport, 380–381
  oxygen uptake, 230, 230f
  during pregnancy
    fetal effects, 533–534
    maternal effects, 533
  in pregnant and nonpregnant women, 533, 533f
  redistribution of blood flow during, 379, 379f
  rehydration methods, 686b
  relationship between stress, illness, immunity, 487–490, 488f
  sedentary behavior guidelines, 534b
  World Health Organization guidelines on, 534b
Physical activity energy spectrum, 185–187, 185f, 186f
Physical Activity Pyramid, 919f
Physical activity ratio (PAR), 221
Physical activity safety, 919–920, 920f
Physical fitness, defined, 913, 913f
Physical inactivity
  diabetes risk factor, 940
  excessive fat accumulation, 871–872
Physical solution, carbon dioxide transport in, 305
Physiologic buffers, 323
Physiologic cross-sectional area (PCSA), 398
Physiologic fluids, solubility coefficients of gases in, 295b
Physiologic responses, effects of exercise on, 930
Physique
  body fat
    anthropometry and percentage total, 841–854, 841f
    bodybuilders, 853–854
    collegiate vs. professional players, 848–852, 849f, 850f, 851f, 859f
    comparisons among elite male sprint, distance, marathon, and decathlon competitors, 843–845, 845t, 845f
    endurance athletes, 845–848, 857t–858t
    field event athletes, 842–843, 843f
    football players, 848
    golfers, 852–853, 860t
    runners, 848
    by sports category, 842, 842f
    swimmers, 848
    weightlifters, 853–854
  fat-free-to-fat ratio, 839–841, 840f
  olympic competitor research, 838–839
  Phelps, Michael, 838–839
  racial differences, 841

upper fat-free body mass limit, 854–855
Picard, August, 707
Picard, Jacques, 708
Pineal gland, 451f, 496t–498t
Pink puffer appearance, 982f
P_1O_2 (partial pressure of oxygen in inspired air), 649f
Pituitary gland, 451f, 455–456, 456f
Pituitary-anterior gland, 496t–498t
Placenta, 496t–498t
Placental hormones, 451f
Plant polysaccharides, 8–9
 fiber, 8
 starch, 8
Plantar flexors, 400f
Plant-based meats, 24b
Plaque, 22
Plasma cortisol, 465, 465f
Plasma volume
 at altitude, 656–657
 cardiovascular adaptations with training, 511
 pre-to postflight changes in, 752–753, 752f
Plasmid, 1048
Plyometric movements, 563–564
Plyometric training, 563–565, 564f, 565f, 566f
Pneumothorax, 720
PNS (Peripheral nervous system), 423f, 427–429, 428f
PO_2
 hemoglobin saturation, 300
 in lungs, 300–303
 peripheral chemoreceptors, 311
 in tissues
  arteriovenous oxygen difference, 303
  Bohr effect, 302–303
  2,3-diphosphoglycerate, 303–304
  overview, 303–304
P/O ratio, 156
Poiseuille, Jean Louis, 360
Poiseuilles law, 360
Polio (poliomyelitis), 548
Polyadenylic acid (poly[A] tail, 1034–1035, 1035f
Polycystic ovary syndrome, 939
Polycythemia, 657
Polydipsia, 469
Polymer, 1018
Polymerase, 1023
Polymerase chain reaction (PCR), 1013
 applications, 1056–1059, 1059f
 DNA amplification, 1054–1056, 1057f
Polynucleotide, 1018
Polypeptides, 28
 chain, 1034
 diagram of, 299f
 elongation and termination, 1037, 1038f
 Golgi complex, 1037–1038, 1039f
 role of tRNA, 1036–1037, 1037f
 sites, 1036
 synthesis, 1036, 1036f
Polyphagia, 469
Polysaccharides, 8
Polyunsaturated fatty acid, 16
Polyuria, 469, 473–475
POMC (proopiomelanocortin), 455–456
Pons, 423
Pores of Kohn, 277
Portable spirometry, 199–200, 200f
Porter, Stephen, 709
Positive nitrogen balance, 33
Posterior pituitary hormones, 496t–498t
 antidiuretic hormone, 458, 480
 overview, 458
Postexercise coughing, 289b
Postexercise oxygen consumption, 191
Postpartum depression, 990
Postsynaptic membrane, 432–433
Posture motion perception, 753, 754f
Potential energy, 136, 136f
Powell, John, 843
Power (P), 141b
Power belts, 232
Powerlifters, aging, 922, 922f
PP output (peak power output), 528
PPARγ (peroxisome proliferation activated receptor gamma) gene, 878
P-R interval, 357f
PRDM16 gene, 879

Preadipocyte cells, 878
Precapillary sphincter, 334
Precompetition meal, 103–104
 benefits of, 104
 liquid and prepackaged bars, 104–106
 liquid meals, 104
 nutrition bars, 104–105
 nutrition powders and drinks, 105
Pre-exercise alkalosis, 618
Pre-exercise fructose, 108
Pre-exercise hyperhydration, 686b
Pregnancy
 effect on energy expenditure, 219
 exercise training during
  current opinion, 534–536
  fetal effects, 533–534
  maternal effects, 533
  predicting VO_{2max} during, 219b
Prehabilitation program, 920
Preliminary exercise (warm-up), 623–625
Preload, 376–377
Premature vascular aging, 911–912
Premature ventricular contractions (PVCs), 964
Preoxygenation, 752
Preparation phase, strength training, 558
Pre-physical activity feedings, 106–108
Presynaptic terminals, 432
Primary RNA transcript, 1029
Primary structure, 1038
Primase, 1023
Primer, 1023
Prinzmetal's angina/variant angina, 972
PRL (prolactin), 458
Professional football players, 848–852, 849f, 850f, 851f, 859t
Progesterone, 465
Progressive resistance exercise (PRE)
 overload principle, 557
 overview, 557
 periodization, 558–559, 558f
 variations, 557–558
Progressive-resistance weight training, 556
Prohormones, 606–607, 640
Project 714, 748
Projections, contractile filaments, 401
Prokaryotes, 1030
Prolactin (PRL), 458, 480
Prolapse, 964
Promoter, 1029
Pronucleus, 1059
Proopiomelanocortin (POMC), 455–456, 1063–1064, 1064f
Proprioceptive neuromuscular facilitation (PNF)
 streching techniques, 440b
Proprioceptors
 Golgi tendon organs, 441–442, 442f
 muscle spindles, 439–441, 439f, 441f
 Pacinian corpuscles, 442
Prostaglandins, 495t
Prostate cancer, 950t
Proteasome, 1039–1041
Protein, 28–29, 125
 associated with muscle fiber sarcomere, 419t
 categories, 29–30
 combustion heat, 126
 complete, 29
 dynamics in physical activity, 35–36, 35f
 energy release from, 172, 172f
 food ratings, 29b
 high-protein diets, 889
 incomplete, 29
 intake, 32b
 malnutrition, 29
 metabolism dynamics, 32–33, 33f
 microgravity, 763–764
 modifying recommended intake, 35–36
 nitrogen balance, 33–35
 Recommended Dietary Allowance for, 31–32
 recommended intake of, 30–32
 requirement for athletes, 31
 respiratory quotient for, 203
 role of, 32
 sources, 29–30, 41t
Protein buffer, 323

Protein conversion to lipid, 174
Protein delivery system, 1037–1038, 1039f
Protein enzymes, 1031
Protein intake during recovery, insulin, 111
Protein kinases, 1027
Protein synthesis
 enzyme turnover number, 1032, 1033f
 enzymes, 1031
 events, 1028
 exercise performance
  exiting nucleus, 1035
  exons and introns, 1033–1035, 1034f
  mRNA packaging, 1034–1035, 1035f
  RNA splicing, 1034
 gene expression, 1031, 1031f
 generalized overview, 1028–1030, 1028f
 human exercise performance, 1032–1033
 transcription
  enzyme turnover number, 1032, 1033f
  gene expression, 1030–1031
  protein enzymes, 1031
  transcription control, 1031–1032
 translation
  defined, 1028
  essential concepts and sequences, 1041, 1086t
  Golgi complex, 1037–1038
  hemoglobin, 1039
  polypeptides, 1037
  proteolysis, 1039–1041, 1041f
  ribosomes, 1036
  stages of, 1035
  termination of protein synthesis, 1038, 1040f, 1085t
  tRNA, 1023
Protein-to-energy pathways, 172f
Proteolysis, 580, 1039–1041, 1041f
Proteomics, 956, 1010
PS (phosphatidylserine), 620, 640
Pseudoanemia, 63–64
Pseudoephedrine, 616–617, 640
Psychologic benefits, physical activity, 517
Psychologic profile, 485
PTH (parathyroid hormone), 460, 481
Pulmonary adaptations, 515–516, 516f
 with training, 751–752, 752f, 782t
Pulmonary congestion, 962
Pulmonary diffusing capacity, 751–752, 752f
Pulmonary diseases
 asthma, 986–987
  area affected and results of, 981b
  environmental impact, 987
  fluid loss, 986
  medication, 987
  thermal gradients and fluid loss, sensitivity to, 986
  warm-up, 987
 chronic obstructive pulmonary disease
  asthma and exercise-induced bronchospasm (see Asthma)
  chronic bronchitis, 981, 981b
  cystic fibrosis, 981b, 982–983
  emphysema, 981–982, 981b, 982f
  major COPD diseases, 981b
  risk factors, 981
 medications, 985
 pulmonary assessments
  computed tomography, 983
  diffusing capacity, 983
  spirometry, 983
  X-ray, 983, 983f
 rehabilitation and physical activity prescription, 984
 restrictive lung dysfunction, 980, 1002t–1003t
Pulmonary function
 aging, 927
 in runners, 291t
 variables, predicting, 285b
Pulmonary oxygen uptake, 182–183
Pulmonary respiration vs. cellular respiration, 276b
Pulmonary system
 acid-base regulation
  buffering, 321–323
  effects of intense exercise, 323–324, 324f
 aerobic fitness, 283–284
 at altitude, 653f
 alveolar minute, 284–287

Pulmonary system (*Continued*)
  anatomy of
    alveoli, 277–278
    lungs, 276–277
    overview, 276–278, 276f
  common symbols, 277, 277t
  during exercise
    aerobic power and endurance, 320–321
    graded exercise to maximum, 314f
    oxygen cost of breathing, 317–320
    steady-rate exercise, 314
  exercise performance, 283
  gas exchange surface, 276
  lung volumes
    dynamic lung volumes, 282–283
    gender differences in, 283
    static lung volumes, 281–282
  in microgravity, 751–752, 782t
  minute, 284
  physical performance, 283–284
  regulation of
    breath holding, 312
    chemical control, 312
    humoral factors, 310–312
    hyperventilation, 312
    integrated regulation, 313
    neural factors, 310
    nonchemical control, 312–313
  respiratory tract during cold-weather exercise, 289, 289b
  variations from normal breathing patterns
    dyspnea, 287
    hyperventilation, 287
    valsalva maneuver, 288, 288f
  ventilation
    alveolar minute, 284–287
    expiration, 280
    inspiration, 279–280
    minute, 284
    overview, 278–279
    surfactant, 280–281
    values, 286f
  ventilation anatomy
    alveoli, 277–278
    lungs, 276–277
    overview, 276
Pulmonary ventilation, 276
Purine, 1023
Purkinje system, 354
Pyramidal (lateral) tract, 425–427, 427f
Pyramiding, 598, 640
Pyrimidine, 1023
Pyruvate, 162, 637–638

Q

QRS complex, 356, 972–973
Quadriceps, muscle architectural properties, 400f
Quantitative trait loci (QTL), 1075
Quaternary structure, 1038
Quiescent, 1042, 1061–1062

R

R group chain, 28
Racewalking, 236f
Racial differences, obesity, 870–871
Racial factors
  life expectancy, 912–913, 912f
  onset of blood lactate accumulation, 317f
  physique, 841
Radiation, 673
  cancer therapy, 956
  effects on Mars and Moon, 773
  heat loss by, 673
Radiation exposure–induced death (REID), 773
Radiculopathy, 567
Radiography, of chest, 968
Radioisotope, 1053
Radionuclide studies, cardiovascular disease, 968–969
Range of motion (ROM), 546–547, 760
Ranvier, Louis Antoine, 431
Rapid loading procedure, 629–630, 630f
Rapture of the deep (nitrogen narcosis), 722–723
Ratcliffe, Bob, 708, 710–711
Rate-pressure product (RPP), 346

Rating of perceived exertion (RPE), 521–523, 617, 921
RDEE (resting daily energy expenditure), 215–216, 216f
Reactive oxygen species (ROS), 1071
Readaptating from microgravity environment, 767, 770f
Real anemia/pseudoanemia, 63–64
Reality check, 896
Reassortment virus vaccines, 1047
Rebound hypoglycemia, 106
Rebound jumping technique, plyometrics, 566f
Recombinant DNA, 1048
Recombinant human EPO (rHuEPO), 622
Recombinant subunit vaccines, 1047
Recommended Dietary Allowance (RDA), 31–32, 46
Recompression chamber, portable, 724, 724f
Recovery
  blood pressure response to, 343–345
  oxygen consumption, 187–191, 187f
  pulmonary ventilation, regulation of, 313
Recovery afterglow, 892–893
Rectal cancer, 950t
Rectal temperature, 693
Red blood cell mass, 657, 752–753, 752f
Red blood cell reinfusion, 621–622, 622f, 640
Red meat diet, 30b
Redox reaction, 145
Redox (oxidation/reduction) reaction, 145, 146f
RED-S (Relative energy deficiency in sport), 61
Reducing agent, 145
Reduction potential, 155
Reduction reactions, 144–145
REE (resting energy expenditure), 870–871
Re-esterification, 169
Reference man/woman, 805–807, 805f
Reflex arc, 429–430, 430f
Refractory period, 356, 987
Regular dietary intake, 609–610
Regular moderate exercise, 932–933
  physiologic factors, influence of, 933
  structured physical activity, 933
Regurgitation. *see* Insufficiency
Rehydration, 683–686
  adequacy of, 684–685, 686b
  electrolyte replacement, 685, 685f, 686b
  exogenous glycerol, 684
  physical activity, 686b
  whole-body precooling, 685–686
Relative body fat, 813
Relative energy deficiency in sport (RED-S), 61
Relative humidity, 72, 674
Relative insulin deficiency, 473
Relative muscle strength, 553–554, 553f
Relaxation, muscle, 407
Releasing factor, 455–456
Relief interval, 529
Remodeling, 53
Renal blood flow, 366
Renal buffer, 323
Renal disease, 988–989
  clinical features, 989
  exercise prescription, 989
Renin, 463
Renin inhibitors, 341
Renin-angiotensin mechanism, 463
Renin-angiotensin system, 463
Replication bubble, DNA, 1026, 1026f
Replication, DNA molecule, 1025–1026, 1026f
Repressor protein, 1032
RER (respiratory exchange ratio), 205–207
Residual lung volume (RLV), 281–282, 715–716
Residual smoking effect, 318
Resistance training, 557
  acute responses and chronic adaptations, 569
  adaptations to, 569
  aerobic training plus, 559–560
  aging, 924–925, 924f
  blood pressure response to, 342–343
  during cancer management, 959–960
  cardiovascular disease, 979
  effect on muscle structure and maximal strength performance, 486f
  effects on body composition of, 903t
  effects on handgrip strength in elderly, 549b
  endocrine system and, 485–486, 486f
  equipment categories, 551

equipment with variable, 563
factors influencing lean tissue synthesis with, 899f
guidelines for health enhancement and disease prevention, 559
interacting factors in developing and maintaining muscle mass, 569, 569f
and joint-flexibility exercise, 583
and metabolic stress, 578
middle-age and older adults, 559
objectives, 548
physiologic adaptations to, 572, 590t
progressive resistance exercise (PRE)
  overload principle, 557
  overview, 557
  periodization, 558–559, 558f
  variations, 557–558
specificity, 561–562
structural and functional adaptations, 569
  circuit resistance training, 578–579
  comparative male and female training responses, 576–577
  detraining effects on muscle, 577–578
  muscle soreness and stiffness, 579–585
  neural and muscular adaptations impact strength improvements, 569–576
  weight control, 893–894, 894f, 903t
Resistance-trained bodybuilders, 853
Respiration, 138–139
Respiratory center, 298
Respiratory (cytochrome) chain, 155
Respiratory compensation, 314
Respiratory disease, 318
Respiratory exchange ratio (RER), 205–207
Respiratory gas exchange, 197, 205–207
Respiratory quotient (RQ)
  calculating, 205
  carbohydrate, 203
  lipid, 203
  mixed diet, 205, 209t
  nonprotein, 203–205, 209t
  protein, 203
Respiratory tract, cold-weather exercise, 695–696
Rest
  a-vO2 difference (AU: Please check symbol), 381
  cardiac output at
    endurance athletes, 375–376
    overview, 375–376
    untrained individuals, 375
  energy expenditure at
    basal metabolic rate, 212, 214
    factors that affect, 216–219
    metabolic rates, 214–216, 214f
    metabolic size concept, 212–213, 213f, 214f
    resting metabolic rate, 212
  oxygen transport at, 380
Resting daily energy expenditure (RDEE), 215–216, 216f
Resting energy expenditure (REE), 870–871
Resting membrane potential, 433–434
Resting metabolic rate (RMR), 212
Resting minute ventilation, 291t
Restriction endonuclease, 1052
Restriction enzyme, 1052
Restriction fragment-length polymorphisms (RFLPs), 1059f
Restrictive lung disease (RLD), 980, 1002t–1003t
Reticular formation, 423, 427
Retrovirus, 1030–1031
Reverse cholesterol transport, 20, 941
Reverse transcriptase, 1048–1051
Rheumatic fever, 964
rHuEPO (recombinant human EPO), 622
Ribosomal RNA (rRNA), 1023
Ribosome, 1036
Rigor mortis, 407
RLV (Residual lung volume), 715–716
RLV (residual lung volume), 281–282
RMR (Resting metabolic rate), 212
RNA (ribonucleic acid)
  defined, 1013
  forms of, 1023
  genetic code, 1025
  phosphodiester bonding, 1020–1021, 1021f
  synthesis of, 1030–1031
    enzyme turnover number, 1032, 1033f
    gene expression, 1031

protein enzymes, 1031
transcription control, 1031–1032
vs. DNA, molecular configuration, 1017–1018, 1018f
RNA polymerase I, 1029
RNA primers, 1026
RNA splicing, 1034
Roberts, Richard John, 1033
Rohrer, Heinrich, 404
Roid rage, 599
ROM (range of motion), 760
Röntgen, Wilhelm Konrad, 983
Rosa, E. B, 196
Roslin method, 1061–1062, 1062f
Rouquayrol, Benoît, 705
RPE (rating of perceived exertion), 521–523, 617, 921
RPP (rate-pressure product), 346
Rubner, Max, 216
Ružička, Leopold, 594
Runners
   body composition, 858t
   body fat, 848
   pulmonary function, 291t
Running
   age factors, 230b
   for different durations, 894, 904t
   energy expenditure during
      air resistance, 237–238, 238f
      competition walking, 236, 236f
      drafting, beneficial outcomes, 238–239
      footwear and other distal leg loads, 232
      marathon running, 239
      net, 234, 245t–246t
      running economy, 230b, 236–237
      speed, 234–236
      stride frequency, 234–236
      stride length, 234–236
      treadmill versus track running, 239, 246t
   guidelines for determining interval-training exercise rates, 529, 541t
   training-sensitive zone, 521
   weight control, 893
Russian Federal Space Agency (RFSA or Roscosmos), 736

S

SA (Sinoatrial) node, 354
Salbutamol, 605
Salt reduction strategy, 66
Saltatory conduction, 431
Salt-sensitive individuals, 66
Sand, walking in, 231
Sandow, Eugen, 547b
S_aO_2 (oxygen saturation of hemoglobin), 651f
Sarcolemma, 391–392, 395
Sarcomas, 956, 1044
Sarcomeres, 390, 396–397, 397f, 419t
   length, 405–406, 406f–407f
   patients with cerebral palsy, 399b
   resting, 401f
   structural position of the filament, 397f
Sarcopenia, 32b, 923
Sarcoplasm, 395
Sarcoplasmic reticulum, 395, 580–581
Satcher, Bobby, 771b
Satellite cells, 395
Satiety gene, 869f
Saturated fatty acid, 15–16
Saturation diving, 726–727, 727f
Sayre, Ann C., 1015b
SBP (systolic blood pressure), 333
Scaleni muscle, 280
Schneider, E.C., 648
Scholander, 201
Scholander technique, 201
Schwann cell, 431
SCNT (somatic cell nuclear transfer), 1013, 1060–1061, 1061f
Scott, Winston E., 771b
Scuba diving
   closed-circuit scuba, 719–720, 719f
   hazards of, 720, 721f
   open-circuit scuba, 718–719, 718f, 719f
   overview, 717–720
Scyllias, 704

Sea-level performance, 661–662, 661f
Seasonal affective disorder, 990
Second law of thermodynamics, 137–138
Second messenger, 453
Second transition phase, strength training, 559
Secondary structure, 1038
Secreted amount, hormone, 454
Secretin, 478, 495t
Sedentary environmental death syndrome (SeDS), 914–918, 1010
   changing fitness trends, 915–918, 949t
   2020 top 10 fitness trends, 918
   U.S. adult population, 914–915
   U.S. children and teenagers, 915
Sedentary lifestyles
   heart disease, 932–933
SEE (standard error of estimate), 264
Selenium, 82t
Self-contained underwater breathing apparatus (scuba), 717–719
Semilunar valves, 328–329
Semistarvation diets, 889
Sensitivity, of test, 971–972
Sensorimotor integration, 753
Sensory function, at altitude, 653, 653f
Sensory neurons, spinal cord, 425, 427
Series-fibered muscle, 400
Serum glutamic oxaloacetic transaminase (SGOT), 968
Set point theory
   biologic feedback mechanism, 886–887
   dieting extremes, 887
   high-protein diets, 889
   low-carbohydrate ketogenic diets, 887–889
   overview, 885
   resting metabolism decreases, 885–886, 886f
   semistarvation diets, 889
Severe lung disease, 985
Sex-specific essential fat, 806
Shallow water blackout (SWB), 715
Sharp, Phillip Allen, 1033
Sheldon, William H., 802, 838
Shell temperature, 670
ShenZhou-3 flight, 748
Shepard, Alan, 748–749
Shivering, 672
Shorter, Frank, 846
Short-term energy system, 250f
Short-term exercise effects, 488
Shoulder and wrist elevation test, 916b, 916f, 917t
Shoulder flexibility, 917, 917t
Shoulder rotation test, 917, 917t
Shoulder-wrist flexibility test, 916b, 916f, 917t
Shuttle Columbia (STS-90), 746
Sickle cell anemia, 1016b
Siebe, Augustus, 705, 718
Simple lipids, 15–20, 16f
Simple sugars, 6, 8
Simpson, Tom, 613f
Single-nucleotide polymorphisms (SNPs), 1042–1044, 1043f, 1074
Single-strand binding protein (SSB), 1026
Sinoatrial (SA) node, 354
Sinus bradycardia, 964
Sinus cavities, skin divers, 716
Sinus tachycardia, 964
Sinuses, blockage of, 721f
Siri equation, 813
Sit-and-reach test, 916t, 916b
Site-specific muscular force effects, 58
Size principle, 437
Skeletal muscle
   actin-myosin orientation, 401–402, 401f, 402f
   chemical and mechanical events during action and relaxation
      actin, myosin, and ATP, linkage among, 406–407
      actomyosin research tools, 404–405
      excitation-contraction coupling, 407, 407f
      mechanical action, of crossbridges, 403–404, 404f
      overview, 403
      relaxation, 407
      sarcomere length, 405–406, 406f–407f
      sliding-filament model, 403–407, 403f
      steps in muscle action events, 407–409, 408f
   connective tissue, 391f
   epigenetic modifications
      with exercise, 1073

      following exercises, 1074
   function, 399b
   genes that define phenotype, 411–412
   gross structure of, 390–396, 391f
      blood supply, 395–396
      membranes, 395
      mitophagy, 392
      muscle composition, 395
      organization, 392, 393f
      tendon structure and trauma, 395
   intracellular cytoskeletal tubule systems, 402–403, 402f
   mass decline with aging, 412b
   muscle fiber
      alignment, 398–401, 398f, 400f
      type of, 409–413, 410f–409f, 419t
   overview, 328
   oxygen treatment, 626f, 627f
   ultrastructure, 393f, 396–403, 397f
Skeletal muscle atrophy, 463
Skin, 496t–498t
Skin friction drag, swimming, 240
Skin, water loss through, 72
Skinfold measurements
   age, 817–818
   athletes, 857t
   and girth, bioelectric impedance, body fat from, 844b
   sites for, 816, 817f
   subcutaneous fat measurement, 815–819
   usefulness of, 816–817, 835t
Skylab missions, 763
Sledge ergometer, 565f
Sleep disorders, 923b
Sliding-filament model, 403–407, 403f
Sling suspension methods, 566–567
Slow component of recovery oxygen consumption, 188
Slow glycolysis, 161
Slow oxidative (SO) fibers, 411
Slow-twitch (ST) muscle fibers, 184–185, 411, 438f
Smeaton, John, 705
Smith, Andrew H., 705
Smithies, Oliver, 1060
Smoke helmet, 705
Smooth muscle, 328
SMS (space motion sickness), 753, 761, 788t
Snorkel, 712
Snorkeling, 712–718
Snow, walking in, 231
SO (slow oxidative) fibers, 411
Sodium, 66–67, 73–74
   high-sodium culprits, 66
   induced hypertension, 67
   optimal intake, 66
Sodium bicarbonate, 322
Sodium-induced hypertension, 67
Soleus, 394b
Solubility, 295
Somatic cell nuclear transfer (SCNT), 1013, 1060–1061, 1061f
Somatic nerves, 429
Somatoliberin, 478
Somatopause, 926–927
Somatostatin, 456–457
Somatotropin, 456, 605
Somatotyping, 838
Soreness, muscle
   cell damage
      altered sarcoplasmic reticulum, 580–581
      current DOMS model, 581, 581f
      overview, 579–580
   eccentric actions, 579, 591t
   overview, 579
Sörensen, Sören, 321–322
South-East Asia, life expectancy, 912f
Southern blotting, 1054, 1056f
Soviet human space program, 747–748
   Chinese astronauts, 748
   early Chinese human space program, 747–748
   manned flight space missions, 747
Space biology research
   budget process for, 773–774
   dividends, 773
   practical benefits from, 774, 789t–790t
Space Medicine Branch, Aeromedical Association, 740
Space motion sickness (SMS), 753, 761, 788t

Space pharmacology, 761, 788t
Space research, 739–740
Space shuttle energy expenditure, 764–765, 765f
Space Shuttle treadmill, 760
Spatial summation, 433–434
Specific adaptations to imposed demands (SAIDs)
    principle, 504
Specific gravity, 810
Specific warm-up, 623–624, 640
Specificity
    aerobic improvement with CRT, 578–579
    cardiac enlargement, 510
    of energy capacities, 250
    of hormone-target cell, 452
    of hypertrophic response, 573
    local muscle–induced, 505–506
    maximum oxygen uptake, 505, 505f
    of metabolic capacity and exercise performance, 250
    of onset of blood lactate accumulation, 317f
    principle, 504–506
    stress testing, 972
    of test, 972
    of training response, 561–562
Speed walking, 230
Spemann, Hans, 1060
Spencer, Herbert, 1012
Spinal nerve cells, 442b
Spirometry
    closed-circuit, 198, 199f
    open-circuit, 198–199
    portable, 199–200, 200f
Sports anemia, 63
Sports drinks, and energy, 105
Sports medicine, 954, 954b
Sports science, 437b
Sports supplement manufacturing, 631b
Sports-related traumatic brain injury (srTBI), 422–423
Spot reduction, 896–897
Sprint performance, aging, 929, 929f
Spurious correlation, 821
Sputnik 1 satellite, 741
Squalus, 707, 710–711, 726
srTBI (sports-related traumatic brain injury), 422–423
SSB (single-strand binding protein), 1026
SSC (stretch-shortening cycle), 564
S–T segment depression, 971
Stacking, 598, 640
Stage decompression, 724
Staleness, 531
Standard American diet, 93
Standard error of estimate (SEE), 264
Starch, 8, 8f
Starling, Ernest Henry, 355, 377, 450b
Starling's law. *see* Frank-Starling law of the heart
Static flexibility, 916b
Static lung volumes, 281–282
Static muscle action, 548f, 556
Statins, 937
Stature
    defined, 796
    and golf driving distance, 852–853, 853f
Steady rate, 182–183
Steady state, 182–183
Steady-rate physical activity, 183, 343
    optimal recovery, 190
Stefens, Whitey, 708
Stenosis, 964
Stenting, 939
Step test, 266–267
Steroid hormone interactions, 596–600, 596f
    leucine, 597
    mTOR, 597
    muscle hypertrophy, 597
    testosterone and growth hormone, 597
Steroid-derived hormones, 450, 494t
Steroids
    abuse and disease precursors, 600–601
    cardiovascular side effects, 468b
    and plasma lipoproteins, 600–601
Sticking point, 562–563
Stiffness, muscle
    cell damage
        altered sarcoplasmic reticulum, 580–581
        current DOMS model, 581, 581f
        overview, 579–580
    eccentric actions, 579, 591t

overview, 579
Stomach, 451f
    cancer, 950t
Stop codons, 1025
Storage fat, 806
Streching techniques, PNF, 440b
Streeter, Tanya, 709, 716
Stress response integrator, 458
Stress testing
    CHD evaluation, 970–971
    contraindications, 971
    graded exercise stress testing, 970–971, 998t
    informed consent, 971, 1000t
    outcomes, 971–972
    pharmacologic, 969
    protocols
        arm-crank ergometer tests, 975
        Bruce and Balke treadmill tests, 974
        safety, 975–976
Stressors, altitude, 648, 649f
Stretch-shortening cycle (SSC), 564
Striated skeletal muscle fibers, 390
Stride frequency, 234–236, 236f
Stride length, 234–236, 236f, 237f
Stroke (cerebrovascular disease), 476b
    clinical features, 987
    effects of physical activity, 950t
    effects of physical activity on, 874f
    exercise prescription, 987
    overview, 987
Stroke volume (SV), 374
    β_1–adrenoceptor, 378f
    cardiovascular adaptations with training, 512–513
    cardiovascular drift, 377–378
    diastolic filling, 376–377
    elite breath-hold diver, 717, 717f
    systolic emptying, 377
    during upright exercise in endurance athletes, 512f
Subcutaneous adipose tissue, 824
Subcutaneous emphysema, 721f
Subcutaneous fat, 815
Submaximal exercise
    at altitude, 660
    blood flow and distribution, 514
Submaximal oxygen consumption, 237f
Suborbital flights, 740–741
Substance Abuse and Mental Health Services
    Administration (SAMHSA), 604b
Substantia, 446t
Substrate-level phosphorylation, 162
Sucrose, 7
Sudden death risk, during physical activity, 919, 920f
Sugars, minute, 6, 8
Sugary beverages, 6b
Sugary soft drink, 7b
Sulfur, 83t
Sumo wrestlers, 854, 854f
Supercoiled DNA, 1028–1029
Superficial veins, 336f
Superior vena cava, 336
Superoxide dismutase, 47
Suprachiasmatic nucleus (SCN), 1029b
Surface area law, 212
Surface tension, 280–281
Surfactant, 280–281
Sweating, 55
    evaporation, 671f
    gender differences, 688–689
    mineral loss through, 67
Swimmers
    body fat, 848
    Phelps, Michael, 838–839
Swimming
    energy cost of underwater, 728, 728f
    energy expenditure during
        buoyancy, 242
        drag, 240–241
        endurance swimmers, 242–243
        measurement methods, 239–240, 240f
        skill, 241
        velocity, 241, 241f
        water temperature effects, 242, 242f
    guidelines for determining interval-training exercise
        rates, 529, 541b
    training-sensitive zone, 521
Swimming treadmill, 239–240
Sympathetic form, 531
Sympathetic influence, 362, 363f
Sympathetic nervous system, 363f, 429
Sympathetic overtraining, 531
Sympathoadrenal activity, 481
Sympathoadrenal response, 460–461
Sympathomimetic β_2-adrenergic agonists, 605, 640
Sympathomimetics, 1004t
Synapse, 429
Synaptic cleft, 432
Synaptic gutter, 432
Systemic circulation, 328
Systole, 328
Systolic blood pressure (SBP), 333
Systolic emptying, 328, 377
Szent-Györgyi, Albert., 390

T

T_3 (Triiodothyronine), 459
T_4 (Thyroxine), 459, 926
T wave, 356
Tabled values, 126–127
Tachycardia, 362, 964
Tapering for peak performance, 527
TBM (total body mineral), 766f
TBP (total body protein), 766f
TBW (total body water), 766, 766f
TDEE (total daily energy expenditure), 212, 212f
Technical diving, 727–728, 728f
Technique, exercise efficiency, 229
TEE (total energy expenditure), 885–886
Teenage obesity, 463
Teenagers, physical activity population, 915
Telencephalon, 422, 425
Telophase, 1027
Temin, Howard, 1048–1051
Temperature, 125, 670
    defined, 127
    versus heat, 122
    of water, 242, 242f
Template, 1015
Template strand, 1015
Temporal summation, 433–434
Tendinitis, 395
Tendon structure, 391–392, 391f
    and trauma, 395
Tendons, 392
Tension characteristics, 437, 438f
Teratogen, 1044
Tereshkova, Valentina, 744–745
Terrain, energy expenditure during walking, 231, 245t
Terrorist Explosive Device Analytical Center
    (TEDAC), 1045
Tertiary structure, 1038
Testes, 451f, 496t–498t
Testosterone, 465, 465f, 466b
    anabolic steroids, 597
    overview, 464–465, 464f, 480
Tethered swimming, 239–240, 505, 505f
Tethered treadmill exercise, 760, 760f
Thallium imaging, 969
Thermal balance, 670–671, 670f, 697t
Thermic effect of food (TEF), 216, 882, 882f
Thermodynamics, 697t
Thermoregulation, 668–701
    body art hindrance to, 674b
    clothing impacts, overview, 675
    in cold stress
        hormonal output, 672
        muscular activity, 672
        vascular adjustments, 672
    effects of clothing on
        clothing insulations, 675, 697t–698t
        cold-weather clothing, 677
        football uniforms, 677–678, 677f
        modern cycling helmet does not thwart heat
            dissipation, 678
        warm-weather clothing, 677
    environment
        cold, 691
        heat, 678
    heat loss
        by conduction, 673
        by convection, 673
        by evaporation, 674–675

heat-dissipating mechanisms, 675
    overview, 672–673, 672f
    by radiation, 673
hypothalamic temperature regulation, 671, 671f
thermal balance, 670–671, 670f, 697t
Thiazide diuretics, 341
Thick protein filaments, 402f
Thin protein filaments, 402f
Thioredoxin, 1071
Third-degree atrioventricular (AV) heart block, 971
Thoracic cavity, 276f
Thoracic squeeze, 715–716
Threshold for excitation, 433–434
Thrombus (blood clot), 346, 936–937, 938f
Thymine (T), 1021
Thymus gland, 451f, 496t–498t
Thyroid gland, 451f, 496t–498t, 926
Thyroid hormones, 459–460, 459f, 481, 494t
Thyroid-stimulating hormone (TSH), 457
Thyrotropin, 457, 926
Thyroxine (T_4), 459, 926
Tidal volume (TV), 281, 281f, 284b, 286f, 287f
Tiselius, Arne Wilhelm, 1052
Tissue synthesis, 456–457
Titin, 419t
TLE (total life expectancy), 913b
TLR-2 (toll-like receptor 2), 935
TNF-alpha (tumor necrosis factor-alpha), 484f
Tofu, 29–30
Tolerable upper intake level (UL), 46
Toll-like receptor 2 (TLR-2), 935
Tongue, 394b
Tonic motor neurons, 436, 436f
Torr, 294
Torricelli, Evangelista, 294
Total body mineral (TBM), 766f
Total body protein (TBP), 766f
Total body water (TBW), 766, 766f
Total daily energy expenditure (TDEE), 212, 212f
Total energy expenditure (TEE), 885–886
Total energy transfer
    from glucose catabolism, 167–168, 167f
    from lipid catabolism, 170
Total life expectancy (TLE), 913b
Total lung capacity (TLC), 281–282
Total peripheral resistance, 333–334
Totipotent, 1061
Tour de France, 99–100, 100f
Trabecular bone, 53
Trace minerals, 67–69
    and physical activity, 67–69, 83t
Trachea, 276
Tracheal air, 295
Track running, 239, 246t
Tract, defined, 446t
Training programs
    for exercise physiologists, 954–955
    organizations that offer, 954
Training volume, 557
Training-induced hypertrophy, 572–573, 572f
Training-induced plasma volume, 510–511
Training-sensitive zone, 520–521, 520f
Transactivating CRISPR RNA (tracrRNA), 1066
Transamination, 32
Transcranial magnetic stimulation (TMS), 435–436
Transcription
    control, 1031–1032, 1032f
    enzyme turnover number, 1032, 1033f
    gene expression, 1030–1031
    protein enzymes, 1031
    transcription control, 1031–1032
Transcription activator–like effector nucleases (TALEN), 1065
Trans-fatty acids, 18
Transfection, 1059
Transfer RNA (tRNA), 1023
Transferases, 148t, 1031
Transgender competitors, 576–577
Transgene, 1059
Transgenic, defined, 1059
Transitional and respiratory zones, ventilatory system, 278, 279f–280f
Translation
    defined, 1028
    essential concepts and sequences, 1041, 1086t
    Golgi complex, 1037–1038

hemoglobin, 1039
polypeptides, 1037
proteolysis, 1039–1041, 1041f
ribosomes, 1036
stages of, 1035
termination of protein synthesis, 1038, 1040f, 1085t
tRNA, 1023
Translocation, 1064–1065
Transport work, 139
Transverse (T)-tubule system, 391–392
Transverse tubule system (T-tubule system), 402
Traumatic brain injury, 422–423
Treadmills
    continuous and discontinous oxygen consumption tests, 269t
    energy expenditure using, 235b, 239, 246t
    protocols, 260, 261f
    work calculation, 141b
Triacylglycerol synthesis (esterification), 17, 18f
Triacylglycerols, 15, 168
    recommendations for, 940–941
Triathletes, body fat, 846–848
Tricuspid valve, 328
Triiodothyronine (T_3), 459
Triosephosphate isomerase, 161f
Tripeptide, 28
TRISH (Translational Research Institute for Space Health), 739–740
Tropomyosin, 419t
Troponin, 419t
Trunk and neck extension test, 916b, 917t
Trunk, flexibility of, 916b, 917t
    and strengthening exercises for, 584b
TSH (thyroid-stimulating hormone), 457
T-tubule system (transverse tubule system), 402
Tubule system, muscle fiber, 402f
Tumor, 1044
Tumor necrosis factor-alpha (TNF-alpha), 484f
Turnover number, 140–142, 1032, 1033f
Turnverein societies, 544–545
Turtle, submarine, 709b
Tvent (ventilatory threshold), 315
T-wave alternans, 973
Twin studies, 1070–1071
Twitch characteristics, 436–437, 436f
Two-component model, 813
Type 1 diabetes, 468–473
    physical activity guidelines for, 485
    stages, 470–473
    vs. type 2 diabetes, 475, 475f
Type 2 diabetes, 471f, 485f
    age factor, 473
    characteristics, 475, 475f
    definition, 468
    exercise training, possible mechanisms of, 483, 484f
    fasting plasma glucose (FPG) test for, 470
    genetic and environmental factors, 469
    metabolic syndrome and, 476b
    physical activity benefits for, 483–485
        glycemic control, 483–484
        improved psychological profile, 485
        occurrence of, 485
        reduced cardiovascular disease risk, 484–485
        weight loss, 485
    reducing risk of, 469b
    regular physical activity, 482–483
    risk factors, 473–475, 474b, 485b
Type I muscle fibers, 411
Type II muscle fibers, 411. *see also* Fast-twitch (type II) muscle fibers

U

UCP2 (uncoupling protein-2 gene), 870
Ultraendurance activities, 100–102
Ultraendurance competitions, 100–102
Ultraendurance Sports, 102–103
Ultrafast CT scan, 970
Ultrafast electron beam CT scan (EBCT), 970
Ultrasound, 823–824
Ultrastructure, 393f, 396–403, 397f
Ultraviolet light, 1054
Uncompensable heat stress, 683
Uncoupling protein-2 gene (UCP2), 870
Underwater swimming energy cost, 728, 728f
Underwater weighing, 809, 811–812

Unipennate fiber arrangement, 398–400
United States obesity epidemic, 865–867, 866f
United States Preventive Services Task Force, 866
Unregulated glucose transport, 111
Unsaturated fatty acids, 15–17, 17f
Upper intake levels (ULs), 80t
Upper respiratory tract infections (URTIs), 50–51, 640
    glutamine, 619–620
    long-term exercise effects, 488–489
    optimizing immune function, 490
    short-term exercise effects, 488
Upper-body exercise
    maximal oxygen consumption, 382
    physiologic response, 382–384
    submaximal oxygen consumption, 382–384, 382f
Upper-body physical activity, 343
Up-regulation, 453
Uracil, 1017–1018
Urea, 32, 35, 35f
Uremia, 989
Urine, water loss thorugh, 71
U.S. Air Force School of Space Medicine, 746
US Anti-Doping Agency (USADA), 623
U.S. Department of Energy (DOE), 1010
U.S. Diets and Federal Recommendations, 867
USADA (US Anti-Doping Agency), 623

V

Vagus nerves, 364
Valsalva maneuver, 288, 288f
van Leeuwenhoek, Antonie., 390
van Tschermak-Seysenegg, Erich, 1013
Vapor, water loss as, 72
Variant angina, 972
Varicose veins, 338
Vascular diseases
    peripheral vascular disease, 950t
    stroke, 950t
Vasculogenesis, 1044
Vasodilation, 366
Vasomotor tone, 362
Vasopressin, 458, 480, 480f
Vasopressin (antidiuretic hormone), 675
Vastus lateralis muscle, human, 410f–409f
VAT (visceral adipose tissue), 826, 826f
Vector, 1052
Vegan approach, 30, 30f
Vegetarians, 30
Vegetative nerves, 429
Venous admixture, 298
Venous system
    active vasculature, 337
    overview, 336–338
    varicose veins, 338
    venous pooling, 338
    venous return, 337
Ventilated Hood technique, 201, 201f
Ventilation
    alveolar
        breathing rate vs. depth, 286–287, 287f
        dead space vs. tidal volume, 284
        overview, 284, 291t
        physiologic dead space, 286, 286f
        ventilation-perfusion ratio, 284–286
    anatomy of
        alveoli, 277–278
        lungs, 276–277
        overview, 276–278, 276f
    common symbols, 277, 277t
    mechanics of
        expiration, 280
        inspiration, 279–280
        overview, 278–279
        surfactant, 280–281
    minute ventilation, 284
Ventilatory buffer, 323
Ventilatory equivalent, 314, 516f
Ventilatory system, 276, 276f
Ventilatory threshold (Tvent), 315
Ventral horn, spinal cord, 425
Ventricular depolarization, 357f
Ventricular ectopy, 971
Ventricular fibrillation, 974
Ventricular or atrial septal defects, 964
Ventricular repolarization, 357f

Ventrolateral medulla, 360
Ventromedial (extrapyramidal) tract, 427, 427f
Venules, 336
Vertical jump test, 252
Very low-calorie diets (VLCD), 889
Very low-density lipoprotein cholesterol (VLDL-C), 941
Very low-density lipoproteins (VLDLs), 20, 21f
Videofluoroscopy, 582
Virus, 1047
Visceral adipose tissue (VAT), 826, 826f
Visceral nerves, 429
Viscous pressure drag, swimming, 240
Vitality, 910
Vitamins
   antioxidants
      exercise and, 49
      role, 47–48
      vitamins as, 49–50
   B_6, 51
   B-complex, 51
   biologic function of, 43, 45, 46f
   C, 51
   dietary reference intakes, 46–47, 46b
   food sources, 48
   free radicals, 49–50
   multivitamin-mineral supplementation, 51
   nature of, 52
   role of, 45, 47–48, 77t–78t
   supplementation, 45b, 50–51
   types
      fat-soluble, 44
      water-soluble, 44
   vitamin A, 48
   vitamin B, 48
   vitamin C, 48, 78t
   vitamin D, 44b, 48, 58b
   vitamin E, 48, 77t
   vitamin K, 48
VLCD (very low-calorie diets), 889
VLDLs (very low-density lipoproteins), 20, 21f
Volume percent (vol%), 300
VO_2max. see Maximal oxygen uptake (VO_{2max})
Vomit Comet, 739
Von Drieberg, Friedrich, 705
von Purkinje, Jan Evangelista, 354

W

WADA (World Anti-Doping Agency), 596, 601
Waist girth, 930f
Waist-to-hip girth ratio, 876–877, 876f
Waist-to-hip ratio, 876f
Walking
   adolescents, 237f
   benefits of, 932–933
   for different durations, 894, 904t
   energy expenditure during
      body mass, influence of, 230–231, 244t
      competition walking, 232–233, 232f–233f
      downhill walking at grades, 231, 231f
      footwear and other distal leg loads, 231–233
      on level surface, 230, 231f
      terrain and walking surface, 231, 245t
   energy expenditure for
      predicting, 235b
   weight control, 893
Walking tests, 264
Walkthrough angina, 961
Walk-through angina. see Chronic stable angina
Wallace, Alfred Russel, 1012
Walsh, Don, 708
Warm-up (preliminary exercise), 623–625
Warm-weather clothing, 677
Water, 44
   balance of
      intake, 70–72
      output, 70–72
   content of, in body, 69
   exercise requirements, 49
   in foods, 70
   functions of, 69–70
   in liquids, 70
   loss of

      at altitude, 652–653
      asthma, 986
      hot-weather exercise, 680–683
      relates to activity intensity and ambient temperature, 681b
   requirements and physical activity, 72–75
   temperature effects, 242, 242f
   weight control, 889–890
Water displacement, 811
Water flow calorimeter, 197
Water intake guidelines during endurance activities, 74–75
Water loss
   in feces, 72
   in sweat, 71–72
   in urine, 71
   in vapor, 72
Water output, 71–72
Water uptake, 112–113
Water vapor transfer, 675
Water-insoluble fibers, 9
Water-soluble fibers, 9
Water-soluble vitamins, 44, 51f
Watson, James Dewey, 1014
Watson, R. Neal, 708
Wave drag, swimming, 240
WB-GT index. see Wet bulb-globe temperature (WB-GT) index
Weakest link training, 567–568
Wearable technology, 918
Weather
   impact on running performance, 681b
   time as a factor, 670
Weight bearing physical activity, 222
Weight control
   dieting for
      classic approach, 883
      extremes in, 883–889, 883f–884f
      long-term success, 883–885, 883f–884f
      set point theory, 885–889, 886f
   exercise for
      adolescents, 891
      children, 891
      dietary restriction, 892b
      increasing energy output, 891
      metabolic inflexibility, 890–891
      misconceptions, 891–893
      obese infants, 891
      overview, 890
   factors affect
      hydration level, 890
      input versus output, 882–883, 882f
      longer-term deficit, 890
      water loss, 889–890
   gaining weight, 898–900
   input versus output, 882–883, 882f
   recommendations for wrestlers and power athletes, 897–898
   regular physical activity effectiveness
      caloric restraint plus exercise, 895–896, 904t
      dose-response relationship of energy expended, 894–895, 904t
      and excess body fat, 893, 903t
      gender difference, 897
      overview, 893, 893f
      resistance training, 893–894, 894f, 903t
      spot reduction, 896–897
Weight gain
   cancer risk, 872–874
   hypertension risk, 874f
Weight loss, 485
   genetics influence and, 869–870
   improves disease risk biomarkers, 884–885, 885f
   reduces knee osteoarthritis, 876b
   with structured assistance, 884
Weightless environment, 736–738. see also Microgravity
   apparent sense of, 738
   associated with free fall, 738
   gravity, 736–737, 736f
   potential deleterious effects of, 742, 780t
Weightlifters and powerlifters, age trends among, 922, 922f
Weightlifters, DNA polymorphisms in, 1074

Weightlifting
   aging, 922
   body fat, 853–854
   in early America, 545–547
   gender differences, 552–553
   versus isokinetic resistance training, 562–563
Weight-supported physical activity, 222
Weir, J. B., 206
Weir method, 206b
Wesley, Claude, 708
Western blotting, 1054, 1056f
Western Pacific, life expectancy, 912f
Wet bulb-globe temperature (WB-GT) index, 676b
Wet suit, 719
White fat, 878–879, 879f
White matter, 446t
White, Ralph, 709
Whitlock, Ed, 928–929
Whitlock, Len, 709
Whole-body precooling, 685–686
Wilkins, M. H. F., 1014, 44, 1015
Wilkins, Mac, 843
Wilson, Danny, 708
Wilson, Stephanie D., 771b
Wind speed, 675
Wind-chill temperature index, 694–695, 695f
Wingate test, 605
Winter sports technology, 775b
Women, 54
   anterior pituitary hormones, 480
   diving risks, 725
   iron loss during, 62–63
   menstruation
      bodybuilders, 853–854
      delayed onset of and cancer risk, 808
      sweating, 688–689
      variations in hydrostatic weighing with, 812
   osteoporosis, 48
   pharmacologic training aid risks, 601
   pregnancy
      effect on energy expenditure, 219
      physical activity and exercise training during, 533–536, 533f
Work (W), 136–137, 141b
Work rate, 229
World Anti-Doping Agency (WADA), 596, 601, 623b
World records, effect of performance-enhancing drugs on, 594–595
World Underwater Federation, 708
Wrestlers, 897–898
Wrist, flexibility of, 916b, 916f, 917t

X

X chromosome, 1016, 1016f
X-1 rocket aircraft, 742
X-2 rocket aircraft, 742
X-15 rocket aircraft, 742
Xenotransplantation, 1061
X-rays
   crystallography, 1014f
   dual-energy X-ray absorptiometry, 764–765, 828–829, 829f
   pulmonary diseases, assessing, 983

Y

Y chromosome, 1016, 1016f
Yiannis Kouros—All-Time Greatest Record-Breaking Ultraendurance Runner, 102b
Yonath, Ada, 1065

Z

Z line, sarcomere, 396–397, 397f
Zander, Dr. Gustav, 546
Zander mechanotherapy machines (late 19th century), 546, 546f
Zero-g, 738
Zinc, 80t
Zinc finger nucleases, 1065
Zumaya, Joel, 437b
Zuntz, Nathan, 199